OXFORD MEDICAL PUBLICATIONS

Brain's
Diseases of the
Nervous System

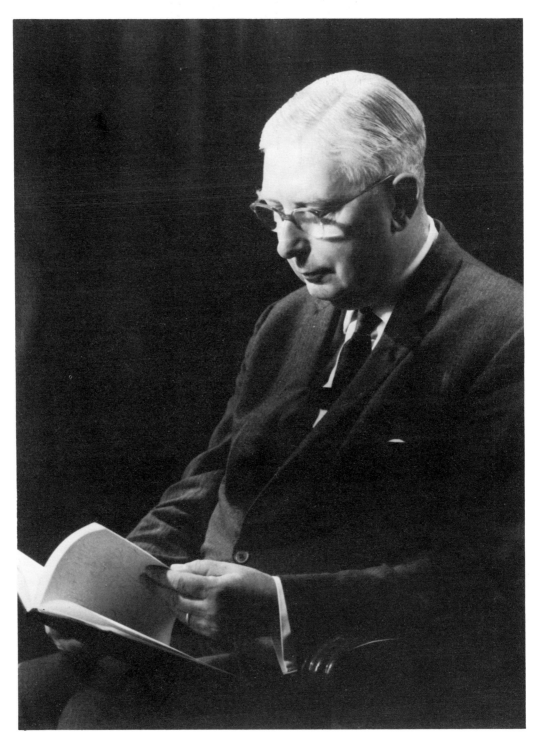

Lord Brain of Eynsham
1895–1966

Brain's Diseases of the Nervous System

NINTH EDITION

Sir John Walton

TD, MA, MD, DSc, FRCP

Warden, Green College, Oxford

Formerly
*Professor of Neurology and Dean of Medicine,
University of Newcastle upon Tyne*
and *Consultant Neurologist,
Newcastle Area Hospitals*

Oxford   New York   Tokyo
OXFORD UNIVERSITY PRESS
1985

Oxford University Press, Walton Street, Oxford OX2 6DP
Oxford New York Toronto
Delhi Bombay Calcutta Madras Karachi
Kuala Lumpur Singapore Hong Kong Tokyo
Nairobi Dar es Salaam Cape Town
Melbourne Auckland
and associated companies in
Beirut Berlin Ibadan Nicosia

Oxford is a trade mark of Oxford University Press

Published in the United States
by Oxford University Press, New York

© *Oxford University Press 1962, 1969, 1977, 1985*

First edition 1933
Ninth edition 1985

British Library Cataloguing in Publication Data
Brain, Walter Russell Brain, Baron
Brain's Diseases of the nervous system.—
9th ed.
1. Nervous system—Diseases
I. Title   II. Walton, Sir John, 1922–
616.8   RC346
ISBN 0-19-261438-X

Library of Congress Cataloging in Publication Data
Brain, W. Russell Brain (Walter Russell Brain),
Baron, 1895–1966.
Brain's Diseases of the nervous system.
(Oxford medical publications)
Includes bibliographies and index.
1. Nervous system—Diseases. I. Walton,
John Nicholas.   II. Title.   III. Title:
Diseases of the nervous system.   IV. Series.
[DNLM: 1. Nervous System Diseases.
WL 100 B814d]
RC346.B67   1985   616.8   85–11612
ISBN 0–19–261438–X

Set by Promenade Graphics, Cheltenham
Printed in Great Britain by
Butler & Tanner Ltd, Frome and London

Preface to the Ninth Edition

IN my preface to the seventh edition, I noted that before Lord Brain's untimely death in 1966 he had revised about one-third of *Diseases of the nervous system* in preparation for that new edition. Inevitably therefore it was something of a hybrid as it was clearly necessary to leave untouched those sections which Lord Brain had revised before his death. Nevertheless, I was able to add an introductory commentary on general principles, based largely upon a part of the opening chapters of my own *Essentials of neurology* (Pitman Medical Publishing Company Ltd.) and I also rewrote the chapter on disorders of muscle, drawing widely upon that which had been written by Dr David Gardner-Medwin and myself in *Disorders of voluntary muscle* (Churchill Livingstone). Many other chapters, too, were extensively revised and new illustrations and references to the neurological literature were added.

While in my preface to the eighth edition I commented that the previous editions of this book will inevitably stand as a permanent monument to Lord Brain's clinical expertise, to his thoughtful approach to neurological medicine, and to his outstanding literary skills, I felt that that edition, though extensively revised, should be one in which the traditional structure of the volume, so carefully conceived by Lord Brain over many years, should be maintained. Nevetheless, every chapter was extensively modified, some were virtually rewritten, and there were substantial additions to the text, new illustrations, and many new references. Many familiar pictures so well known to readers of former editions had to be replaced as the blocks from which they had been made were no longer serviceable; I was able to add new illustrations, particularly of radiographs and of CT scans and others demonstrating the results of electrophysiological techniques of investigation.

In preparing this ninth edition, it seemed that almost twenty years after Lord Brain's death the volume should be largely reconstructed and published in a different two-column format, similar to that in which the highly successful *Oxford Textbook of Medicine* had been published. The whole of the first chapter has been rewritten on pathophysiological principles and has been largely based upon the chapters which I wrote for the *International Textbook of Medicine* (Volume I: Pathophysiology, edited by Sahmy, Smith, and Thier and published by Saunders, 1981), as subsequently republished in *An introduction to clinical neuroscience* (Baillière Tindall, 1983). And similar commentaries on pathophysiology introduce several subsequent chapters. I have drawn extensively upon the text used in these publications and upon some of that utilized in the introductory chapters to the fifth edition of *Essentials of neurology*; I warmly acknowledge the permission of the editors and publishers concerned to include this material, which will, I hope, present the reader with a firm understanding of pathophysiological principles as they relate to the elucidation of disease and dysfunction of the nervous system.

In the remainder of the volume I have also undertaken a great deal of updating and rewriting, as well as substantial rearrangement. Thus descriptions of the many inherited metabolic and storage diseases of the nervous system which were previously considered in Chapter 13 on congenital, developmental, and degenerative disorders have now been transferred to Chapter 15 on intoxications and metabolic disorders. There has also been much additional rearrangement: a new introductory section on neuroimmunology has been added to Chapter 11 on demyelinating disease, and advances in neuro-imaging, in genetics, in molecular biology, new information about neurotransmitters and neuropharmacology have all been given due weight. In every chapter outdated and outmoded material has been deleted and much new information has been included to take note of advances not only in clinical neurology but also in related neuroscientific disciplines. Very many new references have been included in the individual sections, many from 1984 and some from 1985.

In the seventh edition new illustrations were included by kind permission of Dr D. Denny-Brown and the Liverpool University Press, Dr C. S. Hallpike and the editors and publishers of *Proceedings of the Royal Society of Medicine*, Professor W. Blackwood and E. & S. Livingstone Ltd., Dr J. R. Smythies and Blackwell Scientific Publications Ltd., Dr P. Hudgson and the editors and publishers of *Neurology (Minneapolis)*; others were kindly supplied by Dr G. L. Gryspeerdt, Dr G. W. Pearce, Dr James Ambrose, Professor B. E. Tomlinson, Mr L. P. Lassman, Dr R. Madrid, Dr D. D. Barwick and Dr R. Weiser; several illustrations were also reproduced from *An atlas of clinical neurology* (Oxford University Press) by Dr J. D. Spillane, and from *Neuro-*

logical anatomy in relation to clinical medicine (Oxford University Press) by Professor A. Brodal. Professor W. G. Bradley also allowed me to reproduce electrophysiological and histological illustrations previously published in *Disorders of peripheral nerves* (Blackwell Scientific Publications Ltd.), while Dr J. C. Brown and Dr R. J. Johns and the editor of the *Bulletin of the Johns Hopkins Hospital* gave permission for reproduction of a diagram. Inevitably both in the eighth edition and in this, the ninth, I have included many tables, illustrations, and other material which has been previously published either in works of my own or in those of others. Thus the chapter on diseases of muscle includes much material also included in the relevant chapter written by myself for the second edition of *The Oxford Textbook of Medicine*. I have also drawn extensively upon other writings as, for example, from *Child neurology* 2nd edition, by J. L. Menkes, published by Lea & Febiger. Throughout the pages of the book, whenever material is quoted directly or modified from other original sources, full acknowledgement is given in the captions to the illustrations or in footnotes to tables, etc. However, a list follows of the major sources from which material has been included with the permission of authors, editors, and publishers, to whom I am very grateful: *Introduction to basic neurology* by Patton, Sundsten, Crill, and Swanson (1976) and *Fundamentals of Neurology* by Gardner (1975) (both published by W. B. Saunders); *The essentials of neuroanatomy* by Mitchell (Churchill Livingstone, 1971); *The anatomy of the nervous system* by Ranson and Clark (W. B. Saunders, 1959); *A physiological approach to clinical neurology* 2nd edition, by Lance and McLeod (Butterworth, 1975); *Gray's anatomy* 35th British edition, edited by Warwick and Williams (Longman, 1973); *Textbook of medical physiology* 5th edition, by Guyton (W. B. Saunders, 1976); *The biochemical basis of neuropharmacology* 2nd edition, by Cooper, Bloom, and Roth (Oxford University Press, 1974); *Aids to the examination of the peripheral nervous system* by the Medical Research Council (HMSO, 1976); *Scientific approaches to clinical neurology* edited by Goldensohn and Appel (Lea & Febiger, 1977); *Scientific foundations of neurology* edited by Critchley, O'Leary, and Jennett (Heinemann, 1972); *Brain's clinical neurology* by Bannister (Oxford University Press, 1984); *An atlas of clinical neurology* by Spillane and Spillane (Oxford University Press, 1982); *Cerebrovascular disorders* by Toole and Patel (McGraw-Hill, 1974); *Neuroimmunology I: Immunoregulation in neurological disease* by Weiner and Hauser (Annals of Neurology, 1982); an article on neurotransmitters in basal ganglia disease by Marsden, published in *The Lancet* on 20 November 1982; a paper by Barnard published in *Neuropathology and Applied Neurobiology* in 1982; *The cerebrospinal fluid* by Fishman (W. B. Saunders, 1981); *Histological typing of tumours of the central nervous system* edited by Zulch (WHO); and *Head injury* by Cartlidge and Shaw (W. B. Saunders, 1981). To all of these authors and publishers I express my sincere thanks, as I also do to Dr James Bull, Dr D. Gardner-Medwin, Professor L. P. Garrod, Professor A. J. McComas, Professor F. W. O'Grady, and Dr J. B. Selkon, all of whom gave help with the seventh, eighth, or ninth editions in many different ways.

The preparation of this volume would never have been possible but for the efficient and tireless help of my secretary, Miss Rosemary Allan, who typed many hundreds of pages of inserts and corrections and who was a tower of strength throughout. To the staff of Oxford University Press, and to Dr J. Gibson who provided the index, I must express my thanks for their patience, understanding and tolerance during the gestation period. I can but hope that I have done justice to some at least of what Lord Brain's aims and intentions for this edition would have been.

Oxford   John Walton
February 1985

Preface to the First Edition

THE last twenty years have witnessed a remarkable development in neurology. Investigation of the effects of war injuries of the spinal cord has greatly increased our knowledge of reflex action in man. The appearance of encephalitis lethargica and the multiplication of forms of acute disseminated encephalitis have added a new field to clinical neurology and brought it into relationship with the new branch of bacteriology which studies the filterable viruses. The discovery of important metabolic centres in the hypothalamus has enhanced the importance of neurology to general medicine. Advances in the technique of neurological surgery have aroused fresh interest in the symptoms and in the pathology of intracranial tumours. Other developments, scarcely less important, have occurred.

Much of this new knowledge is physiological, and in one respect I have departed from the traditional arrangement of a textbook of nervous diseases. Neurology is more dependent than many other branches of medicine upon anatomy and physiology. These subjects, the essential basis of neurological diagnosis, are usually dismissed in a few introductory pages, with the result that much clinical neurology is apt to be both unintelligible and uninteresting to the student. In the first part of this book, as an introduction to the subject, I have discussed—at greater length than usual—the application of anatomy and physiology to the interpretation of the physical signs of nervous disease. Elsewhere will be found sections dealing with anatomy and physiology as introductions to clinical sections. In planning the clinical sections I have used what seemed the most practical, if not always the most logical, arrangement, for there is no entirely satisfactory way of arranging subjects, many of which might be placed in more than one group.

Limitations of space restrict the number of references which it is possible to quote. I have, therefore, chosen only those of special interest and those which form the best introduction to a subject, or are themselves useful sources of references. To the many other writers upon whose work I have freely drawn I express my indebtedness. I am indebted also to a number of my colleagues for the loan of illustrations.

Finally, I welcome this opportunity of expressing my gratitude to my colleagues at the London Hospital for their teaching, encouragement, and help, expecially to Dr. Charles Miller, Professor Arthur Ellis, and Dr. George Riddoch, under whom I had the privilege of working on the Medical Unit, and to Mr. Hugh Cairns, Dr. Dorothy Russell, and Dr. S. Phillips Bedson.

London   W. Russell Brain
June 1933

Contents

1. **Disorders of function in the light of anatomy and physiology**   1
    Some general considerations   1
    The cerebrum   12
    The motor system   15
    The sensory system   37
    The reflexes   48
    Speech and its disorders   52
    Apraxia and agnosia   62
    The cerebrospinal fluid (CSF)   64
    History and examination   73

2. **The cranial nerves and special senses**   83
    The first or olfactory nerve and the sense of smell   83
    The sense of vision, the visual apparatus, and the second or optic nerve   83
    External ocular movement and its abnormalities   95
    Lesions of the third, fourth, and sixth nerves   106
    The fifth or trigeminal nerve   109
    The seventh or facial nerve   113
    The eighth or vestibulocochlear nerve   117
    The ninth or glossopharyngeal nerve   128
    The sense of taste   128
    The tenth or vagus nerve   129
    The eleventh or accessory nerve   133
    The twelfth or hypoglossal nerve   133

3. **Raised intracranial pressure, cerebral oedema, hydrocephalus, intracranial tumour, and headache**   135
    Raised intracranial pressure — pathophysiology   135
    Cerebral oedema   137
    Hydrocephalus   137
    Intracranial tumour   143
    Headache   175
    Migraine   177

4. **Disorders of the cerebral circulation**   183
    The cerebral arterial circulation   183
    Cerebral ischaemia   188
    Classification of the cerebrovascular diseases   191
    The incidence and epidemiology of 'strokes'   191
    Cerebral infarction   192
    Syndromes of the cerebral arteries   194
    Cerebral embolism   200
    Hypertensive encephalopathy   205
    Intracranial aneurysm   206
    Arteriovenous angioma   208
    Subarachnoid haemorrhage   208
    Cerebral haemorrhage   214
    Other degenerative vasculopathies   218
    Vascular diseases without changes in the brain and strokes of undetermined aetiology   219
    Inflammatory diseases of intracranial arteries   219
    The cerebral venous circulation   221
    Thrombosis of the intracranial venous sinuses and veins   223

5. **Head injury**   226
    Non-penetrating injuries of the brain   226
    Traumatic pneumocephalus and CSF rhinorrhoea   231
    Subdural haematoma   231
    Post-traumatic epilepsy   232
    Intracranial birth injuries   235

6. **Diseases of the meninges**   237
    The anatomy of the meninges   237
    Calcification of the falx   237
    Pachymeningitis   237
    Acute leptomeningitis   237

7. **Suppurative encephalitis: intracranial abscess**   250

8. **Nervous complications of miscellaneous infections**   254
    Acute toxic encephalopathy   254
    Scarlet fever   255
    Whooping cough   255
    Typhoid fever   255
    Typhus fever   256
    Malaria   256
    Trypanosomiasis   257
    Influenza   257
    Infective hepatitis   257
    Infectious mononucleosis   258
    Sarcoidosis   258
    Mycoplasma infection   258
    Toxoplasmosis   258
    Benign myalgic encephalomyelitis   259
    Behçet's disease   259
    Metazoal infections   260
    Whipple's disease   261

9. **Syphilis of the nervous system**   263
    Secondary syphilis   263
    Tertiary meningovascular syphilis   264
    General paresis   267
    Tabes dorsalis   268
    Congenital neurosyphilis   272

10. **Virus infections of the nervous system**   274
    General considerations   274
    Epidemic encephalitis lethargica   275
    Epidemic encephalitis: Japanese type B, St. Louis type, and Murray Valley type   277
    Eastern and Western (equine) encephalomyelitis   278
    Other forms of viral encephalitis   279
    Subacute sclerosing panencephalitis   279
    Herpes simplex encephalitis   280
    Poliomyelitis   282
    Rabies   286
    Virus meningitis   288
    Nervous complications of mumps   289
    The Coxsackie viruses   289
    The Echo viruses   290
    Acute haemorrhagic conjunctivitis   290
    Other viral CNS infections   290
    Herpes zoster   291
    Cytomegalovirus infection   293
    Congenital rubella   293
    'Slow virus' infections   294

11. **Neuroimmunology and the demyelinating diseases of**
   the nervous system   295
      The foundations of neuroimmunology   295
      Classification of the demyelinating diseases   298
      Acute disseminated encephalomyelitis   300
      Acute haemorrhagic leuco-encephalitis   305
      Disseminated myelitis with optic neuritis   306
      Multiple sclerosis (MS)   307
      Central pontine myelinolysis   319
      Diffuse sclerosis (Schilder's disease)   319

12. **Extrapyramidal syndromes**   322
      The basal ganglia   322
      The parkinsonian syndrome   325
      Forms of parkinsonism   329
      Wilson's disease   336
      Hallervordern–Spatz disease and infantile
         neuroaxonal dystrophy   339
      Neuronal intranuclear inclusion disease   339
      Torsion dystonia   339
      Spasmodic torticollis   341
      Athetosis   342
      Chorea   343

13. **Some congenital, developmental, and degenerative**
   disorders   351
      Cerebral palsy   351
      Congenital diplegia and quadriplegia   351
      Congenital and infantile hemiplegia   354
      Minimal cerebral dysfunction   355
      Kernicterus   356
      Cerebral malformations   356
      Tuberous sclerosis (epiloia)   358
      Neurofibromatosis   359
      Ataxia telangiectasia   362
      The hereditary ataxias   362
      Motor-neurone disease   370
      Creutzfeldt–Jakob disease   379
      Familial cerebral amyloidosis   379
      Peroneal muscular atrophy   380
      Infantile spinal muscular atrophy and related
         disorders   383
      Facial hermiatrophy   387
      Hemihypertrophy   388

14. **Disorders of the spinal cord and cauda equina**   390
      Anatomy of the spinal cord and cauda equina   390
      Paraplegia   391
      The innervation of the bladder and rectum   393
      The care of the paraplegic patient   394
      Haematomyelia and acute central cervical-cord injury   398
      Compression of the spinal cord   402
      Syringomyelia   412
      Myelodysplasia (spinal dysraphism)   416
      Caudal dysplasia (sacral agenesis)   417
      The Arnold-Chiari malformation   417
      Congenital cervical spinal atrophy   418
      Spina bifida   418
      Myelitis (myelopathy)   420
      Radiation myelopathy   422
      Subacute necrotic myelitis   422
      'Landry's paralysis'   423
      Infarction and ischaemia of the spinal cord and cauda
         equina   423

15. **Intoxications and metabolic disorders**   426
      Alcohol addiction   426
      Drug addiction   431

      Lead poisoning   435
      Manganese poisoning   437
      Mercury poisoning   438
      Other metals   438
      Poisoning with organophosphorus and
         organochlorine insecticides   439
      Subacute myelo–optico–neuropathy (SMON)   439
      Some other poisons with neurological effects   440
      Oral contraceptives   440
      Cerebral anoxia and hypoxia   440
      Carbon monoxide poisoning   441
      Caisson disease   442
      Electric shock   443
      Heat stroke   444
      Accidental hypothermia   444
      Snake bite   444
      Tetanus   444
      Botulism   447
      Saxitoxin poisoning   448
      Ergotism   448
      The neurological manifestations of acute porphyria   449
      The neurological manifestations of hepatic failure   451
      Inborn errors of metabolism including the neuronal
         storage disorders   452
      Urea-cycle disorders   452
      Amino-acid disorders   453
      The lipidoses (lipid storage diseases)   455
      Disorders of serum lipoproteins   464
      Disorders of purine metabolism   464
      Disorders of carbohydrate metabolism   465
      Disorders of mucopolysaccharide metabolism   467
      Miscellaneous disorders of varied or unknown
         aetiology   467
      Some other metabolic disorders   469
      Some endocrine causes of mental retardation and of
         other neurological symptoms   470
      Some non-metabolic causes of mental retardation   471
      Mental retardation syndromes of undetermined
         cause   471
      Carbon dioxide intoxication   472

16. **Deficiency disorders**   473
      Beriberi   474
      Wernicke's encephalopathy   475
      Pellagra   476
      Nutritional neuropathies of obscure origin   477
      Vitamin B_{12} neuropathy (subacute combined
         degeneration of the spinal cord and brain)   479
      Folate deficiency   482
      Neurological complications of other haematological
         disorders   482

17. **The neurological manifestations of neoplasms arising**
   outside the nervous system   484
      Neurological complications of the reticuloses   485
      Paraneoplastic neurological syndromes   486
      The incidence of non-metastatic complications of
         carcinoma   486
      Neurometabolic disorders associated with neoplasms   488

18. **Disorders of peripheral nerves**   492
      Tumours of nerves   492
      Traumatic and allied lesions of peripheral nerves   492
      Symptoms, signs and treatment of individual nerve
         lesions   499
      Spinal radiculitis and radiculopathy   514
      Other forms of mononeuropathy   520
      Polyneuritis (polyneuropathy)   522

Contents   xi

19. **Disorders of muscle**   551
   The anatomy and physiology of muscle   551
   General comments on disorders of muscle   553
   Progressive muscular dystrophy   553
   Myotonic disorders   557
   Inflammatory disorders of muscle   563
   Myasthenia gravis   567
   Endocrine and metabolic myopathies   574
   The floppy infant syndrome   582
   Some miscellaneous disorders of muscle   584
   Differential diagnosis   585

20. **Disorders of the autonomic nervous system**   593
   The autonomic nervous system   593
   Disorders of autonomic function   598
   Syndromes of the hypothalamus   601

21. **Diseases of the bones of the skull**   604
   Osteitis deformans   604
   Leontiasis ossea, polyostotic fibrous dysplasia, and other craniotubular modelling disorders   606
   Craniostenosis   606
   Cleidocranial dysostosis   607

   Hypertelorism   607
   Basilar impression and other craniovertebral anomalies   607

22. **Paroxysmal and convulsive disorders**   609
   Epilepsy   609
   Myoclonus and the myclonic epilepsies   630
   Tetany   633

23. **Psychological aspects of neurology (including consideration of memory, sleep, coma, and the dementias)**   636
   Anatomy and physiology   636
   Consciousness and unconsciousness   640
   Disorders of memory   653
   Disorders of mood   655
   The investigation of mental changes after cerebral lesions   656
   Dementia   657
   Hysteria   661
   Occupational cramps or neuroses   667

Index   669

1

Disorders of function in the light of anatomy and physiology

Some general considerations

Though there can be no absolute distinction between diseases of the nervous system and those which affect other organs or systems of the human body, by convention the clinical science of neurology embraces those many disorders which affect the functioning of the central and peripheral nervous systems and the voluntary muscles. This first chapter will review briefly current knowledge of the means by which disorders of nervous function may be brought about by various pathological processes. The review is organized on an anatomical and physiological basis so that descriptions of the anatomy and,where necessary of the physiology of certain structures and pathways in the nervous system will be considered, together with the disorders of function which result when they are diseased. But it is also important to recognize that the manifestations of disordered function of the central nervous system may be greatly modified by mental, as by pathological processes, and also by the influence of the individual's constitution and inherited characteristics. Furthermore, before considering the pathophysiology of the more important nervous pathways which are commonly affected by disease, it will be necessary to consider the nature of some important units of structure of the nervous system, as well as to classify some of the pathological processes which commonly influence their behaviour.

There are still many problems in neurology which are not clearly understood. We have, for instance, little evidence as to how the brain controls thought processes; while disordered activity of the mind is often present and is attributed to cerebral dysfunction even when modern techniques demonstrate no abnormality of structure and no measurable disorder of function in physiological terms, conversely the influence of the mind upon the physical activity of bodily organs can also be profound. Mental disorders frequently initiate or accentuate symptoms of physical disease and some organic diseases are regularly accompanied by psychological manifestations. The importance of these mechanisms must be recognized by the physician who deals with sick people, as disease is an abstraction; it is the patient who suffers from the disease who is real and who shows a personal and individual reaction to it. Thus although many physical disorders of the nervous system regularly produce specific symptoms and physical signs independent of the personality and constitution of the individual, the severity of the resultant symptoms and the rate of recovery or of deterioration, depending upon the pathological process involved, can be influenced by factors which are independent of the physical process involving nervous tissue. While a single peripheral nerve lesion usually produces a consistent clinical syndrome, its clinical effects may depend upon the nature of the causal lesion, in that in industrial injuries, for instance, the patient's disability may be excessive and his recovery unduly delayed, particularly if financial compensation is involved.

In disorders of the nervous system, more perhaps than in any other group of diseases, the physical signs discovered on examination often indicate the anatomical localization of the lesion or lesions responsible for the abnormalities of function which are present, while it is the history of the illness, revealing the detailed evolution of the patient's symptoms, which generally indicates the nature of the pathological process. Thus although the intelligent interpretation of physical signs demands an adequate knowledge, first, of neuroanatomy for localization of the lesion, and secondly of neurophysiology in order to assess the means by which function

has been disordered, the student must also have some understanding of neuropathology in order to be able to analyse the nature of the pathological process which is present. Admittedly in many neurological disorders, such as migraine and epilepsy, for instance, the clinical picture is typical but physical examination is negative and diagnosis must rest upon analysis of the history alone. Furthermore, as already indicated, the clinical effects of pathological processes are not immutable and the resultant disease can be greatly influenced by the personality and constitution of the individual and by his state of mind. Some patients are born physically and mentally less perfect than others and yet show no obvious defect, but constitutionally are less capable of resistance to stress, both mental and physical, and are seriously disturbed by environmental influences which would leave others unaffected. Hence the possible effects of fatigue, of ageing processes, and of other contributory influences which cannot easily be measured by scientific parameters must be also stressed. In his analysis of the interplay of these many factors, the doctor may need to deploy all his reserves of experience and understanding. It is also important to consider the concept of 'functional' illness or 'functional' disorder. In the strictest anatomical and physiological terms, it would seem reasonable to regard as 'functional' those diseases in which there is an important disorder of the function of some organ of the body but which do not depend upon any recognizable pathological change in the organ concerned. By convention, however, the term 'functional disorder' is more often applied in medicine to symptoms and signs which result from a disordered state of mind. Thus headaches due to anxiety or nervous tension are 'functional', and so, too, is hysterical aphonia, while other forms of anxiety or hysterical reaction are commonly included in this category. Functional disorders, therefore, are those conditions in which symptoms and signs result not from physical disease but from conscious or subconscious mental processes; it must be appreciated that these processes may profoundly affect the physical bodily function, giving rise to such manifestations as increased cardiac output, tachycardia, perspiration, and insomnia. Hence the clinical use of the term 'functional', if not strictly correct semantically, is hallowed through common usage and can usefully be employed provided the doctor using it understands its meaning and does not regard this as a final diagnosis. The distinction between organic and functional disease is often one of the most difficult to make in medicine since even when there is clear evidence of a primary physical abnormality, symptoms may readily be accentuated or distorted by concurrent psychological factors.

Disordered function depends not only upon the localization of pathological change but also upon its severity, its extent, and the effects it has upon contiguous nervous tissue and upon interconnected though anatomically remote structures in the nervous system. Thus an acute and extensive lesion may affect a greater area of the brain than its anatomical extent would lead one to expect, for around the edge of the lesion itself the activity of the surrounding nervous tissue is disturbed by oedema, vascular changes, and other ill-defined abnormalities. Furthermore, an acute lesion can produce a state of 'shock' or temporary dissolution of function in related areas of the brain or spinal cord. By contrast, lesions of equal extent which are slow to develop produce fewer symptoms and signs as it is only the structures which are actively invaded or destroyed by the lesion whose function is disturbed; the surrounding tissues have more time to adapt to the presence of the lesion. Other forms of adaptation may also occur, particularly in the cerebral cortex, for here, particularly in children rather than in adults, a function which has been lost through a cortical lesion may be 'adopted', though usually much less efficiently, by another area of the brain. The younger the patient, the greater the flexibility of cerebral organization. This type of re-organization is much less likely to occur in the spinal cord for the pathways followed here are more stereotyped and probably less complex. No such adoption of function occurs in peripheral nerves, but peripheral nerves are able to regenerate effectively following injury, while effective regeneration does not occur within the spinal cord or brain.

Constitution and heredity

Some neurological disorders are clearly inherited in a strictly Mendelian manner. Diseases such as migraine, Huntington's chorea, and facioscapulohumeral muscular dystrophy are generally inherited by an autosomal mechanism, meaning that they result from a dominant gene situated on one of the autosomes and are thus passed on by an affected individual to half his or her children of either sex if penetrance or expressivity of the gene is complete. An autosomal recessive gene, however, can only produce its phenotypic effect if it is paired with a similar gene, lying on the other chromosome of the pair. Hence such a disease is only expressed when two unaffected heterozygous carriers have children; usually, therefore, there is no previous history of the disease in the family unless there has been intermarriage between relatives (consanguinity). In such families the disease will affect one in four of a series of brothers and sisters; Friedreich's ataxia, hepatolenticular degeneration (Wilson's disease), and spinal muscular atrophy of infancy are usually inherited in this way. A recessive gene can produce an effect, however, if it is situated on the unpaired portion of the X-chromosome, so that the condition occurs in males and is carried by apparently unaffected females. This is the typical pattern of sex-linked recessive (or X-linked) inheritance when the disease may have been found in maternal uncles and now occurs in half the male children of an apparently normal female carrier. Red-green colour blindness, haemophilia, and muscular dystrophy of the Duchenne type are inherited in this way. Any inherited disease can, of course, appear anew in a family if a previously normal gene has undergone a process of spontaneous change or mutation. However, apart from those diseases which are clearly inherited by recognizable genetic mechanisms, there are many other disorders of the nervous system in which genetic influences are important, though these factors are difficult to define. Recent work has however shown that some diseases, like multiple sclerosis, myasthenia gravis and narcolepsy, occur more often in individuals possessing various histocompatibility (HLA) antigens.

Before discussing individual anatomical pathways in the nervous system and the clinical effects of their dysfunction, we must now consider certain units of nervous structure and some of the ways in which they may be affected by pathological processes. This commentary is simple and introductory in nature and for fuller information the reader is referred to textbooks on neuroanatomy, neurophysiology, and neuropathology.

The neurone and its structure

General morphology

The nerve cell or neurone is one of the few cells in the human body which cannot be replaced once destroyed; it cannot divide nor can it regenerate after the first few weeks of extra-uterine life. The neurone theory first proposed by Cajal and his co-workers in 1889–91 stated that each neurone is a separate cellular entity which consists first of a cell body or soma, secondly of dendrites (processes which extend only a short distance from the cell), and

thirdly of an axon which is usually much longer (though some are short) varying in length from a few millimetres to more than a metre. Axons make contact with dendrites or cell bodies of other neurones or with muscle or other effector cells. Each embryonic neuroblast forms a single adult nerve cell and, in the mature human or animal, synaptic junctions of some kind are always present when axons and dendrites meet, so that neurofibrils never pass from one cell to another. It follows that degenerative change in one nerve cell and its processes does not necessarily spread to other cells with which it is in synaptic contact. Similarly, nerve processes always arise by direct growth from parent cells and never by differentiation from intercellular material.

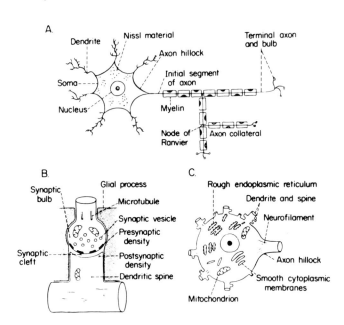

Fig. 1.1. A: a multipolar neurone, as seen under the light microscope. B: a synapse. C: the neurone soma, as shown by light microscopy. (Reproduced from Patton, Sandsten, Crill, and Swanson (1976) by kind permission of the authors and publisher.)

The cell body or soma (Fig. 1.1) contains a nucleus of variable size within which a nucleolus is generally apparent. Nucleoli are rarely multiple; in females there is often a nucleolar satellite made up of heterochromatic X-chromosome material. In the cytoplasm (especially concentrated in synaptic regions) are mitochondria which provide energy and ribosomes which, when aggregated with rough endoplasmic reticulum, form the granules of so-called Nissl substance which stains intensely with basic dyes such as cresyl violet or toluidine blue and these granules may extend for a short distance into the dendrites but never into the axon. Channels and cisternae of endoplasmic reticulum without attached ribosomes, some rough and some smooth, are also present and often connect to form the Golgi apparatus. Even smaller microtubules are also present and probably provide a rapid transport system to distant parts of the cell, while protein threads or neurofilaments, present in the soma, become arranged in a parallel and longitudinal manner in the axons and dendrites. Many different proteins, amines, and enzymes may be synthesized in the cytoplasm of specialized nerve cells and are transported along the axons either to enter the bloodstream through end-feet upon capillaries or to stimulate effector organs or other neurones or synaptic junctions. Some cells form secretory granules or pigment inclusions (e.g. melanin).

There are many millions of neurones in the central nervous system, and they vary greatly in size, shape, and functional characteristics (Fig. 1.2). Unipolar and bipolar neurones are primarily

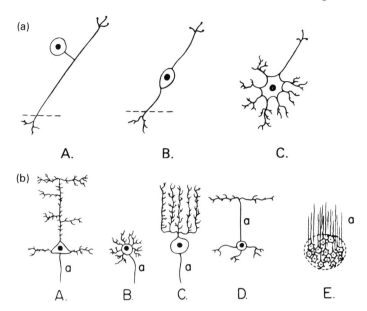

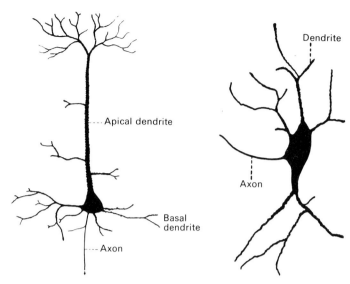

Fig. 1.2. (a) Morphological types of neurones. A: the unipolar (pseudobipolar) neurone is typical of all dorsal root ganglia and general sensory ganglia associated with cranial nerves. B: the bipolar neurone occurs in the cranial nerves for special senses. C: the multipolar neurones differ widely in shape; the motoneurone type is shown here.

(b) Various representative configurations of multipolar neurones. A: pyramidal cell. B: stellate cell. C: Purkinje cell. D: granule cell. E: a nucleus of multipolar cells. a indicates axon. Dendrites have been omitted from E for clarity.

(Reproduced from Patton *et al.* (1976) by kind permission of the authors and publisher.)

Fig. 1.3. (a) Drawing of a pyramidal cell from rabbit cortex. This is a Golgi Type I neurone. Note the surface irregularities of the dendrites (dendritic spines). The axon of this type of cell in man may be 1 m or more in length. Magnification about × 100.

(b) A spindle-shaped neurone from rabbit cortex, about 10 μm in diameter. This is a Golgi Type II neurone. Only the first part of the axon is shown. Magnification about × 500.

(Reproduced from Gardner (1975) by kind permission of the author and publisher.)

afferent and convey sensory information from receptor endings into the central nervous system and are thus largely confined to the spinal dorsal-root ganglia and the cranial nerves. The unipolar (pseudobipolar) neurone has a single process which divides into two parts, one entering the spinal cord, the other extending to the peripheral sensory receptor (as in the skin). Bipolar neurones have an axon which enters the nervous system and a dendrite extending peripherally; these relatively primitive neurones are virtually confined to the sense organs concerned with olfaction, vision, hearing, and equilibrium. Most of the neurones in the central nervous system are of the more complex multipolar type (Fig. 1.2) with a single axon (though this often branches) and multiple branching dendrites. The point of origin of the axon is called the axon hillock. Often these cells are grouped together into conglomerates of uniform function called nuclei (e.g. the motor nucleus of a cranial nerve). There are some neurones which have very large cell bodies (of 50–100 μm diameter) with long axons (such as the anterior horn cell of the spinal cord) and these are often classified as of Golgi Type I. But very many more in both brain and cord are small (with a soma of 5–10 μm diameter) and are called Golgi Type II (Fig. 1.3). Alternatively one may talk of projector neurones (with long axons), interneurones (which play a linking role between other neurones), or motor (effector) or sensory (afferent) neurones. Close to their termination, axons usually divide into fine terminal twigs or telodendria which enter a peripheral end-organ or make synaptic contact with cell bodies or dendrites of other neurones, then forming ring-like endings or *boutons terminaux*. In the central nervous system the mesh of branching axons and dendrites is known as the neuropil.

Dendrites and axons
Dendrites, which are usually short and always branched, often forming a dendritic tree (Fig. 1.2), contain endoplasmic reticulum, microtubules, and neurofilaments but are not myelinated;

they are usually irregular in outline because of their spines (Fig. 1.3) which are devoid of organelles. The dendrites of unipolar and bipolar neurones end in sensory receptors which are sometimes highly specialized (e.g. the rods and cones of the retina and the hair cells of the cochlea and labyrinth).

The axon, sometimes called the axis cylinder (in myelinated fibres) or nerve fibre, is smooth in outline and usually of constant diameter. Its plasma membrane is called the axolemma; its cytoplasm (which contains mitochondria, smooth endoplasmic reticulum, many neurofilaments but few microtubules) is called the axoplasm. Proteins, enzymes, and hormones, and the substances which mediate transmission at the synapses in which the axons terminate, are synthesized in the soma but travel distally along the axoplasm in a process known as axoplasmic flow. The flow of structural proteins and polypeptides is usually slow (1–2 mm a day) while that of transmitter substances and of the hormones produced by some specialized neurones is usually fast (100 mm a day or more). There is also evidence of a reverse flow in many neurones.

The cellular and myelin sheaths

In the peripheral nervous system, all dendrites and axons are surrounded by specialized cellular sheaths, but in the central nervous system dendrites are not so enclosed. In peripheral nerves, axons more than 1–2 μm in diameter are ensheathed by neurilemmal cells (Schwann cells) whose cytoplasmic processes form a spiral enclosing a complex lipoprotein containing sphingomyelin, cerebroside, and cholesterol, called myelin. Unmyelinated axons are also surrounded by neurilemmal cells (Remak cells), one of which may enclose several axons. In myelinated fibres, the investing Schwann cells and myelin are interrupted at regular intervals by short gaps, the nodes of Ranvier, across which so-called saltatory conduction of the nervous impulse occurs. Outside the Schwann cells are the basal lamina (a layer of protein and polysaccharide) and the collagen and reticulum of the endoneurium. The individual axons and their sheaths are bound together into nerves by connective tissue. In the central nervous system, both myelinated and unmyelinated fibres also occur, but it is the oligodendrocyte rather than the Schwann cell which controls the myelin between nodes of Ranvier. The unipolar and bipolar cells of spinal and cranial sensory ganglia are surrounded by satellite cells, some of which can form myelin, and these cells form contact with neurilemmal cells at the origin of the axon. The speed of conduction in myelinated fibres is much faster than in unmyelinated axons, and is indeed faster the greater the diameter of the myelin sheath.

Synapses and neuroeffector junctions

Axons of multipolar neurones either make contact with other neurones in synapses or else they end in an effector organ (e.g. muscle or a secretory gland) or terminate on a blood vessel wall in order to release some substance into the circulation. The telodendria of an axon are unmyelinated and, in both the central nervous system and the ganglia of the autonomic system, they may make contact with a dendrite (axodendritic synapse), with a cell body (axosomatic synapse), or with another axon (axo-axonal synapse), each ending in a *bouton terminal*. Side-to-side contact between individual telodendria can occur at *boutons de passage*; relatively uncommon but found in certain parts of the brain are dendrodendritic, dendrosomatic, and somatosomatic synapses. At most synapses, transmission of the nervous impulse is chemically mediated (chemical synapses) through the release of a transmitter substance (e.g. acetylcholine, noradrenaline, or dopamine) which is stored in synaptic vesicles in the axonal ending, and which passes across the presynaptic membrane and the synaptic cleft to polarize the postsynaptic membrane. The transmitter is stored on only one side of the cleft and transmission is, therefore, unidirectional. In Type I synapses the synaptic vesicles are rounded and the postsynaptic membrane is more dense than the presynaptic, while in Type II the vesicles are smaller and ellipsoid and the presynaptic and postsynaptic membranes are of comparable density. It seems the Type I synapses are excitatory, Type II inhibitory; vesicles containing acetylcholine are usually clear, while those containing catecholamines usually have an electron-dense core. Thousands of synapses may be present on the surface of a single neurone. In invertebrates, in immature mammalian brains, and in a few parts of the adult human nervous system, electrical (nonchemical) synapses or gap junctions are found where there is loose apposition of the plasma membrane of two neurones and synaptic vesicles are absent, so that current flows directly across the junction, at which electrical resistance is low. Tight junctions, at which plasma membranes of two cells adhere, do not occur between neurones but are seen between capillary endothelial cells, ependymal, and Schwann cells. Neuroeffectors are motor end-organs under nervous control, including muscle and secretory glands. The highly specialized myoneural or neuromuscular junction will be considered later.

Receptors

Receptors are specialized structures which respond to changes in their environment by converting the mechanical, electrical, electromagnetic, or chemical information which they receive into an electrical impulse which is either conveyed into the central nervous system as sensory information or which initiates a motor or effector response in the organ upon which the receptor is situated. Some are arrangements of dendrites or neurones, some are not neuronal but are especially sensitive to certain specific stimuli. Some, such as the bipolar olfactory neurones, consist of a cell body with a single modified dendrite, others are highly specialized cells such as the retinal rods and cones, and others are neurones which are sensitive to chemical or physical changes occurring in the circulating blood or extracellular fluid. Many others, and especially those in the skin, tendons, and joints, are specialized structures or complex arrangements of branching nerve fibres in which one branch of the dendrite of a unipolar cell terminates. Sometimes receptors are classified according to whether they are situated in skin (exteroceptors), in muscle and joints (proprioceptors), or in viscera (interoceptors). Comparatively recently, many types of receptors have been identified which are simply specialized areas of cell membranes, such as the postsynaptic membranes, which respond specifically to transmitter release; a good example is the acetylcholine on the surface of the skeletal muscle cell.

The neuroglia

Many differentiating neuroepithelial cells develop into the neuroglia, which neither form synapses nor conduct impulses but which are clearly metabolically active as they contain mitochondria, ribosomes, endoplasmic reticulum, and lysosomes. The so-called macroglia are the oligodendrocytes and astrocytes. Oligodendrocytes are sometimes seen as satellites of large neurones in the grey matter but predominate in the white matter, especially in rows between bundles of nerve fibres (interfascicular oligodendroglia). These cells play the same role in myelination of fibres in the central nervous system as do the Schwann cells in peripheral nerves but, unlike Remak cells, they do not invest but often lie in close relationship to unmyelinated fibres. While Schwann cells individually myelinate a single nerve fibre between internodes, a single oligodendrocyte often myelinates several axons, again between internodes (about 1 mm). When stained with special silver stains, oligodendrocytes are seen to be small with a few short processes (Fig. 1.4); they contain few fibrils and with other stains are difficult to distinguish from small neurones. The astrocytes are larger and stellate, occurring in two forms, called protoplasmic and fibrous. All contain numerous cytoplasmic fibrils and most have at least one process which forms an end-foot on a capillary endothelial cell, so that these end-feet form cuffs around capillaries. Other processes blend with the subpial basal lamina to form a glial limiting membrane, but a basement membrane separates the glial cells from the mesodermal or pial elements. The fibrous astrocytes (Fig. 1.4) predominate in white matter, contain abundant fibrils, and have long, fine, beaded processes which branch less frequently than those of the protoplasmic astrocytes; the latter have thicker, shorter, branching processes, and predominate in grey matter, especially in the neuropil and in relation to synapses, where they seem to separate synaptic zones from one another. Although the astrocytes play an important supporting role in the nervous system, may at times be phagocytic, and can proliferate to form a scar (gliosis) in response to injury, and while they may assume abnormal sizes and shapes in response to various metabolic disturbances or infections (e.g. in hepatic encephalopathy and multifocal leukoencephalopathy), their primary metabolic role and influence upon neuronal activity is not understood.

The cells termed microglia are mesodermal, many being derived from mononuclear cells which migrate from the blood vessels. When inactive, they are small, stain darkly, and have few short processes. When activated in response to disease or injury, they become macrophages (Fig. 1.4).

Ependyma and neurilemma

Ependymal cells, believed by some to be neuroglial, form a single layer of cells with ciliated surfaces lining the cerebral ventricles and the central canal of the spinal cord. Specialized ependymal

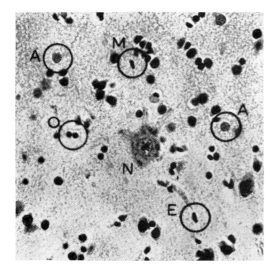

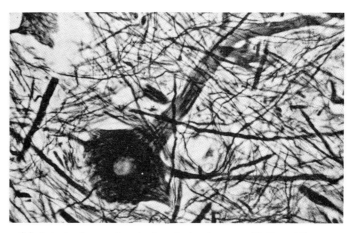

(b) Anterior horn cell, spinal cord, showing neurofibrils and the axon. Hortega's silver, × 350.

Fig. 1.4. (a) Cells of normal precentral cortex stained by Nissl's method. N = nerve cell; A = astrocyte; O = two oligodendrocytes; M = microglial nucleus; E = capillary endothelial cell nucleus. Thionin, × 350.

cells in the choroid plexuses control the production (part diffusion and part secretion) of the cerebrospinal fluid.

The role of the neurilemma in forming myelin sheaths and in investing unmyelinated fibres in the peripheral nervous system has already been mentioned. The neurilemmal sheath is also important in directing regenerating nerve fibres after injury to a nerve. These cells possess other functions which are still poorly understood; thus they may sometimes be phagocytic, ingesting degenerating myelin after disease or injury.

Ground substance

Although grey matter is almost wholly made up of the neuropil, with neuronal cell bodies, their processes and astrocytes and oligodendrocytes along with blood vessels, there appears to be a background substance or intercellular fluid (which is increased in cerebral oedema). Apart from the fact that it probably contains mucopolysaccharides, its nature and function is still unknown.

Some physiological characteristics of the neurone and of synapses and receptors

The neurone

All nerve cells are excitable, reacting or responding to stimuli by undergoing transient physicochemical changes. In the neurone this usually implies a change in the resting potential of the cell, initiating a nerve impulse. The latter then propagates along the cell membrane and is accompanied by an action potential which can be recorded electrically.

The membrane of the nerve cell consists of a bimolecular lipid layer, largely made up of phospholipid, with layers of protein on its inner and outer aspects. While different types of cell membrane often have varying but specific functions, they are not, as their morphology would suggest, fixed and stable structures; on the contrary, they are labile and metabolically active, controlling not only active transmembrane transport in either direction but also relative permeability to different ions. In nerve and skeletal muscle cells, the membrane is relatively impermeable to organic cations, freely permeable to chloride (Cl^-), relatively permeable to potassium (K^+), and much less permeable to sodium (Na^+). In the resting state, the concentration within the cell of K^+ is high

and of Na^+ relatively low, while extracellularly Na^+ and Cl^- are higher and K^+ relatively low. The differences in ionic concentration and electrical charge on either side of the membrane mean that in the resting state the interior of the fibre is negative to the exterior. This state of polarization can be quantified by recording the resting potential through a microelectrode inserted into the neuronal soma (or muscle cell); normally this potential is about -70 mV in nerve and -90 mV in muscle. Some transfer of ions across this membrane in response to a stimulus sufficient to excite the cell occurs by simple diffusion, but normally a state of equilibrium exists so that inward movement of one ion is balanced by a comparable outward movement of another; at equilibrium, the difference in charge across the membrane for a single ion is called the equilibrium potential; it differs from the resting potential slightly because of differences between passive flux and pump flux (see below) for the different ions. It is now known that selective permeability of the membrane to different ions exists, and that passive ionic transfer occurs, but in addition the propagated nerve impulse also involves a process of active transport involving the operation of the sodium (or sodium–potassium) pump and the expenditure of energy, largely derived from adenosine triphosphate (ATP).

Excitation of a neurone giving rise to a propagated action potential is accompanied by the utilization of oxygen and glucose, the formation of carbon dioxide, and the production of heat. Once this potential is initiated, the wave of depolarization spreads at constant speed along the axon, its rate of conduction being dependent upon the diameter of the fibre. Thus in large-diameter axons (such as the giant axon of the squid), a velocity of 25 m a second is achieved but, in man, unmyelinated axons are all much thinner and conduct much more slowly. However, in myelinated nerves, the insulating quality of the myelin decreases capacitance and thus reduces the number of charges held across the membrane at a given resting potential; this allows much more rapid conduction which again depends upon the thickness of the insulation. In such nerves conduction 'jumps' from one node of Ranvier to the next, a process called saltatory conduction. Conduction of the action potential is accompanied by inward movement of sodium and outward movement of potassium, so that in less than 1 ms the polarity of the resting potential is reversed to about $+40$ mV; an electrical 'spike' can be recorded accompanying this event. As the peak of the potential moves on, sodium is pumped out, potassium is pumped back inwards, and the resting potential is eventually restored.

In peripheral nerve axons and their parent nerve-cell bodies, a stimulus applied at above threshold induces an all-or-none response, so that the action potential, once generated, spreads irresistibly with constant amplitude to the termination of the axon;

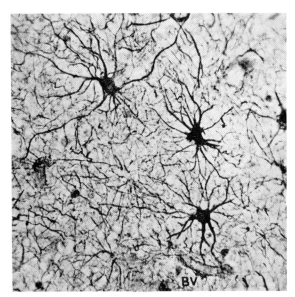

Fig. 1.4. (c) Fibrous astrocytes in the cortex. Cajal's gold sublimate, × 350.

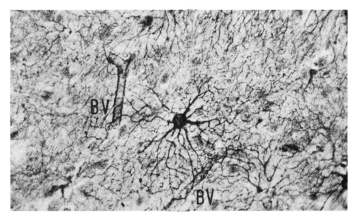

(d) Protoplasmic astrocytes in the cortex. Cajal's gold sublimate, × 350.

thus conduction in nerves and fibre tracts is either 'on' or 'off' and is digital in nature. During the transmission of the action potential, the axon remains insensitive to a further stimulus, however strong this may be (the absolute refractory period); during the period of return to the resting potential, it again becomes excitable, but at a higher threshold (the relative refractory period). Transient hyperpolarization for a few milliseconds follows return to the resting level, producing a brief positive after-potential. However, subthreshold stimuli may produce, even in such structures, localized, non-propagating electrical charges which are graded in intensity until the stimulus increases so as to reach threshold and induce the all-or-none response. Graded responses which diminish decrementally as they spread from the site of stimulation are typically seen in nerve-cell bodies and their dendrites or in peripheral sensory receptors.

Synapses

The arrival of a nerve impulse at a synaptic junction on a cell body may, at those rare electrical synapses which exist in the mature mammalian nervous system, induce a local depolarization in the cell membrane. But transmission at most mammalian synapses is chemically mediated, involving the release of a transmitter substance which crosses the synaptic cleft to combine with receptor sites on the postsynaptic membrane. The synaptic delay (0.6–0.9 ms) required for this process is followed, at excitatory synapses, by a depolarization of the postsynaptic membrane accompanied by the generation of an excitatory postsynaptic potential (EPSP). If this EPSP is subthreshold, no action potential is generated in the postsynaptic cell, but it is rendered temporarily more sensitive to a subsequent stimulus (facilitation); an EPSP above threshold (about 10 mv), by contrast, causes the cell to discharge. If the synapse lies close to the axon hillock, however, the axon may have a lower threshold than the cell body itself, so that initial excitation of the axon may give antidromic conduction of an impulse into the soma and its dendrites. The properties of axodendritic synapses are less well understood; they have a relatively high excitatory threshold but, once excited, depolarization may be relatively prolonged; thus constant stimulation may be applied to the cell body, accounting for the repetitive activity of certain neurones.

There is some similarity between this mechanism of synaptic transmission in the nervous system, with generation of an EPSP, and neuromuscular transmission in which the release of acetylcholine at the motor-nerve ending produces an endplate potential.

However, while acetylcholine is also the transmitter at many synapses in the central nervous system, there are many other central synaptic transmitter substances including noradrenaline, dopamine, and serotonin and various amino acids, probably including glutamic and aspartic acids, and many more. Adenosine may also act as a transmitter in certain spinal-cord synapses. An important difference between neuromuscular and central synaptic transmission is that the former depends upon the sudden massive release of acetylcholine from a single axon on to a single muscle fibre, while in the central nervous system many EPSPs are subthreshold and excitation of the target cell depends upon the summation of the output flow from many presynaptic terminals or synaptic knobs each of which may release subliminal amounts of transmitter substance.

Whereas neuromuscular transmission and that at other neuroeffector junctions, such as those which stimulate glandular secretion, is always excitatory, many synapses in the central nervous system are inhibitory. Presynaptic inhibition is a process which reduces the amount of transmitter released from excitatory presynaptic endings, thus rendering the EPSP subthreshold. This process is probably due, at least in part, to the fact that some excitatory presynaptic terminals actually terminate on other synaptic knobs producing prolonged subthreshold depolarization in the latter with a consequent reduction in transmitter release. In other words, this mechanism diminishes the efficacy of the excitatory input into the postsynaptic cell. Probably commoner is a mechanism which releases an inhibitory, rather than excitatory, transmitter substance; this produces hyperpolarization in the postsynaptic cell, generating an inhibitory postsynaptic potential (IPSP) which has the effect of rendering the cell less excitable. Thus the activity of a cell at any one time may depend upon the balance between excitatory and inhibitory activity in the synapses upon its surface. The principal inhibitory transmitters are gamma-aminobutyric acid, glycine, and alanine.

Thus the passage of information through the nervous system involves alternating electrical and chemical mechanisms. In each neurone, generation and propagation of the impulse (the Hodgkin cycle) either induces an effector response or causes release at a synapse of a transmitter substance which may then initiate the process in another neurone. This process is, however, constantly modulated through the balance existing at any one moment between excitation and inhibition.

Receptors

Many sensory receptors act as transducers which convert the energy to which they respond in a specific manner into an electrical response in that its amplitude depends upon the intensity of the stimulus; if the latter reaches threshold, it elicits an all-or-none response in the form of an action potential which carries sensory

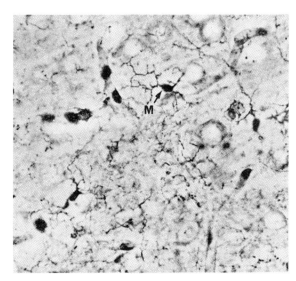

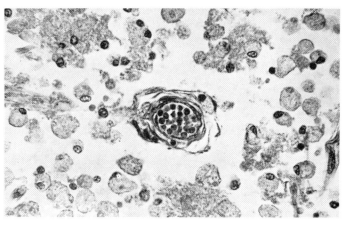

(f) Reactive microglial cells ('compound granular corpuscles' or 'gitter' cells) which are distended with phagocytosed lipid.
(Fig.1.4 (a) – (f) is reproduced from Blackwood, Dodds, and Sommerville (1964) by kind permission of the authors and publisher.)

Fig. 1.4. (e) Normal microglia in the cortex of a rabbit (human cells are similar). Hortega's silver, × 450.

information into the central nervous system. Whereas the generator potential is amplitude-modulated in that its amplitude depends upon the intensity of the sensory input, the action potential is frequency-modulated; as this potential is all-or-none, it can only signify an increased intensity of stimulus by an increased firing frequency.

If a stimulus is prolonged at a steady intensity, then the frequency of discharge becomes progressively less and either ceases or is maintained at a much lower frequency. This phenomenon, known as adaptation, differs in different receptors. The same term, adaptation, is also used to identify a change in the amplitude of the generator potential during a steady stimulus in that the initial peak response is higher than the subsequent plateau potential which resembles a square wave. Physiologically, the first type of adaptation explains why one is conscious of the movement of a part of the body, but awareness of the new posture adopted then declines until further movement occurs.

Receptors in which adaptation leads to a reduced but stable generator potential with a reduced firing rate are called tonic; in these the frequency of repetitive discharge is directly proportional to the magnitude of the generator potential. Such repetitive firing depends upon the fact that, while a constant generator potential persists, a new spike discharge in the axon is generated as soon as the refractory period following the previous spike discharge has passed. In some other receptors, which are called phasic (such as Pacinian corpuscles and hair-follicle receptors), adaptation is rapid and total, so that the generator potential, a transient depolarization, rapidly declines to the baseline even though the stimulus continues. Hence these receptors effectively generate sensory information which reaches perception only during changing stimuli (as in oscillatory or rhythmical stimulation) but not when the stimulus is constant. In some specialized receptors, such as the muscle spindle, sensitivity may be modified by activity in motor-nerve fibres which innervate components of the receptor.

In the earlier section on morphology, we noted that certain specialized nerve cells respond to chemical changes in their extracellular environment (chemoreceptors); little is known of the mechanisms involved. Membrane receptors of many specialized types are found, especially on postsynaptic membranes, which are capable of recognizing, of combining with, and of responding to transmitter substances, such as acetylcholine and the various catecholamines. Some recent progress has been made in isolating and characterizing such receptors. Thus at the neuromuscular junction, using α-bungarotoxin which binds irreversibly to the cholinergic receptor, it appears that there are about 4×10^7 acetylcholine receptors/end-plate and the receptor is probably a lipoprotein with a molecular weight of about 42 000. However, in the neuromuscular junctions of smooth and cardiac muscle, in the neuroeffector junctions in secretory glands, and in cholinergic synapses in the central nervous system and autonomic ganglia, the cholinergic receptors may well be different. Thus, in autonomic ganglia and in certain neuromuscular junctions, they are of two types—nicotinic and muscarinic (see below).

Some neuropharmacological principles

Certain principles of neuropharmacology which relate to processes of nerve conduction and synaptic transmission can usefully be considered here, because of the information we now possess about disordered nervous function which has been derived from studying the effects of various drugs and toxins.

The nerve impulse

Generation and conduction of the neuronal action potential depends upon changes in the permeability of its membrane to Na^+ and K^+ and upon the sodium–potassium pump. There are voltage-sensitive Na^+ and K^+ pores in the membrane and both can be blocked by the local anaesthetic procaine and its analogues. Tetrodotoxin (from the puffer-fish) and tarichotoxin (from certain newts) block only the Na^+ pores, leaving the K^+ channels intact, while saxitoxin (derived from some marine dinoflagellates) has a similar effect. Tetraethylammonium ions, by contrast, block the K^+ but not the Na^+ pores; this does not affect neuronal excitability but prolongs the time-course of action potentials by delaying repolarization.

Synaptic transmission

While the number of chemical substances which can act as neurotransmitters is being added to almost daily, some of the more important will now be described.

Acetylcholine
Acetylcholine is synthesized within neurones from mitochondrial acetyl Co A and extracellular choline through the action of choline acetylase and is then stored in synaptic vesicles. When a nerve impulse arrives, calcium (Ca^{2+}) ions enter the terminal and in some way assist the release mechanism; magnesium ions (Mg^{2+}) may block it. Most of the released acetylcholine then combines

with the acetylcholine receptors in the postsynaptic membrane, but some diffuses away and some is hydrolysed by acetylcholinesterase. This hydrolytic process can be blocked by cholinergic drugs such as physostigmine (eserine), neostigmine, or pyridostigmine, a fact which accounts for the value of these drugs in treating myasthenia gravis, a disease in which some acetylcholine receptors become coated with antibody and are thus unresponsive. The nicotinic effect of acetylcholine is so called because nicotine applied in low concentration to motor end-plates and ganglion cells stimulates and, in high concentration, blocks transmission. Acetylcholine can behave similarly, and the block induced by high concentrations, as may follow overdosage of cholinergic drugs, gives cholinergic paralysis. The action of acetylcholine upon smooth muscle, however, resembles that of muscarine which causes such cells to contract; this action is blocked by atropine. Most synapses in the central nervous system at which acetylcholine is the transmitter are muscarinic in type.

There are many drugs in common clinical use which influence the activity of acetylcholine either by mimicking its action or by blocking its effects. In the central nervous system, atropine, scopolamine, and diisopropyl phosphofluoridate reduce the acetylcholine concentration and may produce confusion, hallucinations, agitation, and slowing of mental processes. Oxotremorine and arecoline have the reverse effect of increasing acetylcholine concentration and increase the amplitude of physiological tremor which then becomes overt. In recent years, cholinergic opiate receptors have also been identified upon those cell bodies in the central nervous system at which it is now known that morphine and its analogues exert their pharmacological effects. Examples of the many drugs which produce muscular weakness or paralysis by acting at the neuromuscular junction are *d*-tubocurarine and suxamethonium, in daily use in anaesthesia; the former blocks the effect of acetylcholine by competing for receptor sites, the latter by mimicking the effects of acetylcholine but by having so prolonged an effect that its action is blocked.

Biogenic amines

The principal biogenic amine transmitters are the catecholamines dopamine, noradrenaline and adrenaline, and serotonin (5-hydroxytryptamine, 5-HT) which is an indole amine. These substances are synthesized within the neuronal soma and transported to the axon terminals. Tyrosine, produced by the hydroxylation of phenylalanine, is the precursor of catecholamine synthesis and is converted by tyrosine hydroxylase into dihydroxyphenylalanine (dopa). Decarboxylation of the latter by dopa-decarboxylase produces dopamine which is a major neurotransmitter, especially in the cells of the substantia nigra; these also contain its pigmentary derivative, melanin. In other cells, dopamine-β-hydroxylase, in the presence of oxygen and ascorbic acid, converts dopamine into noradrenaline. In the adrenal medulla, circulating noradrenaline may be converted by phenylethanolamine-N-methyltransferase into adrenaline which then enters the bloodstream in order to exercise its hormonal effects.

The noradrenaline-containing neurones of the brain originate from cell bodies in the pons and medulla oblongata and connect monosynaptically with various cortical areas, and especially with the limbic system and hypothalamus; some descend into the spinal cord. They appear to be involved in many functions including sleep and wakefulness, emotion, neuroendrocrine function, and temperature regulation. There are three principal systems of dopamine-containing neurones: the nigrostriatal system is largely involved in motor function and the tuberoinfundibular in hypothalamic–pituitary control, but the mesolimbic dopamine system is less well understood, though it probably plays a part in the control of mental and emotional processes. As with acetycholine, the release of these transmitter amines at nerve endings is Ca^{2+}-dependent.

The degradation of catecholamine neurotransmitters is thought to depend largely upon two enzymes, namely monoamine oxidase (MAO) which is largely intraneuronal and is released from mitrochondria, and catechol-*O*-methyltransferase (COMT) which is largely extraneuronal and is probably associated with the adrenergic receptor. Any noradrenaline or adrenaline released into the circulation is metabolized in the liver.

Postsynaptic receptors specifically responding to dopamine and to noradrenaline and adrenaline have been identified. The adrenergic receptors are of two types: alpha receptors, which respond to noradrenaline and to a lesser extent to adrenaline, and are probably regulatory in that the receptor, when activated, inhibits the further release of transmitter; beta receptors, by contrast, activate adenylate cyclase which converts ATP to adenosine 3,5-monophosphate (cAMP) which in turn activates the response in the effector cell.

Serotonin (5-HT) is synthesized from tryptophan via 5-hydroxytryptophan through oxidation prior to decarboxylation. Decarboxylation alone produces pressor agents (tyramine, tryptamine). Serotonin produces contraction in smooth muscle (e.g. in the walls of arteries) and is probably involved in the control of behaviour and in the regulation of sleep and body temperature. It is synthesized in certain neurones of the median raphe of the brainstem and is believed to be the neurotransmitter in some of these cells. In the pineal body, noradrenaline-induced release of cAMP can stimulate the enzymatic conversion of serotonin into melatonin, a hormone which, among other actions, produces lightening of skin pigmentation and may also have an effect upon the sex glands.

There are many drugs which influence the activity of these biogenic amines with consequent profound effects upon brain function. In general, drugs which depress the synthesis or release of noradrenaline or adrenaline have a sedative or depressant effect, while those which similarly depress dopamine tend to produce drug-induced parkinsonism. Reserpine, originally used to treat hypertension but later used as a sedative, may produce severe depression and also parkinsonism; it depletes all brain catecholamines and also serotonin. Certain major tranquillizers, such as the phenothiazines, thioxanthenes, and butyrophenones, interact both with noradrenergic and dopaminergic neurones; it is probably their effect of blocking dopamine receptors which accounts for their antipsychotic action, but which is also responsible for their tendency to produce drug-induced parkinsonism and dyskinesias. The minor tranquillizers used principally to treat anxiety, including the benzodiazepines, appear to act by 'turning off' central noradrenergic neurones. There are two main classes of antidepressant drugs. The MAO inhibitors block the action of MAO in oxidatively deaminating catecholamines, thus increasing the cerebral concentration of both dopamine and noradrenaline. However, the effect of tricyclic antidepressants such as amitriptyline and imipramine is much more selective upon noradrenergic neurones; desimipramine, for instance, is a potent inhibitor of noradrenaline uptake but has only a minimal effect upon dopamine. The tricyclic drugs also have some effect in blocking serotonin. From this it follows that some of these drugs, and especially desimipramine, may have a powerful stimulant effect which is beneficial in the treatment of narcolepsy. Hence they have largely supplanted other stimulants such as the amphetamines and methylphenidate which have also been used as appetite suppressants but which have been widely abused. Amphetamine and its derivatives interact with catecholamine-containing neurones; increased motor activity is thought to be due to stimulation of noradrenergic neurones, its behavioural effects and amphetamine-induced psychosis to its dopaminergic effect. But the effects of amphetamines are not yet fully understood; other dopaminergic drugs such as bromocriptine, which may be beneficial in parkinsonism, as well as levodopa, which restores depleted dopamine stores in the brain, have effects which are similar in some respects to those of amphetamine but very different in others. Another interesting drug, γ-hydroxybutyrate, blocks dopaminergic transmission in the nigrostriatal system, but whether it will prove to be of value in the treatment, say, of phenothiazine-induced tardive dyskinesia has yet to be established.

Another important class of drugs deserving brief consideration here are the hallucinogenic agents such as lysergic acid diethylamide (LSD). It is still not certain whether this and related agents produce their effects by occupying serotonin receptor sites or by direct inhibition of serotoninergic neurones.

Amino acids and polypeptides

The neurotransmitter role of excitatory amino acids such as glutamic and aspartic acids has been inferred from the effects induced when these substances are applied iontophoretically to the surface of postsynaptic neurones. Both are present in high concentration in the cerebral cortex; glutamic acid is the more powerful but their exact localization and function and their putative receptors have not been identified. There is some scanty evidence that glutamic acid may be a sensory afferent transmitter in the spinal cord but here the polypeptide substance P is much more powerful. It is also possible that the latter substance, now isolated not only from dorsal root ganglia but also from the hypothalamus, or some related peptide, may be a neurotransmitter acting in the hypothalamus–pituitary axis.

The inhibitory action of γ-aminobutyric acid (GABA) and of glycine is, however, much better understood and receptors for both have been identified. GABA is derived from glutamic acid by decarboxylation and appears to be the principal inhibitory neurotransmitter in the brain; in the spinal cord, however, it seems to be involved only in presynaptic inhibition. It is directly antagonized by picrotoxin and bicuculline, drugs which consequently produce convulsions in experimental animals. In the spinal cord, and probably in the brainstem, by contrast, the major inhibitory postsynaptic transmitter is glycine, acting particularly at interneurones. The glycine receptors are blocked by strychnine so that poisoning with this drug causes severe muscular spasms which may be precipitated by any sensory stimulus, due to loss of the modulating inhibitory role upon motor activity of these interneurones. Tetanus toxin, which has a similar clinical effect, by contrast, blocks the release of glycine from the same inhibitory nerve endings. The effect of benzodiazepine drugs in producing muscular relaxation and in reducing spasticity appears to result from competition for the glycine receptors where they mimic the effect of glycine.

Histamine

The role of histamine in the brain and in other parts of the central nervous system, as in postganglionic sympathetic fibres where it is present in high concentrations, is still uncertain. It is also present in the hypothalamus, and while a neurotransmitter role has been postulated, proof is still lacking.

cAMP, adenosine, and prostaglandins

cAMP is the intracellular mediator of the action of many substances which interact with cellular receptors, thus influencing cell function; it therefore plays an important part in synaptic transmission. Certainly it mediates the effects of noradrenaline upon postsynaptic neurones. Adenosine can increase cAMP levels experimentally in brain slices and cultured cells by interacting with extracellular receptors linked to adenylate kinase; evidence is accumulating to indicate that it may act as a transmitter in both the central and the peripheral nervous systems but its function has yet to be defined. Prostaglandins (PG) are a class of chemical substances occurring naturally in many tissues and are related derivatives of prostanoic acid. The first to be isolated was an active acidic lipid which caused contracture of uterine muscle. It now appears that PGE_1 and PGE_2 may inhibit sympathetic nervous activity by acting first upon the release of transmitter from adrenergic terminals and by affecting the response in the noradrenaline receptor.

Degeneration and regeneration in the nervous system

An adult nerve cell, once destroyed, can never be replaced. Ageing is associated with a progressive loss of some cortical and spinal neurones. In elderly individuals it is common to find within the cerebral cortex neurofibrillary tangles or so-called senile argyrophilic plaques which develop in relation to degenerating neurones. Such lesions, if seen in profusion in the cerebral cortex at a relatively early age, are virtually diagnostic of presenile dementia and the changes in senile dementia are similar, but it is the age at which they are found and their profusion which is important as they are almost invariably found to some extent as a result of normal ageing processes in the eighth or ninth decades.

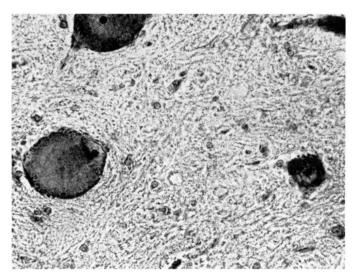

Fig. 1.5. Chromatolysis of an anterior horn cell. The cell is swollen and rounded, the Nissl substance is accumulated at the periphery, and the nucleus is eccentric. H & E, × 350. (Reproduced from Blackwood *et al.* (1964) by kind permission of the authors and publisher.)

When certain processes of a nerve cell are destroyed, the cell body may survive, but if, as a result, say, of peripheral nerve injury, the axon of an anterior horn cell is divided, the Nissl substance in the cell of origin at first aggregates and later disappears (chromatolysis) and the nucleus shifts towards the periphery. These changes are more easily seen in large cells with abundant Nissl substance; their severity is related to the distance of the axonal lesion from the parent cell body, being more severe when the break is close. It is rare for cells with bodies and processes confined to the central nervous system to survive axonal section and hence these cellular changes are sometimes used to locate the cells of origin of degenerating axons in a peripheral nerve or in a specific fibre pathway. However, appearances somewhat similar to those of chromatolysis may occasionally be seen in control material and can result from post-mortem autolysis. When degeneration of a cell body proceeds even further, due either to damage to its axon or to a primary degenerative process, it may be surrounded by microglial cells and later disappears leaving only a small glial cluster (neuronophagia).

An axon that has been severed from its cell body undergoes Wallerian degeneration. Within a few days the terminal part of the axis-cylinder swells; subsequently it becomes beaded and then disintegrates. This process of swelling and disintegration then moves slowly proximally (dying back of the the neurone). If the axon is myelinated, the myelin sheath begins to break down within a few days and the neurilemmal cells then proliferate, subsequently ingesting or enfolding both the disintegrating axis-cylinder and the myelin within Schwann-cell processes. Histiocytes have a phago-cytic role and proliferating connective tissue cells also play a part in the process. Similar axonal changes occur in the central nervous system, except that gliosis results from astrocytic proliferation and the microglia act as phagocytes. The degeneration of myelin secondary to such axonal damage may be identified by specific stains in the Marchi method which demonstrates degenerating myelinated fibres in such a way that these fibres can be traced in microscopic sections.

In peripheral nerves, soon after an axon has been divided, its tip begins to grow out distally into the surviving neurilemmal sheath which directs its growth. Collateral sprouting often occurs alongside the growing axon, though it is usual for one axon to grow distally more rapidly than its collateral sprouts; this distal growth only occurs when the cell body survives and the chromato-lytic process is then reversed. Growth occurs at a rate of a milli-metre or two a day at first, but after a few weeks it slows down; myelin gradually re-forms until eventually the axon re-establishes distal contact. Although profuse axonal sprouting is seen in the brains or spinal cords of very young animals and infants after injury, it is doubtful as to whether it is ever effective as the axonal sprouts rarely, if ever, make contact with any effector cell or organ.

In clinical neurology there are many disease processes which cause demyelination in peripheral nerves or in the central nervous system but which initially leave the axon intact, though incapable of conducting normally. In peripheral nerves such demyelination may begin at or close to the nodes of Ranvier (perinodal demyeli-nation) and may then spread to involve one or many internodal distances. Subsequently, if the disease process is reversed, remye-lination may occur. In teased specimens of nerve fibres obtained by biopsy or at autopsy in such cases, it is often found that the regenerated myelin sheath is thinner than normal and the inter-nodal distances are often irregular and much shorter than normal. A demyelinating neuropathy frequently produces marked slowing of conduction in peripheral nerves, but as the disease process recovers this may eventually return to normal. Demyelination within the central nervous system also affects conduction in the parent axon. The process through which remyelination occurs in the central nervous system is unknown, but presumably accounts for the remissions which occur in demyelinating disorders such as multiple sclerosis.

Some pathological reactions in the nervous system

Pathological changes in the nervous system can be classified into three broad groups, namely focal lesions, which cause a disturb-ance in the function of a strictly localized area; diffuse or genera-lized disorders, whether of metabolic, toxic, vascular, or other aetiology, which affect nervous and supporting elements through-out the nervous system; and systemic nervous diseases, in which the pathological process shows a predilection for a particular neur-onal structure or group of structures such as, for instance, the anterior horn cells, the cerebellum and its connections, or the pyr-amidal tracts. Many focal lesions and diffuse disorders affect ner-vous tissue more or less by accident and are not primarily neurological diseases. Thus cerebral vascular disease, producing ischaemia, infarction, or haemorrhage, is usually a complication of atherosclerosis or hypertension, while the pathological changes which occur in the brain in syphilis, for instance, are only a part of those resulting from infection of the entire human organism. In the systemic nervous diseases, by contrast, as in motor-neurone disease, there is clearly some unknown factor which causes the pathological process to be confined to a particular group of nerve cells or fibre pathways. In this context one must note that the tis-sues of the nervous system vary considerably in their response to many different noxious influences. Thus ischaemia affects nerve cells more severely than myelin and neuroglia, while plaques of demyelination, as in multiple sclerosis, largely affect the nerve fibres of the white matter. There are also considerable differences in the effects of ischaemia, compression, and various toxins upon nerve fibres depending upon axonal and myelin sheath diameter.

Pathological processes may be classified simply on an aetio-logical basis. Thus one can recognize that certain lesions are con-genital or due to developmental abnormality. Others may be traumatic, the lesion then resulting from physical or possibly chemical injury. A third large group is that of the inflammatory disorders which in turn may be subdivided according to whether the inflammation is of infective origin or due to disordered immunity. In either category the inflammation may be acute, subacute, or chronic. Neoplastic disorders must next be con-sidered and these in turn may be benign or malignant, while malig-nant processes may involve the nervous system primarily, or secondarily as a result of metastasis from a tumour elsewhere. Within a further large group of conditions classified at present as being degenerative because their nature is not yet understood, cerebral vascular disease is included, but there are also many other conditions of unknown aetiology which must still be so classified. Finally, many metabolic and endocrine disorders may also affect the functioning of the nervous system.

Of the congenital disorders, these are most often apparent as gross disorders of anatomical development and configuration and include such conditions as anencephaly, hydrocephalus, and men-ingomyelocele. Vascular malformations are almost certainly also of congenital origin. Trauma to the nervous system produces nec-rosis, haemorrhage, and subsequent scar formation, the scar con-sisting of proliferated neuroglial cells and fibrils (gliosis) and of mesenchymal fibrous tissue derived from microglial cells and fibroblasts coming from the supporting tissue of the blood vessels. In the group of acute inflammatory disorders, one must consider the meningitides, producing the typical pathological changes of inflammation and exudation in the meninges. However, men-ingitis may also give rise to superficial degenerative changes in underlying nervous tissue or to ischaemic changes in the nervous parenchyma due to an obliterative endarteritis of those blood ves-sels which traverse the subarachnoid space. Chronic granuloma-tous meningitis (tuberculosis, cryptococcosis, sarcoidosis) produces similar effects but can also cause hydrocephalus due to blockage of circulation of the cerebrospinal fluid (CSF), as well as multiple cranial-nerve lesions due to involvement of the nerve trunks in the inflammatory process. Pyogenic infection in the brain, as elsewhere, begins with diffuse suppuration, but localiza-tion and abscess formation generally follow with the formation of a capsule through gliosis and fibrosis. Most 'neurotropic' viruses, such as those of encephalitis and poliomyelitis, show an affinity for nerve cells, and inflammatory changes with perivascular cellular infiltration and degeneration of nerve cells are therefore seen in the grey matter of the brain and/or spinal cord, sometimes with inclusion bodies in the nucleus or cytoplasm of infected cells. The virus of herpes zoster shows a particular affinity for the cells of the posterior root ganglia, while that of herpes simplex can cause an acute necrotizing encephalitis, involving especially the temporal lobes. The virus can be identified in a biopsy sample of necrotic brain by immunofluorescent methods and/or electron microscopy.

Syphilis, and to a lesser extent tuberculosis, are still two important chronic infections of the nervous system. The patholo-gical changes they produce will be considered under appropriate sections later in this volume as they do not differ significantly from those produced by these diseases elsewhere, except in so far that in general paresis there are degeneration of nerve cells, glio-sis, and minimal inflammatory changes in the cerebral cortex, while in tabes dorsalis the most prominent change is gliosis and meningeal fibrosis of the entry zones of the posterior spinal roots with secondary ascending degeneration of the posterior columns of the spinal cord. In auto-immune or postinfective encephalomyelitis, by contrast to the virus infections, inflammatory changes, consisting largely of perivascular collections of inflammatory cells with loss of myelin, are seen particularly in the white matter. These pathological changes show some resemblance to those observed in the demyelinating disorders of unknown aetiology such as multiple sclerosis and diffuse sclerosis. In these disorders there is patchy loss of myelin of variable extent and severity occurring generally throughout the white matter of the brain and spinal cord. This type of lesion in which the axiscylinders of the nerve fibres are initially preserved is eventually replaced by a glial scar.

In the systemic auto-immune disorders, such as polyarteritis nodosa and systemic lupus erythematosus, the granulomatous vascular lesions may involve the central and/or peripheral nervous system causing multifocal infarction of the brain or infarcts in peripheral nerves with resultant polyneuropathy or mononeuritis multiplex. Other granulomatous arteritides (such as cranial or giant-cell arteritis) can sometimes have similar effects, while thrombotic microangiopathy (thrombotic thrombocytopenic purpura) involves small cortical arterioles and capillaries rather than medium-sized arteries.

The pathology of the neoplastic disorders will be considered in greater detail in the sections on intracranial and intraspinal tumours, but it should be noted here that the commonest benign tumours which compress and distort nervous tissues are the meningioma, which arises from cells of the arachnoid membrane, and the neurofibroma, which grows from the sheath of Schwann of the cranial nerves, spinal roots, or peripheral nerves. The commonest malignant tumour of the central nervous system is the glioma; these are infiltrating and invasive tumours whose relative malignancy depends upon whether the principal constituent cell of the tumour is a relatively mature astrocyte or one of its more rapidly multiplying primitive precursors. Metastatic malignant tumours are also very common; cancer of the lung, breast, and kidney and the malignant melanoma are among those which most often metastasize to the brain. Metastases, which are rarely single, much more often multiple, are often found at the junction of the white and grey matter. Less often, these deposits, or those of lymphadenoma, of leukaemic cells, or of other reticuloses, occur diffusely throughout the meninges giving carcinomatosis of the meninges and a clinical picture like that of granulomatous meningitis. When dural deposits of carcinoma, myeloma, or lymphoma occur in the spinal canal or if a vertebral body collapses following malignant infiltration, spinal cord compression may result.

Vascular disorders are common. Bleeding into the subarachnoid space produces an aseptic meningeal inflammation comparable to that of meningitis and sometimes chronic arachnoiditis may result, while chronic bleeding can cause haemosiderosis of the meninges. Haemorrhage into the nervous parenchyma gives a central area of total necrosis which is eventually walled off by gliosis and fibrosis. Sometimes a scar results, but more often a cavity, filled with a clear straw-coloured fluid containing bilirubin, is left. An infarct shows an area of central ischaemic necrosis but within 24 hours activated microglial cells invade the necrotic area and soon become distended with the fatty remnants of the necrotic myelin which they have ingested. A minute infarct produced by embolic occlusion of a tiny cortical vessel may consist of no more histologically than a small cluster of activated microglial cells, whereas a large one will show an extensive central area of necrosis surrounded by distended phagocytes ('gitter' cells) and proliferating astrocytes. A large infarct may eventually be replaced by a contracted glial scar or cavity, while multifocal infarction sometimes leads to the formation of multiple small cavities (status lacunosus).

There remain many degenerative disorders of the central nervous system whose aetiology is at present unknown, but in some of which specific neuropathological changes are seen. In motor-neurone disease, for instance, the cells of the motor nuclei of the brainstem, the anterior horn cells of the spinal cord, and the corticospinal or pyramidal tracts degenerate progressively. In Huntington's chorea there is selective degeneration of the caudate nucleus and of the nerve cells of the frontal cortex. But in these and in many other disorders which will be considered in later chapters, though the anatomical distribution of the pathological lesions has been well defined, their nature is little understood. Nor do we know why anoxia should affect particularly the cells of the deeper laminae of the cerebral cortex, the Ammon's horn area of the hippocampus, or the Purkinje cells of the cerebellum, nor why hypoglycaemia should involve similar structures save for the Purkinje cells, or even why deficiency of vitamin B_{12}, as in subacute combined degeneration of the spinal cord, should damage so selectively the sensory nerves, posterior columns, and pyramidal tracts.

Many metabolic disorders which seriously disturb nervous function produce relatively little pathological change, but in hepatic failure there is astrocytic proliferation, particularly in the basal ganglia and the brainstem. The pathological changes in many different forms of polyneuropathy are also non-specific as the damage is sometimes primarily axonal swelling and fragmentation of axis-cylinders, but in others it is mainly demyelinating.

The purpose of this section has been to comment briefly upon some of the basic pathological reactions which may occur in the diseased nervous system and not to give comprehensive descriptions of the detailed changes seen in individual disease entities as these will be described later. It will now be convenient to consider the general morphology and organization of the nervous system and some of the important neuronal and fibre systems and pathways as well as the disorders of function which may be produced by disease in these specific structures. The blood supply of the brain and spinal cord will not, however, be considered here, but in Chapters 4 and 14.

References

Behan, P. O. and Currie, S. (1978). *Clinical neuroimmunology*. Saunders, London.

Blackwood, W. and Corsellis, J. A. N. (1976). *Greenfield's neuropathology*, 3rd edn. Arnold, London.

——, Dodds, T. C. and Sommerville, J. C. (1964). *Atlas of neuropathology*. 2nd edn. Livingstone, Edinburgh.

Cooper, J. R. Bloom, F. E., and Roth, R. H. (1978). *The biochemical basis of neuropharmacology*, 3rd edn. Oxford University Press, New York and London.

Davison, A. N. and Thompson, R. H. S. (1981). *The molecular basis of neuropathology*. Arnold, London.

Emery, A. E. H. (1979). *Elements of medical genetics*, 5th edn. Churchill Livingstone, Edinburgh and London.

Gardner, E. (1975). *Fundamentals of neurology*, 6th edn. Saunders, Philadelphia.

Katz, B. (1966). *Nerve, muscle and synapse*. McGraw-Hill, New York.

Kreig, W. J. S. (1966). *Functional neuroanatomy*, 3rd edn. Brain Books, Evanston, Illinois.

Matthews, W. B. (1976). *Practical neurology*, 3rd edn. Blackwell, Oxford.

Patton, H. D., Sundsten, J. W., Crill, W. E., and Swanson, P. D. (1976). *Introduction to basic neurology*. Saunders, Philadelphia.

Pratt, R. T. C. (1967). *The genetics of neurological disorders*. Oxford University Press, London.

Tower, D. B. (ed.) (1975). *The nervous system*, Vol. 1, *The basic neurosciences*. Raven Press, New York.

Walton, J. N. (1982). *Essentials of neurology*, 5th edn. Pitman, London.

Zacks, S. I. (1971). *Atlas of neuropathology*. Harper and Row, New York.

The cerebrum

General morphology

The general morphology of the cerebral hemispheres is illustrated in Fig. 1.6. The longitudinal fissure separating the two hemispheres is largely occupied by a fold of dura mater, the *falx cerebri*. The convolutions are called *gyri*, the fissures between them the *sulci*, and many of both are named (Fig. 1.7). The *frontal lobe*

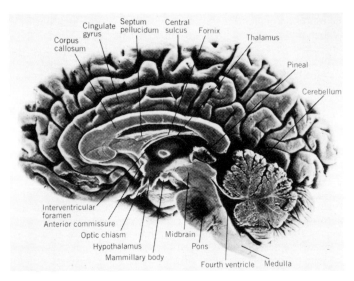

Fig. 1.6. (a) Sagittal view of an adult brain specimen.

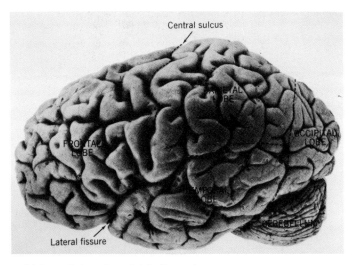

(b) Lateral view of an adult brain specimen.

lies anterior to the *central or Rolandic sulcus*, the *temporal lobe* below the *lateral sulcus* (*fissure of Sylvius*) in the depths of which is the *insula*. The *parietal lobe* lies behind the central sulcus but the division between it and the posterior part of the temporal lobe is not well defined; the transition between both these lobes and the *occipital lobe* is also somewhat arbitrary, not being defined by any single sulcus. The frontal *precentral gyrus* is especially concerned with the control of movement, the *postcentral gyrus* of the parietal lobe with somatic sensation, the middle part of the *superior temporal gyrus* with hearing, and the striate cortex of the *occipital pole* with vision. The prefrontal cortex plays a part in controlling intellect and personality, the *orbital cortex* (and especially its cingulate gyrus) in visceral and emotional activity, and the medial

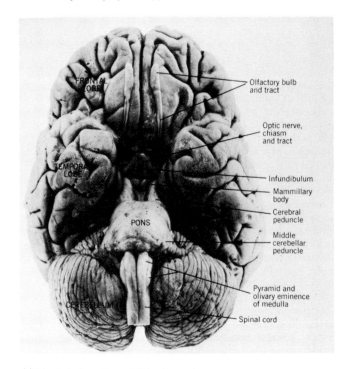

(c) Ventral view of an adult brain specimen.
(Reproduced from Paton, Sundsten, Crill, and Swansen (1976) by kind permission of the authors and publisher.)

temporal cortex (especially the hppocampal gyrus and related structures) in controlling the sense of smell and memory. In man, specialized functions relating to the production and perception of speech and to various executive and cognitive skills (praxis and gnosis) reside in one cerebral hemisphere (usually the left in right-handed persons); this is called the *dominant hemisphere*. Deep in the cerebral cortex are many myelinated fibre tracts forming the central white matter of the hemispheres and joining the various cortical areas to one another. There are also ascending and descending tracts connecting with the central grey matter of the basal ganglia and other nuclei and with the brainstem and spinal cord; yet others cross to the opposite hemisphere in various midline commissures, of which the *corpus callosum* is the most important. The principal grey nuclei in the depths of each hemisphere are the *thalamus* and *hypothalamus*, the *caudate and lenticular nuclei* which together form the *corpus striatum*, the *globus pallidus*, and the *putamen* (Fig. 1.8). The *internal capsule* is an important collection of myelinated fibre tracts, connecting the central white matter above with the *cerebral peduncle* below.

The cerebral cortex

The cerebral cortex or *pallium* is the layer of grey matter covering the cerebral hemisphere. Man is distinguished from the lower vertebrates and invertebrates by the massive development of the *neocortex* of the forebrain. The phylogenetically primitive *paleocortex* (largely olfactory) and *archicortex* (largely embodied in man in the the so-called limbic system, including the hippocampus) together form the so-called *rhinencephalon* or smell brain, though these areas subserve many other functions in man relating to memory and emotion in addition to smell.

Man's neocortex has a surface area of 2000 cm² and varies in thickness from 2 to 4.5 cm. Silver and Nissl stains have revealed that many different cell types are present in the cortex and are usually arranged into six layers (Fig. 1.9). The way in which the

(a)

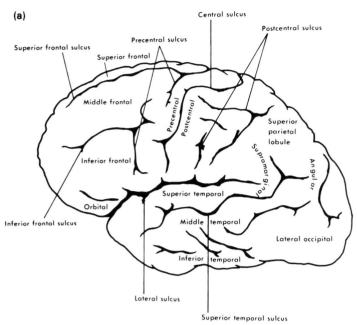

(b)

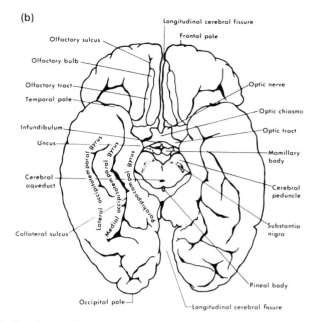

Fig. 1.7. (a) Outline sketch of the lateral surface of the cerebral hemisphere. The gyri are directly labelled (except the superior frontal) and the sulci are indicated by lines.

(b) Outline sketch of the inferior aspect of the brain with the brainstem removed by a section through the midbrain.
(Reproduced from Gardner (1975) by kind permission of the author and publisher.)

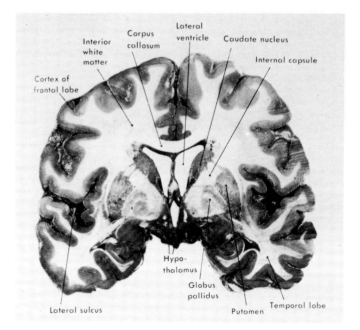

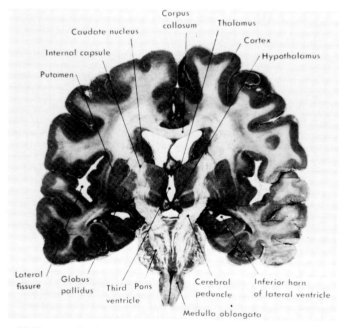

Fig. 1.8. (a) Photograph of a coronal slice of brain, stained by a Berlin blue reaction that accentuates the grey matter and leaves white matter relatively unstained.

(b) Photograph of a coronal slice of brain, posterior to that of Fig.1.8 (a) and stained by the same method.

cells are arranged within these layers varies greatly from one area of cortex to another. The study of this cellular arrangement is known as cytoarchitectonics, of which Brodmann was the principal proponent. He divided the cortex into 52 numbered areas (Fig. 1.10); while some of these are of functional significance (area 4 corresponds roughly to the precentral motor cortex and area 17 to the occipital visual cortex), many such variations in cortical structure have no obvious functional correlates.

Cortical neurones

Four types of neurones have been identified, namely the *pyramidal*, *stellate* (or granule), *fusiform*, and *horizontal* cells. Pyramidal

cells have a soma varying in diameter from 15 to 100 μm, and the largest are the *Betz cells*. They each have an apex with a long dendrite projecting towards the cortical surface, a basal dendritic arborization, and axons which project away from the cortex into white matter but usually have collateral branches which turn back to the surface. Relatively few axons, even of the Betz cells, reach the corticospinal (pyramidal) tract. A few (*Martinotti cells*) have axons which do not leave the cortex. Stellate cells have a star-shaped dendritic tree also confined to the cortex, and the fusiform cells of the deepest cortical layer lie with their bodies perpendicular to the cortical surface. They have short dendrites leaving each pole, and are to be contrasted with Cajal's horizontal cells of the superficial cortical layer, which have bodies lying parallel to the surface and dendrites running in a similar direction.

The cortical layers

The *molecular layer* (I; see Fig. 1.9) consists mostly of dendritic fibres and scattered horizontal cells. The *outer granular layer* (II) contains small pyramidal and stellate cells, while the *pyramidal-cell layer* (III) contains small pyramidal cells. The *inner granular layer* (IV) consists of numerous stellate cells whose axons largely synapse with dendrites of cells in layers V and VI; this layer is also traversed by the axons of pyramidal cells in layer III, most of which enter white matter. The *ganglionic layer* (V) contains pyramidal cells including Betz and Martinotti cells and some stellate neurones. Axons of these cells enter white matter and form corticospinal (or other projection) tracts as well as commissural or association fibres. The deepest or *fusiform layer* (VI) consists mainly of fusiform cells.

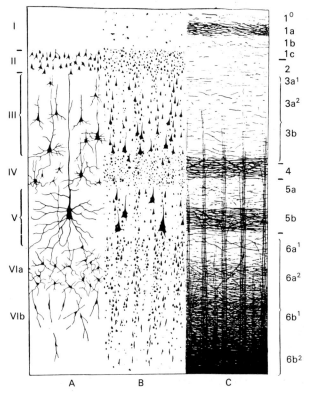

Fig. 1.9. Schematic diagram showing the structure of the cerebral cortex obtained by A: Golgi stain; B: Nissl stain; and C: myelin stain. (Reproduced from Ranson and Clark (1959) by kind permission of the authors and publisher.)

Myelin stains (C in Fig. 1.9) demonstrate horizontal bands of myelinated fibres in layers IV and V (the *lines of Baillarger*),the outer of which is so prominent in the visual cortex that it gives a visible striation (the *line of Gennari*) so that this is known as the *striate cortex*.

When the six layers of cortex are clearly identifiable, the cortex is called *homotypical*. But in some areas the layers are less distinct (*heterotypical cortex*); thus, in the precentral motor cortex, layers II and IV are poorly defined (*agranular cortex*), while in some areas where sensory information is recorded (the postcentral gyrus and especially the occipital striate cortex), layers III and V contain few pyramidal cells and the density of stellate or granular cells in layers II and IV is increased (*granular cortex*). In certain cortical areas, groups of cells in various cortical layers, interconnected by vertical axons or dendrites, appear to form functional units or *columns*. All cortical cells gradually decrease in number with increasing age after the age of 20 years, and this decrease is greatest in

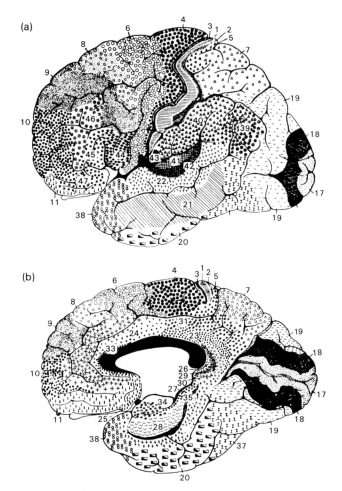

Fig. 1.10. Cerebral cortical cytoarchitectural map of Brodmann. (Reproduced from Ranson and Clark (1959) by kind permission of the authors and publisher.)

'large neurones', less in 'small neurones', and least in glial cells (Henderson, Tomlinson, and Gibson 1980).

Some axons which leave the cortex constitute *corticofugal fibres* which project to the basal ganglia, thalamus, brainstem, cerebellar grey nuclei, and the spinal cord, while others form *commissural fibres* travelling to the opposite hemisphere. Yet others form *association fibres* and project to other areas of cortex; some are short and remain cortical, but others are long and form prominent tangential subcortical tracts (the *arcuate or U-fibres* which are especially prominent in the posterior parts of both hemispheres).

The electrical activity of the cortex

Intracellular recordings from cortical neurones have shown that they have properties similar to those of nerve cells in the spinal cord (see above), but with some important differences (see Patton, Sundsten, Crill, and Swanson 1976). Their resting potential of about -60 mV shows marked fluctuations, presumably resulting from constant bombardment through synaptic connections with other cells. Many also show graded excitatory or depolarizing postsynaptic potentials (EPSPs) and inhibitory, hyperpolarizing postsynaptic potentials (IPSPs), but the IPSPs are often larger and of longer duration than those recorded in spinal cord. A bewildering and complex array of connections (somatodendritic, axodendritic, and many more) interlink the cortical neurones. For example, pyramidal cells may be excited or inhibited by afferent fibres, by interneurones, and by recurrent collaterals. Few generalizations about the physiological activity of cortical neurones are yet possible.

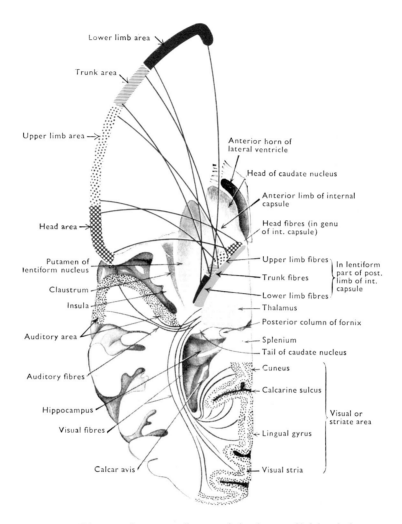

Lower limb area

Trunk area

Upper limb area

Anterior horn of
lateral ventricle

Head of caudate nucleus

Anterior limb of internal
capsule

Head area

Head fibres (in genu
of int. capsule)

Putamen of
lentiform nucleus

Upper limb fibres
Trunk fibres
Lower limb fibres

In lentiform
part of post.
limb of int.
capsule

Claustrum

Insula

Thalamus

Posterior column of fornix

Auditory area

Splenium

Tail of caudate nucleus

Auditory fibres

Cuneus

Calcarine sulcus

Hippocampus

Visual or
striate area

Visual fibres

Lingual gyrus

Calcar avis

Visual stria

Fig. 1.11. Diagram of motor, auditory, and visual areas of left hemisphere
and their relations to the internal capsule.

The *electrocorticogram* (ECoG) is the spontaneous electrical activity of the cerebral cortex recorded through an electrode applied to its surface; the *electroencephalogram* (EEG) is the electrical activity of the brain studied by recording from electrodes applied to the intact skull. Increasingly used of late in clinical neurological practice is the technique of recording *sensory evoked potentials* induced by a sensory stimulus applied to a peripheral receptor which projects to the area of cortex where the afferent impulses are received. While initially these evoked potentials, which represent synchronous potential changes in the neuronal population underlying the recording electrode, were often recorded from the exposed cortex, increasingly sophisticated recording methods and techniques of summating and averaging have made it possible to record somatic, visual, and auditory evoked responses through the intact skull. Individual cortical neuronal spikes, which can be recorded through extracellular electrodes inserted into the cortex, contribute little to these evoked potentials. The initial positive wave of the primary evoked sensory potential appears to reflect summated EPSPs occurring deep in the cortex, while the later negative deflection results from a combination of delayed IPSPs arising deeply and EPSPs arising nearer to the surface. Such evoked-potential recording in clinical practice, demonstrating abnormalities of pattern, amplitude, and latency of response, can give invaluable information concerning the integrity of sensory pathways.

The motor system

Introduction

Disorders of movement of the parts of the body produce some of the commonest symptoms professed by patients with disease or disordered function of the nervous system. Sometimes the ability to move a part voluntarily is impaired (weakness or paresis) and sometimes it is lost completely (paralysis). Alternatively, willed movements are clumsy, ill-directed, or uncontrolled (ataxia or incoordination), or else the part moves spontaneously or independently of the will (involuntary movements). On examination the examiner may be able to confirm these abnormalities and may also find abnormalities of tone in which the normal response to passive stretching of a muscle is altered; it can be reduced (hypotonia) or increased in one of two ways (spasticity, rigidity). Abnormalities of movement, and particularly weakness or paralysis, are sometimes emotionally determined (hysteria); alternatively they can be apraxic, resulting from a cortical lesion which has impaired the ability to recall acquired motor skills.

More often, however, they are due to disordered function of the motor pathway which begins in the motor area of the cerebral cortex and ends in the voluntary musculature. There are many important physical signs which help to localize lesions within this motor apparatus, but in order to appreciate their significance a working knowledge of the organization of movement is essential.

The organization of movement

General considerations

The motor system of man consists first of the descending pathways derived from the cerebral cortex and brainstem which are concerned with the suprasegmental control of movement; second of the basal ganglia and cerebellum; third of the continuation of these pathways within the spinal cord; and fourth of the neuromuscular system, made up of the nuclei of the motor cranial nerves and the muscles which they innervate, as well as the anterior horn cells of the spinal cord along with the segmentally organ-

ized voluntary musculature of the trunk and limbs. Both at the higher and at segmental levels, major afferent pathways project to these motor structures providing an input of information about the relative positions of different parts of the body and about muscle length (through the fusimotor spindle system of the muscles); this input modulates movement. The basal ganglia and cerebellum do not project directly to the segmental motor structures of the brainstem and spinal cord but process information from other parts of the nervous system and project backwards on to the cortical and brainstem structures from which the suprasegmental pathways arise.

The components of the motor system

The corticospinal and corticobulbar (pyramidal) system

While, strictly speaking, the pyramidal tract is that bundle of descending motor nerve fibres which traverses the medullary pyramid to enter the spinal cord and thus contains both corticospinal fibres and others derived from brainstem structures, it has been conventional, if slightly inaccurate, to regard the terms corticospinal and pyramidal as being synonymous in referring to descending motor pathways.

Structure. The *upper motor neurones*, which constitute this pathway, arise in part from nerve cells in the precentral motor cortex of the cerebrum (see above and Fig. 1.11). Whereas some of these neurones arise from the giant Betz cells which are common in this area, there are far more fibres in the pyramidal tracts than could be accounted for by the axons of all the Betz cells, so that many of the other motor neurones must arise from nerve cells in or near this area which are not structurally distinctive. In man, the pyramidal tract contains about 1 000 000 fibres, of which 94 per cent are myelinated but only 10 per cent have a diameter of more than 4 μm and only 2 per cent originate from Betz cells and are more than 10 μm in diameter. Thus most fibres of this tract are small myelinated fibres which arise from neurones (mostly frontal, but some parietal) lying around the central or Rolandic sulcus (Walshe 1943). Stimulation experiments have revealed that activation of cells in the lower end of the precentral gyrus will cause bilateral movement of the pharynx and larynx, while just above are others which, if stimulated, give rise to movement of the contralateral half of the tongue (Figs. 1.11 and 1.12). Facial movement can be elicited at a point slightly higher still and stimulation will give bilateral movement of the upper face but unilateral movement only of the lower face. Movement of the contralateral hand, arm, trunk, leg, and foot are then produced in turn as one ascends the gyrus, and in each case 'representation' is strictly unilateral. The leg and foot 'area' lies partly on the medial surface of the hemisphere and partly on its superior aspect (Fig. 1.12). Nerve fibres arising from these cortical cells then come together in the corona radiata and converge upon the internal capsule which lies deep in the hemisphere between the thalamus and caudate nucleus medially and the lenticular nucleus laterally (Fig. 1.13). The pyramidal tract has long been thought to occupy the posterior one-third of the anterior limb, the genu, and the anterior two-thirds of the posterior limb of the capsule (Fig. 1.12); however, there is some recent evidence to suggest that most of its fibres lie in the middle third of the posterior limb (Nathan and Smith 1955; Englander, Netsky and Adelman 1975). Behind it lie sensory fibres travelling to the postcentral sensory cortex and other fibres forming the optic radiation, while anteriorly are frontopontine fibres. From the internal capsule the tract passes down in the middle three-fifths of the cerebral peduncle to enter the midbrain; in the pons it is broken into bundles by transverse pontine fibres, but in the medulla it again becomes a compact tract, the pyramid, which forms an anterior prominence. Throughout the brainstem, the tract gives off corticobulbar fibres which travel to the contralateral motor nuclei of the cranial nerves. In the lower part of the medulla, most fibres of the pyramidal tract decussate to form the crossed pyramidal tract which descends in the lateral column of the spinal cord on the opposite side, but a small proportion do not do so and continue downwards in the anterior column, forming the direct or uncrossed pyramidal tract which extends downwards only as far as the dorsal spinal cord; there is, however, a good deal of individual variation (Nathan and Smith 1955; Nyberg-Hansen and Rinvik 1963). Fibres of the pyramidal tract do not as a rule synapse directly with the anterior horn cells from which the lower motor neurones arise (Hoff and Hoff 1934) but rather with inter-nuncial neurones in the grey matter of the spinal cord, which in turn pass on to synapse in the anterior horns.

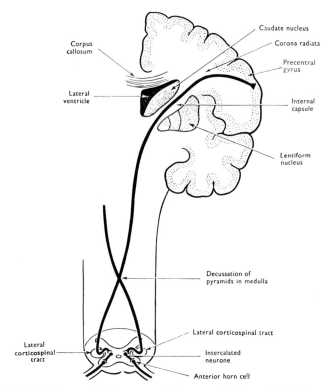

Fig. 1.13. Diagram showing course of the crossed corticospinal tracts.

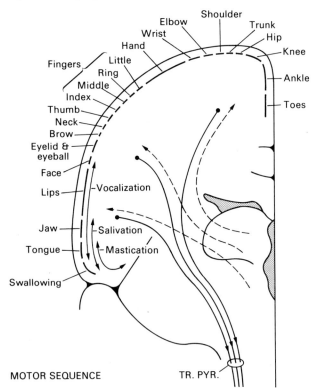

Fig. 1.12. Corticospinal motor pathway (pyramidal tract). Cross-section through right hemisphere along the plane of the precentral gyrus. The sequence of responses to electrical stimulation of the surface of the cortex (from above down, along the motor strip from toes through arm and face to swallowing) is unvaried from one individual to another.

The *lower motor neurones* (alpha neurones), which transmit impulses from the motor nuclei of the cranial nerves and from anterior horn cells of the spinal cord to the voluntary muscles, constitute the final common path of motor activity. In other words, all nervous mechanisms which influence muscular activity must produce their final effects through impulses which travel along these fibres. Their structure and function and that of the motor unit will be considered later.

Other small motor neurones (gamma neurones) innervate only the intrafusal fibres of the muscle spindle and form part of the reflex mechanism concerned with the control of muscle tone.

Function. The basic functional units through which a muscular movement is initiated and performed are outlined in the anatomical schema laid out above. However, the organization of movement is much more complex than this outline would suggest. Thus no single cell in the motor area of the cerebral cortex can be said to innervate any single muscle. Stimulation experiments (Denny-Brown 1966) have revealed that it is not single muscle twitches, but organized movements, which are initiated in the motor cortex. These movements involve several muscles or muscle groups, of which only some act as *prime movers* or *agonists*. Others, the

antagonists, must be enabled to relax smoothly as the agonists contract, while yet others (*fixators*) are required to fix a limb proximally, say, in order to allow a movement occurring distally to be efficient. Other muscles (*synergists*) counteract unwanted effects which would be produced by the unmodified action of the agonists. In general, stimulation of pyramidal-tract neurones excites those groups of muscles which fulfil physiologically a flexor role, and inhibits the antigravity or extensor muscles, so that those neurones primarily concerned with voluntary movement excite the agonists concerned with fine or precise movements while inhibiting the antagonists, many of which are concerned with segmental postural mechanisms. The descending fibres of the tract also exercise an effect upon gamma as well as alpha motor neurones. The profuse internuncial neurones in the spinal cord, which receive impulses from many pyramidal axons and influence the activity of many anterior horn cells, are clearly important in this organization. However, incoming sensory impulses from stretch receptors (muscle spindles) in the muscles themselves, as well as other proprioceptive input which continually informs the individual of the position of the part which is being moved, also modifies this activity through various spinal reflexes. Additional modifying influences are exerted through sensory impulses from the eyes and labyrinths which enter the brainstem and initiate activity in the vestibulospinal tracts.

Not only can sensory impulses influence movement in this way, but other important effects are exerted by the so-called *extrapyramidal motor system* and by the *cerebellum*, which will be considered below. These structures exercise their effects through a series of descending pathways which, though they may influence profoundly the activity of the pyramidal tract, are yet independent of it.

The rubrospinal, vestibulospinal, and reticulospinal tracts
Axons arising from the red nucleus which lies in the tegmentum of the midbrain cross the midline immediately and then descend through the lateral brainstem and lateral column of the spinal cord, where they are closely related to fibres of the pyramidal

tract, and synapse with internuncial neurones in the lateral part of the ventral grey matter, Excitation of these fibres gives facilitation of both alpha and gamma neurones supplying distal limb muscles. The red nucleus itself receives an input from the cerebral cortex, largely through corticospinal-tract collaterals, and from the cerebellum; while in primates division of this *rubrospinal tract* causes paresis of distal limb muscles, there is no clinical syndrome in man recognized as being due to interruption of this pathway.

The *lateral vestibulospinal tract* originates in neurones of the lateral vestibular (Deiters') nucleus of the pons, which receives an input from vestibular neurones and from cerebellar Purkinje cells as well as midline cerebellar nuclei. The fibres of this tract synapse with alpha and gamma neurones and with internuncial neurones in the ipsilateral anterior horns of the cord, and especially with those which supply axial and proximal limb muscles. Stimulation of this tract excites the neurones which innervate extensor or postural muscles and inhibits those which fulfil a flexor role. The shorter *medial vestibulospinal tract* arising from the medial vestibular nuclei only extends downwards to the mid-dorsal level and appears to subserve a similar function in relation to neck and paraspinal muscles.

Descending *reticulospinal tracts*, originating respectively in the pontine and medullary reticular systems, excite both alpha and gamma neurones supplying extensor muscles. The anatomy of these descending tracts has been reviewed in man by Nathan and Smith (1955) and in the cat by Nyberg-Hansen and Brodal (1963, 1964) and by Nyberg-Hansen (1965).

Conclusions

It thus appears that a particular movement is initiated when the idea of the movement is first invoked in the 'association' areas of the cortex in which acquired motor skills (praxis) are stored (see below). The appropriate motor cells of the precentral cortex are then activated and impulses travel down the pyramidal tracts, in order to activate the appropriate anterior horn cells and the motor units which they supply. Simultaneously the movement is influenced and controlled by the activity of the cerebellum and of the components of the extrapyramidal motor system; at the same time as the agonists are being stimulated to contract, the synergists to assist, and the fixators to fix, an inhibitory mechanism must be invoked to produce controlled relaxation of the antagonists. Once the movement has begun it is then continuously modified through sensory impulses arriving from the proprioceptors, or from the eyes and labyrinths. Clearly, therefore, in view of its complexity, movement can be disorganized by lesions of many different nervous pathways, and some of the principles which aid in deciding which pathway or pathways are diseased will be considered below.

The basal ganglia

Structure. The basal ganglia, a group of nuclei situated deep within the substance of the cerebral hemispheres and brainstem, include the *caudate nucleus, putamen, globus pallidus* or *pallidum*, the *claustrum, subthalamic nucleus*, and *substantia nigra* (see Mettler 1968). The putamen and pallidum together form the *lentiform nucleus*, while the streaky appearance of the caudate, putamen, pallidum, and claustrum in myelin-stained sections has resulted in these nuclei being referred to collectively as the *corpus striatum*. The *thalamus*, in addition to its important sensory functions, plays a part in the control of movement; it and the caudate nucleus lie medially in close relationship to the lateral ventricle and they are separated from the lenticular nucleus by the internal capsule, while the claustrum, lying deep to the insula, is separated from the lenticular nucleus by the external capsule. Phylogenetically, the pallidum or *paleostriatum* is older than the caudate nucleus and putamen or *neostriatum*. Some of the principal interconnections of the basal ganglia are shown in Fig. 1.14.

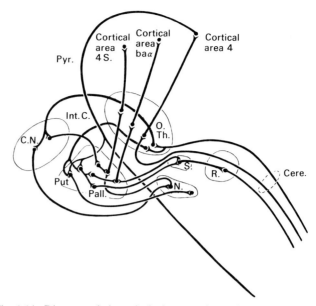

Fig. 1.14. Diagram of the principal connections of the basal ganglia. Abbreviations: Pyr., corticospinal tract; Int. C., internal capsule; C.N., caudate nucleus; Put., putamen; Pall., globus pallidus; O.Th., optic thalamus; S., subthalamic nucleus; N., substantia nigra; R., red nucleus; Cere., ascending cerebellar pathways.

The principal connections of the basal ganglia, organized topographically, are from the cerebral cortex to the striatum, to the pallidum and onwards to the thalamus, with further projections rostrally from the nucleus ventralis anterior (VA) and nucleus ventralis lateralis (VL) back to the motor areas of the cortex. Efferent pathways also connect the striatum, but more particularly the pallidum, with the subthalamic nucleus and substantia nigra. Recent work has also demonstrated an important reverse pathway (not shown in Fig 1.14) from the substantia nigra to the striatum. It now seems that the basal ganglia influence movement largely through thalamic relays which project to the motor cortex, by integrating their output with cerebellar input to the VL nucleus, and by descending impulses conveyed by the rubrospinal and reticulospinal tracts.

Function. While the function of the basal ganglia is complex and much more remains to be elucidated, the corpus striatum clearly plays an important role in the regulation of posture and the globus pallidus (pallidum) is the final efferent-cell station of the basal ganglia, its activity being influenced by inputs from the cortex, striatum, substantia nigra, and subthalamic nucleus. The principal efferent pathway from the pallidum passes rostrally via the VL nucleus of the thalamus and caudally via the subthalamic and red nuclei; it plays a vital role in initiating movement and lesions of this nucleus can give severe akinesia (inability to initiate movement) or bradykinesia (excessively slow movement). Clearly, too, the basal ganglia exert a controlling influence upon the balance of alpha and gamma motor neurone activity; when disease causes imbalance, abnormalities of muscle tone or tremor may result. The concerted activity of the basal ganglia gives a smooth co-ordination of voluntary movement, depending upon a delicate physiological balance; certain lesions of individual components of the system distort this balance, allowing the release, due to removal of inhibitory mechanisms, of various involuntary movements (chorea, athetosis, dystonia, hemiballismus) which will be described in Chapter 12.

Neuropharmacological studies (see Yahr 1976) have shown that in parkinsonism the concentration of dopamine in some nuclei of the basal ganglia is reduced and that many of the neurones of the substantia nigra, and especially those of the nigrostriatal pathway, are dopaminergic, while striatonigral neurones, by contrast, appear to employ GABA as their transmitter. Reserpine and some phenothiazine drugs can deplete dopamine stores and give rise to drug-induced parkinsonism, while phenothiazines can also produce facial dyskinetic movements (tardive dyskinesia) or dystonic phenomena. Similarly, levodopa, a dopamine precursor, while it restores dopamine stores and ameliorates parkinsonism, can produce, as a troublesome side-effect, movements resembling athetosis. It is also known that many neurones in the striatum are cholinergic and that cholinergic activation can enhance the manifestations of parkinsonism. Hence it seems that many of the clinical features of disease or dysfunction of the basal ganglia are due an imbalance in the relative activities of cholinergic and dopaminergic neurones and their receptors.

The cerebellum

It has been suggested that the cerebellum is responsible for modulating afferent somatic sensory information and for correlating this with the motor output from the cerebrum and brainstem in order to co-ordinate movements of greater precision.

General morphology. The cerebellum occupies the greater part of the posterior cranial fossa, being separated from the cerebral hemispheres above by a fold of dura mater, the tentorium cerebelli, whose free medial border virtually encircles the midbrain. It consists of two *cerebellar hemispheres* united by the median *vermis*; on its surface is a midline hollow, the vallecula, into which the inferior part of the vermis projects. The superior, middle, and inferior *cerebellar peduncles* join the cerebellum to the brainstem.

The cerebellar surface shows gyri and sulci which are much narrower than those of the cerebral cortex, together with several deeper fissures. The *horizontal fissures* separate the upper and lower parts of the cerebellar hemispheres. The *primary fissure* separates the anterior and middle lobes of the hemispheres, and the *retrotonsillar fissure* defines two tongues of cerebellar tissue close to the midline and just above the foramen magnum; these are the cerebellar tonsils. The *secondary fissure* separates two parts of the vermis known as the uvula and pyramid.

The *anterior lobe* includes most of the superior vermis and the anterosuperior parts of the cerebellar hemisphere. The *posterior lobe* includes the *flocculus*, a small ovoid portion of cerebellum lying between the tonsil and the middle cerebellar peduncle, and the *nodule*, a part of the vermis lying anterior to the uvula. Phylogenetically this posterior or *flocculonodular lobe* is the oldest part of the cerebellum and has extensive connections to the vestibular nuclei of the brainstem through vestibulocerebellar fibres. The remainder of the cerebellum not included in the anterior and posterior lobes forms the *middle lobes*; together the anterior and middle lobes, which include the hemispheres and part of the vermis, are often called the *neocerebellum*.

In contrast to the brainstem with its external white matter and internal grey matter, the cerebellum, like the cerebrum, has a core of white matter and an outer cortex of grey. Deep in the white matter lie a series of grey nuclei, the *lateral (or dentate)*, the *intermediate*, and the *medial or fastigial*; the intermediate and medial nuclei are often called the roof nuclei. Axons from the cells of the cortex and of the nuclei connect cortex to cortex (association fibres), cortex to nuclei and vice versa, and cerebellum to brainstem or spinal cord (projection fibres) as well as hemisphere to hemisphere (commissural fibres). Thus efferent fibres from the dentate nuclei constitute the major part of the superior cerebellar peduncles.

Cellular structure and organization. The cerebellar cortex, unlike the cerebral, is of uniform thickness and shows a regular cellular and synaptic organization. In the deepest part of the outer *molecular layer* lie the *Purkinje cells* with related *basket, Golgi, and stellate cells*; beneath these is the *granular layer* made up largely of small granular neurones.

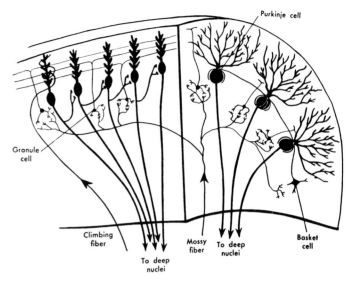

Fig. 1.15. Diagram of cells in a folium of the cerebellum. The Purkinje cells have a large dendritic tree across the plane of the folium; hence in the view on the right they are much more extensive than in the plane parallel to the length of the folium on the left. Mossy fibres synapse with many granule cells in the cerebellar glomeruli. The axons of granule cells enter the molecular layer and divide, each branch running lengthwise in the folium as a parallel fibre, synapsing with Purkinje cells and basket cells. Climbing fibres synapse directly with Purkinje cells. Axons of Purkinje cells have recurrent branches to adjacent Purkinje cells and to other cells (not shown). (Reproduced from Gardner (1975) by kind permission of the author and publisher.)

The Purkinje cells have an extensive dendritic arborization (Fig. 1.15) in the molecular layer; their axons project into white matter but give off collaterals to other Purkinje cells and Golgi cells. Two main types of afferent fibres enter the cerebellum through the inferior and middle peduncles. *Mossy fibres*, derived from many sources, synapse with granule cells forming *synaptic glomeruli* in islands of the granular layer. Axons of granule cells enter the molecular layer and bifurcate forming *parallel fibres* which synapse with many Purkinje-cell dendrites thus enabling a single mossy fibre to influence the activity of many Purkinje cells. *Climbing fibres* arise from the inferior olives in the medulla and synapse with the dendrites of not more than 10 Purkinje cells. Mossy-fibre input to granular cells is excitatory, as is the parallel fibre system, and each Purkinje cell may receive synaptic input from up to 100 000 parallel fibres, allowing a finely graded excitatory input which evokes repetitive firing represented by single spikes when action potentials are produced in Purkinje cells. The stellate and basket cells, by contrast, are inhibitory interneurones which inhibit Purkinje-cell activity, while the Golgi cells fulfil a similar inhibitory role upon granule cells by synapsing with their dendrites. By contrast, the climbing fibres, which enter by the inferior cerebellar peduncle, may synapse with several Purkinje cells but each of the latter receives an excitatory input from only one such fibre; however, each winds around many dendrites of a single cell, making up to 200 synaptic contacts, thus fulfilling a powerful excitatory role. The EPSP of a climbing fibre has an amplitude of more than 25 mV, well above the threshold of the Purkinje cell. Excitation through climbing fibres, in contrast to that evoked through parallel fibres, evokes complex spike discharges. It has been suggested that the climbing-fibre system is concerned with the control of rapid, phasic movements, while that of the mossy-fibre system is involved in the control of slow tonic movements.

Function. The *archicerebellum*, consisting of the flocculonodular lobe and uvula, receives afferent fibres from the vestibular neurones direct and also via the vestibular nuclei; in turn, efferent fibres from this lobe derived from Purkinje cells travel via the fastigial nucleus and the inferior cerebellar peduncle to the vestibular nuclei. This area is concerned with the control of eye movements and with postural reflexes involving neck and axial muscles and thus with equilibrium. Lesions in this midline area give dysequilibrium without vertigo (truncal ataxia) and often positional nystagmus.

The *palaeocerebellum*, the next oldest, consists of the vermis and of contiguous portions of the cerebellar hemispheres. The spinocerebellar and cuneocerebellar tracts end in mossy fibres which enter this structure. The *dorsal spinocerebellar tract* originates in Clarke's column of cells near the lateral horn area of spinal grey matter in segments T1–L2, which receive afferents from the muscle spindles and Golgi tendon organs. The fibres of this tract enter the cerebellum through the inferior cerebellar peduncle and project to the palaeocerebellar cortex, carrying especially information conveyed by muscle spindle Group Ia afferents concerned with the control of muscle tone, and derived from specific muscles and muscle groups on the same side of the body. The *cuneocerebellar tract* conveys similar information from the head and neck musculature. The *ventral* (from the legs and trunk) and *rostral* (from the arms) *spinocerebellar tracts* project similarly to the palaeocerebellum but enter via the superior cerebellar peduncles and carry incoming information from the Group Ib spindles afferents and from cutaneous sensory receptors. There is also an efferent pathway from the palaeocerebellum via the fastigial nucleus to vestibular and reticular neurones which travels onwards in the vestibulospinal and reticulospinal tracts. These pathways exercise a modulating effect upon muscle spindle activity and integrate many afferent signals relating to the length of muscle fibres, thus providing a kind of positive servo-mechanism. Clinical lesions of this part of the cerebellum may increase decerebrate rigidity causing a shift from a gamma- to an alpha-type of rigidity (see below) and, like some lesions of the archicerebellum, selective damage to this area may (as in alcoholic cerebellar degeneration) cause truncal ataxia with a broad-based unsteady gait.

The remainder of the cerebellum, constituting the major part of the cerebellar hemispheres (the *neocerebellum*) receives collateral branches from pyramidal neurones and mossy pontocerebellar fibres originating in contralateral pontine nuclei. Efferent fibres from the deep nuclei of the cerebellar hemispheres (which receive afferents from cortical Purkinje cells) leave the cerebellum through the superior peduncles, cross the midline, and then project to the VL nucleus of the thalamus. This part of the cerebellum is especially concerned with the regulation and smooth co-ordination of limb movements, fulfilling a graduating and harmonizing role and also playing a part in the control of posture. Neurophysiological studies have confirmed that striking differences in firing rates (some increasing, some decreasing) occur in the Purkinje cells and in the neurones of cerebellar nuclei during voluntary activity.

The brainstem

General organization

The *midbrain*, *pons*, and *medulla oblongata* together constitute the brainstem which is largely made up of ascending, descending, and decussating myelinated-fibre tracts which join the different parts of the brain and the spinal cord, together with other tracts which interconnect various nuclei of the brainstem itself. But in addition, the brainstem contains numerous grey nuclei which form the afferent and efferent nuclei of the cranial nerves as well as others such as the *substantia nigra* and *red nucleus* of the midbrain and the *inferior olivary nuclei* of the medulla which play important roles in the control of movement and, in effect therefore, are related to the extrapyramidal motor and cerebellar systems. Other nuclei, such as the *geniculate bodies* of the midbrain (visual and

auditory) and the *gracile* and *cuneate nuclei* of the medulla (somatic sensory), constitute important relay stations in sensory pathways; the relay function of the many grey nuclei in the basis pontis (*pontine grey matter*) is less well understood, but myelinated axons from these nuclei form much of the middle cerebellar peduncle. The nuclear groups receiving primary afferent fibres from the cranial nerves are generally situated in the posterolateral part or tegmentum of the brainstem while the efferent (largely motor) neurones are situated more anteriorly, but instead of forming continuous columns of cells as in the anterior horns of the cord, they are divided into discrete nuclei. Diagrammatic representations of various structures seen in sections of the brainstem at different levels are given in Fig. 1.16.

Another important component of brainstem structure is the *reticular formation* which contains, in a physiological rather than an anatomical sense, both activating and inhibitory systems concerned with sleep, consciousness, and arousal, with activation and inhibition of movement, and with control of behaviour and memory via connections with the cerebral limbic system. It is continuous above with the intralaminar nuclei of the thalamus which form another part of the system. This formation is represented by a group of cells and fibres which form the central portion or core of the brainstem, lying largely between the anterior motor nuclei and tracts and those situated more posteriorly which are more often sensory or afferent. It receives multisynaptic inputs from the spinal cord and its axons project both to the spinal cord and to more rostral structures in the brain. Within the reticular system of the medulla oblongata are small groups of neurones which constitute the *respiratory* and *cardiac centres*, which exercise profound controlling influences through somatic, but more particularly autonomic, efferents upon respiration and upon the cardiovascular system. There is also a less well-defined centre controlling peristaltic and other motor and secretory activity in the gastrointestinal tract, sometimes loosely referred to, because of one of its functions, as the vomiting centre.

So far as the cranial nerves are concerned, many of the 12 pairs are comparable in many respects to spinal nerves, except that some are purely motor or purely sensory, unlike spinal nerves, each of which contains motor (anterior roots) and sensory (posterior roots) components. The *second or optic nerve* is in fact a myelinated-fibre tract extruded from the central nervous system during development and the *olfactory bulb and tract* (the first nerve) is somewhat similar, as its ganglion cells lie in the nasal mucosa. The *eighth* (*vestibulocochlear*) nerve is concerned with hearing and equilibrium, the *third* (*oculomotor*), *fourth* (*trochlear*), and *sixth* (*abducens*) nerves with ocular movement and the pupillary reactions. The *fifth nerve* (*trigeminal*) has a sensory root and ganglion (Gasserian) which carries somatic sensation from the face and a motor root which innervates the muscles of mastication (temporales, masseters, and pterygoids). The *seventh* (*facial*) nerve is motor to the facial muscles, but also includes the *chorda tympani* which carries taste from the anterior two-thirds of the tongue to the tractus solitarius (solitary nucleus) in the pons; the *eleventh* (*spinal accessory*) innervates the sternomastoids and trapezii, and the *twelfth* (*hypoglossal*) the muscles of the tongue. The *ninth or glossopharyngeal* is motor to the cricopharyngeus (pharyngeal sphincter) but also carries taste from the posterior one-third of the tongue, while the *tenth or vagus* innervates the muscles of the soft palate, pharynx, and larynx but also carries the principal cranial parasympathetic outflow to the lungs, heart, and abdominal viscera. The cranial nerves are considered in detail in Chapter 2.

The spinal cord and ganglia

General morphology

The spinal cord begins where the medulla oblongata ends at the foramen magnum and extends to the lower border of the first lumbar vertebra, where it terminates in a thin terminal fibrous extension of the pia mater, the *filum terminale*, which lies among the

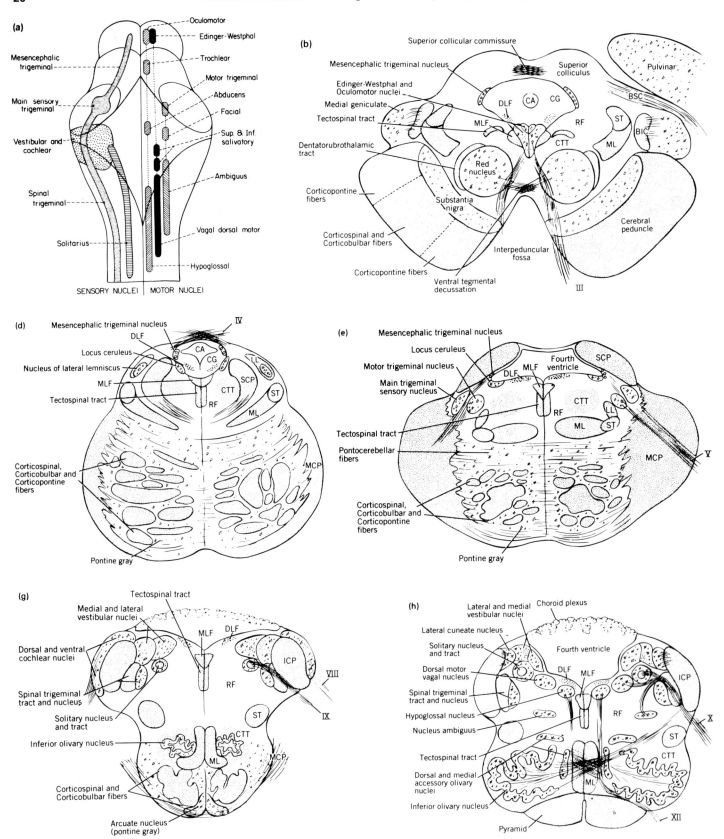

Fig. 1.16. (a) Cranial-nerve nuclei in surface projection on a schematic posterior view of the brainstem. The cerebellum has been removed by a cut through the cerebellar peduncles, so that the floor of the fourth ventricle is revealed. Caudally, the medulla is severed at about the transition to the spinal cord. Rostrally, the superior and inferior colliculi of the midbrain are indicated. The cranial-nerve sensory nuclei are shown on the left side and the motor nuclei on the right. These motor and sensory nuclei are grouped according to the functional categories of their efferent and afferent fibres and associated brainstem nuclei.

(b) The midbrain at the level of the superior colliculus and oculomotor nerve (III). Fibres of the oculomotor nerve are leaving to enter the interpeduncular fossa. The medial lemniscus (ML) is in the lateral part of the

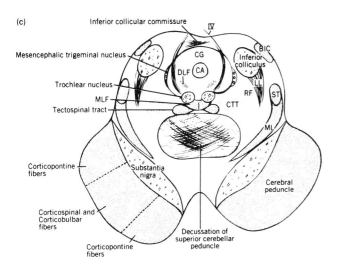

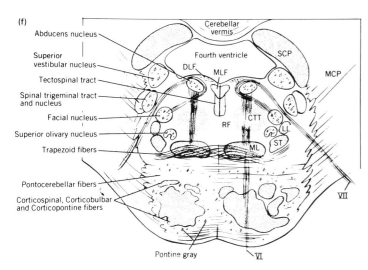

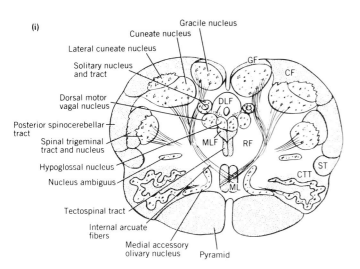

from the red nucleus cross at the ventral tegmental decussation, and at a more caudal level will join the fibres in the central tegmental tract (CTT), finally ending in the spinal cord. CA, cerebral aqueduct; CG, central grey matter; MG, medial geniculate; MLF, medial longitudinal fasciculus; RF, reticular formation; ST, spinothalamic tract.

(c) The midbrain at the level of the inferior colliculus and the trochlear nerve (IV). Fibres of the trochlear nerve are leaving dorsally. The medial lemniscus (ML) is rotating into a dorsoventral position in the lateral tegmental field. The lateral lemniscus (LL) is entering the nucleus of the inferior colliculus. Fibres from the cerebellum are crossing through the tegmentum as the decussation of the superior cerebellar peduncle. BIC, brachium of the inferior colliculus; CA, cerebral aqueduct; CG, central grey matter; CTT, central tegmental tract; DLF, dorsal longitudinal fasciculus; MLF, medial longitudinal fasciculus; RF, reticular formation, ST, spinothalamic tract.

(d) The rostral pons at the isthmus. Fibres of the trochlear nerve (IV) are crossing as they leave dorsally. The medial lemniscus (ML) is moving laterally and beginning to rotate to a dorsoventral position. The superior cerebellar peduncle (SCP) is moving towards the midline. The rostralmost edge of the middle cerebellar peduncle (MCP) is present. The corticospinal, corticobulbar, and corticopontine fibres, which constitute the cerebral peduncle, are separating as they plunge into the basilar pontine grey matter. CA, cerebral aqueduct; CG, central grey matter; CTT, central tegmental tract; DLF, dorsal longitudinal tract; LL, lateral lemniscus; MLF, medial longitudinal fasciculus; RF, reticular formation; ST, spinothalamic tract.

(e) The midpons at the level of the trigeminal nerve (V). Fibres of the trigeminal nerve separate the main sensory trigeminal and motor trigeminal nuclei. The cell bodies of proprioceptive trigeminal afferents constitute the mesencephalic nucleus. The trigeminal nerve leaves throught the middle cerebellar peduncle (MCP). The medial lemniscus (ML) has begun to move laterally towards the spinothalamic tract (ST). The superior cerebellar peduncle (SCP) forms the lateral wall of the fourth ventricle as it descends from the cerebellum towards the midbrain tegmentum. Pontocerebellar fibres (receiving input from the corticopontine fibres) are streaming across the midline to form the middle cerebellar peduncle. The corticospinal, corticobulbar, and corticopontine fibres are scattered throughout the basilar pontine grey matter. CCT, central tegmental tract; DLF, dorsal longitudinal fasciculus; LL, lateral lemniscus; MLF, medial longitudinal fasciculus; RF, reticular formation.

(f) The caudal pons at the level of the abducens (VI) and facial (VII) nerves. The abducens nerve leaves ventrally through the basal pons near the midline; the facial nerve loops medially around the abducens nucleus and then courses laterally to emerge at the caudal edge of the middle cerebellar peduncle (MCP). The pontine grey matter is sending pontocerebellar fibres across the midline to form the middle cerebellar peduncle. The superior cerebellar peduncle (SCP) is projecting towards the midbrain. The medial lemniscus (ML) has rotated to a mediolateral position and is obscured by trapezoid fibres of the auditory system that cross the midline; the trapezoid fibres will turn rostrally to ascend in the lateral lemniscus. Primary afferents from the trigeminal nerve have formed the spinal trigeminal tract. CTT, central tegmental tract; DLF, dorsal longitudinal fasciculus; LL, lateral lemniscus; MLF, medial longitudinal fasciculus; RF, reticular formation; ST, spinothalamic tract.

(g) The rostral medulla at the level of the vestibulocochlear (VIII) and glosopharyngeal (IX) nerves. The cochlear nuclei cap the lateral surface of the inferior cerebellar peduncle (ICP). The medial lemniscus (ML) is still situated medially along the midline. Its trigeminolemniscal components (not shown) would be in its most dorsal part; the laterally placed spinothalamic tract (ST) would also contain trigeminothalamic components. The rostral pole of the inferior olivary nucleus appears in the course of the descending central tegmental tract (CTT), some of whose fibres terminate there; another component of the central tegmental tract will continue its descent to the spinal cord (rubrospinal tract). The corticospinal and corticobulbar fibres are closely grouped as the pontine grey matter thins out; just caudal to this section they will form the medullary pyramids. The caudalmost edge of the middle cerebellar peduncle (MCP) is present. DLF, dorsal longitudinal fasciculus; MLF, medial longitudinal fasciculus; RF, reticular formation.

(h) The midmedulla at the level of the vagus (X) and hypoglossal (XII) nerves. The vagus nerve leaves lateral to the inferior olivary nucleus, whereas the hypoglossal nerve does so between it and the pyramid. Motor components of the vagus are shown coming from the dorsal motor vagal nucleus and nucleus ambiguus; visceral afferents are forming the tractus solitarius. The medial lemniscus is orientated dorsoventrally along the

tegmental field. The brachium of the inferior colliculus (BIC) is entering the medial geniculate and the brachium of the superior colliculus (BSC) is entering the superior colliculus. Fibres from the decussation of the superior cerebellar peduncle have formed at the lateral margin of the red nucleus as the dentatorubrothalamic tract; it sends fibres to the red nucleus and to the ventralis lateralis nucleus of the thalamus. Rubrospinal fibres midline above the pyramid; the spinothalamic tract (ST) is in the lateral part of the tegmental field. Olivocerebellar fibres are crossing and will enter the inferior cerebellar peduncle (ICP). The lateral cuneate nucleus is also sending fibres into the inferior cerebellar peduncle. The descending corticospinal and corticobulbar fibres have grouped together to form the pyramids. CTT, central tegmental tract; DLF, dorsal longitudinal fasciculus; ML, medial lemniscus; MLF, medial longitudinal fasciculus; RF, reticular formation.

(i) The caudal medulla at the level of the sensory decussation. Most of the fibres of the gracile fasciculus (GF) have already synapsed in the gracile nucleus. Internal arcuate fibres from the cuneate and gracile nucleus are crossing to form the medial lemniscus (ML). Second-order fibres from the spinal trigeminal nucleus are extending towards the midline. They will cross, some forming a component of the medial lemniscus and others mixing with the spinothalamic fibres. The spinothalamic tract (ST) is in the lateral tegmental field. The posterior spinocerebellar tract is lateral to the spinal trigeminal tract and will enter the inferior cerebellar peduncle rostral to this level. CF, cuneate fasciculus; CTT, central tegmental tract; DLF, dorsal longitudinal fasciculus; MLF, medial longitudinal fasciculus; RF, reticular formation.

(Fig. 1.16(a)–(i) is reproduced from Patton *et al.* (1976) by kind permission of the authors and publisher.)

many roots of the *cauda equina* which fill the spinal canal below the termination of the cord, eventually fusing with the coccygeal dura mater and thus in a sense tethering the cord. The tapering terminal portion of the cord is known as the *conus medullaris*.

There is a posterior median longitudinal groove on the surface of the cord, the *posterior median sulcus*, with two less clearly defined *posterior intermediate sulci* lateral to it and a deep anterior fissure, the *anterior median fissure*, in the depths of which lies the anterior spinal artery. The *central gray matter* of the cord, in which lies the *central canal*, is approximately H-shaped but varies considerably in its extent and shape in different segments, being considerably larger in the *cervical* and *lumbar enlargements*; it is surrounded by myelinated columns of fibres which are organized into *columns* or *funiculi*, the *anterior, lateral,* and *posterior*, which again vary in configuration depending upon the segmental level at which a transverse section is examined. A spinal cord *segment* is that portion of the cord giving rise to a single spinal nerve on each side. Since the cord is much shorter than the spinal column, it follows that the individual segments of the cord do not correspond to the vertebrae in relation to which they lie, so that, for instance, the sixth dorsal segment of the cord lies approximately at the level of the fourth dorsal spinous process, while all of the lumbar, spinal, and coccygeal segments occupy that part of the cord lying behind the tenth dorsal to the first lumbar vertebrae inclusive. The segmental organization of the cord is illustrated in Fig. 1.17 and the appearance of the cord in transverse section at different levels in Fig. 1.18.

In the spinal-cord grey matter, the *posterior horns* are particularly concerned with the reception of afferent fibres of various kinds and many cells within them are interneurones, while in the *anterior horns* the neurones are almost wholly efferent, being largely *alpha* and *gamma* motor neurones. The *intermediolateral grey matter* in the dorsal region gives rise to sympathetic efferent fibres, in the sacral region to parasympathetic efferents, while in the dorsal region there is a lateral horn occupied by a column of cells (Clarke's column) from which the dorsal spinocerebellar tract arises.

The posterior columns of grey matter, divided in the cervical cord into the gracile (medial) and cuneate (lateral) fasciculi, largely convey fine tactile and proprioceptive sensation rostrally, the gracile from the lower limbs, the cuneate from the upper, while the more important tracts in the lateral columns are the *lateral corticospinal* (pyramidal) (motor efferent), spinocerebellar, and *lateral spinothalamic* tracts (sensory afferent for pain and temperature sensation). There is also an *anterior corticospinal* tract and an *anterior spinothalamic* which conveys crude touch sensation (Fig. 1.19); in the rostral cervical cord one may also find the

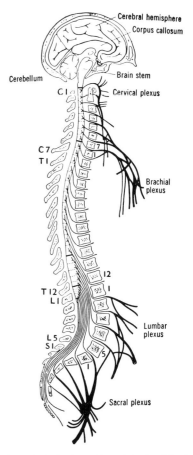

Fig. 1.17. Drawing of the brain and cord *in situ*. The brain is shown sectioned in the median plane. Although not illustrated, the first cervical vertebra articulates with the base of the skull. The letters along the vertebral column indicate cervical, thoracic, lumber, and sacral. Note that the cord ends at the upper border of the second lumbar vertebra. (Reproduced from Gardner (1975) by kind permission of the author and publisher.)

lower part of the spinal accessory (eleventh cranial nerve) nucleus and a downward extension of the medial longitudinal fasciculus, an important interconnecting pathway, largely confined to the brainstem, and principally concerned with the co-ordination of ocular movement and with binocular vision.

The spinal nerve and ganglia. The spinal nerves are formed by the fusion of the *posterior roots* which enter the cord close to the posterior horns of grey matter upon which lie the *posterior root ganglia*, and of the *anterior roots* which emerge from the surface of the cord close to the anterior horns. The anterior roots are wholly efferent, containing both *somatic and visceral efferent fibres* arising from the anterior horn and intermediolateral cells respectively. Similarly, the posterior roots receive both somatic and visceral *afferents*, but their pseudounipolar ganglion cells lie in the posterior root ganglia (Fig. 1.20).

The anatomy of the motor efferent system, the organization of the spinal nerves into plexuses and/or peripheral nerves, and the principles governing the innervation and activity of the limb and trunk musculature, and similar considerations relating to the sensory system, will be considered later, while the structure and function of the autonomic nervous system are described in Chapter 20. However, certain general principles deserve consideration here. Thus, each spinal nerve, containing afferent and efferent fibres, divides into a *posterior ramus* innervating the muscles and skin of the back and an *anterior ramus* supplying the anterior body wall, limbs, and other appendages. The individual muscles or muscle

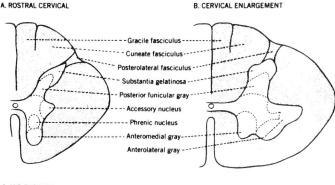

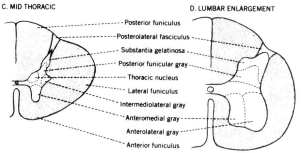

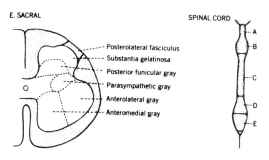

Fig. 1.18. Grey matter and white matter of the spinal cord, as seen in representative cross-sections. The inset at the lower right indicates the approximate level in the spinal cord for each of the sections. (Reproduced from Patton *et al.* (1976) by kind permission of the authors and publisher.)

groups innervated by a single anterior root may be referred to as a *myotome*, in developmental terms, but such is the complexity of the arrangement of spinal nerves and plexuses and peripheral nerves that with the exception of the intercostal muscles, each of which is supplied by a single dorsal segment, most muscles of the trunk and limbs receive contributions from several spinal nerves. Similarly, cutaneous areas which send sensory afferents to a single cord segment are called *dermatomes* and, while on the trunk, despite substantial overlap, a segmental arrangement of dermatomes is well preserved (see below), sensory segmentation in the limbs is much less clear cut. In the autonomic system, preganglionic efferent fibres travel to the various sympathetic and parasympathetic ganglia via *white rami communicantes*, while some of the postganglionic fibres which arise from the latter re-enter peripheral nerves via *grey rami* in order to travel distally to effector organs (Fig. 1.20).

Motor and sensory organization in the spinal cord. The *primary afferent neurones* of the posterior roots enter the spinal cord in a series of rootlets; the thinly myelinated fibres and the unmyelinated ones become grouped more laterally, the heavily myelinated fibres destined for the posterior columns more medially. In the *posterolateral fasciculus* which caps the posterior horn (Fig. 1.19), many of these fibres especially give off ascending and descending collaterals, some long and ascending to the medulla, some short which later enter the posterior horns to synapse with a variety of interneurones at different segments. The result is that afferent input at one level can be rapidly transmitted to many different cord segments. Some fibres then traverse the posterior horns intact in order to synapse with motor neurones forming a simple reflex arc, but others synapse with interneurones in the posterior horn. In the posterior horn of grey matter itself, many poorly defined layers of cells have been identified including the *substantia gelatinosa* (posterior) and the *nucleus proprius* (near the base of the horn). The role of these cells, of the ascending, descending, commissural, and interneuronal connections which they make and of their function in modulating various forms of sensation and of movement and reflex activity will be considered later.

The principal cells of the anterior horn are the small *gamma motor neurones* which innervate the intrafusal fibres of the muscle spindles, the large *alpha motor neurones* which innervate the voluntary muscles, and the *Renshaw cells*, interneurones which through recurrent axons synapsing with anterior horn cells, produce an inhibitory 'negative feed-back' which limits the discharge of alpha motor neurones. Anatomical studies have demonstrated

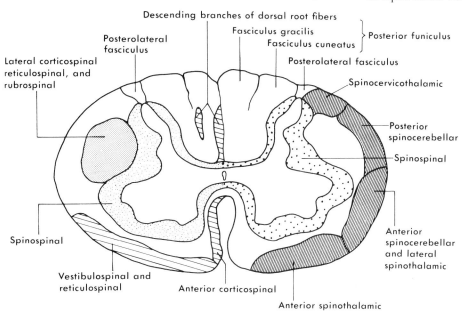

Fig. 1.19. The main tracts of the spinal cord. Ascending tracts are shown on the right and descending tracts on the left. (Reproduced from Gardner (1975) by kind permission of the author and publisher.)

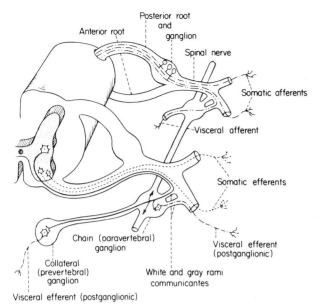

Fig. 1.20. Diagram of spinal cord, spinal nerves, and sympathetic components, emphasizing the route taken by somatic efferent and afferent fibres, and visceral efferent and afferent fibres. For clarity, afferent paths are shown in the upper and efferent paths in the lower spinal nerve. (Reproduced from Patton *et al.* (1976) by kind permission of the authors and publisher.)

not only that the number of alpha motor neurones in different segments of the cord and on the two sides is remarkably constant in different individuals and throughout life (Tomlinson, Irving, and Rebeiz 1973; except for evidence that there is a progressive decline in number in advanced age—Tomlinson and Irving 1977), but also that they are organized consistently into groups which can be shown to innervate specific muscles and muscle groups (Sharrard 1955). Physiologically, too, alpha motor neurones innervating flexor muscles can be distinguished in certain aspects of their behaviour from those which have an extensor function. The heavily myelinated fibres of the anterior roots which carry the axons of the alpha motor neurones traverse the peripheral nerves to end in the voluntary muscles where they branch and each terminal branch, which loses its myelin sheath, ends at a *neuromuscular junction* or *end-plate* upon a single striated muscle fibre. A single anterior horn cell (alpha neurone), its axon, and the many muscle fibres which it supplies form one *motor unit*.

The peripheral nerves

Strictly speaking, the peripheral nervous system begins in the anterior and posterior roots as they enter or leave the cord, at which point the Schwann cells which invest them begin. However, in everyday clinical practice peripheral nerves are usually regarded as those nerves which are formed from individual spinal nerves or groups of them or which emerge, for instance, from the brachial and lumbosacral plexuses. *Unmyelinated nerve fibres* are axons 0.2–3.0 μm in diameter, of which up to 10 lie within each Remak cell. *Myelinated fibres* range from 1 to 15 μm in diameter and each lies within a chain of Schwann cells, each of which forms a segment of the myelin sheath. The boundary between one Schwann cell and the next in a myelinated fibre is demarcated in a *node of Ranvier* (Fig. 1.21) but the boundaries between Remak cells are less clearly defined because of interdigitations of the cytoplasm. The *myelin sheath* is concentrically laminated with a periodicity of about 18 nm; this periodicity refers to the distance between the *major dense lines* between which is a less electron-dense *intraperiod line*; the clear space on either side of the latter is believed to contain hydrophobic lipids of the membrane. The number of myelin lamellae and hence the thickness of the sheath is

related to the diameter of the axon, and so too is the *internodal length* (the distance between individual nodes of Ranvier). In an adult limb nerve fibre with an axonal diameter of about 12 μm, each internodal length is about 1.0 mm, but there is a good deal of variation between different nerves. In many areas small pockets of Schwann-cell cytoplasm split the major dense line of the myelin sheath and sometimes several such clefts are seen at a point where the myelin sheath shows funnel-shaped clefts (the *Schmidt–Lantermann incisures*). These may be points at which substances pass from the Schwann-cell cytoplasm through the myelin into the axon; they are especially frequent in young and regenerating nerves and are only seen as a rule in those with more than 20 myelin lamellae.

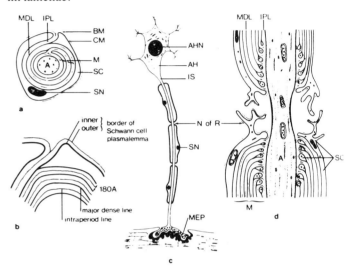

Fig. 1.21. Diagrams of the structure of a myelinated nerve fibre. a: Formation of the myelin sheath (M) by wrapping of the Schwann cell (SC) membrane (CM) around the axon (A): SN = Schwann cell nucleus, MDL = major dense line, IPL = intraperiod line, BM = basement membrane. b: High-power drawing of the inner mesaxon to show the formation of the major dense line from the union of two inner borders of the Schwann-cell plasmalemma, and the intraperiod line by the union of two outer borders of the Schwann-cell plasmalemma. c: Diagram of an α-motor neurone. The anterior horn cell (AH), with its nucleus (AHN) and initial segment (IS), lies in the spinal cord. The axon is invested with Schwann cells separated by nodes of Ranvier (N of R), and the terminal ramification lies in the motor end plate (MEP). d: Diagram of the structure of a node of Ranvier. The interdigitating processes from adjacent Schwann cells almost occlude the nodal gap. Schwann-cell cytoplasm (SC) lies superficial to the myelin sheath, and also in pockets splitting the major dense lines where the myelin becomes applied to the axon. (Reproduced from Bradley (1974) by kind permission of the author and publisher.)

The characteristic *compound nerve action potential* which can be recorded along the course of a mixed motor and sensory peripheral nerve following supramaximal electrical stimulation shows that this is divided into the *A wave*, the largest, which has three components, alpha, beta, and gamma, conducting at 90, 50, and 30 m/s, respectively, a smaller *B wave* with a velocity of 10 m/s, and the smallest *C wave*, with a velocity of about 2 m/s. The velocity of conduction can be correlated precisely with axonal diameter (in unmyelinated fibres) and with myelin-sheath thickness (in myelinated fibres) which, as we have seen, correlates well with the latter. The fibres of largest diameter conduct most rapidly. On this basis, the fibres of peripheral nerves can be divided similarly into *A, B, and C fibres*, depending upon their axonal and myelin-sheath diameter and their speed of conduction. The A fibres (diameter 10–18 μm) are the largest, the alpha wave being produced by alpha motor neurones and by group Ia sensory fibres from the muscle spindles and tendon organ receptors; the beta wave is produced by group II sensory fibres (6–12 μm) such as those from the

Pacinian corpuscles, and the gamma wave by gamma motor neurones innervating intrafusal muscle fibres in the spindles and by group II afferents from the spindles (4–18 μm). The B potential is derived from small myelinated fibres of 2–6 μm diameter which include slow gamma efferents and group III sensory afferents from pain and hair receptors. Finally the C potential comes from unmyelinated fibres (diameter 0.2–3 μm) which are mainly group III pain and temperature afferent fibres and postganglionic fibres of the autonomic nervous system. In a sensory nerve such as the sural, unmyelinated fibres outnumber the myelinated ones by about four to one.

Finally, in considering the macroscopic structure of peripheral nerves, each large mixed nerve comprises thousands of nerve fibres grouped into *fasciculi*, each surrounded by a sheath of *perineurium*, consisting of three or four layers of specialized cells which form a blood–nerve barrier, similar in certain respects to the blood–brain barrier and acting as a major barrier against the passage into nerves of large molecular weight substances. The fact that the blood–brain barrier is less efficient in the spinal-nerve roots may account for the selective involvement of the latter in some disease processes, especially auto-immune polyneuropathies. Within the fasciculi themselves are strands of *endoneurial connective tissue*, while the fasciculi themselves are bound together by the collagen of the *epineurium*. Blood is supplied to peripheral nerves by small *vasa nervorum*; blockage of these arteries resulting from disease or compression may give rise to infarction of peripheral nerves or to various forms of ischaemic neuropathy.

The neuromuscular system

The lower motor neurones
As indicated above, the cell bodies of the lower motor neurones are situated in the motor nuclei of the brainstem and in the anterior horns of grey matter of the spinal cord (see above). There are several morphological characteristics relating to size, density of Nissl substance, etc., through which the larger cell bodies, most of which are alpha motor neurones, can be distinguished from the smaller gamma neurones. The axons of the motor neurones leave the central nervous system via the cranial nerves or the spinal ventral roots, and from the latter enter the peripheral nerves, those destined for the limbs being organized into the brachial and lumbosacral plexuses.

The structure and function of voluntary muscle
A voluntary muscle is composed of muscle fibres, each of which is a multinucleate cell, consisting of myofibrils, sarcoplasm, and certain discrete intracellular organelles including mitochondria, ribosomes, and the sarcotubular system. Each fibre is enclosed within a sarcolemmal sheath, deep to which the muscle nuclei are situated, and each has a motor end-plate in which the nerve fibre terminates. Under normal conditions muscle fibres never contract singly, but the functional unit of muscle fibre activity is known as the motor unit, being that group of fibres supplied by a single alpha neurone and its axon. Discharge of such a single anterior horn cell results in the simultaneous contraction of all of the muscle fibres which it innervates. In most human limb muscles each motor unit contains between 500 and 200 such fibres (see Lewis and Ridge 1981).

The motor unit. For many years it was thought that the constituent fibres of motor units in mammalian skeletal muscle were gathered into groups or subunits, but the work of Edstrom and Kugelberg (1968) and others has shown that the fibres of a single unit are usually widely scattered throughout a muscle when examined in transverse section. Only after denervation and subsequent reinnervation by regenerating neurones are fibres innervated by a single anterior horn cell or by one of its axonal branches gathered together into groups. Contraction of the muscle fibres which make up a motor unit is preceded by electrical excitation of the fibre membranes. The appearance of this electrical activity in the electromyogram (EMG) depends on physical factors such as the dimensions of the electrode used, as well as on the muscle chosen for examination. For example, in the biceps brachii of a healthy young adult, the electrical activity of a single motor unit usually appears as a di- or triphasic wave with a duration of 5–10 ms and an amplitude of less than 500 μV; however, the variation in form, amplitude, and duration is considerable.

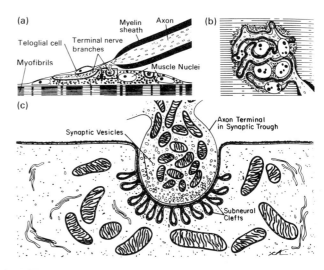

Fig. 1.22. Schematic drawings of motor end plates. (a) and (b): Views from the side and from above, respectively. (c): Enlarged view (as seen in electron micrographs) of the region outlined by the rectangle in (a). (Reproduced from Patton *et al.* (1976) and previously published in Bloom and Fawcett (1970), by kind permission of the authors and publisher.)

Neuromuscular transmission. An important advance in our knowledge of the physiology of muscular contraction was the discovery that the release of acetylcholine (ACh) is responsible for transmission of the nerve impulse at the myoneural junction (Fig. 1.22). The synaptic vesicles in the motor nerve terminal contain packets of ACh. Single packets of ACh are continually being released spontaneously and give rise to small depolarizations (miniature end-plate potentials) which can be recorded electrically with a micro-electrode in the region of the end-plate. The ACh so released combines with specific ACh receptors on the postjunctional membrane. The arrival of a nerve impulse at the motor end-plate causes the synchronous release of many packets or quanta of ACh, giving a localized depolarization of the muscle fibre membrane in the end-plate region; this is the end-plate potential. When this potential reaches a certain critical size, it triggers off an excitatory wave, the action potential, which then travels away from the end-plate along the surface membrane of the fibre. Under normal circumstances ACh receptors are confined to the area of the end-plate. After denervation extra-junctional receptors may be identified on other parts of the sarcolemmal membrane. This is accompanied by a 100-fold increase in sensitivity of the muscle fibre to ACh (denervation hypersensitivity). At rest, the inside of the fibre membrane is some 80 mV negative with respect to the outside, but, during the action potential, the polarization of the membrane momentarily reverses, so that for about 1 ms the inside of the fibre becomes positive. This reversal of electrical polarity is caused by increased sodium permeability of the fibre membrane. There is evidence that the wave of excitation spreads inwards into the substance of the muscle fibre along the transverse system of tubules, the 'T' system (Fig. 1.23) and that the consequent mobilization of calcium ions in the sarcoplasmic reticulum initiates contraction of the myofibrils.

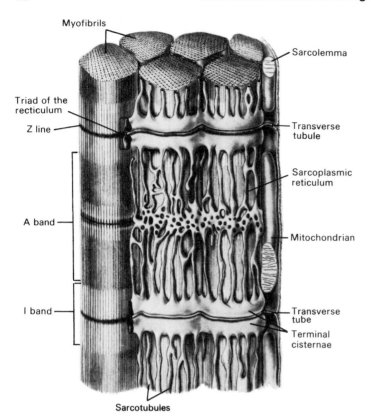

Fig. 1.23. Muscle structure, showing relation of endoplasmic reticulum and of transverse tubular system to fibrils. (Reproduced from Patton *et al.* (1976) and previously published in Bloom and Fawcett (1970), by kind permission of the authors and publisher.)

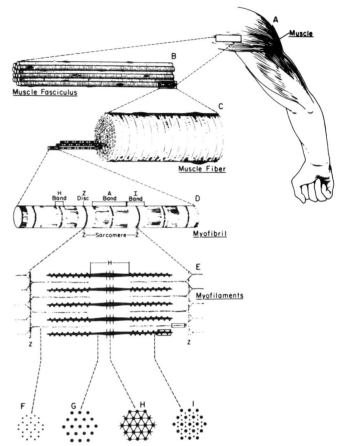

Fig. 1.24. Histological and molecular structure of skeletal muscle. (Reproduced from Patton *et al.* (1976) and modified from by Bloom and Fawcett (1970) by kind permission of the authors and publisher.)

Muscle ultrastructure. Ultrastructural studies of skeletal muscle have demonstrated that the unit structure of the individual myofibril is the sarcomere (Fig 1.24), extending from one Z-line (situated in the midst of the 'I'-band) to the next. Attached to each Z-line are thin filaments of the protein actin. There is also a second thicker type of filament which is composed of myosin; these filaments correspond to the dark (birefringent) A-bands of the myofibrils. Each filament of myosin is surrounded by a hexagonal array of actin filaments; in addition, molecular cross-bridges reach out from the myosin to the actin filaments. During contraction, the cross-bridges repeatedly disengage and re-engage at successive sites on the actin filaments. The propulsion imparted to the actin filaments causes them to slide over the myosin filaments so as to interdigitate more fully with the latter; in this way the whole myofibril, and consequently its parent fibre, shortens (see Huxley 1980). The biochemical changes which accompany muscle contraction are complicated but it is plain that among the many biochemical reactions which occur, creatine phosphate is broken down in the presence of calcium to creatine and phosphate, and adenosine triphosphate (ATP) is broken down to adenosine diphosphate (ADP) (Gergely 1981). The release of high-energy phosphate bonds provides much of the energy required for muscular contraction.

Types of muscle fibre. Skeletal muscles are not homogeneous in that in man they contain at least two main types of muscle fibre which are morphologically and histochemically distinct (see Dubowitz and Brooke 1973; Mastaglia and Walton 1982). One type of fibre, the so-called Type I fibre, tends to be somewhat smaller than the second type; it contains myofibrils which are somewhat slender and a high concentration of mitochondria. Histochemical stains show that this type of fibre contains a high concentration of enzymes, such as succinic dehydrogenase, which are

concerned with aerobic metabolism. In the larger Type II fibre, whose myofibrils are slightly more coarse and more widely dispersed, there are fewer mitochondria and histochemical studies indicate that these fibres contain a higher concentration of glycogen and of enzymes such as phosphorylase and myofibrillar adenosine triphosphatase (ATPase) which are concerned with anaerobic metabolism. In man, all skeletal muscles contain an admixture of Type I and Type II fibres, so that, in transverse sections stained histochemically, a characteristic checkerboard pattern is observed. Refinements of histochemical technique have shown that each major fibre type can be further subdivided according to the intensity of staining demonstrated, for instance, with myofibrillar ATPase at varying pH. Physiological experiments also indicate that these fibres are functionally different. Thus in many mammals other than man there are certain muscles such as soleus which are made up predominantly of Type I fibres (so-called red muscle). These muscles are concerned largely with the maintenance of posture and, upon stimulation, are found to contract and relax relatively slowly. By contrast, other muscles concerned more directly with phasic motor activity, such as the flexor digitorum longus, are made up predominantly of Type II fibres (white muscle) and are more rapidly contracting (fast 'twitch' muscles). It is now known that the motor nerve appears to control, through its rate of stimulus delivery, not only the physiological behaviour, but also the histochemical structure of the muscle fibres in that transposition of the motor nerve supply from a fast muscle to a slow muscle, and vice versa, may completely alter the physiological and histochemical characteristics of the muscle fibres. Thus in a sense it is the neurones which control the constituent muscle fibres of motor units so that one can speak of Type I and Type II alpha neurones. Thus when a group of muscle fibres which have lost their nerve supply are reinnervated by a sprouting neurone they become of uniform histochemical type (so-called 'type-grouping').

The effect of drugs. Finally, it is important to mention briefly a number of drugs which act upon the neuromuscular junction. ACh, when released at the neuromuscular junction, is broken down by cholinesterase which is normally present in the subneural apparatus and can be demonstrated histochemically. The drug curare acts on the post-junctional membrane, where it reduces or prevents the depolarizing effect of the transmitter excited by the nerve impulse. Botulinum toxin blocks ACh release. Drugs such as physostigmine and neostigmine destroy cholinesterase and allow ACh liberated at the myoneural junction to accumulate. Guanidine hydrochloride acts by increasing the output of ACh at the nerve endings and may thus be helpful in botulism. However, while initially the accumulation of ACh produces muscular contraction as a result of depolarization of the muscle fibre membrane, if this substance is allowed to accumulate in excess, as in overdosage with neostigmine or guanidine, the depolarization persists and may result in blockage of the muscle action potential (depolarization block). Whereas drugs such as tubocurarine and gallamine complete with ACh for the end-plate chemical receptors and are thus known as competitive inhibitors, drugs such as decamethonium and suxamethonium produce muscle paralysis first through depolarization block but subsequently they also produce competitive block so that they are said to have a 'dual' action. In myasthenia gravis it is now known that ACh receptors become coated with antibodies, thus preventing ACh from having its full normal effect.

The muscle spindles (the fusimotor system) and other muscle and tendon receptors

The stretch receptors of muscle and tendon are the *Golgi tendon organs* and the *muscle spindles*. The *Golgi organs or neurotendinous endings* lie most often on tendons, less often on the tendinous endings of muscle which terminate on the perimysium of other fibres short of the musculotendinous junction. They give origin to large myelinated Group I afferent axons (12–20 μm); they are excited by stretch (as in tension applied to the tendon during muscular contraction, or to a lesser extent by passive stretching of the muscle). These stimuli produce a tonic generator potential and repetitive spike discharge in the afferent fibres; the effect of such discharge is to inhibit alpha neurone activity.

The *muscle spindles* (Figs. 1.25 and 1.26) which are present in all voluntary muscles but are scanty in the extraocular muscles, contain on average seven or eight muscle fibres, called intrafusal because they are enclosed in a fluid-containing connective tissue capsule. These fibres are of two types, *nuclear bag fibres* which are few, larger in diameter, and show a collection of nuclei at their equator, and the narrower and often more numerous *nuclear chain fibres* each of which contains a single row of nuclei. Axons (2–7 μm in diameter) of gamma (effector) neurones enter the striated poles of these fibres, while at the equatorial unstriated and presumably non-contractile region of the fibres there are two types of sensory endings: these are the *primary or annulospiral endings* giving rise to Group I myelinated axons (12–20 μm) and the *secondary or flower-spray endings* which give origin to Group II myelinated axons (6–12 μm). Both types of receptor are tonic receptors which are depolarized by stretch, which, if sustained, gives rise to repetitive discharge in the relevant afferent neurones. The tendinous ends of the intrafusal muscle fibres project beyond the capsule at each end of the spindle and are attached either to the tendon of the muscle or to the perimysium of nearby extrafusal fibres, so that stretching of the extrafusal fibres applies tension to the intrafusal ones, while contraction of the muscle causes them to relax.

Sensory endings in the spindle are arranged in parallel with the

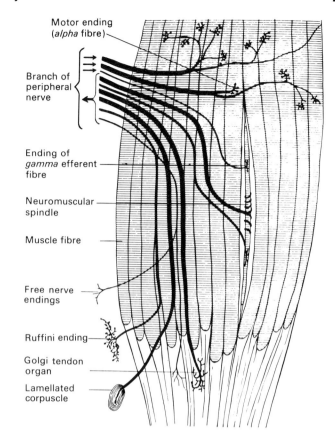

Fig. 1.25. Schematic representation of a muscle and its nerve supply. Arrows indicate direction of conduction. Each muscle fibre has a motor ending from a large myelinated (alpha) fibre. The muscle fibres within a spindle have motor endings from small myelinated (gamma) fibres. Muscle nerves contain many sensory fibres. Some are large myelinated fibres from primary (annulospiral) endings in spindles, from neurotendinous spindles (Golgi tendon organs), and from pacinian corpuscles in the connective tissue within and external to the muscle. Smaller myelinated and non-myelinated fibres arise from Ruffini endings in the connective tissue in and around muscle, and in joints. Finally there are small myelinated and non-myelinated fibres that form free endings in the connective tissue in and around muscle. (Reproduced from Gardner (1975) by kind permission of the author and publisher.)

extrafusal muscle fibres, while tendon endings are in series. The Group I afferent fibres from these two receptors are thus conventionally divided into IA afferents (from the annulospiral spindle endings) and IB afferents (from the tendon endings). The respective arrangement of these receptors determines the fact that, during muscular contraction, IA afferents are silent due to relaxation of intrafusal fibres, while IB afferents discharge. These afferent fibres play a crucial role in the control of monosynaptic spinal reflexes, while the Group II afferents from the flower-spray endings of the spindles are more concerned with polysynaptic reflex activity. In general, therefore, Golgi tendon organs are more sensitive to changes in *tension*, spindle receptors to changes in muscle fibre *length*. However, the gamma neurones also influence this process as, when these discharge causing the intrafusal fibres to contract, the sensory receptors in the equatorial region are stretched so that increased gamma-neurone discharge also increases the sensitivity of the muscle to tension. These fusimotor fibres are of two types—dynamic fibres which respond to afferent stimuli concerned with the *velocity* of stretch and static fibres concerned with changes solely in *length* (see Lewis and Ridge 1981).

Thus passive stretching of a muscle gives rise to afferent impulses which reach the spinal cord, stimulating the alpha neurones which then discharge causing the muscle to contract and

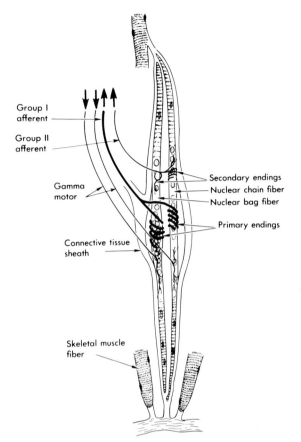

Fig. 1.26. Schematic representation of a neuromuscular spindle. Parts of three skeletal muscle fibres are shown (cross-striated, nuclei at edge). Inside the connective tissue sheath of the spindle are three muscle fibres (thinner than extrafusal skeletal muscle fibres, with central nuclei, and striations minimal or absent in the region of the sensory endings). Sensory nerve fibres form primary (annulospiral) and secondary (flower-spray) endings, the primary arising from the large fibres. (The form of primary and secondary endings varies according to species. In some, such as rabbit and man, the primary endings of the large fibre may be flower-spray in type, not winding around the muscle fibre). Small nerve fibres (gamma efferents) form motor endings at each end of the spindle muscle fibres. Motor discharges over gamma efferents cause the muscle spindle fibres to contract at each end, thus stretching the intervening, non-contractile sensory region and activating the sensory endings. Arrows indicate direction of conduction. (Reproduced from Gardner (1975) by kind permission of the author and publisher, and based on Barker, D. (1948). *Quart, J. Micr. Sci.* 89, 143–86; Boyd, I.A. (1962). *Phil. Trans. Soc., Lond.* B 245, 81–136; and Matthews, P.B.C. (1964). *Physiol. Rev.* 4, 219–88.)

regain its former length; this process is responsible for monosynaptic spinal reflex activity as in the *tendon jerks* (see below). However, sensory impulses from the spindles also reach the brainstem, cerebellum, and cerebral cortex by a number of ascending pathways, and in turn the descending pathways from these structures, as described above, influence the excitability of gamma neurones, thus exercising important controlling influences over muscle tone. Sudden and transient stretching of a muscle, as in the tendon jerks, causes selective discharge in Group IA afferents, thus eliciting a monosynaptic reflex, but steady stretch or vibration applied to the muscle, by contrast (see Lance and McLeod 1981), excite Groups IA and B and Group II afferents from all of the receptors in the muscle, eliciting stretch reflexes which are more complex, often polysynaptic, and which are modulated by activity in many descending pathways concerned in the control of posture and of muscle tone; essentially the response consists of tonic or continuous muscle contraction (the *tonic stretch reflex*).

Segmental and peripheral organization of the neuromuscular system

The motor nuclei of the cranial nerves are derived from *branchial columns* of cells in the brainstem which innervate structures derived from the *branchial arches*. In the adult, the anatomical organization of these nuclei in the brainstem retains some semblance of segmental organization but this is much less clear than is the segmental or metameric arrangement of the spinal cord. Corresponding to each spinal segment is one pair of spinal nerves composed of the ventral and dorsal roots derived from the segment. The sensory neurones in the dorsal root ganglia are completely separated in each segment from those of the contiguous segments, but the organization of the alpha motor neurones is less distinct in that their cell bodies are arranged in longitudinal columns and those innervating a single muscle often extend over more than one segment. Thus several muscles may be represented in one segment; hence a lesion of the anterior horn of a single segment gives weakness of all muscles innervated by that segment but paralyses completely only those which have no nerve supply from adjacent segments.

The innervation and organization of the voluntary muscles of the trunk and limbs. As described above, the axons derived from the alpha and gamma motor neurones in each spinal cord segment leave that segment in the anterior or ventral root which joins with the posterior root in the spinal nerve of that segment. Each spinal nerve, after leaving the spinal column via the intervertebral foramina, divides into dorsal and ventral rami. The dorsal rami largely supply the muscles of the trunk; the larger ventral rami those of the limbs. But in the brachial and lumbosacral plexuses the axons are redistributed and enter into new groupings in the peripheral nerves. Hence the fibres from a single spinal segment may reach several peripheral nerves, and conversely a single peripheral nerve often receives fibres from several spinal segments; in addition, many peripheral nerves divide into several branches, each supplying one or more voluntary muscles. Thus in clinical neurology a working knowledge of anatomy of the peripheral neuromuscular system is necessary in order to be able to distinguish between lesions involving

1. A spinal-cord segment or anterior horn or one ventral root;
2. A spinal nerve, in which case somatic afferent fibres are also involved;
3. One or more components (e.g. cords) of the brachial or lumbosacral plexus;
4. A single peripheral nerve or one of its branches;
5. The voluntary muscles themselves.

To assist the reader in this differential diagnostic process, the brachial plexus is illustrated in Fig. 1.27, the distribution to the musculature of various peripheral nerves is given in Fig. 1.28, and the root and nerve supplies of the muscles commonly examined in clinical practice are listed in Table 1.1. The principles governing the examination of the individual skeletal muscles will be described later; for illustrations of the technique the reader is referred to Medical Research Council (1976).

Disorders of the motor system

Weakness and paralysis

Weakness (paresis) of a group of muscles implies that the power produced on voluntary contraction of the affected muscles is reduced, whereas complete paralysis indicates that the power to move the part concerned is totally lost. Weakness of one limb is referred to as a *monoparesis*, while total paralysis of a limb is called *monoplegia*. Hemiplegia is the term utilized to identify paralysis which afflicts one side of the body, and particularly the arm and leg, while *paraplegia* signifies a paralysis of both lower limbs. When all four limbs are paralysed, the terms *quadriplegia* or *tetraplegia* are used; a symmetrical weakness of all four limbs, affecting the lower more markedly than the upper, and occurring in children with cerebral palsy, is often called a *diplegia*. The term 'palsy' can be used interchangeably with 'paralysis', but is more often utilized in modern neurological practice to identify the paralysis of individual muscles or muscle groups which results from a single peripheral nerve lesion.

Paralysis may result from a lesion of the upper motor neurone or of the lower motor neurone, and under certain circumstances it can be due to a defect in conduction at the neuromuscular junction or to a biochemical or structural abnormality of the muscle fibres themselves. Some principles governing the differentiation of these causes of paralysis will be discussed below.

Muscle 'tone' and its disorders

General considerations

The tone of a muscle can be regarded as the response it shows to passive stretching. Contrary to the views once held, a completely relaxed and resting muscle is not in a state of continuous partial contraction and is silent electrically; it has elasticity, but no tone. Tone can only therefore be assessed when the muscle is moved or when it is concerned with maintaining a posture against an applied force such as that of gravity. *Postural tone* can thus be considered to be that state of partial contraction of certain muscles which is needed to maintain the posture of the parts of the body; clearly the muscles involved and the force of muscular contraction required will depend upon the position of the parts concerned at any one time.

In neurological practice, tone is usually assessed by moving a limb or some other part passively and by observing the reaction which occurs in the muscles which are being stretched. The moment this stretching begins, stretch receptors in the muscle concerned, and particularly the muscle spindles, give out afferent stimuli and reflex partial contraction of the muscle results. As noted above, the responses to momentary and to more prolonged stretching are different—the former being responsible, for instance, for the tendon jerks, the latter eliciting more complex responses, often in the form of tonic contraction. Variations in the degree of sensitivity of these reflexes account for the alterations in tone which occur as a result of nervous disease. Forceful continued contraction of a group of muscles (e.g. clenching one hand or pulling firmly with the flexed fingers of both hands opposed to

one another) temporarily causes an increased flow of afferent impulses in the sensory fibres from the spindles. This in turn gives an increased rate of discharge in gamma neurones throughout the body, thus causing a generalized slight increase in sensitivity of the spindles to stretch, and the tendon reflexes become more brisk as the 'set' of the spindle (the state of contraction of its intrafusal fibres) is altered. This phenomenon, also known as reinforcement, or Jendrassik's manoeuvre, is often used to elicit tendon reflexes which at first seem to be absent. In spasticity and in extrapyramidal rigidity, the 'set' of the spindles is continuously abnormal.

On stretching, the tone of the muscle may be increased (*spasticity* or *rigidity* or *hypertonia*) or it may be reduced (*flaccidity* or *hypotonia*) and these alterations are of great value in neurological diagnosis.

Muscle tone is normally regulated by reticulospinal fibres which accompany the pyramidal tract throughout its course and which have an inhibitory effect upon the stretch reflex. This inhibition balances the background facilitatory impulses conveyed by the pontine reticulospinal and lateral vestibulospinal pathways, and these influences are in turn influenced by multisynaptic reflex arcs traversing the cerebellum, basal ganglia, and brainstem. Dorsal reticulospinal fibres appear specifically to inhibit flexor lower-limb reflexes. There is evidence that when lesions of the pyramidal and reticulospinal tracts release stretch reflexes from inhibition, the increased tone which results is initially associated with hyperactivity of dynamic fusimotor neurones but, if such increased tone persists (*spasticity*), increased alpha-neurone discharge develops so that spasticity in man at different stages may be associated with both increased gamma (dynamic fusimotor) and alpha-neurone activity. The role of the basal ganglia appears to be of particular importance in balancing alpha and gamma neurone activity. The fact that negative feed-back through the Renshaw-cell system in the spinal grey matter, which inhibits alpha-neurone discharge, is also of importance in controlling excessive discharge in these neurones indicates something of the complexity of the many mechanisms which control tone.

Spasticity

In one form of increased tone or hypertonia, called spasticity, resulting from lesions of the pyramidal and often of the reticulospinal pathways, the stretch reflexes, released from descending inhibitory influences, become hyperactive as a consequence of increased excitability of dynamic fusimotor neurones and alpha neurones, as mentioned above. If the dorsal reticulospinal system, closely related anatomically to the pyramidal tract in the spinal

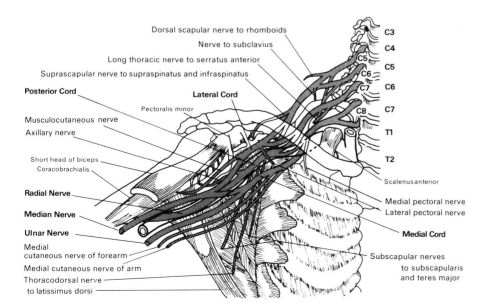

Dorsal scapular nerve to rhomboids
Nerve to subclavius
Long thoracic nerve to serratus anterior
Suprascapular nerve to supraspinatus and infraspinatus
Posterior Cord
Lateral Cord
Pectoralis minor
Musculocutaneous nerve
Axillary nerve
Short head of biceps
Coracobrachialis
Radial Nerve
Median Nerve
Ulnar Nerve
Medial cutaneous nerve of forearm
Medial cutaneous nerve of arm
Thoracodorsal nerve to latissimus dorsi

C3
C4
C5 C5
C6 C6
C7 C7
C8
T1
T2
Scalenus anterior
Medial pectoral nerve
Lateral pectoral nerve
Medial Cord
Subscapular nerves to subscapularis and teres major

Fig. 1.27. Diagram of the brachial plexus, its branches, and the muscles which they supply. (Reproduced from Medical Research Council (1976) by kind permission of the authors and publisher.)

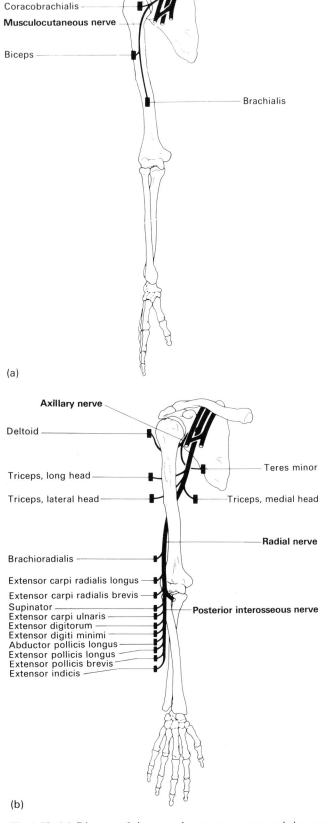

(a)

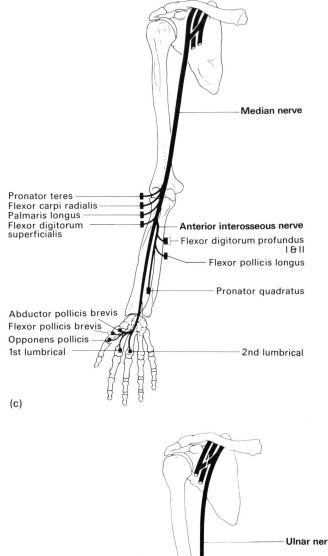

(c)

(b)

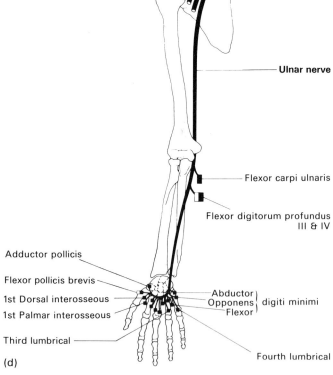

(d)

Fig. 1.28. (a) Diagram of the musculocutaneous nerve and the muscles which it supplies.

(b) Diagram of the axillary and radial nerves and the muscles which they supply.

(c) Diagram of the median nerve and the muscles which it supplies. Note: the white rectangle signifies that the muscle indicated receives a part of its nerve supply from another peripheral nerve (see (d), (e), and (f)).

(d) Diagram of the ulnar nerve and the muscles which it supplies.

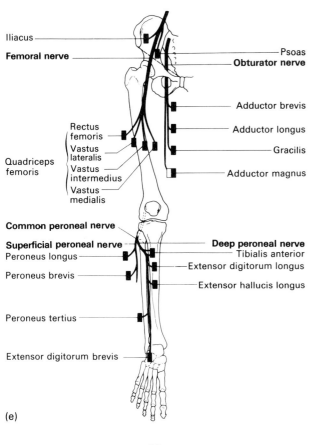

Iliacus

Femoral nerve

Psoas
Obturator nerve

Adductor brevis

Adductor longus

Rectus femoris
Vastus lateralis
Quadriceps femoris
Vastus intermedius
Vastus medialis

Gracilis

Adductor magnus

Common peroneal nerve

Superficial peroneal nerve
Peroneus longus

Deep peroneal nerve
Tibialis anterior
Extensor digitorum longus

Peroneus brevis

Extensor hallucis longus

Peroneus tertius

Extensor digitorum brevis

(e)

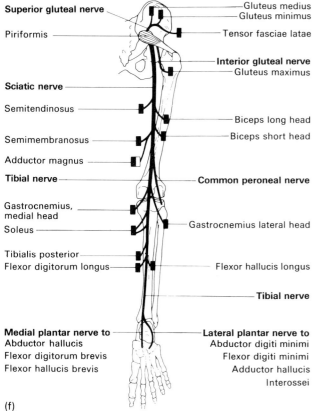

Superior gluteal nerve

Gluteus medius
Gluteus minimus

Piriformis

Tensor fasciae latae

Interior gluteal nerve
Gluteus maximus

Sciatic nerve

Semitendinosus

Biceps long head
Biceps short head

Semimembranosus

Adductor magnus

Tibial nerve

Common peroneal nerve

Gastrocnemius, medial head
Soleus

Gastrocnemius lateral head

Tibialis posterior
Flexor digitorum longus

Flexor hallucis longus

Tibial nerve

Medial plantar nerve to
Abductor hallucis
Flexor digitorum brevis
Flexor hallucis brevis

Lateral plantar nerve to
Abductor digiti minimi
Flexor digiti minimi
Adductor hallucis
Interossei

(f)

(e) Diagram of the nerves on the anterior aspect of the lower limb, and the muscles which they supply.

(f) Diagram of the nerves on the posterior aspect of the lower limb, and the muscles which they supply.

cord, is also damaged, there is disinhibition of afferent flexor reflex pathways. Release of such flexor reflexes may give flexor spasms in the lower limbs in response to stimulation of the legs, bladder, or bowels, and the 'extensor' plantar or Babinski reflex is one component of the primitive flexor withdrawal reflex, similarly released. Usually in spasticity the affected limb or limbs show an increase in resistance to passive stretching; this resistance is particularly severe initially, but then tends to 'give' suddenly as the movement is continued. Hence this sign, seen particularly well in the legs of a patient with a spastic paraplegia due to bilateral pyramidal-tract disease, is known as 'clasp-knife' rigidity. In individuals with spastic weakness, movement is impaired owing to defective conduction of motor impulses by the pyramidal tracts, while there is also 'clasp-knife' rigidity on passive movement. Hyperactivity of tendon reflexes is often accompanied by *clonus*, a phenomenon in which sustained stretch of a muscle evokes repetitive contraction and relaxation due to reverberating activity in the hyperexcitable fusimotor system.

Extrapyramidal hypertonia

Rigidity of extrapyramidal type, in patients with disease of the basal ganglia or substantia nigra, is essentially different from spasticity. It is seen characteristically in parkinsonism. In such cases the rigidity is either uniform in degree throughout the entire range of passive movement, when it is known as 'plastic' or 'lead-pipe' rigidity, or else it intermittently 'gives' and returns throughout the movement, being then referred to as 'cog-wheel' in type. Physiological evidence indicates that, in contrast to spasticity, alpha-neurone discharge predominates over gamma in extrapyramidal rigidity but there is usually increased activity as well in static fusimotor fibres and not in the dynamic ones which are involved in spasticity. In dystonia, which may be an end-stage of many extrapyramidal disorders but which is also the presenting feature of torsion spasm or dystonia musculorum deformans, there is simultaneous contraction of agonists and synergists so that the reciprocal inhibition of antagonists is seriously deranged and there is greatly increased alpha-neurone discharge. The consequence is that parts of the body become virtually fixed in an abnormal posture.

Decerebrate rigidity

In animals a transverse lesion across the midbrain at about the level of the superior colliculus or red nucleus releases the brainstem, cerebellum, and spinal cord from cerebral control. There is then strong continuous contraction in extensor groups of muscles, so that the animal placed upright with support will remain standing, but if pushed over cannot rise. In this state excitatory mechanisms controlling posture of extensor muscles predominate and inhibitory mechanisms as well as those excitatory to the flexor muscles are suppressed. These mechanisms are clearly mediated by the reticulospinal and vestibulospinal pathways, and a further lesion induced at the level of the vestibular nuclei, as Sherrington showed (Denny-Brown 1966), abolishes this rigidity. In this decerebrate state, tonic rather than phasic stretch reflexes are increased and there is increased gamma efferent discharge to extensor muscles, especially involving static fusimotor fibres. In man, a somewhat similar state may accompany severe midbrain lesions which almost invariably cause loss of consciousness. In such a case all four limbs are rigidly extended, the back is arched, and there may be neck retraction so that the patient, if lying supine, is virtually supported by the back of the head and the heels. This posture is known as *opisthotonos*; the arching of the back can be increased by any sensory stimulus and there is striking resistance to any attempt at flexing the limbs passively. In such

(Reproduced from Medical Research Council (1976) by kind permission of the authors and publisher, and modified from Pitres and Testut (1925)).

Table 1.1. *Nerve and main root supply of muscles*

Upper limb	Spinal Roots
Spinal accessory nerve	
Trapezius	C3, C4
Brachial Plexus	
Rhomboids	C4, C5
Serratus anterior	C5, C6, C7
Pectoralis major	
Clavicular ⎤	**C5**, C6
Sternal ⎦	C6, **C7**, C8
Supraspinatus	**C5**, C6
Infraspinatus	**C5**, C6
Latissimus dorsi	C6, **C7**, C8
Teres major	C5, 6, 7
Axillary nerve	
Deltoid	**C5**, C6
Musculocutaneous nerve	
Biceps	C5, C6
Brachialis	C5, C6
Radial nerve	
Triceps ⎰ Long head ⎱	
⎨ Lateral head ⎬	C6, **C7**, C8
⎱ Medial head ⎰	
Brachioradialis	C5, **C6**
Extensor carpi radialis longus	C5, **C6**
Posterior interosseous nerve	
Supinator	C6, C7
Extensor carpi ulnaris	**C7**, C8
Extensor digitorum	**C7**, C8
Abductor pollicis longus	**C7**, C8
Extensor pollicis longus	**C7**, C8
Extensor pollicis brevis	**C7**, C8
Extensor indicis	**C7**, C8
Median nerve	
Pronator teres	C6, C7
Flexor carpi radialis	C6, C7
Flexor digitorum superficialis	C7, **C8**, T1
Abductor pollicis brevis	C8, **T1**
Flexor pollicis brevis*	C8, **T1**
Opponens pollicis	C8, **T1**
Lumbricals I & II	C8, **T1**
Anterior interosseous nerve	
Flexor digitorum profundus I & II	C7, **C8**
Flexor pollicis longus	C7, **C8**
Ulnar nerve	
Flexor carpi ulnaris	C7, **C8**, T1
Flexor digitorum profundus III & IV	C7, **C8**
Hypothenar muscles	C8, **T1**
Adductor pollicis	C8, **T1**
Flexis pollicis brevis	C8, **T1**
Palmar interossei	C8, **T1**
Dorsal interossei	C8, **T1**
Lumbricals III & IV	C8, **T1**

Lower limb	Spinal Roots
Femoral nerve	
Iliopsoas	**L1, L2**, L3
Rectus femoris ⎤	
Vastus lateralis ⎫ Quadriceps	
Vastus intermedius ⎬ femoris	L2, **L3, L4**
Vastus medialis ⎭	
Obturator nerve	
Adductor longus ⎱	**L2, L3**, L4
Adductor magnus ⎰	
Superior gluteal nerve	
Gluteus medius and minimus ⎱	**L4, L5**, S1
Tensor fasciae latae ⎰	
Inferior gluteal nerve	
Gluteus maximus	**L5, S1**, S2
Sciatic and tibial nerves	
Semitendinosus	L5, **S1**, S2
Biceps	L5, **S1**, S2
Semimembranosus	L5, **S1**, S2
Gastrocnemius and soleus	S1, S2
Tibialis posterior	L4, L5
Flexor digitorum longus	L5, **S1**, S2
Flexor hallucis longus	L5, **S1**, S2
Abductor hallucis ⎱	S1, S2
Abductor digiti minimi ⎬ Small muscles	
Interossei ⎰ of foot	
Sciatic and common peroneal nerves	
Tibialis anterior	**L4**, L5
Extensor digitorum longus	**L5**, S1
Extensor hallucis longus	**L5**, S1
Extensor digitorum brevis	L5, S1
Peroneus longus	L5, S1
Peroneus brevis	L5, S1

The list given in Table 1.1 does not include all the muscles innervated by these nerves, but only those more commonly tested, either clinically or electrically, and shows the order of innervation. (Reproduced from Medical Research Council, 1976)

*Flexor pollicis brevis is often supplied wholly or partially by the ulnar nerve.

cases, *tonic neck reflexes* may often be elicited; thus turning the head to one side gives extension of the limbs on that side and flexion on the other.

Hypotonia

Flaccidity, or hypotonia, is a reduction in tone. It may be due to cerebral or spinal shock, a phenomenon which may result from acute and extensive lesions of the brain or spinal cord which have the effect of suppressing transiently all motor reflex activity, and hence there is temporary loss of muscle tone; it is a common manifestation of cerebellar disease, being then associated with diminished gamma efferent activity; and it occurs whenever a lesion of the afferent or efferent pathway interrupts the spinal reflex arc. In severe degrees of the phenomenon, as in patients with total flaccid paralysis, all resistance to passive stretch is lost and the limbs are limp and flail-like. Lesser degrees of hypotonia in the upper limbs, for instance, can be elicited by asking the patient to hold out his arms horizontally in front of him. The forearms are then tapped briskly; when tone is increased (spasticity) the recoil is sharp, immediate, and exaggerated. When one limb is hypotonic, the recoil is slower and the arm swings through a wider range. If the patient is asked to contract the biceps brachii against resistance, by bending the arm towards his face, and the examiner's restraining hand is suddenly removed, the patient's hand may strike his face if the limb is hypotonic, whereas if the tone is normal he will be able to stop the movement before it does so. Furthermore, if the subject is asked to raise his arms above his head with the palms facing forwards, the palm of a hypotonic limb will be seen to be externally rotated and facing more laterally than the other. In the lower limbs it is useful to place one's hands beneath the knee and to lift the leg from the bed, then to allow it to fall back quickly; with experience it will soon be possible to judge from the resistance which the limb shows to this movement whether tone is increased or reduced.

The clinical features of upper motor-neurone lesions

Let us take an example of the effects of an *upper motor-neurone lesion* the hemiplegia which is produced by an extensive lesion of the contralateral motor area of the cerebral cortex, or of the internal capsule. If the lesion is an acute one, say, a massive haemorrhage, the paralysed limbs are at first limp and flaccid, immobile, and without tone, owing to the phenomenon of so-called 'shock', through which a sudden and extensive lesion produces an abrupt depression of reflexes subserved by relatively remote areas of the nervous system, even though the reflex arc or arcs concerned remain intact. All reflexes are absent at this stage on the affected side. Gradually over the course of a few days or weeks this flaccidity lessens and the affected limbs become spastic, though there are some few cases in which, particularly if there is also an extensive parietal-lobe lesion, the hemiplegia remains permanently flaccid. Whereas the affected arm and leg are completely paralysed, those parts of the body which are bilaterally 'represented' in the cerebral cortex can still be moved voluntarily, even on the paralysed side. Thus facial weakness affects mainly the lower part of the face and the upper part slightly or not at all, while no defect in palatal movement will be apparent. Furthermore, since emotional movement of the face, as in smiling, appears to be controlled not by the cerebral cortex but by more deeply situated structures, a patient who is completely unable to move the lower half of one side of the face at will may yet smile symmetrically.

If the lesion involves Brodmann's area 8 of the frontal cortex (the frontal eye field), its irritative effects may cause deviation of the eyes and sometimes of the head as a whole to the opposite side. A more extensive destructive lesion involving this area may cause deviation of the head and eyes towards the side of the lesion and, if the patient regains consciousness, voluntary movements of the head and eyes to the opposite side may be temporarily impaired. There may also be slight weakness of mandibular and lingual movement with minimal deviation of the jaw and tongue on opening the mouth and protruding the tongue towards the paralysed side. Respiratory movements may also be slightly reduced on that side.

As flaccidity passes off in the paralysed limbs and spasticity makes its appearance, so the tendon reflexes return, become greatly exaggerated, and may be accompanied by clonus. The abdominal and cremasteric reflexes on the affected side remain absent and the plantar response is clearly extensor. Spasticity is often greatest in the flexor muscles of the upper limbs and in the extensor muscles of the lower so that, in a patient with a long-standing hemiplegia, the arm is flexed at the elbow and at the wrist and fingers, while the leg remains fully extended. In *hemiplegic spasticity*, unlike that resulting from lesions in the brainstem or spinal cord in which reticulospinal pathways are commonly

involved in the lesion, dynamic fusimotor drive (gamma discharge) predominates, though alpha-neurone hyperexcitability may develop later in longstanding cases.

When the pyramidal-tract lesion is not sufficiently severe to cause total paralysis but only causes a relatively minor degree of weakness, it is the finer and more skilful movements, those most recently acquired by man in the process of evolution, which are most severely impaired. Thus independent finger and toe movements are very poor, though the strength of movement at proximal joints such as the elbow and knee remains good. Hughlings Jackson's law of dissolution states that the movements most recently acquired in the process of evolution are the first to be lost following a corticospinal-tract lesion. Thus the 'precision grip' which depends upon opposition of the thumb and the individual fingers, a pattern of movement not well developed in primates, is impaired when the 'power grip' produced by flexion of the thumb and fingers is relatively unaffected. It also becomes difficult to move the thumb or other individual digits. If a normal individual is asked to flex the terminal phalanges of the fingers of one hand against the flexed fingers of the examiner, the thumb remains abducted and extended; after a corticospinal-tract lesion, however, the thumb flexes and adducts (Wartenberg's sign). Another useful sign of early pyramidal-tract dysfunction is to observe the hands and arms outstretched in front of the patient when the eyes are closed; a downward 'drift' may be an early sign of upper motor-neurone weakness. Furthermore, while difficulty in opposing the thumb and individual fingers may be an early sign, objective testing of muscle power often shows that 'pyramidal' weakness is first apparent on abduction of the shoulder and in the hand-grip in the upper limbs and in hip flexion and foot dorsiflexion in the lower. So, too, during the process of recovery from a pyramidal-tract lesion, movement usually returns first at the proximal joints; it is the cruder movements which are first regained, while the more delicate activity of he fingers and toes is the last to return. A patient who is recovering from a hemiplegia resulting from, say, cerebral thrombosis, may be able to use his hand to grip or lift objects, but will often be quite unable to write or to fasten buttons or shoelaces. He walks with his arm flexed across the front of his chest and with stiffness, dragging, and circumduction of the affected leg.

Similar physical signs are apparent in patients with bilateral pyramidal-tract lesions giving rise to spastic paraplegia but, if the lesion responsible is in the brainstem or spinal cord, concomitant involvement of reticulospinal and other descending pathways modifies the nature of the spasticity so that increased alpha-neurone excitability as well as dynamic fusimotor drive often appear earlier and the primitive flexor withdrawal reflex may be released from inhibition. If the lesion responsible is an acute transverse lesion of the cord, say, from infection or injury, there is a total flaccid paralysis of the limbs below the affected segment during the initial stage of spinal shock; subsequently spasticity, increased tendon reflexes, and extensor plantar responses appear. As the lower motor-neurone and the spinal reflex arc are intact, severe wasting of muscles does not occur although, when paralysis has been present for some time, some degree of disuse atrophy, affecting all muscles of the limb or limbs, appears. There is also evidence to suggest that trans-synaptic changes in alpha motor neurones may follow degeneration of corticospinal-tract fibres (McComas, Sica, Upton, and Aguilera 1973). When the spinal-cord lesion is incomplete and affects principally the pyramidal tracts, the tone of the spastic lower limbs is particularly increased in the extensor muscles (*paraplegia-in-extension*) but, when both pyramidal tracts are severely diseased and there are also lesions of other descending spinal pathways as mentioned above, the legs become progressively more flexed at the knees and hips and stimulation will provoke painful flexor spasms (*paraplegia-in-flexion*).

The clinical features of an upper motor-neurone lesion may, however, vary considerably in individual cases, depending upon the rate of evolution. Whereas an acute lesion, e.g. cerebral haemorrhage or cord transection, will give a total flaccid paralysis initially with spasticity slowly evolving over the subsequent days or weeks, a chronic or slowly progressive lesion such as a tumour may give little more initially than a slight impairment of fine finger movement in one hand, or simply a minimal increase in tendon reflexes in the affected arm; subsequently, however, a spastic monoparesis or hemiparesis slowly develops.

The pathological causes of upper motor-neurone lesions are many and varied—too many for their differential diagnosis to be considered in detail here. Once the lesion has been localized by means of the physical signs, the clinical history should again be analysed carefully to see if any clue can be obtained as to the nature of the pahological process. In this context, the scheme of pathological classification already described (p. 10) is often useful. Thus if we take the cerebral causes of spastic weakness, these may include traumatic (cerebral contusion, extradural haematoma), developmental (cerebral palsy), inflammatory (cerebral abscess, encephalomyelitis), neoplastic (meningioma, glioma, metastases), and degenerative (cerebral thrombosis or haemorrhage) causes.

The natural histories of these and of the many other conditions which give corticospinal-tract lesions differ considerably, and associated physical signs indicating involvement of other nervous structures or of other systems may be invaluable. Similarly, in spinal-cord disease giving rise to spastic paraplegia, many causes are possible. These include developmental causes (basilar impression, Chiari malformation), trauma (fracture dislocation of spine, haematomyelia), inflammation, either extradural (abscess) or intramedullary (transverse myelitis), neoplasia (meningioma, neurofibroma, glioma, metastases, reticulosis), and a group of common degenerative, demyelinating, and metabolic disorders. Of these, multiple sclerosis is characterized by a remittent course and often by involvement of brainstem structures; it sometimes gives temporal pallor of the optic discs, nystagmus, or diplopia and cerebellar signs as well as signs of a spastic paraplegia with impaired appreciation of 'posterior column' type sensation in the lower limbs. Some few cases, however, run a progressive course with only a spastic paraplegia and no signs of involvement of brainstem structures. In these cases the condition is difficult to distinguish from cervical-cord compression due to tumour or cervical spondylosis. In the latter disorder, however, particularly if the longstanding disc protusions extend laterally, spinal roots are often compressed as well as the cord, and there may be amyotrophy or 'inversion' of upper limb reflexes (see below) as well as a spastic paraplegia. Patients with motor-neurone disease will usually demonstrate some wasting, weakness, and fasciculation of muscles in the limbs, as well as signs of a spastic paraparesis, while in this condition there is no sensory impairment whatever. In syringomyelia, on the other hand, dissociated anaesthesia to pain and temperature sensation with retention of touch and loss of tendon reflexes are often present in one upper limb, combined with some wasting and weakness of muscles due to a lower motor-neurone lesion, while in the lower limbs there are usually signs of a spastic paraparesis. Spastic weakness of the lower limbs is also present in some cases of subacute combined degeneration of the cord (combined system disease), but here sensory symptoms and signs indicating dysfunction of the posterior columns of the cord and sensory peripheral nerves are usually predominant; there may be tenderness of the calves and absence of certain tendon reflexes owing to a neuropathy interrupting the sensory side of the reflex arc, while signs of pyramidal-tract disease, though present, are often relatively unobtrusive.

The localization of lesions in the corticospinal tract

The following are some distinctive symptoms of lesions of the corticospinal tract at different points in its course.

Cortical lesions
The chief characteristic of cortical corticospinal lesions arises out of the wide surface distribution of the cells of origin of this tract. As a result a lesion of moderate size involves only a part of the motor cortex. In contrast to the internal capsule, where the fibres are so crowded that even a small lesion usually produces a complete hemiplegia, cortical corticospinal lesions usually produce a monoplegia, that is, paralysis of the face or of one limb only, without, or with only slight, involvement of parts of the body controlled by adjoining cortical areas.

Jacksonian attacks. Since the precentral cortex contains the bodies of the corticospinal cells, a lesion here often excites corticospinal fibres, causing a focal epileptic attack. This is of the well-recognized type described by Hughlings Jackson and hence known as Jacksonian. Such an attack begins as a rule with clonic movements, rarely with tonic spasm, of a small part of the opposite side of the body, usually the thumb and index finger, the angle of the mouth, or the great toe, these movements being 'those that have the widest fields of low threshold excitability' (Walshe 1943). As the convulsion becomes more severe, the initial movement becomes more violent and the movement spreads, in the case of a limb, centripetally, involving the flexor muscles predominantly. A convulsion beginning in a limb then involves the other limb on the same side centrifugally, and the face, and finally may become bilateral, when consciousness is usually lost. The spread of the convulsion corresponds generally to the representation of movements in the motor cortex.

Subcortical lesions
In the corona radiata the corticospinal fibres converge towards the internal capsule and are closer together than in the cortex. Subcortical lesions tend therefore to involve more fibres than cortical lesions of equal size, and hence although the weakness usually predominates in one limb, the whole of the opposite side of the body is affected to some extent. Adjacent thalamocortical sensory fibres may also be involved, causing impairment of postural sensibility and tactile discrimination in the affected limbs. Damage to the optic radiation causes crossed homonymous hemianopia. A lesion in the internal capsule itself is likely to cause motor symptoms on the whole of the opposite side.

Lesions in the midbrain
Here the proximity of the corticospinal fibres to the third nerve sometimes adds signs of localizing value. One example is paralysis of one third nerve with a contralateral hemiplegia (*Weber's syndrome*). Throughout the brainstem the two corticospinal tracts lie close together. Vascular lesions are often strictly unilateral, but space-occupying lesions, such as tumours, frequently involve both corticospinal tracts. The corticospinal fibres decussate at different levels, those destined for the opposite facial nucleus, for example, crossing at the junction of the midbrain and the pons, while those which are concerned in the movements of the limbs do not cross till they reach the corticospinal decussation in the medulla. A lesion in the midline situated anteriorly at the junction of the midbrain and pons may thus involve only the decussating fibres running to the facial nuclei, and so produce facial diplegia of the supranuclear type. This may be associated with bilateral paralysis of lateral conjugate ocular deviation, the supranuclear fibres for this movement crossing the midline at the same level.

Lesions in the pons
Owing to the higher level of the corticofacial fibres, a unilateral corticospinal lesion in the pons does not cause weakness of the opposite side of the face, but only of the opposite bulbar muscles and limbs. But the lesion may also involve the facial nucleus or the intrapontine fibres of the facial nerve on the same side, thus causing one form of 'crossed hemiplegia'. Many forms of this have been described and named after those who first described them.

The *Millard-Gubler syndrome* consists of paralysis of one lateral rectus, due to involvement of the sixth-nerve nucleus with or without facial paralysis of the lower motor-neurone type on the same side and supranuclear paralysis of the bulbar muscles and limbs on the opposite side.

Foville's syndrome is similar to the Millard-Gubler syndrome, except that paralysis of conjugate ocular deviation to the side of the lesion takes the place of lateral rectus paralysis.

Ipsilateral paralysis of the jaw muscles due to involvement of the motor nucleus of the fifth nerve may be associated with either of these syndromes. When the lesion is situated deeply in the pons, near the midline, involvement of the medial lemniscus causes impairment of postural sensibility on the opposite side of the body. When the lesion lies mainly in the lateral part of the pons, the lemniscus escapes, but damage to the spinothalamic tract causes crossed analgesia and thermo-anaesthesia, with or without some impairment of sensibility in the trigeminal area on the side of the lesion, owing to involvement of the trigeminal fibres within the pons. *Horner's syndrome*, paralysis of the ocular sympathetic, may also result from a lesion in the tegmentum of the pons.

Lesions in the medulla

Many varieties of crossed hemiplegia have been described as a result of unilateral medullary lesions. A lesion near the midline will involve the corticospinal fibres to the limbs above their decussation, together with the fibres of the hypoglossal nerve, causing unilateral paralysis of half of the tongue, with contralateral hemiplegia, to which loss of postural sensibility in the paralysed limbs may be added. When the lateral part of the medulla is affected as well, there will also be unilateral paralysis of the soft palate and vocal cord, due to involvement of the vagal nucleus with Horner's syndrome and trigeminal analgesia and some cerebellar deficiency, all on the side of the lesion, and with loss of appreciation of pain, heat, and cold in the limbs and trunk on the opposite side. Vascular lesions in the midline of the medulla may involve both corticospinal tracts, leading to quadriplegia, sometimes with unilateral or bilateral paralysis of the tongue.

Spinal hemiplegia

A unilateral lesion of the corticospinal tract in the spinal cord below the medulla and above the fifth cervical segment causes hemiplegia on the affected side but spares, of course, the muscles innervated by the cranial nerves.

Lesions of the lower motor neurone

In lower motor-neurone lesions, as there is an interruption of the final common path of all forms of motor activity, the muscle or muscle groups involved become paralysed and flaccid (hypotonic) and remain so. Any reflex movement for which the paralysed muscles are necessary will be lost. Another invariable feature is that all muscles which are deprived of their motor nerve supply undergo rapid atrophy; they may shrink to half the normal size within about six weeks and will eventually disappear almost completely, being virtually replaced by fibrous connective tissue. Before this stage of total atrophy is reached, and particularly if the lesion responsible lies in the anterior horn cells of the spinal cord (e.g. motor-neurone disease), *fasciculation* is commonly seen. The latter is a phenomenon, visible through the intact skin unless the subject is very obese, in which individual muscle fasciculi contract spontaneously, and an irregular but continuous flickering of these fibre bundles can be seen to be occurring in a muscle which is apparently completely at rest. Fasciculation, though most often seen in patients with motor-neurone disease, is not diagnostic of this condition, as it may occur, for example, following old poliomyelitis, and is also observed occasionally in polyneuropathy and as a result of other lesions of the peripheral nerves. Furthermore,

it may be benign and of no pathological significance; it is sometimes observed by doctors in their calf and small hand muscles. A benign condition in which very widespread and coarse fasciculation occurs along with profuse sweating and severe muscular cramps is sometimes known as *myokymia* but other disorders have also been given this name (see Chapter 19).

Fibrillation, or spontaneous contraction of individual muscle fibres, also occurs following a lesion of the lower motor neurone, but cannot be seen through the skin, though it can be recorded electromyographically. Hence, the clinical features of an acute lower motor-neurone lesion are total flaccid paralysis with absence of all reflexes and rapid atrophy of the affected muscle or group of muscles. Following such atrophy, fibrous contractures with shortening of muscles and tendons may occur in less severely affected muscles, especially if, at a joint, their antagonists are very weak. Trophic changes (atrophy of bones and finger nails, cyanosis, shiny atrophic skin, and even sometimes oedema), largely resulting from disuse, are often seen eventually, especially in paralysed extremities.

In a slowly progressive lesion, weakness and atrophy increase gradually and eventually the reflexes are lost. In such a case it can be difficult to decide whether the lesion involves a single peripheral nerve, several peripheral nerves, a group of spinal anterior roots, or the anterior horn cells of the cord. All-important in making this distinction is a knowledge of the anatomy and innervation of muscles. If more muscles are affected than could be supplied by a single peripheral nerve, it must then be asked whether lesions of a cord of the brachial or lumbosacral plexus or of one group of spinal roots could be responsible, in which latter case there may also be evidence of spinal-cord disease or dysfunction. If the muscular weakness and wasting is more widespread still and particularly if it occurs symmetrically in the peripheral muscles of the limbs, the two commonest conditions to be considered are polyneuropathy (polyneuritis) and motor-neurone disease (progressive muscular atrophy). The presence of sensory loss, particularly if present symmetrically in the periphery of the limbs, will confirm the former diagnosis, while if there is widespread fasciculation of muscles, no sensory loss, and some evidence of corticospinal-tract disease, motor-neurone disease can be diagnosed with reasonable confidence. In this disease, because of associated corticospinal-tract dysfunction, the tendon reflexes may be exaggerated even when the muscles responsible for the individual reflexes are weak and wasted.

Muscular weakness and wasting which can mimic that due to a lower motor-neurone lesion may result from a primary disease of the muscles themselves, a myopathy. Here, too, there is flaccid weakness with atrophy and absence of tendon reflexes. Even in disorders of conduction at the motor end-plate, such as myasthenia gravis, the muscles may be weak and hypotonic, though atrophy is uncommon. In general, however, myopathic as distinct from neuropathic disorders tend to affect the proximal rather than the distal muscles of the limbs; fasciculation does not occur. The clinical effects of disease in the plexuses and peripheral nerves are described in Chapter 18 and diseases of muscle in Chapter 19, along with relevant diagnostic techniques including electromyography and measurement of nerve conduction velocity.

Dysfunction of the basal ganglia

Involuntary movements and the many other clinical syndromes which result from dysfunction of the basal ganglia are described in Chapter 12.

Cerebellar dysfunction

Ataxia and incoordination

Ataxia, unsteadiness, or incoordination is essentially a clumsiness of motor activity, resulting from an inability to control accurately the range and precision of movement. It can result from a defect in the sensory pathways responsible for the transmission of proprioceptive information from sensory receptors in the periphery. Under such circumstances the appreciation of the position of the parts of the body in space is impaired and, since controlled movement requires continuous and accurate information of this nature for its performance, it may be seriously deranged. This phenomenon, known as *sensory ataxia*, will be considered shortly. In such a case, the cause of the unsteadiness will be apparent on sensory examination. Similarly, sensory stimuli from the labyrinths are important in the maintenance of posture. If, as a result of disease of the labyrinths, of the vestibular nerves, or of their central connections, distorted information concerning the position of the head is received, the patient's gait will become grossly unsteady and the movements of his limbs clumsy and poorly controlled. Thus ataxia may also be the result of *labyrinthine dysfunction*. Usually, however, it results from cerebellar dysfunction.

As we have seen, the controlling activity of the cerebellum upon the motor system is concerned particularly with the fine co-ordination of movement and with the judgement of distance; it is these faculties which are selectively impaired as a result of cerebellar disease. In general, the central cerebellar structures, the vermis and flocculonodular lobe (the palaeocerebellum), have predominantly vestibular connections and are concerned particularly with equilibration. Hence lesions in this situation produce an ataxia which involves central structures of the body and is thus particularly apparent when the patient walks. The patient is unsteady and staggers in a drunken manner: he walks on a wide base and has considerable difficulty in stopping suddenly or in turning. Lesser degrees of ataxia can be brought out by asking the patient to walk 'heel-to-toe'; even in mildly ataxic individuals this is usually impossible. There may also occasionally be a rhythmical nodding or 'titubating' tremor of the head. In such case the tests of cerebellar function to be described below, which are concerned with the demonstration of ataxia in lateral structures, such as the limbs, may be singularly uninformative. Because these tests are negative, it is a common pitfall to regard such patients as hysterical, particularly if the doctor fails to recognize that a cerebellar lesion which is centrally situated gives this particular type of so-called *truncal or central ataxia*. This type of disturbance is particularly well seen in children with medulloblastomas. Cerebellar dysarthria is also characteristic, and is more common in lesions involving central structures. Articulation is slow but jerky, the individual syllables are slurred but they are also separated abnormally, a phenomenon sometimes called 'scanning speech'.

Lesions of the lateral cerebellar hemispheres, affecting the so-called neocerebellum, give rise to a number of physical signs which are more readily identifiable. If the lesion is predominantly unilateral, these signs are apparent in the limbs on the same side as the lesion. There may also be *ocular signs*; thus in an acute cerebellar lesion *skew deviation* is occasionally seen, in which the eye on the affected side is deviated downwards and inwards, while the contralateral eye is turned upwards and out; however, this rare manifestation is more common in upper brainstem lesions. *Nystagmus* is much more common and usually it is prominent, being of greatest amplitude on looking to the side of the lesion. Less often it is rotary in type and vertical nystagmus may be seen as a result of lesions of the cerebellar tonsils near the foramen magnum. Occasionally the head is tilted to the side of the lesion and there may be transient impairment of conjugate ocular deviation to the affected side. *Hypotonia* is often present in the ipsilateral limbs. This is shown first by diminished resistance to passive joint movement and secondly by the wide excursions occurring at terminal joints when a limb is shaken vigorously. If the upper limb is held outstretched and is tapped sharply, it shows a greater degree of temporary displacement than a normal limb. When the lesion is unilateral, then hypotonia may be seen on only one side. In the rebound phenomenon, if the patient flexes the forearm at the elbow against the examiner's resistance and the examiner then lets go, a normal individual can arrest the sudden further flexion but a patient with cerebellar hypotonia cannot do so and the hand may strike the patient's face. In a limb or limbs which are hypotonic due to cerebellar disease, the tendon reflexes are preserved but the knee jerk may be pendular, showing recurring oscillations of the dependent limb after the initial quadriceps contraction due to lack of cerebellar inhibition of the reflex contraction.

Ataxia is evidenced by a striking clumsiness and incoordination of movement. The patient is unable to button his clothes and his handwriting is scrawling and illegible. Judgement of distance is grossly impaired, a phenomenon known as *dysmetria*, and the hand performing a movement may wildly overshoot the mark (*past-pointing*). Tremor of the limbs may be apparent at rest but is sometimes greatly accentuated by movement, especially in disease of the cerebellar connections in the brainstem, when it may be much worse towards the end of an action (*intention tremor*). These signs are particularly apparent on carrying on carrying out the 'finger–nose' and 'heel–knee' tests and there will also be a gross irregularity of movement if the patient is asked to tap quickly and repetitively upon a smooth surface, or to make dots within a small circle with a pencil. Rapid alternating movements of the limbs, such as pronation and supination of the forearms, are poorly and jerkily performed (*dysdiadochokinesis*). The patient with a unilateral cerebellar lesion shows outward deviation of the outstretched arm and hand on the side of the lesion (Baràny's pointing test) and also tends to stagger and to deviate towards the affected side when walking. A minimal cerebellar lesion on one side can sometimes be identified most easily by asking the patient to walk a few paces with his eyes closed, when he will deviate to the affected side. Alternatively, if asked to walk in a circle around the examiner first clockwise then anticlockwise, the deviation away from the examiner in one direction and towards him in the other will be apparent.

Vertigo is a not infrequent symptom of an acute cerebellar lesion; symptoms and signs are always more striking when the lesion is acute, whether vascular or inflammatory. The nervous system seems able to adapt to the presence of a slowly-developing lesion such as a cerebellar tumour, so that lesions of the latter type may be present for some time before producing overt symptoms.

References

Adams, R. D. and Victor, M. (1981). *Principles of neurology*, 2nd edn. McGraw Hill, New York.

Bloom, W. and Fawcett, D. W. (1970). *A textbook of histology*, 10th edn. Saunders, Philadelphia.

Bradley, W. G. (1974). *Disorders of peripheral nerves*. Blackwell, Oxford.

Brain, W. R. (1927). On the significance of the flexor posture of the upper limb in hemiplegia, with an account of a quadrupedal extensor reflex. *Brain*, **50**, 113.

Brodal, A. (1981). *Neurological anatomy in relation to clinical medicine*, 3rd edn. Oxford University Press, Oxford.

Bull, J. W. D. (1969). The tentorium cerebelli. *Proc. R. Soc. Med.* **62**, 1301.

Burke, D. and others (1980). Control of movement. *Trends Neurosci*, special issue.

Clarke, E. and O'Malley, C. D. (1968). *The human brain and spinal cord*. University of California Press, Berkeley.

Cooper, J. R., Bloom, F. E., and Roth, R. H. (1978) *The biochemical basis of neuropharmacology*, 3rd edn. Oxford University Press, Oxford.

Curtis, B. A., Jacobson, S., and Marcus, E. M. (1972) *An introduction to the neurosciences*. Saunders, Philadelphia.

Denny-Brown, D. (1966). *The cerebral control of movement*. Liverpool University Press, Liverpool.

Dubowitz, V. and Brooke, M. H. (1973). *Muscle biopsy: a modern approach*, Saunders, London.

Eccles, J. C. (1957). *The physiology of nerve cells*. Johns Hopkins Press, Baltimore.

Edström, L. and Kugelberg, E. (1968). Histochemical composition, distribution of fibres and fatiguability of single motor units. *J. Neurol. Neurosurg. Psychiat.* **31**, 424.

Englander, R. N., Netsky, M., and Adelman, L. S. (1975). Location of human pyramidal tract in the internal capsule: anatomic evidence. *Neurology (Minneapolis)* **25**, 823.

Gardner, E. (1975). *Fundamentals of neurology*, 6th edn. Saunders, Philadelphia.

Gergely, J. (1981). Biochemical aspects of muscular structure and function. Chapter 1 in *Disorders of voluntary muscle*, 4th edn. J. N. Walton, Churchill-Livingstone, Edinburgh and London.

Goldensohn, E. and Appel, S. (1977). *Scientific approaches to clinical neurology*. Lea and Febiger, Philadelphia.

Granit, R. (1970). *The basis of motor control*. Academic Press, New York and London.

Henderson, G., Tomlinson, B. E., and Gibson, P. H. (1980). Cell counts in human cerebral cortex in normal adults throughout life using an image analysing computer. *J. neurol. Sci.* **46**, 113.

Hoff, E. C. and Hoff, H. E. (1934). Spinal terminations of the projection fibres from the motor cortex of primates. *Brain* **57**, 454.

Holmes, G. (1917). The symptoms of acute cerebellar injuries due to gunshot injuries, *Brain* **40**, 461.

—— (1939). The cerebellum of man. *Brain* **62**, 1.

Huxley, A. (1980). *Reflections on muscle*. Liverpool University Press, Liverpool.

Kandel, E. R. and Schwartz, J. H. (1981). *Principles of neural science*. Elsevier North-Holland, New York.

Keynes, R. D. and Aidley, D. J. (1981). *Nerve and muscle*. Cambridge Texts in the Physiological Sciences, Vol. 2. Cambridge University Press, Cambridge.

Kuffler, S. W. and Nicholls, J. G. (1976). *From neuron to brain*. Sinauer Associates, Sunderland, Massachusetts.

Lance, J. W. (1980). The control of muscle tone, reflexes, and movement: Robert Wartenberg Lecture. *Neurology, Minneapolis* **30**, 1303.

—— and McLeod, J. G. (1981). *A physiological approach to clinical neurology*, 3rd edn. Butterworth, London.

Lenman, J. A. R. (1975). *Clinical neurophysiology*. Blackwell, Oxford.

Lewis, D. M. and Ridge, R. M. A. P. (1981). The anatomy and physiology of the motor unit, in *Disorders of voluntary muscle*, 4th edn (ed. J. N. Walton). Churchill-Livingstone, Edinburgh and London.

Mastaglia, F. L. and Walton, J. N. (1982). *Skeletal muscle pathology*. Churchill-Livingstone, Edinburgh and London.

McComas, A. J. Sica, R. E. P., Upton, A. R. M., and Aguilera, N. (1973). Functional changes in motoneurones of hemiparetic patients. *J. Neurol. Neurosurg. Psychiat.* **36**, 183.

Medical Research Council (1976). *Aids to the examination of the peripheral nervous system*, MRC Memorandum No. 45, HMSO, London.

Mettler, F. A. (1968). Anatomy of the basal ganglia. Chapter 1 in *Handbook of clinical neurology* (ed. P. J. Vinken and G. W. Bruyn) Vol. 6. North-Holland, Amsterdam.

Nathan, P. W. and Smith, M. C. (1955). Long descending tracts in man. I. Review of present knowledge. *Brain* **78**, 248.

Newman, P. P. (1980). *Neurophysiology*. Spectrum, New York.

Nyberg-Hansen, R. (1965). Sites and mode of termination of reticulo-spinal fibers in the cat: an experimental study with silver impregnation methods, *J. comp. Neurol.* **124**, 71.

—— and Brodal, A. (1963). Sites of termination of corticospinal fibers in the cat: an experimental study with silver impregnation methods. *J. comp. neurol.* **120**, 369.

—— and —— (1964). Sites and mode of termination of rubrospinal fibers in the cat: an experimental study with silver impregnation methods, *J. Anat., Lond.* **98**, 235.

—— and Rinvik, E. (1963). Some comments on the pyramidal tract, with special reference to its individual variations in man, *Acta neurol. scand.* **39**, 1.

Patton, H. D., Sundsten, J. W., Crill, W. E., and Swanson, P. D. (1976). *Introduction to basic neurology*. Saunders, Philadelphia.

Penfield, W. and Jasper, H. (1954). *Epilepsy and the functional anatomy of the human brain*. Little Brown & Co., Boston.

Peters, A., Palay, S. L., and Webster, H. de F. (1976). *The fine structures of the nervous system: the neurons and supporting cells*. Saunders, Philadelphia.

Pitres and Testut (1925). *Les neufs en schemes*. Doin, Paris.

Price, H. M. and Van de Velde, R. L. (1981) Ultrastructure of the skeletal muscle fibre. In *Disorders of voluntary muscle*, 4th edn (ed. J. N. Walton). Churchill-Livingstone, Edinburgh and London.

Ransom, S. W. and Clark, S. L. (1960). *The anatomy of the nervous system*. Saunders, Philadelphia.

Sharrard, W. J. W. (1955). The distribution of the permanent paralysis in the lower limb in poliomyelitis, *J. Bone Joint Surg.* **37B**, 540.

Sidman, S., Bloedel, J. R., and Lechtenberg, R. (1981). *Disorders of the cerebellum*, Contemporary Neurology Series, Vol. 21. F. A. Davis, Philadelphia.

Snider, R. S. (1972). The cerebellum. Chapter III. 2 In *scientific foundations of neurology* (ed. M. Critchley, J. L. O'Leary, and W. B. Jennett). Heinemann, London.

Spillane, J. D. and Spillane, J.A. (1982). *An atlas of clinical neurology*, 3rd edn. Oxford University Press, Oxford.

Tomlinson, B. E. and Irving, D. (1977). The numbers of limb motor neurons in the human lumbosacral cord throughout life. *J.neurol. Sci.* **34**, 213.

——, ——, and Rebeiz, J. J. (1973). Total numbers of limb motor neurones in the human lumbosacral cord and an analysis of the accuracy of various sampling procedures. *J. neurol. Sci.* **20**, 313.

Tower, D. B. and Brady, R. O. (1975). *The nervous system. Vol. 1: the basic neurosciences*, Raven Press, New York.

Walshe, F. M. R. (1943). On the mode of representation of movements in the motor cortex, with special reference to 'convulsions beginning unilaterally' (Jackson), *Brain* **66**, 104.

—— (1965). *Further critical studies in neurology*. Livingstone, Edinburgh.

Walton, J. N. (1981a). Neurology (Section XII) in *Pathophysiology—the biological principles of disease* (ed. L. H. Smith, Jr and S. O. Thier) International Textbook of Medicine. Saunders, Philadelphia.

—— (1983). *An introduction to clinical neuroscience*. Baillière Tindall, London.

—— (Ed.) (1981b). *Disorders of voluntary muscle*, 4th edn. Churchill-Livingstone, Edinburgh and London.

—— (1982). *Essentials of neurology*, 5th edn. Pitman, London.

Yahr, M. D. (Ed.) (1976). *The basal ganglia*. Association for Research in Nervous and Mental Disease vol. 55. Raven Press, New York.

Zaimis, E. and Wray, D. (1981). General physiology and pharmacology of neuromuscular transmission. Chapter 3 In *Disorders of voluntary muscle* 4th edn (ed. J. N. Walton). Churchill-Livingstone, Edinburgh and London.

The sensory system

Introduction

The nature of sensory receptors and of afferent pathways in the nervous system which carry somatic sensory impulses have already been mentioned and will be amplified here. In general, sensory input is of two principal types: first, there are impulses which lead to *motor responses* through segmental reflex systems, and second there are those which ascend either directly or via interneurones to reach centres (mainly the thalamus and sensory cortex) in which sensory experiences are recorded and enter perception. The latter are known as *sensory responses*. These two processes are not totally independent as a single primary afferent nerve fibre may initiate a reflex response, while its long ascending collateral branches may also convey sensory information which reaches consciousness (sensory awareness). Nevertheless, it has become conventional to accept that the term 'sensory' relates only to those neurones and pathways which convey impulses to levels of the nervous system (thalamus and cortex) at which the sensation conveyed evokes conscious awareness and not to those afferents which excite reflex activity only and do not contribute to conscious experience. While this distinction is a useful concept in sensory physiology, in clinical neurological practice it is difficult to adopt totally since proprioceptive sensory information, for instance, relating to the position and interrelationship of the parts of the body, does not as a rule enter consciousness and yet defects of this sense, as we shall see, produce striking clinical manifestations, of which many are due to the impairment of reflex mechanisms concerned with motor control. Hence in this section we must consider not only sensory mechanisms in the strict sense outlined above but also some of the pathophysiological consequences of impaired reflex responses due to dysfunction of afferent pathways.

The anatomical and physiological organization of somatic sensation

General organization

The sensory apparatus consists first of a series of sensory receptors in the skin and other organs, second of the first sensory neurone, whose bipolar cells are located in the posterior root ganglia, and third of secondary sensory neurones which conduct impulses through the spinal cord and brainstem to the thalamus and thence, sometimes, to the cerebral cortex. Cells in the substantia gelatinosa of the spinal cord and the internuncial neurones which arise from them probably play a major role in modulating sensory input (Cervero and Iggo 1980). Visceral sensation, which is conveyed initially alongside fibres of the autonomic nervous system, enters the spinal cord along with somatic sensory impulses and is conveyed centrally in a similar manner.

Receptors

Sensory receptors can be divided into *exteroceptors*, which are largely situated in the skin and are concerned with recording information about the external environment of the body, and *proprioceptors*, which are situated in muscles, tendons, and viscera and which inform us of the position and condition of these deeper structures. Many of the exteroceptors consist simply of a network of fine nerve endings which terminate in the skin, but there are also more specialized receptors such as the basket-like nerve endings which surround hair follicles, as well as Merkel's discs and Meissner's corpuscles which are believed to record touch sensation, and Krause's bulbs and Ruffini's corpuscles which respond to thermal stimuli. Indeed it was once believed that specific sensory receptors were necessary for the recording of each form of sensation, but work on the cornea (Weddell, Sinclair, and Feindel 1948) showed that touch, pain, and thermal sensations can all be appreciated through undifferentiated nerve endings. However, it is now recognized that many terminations of what are apparently at first sight undifferentiated endings in the skin and indeed in all organs, constitute specific *nociceptors* concerned with the perception of pain (see Zimmerman 1981). Each so-called 'sensory spot' on the skin may receive filaments from several branches of a nerve and it has been suggested that it is the pattern of stimulation and the frequency of discharge in these fibres which determines the nature of the sensation which is perceived, rather than total specificity of the nerve endings themselves. However, certain cutaneous 'spots' are particularly sensitive to pain (the nociceptors), and others to cold or warmth. This is why there is considerable variation in the sensation evoked by uniform stimuli in contiguous skin areas. Thus a touch on a cold spot will feel cold, or a pin-prick on a pain spot may be more painful than one applied with similar force nearby. Muller's law states that the quality of sensory experiences depends upon *which* receptors are excited and not *how* the excitation takes place. Fortunately these fine distinctions are of comparatively little significance in clinical neurology, since sensory abnormalities, to be of practical importance, must generally be relatively crude.

The *proprioceptive receptors* consist of the muscle spindles and the Golgi–Mazzoni tendon organs, which respond to tension or stretching of muscles, and the Pacinian corpuscles which are probably responsive to pressure. Comparatively few proprioceptive stimuli reach consciousness; as we have seen, many are concerned with reflex activity mediated through the spinal cord or cerebellum, by means of which posture and movement are controlled.

Somatic sensation: its nature, coding and measurement

Sensory parameters

Somatic sensation is not a uniform sensory experience but is a fusion of several qualities or parameters which cannot be consciously dissociated but may be differentially affected by disease or dysfunction. Thus each sensory experience has a *quality* or *modality* (touch, pain, heat, and cold etc.) and the various sensory modalities will be considered below. As described above, different receptors respond to different modalities and there is evidence to indicate that some secondary sensory neurones in the posterior horn of spinal-cord grey matter, some fibres in the ascending sensory tracts, some thalamic neurones, and to a lesser extent those in the cortex are modality-specific. *Intensity* is another parameter of importance, enabling us to distinguish between a light pin-prick and a fierce jab. There is also clear neurophysiological evidence indicating that intensity discrimination is pattern-coded, i.e. it depends upon frequency of firing in tonic sensory receptors and in neurones and afferent fibres at all levels of the nervous system; the position with respect to phasic (on–off) receptors, such as those concerned with light touch, is more complex, intensity being little if at all related to frequency, but again the pattern of discharge is fundamental. The normal human subject is also skilled at the *localization* of sensory stimuli. This faculty is clearly related to the segmental organization of cutaneous sensory input as we shall see below; localization of visceral sensation is less accurate, though even this may be aided by the interpretation, for instance, of referred pain. In the posterior roots of the spinal cord and their ganglia, in the posterior horns of grey matter, in the ascending pathways in the spinal cord, in the peripheral sensory nuclei of the brainstem, in the thalamus, and in the sensory cortex, as we shall see, there is a clear, consistent, and precise somatotopic localization in that specific groups of neurones can be excited by specific sensory stimuli applied to particular areas of the body surface. Another factor of importance is the density of sensory receptors in different areas of skin; this variability of distribution accounts for the striking differences observed, for instance, in the ability to discriminate between two points applied at set distances apart (two-point discrimination). This variation explains why the receptive fields of somatosensory cortical neurones show an inverse relationship to sensory acuity in that these fields are small, for instance, in respect to sensory input from the tips of the fingers and large for many areas of the trunk.

The nervous system is also capable of recognizing the *duration and temporal pattern* of sensory stimuli. Thus the onset and the termination of a stimulus and its reaction time (the time taken for its conscious perception) can be recognized, as can recurring stimuli such as the perception of vibration. As already indicated, different fibres in peripheral nerves conduct at different rates, depending upon their diameter and upon whether or not they are myelinated, and different modalities of sensation are therefore conducted at different rates; reaction time is directly related to conduction velocity in both the peripheral and the central nervous system. The mechanism of perception of vibration is more complex; such recurrent stimuli specifically excite phasic (on–off) receptors, each oscillation exciting a single spike, but there is also evidence that different thalamic and cortical neurones may respond to different frequencies so that both place and pattern coding are involved.

Finally, it should be noted that most sensations evoke *affective responses* which determine whether the sensation perceived is pleasant (warmth), unpleasant (pain, excessive heat or cold), or neutral (touch, change of position, etc.). The influence of cerebral and hypothalamic centres concerned with pleasure, reward, and punishment upon somatic sensation will be considered in Chapters 20 and 23. Sedative drugs, such as barbiturates and phenothiazines, for example, and surgical procedures, such as prefrontal leucotomy or lesions which interrupt connections between the prefrontal cortex and subcortical centres, may all diminish or even abolish affect, while leaving intact the ability to recognize sensory modalities. Thus the patient continues to feel and to recognize pain but it no longer disturbs him.

From this evidence it follows that the coding of sensory information allows the subject to recognize the nature of the somatic stimulus which he perceives, its intensity, where it is situated, how long it lasts, and whether it is repetitive, and its character and emotional connotations.

Examinations and measurement
Methods of examining the commoner sensory modalities in clinical practice will be described later, but it is important to recognize that much depends upon the co-operation of the subject, upon his state of consciousness, intellectual capacity, and emotional state. Areas of cutaneous sensory impairment, especially for light touch and pin-prick, subsequently shown on re-examination to be spurious, are often elicited by even skilled observers, and intelligent, obsessional, or introspective patients often perceive relatively slight variations in intensity of stimulation which the examiner cannot avoid and which ultimately prove to be of no pathological significance. In addition, individuals vary in their affective response to sensory stimuli, a sensation which appears acutely painful to one being well tolerated by another.

Considerable advances have been made in methods of measuring somatic sensory perception, both in animals and in man, but the techniques involved are generally too complex for use in clinical practice. However, many years ago Weber, assessing the ability of subjects to recognize differences in the weights of a series of test objects which they lifted, introduced the concept of 'just noticeable difference' (j.n.d.) and Weber's law stated that

$$\frac{\text{j.n.d.}}{I} = k$$

where I was the weight of a reference object and k a constant found to be 1/30. Thus with a 30-g reference weight, the difference between weights of 29 and 31 g could be perceived but, if the reference weight was 60 g, the subject could only discriminate between objects weighing 58 and 62 g. Subsequently Fechner, extending Weber's observations, concluded that the magnitude of the sensation perceived is directly proportional to the log of the physical stimulus. While the accuracy of this postulate has subsequently been called into question, Fechner's law remains a useful guide. More recently, reliable and reproducible methods of measuring, for example, touch pressure, vibration, and thermal cutaneous sensation in man (Dyck, Schultz, and O'Brien 1972; Dyck, Zimmerman, O'Brien, Ness, Caskey, Karnes, and Bushek 1978) as well as pain perception (Huskisson 1974) have been introduced.

The simpler sensory modalities
While all forms of sensory experience are interrelated, several clearly definable forms of somatic sensation can be recognized whose integrity is customarily assessed during neurological examination. The first is *touch*, commonly tested with a light application to the skin of a pledget of cotton wool. Touch may be assessed quantitatively with von Frey hairs, so graduated that differing pressures are needed to bend them. The threshold for touch appreciation varies considerably on different parts of the surface of the body, depending upon such variables as the thickness of the epidermis and the number of hair follicles present. *Pain* sensation is generally assessed by pin-prick, which can also be of graduated severity if an algesimeter is used. The patient must be asked to assess the painful quality of this stimulus and not the sensations of pressure or touch which may be simultaneously evoked. Squeezing of the tendon of Achilles or of other deep tendons will determine whether the appreciation of *deep pressure* is intact, but this sensation can also be painful. *Thermal sensation* is generally tested by applying metal test-tubes to the skin, one filled with ice, the other with water at 45 °C. Again the patient is told that it is the feeling of heat or cold he is being asked to note and not that of touch or pressure. The assessment of *position and joint sense* is carried out by moving the terminal phalanx of the forefinger or the great toe in a vertical plane and by asking the patient, whose eyes are closed, to describe the direction of movement each time the

digit is moved. After making an initial movement of substantial amplitude, it must then be determined whether the patient can appreciate movements through a very small range (about 1 mm). Another useful test of positional sensibility is to ask the patient, with his eyes closed, to point towards a part of his body, when the position of the part in space has been altered by the examiner. *Vibration sense*, as tested with a tuning fork of 128-frequency applied to bony prominences, is not a physiological sensation, being compounded of both touch and pressure, but nevertheless absence of the perception of this form of somatic sensibility is very significant in clinical neurology. *Tactile discrimination* is assessed by recording the threshold distance at which the two blunt points of a compass, simultaneously applied, are independently perceived (Fig. 1.29). The normal threshold for two-point discrimination on the tip of the tongue is 1 mm, on the tips of the fingers 2–3 mm, on the palm of the hand or sole of the foot 1.5–3 cm, and in the centre of the back 6–7 cm. The appreciation of *texture*, *weight*, *size*, and *shape* of objects can also be assessed, somewhat crudely, by asking the patient, with his eyes closed, to identify objects placed in the hand, while tactile localization is tested by asking him to identify on a diagram or model, or on the examiner, the point or points on his body which had been stimulated. He may also be asked to identify figures or letters which are traced with a blunt point on his skin (*graphaesthesia*). There is considerable individual variation in the ability to perceive and interpret these more comlex sensations, but retention of these functions on one side of the body and their absence on the other is always a finding of pathological significance. Inability to perceive one of a pair of tactile stimuli simultaneously applied to comparable points on opposite sides of the body (tactile inattention) is also a useful sign, as will be seen.

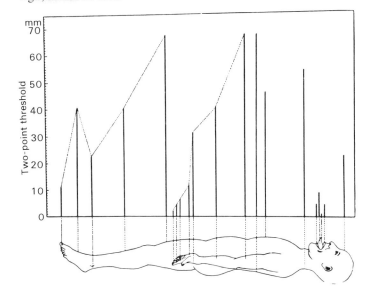

Fig. 1.29. Regional variation in tactile two-point discrimination threshold in man. (Reproduced from Patton *et al.* (1976) and previously published in Ruch and Patton (1965), by kind permission of the authors and publisher.)

The sensory pathways

The cells of the first sensory neurone are situated in the posterior root ganglia and are bipolar in type, having peripheral axons which convey afferent impulses from the sensory receptors, and central axons which enter the spinal cord in the posterior-nerve roots. As previously noted, the sensory fibres in the *peripheral nerves* vary in diameter and in their rate of conduction; the large, heavily-myelinated, rapidly-conducting A fibres are primarily concerned with the conduction of impulses subserving touch, pressure, and proprioceptive sensation, but some undoubtedly transmit painful and thermal sensations. The most slowly-conducting unmyelinated *C* fibres are largely concerned with temperature and pain sensation, but some also convey touch, so that there is no exact relationship between the size and myelination of sensory axons on the one hand and their function on the other. However, since certain diseases of the peripheral nerves, and particularly various forms of peripheral neuropathy, may have a selective effect upon fibres of one particular size or degree of myelination, there are some cases in which the appreciation of painful stimulation is more severely affected than that of touch and vice versa. And while cutaneous and pressure sensations travel in pure sensory (cutaneous) and later in mixed sensory and motor nerves, some proprioceptive stimuli, especially those concerned in reflex activity, and particularly those coming from the muscle spindles, travel centrally first of all in motor nerves.

As the central axons of the first sensory neurone enter the spinal cord, some degree of regrouping of these fibres occurs, according to their function. Initially many of them enter the posterior column, lying just medially to the posterior horn of grey matter. At this point internuncial neurones arising from cells in the substantia gelatinosa exert a modifying or 'gating' influence (see below), especially upon painful sensations. Many of the fibres concerned with proprioception, position and joint-sense, vibration sense, and tactile discrimination, as well as some of those conveying touch, turn immediately upwards in the *posterior columns* and travel to the nuclei of Goll and Burdach in the medulla. Since entering fibres continually displace medially those which have entered the cord at a lower level, it follows that the fibres from the lower limbs lie in the medial part of the posterior column (the fasciculus graci-

lis or column of Goll), while those from the upper limbs lie more laterally (the fasciculus cuneatus or column of Burdach (Fig. 1.30)). Recent studies have indicated that the posterior columns are concerned with the conduction of impulses relating to the simultaneous analysis of spatial and temporal characteristics of somatosensory stimuli, since complete transection of a dorsal column does not abolish all fine tactile appreciation and position and joint sense (Wall 1970; Wall and Noordenbos 1977; *The Lancet* 1978*a*).

A second group of entering fibres, concerned with the appreciation of touch, also enters the most lateral part of the posterior column and these ascend for several segments, then entering the posterior horn of grey matter to synapse with cells in this area. The axons of these cells then cross the midline close to the central canal to end in the *ventral spinothalamic tract*. Fibres subserving pain and temperature sensation run a very similar course, except that they only ascend in the posterior column for a few segments before crossing the midline in the grey matter close to the central canal to end in the more *lateral spinothalamic tract* in the opposite lateral column of the cord (Fig. 1.30). As in the posterior columns, there is some lamination of sensory fibres in these tracts, those from the lower limbs lying nearest the surface of the cord and those from the upper limbs being situated more centrally. This probably explains why a lesion giving rise to spinal-cord compression may impair pain sensation first in the lower limbs; the sensory 'level' then ascends steadily but finally becomes arrested on the trunk several segments below the situation of the lesion; presumably the fibres situated nearest to the surface of the cord are the first to be affected by pressure (White and Sweet 1955).

When the sensory fibres of the spinal cord reach the medulla oblongata, the spinothalamic fibres enter it laterally and travel upwards through the pons and midbrain to reach the thalamus. The fibres of the posterior columns, however, terminate in synapses in the nuclei of Goll (nucleus gracilis) and Burdach (nucleus cuneatus). From the cells of these nuclei, new axons arise

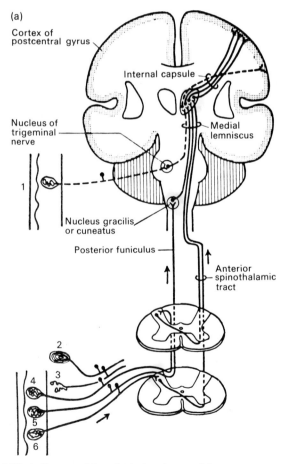

(a)

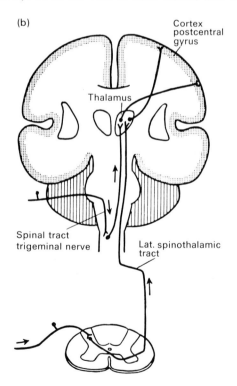

(b)

Fig. 1.30. A diagram of the principal pathways of the sensory system.

(a) The pathways followed by impulses subserving touch, tactile discrimination position and joint sense, and related sensations. 1, 4, 5, and 6 represent Meissner's corpuscles; the pathways from 2 (Pacinian corpuscle) and 3 (joint receptor) are similar to those followed by impulses from 5.

(b) The pathways followed by impulses subserving pain and temperature sensation.

(Reproduced from Walton (1982) and previously published in Gardner (1975) by kind permission of the authors and publishers.)

which immediately cross the midline and then travel upwards as the *medial fillet* or *lemniscus*, again to enter the thalamus.

The pathway followed by sensory impulses from the face deserves special mention. The fibres of the trigeminal nerve which carry touch and tactile discrimination enter the main trigeminal nucleus and then, in the *quintothalamic or trigeminothalamic tract*, cross the midline to join the medial fillet. Those subserving pain and thermal sensation enter the pons but then travel downwards in the *descending root of the trigeminal nerve* to end in a nuclear mass which extends downwards as far as the second cervical segment of the cord; then they, too, forming another part of the quintothalamic tract, cross the midline and travel upwards in the spinothalamic tract. 'Representation' of the parts of the face in the descending root of the trigeminal nerve is inverted; thus a lesion of the lower end of the root in the upper cervical cord will give loss of pain and temperature sensation only, but not of touch, over the area supplied by the ophthalmic division on the same side of the face. Furthermore, as in the limbs, proprioceptive stimuli from the face travel centrally in the facial nerve, so that sense of position in the facial muscles (a difficult faculty to test) is not abolished by a lesion of the trigeminus.

Thus all sensory pathways which ascend as far as the brainstem terminate in the thalamus. Throughout their course in the spinal cord and brainstem many, indeed most, of these fibres have given off collaterals or have synapsed with internuncial neurones. These connections have completed the sensory side of the arcs concerned with those spinal and brainstem reflexes which are necessary for the maintenance of posture and other functions. There are, for instance, many sensory fibres, some of which synapse in Clarke's columns of the posterior horn of grey matter, which ascend the spinal cord in the dorsal and ventral spinocerebellar tracts and which are largely concerned with supplying the information through which the cerebellum exerts control over posture and movement.

Studies of evoked somatosensory potentials which can be recorded from surface electrodes applied over the spine or from electrodes inserted into the epidural space, after stimulation, for example, of median and tibial nerves, have cast considerable light on the function of sensory pathways in the spinal cord in health and disease (Mathews, Beauchamp, and Small 1974; Caccia, Ubiali, and Andreussi 1976; el-Negamy and Sedgwick 1978; Delbeke, McComas, and Kopec 1978). Similarly, measurement of cerebral evoked potentials, using surface scalp electrodes and averaging techniques, gives useful information about function and dysfunction at higher levels (Desmedt 1971; Shibasaki, Yamashita, and Tsuji 1977; Halliday 1980).

The thalamus

This is the principal sensory relay station of the brain. The principal nuclei of the thalamus and their cortical projections in the cerebral hemisphere are illustrated diagrammatically in Fig. 1.31. The sensory relay nuclei which receive input from the ascending pathways conveying somatic and visceral sensation are the nucleus ventralis posterolateralis (VPL), which receives afferent stimuli from the trunk and limbs, and the ventralis posteromedialis (VPM), which is similarly concerned with input from the face. Both in turn send corticothalamic neuronal projections to the somatosensory and parietal association areas of the cortex and receive corticothalamic projections from the same area. The lateral and medial geniculate bodies are concerned with vision and audition, respectively; the ventralis lateralis (VL) with cerebellar and extrapyramidal function; the ventralis anterior (VA) with activity of the basal ganglia; and the nucleus anterior (A) with hypothalamic function. The dorsomedial nucleus (MD), which projects to the prefrontal cortex, is not primarily concerned with the awareness of somatic sensation but appears to have a role relating to the affective response to sensory input, especially of pain (see Henson 1949). Electrical recording from the sensory

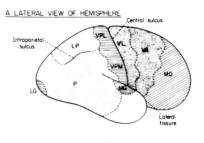

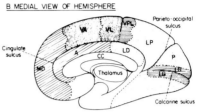

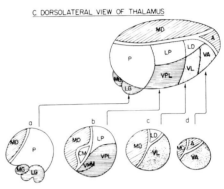

Fig. 1.31. Thalamic nuclei and their cerebral cortical projection sites. A and B: The right cerebral hemisphere; the dotted lines represent approximate projection boundaries that cut across different cortical gyri. C: The right thalamus and representative frontal sections (a–d) through it. The thalamic nuclei and their projection areas are shaded according to categories as follows: Somatosensory and special sensory, *horizontal shading*, cerebellar and striatal, *dense stippling*; hypothalamic, *oblique shading*; and 'association', *light stippling*. Thalamic nuclei: A, anterior; CM, centromedian; LD, lateralis dorsalis; LG, lateral geniculate; LP, lateralis posterior; MD, medialis dorsalis; MG, medial geniculate; P, pulvinar; VA, ventralis anterior; VL, ventralis lateralis; VPL, ventralis posterolateralis; VPM, ventralis posteromedialis. (Reproduced from Patton *et al.* (1976) by kind permission of the authors and publisher.)

relay nuclei has shown that there is a clear somatotopic representation of parts of the body, with caudal areas projecting to the lateral part of VPL, rostral segments more medially, and the face most medially in VPM (Jasper and Bertrand 1966; Tasker and Organ 1972).

The somatosensory cortex

A similar and precise somatotopic representation continues in the thalamocortical neuronal projections and even more so in the *primary sensory cortex* of the postcentral gyrus (Fig. 1.32) and to a lesser extent in projections to the other (association) areas of the parietal lobe.

It is apparent that the cortex is concerned with the appreciation of most of those stimuli which enter consciousness. The integrity of the sensory cortex is particularly important if we are to recognize form, texture, size, weight, and consistency of objects, or changes in position of parts of the body (Head 1920). It is also essential for the accurate localization and recognition of the nature of stimuli applied to the body, for discrimination between two simultaneously applied stimuli, and even more for the ability to relate sensory experiences to others experienced previously, or to sense data perceived through the special senses. Clearly, numerous association pathways are concerned in the interpretation and recognition of these more complex sensory experiences which may nevertheless be grossly deranged if there is a lesion of the primary sensory cortex, an important cell station in all sensory association mechanisms. As with the motor cortex (Penfield and Rasmussen 1950; Fig. 1.32), specific portions of the postcentral gyrus are concerned with the appreciation of sensations from particular areas of the opposite side of the body. 'Representation' in the sensory cortex corresponds topographically to that in the motor area; thus a lesion of the lower end of the postcentral gyrus will impair sensory perception in the contralateral face and hand, while a lesion on the superior and medial aspect of the hemisphere will result in a failure to appreciate 'cortical' forms of sensation in the opposite leg.

It is important to recognize that cortical or subcortical lesions, even if they divide all thalamocortical fibres, do not destroy completely the ability to perceive sensory experiences in the opposite half of the body. When such a lesion is present, sensitivity to pain and temperature is affected comparatively little, while crude touch will still be felt, though finer forms of sensory experience may be greatly impaired. Hence it is apparent that the cruder varieties of sensation are in some way recorded in consciousness at a thalamic level. Nevertheless, it is clear that the cortex plays some part in the perception of pain and temperature, at least in a qualitative sense, but cortical lesions also impair quantitative aspects of such perception (see Patton, Sundsten, Crill, and Swanson 1976).

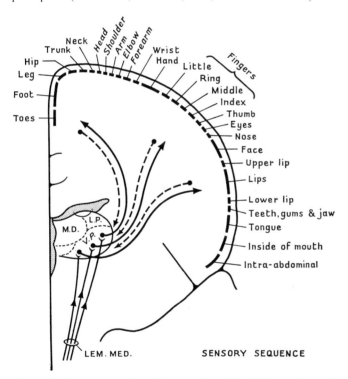

Fig. 1.32. Somatic sensation. Cross-section of the left hemisphere along the plane of the postcentral gyrus. The afferent pathway for tactile and kinaesthetic sensation is indicated by the unbroken lines coming up, through the medial lemniscus, and the posterolateral ventral nucleus of the thalamus, to the postcentral gyrus.

Cutaneous sensory segmentation

As we have seen, the human fetus, early in its development, demonstrates metameric segmentation and each somatic segment or metamere is linked to the corresponding segment of the neuraxis by a pair of spinal nerves. But in the course of evolution with specialization of the anterior end of the human organism to form the head and the growth of the complicated motor and sensory functions of the limbs, this metameric segmentation of the nervous system has been disrupted, persisting in the mature human only in the dorsal region. After the fusion of ventral and dorsal roots to form a spinal nerve, the dorsal primary division conveys motor fibres to the spinal muscles and sensory fibres to the overlying cutaneous area. In the mid-dorsal region, the ventral primary division supplies motor fibres to the intercostal muscles and sensory fibres to a narrow zone extending more or less horizontally around the thorax on one side as far as the midline. In the cervical and lumbosacral regions, the arrangement is complicated by the formation of the limb plexuses in which several ventral primary divisions unite and subsequently subdivide to form the peripheral nerves supplying the limbs. Through the intervention of the plexuses a single spinal nerve may send both motor and sensory contributions to several peripheral nerves and, conversely a single peripheral nerve may receive contributions from several spinal nerves. It follows that the sensory loss resulting from interruption of a peripheral nerve differs in its distribution from that produced by interruption of a posterior root or spinal nerve. A segmental or radicular cutaneous area—a dermatome—is an area of skin which receives its sensory supply from a single dorsal root and spinal nerve. In the trunk these segmental areas still exhibit a metameric arrangement. In the limbs this has been modified, but as a rule the segmental areas occupy elongated zones in the long axis of the limb (Fig. 1.33). Much information we now possess about the cutaneous areas of the individual dermatomes comes from the work of Foerster (1933) based upon his observations upon effects of posterior root section in human subjects, but electrophysiological methods are now available to check upon the sensory contributions made by individual posterior roots to limb peripheral nerves (Inouye and Buchthal 1977).

Owing to the specialization of the ventral primary divisions of the lower cervical and first thoracic spinal nerves in the innervation of the upper limb, these have lost their cutaneous supply to the trunk anteriorly and, at the level of the second rib, the fourth cervical segmental cutaneous area is contiguous with the second thoracic. The lower six thoracic spinal nerves supply the abdominal wall as far as the inguinal ligament. Probably owing to the fact that the dorsal divisions of the spinal nerves take no part in the formation of the limb plexuses, all spinal segments appear to be represented in the cutaneous supply of the back.

There is considerable overlapping of contiguous segmental cutaneous areas; hence the division of a single dorsal root does not cause any sensory loss detectable by ordinary clinical methods. Each root seems to supply fibres for pain, heat, and cold to a larger area than that to which it supplies those subserving light touch.

In the sensory innervation of the head, the trigeminal nerve represents a fusion of the sensory supply of several segments, though the seventh and tenth cranial nerves still possess rudimentary sensory branches distributed to the neighbourhood of the auricle. The posterior and inferior boundary of the trigeminal cutaneous area is contiguous with those of the first and second cervical segments respectively.

Some common abnormalities of sensation

Symptoms

In clinical neurology, it is necessary to appreciate the meaning of several terms commonly utilized to describe disorders of sensation. The word *numbness* can have many meanings; when a patient says that a part of the body is numb, he may mean that sensation in the part is abnormal, but sometimes the term is used to denote weakness or clumsiness. Hence careful enquiry is needed in order to determine the significance of this symptom. Many

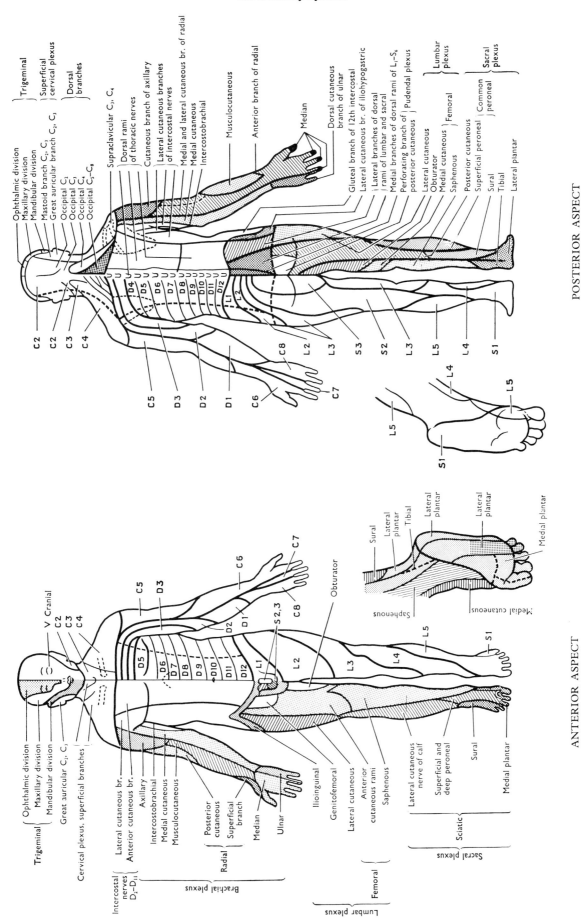

Fig. 1.33. Cutaneous areas of distribution of spinal segments and of sensory fibres of the peripheral nerves.

POSTERIOR ASPECT

ANTERIOR ASPECT

other types of spontaneous, subjective sensory abnormalities are professed in patients with neurological disease. Of these, one of the commonest is *pain*, which we shall consider in detail later. It can result from inflammation or compression of any pain-sensitive structure; if, for instance, it is due to irritation of a sensory root, the distribution of the pain will be in the cutaneous area supplied by the nerve or root concerned. Pain can alternatively be felt in the organ or organs which are diseased, while if it arises in a viscus or in a muscle, it can be referred to an area of skin which sometimes overlies the viscus but may be anatomically remote. The mechanism of such referred pain is not fully understood, though it seems to be due to a spread of impulses to contiguous sensory neurones within the cord (see below). Spontaneous pain in the limbs or trunk can result from discrete thalamic lesions, usually due to infarction, when it has a peculiarly unpleasant burning character, often with additional 'grinding' or 'tearing' qualities. This so-called *thalamic pain* is most often felt in the face, around one angle of the mouth, and in the hand and foot on the affected side. A closely-related sensation of continuous burning, of pricking, of warmth, or even cold, may result from a spinothalamic-tract lesion, but tends to be more diffusely felt in the area of altered cutaneous sensation. Disordered sensations of this type, occurring spontaneously, are often referred to as *dysaesthesiae*. In addition to these abnormal sensations, patients with lesions of the spinothalamic tract often note that they cannot feel pain or temperature in the affected part. They may perhaps injure or burn a limb without discomfort or may recognize that they are unable to assess the temperature of bath water.

Other spontaneous abnormal sensations which the patient may experience are called *paraesthesiae*. These include feelings of tingling, pins and needles, of swelling of a limb, and sensations suggesting that tight strings or bands are tied around a part of the body, or as if water were trickling over the skin. Sensory experiences of this type result from disordered function in the pathways conducting the finer and discriminative aspects of sensibility. Thus tingling or pins and needles can result from ischaemia of peripheral nerves, from polyneuropathy, from transient ischaemia of the sensory cortex, or from sensory Jacksonian epilepsy due to a cortical lesion. Similar symptoms are experienced by patients with lesions of the posterior columns of the cord and it is usually in such individuals that the 'tight, constricting band' or the 'trickling' type of sensation is felt. Often the affected part feels swollen, although inspection shows that this is not the case, or the patient may feel, for instance, as if the limb were encased in a firm glove or plaster cast. If there is a lesion of the posterior columns in the cervical region, sudden flexion or extension of the neck may give an 'electric shock' sensation which travels rapidly down the trunk or even to the hands and feet; this sign (*Lhermitte's sign*) is commonly observed in multiple sclerosis and in cervical spondylosis. Similarly, tapping or pressure over the trunk of an ischaemic nerve (as in patients with median-nerve compression in the carpal tunnel) or over a sensory nerve which has been injured in some other way, will often give paraesthesiae which shoot along the cutaneous distribution of the nerve concerned. A comparable sign produced by tapping a nerve in which regeneration is occurring is known as Tinel's sign.

As well as spontaneous paraesthesiae, patients with disordered function of the posterior columns of the cord or of the sensory cortex often observe that the affected part has become clumsy or even useless. If a hand is affected (the 'useless hand syndrome'), the subject may be unable to use it except under careful visual supervision and cannot recognize objects felt in a pocket or handbag, unless they can be taken out and examined visually. Fine movements such as fastening buttons or threading needles are grossly impaired. If both lower limbs are affected, the patient is unsteady; he feels as if he were walking on cotton wool, and is worse in the dark. When the eyes are covered while washing the face, he will tend to fall forwards into the washbasin.

Signs

Turning now to sensory abnormalities which may be discovered on physical examination, anaesthesia is generally used in describing a cutaneous area in which touch sensibility is totally lost, while *hypaesthesia* implies impaired appreciation of this sense. Similarly, *analgesia* refers to absence and *hypalgesia* to diminution of the appreciation of painful sensations. When thermal sensations cannot be appreciated, the term *thermoanaesthesia* is sometimes utilized, but this very rarely occurs unless hypalgesia is also present. *Hyperalgesia* is allegedly an increased sensitivity to painful stimuli and *hyperaesthesia* a heightened perception of touch. In fact, however, careful examination will generally reveal that in the one case the pain threshold, and in the other the touch threshold, is actually raised above normal, owing to a disorder of the pain or touch pathways. The apparent over-reaction is due to some abnormal and often unpleasant additional quality added to the primary sensation which is in itself impaired; for this reason, the term *hyperpathia* (Head's protopathic pain) is generally preferred to hyperalgesia which is semantically incorrect.

Romberg's sign is an important sign of impaired position and joint sense in the lower limbs. The preservation of the upright position depends upon labyrinthine, cerebellar, and visual postural reflexes, as well as upon those reflexes whose afferent pathway is from the proprioceptors of the lower limbs. As long as the eyes are open and even if the conduction of proprioceptive stimuli from the lower limbs is grossly impaired, the patient can maintain his position, but once the eyes are closed he will sway or fall. Cerebellar or labyrinthine disease may also cause him to sway excessively, but severe instability and a tendency to fall results only from a severe impairment of position and joint sense in the lower limbs. The same patient will show *sensory ataxia* when walking; being unaware of the position of his feet in relation to the ground, he lifts them unusually high and then bangs them down heavily (the steppage gait). He is also unsteady and, owing to loss of visual control of posture, is much more so in the dark.

Ataxia of sensory type is also apparent in the upper limbs if they are affected by similar lesions. The hands are clumsy, and fine movements cannot be performed, particularly when the hands are out of sight (e.g. fastening a button). If the affected arm is held outstretched with the eyes closed, the hands and fingers tend to 'wander' in space, upwards or sideways or indeed in any direction, unlike the downward drift of the limb showing motor weakness due to corticospinal-tract disease. Often there are also purposeless movements of the fingers, of which the patient is unaware, and these may have a 'writhing' character (*pseudoathetosis*).

Abnormalities of the finer discriminative aspects of sensibility are more difficult to assess, although in a patient with a lesion of the sensory cortex, the threshold for two-point discrimination is much greater on the abnormal than on the normal side, and there may be a total inability to recognize figures or letters drawn on the skin. Sensory stimuli are also incorrectly localized on the affected side. Lesions of the parietal lobe of less severity can be demonstrated by the phenomenon of so-called *sensory inattention* due to perceptual rivalry. The patient is well able to appreciate stimuli when applied independently to the two sides of the body, but when two similar stimuli are applied simultaneously to homologous points on the skin of the two sides, one may then be ignored, a finding which implies a disturbance in function of the sensory area of the contralateral cerebral cortex. The phenomenon does not occur if the interval between the two contacts is more than three seconds (Denny-Brown, Meyer, and Horenstein 1952; Critchley 1953). It is also well appreciated that, following amputation of a limb or of some other member, it takes time, in a sense, for the brain to realize that the limb is no longer there, and there is generally a clear-cut 'phantom' sensation as if the amputated part were still present and were able to move; sometimes the phantom is painful. A *phantom limb* can be abolished by a lesion of the contralateral sensory cortex.

Another defect which can be observed in patients with lesions of the arm area of the opposite sensory cortex is an inability to appreciate the form and texture of objects placed in the hand. Correctly this abnormality should be entitled *stereoanaesthesia*, but the term *astereognosis* is more often used. Strictly speaking, the latter term should be reserved for a failure to recognize the nature of objects when the primary sensory modalities are intact. This is an agnosic defect, due to a disorder of sensory association and akin to the other more complex disorders of parietal-lobe function which will be described later in this chapter.

The pathophysiology and clinical significance of sensory abnormalities

In order to localize the situation of the lesion responsible for disordered sensation, it must be asked whether the sensory changes elicited could be due to a lesion of one or several peripheral nerves, to one of sensory roots, of the spinal cord, of the brainstem, of the thalamus, or of the sensory cortex.

Identification of the sensory abnormalities which result from *peripheral-nerve lesions* or from lesions of the brachial and lumbosacral plexuses can only stem from a knowledge of the cutaneous distribution of the various peripheral nerves and of the components of the plexuses (Fig. 1.33). If a nerve is divided and if it has an extensive cutaneous area of supply, there will be a central area of sensory loss to all forms of sensation and a surrounding zone in which tactile loss is more extensive than that for pain and temperature sensibility. There is considerable overlap in the cutaneous supply of the individual peripheral nerves so that section of a small cutaneous nerve may produce no definable sensory abnormality. This fact is even more true of the dermatomes innervated by the individual sensory roots; these have a strictly segmental distribution (Fig. 1.33) but, as we have seen, if a single root is sectioned, no area of sensory impairment can be distinguished. When more than one root is interrupted, however, there is usually some cutaneous sensory loss whose distribution will clearly indicate which roots are involved. With a working knowledge of the dermatomes it is relatively easy to distinguish on clinical grounds the sensory loss resulting from a root lesion from that due to abnormality of a peripheral nerve. Associated signs of a lower motor-neurone lesion can be very helpful in confirming the distinction.

In clinical practice, for instance, the sensory loss resulting from an ulnar-nerve lesion affects mainly the little finger and the ulnar half of the ring finger, while that due to a disorder of the median nerve involves chiefly the thumb, the first two fingers, and the radial half of the ring finger. An ulnar-nerve lesion will also give wasting of most of the small hand muscles, while median-nerve damage will affect only those in the lateral part of the thenar eminence. By contrast, compression of the medial or inner cord of the brachial plexus, which can also give wasting and weakness of the small hand muscles, produces sensory impairment in the medial aspect of the arm and forearm and only occasionally in the little finger.

When multiple peripheral nerves are symmetrically involved, as in *polyneuropathy*, it is the longest sensory fibres which tend to be most severely affected. Hence sensory impairment, which generally affects all forms of sensation but may affect one more severely than the others, is most severe in the periphery of the limbs. Although this type of sensory impairment is often described as of 'glove and stocking' distribution, the borderline between normal and abnormal areas of sensory perception is not usually abrupt, but there is a gradual transition between the two. When there is widespread disease of posterior spinal roots (as in the Guillain–Barré syndrome of postinfective polyneuropathy) there is occasionally an ascending level of sensory loss which eventually involves the entire trunk and all four limbs, but the disease can arrest at any stage. The condition may mimic a transverse lesion of the spinal cord, as motor paralysis is often severe. Indeed in many

such cases, motor weakness predominates and sensory impairment is slight or absent. A rare variety of hereditary sensory neuropathy exists (one of the so-called acrodystrophic neuropathies) in which pain fibres are affected almost exclusively and there is a peripheral insensitivity to pain, often resulting in perforating ulcers of the feet and in extensive destruction of bones and joints (Morvan's syndrome).

Sensory abnormalities resulting from *spinal-cord disease* depend upon which sensory pathways are principally affected. Total transection of the spinal cord will give rise to a total loss of all forms of sensation below the dermatome level on the trunk corresponding to the segment at which the cord transection took place. Often there is a zone of so-called 'hyperaesthesia' in the skin area supplied by the segment immediately above the lesion. In hemisection of the spinal cord (the Brown–Séquard syndrome), there is loss of tactile discrimination, impaired touch perception, and loss of position and joint sense on the same side of the body as that on which the cord has been divided, and these sensory faculties are impaired on the trunk up to the dermatome of the cord segment at which the lesion is present. There are also signs of pyramidal-tract dysfunction on the same side. On the opposite side of the body there is loss of pain and temperature sensation, but the sensory level for these modalities is a few segments lower, in view of the fact that pain fibres ascend in the posterior horn for a few segments before crossing to the spinothalamic tract on the opposite side. A Brown–Séquard syndrome can result from trauma or from asymmetrical cord compression by a neoplasm, and in young adults is often an initial manifestation of multiple sclerosis.

The principal pathological changes of *tabes dorsalis* involve the root entry zone of the posterior nerve roots; there is ascending degeneration of the posterior columns and to a lesser extent of the spinothalamic tracts. Hence patients with this disease show severe sensory ataxia and there is often pain loss, and impairment of deep pressure sensation, over the bridge of the nose, centre of sternum, perineum, and tendons of Achilles, while position and joint sense and vibration sense are greatly impaired in the lower limbs. The tendon reflexes are lost owing to a break on the sensory side of the reflex arc. Similar impairment of deep reflexes in the lower limbs with other evidence of sensory neuropathy may be seen in *subacute combined degeneration of the cord* (combined system disease or B_{12} deficiency neuropathy), in which disease sensory ataxia is also usual and vibration and position sense are commonly lost in the lower limbs; signs of corticospinal-tract disease are often also present. The cavity of *syringomyelia* usually develops in the central grey matter of the spinal cord in the cervical region; hence the decussating pain and temperature fibres are interrupted, resulting in *dissociated anaesthesia*, i.e. loss of pain and temperature sensation but preservation of touch and of position and joint sense. Commonly, this sensory loss is unilateral, affecting the whole of one upper limb and shoulder and ending on the trunk at the midline and with a sharp lower level like the edge of a cape. As the anterior horns of the cord and the pyramidal tracts may also be compressed or invaded by the cavity, there is often wasting of upper limb muscles with loss of reflexes in the affected arm or arms and a spastic paraparesis. The sensory changes of *multiple sclerosis* are usually due to lesions of the posterior columns, giving impaired tactile discrimination, vibration sense, and sense of position, sometimes in one arm, in both lower limbs, or even in all four limbs. Occasionally, however, a plaque of demyelination affects one trigeminal nucleus to give facial hemianaesthesia and sometimes, though rarely, a unilateral lesion of the cord involves the spinothalamic tract and gives loss of pain and temperature sensation in one lower limb.

Lesions of the brainstem may give sensory abnormalities which can easily be interpreted on an anatomical basis. Dissociated sensory loss in the face can result from syringobulbia, due to involvement of the descending root of the trigeminal nerve, while lesions of the pons and medulla can give facial sensory impairment on one side (due to a lesion of the trigeminal nucleus) with hemianaesthesia and/or hemianalgesia of the trunk and limbs on the opposite side due to involvement of the ascending sensory tracts. A lesion of the upper pons or midbrain, however, may give complete contralateral sensory loss. An infarct in the midbrain involving the third-nerve nucleus, red nucleus, and medial lemniscus may give a unilateral third-nerve palsy with contralateral static tremor, hemianaesthesia (*Benedikt's syndrome*), and hemianalgesia. More often such unilateral sensory loss is dissociated, involving only pain and temperature sensation, owing to selective involvement of ascending fibres of the spinothalamic tract, as in the *lateral-medullary (Wallenberg's) syndrome* due to vertebral or posterior inferior cerebellar-artery thrombosis.

A patchy contralateral hemianaesthesia and hemianalgesia can also result from a *thalamic lesion* and there will often be in addition spontaneous pain of a peculiarly unpleasant and disturbing nature on the partially anaesthetic side. Fortunately, this *thalamic syndrome*, which usually results from cerebral infarction, is rare. The pain most commonly affects the face, arm, and foot. Surprisingly, however, extensive thalamic lesions such as neoplasms often produce comparatively little sensory loss, while thalamic infarcts may also, on occasion, impair appreciation of posture, passive movement, light touch, and tactile discrimination with little effect upon pain and thermal sensibility. In one patient with 'pure sensory stroke' who had a contralateral hemianaesthesia but not hemianalgesia (Fisher 1965) a small lacune was found in VPL at autopsy.

Lesions of the *sensory cortex*, if irritative in nature, give rise to sensory Jacksonian epilepsy, often taking the form of spreading paraesthesiae whose 'march' corresponds closely to the anatomical 'representation' of the parts of the body in the sensory cortex (Fig. 1.32). This symptom is easy to confuse with the paraesthesiae which often occur during the aura of migraine, or during transient cerebral ischaemic attacks. When there is destruction of a part of the postcentral gyrus, then in the corresponding part of the opposite half of the body there is no impairment of pain sensibility and comparatively little of touch, but the appreciation of position, of tactile discrimination and localization, and of form and texture is profoundly impaired. Figures written upon the skin cannot be recognized and the threshold for two-point discrimination is raised. In a less severe cortical lesion, there may simply be tactile inattention on the affected side. Defects of recognition and interpretation of sense data which may be noted in parietal-lobe lesions will be discussed later.

One final diagnosis to be considered as a possible cause of sensory abnormalities discovered on clinical examination is *hysteria*. In a suggestible patient it is only too easy to discover areas of spurious sensory loss. A total hemianaesthesia affecting all modalities of sensation and even vibration sense over one-half of the skull, is a common hysterical manifestation, as is anaesthesia of the palate or of the limbs in 'glove and stocking' distribution. Commonly such sensory loss is found in one limb only, particularly after minor injury in a compensation setting, when there is usually associated hysterical weakness and the sensory impairment often ends at the level of a joint (e.g. the elbow, shoulder, knee, or hip). In such cases, unlike the findings in polyneuropathy, there is an abrupt line of demarcation between the area of complete sensory loss and that where all sensation is normal. In a patient with hysterical sensory loss it may be possible to 'find' (with suggestion) a small area within the anaesthetic region (impossible to explain on an anatomical basis) where a pin-prick is felt acutely. Another useful pointer is that the patient, though claiming that all forms of sensation are impaired in the affected part, is yet able to localize in space one finger or toe, say, quite accurately with his eyes closed, indicating that the sense of position is well preserved.

Sensory examination is a technique which can only be learned by experience and which even so is full of pitfalls, particularly with an anxious and suggestible patient. Nevertheless, consistent and clear-cut sensory abnormalities can be of great value in achieving accurate anatomical localization of a lesion within the nervous system, while the precise nature and evolution of the changes may give invaluable aid in determining the character of the lesion.

Pain

General considerations

Pain is one of the most common and disturbing of human experiences (see *British Medical Journal* 1977). While it has many causes, the appreciation of painful sensations depends upon the stimulation of pain-sensitive nerve endings in the skin, muscles, skeleton, blood vessels, viscera, and membranes, and upon the conduction of nerve impulses into the central nervous system where the sensation finally enters consciousness. The central pathways along which impulses conveying painful sensations travel and the effect of disease of the central nervous system upon its appreciation have been considered above. In this section a number of common neurological syndromes, of which pain is a prominent symptom, will be mentioned, with particular reference to the pathophysiological mechanisms involved. It must also be remembered that patients vary widely in their response to painful experiences, some remaining relatively impassive when experiencing sensations which produce in others an intense reaction. This individuality of emotional response to painful stimuli means that although the threshold intensity of stimulus required to give the appreciation of pain (the pain threshold) is relatively constant, the reaction to painful stimuli which exceed the threshold intensity may be specific to the individual and can even vary in the same patient, depending upon circumstances.

Painful sensations: their recording and modulation

As we have seen, it is the nociceptors in the skin and other organs which are concerned with the perception of pain; these painful stimuli are then transmitted by multiple fine afferent nerve fibres (see Zimmermann 1981). In general, nerve-fibre networks of this type are most luxurious in those areas of skin which are most sensitive. We have also noted that pain sensation is conveyed in peripheral nerves both by large heavily-myelinated A fibres and/or by small unmyelinated C fibres.

There are two principal opposing theories relating to pain sensation: one, the specificity theory, suggests that pain is a specific modality with its own specific central and peripheral apparatus for recording its perception; the other, the pattern theory, suggests that the nerve-impulse pattern subserving pain is caused by excessive stimulation of non-specific receptors. As Melzack and Wall (1965) pointed out, neither theory satisfactorily explains the observed facts. In their so-called 'gate theory', they proposed that interneurones in the substantia gelatinosa of the spinal cord exercise a modulating effect upon sensory input, before this activates the first central transmission (T) cells in the dorsal horn of the cord which stimulate central mechanisms responsible for response and perception. They suggested that tonic activity in small C fibres keeps open the gate and allows the onwards transmission of painful sensation. Activity in large A fibres is, by contrast, essentially inhibitory and tends to close the gate. Descending impulses from the brain may also influence the opening and closing of 'the gate' (Wall 1978). Hence the final discharge from the T cells and the perception of pain is dependent upon the relative activity in large and small fibres. Counter-irritation, as by scratching or rubbing, increases large-fibre discharge and so reduces pain. Repeated percutaneous electrical stimulation of large-diameter A fibres has been found to be an effective method of relieving chronic pain, a finding which gives some support to the gate control hypothesis, but some other evidence derived from electrical stimulation in human subjects has given conflicting results (Nathan and Rudge

1974). Similarly, not all the recent physiological evidence supports the gate theory in its entirety (Iggo 1972; Nathan 1976; Bonica 1986) but it is a useful working hypothesis.

On the basis of this theory, so-called hyperalgesia, better called hyperpathia, for reasons given above, can be explained by an excessive continuing stimulation of C fibres, thus keeping the gate open, or by a selective loss of A fibres, thus reducing inhibition, as may be seen in post-herpetic neuralgia. Similarly, the phenomenon of referred pain (see below) can be explained by central summation effects as there is a widespread, diffuse monosynaptic input to the T cells, often from relatively distant afferents.

The role of the cerebral cortex in the perception and localization of pain must also be considered. While cortical lesions which impair the ability to localize touch sensation similarly disrupt the faculty of localizing painful stimuli, there are few cortical neurones which show any selective response to painful stimuli. Similarly, electrical stimulation of the sensory cortex fails to evoke painful sensations, though similar stimulation of cells in the posterior thalamus and intralaminar reticular substance may do so. However, the receptive fields of the latter cells are immense and would appear to be incapable of recording spatial information, even though the perception of pain probably occurs at this level. It is likely that the localization of painful stimuli recorded by nociceptors with high stimulus thresholds depends upon the simultaneous activation of other contiguous receptors of lower threshold which, with their central pathways, have precise localizing capabilities. In other words, our ability to localize painful sensations appears to depend upon the fact that nociceptive stimuli such as pain invariably stimulate other nearby receptors concerned with touch.

Some recent developments in the neuropharmacology of pain

There is now good evidence that many neurones concerned with pain perception possess morphine (or other opiate) receptors with which morphine and its analogues combine to produce their analgesic effects. The cells of the periaqueductal grey matter of the brainstem seem to possess many such receptors and it is believed that this area is a principal site of action of these analgesic drugs. It is thought that the action of morphine upon these neurones produces analgesia by activating a descending serotoninergic system which inhibits the transmission of pain sensation in the spinal cord; however, the exact mechanism of this action is still poorly understood. It also seems that the brain produces its own endogenous analgesic in the form of a pentapeptide called enkephalin (see *The Lancet* 1978b; Terenius 1981; Kandel and Schwartz 1981; Fields 1981) which has an action similar to morphine. The naturally-occurring C-fragment of β-lipoprotein (also called β-endorphin), which contains the enkaphalin sequence, and which has been isolated from the pituitary, has been shown to have a particularly powerful analgesic effect when administered intraventricularly in animals. There is some evidence that acupuncture used in the treatment of pain may increase CSF β-endorphin (Clement-Jones, McLoughlin, Tomlin, Besser, Rees, and Wen 1980). The part played by enkephalin and the endogenous ligands which are formed when it is combined with various cerebral lipoproteins in those disorders of the central nervous system which cause abnormalities of pain perception remains to be determined.

Types of pain and their causation

Analysis of the pain which follows cutaneous stimulation has shown that it has two components—the first immediate and the second delayed; probably these two forms of the sensation are conveyed by nerve fibres which conduct at different rates. A sensation of deep pain is also felt after stimulation of deeper structures such as tendons, blood vessels, and the periosteum. Painful lesions of the muscles or viscera sometimes give pain in the over-lying skin, or else it may be felt in a cutaneous area which is comparatively remote (*referred pain*). In other words, such painful sensations seem not to be coming from the viscus involved (see below) but from the body surface. But this apparent error in localization, giving what is sometimes called alternatively *pseudovisceral pain*, is systematic and not random as the reference is always to the dermatomes innervated by those dorsal roots that supply the diseased viscus. Thus afferent pain fibres from the myocardium enter the T1-5 dorsal root ganglia and myocardial pain is therefore referred to the anterior chest wall and down the inner aspect of the left or of both arms. Similarly, pain fibres from the diaphragm travel in the phrenic nerve (C3-4) so that diaphragmatic pain is often referred to the C3 and 4 dermatomes in the neck and shoulder.

Many different types of pathological change can cause pain, through stimulation of pain-sensitive nerve endings in the diseased organ or organs. Thus, trauma and inflammation are two important causes of cutaneous pain, while pain of skeletal origin is often similarly produced; malignant disease, including metastases in bone, can also be very painful. *Visceral pain*, particularly that arising in abdominal organs, usually results from excessive contraction of plain muscle, resulting in the passage of pain-carrying impulses along afferent fibres accompanying sympathetic nerves, though distension of hollow organs or inflammation of their enveloping membranes (such as the peritoneum) may also be painful; in the latter case, the impulses are carried by somatic afferents. Pain arising in skeletal muscle is commonly due to prolonged overactivity, cramp, or fatigue, though repeated activity of a muscle with an inadequate blood supply (ischaemic work) can also be responsible; this principle applies also to cardiac muscle (angina of effort).

Since the sensory nerve fibres and central structures concerned in the reception and appreciation of painful stimuli are themselves sensitive to inflammation or irritation and since there are a number of other pain-sensitive structures within the cranium and spinal canal, pain is a relatively common symptom of disease of the nervous system. The many painful neurological syndromes observed in clinical practice will be considered later.

References

Adams, R. D. Victor, M. (1981). *Principles of neurology*, 2nd edn. McGraw-Hill, New York.

Bonica, J. J. (1986). Pain, in *Oxford Companion to Medicine*, Oxford University Press, Oxford.

British Medical Journal (1977). Pain sensation in man. *Br. med. J.* **2**, 783.

Brodal, A. (1981). *Neurological anatomy in relation to clinical medicine*, 3rd edn. Oxford University Press, Oxford.

Caccia, M. R., Ubiali, E., and Andreussi, L. (1976). Spinal evoked potentials recorded from the epidural space in normal and diseased humans. *J. Neurol. Neurosurg. Psychiat.* **39**, 962.

Cervero, F. and Iggo, A. (1980). The substantia gelatinosa of the spinal cord: a critical review. *Brain* **103**, 717.

Clement-Jones, V., McLoughlin, L., Tomlin, S., Besser, G. M., Rees, L. H., and Wen, H. L. (1980). Increased β-endorphin but not metenkephalin levels in human cerebrospinal fluid after acupuncture pain. *Lancet* **ii**, 946.

Critchley, M. (1953). *The parietal lobes*. Arnold, London.

Delbeke, J., McComas, A. J., and Kopec, S. J. (1978). Analysis of evoked lumbosacral potentials in man. *J. Neurol. Neurosurg. Psychiat* **41**, 293.

Denny-Brown, D. (1966). *The cerebral control of movement*. Liverpool University Press, Liverpool.

—— Meyer, J. S., and Horenstein, S. (1952). The significance of perceptual rivalry resulting from parietal lesion. *Brain* **75**, 433.

Desmedt, J. E. (1971). Somatosensory cerebral evoked potentials in man. In *Handbook of electroencephalography and clinical neurophysiology*, Vol. 9. (ed. A. Rémond). Elsevier, Amsterdam.

Dyck, P. J., Schultz, P. W., and O'Brien, P. C. (1972). Quantitation of touch-pressure sensation. *Arch. Neurol., Chicago* **26**, 465.

——, Zimmerman, I. R., O'Brien, P. C., Ness, A., Caskey, P. E., Karnes, J., and Bushek, W. (1978). Introduction of automated systems to evaluate touch-pressure, vibration, and thermal cutaneous sensation in man. *Ann. Neurol.* **4**, 502.

El-Negamy, E. and Sedgwick, E. M. (1978). Properties of a spinal somatosensory evoked potential recorded in man, *J. Neurol. Neurosurg. Psychiat.* **41**, 762.

Fields, H. L. (1981). Pain II: new approaches to management, *Ann. Neurol.* **9**, 101.

Fisher, C. M. (1965). Pure sensory stroke involving face, arm and leg, *Neurology, (Minneapolis)*. **15**, 76.

Foerster, O. (1933). The dermatomes in man. *Brain.* **56**, 1.

Gardner, E. (1975). *Fundamentals of neurology*, 6th edn. Saunders, Philadelphia.

Halliday, A. M. (1980). Evoked brain potentials: how far have we come since 1875? In *Evoked potentials*. (ed. C. Barber). MTP Press, Lancaster.

Head, H. (1920). *Studies in neurology*, Vols. i and ii. Oxford University Press, London.

Henson, R. A. (1949). On thalamic dysaesthesiae and their suppression by bilateral stimulation. *Brain* **72**, 576.

Huskisson, E. C. (1974). Measurement of pain. *Lancet* **ii**, 1127.

Iggo, A. (1972). The case for pain receptors, and critical remarks on the gate control theory. in *Pain* (ed. R. Janzen, W. D. Keidel, A. Herz, C. Steichele, J. P. Payne, and R. A. P. Burt), pp. 60 and 127. Georg Thieme, Stuttgart and London.

Inouye, Y. and Buchthal, F. (1977). Segmental sensory innervation determined by potentials recorded from cervical spinal nerves. *Brain* **100**, 731.

Jasper, H. H. and Bertrand G. (1966). Thalamic units involved in somatic sensation and voluntary and involuntary movements in man. In *The thalamus* (ed. D. P. Purpura and M. D. Yahr). Columbia University Press, New York.

Kandel, E. R. and Schwartz, J. H. (1981). *Principles of neural science*. Elsevier North–Holland, New York.

Lance, J. W. and McLeod, J. G. (1981). *A physiological approach to clinical neurology*, 3rd edn. Butterworths, London.

The Lancet (1978*a*). The dorsal columns revisited. *Lancet* **i**, 918.

—— (1978*b*). Enkephalins: the search for a functional role. *Lancet* **ii**, 819.

Lenman, J. A. R. (1975). *Clinical neurophysiology*. Blackwell, Oxford.

Matthews, W. B., Beauchamp, M., and Small, D. G. (1974). Cervical somato-sensory evoked responses in man. *Nature* **252**, 230.

Medical Research Council (1976). *Aids to the examination of the peripheral nervous system*. MRC Memorandum No. 45, HMSO, London.

Melzack, R. and Wall, P. D. (1965). Pain mechanisms: a new theory. *Science* **150**, 971.

Mendall, L. M. and Wall, P. D. (1965). Responses of single dorsal cord cells to peripheral cutaneous unmyelinated fibres. *Nature, Lond.* **206**, 97.

Nathan, P. W. (1976). The gate–control theory of pain: a critical review. *Brain* **99**, 123.

—— and Rudge, P. (1974). Testing the gate-control theory of pain in man. *J. Neurol. Neurosurg. Psychiat.* **37**, 1366.

Newman, P. P. (1980). *Neurophysiology*. Spectrum, New York.

Patton, H. D., Sundsten, J. W., Crill, W. E., and Swanson, P. D. (1976). *Introduction to basic neurology*. Saunders, Philadelphia.

Penfield, W. and Rasmussen, T. (1950). *The cerebral cortex of man*. McMillan, New York.

Riddoch, G. 81938). The clinical features of central pain. *Lancet* **i**, 1093, 1150, 1205.

Ruch, T. C. and Patton, H. D. (Eds.)(1965). *Physiology and biophysics*. Saunders, Philadelphia.

Schneider, R. J., Kulics, A. T., and Ducker, T. B. (1977). Proprioceptive pathways of the spinal cord. *J. Neurol. Neurosurg. Psychiat.* **40**, 417.

Shibasaki, H., Yamashita, Y., and Tsuji, S. (1977). Somatosensory evoked potentials: diagnostic criteria and abnormalities in cerebral lesions. *J. neurol. Sci.* **34**, 427.

Sinclair, D. C. (1955). Cutaneous sensation and the doctrine of perceptual rivalry. *Brain* **78**, 584.

——, Weddell, G., and Feindel, W. H. (1948). Referred pain and associated phenomena. *Brain* **71**, 184.

Tasker, R. R. and Organ, L. W. (1972). Mapping of the somatosensory and auditory pathways in the upper midbrain and thalamus in man. In *Neurophysiology studied in man* (ed. G. G. Somjen) p. 169. Elsevier, Amsterdam.

Terenius, L. (1981). Biochemical mediators in pain. *Triangle* **20**, 19.

Wall, P. D. (1970). The sensory and motor role of impulses travelling in the dorsal columns towards cerebral cortex, *Brain* **93**, 505.

—— and Noordenbos, W. (1977). Sensory functions which remain in man after complete transection of dorsal columns. *Brain* **100**, 641.

Walshe, F. M. R. (1942). The anatomy and physiology of cutaneous sensibility: a critical review. *Brain* **65**, 48.

Weddell, G., Sinclair, D. C., and Feindel, W. H. (1948). An anatomical basis for alterations in quality of pain sensibility. *J. Neurophysiol* **2**, 99.

—— and Verrillo, R. T. (1972). Common sensibility. In *Scientific foundations of neurology* (ed. M. Critchley, J. L. O'Leary, and W. B. Jennett) p. 117. Heinemann, London.

White, J. C. and Sweet, W. H. (1955). *Pain, its mechanisms and neurosurgical control*. C. C. Thomas, Springfield, Illinois.

Zimmermann, M. (1981). Physiological mechanisms of pain and pain therapy. *Triangle* **20**, 7.

The reflexes

General considerations

A reflex is the simplest form of involuntary response to a stimulus. The anatomical basis of a reflex arc, which consists of: (*1*), a receptor organ; (*2*) an afferent path running from the periphery to the brainstem or spinal cord; (*3*) one or more intercalated neurones in the central nervous system linking the afferent path to (*4*), the afferent path which leaves the neuraxis by the lower motor neurones to reach (*5*), the effector organ. The reflex is elicited by a stimulus which may be touch, prick, the sudden stretching of a muscle, or some other event which excites an appropriate afferent impulse. The response is a muscular contraction, a modification in muscle tone, glandular secretion, etc., depending upon the nature of the reflex. Important though visceral reflexes are, the neurologist investigating the state of the nervous system is mainly concerned with reflexes which excite responses in the somatic musculature. Reflex action, conceived by Descartes, was first observed by Stephen Hales in a pithed frog about 1730. The concept was elaborated by Robert Whytt in 1755, and later by Marshall Hall in 1833.

A reflex is dependent upon the integrity of its arc. Lesions which interrupt this at any point abolish it. Loss of a reflex may thus be due to interruption of the afferent path by a lesion involving the first sensory neurone in the peripheral nerves, plexuses, spinal nerves, or dorsal roots, by damage to the central paths of the arc in the brainstem or spinal cord, or by lesions of the lower motor neurone at any point between the anterior horn cells and the muscles, or of the muscles themselves, or by the depression produced by neural shock. The activity of many bulbar and spinal reflexes is also profoundly influenced by the state of the muscle spindles and of the gamma efferent system of motor nerve fibres. In conditions causing hypotonia (e.g. cerebellar lesions) the tendon reflexes are depressed, but hypertonia associated with increased gamma efferent discharge gives exaggeration of these reflexes; this enhancement is greater in spasticity than in extrapyramidal rigidity. Anxiety, tension, and painful conditions may also give rise to some increase in the deep tendon reflexes. Paradoxically in severe long-standing spinal cord lesions—or spastic diplegia—spasticity is sometimes so severe that the tendon reflexes in the lower limbs may be difficult to elicit, perhaps due to irreversible muscular shortening due to chronic spasticity, or else the flexor withdrawal reflex may be so dominant as to inhibit the tendon reflexes.

Reflexes involving the cranial nerves

The pupillary reflexes. These are described on page 102.

The corneal reflex. The stimulus which evokes the corneal reflex is a light touch upon the cornea, e.g. with a wisp of cotton wool, and the response is bilateral blinking. The afferent path is through the first division of the fifth cranial nerve; the central path consists of fibres uniting the spinal nucleus of the fifth nerve with both facial nuclei, and the efferent path passes through the facial nerves to both orbiculares oculi muscles. A lesion involving the fifth nerve or its spinal nucleus, since it interrupts the afferent path, causes bilateral loss of blinking in response to stimulation of the cornea on the side of the lesion. A lesion involving the nucleus or fibres of the seventh nerve interrupts the efferent path and hence causes loss of the reflex on the side of the lesion only, and blinking occurs on the opposite side. Loss of the corneal reflex is often an early sign of a lesion of the fifth nerve and may occur before any cutaneous anaesthesia can be detected. Apart from lesions involving the reflex arc, the corneal reflex is lost in states of deep coma.

Facial reflexes. A brisk tap on the glabella above the bridge of the nose causes bilateral blinking. In the normal individual, on repeated tapping the blinking ceases after two or three taps, but in patients with parkinsonism it may continue in time with the taps (the 'glabellar tap' sign). Electrophysiological recordings from the orbicularis oculi have shown that there is an initial monosynaptic reflex response of low amplitude, followed by a larger response of longer latency which is clearly polysynaptic (Kugelberg 1952; Gandiglio and Fra 1967) and which habituates in normal individuals but not in parkinsonism.

The oculocephalic reflex (the doll's head phenomenon). When the eyelids are held open and the head is rotated sharply from side to side, the eyes show conjugate deviation away from the side to which the head is moved and on flexion of the neck they move upwards; after each such movement they return rapidly to the mid position even if the head remains rotated or flexed. The exact physiological basis of this reflex is unknown but persists in blind individuals and after occipital lobectomy (Plum and Posner 1972); it is however, impaired when there are lesions of the oculomotor nerves. While it is sometimes preserved in comatose patients, when it and the oculovestibular reflex are absent, this is usually indicative of an irreversible brainstem lesion and is useful in the diagnosis of 'brain death'.

The oculovestibular caloric reflex. Irrigation of an external auditory meatus with warm or cold water causes nystagmus in normal individuals (see p. 122). As this reflex depends upon the integrity of the vestibular nuclei, loss of this reflex may be a valuable sign of pontine damage if there is no reason to suspect a labyrinthine or eighth-nerve lesion.

The jaw reflex. In response to a tap upon the chin, depressing the lower jaw, there is a bilateral contraction of the elevators of the jaw. Both afferent and efferent paths pass through the trigeminal nerve. This reflex is a stretch reflex, and, like other such reflexes, becomes exaggerated as a result of bilateral corticospinal-tract lesions.

The sucking reflex. In the infant the contact of an object with the lips evokes sucking movement of the lips, tongue, and jaw. This sucking reflex is lost after infancy but may reappear in states of severe cerebral degeneration, for example, the presenile and senile dementias (Paulson and Gottlieb 1968). It may be unilateral, and associated with a grasp reflex on the same side. When the lips follow the stimulating object, this is sometimes called the 'rooting reflex'.

The 'snout' reflex. A tap on the centre of the closed lips will, in normal infants, provoke a pouting movement of the lips like the formation of a 'snout'. This reflex normally disappears with maturation but may reappear in the presence of bilateral corticospinal-tract lesions in or above the upper brainstem and in cerebral degenerative disorders such as those in which the sucking reflex is re-established.

The palatal reflex. The palatal ('gag') reflex consists of elevation of the soft palate in response to a touch. The afferent path is by the second division of the fifth nerve; the efferent by the vagus.

The palatal reflex is variable in intensity in normal individuals. It is abolished by lesions causing anaesthesia of the palate and by lesions of the vagus nuclei and, in lesions of one vagus nerve, the response is unilateral and the uvula is displaced towards the normal side.

The pharyngeal reflex. The pharyngeal reflex consists of constriction of the pharynx in response to a touch upon the posterior pharyngeal wall. Its afferent path runs in the glossopharyngeal nerve, its efferent path in the vagus. Like the palatal reflex, it is abolished by lesions causing pharyngeal anaesthesia and by lesions of the vagus nuclei. In cases of unilateral paralysis of the vagus, the response is confined to the opposite half of the pharynx.

Reflexes of the limbs and trunk

The tendon reflexes

Physiology
The basis of the tendon reflex is the myotatic reflex which is the reflex contraction of a muscle or part of a muscle in response to stretch. It is monosynaptic, i.e. it is mediated by a reflex arc consisting of two neurones with one synapse between them (Lloyd 1952). While it is a form of stretch reflex, it must be distinguished from the tonic stretch reflex which results from slow or prolonged stretch of a muscle and which is undoubtedly a polysynaptic response, probably involving cortical pathways (Marsden, Merton, and Morton 1973).

A so-called 'tendon reflex' or jerk is a sharp muscular contraction evoked by suddenly stretching the muscle. The sudden stretch may be brought about by tapping the tendon, or by suddenly displacing the segment of a limb into which the muscle is inserted. The response, a muscular contraction, is most evident in the muscle stretched, but may not be confined to this muscle. A tendon reflex is diminished or abolished by a lesion interrupting either the afferent, central, or efferent paths of the reflex arc or a disorder which makes the muscle incapable of responding to the nervous impulse. Reinforcement of the tendon jerks may be achieved by clenching the fists or by pulling the flexed fingers of the two hands against each other (Jendrassik's manoeuvre), movements which cause increased activity of the gamma efferent system. Reflex activity in the legs may be studied electrically by recording the 'H' reflex, a contraction in the calf muscles which may be elicited by stimulating electrically the medial popiteal nerve. The H response, which is a monosynaptic reflex evoked by stimulation of Group I afferent fibres in the nerve, follows the so-called M response evoked in the muscle by the direct effect of the nerve stimulus upon alpha efferent fibres. In early polyneuropathy the tendon reflexes may be lost before sensory loss is detectable clinically, but in such cases abnormalities of conduction may be detectable electrically. Rarely, the tendon reflexes are congenitally absent. Table 1.2 gives the principal tendon reflexes, the mode of elicitation, and their innervation.

Clonus. Clonus, a rhythmical series of contractions in response to the maintenance of tension in a muscle, associated with increased gamma efferent discharge, is often elicitable when the tendon reflexes are exaggerated after a corticospinal lesion. Clonus of the quadriceps, patellar clonus, is best elicited by a sudden sharp downward displacement of the patella. Ankle clonus is obtained by sharply dorsiflexing the ankle. Clonus of the flexors of the fingers can sometimes be elicited by suddenly extending the fingers.

Hoffmann's reflex. The patient's hand is pronated and the observer grasps the terminal phalanx of the middle finger between his forefinger and thumb. With a sharp flick the phalanx is passively flexed and suddenly released. A positive response consists of a sharp twitch of adduction and flexion of the thumb and flexion of the fingers. This reflex is physiologically identical with the *flexor*

Table 1.2 *The tendon reflexes*

Reflex	Mode of elicitation	Response	Spinal segment	Peripheral nerve
Biceps-jerk	A blow upon the biceps tendon	Flexion of the elbow	Cervical 5–6	Musculocutaneous
Triceps-jerk	A blow upon the triceps tendon	Extension of the elbow	Cervical 6–7	Radial
Supinator-jerk or radial reflex	A blow upon the tendon of brachioradialis at the distal end of the radius	Flexion of the elbow	Cervical 5–6	Radial
Flexor finger-jerk	A blow upon the palmar surface of the semiflexed fingers	Flexion of the fingers and thumb	Cervical 7–8	Median and ulnar
Knee-jerk	A blow upon the quadriceps tendon	Extension of the knee	Lumbar 2–4	Femoral
Ankle-jerk	A blow upon the tendo calcaneus	Plantar flexion of the anxle	Sacral 1–2	Sciatic

finger-jerk, which is elicited by tapping the palmar surface of the slightly flexed fingers. It is an index of muscular hypertonia rather than of a corticospinal lesion as such. It is not always positive in the presence of such a lesion, and may be elicitable in a nervous individual with no organic disease; if present unilaterally, however, it is likely to be significant.

Reflex spread and inverted reflexes. In states of muscular hypertonia a reflex response may spread beyond the muscles stretched, as when a tap on the styloid process of the radius elicits a contraction not only of the brachioradialis, but also of the long flexors of the fingers.

In the upper limbs, so-called 'inverted reflexes' may be a useful sign of lesions of the cervical cord. If there is a lesion at C5–6 which interrupts the arc for reflexes innervated by that segment, but which is also compressing the corticospinal tracts to give exaggeration of reflexes subserved by lower segments, tapping the biceps tendon may fail to elicit the biceps jerk but gives contraction of triceps (the inverted biceps jerk); similarly, the radial jerk may be absent but the appropriate stimulus causes finger flexion (the inverted radial jerk). An inverted knee jerk (contraction of the hamstrings with knee flexion when the quadriceps tendon is tapped) may also be a sign of a spinal-cord lesion at L2–4 (Boyle, Shakir, Weir, and McInnes 1979) but is much less common.

The palmomental reflex. To elicit this reflex, a pin is used to apply a scratch across the base of the thenar eminence. A positive response consists of contraction of the ipsilateral mentalis muscle giving a dimpling of the chin. The reflex may be present bilaterally in normal individuals or in states of reflex hyperexcitability but, when present on one side only, it may be indicative of a corticospinal-tract lesion (see Wartenberg 1945).

Cutaneous superficial reflexes

The nociceptive abdominal reflexes. These are cutaneous reflexes consisting of a brisk unilateral contraction of a part of the abdominal wall in response to a cutaneous stimulus, such as a touch or a light scratch with a pin. It is convenient to elicit them at three levels on each side—just below the costal margin, at the level of the umbilicus, and at the level of the iliac fossa. Kugelberg and Hagbarth (1958) have shown that the abdominal and erector spinae reflexes are polysynaptic, and are reactions of the trunk to potential injury. They are plurisegmental, and lead to a local withdrawal from the stimulus. They are normally dependent, for reasons not fully understood, upon the integrity of the cortico-

spinal tract. Hence a corticospinal lesion is usually associated with diminution or loss of the superficial abdominal reflexes upon the same side. If the lesion is slight, the reflexes may be reduced but not completely abolished, the reflexes of the lowest segments being most impaired. Loss of the abdominal reflexes is not always proportional to the severity of the lesion. In multiple sclerosis, for example, they may be lost early, at a stage of the disease when other signs of corticospinal-tract dysfunction are slight. In spastic diplegia and motor-neurone disease, on the other hand, they are often retained.

The reflex arcs of the superficial abdominal reflexes are localized in the spinal cord from the seventh to the twelfth dorsal segments. Lesions involving the arcs themselves may produce diminution or loss of the reflexes. One such lesion is damage to the lower motor neurone by poliomyelitis. These reflexes may, however, be absent in some normal people, especially women, and especially in the aged; obesity, abdominal scars, and repeated pregnancies are not always responsible (Madonick 1957).

The cremasteric reflex. The cremasteric reflex is a cutaneous reflex closely related to the abdominal reflexes. The appropriate stimulus is a light scratch along the inner aspect of the upper part of the thigh, and the response is a contraction of the cremaster muscle, with elevation of the testicle. This reflex, the arc of which runs through the first lumbar spinal segment, is diminished or abolished by a lesion of the corticospinal tract. It is usually extremely brisk in children, in whom it may sometimes be elicited by a stimulus applied to any part of the lower limb. It is often diminished or absent on the affected side in a patient with varicocele.

The gluteal reflex. The gluteal reflex is physiologically akin to the abdominal reflexes. A scratch on the buttock evokes contraction of the glutei. The spinal segments concerned are lumbar 4 and 5.

The plantar reflex or response. The plantar reflex is one of the most important of all reflexes to the neurologist, because its meaning is unequivocal.

1. *The flexor plantar reflex.* The flexor plantar reflex is normal after the first year of life. The stimulus which evokes it is a longitudinal scratch upon the lateral aspect of the sole of the foot from the heel towards the toes, and the response is plantar flexion of the toes sometimes associated with dorsiflexion of the foot at the ankle, contraction of the tensor fasciae latae muscle, and other variable muscular contractions. It is a spinal segmental reflex

mediated by the first sacral segment of the cord and akin to the abdominal reflexes.

2. *The extensor plantar reflex.* Babinski in 1896 first pointed out that, in the presence of a corticospinal lesion, the normal flexor plantar reflex did not occur, but its place was taken by an upward, extensor movement of the great toe. Riddoch, Walshe, and others showed that the extensor plantar reflex is not an isolated phenomenon, but is part of a general reflex flexion of the whole lower limb, related to the primitive flexor withdrawal reflex in response to a nociceptive stimulus to the lower limb seen in animals after division of the spinal cord. Clinical and physiological studies in man (Brain and Wilkinson 1959; Landau and Clare 1959; and Kugelberg, Ekland, and Grimby 1960) have shown that the distinction between the flexor and extensor plantar reflexes is not absolute. Both are nociceptive reflexes, but 'the unique feature of the pathological extensor response is the recruitment of extensor hallucis longus into contraction with tibialis anterior and extensor digitorum longus' (Kugelberg and Hagbarth 1958). The afferent focus, i.e. the region of easiest elicitation of this reflex, is the outer border of the sole and the transverse arch of the foot (Dohrmann and Nowack 1973). The motor focus, or minimal response, is a contraction of the inner hamstring muscles. When fully developed, the reflex consists of flexion at all joints of the lower limb with dorsiflexion of the great toe and abduction or fanning of the other toes.

Confusion has arisen from the application of the term extensor plantar reflex to a movement which forms part of a flexor reflex of the lower limb. The explanation of this misnomer is that the extensor hallucis longus muscle, though named extensor by the anatomists, is in fact a flexor muscle, since its action is to shorten the limb, and it contracts reflexly in association with other flexor muscles. The term extensor plantar reflex, however, appears to be too firmly established to be altered. 'Positive Babinski reflex' and 'upgoing toe' are alternative terms which are sometimes employed.

Physiological understanding illuminates several points of practical importance in the elicitation of the plantar reflex. The stimulus should always be applied first along the outer border of the sole; an extensor response may sometimes be obtained from this region when the inner border of the sole yields a flexor response. Dohrmann and Nowack (1973) have shown that the response is more consistently obtained if the stimulus is then continued medially across the anterior arch of the foot. Oppenheim's reflex, dorsiflexion of the great toe, evoked by firm moving pressure on the skin over the tibia, is physiologically the same as Babinski's reflex, differing only in the site of the stimulus. The same is true of Chaddock's and Gordon's reflexes. Chaddock's reflex or sign (also called the external malleolar sign) consists of an extensor plantar response elicited by scratching the skin in the region of the external malleolus, while in Gordon's sign or reflex (also called the paradoxical flexor reflex) the stimulus consists of squeezing the calf muscles. The extensor plantar reflex is not an all-or-none reaction: minor degrees of corticospinal-tract damage lead to an incomplete flexor response or a failure of the great toe to move up or down (an 'equivocal' response).

Bilateral extensor plantar reflexes are often observed during sleep and deep coma from any cause, for a short time after an epileptic convulsion and usually in the first year of life, that is, when the corticospinal fibres are either functionally depressed or incompletely developed. Although this response has sometimes been noted in cases in which no anatomical lesion of the corticospinal tract was subsequently discovered, and is occasionally absent in the presence of such a lesion (Nathan and Smith 1955; van Gijn 1978), and, although it may occur transiently as a result of physical fatigue, it can with confidence be accepted in clinical practice as indicating an organic lesion or dysfunction of this tract. In the presence of such a lesion, however, it may be lost if an associated lower motor-neurone lesion paralyses the extensor hallucis.

The bulbocavernosus reflex. The bulbocavernosus reflex consists of contraction of the bulbocavernosus muscle, which can be detected by palpation, in response to squeezing the glans penis. The spinal segments concerned are sacral 2, 3, and 4. This reflex is frequently abolished in tabes and in lesions of the cauda equina.

The anal reflex. The anal reflex consists of contraction of the external sphincter ani in response to a scratch in the perianal region. The spinal segments concerned are sacral 4 and 5.

Postural reflexes

'Postural reflexes' is a convenient term to apply to reflexes in which the response consists not of a brief muscular contraction but of a sustained modification in the posture of one or more segments of the body.

Tonic neck reflexes. In the decerebrate animal it was found by Magnus and de Kleijn that changes in the position of the head relative to the body caused reflex modifications of the tonus and posture of the limbs. These reflexes, which are excited from the proprioceptors of the cervical spine, are known as *tonic neck reflexes* and may sometimes be observed in severe cerebral diplegia. Passive turning of the head to one side may then evoke extension of the arm and leg on the side to which the head is turned with flexion of the contralateral limbs.

Associated reactions. Associated reactions, or associated movements, are automatic modifications of the posture of parts of the body when vigorous voluntary or reflex movement of some other part occurs. They are best observed in the paralysed upper limb in hemiplegia, following a vigorous grasping movement with the sound hand. Other patterns of associated movement occur. Such semi-voluntary activities as yawning, stretching, and coughing often evoke associated movements in the paralysed limbs in hemiplegia, and may arouse in the patient or his friends false hopes of recovery.

Forced grasping, groping, and avoiding

The grasp reflex of the hand. In certain patients the contact of an object with the palmar surface of the fingers, especially the region between the thumb and the index finger, causes reflex flexion of the fingers and thumb so that the hand involuntarily grasps the object. The patient is unable voluntarily to relax his grasp, and efforts to pull the object away only cause it to be more firmly held. The patient may notice that when he is holding an object he is unable to relinquish his hold of it in order to put it down. This phenomenon is known as the *grasp reflex.* In some cases, when the patient's eyes are closed, if the palmar surface of the hand or fingers is lightly touched, the fingers close upon the object and the hand and arm move towards the stimulus and in this way may be drawn in any direction – *forced groping* or the *instinctive grasp reaction.* Even an object presented to vision may be groped for (Seyffarth and Denny-Brown 1948).

Forced grasping and groping, which have been considered a regression to the infantile stage of the function of grasping, usually indicate a lesion involving the upper part of the opposite frontal lobe, particularly areas 8s and 24s (Denny-Brown 1951). A unilateral grasp reflex in a fully conscious patient is of localizing value. When the reflex is bilateral or the patient semi-comatose its value is much less. When the causative lesion produces a progressive hemiplegia, the grasp reflex disappears when paralysis becomes complete; this appears to indicate that it utilizes the corticospinal tract as part of its motor path.

The grasp reflex of the foot. An allied grasp reflex may sometimes be observed in the foot, light pressure or a stroking movement applied to the distal half of the sole and plantar surface of the toes evoking tonic flexion and adduction of the toes without other associated movements. Like the fingers, the toes may grasp and hold an object. This reflex is present in the normal infant up to the end of the first year, and in 50 per cent of children with Down's syndrome (mongolism). It may occur either with or without the hand-grasp reflex, and is caused by similar lesions.

The avoiding and grab reflexes. The avoiding reflex, which is in many respects the converse of the grasp reflex, is seen in animals with lesions induced experimentally in the parietal lobe. When an object is brought close to the hand on the affected side, the limb is drawn away instead of grasping the object. While phenomena similar to avoiding are sometimes seen in human subjects with parietal-lobe lesions, this reflex is rarely seen in clinical practice and is thus of little value. The question as to whether the so-called 'grab reflex' which causes flexion of the terminal phalanx of the thumb when the hand is passively displaced radially at the wrist (Traub, Rothwell, and Marsden 1980) is likely to be of clinical significance is still uncertain.

References

Adie, W. J. and Critchley, M. (1927). Forced grasping and groping. *Brain*, **50**, 142.

Babinski, J. (1922). Reflexes de defense. *Brain* **45**, 149.

Bickerstaff, E. R. (1980). *Neurological examination in clinical practice*, 4th edn. Blackwell, Oxford.

Boyle, R. S., Shakir, R. A., Weir, A. I., and McInnes, A. (1979). Inverted knee jerk: a neglected localizing sign in spinal cord disease. *J. Neurol. Neurosurg. Psychiat.*, **42**, 1005.

Brain, W. R. and Curran, R. D. (1932). The grasp reflex of the foot. *Brain* **55**, 347.

—— and Wilkinson, M. (1959). Observations on the extensor plantar reflex and its relationship to the functions of the pyramidal tract. *Brain* **82**, 297.

Denny-Brown, D. (1951). Chapter 1 in *Modern trends in neurology* (ed. A. Feiling). Butterworths, London.

Dohrmann, G. J. and Nowack, W. J. (1973). The upgoing great toe: optimal method of elicitation. *Lancet* **i**, 339.

Gandiglio, G. and Fra, L. (1967). Further observations on facial reflexes. *J. neurol. Sci.* **5**, 273.

Granit, R. (1970). *The basis of motor control*. Academic Press, New York.

Head, H. and Riddoch, G. (1917). The automatic bladder, excessive sweating and some other reflex conditions in gross injuries of the spinal cord. *Brain* **40**, 188.

de Jong, R. N. (1979). *The neurologic examination*, 4th edn. Hoeber, New York.

Kugelberg, E. (1952). Facial reflexes. *Brain* **75**, 385.

——, Eklund, K., and Grimby, L. (1960). An electromyographic study of the nociceptive reflexes of the lower limb. *Brain* **83**, 394.

—— and Hagbarth, K. E. (1958). Spinal mechanism of the abdominal and erector spinae skin reflexes. *Brain* **81**, 290.

Lance, J. W. and McLeod, J. G. (1980). *A physiological approach to clinical neurology*, 3rd edn. Butterworths, London.

Landau, W. M. and Clare, M. H. (1959). The plantar reflex in man. *Brain* **82**, 321.

Lenman, J. A. R. (1981). Integration and analysis of the electromyogram and related techniques. Chapter 29 in *Disorders of voluntary muscle*, 4th edn. (ed. J. N. Walton). Churchill Livingstone, Edinburgh.

Lloyd, D. P. C. (1952). On reflex action of muscular origin. *Res. Publ. Ass. nerv. ment. Dis.* **30**, 48.

Madonick, M. J. (1957). Statistical control studies in neurology:8. The cutaneous abdominal reflex. *Neurology, Minneapolis* **7**, 459.

Marsden, C. D., Merton, P. A., and Morton, H. B. (1973). Is the human stretch reflex cortical rather than spinal? *Lancet* **i**, 759.

Monrad-Krohn, G. H. (1925). Reflexes of different order elicitable from the abdominal region. *Arch. Neurol. Psychiat., Chicago* **13**, 750.

Nathan, P. W. and Smith, M. C. (1955). The Babinski response: a review and new observations. *J. Neurol. Neurosurg. Psychiat.* **18**, 250.

Paine, K. S. and Oppé, T. E. (1966). *Neurological examination of children*. Spastics International Publications, Heinemann, London.

Paulson, G. and Gottlieb, G. (1968). Developmental reflexes; the reappearance of foetal and neonatal reflexes in aged patients. *Brain* **91**, 37.

Plum, F. and Posner, J. B. (1980). *The diagnosis of stupor and coma*, 3rd edn. Blackwell, Oxford and Philadelphia.

Riddoch, G. and Buzzard, E. F. (1921). Reflex movements and postural reactions in quadriplegia and hemiplegia, with especial reference to those of the upper limb. *Brain* **44**, 397.

Seyffarth, H. and Denny-Brown, D. (1948). The grasp reflex and the instinctive grasp reaction. *Brain* **71**, 109.

Traub, M. M., Rothwell, J. C., and Marsden, C. D. (1980). A grab reflex in the human hand. *Brain* **103**, 869.

van Gijn, J. (1977). *The plantar reflex*. Krips Repro, Meppel.

—— (1978). The Babinski sign and the pyramidal syndrome. *J. Neurol. Neurosurg. Psychiat.* **41**, 865.

Walshe, F. M. R. (1914–15). The physiological significance of the reflex phenomena in spastic paralysis of the lower limbs. *Brain* **37**, 269.

—— (1919). On the genesis and physiological significance of spasticity and other disorders of motor innervation, with a consideration of the functional relationships of the pyramidal system. *Brain* **42**, 1.

—— (1965). *Further critical studies in neurology*. Livingstone, Edinburgh.

Wartenberg, R. (1945). *The examination of reflexes*. Year Book Publishers, Chicago.

Speech and its disorders

The nature of speech

Psychological considerations

Speech is an extremely complex activity. In order to understand its nature it is necessary to trace its development in the individual from infancy. Infant speech goes through several phases including babbling, which is the spontaneous production of sounds, and echolalia, which is the imitation of sounds made by others. The foundation of speech is thus sensorimotor—the sounds produced by others cause the child to reproduce sounds which it hears itself and which are linked with proprioceptor impulses from its own muscles of articulation. The next stage is the long one of learning the meanings of words; this involves associating sounds of the words with objects which are perceived in abstraction from their environment; later increasing abstraction is involved in naming qualities, actions, and relationships. The meaning of words is also influenced by their arrangements in sentences, i.e. by their grammatical and syntactical modifications.

When the child learns to read it does so by associating visual signs, i.e. letters and words, with the sounds which it has already learned. Through reading aloud, written words become linked with heard words, and with the kinaesthetic sensations of speech. In writing, movements of the hand are employed to reproduce visual signs similar to those which form the basis of reading. Since in writing one reads as one writes, there exists a close link between the perception of the visual signs which constitute letters and words and the kinaesthetic sensations derived from the fingers.

Words therefore are symbols. A spoken word is to the hearer an auditory symbol of an object, action, or relationship; a written word in the first instance acquires its symbolic significance through its association with heard speech, that is, symbolic sounds. Words as symbols possess meanings, but these meanings are of an elementary nature. In fully developed speech, individual words possess significance only in relationship with other words. The unit of meaning is then a phrase or sentence or even a series of sentences. Speech, therefore, is the communication of meanings by means of symbols, which usually take the form of spoken or written words. Meaning may, however, be communicated by facial expression or gesture ('silent language') and gesture meanings have been especially elaborated in the manual speech of the deaf and dumb. In reading Braille print, the blind utilize tactile instead of visual sensations. Mathematics and music also involve the use of written symbols.

Hughlings Jackson first pointed out that speech is not always used to communicate meanings—propositional speech, as he called it—but may also constitute the expression of feeling, in which case it may have no propositional value.

How far is thought dependent upon speech? It has been maintained that we think in words and that normal speech functions are therefore necessary for thought. The process of logical thought is probably subject to large individual variations depending upon whether the thinker chiefly utilizes visual or auditory images. It appears, however, that internal verbal formulation is not always necessary, at least for the simpler forms of logical thought. It is probably required for more abstract thinking and is necessary for the communication of the products of thought to others.

Physiological and anatomical considerations

At the psychological level, the meaning of a written or a spoken word is the outcome of the association of the given visual and auditory sensations with other forms of sensation in the past. A meaning is thus based upon a constellation of associations built up by experience. At the physiological and anatomical levels, the basis of such meanings is presumably a linkage of neurones, with progressive facilitation of synapses underlying the learning process. Visual impulses reach the cerebral cortex in the region of the calcarine sulcus of the occipital lobes, auditory impulses in the posterior part of the superior temporal gyrus. Kinaesthetic impulses from the muscles of articulation and from the upper limb terminate in the lower half of the postcentral gyrus. It is to be expected therefore that the anatomical linkages of neurones upon which verbal meanings depend will join together these regions of the cerebral cortex, and these connections are found in the tracts of white matter known as association fibres, which underlie the grey matter of the cerebral cortex.

For reasons which are little understood, about 93 per cent of persons are right-handed, and in these the left cerebral hemisphere plays the predominant role in speech and is known as the dominant or major hemisphere: it is the site of the speech functions in about 40 per cent of left-handed people also. In the remainder of the left-handed, the right hemisphere is the dominant one for speech, or speech functions may be bilaterally represented. There is evidence from cases of hemispherectomy in childhood that, up to the age of four or five years, speech function can, after an extensive lesion of the dominant hemisphere, be transferred to the other, but little or no such adaptation can occur in older children or adults (Subirana 1969). The important associational paths just described are therefore situated in the left hemisphere in right-handed persons, but sensory impulses concerned in the reception of spoken and written speech also reach the auditory and visual regions of the right cerebral cortex, which are linked to the left hemisphere by paths passing through the corpus callosum. Their importance was demonstrated by Gazzaniga (1965), who found that, after division of the corpus callosum and the other commissural connections in man, speech could deal only with perceptual information reaching the left cerebral hemisphere. The right cerebral hemisphere still had capacities of its own but was isolated from verbal expression (see also Geschwind 1965).

Recent work has shown first that cerebral dominance for speech and related functions is not absolutely complete in that further work on patients submitted to surgical commissurotomy for the treatment of intractable epilepsy (Bogen and Vogel 1975; Gazzaniga, Le Doux, and Wilson 1977) has indicated, for example, that while the right hemisphere is incapable, in right-handed individuals, of initiating expressive speech, it can comprehend nouns and verbs and can spell the names of items presented visually as well as controlling writing with the left hand (Gazzaniga et al. 1977). Many patients can also spell out answers to questions by manipulating cardboard letters with the left hand (see The Lancet 1979). Division of the corpus callosum, by contrast, does not impair the ability to assess the sensation of heaviness of objects in either hand (Gandevia 1978), but it does impair severely the awareness of and attention to visual stimuli presented independently to the two hemispheres (Dimond 1976, 1978). In general the right hemisphere appears to be dominant for the visual recognition of words when no semantic or phonetic decoding is required. It is also dominant in respect of visual localization, and directional and

topographical sense of visuospatial judgement (Benton, Varney, and Hamsher 1978). However, the left hemisphere assumes control of behaviour when written words have to be matched semantically to pictures and when complex verbal skills, as in tests of rhyming ability, are needed (Levy and Trevarthen 1977). It is also known that mild aphasia is seen very rarely in apparently right-handed individuals with right-hemisphere lesions (Archibald and Wepman 1968). Admittedly, psychological tests for hemisphere dominance (Benton 1976) involving methods of determining which hand, foot, and eye is dominant in a variety of tasks (Annett 1967) are not totally reliable, and the intracarotid injection of sodium amylobarbitone which was often used in the past to determine dominance prior to neurosurgical operations involving cortical ablation for the treatment of focal epilepsy (Branch, Milner, and Rasmussen 1964) is not without risk and has also been found to give inconsistent results. Methods of spectral analysis of visual and auditory evoked potentials (Davis and Wada 1977) appear to give a more consistent and reliable indication of hemisphere dominance. This may be important if unilateral electroconvulsion therapy is to be used for the treatment of depression (Fleminger and Bunce 1975).

While handedness is almost certainly genetically determined, there is some evidence to indicate that left-handedness sometimes results from a disorder of development or from an acquired lesion of the left hemisphere arising in early life in an individual destined genetically to be right-handed (Bishop 1980; British Medical Journal 1981). In left-handed or ambidextrous individuals and in their children, a temporary phase of mirror-writing and of right-left disorientation is not uncommon during early childhood. There is also recent interesting morphological and cytoarchitectonic information indicating the presence of physical asymmetries observed between the dominant and non-dominant hemispheres, especially in the areas controlling speech, even from the twentieth week of intrauterine life (Galaburda, Le May, Kemper, and Geschwind 1978a; Galaburda, Sanides, and Geschwind 1978b) and there is evidence that cerebral blood-flow increases more rapidly during development in Broca's area in children who are left-hemisphere dominant, than in the comparable cortical area on the opposite side (British Medical Journal 1981).

The posterior half of the left cerebral hemisphere is the site of those neuronal linkages which underlie the elaboration of meanings in response to auditory and visual stimuli, i.e. the comprehension of heard and written speech. Since articulated speech is the expression of meanings, it must be the outcome of the activity of a part of the brain which at least overlaps that concerned in the reception of speech, for the anatomical basis of meanings is common to both. Articulation involves movements of the jaw, lips, tongue, palate, pharynx, and phonation involves the respiratory muscles, which are all represented in the lowest part of the precentral gyrus. If meanings are to gain articulate expression, the posterior half of the left hemisphere must be linked to the lowest part of the precentral gyrus. An important part in this association is played by the arcuate fasciculus and the external capsule, which is a band of white matter running from the temporal lobe beneath the cortex of the inferior parietal lobe and insula to the lower part of the precentral gyrus and the posterior part of the middle and inferior frontal gyri. Speech requires co-ordinated bilateral movements of the muscles of articulation, and this co-ordination is effected by fibres passing from the lower part of the left frontal lobe to the corresponding region of the right hemisphere by the corpus callosum. From the lower part of the precentral gyri the motor fibres concerned in phonation and articulation pass downwards in the corticospinal tracts and after decussation end in the trigeminal and facial nuclei, the nuclei ambigui, and the hypoglossal nuclei in the pons and medulla, whence the lower motor neurones run in the corresponding cranial nerves to the lips, soft palate, tongue, and larynx. Corticospinal fibres similarly innervate the diaphragm and intercostal muscles. As with other motor activities, the cerebellum and striatum exercise a regulating influence upon articulation.

Dysarthria

We are now in a position to draw a distinction between speech, phonation, and articulation. Speech is the term employed for the whole process by which meanings are comprehended, conceived, and expressed in words. Phonation is the process of driving a column of air across the vocal cords, with resonance in the larynx and pharynx, in order to produce a sound, and articulation is the process of moulding this sound into words. Aphonia means loss, and dysphonia impairment, of phonation. Dysarthria is a disorder of articulation. It does not therefore involve any disturbance in the proper construction and use of words. In the dysarthric patient symbolic verbal formulation is normal: only the mechanism of verbal sound production is faulty. When this is so severely affected that the patient is totally unable to articulate, he is said to be anarthric.

The following are the principal causes of dysarthria:

Upper motor-neurone lesions

The articulatory muscles on each side appear to be innervated by both cerebral hemispheres. Hence a unilateral corticospinal lesion, for example in the internal capsule, may cause temporary but not permanent dysarthria; however, an extensive unilateral lesion involving the motor cortex may cause persistent dysarthria, especially when the dominant hemisphere is involved, when the dysarthria is often associated with some degree of Broca's aphasia (see below). Dysarthria is consistently produced, however, by bilateral corticospinal lesions, due, for example, to congenital diplegia, vascular lesions of both internal capsules, degeneration of both corticospinal tracts, as in motor-neurone disease, and lesions such as tumours involving both corticospinal tracts together in the midbrain. With such lesions the articulatory muscles are weak and spastic and the tongue appears smaller, firmer and less mobile than normal. The jaw-jerk and the palatal and pharyngeal reflexes are exaggerated. Speech is slurred and often explosive, production of consonants, especially labials and dentals, being severely affected. Spastic dysarthria is usually associated with dysphagia and often with impairment of voluntary control over emotional expression, a syndrome which is often called 'pseudobulbar palsy'

Extrapyramidal lesions

With lesions of the corpus striatum, articulation is impaired, partly, at least, as a result of muscular rigidity. Thus in hepatolenticular degeneration and in parkinsonism, articulation is slow and slurred owing to immobility of the lips and tongue and the pitch of the voice is monotonous. In cases of athetosis, torsion dystonia, and Huntington's chorea, too, dysarthria is common; indeed in severe cases speech may be unintelligible. Irregular respiration may contribute to the dysarthria.

Cerebellar lesions

The co-ordination of articulation suffers severely when the vermis is damaged and also when lesions involve the cerebellar connections in the brainstem. Speech in such cases is often explosive with slurring and undue separation of individual syllables—scanning or syllabic speech. Ataxic dysarthria of this character is seen after acute cerebellar lesions and in multiple sclerosis and the hereditary ataxias.

Lower motor-neurone lesions

Lower motor-neurone lesions cause wasting and weakness, and often fasciculation, of the muscles of articulation (true bulbar palsy). In the early stages the pronunciation of labials suffers most. Later, progressive weakness of the tongue impairs the production of dentals and gutturals, and weakness of the soft palate gives the voice a nasal quality. There is often associated dysphonia and finally total anarthria. Progressive bulbar palsy is the commonest cause, but paresis of the bulbar muscles may also be seen in syringobulbia, bulbar poliomyelitis, cranial polyneuritis, and brainstem tumours.

Combinations of these varieties of dysarthria are common; for example, in multiple sclerosis the articulatory muscles may be both spastic and ataxic and in motor-neurone disease a combination of upper and lower motor-neurone lesions may be present.

Myopathies

Disease of the muscles, such as myasthenia gravis, polymyositis, and muscular dystrophy involving facial muscles, leads to dysarthria similar to that resulting from lesions of the lower motor neurones. In myasthenia fatigability may cause increased slurring if the patient is asked to count aloud. In the myotonias impaired muscular relaxation may add a spastic quality to the speech.

Treatment

Little can be done when dysarthria is due to a progressive disorder but, in children suffering from congenital dysarthria or dysarthria due to diplegia, athetosis, and chorea, much can be accomplished by speech therapy.

Palilalia

Palilalia is a rare disorder of speech, the nature of which is obscure. As its name implies (from the Greek *palin*, again; *lalein*, to chatter), it is characterized by repetition of a phrase which the patient reiterates with increasing rapidity. Palilalia most frequently occurs in post-encephalitic parkinsonism, in general paresis, and in pseudobulbar palsy due to vascular lesions. Boller, Denes, Timberlake, Zieper, and Albert (1973), who reported palilalia occurring in a mother and son who also had chorea, dementia, and symmetrical intracerebral calcification, suggest that this phenomenon is the speech counterpart of other disinhibition phenomena such as the emotional incontinence of pseudobulbar palsy.

Mutism

Mutism is a term usually applied to a complete loss of speech in a conscious patient. It differs from Broca's aphasia (see below) in that phonation and articulation are also lost. It occurs in congenital deaf-mutes and also in akinetic mutism in which there is, however, an abnormal state of consciousness (see p. 645) but also in some cerebral lesions with preservation of consciousness, e.g. after severe head injury, after certain cerebrovascular lesions, in advanced parkinsonism, after bilateral thalamotomy, and after anoxic states due to many causes, e.g. carbon monoxide poisoning. It is also seen in psychiatric disorders, such as psychotic depression, schizophrenia, mental retardation, 'compensation neurosis', and hysteria. In psychosis the severity of the mental disorder is always apparent and the mute patient is usually unable to write. In hysterical mutism other hysterical symptoms are usually present. Elective or voluntary mutism is occasionally seen in children, more often in boys than girls; the child is persistently mute in many selected circumstances but not in all and there are usually other features indicating emotional maladjustment (see Ingram 1969).

Hysterical mutism is usually transient; it often resolves following abreaction during intravenous anaesthesia or after speech therapy.

Aphonia

In aphonia phonation is lost but articulation is preserved; hence the patient talks in a whisper. Aphonia may be due to organic disease causing bilateral paralysis of the adductors of the vocal cords (see p. 131) or disease of the larynx, for example, laryngitis. It is most commonly a symptom of hysteria, in which case the patient, though unable to phonate when speaking, can do so when coughing. Like hysterical mutism, hysterical aphonia (see p. 667) often resolves spontaneously once the precipitating stress is removed as in the singer or actress who loses her voice before an important performance; otherwise, it too may be helped by abreaction or speech therapy.

Aphasia

Whereas dysarthria is a disorder of the motor mechanism of articulation, aphasia is a disturbance of the higher and much more complex functions, described on pages 52–3, by which meanings are comprehended and expressed. It is thus a disorder of the use of symbols in speech. Since aphasia strictly interpreted means absence of speech, the term dysphasia, meaning disorder of speech, is sometimes employed when the deficit is incomplete. Some of the terminology used in the description of aphasia was formerly based upon old-fashioned views concerning the psychological nature of speech and outworn conceptions of cerebral localization. Confusion sprang from a failure to distinguish between psychological, physiological, and anatomical speech and its disorders, and to recognize the complexity of the relations between them.

The development of thought about aphasia

The earliest historical concepts of aphasia were well reviewed by Head (1926) and Weisenburg and McBride (1935).

The first attempt to localize functions in different parts of the brain was made by Gall (1758–1828), who distinguished six varieties of memory, including name-memory, verbal, and grammatical memory, all of which he localized in the frontal lobes. Dax in 1836 first drew attention to the special importance of the left cerebral hemisphere for speech. Broca (1824–80) reported two cases which led him to take the view that articulation was controlled by the inferior frontal gyrus (Broca's area). Damage to this area caused what he called 'aphemia'—a term altered by Trousseau to 'aphasia'. Broca distinguished two forms of speech disturbance—aphemia and verbal amnesia, the former being a defect of verbal expresson and the latter a loss of memory for both spoken and written words.

Hughlings Jackson's (1835–1911) first paper on speech was published in 1864. His great contribution was the introduction of a dynamic concept. Like Broca he recognized two main groups of aphasic patients. In one group speech was lost or gravely damaged; in the other the patient had numerous words but used them wrongly. He pointed out that the higher control of speech tended to suffer more than the lower and automatic, and he distinguished what he called 'propositional' from emotional speech. Aphasia was essentially an inability to 'propositionize' in speech, and the same fundamental difficulty underlay spoken speech, reading, and writing. Internal speech was affected like external speech and the thinking of the aphasic patient was therefore disturbed, but in most cases of aphasia mental images were unimpaired.

Hughlings Jackson's work was little appreciated at the time and most published work on aphasia emphasized increasing localization of function. Bastian (1837–1915) in 1869 maintained that we think in words and that words are revived in the cerebral hemispheres as remembered sounds. He localized auditory and visual word centres as well as other centres linked by association paths. He was thus the most notable of the 'diagram-makers' as Head called them. He prepared the way for the concept of word-deafness and word-blindness—terms introduced by Kussmaul—caused by lesions of these centres. Wernicke (1848–1905) in 1874 localized the centre for auditory images in the left superior temporal gyrus and described three varieties of aphasia—sensory, due to destruction of this centre, motor, due to a lesion of Broca's area, and a third due to interference with conduction between these two centres. When both centres were destroyed there was total aphasia.

Henry Head (1861–1940) returned to and developed the dynamic concepts of Jackson. He expressly avoided the question of localization and developed a functional approach, seeking to discover by a specially devised series of tests how the function of speech broke down in aphasia, which he regarded as a disorder of 'symbolic formulation and expression'. In Head's (1926) view, 'disorders of language of this kind cannot be classified as isolated affections of speaking, reading, and writing, for these acts are more or less disturbed whatever the primary nature of the defect. Nor can they be attributed directly to destruction of auditory or visual images or to any other analogous processes, which belong to a relatively low order in the psychical hierarchy. Each clinical variety represents some partial affection of symbolic formulation and expression; the form it assumes depends upon the particular modes of behaviour which are disturbed or remain intact.' Head recognized four such forms of disturbance, which he termed verbal, nominal, syntactical, and semantic.

More recently, aphasic patients have been studied by applying many techniques including phonetic analysis (Alajouanine and Mozziconacci 1948; Alajouanine 1956; Bay 1957), psychological testing (Bay 1960), and the Gestalt theory (Conrad 1954). Most recent work, as will be seen below, has indicated that the original concepts formulated by Wernicke relating to the localization of various speech functions in specific parts of the dominant hemisphere with complex interrelationships between them are still basically sound. For detailed reviews see Brain (1965), Lhermitte and Gautier (1969), Geschwind (1970), Critchley (1970), Goodglass and Kaplan (1972), Lesser and Watt (1978), and Marin and Gordon (1979).

The nature and classification of aphasia

Aphasia is a disorder of function and must therefore be interpreted in functional terms. Neuropsychological studies speak of word concepts (ideograms) and of visual (graphemes) and auditory (phonemes) images of words, phrases, and sentences and of their impairment in aphasic disorders (Marin and Gordon 1979; Sarno and Höök 1980). It rarely happens, however, that a localized cerebral lesion disturbs only one physiological function, and the same psychological disorder may be the result of more than one kind of physiological disturbance. This is why psychological classifications of aphasia have proved inadequate and why attempts to correlate anatomical lesions with clear-cut disorders of function have not always been successful (Goldstein 1948; Brain 1965). However, experience has shown that, on the whole, a lesion in one part of the brain disturbs speech in certain ways and a lesion in another situation in different ways. Hence, there exists an anatomical classification of aphasia which roughly corresponds to a functional one. Thus, modified from Geschwind (1970), the principal forms of aphasia and related disorders can be classified as follows:

1. Broca's aphasia (expressive or motor aphasia, anterior aphasia);
2. Wernicke's aphasia (sensory or receptive aphasia);
   (a) pure word-deafness;
3. Global or total aphasia;

4. Conduction aphasia (central aphasia of Goldstein, syntactical aphasia);
5. The posterior (association) aphasias:
   (a) the syndrome of the isolated speech area;
   (b) nominal, anomic, or amnestic aphasia;
6. Related disorders of language: agraphia, alexia, acalculia, amusia.

Broca's aphasia

A lesion of Broca's area has been thought to cause an inability to translate speech concepts into meaningful articulated sounds so that the content of speech is greatly reduced. However, careful clinicopathological studies by Mohr, Pessin, Finkelstein, Funkenstein, Duncan, and Davis (1978) have suggested that infarction restricted to Broca's area and its surroundings causes transient mutism followed by dyspraxic and laboured articulation without impairment of language. The syndrome traditionally called Broca's aphasia is characterized initially by mutism and then by poverty of language with verbal stereotypy and agrammatism; it is generally associated with a much larger infarct involving not only Broca's area but also the operculum, insula, and adjacent cerebrum. 'Propositional' speech suffers more than emotional so that other emotional expressions may be repeated spontaneously. Questions are often answered appropriately, but only in monosyllables, and spontaneous speech, when present, is telegraphic with lack of intonation, though word repetition is better than spontaneous formulation of thought concepts and the patient who is unable to think of a word readily recognizes it when offered to him. Comprehension of both written and spoken language is unimpaired, but reading aloud produces the same defective utterances as spontaneous speech. Singing, however, may be surprisingly unaffected both in relation to the words and the melody (Yamodori, Osumi, Masuhara, and Okubo 1977).

As Broca's area lies close to the motor cortex, many patients have an associated hemiparesis so that, if writing is to be tested, this must be attempted with the unaffected hand (usually the left). The handwriting is usually defective and there is poverty and lack of precision of written language, though copying is relatively unimpaired. The rare condition of *pure word-dumbness* or subcortical motor aphasia, thought to be due to a lesion in the subcortical white matter deep to Broca's area, is characterized by a similar impairment of spoken speech but writing is unimpaired.

It has often been suggested that, during recovery from Broca's aphasia in polyglots, ability to converse in the patient's mother tongue returns before the language subsequently acquired, but van Thal (1960) and others have shown that this is uncommon. More often the language most used is the first to recover (Silverberg and Gordon 1979).

Wernicke's aphasia

Lesions of Wernicke's area impair the comprehension of speech, as the meaning and significance of spoken words, received and recorded in the auditory cortex, are not understood. As Broca's area is unaffected, the production of speech is unimpaired so that the patient can produce fluent speech with normal rhythms and cadences, but its content is abnormal as he is also unaware of the meaning of many words which he himself produces. Paraphasias (incorrect word usage) are invariable in this form of aphasia and are either literal (the use of incorrect vowels or consonants within a word) or verbal (the use of incorrect words). In severe cases the patient produces meaningless jargon (*jargon aphasia*); it should, however, be noted that similar spontaneous speech occurs in conduction aphasia (see below). The repetition of words offered by the examiner is also impaired, as is the naming of objects; handwriting is usually normal but the content of written, as of spoken spontaneous language, is abnormal, though copying is relatively unaffected. The appreciation of musical sounds may be lost (amu-

sia); while the comprehension of written or printed language is often impaired (alexia), this is not invariably so (Heilman, Rothi, Campanella, and Wolfson 1979). Word-retrieval as well as word comprehension is usually severely affected (Coughlan and Warrington 1978). The patient often shows striking lack of insight, being unaware that his speech is abnormal, and he is commonly frustrated by his inability to make himself understood.

Pure or *subcortical word-deafness* (auditory aphasia) is a rare and fractional form of Wernicke's aphasia, thought to be due to a lesion of the white matter deep to the posterior part of the left superior temporal gyrus (Hemphill and Stengel 1940). The patient distinguishes words from other sounds but cannot understand them so that his own language, even when he uses words appropriately, sounds to him like a foreign tongue. He cannot repeat words or write to dictation but spontaneous speech, writing, and reading are unimpaired. Similarly, in word-blindness the subject cannot recognize words or letters; in 'pure' word-blindness, the defect involves only literal and verbal symbols, but sometimes the significance of numbers and even of colours cannot be appreciated either. In such cases, the lesion is also subcortical but more posterior.

Global aphasia

An extensive lesion of the dominant hemisphere involving both the frontal and temporal lobes often gives global aphasia (Mohr 1973) in which both the production of speech and the comprehension of spoken and written language are impaired.

Conduction aphasia

A lesion in the arcuate fasciculus or external capsule which interrupts the main association pathway between Broca's and Wernicke's areas gives this form of aphasia (Damasio and Damasio 1980) in which speech is again fluent but with many paraphasic errors, usually of the literal type (see above). There may be slight impairment of articulation and object-naming is usually, but not invariably impaired (Heilman, Tucker, and Valenstein 1976) as is written spontaneous language, though the handwriting is usually normal. Hence, as in Wernicke's aphasia, the patient's fluent but inappropriate speech is usually that of jargon aphasia and the ability to repeat words or to read aloud is markedly impaired. The only real distinction between this and Wernicke's aphasia is that, in this variety, the comprehension of spoken language is excellent as is that of written commands.

The posterior association aphasias

Lesions in or near the angular gyrus of the dominant hemisphere may interrupt connections between Wernicke's area and most other areas of the brain but leave intact the association pathway to Broca's area via the arcuate fasciculus and external capsule.

A large lesion may produce '*the syndrome of the isolated speech area*' (Geschwind, Quadfasel, and Segarra 1968) in which speech is fluent but paraphasic, while object-naming, spontaneous writing, and comprehension of both oral and written language are impaired. However, repetition of words spoken by the examiner is normal and the patient may show parrot-like repetition of a word or phrase ('echolalia').

If the lesion is less extensive, then speech may be fluent with only occasional paraphasia, and comprehension of written and spoken language as well as repetition are all normal, though written speech may be impaired. However, the most striking abnormality is often difficulty in naming objects and people (*anomia, nominal, or amnestic aphasia*). Typically the difficulty is most evident if the subject is asked to name unfamiliar rather than familiar objects, and proper names, even of close friends, may be especially difficult to recall. It is also characteristic that the patient rejects a wrong name suggested by the examiner and insists that he knows the object and its purpose (which he may demonstrate by writing, say, with a pencil, or putting on spectacles), even though he is unable to name it. One subvariety of this condition, also resulting from a parieto–occipital lesion, is *tactile aphasia* (Beauvois, Saillant, Meininger, and Lhermitte 1978). The subject, who is not dysphasic and shows no cortical sensory loss in the hands, misnames objects presented tactually in either hand but recognizes them at once when presented visually or auditorily.

Related disorders of language

Agraphia is an inability to produce written language (see Shallice 1981), *alexia* an inability to understand written or printed speech. As we have seen, agraphia usually accompanies Broca's aphasia, being a defect in the production of written as distinct from verbal language. However, *alexia with agraphia*, so-called *visual asymbolia*, or *cortical word-blindness* (total inability both to read and write and copy, also called Dejerine's first type of alexia—Dejerine 1891) usually results from a lesion of the angular gyrus region which divides the pathways between the visual association and speech areas *(British Medical Journal* 1979). Alexia without agraphia (Dejerine's second type—Dejerine 1892, and see below) is produced by a lesion situated more posteriorly. However, Benson, Brown, and Tomlinson (1971) and Benson (1977) have also described a third type of alexia due to a lesion of the dominant frontal lobe, commonly in association with Broca's aphasia, in which the patient has difficulty in comprehending the syntactical structure of written or printed speech rather than its meaningful content. Warrington and Shallice (1980) have described a rare form of 'word-form' or 'spelling' dyslexia in which the reading of whole words is impossible but the subject can read letter by letter. The lesion in such cases is posterior in the dominant hemisphere, as in alexia and agraphia and agraphia for musical symbols (Brust 1980).

Pure alexia without agraphia has also been called pure *subcortical word-blindness* or visual aphasia as the patient cannot recognize words, letters, or colours but can visualize colours. He cannot copy but can write and speak spontaneously and normally. The lesion responsible usually involves the visual cortex of the dominant hemisphere and the splenium of the corpus callosum, thus disconnecting the intact visual cortex of the opposite hemisphere from Wernicke's and Broca's areas (Cumming, Hurwitz, and Perl 1970; Caplan and Hedley-Whyte 1974; Cohen, Salanga, Hully, Steinberg, and Hardy 1976). A contralateral homonymous hemianopia is invariably present.

Acalculia is a term applied to a defect in the ability to use mathematical symbols; a patient with Broca's aphasia may be unable to carry out mental arithmetic, but loss of the ability to understand and use mathematical symbols whether verbal or written is more often seen in lesions of the dominant parietal lobe, in association with other features of Gerstmann's syndrome (p. 64).

Amusia is the term given to a defect of musical expression or appreciation and, like aphasia, can be either expressive (in association with Broca's aphasia) or receptive (in association with Wernicke's aphasia) (see Brust 1980).

Examination of a patient with aphasia

Examination of a patient with aphasia requires care and patience and should be carried out in a systematic manner. The following scheme of investigation fulfils most clinical requirements.

(1) Is the patient right-or left-handed, and, if the latter, did he write with the right hand? (2) What was his state of education as regards reading, writing, and foreign languages? (3) Does he understand the nature and uses of objects, and can he understand pantomime and gesture, or express his wants thereby? (4) Is he deaf? If so, to what extent and on one or both sides? (5) Can he recognize ordinary sounds and noises? (6) Can he comprehend spoken language? If so, does he at once attempt to answer a question? (7) Is spontaneous speech good? If not, to what extent and in what manner is it impaired? Does he make use of paraphasias,

either literal or verbal recurring utterances, or jargon? (8) Can he repeat words uttered in his hearing? (9) Is the sight good or bad; is there hemianopia, or impaired acuity? (10) Does he recognize written or printed speech and obey a written command? If not, does he recognize words, letters, or numerals? (11) Can he write spontaneously? What mistakes occur in writing? Is there paragraphia? Can he read his own writing some time after he has written it? (12) Can he copy written words, or from print into printing? Can he write numerals or perform simple mathematical calculations? (13) Can he read aloud? (14) Can he name at sight words. letters, numerals, and common objects? (15) Can he write from dictation? (16) Can he match an object with its name, spoken or written, when a series of objects and names are simultaneously presented?

For more precise and detailed assessment, many specific neuro-psychological tests and batteries of tests have been devised. These have included the Boston Diagnostic Aphasia Examination (Goodglass and Kaplan 1972; Naeser and Hayward 1978), the Western Aphasia Battery and Aphasia Quotient (Kertesz and Poole 1974), based upon numerical scores for fluency, comprehension, repetition, and naming, etc., and a graded naming test (McKenna and Warrington 1980) specifically designed for the assessment of nominal dysphasia.

Conclusions

In general, a fluent syndrome with paraphasia suggests that Broca's area is intact and suggests a posterior lesion, while speech which is slow, telegraphic, and dysarthric indicates one situated anteriorly. Impaired comprehension and repetition suggest Wernicke's aphasia, good comprehension and poor repetition conduction aphasia; conversely, good repetition and poor comprehension favour a lesion in the angular gyrus region isolating the speech area. In global aphasia, spontaneous speech, writing, reading, comprehension, repetition, and object-naming are all impaired, while in nominal aphasia the latter capacity is abnormal but comprehension is good and spontaneous speech relatively unaffected. It must be remembered that comprehension should not be tested simply by asking the patient to obey commands, as an individual with apraxia (see p. 62) may understand the command but be unable to comply.

Associated neurological signs may also be helpful. A contralateral hemiparesis is usually present in Broca's aphasia, less often in Wernicke's; a visual-field defect, on the contrary, is commonly present in association with the latter, rarely with the former.

The causes of aphasia

Apart from developmental disturbances of speech described below, aphasia is rare in childhood and increases in frequency with increasing age. A rare syndrome of 'acquired aphasia with convulsive disorder' was first described by Landau and Kleffner (1957); it develops in otherwise normal children and is usually associated with paroxysmal discharges in the EEG. About half the affected children recover after anticonvulsant drugs are introduced, but in the remainder some language disturbance persists; the cause is unknown (Gascon, Victor, Lombroso, and Goodglass 1973; Mantovani and Landau 1980). Acquired aphasia more often develops after middle life, since the commonest cause is a vascular lesion, especially an ischaemic one. Cerebral haemorrhage causes aphasia less often, because haemorrhage occurs deep in the white matter of the hemisphere more often than in the cortex or subcortical regions. Transitory attacks of aphasia may result from transient cerebral ischaemia, whether due to micro-embolism consequent upon arterial atheroma and stenosis or upon embolism from cardiac lesions. Aphasia may be a feature of the migrainous aura. The varieties of aphasia due to obstruction of the different cerebral arteries are described elsewhere (see pp. 194–5).

Intracranial tumour is a common cause of aphasia during the

first half of adult life, when cerebral vascular lesions are rare. Abscess of the left temporal lobe may also cause aphasia, as may traumatic lesions involving the 'speech areas' (Luria 1970). Apart from abscess, infective cerebral lesions rarely cause aphasia, though it occurs occasionally in acute necrotizing encephalitis, while acute cerebral lesions causing hemiplegia and attributed to encephalitis or vascular occlusion are almost the only causes of aphasia in childhood. Neurosyphilis may cause aphasia, by causing either cerebral infarction or general paresis. In the latter, transitory aphasia may occur early, while a profound disintegration of speech may develop as a result of the widespread deterioration of cortical function in the later stages, comparable to that seen in the presenile and senile dementias.

Prognosis

The prognosis of aphasia depends largely upon its cause. When it is due to a vascular lesion, neural shock is responsible for part of the immediate disturbance of function. Consequently considerable improvement may be anticipated as this passes off. The prognosis seems rather better in Broca's and in conduction aphasia, less good in Wernicke's and least good in global aphasia (Kertesz and McCabe 1977); it also appears better in the left-handed than in the right-handed. The prognosis is also good when aphasia is due to a removable extracerebral tumour, such as a meningioma, which has compressed but not invaded the brain. Recovery often occurs from aphasia due to acute inflammatory lesions, and from any lesion of the dominant hemisphere developing during the first four years of life.

Treatment

The treatment of aphasia requires unlimited patience and is likely to be more successful when the disturbance of speech affects the expressive rather than the receptive function. In the latter type of aphasia the patient not only has difficulty in understanding what is required of him, but he also fails to understand his own attempts at speech. There is good evidence to indicate that speech therapy is much more successful in promoting more effective rehabilitation and even ultimate recovery in the less severe cases and when it is begun as soon as possible after the onset (Basso, Capitani, and Vignoli 1979; Sarno and Höök 1980). The use of untrained volunteers who are prepared to talk with stroke sufferers with language disorders produces little if any improvement in language but increases social confidence (Lesser and Watt 1978). The scheme of instruction must be adapted to meet the requirements of each individual case and to utilize to the best effect those elements of speech which are least seriously impaired.

References

Alajouanine, T. (1956). Verbal realization in aphasia. *Brain* **79**, 1.
—— and Mozziconacci, P. (1948). *L'aphasie et la désintégration fonctionnelle du langage*. Masson, Paris.
Annett, M. (1967). The binomial distribution of right, mixed and left handedness. *Quart. J. exp. Psychol.* **19**, 327.
Archibald, Y. M. and Wepman, J. M. (1968). Language disturbance and nonverbal cognitive performance in eight patients following injury to the right hemisphere. *Brain* **91**, 117.
Basso, A., Capitani, E., and Vignoli, L. A. (1979). Influence of rehabilitation on language skills in aphasic patients: a controlled study. *Arch. Neurol., Chicago* **36**, 190.
Bay, E. (1957). Die corticale Dysarthrie und irhe Beziehungen zur sog. motorischen Aphasie. *Dtsch. Z. Nervenheilk.* **176**, 553.
—— (1960). Zur Methodik der Aphasie-Untersuchung *Nervenarzt* **31**, 145.
Beauvois, M.-F., Saillant, B., Meininger, V., and Lhermitte, F. (1978). Bilateral tactile aphasia: a tacto-verbal dysfunction, *Brain* **101**, 381.
Benson, D. F. (1977). The third alexia. *Arch. Neurol., Chicago* **34**, 327.
—— Brown, J., and Tomlinson, E. B. (1971). Varieties of alexia—word and letter blindness. *Neurology, Minneapolis* **21**, 951.

Benton, A. L. (1976). Historical development of the concept of hemisphere cerebral dominance. In *Philosophical dimensions of the neuromedical sciences* (ed. S. F. Spicker and H. T. Engelhardt), Reidel, Dordrecht, Holland.
—— Varney, N. R., and Hamsher, K.deS. (1978). Visuospatial judgement. *Arch. Neurol., Chicago* **35**, 364.
Bishop, D. V. M. (1980). Handedness, clumsiness and cognitive ability. *Dev. Med. child Neurol.* **22**, 569.
Bogen, J. E. and Vogel, P. J. (1975). Neurological status in the long term following complete cerebral commissurotomy. In *Les syndromes de disconnexion calleuse chez l'homme* (ed. F. Michel, and B. Schott,). Colloque International de Lyon.
Boller, F., Boller, M., Denes, G., Timberlake, W. H., Zieper, I., and Albert, M. (1973). Familial palilalia. *Neurology, Minneapolis* **23**, 1117.
Brain, Lord (1965). *Speech disorders*, 2nd edn. Butterworths, London.
—— (1945). Speech, and handedness. *Lancet* **ii**, 837.
Branch, C., Milner, B., and Rasmussen, T. (1964). Intracarotid sodium amytal for the lateralization of cerebral speech dominance. *J. Neurosurg.* **21**, 399.
British Medical Journal (1979). Acquired cerebral disorders of reading. *Br. med. J.* **2**, 350.
—— (1981). Left hand, right hand. *Br. med. J.* **282**, 588.
Brust, J. C. M. (1980). Music and language: musical alexia and agraphia. *Brain*, **103**, 367.
Caplan, L. R. and Hedley-Whyte, T. (1974). Cuing and memory dysfunction in alexia without agraphia—a case report. *Brain* **97**, 251.
Cohen, D. N., Salanga, V. D., Hully, W., Steinberg, M. C., and Hardy, R. W. (1976). Alexia without agraphia. *Neurology, Minneapolis*, **26**, 455.
Conrad, K. (1954). Some problems of aphasia. *Brain* **77**, 491.
Coughlan, A. K. and Warrington, E. K. (1978). Word-comprehension and word-retrieval in patients with localized cerebral lesions. *Brain* **101**, 163.
Critchley, M. (1927–8). On palilalia. *J. Neurol. Psychopath.* **8**, 23.
—— (1970). *Asphasiology and other aspects of language*. Arnold, London.
—— (1975). *Silent language*. Arnold, London.
Cumming, W. J. K., Hurwitz, L. H., and Perl, N. T. (1970). A study of a patient who had alexia without agraphia. *J. Neurol. Neurosurg. Psychiat.* **33**, 34.
Damasio, H. and Damasio, A. R. (1980). The anatomical basis of conduction aphasia. *Brain* **203**, 337.
Davis, A. E. and Wada, J. A. (1977). Lateralisation of speech dominance by spectral analysis of evoked potentials. *J. Neurol. Neurosurg. Psychiat.* **40**, 1.
Dejerine, J. (1981). Sur un cas de cecité verbale avec agraphie, suivi d'autopsie. *Mem. Soc. Biol.* **3**, 197.
—— (1892). Contribution a l'étude anatomopathologique et clinique des differentes varietés de cecité verbale. *Mem. Soc. Biol.* **4**, 61.
Dimond, S. J. (1976). Depletion of attentional capacity after total commissurotomy in man. *Brain* **99**, 347.
—— (1978). *Introducing neuropsychology*. Thomas, Springfield, Illinois.
Fleminger, J. J. and Bunce, L. (1975). Investigation of cerebral dominance in 'left-handers' and 'right-handers' using unilateral electroconvulsive therapy. *J. Neurol. Neurosurg. Psychiat.* **38**, 541.
Galaburda, A. M., LeMay, M., Kemper, T. L., and Geschwind, N. (1978a). Right–left asymmetries in the brain. *Science* **199**, 852.
—— Sanides, F., and Geschwind, N. (1978b). Human brain: cytoarchitectonic left–right asymmetries in the temporal speech region. *Arch. Neurol., Chicago*, **35**, 812.
Gandevia, S. C. (1978). The sensation of heaviness after surgical disconnection of the cerebral hemispheres in man. *Brain* **101**, 295.
Gascon G., Victor, D., Lombroso, C. T., and Goodglass, H. (1973). Language disorder, convulsive disorder, and electroencephalographic abnormalities: acquired syndrome in children. *Arch. Neurol., Chicago* **28**, 156.
Gazzaniga, M. S., Bogen, J. E., and Sperry, R. W. (1965). Observations on visual perception after disconnexion of the cerebral hemispheres in man. *Brian* **88**, 221.
—— LeDoux, J. E., and Wilson, D. H. (1977). Language, praxis, and the right hemisphere: clues to some mechanisms of consciousness. *Neurology, Minneapolis* **27**, 1144.
Geschwind, N. (1965). Disconnexion syndromes in animals and man, *Brain* **88**, 237, 585.
—— (1970). The organization of language and the brain, *Science* **170**, 940.

—— (1974). *Selected papers on language and the brain*, Boston Studies on the Philosophy of Science, Vol. xvi. Reidel, Dordrecht, Holland and Boston.

—— Quadfasel, F. A., and Segarra, J. M. (1968). Isolation of the speech area. *Neuropsychologia* **6**, 327.

Goldstein, K. (1948). *Language and language disturbances*. Grune & Stratton, New York.

Goodglass, H. and Kaplan, E. (1972). *The assessment of aphasia*. Lea & Febiger, New York.

Head, H. (1926). *Aphasia and kindred disorders of speech* (2 vols.). Cambridge University Press, Cambridge.

Heilman, K. M., Rothi, L., Campanella, D., and Wolfson, S. (1979). Wernicke's and global aphasia without alexia, *Arch. Neurol., Chicago* **36**, 129.

—— Tucker, D. M., and Valenstein, E. (1976). A case of mixed transcortical aphasia with intact naming. *Brain* **99**, 425.

Hemphill, R. E. and Stengel, E. (1940). A study on pure word-deafness. *J. Neurol. Psychiat.* **3**, 251.

Hermann, G. and Pötzl, O. (1926). Über die Agraphie. *Abhandlung aus der Neurol. Pshchiat., Psychol. und ihr Grenzgetret*, Berlin.

Ingram, T. T. S. (1969). Developmental disorders of speech. In *Handbook of clinical neurology* (ed. P. J. Vinken and G. W. Bruyn) Vol. 4, Chapter 21. North-Holland, Amsterdam.

Jackson, J. H. (1932). *Selected Writings*, Vol. ii. Staples, London.

Kertesz, A. and McCabe, P. (1977). Recovery patterns and prognosis in aphasia. *Brain*, **100**, 1.

—— and Poole, E. (1974). The aphasia quotient: the taxonomic approach to measurement of aphasic disability. *Can. J. neurol. Sci.* **1**, 7.

The Lancet (1979). Life with a split brain, *Lancet* **i**, 479.

Landau, W. M. and Kleffner, F. R. (1957). Syndrome of acquired aphasia with convulsive disorder in children. *Neurology, Minneapolis* **7**, 523.

Lesser, R. (1978). *Linguistic investigations of aphasia*. Arnold, London.

—— and Watt, M. (1978). Untrained community help in the rehabilitation of stroke sufferers with language disorder. *Br. med. J.* **2**, 1045.

Levy, J. and Trevarthen, C. (1977). Perceptual, semantic and phonetic aspects of elementary language processes in split-brain patients. *Brain* **100**, 105.

Lhermitte, F. and Gautier, J. C. (1969). Aphasia. In *Handbook of clinical neurology*, (ed. P. J. Vinken and G. W. Bruyn), North-Holland, Amsterdam.

Luria, A. R. (1970). *Traumatic aphasia*. Mouton, The Hague and Paris.

McKenna, P. and Warrington, E. K. (1980). Testing for nominal dysphasia. *J. Neurol. Neurosurg. Psychiat.* **43**, 781.

Mantovani, J. F. and Landau, W. M. (1980). Acquired aphasia with convulsive disorder: course and prognosis. *Neurology, Minneapolis* **30**, 524.

Marine, O. S. and Gordon, B. (1979). Neuropsychologic aspects of aphasia. In *Current neurology* (ed. H. R. Tyler and D. M. Dawson), Vol. 2, Chapter 19. Houghton Mifflin, Boston.

Meyer, A. (1974). The frontal syndrome, the aphasias and related conditions—a contribution to the history of cortical localization, *Brain* **97**, 565.

Mohr, J. P., Pessin, M. S., Finkelstein, A., Funkenstein, H. H., Duncan, G. W., and Davis, K. R. (1978). Broca aphasia: pathologic and clinical, *Neurology, Minneapolis* **28**, 311.

—— Sidman, M., Stoddart, L. T., Leicester, J., and Rosenberger, P. B. (1973). Evolution of the deficit in total aphasia. *Neurology, Minnneapolis* **23**, 1302.

Naeser, M. A. and Hayward, R. W. (1978). Lesion localization in aphasia with cranial computed tomography and the Boston Diagnostic Aphasia Exam. *Neurology, Minneapolis* **28**, 545.

Sarno, M. T. and Höök, O. (1980). *Aphasia: assessment and treatment*, Almqvist and Wiksell, Stockholm.

Shallice, T. (1981). Phonological agraphia and the lexical route in writing. *Brain* **104**, 413.

Silverberg, R. and Gordon, H. W. (1979). Differential aphasia in two bilingual individuals. *Neurology, Minneapolis*, **29**, 51.

Subirana, A. (1969). Handedness and cerebral dominance. In *Handbook of clinical neurology* (ed P. J. Vinken and G. W. Bruyn) Vol. 4, Chapter 13. North-Holland, Amsterdam.

Van Thal, J. H. (1960). Polygot aphasics. *Folia phoniat.* **12**, 123.

Warrington, E. K. and Shallice, T. (1980). Word-form dyslexia, *Brain* **103**, 99.

Weisenburg, T. H. and McBride, K. E. (1935). *Aphasia*. The Commonwealth Fund, New York.

Yamadori, A., Osumi, Y., Masuhara, S., and Okubo, M. (1977). Preservation of singing in Broca's aphasia. *J. Neurol. Neurosurg. Psychiat.* **40**, 221.

Developmental speech disorders

Developmental speech disorders are important, since, unless a correct diagnosis is made, the sufferer may be wrongly regarded as mentally retarded, and valuable opportunities of treatment may be missed. It is also essential to exclude congenital nerve deafness, which may cause severe delay in the acquisition of language, before concluding that a child with defective speech is suffering from a cerebral disorder of language or articulation. Lesser degrees of hearing loss may result in defective articulation; in particular, high-tone deafness causes difficulty in using high-tone consonants such as 'f' and 's'.

Developmental expressive aphasia is rare, developmental aphasia usually being of receptive type. Two varieties, congenital word-deafness and developmental dyslexia, are distinguished, but combined forms occur (Orton 1937; Ingram 1969). All varieties of developmental speech defect are commoner in males and in those of poorer family backgrounds and many are born towards the end of a large sibship. These children are often disadvantaged educationally and show more evidence of clumsiness and of visuomotor incoordination than their peers (Butler, Peckham, and Sheridan 1973).

Developmental receptive aphasia

Congenital word-deafness, or congenital auditory imperception, as it has also been called, is a rare inborn defect of speech. It is often familial and affects different members of successive generations of a family. Males are affected more frequently than females in the proportion of 5 to 1. The essential disturbance of function appears to be an inability to appreciate the significance of sounds, although hearing is normal. It seems that there is a lack of the anatomical or physiological mechanism whereby sounds become associated with other sensory impressions and with kinaesthetic sensations produced by speech and so acquire meanings. Since the disorder is more profound than merely a lack of appreciation of the significance of words, the term 'congenital auditory imperception' was proposed by Worster-Drought and Allen (1928–9).

The defect is present from birth but is not as a rule noticed until the age at which a normal child begins to understand speech and to learn to speak. It is then found that the patient takes no notice when spoken to and does not learn to repeat words. Hearing, however, is normal and he responds to noises. Spoken language is not understood unless he has learned to lip-read. The appreciation of musical sounds may or may not be defective. Worster-Drought and Allen pointed out that along with word-deafness there may be a defect in appreciating the meaning of written and printed symbols. This is not surprising in view of the part played by hearing in learning to read in normal individuals. Speech suffers seriously as a result of auditory imperception. For a number of years the child may not speak at all. Sooner or later, however, most patients acquire a vocabulary of their own, which is comprehensible only to those closely associated with them. The words spoken bear little resemblance to normal words, but possess meaning for the speaker. This defective form of speech has been identified by the now outdated terms 'idioglossia' and 'lalling'.

Although sufferers from congenital word-deafness are frequently found in institutions for the mentally subnormal, they do not necessarily suffer from mental retardation but are severely handicapped by the inadequacy of the primary channel through which we learn the meaning of things around us. It is not surprising therefore that sufferers tend to develop abnormal psychological reactions to their surroundings, especially when they are treated as mentally retarded. The diagnosis is from general mental retardation, and from high-tone deafness which can be excluded by audiometry.

The education of the congenitally word-deaf requires much care, and an intelligent appreciation of the nature of their disorder. As in the case of the deaf, they are educated principally through the sense of sight and are taught lip-reading, while their sense of touch may also be used to teach them correct articulation. The nature of the disability must be taken into account in planning an occupation.

Developmental dyslexia

Developmental dyslexia seems the best term to apply to a mixed group of individuals who possess in common a defect in learning to read. This condition has been called congenital word-blindness (Drew 1956), but a defect which can rightly be so described is the cause in only a small proportion of cases.

Developmental dyslexia is much commoner than congenital word-deafness, and Thomas (1905) estimated that it was present in 1 in every 2 000 London school-children. Like congenital word-deafness it is familial and may occur in more than one generation of the same family. In some cases it may be due to a congenital lack of the ability to appreciate the significance of visual symbols. In many patients, however, visual symbolization appears to be normal, and the defect appears to consist in an ability to differentiate the spoken word into its sounds and to break up a written word into its sounds and letters (Schilder 1944). Consequently the printed word is wrongly pronounced and conversely a dictated word is wrongly spelt. In one reported case studied in depth at post-mortem using cytoarchitectonic techniques, there was polymicrogyria in the left temporal speech area and various cortical dysplasias were found elsewhere in various association areas of the left hemisphere (Galaburda and Kemper 1979). This finding, the results of CT scanning (Haslam, Dalby, Johns, and Rodemaker 1981), and the abnormalities of visual evoked responses which have been found in some such cases (Symann-Louett, Gascon, Matsumiya, and Lombroso 1977) favour the suggestion that the condition is more probably dependent upon anatomical abnormalities in the brain than upon the defective establishment, in a physiological sense, of dominance in the left hemisphere. The writing of dyslexic children is often very abnormal. The subject was reviewed by Money (1962) and Critchley (1964).

Developmental dyslexia usually becomes apparent owing to the child's backwardness in learning to read. This may be wrongly attributed to a general defect of intelligence or to laziness. Yet by intelligence tests these children are frequently normal and their power of visual imagery is unimpaired. Such children are apt to develop psychoneurotic reactions owing to lack of understanding of their disability. Even adults who are otherwise of normal intelligence often make strenuous efforts to conceal their illiteracy, are resistant to remedial therapy, and may become psychiatrically disturbed (Saunders and Barker 1972).

Children with congenital auditory imperception frequently have some difficulty in learning to read as well as to speak (Ingram 1959, 1969), but in those with developmental dyslexia, spontaneous speech is usually normal in fluency and content.

Mirror-writing

This is the term applied to script which runs from right to left, the letters being reversed and forming mirror-images of normal script. Some normal individuals can carry out mirror-writing with the left hand, either when writing with the left hand alone or with both hands simultaneously. Such mirror-writing with the left hand may become evident in right-handed individuals who have developed right hemiplegia and has been known to follow an injury of the occipital region of the brain.

The situation is more complicated, however, in patients with developmental dyslexia who exhibit mirror-writing, for in such individuals mirror-writing appears secondary to mirror-reading (Orton 1937). These children tend to read words from right to left and pronounce them accordingly. For example, 'not' is pronounced 'ton' and, if asked to copy words, they frequently do so in the reversed order, with or without reversal of single letters. The frequent association of left-handedness with mirror-reading and writing suggests that these disorders may be secondary to a lesion of the left hemisphere which is normally dominant and to a substituted dominance of the right hemisphere. Many normal children pass through a temporary phase of mirror-writing, at least of certain letters, when first learning to write, especially when there is a family history of left-handedness or ambidexterity. This favours, by contrast, a phase of temporary difficulty in establishing cerebral dominance for this specific skill.

Treatment

Treatment of dyslexia must be based upon an understanding of the nature of the disability. The child must be taught association of syllables with the articulatory movements employed in their pronunciation. The phonetic method of teaching spelling, in which letters are learned by their sounds and not by their names, should be employed. Special care must be taken in teaching the child to read from left to right. The teacher points to the letters in this order and the child is encouraged to do the same with the forefinger of the right hand (for details see Schonell 1948 and Schiffman 1962). Similar principles apply in teaching dyslexic adults.

Stress should be laid upon reading for amusement and, in dictation, the patient should sit by a normal individual and be allowed to see what he has written. Educational authorities throughout an affected child's career should be briefed in order that appropriate allowances may be made, especially in examinations.

Developmental dysarthria

Although dysarthria may be a striking feature of the various forms of cerebral palsy and may even occur in some cases of 'minimal cerebral dysfunction' (p. 63), Morley, Court, and Miller (1954) and Morley (1972) have pointed out that some children who show a relatively normal development of language and who have no evidence of spasticity, paresis, or dystonia of the articulatory muscles, demonstrate slow and clumsy articulation, associated with clumsiness of movement of the lips, tongue, and palate. They suggest that in some cases the defect is a form of articulatory dyspraxia. Some affected individuals also show associated clumsiness of limb movements or developmental apraxia (p. 63). Ingram (1959, 1969) found that developmental dysarthria is often associated with variable defects in the acquisition of language and suggests that this syndrome rarely occurs in a 'pure' form.

Dyslalia

This term was used by Morley (1957) to identify a syndrome in which speech is acquired at the normal age and soon becomes fluent but the child demonstrates many defects of consonant substitution and omission. The condition quickly responds to speech therapy and speech usually becomes normal in a few months. This is probably a syndrome of multiple aetiology (Ingram 1959, 1969; Morley 1972); in some cases the child imitates the defective articulation of other family members, in some there is mild mental retardation, and in yet others the condition may be a mild and rapidly reversible form of developmental receptive aphasia or developmental dysarthria.

Stuttering (Stammmering)

Definition. A dysrhythmia of speech leading to a disturbance of articulation characterized by abrupt interruptions of the flow of speech, or the repetition of sounds or syllables.

Aetiology

There is still much controversy about the aetiology of stuttering. Orton (1937) suggested that this disorder is due to a defect in the establishment of dominance with respect to speech function in one or other cerebral hemisphere and found that it was commoner in left-handed persons and in shifted sinistrals. Others have suggested that the condition is of psychoneurotic origin. However, many studies have confirmed an association with partial or complete left-handedness or ambidexterity though this has been disputed (Luessenhop, Boggs, La Borwit, and Walle 1973). Fransella (1970) has pointed out that stutterers do not have neurotic personalities or behaviour characteristics according to accepted psychological criteria. Transient stuttering may occur in adults as a result of dominant hemispheric lesions giving mild Broca's aphasia. Thus it is sometimes seen as a manifestation of head injury, stroke, or progressive neurological disease (Quinn and Andrews 1977); when the lesion responsible is unilateral in the dominant hemisphere, stuttering is usually transient, but may be more persistent when there is bilateral pathological change (Helm, Butler, and Benson 1978). The 'idiopathic' condition is much commoner in males, rarely develops after 7–8 years, and has been found in about 1 per cent of British schoolchildren (Andrews and Harris 1964; Butler, Packham, and Sheridan 1973). There is a strong familial incidence (Johnson, Brown, Curtis, Edney, and Keaster 1948; Jameson 1955) and the condition sometimes occurs in children with mild developmental dysarthria or apraxia or other evidence of minimal cerebral dysfunction. Morley (1972) suggests that the defect begins inadvertently in early life when neuromuscular control of speech is still unstable. The normal hesitations and repetitions of early childhood may be regarded as abnormal by adults in the child's environment, and parental anxiety, communicated to the child, results in perpetuation of the defect. Anxiety, frustration, self-consciousness, and increasing attempts to correct the defect often make it worse.

Symptoms

The flow of speech may be broken by pauses, during which it is entirely arrested, or by the repetition of sounds or syllables. The pause may be filled with grunts or hisses, and stuttering is frequently associated with facial contractions or tics involving the limbs or even the whole body. The spastic element is usually called *tonus* and the repetitive *clonus*. Dentals (*t,d*), labials (*p,b*), and gutturals (*k* and hard *g*) are the consonants which are usually the most troublesome to the stutterer, especially when they occur at the beginning of a word. Stutterers often go out of their way to avoid certain words by reconstructing sentences and may employ tricks to enable them to achieve correct pronunciation, for example, spelling a word before pronouncing it. They can usually sing, may be able to recite without hesitancy, and sometimes speak fluently when angry or when alone.

Prognosis

Mild stuttering tends to disappear spontaneously. In some severe cases considerable improvement and even complete cure can be achieved by thorough treatment.

Treatment

When stuttering occurs in a left-handed child who has been made to use the right hand, a return to left-handedness occasionally produces improvement. Re-education of speech by a trained therapist is helpful. The patient should be taught to practise relaxation of the muscles concerned in speech. Relaxation is followed by breathing exercises and by exercises in which the lips, tongue, jaw, and palate are moved without the production of sounds. Later the patient begins to practise words, and articulation may be facilitated by various devices such as singing, or speaking through a megaphone or in time with a metronome. The use of syllabic speech under the supervision of a trained speech therapist has proved to be remarkably successful in some cases. Other techniques such as delayed auditory feedback, masking and syllable-timed, prolonged or slowed speech, as well as behaviour therapy and tranquillizing drugs have been used (Martin and Haroldson 1979; Azrin, Nunn, and Frantz 1979), but oxprenolol, for example, has been shown to be less effective than skilled speech therapy (Rustin, Kuhr, Cook, and James 1981).

In children psychological problems at home and at school should be dealt with if possible. In the pre-school child, treatment largely depends upon the mother, while in school, a teacher who understands and is prepared to be patient can do a great deal. At all ages suggestion and the enthusiasm of the therapist play a vital role (Travis 1959; Andrews and Harris 1964; Morley 1972).

References

Andrews, G. and Harris, M. (1964). *The syndrome of stuttering*, Clinics in Developmental Medicine, no. 17. The Spastics Society. Heinemann, London.

Azrin, N. H., Nunn, R. G., and Frantz, S. E. (1979). Comparison of regulated breathing versus abbreviated desensitisation on reported stuttering episodes. *J. Speech Hear. Disord.* **44**, 331.

Brain, W. R. (1945). Speech and handedness. *Lancet* **ii**, 837.

Butler, N. R., Peckham, C., and Sheridan, M. (1973). Speech defects in children aged 7 years: a national study, *Br. med. J.* **1**, 253.

Critchley, M. (1964). *Developmental dyslexia*. Heinemann, London.

Drew, A. L. (1956). A neurological appraisal of familial congenital word-blindness. *Brain* **79**, 440.

Fransella, F. (1970). Stuttering—not a symptom but a way of life. *Br. J. Dis. Commun.* **5**, 22.

Galaburda, A. M. and Kemper, T. L. (1979). Cytoarchitectonic abnormalities in developmental dyslexia: a case study. *Ann. Neurol.* **6**, 94.

Haslam, R. H. A., Dalby, J. T., Johns, R. D., and Rademaker, A. W. (1981). Cerebral asymmetry in developmental dyslexia. *Arch. Neurol. Chicago* **38**, 679.

Helm, N. A., Butler, R. B., and Benson, D. F. (1978). Acquired stuttering. *Neurology, Minneapolis* **28**, 1159.

Ingram, T. T. S. (1959). Specific developmental disorders of speech in childhood. *Brain*, **82**, 450.

—— (1969). Developmental disorders of speech. In *Handbook of clinical neurology* (ed. P. J. Vinken and G. W. Bruyn), vol. 4, Chapter 21. North-Holland, Amsterdam.

Jameson, A. M. (1955). Stammering in children. Some factors in the prognosis. *Speech* **19** (2), 60.

Johnson, W. (1959). In *Handbook of speech pathology* (ed. L. E. Travis) p. 897. Appleton, New York.

—— Brown, S. F., Curtis, J. F., Edney, J. C., and Keaster, J. (1948). *Speech handicapped school children*. Harper, New York.

Lesser, R. (1978). *Linguistic investigations of aphasia*. Arnold, London.

Luessenhop, A. J., Boggs, J. S., Laborwit, L. J., and Walle, E. L. (1973). Cerebral dominance in stutterers determined by Wada testing, *Neurology, Minneapolis* **23**, 1190.

Martin, R. and Haroldson, S. (1979). Effects of five experimental treatments on stuttering. *J. Speech Hear. Res.* **22**, 132.

Money, J. (Ed.) (1962). *Reading disability. Progress and research needs in dyslexia*. Johns Hopkins Press, Baltimore.

Morley, M. E. (1957 and 1972). *The development and disorders of speech in childhood*, 1st and 2nd edns. Livingstone, Edinburgh.

—— Court, S. D. M., and Miller H. (1954). Developmental dysarthria. *Br. med. J.* **1**, 8.

Orton, S. T. (1937). *Reading, writing and speech problems in children*. Norton, New York.

Quinn, P. T. and Andrews, G. (1977). Neurological stuttering—a clinical entity? *J. Neurol. Neurosurg. Psychiat.* **40**, 699.

Rustin, L., Kuhr, A., Cook, P. J., and James, I. M. (1981). Controlled trial of speech therapy versus oxprenolol for stammering, *Br. med. J.* **283**, 517.

Saunders, W. A. and Barker, M. G. (1972). Dyslexia as cause of psychiatric disorder in adults. *Br. med. J.* **4**, 759.

Schiffman, G. (1962). In *Reading disability. Progress and research needs in dyslexia* (ed. J. Money). Johns Hopkins Press, Baltimore.

Schilder, P. (1944). Congenital alexia and its relation to optic perception. *J. genet. psychol.* **65**, 67.

Schonell, F. J. (1948). *Backwardness in the basic subjects*, 4th edn. Oliver & Boyd, Edinburgh.

Symann-Louett, N., Gascon, G. G., Matsumiya, Y., and Lombroso, C. T. (1977). Wave form difference in visual evoked responses between normal and reading disabled children, *Neurology, Minneapolis* **27**, 156.

Thomas, C. J. (1905). Congenital word-blindness and its treatment. *Opthalmoscope* **3**, 380.

Travis, L. E. (Ed.) (1959). *Handbook of speech pathology*. Appleton, New York.

Worster-Drought, C. and Allen, I. M. (1928–9). Congenital auditory imperception. *J. Neurol. Psychopathol.* **60**, 193, 289.

Apraxia and agnosia

Apraxia

Apraxia may be defined as an inability to carry out a purposive movement, the nature of which the patient understands, in the absence of severe motor weakness or paralysis, sensory loss, or ataxia. For example, a patient who is asked to protrude his tongue is unable to do so on request, though he may carry out inappropriate movements such as opening his mouth. A moment later he spontaneously protrudes his tongue to lick his lips. Apraxia may involve any movement which is normally initiated voluntarily—movements of the eyes, face, muscles of articulation, chewing and swallowing, manipulation of objects, gestures with the upper limb, walking, or sitting down.

Normal purposive movements depend upon the integrity not only of the corticobulbar and corticospinal tracts, but also of association tracts whereby these efferent paths are excited. The idea of the movement, whether formulated spontaneously or in response to an external command thus passes into action. Apraxia is the result of interruption of the pathways which thus act as ideomotor links. In right-handed individuals purposive motor activity appears thus to be controlled by the posterior part of the left hemisphere, especially by the supramarginal gyrus. Thence fibres pass forwards to the precentral gyrus and cross to the same gyrus on the right side, through the corpus callosum. Lesions in the left parietal lobe often therefore produce bilateral apraxia. Lesions between this region and the left precentral gyrus may lead to apraxia of the limbs on the right side, and lesions involving the anterior part of the corpus callosum or of the subcortical white matter on the right side may cause left-sided apraxia. A common form of apraxia is that involving the lips and tongue, which is frequently encountered in association with right hemiplegia due to a lesion of the left hemisphere. *Dressing apraxia*, in which the patient cannot dress because he is unable to relate the parts of his body to the parts of a garment, is due to a disturbance of the body image (see below) and is usually the result of a lesion of the right parietal lobe.

Apraxia was classified by Liepmann (1908) into limb-kinetic apraxia, due to loss of kinetic memories of limb movements, ideokinetic (or ideomotor) apraxia, due to a dissociation between ideational and kinaesthetic processes, and ideational apraxia, in which the general concept of the movement is imperfect, its component parts being correctly carried out but wrongly combined. *Ideomotor apraxia*, where there is a disconnection between the idea of a movement and its execution or recognition, appears to be due to a destruction of engrams, established through learning and experience, of specific motor sequences or skills and is associated with inability to relearn as well as to retain such skills (Heilman, Schwartz, and Geschwind 1975). In *ideational apraxia*, by contrast, patients will look at their hands in a perplexed manner and will make irrelevant movements even though they confirm verbally that they understand the nature of the movement required and can pick it out correctly from a series of movements performed by the examiner. CT scanning in patients with such apraxia after strokes (Basso, Luzzatti, and Spinnler 1980) has shown that there is a marked inconsistency in the exact location of the causal lesion in the dominant hemisphere but it is usually superficial and cortical rather than deeply situated. Apraxia is usually associated with an impairment of the power to imitate movements. The disturbance of function is essentially similar to that responsible for motor aphasia, which may justly be regarded as an apraxia of the purposive movements concerned in speech. The nature of apraxia has been discussed by Geschwind (1975).

A special form of apraxia was named by Kleist (1922) *constructional or optical apraxia*. There is no apraxia of single movements but the spatial disposition of the action is disordered. The patient, for example, cannot copy a simple arrangement of matches, but recognizes his mistakes. Constructional apraxia may occur in association with lesions of either parietal lobe; when the dominant hemisphere is involved it is often associated with the other features of Gerstmann's syndrome (p. 64), but as an isolated defect it is commoner in lesions of the non-dominant hemisphere (Piercy, Hécaen, and Ajuriaguerra 1960). *Apraxia of gait* is usually the result of bilateral frontal lesions (Meyer and Barron 1960) and is sometimes seen in presenile dementia. Apraxia of ocular movements (Altrocchi and Menkes 1960) will be described on page 98.

Apraxia is most frequently seen as a result of localized lesions of the brain, especially vascular lesions and tumours. It may also be a symptom of diffuse cerebral inflammatory or degenerative states, such as general paresis and the presenile or senile dementias.

Agnosia

The arrival of nerve impulses at the cortical areas concerned with vision, hearing, and cutaneous and postural sensibility excites crude sensations which have not yet attained the perceptual level involved in the recognition of objects. Recognition is brought about by the association of the sensations excited through one sensory channel with memories of sensations derived from other sensory channels during previous experiences of the object, which include our actions in regard to it. The perception of an object seen or felt is thus a constellation of sensory images and memories directed towards action, and the recognition of an object as having been seen before, and of its use, depends upon the capacity of the primary visual or tactile sensation which it evokes to excite the correct motor or sensory associations. When, by reason of disease of the brain, this secondary process fails to occur, the patient fails to recognize the object. This defect is known as agnosia or mind-blindness. Its nature has been discussed by Geschwind (1965).

Visual agnosia is present when the patient, in whom the paths from the retina to the occipital cortex are intact and the latter is undamaged, nevertheless fails to recognize common objects which he clearly sees. This condition may result from lesions in the left parieto-occipital region in right-handed persons. Bender and Feldman (1972) point out that visual agnosias for form (Benson and Greenberg 1969) and colour and object recognition (Rubens and Benson 1971) rarely occur in 'pure' form but are usually associated with a contralateral hemianopia and with various other deficits of mental and cognitive function. *Prosopagnosia* is a restricted form of visual agnosia in which the patient is unable to recognize faces (Meadows, 1974a); it is sometimes associated with non-dominant occipital-lobe lesions (Whiteley and Warrington 1977) but more often there are bilateral lesions specifically involving the fusiform gyri (Cohn, Neumann, and Wood 1977). It may also be associated, though not invariably, with defective colour perception (*achromatopsia*) (Meadows 1974b). *Auditory agnosia* implies the failure to recognize sounds in a patient who is nevertheless not deaf. An individual suffering from this disability in a severe form will fail to appreciate not only the nature of words but also musical tunes. This results from a lesion of the left temporal lobe in right-handed persons. Word-deafness (p. 59) can be considered to be a form of auditory agnosia for spoken verbal symbols. *Tactile agnosia* is one of the group of disorders comprised under the more general term *astereognosis*. The patient, though not suffering from a gross sensory defect in the fingers or hand, is nevertheless unable to recognize an object placed in the hand. This may be produced by a lesion of the parietal lobe situated deep to or just behind the postcentral gyrus at the level of the hand area. Astereognosis, which is a defect of tactile object recognition (Roland 1976), must be distinguished from stereoanaesthesia which is an abnormality of the appreciation of the size, shape, and texture of objects held in the hand due to loss of the finer and discriminative aspects of sensibility; the latter may be identified by other methods such as measurement of two-point discrimination and results from a lesion of the postcentral gyrus itself. One form of congenital indifference to pain (*pain asymbolia*) is thought to be an agnosia for painful sensations; it has been described in association with congenital auditory imperception (Osuntokun, Odeku, and Luzzato 1968).

Agnosia usually affects only the recognition of objects through one sensory channel. Thus a patient suffering from visual agnosia, who cannot recognize a key when he sees it, can usually recognize it when it is placed in his hand. Conversely, a patient who cannot recognize objects placed in his hand recognizes them readily when he sees them. The various forms of agnosia, like apraxia, may result from focal vascular or neoplastic lesions and are sometimes seen in the presenile dementias. Visual agnosia is especially common as a consequence of cerebral anoxia, as in carbon monoxide poisoning.

References

Altrocchi, P. H. and Menkes, J. H. (1960). Congenital ocular motor apraxia. *Brain* **83**, 579.

Basso, A., Luzzatti, C., and Spinnler, H. (1980). Is ideomotor apraxia the outcome of damage to well-defined regions of the left hemisphere? *J. Neurol. Neurosurg. Psychiat.* **43**, 118.

Bender, M. B. and Feldman, M. (1972). The so-called 'visual agnosias'. *Brain* **95**, 173.

Benson, D. F. and Greenberg, J. P. (1969). Visual form agnosia. A specific defect in visual discrimination. *Arch. Neurol., Chicago* **20**, 82.

Brain, Lord (1965). *Speech disorders*, 2nd ed. Butterworth, London.

—— (1941). Visual object-agnosia, with special reference to the Gestalt theory. *Brain* **64**, 43.

Cohn, R., Neumann, M. A., and Wood, D. H. (1977). Prosopagnosia: a clinicopathological study. *Ann. Neurol.* **1**, 177.

Geschwind, N. (1965). Disconnexion syndromes in animals and man. *Brain* **88**, 237, 585.

—— (1975). The apraxias: neural mechanisms of disorders of learned movements. *Am. Scientist* **63**, 188.

Heilman, K. M., Schwartz, H. D., and Geschwind, N. (1975). Defective motor learning in ideomotor apraxia. *Neurology, Minneapolis* **25**, 1018.

Kleist, K. (1922). Die psychomotorischen Störungen und ihr Verhältnis zu den Motilitätsstörungen bei Erkrankungen der Stammganglien. *Mschr. Psychiat. Neurol.* **52**, 253.

Liepmann, H. (1908). *Drei Aufsatze aus dem Apraxiegebiet*. Karger, Berlin.

Meadows, J. C. (1974*a*). The anatomical basis of prosopagnosia. *J. Neurol. Neurosurg. Psychiat.* **37**, 489.

—— (1974*b*). Disturbed perception of colours associated with localized cerebral lesions. *Brain* **97**, 615.

Meyer, J. S. and Barron, D. W. (1960) Apraxia of gait: a clinico-physiological study. *Brain* **83**, 261.

Nathan, P. W. (1947). Facial apraxia and apraxic dysarthria. *Brain* **70**, 449.

Nielsen, J. M. (1946). *Agnosia, apraxia, aphasia. Their value in cerebral localization*, 2nd edn. Hoeber, New York.

Osuntokun, B. O., Odeku, E. L., and Luzzato, L. (1968). Congenital pain asymbolia and auditory imperception. *J. Neurol. Neurosurg. Psychiat.* **31**, 291.

Piercy, M., Hécaen, H., and Ajuriaguerra, J. de (1960). Constructional apraxia associated with unilateral cerebral lesions—left and right sided cases compared. *Brain* **83**, 225.

Roland, P. E. (1976). Astereognosis: tactile discrimination after localized hemispheric lesions in man. *Arch. Neurol., Chicago* **33**, 543.

Rubens, A. B. and Benson, D. F. (1971). Associative visual agnosia. *Arch. Neurol., Chicago* **24**, 305.

Whiteley, A. M. and Warrington, E. K. (1977). Prosopagnosia: a clinical, psychological and anatomical study of three patients. *J. Neurol. Neurosurg. Psychiat.* **40**, 395.

Developmental apraxia and agnosia

Gubbay, Ellis, Walton, and Court (1965) showed that some 'clumsy children' who presented with poor school performance due to delay in the development of motor skills could be shown to have defects of cognitive and executive performance which could be classified as various forms of apraxia and agnosia. Many such children also showed variable involuntary limb movements which superficially resembled chorea. In some children collateral clinical evidence suggested that perinatal brain damage may have been the cause, but in others the condition may have been due to a physiological disorder of the establishment of dominance in one or other hemisphere as there was evidence of crossed laterality. Most such children showed a discrepancy between a high verbal and low performance score on the Wechsler Intelligence Scale for Children. Improvement occurred with maturation but in several cases patient individual tuition was needed to overcome the disability. Minor degrees of this syndrome often go unrecognized and uncorrected in apparently normal schoolchildren (Walton, Ellis, and Court 1962; Brenner, Gillman, Zangwill, and Farrell 1967) and others are loosely classified as examples of 'minimal brain dysfunction' (*The Lancet* 1973). A developmental form of Gerstmann's syndrome has been described (Benson and Geschwind 1970).

References

Benson, D. F. and Geschwind, N. (1970). Developmental Gerstmann syndrome. *Neurology, Minneapolis* **20**, 293.

Brenner, M. W., Gillman, S. Zangwill, O. L., and Farrell, M. (1967). Visuo-motor disability in schoolchildren. (*Br. med. J.* **4**, 259.

Gubbay, S. S. (1976). *Clumsy children*. Saunders, London.

——, Ellis, E., Walton, J. N., and Court, S. D. M. (1965). Clumsy children: a study of apraxic and agnosic defects in 21 children. *Brain* **88**, 295.

The Lancet (1973). Minimal brain dysfunction. *Lancet* ii, 487.

Walton, J. N., Ellis, E., and Court, S. D. M. (1962). Clumsy children: a study of developmental apraxia and agnosia. *Brain* **85**, 603.

Disorders of the body-image

We are aware of the existence of our bodies, their position in space, and the relation of their parts to one another because we receive sense-data through numerous sensory channels, which include vision, cutaneous sensibility, and proprioceptor impulses from the muscles, joints, and labyrinths. The somatic impulses pass via the ventral nucleus of the thalamus to the supramarginal gyrus which is thus concerned with awareness of the opposite half of the body. This concept of the body in consciousness is known as the body-image or body-schema.

Symptoms of disorders of the body-image may be positive or negative. The chief positive symptom is the phantom—an illusion of the persistence of a part of the body lost by amputation, e.g. a phantom limb, or an illusory awareness of a part from which sensation has been lost through interruption of afferent pathways. Phantom limbs after amputation may be painless or painful (Riddoch 1941). The painless phantom soon becomes less obtrusive, and gradually shortens, eventually to disappear. A painful phantom is usually associated with abnormalities of the stump, such as large, tender terminal neuromas on the divided nerves. Painful phantoms may persist indefinitely and cause much distress. A phantom limb may be abolished by a lesion of sensory pathways in the spinal cord or of the opposite parietal cortex (Appenzeller and Bicknell 1969).

Defects of the body-image are less easily demonstrated in patients with lesions of the dominant hemisphere as they are often obscured by associated aphasia or other related phenomena. They are certainly more common in lesions of the non-dominant hemisphere but bilateral defects of the 'body-schema' are also seen in damage to the dominant parietal lobe (Sauguet, Benton, and Hécaen 1971). However, in *Gerstmann's syndrome* (Gerstmann 1924, 1940, 1970), a lesion of the dominant angular gyrus gives finger agnosia, an inability to name or select individual fingers in the patient himself or in the examiner. In the syndrome as classically described, this abnormality is associated with agraphia, acalculia, and right-left disorientation; in some otherwise typical cases, constructional apraxia and/or alexia are also present

Whereas visual agnosia for form and object recognition is also most often seen in lesions of the visual association areas of the dominant hemisphere, the most striking abnormalities of the body-image occur as a result of lesions of the non-dominant parieto-occipital region and can be regarded as various forms of visuo-spatial agnosia (Ettlinger, Warrington, and Zangwill 1957).Thus the patient may be unaware of the opposite half of his body and of extrapersonal space on that side—*autotopagnosia*, or contralateral visual neglect (Leicester, Sidman, Stoddart, and Mohr 1969). He ignores people and objects in that half of the visual field, may deny that his limbs on the affected side, even if hemiplegic, belong to him, and, and if he attempts to draw a clock face, will crowd all the figures into the opposite half of the circle. When there is an associated visual-field defect, contralateral visual neglect is often more severe (Chedru 1976). In severe cases, visual disorientation may be so severe that the patient is unable to find his way about, even in familiar surroundings (*topographical agnosia*). There is often some dissociation between visual perceptual and spatial deficits in lesions of the right parietal lobe (Newcombe and Russell 1969) but these commonly impair the ability to localize visual stimuli, while dominant-hemisphere lesions do not (Hannay, Varney, and Benton 1976). Contralateral *auditory neglect* may also result from lesions of the inferior parietal lobe in both animals and man (Heilman, Pandya, Kanol, and Geschwind 1971; Heilman and Valenstein 1972). *Global contralateral hemianaesthesia*, superficially suggesting an hysterical phenomenon, is also a rare consequence of parietal-lobe lesions (Yarnell, Melamed, and Silverberg 1978); in such cases there is a marked discrepancy between the complaint of limb anaesthesia and the preservation of motor and postural control. Denial of evidence of bodily disease, e.g. hemiplegia, is known as *anosognosia*, while denial of blindness has been identified as Anton's syndrome. In anosognosia for hemiplegia there is often diffuse slowing of the EEG rhythms over the affected hemisphere (Watson, Andriola, and Heilman 1977) and somatosensory evoked potentials are generally absent bilaterally after unilateral stimulation of the neglected limb (Green and Hamilton 1976) suggesting impairment of arousal and of cortical processing of sensory information.

In parieto-occipital lesions of lesser severity the patient may be unable to localize accurately visual or auditory stimuli in the opposite half-field or tactile stimuli on the opposite side of the body. When a stimulus, whether visual, auditory, or tactile, is perceived when delivered independently on either side, but when one of two such stimuli presented simultaneously on the two sides is ignored, this is known as visual, auditory, or tactile inattention (p. 44).

References

Appenzeller, O. and Bicknell, J. M. (1969). Effects of nervous system lesions on phantom experience in amputees. *Neurology, Minneapolis* **19**, 141.

Chedru, F. (1976). Space representation in unilateral spatial neglect. *J. Neurol. Neurosurg. Psychiat.* **9**, 1057.

Critchley, M. (1953). *The parietal lobes*. Arnold, London.

Ettlinger, G. Warrington, E., and Zangwill, O. L. (1957). A further study of visual–spatial agnosia. *Brain* **80**, 335.

Fredericks, J. A. M. (1969). Disorders of the body schema. In *Handbook of clinical neurology* (ed. P. J. Vinken and G. W. Bruyn) Vol. 4, Chapter 11. North-Holland, Amsterdam.

Gerstmann, J. (1924). Fingeragnosie. Eine umschriebene Störung der Orientierung am eigenen Körper. *Wien. klin. Wschr.* **37**, 1010.

——(1940). Syndrome of finger agnosia, disorientation for right and left; agraphia and acalculia. *Arch. Neurol. Psychiat., Chicago* **44**, 398.

——(1970). Some posthumous notes on the Gerstmann syndrome. *Wien. Z. Nervenheilkunde* **28**, 12.

Green, J. B. and Hamilton, W. J. (1976). Anosognosia for hemiplegia: somatosensory evoked potential studies. *Neurology, Minneapolis* **26**, 1141.

Hannay, H. J., Varney, N. R., and Benton, A. L. (1976). Visual localization in patients with unilateral brain disease. *J. Neurol. Neurosurg. Psychiat.* **39**, 307.

Heilman, K. M. and Valenstein, E.(1972). Auditory neglect in man. *Arch. Neurol., Chicago* **26**, 32.

——, Pandya, D. N., Karol, E. A., and Geschwind, N. (1971). Auditory inattention. *Arch. Neurol., Chicago* **24**, 323.

Leicester, J., Sidman, M., Stoddart, L. T., and Mohr, J. P. (1969). Some determinants of visual neglect. *J. Neurol. Neurosurg. Psychiat.* **32**, 580.

Lhermitte, J. (1939). *L'image de notre corps*. Nouvelle Revue Critique, Paris.

Newcombe, F. and Russell, W. R. (1969). Dissociated visual perceptual and spatial deficits in focal lesions of the right hemisphere. *J. Neurol. Neurosurg. Psychiat.* **32**, 73.

Raney, A. A. and Nielsen, J. M.(1942). Denial of blindness (Anton's syndrome). *Bull. Los Angeles Neurol. Soc.* **7**, 150.

Redlich, F. C. and Dorsey, J. F. (1945). Denial of blindness by patients with cerebral disease. *Arch. Neurol. Psychiat., Chicago* **53**, 407.

Riddoch, G. (1941). Phantom limbs and body shape. *Brain* **64**, 197.

Sauguet, J., Benton, A. L., and Hécaen, H. (1971). Disturbances of the body schema in relation to language impairment and hemispheric locus of lesion. *J. Neurol. Neurosurg. Psychiat.* **34**, 496.

Schilder, P. (1935). *The image and appearance of the human body*. International Universities Press, London.

Watson, R. T., Andriola, M., and Heilman, K. M. (1977). The electroencephalogram in neglect. *J. Neurol. Sci.* **34**, 343.

Yarnell, P., Melamed, E., and Silverberg, R. (1978). Global hemianaesthesia: a parietal perceptual distortion suggesting non-organic illness. *J. Neurol. Neurosurg. Psychiat.* **41**, 843.

The cerebrospinal fluid (CSF)

Anatomy and physiology

Formation, circulation, and absorption

Clinical and experimental observation has established that the cerebrospinal fluid (CSF) is mainly formed by secretion from the choroid plexuses of the cerebral ventricles. That formed by the plexuses of the lateral ventricles passes through the interventricular foramina into the third ventricle. Thence the fluid flows through the cerebral aqueduct into the fourth ventricle, which it leaves by the median and two lateral foramina (of Magendie and Luschka) of the fourth ventricle to reach the subarachnoid space covering the cerebrum and also the spinal cord. The subarachnoid space, which lies between the arachnoid membrane externally and the pia mater internally, carries the fluid from the cerebral ventricles to its points of absorption. The inner surface of the arachnoid and the outer surface of the pia are covered with flattened mesothelial cells; these also cover the numerous trabeculae, which bridge the subarachnoid space, and the nerves and blood vessels which pass across it. The subarachnoid space is deepest at the base of the brain; its expansions constitute the various cisterns, the largest of which is the cerebellomedullary cistern or cisterna magna which lies between the cerebellum and medulla and extends downwards below the foramen magnum behind the spinal cord.

The subarachnoid space extends superficially over the whole surface of the brain and spinal cord. Every blood vessel entering or leaving the nervous system must pass across it. In so doing, it carries with it into the nervous system a sleeve of arachnoid immediately surrounding the vessel and a sleeve of pia mater more externally. Between the two lies an extension of the subarachnoid space, known as the perivascular or Virchow–Robin space which subdivides with each division of the vessel to terminate where the pia mater and arachnoid become continuous. Probably, products of metabolism and cell-containing inflammatory exudates pass from the perivascular spaces to enter the CSF in the subarachnoid space, but must cross the tight junctions of the capillary endothelial cells which largely constitute the blood/CSF and blood/brain barriers in order to do so. These barriers may be damaged by inflammation and other processes and it is in the perivascular spaces that cuffs of inflammatory cells are found in inflammatory disorders of the nervous system.

Much work involving clinical observations in man and experimental studies in animals using studies of spinal drainage, of isotopic exchange, of ventriculo–cisternal perfusion (see Fishman 1980), manometric infusion techniques (Ekstedt 1977), and radiographic contrast studies, most recently employing metrizamide washout to measure CSF bulk flow (Rottenberg, Howieson, and Deck 1977) as well as biochemical investigations upon the composition of ventricular, cisternal, and spinal samples of fluid have shown that the fluid is largely formed by active secretion and transport via the choroid plexuses. Vesicular transport is probably also involved. The total *volume* of the fluid at any one time probably varies between 70 and 120 ml in different subjects and its *rate of formation* is about 0.35 ml/min. It is thus replaced several times each day. There is also known to be a constant process of dialysis, with exchange of various chemical constituents between the CSF and the blood across the ventricular ependyma, the perivascular spaces, and the arachnoid membrane at all levels. Large molecules fail to enter the CSF from the blood because of the interposition of the vascular endothelium (the blood/CSF barrier) but there is a rapid exchange of small-molecular-weight substances between the CSF and the extracellular fluid of the brain and cord. The fluid acts in some respect as a 'sink', preventing the extracellular fluid of the brain from achieving a true equilibrium with the blood plasma. The composition of ventricular CSF is very different from that of cisternal and spinal fluid, indicating that some components are added to the fluid across the spinal arachnoid.

After bathing the surface of the spinal cord and the base of the brain, CSF passes upwards over the convexity of the hemispheres, to be absorbed into the intracranial venous sinuses. Studies of bulk flow have shown that absorption takes place through the microscopic arachnoid villi, which are minute projections of the subarachnoid space into the lumen of the sinuses. The work of Welch and Friedman(1960) suggested that these operated as valves, but electron-microscopic studies by Tripathi (1973, 1974) demonstrated vacuoles within the cells of the villi which suggested that there is a dynamic system of transcellular channels or pores which allow the bulk outflow of CSF across the mesothelial barrier.

Appearance and chemical composition of CSF

Normal CSF is crystal-clear and colourless. Any visible discoloration is due to the presence of pigment and is pathological. The fluid becomes turbid when it contains about 400 cells/mm^3 but a pleocytosis (see below) of much less than this number may produce cloudiness visible with the naked eye if one makes use of the Tyndall effect (see Fishman 1980; Wood 1980a) by examining a glass tube of the fluid against direct sunlight. In Table 1.3 (from Fishman 1980), the composition of the normal lumbar CSF is compared with that of the serum.

Table 1.3. *Composition of normal lumbar cerebrospinal fluid and serum*[*]

	Cerebrospinal fluid		Serum		
Osmolarity	295	mOsm/l	295	mOsm/l	
Water content	99	%	93	%	
Sodium	138.0	mEq/l	138.0	mEq/1	
Potassium	2.8	mEq/l	4.5	mEq/l	
Calcium	2.1	mEq/l	4.8	mEq/l	
Magnesium	2.3	mEq/l	1.7	mEq/l	
Chloride	119.0	mEq/l	102.0	mEq/l	
Bicarbonate	22.0	mEq/l	24.0	mEq/l	(arterial)
CO_2 tension	47.0	mm Hg	41.0	mm Hg	(arterial)
pH	7.33		7.41		(arterial)
Oxygen	43.0	mm Hg	104.0	mm Hg	(arterial)
Glucose	60.0	mg/dl	90.0	mg/dl	
Lactate	1.6	mEq/l	1.0	mEq/l	(arterial)
Pyruvate	0.08	mEq/1	0.11	mEq/1	(arterial)
Lactate/pyruvate ratio	26.0		17.6		(arterial)
Fructose	4.0	mg/dl	2.0	mg/dl	
Polyols	340	μmol/1	148.0	μmol/l	
Myoinositol	2.6	mg/dl	1.0	mg/dl	
Total protein	35.0	mg/dl	7.0	g/dl	
prealbumin	4	%	trace		
albumin	65	%	60	%	
alpha$_1$ globulin	4	%	5	%	
alpha$_2$ globulin	8	%	9	%	
beta globulin (beta$_1$+tau)	12	%	12	%	
gamma globulin	7	%	14	%	
IgG	1.2	mg/dl	987	mg/dl	
IgA	0.2	mg/dl	175	mg/dl	
IgM	0.06	mg/dl	70	mg/dl	
kappa/lambda ratio	1.0		1.0		
beta-trace protein	2.0	mg/dl	0.5	mg/dl	
fibronectin	3.0	μg/ml	300	μg/ml	
Total free amino acids	80.9	μmol/dl	228.0	μmol/dl	
Ammonia	24.0	μg/dl	37.0	μg/dl	(arterial)
Urea	4.7	mmol/l	5.4	mmol/l	
Creatinine	1.2	mg/dl	1.8	mg/dl	
Uric acid	0.25	mg/dl	5.50	mg/dl	
Putrescine	184.0	pmol/ml			
Spermidine	150.0	pmol/ml			
Total lipids	1.5	mg/dl	750.0	mg/dl	
free cholesterol	0.4	mg/dl	180.0	mg/dl	
cholesterol esters	0.3	mg/dl	126.0	mg/dl	
cAMP	20.0	nmol/l			
cGMP	0.68	nmol/l			
HVA	60.0	μg/ml			
5-HIAA	0.04	μg/ml			
Norepinephrine	200.0	pg/ml	350.0	pg/ml	
MHGP	15.0	pg/ml			
Acetylcholine	1.8	mg/dl			
Choline	2.5	mM/ml			
Prostaglandin PGF$_2$ alpha	92.0	pg/ml			
Insulin	3.7	mμ/ml	36.0	mμ/ml	
Gastrin	3.4	pmol/l			
Cholecystokinin	14.0	pmol/l			
Beta endorphin	145.0	pmol/l	10.0	pmol/l	
Phosphorus	1.6	mg/dl	4.0	mg/dl	
Iron	1.5	μg/dl	15.0	mg/dl	

[*]Average or representative values are given. (Reproduced from Fishman (1980) by kind permission of the author and publisher.)

Functions of the CSF

The CSF provides physical support for the brain, acting as a cushion and protecting it from jars and shocks. It also assists in regulating the intracranial pressure, supports the intracranial venous sinuses, and absorbs much of the pressure waves transmitted to it by pulsations of the arteries within the cranial and spinal subarachnoid space (Bowsher 1953, 1957; O'Connell 1970). The spinal dural sac is a distensible reservoir which readily changes its capacity in response to pressure gradients developed in the subarachnoid space as determined, for example, by pressure changes in intracranial venous sinuses and in the spinal venous plexuses (Martins, Wiley, and Myers 1972).

Undoubtedly the fluid also possesses an excretory function, being concerned with the removal of products of cerebral metabolism such as carbon dioxide, lactate, and hydrogen ions. Its sink action (Davson 1967) is evident from the fact that the concentration of some polar (water-soluble) markers, such as iodide, bromide, thiocyanate, and sucrose, is lower in the CSF than in the brain. It appears that they enter the brain slowly from the blood and then diffuse slowly into the CSF from which they are rapidly removed by bulk flow. There is also evidence that the CSF distributes, by intracerebral transport, biologically active substances within the central nervous system. For example, certain hormones such as thyrotropin-releasing factor originate in the hypothalamus, enter the third ventricular CSF, and are then conveyed to the pituitary gland (Knigge, Scott, Kobayashi, and Ishii 1975; Fishman 1980). The CSF also contributes to the functions of the blood–brain barrier by regulating the composition of the extracellular fluid of the brain both under normal circumstances and in disease states. The pH of the fluid, which is normally maintained at about 7.31, and which is largely determined by its CO_2 tension, probably plays a part in the central regulation of respiration (Cameron 1969; Johnson 1972).

Methods of obtaining CSF

To obtain CSF for examination it is necessary to puncture either the cerebral ventricles or the subarachnoid space, either in the cisterna magna or in the lumbar theca beyond the termination of the spinal cord.

Lumbar puncture

Lumbar puncture is the simplest method of obtaining CSF and is so frequently used that every practitioner of medicine should be capable of carrying it out. The spinal cord terminates at the lower border of the first lumbar vertebra in the adult, and at a slightly lower level in the child. The arachnoid continues downwards below the termination of the spinal cord as far as the second sacral vertebra, and forms a lumbar cul-de-sac of the subarachnoid space normally containing CSF and crossed by the roots of the cauda equina. A needle can be introduced into this space without risk of injuring the cord.

Indications and contra-indications

Lumbar puncture is carried out in order to: (1) obtain CSF for cytological, chemical, and other investigations and to estimate its pressure; (2) introduce into the subarachnoid space therapeutic substances or local anaesthetics; (3) introduce air into the subarachnoid space for encephalography or myelography; (4) introduce opaque media for myelography.

There are several important contra-indications. When the intracranial pressure is raised and especially when there is reason to suspect a tumour in the posterior fossa of the skull, sudden withdrawal of fluid from the spinal canal may cause herniation of the medulla and cerebellar tonsils into the foramen magnum—the 'cerebellar pressure cone'—with fatal results. When a space-occupying lesion is present or suspected in one cerebral hemisphere, herniation of the medial part of the temporal lobe through the tentorial hiatus and the resultant compression and distortion of the upper brainstem may be equally disastrous. However, in cases of benign intracranial hypertension, lumbar puncture is safe and may even be beneficial as it temporarily reduces the pressure. Thus papilloedema is not necessarily a contra-indication. A CT scan (p. 80) should be done first in all patients with papilloedema and if this reveals no evidence of a mass lesion or of obstruction to, or displacement of, the ventricular system, lumbar puncture can then generally be considered safe. Skin sepsis or extradural suppuration in the lumbar region is also a contra-indication to lumbar puncture, owing to the risk of infecting the spinal canal. Marked spinal deformity in the dorsal or lumbar regions may render it difficult or impossible.

Method of puncture

Lumbar puncture may be performed with the patient either sitting or lying on one side. As many patients cannot sit up, it is common to perform the procedure with the patient lying on his left side. In either position the most important point is to secure the greatest possible degree of flexion of the lumbar spine. If the patient is conscious and co-operative, he is asked to bend his legs until his knees approach his chin and then to clasp his hands beneath his knees, or an assistant can aid flexion of the spine by applying pressure with one hand behind the neck and the other beneath the knees. With the patient in position, the next step is to find the landmarks. A line joining the highest points of the iliac crests, which may be marked with a swab dipped in a suitable antiseptic, usually passes between the third and fourth lumbar spinous processes, and the puncture is performed either at this point or preferably between the fourth and fifth spines, especially in children in whom the conus extends further down the lumbar canal than in adults. The skin is now cleaned and may be anaesthetized with local anaesthetic such as procaine. A general anaesthetic is necessary only in the case of delirious or excitable patients who cannot be maintained in position. Many suitable needles, about 8 cm in length, and of gauge 18–22, with an internal stylet, are available. A sterile technique is essential and gloves should be worn.

The needle, with the stylet in position, is now introduced midway between the spinous processes in the selected interspace in the midline. The cutting edges of the bevelled point should be directed upwards and downwards and not transversely, since the fibres of the ligamenta flava and of the dura run longitudinally. After its point has entered the skin the needle is passed forwards and slightly upwards in the sagittal plane. At an average depth of about 4.5 cm the point of the needle encounters the increased resistance of the ligamentum subflavum and, after penetrating a further 0.5 cm, it should enter the subarachnoid space. The stylet is now withdrawn and laid upon a sterile towel and, if the puncture has been successful, CSF drips from the butt of the needle. After the pressure has been measured as described below, the fluid is collected in two sterile test-tubes consecutively, about 3 ml being allowed to run into each. One sample is used for microbiological examination, the other for cytology and chemistry. The needle is then withdrawn. The patient may complain of pain in one leg when the needle enters the subarachnoid space. This is due to the point coming into contact with one of the roots of the cauda equina, which, however, is not likely to be damaged. Care should be taken not to introduce the needle too far lest a paravertebral vein or an intervertebral disc should be injured.

A dry tap

Often a failure to obtain fluid means that the puncure has been incorrectly carried out. The point of the needle may not have entered the subarachnoid space either because it has been introduced too obliquely in the longitudinal plane, because it has deviated to one side, or because, on account of scoliosis or arthritis, the interspace is difficult to find. It may not have penetrated far enough, or may have gone too far, the point coming into contact with the posterior wall of the vertebral body where puncture of a vein is the commonest cause of blood in the fluid. The stylet should be passed into the needle again to remove any possible obstruction and the depth of the point varied. Gentle suction with a syringe is then applied. If no fluid comes, the needle should be withdrawn and reinserted either in the same interspace or in the one above or below. A genuine dry tap, when the point of the needle is in the subarachnoid space, may occur when the spinal subarachnoid space is blocked at a higher level and hence the pressure of the fluid in the lumbar sac is low, or when the lumbar sac itself is filled by a neoplasm or by a developmental lesion (lipoma or epidermoid), as in spina bifida.

Sequelae of lumbar puncture
The commonest sequel of lumbar puncture is headache, which comes on after a few hours, is throbbing in character, and may be associated with nausea, vomiting, giddiness, and pain in the neck and back. In severe cases it is literally prostrating, being much intensified by sitting up, and lasting for days or even exceptionally for weeks. It is due to lowered intracranial tension produced by a continued leakage of CSF through the puncture wound in the theca. Certain precautions may help to prevent 'lumbar puncture headache'. The needle used should be as small as possible in calibre, and introduced with the cutting edges in the sagittal plane. As little fluid as is needed should be withdrawn and it has been thought to be helpful if the patient lies down for a few hours afterwards. Brocker (1958) suggested that if the patient lies prone rather than supine, a positive rather than a negative pressure in the extradural space is produced and discourages leakage of fluid. However, Smith, Perkin, and Rose(1980) found rest in the prone position to be of no value and Carbaat and van Crevel (1981), in a careful trial, found that the incidence of headaches was the same in 50 patients who were up and about immediately after the procedure as in another 50 who received 24 hours' bed rest. If in spite of all precautions headache develops, analgesics may be needed. Hydration with intravenous fluid is of no value (Tourtellotte, Haever, Heller, and Somers 1964) but the use of a 'blood patch' (Ostheimer, Palahniak, and Shnider 1974), involving the epidural injection of homologous blood to seal the puncture hole in the dura is sometimes helpful (see Fishman 1980).

Lumbar puncture occasionally causes an intensification of symptoms of the disease from which the patient is suffering. Root pains, if present, may be intensified; this is especially liable to occur when a lesion is compressing the spinal cord, as symptoms may then be exacerbated by the alterations of pressure induced by the withdrawal of fluid. In multiple sclerosis, relapses have been attributed to lumbar puncture, but there is no convincing evidence to indicate that this is a significant risk. The risks of lumbar puncture when the intracranial pressure is greatly increased have already been described. Rare complications include diplopia (due to transient unilateral or bilateral sixth-nerve palsy, presumably consequent upon intracranial hypotension),subarachnoid bleeding or spinal subdural haematoma (especially in patients with thrombocytopenia or other haemorrhagic disorders, in whom the procedure is best avoided), introduction of leukaemic cells or of micro-organisms into the subarachnoid space, and prolapsed intervertebral disc following puncture of the annulus fibrosis. Intrathecal seeding of epidermal cells leading to the formation of an epidermoid is avoided by using a needle with a stylet (see Fishman 1980). Meningitis following lumbar puncture is fortunately rare and is due to a failure to preserve asepsis during the procedure.

Ventricular puncture

While ventricular puncture, via a burr hole (in older children and adults) or via the lateral angle of the anterior fontanelle (in young infants), was used commonly in the past to reduce the intracranial pressure prior to operation in patients with intracranial tumour, or to inject air for ventriculography, it was also sometimes used in order to inject an antibiotic into the lateral ventricle in some cases of meningitis. Because of improvements in the technique of reducing intracranial pressure, and the advent of the CT scan and newer antibiotics, it is now very rarely used.

Cisternal puncture

The cisterna magna (cerebellomedullary cistern) which is penetrated in cisternal puncture is a dilatation of the subarachnoid space lying between the inferior surface of the cerebellum above, the posterior surface of the medulla and spinal cord in front, and the dura mater of the posterior atlanto-occipital membrane and upper cervical canal below and behind.

Indications and contra-indications for cisternal puncture
The principal indications for cisternal puncture are: (1) to obtain CSF for examination when lumbar puncture is impossible, for example, on account of lumbar suppuration or disease or deformity of the spine; (2) to compare the composition or pressure of the cisternal and lumbar fluids; (3) to inject opaque media when lumbar myelography is impossible, or when the upper as well as the lower limits of a spinal lesion must be defined; (4) to introduce therapeutic substances, such as an antibiotic; (5) very rarely, to introduce air for encephalography. Cisternal puncture should never be carried out when there is reason to suspect a tumour or abscess in the posterior fossa, when there is a marked rise of intracranial pressure, or when the cistern is likely to be obliterated by inflammatory adhesions, or to be the site of a congenital abnormality (e.g. a Chiari malformation).

Method of cisternal puncture
The patient is prepared by shaving the scalp up to a horizontal line at the level of the external occipital protuberance. The skin is then cleaned with a suitable antiseptic. The patient should be seated and his head is held by an assistant with both hands and well flexed. The operator places the tip of the forefinger of his left hand upon the spinous process of the second cervical vertebra, which is the highest palpable spinous process. A spot 1 cm above this point is anaesthetized with procaine. A lumbar puncture needle with the stylet in position is then inserted at this point and passed forwards in a plane which passes through the point of introduction, the middle of the external acoustic meatus, and the nasion. At a depth of about 3 cm the point of the needle will encounter the posterior atlanto-occipital membrane, which offers considerable resistance. On gently introducing it a further 0.5 cm it should penetrate the cistern, and on withdrawal of the stylet CSF usually drips from the needle. Often, however, although the point of the needle is in the cistern, there is no flow of fluid. This may be promoted by exerting gentle suction with a syringe. The medulla lies at a depth of about 4 cm in front of the posterior atlanto-occipital membrane. With care, therefore, there is no risk that the point of the needle will enter the medulla. It should not, however, be introduced more than 6–7 cm from the surface of the skin. If the operator is unaccustomed to cisternal puncture, it may be made easier if the point of the needle is directed slightly above the plane described, so that it strikes the occipital bone. It is then slightly depressed to pass through the membrane. Headache may follow cisternal puncture. Its prophylaxis and treatment are the same as those described above for lumbar puncture.

Lateral cervical puncture

This technique, introduced in recent years (Zivin 1978), is a useful alternative to cisternal puncture and is used especially as a method of myelography for the demonstration of cervical spinal lesions, using water-soluble media such as metrizamide. The patient lies in bed supine without a pillow and, after preparation of the skin and the injection of local anaesthetic, a lumbar puncture needle is inserted 1 cm caudal and 1 cm posterior to the tip of the mastoid process. It is then advanced slowly parallel to the bed and at right angles to the neck until it passes through the C1–2 interface and enters the spinal canal. The stylet must be removed frequently to see whether fluid is flowing and suction may be applied. Care must be taken not to advance the needle too far, otherwise it will enter the spinal cord, and it must be carefully supported throughout. Fluoroscopic control may be used to ensure correct positioning of the needle (Grainger and Lamb 1980).

Measurement of the CSF pressure

Method of determination. The pressure of the CSF can be measured with a simple manometer. A graduated glass tube is attached to the lumbar puncture needle and the observer reads the height in mm to which the fluid ascends in the tube. Various instruments include two-way stopcocks which permit fluid to be withdrawn without removing the manometer. For routine purposes the pressure is determined with the patient lying on the left side, and it is important to see that the head is at the same level as the lumbar spine. Lumbar puncture having been performed, the tap is turned so that the fluid rises in the manometer. The patient should then be allowed to straighten his spine, relax his muscles, and breathe quietly and regularly, as muscular tension and holding the breath raise the pressure. Pressure is measured in mm of CSF and normally shows oscillations corresponding to respiration and finer variations synchronous with the arterial pulse. The normal CSF pressure in adults in the horizontal position is 60-150 mm of fluid. It is often lower in children, in whom it is normally from 45 to 90 mm of fluid, which is usually less than the height of the vertex above the needle. Hence in the sitting posture the pressure in the ventricles and cerebellomedullary cistern may be negative. Various techniques including differential-pressure manometry and electromanometry (Gilland and Nelson 1970) have been introduced in order to measure rapid changes in pressure, and Avezaat, Van Eijndhoven, and Wyper (1979) have shown that measurement of the CSF pulse pressure may be helpful in assessing intracranial volume–pressure relationships. Significant changes occur with arterial hypertension, physical exertion, postural alterations, and coughing (Williams 1976).

Pathological variations of pressure. An abnormally high pressure is found, for example, in cases of intracranial tumour and haemorrhage, hypertensive encephalopathy, benign intracranial hypertension, hypervitaminosis A, hydrocephalus, intracranial sinus thrombosis, meningism, and in various forms of meningitis, encephalitis, and encephalopathy. The pressure may also be raised in uraemia and in cor pulmonale. In a relaxed patient a pressure exceeding 300 ml of fluid is abnormal; except in benign intracranial hypertension or meningitis the needle should be withdrawn if the pressure exceeds this level and there will then be sufficient fluid in the manometer for examination.

A subnormal pressure occasionally follows head injury and may result from dehydration; a syndrome of idiopathic intracranial hypotension is no longer thought to exist. A subnormal pressure is also seen when the lumbar subarachnoid space cannot communicate with the cerebral space. This is commonest in cases of spinal subarachnoid block due to spinal tumour or localized spinal meningitis. It may also occur when a block exists at or near the foramen magnum due to a tumour, syrinx, congenital anomaly, or arachnoiditis in this situation. The pressure may also be abnormally low if a second lumbar puncture is performed shortly after a previous one.

Queckenstedt's test. Normally, if one compresses the jugular veins digitally or with a cuff (cuff manometrics see Fishman 1980) during lumbar puncture, there is an immediate and rapid rise in the pressure of the CSF which quickly reaches 300 mm of fluid and almost as rapidly falls to normal when compression

ceases. Venous compression causes raised pressure in the intracranial venous sinuses and hence in the cranium. Communication of this raised pressure with displacement of fluid into the manometer attached to the lumbar puncture needle (Bowsher 1953) depends upon the patency of the subarachnoid space between the cranial cavity and the lumbar sac. When the subarachnoid space is obstructed in the region of the foramen magnum or within the spinal canal, the rise of pressure is either absent or slight in extent and slow in appearing, according to whether the block is complete or incomplete. In cervical lesions the accuracy of the test may be improved by flexion or hyperextension of the neck as the block may vary in different positions of the head (Kaplan and Foster Kennedy 1950). When there is a block, the normal variations in pressure due to respiration and the arterial pulse are also diminished or absent, but abdominal compression may cause an exaggerated rise as raised intra-abdominal pressure is transmitted to spinal veins.

Compression of each jugular vein separately may help to identify thrombosis of one transverse sinus for if a sinus is obstructed, there will usually be no rise of CSF when the jugular vein on the affected side is compressed (the Tobey–Ayer test).

Clinical experience has, however, shown that Queckenstedt's test is often unreliable and, with the increasing use of contrast methods of radiological investigation, it is now used less frequently. Its accuracy can, however, be improved by using electromanometrics.

Naked-eye appearance

Turbidity. Turbidity of the CSF is usually due to an excess of polymorphonuclear cells. In acute meningitis these may be present in such numbers that a purulent deposit forms and the supernatant fluid may be yellow. Only rarely does a lymphocytic pleocytosis cause turbidity, but malignant cells can do so in carcinomatous meningitis.

Fibrin clot. A clot of fibrin in a specimen of fluid implies the presence of fibrinogen. Such a clot may occur either in a fluid of which the protein content is only slightly raised or in fluids with a very high protein content as in spinal subarachnoid block or the Guillain–Barré syndrome. In the former situation the clot forms a faint 'cobweb' which takes from 12 to 24 hours to appear. It is most typical of tuberculous meningitis, but also occurs occasionally in other forms of meningitis and in neurosyphilis or poliomyelitis. The clot which forms in fluids containing large amounts of protein may solidify the whole specimen.

Blood. Blood may be present in the CSF, either as an accidental result of injury to an intrathecal vein by the lumbar puncture needle, or as the product of previous haemorrhage into the subarachnoid space. This distinction is obviously of great importance. When a vein is injured at lumbar puncture, the specimen collected in the first tube is often blood-stained, but the second or third usually shows little or no visible blood, whereas after subarachnoid haemorrhage both specimens are uniformly blood-stained. Further, in the former case, if the specimen is centrifuged, the supernatant fluid is seen to be colourless, whereas within a few hours of subarachnoid haemorrhage the supernatant fluid is discoloured (see below). In cases of doubt, spectrophotometry and cytological study of the fluid using the Sayk technique (see below) usually resolve the matter (Buruma, Janson, Van den Bergh, and Bots 1981). *Subarachnoid haemorrhage* may be due to head injury, to the rupture of an intracranial aneurysm or angioma, or to the spread of an intracerebral haemorrhage into either the ventricular system or the subarachnoid space; other causes are uncommon (p. 209). After subarachnoid haemorrhage xanthochromia (see below) appears in a few hours and reaches it greatest intensity at the end of about a week. It has usually disappeared in two to four weeks. The red cells generally disappear from the fluid in three to seven days. Blood in contact with the leptomeninges excites a cellular reaction, and the fluid therefore usually contains a moderate excess of white cells. As a rule these are all mononuclear, but excess polymorphonuclear cells may be found in the early stages.

Xanthochromia. Xanthochromia, or yellow discoloration of the CSF, is found, as described above, after subarachnoid haemorrhage and also when pus is present in considerable amount in the fluid. In subarachnoid haemorrhage, faint xanthochromia due to oxyhaemoglobin appears within four to six hours, the deeper yellow coloration due to bilirubin in about two days; methaemoglobin is present only if there is extensive brain destruction (Barrows, Hunter, and Banker 1955). Xanthochromic fluid is also often found after intracerebral haemorrhage, less often after cerebral infarction, and in some cases of intracranial tumour, especially when the tumour lies near the ventricular system, or arises from the sheath of the eighth nerve. It is also seen in fluid obtained below an obstruction of the spinal subarachnoid space and sometimes in fluid removed above a tumour of the cauda equina or in polyneuritis. A slight yellow coloration may be present in cases of severe jaundice.

Kjellin and Söderström (1974) have shown that the spectrophotometric identification of pigments in the fluid may be of some value in the differential diagnosis of cerebral vascular disease.

Cytological and chemical abnormalities

For details of the techniques normally employed in staining, counting, and identifying cells in the CSF, see Davson (1967) and Fishman (1980). While the counting of cells stained with the Wright or May–Grünwald/Giemsa stains in a Neubauer or Fuchs–Rosenthal haemocytometer is still commonly used in routine clinical practice, many specialized cytological techniques (Sayk 1966), using various forms of cytocentrifuge, and many techniques of sedimentation cytomorphology (Marks and Marrack 1960; Jager 1969; Dyken 1975), fixation and staining (Stokes, O'Hara, Buchanan, and Olson 1975), as well as methods of characterizing lymphocyte subtypes (B and T cells) using immunological techniques (Levinson, Lisak, and Zweiman 1976; Kam-Hansen 1979) are now widely employed.

Cells

The normal CSF contains not more than four or five lymphocytes/mm^3. In disease, many types of cell may be present sometimes in very large numbers. Those most frequently encountered are lymphocytes, large mononuclear cells, and polymorphonuclear cells. Less frequently eosinophils, plasma cells, macrophages, basophils, choroidal, ependymal, and arachnoidal cells, or, in neoplastic conditions, malignant cells of many kinds may be found. Yeasts, amoebae, echinococci, and cysticerci may be found in cases of infection of the nervous system with these organisms.

Significance of cell content. Radioactive labelling has shown that the various leucocytes and even the macrophages are derived from the circulating blood and presumably enter the CSF via the perivascular spaces (Fishman 1980). In general, a pleocytosis, or excess of cells in the spinal fluid, indicates meningeal irritation, though not necessarily meningeal infection. Whether the cellular increase is polymorphonuclear depends partly upon the acuteness of the pathological process and partly, in infective conditions, upon the nature of the infecting organism. A predominantly polymorphonuclear count is usually found in acute infections and in acute exacerbations of chronic infections. But while pyogenic organisms excite a mainly polymorphonuclear reaction, except when chronic, a mononuclear pleocytosis is seen in infections with most viruses, though polymorphonuclear cells are sometimes present when the infection is most acute. We thus encounter predominantly polymorphonuclear, predominantly mononuclear, and mixed cell counts.

A predominantly polymorphonuclear pleocytosis is found in meningitis due to pyogenic organisms, including the meningococcus, staphylococcus, streptococcus, pneumococcus, *Escherichia coli*, *Salmonella typhi*, *Listeria monocytogenes*, and *Haemophilus influenzae*. In these conditions the cells are usually present in very large numbers. Acute syphilitic meningitis may also excite a polymorphonuclear reaction with several thousand cells/mm^3. Mononuclear pleocytosis rarely exceeds 200 cells/mm^3 and more commonly lies between 10 and 50 cells/mm^3. Counts of up to 1000 per mm^3, however, may occur in various forms of virus meningitis. A mononuclear reaction is characteristic of syphilis of the nervous system, encephalitis, multiple sclerosis, poliomyelitis (after the first few days), herpes zoster, acute lymphocytic choriomeningitis, and some cases of tuberculous meningitis. It may also be found in mumps, infectious mononucleosis, whooping cough, malaria, trypanosomiasis, relapsing fever, and leptospirosis canicola or icterohaemorrhagica. In the normal individual the few mononuclear cells in the CSF are mostly round immunocompetent lymphocytes, but in inflammatory disorders, whether infective or auto-immune, these cells become activated and are mostly large lymphoid cells but some are activated monocytes. Macrophages are seen especially after destruction of cerebral tissue as in infarction, siderophages (containing iron) following haemorrhage, and eosinophils in various parasitic and granulomatous inflammatory states (see Fishman 1980). Cerebral tumour may cause a slight mononuclear pleocytosis, especially when the tumour lies close to the meninges. So also may cerebral abscess, intracranial sinus thrombosis, and subarachnoid haemorrhage. The mixed type of pleocytosis, in which polymorphonuclear and mononuclear cells are present in approximately equal numbers, is also found in cerebral abscess, in which case the number of cells is often small, and in cases of infection of the bones of the skull in the neighbourhood of the meninges. A mixed cell count is also present in many cases of tuberculous meningitis, in poliomyelitis during the first few days, and in the more acute forms of syphilitic meningitis. A transient slight pleocytosis, sometimes containing polymorphonuclear cells or even eosinophils but more often mononuclears, may follow lumbar puncture, myelography, or pneumoencephalography.

Plasma cells, as well as the mononuclear forms mentioned above, are sometimes found in the fluid, usually in inflammatory disorders but sometimes in malignant disease (Péter 1967; Oehmichen 1976). Specialized cytological techniques (see above) are now employed increasingly and usually detect malignant cells in cases of carcinomatosis of the meninges, or meningeal leukaemia or lymphoma. Even in cases of cerebral tumour, malignant cells may be found, but positive findings are obtained in only about 10–20 per cent of cases of glioma and 20–30 per cent with intracranial metastases (Marks and Marrack 1960; Jager 1969). False positive results are very rare, false negatives more common; a positive result almost always reflects leptomeningeal tumour (Glass, Melamed, Chernik, and Posner 1979). Immunofluorescent techniques of examining fresh or cultured cells obtained from the fluid have proved helpful in the rapid diagnosis of viral encephalitis, meningitis, and cryptococcosis (Dayan and Stokes 1973; Lindeman 1974, Muller, Versteeg, Bots, and Peters 1974) and in differentiating B and T lymphocytes.

Protein

The total protein content of the normal CSF is 0.15–0.45 g/l. This consists of albumin and globulin in a ratio of 8 to 1. Increase of the protein of the fluid is extremely common. A moderate increase, usually to below 2.0 g/l, is found in inflammatory disorders of the brain and meninges, such as the various forms of meningitis, encephalitis, poliomyelitis, multiple sclerosis, and neurosyphilis. Intracranial tumour and cerebral haemorrhage or infarction may also cause a moderate rise of protein content. In cases of acoustic neuroma the protein often rises to more than 1.0 g/l, while in the Guillain-Barré syndrome increases to 10 g/l or more may occur.

Froin's syndrome is the name originally given to a condition in which the spinal fluid is xanthochromic, contains, as a rule, more than 5.0 g/l of protein, and rapidly clots on standing. It is a phenomenon of multiple aetiology and may even be seen in polyneuropathy, but more often results from a spinal block due to tumour, localized spinal meningitis, or epidural abscess. The block causes stagnation of the CSF in the lumbar dural sac distal to the block with exudation or transudation of proteinaceous material from the tumour itself or from the blood. Similar fluid is sometimes obtained when lumbar puncture is performed above a cauda equina tumour. In Froin's original cases there was also pleocytosis as his patients were suffering from localized spinal meningitis.

Fractionation of CSF proteins
Many reactions were used in the past to identify an excess of globulin in the CSF. Various reagents (ammonium sulphate in the *Nonne-Apelt reaction*, butyric acid in the *Noguchi reaction*, carbolic acid in *Pandy's reaction*, and mercuric chloride in *Weichbrodt's reaction*) were used to precipitate the globulin, giving varying degrees of opalescence of the fluid. *Lange's colloidal gold reaction* was more precise and, until largely superseded by modern quantitative techniques of estimating immunoglobulins, it proved to be of great diagnostic value. In carrying out the test, increasing dilutions of CSF were added to a series of 10 test-tubes containing the reagent and the resultant colorimetric change from cherry-red to blue was graded on a six-point scale from 0 to 5 in each tube. Normal samples of fluid gave little or no precipitation and consequent colour change. The so-called *'paretic' curve* (5555432100) was characteristic of general paresis and sometimes occurred in meningovascular syphilis and tabes; it was also found in up to 50 per cent of cases of multiple sclerosis and sometimes after subarachnoid haemorrhage. The luetic or tabetic curve (1233321000) was more typical of tabes dorsalis, while the meningitic curve (0012344310) was often seen in syphilitic and bacterial meningitis.

More recently many newer techniques have been used to estimate CSF protein fractions in health and disease. These have included chemical precipitation, immunoprecipitation, paper and agar gel electrophoresis, immunoelectrophoresis, and isoelectric focusing. Prealbumin, albumin, alpha$_1$-globulin, alpha$_2$-globulin, betaglobulin (and their subfractions), as well as gammaglobulin (IgG, IgA, IgM, IgD, and a trace of IgF) are all present in normal CSF. Alpha$_2$-globulin is lower in CSF than in serum, as is gammaglobulin (12 per cent of total CSF protein, 18 per cent of total serum protein) and almost all the gammaglobulin in normal CSF is IgG (see Table 1.3). In disease states which alter the blood–brain barrier and cause a rise in total CSF protein or in those such as multiple sclerosis, neurosyphilis, or auto-immune disorders, in which immunoglobulins are manufactured in the nervous system (Dencker and Swahn 1961; Link 1967), various macromolecules not normally present in CSF or present in very small quantities may pass into the CSF from the serum or from the nervous parenchyma (see Fishman 1980). There is now a voluminous literature on changes in the major immunoglobulins, IgG, IgA, and IgM, measured by radioimmunoassay or immunochemical assay in various diseases (Tourtellotte 1970; Lumsden 1972; Laterre 1975; Fishman 1980). Riddoch and Thompson (1970) found that the IgG was raised above the normal upper limit (more than 13 per cent of total protein) in 63 per cent of patients with multiple sclerosis and in only 14 per cent of patients with other neurological diseases, including neurosyphilis. However, Fischer-Williams and Roberts (1971) found that measurement of the total gammaglobulin electrophoretic fraction on concentrated fluid correlated better (over 14 per cent of total protein in 94 per cent of cases) with the diagnosis of multiple sclerosis than did the measurement of IgG by electroimmunodiffusion (over 14 per cent of total protein in 75 per

cent of cases). The typical quantitative change in the immunoglobulins seen in multiple sclerosis has been called oligoclonal banding (Paty, Donnelly, and Bernardo 1978). Isoelectric focusing on thin-layer polyacrylamide gel has been used to add precision to this technique (Latner 1973; Kjellin and Vesterberg 1974) and has shown that, whereas polyclonal IgG migrates as multiple bands between pH 4.7 and 8.6, oligoclonal IgG in multiple sclerosis and neurosyphilis migrates between pH 8.6 and 9.5 and is easily discriminated from other proteins (Laurenzi and Link 1979). In all forms of acute meningitis, IgA and IgG levels are increased in the fluid (Smith, Bannister, and O'Shea 1973). The percentage of IgG in the fluid is lower in children (usually less than 8 per cent of total protein) (Nellhaus 1971; Harms 1975). There is also increasing evidence, using isoelectric focusing and immunofixation, that oligoclonal bands are found in various forms of meningoencephalitis, in subacute sclerosing panencephalitis, and in the Guillain-Barré syndrome (Sidén and Kjellin 1979) and minor abnormalities have also been detected in cases of hereditary ataxia (Kjellin and Stibler 1975). Variations in the kappa/lambda ratios of IgG light chains may also prove to be of diagnostic value (Fishman 1980). The terminal component of complement (C9) is also increased often in the fluid in multiple sclerosis (Morgan, Campbell, and Compston 1984).

Myelin basic protein may also appear in the CSF in demyelination (McKhann 1978); fibronectin is greatly increased in the fluid in some patients with glioma, interferon is also present in some patients with viral infections, and various other trace proteins have been found in a variety of diseases (see Fishman 1980). Ferritin, the major iron storage protein, is increased in the fluid in patients with meningoencephalitis, in cerebral vascular disease, and in some patients with dementia (Sindic, Collet-Cassart, Cambiaso, Masson, and Laterre 1981).

Phospholipids
The total phospholipid content of the fluid may be increased in a number of neurological diseases but a relative rise in the content of cephalin is seen in patients with demyelinating processes (Zilkha and McArdle 1963).

Glucose
The normal glucose content of the CSF is somewhat lower than that of the blood and lies between 0.5 and 0.85 g/l. The glucose content of the fluid is diminished in meningitis and indeed in pyogenic meningitis sugar is usually absent. A moderate decrease to 0.1–0.5 g/l is characteristic of tuberculous meningitis, certain other chronic meningitides (e.g. cryptococcosis, sarcoidosis), and carcinomatosis of the meninges. The low CSF glucose results from increased glucose utilization by the nervous system and by polymorphonuclear cells and from alterations in the membrane carrier system normally concerned with transfer of glucose from the blood to CSF. A low CSF glucose level in the absence of hypoglycaemia is indicative of a diffuse generalized meningeal disorder (Fishman 1980). A rise in the glucose content of the fluid is found in diabetes parallel to that in the blood.

Electrolytes
In hyponatraemia and hypernatraemia, the CSF *sodium* level changes in the same direction as the plasma level but the CSF changes are often less in degree. The CSF *potassium* concentration is very stable and is little affected by changes in the plasma level; there are no significant changes in disease. *Chloride* is the only chemical constituent, other than folate, to be maintained at a higher concentration in the CSF than in the blood; the normal concentration is 7.2–7.5 g/l, estimated as sodium chloride. It was once thought that a fall in chloride concentration was a useful guide to the diagnosis of tuberculous meningitis (Merritt and Fremont-Smith 1937) but it is now known that this change is simply a

consequence of repeated vomiting and that measurement of CSF chloride is of no value in clinical practice (Fishman 1980). Changes in CSF calcium, phosphorus, and magnesium usually follow those in the blood.

Acid–base balance
As already mentioned, the pH of CSF may play a role in regulating respiration. Respiratory and metabolic acidosis and alkalosis are normally accompanied by changes in the pH of the CSF; on the other hand, primary acidosis of the CSF in the presence of normal arterial blood pH has been found in subarachnoid haemorrhage, head injury, infarction, and meningitis (Sambrook, Hutchison, and Aber 1973 *a, b*; Brook, Bricknell, Overturf 1978). However, lumbar CSF analyses do not necessarily reflect changes in the brain (Plum and Price 1973) and the CSF data are much less reliable than measurement of arterial blood gases in guiding clinical management. Measurement of CSF lactate and pyruvate has also failed to yield useful diagnostic information.

Enzymes
Much work has been done in recent years upon the estimation of various enzymes in the CSF. Among others, Green, Oldewurtel, O'Doherty, Forster, and Sanchez-Longo (1957) and Katzman, Fishman, and Goldensohn (1957) found that *glutamic-oxalacetic transaminase* (aspartate aminotransferase) activity was raised in the fluid in some cases of cerebral infarction and multiple sclerosis, but Davies-Jones (1970), who studied that enzyme and *lactic dehydrogenase*, found normal activity in those conditions and in many other neurological disorders although the activity was raised in cases of carcinomatous neuropathy and of metastatic carcinoma in the nervous system. However, Wilcock, Sharpe, and Goldberg 1973 concluded that these enzymes in the fluid derived from those of the serum.

CSF *creatine kinase* activity is raised in cases of muscular dystrophy of the Duchenne type (Banerji, Jayam, and Desai 1969). Sherwin, Norris, and Bulcke (1969) found the activity of this enzyme to be raised in the fluid in 70 of 185 patients with neurological disease, and isoenzyme studies suggested that it was derived from brain and not muscle. However, an elevated activity of this enzyme was of no diagnostic value.

Riekkinen and Rinne (1970) also studied *non-specific esterases* and various *acid and alkaline proteinases* in the fluid. While increased activity of several of these enzymes was found in acute multiple sclerosis and in some cases of cerebral tumour, information of diagnostic value was not obtained. The myelin marker enzyme 2', 3'–cyclic nucleotide 3'-phosphohydrolase may also be raised in demyelinating diseases (Banik, Mauldin, and Hogan 1979). Fishman (1980) concludes that enzyme studies lack specificity and are of no value as routine diagnostic tests.

Sterols
The cholesterol and cholesterol ester content of the CSF is raised in some neurological diseases, especially in multiple sclerosis (Cumings 1953; Green, Papadopoulos, Cevallos, Forster, and Hess 1959) but this change is non-specific. Paoletti, Vandenheuvel, and Fumagalli (1969) showed that desmosterol (24-dehydrocholesterol) appeared in the fluid of many patients with gliomas after the administration of triparanol. Weiss, Ransohoff, and Kayden (1972) found more cholesterol in the fluid of patients with gliomas than in controls and confirmed an increase in CSF desmosterol in about 60 per cent of patients with glioma. Unfortunately, these measurements have proved to be of little diagnostic value (Fishman 1980).

Amino acids, GABA, and glutamine
While changes in the relative proportions of various amino acids in the CSF have been described in parkinsonism and in meningitis and febrile convulsions (van Sande, Mardens, Adriaenssens, and Lowenthal 1970; Heiblim, Evans, Glass, and Agbayani 1978), these changes lack specificity. The assay of CSF GABA, too, has not as yet proved to be of diagnostic value (Wood 1980*b*) but the measurement of CSF glutamine (mean normal level 126 ± 5.1 mg/l) has proved to be a valuable and reliable diagnostic test in suspected hepatic encephalopathy.

Biogenic amines
The CSF contains 5-hydroxyindoleacetic acid (5-HIAA), a metabolite of 5-hydroxytryptamine (serotonin or 5-HT), and also homovanillic acid (HVA), a metabolite of dopamine. Patients with parkinsonism in whom HVA is high in the fluid do not respond as well to treatment with levodopa as do those in whom it is low (Gumpert, Sharpe, and Curzon 1973). While blood levels of 5-HT are low in patients with Down's syndrome (mongolism), the 5-HIAA in the fluid is normal (Dubowitz and Rogers 1969). Studies of these metabolites in the fluid are throwing new light upon the biochemical basis of nervous disorders associated with abnormalities of the cerebral amines, perhaps even including endogenous depression (Moir, Ashcroft, Crawford, Eccleston, and Guldberg 1970) and schizophrenia, but many neurotransmitters do not cross the blood–brain barrier (Wood 1980*b*) and no place for these estimations in clinical diagnosis and management has yet been established.

Other metabolites
Among the many other substances measured in the CSF in various disease states have been histamine, acetylcholine, choline, prostaglandins, polyamines, creatine and creatinine, uric acid, hormones and peptides, vitamins (including B_{12} and folate), many other solutes and cyclic AMP (Fishman 1980; Wood 1980*b*), but these studies have to date failed to yield information of diagnostic value.

Keratin
The presence of keratin in the CSF may indicate the presence of an intracranial epidermoid cyst (Tomlinson and Walton 1967).

Serological reactions
Serological diagnostic tests used in the diagnosis of neurosyphilis are discussed in the section on syphilis.

Microbiological examination
In most forms of pyogenic meningitis the direct staining of a smear of a centrifuged deposit of cells obtained from the fluid will reveal the infecting organism, but meningococci are often curiously difficult to find, whereas pneumococci, for instance, are usually found in profusion. For the detection of tubercle bacilli the Ziehl-Neilsen technique is required. Viruses in the fluid may be detected by direct immunofluorescent techniques. Culture of the fluid, using a variety of different techniques, or sometimes animal inoculation, may be required in order to confirm the nature of the infecting organism, whether this is a bacterium, a virus, or some other form of pathogen. For details the reader is referred to texts on microbiology (e.g. Braude 1981).

CSF fistulae

Following head injury, raised intracranial pressure due to pituitary tumour, or to persistence of a craniopharyngeal canal (Kaufman 1969), fistulous communications may develop between the subarachnoid space and the paranasal sinuses or middle ear, resulting in a leakage of CSF, often giving rhinorrhoea. These fistulae may be detected and localized by means of a variety of biochemical and radiological techniques using such agents as radiosodium and radio-iodinated serum albumin (Crow, Keogh, and Northfield 1956; Ommaya, DiChiro, Baldwin, and Pennybacker 1968; Brisman, Hughes, and Mount 1970).

References

Avezaat, C. J. J., Van Eijndhoven, J. H. M., and Wyper, D. J. (1979).Cerebrospinal fluid pulse pressure and intracranial volume–pressure relationships. *J. Neurol. Neurosurg. Psychiat.* **42**, 687.

Banerji, A. P., Jayam, A. V., and Desai, A. D. (1969). Creatine phosphokinase activity of cerebrospinal fluid in muscular dystrophy and other neurological disorders. *Neurology, Bombay* **17**, 123.

Banik, N. L., Mauldin, L. B., and Hogan, E. L. (1979). Activity of 2', 3'-cyclic nucleotide 3'–phosphohydrolase in human cerebrospinal fluid. *Ann. Neurol.*. **5**, 539.

Barrows, L. T., Hunter, F.T., and Banker, B. Q. (1955). The nature and significance of pigment in the cerebrospinal fluid. *Brain* **78**, 59.

Bowsher, D. (1953). The cerebrospinal fluid pressure. *Brit. med. J.* **1**, 863.

—— (1957). Further considerations on cerebrospinal fluid dynamics. *Brit. med. J.* **2**, 971.

Braude, A. I. (1981). *Medical microbiology and infectious diseases. International textbook of medicine*, Vol II (ed. A. H. Samiy, L. H. Smith, and J. B. Wijngaarden). Saunders, Philadelphia.

Brisman, R., Hughes, J. E. O., and Mount, L. A. (1970). Cerebrospinal fluid rhinorrhea. *Arch. Neurol., Chicago.* **22**, 245.

Brocker, R. J. (1958). Technique to avoid spinal-tap headache. *J. Am. med. Ass.* **168**, 261.

Brook, I., Bricknell, K. S, and Overturf, G. D. (1978). Measurement of lactic acid in cerebrospinal fluid of patients with infections of the central nervous system, *J. infect. Dis.* **137**, 384.

Buruma, O. J. S., Janson, H. L. F., Van den Bergh, F. A. J. T. M., and Bots, G. Th. A. M. (1981). Blood-stained cerebrospinal fluid: traumatic puncture or haemorrhage? *J. Neurol. Neurosurg. Psychiat.* **44**, 144.

Cameron, I. R. (1969). Acid–base changes in cerebrospinal fluid. *Br. J. Anaesthiol.* **41**, 213.

Carbaat, P. A. T. and Van Crevel, H. (1981). Lumbar puncture headache: controlled study on the preventive effect of 24 hours' bed rest. *Lancet* **ii**, 1133.

Crow, H. J., Keogh, C., and Northfield, D. W. C. (1956). The localisation of cerebrospinal-fluid fistulae. *Lancet* **ii**, 325.

Cumings, J. N. (1953). The cerebral lipids in disseminated sclerosis and in amaurotic family idiocy. *Brain* **76**, 551.

Davies-Jones, G. A. B.(1970). Lactate dehydrogenase and glutamic oxalacetic transaminase of the cerebrospinal fluid in neurological disease. *J. neurol. Sci.* **11**, 583.

Davson, H. (1967). *The physiology of the cerebrospinal fluid*. Churchill, London.

Dayan, A. D. and Stokes, M. I (1973). Rapid diagnosis of encephalitis by immunofluorescent examination of cerebrospinal-fluid cells. *Lancet* **i**, 177.

Dencker, S. J. and Swahn, B. (1961). *Clinical value of protein analysis in cerebrospinal fluid*. Lund Universitets Aarskrift, Lund.

Dubowitz, V. and Rogers, K. J. (1969). 5-hydroxyindoles in the cerebrospinal fluid of infants with Down's syndrome and muscle hypotonia. *Develop Med. child Neurol.* **11**, 730.

Dyken, P. R. (1975). Cerebrospinal fluid cytology: practical clinical usefulness. *Neurology, Minneapolis.* **25**, 210.

Ekstedt, J. (1977). CSF hydrodynamic studies in man. 1. Method of constant pressure CSF infusion. *J. Neurol. Neurosurg. Psychiat.* **40**, 105.

Fischer-Williams, M. and Roberts, R. C. (1971). Cerebrospinal fluid proteins and serum immunoglobulins: occurrence in multiple sclerosis and other neurological diseases. *Arch. Neurol., Chicago.* **25**, 526.

Fishman, R. A. (1980). *Cerebrospinal fluid in diseases of the nervous system*. Saunders, Philadelphia.

Gilland, O. and Nelson, J. R. (1970). Lumbar cerebrospinal fluid electromanometrics with a minitransducer. *Neurology, Minneapolis*, **20**, 103.

Glass, J. P., Melamed, M., Chernik, N. L., and Posner, J. B. (1979). Malignant cells in cerebrospinal fluid (CSF): the meaning of a positive CSF cytology. *Neurology, Minneapolis.* **29**, 1369.

Grainger, R. G. and Lamb, J. T. (1980). *Myelographic technique with metrizamide*. Nyegaard, Birmingham.

Green, J. B., Oldewurtel, H., O'Doherty, D. S., Foster, F. M., and Sanchez-Longo, L. P. (1957). Cerebrospinal fluid glutamic oxalacetic transaminase activity in neurologic disease. *Neurology, Minneapolis.* **7**, 313.

—— Papadopoulos, N., Cevallos, W., Foster, F. M., and Hess, W. C. (1959). The cholesterol and cholesterol ester content of cerebrospinal

fluid in patients with multiple sclerosis and other neurological diseases. *J. Neurol. Neurosurg. Psychiat.* **22**, 117.

Gumpert, J., Sharpe, D., and Curzon, G. (1973). Amine metabolites in the cerebrospinal fluid in Parkinson's disease and the response to levodopa. *J. neurol. Sci.* **19**, 1.

Harms, D. (1975). Comparative quantitation of immunoglobulin G (IgG) in cerebrospinal fluid and serum of children. *Eur. Neurol.* **13**, 54.

Heiblim, D. I., Evans, H. E., Glass, L., and Agbayani, M. M. (1978). Amino acid concentrations in cerebrospinal fluid. *Arch. Neurol., Chicago.* **35**, 765.

Jager, W. A. D. H. (1969). Cytopathology of the cerebrospinal fluid examined with the sedimentation technique after Sayk. *J. neurol. Sci.* **9**, 155.

Johnson, R. H. (1972). Cerebrospinal fluid. Chapter VIII.1 in *Scientific foundations of neurology*. (ed. M. Critchley, J. L. O'Leary, and W. B. Jennett). Heinemann, London.

Kabat, E. A., Moore, D. H., and Landow, H. (1942). An electrophoretic study of the protein components in cerebrospinal fluid and their relationship to the serum proteins. *J. clin. Invest.* **21**, 571.

Kam-Hansen, S. (1979). Reduced number of active T cells in cerebrospinal fluid in multiple sclerosis. *Neurology, Minneapolis* **29**, 897.

Kaplan, L. and Kennedy, F. (1950). The effect of head posture on the manometrics of the cerebrospinal fluid in cervical lesions: a new diagnostic test. *Brain* **73**, 337.

Katzman, R., Fishman, R. A., and Goldensohn, E. S. (1957). Glutamic-oxalacetic transaminase activity in spinal fluid. *Neurology, Minneapolis.* **7**, 853.

Kaufman, H. H. (1969). Nontraumatic cerebrospinal fluid rhinorrhea. *Arch. Neurol., Chicago.* **21**, 59.

Kjellin, K. G. and Söderström, C. E. (1974). Diagnostic significance of CSF spectrophotometry in cerebrovascular diseases. *J. neurol. Sci.* **23**, 359.

—— and Stibler, H. (1975). Protein patterns of cerebrospinal fluid in hereditary ataxias and hereditary spastic paraplegia. *J. neurol. Sci.* **25**, 65.

—— and Vesterberg, O. (1974). Isoelectric focusing of CSF proteins in neurological diseases. *J. neurol. Sci.* **23**, 199.

Knigge, K. M., Scott, D. E., Kobayashi, H., and Ishii, S. (Eds.) (1975). *Brain–Endocrine interaction*, Vol. II. Karger, Basle.

Laterre, E. C. (1975). Cerebrospinal fluid. In *Handbook of clinical neurology* (ed. P. J. Vinken and G. W. Bruyn) Vol. 19. North Holland, Amsterdam.

Latner, A. L. (1973). Some clinical biochemical aspects of isoelectric focusing. *Ann. NY Acad. Sci.* **209**, 281.

Laurenzi, M. A. and Link, H. (1979). Characterisation of the mobility on isoelectric focusing of individual proteins in CSF and serum by immunofixation. *J. Neurol. Neurosurg. Psychiat.* **42**, 368.

Levinson, A. I., Lisak, R. P., and Zweiman, B. (1976).Immunologic characterization of cerebrospinal fluid lymphocytes: preliminary report. *Neurology, Minneapolis.* **26**, 693.

Lindeman, J., Muller, W. K., Versteeg, J., Bots, G. T. A. M., and Peters, A. C. B. (1974). Rapid diagnosis of meningoencephalitis, encephalitis. Immunofluorescent examination of fresh and in vitro cultured cerebrospinal fluid cells. *Neurology, Minneapolis.* **24**, 143.

Link, H. (1967). Immunoglobulin G. and low molecular weight proteins in human cerebrospinal fluid. *Acta neurol. scand.* **43**, suppl. 28.

Lumsden, C. (1972). The clinical pathology of multiple sclerosis. In *Multiple sclerosis: a reappraisal*, 2nd edn. (ed. D. McAlpine, C. Lumsden, and E. D. Acheson), Part III. Churchill Livingstone, London.

Marks, V. and Marrack, D. (1960). Tumour cells in the cerebrospinal fluid. *J. Neurol. Neurosurg. Psychiat.* **23**, 194.

Martins, A. N., Wiley, J. K., and Myers, P. W. (1972). Dynamics of the cerebrospinal fluid and the spinal dura mater. *J. Neurol. Neurosurg. Psychiat.* **35**, 468.

McKhann, G. M. (1978). A cellular approach to neurological disease. *Johns Hopkins med. J.* **143**, 48.

Merritt, H. H. and Fremont-Smith, F. (1937). *The cerebrospinal fluid*. Saunders, Philadelphia.

Millen, J. W. and Woollam, D. H. M. (1962) *The anatomy of the cerebrospinal fluid*. Oxford University Press, London.

Moir, A. T. B., Ashcroft, G. W., Crawford, T. B. B., Eccleston, D., and Guldberg, H. C. (1970). Cerebral metabolites in cerebrospinal fluid as a biochemical approach to the brain. *Brain* **93**, 357.

Morgan, B. P., Campbell, A. K., and Compston, D. A. S. (1984). Terminal component of complement (C9) in cerebrospinal fluid of patients with multiple sclerosis. *Lancet* **ii**, 251.

Nellhaus, G. (1971). Cerebrospinal fluid immunoglobulin G in childhood: measurement by electroimmunodiffusion. *Arch. Neurol., Chicago*. **24**, 441.

O'Connell, J. E. A. (1970). Cerebrospinal fluid mechanics. *Proc. R. Soc. Med.* **63**, 507.

Oehmichen, M. (1976). *Cerebrospinal fluid cytology: an introduction and atlas*. Saunders, Philadelphia.

Ommaya, A. K., Di Chiro, G., Baldwin, M., and Pennybacker, J. B. (1968). Non–traumatic cerebrospinal fluid rhinorrhoea. *J. Neurol. Psychiat.* **3l**, 214.

Ostheimer, G. W., Palahniuk, R. J., and Shnider, S. M. (1974). Epidural blood patch for post-lumbar-puncture headache. *Anesthesiology*, **41**, 307.

Paoletti, P., Vandenheuvel, F. A., and Fumagalli, R. (1969). The sterol test for the diagnosis of human brain tumors, *Neurology, Minneapolis*. **19**, 19.

Paty, D. W., Donnelly, M., and Bernardo, M. E. (1978). CSF electrophoresis: an adaptation using cellulose acetate for the identification of oligoclonal binding. *Can. J. neurol. Sci.* **5**, 297.

Péter, A. (1967). The plasma cells of the cerebrospinal fluid. *J. neurol. Sci.* **4**, 22.

Plum, F. and Price, R. W. (1973). Acid–base balance of cisternal and lumbar cerebrospinal fluid. *New Engl. J. Med.* **289**, 1346.

Riddoch, D. and Thompson, R. A. (1970). Immunoglobulin levels in the cerebrospinal fluid. *Br. med. J.*, **1**, 396.

Riekkinen, P. J. and Rinne, U. K. (1970). Enzymes of human cerebrospinal fluid in normal conditions and neurological disorders. *Annales Universitatis Turkuensis*, suppl. 44.

Rottenberg, D. A., Howieson, J., and Deck, M. D. F. (1977). The rate of CSF formation in man: preliminary observations on metrizamide washout as a measure of CSF bulk flow. *Ann. Neurol.* **2**, 503.

Sambrook, M. A., Hutchison, E. C., and Aber, G. M. (1973a). Metabolic studies in subarachnoid haemorrhage and strokes. I. Serial changes in acid–base values in blood and cerebrospinal fluid. *Brain* **96**, 171.

——, ——, and —— (1973b). Metabolic studies in subarachnoid haemorrhage and strokes. II. Serial changes in cerebrospinal fluid and plasma urea, electrolytes and osmolality. *Brain* **96**, 191.

Sayk, J. (1966). Cytologie der Cerebrospinalflüssigkeit. *Wien. Z. Nervenheilk.*, suppl. 1.

Sherwin, A. L., Norris, J. W., and Bulcke, J. A. (1969). Spinal fluid creatine kinase in neurologic disease. *Neurology, Minneapolis*. **19**, 993.

Sidén, A. and Kjellin, K. G. (1979). Isoelectric focusing of csf proteins in known or probable infectious neurological diseases and the Guillain–Barré syndrome. *J. neurol. Sci.* **42**, 139.

Sindic, C. J. M., Collet-Cassart, D., Cambiaso, C. L., Masson, P. L., and Laterre, E. C. (1981). The clinical relevance of ferritin concentration in the cerebrospinal fluid. *J. Neurol. Neurosurg. Psychiat.* **44**, 329.

Smith, F. R, Perkin, G. D., and Rose, F. C. (1980). Posture and headache after lumbar puncture. *Lancet* **i**, 1245.

Smith, H., Bannister, B., and O'Shea, M. J. (1973). Cerebrospinal-fluid immunoglobulins in meningitis. *Lancet* **ii**, 591.

Stokes, H. B., O'Hara, C. M., Buchanan, R. D., and Olson, W. H. (1975). An improved method for examination of cerebrospinal fluid cells. *Neurology, Minneapolis*. **25**, 901.

Tomlinson, B. E. and Walton, J. N. (1967). Granulomatous meningitis and diffuse parenchymatous degeneration of the nervous system due to an intracranial epidermoid cyst. *J. Neurol. Neurosurg. Psychiat.* **30**, 341.

Tourtellotte, W. W. (1970). On cerebrospinal fluid immunoglobulin-G (IgG) quotients in multiple sclerosis and other diseases. A review and a new formula to estimate the amount of IgG synthesized per day by the central nervous system. *J. neurol. Sci.* **10**, 279.

——, Haerer, A. F., Heller, G. L., and Somers, J. E. (1964). *Post-lumbar puncture headaches*. Charles C. Thomas, Springfield, Illinois.

Tripathi, R. C. (1973). Ultrastructure of the arachnoid mater in relation to outflow of cerebrospinal fluid: a new concept. *Lancet* **ii**, 8.

—— (1974). Tracing the bulk outflow route of cerebrospinal fluid by transmission and scanning electron microscopy. *Brain Res.* **80**, 503.

Van Sande, M., Mardens, Y., Adriaenssens, K., and Lowenthal, A. (1970). The free amino acids in human cerebrospinal fluid. *J. Neurochem.* **17**, 125.

Walton, J. N. (1981). The cerebrospinal fluid, raised intracranial pressure, cerebral edema,craniocerebral and spinal trauma, spinal cord compression and relevant investigations—some pathophysiologic principles. In Neurology (Section XII) by J. N. Walton of *Pathophysiology—The biological principles of disease* (ed. L. H. Smith and S. O. Thier) Vol. I, *International Textbook of Medicine*. Saunders, Philadelphia.

Weiss, J. F., Ransohoff, J., and Kayden, H. J. (1972). Cerebrospinal fluid sterols in patients undergoing treatment for gliomas, *Neurology, Minneapolis*.**22**, 187.

Welch, K. and Friedman, V. (1960). The cerebrospinal fluid valves. *Brain* **83**, 454.

Wilcock, A. R., Sharpe, D. M., and Goldberg, D. M. (1973). Kinetic similarity of enzymes in human blood serum and cerebrospinal fluid: aspartate aminotransferase and lactate dehydrogenase, *J. neurol. Sci.* **20**, 97.

Williams, B. (1976). Cerebrospinal fluid pressure changes in response to coughing. *Brain* **99**, 331.

Wolstenholme, G. E. W. and O'Connor, C. M. (1958). *Ciba Foundation Symposium on the cerebrospinal fluid production, circulation and absorption*. Ciba Foundation, London.

Wood, J. H. (Ed.) (1980a). *Neurobiology of the cerebrospinal fluid*. Plenum, New York.

—— (1980b). Neurochemical analysis of cerebrospinal fluid, *Neurology, Minneapolis*. **30**, 645.

Zilkha, K. J. and McArdle, B. (1963). The phospholipid composition of cerebrospinal fluid in diseases associated with demyelination. *Quart. J. Med.* **32**, 79.

Zivin, J. A. (1978). Lateral cervical puncture: an alternative to lumbar puncture. *Neurology, Minneapolis*. **28**, 616.

History and examination

The history of the illness

General considerations

In the diagnosis of nervous disease, the history of the patient's illness is just as important and indeed often more so than the elicitation of physical signs. Thus in disorders such as migraine and epilepsy the diagnosis will often be made on the history alone, though examination must not be neglected lest the symptoms be symptomatic of an underlying structural abnormality such as an intracranial vascular malformation or neoplasm. On the other hand, a particular combination of abnormal physical signs (e.g. those of hemiplegia) may indicate that the pathological process responsible lies in the opposite cerebral hemisphere, but the history is then all-important in assessing its nature; thus a sudden onset may suggest that the lesion is vascular, a gradual evolution that it is neoplastic.

The history obtained from the patient should always be supplemented, if possible, by an account of his illness given by a relative or friend who knows him well. This is essential when the patient suffers from mental symptoms or attacks of loss of consciousness, but it is always desirable, since a relative or friend may remember important points which the patient himself has forgotten to mention.

First note the patient's name and address, age, and exact details of his occupation. The last-named is often of importance as a source of exposure to injury or to toxic substances. Ascertain if he is right-handed. Next ask the patient of what he complains and when he was last in normal health, in this fixing, at least provisionally, the date of onset of his symptoms. He should then be allowed to relate the story of his illness as far as possible without interruption, questions being posed afterwards to expand his statements and to elicit additional information. It is also important to ascertain not only the date but also the mode of onset of all symptoms, whether sudden, rapid, or gradual, and whether each symptom since first appearing has fluctuated in intensity and whether the patient's condition is improving, stationary, or deteriorating at the time of examination.

History of present illness

Inquiry should always be made with regard to the following symptoms, whether or not the patient mentions them spontaneously:

Mental state. The patient's mental history should be ascertained, not only as far as possible from himself, but also from relatives or friends, on the lines laid down below for the examination of his mental condition. If there are mental symptoms, it may be important to assess the patient's premorbid intelligence and personality.

Sleep. Has he suffered from disturbances of sleep, either from paroxysmal or persistent sleepiness or from insomnia?

Speech. Has he had difficulty in speaking? If so, of what nature? Has he been able to understand what is said to him and to read? Has his writing been affected? (see p. 57). If his speech has been slurred, has there been associated dysphagia or difficulty in chewing?

Attacks of loss of consciousness. Has he suffered from attacks of loss or impairment of consciousness? If so, for further inquiries see page 611.

Headache. Has he suffered from headache? If so, further inquiries should be made as described on page 175. Has there been associated vomiting? If so, of what character?

Pain. Has he suffered pain in the face, trunk, or limbs? If so, what is its character, distribution, time of occurrence, constancy, or intermittency? Are there any precipitating or aggravating factors?

Special senses. Has he had hallucinations of smell or taste or noticed an impairment of these senses? Has he had visual hallucinations? If so, what has been their character and distribution in the visual fields? Has there been any visual impairment: if so, of one or both eyes and of what nature? Has it been transitory or progressive? Has he had double vision? If so, has this been transient or persistent and is the symptom present when looking in any special direction? Is his hearing impaired? If so, is this unilateral or bilateral and is there associated tinnitus? Does he suffer from giddiness? If so, he should describe its nature and state whether it is associated with a sense of rotation of himself or of his surroundings, and with deafness, tinnitus, or vomiting.

Movement and sensibility. Does he complain of muscular weakness or wasting, of loss of control over the limbs or of involuntary movements, and if so, what is the distribution of these symptoms? Has his gait been abnormal, and if so, how? Has he tended to stagger, deviate, or fall, and if so, in what direction? Has he had any spontaneous sensory disturbances, especially pain, numbness, or tingling? If so, the symptoms should be further analysed, as described on pages 42–4.

The sphincters and reproductive functions. Has there been any disturbance of sphincter control. Has he experienced difficulty in holding or passing urine or faeces? Has he had polyuria? In the case of a man, is his potency and libido normal for his age? In the case of a woman, has there been any abnormality in menstruation, especially amenorrhoea?

Disorders of other systems. Are there any symptoms of respiratory disease or insufficiency, of cardiac or arterial disease or any complaints to suggest renal, hepatic, gastrointestinal, or endocrine dysfunction?

Nutrition. Is the appetite normal and the weight stationary, diminishing, or increasing?

History of previous illnesses

A difficult birth may be significant in relation to cerebral palsy or epilepsy. A history of aural discharge or of tuberculosis may be important in relation to intracranial abscess or tuberculous meningitis. A history of convulsions or of meningitis in childhood or of encephalitis or venereal disease may be significant in relation to a later illness. Inquiry should always be made for a history of accidental injury, especially to the head and spine.

Social history

This should include the patient's educational and occupational career, adjustments to family life, military service, residence abroad, and personal habits in respect of recreation, tobacco, alcohol, and other drugs. Patients addicted to alcohol or other drugs commonly conceal or underestimate their consumption.

Family history

Many diseases of the nervous system are hereditary. The patient should always be asked whether cases of nervous or mental disease have occurred among his relatives and if so the precise nature of the illness should, if possible, be ascertained and a pedigree constructed, including miscarriages and stillbirths. Consanguinity in the parents should be inquired for. If the patient is married, the state of health of the spouse should be assessed, seeking clues to communicable disease, such as syphilis.

Examination of the patient

The brief commentary given below will serve as a general guide to some important principles to be followed in examining the nervous system. Detailed descriptions of methods of testing the motor and sensory systems have already been given and methods of eliciting other signs of nervous dysfunction are given in other appropriate sections of this book. Techniques of neurological examination are described in greater detail by de Jong (1979) and Bickerstaff (1980). Useful guides to the neurological assessment of neonates, infants, and children are given by André-Thomas, Chesni, and St-Anne Dargassies (1955), Paine and Oppé (1966), Prechtl (1977) and Fenichel (1980).

State of consciousness

Is the patient conscious or unconscious? If unconscious, how far does he respond to stimuli, such as pinching the skin? Can he be roused, and if so, when roused is his mental condition normal or abnormal? Detailed methods of assessment in stupor and coma are described on pages 648–50. If conscious, can he think quickly and clearly; are his responses appropriate? Can he swallow? The following psychological investigations are, of course, applicable only to conscious patients.

Intellectual and memory functions

Is the patient orientated in space and time? Does he recognize his surroundings and does he know the day of the week and date? Is his memory normal? If impaired, is it better for remote than for recent events? Does he fill gaps in his memory by confabulating, that is, by describing imaginary events or others taken out of their temporal context? Retentiveness may be tested by asking the patient to retain and repeat a series of digits—normally seven can be repeated forwards and five backwards—or retain a name, address, and the name of a flower for five minutes. Concentration and immediate recall can also be tested by asking the patient to repeat a Babcock sentence—'One thing a nation must have to be rich and great is a large secure supply of wood'; normally this can be repeated accurately in not more than three attempts. It is also usual to ask for the names of well-known people (e.g. the last three prime ministers or US Presidents) and to test simple calculation by requesting the patient to subtract serial sevens from 100.

What is his level of intelligence? Is he in touch with current events? Can he grasp the meaning of a passage which he reads from a newspaper, or of a picture depicting an incident?

Does he suffer from delusions or hallucinations? A delusion is an erroneous belief which cannot be corrected by an appeal to reason and is not shared by others of the patient's education and status. A hallucination is a sensory impression occurring without a corresponding external stimulus. A patient may conceal both delusions and hallucinations. The latter may sometimes be suspected through his behaviour. For example, a patient with visual hallucinations may seem to be manipulating invisible objects, while one experiencing auditory hallucinations, such as voices, may adopt a listening attitude.

Emotional state

Is the patient's emotional state normal? Is he excited or depressed? If excited, is his condition one of elation (excitement associated with a sense of well-being or of fear and anxiety? Apart from excitement, does he experience an abnormal sense of well-being—euphoria? Is he anxious and, if so, to what does he attribute his anxiety? Is he irritable? Is he emotionally indifferent and apathetic? Does he take care of his dress and appearance, or is he indifferent and dirty? Personal neglect may be due to an affective disorder such as depression but is more often the result of disintegration of the personality and intellect (i.e. dementia).

Speech and articulation

Are speech and articulation normal? If aphasia is suspected the appropriate tests must be carried out (see p. 57).

The cranial nerves

Test the sense of smell in each nostril separately (see p. 83).
Test the visual acuity and visual fields (see pp. 85–7)
Examine the ocular fundi (see p. 89).
Are the pupils equal, central, and regular? Are they abnormally dilated or contracted? Test the reactions to light, both direct and consensual, of each eye separately, and the reaction on accommodation/convergence.
Test the ocular movements, upwards and downwards and to either side, and ocular convergence. Is squint, diplopia, or nystagmus present? If there is nystagmus, is it sustained and is it altered by the position of the head? Note the size of the palpebral fissures. Is there ptosis or retraction of the upper lids? Is exophthalmos present?
Is there wasting of the temporal muscles and masseters? Test the jaw movements and the jaw-jerk.
Examine sensibility to light touch, pin-prick, heat and cold over the trigeminal area, and test the corneal reflexes.
Is the facial expression normal? Is there wasting of the facial muscles? Are there involuntary movements? Test the voluntary movements of eye closure, elevation of the eyebrows, frowning, retraction of the lips, pursing the lips, whistling or the ability to retain air in the cheeks under pressure. Test emotional facial movements as in smiling. In some cases of facial paralysis it is necessary to test the sense of taste (see p. 128).
Test the hearing for both air-conduction and bone-conduction. If hearing is defective, apply both Weber's and Rinne's tests (see p. 120). In certain cases it may be necessary to test the vestibular reactions (see p. 122).
Is the soft palate elevated normally on phonation? Test the palatal and pharyngeal reflexes.
Examine the movements of the vocal cords, if necessary.
Test the movements of the sternomastoids and trapezii.
Examine the tongue. Is it wasted? Is fasciculation present? Is it tremulous? Is it protruded normally or does it deviate to one or other side?
Note the presence or absence of head retraction and test for cervical rigidity.

The skull and skeleton

Inspect and then palpate the skull and spine, noting any evidence of abnormal configuration, local tenderness, or deformity. Note if there are any deformities of the limbs (e.g. contractures or pes cavus). Auscultate over the temporal fossae, over both orbits, and over the great vessels in the neck, noting the presence of bruits; on occasion it may be necessary to auscultate over the spinal column in an attempt to detect a spinal bruit.

Gait

If the patient is well enough, observe whether he can stand without support with the feet together, and whether the steadiness of his stance is affected when he closes his eyes. Ask him to walk, if necessary with support, and note the presence of spasticity or ataxia of the lower limbs in walking. Slight disturbances of stance and gait may be detected by asking the patient to stand first on one foot and then on the other, first with the eyes open and then with the eyes closed; and to walk along a line, placing one heel in front of the toes of the other foot. The 'scissors' gait of spastic diplegia, the hemiplegic gait, the stiff gait with dragging of both feet in spastic paraparesis, the high steppage gait of tabes dorsalis, the slow shuffle or festinant gait of parkinsonism, the broad-based, staggering gait of central cerebellar lesions, the waddling gait of some neuromuscular disorders such as muscular dystrophy, and the footslapping gait of bilateral foot drop, to name but a few, are distinctive.

The limbs and trunk

Different observers employ different methods of examination; some begin with the patient sitting up, others with him lying supine. All methods are satisfactory, if complete. It is normal to begin with inspection, looking for involuntary movements, atrophy, hypertrophy, deformity, or contracture and then to examine successively muscle power, tone, co-ordination, reflexes, and sensation.

Muscular power and co-ordination. In examining the limbs note first their *posture* and the presence or absence of *muscular wasting* and *fasciculation*. Next note the presence or absence of *involuntary movements*, of which the following are those most commonly encountered. A tic is a co-ordinated, repetitive movement involving as a rule a number of muscles in their normal synergic relationships. Choreic movements are quasi-purposive, jerky, irregular, and non-repetitive, and are characterized by dissociation of normal muscular synergy. Athetosis consists of slow, writhing movements, which are most marked in the peripheral segments of the limbs. Tremor is a rhythmical movement at a joint, brought about by alternating contractions of antagonistic groups of muscles. Myoclonus is a shock-like muscular contraction affecting part or the whole of the muscle independently of its antagonists. If involuntary movements are present, note their relationship to rest, posture, and voluntary movement. Also note whether there is any *skeletal deformity* of the skull, spine, or extremities and whether there is any shortening or *contracture* of specific muscles.
Next test *voluntary power* by asking the patient to carry out against resistance the movements possible at the various joints, comparing the same movement on the two sides of the body. Power of individual muscles can be recorded on the following scale: no contraction, 0; flicker or trace of contraction, 1; active movement, with gravity elimated, 2; active movement against gravity, 3; active movement against gravity and resistance, 4; normal power, 5. When assessing weakness due to upper motor-neurone lesions, it may be sufficient to examine the power of a few selected muscles only (e.g. deltoid, biceps, finger flexors, and extensors in the upper limbs, hip flexors, quadriceps, and tibialis anterior in the lower). In the assessment of suspected peripheral nerve lesions and in cases of neuromuscular disease, however, a more extensive examination of individual muscles is needed; full details are given in the Medical Research Council Memorandum 'Aids to the Examination of the Peripheral Nervous System' (1976). In such an examination, grade 4 power as defined above may have to be

divided into two subgroups (e.g. 4+, 4−). The detection of early corticospinal-tract lesions may require the testing of manual dexterity and the ability to move the various fingers independently. It is also useful to ask the patient to hold the hands and fingers outstretched with and without the eyes closed. Downward drift of one hand may indicate weakness due to a corticospinal-tract lesion; wandering of the fingers in space may indicate impairment of position and joint sense. A brisk tap on the limb with observation of the recoil gives a useful indication of muscle *tone* as does the assessment of passive movement at several joints.

Muscular co-ordination is tested in the upper limbs by asking the patient to touch the tip of his nose with the tip of his forefinger, first with the eyes open and then with the eyes closed. He should also be asked to carry out alternating movements of pronation and supination of the hands and forearms simultaneously on both sides. When in bed, lower-limb co-ordination is tested by asking him to place one heel on the opposite knee, or to raise the leg from the bed and touch the observer's finger with his toe.

Movements of the abdominal wall are tested by asking the patient to raise his head from the bed against resistance while noting by palpation contraction of the abdominal muscles and whether displacement of the umbilicus occurs.

Sensation. As a routine, the patient's appreciation of light touch, pin-prick, heat and cold, posture, passive movement, and vibration should be tested, attention being paid not only to sensory defects but also to the presence of tenderness or undue sensitivity to pressure of superficial and deep structures. In some cases additional tests may be needed (see p. 44). Since the spinal segmental areas run longitudinally along the long axis of the upper limbs, sensibility on the ulnar border should be compared with that on the radial border, either by applying successive stimuli transversely to the limb, or by dragging the stimulus, for example a pin, along the skin. On the trunk the segmental areas are distributed almost horizontally. Changes of sensibility are therefore best detected by moving the stimulus from below upwards or vice versa. In the lower limbs the sacral segmental areas, which are represented on the sole and the posterior aspect of the limb and in the perianal area, should always be tested.

The reflexes. The deep tendon reflexes as described on p. 49 are invariably examined and attempts are made to elicit other reflexes as described in that section when appropriate; at the same time tests for patellar and ankle clonus should be carried out.

The sphincters. Note the state of the sphincters and examine the abdomen for evidence of distension of the bladder.

Trophic disturbances. Note the state of the patient's nutrition, especially the presence of wasting or excessive obesity and the condition of the external genitalia. Note the distribution of hair on the body, anomalies of sweating, and the presence or absence of cutaneous pigmentation and trophic lesions of the skin, nails, and joints.

A complete general physical examination of the heart, chest, and abdomen should always be made. Examination of the peripheral blood vessels is important. Inequality of carotid or radial pulsation and bruits should be noted and if there is any difference the blood pressure should be recorded in both arms.

Investigation of the patient with neurological disease

In considering the ancillary investigations which may be used as aids to diagnosis in a patient whose symptoms and signs suggest a disorder of the nervous system, one must appreciate that symptons of neurological dysfunction may result from disease in some other part of the body. The patient must therefore be viewed as a whole if he is not to be subjected to unpleasant tests designed to demonstrate an abnormality in the nervous system when the lesion responsible may be in some other organ apart from the brain and spinal cord. A second important principle is that investigations should always be planned to give the maximum required information about the patient's illness with the least possible discomfort and risk. In some patients with neurological symptoms, there may be no need for investigations either for diagnosis or to give guidance on management. Migraine, for instance, is a condition in which the diagnosis is usually made on the clinical history alone and in which ancillary tests are rarely indicated. In other cases, investigation should be carefully designed in order to establish or exclude the diagnoses brought to mind by the patient's symptoms and signs. It is reasonable to begin with the simpler tests which the doctor is able to do himself before proceeding, if the diagnosis remains in doubt, to the more difficult investigations which require specialized apparatus and skilled technical help.

It follows that in many patients it will be necessary to carry out urinalysis and various haematological and biochemical tests on blood samples, whereas biopsy of muscle, peripheral nerve, or of other tissues and organs may be required in order to clarify the nature of the patient's illness. A detailed commentary upon these tests would be out of place here, but where appropriate these studies are mentioned in subsequent chapters. Indications for, and methods of examination of, the CSF have already been considered (pp. 66–71). Some specialized neurophysiological and radiological techniques are also considered in later chapters, as are methods of investigation of particular relevance in the assessment of the special senses. In addition, methods of masurement of nerve conduction velocity, studies of neuromuscular transmission, and electromyography are described in the sections on disorders of the peripheral nerves and muscle. It would, however, be appropriate here to consider some general principles underlying the use of electroencephalography and related techniques and various methods of neuroimaging.

Electroencephalography (EEG)

Electroencephalography is a technique of recording the electrical activity of the brain through the intact skull. Electrodes are applied to the scalp and the potentials so recorded are amplified and presented for interpretation as an ink-trace on moving paper. Machines in common use today have 16 or more channels so that the activity from many different areas of the head can be recorded simultaneously. The technique is simple and harmless (see Hess 1966). Many modifications or adaptations of the technique have been introduced to meet special requirements (see Kiloh, McComas, Osselton, and Upton 1981), including the development of a portable cerebral-function monitor for use, for example, in intensive-care departments (Prior, Maynard, Sheaff, Simpson, Strunin, Weaver, and Scott 1971), and computer-controlled topographic display of data derived both from the EEG and from evoked potential studies, called brain electrical activity mapping (Duffy, Burchiel, and Lombroso 1979).

In the normal adult the dominant electrical activity in the EEG from the post-central areas is usually a sinusoidal wave form with a frequency of 8–13 Hz (Fig. 1.34 (a)). This is the alpha rhythm; it commonly disappears on attention, as when the eyes open (Fig. 1.34 (b)). Normally there is some faster so-called beta activity (14–22 Hz) in the frontal regions; this is greatly accentuated by the administration of barbiturates and sometimes by anxiety. In young infants the EEG is dominated by generalized slow activity of so-called delta frequency (up to 3–5 Hz); gradually during the processes of maturation this is replaced by theta activity (4–5 Hz) and subsequently by the alpha rhythm. Theta activity disappears last from the posterior temporal regions and the record is usually completely mature, showing no such activity, by the age of 12–14 years. During drowsiness and sleep in the normal individual, theta activity and later delta activity reappear.

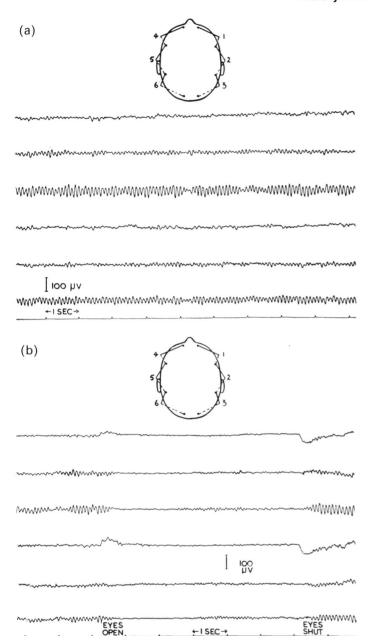

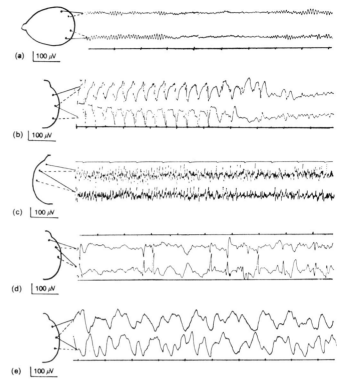

Fig. 1.34. (a) Female, aged 23. Normal electroencephalogram. Dominant 10 Hz alpha activity in the posterocentral regions.

(b) Female, aged 23. Normal electroencephalogram. Almost complete blocking of the dominant alpha rhythm to eye opening.

Fig. 1.35. Some common appearances in electroencephalographic (EEG) recordings (from Walton (1982)). a: A normal alpha rhythm recorded from both occipital regions and disappearing (in the centre of the recording) when the eyes are open; b: a 3 Hz spike and wave discharge of petit mal epilepsy, recorded in this illustration from the right temporal region; c: high-frequency discharges (mainly muscle artefact) recorded from the left fronto-temporal region during a major epileptic seizure; d: a right anterior temporal focus of spike discharge in a patient suffering from temporal-lobe epilepsy; e: a focus of high-amplitude delta activity seen in the right mid–temporal region in a patient suffering from a cerebral abscess in this situation.

The EEG is of particular value in the diagnosis of epilepsy (Fig. 1.35). In cases of petit mal it may show regular rhythmical generalized outbursts of repetitive complexes, each consisting of a spike and a delta wave (spike-and-wave), and recurring at a frequency of about 3 Hz. In idiopathic or centrencephalic major epilepsy, the interseizure record sometimes shows brief generalized outbursts of spikes or sharp waves or of mixed spikes and slow activity. Similarly in patients with partial epilepsy, including temporal-lobe attacks, there may be spikes, sharp waves, or rhythmical outbursts of slow delta or theta activity arising in the epileptogenic area of the cortex. It is important, however, to note that positive sharp waves seen in the occipital regions during visual attention (so-called lambda waves) and negative sharp waves seen at the vertex (V-waves), especially when the individual is drowsy, are normal phenomena (Kiloh *et al.* 1981). Similarly, so-called 'wicket spikes' which may occur in trains and which resemble, in a

sense, transient increases in alpha rhythm amplitude, often relatively sharp in outline (Reiher and Lebel 1977), bear no relationship to epilepsy. Unfortunately, a single record taken in an epileptic patient is often normal; positive findings are more common in children and less common the older the patient. Many patients show only non-specific abnormalities between attacks such as excessive temporal theta activity. Hence it is often necessary to take repeated recordings or alternatively to use various activation techniques in order to uncover epileptic discharges. Overbreathing for two to three minutes is particularly effective in evoking the discharges of petit mal, while photic stimulation (repetitive light flashes of variable frequency) can also bring out epileptic discharges. Since temporal spikes or sharp waves often appear in early sleep, it is usual to carry out recordings after oral or intravenous sedation with barbiturates or other appropriate drugs in cases of suspected temporal-lobe epilepsy. In some such cases, recordings with a needle electrode inserted to lie in contact with the basi-sphenoid underneath the medial surface of the temporal lobe are helpful. Thus a single routine EEG is of limited value but should generally be performed, using simple activating techniques if necessary, in most patients suspected to be suffering from epilepsy. If epileptic discharges are found, this will confirm the diagnosis and the nature of the discharge may help in deciding upon appropriate treatment. Negative findings, however, do not exclude this diagnosis.

The EEG is also of limited value in the diagnosis of focal cerebral lesions. A relatively acute lesion of one cerebral hemisphere usually gives a focus of delta activity in or around the area of the lesion (Fig. 1.35). It is not the lesion itself which produces this abnormal discharge, but the changes which it has caused in the surrounding brain. A cerebral abscess usually gives a slow-wave focus of high amplitude, and similar though less striking abnormalities may result from tumour, haemorrhage, local injury, or infarction. Thus the EEG may help in localization but only rarely gives a clue to the pathological diagnosis, which must depend upon clinical or other information. An abnormality due to a tumour will usually become worse, while that due to an infarct often improves. With lesions which are more chronic or more deeply situated in the cerebral hemisphere, focal theta activity of low amplitude or even an absence of alpha or beta activity on one side may be the only abnormality. Indeed, in some patients with intracranial tumour the record is consistently normal. Whereas some localized abnormality may be found in up to 70 per cent of such patients, the EEG is never sufficiently accurate in localization to be a safe guide to subsequent surgery and the neurosurgeon will invariably require information derived from other diagnostic methods.

A subdural haematoma sometimes produces unilateral suppression of the alpha rhythm and irregular slow activity on the affected side. In many chronic neurological disorders such as parkinsonism and multiple sclerosis the EEG is often normal. In subacute sclerosing panencephalitis, isolated bizarre slow-wave complexes occur simultaneously in all channels against a background of comparative electrical silence, while, in some children with cerebral lipidosis or in adults with Creutzfeldt-Jakob disease, generalized and almost continuous irregular spike and wave discharge may be seen. A similar severe abnormality, often called hypsarrhythmia, may be found in records from infants suffering from infantile spasms. In severe acute necrotizing encephalitis due to herpes simplex virus, repetitive triphasic complexes sometimes occur, especially over the necrotic temporal lobe. Tumours in the posterior fossa or deeply situated lesions near the midline may give paroxysmal outbursts of theta or delta activity at the surface, but these changes are not specific as they occur in patients with many diffuse disorders including meningitis, subarachnoid haemorrhage, and encephalitis or conditions giving a generalized disorder of cerebral metabolism such as anoxia, uraemia, hyperglycaemia, hepatic coma, or pernicious anaemia. Indeed such discharges are most often indicative of diffuse encephalopathy (Schaul, Lueders, and Sachder 1981); in hepatic coma (portal-systemic encephalopathy) diffuse triphasic waves or so-called 'blunt spike-wave discharges' may alternate with diffuse paroxysmal delta activity. The EEG is also widely used in the diagnosis of brain death; total electrocerebral silence (the isoelectric EEG) is a useful criterion of irreversible coma due to organic cerebral damage resulting, say, from cardiac arrest (Binnie, Prior, Lloyd, Scott, and Margerison 1970; Silverman, Masland, Saunders, and Schwab 1970) but unfortunately similar EEG changes occasionally occur in reversible drug-induced coma. Most internationally accepted criteria no longer require an EEG recording in the diagnosis of brain death (see p. 650 and Kiloh *et al.* 1981).

The EEG is of little value in psychiatric diagnosis, though anxious obsessional patients may show excess frontal activity, while psychopaths, and children with behaviour disorders have immature records with excess temporal slow activity. Patients with organic dementia often show a dominant rhythm of theta rather than alpha frequency; this represents a reversion to a childhood pattern and can also occur as a result of ageing.

Hence the EEG is helpful in the diagnosis of epilepsy and of a few brain diseases in which relatively specific changes are sometimes found. It is also of limited value in the investigation of patients with cerebral vascular disease and intracranial space-occupying lesions. It must not, however, be expected to give information which it cannot provide, and a single negative recording is of no value.

Evoked potential techniques

In the late 1960s the scope of clinical neurophysiological studies was greatly increased by the development of various methods of sensory evoked potential recording. Thus measurement of the latency and form of pattern-evoked visual responses, recording from the scalp over the occipital pole and using a computer-controlled averaging technique for the analysis of the potentials evoked, has proved to be of considerable value in assessing the integrity of the visual pathways. These responses correlate well with the visual acuity and are sensitive to the effects of pathological lesions such as compression or demyelination when clinical signs are minimal or absent (Halliday 1978). Methods of recording brainstem auditory evoked responses after monaural or binaural stimulation have also been developed and have proved to be of particular value in investigating neurological disease in infants and children (Hecox, Cone, and Blaw 1981), but the technique is also helpful in localizing brainstem haemorrhage, infarction, or tumour (Oh, Kuba, Soyer, Choi, Bonikowski, and Vitek 1981). Evoked response audiometry (Chapter 2) is also used increasingly. So-called 'far-field' recording has also been used to record somatosensory evoked potentials from the scalp overlying the sensory cortex and over the cervical and lumbosacral spine (Matthews, Beauchamp, and Small 1974; Phillips and Daube 1980); these methods have been helpful in assessing delayed conduction, for example, in the spinal cord or cerebral sensory pathways in disorders such as multiple sclerosis (see Courjon, Maugière, and Revol 1982).

Echo-encephalography

Many simple and inexpensive machines using ultrasonics for neurological diagnosis are now available commercially. An ultrasonic beam is passed horizontally through the intact skull and an 'echo' can be recorded from midline structres (the A-scan). A 'shift' of the midline is easily demonstrated and this method was often used to confirm rapidly the presence of a space-occupying lesion in or overlying one cerebral hemisphere. It was particularly useful for the rapid screening of patients in whom a subdural or extradural haematoma or a tumour in one cerebral hemisphere was suspected (Tanaka 1969). More complicated and refined techniques (the B-scan) have been introduced in order to define echoes arising from intracranial structures other than those in the midline but this method has been largely supplanted by computerized transaxial tomography (see below). However, echo-tomography may still be useful in identifying arterial stenosis, say at the carotid bifurcation (Mikol, Monge-Strauss, Berges, Aubin, and Vignaud 1981).

Gamma-encephalography

Scanning of the radioactivity recorded over the surface of the skull following the intravenous injection of a suitable isotope (^{99}Technetium is now most commonly used) has been widely used in many neurological units as an aid to the diagnosis of intracranial lesions. The blood vessels, and probably the cells of certain tumours, show a selective affinity for such isotopes so that the tumour is shown as an area of increased radioactivity. With lateral and antero-posterior scans, localization may be quite accurate. Increased uptake is also seen in cerebral abscesses and in areas of infarction. Thus a single scan may not give a firm pathological diagnosis, but the technique is helpful in demonstrating multiple intracranial lesions (e.g. metastases). It, too, is used much less often since the advent of the CT scan (Oldendorf 1980, 1981), but is still occasionally helpful (Alderson, Mikhael, Coleman, and Gado 1976).

Isotope ventriculography

If a small amount of radio-iodinated serum albumin (RISA) is injected by lumbar puncture in a normal individual and the skull is scanned a few hours later, radioactivity is demonstrated in the subarachnoid space over the surface of the brain and not, as a rule, in the cerebral ventricles. If, however, the lateral ventricles soon show evidence of radioactivity and little or no isotope flows over the brain surface towards the superior longitudinal sinus, some degree of communicating hydrocephalus is probably present. This method has been of help in detecting cases of so-called low-pressure hydrocephalus (Bannister 1970) and in detecting fistulous communications between the subarachnoid space and the middle ear or paranasal sinuses such as may occur after head injury, otitis media, or sinusitis. Measurement of the rate of clearance of the isotope into the systemic circulation may also be used as a means of detecting the rate of CSF absorption in a case of suspected hydrocephalus (Brocklehurst 1968). The method is now used infrequently.

Radiology

Radiological methods are mong the most helpful and widely used of all the ancillary techniques used in neurological diagnosis. While final diagnosis may depend upon the use of specialized methods involving the injection of contrast media, these techniques are time-consuming, expensive, and sometimes disturbing to the patient. It is therefore important to remember that valuable and sometimes even conclusive information may be obtained from plain radiographs of the skull and/or spine and of other parts of the body. Thus in patients with a clinical picture suggesting intracranial neoplasm or a subacute meningitic illness, X-rays of the chest are all-important, perhaps revealing a bronchogenic carcinoma or pulmonary tuberculosis. Or else changes in the skeleton may cast light upon the significance of neurological symptoms and signs, as in cases of prostatic carcinoma or multiple myelomatosis.

Straight radiography of the skull. It is usual to take routine antero-posterioor and lateral views of the skull, while in most centres an antero-posterior view is also taken with the brow depressed some 35 degrees so that the petrous temporal bones become visible (Towne's view) and another of the skull base. Stenver's view is also used to examine the petrous temporal bone. Usually the skull vault is first examined to see if there is reasonable uniformity of bony thickness or whether there is any erosion or bony overgrowth such as may result from a meningioma, or abnormal vascular markings due to dilatation of the middle meningeal artery supplying a meningeal tumour or vascular malformation. Sometimes, as in carcinomatosis or myelomatosis, there may be multiple areas of bony rarefaction in the skull vault or a general thickening or 'woolliness' of the bone as in Paget's disease. In young children, hydrocephalus due to any cause may give separation of the cranial sutures and a characteristic 'beaten copper' mottling of the bone; however, the latter appearance is so often seen in normal individuals, even in adult life, that in itself it is not diagnostic. Fractures of the vault are noted if present, and it is also wise to examine the frontal, maxillary, and sphenoidal paranasal sinuses for opacities which may suggest infection or neoplasia. Hyperostosis of the inner table of the frontal bone is not uncommon but is of no pathological significance.

The base of the skull is next examined, first in the lateral projection. Here the relationship of the upper cervical spine to the foramen magnum is observed and it is noted whether there is any protrusion of the odontoid process of the axis above a line joining the posterior margin of the hard palate to the posterior lip of the foramen magnum (Chamberlain's line). If the odontoid extends above this line, or if there is an abnormal tilt of the body of the atlas implying invagination of the basi-occiput, then basilar impression is present. The most important structure at the base of the skull visible on the lateral projection is the sella turcica. Its size and shape and the integrity and density of the anterior and posterior clinoid processes which form its lips are noted. In patients with primary pituitary neoplasms, the sella is expanded or ballooned and partially decalcified, while in those with suprasellar lesions it is also expanded but is shallower and flattened and there is often erosion of the clinoid processes. Moderate flattening and expansion of the sella with decalcification of the posterior clinoid processes may occur in any patient with increased intracranial pressure.

Also to be noted on the lateral projection is the presence or absence of intracranial calcification. If present, such calcification can then be more accurately localized by means of antero-posterior views or by stereoscopic lateral projections. In about 50 per cent of adults and even in some normal children, the pineal gland is calcified and may measure up to 0.5 cm in diameter. If the gland is calcified, its distance from the inner table of the skull on anteroposterior radiographs should be measured, as displacement to one or other side may indicate the presence of a space-occupying lesion in one cerebral hemisphere. Other intracranial structures which occasionally calcify in normal individuals are the choroid plexuses, the falx cerebri, and the petro-clinoid ligaments. Pathological intracranial calcification, if mottled in type and suprasellar in situation, often indicates a craniopharyngioma, but many other intracranial tumours including meningiomas, gliomas, and oligodendrogliomas occasionally show a fine spidery pattern of calcification. Fine curvilinear lines of calcification may be seen in the wall of a large aneurysm, while calcific stippling can occur in a haematoma or arteriovenous angioma. Rare additional causes of intracranial calcification include cysticercosis, toxoplasmosis, and hypoparathyroidism. A form of widespread calcification outlining the gyri of one occipital and/or parietal lobe is seen in diffuse cortical angiomatosis associated with a port-wine naevus of the face (the Sturge-Weber syndrome).

In antero-posterior, Towne's, Stenver's, and the basal views, the most important feature to look for is enlargement or erosion of cranial exit foramina. Sclerosis and overgrowth of bone may also occur, particularly in the wings of the sphenoid in patients with a meningioma in this region. It is usual to examine the optic foramina, superior orbital fissures, and internal auditory meati in particular. A funnel-shaped erosion of an internal auditory meatus, revealed by Towne's and Stenver's views, is characteristic of an acoustic neuroma. The basal view may also reveal bony erosion due to malignant infiltration or enlargement of one foramen spinosum in a patient with a meningioma producing dilatation of the middle meningeal artery supplying it.

Radiology of the spinal column. In examining radiographs of the spine, we are concerned first with changes in the vertebrae themselves, secondly with the intervertebral discs, and thirdly with the intervertebral foramina. It is usual to carry out anteroposterior and lateral views to study the vertebrae and discs but, for examination of the intervertebral foramina, oblique views are necessary. In the vertebrae themselves, one may first observe congenital abnormalities such as fusion of several vertebral bodies (if in the cervical region this may be called the Klippel–Feil syndrome) or spina bifida, either of which may be responsible for or associated with neurological signs. Fracture, fracture-dislocation, Paget's disease, osteomyelitis, neoplasia, either benign or malignant, of vertebral bodies, any one of which might give vertebral collapse and spinal cord compression, will generally be revealed by routine X-rays. Bony erosion and in particular enlargement of the relevant intervertebral foramen is typically seen, often with the extraspinal soft tissue shadow of a dumb-bell tumour, in cases of spinal neurofibroma. Less striking but of equal diagnostic importance is a variation in interpedicular distance. The distance between the vertebral pedicles is large in the cervical region, gradually diminishes to a minimum in the mid-dorsal region, and then expands again in the lumbar region, corresponding to the cervical and lumbar enlargements of the spinal cord. If successive interpedicular distances are measured and one or more measurements falls outside the expected arithmetical progression, this indicates the presence of an expanding lesion within the spinal cord or canal in this region. Dorsal meningiomas may produce no more radiological change than this, whereas neurofibromas often give bony erosion as well. Measurement of the antero-posterior diameter of the spinal canal is also of value, particularly in the cervical region; an unduly wide canal is seen, for instance, in some cases of syringomyelia.

In a patient with an acute intervertebral-disc prolapse, radiographs of the spine are often normal or reveal simply a narrowing of the disc space concerned. The prolapsed disc is not itself radio-opaque. If one or more disc protrusions have been present for months or years, the margins of the prolapsed tissue gradually become calcified, giving posterior (and often anterior) osteophyte formation at the upper and lower borders of the contiguous vertebrae. As the prolapsed tissue often projects laterally as well, osteophytes also tend to encroach upon the intervertebral foramina and this change is shown on oblique views. A combination of changes of this type, which are most often observed in the cervical and lumbar regions, is referred to as spondylosis.

Computerized transaxial tomography (the CT scan) and other tomographic techniques

This exciting technique of radiological diagnosis (Gawler, du Boulay, Bull, and Marshall 1974; *The Lancet* 1974; *British Medical Journal* 1974) has already transformed the practice of neuroradiology and is supplanting progressively some of the more traditional contrast methods (Weisberg, Nice, and Katz 1978; Oldendorf 1980, 1981). However, the equipment required is costly and requires considerable technical skill for its operation and maintenance, so that it will be some time before it is available for general use in all parts of the world. It depends upon the transmission of photon beams across the head and recording with crystals instead of X-ray film. The results can be seen visually on a cathode-ray screen, and photographed, and can also be stored on magnetic tape or floppy discs. While the early scanners to be introduced could only scan the head, new-generation whole-body scanners can also be used to scan the head as well as the body cavities and spinal canal. The technique allows one to carry out rapid serial tomographic 'cuts' in multiple planes through the intact skull with no discomfort to the patient and no risk as the radiation exposure is minimal. The entire procedure takes about 20 minutes; confused or restless patients and children may require sedation as the head must be held still during the recording. Accurate outlines of the brain parenchyma, cerebral ventricles, CSF cisterns, subarachnoid space, the pineal, falx cerebri, brainstem, cerebellar hemispheres, and orbital contents can be obtained, and intracranial vascular and space-occupying lesions can be rapidly localized and are often identified in a pathological sense through changes in their density (Fig. 1.36). Enhancement of the images produced by the intravenous injection of contrast medium such as meglamine iothalamate (Conray) may add considerable precision to diagnosis. In general, most neoplasms are seen as areas of increased density unless their centre is necrotic or cystic when a rim of dense tumour around a translucent area is seen, an appearance which may resemble that of an abscess. Areas of haemorrhage, too, usually show typical increased density, whether in the brain substance, ventricles, subdural or subarachnoid space. Infarcts are usually shown as areas of reduced density, as are plaques of demyelination. For a lesion to be visualized it must have a density different from that of the surrounding brain and must be 5 mm or more in diameter. The technique has been widely used not only to investigate and identify focal cerebral lesions (Jacobs, Kinkel, and Heffner 1976; Weisberg 1979) but also to assess the presence or absence of cortical atrophy or ventricular dilatation resulting from ageing (Barron, Jacobs, and Kinkel 1976) or mental disease (Johnstone, Crow, Frith, Husband, and Kreel 1976) and asymmetries of the cerebral hemispheres related to handedness (Chui and Damasio 1980). The whole-body scanner is now being widely used in the investigation of lesions in the spinal canal.

A more recent development has been the introduction of *emission computerized tomography* (Ell, Jaritt, Deacon, Brown, and Williams 1978; Ell, Deacon, Ducasson, and Brandel 1980) in which a CT type of scan is carried out after the intravenous injection of ^{99m}technetium pertechnetate as in gamma-encephalography. This has been thought to improve the visualization of brain tumours and digital imaging techniques are also being explored. *Positron emission tomography* demonstrates not only focal lesions but simultaneously indicates both regional glycolysis and local blood flow, thus giving metabolic as well as morphological information (Phelps, Mazziotta, Kuhl, Nuwer, Packwood, Metter, and Engel 1981; Mazziotta, Phelps, Miller, and Kuhl 1981); unfortunately this method requires access to a cyclotron and is thus very expensive so that for the present it remains a research tool (Oldendorf 1981). *Nuclear magnetic resonance* brain imaging (Doyle, Gore, Pennock, Bydder, Orr, Steiner, Young, Burl, Clow, Gildendale, Bailes, and Walters 1981) is another technique still in the research and development stage which shows considerable promise for the future (see Rosenberg 1984). This method not only gives images which are in some respects superior to those obtained by CT scanning but also provides information about dynamic aspects of cerebral metabolism and is being used increasingly.

Contrast methods. The contrast methods most often used in neurological diagnosis are air encephalography, ventriculography with air or myodil (pantopaque), carotid, vertebral, spinal, and aortic arch angiography, and myelography. Each of these methods carries certain possible hazards to the patient and all involve some pain or discomfort; hence they must not be regarded as routine methods of investigation but should only be utilized when an accurate diagnosis can be reached in no other way. When this is the case, it must be decided which method is likely to give the most helpful information and whether the one chosen is likely to be safe or whether there are contra-indications. Since the advent of the CT scan, very few air encephalograms and ventriculograms are now needed but angiography is often required to demonstrate vascular occlusion or stenosis, aneurysms, or vascular malformations.

The place of these investigations in the diagnosis of cerebral vascular disease, of intracranial space-occupying lesions, and other disease processes, and the place of myelography in the diagnosis of spinal lesions will be considered later in appropriate chapters.

References

Alderson, P. O., Mikhael, M., Coleman, R. E., and Gado, M. (1976). Optimal utilization of computerized cranial tomography and radionuclide brain imaging. *Neurology, Minneapolis* **26**, 803.

André-Thomas, Chesni, Y., and St-Anne Dargassies, S. (1955). *Examen neurologique du nourrisson*. Masson, Paris.

Bannister, R. (1970). The place of isotope encephalography by the lumbar route in neurological diagnosis. *Proc. Roy. Soc. Med.* **63**, 921.

Barron, S. A., Jacobs, L., and Kinkel, W. R. (1976). Changes in size of normal lateral ventricles during aging determined by computerized tomography. *Neurology, Minneapolis* **26**, 1011.

Bickerstaff, E. R. (1980). *Neurological examination in clinical practice*, 4th edn. Blackwell, Oxford.

Binnie, C. D., Prior, P. F., Lloyd, D. S. L., Scott, D. F., and Margerison, J. H. (1970). Electroencephalographic prediction of fatal anoxic brain damage after resuscitation from cardiac arrest. *Br. med. J.* **4**, 265.

British Medical Journal (1974). Computer assisted tomography. *Br. med. J.* **31**, 162.

Brocklehurst, G. (1968). Use of radio-iodinated serum albumin in the study of cerebrospinal fluid flow. *J. Neurol. Neurosurg. Psychiat.* **31**, 162.

Chui, H. C. and Damasio, A. R. (1980). Human cerebral asymmetries evaluated by computed tomography. *J. Neurol. Neurosurg. Psychiat.* **43**, 873.

Courjon, J., Mauguière, F., and Revol, M. (Eds.) (1982). *Clinical applications of evoked potentials in neurology*. Advances in Neurology, Vol. 32. Raven Press, New York.

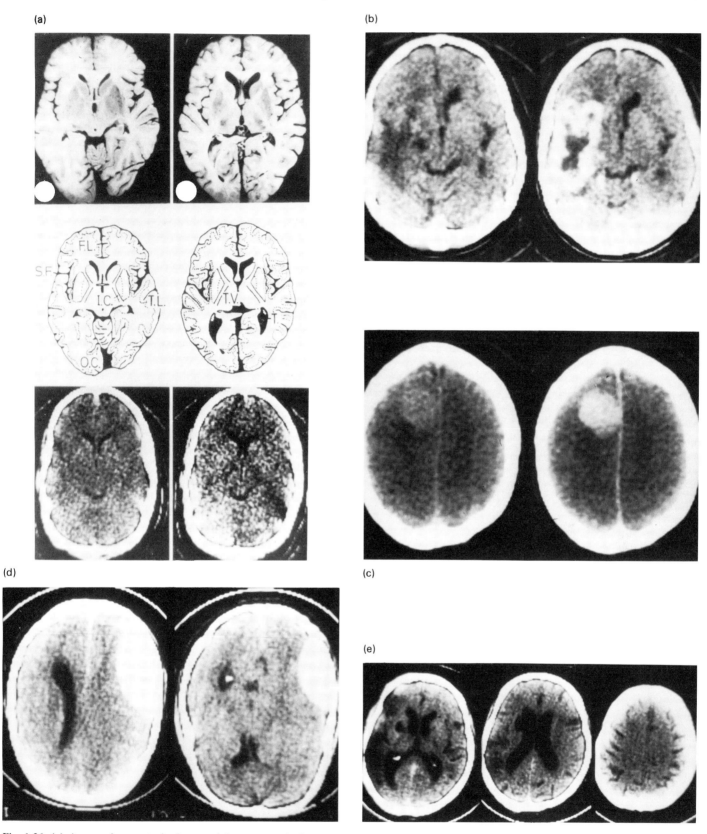

Fig. 1.36. (a) A normal computerized transaxial tomogram (a CT scan) above, showing the cerebral ventricular outlines at different sagittal planes, as seen in the brain slices below and the diagram in between.

(b) A CT scan showing an encapsulated cerebral abscess in the left temporal region. This is seen as an area of reduced density in the left-hand scan. The scan on the right, after contrast enhancement, shows the capsule of the abscess clearly.

(c) A CT scan showing a left frontal haematoma due to head injury, without (on the left) and with (on the right) contrast enhancement.

(d) A CT scan of a large right frontal subdural haematoma.

(e) A CT scan showing ventricular dilatation and widened sulci due to cortical atrophy in a patient with presenile dementia.

Fig. 1.36. (a)–(e) is reproduced, with permission, from Walton (1982).

de Jong, R. N. (1979). *The neurological examination*, 4th ed. Hoeber, New York.

Doyle, F. H., Gore, J. C., Pennock, J. M., Bydder, G. M., Orr, J. S., Steiner, R. E., Young, I. R., Burl, M., Clow, H., Gilderdale, D. J., Bailes, D. R.,, and Walters, P. E. (1981). Imaging of the brain by nuclear magnetic resonance. *Lancet* **ii**, 53.

Duffy, F. H., Burchfiel, J. L., and Lombroso, C. T. (1979). Brain electrical activity mapping (BEAM): a method for extending the clinical utility of EEG and evoked potential data. *Ann. Neurol.* **5**, 309.

Ell, P. J., Deacon, J. M., Ducassou, D., and Brendel, A. (1980). Emission and transmission brain tomography. *Br. med. J.* **1**. 438.

—— Jarritt, P. H., Deacon, J., Brown, N. J. G., and Williams, E. S. (1978). Emission computerised tomography: a new diagnostic imaging technique. *Lancet* **ii**, 608.

Fenichel, G. M. (1980). *Neonatal neurology*. Churchill Livingstone, Edinburgh.

Gawler, J., Du Boulay, G. H., Bull, J. W. D., and Marshall, J. (1974). Computer-assisted tomography (EMI scanner): its place in investigation of suspected intracranial tumours, *Lancet* **ii**, 419.

Halliday, A. M. (1978). New developments in the clinical application of evoked potentials. In *Contemporary clinical neurophysiology* (EEG Suppl. No. 34) (ed. W. A. Cobb and H. Van Duijn). Elsevier, Amsterdam.

Hecox, K. E., Cone, B., and Blaw, M. E. (1981). Brainstem auditory evoked response in the diagnosis of pediatric neurologic diseases. *Neurology, Minneapolis* **31**, 832.

Hess, R. (1966). *EEG handbook*, (Sandoz Monograph). Sandoz, Basle.

Hill, D. and Parr, G. (1963). *Electro-encephalography*, 2nd ed. Macdonald, London.

Jacobs, L., Kinkel, W. R., and Heffner, R. R. (1976). Autopsy correlations of computerized tomography: experience with 6 000 CT scans. *Neurology, Minneapolis* **26**, 1111.

Johnstone, E. C., Crow, T. J., Frith, C. D., Husband, J., and Kreel, L. (1976). Cerebral ventricular size and cognitive impairment in chronic schizophrenia. *Lancet*, **ii**, 924.

Kiloh, L. G., McComas, A. J., Osselton, J. W., and Upton, A. R. M. (1981). *Clinical electroencephalography*, 4th edn. Butterworths, London.

The Lancet (1974). Computer-assisted tomography of the brain. *Lancet* **ii**, 1052.

McKinney, W. M. (1969). Echoencephalography. Chapter 3 in *Special techniques for neurologic diagnosis* (ed. J. F. Toole), Contemporary Neurology Series, Vol. 3. F. A. Davis, Philadelphia.

Matthews, W. B., Beauchamp, M., and Small, D. G. (1974). Cervical somatosensory evoked responses in man. *Nature, London* **252**, 230.

Maynard, C. D. and Janeway, R. (1969). Radioisotope studies in diagnosis. Chapter 2 in *Special techniques for neurologic diagnosis*, (ed. J. F. Toole), Contemporary Neurology Series, Vol. 3. F. A. Davis, Philadelphia.

Mayo Clinic (1976). *Clinical examinations in Neurology*, 4th edn. Saunders, Philadelphia.

Mazziotta, J. C., Phelps, M. E., Miller, J., and Kuhl, D. E. (1981). Tomographic mapping of human cerebral metabolism: normal unstimulated state. *Neurology, Minneapolis* **31**, 502.

Mikol, F., Monge-Strauss, M. F., Berges, O., Augin, M. L., and Vignaud, J. (1981). Examen de la bifurcation carotidienne par echotomographie. *Rev. Neurol.* **137**, 661.

Newton, T. H. and Potts, D. G. (1974). *Radiology of the skull and brain*. Mosby, St. Louis.

Oh, S. J., Kuba, T., Soyer, A., Choi, I. S., Bonikowski, F. P., and Vitek, J. (1981). Lateralization of brainstem lesions by brainstem auditory evoked potentials. *Neurology, Minneapolis* **31**, 14.

Oldendorf, W. H. (1980). *The quest for an image of brain*. Raven Press, New York.

—— (1981). Nuclear medicine in clinical neurology: an update. *Ann. Neurol.* **10**, 207.

Paine, R. S. and Oppé, T. E. (1966). *Neurological examination of children*, Clinics in Developmental Medicine, Vol. 20–1. The Spastics Society, Heinemann, London.

Phelps, M. E., Mazziotta, J. C., Kihl, D. E., Nuwer, M., Packwood, J., Metter, J., and Engel, J. (1981). Tomographic mapping of human cerebral metabolism: visual stimulation and deprivation. *Neurology, Minneapolis.* **31**, 1175.

Phillips, L. H. and Daube, J. R. (1980), Lumbosacral spinal evoked potentials in humans. *Neurology, Minneapolis*. *30*, 1175.

Prechtl, H. (1977). *The neurological examination of the full-term newborn infant*, 2nd edn. Spastics International, Heinemann, London.

Prior, P. F., Maynard, D. E., Sheaff, P. C., Simpson, B. R., Strunin, L., Weaver, E. J. M., and Scott, D. F. (1971). Monitoring cerebral function: clinical experience with new device for continuous recording of electrical activity of brain, *Br. med. J.* **2**, 736.

Reiher, J. and Lebel, M. (1977). Wicket spikes: clinical correlates of a previously undescribed EEG pattern, *Can. J. neurol. Sci.* **4**, 39.

Rosenberg, R. (ed.) (1984). *The clinical neurosciences*. Churchill-Livingstone, Edinburgh.

Schaul, N., Lueders, H., and Sachdev, K. (1981). Generalized, bilaterally synchronous bursts of slow waves in the EEG, *Arch. Neurol., Chicago*. **38**, 690.

Silverman, D., Masland, R. L., Saunders, M. G., and Schwab, R. S. (1970). Irreversible coma associated with electrocerebral silence. *Neurology, Minneapolis.* **20**, 525.

Tanaka, K. (1969). *Diagnosis of brain disease by ultrasound*. Shindan-To-Chiriyo Sho Co, Tokyo.

Walton, J. N. (1982). *Essentials of neurology*, 5th edn. Pitman Medical, London.

Weisberg, L. A. (1979). Computed tomography in the diagnosis of intracranial disease, *Ann. intern. Med.* **91**, 87.

—— Nice, C., and Katz, M. (1978). *Cerebral computed tomography*. Saunders, Philadelphia.

2

The cranial nerves and special senses

The first or olfactory nerve and the sense of smell

The olfactory receptors are a series of bipolar nerve cells situated in the upper part of the mucous membrane on either side of the nasal cavity. Inhaled gases given off by all odorous materials become dissolved in the nasal secretions which continually bathe the surface of these sensitive cells. Impulses so produced are conveyed by nerve fibres through the cribiform plate of the ethmoid bone into the cranial cavity to join the olfactory bulb which lies on the under surface of the ipsilateral frontal lobe. Thence impulses travel posteriorly to the olfactory tracts to reach the prepyriform cortex and uncus in the rostral part of the parahippocampal gyrus of the temporal lobe which can be regarded as the primary rhinencephalic (olfactory) area of the cerebral cortex. The anterior commissure unites the olfactory cortical regions of the two hemispheres and carries fibres from each olfactory tract to the opposite side.

Disorders of olfaction

There is a strong relationship between the faculties of smell and taste, which combined give the sensation of flavour. Thus, if either faculty is impaired, so too may be the ability to appreciate flavours; in such a patient it is not sufficient to test taste sensation alone, as an inability to perceive olfactory sensations may be the primary abnormality.

In testing the sense of smell bottles containing coffee, oil of peppermint, oil of cloves, and camphorated oil are held in turn beneath each nostril, and the patient is asked if he recognizes them. Many normal individuals with an acute sense of smell find difficulty in naming scents. Pinching (1977) suggests that musks and floral odours are more reliable than conventional test substances. After head injury, especially in a compensation setting, anosmia (see below) may be feigned in the hope of material gain; it is therefore useful to ask the patient to smell concentrated ammonia which stimulates the trigeminal sensory terminals in the nose as well as the olfactory; if a patient claims not to be affected by ammonia, it is likely that the anosmia is spurious.

Anosmia, or loss of the olfactory sense, is occasionally congenital, and sometimes hereditary. It may occur either temporarily or permanently as a result of rhinitis, severe coryza, or even heavy smoking. Total anosmia is a rare complication of anoxia; it more often results from division or compression of olfactory nerve fibres as they pass through the cribriform plate of the ethmoid. Complete or partial loss may occur on one or both sides as a result of head injury either with or without fracture of the base of the skull in the anterior fossa. Sumner (1964) found an incidence of 7.5 per cent, the liability increasing with increasing severity of the head injury. Anosmia may be temporary, lasting for only a few days, weeks, or months, but if it persists for more than a year it is unlikely to recover. Even trivial injuries occasionally produce this sign; recovery is much more likely to occur, however, after minor injury than after injuries giving 24 hours or more of post-traumatic amnesia (Sumner 1972). The olfactory tract may be compressed by tumours, especially meningiomas growing from the olfactory groove, or less frequently by tumours of the frontal lobe or in the region of the optic chiasm, or by the distended cerebral hemispheres in obstructive hydrocephalus. Thus unilateral anosmia can be a useful sign of an anteriorly situated space-occupying lesion. The tract may also be damaged by meningitis or rarely by neurosyphilis. It is doubtful whether complete anosmia is ever produced by lesions of one olfactory cortex because fibres from each olfactory tract reach both cerebral hemispheres. Irritative lesions in the neighbourhood of the uncus may cause olfactory hallucinations, often associated with disturbance of consciousness and involuntary convulsive movements of the lips, jaws, tongue, and pharynx–uncinate fits (see p. 616).

Parosmia may occur especially after head injury. Strong scents then smell abnormal, usually unpleasant, and a persistent unpleasant olfactory hallucination may be experienced. A similar symptom sometimes occurs in depressive illness.

References

Brodal, A. (1947). The hippocampus and the sense of smell. *Brain* **70**, 179.

Elsberg, C. A. and Stewart, J. (1938). Quantitive olfactory tests: value in localization and diagnosis of tumours of the brain with analysis of results in three hundred patients. *Arch. Neurol. Psychiat., Chicago* **40**, 471.

Leigh, A. D. (1943). Defects of smell after head injury. *Lancet* **i**, 38.

McCartney, W. (1972). Olfaction. In *Scientific foundations of neurology* (ed. M. Critchley, J. L. O'Leary, and W. B. Jennett), Section V, Chapter 4. Heinemann, London.

Pinching, A. J. (1977). Clinical testing of olfaction reassessed. *Brain* **100**, 377.

Sumner, D. (1964). Post-traumatic anosmia. *Brain* **87**, 107.

—— (1972). Clinical aspects of anosmia. In *Scientific foundations of neurology* (ed. M. Critchley, J. L. O'Leary, and W. B. Jennett), Section V, Chapter 5. Heinemann, London.

The sense of vision, the visual apparatus, and the second or optic nerve

General considerations

The sense of vision exemplifies the remark that, in the case of the special senses, physical stimuli are extensively modified or transduced as they are transmitted through non-neural tissue before reaching the neural sensory receptor specifically designed to record them. Thus the eye can be likened superficially to a camera in that light rays pass through an aperture which can be varied at will, then pass through a lens of variable focus, and are eventually recorded upon a light-sensitive receptor surface (the retina). The neural process of visual perception is, however, much more complex than the simple recording of a single visual image upon a light-sensitive film.

A detailed consideration of physiological optics would be out of place here, but a knowledge of simple principles is useful. Thus the process by means of which the lens focuses images upon the retina is known as *refraction*. The human eye focuses upon near objects by increasing the refractive power of the lens through the process of *accommodation*. As a light source moves closer to the eye, contraction of both the circular and longitudinal fibres of the ciliary muscle allows the lens to bulge passively and to become more nearly spherical; the degree of change is proportional to the strength of ciliary muscle contraction. This change in shape shortens the focal length of the lens, thus bringing the near object into focus; it is accompanied by ocular *convergence*, a reflex action due to contraction of the medial recti which ensures that the images recorded by each eye are focused on the macular area of each retina at the fovea centralis. This process is accompanied by reflex pupillary constriction or *miosis* (see below); this helps to blot out light rays which would otherwise fall upon the periphery of the lens, thus preventing the distortion of images due to *chromatic and spherical aberration*, which would otherwise occur as the lens approaches a more nearly spherical shape.

Among the common disorders of visual refraction are *myopia* (short sight, due to abnormal length of the globe of the eye, which is usually constitutional or developmental) requiring concave lenses for its correction and *hypermetropia* or *hyperopia* (long sight, due to abnormal shortness of the globe) which is somewhat less common. Long-sightedness commonly develops with increasing age (*presbyopia*) at the rate of about one-quarter of a diopter per year after the age of about 25 years, and can be corrected by the use of convex lenses. Presbyopia, however, is due to increasing impairment of the accommodation process resulting from progressive lack of elasticity of the lens. *Astigmatism* is a more complex defect due to asymmetry in its curvature or shape.

The retina

Structure

The retina contains two types of receptor, the rods and the cones, which have entirely different properties. The *cones* are found throughout the retina but are most heavily concentrated in the fovea or macular region which subserves central vision; they have a high stimulus threshold, function mainly in daylight or conditions of high illumination (*photopic illumination*), and are responsible for high-acuity vision and colour vision. The *rods*, by contrast, are absent from the fovea, have very low thresholds of stimulation, are insensitive to colour and relatively insensitive to visual detail, and subserve vision in conditions of poor illumination (night vision, *scotopic illumination*).

The retina lines the inside of the globe of the eye as far forward as the ciliary body where it terminates in a serrated border (the ora serrata); posteriorly, lateral to the macula, it is interrupted by the optic nerve head or disc where the axons of the retinal ganglion cells come together to form the optic nerve.

The retina is strikingly laminated in cross-section. Its outer pigment layer contains a single layer of epithelial cells with finger-like processes pentrating between the outer segments of the receptor cells. The rods and cones possess outer and inner segments connected by an eccentric waist-like constriction. Each outer segment contains free floating discs to which are attached the light-sensitive pigments (*rhodopsin* or visual purple in the rods, and three pigments not yet fully characterized in the cones, of which one may be *iodopsin*). In the rods new discs are constantly being formed at the base of the outer segment while others at the tip bud off and are integrated by pigment cells. This may also occur in the cones but the cone discs have a longer life than those of the rods.

The inner segments of these receptors contain many mitochondria and nuclei which are larger in the cones than in the rods and which constitute the *outer nuclear layer* of the retina. Beyond the nuclei the inner segments continue through the *outer plexiform layer*, terminating in expansions (the *rod spherule* and *cone pedicle*); these make synaptic contacts with the dendrites of bipolar cells, which in turn constitute the *inner nuclear layer*. In this layer there are flat or diffuse bipolar cells, especially in the periphery of the retina, each of which receives connections from about seven cones, but there are also midget bipolar cells, especially in the foveal region, connecting with a single cone, while rod bipolar cells receive impulses from rods exclusively. There are also retinal interneurones, the *horizontal cells* which connect rods and cones, and *amacrine cells* (neurones without identifiable axons) which form connections between bipolar terminals and dendrites of ganglion cells. The ganglion cells form the *innermost cell layer* of the retina and their dendrites synapse with axons of the bipolar cells in the inner plexiform layer; their axons traverse the retina to enter the optic nerve. The photosensitive receptors lie deep in the retina so that light must traverse several retinal layers to excite them; but in the foveal (macular) region there is a cup-shaped shallow depression in the retina where the ganglion and bipolar cells are pushed aside, exposing the receptors. This area is concerned with central vision, with maximal acuity, clarity, and discrimination of visual images.

Ganglion-cell responses to diffuse retinal illumination include *on* responses, *off* responses, and *on–off* responses. On cells discharge with increasing frequency during illumination, off cells do so when light stimulation ends, and on–off cells discharge at the beginning and end of photic stimulation. Stimulation of the retina with minute light spots has shown that many ganglion cells have receptive fields with 'on-centre, off-surround' characteristics, while others show the reverse arrangement. Receptive fields for foveal cells are very small and may correspond to the on response of a single cone, the 'off surround' being mediated by interneurones. The latter cells (the horizontal and amacrine neurones) appear to be responsible for lateral inhibitory responses which enhance the contrast generated by visual images. Synaptic chemical transmitters in the retina have not yet been fully characterized, although acetycholine, dopamine, and GABA are all known to be present.

Function

Photochemical and electrophysiological mechanisms

Retinal photoreceptors are sensitive to light with wavelengths from 400 to 700 nm, that is from blue through green to red; light stimuli falling upon such receptors ultimately lead to firing in ganglion cells as mentioned above. Vitamin A is taken up from the blood stream by retinal epithelial cells, being converted into *retinol* which then combines with opsin to form *rhodopsin* (see above) which is then stored in the outer segments of the rods. When light falls upon the rods, rhodopsin is bleached, the amount being dependent upon the intensity of the light, and, when the stimulus ceases, it is resynthesized. Vitamin A, therefore, is essential for rod function and dietary deficiency of this vitamin causes night-blindness. A similar process of bleaching of pigment followed by resynthesis is presumed to occur with respect to cone pigments.

These photochemical changes initiate the generation of graded responses in bipolar cells, which in turn excite action potentials in ganglion cells; these are then conveyed by optic-nerve axons to the lateral geniculate body (see below). The accompanying electrical changes can be recorded in the electroretinogram (ERG) through an electrode (such as a conducting contact lens) applied to the globe of the eye. It consists of an A-wave, presumed to be due to late photoreceptor activity, a B-wave representing postsynaptic activity, and a C-wave, thought to arise in the pigment epithelium. There may also be an off-effect called a D-wave.

Dark and light adaptation

After 30 to 40 minutes in complete darkness, the sensitivity of the eye to light is increased almost a thousandfold but this sensitivity is almost wholly in the green portion of the spectrum where the greatest absorption by rhodopsin occurs, though light is seen as grey rather than green and all perception of colour is lost. Stimulation with light of other wavelengths reveals reduced sensitivity; some of the decreased sensitivity at the violet end of the spectrum is due to absorption of light of shorter wavelengths by the lens, so that patients whose lenses have been removed for cataract (aphakia) can sometimes see objects in the ultraviolet spectral range which are invisible to others. By contrast, the dark-adapted eye is totally insensitive to light of longer wavelength (i.e. red). Thus dark adaptation can be achieved at least in part by wearing dark red goggles in daylight. By contrast, if an eye is exposed to daylight or strong artificial light, it becomes light-adapted with a shift in sensitivity to the yellow–red end of the spectrum called the *Purkinje shift*.

Visual sensitivity and acuity

It is thus evident that the rods are primarily concerned with visual sensitivity in conditions of dark adaptation, the cones with visual acuity in the light-adapted eye and with colour vision, but the distinction is not absolute as the rods also function in daylight and nocturnal animals can see during the day.

Visual acuity is concerned with the ability to see minute objects in sharp outline. In clinical practice this is measured (see below) by asking the patient to read letters of diminishing size at a standard distance from the eye (distance vision) or to read lines of print held at reading distance (reading acuity). Physiologically it may also be tested by measuring the eye's resolving power, that is the smallest visual angle, say between two vertical lines, at which their separation can be clearly recognized. This is determined by the *grain* of the retina, i.e. the density of its photoreceptors. If these lie far apart, then light from either of the vertical lines or from the contrasting area between them can fall upon an insensitive part of the retina, thus preventing clear resolution of the two lines. Intensity of stimulation is also important; continuing the analogy, if the two vertical lines are dark on a white background, the white area between them gives stimuli of greater intensity than the dark lines themselves, so that acuity also involves a process of intensity discrimination. This is a function of the cerebral cortex rather than of the cone receptors themselves.

Not only, however, is intensity important but also frequency. A single flash of light evokes a burst of electrical impulses in the optic nerve and visual cortex, but, if such flashes are applied with increasing frequency, then a critical fusion frequency, which varies according to the intensity of the stimulus, can be determined, at which point the flashes are no longer distinguished and a single continuous image is perceived. Motion pictures and television make use of this faculty in that the frequency of the visual images is so great that there is no sensation of 'flicker'.

Colour vision

The eyes are sensitive to light of wavelength varying from 400 to 700 nm, from violet through green to red. Coloured objects absorb light of varying wavelength, the colour or hue being a function of wavelength, whereas the brightness or brilliance of a colour is a function of stimulus intensity and purity or saturation of a colour depends upon the extent to which it is diluted by the admixture of white light. The three primary colours of the visual spectrum are red, green and blue, intervening hues or shades being due to mixtures of the primary colours. The widely-accepted Young–Helmholtz theory of colour vision suggests that there are three different types of cones, each responsive to one of the primary colours, and the fact that there are known to be three cone pigments which absorb light of three different wavelengths supports this concept. Colour perception is affected by the point or area of the retina upon which the stimulus falls, so that a stimulus falling on the fovea, for instance, may be perceived as different in a colour sense from the same stimulus striking a more peripheral part of the retina. There is also evidence that the interpretation of colour is not a simple all-or-none phenomenon due to the direct transmission of impulses from colour-sensitive cones to the visual cortex. It is affected by patterns of firing from colour-coded receptors but also by the integration of excitatory and inhibitory signals from populations of cones with different spectral sensitivities both in the ganglion-cell layer of the retina and at subsequent cellular relay stations on the way to the cortex.

Visual acuity (clinical aspects)

The visual acuity is essentially a measurement of the efficiency of macular or central vision as it depends largely upon the function of this part of the retina and of its nervous connections, provided the mechanism for focusing light upon the retina is intact. Visual fixation is so organized that the image of any object at which we look normally falls on the macula. Peripheral retinal lesions rarely influence it, but a small lesion of the macula or of the optic nerve fibres coming from the macular area may seriously impair the ability to read or to distinguish small objects. This is seen particularly in retrobulbar neuritis (see below). Disorders of refraction (myopia, presbyopia, astigmatism) can also impair visual acuity as may other primary abnormalities of the eye (iridocyclitis, cataract, vitreous haemorrhage) which influence the passage of light to the retina, as well as disorders which damage retinal sensitivity (retinal detachment, glaucoma, etc.). These local causes are usually self-evident (see Frisen 1980) and refractive errors can be corrected by the use of appropriate lenses.

Colour blindness

Colour blindness is an inherited defect which occurs in 8 per cent of the male population and in less than 0.5 per cent of females. It is inherited as a sex-linked (X-linked) recessive character; though it occurs in many forms, the commonest variety is red–green blindness, either partial or complete, in which the affected individual finds it difficult to distinguish reds from greens. Many complex defects have been described. Thus *trichromats* (three-colour vision) include normal individuals but also some with weak red vision (protanomaly) or weak green vision (deuteranomaly). *Dichromats* are those who are unable to perceive red (protanopia) or green (deuteranopia): blue-violet colour blindness (tritanopia) is extremely rare. *Monochromats* (with total colour blindness) are also very rare indeed and some also show severe photophobia. Many patients are unaware of their colour blindness as they recognize 'colours' by their brightness, but the diagnosis can be confirmed with the Ishihara charts. The defect is usually of no significance except in occupations where the recognition of coloured lights or signals, say, is important. However, as will be appreciated from the physiological principles previously considered, in patients with minimal lesions of the visual pathways, field defects for coloured objects (red is commonly used) can often be demonstrated at a time when the field for white objects is complete. The field for red is normally smaller than that for white. There is also some evidence to suggest that, very rarely, colour blindness may be an acquired defect consequent upon bilateral occipital-lobe lesions, though there is no evidence that it ever occurs in isolation due to such a cause (Pearlman, Birch, and Meadows 1979).

The visual pathways and the visual fields

Testing visual acuity

The visual acuity is normally tested for both distant and near vision and if a refractive error is present it is reasonable in the neurological examination to allow the patient to wear his spectacles so that the 'corrected' acuity is assessed. To test distant vision, Snellen's test types are used at a distance of 6 metres and the patient is asked to read the letters with each eye covered. The lines of type are numbered; the patient with normal vision can read the line numbered 6 at a distance of 6 metres so that his acuity is recorded as 6/6. When the acuity is grossly impaired, it may be recorded as 6/60; if a patient cannot read the largest type, then his acuity is recorded as 'hand movements', or 'light perception' only, or total blindness (amblyopia). For testing near vision, which depends upon the integrity of the macular area of the retina and the fibres derived from it, many reading types, including Jaeger's, are available. With those approved by the Faculty of Ophthalmologists, London, the smallest type is classified as N5, the largest N48. When testing the visual fields it should be noted that the results of perimetry may be prejudiced if visual acuity is grossly impaired in one or other eye, so that the results may be unreliable if the acuity is 6/60 or worse.

The visual pathways (from the retina to the primary visual centres)

The optic nerves
The fibres of the optic nerve are the axons of the retinal ganglion cells. The macular fibres are the most important part of the visual afferent systems. In the retina these fibres run from the macula to the temporal side of the optic disc. Fibres from the upper and lower temporal quadrants of the retina are displaced by macular fibres to the upper and lower parts of the disc, and those from the nasal quadrants occupy the nasal side. The optic nerves pass backwards and inwards through the optic foramina and terminate posteriorly in the optic chiasm.

The optic chiasm
At the chiasm the two optic nerves unite and the fibres derived from the nasal halves of the retinae decussate (Fig. 2.1). The position of the chiasm is variable and is important in relation to the field defects produced when it is compressed by tumours in this region. It is usually situated a little behind the tuberculum sellae. It is rarely as far forward as the sulcus chiasmatis and is sometimes much further back behind the dorsum sellae, then being related to the posterior pituitary. The relationship of the chiasm to the sella turcica, pituitary, and infundibulum is thus variable. The most important of its other relations are, above, the floor of the third ventricle and, laterally, the internal carotid arteries.

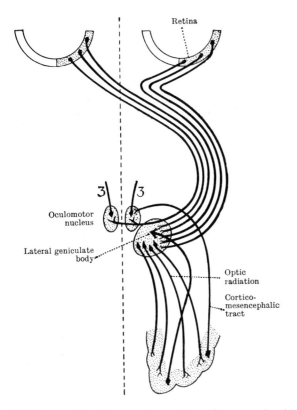

Fig. 2.1. Diagram of central connections of the optic nerve and optic tract.

The decussating fibres from the nasal half of each retina pass backwards to the opposite optic tract. The fibres from the temporal halves of the retinae do not decussate, but continue backwards on the same side in the tract. The blood supply of the chiasm is derived from prechiasmal branches of the ophthalmic artery, a few superior chiasmal branches from the anterior cerebrals, and inferior chiasmal arteries which are branches of the internal carotids (Dawson 1958).

The optic tract
Each optic tract is thus composed of fibres from the temporal half of the retina on the same side and from the nasal half of the retina on the opposite side. Within the tract uncrossed fibres lie dorsolaterally and crossed fibres ventromesially. Each optic tract sweeps outwards and backwards between the cerebral peduncle and the gyrus parahippocampalis, and finally inwards to terminate in the superior colliculus and the lateral geniculate body. The lateral geniculate body appears to receive the fibres concerned in visual perception, and the superior colliculus those destined to excite reflex activity. Besides the localization in a lateral plane already described, there is in the optic nerves, chiasm, and tracts a considerable degree of localization of the fibres in the vertical plane also, fibres from the lower halves of the retinae lying below, and those from the upper halves above.

The geniculocalcarine pathway

From the lateral geniculate body, the visual fibres enter the posterior limb of the internal capsule, where they lie behind the somatic sensory fibres and medial to those of the auditory radiation. They emerge from the capsule as the optic radiation, or geniculocalcarine pathway, which runs to the area striata of the occipital lobe. The more dorsal fibres pass directly to the visual cortex, but those situated more ventrally in the radiation turn downwards and forwards into the uncinate region of the temporal lobe (Meyer's loop), and there spread out over the tip of the temporal horn of the lateral ventricle before turning back beneath the ventricle to reach the inferior lip of the calcarine sulcus (Falconer and Wilson 1958; van Buren and Baldwin 1958). As we have seen, fibres from the lower half of the retina remain below those from the upper half throughout the optic chiasm and tracts, and this relationship persists in the radiation. Hence the more direct upper fibres are derived from the upper halves of the retinae and are excited by images from the lower halves of the visual fields, and the reverse is true of the lower fibres, which pass close to the tip of the temporal lobe.

The visual cortex

The cortical visual area or 'area striata' is situated within the depths of and also above and below the calcarine sulcus and in adjacent portions of the cuneus and lingual gyrus; it may extend slightly on to the lateral surface of the occipital pole. From descriptions given above it will be evident that the visual cortex on one side receives impulses from the temporal half of the retina on the same side and the nasal half of the opposite retina, that is, from those halves of the retinae which are excited by images derived from the opposite halves of the visual fields. The retinae may be regarded as being projected upon the visual cortex as follows. The macular area occupies the depths of the calcarine fissure and a wedge-shaped area of the most posterior part of the visual cortex, extending slightly on to the lateral surface of the occipital lobe, the apex of the wedge being 2 or 3 cm anterior to the occipital pole. The periphery of the retina is represented in front of the macular area of the cortex, concentric zones of the retina from macula to periphery probably being represented from behind forwards in the visual area. The upper quadrants of the retina are represented in the upper part of the visual cortex, above the calcarine sulcus, and the lower quadrants below. From these facts the effects of lesions involving the visual cortex can readily be deduced.

Charting the visual fields

Mapping the fields of vision and the visual acuity within them plays an important part in the routine examination of patients suffering from nervous diseases. Many methods of mapping the fields (perimetry) have been described, of which the following are some.

Confrontation perimetry

This method is crude and only gross defects of the visual fields are likely to be detected by it. The observer stands or sits opposite to the patient and about a metre away from him. The patient is asked to cover one eye with his hand and to fix the gaze of his other eye upon the bridge of the observer's nose. The observer then moves a test object, such as a hat-pin with a small white head, inwards from beyond the limits of his own visual field, midway between himself and the patient, who is asked to say when he first sees it. This procedure is carried out above, below, and to either side, and the observer can thus determine the extent of the patient's visual field relative to his own. The test object should also be moved across the field in various directions and the patient is asked to state if it disappears from view and when it reappears. In this way a *scotoma* (an area of defective vision within the field) may be detected. The 'blind spot' is a scotoma produced by the optic disc which does not contain any visual receptors.

In young children and unco-operative patients a field defect is sometimes detected by observing whether the patient notices an object brought in from the periphery in various directions, or whether he blinks in response to a feint with the hand towards the eye—the *menace reflex*.

Mechanical perimetry

There are many types of perimeter in common use. The patient gazes at a fixation point and the test object is then moved in the arc of a circle towards that point. The object is at a distance of from 250 to 330 mm from the eye and is usually between 3 and 10 mm in diameter. The visual acuity differs in different parts of the visual field. Although a moving object is readily perceived in the peripheral part, central vision for a stationary object is more acute than peripheral vision. Hence the smaller the test object the smaller the field in which it is perceptible. The conditions of the test are indicated by the fraction

diameter of object/distance

If a 3-mm test object is used at a distance of 330 mm, this fraction is 3/330. Boundaries of the normal visual field of 3/330 are situated at about 60 degrees up, 60 degrees in, 75 degrees down, and 100 degrees, or a little more, out. The field for colours is smaller than that for white, that for blue and yellow being somewhat larger than that for red and green.

Scotoma charting with Bjerrum's screen

A mechanical perimeter is useful for determining the boundaries of the visual fields but more refined methods are often necessary for mapping the central fields. Bjerrum's screen enables test objects of 1 and 2 mm to be used at a distance of 2 metres—1/2000 and 2/2000. In this way very slight defects of central vision may be detected and, since they are projected upon a large area, accurately mapped. Reduced visual acuity in the centre of the field is not always demonstrable with reading types. Bjerrum's screen is of special value in detecting such defects. The normal field for a 1/2000 test object by this method extends to nearly 26 degrees in all directions. If a defect exists to 1/2000 or 2/2000 objects, larger objects should be used until one is seen in the area of impaired vision. Other perimeters such as the Goldmann and Tübingen instruments (see Ashworth and Isherwood 1981) are also available for charting both the peripheral fields and central scotomata but none has yet supplanted the Bjerrum screen.

Abnormalities of the visual fields

The term 'hemianopia' indicates a loss of vision in half of the visual field. When this affects the same half of both fields, for example both right halves, we speak of 'homonymous hemianopia'. When the defect on one side is a mirror image of that on the other, the hemianopia is said to be bitemporal or binasal, according to the halves affected. A defect limited to one quadrant is described as 'quadrantic hemianopia' or 'quadrantanopia'. When homonymous field defects can be accurately superimposed one upon another, they are called congruous; when their corresponding boundaries differ, they are called incongruous.

Closely related disturbances of visual function are visual inattention, indicated by a failure to notice movement of an object such as the observer's finger in one half-field, when there is a competing stimulus in the opposite half-field, and visual disorientation, which is inability to localize objects seen, especially to estimate relative distance (see p. 64). Some patients with field defects due to cortical lesions experience simple formed hallucinations in the area of the defect, presumably resulting from irritation of contiguous association cortex (Lance 1976).

Many more precise methods of assessing visual function are now available. Tachistoscopy is a complex method of assessing responses to and perception of visual stimuli presented independently or simultaneously in many parts of the visual field and is especially useful in investigating defects of attention. The electro-retinogram (ERG) is an electrical response of visual receptors in the retina which can be recorded with corneal electrodes, and the visual evoked response (VER) is an electrical potential arriving at the occipital cortex after stimulation of the retina by a flash of light or patterned stimuli; it can be recorded through the intact skull. Measurement of these electrical events and of the character and latency of the VER may be of considerable value in the differential diagnosis of disorders of visual function (Walsh and Hoyt 1969; Harden and Pampiglione 1970; Halliday, McDonald, and Mushin 1972; Halliday, Halliday, Kriss, McDonald, and Mushin 1976; Halliday and Mushin 1980).

Visual-field defects due to lesions of the visual pathways

Lesions of the optic nerve

A lesion of one optic nerve produces a field defect limited to the same eye, since it lies anterior to the chiasmal decussation. The type of defect produced varies according to the pathology of the lesion and is more fully discussed below. In general, inflammatory and compressive lesions of the optic nerve often give a central scotoma (Fig. 2.2) or a sector defect of irregular shape, but in papilloedema due to increased intracranial pressure the characteristic field defect is an enlargement of the blind spot, together with peripheral concentric constriction.

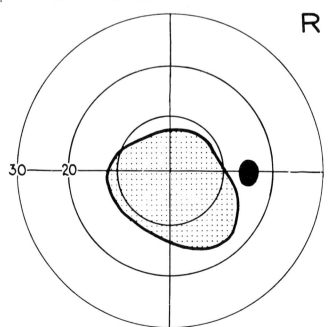

Fig. 2.2. A central scotoma due to retrobulbar neuritis.

Lesions of the chiasm

The commonest lesions of the optic chiasm are those due to pressure, either from tumours of the pituitary or those lying above the sella turcica, such as craniopharyngiomas and meningiomas. In addition, the chiasm itself may be the site of a glioma; it may be compressed by a tumour arising in the third ventricle, by distension of the third ventricle in hydrocephalus, by an intracranial aneurysm, or by a mucocele of the sphenoid sinus (Goodwin and Glaser 1978). It may be involved in chronic arachnoiditis, in granulomatous meningitis due to syphilis, tuberculosis, or sarcoidosis, in demyelinating disorders such as multiple sclerosis and neuromyelitis optica; rarely, it is damaged by ischaemia or head injury.

When the point of maximal pressure is in the midline, the decussating fibres are first compressed, so that at some stage there is bitemporal hemianopia, for, as we have seen, the decussating fibres are derived from the nasal halves of both retinae, which receive images from the temporal halves of the visual fields. Binasal hemianopia may result from compression of the lateral aspects of the chiasm by atherosclerotic internal carotid or anterior cerebral arteries (O'Connell and du Boulay 1973); O'Connell (1973) suggested that the medial fibres of the chiasm are most sensitive to the effects of tension, the lateral ones to pressure. When there is pressure upon the chiasm from below, the fibres from the lower nasal quadrants of the retinae are first affected. Hence the field defect begins in the upper temporal quadrants. When the pressure comes from above, the reverse is the case. This schematic explanation must now be qualified by the statement that pituitary and suprasellar tumours rarely exert symmetrical pressure in the midline. Hence the decussating fibres are usually involved on one side before the other. Consequently, in the case of pituitary tumours,

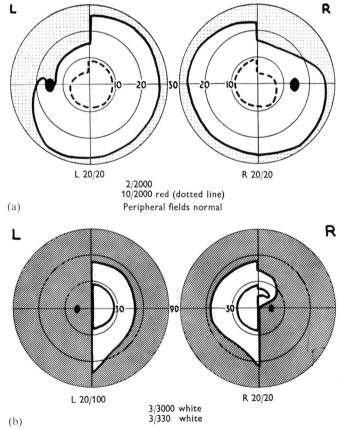

L   R

L 20/20   R 20/20
2/2000
10/2000 red (dotted line)
(a)   Peripheral fields normal

L   R

L 20/100   R 20/20
3/3000 white
(b)   3/330 white

Fig. 2.3. (a) Visual fields of a patient with a chromophobe adenoma of the pituitary, showing early changes in the upper temporal quadrants.
   (b) Field changes in a patient with a chromophobe adenoma of the pituitary. There is an almost complete bitemporal hemianopia.

the field defect begins as a rule in the upper temporal quadrant on one side as an indentation which may be associated with a paracentral scotoma with which it subsequently fuses. It then spreads to the lower quadrant, while a similar change occurs a little later on the opposite side (Fig. 2.3). Further pressure leads to involvement of the nasal field of the eye first affected so that eventually there is blindness of one eye with temporal hemianopia of the other. Finally the remaining nasal field is lost. Since pressure may involve also either the optic nerve or tract, many forms of visual field change are encountered. The most characteristic feature of the visual-field defects associated with lesions of the chiasm is their asymmetry compared with the more symmetrical defects due to lesions of the optic tracts and radiation. Early compression of the optic nerve and chiasm is often misdiagnosed as optic neuritis (Garfield and Neil-Dwyer 1975).

Lesions of the optic tract

Since the optic tracts receive fibres from the temporal half of the retina of the same side and the nasal half of the opposite retina, they carry impulses derived from visual images of objects in the opposite half of the visual field. Lesions of one optic tract, therefore, result in a crossed homonymous field defect which usually begins in one quadrant and rarely extends to a complete homonymous hemianopia. Sometimes there are homonymous central scotomas (Bender and Bodis-Wollner 1978). The defects in the two visual fields are not as a rule totally congruous, the defect being usually slightly greater upon the side of the lesion than upon the opposite side. A homonymous field defect occurs in cases of pituitary tumour about half as frequently as bitemporal hemianopia, and the optic tract may also be compressed by other tumours at the base of the brain, including those of the anterior temporal lobe, by aneurysm of the internal carotid and posterior communicating arteries; it may also be involved in inflammatory lesions, such as granulomatous meningitis.

Lesions of the optic radiation

Complete destruction of one optic radiation produces a contralateral homonymous hemianopia, while less extensive lesions produce contralateral homonymous defects which are congruous. There is often apparent sparing of a small area around the fixation point ('sparing of the macula') but this may be an artefact (see below). Lesions in the lower part of the radiation such as temporal-lobe tumours produce a contralateral homonymous superior quadrantopia (Fig. 2.4) while lesions in the parietal lobe produce conversely a crossed inferior quadrantic loss. The commonest lesions involving the radiation are infarction, haemorrhage, or tumour (Fig. 2.5), but abscesses and many other pathological processes may involve the optic radiations. Thus they affected early in various forms of diffuse cerebral sclerosis such as Schilder's disease.

Lesions of the visual cortex

There is still dispute about the significance of 'macular sparing' and some continue to believe that the macula is bilaterally represented at the visual cortex, others that each half of it projects to the opposite side. Gassel and Williams (1962) suggested that macular sparing was an artefact resulting from defective ocular fixation during charting of the fields, but Walsh and Hoyt (1969) disagreed. The majority view now, however, suggests that macular representation is split between the two hemispheres. Nevertheless, true macular sparing may be seen when a lesion of the visual cortex spares the tip of the occipital pole (Safran, Babel, and Werner 1978; Bynke 1980).

Lesions of one visual cortex cause crossed homonymous field defects which are always congruous. Lesions involving the upper half, i.e. the area above the calcarine sulcus, produce inferior quadrantic field defects, and vice versa. Complete destruction of the visual cortex on one side produces a crossed homonymous hemianopia.

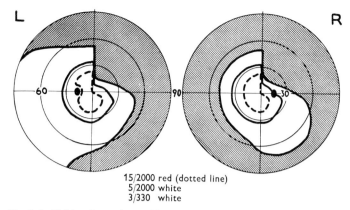

15/2000 red (dotted line)
5/2000 white
3/330 white

Fig. 2.4. Fields of a patient with a glioma in the left temporo-occipital region.

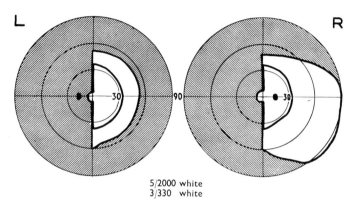

5/2000 white
3/330 white

Fig. 2.5. Fields of a patient with a metastasis from a breast carcinoma involving the right geniculocalcarine pathway.

The main arterial supply of the visual cortex is the posterior cerebral artery. Thrombosis of the posterior cerebral artery therefore causes a crossed homonymous hemianopia. Bilateral posterior cerebral artery occlusion usually gives total cerebral or cortical blindness (Symonds and Mackenzie 1957); transient cortical blindness is also a common manifestation of cerebral anoxia, especially in children (Barnet, Manson, and Wilner 1970), and recovery is often incomplete. The commonest lesions of the visual cortex are vascular lesions and tumours. Many cases of gunshot wound of this part of the brain were observed during the first World War (Holmes 1918). In occasional cases, intensive retraining using visual stimuli delivered around the edges of the field defect produces limited improvement (Zihl and von Cramon 1979).

References

Ashworth, B. and Isherwood, I. (1981). *Clinical neuro-ophthalmology*, 2nd edn. Blackwell, Oxford.

Barnet, A. B., Manson, J. I., and Wilner, E. (1970). Acute cerebral blindness in childhood. *Neurology, Minneapolis* **20**, 1147.

Bender, M. C. and Bodis-Wollner, I. (1978). Visual dysfunctions in optic tract lesions. *Ann. Neurol.* **3**, 187.

Bynke, H. (1980). Visual fields. In *Neuro-ophthalmology*, ed. S. Lessell and J. T. W. van Dalen, Vol. 1, Chapter 21. Excerpta Medica, Amsterdam.

Cogan, D. (1977). *Neurology of the visual system*, 2nd edn. Thomas, Springfield, Illinois.

Cushing, H. and Walker, C. B. (1914–15). Distortion of the visual fields in cases of brain tumour (4); chiasmal lesions with especial reference to bitemporal hemianopsia. *Brain* **37**, 341.

Dawson, B. H. (1958). The blood vessels of the human optic chiasma and their relation to those of the hypophysis and hypothalamus. *Brain* **81**, 207.

Falconer, M. A. and Wilson, J. L. (1958). Visual field changes following anterior temporal lobectomy; their significance in relation to 'Meyer's loop' of the optic radiation. *Brain* **81**, 1.

Frisen, L. (1980). The neurology of visual acuity. *Brain* **103**, 639.

Garfield, J. and Neil-Dwyer, G. (1975). Delay in diagnosis of optic nerve and chiasmal compression presenting with unilateral failing vision. *Br. med. J.* **1**, 22.

Gassel, M. M. and Williams, D. (1962). Visual function in patients with homonymous hemianopia. Part I. The visual fields. *Brain* **85**, 175.

Goodwin, J. A. and Glaser, J. S. (1978). Chiasmal syndrome in sphenoid sinus mucocele. *Ann. Neurol.* **4**, 440.

Halliday, A. M., Halliday, E., Kriss, A. McDonald, W. I., and Mushin, J. (1976). The pattern-evoked potential in compression of the anterior visual pathways. *Brain* **99**, 357.

——, McDonald, W. I., and Mushin, J. (1972). Delayed visual evoked response in optic neuritis. *Lancet* **ii**, 982.

—— and Mushin, J. (1980). The visual evoked potential in neuroophthalmology. *Inter. Ophthalmol. Clinics* **20**, 155.

Harden, A. and Pampiglione, G. (1970). Neurophysiological approach to disorders of vision. *Lancet* **ii**, 805.

Holmes, G. (1918). Disturbances of vision by cerebral lesions, *Br. J. Ophthal.* **2**, 353.

—— (1931). A contribution to the cortical representation of vision. *Brain* **54**, 470.

Horrax, G. and Putnam, T. J. (1932). Distortion of the visual fields in cases of brain tumour. The field defects and hallucinations produced by tumours of the occipital lobe. *Brain* **55**, 499.

Kandel, E. R. and Schwartz, J. H. (1981). *Principles of neural science*. Elsevier North-Holland, New York.

Lance, J. W. (1976). Simple formed hallucinations confined to the area of a specific visual field defect. *Brain* **99**, 719.

Lessell, S. and van Dalen, J. T. W. (Eds.) (1980). *Neuro-ophthalmology*, Vol. 1. Excerpt Medica, Amsterdam.

O'Connell, J. E. A. (1973). The anatomy of the optic chiasm and heteronymous hemianopia. *J. Neurol. Neurosurg. Psychiat.* **36**, 710.

—— and du Boulay, E. P. G. H. (1973). Bisnasal hemianopia. *J. Neurol. Neurosurg. Psychiat.* **36**, 697.

Patton, H. D., Sundsten, J. W., Crill, W. E., and Swanson, P. D. (1976). *Introduction to basic neurology*. Sanders, Philadelphia.

Pearlman, A. L., Birch, J., and Meadows, J. C. (1979). Cerebral color blindness: an acquired defect in hue discrimination. *Ann. Neurol.* **5**, 253.

Safran, A. B., Babel, J., and Werner, A. (1978). Aspects campimétriques des lésions occipitales. *J. franç. Ophtal.* **1**, 9.

Symonds, C. P. and Mackenzie, I. (1957) Bilateral loss of vision from cerebral infarction. *Brain* **80**, 415.

Traquair, H. M., Dott, N. M., and Russell, W. R. (1935). Traumatic lesions of the optic chiasma. *Brain* **58**, 398.

van Buren, J. M. and Baldwin, M. (1958). The architecture of the optic radiation in the temporal lobe of man. *Brain* **81**, 15.

Walsh, F. B. and Hoyt, W. F. (1969). The visual sensory system; anatomy, physiology and topographic diagnosis. In *Handbook of clinical neurology* (ed. P. J. Vinken and G. W. Bruyn) Vol. 2, Chapter 19. North-Holland, Amsterdam.

Walton, J. N. (1981). The special senses, in Neurology (Section XII) by J. N. Walton. In *Pathophysiology—the biological principles of disease* (ed. L. H. Smith Jr. and S. O. Thier), *International Textbook of Medicine*. Saunders, Philadelphia.

Zihl, J. and von Cramon, D. (1979). Restitution of visual function in patients with cerebral blindness. *J. Neurol. Neurosurg. Psychiat.* **42**, 312.

Examination of the optic fundus (ophthalmoscopy)

Examination of the fundus oculi is so important that it should form part of the routine examination of every patient. Except when the pupil is greatly contracted, it is usually possible to examine the optic disc; but to examine completely the macular region and the periphery of the retina, the pupil should previously be dilated with homatropine. The normal optic disc is circular and rosy pink in colour, though slightly paler than the surrounding retina. It possesses a well-defined edge and a depression—the physiological cup—from which the arteries and veins emerge. The normal appearance of the disc and vessels can be learned only from experience. The following are the most important abnormalities. The disc may be pinker than normal, from hyperaemia, or abnormally pale from optic atrophy. Its edge may be indistinct. The physiological cup may be filled or the disc may be actually swollen above the level of the surrounding retina, the swelling being measured in dioptres. Abnormal 'cupping' of the entire disc is typical of glaucoma. Streaks of white medullated nerve fibres extending on to the retina from one part of the disc are occasionally seen but have no pathological significance. A white crescentic area to one side (a myopic crescent) is often present in myopic individuals. The veins may be congested, the arteries may be thickened and tortuous, or both arteries and veins may be abnormally fine and narrow. Visible pulsation of arteries is abnormal, but venous pulsation is sometimes seen in normal idividuals. Finally, the disc and surrounding area of the retina may be the site of exudate or haemorrhages.

The macular region lies about two disc-breadths horizontally outwards from the outer edge of the disc. It is somewhat darker than the rest of the fundus and is almost devoid of blood vessels. The principal abnormalities to be seen in the macula are an extension of oedema from the disc—the macular 'fan'—and a stippled, star-shaped, or haemorrhagic exudate in cases of hypertensive retinopathy. A cherry-red spot is seen at the macula in some cases of occlusion of the central retinal artery and in infantile cerebromacular degeneration, and pigmentation is seen in the late infantile and juvenile forms. Since the macula is concerned with central vision, macular lesions cause severe impairment of visual acuity.

Finally the periphery of the retina should be inspected. The condition of the arteries and the veins is noted. Retinal arteriosclerosis first manifests itself in constriction of veins at the point where they are crossed by the arteries, with congestion of the portion distal to the crossing. Greater degrees of arterial thickening lead to tortuosity and irregularity of the arteries, with increased light refraction from their surface—silver-wire arteries. In retinal arteriosclerosis and hypertensive retinopathy haemorrhages and exudate may be seen in the peripheral parts of the retina and, in diabetic retinopathy, similar patches of white exudate may be seen, sometimes associated with microaneurysms though, for the accurate demonstration of the latter, fluorescein retinal angiography is needed. In cases of recurrent retinal micro-embolism, as in carotid stenosis, it is sometimes possible to visualize micro-emboli of platelets or cholesterol in smaller retinal arteries. Occlusion of individual arterial branches may occasionally occur in migraine; marked narrowing of all of the retinal arteries with pallor of the fundus can result from central retinal artery occlusion in cranial arteries. Patchy black pigmentation of the retina may be seen in choroidoretinitis, but longitudinal streaks of pigment lying between the vessels, when accompanied by optic atrophy and attenuation of arteries, are typical of retinitis pigmentosa, while similar pigmentary degeneration without changes in the disc and vessels is found in some hereditary ataxias and in the Kearns–Sayre syndrome. A retinal angioblastoma may sometimes be seen in cases of Lindau's disease and a phakoma in tuberous sclerosis or neurofibromatosis while, in cases of miliary tuberculosis or tuberculous meningitis, tubercles may be seen in the retina as roundish, yellow bodies about half the size of the disc.

Lesions of the optic nerve

Papilloedema (choked disc)

Papilloedema simply means oedema of the optic disc, without reference to its underlying cause. It may be due to different pathological states, of which the following are the most important:

1. Increased intracranial pressure (tumour, haemorrhage, infarction, abscess, oedema).
2. Inflammation of the optic nerve as in optic or retrobulbar neuritis.

3. Oedema associated with disease of the retinal arteries and retinal exudation, as in malignant hypertension and giant-cell arteritis.
4. Venous obstruction, due to space-occupying lesions in the orbit, thrombosis of the central retinal vein, cavernous sinus thrombosis, cortico-cavernous fistula, intrathoracic venous obstruction, as by neoplasms, aneurysm of the aorta.
5. Conditions associated with a massive increase in the protein content of the CSF (e.g. some cases of the Guillain-Barré syndrome).
6. Changes in the blood, as in severe anaemia or primary or secondary polycythaemia.
7. Miscellaneous causes. Connective-tissue disease, carcinomatous neuropathy, the reticuloses, infective endocarditis, low intraocular pressure as in uveitis or ischaemic optic neuropathy, and Graves' disease with severe exophthalmos.

In neurology, the papilloedema due to increased intracranial pressure and that associated with optic neuritis are of greatest importance. The single most useful distinguishing feature is that, in papilloedema due to raised pressure, visual failure occurs late if at all, while in that due to optic neuritis severe loss of visual acuity is usually the first manifestation.

Papilloedema due to increased intracranial pressure

The optic nerve, which developmentally and histologically is part of the brain, is surrounded like it by the three meninges. Immediately covering the nerve is the pia mater and superficial to that the arachnoid; both extend forwards to fuse with the sclera. Outside both is the dura mater, which is continuous anteriorly with the orbital periosteum. The optic nerve, therefore, is surrounded by a subarachnoid space which is continuous with the cerebral subarachnoid space. A rise in the pressure in the subarachnoid space therefore has a double effect, causing compression of the central vein of the retina where it crosses the space, and impeding lymphatic drainage from the retina and optic nerve. The combined result of this venous and lymphatic obstruction is congestion and oedema of the optic disc and retina. Diffuse cerebral oedema also involving the optic nerves themselves may sometimes be a factor (Behrman 1966) as may impaired axoplasmic flow and blockage of extra-axonal centripetal transport of tissue fluid (Bradley 1976; *British Medical Journal* 1978). The following are the principal causes of increased intracranial pressure leading to papilloedema.

Intracranial tumour. Not all intracranial tumours cause papilloedema (see Wolfe and Bird 1980). Generally speaking, the occurrence of papilloedema depends upon whether the tumour is so placed as to cause a rise in the tension of the CSF, and also upon its rate of growth. It almost invariably develops eventually in the case of tumours of the cerebellum and the fourth ventricle, but is absent in many cases of temporal subcortical and pontine tumours. It is frequently late in developing when the tumour is in the prefrontal region or arises near the vertex. Posterior fossa tumours give rise to papilloedema of the greatest severity. The more rapidly a tumour grows the more likely it is to cause this sign. Inequality of the oedema in the two eyes is not uncommon, but if the difference is not great it is of no localizing value. A tumour arising near one optic foramen may prevent the development of papilloedema in that eye by cutting off the optic sheath from communication with the cerebral subarachnoid space. In such cases primary optic atrophy may develop on the side of the tumour, often with papilloedema on the opposite side (syndrome of Gowers, Paton, and Foster Kennedy).

Cerebral abscess. Papilloedema is inconstant and late in developing.

Hydrocephalus. Hydrocephalus from any cause may led to papilloedema, but the pressure of the distended floor of the third ventricle upon the optic chiasm may cause optic atrophy.

Meningitis. Meningitis causes papilloedema less often then might be expected, possibly because the condition is often acute and rapidly responsive to treatment or because meningeal exudates tend to wall off the optic sheaths. Papilloedema is commonest in tuberculous and other forms of granulomatous meningitis.

Intracranial sinus thrombosis. This increases the pressure of the CSF by diminishing its rate of absorption.

Cerebral oedema. Generalized brain swelling (as in head injury or various toxic and metabolic states) or focal oedema (as after massive infarction or cerebral haemorrhage) sometimes causes papilloedema. The sign is almost invariable in benign intracranial hypertension, a syndrome of diffuse cerebral oedema of multiple (often unknown) aetiology (p. 137).

Subarachnoid haemorrhage. Haemorrhage into the subarachnoid space may cause papilloedema, as the blood distends the subarachnoid space of the optic sheaths.

Some unusual causes. Rarely emphysema leads to papilloedema by raising the venous and CSF pressure; various toxic and metabolic encephalopathies may also give raised pressure (p. 254).

Ophthalmoscopic appearances of papilloedema
In the earliest stage of papilloedema the retinal veins are congested and the optic disc is pinker than normal. The disc edge is blurred at its upper and lower margins, and this blurring extends to the nasal side before the temporal. Increasing oedema fills the physiological cup, and later the nerve head becomes elevated above the retina, sometimes by as much as 8 or even 10 dioptres. The oedema in severe cases spreads into the retina causing a macular 'fan'. Distension of retinal veins is extreme, and haemorrhages may develop in the retina and on the disc itself. In severe papilloedema, transient amblyopic episodes or other obscurations of vision may occur, especially on stooping or on coughing, and the patient may see 'haloes' around lights. These symptoms demand urgent measures to reduce the intracranial pressure as they indicate ischaemia due to pressure upon the central retinal artery; if they continue unchecked, the artery may be permanently occluded, giving irreversible blindness. If chronic papilloedema persists, the condition may progress to so-called secondary optic atrophy. The swelling of the disc diminishes, it becomes paler, and the arteries become constricted. Finally, in a typical case, the disc is pale and flat, the physiological cup remains filled, and the edges of the disc are less distinct than formerly. The arteries are constricted, but the veins often remain congested for some time.

The visual fields in papilloedema
In the earlier stages the only change may be enlargement of the blind spots. Later there is concentric constriction of the fields. Papilloedema may, of course, be associated with field changes due to lesions involving other parts of the visual system.

Pseudopapilloedema: diagnosis from true papilloedema.
Slight elevation of the optic disc due to increased myelin anterior to the lamina cribrosa is sometimes seen in hypermetropic individuals and is one cause of pseudopapilloedema. More difficult to distinguish are hyaline bodies or drusen, congenital lesions of no pathological significance, which may be buried in the disc and may cause it to be elevated with blurred margins. They may also enlarge the blind spot (Wolfe and Bird 1980) and rarely cause small peri-papillary haemorrhages (Hitchings, Corbett, Winkleman and Schatz 1976). The absence of venous congestion is a valuable sign in distinguishing this change from true papilloedema but, when doubt persists, fluorescein retinal angiography (Dollery, Hodge and Engel 1962; Hoyt 1963, Haining 1966) is helpful as in true papilloedema this usually shows swollen and proliferated capillaries around the disc margin and fluorescence in the swollen disc itself; however, the method is not infallible (*British Medical Journal* 1978). It is also valuable in diagnosing anterior ischaemic optic neuropathy (see below and Hayreh 1981).

Optic neuritis and retrobulbar neuritis
The term 'optic neuritis' was once employed for all conditions giving oedema of the optic disc, even including intracranial tumour. Since neuritis implies inflammation this was a misnomer, and the name is now confined to infective, demyelinating, or toxi-infective conditions of the optic nerve giving acute unilateral or bilateral visual loss. The distinction between optic and retrobulbar neuritis is based upon an opthalmoscopic rather than a pathological difference, and is apt to be misleading. If a neuritis of the nerve is sufficiently anterior to cause oedema of the disc, it is described as optic neuritis or papillitis; if it is more posteriorly situated so that the direct effects of the inflammation are not visible ophthalmoscopically, it is called retrobulbar neuritis. This distinction is of no pathological significance.

Terminology and aetiology
Even the definition given above lacks clarity. While local inflammation (e.g. in orbital cellulitis or paranasal sinusitis) may spread to involve the optic nerve (Bradley 1968) and this is plainly neuritis in a pathological sense, the term is now generally used to identify a syndrome of unilateral visual failure of rapid onset, not shown to be due to local inflammation in the eye or orbital tissues, to vascular occlusion, or to toxic or metabolic causes. In most such cases the pathological process is one of acute demyelination in the optic nerve, associated with distortion of the waveform, as well as delay in conduction of pattern-evoked visual potentials (Halliday, McDonald and Mushin 1972, 1973; Heron, Regan, and Milner 1974; Halliday 1978); the changes in these responses when a reversing checkerboard of black and white squares is used as the stimulus generally differ from the abnormalities resulting from compression of the anterior visual pathways (Halliday, Halliday, Kriss, McDonald and Mushin 1976). This form of optic neuritis is a manifestation of multiple sclerosis in about 50 per cent of cases, the risk of subsequent development of the latter disease varying from 17 per cent to 87 per cent in different series (Wray 1980). In many other cases, however, the condition remains unexplained, even after detailed investigation and prolonged follow-up (Bradley and Whitty 1968; Ellenberger, Keltner and Burde 1973).

In many previous reports, confusion has resulted from the inclusion in various series of cases of acute unilateral or bilateral visual failure resulting from vascular occlusion, toxins, drugs, or metabolic and hereditary causes. Some of these give rise to irreversible optic atrophy. It is preferable that these conditions should be classified as optic neuropathies, with their individual causes being indentified wherever possible.

Multiple sclerosis (MS)
Optic neuritis is the presenting symptom of this disease, sometimes preceding other manifestations by many years, in about 15 per cent of cases, while about 50 per cent of patients with established MS experience an attack during the course of the illness (Wray 1980). Rarely, except in neuromyelitis optica (see below), the condition affects both eyes simultaneously; more often there are successive attacks affecting one eye first and the other much later, but in most cases a single attack is experienced involving only one eye. However, visual evoked-response recording has shown that many patients with MS must have experienced previous asymptomatic episodes of optic-nerve demyelination. Recovery of vision following an attack is usually complete but a permanent central scotoma sometimes persists; the size of the scotoma may increase with a corresponding transient diminution in reading acuity during exercise or on exposure to heat (e.g. a hot bath) or vasodilator drugs such as alcohol (Uhthoff's symptom). Often after recovery, even if clinically complete, there is pallor of the temporal half of the affected optic disc. The finding of an

increased relative proportion of IgG and of an abnormal electrophoretic pattern in the CSF in cases of optic neuritis implies a high risk of subsequently developing MS, but a normal CSF does not exclude this possibility (Nikoskelainen, Frey and Salmi 1981). While both optic neuritis and MS are associated with the HLA-DR2 antigen, it seems that the polymorphic properdin factor Bf shows a lower incidence in those patients with clinically definite MS (Fielder, Batchelor, Nason Vakarelis, Compston and McDonald 1981).

Neuromyelitis optica (Devic's disease)
This syndrome, in which an acute transverse myelitis is associated with bilateral optic neuritis, may occur at any age from childhood until late life. Sometimes the optic neuritis affects one eye before the other, sometimes the two simultaneously. On occasion the ocular symtoms come first, in other cases those of the spinal-cord affliction, or again all may begin together. Recovery may ultimately be complete or the patient may be left with bilateral central scotomata and residual paralysis (p. 306). The condition seems to be unusually frequent in Japan. Most authorities accept that while this syndrome may be due to a self-limiting encephalomyelitis also involving the optic nerve, a condition which can also give bilateral optic neuritis without spinal-cord involvement (Hierons and Lyle 1959), it usually represents only one of the symptom complexes with which MS may become manifest (McAlpine, Lumsden and Acheson 1972).

Clinical features of optic and retrobulbar neuritis
In acute optic neuritis there is often pain in the affected eye increased by ocular movement or by pressure on the eyeball and visual acuity declines rapidly, often giving total blindness in the eye within hours or days. Demyelination close to the disc often causes disc swelling but this is rarely severe and haemorrhages are uncommon. A lesion situated more posteriorly may give no change in the disc. Usually recovery begins in a week or two and is complete in six to 12 weeks, but in severe cases there may be residual optic atrophy involving either the whole disc or its temporal half. Macular fibres suffer most, either because the central part of the nerve is most involved or because, being the most highly evolved part of the visual afferent system, they are most susceptible to damage. Hence the characteristic visual-field defect is a central scotoma, the loss for red and green objects being greater than that for white. When there is residual atrophy, a central scotoma often persists, much smaller than that of the acute phase. Helpful points of distinction between optic neuritis with papillitis on the one hand and papilloedema on the other are that in the former the swelling of the disc is slight in comparison with the loss of vision, in the latter the reverse is usually the case; and in optic neuritis the usual field defect is a central scotoma, in papilloedema a peripheral concentric constriction. The so-called retrobulbar pupil reaction is also helpful; direct light stimulation of the affected eye gives a sluggish reaction while stimulation of the unaffected eye elicits a brisk response in both eyes. Alternatively, in less severe cases, a reasonably brisk direct reaction in the affected eye is followed by slow pupillary dilatation.

Treatment. Controlled trials have shown that prednisone 60 mg daily or corticotrophin 80 units daily by injection given for two to three weeks early in the course of acute optic or retrobulbar neuritis may relieve pain and shorten the course of the illness. However, neither these remedies nor retrobulbar injections of steroid (Gould, Bird, Leaver and McDonald 1977) seem to influence the eventual outcome, though there is some evidence that high-dose intravenous steroids given early may have a favourable influence upon prognosis (Wray 1980).

Optic and retrobulbar neuropathy

Miscellaneous causes
Among the many conditions which have been known to give rise to acute unilateral or bilateral visual failure, resembling optic neuritis, and which were formerly included as possible causes of that syndrome, are granulomatous meningitis (in syphilis, tuberculosis, sarcoid, and cryptococcosis), carcinomatosis of the meninges, ophthalmic herpes zoster, vaccination against smallpox, rabies, and influenza, and viral infections including infective mononucleoisis (see Wray 1980). In these conditions the prognosis and treatment is that of the primary disease. The same applies to drug-induced acute visual failure as in methyl alcohol poisoning; most drugs which damage the optic nerves give optic atrophy. In addition, the acute onset of Leber's optic atrophy (see below) is also reminiscent of that of optic neuritis.

Vascular causes
Granulomatosis or obliterative endarteritis due to syphilis or to connective-tissue disease may cause sudden unilateral or bilateral visual failure due to occlusion of the central retinal or posterior ciliary arteries (Hayreh 1981). Anterior ischaemic optic neuropathy is most often due, especially after the age of 55 years, to cranial or giant-cell arteritis and this may give swelling of the affected disc. Acute ischaemic optic neuropathy also occurs in elderly patients with diabetes, hypertension, and atherosclerosis (Ellenberger et al, 1973), while chronic posterior ischaemic neuropathy or severe blood loss can give bilateral or unilateral visual loss and low-tension glaucoma (Drance, Morgan, and Sweeney 1973). Ischaemic optic neuropathy has also been reported as a consequence of micro-embolism, Behcet's disease, and acute porphyria (see Behrens 1980).

Metabolic, toxic, and nutritional causes
It has long been thought in Britain that there is a clear association between the smoking of strong dark pipe tobacco and sudden bilateral visual failure characterized by centrocaecal scotomas. The condition was entitled tobacco amblyopia in Britain and tobacco/ alcohol amblyopia in the United States because there was usually a history of heavy alcohol consumption as well. Heaton, McCormick, and Freeman (1958) suggested that cyanide in the pipe tobacco interfered with vitamin B12 metabolism. However, while some neurologists and ophthalmologists continue to hold the view that tobacco plays a part, it is now generally believed that this is in fact one form of nutritional amblyopia due to vitamin B deficiency (Adams and Victor 1981). Nevertheless, cessation of pipe smoking and treatment with hydroxocobalamin may produce improvement (Davies 1981). Vitamin B_1 deficiency may rarely cause optic neuropathy but visual failure is well-recognized to occur as a result of malabsorption of Vitamin B_{12} in pernicious anaemia or of a primary dietary deficiency of this vitamin in vegans (who eat no meat products). Cyanide in cassava root is clearly the cause of optic neuropathy in the tropical ataxic neuropathy syndrome seen in Nigeria (Williams and Osuntokun 1969) but it is probable that not all the causes of nutritional amblyopia have yet been fully defined (p. 478). Among the many toxic factors which may damage the optic nerve are drugs such as tetramisole, clioquinol (in subacute myelo-optico-neuropathy), other iodoquinoline derivatives, and remedies as diverse as chloramphenicol, ethambutol, disulfiram, chloroquine, ibuprofen, and many more. Davies (1981) lists 40 classes of drugs which have been implicated.

Amaurosis fugax

Transient monocular blindness, lasting for seconds, minutes, or occasionally for hours, sometimes occurs in the aura of migraine or as a consequence of atherosclerosis but is most often due to micro-embolism of the central retinal artery with platelet or cholesterol emboli resulting from occlusion or stenosis of the ipsilateral internal carotid artery (Fisher 1959; Marshall and Meadows 1968; Ross 1977). However, in many patients no cause is ever discovered and in young patients particularly the prognosis may be excellent though the aetiology remains obscure (Eadie 1968).

Optic atrophy

Symptoms and signs. The usual symptom of optic atrophy is one of slow progressive visual failure in one or both eyes depending upon the cause but, when it is the result of vascular occlusion, trauma, or severe optic neuritis, the onset may be abrupt. The affected optic disc (or both discs when the condition is bilateral) is chalky-white in colour with clearly defined margins. The types of visual-field defect seen in such cases are considered below.

'Primary' and 'secondary' optic atrophy
Optic atrophy may result from many lesions or pathological processes. When these were less well understood, a confusing distinction was often drawn between 'primary' and 'secondary' optic atrophy. This was purely an ophthalmoscopic distinction, 'secondary' or 'consecutive' atrophy being the term used when it followed some observable change in the optic disc or retina and 'primary' atrophy when no such cause was ophthalmoscopically obvious. We now know that even the 'primary' atrophies are secondary to some pathological process such as pressure upon, demyelination of, or toxic damage to the optic nerve.

Causes of optic atrophy
Optic-nerve hypoplasia. Congenital hypoplasia of the optic nerve may be mild and clinically undetectable or severe and associated with markedly impaired vision and pallor of the hypoplastic optic discs. There may be associated nerve-fibre layer defects in the retina, either generally or in one segment of the retina which is also hypopigmented (see Behrens 1980). The condition sometimes occurs as a result of maternal diabetes or quinine ingestion or in association with developmental hypoplasia of the septum pellucidum.

Heredofamilial disorders. There are many genetically determined diseases in which there is degeneration of many parts of the nervous system including the retinae and optic nerves.
1. *Cerebromacular degeneration.* In this group of disorders (p. 455), optic atrophy is secondary to the storage of abnormal lipid in retinal ganglion cells. In the infantile variety (Tay–Sachs disease) there is also a cherry-red spot at the macula but this is often absent in the late infantile and juvenile forms.
2. *Hereditary ataxias.* Optic atrophy with or without pigmentary retinal degeneration (see below) has been described as occurring sometimes in association with virtually all of the diseases of the hereditary ataxia group (pp. 362–70). Behr's syndrome is a name which has been given to a disorder due to an autosomal recessive gene in which there is bilateral progressive optic atrophy associated with spastic paraparesis, inconstant and mild cerebellar ataxia, and evidence of posterior column degeneration, but there is doubt as to whether this is an independent entity (Horoupian, Zucker, Moshe, and Peterson 1979).
3. *Dominant optic atrophy.* Insidiously progressive optic atrophy not usually leading to complete blindness but giving bilateral centrocaecal scotomas and demonstrating autosomal dominant inheritance is one of the commonest varieties of hereditary optic atrophy (Kline and Glaser 1979).
4. *Stargardt's disease.* This is one of the many tapetoretinal degenerations or retinal dystrophies, usually of autosomal recessive inheritance and giving rise to a progressive loss of central vision, usually in individuals between six and 20 years of age. The macula is grey or brown with pigmented spots and there are central scotomata.
5. *Retinitis pigmentosa.* This is the commonest tapetoretinal degeneration which is usually recessive, occasionally dominant, and very rarely X-linked. There is degeneration of all retinal layers with initially spidery black and linear pigmentation of the retina between the vessels, ultimately with clumping of pigment (bone corpuscles); the fovea is often spared at least initially and the retinal vessels become progessively attenuated. There is pro-gressive visual impairment and constriction of the visual fields leading to tunnel vision; often the patients become totally blind but sometimes limited central vision is retained indefinitely. The retinal degeneration leads to progressive optic atrophy and the electroretinogram diminishes progressively and is eventually lost.

The condition may be associated with mental retardation, obesity, and hypogonadism (Laurence–Moon–Biedl syndrome) or with those features and syndactyly (Bardet–Biedl syndrome), with epilepsy (Cohan, Kattah, and Limaye 1979), hereditary nerve deafness, and/or many other conditions of the hereditary ataxia group. Similar retinal pigmentation is seen in Refsum's disease and in the Kearns–Sayre syndrome but without, as a rule, vascular attenuation or progressive visual failure.

6. *Leber's optic atrophy.* This condition is usually due to an X-linked recessive gene although transmission is not totally consistent in all families and female carriers rarely develop the condition (François 1961; *British Medical Journal* 1980). Mitochondrial inheritance is possible (Nikoskelainen 1984). Usually there is a relatively sudden onset in a young adult male of bilateral visual impairment lasting for weeks or months, but remissions sometimes occur so that the clinical picture resembles that of optic neuritis. Following remission, further episodes of sudden deterioration in vision may be experienced, but in many cases visual failure is progressive from the onset. Occasionally symptoms begin in one eye and the other is affected weeks or months later, but in very occasional cases the affliction remains monocular for many years (Carroll and Mastaglia 1979). In the acute phase there may be disc swelling and abnormal vascular permeability demonstrated by fluorescein angiography (Smith, Hoyt, and Susac 1973), but eventually there is pallor of the discs. Visually evoked potentials show an abnormal morphology (with a double positive peak) and increased latency; Dorfman, Nikoskelainen, Rosenthal, and Sogg (1977) found such studies to be of no value in detecting preclinical cases or female carriers, but Carroll and Mastaglia (1979) did find small central scotomata or minor abnormalities of the VEP in asymptomatic individuals in affected families.

Leber's disease has been described in patients with hereditary ataxia and Charcot–Marie–Tooth disease (McLeod, Low, and Morgan 1978) but the relationship may be coincidental, and a suggestion that a slow virus may be implicated (Wallace 1970) has not been confirmed. Some patients with the classical syndrome do have evidence of minor dysfunction of the cerebellum, and of the lateral and posterior columns of the spinal cord. Low plasma and urinary concentrations of thiocyanate have been found in some patients (Adams, Blackwood, and Wilson 1966; Rogers 1977) and smoking may aggravate the condition, so that an inborn metabolic inability to detoxicate cyanide has been postulated but remains unproven. Neither treatment with hydroxocobalamin (which detoxicates cyanide) nor steroids have been shown to halt visual failure in the first affected eye or to prevent its development in the other (*British Medical Journal* 1980).

Secondary optic atrophy
As already mentioned, optic atrophy may be a consequence of severe papilloedema, ischaemic optic neuropathy, or severe optic neuritis and can also follow glaucoma, choroidoretinitis, and other primary ocular disorders.

Syphilitic optic atrophy. Syphilis once accounted for 40 per cent of cases of optic atrophy but is now a rare cause. It used to be seen in 10 to 15 per cent of cases of tabes dorsalis, was rare in acquired general paresis, but occurred in up to 50 per cent of cases of congenital taboparesis. The process begins in the superficial fibres of the optic nerve, giving peripheral constriction of the visual fields, but is not due to arachnoiditis (Bruetsch 1948). Optic atrophy due to obliterative endarteritis and ischaemia or to granulomatous meningitis occurs rarely in meningovascular syphilis (p. 264).

Toxic optic atrophy. The optic nerve fibres are susceptible to a number of poisons and drugs, though their mode and site of action are little understood. Among these are cyanide, lead, arsenic, (especially tryparsamide), methyl mercuric iodide, methyl alcohol, carbon bisulphide, thallium, certain insecticides, clioquinol and other related remedies, chloramphenicol, ethambutol, chlorpropamide, penicillamine, disulfiram, phenylbutazone, indomethacin, cardiac glycosides, ibuprofen, antihelmithics such as tetramisole, and quinine. Many of the drugs listed produce this complication very rarely and then only after prolonged administration. A full list of those remedies which have been implicated is given by Davies (1981) who also points out that xanthopsia (yellow vision) may be produced by drugs such as santonin, sulphonamides, streptomycin, methaqualone, and thiazide diuretics. Troxidone and related anticonvulsants produce a sensation of glare and impaired colour vision but not optic atrophy. The optic atrophy which rarely results from isoniazid administration is probably due to vitamin B_6 deficiency, while the retinopathy resulting from sensitivity to chloroquine may be accompanied by pallor of the optic discs.

Pressure. Pressure is a common and important cause. In the eye itself it is produced by glaucoma. It may occur in the optic foramen, if narrowed by bony overgrowth, as in Paget's disease, or if there is a glioma within the optic nerve, or even as the result of a sclerotic ophthalmic artery. Behind the foramen, the commonest cause is a tumour, either of the pituitary, a craniopharyngioma, a meningioma arising above the sella or in the olfactory groove, or a glioma of the optic chiasm, of the frontal lobe, or of the tip of the temporal lobe. Pressure may also result from chiasmal arachnoiditis, the distended floor of the third ventricle in obstructive hydrocephalus, an intracranial aneurysm, or from arteriosclerotic internal carotid arteries. Radiography of the optic foramina is often of value.

Trauma. Primary optic atrophy may result from direct injury, usually to one, rarely to both optic nerves in head injury. There is often no radiographic evidence of fracture. The eye is usually completely blind, but rarely an incomplete lesion gives a localized visual–field defect.

Visual fields in optic atrophy

No generalization about the visual fields in optic atrophy is possible, since they depend entirely upon the cause. After papilloedema there is usually enlargement of the blind spot with peripheral concentric constriction. Optic neuritis and the toxic or metabolic amblyopias are usually associated with central, paracentral, or centrocaecal scotomas. Pressure lesions may produce central scotomata or other partial field defects. In Leber's optic atrophy and the other hereditary forms, central scotomas are also usual, while in retinitis pigmentosa there is usually severe concentric constriction of the fields with 'tunnel vision'. The latter sign, however, when unaccompanied by ophthalmoscopic abnormality of the disc or retina, is usually hysterical. And, of course, lesions which give rise to secondary optic atrophy following papilloedema due to raised pressure may involve the visual pathways more posteriorly, producing other types of field defect.

Prognosis of optic-nerve lesions

The prognosis of lesions of the optic nerve depends chiefly upon the extent to which the cause can be removed. When papilloedema is due to increased intracranial pressure, relief of this is usually followed by marked improvement in vision, provided optic atrophy due to retinal-artery occlusion has not already developed. Similarly, improvement in vision often follows rapidly upon the removal of direct pressure upon the optic nerve. Substantial and even complete recovery can usually be expected in optic neuritis due to multiple sclerosis, and also in most sporadic cases of acute optic neuritis, though occasionally vision is permanently impaired or rarely lost. The outlook is less satisfactory in toxic or metabolic

optic atrophy, though some improvement may occur if exposure to the toxin can be terminated or the nutritional defect corrected. Tabetic optic atrophy often progresses in spite of treament. Unfortunately, no form of treatment has any beneficial effect in the hereditary optic atrophies or in the tapetoretinal degenerations.

References

Acheson, D., Matthews, W. B., Batchelor, J. R., and Weller, R. (ed.) (1982). *McAlpine's multiple sclerosis*, 3rd edn. Churchill-Livingstone, Edinburgh.

Adams, J. H., Blackwood, W., and Wilson, J. (1966). Further clinical and pathological observations on Leber's optic atrophy. *Brain* **89**, 15.

Adams, R. D. and Victor, M. (1981). *Principles of neurology*, 2nd edn. McGraw-Hill, New York.

Ashworth, B. and Isherwood, I. (1981). *Clinical neuro-ophthalmology*, 2nd edn. Blackwell, Oxford.

Behrens, M. (1980). Other optic nerve disease. In *Neuro-ophthalmology*, (ed. S. Lessell and J. T. W. van Dalen) Vol. 1, Chapter 4. Excerpta Medica, Amsterdam.

Behrman, S. (1966). Pathology of papilloedema. *Brain* **89**, 1.

Bell, J. (1931). Hereditary optic atrophy (Leber's disease).*Treasury of human inheritance*, Vol. ii, Part iv. University Press, Cambridge.

Bradley, W. G. (1968). Symptomatic optic neuritis (aetiological factors in acute optic neuritis). *Dis. nerv. System* **29**, 668.

—— (1976). Axonal transport and the eye. *Br. J. Ophthal* **60**, 547.

—— and Whitty, C. W. M. (1968). Acute optic neuritis: prognosis for development of multiple sclerosis. *J. Neurol. Neurosurg. Psychiat.* **31**, 10.

British Medical Journal (1978). Parsons' papilloedema 70 years on. *Br. med. J.* **1**, 263.

—— (1980). Leber's optic neuropathy. *Br. med. J.* **1**, 1097.

Bruetsch, W. L. (1948). Surgical treatment of syphilitic primary atrophy of the optic nerves (syphilitic optochiasmatic arachnoiditis). *Arch. Ophthal., Chicago* **38**, 735.

Carroll, W. M. and Mastaglia, F. L. (1979). Leber's optic neuropathy. A clinical and visual evoked potential study of affected and asymptomatic members of a six generation family. *Brain* **102**, 559.

Cohan, S. L., Kattah, J. C., and Limaye, S. R. (1979). Familial tapetoretinal degeneration and epilepsy. *Arch. Neurol., Chicago* **36**, 544.

Davies, D. M. (1981). *Textbook of adverse drug reactions*, 2nd edn. Oxford Medical Publications, Oxford.

Dollery, C. T., Hodge, J. V., and Engel, M. (1962). Studies of the retinal circulation with fluorescein. *Br. med. J.* **2**, 1210.

Dorfman, L. J., Nikoskelainen, E., Rosenthal, A. R., and Sogg, R. L. (1977). Visual evoked potentials in Leber's hereditary optic neuropathy. *Ann. Neurol.* **1**, 565.

Drance, S. M., Morgan, R. W., and Sweeney, V. P. (1973). Shock-induced optic neuropathy: cause of nonprogressive glaucoma. *New Engl. J. Med.* **288**, 392.

Eadie, M. J., Sutherland, J. M., and Tyrer, J. H. (1968). Recurrent monocular blindness of uncertain cause. *Lancet* **i**, 319.

Ellenberger, C., Jr., Keltner, J. l., and Burde, R. M. (1973). Acute optic neuropathy in older patients. *Arch. Neurol., Chicago* **28**, 182.

Ferguson, F. R. and Critchley, M. (1928–9). Leber's optic atrophy and its relationship with the heredo-familial ataxias. *J. Neurol. Psychopathol* **9**, 120.

Fielder, A. H. L., Batchelor, J. R., Nason Vakarelis, B., Compston, D. A. S., and McDonald, W. I. (1981). Optic neuritis and multiple sclerosis: do factor B alleles influence progression of disease? *Lancet* **ii**, 1246.

Fisher, C. M. (1959). Observations of the fundus oculi in transient monocular blindness. *Neurology, Minneapolis* **9**, 333.

François, J. (1961). *Heredity in ophthalmology*. Mosby, St. Louis, Missouri.

Freeman, A. G. and Heaton, J. M. (1961). The aetiology of retrobulbar neuritis in Addisonian pernicious anaemia. *Lancet* **i**, 908.

Gould, E. S., Bird, A. C., Leaver, P. K., and McDonald, W. I. (1977). Treatment of optic neuritis by retrobular injection of triamcinolone. *Br. med. J.* **1**, 1495.

Graveson, G. S. (1950). Syphilitic optic neuritis. *J. Neurol. Neurosurg. Psychiat.* **13**, 216.

Haining, W. M. (1966). Diagnostic value of intravenous fluorescein studies. *Br. J. Ophthal.* **40**, 587.

Halliday, A. M. (1978). New developments in the clinical application of evoked potentials. In *Contemporary clinical neurophysiology* (ed. W.

A. Cobb and H. Van Duijn), EEC Supplement No. 34. Elsevier, Amsterdam.

——, Halliday, E., Kriss, A., McDonald, W. I., and Mushin, J. (1976). The pattern-evoked potential in compression of the anterior visual pathways. *Brain* **99**, 357.

——, McDonald, W. I., and Mushin, J. (1972). Delayed visual evoked response in optic neuritis. *Lancet* **i**, 982.

——, ——, and —— (1973). Delayed pattern-evoked responses in optic neuritis in relation to visual acuity. *Trans. Ophthal. Soc.* **93**, 315.

Hayreh, S. S. (1981). Anterior ischemic optic neuropathy. *Arch. Neurol., Chicago* **38**, 675.

Heaton, J. M., McCormick, A. J. A., and Freeman, A. G. (1958). Tobacco amblyopia: a clinical manifestation of vitamin-B12 deficiency. *Lancet* **ii**, 286.

Heron, J. R., Regan, D., and Milner, B. A. (1974). Delay in visual perception in unilateral optic atrophy after retrobulbar neuritis. *Brain* **97**, 69.

Hierons, R. and Lyle, T. K. (1959). Bilateral retrobulbar optic neuritis. *Brain* **82**, 56.

Hitchings, R. A., Corbett, J. J., Winkleman, J., and Schatz, N. J. (1976). Hemorrhages with optic nerve drusen. A differentiation from early papilledema. *Arch. Neurol., Chicago* **33**, 675.

Horoupian, D. S., Zucker, D. K., Moshe, S., and Peterson, H. (1979). Behr syndrome: a clinicopathologic report. *Neurology, Minneapolis* **29**, 323.

Hoyt, W. F. (1963). Neuro-ophthalmology. *Arch. Ophthal.* **70**, 679.

Kline, L. B. and Glaser, J. S. (1979). Dominant optic atrophy: the clinical profile. *Arch. Ophthal.* **97**, 1680.

Marshall, J. and Meadows, S. (1968). The natural history of amaurosis fugax. *Brain* **91**, 419.

McAlpine, D., Lumsden, C. E., and Acheson, E. D. (1972). *Multiple sclerosis: a reappraisal* 2nd ed. Churchill Livingstone, Edinburgh.

McLeod, J. G., Low, P. A., and Morgan, J. A. (1978). Charcot–Marie–Tooth disease with Leber optic atrophy. *Neurology, Minneapolis* **28**, 179.

Nikoskelainen, E. (1984). New aspects of the puzzle of Leber's disease. *Neurology (Cleveland)* **34**, 1482.

——, Frey, H., and Salmi, A. (1981). Prognosis of optic neuritis with special reference to cerebrospinal fluid immunoglobulins and measles virus antibodies. *Ann. Neurol.* **9**, 545.

Rogers, J. A. (1977). Leber's disease. *Aust. J. Ophthal.* **5**, 111.

Ross, R. T. (1977). Transient monocular blindness. *Can. J. neurol. Sci.* **4**, 143.

Smith, J. L., Hoyt, W. F., and Susac, J. O. (1973). Ocular fundus in acute Leber optic neuropathy. *Arch. Ophthal.* **90**, 349.

Wadia, N. H., Desai, M. M., Quadros, E. V., and Dastur, D. K. (1972). Role of vegetarianism, smoking and hydroxocobalamin in optic neuritis. *Br. med. J.* **3**, 264.

Wallace, D. C. (1970). A new manifestation of Leber's disease and a new explanation for the agency responsible for its unusual pattern of inheritance. *Brain* **93**, 121.

Williams, A. O. and Osuntokun, B. O. (1969). Peripheral neuropathy in tropical (nutritional) ataxia in Nigeria: light and electron microscopic study. *Arch. Neurol., Chicago* **21**, 475.

Wolf, R. and Bird, A. C. (1980). Fundus. In *Neuro–ophthalmology* (ed. S. Lessell and J. T. W. van Dalen, Vol. 1, Chapter 1. Excerpta Medica, Amsterdam.

Wray, S. H. (1980). Optic neuritis. In *Neuro-ophthalmology* (ed. S. Lessell and J. T. W. van Dalen), Vol. 1, Chapter 2. Excerpta Medica, Amsterdam.

External ocular movement and its abnormalities

The nature and control of ocular movements

The ocular movements are described as horizontal movement outwards, or abduction; horizontal movement inwards, or adduction; vertical movement upwards, or elevation; vertical movement downwards, or depression. The eye is, of course, capable of diagonal movements at any intermediate angle. The term 'rotation' should be reserved for wheel-like movements around an imaginary pivot passing from before backwards through the centre of the pupil. Such movements of rotation do not normally occur, but are

observed only as a result of the unbalanced action of certain muscles. Inward rotation is a movement similar to that of a wheel rolling towards the nose, and outward rotation is the opposite rotatory movement. Normally the movements of the two eyes are harmoniously symmetrical and we then speak of conjugate ocular movements or deviation. Conjugate ocular deviation is described as horizontal or lateral, upward and downward. Conjugate adduction of the two eyes is known as convergence.

The nuclei which innervate the ocular muscles

The lower motor neurones which innervate the ocular muscles originate in the nuclei of the third, fourth, and sixth cranial nerves. The first two lie in the midbrain just anterior to the cerebral aqueduct at the level of the superior and inferior colliculi. The nuclei of the sixth nerve lie in the pons beneath the floor of the upper part of the fourth ventricle and partly encircled by the fibres of the seventh nerve.

The representation of muscles in the nucleus of the third-nerve is illustrated diagrammatically in Fig. 2.6. The median, unpaired, small-celled nucleus of Perlia is the centre for convergence and accommodation, while the lateral, paired, small-celled nucleus of Edinger-Westphal innervates the parasympathetic constrictor of the pupil. The remainder of the nucleus is the paired, large-celled, lateral nucleus in which the muscles are represented from above downwards as follows: levator palpebrae, superior rectus, inferior oblique, medial rectus, inferior rectus. Decussating fibres unite the lower parts of the nuclei. Immediately below the third-nerve nucleus lies that of the fourth nerve which innervates the opposite superior oblique. This nucleus and the adjacent lowest part of that of the third nerve innervate the two muscles concerned in depression of the eye, and the two elevating muscles are innervated by mutually adjacent portions of the upper half of the third-nerve nucleus.

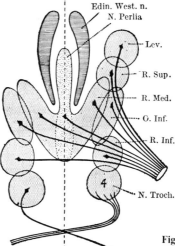

Fig. 2.6. Diagram of the oculomotor nucleus.

The extrinsic ocular muscles

The extrinsic ocular muscles are the four recti, superior and inferior, lateral and medial, and the two obliques, superior and inferior. The action of each of these muscles is shown in Fig. 2.7.

It will be seen that only the lateral and medial recti act in a single plane. The other muscles always act in concert in such a way that their conflicting tendencies cancel and a harmonious resultant is produced. Thus when the two obliques aid the lateral rectus in adduction, their vertical and rotatory forces cancel and, when the superior rectus and inferior oblique contract together to elevate the eye, their horizontal and rotatory components also cancel.

But, owing to the planes in which the superior and inferior recti and the obliques are placed, their actions are influenced by the

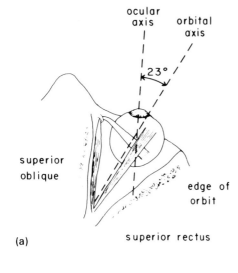

(a)

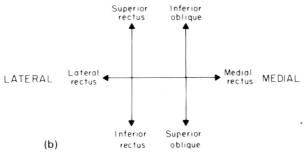

(b)

Fig. 2.7. A: Dorsal view of the orbit, globe, superior rectus muscle, and superior oblique muscle. Note the relationship of the ocular axis to the orbital axis with regard to insertion of eachmuscle. B: Primary direction of pull by each of the six extraocular muscles. B: Primary direction of pull by each of the six extraocular muscles. (Reproduced from Patton, Sundsten, Crill, and Swanson (1976) by kind permission of the authors and publisher.)

position of the eye in the orbit. When it is rotated outwards 23 degrees, the superior rectus is a pure elevator and the inferior rectus a pure depressor. The more it is turned inwards the more they act as internal and external rotators. The converse is true of the obliques. In conjugate deviation there is harmonious contraction of the appropriate muscles of both eyes. In lateral conjugate deviation the lateral rectus of one eye and the medial rectus of the other are associated; in conjugate deviation upwards and downwards, the elevators and depressors of the two eyes respectively; and in convergence, the medial recti. Ocular movements must not be regarded as consisting merely of contractions of the prime movers, the muscles actively displacing the eye. Graded contraction and relaxation of their antagonists play an important part in orderly movement.

Paralysis of individual ocular muscles

The more important results of paralysis of an ocular muscle are: (1) defective ocular movement; (2) squint; (3) erroneous projection of the visual field; and (4) diplopia.

Defective ocular movement

Defective ocular movement is demonstrated by asking the patient to fix his gaze on an object, such as the observer's finger, which is then moved upwards and downwards and to either side, convergence being tested by bringing it towards the patient. The movement is defective in the direction in which the eye is normally moved by the muscle which is paralysed. Slight weakness may not give any defect of ocular movement evident to the observer.

Squint

Squint, or strabismus, is the term applied to a failure of the normal co-ordination of the ocular axes. It is necessary to distinguish paralytic squint from concomitant squint. Paralytic squint may be present when the eyes are at rest, due to the unbalanced action of the normal antagonist of the paralysed muscle; for example, the affected eye may be slightly adducted when the lateral rectus is paralysed. More often it is apparent only when the eyes move in the direction in which the eye should be pulled by the paralysed muscle, or else squint present at rest is increased by such a movement. Concomitant squint, however, is present at rest and is equal for all positions of the eyes, and, if the fixing eye is covered, the movements of the squinting eye are found to be full. Concomitant squint is not usually associated with diplopia; paralytic squint, at least in the early stages, usually is. However, when there is long-standing ocular muscle imbalance (latent concomitant squint or heterophoria), the patient may be able for many years to contract the ocular muscles so as to fuse the images from the two eyes; as he becomes older the effort may no longer be possible so that the latent squint breaks down and diplopia results. Similarly, in long-standing paralytic squint, one image may ultimately be suppressed so that diplopia disappears; suppression of this type often results in one eye becoming amblyopic as a result of untreated concomitant squint in early childhood.

When the lateral rectus is paralysed, the ocular axes converge and the squint is said to be convergent. Paralysis of the medial rectus causes divergent squint. The deviation of the axis of the affected eye from the parallelism with that of the normal eye is called the 'primary deviation'. If the patient is made to fix an object in a direction requiring the action of the affected muscle and at the same time is prevented from seeing it with his normal eye, the latter deviates too far in the required direction. This is called 'secondary deviation', and is due to the increased effort evoked by his attempt to move the affected eye.

Erroneous projection of the visual field

If we look at a light in any position of the eyes, its image falls upon the macula. When the right lateral rectus is paralysed, on conjugate deviation to the right the left eye moves normally and the right eye remains directed forwards. The image of the object falls in the left eye upon the macula, in the right eye upon the nasal half of the retina. The patient is accustomed to regarding an object, the image of which falls upon the nasal half of the right retina, as situated to the right of one of which the image falls upon the macula. Consequently, he sees two images and projects the false image perceived by his affected eye to the right of the true image perceived by his normal eye. If his normal eye is then covered and he is asked to touch the object, he will direct his finger to the right of its true position. The erroneous projection is always in the normal direction of action of the affected muscle. The spatial disorientation it causes may give subjective giddiness. Hess's screen can be used to record the position of the false image.

Diplopia

Erroneous projection of the visual field of the affected eye is responsible for double vision or diplopia. When both eyes are used, two images are seen, one correctly and one erroneously projected, the true and the false images.

In paralysis of the right lateral rectus the right eye cannot be abducted. If the patient attempts to deviate his eyes horizontally to the right, the image of a small object falls in the left eye upon the macula. In the right eye, it falls upon the nasal half of the retina and hence is seen in (or projected into) the temporal field of the right eye. The false image is parallel with and to the right of the true image. The further the test object is moved to the right, the further into the nasal half of the right retina its image moves, and the further the false image appears to move to the right. From these facts two simple rules about diplopia can be deduced:

1. The separation of the images increases the further the eyes are moved in the normal direction of pull of the paralysed muscle.

2. The false image is displaced in the direction of the plane or planes of action of the paralysed muscle.

It follows that when the gaze is so directed that the separation of the images is greatest, the more peripherally situated image is the false one, derived from the affected eye. A useful method is to cover one eye with a red, and the other with a green, glass. The patient then looks at a light, which is moved until the maximal separation of the images is obtained; they are then distinguishable by their colour and the affected eye is identified. If coloured glass is not available, an intelligent and co-operative patient can usually distinguish the images by noticing which disappears when each eye is covered separately.

When the affected eye is identified, the paralysed muscle can be determined. It is the one which normally displaces the eye in the direction of displacement of the false image. The positions of the false images resulting from paralysis of the various ocular muscles are described below for the right eye. The description will apply to the left eye if right be substituted for left and vice versa. The diplopia is said to be simple, or uncrossed, when the false image lies on the same side of the true image as the affected eye, and crossed when it lies on the opposite side.

Position of false image in paralysis of the ocular muscles of the right eye

Lateral rectus. The diplopia is uncrossed; there is maximal separation of the images on abduction, when the false image is level with, and parallel with, the true.

Medial rectus. The diplopia is crossed; there is maximal separation of the images on abduction, when the false image is level with, and parallel with, the true.

Superior rectus. The false image is above and to the left of the true and tilted away from it. Vertical separation of the images is greatest on abduction, the tilting greatest on adduction. The diplopia is crossed.

Inferior rectus. The false image is below and to the left of the true and tilted towards it. Vertical separation of the images is greatest on abduction, and tilting on adduction. The diplopia is crossed.

Inferior oblique. The false image is above and to the right of the true and tilted away from it. The diplopia is uncrossed. Vertical separation of the images is greatest on adduction, and tilting on abduction.

Superior oblique. The false image is below and to the right of the true and tilted towards it. The diplopia is uncrossed. Vertical separation of the images is greatest on adduction, and tilting on abduction. Since the diplopia occurs on looking downwards, it is particularly troublesome to the patient when walking downstairs.

A patient suffering from diplopia usually rotates or tilts the head into the position in which the least demand is made upon the paralysed muscle.

The supranuclear and internuclear control of ocular movement

Types of ocular movement

During *conjugate* or *version* movements of the eyes, the visual axes remain parallel, while, during *disconjugate* or *vergence* movements, the axes intersect. Version movements are of two types; in one (*saccades* or *saccadic movements*) the eyes jump rapidly and successively from one point of fixation to another, while in the other (*smooth-pursuit movements*) the eyes follow smoothly a moving object. Saccadic movements are fast in that the eyes can move 40° in 100 ms. All voluntary eye movements (except when viewing a moving object) take the form of saccades; thus, in reading a line of print, the eyes read one to four words in the course of a single fixation and then jump to the next series of words. Speed and efficiency of reading depend upon the number of words read during each fixation. Saccadic movements can be recorded by an eye movement camera. The latency of successive saccades is 200–500 ms; during each movement visual acuity is reflexly suppressed via a pathway which appears to involve the lateral geniculate body. Physiological studies in animals have demonstrated bursts of 400–600 spike discharges per second in the oculomotor, trochlear, and abducens nuclei immediately prior to the onset and throughout each saccade, with steady firing at a slower rate during the intervening periods of fixation. Saccadic movements are little influenced by drugs but are selectively impaired in some diseases such as Huntington's chorea and progressive supranuclear palsy.

Smooth pursuit movements, used to track moving targets, are slower than saccades, having a maximum velocity of about 50° per second. During such movements, unlike saccades, visual acuity is unimpaired; such movements cannot be performed at will without the stimulus of a moving target. The latency between displacement of the target and the pursuit movement is 130 ms. Drugs such as barbiturates and anticonvulsants (Bittencourt, Gresty, and Richens 1980) depress this type of movement, breaking it down into saccades.

By contrast to saccadic and smooth pursuit (version) movements which involve conjugate deviation of the eyes, vergence movements, which are slow (20° per second), track approaching (convergence) or receding (divergence) objects, and during these the eyes move in opposite directions. The vestibular system also plays a part in the control of ocular movement in reflexly maintaining ocular fixation upon a visual target during head movement; thus lesions of the labyrinth or vestibular nerve or nucleus may result in impaired ocular fixation and consequent blurred vision when the head is moved.

Supranuclear and internuclear pathways

The supranuclear pathway concerned with voluntary conjugate eye movement (saccades) in a lateral direction originates in the frontal eye field in the contralateral middle frontal gyrus (Brodmann's area 8). Stimulation in this area gives contralateral saccades with a latency of about 25 ms, while destructive lesions give difficulty in carrying out voluntary version movements of the eyes to the opposite side. The pathway from the cortical area descends through the corona radiata, internal capsule, and cerebral peduncle, subsequently decussating in the midbrain and descending in the pons to join the medial longitudinal fasciculus at about the level of the sixth-nerve nucleus. Thus stimulation in the pons, below the decussation of this pathway, causes conjugate deviation of the eyes *towards* the lesion or point of stimulation, while a unilateral lesion of the ponto–mesencephalic reticular formation may cause paralysis of conjugate gaze towards the affected side. There is also evidence that visual input into the superior colliculus has a powerful controlling influence upon this fronto–mesencephalic–pontine (supranuclear) pathway as bursts of spikes can be recorded from collicular neurones during saccades.

Another important cortical centre controlling ocular movements lies in or near the visual cortex in the occipital lobe. Recent neurophysiological evidence suggests that occipito–mesencephalic pathways are concerned especially with smooth pursuit movements and occipito–pretectal pathways with vergence (Bender, Postel, and Krieger 1957; Gay and Newman 1972).

Less is known about supranuclear pathways controlling vertical conjugate deviation (Bender 1980); probably they also originate in the middle frontal gyrus but bilateral activation may be needed to evoke vertical movements, so that defective vertical conjugate gaze of cerebral origin only occurs as a rule as a result of massive bifrontal lesions. On the other hand, recent evidence suggests that lesions in the neighbourhood of the posterior commissure may also paralyse vertical gaze.

Because co-ordination of the movement of the two eyes is

essential for binocular vision, the nuclei of the individual third, fourth, and sixth cranial nerves are linked together in the *medial longitudinal fasciculus* (also sometimes called the posterior longitudinal bundle) which is the principal internuclear pathway controlling ocular movement, and which also receives an extensive input from vestibular, cerebellar, and other nuclei and pathways concerned with reflex ocular movement. Supranuclear pathways as described above all feed into this fasciculus. The influence of the cerebellum is indicated by the fact that cerebellar lesions often cause over- or undershoot of saccadic movements and/or the breaking down of smooth pursuit movements into saccades.

Reflex ocular movement

In voluntary conjugate deviation of the eyes, the patient may turn his eyes spontaneously or on command, but some ocular movements are reflexly induced. Visual stimuli usually result in movement of the head (or, if the head is held fixed in one position, of the eyes) in order to keep the image of the stimulus upon the macula. Continuous movement of a series of objects or lines in one direction evokes optokinetic nystagmus (see below). Similarly, auditory stimulation may give deviation of the eyes towards the origin of the sound, while caloric or electrical excitation of one labyrinth evokes conjugate ocular deviation and nystagmus (see below). If the patient fixes his gaze upon an object and the head is then flexed, rotated, or extended at the neck, reflex ocular deviation occurs in an attempt to keep the image of the object upon the macula. This oculocephalic reflex (the doll's head manoeuvre) is dependent upon the integrity of the medial longitudinal fasciculus and of its connections with the vestibular system, and is thus valuable in determining whether pontine vestibulo–ocular connections are intact in patients in coma. Absence of this reflex is almost invariably an indication of irreversible brainstem injury but is seen exceptionally in patients with supratentorial lesions receiving therapeutic doses of anticonvulsant drugs (Rosenberg, Sharpe, and Hoyt 1975).

Supranuclear and internuclear lesions

Spasmodic conjugate lateral movement of the eyes may occur in focal attacks of epilepsy due to lesions involving the contralateral frontal eye field, and less often the contralateral occipital cortex. It is also an occasional consequence of deep contralateral intracerebral haemorrhage involving the thalamus and basal ganglia (Keane 1975a). Periodic alternating movements in which the eyes rove from one extreme of horizontal gaze to the other every 2 to 5 s ('ping-pong gaze') is a rare consequence of bilateral cerebral infarction (Fisher 1967; Stewart, Kirkham, and Mathieson 1979).

Paralysis of conjugate lateral movement may occur as the result of a lesion at any point in the supranuclear pathway described above but this effect is always transient in lesions situated above the pons, though one involving the decussation of the pathways at the ponto–mesencephalic junction can give paralysis of conjugate gaze to both sides. However, a unilateral pontine lesion may give long-lasting paralysis of both voluntary and reflex conjugate gaze to the affected side (Halsey, Ceballos, and Crosby 1967; Goebel, Komatsuzaki, Bender, and Cohen 1971). This can result from encephalomyelitis or Wernicke's disease but is more often due to brainstem infarction.

Dissociation of conjugate lateral movement is usually a consequence of a lesion of the medial longitudinal fasciculus (an internuclear lesion). Much the commonest effect is the so-called *anterior internuclear ophthalmoplegia* (Harris's sign or '*ataxic nystagmus*') in which there is phasic nystagmus confined to the abducting eye associated with failure of medial movement of the adducting eye. While this sign can rarely be a consequence of brainstem tumour (Cogan and Wray 1970) or infarction (Gonyea 1974), it is much more often due to multiple sclerosis and can be unilateral or bilateral. When such cases are examined with electro-oculographic recording and computer simulation, there is evi-

dence first that adducting saccades on the side of the lesion are slowed while abducting saccades in the contralateral eye are of normal velocity but consistently overshoot (Baloh, Yee, and Honrubia 1978 a, b); the evidence suggests that there is disordered inhibitory and excitatory control of the medial rectus motor pool during rapid eye movements and eccentric gaze (Feldon, Hoyt, and Stark 1980). Very rarely a *posterior internuclear ophthalmoplegia* resulting from a lesion (usually an infarct—Rothstein and Alvord 1971) of the fasciculus just rostral to the abducens nucleus may occur, giving paralysis of abduction of one eye with normal adduction of the other, and with nystagmus, thus differentiating this sign from the effects of a sixth-nerve lesion. Another rare manifestation of an acute brainstem lesion involving the paramedian pontine reticular formation and the medial longitudinal fasciculus is *paralytic pontine exotropia* (Sharpe, Rosenburg, Hoyt, and Daroff 1974) in which there is external deviation of the contralateral eye with total horizontal immobility of the ipsilateral eye.

Skew deviation of the eyes, in which one eye is deviated upwards and outwards, the other downwards and out, is a rare consequence of an acute brainstem lesion, usually in the pons on the side of the lower eye, less often in the midbrain, medulla, or cerebellum and usually resulting from infarction (Keane 1975b).

Spasmodic conjugate vertical movement of the eyes upwards is a rare phenomenon, occasionally occurring in an attack of epilepsy, especially petit mal, but it is also seen in the oculogyric crises of post-encephalitic parkinsonism.

Paralysis of conjugate vertical deviation in an upward direction is not uncommon, but paralysis of downward movement is very rare; when it does occur, it usually results from an infarct involving the region of the thalamo–mesencephalic junction bordering the dorsomedial aspect of the red nucleus (Trojanowski and Wray 1980; Trojanowski and Lafontaine 1981). In midbrain lesions involving the region of the superior colliculus, voluntary upward deviation can be lost even though the movement can still be excited reflexly. Usually the lesions are bilateral, involving the pretectum, posterior commissure, or dorsal midbrain tegmentum; unilateral lesions only impair upward gaze when the posterior commissure is involved (Christoff 1974). The term 'Parinaud's syndrome' is often applied to isolated defects of upward conjugate gaze, which can rarely be congenital but, in the fully-developed syndrome due to lesions of the midbrain tectum, there is often loss of the pupillary light reflexes and paralysis of convergence in addition. This may result from encephalitis, from tumours of the third ventricle, midbrain, or pineal body, from Wernicke's disease, or from infarction.

Paralysis of convergence is occasionally seen in post-encephalitic parkinsonism, as a result of head injury or midbrain infarction, and rarely results from ageing. Loss of convergence is occasionally, and spasm of convergence invariably, hysterical.

Ocular motor apraxia

Just as apraxia of limb movement identifies an inability to carry out skilled movements in the absence of paralysis (see p. 62), so ocular motor apraxia (Cogan and Adams 1953) is an inability to move the eyes voluntarily in the desired direction when random and reflex eye movements are intact. The condition is usually congenital; the patients show increased latencies and decreased amplitudes of voluntary saccadic eye movements in the horizontal plane, especially when the head is held fixed but, when their heads are free to move, they make conspicuous, thrusting, compensatory head movements in the direction they wish to look (Zee, Yee, and Singer 1977). Rarely a similar phenomenon may develop as a consequence of an acquired lesion of the prefrontal motor cortex, and a somewhat similar supranuclear pseudo-ophthalmoplegia with inability to initiate saccadic eye movement, with preservation of slow pursuit and reflex movements has been described in olivopontocerebellar degeneration (Koeppen and Hans 1976).

Progressive supranuclear degeneration

In 1964, Steele, Richardson, and Olszewski described a rare degenerative disorder characterised by ophthalmoplegia affecting vertical and especially downward gaze with early loss of saccadic movements. The ophthalmoplegia is associated with variable parkinsonian and dystonic features as well as dysarthria, pseudobulbar palsy, inconstant cerebellar and pyramidal signs, and, exceptionally, dementia. Pathologically, such cases have shown neurofibrillary and granulovacuolar degeneration of neurones with gliosis and demyelination, especially in the brainstem, basal ganglia, and cerebellum, and the oculomotor nuclei are sometimes involved as well (Blumenthal and Miller 1969). The disease is progressive and generally uninfluenced by levodopa or any other form of treatment.

Nuclear ophthalmoplegia

Nuclear ophthalmoplegia means paralysis of ocular muscles due to a lesion of the nuclei of the oculomotor nerves. When the extrinsic ocular muscles are involved, this is external ophthalmoplegia: paralysis of the pupillary and ciliary muscles is known as internal ophthalmoplegia. When both are affected, there is total ophthalmoplegia. Internal ophthalmoplegia is dealt with later. We are here concerned only with external ophthalmoplegia, excluding ptosis (see p. 105).

Nuclear ophthalmoplegia must be distinguished from supranuclear lesions and from lesions of the oculomotor nerve trunks. Supranuclear lesions disturb conjugate ocular movement so that the ocular axes remain parallel and diplopia is not produced. Nuclear lesions may be unilateral, but are more often bilateral. When bilateral they are not always symmetrical, and loss of parallelism of the ocular axes and diplopia occur. The unequal paralysis of the muscles of both eyes, with or without internal ophthalmoplegia, gives a picture, therefore, which is different from that due to a lesion of the trunk of one third nerve. Nuclear ophthalmoplegia involving only the fourth nerve is unknown. Since the sixth nerve supplies only one muscle, an isolated lesion of the sixth-nerve nucleus can only be distinguished from one of the nerve trunk by the presence of associated signs of a pontine lesion.

The following are the principal causes of nuclear ophthalmoplegia:

1. *Massive lesions of the brainstem*, especially tumours of the midbrain, pineal region, and pons, and vascular lesions (haemorrhage or infarction).

2. *Nutritional deficiency and metabolic disorders.* Bilateral external ophthalmoplegia due to pathological changes in the brainstem is common in Wernicke's encephalopathy due to vitamin B$_1$ deficiency (p. 475) and may also occur in central pontine myelinolysis (p. 319).

3. *Infections.* Nuclear ophthalmoplegia was often seen in encephalitis lethargica; it occurs rarely in viral and in post-infective encephalitis and encephalomyelitis. It is a rare manifestation of parenchymal neurosyphilis; syphilitic ophthalmoplegia is much more often due to involvement of nerve trunks in meningovascular inflammation.

4. *Demyelination.* An isolated third- or sixth-nerve palsy is an occasional manifestation of multiple sclerosis, but internuclear ophthalmoplegia is more common. The syndrome of so-called acute idiopathic ophthalmoplegia with ataxia and areflexia (Fisher 1956; Elizan 1971) is clearly a form of polyneuropathy, involving the oculomotor nerve trunks and akin to the Guillain-Barré syndrome; hence the lesion is not nuclear (Sauron, Bouche, Cathala, Chain, and Castayne 1984).

5. *Progressive ophthalmoplegia* is the term which has been applied to a group of ophthalmoplegias of mixed aetiology, characterized by the insidious onset and slowly progressive course of ptosis and external ophthalmoplegia. The disorder may start at any age and is sometimes familial. Muscular dystrophy of the external ocular muscles accounts for some cases, but in others there is pigmentary retinal degeneration and cardiomyopathy with cerebellar and pyramidal-tract signs, and the lesion may well involve brainstem nuclei as well as the ocular muscles in some cases (Kearns and Sayre 1958; Drachman 1968; Mills, Bowen, and Thomson 1971) (also see p. 579); mitochondrial abnormalities have been found in muscle and cerebellum in some such cases (Schneck, Adachi, Briet, Wolnitz, and Volk 1973) and CT scanning has shown periventricular areas of low density in some (Okamoto, Mizuno, Iido, Sobue, and Mukoyama 1981). External ophthalmoplegia has also been reported as a consequence of phenytoin toxicity (Spector, Davidoff, and Schwartzman 1976) and may also occur in various inborn errors of metabolism such as maple-syrup urine disease (Zee, Freeman, and Holtzmann 1974).

6. *Syringobulbia* rarely produces ophthalmoplegia.

7. *Head injury* is a rare cause of nuclear ophthalmoplegia, which may result from contusion of the brainstem.

8. *Congenital defects* of ocular movement occur. Some are supranuclear (e.g. ocular motor apraxia) and others represent developmental synkinesias such as contraction of the superior oblique muscle during swallowing (McLeod and Glaser 1974). Unilateral or bilateral aplasia of the third and less often of other oculomotor nuclei has been described as a consequence of intra-uterine hypoxia or ischaemia (Norman 1974). However, most of the congenital abnormalities are not nuclear. Thus congenital unilateral third-nerve palsy is probably due to birth injury (Victor 1976). Others may occur sporadically or may affect more than one family member. One of the commonest of these is *Duane's syndrome*, in which there is paralysis of abduction of the affected eye and on attempted adduction the globe retracts and the palpebral fissure narrows; the lateral rectus muscle is usually fibrotic. The condition may be bilateral. *Brown's syndrome* is one in which there is a mechanical obstruction to fine movement of the superior oblique tendon so that the clinical picture suggests an isolated palsy of the inferior oblique. The condition is often congenital but may be acquired (Goldhammer and Lawton Smith 1974) when it gives rise to diplopia and may at first suggest neurological disease.

Nystagmus and other spontaneous movements

Nystagmus is a disturbance of ocular posture characterized by a more or less rhythmical oscillation of the eyes. This movement may be of the same rate in both directions, or quicker in one direction than in the other. In the latter case the movement is divided into the quick and the slow phases (phasic nystagmus). The quick phase is taken to indicate the direction of the nystagmus, so that if the slow phase is to the left and the quick to the right, the patient is said to exhibit nystagmus to the right. Nystagmus may occur when the eyes are in the position of rest, or only on deviation in certain directions or on convergence, or only when the head is in a certain position—positional nystagmus. The movement may be confined to one plane, horizontal or vertical, or occur in more than one plane—rotary nystagmus. Nystagmus is described as *first-degree* when present on lateral gaze to one side only, *second-degree* when present on looking ahead but accentuated on looking to one side, and *third-degree* when present on fixation and on looking to both sides but much more striking to one of the two sides. The acquired forms may cause an apparent movement of objects seen by the patient (oscillopsia). Nystagmus can be recorded by electronystagmography.

The nature of nystagmus can be best appreciated by recalling (p. 98) that the posture of the eyes is influenced reflexly by several factors of which the most important are impulses derived from the retinae, the labyrinths, and the cervical spine. Nystagmus may therefore be due to: (1) defective or abnormal retinal impulses; (2) disease or dysfunction of the labyrinths or of the vestibular nuclei or vestibular connections in the brainstem; (3) lesions of the cervical spinal cord; (4) lesions involving central pathways controlling ocular posture; (5) it may be congenital and of unknown aetiology; (6) it has been said to occur in hysteria, but the irregular vertical ocular movements seen in some hysterical subjects are not true nystagmus; (7) it may be toxic; and (8) it may be mimicked voluntarily.

Nystagmus of retinal origin

1. *Amblyopia* developing in early life may cause nystagmus if some vision is retained, and especially if macular vision is impaired. The visual impairment renders ocular fixation defective, and a pendular nystagmus results. Similar pendular nystagmus may be seen as central vision deteriorates progressively in patients with retinitis pigmentosa or progressive optic atrophy.

2. *Miners' nystagmus* was due to the relative inefficiency of macular vision in a dim light because of the absence of rods in the macula. The defective macular vision caused defective fixation. Patients with this disorder often showed in addition variable features of anxiety and even hysteria, especially in a compensation setting. The condition has virtually disappeared since underground lighting was improved.

Optokinetic nystagmus

Optokinetic nystagmus is that type of nystagmus evoked when a series of moving objects passes before the eyes. A familiar example is the nystagmus which occurs in an individual looking out of the window of a moving train. The slow phase is in the direction in which the landscape appears to move and the quick phase is in the direction in which the train moves. To test for optokinetic nystagmus a Bárány drum is used. This is a revolving, striped cylinder, the speed and direction of which can be altered easily. Horizontal or vertical nystagmus can be produced by revolving the drum laterally or vertically. The amplitude and regularity of the nystagmus in each direction is noted.

Optokinetic nystagmus is a brainstem reflex, distinct from that for vestibular nystagmus and independent of the vestibular nuclei (Dix, Hallpike, and Harrison 1949). The cortical centre for optokinetic nystagmus is in the supramarginal and angular gyri (Carmichael, Dix, and Hallpike 1956). Optokinetic nystagmus to the opposite side is suppressed by lesions of this area. Indeed, directional preponderance of optokinetic nystagmus towards the side of the lesion may occur not only with parieto-occipital cortical or subcortical lesions but also with lesions of the upper brainstem. The test may be unreliable in the presence of a homonymous hemianopia, but absent, sluggish, or irregular optokinetic responses usually indicate a pontine lesion (e.g. tumour, infarct, or demyelination) (Cawthorne, Dix, Hood, and Harrison 1969).

Labyrinthine nystagmus

The clinical aspects of labyrinthine nystagmus are considered on page 122. Appropriate stimulation of the horizontal semicircular canals evokes horizontal nystagmus, and of the vertical canals, rotary nystagmus. Acute lesions of the internal ear, whether primary or secondary to middle-ear disease, cause nystagmus, usually rotary, and with the quick phase as a rule towards the opposite side. The amplitude of the oscilliation is increased when the eyes are deviated in the direction of the quick phase and diminished on fixation in the direction of the slow phase. Chronic labyrinthine lesions often give fine rotary nystagmus on lateral fixation to one or both sides, especially to the side of the lesion.

Nystagmus due to spinal-cord lesions

Nystagmus is very rarely seen after cervical-cord lesions and has then been attributed to a defect of afferent impulses from the cervical spine (Biemond and de Jong 1969). It may be due to loss of cerebellar inhibition on the cervico-ocular reflex (Bronstein and Hood 1985). Vertical nystagmus commonly occurs as a result of lesions in the neighbourhood of the foramen magnum, especially in cases of the Chiari malformation, with or without syringomyelia (Barnett, Foster, and Hudgson 1973).

Nystagmus due to central lesions

Nystagmus is a common sign of brainstem and cerebellar lesions. With cerebellar lesions, nystagmus may occur on fixation in any direction, the slow phase being towards the position of rest, and the quick phase towards the periphery. With a unilateral cerebellar lesion, it is present in both eyes but is most marked on conjugate deviation to the side of the lesion. It may result from lesions involving the cerebellar connections within the brainstem, the vestibular nucleus, and the posterior longitudinal bundle. Multiple sclerosis is the commonest cause. Nystagmus of central origin also occurs in cases of hereditary ataxia, encephalitis, syringomyelia, tumours, and vascular lesions of the brainstem and cerebellum.

Positional nystagmus (see p. 124) has been used to distinguish central from labyrinthine lesions. A change in the direction of the nystagmus produced by a change in the position of the head favours a central lesion. Positional nystagmus elicited by rotation of the head to one side only is often seen in benign positional nystagmus (Nylén 1950), due to a lesion of the utricle and saccule of one labyrinth. Similar nystagmus occurring to both sides due to labyrinthine damage is a common temporary sequel of concussive head injury (Cartlidge and Shaw 1981). The positional nystagmus which may result from brainstem lesions (e.g. multiple sclerosis) but which is more often due to posterior fossa tumours (especially ependymomas of the fourth ventricle or medulloblastomas in children and young adults or metastases in the elderly) is usually elicited by rotation to either side or by flexion or extension (Grand 1971).

Rebound nystagmus

Rebound nystagmus is an uncommon variety in which nystagmus of phasic type occurs on looking laterally but fatigues after about 20 seconds; when the eyes are then returned to the midline, phasic nystagmus to the opposite side develops and also quickly fatigues. The underlying pathology appears to be cerebellar degeneration (Hood, Kayan, and Leech 1973).

Primary position upbeat nystagmus

This is a form of vertical nystagmus which occurs in an upward direction during ocular fixation, is increased by looking upwards, but decreased by downward gaze. It appears to be due to a defect in the upward smooth pursuit system and can result from lesions of the vermis or of interconnecting pathways in the caudal brainstem at the level of the inferior olives (Gilman, Baloh, and Tomiyasu 1977).

Horizontal pursuit defect nystagmus

This rare phenomenon is a form of nystagmus seen to occur in one lateral direction when the eyes are in the primary position and in which the slow phase has a constant velocity. It is associated with a defect of smooth pursuit movements in the direction in which the nystagmus occurs and is usually due to large posterior fossa lesions (Abel, Daroff, and Dell'Osso 1979).

Periodic alternating nystagmus

This is a form of spontaneous nystagmus which alternates in direction, occurring periodically in one direction, then in the opposite direction (Baloh, Honrubia, and Konrad 1976). It may be associated with lesions of the vestibular nuclei and vestibulocerebellum, multiple sclerosis, posterior fossa malformations, spinocerebellar degeneration, and even congenital nystagmus (see below); it is reduced in some cases by treatment with baclofen (Halmagi, Rudge, Gresty, Leigh, and Zee 1980). It causes oscillopsia and usually impairs vision.

See-saw nystagmus

In this rare form of nystagmus one eye moves up while the other moves down; this disjunctive variety has been seen in patients with tumours of the third ventricular region but may also be a rare consequence of a pontine lesion (Mastaglia 1974).

Congenital and familial nystagmus

Nystagmus may be present from birth, and in several members of the same family, sometimes in successive generations. Congenital nystagmus is usually a fine pendular oscillation present at rest and increased on deviation in all directions, but more than one variety occurs. There may be associated head movement but eye closure may suppress the movements of both eyes and head (Shibasaki, Yamashita, and Motomura 1978). There is usually no subjective oscillopsia. Its cause is unknown, but it may be associated with other ocular defects involving poor vision such as albinism, astigmatism, or amblyopia. It may be inherited as a Mendelian dominant or as a sex-linked recessive trait, and males are affected three times as often as females.

Hysterical 'nystagmus'

Hysterical eye movements superficially resembling nystagmus disappear when ocular fixation is unconscious and reappear on testing the eye movements. They may be associated with spasm of convergence or blepharospasm. *Pseudonystagmus*, often monocular, is also occasionally seen when there is weakness of external ocular muscles, as in myasthenia gravis. *Voluntary nystagmus* (the ability to 'jiggle the eyes') could be produced by 8 per cent of a group of college students studied by Zahn (1978). It resembled pendular nystagmus in waveform and ocular flutter or opsoclonus (see below) in frequency but could be easily differentiated from other forms.

Toxic nystagmus

Phasic nystagmus occurring on lateral gaze to both sides is seen in alcoholic intoxication and as a result of many other drugs, including anticonvulsants and barbiturates.

Other spontaneous ocular movements

Opsoclonus is a term which has been given to rapid fluttering oscillations of the eyes, often interrupted by sudden, jerk-like myoclonic movements. It is seen most often in association with limb myoclonus in association with so-called acute myoclonic encephalopathy of infancy (Kinsbourne 1962) but can also be a manifestation of encephalopathy or encephalitis in adults (Baringer, Sweeney, and Winkler 1968; McLean 1970). So-called *ocular flutter* is similar; these abnormal movements are closely related to ocular dysmetria, in which the eyes during conjugate movement overshoot and briefly oscillate about the target upon which they ultimately fix (Ellenberger, Keltner, and Stroud 1972) and which is invariably a manifestation of cerebellar disease (Selhorst, Start, Ochs, and Hoyt 1976 a, b). These ocular macro-oscillations have also been called *macrosaccadic oscillations* since they clearly represent abnormal saccades in which the normal 'damping' action of the cerebellum is impaired.

Ocular bobbing is a syndrome of brisk, repetitive, downward conjugate deviation of the eyes, associated usually with pontine lesions in comatose patients (Fisher 1964; Nelson and Johnston 1970); however, it has been described in a patient with an acute cerebellar haemorrhage with no evidence of a pontine lesion (Bosch, Kennedy, and Aschenbrener 1975). Recovery has been reported (Newman, Gay, and Heilbrun 1971).

References

Abel, L. A., Daroff, R. B., and Dell'Osso, L. F. (1979). Horizontal pursuit defect nystagmus *Ann. Neurol.* **5**, 449.

Baloh, R. W., Honrubia, V., and Konrad, H. R. (1976). Periodic alternating nystagmus. *Brain*, **99**, 11.

——, Yee, R. D., and Honrubia, V. (1978a). Internuclear ophthalmoplegia. I. Saccades and dissociated nystagmus. *Arch. Neurol., Chicago* **35**, 484.

——, ——, and ——, (1978b). Internuclear ophthalmoplegia. II. Pursuit, optokinetic nystagmus, and vestibulo-ocular reflex. *Arch. Neurol., Chicago*, **35**, 490.

Baringer, J. R., Sweeney, V. P., and Winkler, G. F. (1968). An acute syndrome of ocular oscillations and truncal myoclonus. *Brain* **91**, 473.

Barnett, H. J. M., Foster, J. B., and Hudgson, P. (1973). *Syringomyelia*. Saunders, London.

Bender, M. B. (1964). *The oculomotor system*. Hoeber, New York.

——, (1980). Brain control of conjugate horizontal and vertical eye movements. A survey of the structural and functional correlates. *Brain* **103**, 23.

——, Postel, D. M., and Krieger, H. P. (1957). Disorders of oculomotor function in lesions of the occipital lobe, *J. Neurol. Neurosurg. Psychiat.* **20**, 139.

Biemond, A. and De Jong, J. M. B. V (1969). On cervical nystagmus and related disorders. *Brain* **92**, 437.

Bittencourt, P., Gresty, M. A., and Richens, A. (1980). Quantitative assessment of smooth-pursuit eye movements in healthy and epileptic subjects. *J. Neurol. Neursurg. Psychiat.* **43**, 1119.

Blumenthal, H. and Miller, C. (1969). Motor nuclear involvement in progressive supranuclear palsy. *Arch. Neurol., Chicago* **20**, 362.

Bosch, E. P., Kennedy, S. S., and Aschenbrener, C. A. (1975). Ocular bobbing: the myth of its localizing value. *Neurology, (Minneapolis)* **25**, 949.

Bronstein, A. M. and Hood, J. D. (1985). Cervical nystagmus: a case report. *J. Neurol. Neurosurg. Psychiat.* **48**, 128.

Carmichael, F. A., Dix, M. R., and Hallpike, C. S. (1956). Pathology, symptomatology, and diagnosis of organic affections of the eighth nerve system. *Br. med. Bull.* **12**, 146.

Cartlidge, N. E. F. and Shaw, D. A. (1981). *Head injury*. Saunders, London.

Cawthorne, T., Dix, M. R., Hood, J. D., and Harrison, M. S. (1969). Vestibular syndromes and vertigo. In *Handbook of clinical neurology*, (ed. P. J. Vinken and G. W. Bruyn), Vol. 2. North-Holland, Amsterdam.

Christoff, N. (1974). A clinicopathologic study of vertical eye movements. *Arch. Neurol., Chicago* **31**, 1.

Cogan, D. G. and Adams, R. D. (1953). A type of paralysis of conjugate gaze (ocular motor apraxia). *Arch. Ophthalmol.* **50**, 434.

—— and Williams, H. W. (1966). *Neurology of the visual system*. Thomas, Springfield. Illinois.

—— and Wray, S. H. (1970). Internuclear ophthalmoplegia as an early sign of brainstem tumours. *Neurology, Minneapolis* **20**, 629.

Dix, M. R., Hallpike, C. S., and Harrison, W. S. (1949). Some observations on the otological effects of streptomycin intoxication. *Brain* **72**, 241.

Drachman, D. A. (1968). Ophthalmoplegia plus. The neurodegenerative disorders associated with progressive external ophthalmoplegia. *Arch. Neurol., Chicago* **18**, 654.

Elizan, T. S., Spire, J. P., Andiman, R. M., Baughman, F. A., and Lloyd-Smith, D. L. (1971). Syndrome of acute idiopathic ophthalmoplegia with ataxia and areflexia. *Neurology, Minneapolis* **21**, 281.

Ellenberger, C., Keltner, J. L., and Stroud, M. H. (1972). Ocular dyskinesia in cerebellar disease: evidence for the similarity of opsoclonus, ocular dysmetria and flutter-like oscillations. *Brain* **95**, 685.

Feldon, S. E., Hoyt, W. F., and Stark, L. (1980). Disordered inhibition in internuclear ophthalmoplegia. Analysis of eye movement recordings with computer simulations. *Brain* **103**, 113.

Fisher, C. M. (1956). An unusual variant of acute idiopathic polyneuritis (syndrome of ophthalmoplegia, ataxia, and areflexia). *New Engl. J. Med.* **255**, 57.

—— (1964). Ocular bobbing. *Arch. Neurol., Chicago* **11**, 543.

—— (1967). Some neuro-ophthalmological observations. *J. Neurol. Neursurg. Psychiat.* **30**, 383.

Gay, A. J. and Newman, N. M. (1972). Eye movements and their disorders. In *Scientific foundations of neurology* (ed. M. Critchley, J. L. O'Leary, and W. B. Jennett). Heinemann, London.

Gilman, N., Baloh, R. W., and Tomiyasu, U. (1977). Primary position upbeat nystagmus: a clinicopathologic study, *Neurology, Minneapolis* **27**, 294.

Goebel, H. H., Komatsuzaki, A., Bender, M. B., and Cohen, B. (1971). Lesions of the pontine tegmentum and conjugate gaze paralysis. *Arch. Neurol. Chicago* **24**, 431.

Goldhammer, Y. and Lawton Smith, J. (1974). Acquired intermittent Brown's syndrome. *Neurology, Minneapolis* **24**, 666.

Gonyea, E. F. (1974). Bilateral internuclear ophthalmoplegia. Association with occlusive cerebrovascular disease. *Arch. Neurol., Chicago* **31**, 168.

Grand, W. (1971). Positional nystagmus: an early sign in medulloblastoma. *Neurology, Minneapolis* **21**, 1157.

Halmagyi, G. M., Rudge, P., Gresty, M. A., Leigh, R. J., and Zee, D. S. (1980). Treatment of periodic alternating nystagmus. *Ann. Neurol.* **8**, 609.

Halsey, J. H., Ceballos, R., and Crosby, E. C. (1967). The supranuclear control of voluntary lateral gaze. Clinical and anatomic correlation in a case of ventral pontine infarction. *Neurology, Minneapolis* **17**, 928.

Hood, J. D., Kayan, A., and Leech, J. (1973). Rebound nystagmus. *Brain* **96**, 507.

Keane, J. R. (1975a). Contralateral gaze deviation with supratentorial hemorrhage: three pathologically verified cases. *Arch. Neurol., Chicago* **32**, 119.

——, (1975b). Ocular skew deviation: analysis of 100 cases. *Arch. Neurol., Chicago* **32**, 185.

Kearns, T. P. and Sayre, G. P., (1958). Retinitis pigmentosa, external ophthalmoplegia, and complete heart block: unusual syndrome with histologic study in one of two cases. *Arch. Ophthalmol.* **60**, 280.

Kinsbourne, M. (1962). Myoclonic encephalopathy of infants, *J. Neurol. Neursurg. Psychiat.* **25**, 271.

Koeppen, A. H. and Hans M. B. (1976). Supranuclear ophthalmoplegia in olivopontocerebellar degeneration. *Neurology, Minneapolis* **26**, 764.

Mastaglia, F. L. (1974). See-saw nystagmus: an unusual sign of brain-stem infarction. *J. neurol. Sci.* **22**, 439.

McLean, D. R. (1970). Polymyoclonia with opsclonus. *Neurology, Minneapolis* **20**, 508.

McLeod, A. R. and Glaser, J. S. (1974). Deglutition-trochlear synkinesis. *Arch. Ophthalmol.* **92**, 171.

Mills, P. V., Bowen, D. I., and Thomson, D. S. (1971). Chronic progressive external ophthalmoplegia and pigmentary degeneration of the retina. *Br. J. Ophthal.* **55**, 302.

Nelson, J. R. and Johnston, C. H. (1970). Ocular bobbing. *Arch. Neurol., Chicago* **22**, 348.

Newman, N., Gay, A. J., and Heilbrun, M. P. (1971). Disjugate ocular bobbing: its relation to midbrain, pontine and medullary function in a surviving patient. *Neurology, Minneapolis* **21**, 633.

Norman, M. G. (1974). Unilateral encephalomalacia in cranial nerve nuclei in neonates: report of two cases. *Neurology, Minneapolis* **24**, 424.

Nylén, C. O. (1950). Positional nystagmus: a review and future prospects. *J. Laryngol* **64**, 295.

Okamoto, T., Mizuno, K., Iida, M., Sobue, I., and Mukoyama, M. (1981). Ophthalmoplegia-plus: its occurrence with periventricular diffuse low density on computed tomography scan, *Arch. Neurol., Chicago* **38**, 423.

Patton, H. D., Sandsten, J. W., Crill, W. E., and Swanson, P. D. (1976). *Introduction to basic neurology*. Saunders, Philadelphia.

Rosenburg, M., Sharpe, J., and Hoyt, W. F. (1975). Absent vestibulo-ocular reflexes and acute supratentorial lesions. *J. Neurol. Neurosurg. Psychiat.* **38**, 6.

Rothstein, T. L. and Alvord, E. C. (1971). Posterior internuclear opthalmopegia: a clinicopathologic study. *Arch. Neurol., Chicago* **24**, 191.

Sachsenweger, R. (1969). Clinical localisation of oculomotor disturbances. In *Handbook of clinical neurology* (ed. P. J. Vinken and G. W. Bruyn), Chapter 13, Vol. 2. North-Holland, Amsterdam.

Schneck, L., Adachi, M., Briet, P., Wolintz, A., and Volk, B. W. (1973). Ophthalmoplegia plus with morphological and chemical studies of cerebellar and muscle tissue. *J. neurol. Sci.* **19**, 37.

Sauron, B., Bouche, P., Cathala, H.-P., Chain, F., and Castayne, P. (1984). Miller Fisher syndrome: clinical and electrophysiologic evidence of peripheral origin in 10 cases. *Neurology, Minneapolis* **34**, 953.

Selhorst, J. B. Stark L., Ochs, A. L., and Hoyt, W. F. (1976a). Disorders in cerebellar ocular motor control.I. Saccadic overshoot dysmetria: an oculographic, control system and clinico-anatomical analysis. *Brain* **99**, 497.

——, ——, ——, and —— (1976b). Disorders in cerebellar ocular motor control. II. Macrosaccadic oscillation: an oculographic, control system and clinico-anatomical analysis. *Brain*, **99**, 509.

Sharpe, J. A., Rosenburg, M. A., Hoyt, W. F., and Daroff, R. B. (1974). Paralytic pontine exotropia. A sign of acute unilateral pontine gaze palsy and internuclear ophthalmoplegia. *Neurology, Minneapolis* **24**, 1076.

Shibasaki, H., Yamashita, Y., and Motomura, S. (1978). Suppression of congenital nystagmus. *J. Neurol. Neurosurg. Psychiat.* **41**, 1078.

Smith, J. Lawton (1963). *Optokinetic nystagmus*. Thomas, Springfield, Illinois.

Spector,R. H., Davidoff, R. A., and Schwartzman, R. J. (1976). Phenytoin-induced ophthalmoplegia. *Neurology, Minneapolis* **26**, 1031.

Steele, J. C., Richardson, J. C., and Olszewski, J. (1964). Progressive supranuclear palsy: a heterogeneous degeneration involving the brain stem, basal ganglia and cerebellum with vertical gaze and pseudobulbar palsy, nuchal dystonia and dementia. *Arch. Neurol., Chicago* **10**, 333.

Stewart, J. D., Kirkham, T. H., and Mathieson, G. (1979). Periodic alternating gaze. *Neurology, Minneapolis* **29**, 222.

Trojanowski, J. Q. and Lafontaine, M. H. (1981). Neuroanatomical correlates of selective downgaze paralysis. *J. neurol. Sci.* **52**, 91.

—— and Wray, S. H. (1980). Vertical gaze ophthalmoplegia: selective paralysis of downgaze. *Neurology, Minneapolis* **30**, 605.

Victor, D. I. (1976). The diagnosis of congenital unilateral third-nerve palsy. *Brain* **99**, 711.

Walton, J. N. (1981). The special senses. In Neurology (Section XII) by J. N. Walton. In *Pathophysiology—the biological principles of disease* (ed. L. H. Smith, Jr. and S. O. Thier), Vol. I, *International Textbook of Medicine*. Saunders, Philadelphia.

Zahn, J. R. (1978). Incidence and characteristics of voluntary nystagmus. *J. Neurol. Neurosurg. Psychiat.* **41**, 617.

Zee, D. S., Freeman, J. M., and Holtzman, N. A. (1974). Ophthalmoplegia in maple syrup urine disease. *J. Pediat.* **84**, 113.

——, Yee, R. D., and Singer, H. S. (1977). Congenital ocular motor apraxia. *Brain*, **100**, 581.

The pupils, eyelids, and orbital contents

The innervation of the pupils

The size of the pupil is under the control of two mutually antagonistic muscles: the circular muscle of the iris, the sphincter pupillae, which causes contraction and is innervated by the third nerve, and the radial fibres of the iris which cause dilatation and receive their nerve supply from the cervical sympathetic.

The iridodilator fibres

The sympathetic fibres which control pupillary dilatation (p. 594) arise in the sympathetic nuclei of the hypothalamus; there is clearly a pathway from the frontotemporal cortex which influences hypothalamic activity and which accounts, for example, for pupillary dilatation induced by emotion, but this is poorly defined. The iridodilator fibres continue downwards in the tegmentum of the pons, medulla, and the cervical cord to synapse with the cells of the lateral horn of grey matter of the eighth cervical and first and second thoracic segments. From these cells the preganglionic fibres arise and leave the cord by the corresponding ventral roots. From the spinal nerves they pass by the white rami communicantes to the cervical sympathetic nerve trunk to end in the superior cervical ganglion. The postganglionic fibres start from this ganglion and join the plexus in the coat of the internal carotid artery with which they enter the skull; some then pass to the ophthalmic division of the trigeminal nerve and reach the pupil by the nasociliary and long ciliary nerves, while others go from the carotid plexus through the ciliary ganglion without interruption, and into the short ciliary nerves.

The iridoconstrictor and ciliary fibres

The iridoconstrictor fibres originate in the Edinger-Westphal nuclei (see Fig. 2.6, p. 95). Entering the third nerve, they terminate in the ciliary ganglion, from which postganglionic fibres arise which pass by the short ciliary nerves to the circular muscle of the iris. This may be true only of the fibres concerned in the reaction to light and those involved in the reaction on accommodation may bypass the ciliary ganglion (see below). The ciliary fibres follow the same route except that they arise in the median nucleus of Perlia and terminate in the ciliary muscle, contraction of which allows the lens to become more convex, thus accommodating the eye for near vision.

Paralysis of the sphincter pupillae

The constrictor muscle of the iris may be paralysed due to a lesion of the iridoconstrictor fibres at any point between the Edinger-Westphal nucleus and the eye. The pupil is widely dilated owing to the unantagonized action of the iridodilator muscle, and the reaction to both light and accommodation is lost. Paralysis of the sphincter pupillae occurring without paralysis of the extra-ocular muscles may be due to a lesion either of the Edinger-Westphal nucleus or of the ciliary ganglion but can also be the first manifestation of compression of the third-nerve trunk as in herniation of one temporal lobe through the tentorial hiatus, as the pupillo-constrictor fibres lie superficially in the nerve trunk.

Pupillary size and inequality

The size of the pupil can be measured accurately by electronic pupillometry. This technique has shown that minor inequalities in pupillary diameter (*anisocoria*) of up to 4 mm are common in the normal population and increase over the age of 60 years (Thompson 1980). Inequality greater than this is seen when a pupil is pathologically dilated or constricted or when one of moderate size fails to react to light; then the normal eye is the larger in dark and the smaller in bright illumination. Pupillary inequality may also at times be the result of local lesions of the eye such as iridocyclitis.

Paralysis of the dilator pupillae: ocular-sympathetic paralysis

Paralysis of pupillary dilatation is due to a lesion of the iridodilator fibres of the sympathetic. The pupil is constricted—myosis—by the unopposed iridoconstrictor muscle, and does not dilate in the dark or to emotion, while the ciliospinal reflex (see below) is lost. The iridodilator fibres lie close to the other fibres of the ocular sympathetic, viz. those which produce tonic elevation of the upper lid and tonic protrusion of the eyeball by means of the unstriped muscle of the orbit. Paralysis of the dilator is usually therefore associated with paralysis of these muscles, giving slight ptosis and enophthalmos (Horner's syndrome).

The myosis of the Argyll Robertson pupil has been attributed to a lesion of the iridodilator fibres in the midbrain but afferent fibres must also be involved (Ashworth and Isherwood 1981). Nevertheless, neuropathological evidence plainly indicates a lesion in the periaqueductal region of the midbrain (Poole 1984). Myosis may also occur with pontine lesions, as in the pin-point pupils of pontine haemorrhage, and of the lateral part of the medulla which interrupt descending fibres of the sympathetic, as in lateral medullary infarction. In the spinal cord the lateral horns of the upper dorsal region may be involved in a variety of lesions. The sympathetic white rami may be destroyed by trauma, as in the Klumpke type of birth palsy of the brachial plexus; and the cervical sympathetic may be damaged in the neck by trauma or pressure, especially from enlarged cervical lymph nodes.

Within the cranium postganglionic fibres may be damaged by the pressure of a retro-orbital tumour or aneurysm. In *Raeder's paratrigeminal syndrome*, division of the sympathetic fibres in the coat of the internal carotid artery gives the ocular manifestation of Horner's syndrome without loss of sweating on the affected side of the face as the fibres controlling the latter travel in the external carotid.

Paralysis of accommodation

Paralysis of accommodation may be produced by lesions involving the median nucleus of Perlia, the third nerve, or the ciliary ganglion. As an isolated ocular phenomenon it was once seen in diphtheritic neuropathy but is otherwise rare.

Action of drugs on the pupil and ciliary muscle

Many drugs influence pupil size and accommodation whether given systematically or in eye-drops. Pilocarpine and physostigmine (eserine) cause constriction of the pupil and spasm of accommodation by stimulating the nerve endings of the third nerve in the pupil and ciliary muscle. Atropine, homatropine, propantheline, and their analogues, including many anticholinergic drugs used in parkinsonism as well as many psychotropic antidepressive remedies, cause dilatation of the pupil and paralysis of accommodation by paralysing the same nerve endings. Cocaine causes dilatation by stimulating sympathetic nerve endings. The action of morphine in causing iridoconstriction is central, not peripheral. Ishikawa, Oono and Hikita (1977) reviewed the effects of many drugs on the pupil.

The pupillary reactions

The light reflex

If one eye is exposed to light, a constriction of both pupils normally occurs. The response of the pupil of the eye upon which the light falls is called the direct reaction, that of the opposite pupil the consensual reaction. *Hippus* (a phenomenon of transient rhythmical contraction and dilatation of the pupil exposed to light) is of no pathological significance. In eliciting the light reflex, the patient should be asked to look at a distant object in order to eliminate the contraction of the pupil on accommodation, and the eye not being tested should be covered in order to eliminate the consensual reaction. The afferent impulses from the retina follow the path of the visual afferent fibres as far as the optic tracts, with a similar decussation of those from the nasal halves of the retina at the optic chiasm, although it seems that more afferent pupillomotor fibres cross than remain uncrossed so that the consensual reaction is very slightly weaker than the direct (Thompson 1980). On leaving the optic tracts the reflex fibres separate from the visual and appear to pass through the brachium of the superior colliculus, but do not enter it, turning rostrally and medially into the pretectal region and then descending to the oculomotor nuclei. The decussating fibres cross, some in the posterior commissure and some ventral to the aqueduct near the nuclei. Both optic tracts must be connected with both oculomotor nuclei since a beam of light falling upon either half of either retina evokes a contraction of both pupils. The efferent path of the reflex runs from the Edinger–Westphal nuclei by the iridoconstrictor fibres already described.

Reaction on accommodation/convergence

When the gaze is directed from a distant to a near object, contraction of the medial recti causes convergence of the ocular axes; accommodation results from contraction of the ciliary muscle, and the pupil contracts. In eliciting this reaction the patient is asked to look at a distant object and then at the examiner's finger, which is gradually brought to within 50 mm of the eyes.

Constriction of the pupil may be associated with either convergence or accommodation, as it occurs on accommodation when convergence is paralysed and vice versa. Usually the two actions cannot be dissociated but in post-encephalitic parkinsonism, when convergence is lost, the accommodation reaction on focusing on a near object may be preserved, though it is often less brisk than normal. The reaction on accommodation/convergence is impaired by any lesion which involves iridoconstrictor fibres; very rarely, in midbrain lesions this reaction is lost when that to light is impaired.

The ciliospinal reflex

Pinching the skin of the face, neck, or upper trunk causes rapid bilateral pupillary dilatation. This polysynaptic reflex, of which the afferent limb consists of somatic fibres, the efferent of sympathetic ones, is preserved in lesions of the central nervous system but is lost in lesions of the afferent somatosensory or efferent sympathetic pathways.

Reflex iridoplegia and the Argyll Robertson pupil.
The term 'reflex iridoplegia' indicates a failure of the pupil to react to light and/or other stimuli which normally produce a change in its diameter. The term 'Argyll Robertson pupil' should be reserved for a form of reflex iridoplegia in which, as described by Argyll Robertson, the pupil 'is small . . . constant in size, and unaltered by light or shade; it contracts promptly and fully on convergence and dilates again promptly when the effort to converge is relaxed; it dilates slowly and imperfectly to mydriatics'. Most of the features were described by Romberg many years before Argyll Robertson. Very rarely the affected pupil reacts paradoxically to light by a slight dilatation. In addition to loss of the light reaction, the typical Argyll Robertson pupils of syphilis are irregular and unequal, and there is atrophy and depigmentation of the iris and loss of the ciliospinal reflex. In congenital neurosyphilis the pupils are often dilated but unresponsive to light and so are not of the Argyll Robertson type. Pupils showing most if not all of these typical Argyll Robertson features may also be seen rarely in diabetes, in alcoholic polyneuropathy, in hypertrophic polyneuropathy, and in tumours of the pineal region when there is also, as a rule, a defect of upward conjugate gaze. Reflex iridoplegia may also occur as a result of lesions in the following situations.

Lesions of the optic nerve. Accommodation, convergence, and the associated iridoconstriction can occur in the absence of vision, as when an individual who has become blind tries to look at the end of his nose. Consequently a lesion of the optic nerve severe enough to impair the conduction of the afferent impulses concerned in the light reflex can cause loss of that reflex with retention of the reaction on accommodation. The so-called *retrobulbar pupil reaction* (sometimes called the Marcus Gunn response) is seen in unilateral retrobulbar neuritis or neuropathy. In the affected eye a strong light stimulus may cause only minimal pupillary contraction or even slow dilatation, while the consensual reaction in that pupil elicited by applying the same stimulus to the other (normal) eye is brisk.

Lesions of the optic tract. Destruction of one optic tract causes loss of the light reflex when the temporal half of the ipsilateral retina and the nasal half of the contralateral retina are illuminated, though the reflex can be elicited from the other half of each retina. Homonymous hemianopia due to a tract lesion can thus be distinguished from that due to a lesion of the optic radiation which does not interrupt the light reflex (Wernicke's hemianopic reaction). Since more than half the afferent pupillomotor fibres decussate in the optic chiasm, it follows that in optic-tract lesions the light reflex is relatively less strong in the contralateral than in the ipsilateral eye (Behr's pupil). This has been shown to be the case, but the difference is so slight as only to be detectable with pupillometry (Thompson 1980).

Central lesions. There is abundant evidence that reflex iridoplegia may be produced by lesions of the upper midbrain. It has been observed in cases of pineal tumour, as a result of vascular lesions, in encephalitis lethargica, as a rare manifestation of multiple sclerosis and syringobulbia, and due to trauma to the upper midbrain. Syphilis is, of course, far the commonest cause of the Argyll Robertson pupil, which is usually present in general paresis and tabes and less often in meningovascular syphilis. The site of the lesion responsible for this sign has been disputed. It is now generally agreed to be in the upper half of the midbrain, near the aqueduct, where it interrupts the fibres approaching the iridoconstrictor nucleus (Lowenstein 1956; Poole 1984).

Lesions of the motor path. An alternative view previously expressed was that the lesion of the Argyll Robertson pupil lay in the ciliary ganglion, the fibres concerned in the accommodation reaction reaching the ciliary body without passing through the ganglion and so escaping damage (Nathan and Turner 1942; Naquin 1954). However, it is now known that this is the site of the lesion in the Holmes–Adie syndrome (see below) which has different clinical features. Lesions of the third nerve occasionally abolish the reaction to light but not that to accommodation. Such a dissociation can unquestionably occur as a result of lesions in or behind the eye, and has been described in cases of ocular trauma and of ophthalmic herpes zoster.

References

Ashworth, B. and Isherwood, I. (1981). *Clinical neuro-ophthalmology*, 2nd edn. Blackwell, Oxford.
Cogan, D. G. and Williams, H. W. (1966). *Neurology of the visual system*. Thomas, Springfield, Illinois.
Harris W. (1935). The fibres of the pupillary reflex and the Argyll Robertson pupil. *Arch. Neurol. Psychiat., Chicago* **39**, 1195.
Ishikawa, S., Oono, S., and Hikita, H. (1977). Drugs affecting the iris muscle. In *Drugs and ocular tissues* (ed. S. Dickstein), Chapter 5a. Karger, Basle.
Lowenstein, O. (1956). The Argyll Robertson pupillary syndrome: mechanism and localisation. *Am. J. Ophthal.* **42**, 105.
Merritt, H. H. and Moore, M. (1933). The Argyll Robertson pupil: an anatomic–physiologic explanation of the phenomenon, with a survey of its occurrence in neurosyphilis. *Arch. Neurol. Psychiat., Chicago* **30**, 357.
Naquin, H. A. (1954). Argyll Robertson pupil following herpes zoster ophthalmicus with remarks on efferent pupillary pathways. *Am. J. Ophthal.* **38**, 23.
Nathan, P. W. and Turner, J. S. A. (1942). The efferent pathway for pupillary contraction. *Brain* **65**, 343.
Poole, C. J. M. (1984). Argyll Robertson pupils due to neurosarcoidosis: evidence for site of lesion. *Br. med. J.* **ii**, 356.
Thompson, H. S. (1980). The pupil and accommodation. In *Neuro-ophthalmology* (ed. S. Lessell and J. T. W. van Dalen) Vol. 1, Chapter 15. Excerpta Medica, Amsterdam.

Tonic pupils and absent tendon reflexes

Definition. A syndrome of unknown aetiology characterized in its fully developed form by abnormalities in the reaction of one or both pupils to light and accommodation and absence of the tendon reflexes. Our present knowledge is based chiefly upon clinical observations of Moore (1924, 1931), Holmes (1931), Adie, 1931 *a*, *b*, 1932), Russell (1956, 1958), and Thompson (1980).

Synonym. The Holmes–Adie syndrome.

Aetiology and pathology
The disorder occurs in females much more often than in males and usually develops during the third decade. A slow virus infection has been postulated as a possible cause but viral antibody studies have been negative (Thompson 1980). Russell's (1956) work suggested that the lesion is in the efferent parasympathetic pathway to the eye, probably postganglionic. Harriman and Garland (1968) and Harriman (1976) reported cases of tonic pupil which came to autopsy. The pupils affected were the right ones and the right ciliary ganglia, in contrast to the left, showed degeneration of neurones, most of which were replaced by clumps of capsular cells. There was also a loss of large axons though many fine axons still traversed the ganglion. Some loss of neurones in dorsal root ganglia was also found.

Symptoms
The onset is usually sudden, the patient or her friends noticing that one pupil has become larger than the other. Sometimes the first complaint is of mistiness of vision in one eye. The pupillary abnormality is unilateral in about 80 per cent of cases. The affected pupil is moderately dilated and is therefore usually larger than its fellow. The reaction of the affected pupil to light, both direct and consensual, is either completely or almost completely absent but a sluggish reaction to light can sometimes be elicited after the patient has remained in a dark room for about half an hour. The characteristic feature, however, is the response to accommodation. Whereas a hasty examination may suggest that the pupil

does not react at all, nevertheless, if the patient is made to gaze fixedly at a near object, the pupil, sometimes after a slight delay, contracts very slowly through a range which is often greater than normal, so that it actually becomes smaller than the normal one. When accommodation is relaxed, dilatation begins either at once or after a slight delay and proceeds even more slowly than contraction. This is the tonic pupillary reaction.

This reaction, however, is not always present, and the pupil may thus be fixed to light and accommodation. Russell (1956, 1958) distinguished a 'paralytic' type of pupil attributed to parasympathetic denervation and a 'tonic' type, due to supersensitization of the denervated sphincter pupillae to acetylcholine liberated by intact parasympathetic fibres. Accommodation may also be tonic. It has been known for some years that the affected pupillary muscle shows cholinergic denervation supersensitivity, contracting in response to drops of 2.5 per cent methacholine, unlike normal pupils (Bourgon, Pilley, and Thompson 1978). Wirtschafter, Volk, and Sawchuk (1978) suggested that the dissociation between the light and accommodation reflexes is due to diffusion in the posterior chamber of the eye of acetylcholine derived from the ciliary muscle which then reaches the denervated supersensitive pupillary muscle, but Thompson (1980) feels that aberrant regeneration of fibres subserving accommodation into the pupillary muscle may also be a factor.

Some abnormality of the tendon reflexes is usually present, the ankle-jerks, knee-jerks, and arm-jerks being diminished or lost in this order of frequency. H-reflex studies suggest that there is depression of the monosynaptic spinal reflex arc (McComas and Payan 1966). Occasionally the tonic pupil occurs with normal reflexes, or, less frequently, normal pupils with absent tendon reflexes.

Diagnosis

It is important to distinguish the tonic pupil from the Argyll Robertson pupil, but this is not difficult as the Argyll Robertson pupil is smaller than normal, does not react to light, reacts promptly and fully on convergence, and dilates incompletely to mydriatics, differing in all these respects from the typical tonic pupil. Contraction of the affected pupil in response to methacholine is virtually diagnostic. Rarely, however, similar bilateral pupillary changes are seen in diabetic or postinfective polyneuropathy (Thompson 1980).

Prognosis

The syndrome is permanent but has no ill effect beyond the inconvenience attaching to tonic accommodation. Patients have been seen in whom the condition of the pupil has remained unchanged for 30 or 40 years. With the passage of time there is progressive miosis in the affected eye, the other is often affected, and eventually both pupils usually become small and react poorly to light (Thompson, Bell, Bourgon, Meek, Purcell, and Val Allen 1979).

Treatment

No treatment is consistently of value, but eserine drops may be used if the dilated pupil leads to discomfort.

Reference

Adie, W. J. (1931a). Pseudo-Argyll Robertson pupils with absent tendon reflexes. *Br. med. J.* **1**, 928.
—— (1931b). Argyll Robertson pupils true and false. *Br. med. J.* **2**, 136.
—— (1932). Tonic pupils and absent tendon reflexes. A benign disorder *sui generis*; its complete and incomplete forms. *Brain* **55**, 98.
Bourgon, P., Pilley, S. F. J., añ Thompson, H. S. (1978). Cholinergic supersensitivity of the iris sphincter in Adie's tonic pupil. *Am. J. Ophthal.* **85**, 373.
Harriman, D. G. F. (1970). Pathological aspects of Adie's syndrome. *Adv. Ophthal.* **23**, 55.
—— and Garland, H. G. (1968). The pathology of Adie's syndrome. *Brain* **91**, 401.
Holmes, G. (1931). Partial iridoplegia associated with symptoms of other disease of the nervous system. *Trans. ophthal. Soc. UK* **41**, 209.
McComas, A. J. and Payan, J. (1966). Motoneurone excitability in the Holmes-Adie syndrome. In *Control and innervation of skeletal muscle* (ed. B. L. Andrews). Churchill-Livingstone, Edinburgh and London.
Moore, R. F. (1924). Discussion on the pupil from the ophthalmological point of view. *Trans. ophthal. Soc. UK* **44**, 38.
—— (1931). The non-luetic Argyll Robertson pupil. *Trans. ophthal. Soc. UK* **51**, 203.
Russell, G. F. M. (1956). The pupillary changes in the Holmes–Adie syndrome. *J. Neurol. Neurosurg. Psychiat.* **19**, 289.
—— (1958). Accommodation in the Holmes–Adie syndrome. *J. Neurol. Neurosurg. Psychiat.* **21**, 290.
Thompson, H. S. (1980). The pupil and accommodation. In *Neuro-ophthalmology* (ed. S. Lessell and J. T. W. van Dalen) Vol. 1, Chapter 15. Excerpta Medica, Amsterdam.
——, Bell, R. A., Bourgon, P., Meek, E. S., Purcell, J. J. Jr., and van Allen, M. W. (1979). Seven papers on Adie's syndrome. In *Topics in neuro-ophthalmology* (ed. H. S. Thompson), Section 2, pp. 95–123. Williams and Wilkins, Baltimore, Maryland.
Wirtschafter, J. D., Volk, C. R., and Sawchuk, R. J. (1978). Transaqueous diffusion of acetylcholine to denervated iris sphincter muscle: a mechanism for the tonic pupil syndrome (Adie syndrome). *Ann. Neurol.* **4**, 1.

The innervation of the eyelids

Two muscles elevate the upper eyelid, the striated levator palpebrae superioris, innervated by the third nerve, and Müller's palpebral muscle, part of the unstriated muscle of the orbit, which is supplied by the cervical sympathetic. Lid closure depends upon the orbicularis oculi, the motor nerve of which is the facial.

Retraction of the upper lid

Retraction of the upper lid results from relative or absolute shortening of the elevating muscles, especially of the unstriated muscle. It is exaggerated when the patient looks upwards and causes the lag of the upper lid in following downward movement of the eye, known as von Graefe's sign. Lid retraction is most often seen in ophthalmic Graves' disease, but it may also be produced by a lesion in the upper midbrain, especially one involving the posterior commissure. It may follow a vascular lesion in this situation and it is also sometimes seen in tabes, multiple sclerosis, postencephalitic parkinsonism, myasthenia gravis, and as a congenital abnormality. It may be unilateral or bilateral and can occur with or without exophthalmos. When due to a lesion (such as a tumour) in the upper midbrain it may be associated with impaired conjugate elevation of the eyes or with reflex iridoplegia.

Ptosis

Ptosis (drooping of the upper lid) may be the result of paralysis of either the levator palpebrae superioris or of the orbital smooth muscle. In the latter case the drooping is comparatively slight. Complete paralysis of the levator, however, causes closure of the eye. It is necessary to distinguish ptosis due to a sympathetic lesion from that due to paresis of the levator. This may be done by observing the lid when the patient looks upwards; normally, elevation of the upper lid then occurs as an associated movement. In ptosis of sympathetic origin the amplitude of this associated movement is normal. In ptosis due to paresis of the levator it is diminished. Over-action of the occipitofrontalis muscle giving compensatory wrinkling of the forehead is commonly present. Paralysis of the levator may be due to a lesion involving the nucleus of the third nerve, of the third-nerve trunk, or its superior division within the orbit, to a disorder of function at the myoneural junction in myasthenia gravis, or to involvement of the muscle itself in ocular myopathy (see *British Medical Journal* 1973). Slight bilateral ptosis may occur as a result of acute infarction in one cerebral hemisphere and is sometimes worse on the hemiparetic side, presumably due to the effects of the upper motor-neurone lesion upon the levator muscles (Caplan 1974). It may be congenital (and sometimes of dominant inheritance) and may occur intermittently on one side as a congenital synkinetic phenomenon with each movement of the jaw on chewing in the Marcus Gunn jaw-winking phenomenon (Gunn 1883). A lesion of the ocular sympathetic responsible for ptosis may occur within the brainstem, spinal cord, the eighth cervical and first and second thoracic ventral roots and spinal nerves, or the cervical sympathetic trunk. It is usually associated with other signs of Horner's syndrome (see Chapter 20).

Exophthalmos and enophthalmos

The smooth muscle of the orbit is normally in a state of sufficient tonic contraction to produce some protrusion of the eyeball. Paralysis of this muscle causes slight enophthalmos: exophthalmos is never due to its over-activity. The commoner causes of exophthalmos are : (1) ophthalmic Graves' disease; (2) pseudotumour of the orbit and orbital myositis; (3) primary tumours within the orbit, especially of the optic nerve and its sheath; (4) diseases of the nasal air sinuses, empyema, mucocele, and carcinoma; (5) retro-orbital intracranial tumours, especially meningiomas and aneurysms; (6) primary or secondary tumours of the bones forming the walls of the orbit; (7) orbital arteriovenous or venous angioma. Less common causes are carotid-cavernous sinus aneurysm, craniostenosis, xanthomatosis, Wegener's granulomatosis, chloroma, and metastatic tumour from the suprarenal (Hutchinson type) or breast (van Buren, Poppen, and Horrax 1957; Bedford and Daniel 1960). The detailed effects of these lesions are considered in later appropriate sections of this book. However, it should be noted that the diagnosis of orbital lesions has been greatly improved by the use of diagnostic ultrasound (Restori, McLeod, and Wright 1980) and CT scanning (Lloyd 1980; Sanders 1980).

References

Bedford, P. D. and Daniel, P. M. (1960). Discrete carcinomatous metastases in the extrinsic ocular muscles. *Am. J. Ophthal.* **49**, 723.

Brain, W. R. (1955). Exophthalmic ophthalmoplegia. *Trans. ophthal. Soc. UK* **55**, 351.

British Medical Journal (1973). Ptosis. *Br. med. J.* **1**, 679.

Caplan, L. R. (1974). Ptosis. *J. Neurol. Neurosurg. Psychiat* **37**, 1.

Gunn, R. M. (1883). The jaw-winking phenomenon. *Trans. ophthal Soc. UK* **3**, 283.

Lloyd, G. A. S. (1980). Computerized tomography in orbital lesions. *J. R. Soc. Med.* **73**, 279.

Pochin, E. E. (1939*a*). Ocular effects of sympathetic stimulation in man. *Clin. Sci.* **4**, 79.

—— (1939*b*). The mechanism of lid retraction in Graves' disease. *Clin. Sci.* **4**, 91.

Restori, M., McLeod, D., and Wright, J. E. (1980). Diagnostic ultrasound in ophthalmology. *J. R. Soc. Med.* **73**, 273.

Sanders, M. D. (1980). CT scanning in diagnosis of orbital disease. *J. R. Soc. Med.* **73**, 284

van Buren, J., Poppen, J. L., and Horrax, G. (1957). Unilateral exophthalmos. *Brain* **80**, 139.

Lesions of the third, fourth, and sixth nerves

The control of ocular movements, movement of the eyelids, the pupillary reactions, and nystagmus have already been considered.

Third-nerve paralysis

After leaving the nucleus, the fibres of the third nerve sweep outwards and forwards through the red nucleus and the medial margin of the substantia nigra to emerge from the brainstem along the oculomotor sulcus on the medial aspect of the crus cerebri. The nerve passes forwards between the posterior cerebral and superior cerebellar arteries, close to the posterior communicating artery, and pierces the dura mater beside the posterior clinoid process in a small triangular space between the free and attached borders of the tentorium cerebelli. It then passes through the lateral part of the cavernous sinus, lying close to the fourth and sixth nerves and the first division of the fifth, and enters the orbit through the superior orbital fissure between the two heads of the lateral rectus muscle. Here it divides into two branches, the upper supplying the levator palpebrae and the superior rectus, and the lower the medial and inferior recti and the inferior oblique, the nerve to which gives off the short root to the ciliary ganglion.

Paralysis of the third nerve causes ptosis, complete internal ophthalmoplegia, and paralysis of the superior, medial, and inferior recti, and inferior oblique. The pupil is widely dilated and fixed owing to paralysis of the sphincter pupillae and the unantagonized action of the dilator. Accommodation is also paralysed. The unantagonized lateral rectus causes outward deviation of the eye, and the only ocular movements possible are abduction, carried out by the lateral rectus, and some depression and internal rotation by the superior oblique. Paralysis of the levator palpebrae causes ptosis; the resulting closure of the eye masks the diplopia, which is evident to the patient only when the lid is passively raised (Fig. 2.8).

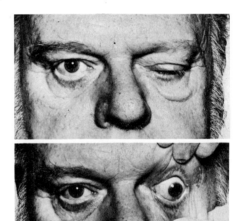

Fig. 2.8. A left third-nerve palsy in a diabetic subject who also had a carcinoma of the left ethmoid sinus (figure kindly supplied by Dr J.D. Spillane). Note the ptosis and the abduction of the eye due to the unopposed action of the lateral rectus.

Although lesions of this nerve usually cause both external and internal ophthalmoplegia, in a partial lesion the iridoconstrictor fibres may escape or in recovery from a complete lesion the intrinsic fibres may recover before the extrinsic. When both the third nerve and the ocular sympathetic are injured, as may happen with a lesion just behind the orbit, the pupil is not dilated but is fixed in the mid-position and unreacting. As the pupilloconstrictor fibres and those innervating the levator palpebrae lie superficially in the trunk of the nerve, a fixed dilated pupil is often the first sign of third-nerve compression and ptosis the second, before external ophthalmoplegia develops (Sunderland and Hughes 1946).

Fourth-nerve paralysis

The fibres of the fourth nerve, after leaving the nucleus, turn backwards through the peri-aqueductal grey matter medial to the mesencephalic root of the trigeminal nerve, and then downwards and medially to decussate in the anterior medullary velum, whence the nerve emerges just behind the colliculi. It then passes round the cerebral peduncle, lying between it and the temporal lobe, and pierces the free border of the tentorium cerebelli lateral to the third nerve to enter the lateral wall of the cavernous sinus.

It enters the orbit through the superior fissure and terminates in the superior oblique. A lesion of the fourth nerve causes paralysis of this muscle with weakness of downward and inward movement of the eye. For the character of the resulting diplopia, see page 97. When the lesion involves the nucleus or the fibres of the nerve within the midbrain before their decussation, the paralysis of the superior oblique is on the opposite side to the lesion. When the nerve is damaged in its extracerebral course the paralysis is ipsilateral.

Sixth-nerve paralysis

The fibres of the sixth nerve, after leaving the nucleus just below the floor of the fourth ventricle, pass forwards through the pons to emerge at its inferior border above the lateral side of the medullary pyramid. It has a long extracerebral course along the base of the brain and over the apex of the petrous temporal bone before it pierces the dura mater of the posterior fossa, just below the dorsum sellae. Like the third and fourth nerves, it lies in the lateral wall of the cavernous sinus, and then passes through the superior orbital fissure to terminate in the lateral rectus. A lesion of the sixth nerve causes paralysis of this muscle with loss of abduction of the eye, which is deviated inwards by the unantagonized medial rectus (Fig. 2.9). For the character of the resulting diplopia, see page 97.

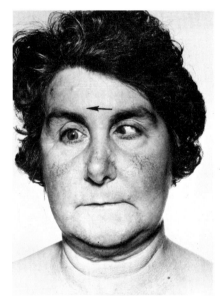

Fig. 2.9. A right sixth-nerve palsy, evident on right lateral gaze. (Reproduced from Spillane (1975) by kind permission of the author and publisher.)

Causes of paralysis of the third, fourth, and sixth nerves

The third, fourth, and sixth nerves may be damaged singly or together, and on one or both sides.

Within the brainstem their nuclei or intracerebral fibres may be damaged by trauma, neoplasms, vascular lesions, encephalitis, poliomyelitis, or multiple sclerosis, and in the case of the sixth nerve, syringobulbia. Thiamine deficiency giving Wernicke's encephalopathy is another cause of ophthalmoplegia and nystagmus. Congenital aplasia of the nuclei may cause bilateral ptosis, absence of elevation of the eyes, or lateral rectus paralysis with or without facial paralysis (Moebius syndrome). While most cases of what used to be called progressive nuclear ophthalmoplegia are known to be due to a progressive ocular myopathy often associated with abnormal mitochondria (see Chapter 19), it is possible that, in some cases of ophthalmoplegia associated with hereditary ataxia, nuclear degeneration does in fact occur (see p. 366).

Duane's syndrome is a benign congenital abnormality of ocular movement, commoner in females and often familial, in which there is impaired abduction of the eye; on attempted adduction there is retraction of the globe and narrowing of the palpebral fissure. The condition is due to fibrous replacement of the lateral rectus muscle; though it resembles a sixth-nerve palsy, there is probably no abnormality of the sixth nerve or its nucleus. Congenital third-nerve palsy and *Brown's syndrome* have been described on p. 99.

Intracranial tumour may cause direct compression of the nerves at any point in their course, but, in addition, *increased intracranial pressure* due to intracranial tumour or abscess remote from the nerves, or to hydrocephalus, may indirectly impair their conductivity. The sixth nerve most often suffers in this way, and sixth-nerve paralysis may occur as a false localizing sign of a tumour in any situation. Supratentorial tumours probably cause this by displacing the brainstem downwards and so stretching the nerve across the petrous apex. It may be unilateral or bilateral (Keane 1976). The third nerve may also suffer, especially with tumours of the temporal lobe. The nerve may then be compressed as it crosses the free edge of the tentorium cerebelli; a partial or complete third-nerve palsy is an important warning sign of herniation of the temporal lobe through the tentorial hiatus; a fixed dilated pupil is an important early sign. The fourth nerve escapes. An isolated third-nerve palsy is an occasional sign of a rapidly expanding *chromophobe adenoma of the pituitary* (see p. 164). Aberrant regeneration of one third nerve is thought to be typical of a cavernous sinus meningioma (Boghen, Chartrand, La Flamme, Kirkham, Hardy, and Aube 1979).

Neoplastic infiltration of the meninges may involve the nerves in their passage across the base of the skull and through the dura mater. Such meningeal metastases may be due to extension of a primary growth in the nasopharynx, or there may be diffuse carcinomatosis of the meninges due to metastasis from a tumour elsewhere, e.g. in the lung, breast, stomach, or prostate.

Intracranial aneurysm, especially when arising near the circle of Willis, may directly compress one or more of the oculomotor nerves, especially the third nerve, or they may be subjected to pressure by extravasated blood or clot after rupture of the aneurysmal sac. Compression may also arise from a normal vessel which is congenitally abnormal in position (Sunderland 1948). A unilateral third-nerve palsy, often developing rapidly with pain behind the eye, is a common sign of a supraclinoid aneurysm of the internal carotid or posterior communicating arteries. An infraclinoid aneurysm of the internal carotid, by contrast, lying within the walls of the cavernous sinus, more often causes paralysis of the third, fourth, and sixth nerves, and involvement of the first division of the fifth; the second division of the fifth nerve, which passes through the inferior part of the sinus, sometimes but not invariably, escapes.

Ophthalmoplegic migraine is a term applied to cases of recurrent third- or sixth-nerve palsies, the onset of which is associated with severe headache, and which tend to recover in the course of days or weeks, only to relapse subsequently, sometimes becoming permanent. The relationship of this condition to true migraine is doubtful (see p. 179).

Inflammatory disorders of the meninges may involve any or all of the oculomotor nerves, most often the third and the sixth. Sixth-nerve palsies are common in some severe cases of *pyogenic meningitis*, whereas unilateral or bilateral third- or sixth-nerve palsies may also develop in *meningovascular syphilis*, in *tuberculous or cryptococcal meningitis*, or in *sarcoidosis*.

Osteitis of the base of the skull and particularly of the apex of the petrous temporal bone due to otitis media may give a unilateral sixth-nerve palsy; there is often thrombosis of the inferior petrosal sinus. In this condition (Gradenigo's syndrome) there may also be facial pain and paraesthesiae due to involvement of the Gasserian ganglion. A transient third- or sixth-nerve palsy may be due to a misplaced alcohol injection intended for the Gasserian ganglion and is an occasional complication of *spinal anaesthesia*.

Polyneuritis cranialis is a term used to identify a syndrome of multiple unilateral or bilateral cranial-nerve palsies, often involving the third, fourth, and sixth nerves as well as others. Certainly any form of polyneuropathy, and particularly that of diphtheria or the Guillain-Barré syndrome, may involve the cranial nerves as well as the limbs and occasionally cranial nerves only are involved, as may also be the case in cephalic tetanus. Usually the CSF protein content is raised. It is, however, important to exclude in such cases other causes of multiple cranial-nerve palsies (e.g. nasopharyngeal carcinoma). Rarely multiple recurrent cranial-nerve palsies occur and are unexplained (Symonds 1958). A combination of bilateral external ophthalmoplegia of acute or subacute onset associated with areflexia and impairment of proprioceptive and vibration sense in the extremities but without limb weakness has been called the *Miller–Fisher syndrome* (Fisher 1956; Adams and Victor 1981); it probably represents a variant of cranial polyneuritis, related to the Guillain-Barré syndrome (see p. 526). Transient total ophthalmoplegia has also been reported as a consequence of phenytoin intoxication (Spector, Davidoff, and Schwartzman 1976). Isolated unilateral sixth-nerve palsy developing in childhood 7–21 days after a respiratory infection has been reported as a benign syndrome which usually recovers in three months (Knox, Clark, and Schuster 1967). The possible role of viral infection has been underlined by a report of an acute unilateral third-nerve palsy in an infant associated with systemic ECHO 9 viral infection (Hertenstein, Sarnat, and O'Connor 1976).

Vascular lesions of the oculomotor nerves are not uncommon, especially in diabetic and in other individuals with hypertension and atherosclerosis. An isolated painless third- or sixth-nerve palsy is the most usual presentation, often followed by complete recovery in three to six months; in some patients attacks of ophthalmoplegia recur and facial pain has also been described (Currie 1970). Pathological evidence indicates that these attacks are due to ischaemic infarction of the trunk of the nerve (Dreyfus, Hakim, and Adams 1957; Weber, Daroff, and Mackey 1970; Asbury, Aldridge, Hershberg, and Fisher 1970). *Thrombosis of the cavernous sinus* may also damage the third, fourth, and sixth nerves, and these nerves can also be contused or divided in their intracranial course by *head injury*. A palsy of the inferior branch of the third nerve can result from trauma or possibly (when transient) from viral infection (Susac and Hoyt 1977); this gives paralysis of the medial and inferior recti, the inferior oblique, and the sphincter pupillae.

Finally, *orbital lesions* must be considered. A syndrome of the superior orbital fissure, or so-called *painful ophthalmoplegia*, has been attributed to orbital periostitis or to granulomatous vasculitis in the cavernous sinus (the Tolosa–Hunt syndrome). It is characterized by pain in the eye and by the development of a unilateral third-, fourth-, and sixth-nerve palsy, often with involvement of the first division of the fifth. The erythrocyte sedimentation rate is usually raised and there is a rapid response to prednisone. In some such cases deformity of the carotid sinus suggesting periarteritis is demonstrated angiographically (Kettler and Martin 1975). The condition can sometimes remit and relapse spontaneously (Dornan, Espir, Gale, Tattersall, and Worthington 1979) and a similar acute disorder, sometimes giving not only palsy of the third, fourth, and sixth nerves but also involvement of the first and second divisions of the fifth, is especially common in India and South-east Asia (Tay, Tan, Cheah, and Ransome 1974). External (and sometimes internal) ophthalmoplegia is also well-recognized to occur in 10–15 per cent of patients with temporal or cranial arteritis (Barricks, Travesia, Glaser, and Levy 1977; Dimant, Grob, and Brunner 1980). Orbital tumours or pseudotumours due

to orbital granuloma or myositis (see Chapter 19) of multiple aetiology (Jellinek 1969; *British Medical Journal* 1974) may also give ophthalmoplegia, as may ophthalmic Graves's disease and *paranasal sinusitis* (Dimsdale and Phillips 1950). A mucocele of the ethmoid sinus can give asymmetrical painless proptosis and ophthalmoplegia; carcinoma of the paranasal sinuses will give a similar picture but with considerable local pain.

Treatment of lesions of the oculomotor nerves

Treatment is primarily that of the causal condition. When diplopia is present the patient may be helped by wearing a shade or a frosted glass in front of the eye. Orthoptic exercises are helpful during the recovery phase and it is sometimes possible to diminish diplopia by the use of a prism.

References

Adams, R. D. and Victor, M. (1981). *Principles of neurology*, 2nd edn. McGraw-Hill, New York.

Asbury, A. K., Aldredge, H., Hershberg, R., and Fisher, C. M. (1970). Oculomotor palsy in diabetes mellitus: a clinico-pathological study. *Brain* 93, 555.

Ashworth, B. and Isherwood, I. (1981). *Clinical neuro-ophthalmology*, 2nd edn. Blackwell, Oxford.

Barricks, M. E., Traviesa, D. B., Glaser, J. S., and Levy, I. S. (1977). Ophthalmoplegia in cranial arteritis. *Brain* 100, 209.

Boghen, D., Chartand, J. P., La Flamme, P., Kirkham, T., Hardy, J., and Aube, M. (1979). Primary aberrant third nerve regeneration. *Ann. Neurol.* 6, 415.

British Medical Journal (1974). Pseudotumours of the orbit. *Brit. med. J.* 1, 5.

Cogan, D. G. and Williams, H. W. (1966). *Neurology of the visual system*. Thomas, Springfield, Illinois.

Currie, S. (1970). Familial oculomotor palsy with Bell's palsy. *Brain* 93, 193.

Dimant, J., Grob, D., and Brunner, N. G. (1980). Ophthalmoplegia, ptosis, and miosis in temporal arteritis. *Neurology, Minneapolis* 30, 1054.

Dimsdale, H. and Phillips, D. G. (1950). Ocular palsies with nasal sinusitis. *J. Neurol. Neurosurg. Psychiat.* 13, 225.

Dornan, T. L., Espir, M. L. E., Gale, E. A. M., Tattersall, R. B., and Worthington, B. S. (1979). Remittent painful ophthalmoplegia: the Tolosa–Hunt syndrome? *J. Neurol. Neurosurg. Psychiat.* 42, 270.

Dreyfus, P. M., Hakim, S., and Adams, R. D. (1957). Diabetic ophthalmoplegia. *Arch. Neurol. Psychiat.* 77, 337.

Fisher, M. (1956). A syndrome of ophthalmoplegia, ataxia, and areflexia. An unusual variant of acute idiopathic polyneuritis. *New Engl. J. Med.* 255, 57.

Hertenstein, J. R., Sarnat, H. B., and O'Connor, D. M. (1976). Acute unilateral oculomotor palsy associated with ECHO 9 viral infection. *J. Pediat.* 89, 79.

Jellinek, E. H. (1969). The orbital pseudotumour syndrome and its differentiation from endocrine exophthalmos. *Brain* 92, 35.

Keane, J. R. (1976). Bilateral sixth nerve palsy: analysis of 125 cases. *Arch Neurol., Chicago* 33, 681.

Kettler, H. L. and Martin, J. D. (1975). Arterial stationary wave phenomenon in Tolosa–Hunt syndrome. *Neurology, Minneapolis* 25, 765.

Knox, D. L., Clark, D. B., and Schuster, F. F. (1967). Benign sixth nerve palsies in children. *Pediatrics* 40, 560.

Spector, R. H., Davidoff, R. A., and Schwartzman, R. J. (1976). Phenytoin-induced ophthalmoplegia. *Neurology, Minneapolis* 26, 1031.

Spillane, J. D. and Spillane, J.A. (1982). *An atlas of clinical neurology*, 3rd edn. Oxford University Press, Oxford.

Sunderland, S. (1948). Neurovascular relations and anomalies at the base of the brain. *J. Neurol. Neurosurg. Psychiat.* 11, 243.

—— and Hughes, E. S. R. (1946). The pupillo-constrictor pathway and the nerves to the ocular muscles in man. *Brain* 69, 301.

Susac, J. O. and Hoyt, W. F. (1977). Inferior branch palsy of the oculomotor nerve. *Ann. Neurol.* 2, 336.

Symonds, C. (1958). Recurrent multiple cranial nerve palsies. *J. Neurol. Neurosurg. Psychiat.* 21, 95.

Tay, C. H., Tan, Y. T., Cheah, J. S., and Ransome, G. A. (1974). Ocular palsies of obscure origin in south east Asia, *J. Neurol. Neurosurg. Psychiat.* 37 739.

Walsh, F. B. and Hoyt, W. F. (1969). *Clinical neuroophthalmology*, 3rd edn. Williams and Wilkins, Baltimore, Maryland.

Weber, T. B., Daroff, R. B., and Mackey, E. A. (1970). Pathology of oculomotor nerve palsy in diabetics. *Neurology, Minneapolis* **20**, 835.

The fifth or trigeminal nerve

Peripheral distribution

The fifth nerve contains both motor and sensory fibres. It is the principal sensory cranial nerve and represents a fusion of the sensory nerves of a number of metameric segments. It arises from the inferior surface of the pons on its lateral aspect by two roots, a large sensory root and a small motor root. The two roots pass forwards in the posterior fossa and, piercing the dura mater beneath the attachment of the tentorium to the tip of the petrous temporal bone, enter a cavity in the dura overlying its apex. Here the sensory root expands to form the trigeminal or Gasserian ganglion, which contains the sensory ganglion cells and is homologous with the dorsal root ganglia of the spinal nerves. The ganglion gives rise to three large nerve trunks, which constitute the three divisions of the nerve, namely the ophthalmic or first division, the maxillary or second, and the mandibular or third (Fig. 2.10). The motor root of the nerve passes forwards beneath the ganglion and fuses with the third division.

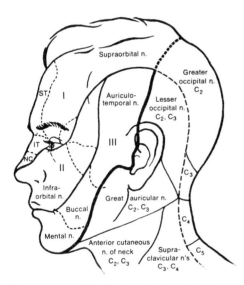

Fig. 2.10. The cutaneous distribution of the trigeminal nerve and its branches. ST = supratrochlear nerve; IT = intratrochlear nerve; NC = nasociliary nerve. (Reproduced from Brodal (1981) by kind permission of the authors and publisher.)

The ophthalmic nerve

The ophthalmic nerve, after lying in the lateral wall of the cavernous sinus together with the third, fourth, and sixth nerves, enters the orbit through the superior orbital fissure. It supplies a narrow zone adjacent to the midline throughout the length of the nose; the upper eyelid and the scalp from the base of the nose and the eyelid as far back as the lambdoidal suture in the midline and for about 8 cm laterally to this. The first division also supplies sensory fibres to the eye, including the conjunctiva and cornea, to the iris, and to the mucous membrane of the frontal sinuses and the upper nasal cavity.

The maxillary nerve

The maxillary nerve passes through the inferior part of the cavernous sinus and then via the foramen rotundum into the sphenopala-tine fossa. Here it is joined by postganglionic parasympathetic fibres from the sphenopalatine ganglion which are secretory to the lacrimal gland. It enters the orbit as the infra-orbital nerve through the inferior orbital fissure, and via the infra-orbital canal reaches the face through the infra-orbital foramen. It supplies the skin of the upper lip as far as the midline and that of the cheek between the area on the nose supplied by the ophthalmic nerve and a line down from the angle of the mouth, crossing the zygoma about midway between the outer canthus of the eye and the ear, and continuing upwards to join the lateral boundary of the area of supply of the first division on the scalp, at about the middle of the temporal ridge. The maxillary division also supplies the mucous membrane of the maxillary sinus and of the lower nasal cavity, together with that of the upper lip, the hard and soft palate (except its posterior aspect), together with the teeth of the upper jaw.

The mandibular nerve

The mandibular nerve is formed by fusion of the third sensory division with the motor root. These two roots pass out of the skull by the foramen ovale and unite to form a single trunk in the infratemporal fossa. The mandibular nerve supplies the skin of the lower lip and chin, together with a zone of the cheek about 2.5 cm wide below the infralateral boundary of the cutaneous supply of the maxillary nerve and bounded below by the border of the area supplied by the cervical plexus. Its distribution includes the tympanic membrane, the external auditory meatus, and the skin of the temple, where its distribution is bounded anteriorly by the lateral border of the second division, above by the lateral border of the first division, and behind by a line drawn upwards from the external meatus to the vertex in the region of the lambdoid suture. The tragus and upper part of the pinna are supplied by the auriculotemporal branch of the mandibular divsion. Clinical evidence suggests that there is some variation in precise distribution and there is often some overlap. In addition, the mandibular nerve supplies the mucous membrane of the cheek, lower jaw, floor of the mouth, and anterior two-thirds of the tongue, and the teeth of the lower jaw. From the chorda tympani, taste fibres pass to the anterior two-thirds of the tongue by the lingual nerve, a branch of the mandibular; postganglionic parasympathetic fibres destined via the submaxillary ganglion for the submaxillary and sublingual glands also travel in it. Meningeal branches of the trigeminal nerve supply the dura mater of the greater part of the skull above the tentorium and of the tentorium itself.

The cervical plexus supplies a zone of the cheek about 2.5 cm wide overlying the angle of the jaw.

The motor root

The motor root of the trigeminal nerve innervates the following muscles: temporalis, masseter, the medial and lateral pterygoids, the anterior belly of the digastric and mylohyoid, the tensor tympani, and the tensor veli palatini.

Central connections

The motor nucleus of the trigeminal nerve lies in the lateral part of the pontine tegmentum. The mesencephalic root is probably also motor. Incoming sensory fibres of the trigeminal divide, some passing into the principal sensory nucleus, which is situated in the substantia gelatinosa in the lateral pontine tegmentum, while others turn downwards to form the spinal tract which descends lateral to the substantia gelatinosa. As the spinal tract passes downwards its fibres gradually terminate in the substantia gelatinosa which constitutes the nucleus of the spinal tract. In a sense, therefore, the trigeminal sensory nucleus consists of two parts, the nucleus spongiosus or principal nucleus which is like an upward extension of the stratum spongiosum of the cord, receiving impulses from the posterior columns, and the nucleus gelatinosus corresponding to an upward extension of the substantia gelatinosa of the dorsal horn of spinal grey matter. Both the spinal tract and its nucleus end in the upper cervical cord at about the level of the second spinal nerve. The sensory fibres entering the principal sensory nucleus carry tactile and postural sensibility. From this nucleus, relay fibres cross the midline to form the quintothalamic tract or trigeminal lemniscus at the inner end of the medial lemniscus. The descending fibres of the spinal tract convey pain and thermal sensibility and assist in the co-ordination of stimuli arising in areas of overlapping innervation on the surface of the head supplied by the fifth, seventh, and tenth cranial nerves and the second and third cervical sensory roots (Denny-Brown and Yanagisawa 1973). Fibres from the ophthalmic division end in the lowest part of the spinal nucleus, those from the mandibular division in the highest part, and those from the maxillary intermediately so that 'representation' of cutaneous sensation on the face is inverted. Relay fibres from this nucleus cross the midline and pass upwards close to the medial lemniscus to join the spinothalamic tract in the pons.

Lesions of the trigeminal nerve

Peripheral lesions

The nerve may be involved between the pons and the trigeminal ganglion in granulomatous meningitis, or it may be compressed by a tumour or an aneurysm. This part of the nerve commonly degenerates in tabes. In the trigeminal ganglion it may be compressed by a tumour of the ganglion itself, or by a meningioma or acoustic neuroma arising in its neighbourhood, or damaged by a basal skull fracture involving the middle fossa. With the sixth nerve it may be involved in inflammation spreading from the petrous apex to the inferior petrosal sinus—Gradenigo's syndrome. Inflammation of the ganglion occurs in trigeminal herpes zoster. Unilateral facial sensory loss is sometimes a false localizing sign resulting from distortion of the trigeminal sensory root caused by brainstem displacement (O'Connell 1978), whether this is due to supratentorial or posterior fossa lesions; thus a diminished corneal reflex is an occasional sign of a contralateral parietal-lobe lesion (Ross 1972). Like the third, fourth, and sixth nerves (p. 106), its upper two divisions may be damaged by lesions in the cavernous sinus or its first division in the superior orbital fissure; more peripherally still its divisions and their major branches may be injured as a result of fracture of the facial bones; this is particularly true of the supraorbital and infraorbital nerves. Lesions of the nerve often cause pain referred to the cutaneous area it supplies, and may be associated with cutaneous anaesthesia and analgesia. When the nerve is involved between the pons and the ganglion, all three divisions are likely to be affected, but lesions of the ganglion itself may lead to symptoms confined to one division, most often the first. Lesions of the motor root cause weakness and wasting of the muscles of mastication on the affected side. Wasting of temporalis and of masseter leads to hollowing above and below the zygoma, and, when the patient clenches his teeth, palpation reveals that contraction of these muscles is less vigorous than on the normal side. When the mouth is opened, the jaw deviates to the paralysed side as a result of the unantagonized action of the opposite lateral pterygoid.

Central lesions

The central connections of the trigeminal nerve may be involved in lesions, especially tumours, syringobulbia, and vascular lesions, affecting the pons, medulla, and the upper cervical cord. A plaque of demyelination may occur at the point of entry of the sensory root into the brainstem in multiple sclerosis so that trigeminal neuralgia or unilateral facial sensory loss involving all modalities of sensation, subsequently remitting, are among the less common manifestations of this disease. The motor nucleus can be affected by a lesion in the lateral pontine tegmentum, in which case weakness of the masticatory muscles is usually associated with paresis of the lateral rectus and facial muscles on the affected side. Owing to the divergence of the sensory fibres of the trigeminal nerve within the brainstem, dissociated facial sensory loss often results from central lesions. A pontine lesion involving the principal sensory nucleus will give anaesthesia to light touch in trigeminal distribution, with preservation of pain, heat, and cold. On the other hand, lesions involving the medulla and the upper cervical cord, by injuring the spinal tract and its nucleus, will cause analgesia and thermo-anaesthesia, with preservation of light touch; sometimes there is severe and persistent spontaneous pain referred to the trigeminal area. This latter dissociation is characteristic of syringobulbia and of the lateral medullary syndrome due to thrombosis of one vertebral or posterior inferior cerebellar artery. Since the first division is represented lowest and the third division highest in the nucleus of the spinal tract a lesion of the lowest part of the medulla will cause analgesia limited to the first and second divisions only. Syringobulbia, however, often gives a typical progressive advance of the analgesia, which begins posteriorly in so-called 'onion skin' distribution, gradually converging upon the tip of the nose and upper lip, these usually being the last places to lose painful sensibility.

A lesion of the pons may also cause analgesia and thermo-anaesthesia on the opposite side of the face through damage to the crossed quintothalamic tract.

Neuropathic keratitis

Neuropathic keratitis is a change in the cornea which may follow any lesion of the fifth nerve if corneal analgesia results. It was often seen in the past after alcoholic injection of the trigeminal ganglion. It is due to recurrent trauma to the insensitive cornea and can usually be avoided by the use of protective drops or, if necessary, tarsorrhaphy. The corneal surface becomes hazy; if unchecked, loss of the surface epithelium, ulceration, and secondary infection may develop.

Trigeminal neuralgia

Synonym. Tic douloureux.

Definition. A disorder characterized by paroxysmal brief attacks of severe pain within the distribution of one or more divisions of the trigeminal nerve, usually without evidence of organic disease of the nerve.

Aetiology, incidence, and pathology

The aetiology of the 'idiopathic' condition is unknown (Penman 1968). However, symptomatic cases, secondary to an identifiable organic lesion, are commoner than was formerly realized and compression of the sensory root by an ectatic artery probably accounts for many cases (see below and *The Lancet* 1984). While it is rarely a presenting symptom of multiple sclerosis (Harris 1926) or develops during the course of this disease, which is therefore the commonest cause of the condition in young patients, and while it rarely develops in patients with ipsilateral or contralateral tumours in the posterior fossa (Hamby 1947), in which case traction on the sensory root is postulated, many cases are 'idiopathic'. The condition is slightly commoner in females than males and usually develops after the age of 50 years, not uncommonly in those over 70. There is slightly greater familial incidence (2 per cent) than could be accounted for by chance, and rarely it is bilateral. Traction upon the sensory root of the nerve, not only due to tumour but also to hydrocephalus in aqueduct stenosis (Tucker, Fleming, Taylor, and Schutz 1978) or to basilar aneurysm or compression of the nerve trunk in the posterior fossa by an ectatic vertebrobasilar arterial system (Pulsinelli and Rottenberg 1977); nonspecific inflammation of the ganglion, dental malocclusion (Carney 1967), and ischaemia have all been postulated as the cause, but this is often a disease without a specific pathology. Epidemiological risk factors (age, race, smoking, and drinking habits) have been postulated as being of significance in relation to whether the upper or lower face is involved (Rothman and Beckman 1974). Kugelberg and Lindblom (1959) suggest that the pain is due to central dysfunction in the substantia gelatinosa comparable to a disorder of the spinal cord 'gating' mechanism (p. 46).

Symptoms

Typical of trigeminal neuralgia are brief, lancinating paroxysms of pain, which are usually for a long time confined to the distribution of one division of the nerve. When confined to the area of supply of a single division, the condition may be called supraorbital, infraorbital or mandibular neuralgia respectively. The second and third divisions are the site with approximately equal frequency. The first division is affected less often and sometimes only after the second division has been involved. Whether the pain begins in the second or third division, it usually spreads later to the other of the two lower divisions. In a few cases it is bilateral, though rarely from the onset. By definition, there is freedom from pain between paroxysms, though a slight background ache is occasionally present; the pain is confined to the cutaneous distribution of the trigeminal nerve, does not cross the midline, and is precipitated by more than one 'trigger' (see below).

In an attack the pain is usually most intense in, and may be confined to, part of the region supplied by the affected division. Thus it may be most marked in the forehead, cheek, the upper or lower jaw, or the tongue. It tends to spread, however, through the rest of the divisional area. It is usually described as stabbing (like a 'red-hot needle'). A striking feature is that the attacks tend to be precipitated by chill, by touching the face, as in washing or shaving, by talking, mastication, and swallowing. Many patients describe 'trigger zones', touching of which invariably excites an attack. The attacks are always brief and do not last longer than one or two minutes. The pain is very severe and the patient may be in agony. The pain often evokes reflex spasm of the facial muscles on the affected side, hence the term 'tic douloureux'. Flushing of the skin, lacrimation, and salivation may also occur.

In trigeminal neuralgia there is usually no reduction of sensibility but minimal blunting of touch or a diminished corneal reflex is rarely found. The attacks may interfere with eating, and the recurrence of severe pain over a long period may cause loss of weight, depression, and even suicide. Fortunately the attacks usually cease at night, though they sometimes awaken the patient from sleep. Long remissions of pain, lasting weeks or months, are the rule in the early stages.

Diagnosis

There is usually little difficulty in diagnosis if attention is paid to the cardinal symptoms, especially the paroxysmal attacks with intervening freedom from pain, the factors which precipitate them, and the absence of signs of an organic lesion. In the rare cases in which this syndrome is associated with organic disease, for example, multiple sclerosis or posterior fossa tumour, other signs of these disorders are usually present. Electrophysiological measurement of the latency of the blink and jaw reflexes combined with electromyography of the masseter has proved helpful in distinguishing idiopathic from symptomatic cases (de Visser and Goor 1974). The measurement of somatosensory evoked potentials following trigeminal nerve stimulation may also be of value in detecting those cases in which the nerve is being compressed by ectatic blood vessels and who may therefore benefit from operative decompression of the nerve trunk in the posterior fossa (Stöhr, Petruch, and Scheglmann 1981). Trigeminal neuralgia must also be distinguished from the pain due to compression by a tumour or aneurysm. In such cases the pain is more persistent and

is usually associated with impairment of sensibility in the distribution of the nerve; weakness of the muscles supplied by the motor root is often present. Trigeminal pain may follow central lesions, for example, lateral medullary infarction or syringobulbia. In such cases, however, other signs of a brainstem lesion are present. Post-herpetic trigeminal pain is distinguished by the history of zoster with the characteristic residual cutaneous scars, by the constant pain, and by the impairment of sensibility. Tabes dorsalis is an occasional cause of paroxysmal facial pain. The characteristic signs of tabes, however, render the diagnosis easy. Attacks of similar neuralgic pain confined to the distribution of the supraorbital and infraorbital nerves sometimes occur and are often similar in aetiology to the more fully developed syndrome, but are sometimes due to local irritative lesions of these nerves in or near their foramina of exit from the skull, in which case there may be local tenderness over the upper margin of the orbit or maxilla. Costen's syndrome (pain radiating into the lower jaw and temple on chewing) may resemble trigeminal neuralgia but is provoked by chewing and no other trigger; it is usually due to temporomandibular arthrosis and dental malocclusion and may be relieved by building up the bite.

Referred pain is common in the trigeminal distribution and must always be excluded. Frontal and maxillary sinusitis tend to cause pain referred to the areas of the first and second divisions respectively. In such cases there may be oedema of the tissues overlying the infected sinus and, in addition to tenderness of the supraorbital and infraorbital nerves, the bone is also tender. Radiography of the sinuses and examination of the nose may be necessary for diagnosis. Similar facial pain can result from malignant disease of the head and neck. Disease of the eye may cause severe referred pain, especially glaucoma, in which the pain is referred to the temple. Examination of the eye will reveal the cause of the trouble. The teeth are another common source. In addition to dental caries, which is easily detected, pain may be due to a peri-apical abscess or an unerupted wisdom tooth. In case of doubt, radiograms of the teeth should be taken. Pain provoked by hot or cold fluids or food is usually dental. Severe pain in the lower jaw developing on exertion is sometimes experienced in angina of effort.

Psychogenic pain in the face often leads to diagnostic difficulties. In this syndrome of so-called atypical facial neuralgia, most often seen in young and middle-aged women, the pain is dull and constant, often occurring unilaterally in the upper jaw (though it may spread to other parts of the head and neck) and there are usually associated manifestations of chronic anxiety and depression. It does not conform to the characteristics of either trigeminal neuralgia or of the pain due to any organic disease. Physical signs are absent and it does not respond to analgesic drugs. Improvement is often achieved with antidepressive and tranquillizing remedies (Feinmann, Harris, and Cawley 1984).

Migrainous neuralgia ('cluster headache') causes severe paroxysmal pain within the trigeminal distribution (p. 182), but is distinguished from trigeminal neuralgia by its periodicity, the absence of precipitating factors, and the much longer duration of each paroxysm.

Prognosis

Spontaneous recovery from trigeminal neuralgia is rare. The interval between the bouts of pain may be long, remissions lasting months or even years. As a rule, however, once the disorder is established attacks follow each other fairly frequently and the intervals between them become shorter. Trigeminal neuralgia caused by multiple sclerosis may cease spontaneously.

Treatment

The most effective drug is carbamazepine (*Tegretol*) in doses of 100–200 mg three or four times daily depending upon tolerance (Blom 1962; Campbell, Graham, and Zilkhal 1966; Killian and

Fromm 1968). This drug, an anticonvulsant, is effective in most cases, but causes dizziness and nausea in some, while in others skin rashes and leucopenia develop and occasionally necessitate withdrawal. Often after a few weeks or months of treatment the drug can be withdrawn but must be reintroduced when the pain recurs. Baclofen has been shown to be an effective alternative in a daily dose of 30–80 mg (Fromm, Terrence, and Chattha 1984).

For patients who do not respond or who are intolerant of carbamazepine, injection or surgical treatment may be required. When pain is limited to the distribution of the supraorbital or infraorbital nerves, alcohol or phenol injection or surgical division of these nerves sometimes gives relief for months or years. Pain corresponding to the distribution of the third division, too, is occasionally relieved by providing improved dentures or by injecting the inferior dental nerve. If these relatively minor measures fail, then it is necessary to consider alcohol or phenol injection of the Gasserian ganglion (Harris 1937, 1938) or surgical division of the sensory root intracranially. Radiofrequency thermocoagulation of the Gasserian ganglion and its posterior rootlets has also been used successfully (Sengupta and Stunden 1977) (see *British Medical Journal* 1977). Osmolytic neurolysis, performed by injecting hypertonic saline into the cisterna magna, has been used for the treatment of intractable facial pain in facial carcinoma (Hitchcock 1969); its mode of action is uncertain. Surgical treatment is usually preferred to injection in younger patients, first because pain may return after injection in 1–3 years and secondly because with injection in the hands of the inexperienced it may be difficult to spare the cornea. Hence many workers reserve injection of the ganglion for use in the elderly, though the method using radiological control devised by Penman (1949, 1950), though time-consuming, was shown to be very effective and gave long-lasting relief in experienced hands. The surgical operation usually employed has been partial extradural division of the sensory root, approached via the middle fossa; care can be taken, when appropriate, to spare corneal fibres. Many surgeons now prefer an approach via the posterior fossa; the operation is more hazardous; however this method is much preferred if there is any reason to consider that the sensory root is being compressed by an aberrant vessel (Stöhr *et al.* 1981). In such cases, ligation or displacement of the artery may alone be effective, there being no need to divide the trigeminal root. Division of the spinal tract of the nerve in the medulla (Sjöqvist 1937) is now outmoded. An occasional troublesome sequel of partial division of the root is dull aching pain in the anaesthetic area (anaesthesia dolorosa) but in most cases the operation is successful and relief permanent. It is, however, important to warn the patient in advance that the affected side of the face will be permanently numb; before the operation is performed it is important to be sure that the pain is severe enough to justify this inevitable consequence.

Trigeminal neuropathy

This term was used by Spillane and Wells (1959) to describe a disorder characterized by 'persistent sensory disturbance of the face, usually numbness in the territory of one or more divisions of the trigeminus'. Pain may occur, and sometimes trophic ulceration of the nose. Hughes (1958) found at operation on similar cases evidence of a chronic inflammatory process causing atrophy of the sensory root and Ashworth and Tait (1971) described persistent unilateral facial sensory loss in cases of progressive systemic sclerosis and systemic lupus erythematosus. At autopsy one patient was found to have amyloid-like deposits in the trigeminal root (Spillane and Urich 1976). A similar picture in Sjögren's syndrome (keratoconjunctivitis sicca) has been described (Kaltreider and Talal, Harris, and Kennett 1969), but Blau, Harris, and Kennett (1969) have shown that many such cases remain unexplained and run a benign course. Even so, some prove after prolonged follow-up to have lesions such as nasopharyngeal carcinoma, men-

ingioma, or intracranial metastases (*The Lancet* 1974). As already mentioned, a transient trigeminal neuropathy is sometimes seen in multiple sclerosis.

References

Ashworth, B. and Tait, G. B. W. (1971). Trigeminal neuropathy in connective tissue disease. *Neurology, Minneapolis* **21**, 609.

Blau, J. N., Harris, M., and Kennett, S. (1969). Trigeminal sensory neuropathy. *New Engl. J. Med.* **281**, 873.

Blom, S. (1962). Trigeminal neuralgia; its treatment with a new anticonvulsant drug (G32883). *Lancet* **ii**, 839.

British Medical Journal (1977). Surgical treatment of trigeminal neuralgia. *Brit. med. J.* **2**, 718.

Brodal, A. (1981). *Neurological anatomy in relation to clinical medicine*, 3rd edn. Oxford University Press, Oxford.

Campbell, F. G., Graham, T. G., and Zilkha, K. J. (1966). Clinical trial of carbamazepine (Tegretol) in trigeminal neuralgia. *J. Neurol. Neurosurg. Psychiat* **29**, 265.

Carney, L. R. (1967). Considerations of the cause and treatment of trigeminal neuralgia. *Neurology, Minneapolis* **17**, 1143.

Dandy, W. E. (1929). An operation for the cure of tic douloureux. *Arch. Surg.* **18**, 687.

Denny-Brown, D. and Yanagisawa, N. (1973). The function of the descending root of the fifth nerve. *Brain* **96**, 783.

de Visser, B. W. O. and Goor, C. (1974). Electromyographic and reflex study in idiopathic and symptomatic trigeminal neuralgias: latency of the jaw and blink reflexes. *J. Neurol. Neurosurg. Psychiat* **37**, 1225.

Feinmann, C., Harris, M., and Cawley, R. (1984). Psychogenic facial pain: presentation and treatment. *Br. med. J.* **i**, 436.

Fromm, G. H., Terrence, C. F., and Chattha, A. S. (1984). Baclofen in the treatment of trigeminal neuralgia: double-blind study and long-term follow-up. *Ann. neurol.* **15**, 240.

Goldstein, N. P., Gibilisco, J. A., and Rushton, J. G. (1963). Trigeminal neuropathy and neuritis. *J. Am. med. Ass.* **184**, 458.

Hamby, W. B. (1947). Trigeminal neuralgia due to contralateral tumours of the posterior fossa. Report of 2 cases. *J. Neurosurg.* **4**, 179.

Harris, W. (1937). *The facial neuralgias*. Oxford University Press, London.

—— (1938). Alcohol injection in inoperable malignant growths of the jaws and tongue. *Br. med. J.* **2**, 831.

Hitchcock, E. (1969). Osmolytic neurolysis for intractable facial pain. *Lancet* **i**, 434.

Hughes, B. (1958). Chronic benign trigeminal paresis. *Proc. R. Soc. Med.* **51**, 529.

Jefferson, G. (1931). Surgical treatment of trigeminal neuralgia. *Br. med. J.* **2**, 309.

Kaltreider, H. B. and Talal, N. (1969). The neuropathy of Sjögren's syndrome: trigeminal nerve involvement. *Ann. intern. Med.* **70**, 751.

Killian, J. M. and Fromm, G. H. (1968). Carbamazepine in the treatment of neuralgia: use and side effects. *Arch. Neurol., Chicago* **19**, 129.

Kugelberg, E. and Lindblom, U. (1959). The mechanism of the pain in trigeminal neuralgia. *J. Neurol. Neurosurg. Psychiat.* **22**, 36.

The Lancet (1974). Trigeminal neuropathy. *Lancet* **i**, 1326.

The Lancet (1984). Management of trigeminal neuralgia. *Lancet* **i**, 662.

O'Connell, J. E. A. (1978). Trigeminal false localizing signs and their causation. *Brain* **101**, 119.

Penman, J. (1949). A simple radiological aid to Gasserian injection. *Lancet* **ii**, 268.

—— (1950). The differential diagnosis and treatment of tic douloureux. *Postgrad. med. J.*, **26**, 627.

—— (1968). Trigeminal neuralgia. In *Handbook of clinical neurology* (ed. P. J. Vinken and G. W. Bruyn) Vol. 5, Chapter 28. North-Holland, Amsterdam.

—— and Smith, M. C. (1950). Degeneration of the primary and secondary sensory nerves after trigeminal injection. *J. Neurol. Neurosurg. Psychiat* **13**, 36.

Pulsinelli, W. A. and Rottenberg, D. A. (1977). Painful tic convulsif. *J. Neurol. Neurosurg. Psychiat.* **40**, 192.

Ross, R. T. (1972). Corneal reflex in hemisphere disease. *J. Neurol. Neurosurg. Psychiat* **35**, 877.

Rothman, K. J. and Beckman, T. M. (1974). Epidemiological evidence for two types of trigeminal neuralgia. *Lancet* **i**, 7.

Sengupta, R. P. and Stunden, R. J. (1977). Radiofrequency thermocoagulation of Gasserian ganglion and its rootlets for trigeminal neuralgia. *Br. med. J.* **1**, 142.

Sjöqvist, O. (1937). Eine neue Operationsmethode bei Trigeminusneural-gie: Durchschneidung des Tractus spinalis trigemini. *Zbl. Neurochir.* **i–ii**, 274.

Smyth, G. E. (1939). The systematization and central connections of the spinal tract and nucleus of the trigeminal nerve. *Brain* **62**, 41.

Spillane, J. D. and Urich, H. (1976). Trigeminal neuropathy with nasal ulceration: report of two cases and one necropsy, *J. Neurol. Neurosurg. Psychiat.* **39**, 105.

—— and Wells, C. E. C. (1959). Isolated trigeminal neuropathy. *Brain* **82**, 391.

Stöhr, M., Petruch, F., and Scheglmann, K. (1981). Somatosensory evoked potentials following trigeminal nerve stimulation in trigeminal neuralgia. *Ann. Neurol.* **9**, 63.

Tucker, W. S., Fleming, R., Taylor, F. A., and Schutz, H. (1978). Trige-minal neuralgia in aqueduct stenosis. *Can. J. Neurol. Sci.* **5**, 331.

The seventh or facial nerve

Origin, course, and distribution

The seventh cranial nerve consists largely of motor fibres, though it has a sensory root (the nervus intermedius) which contains a small number of sensory fibres from the external acoustic meatus, fibres which excite salivary secretion, and others which convey taste impulses from the anterior two-thirds of the tongue. The motor nucleus is situated in the ventral part of the pontine teg-mentum. The fibres arising from this nucleus pass backwards in the pons almost as far as the floor of the fourth ventricle, where they loop around the nucleus of the sixth nerve before turning for-wards to emerge from the lateral aspect of the lower border of the pons, on the medial side of the eighth nerve, from which the seventh is separated by the nervus intermedius (Fig. 2.11). The three nerves then pass together from the pons to the internal acoustic meatus. Within the petrous temporal bone the facial nerve traverses the aqueductus Fallopii or facial canal. After pass-ing outwards it turns sharply backwards on the medial side of the middle ear and then downwards behind it to emerge from the skull at the stylomastoid foramen. At the backward turn of the nerve it expands in the geniculate ganglion which receives the nervus inter-medius and which contains the ganglion cells of the taste fibres of the chorda tympani. It sends branches to the pterygopalatine and otic ganglia, carrying fibres which excite salivary secretion. Within the facial canal the nerve gives off a nerve to the stapedius muscle, and the chorda tympani nerve which carries gustatory fibres from the anterior two-thirds of the tongue. The chorda tympani crosses the tympanic cavity and emerges from the skull by the anterior canaliculus of the chorda tympani; it unites with the lingual nerve, a branch of the mandibular, beneath the lateral pterygoid muscle. The facial nerve after leaving the stylomastoid foramen gives branches to the stylohyoid muscle, the posterior belly of the digas-tric, and the occipital belly of the occipitofrontalis, and then turns forwards to divide within the parotid gland into a number of branches which innervate the muscles of expression, including the buccinator and platysma.

Facial reflexes

The reflexes mediated by the facial nerve include the *naso-lacri-mal reflex* (secretion of tears produced by stimulation of the nasal mucosa, with the afferent pathway via the trigeminus and the efferent via the greater petrosal), the *corneal reflex* (p. 48), the *stapedius reflex* (reflex contraction of stapedius with consequential reduction of transmission of sound stimuli via the stapes evoked by loud noise), and the *nasomental reflex* in which tapping the side

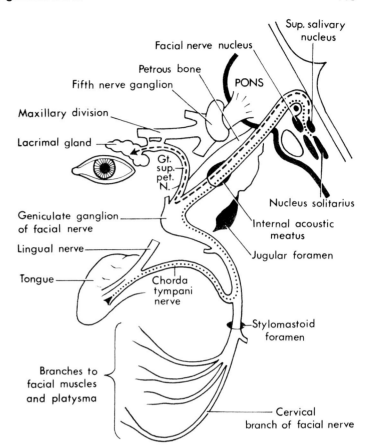

Fig. 2.11. The facial nerve. Lesions involving the facial-nerve trunk above the geniculate ganglion will cause loss of lacrimation (greater petrosal nerve), and loss of taste in the anterior two-thirds of the tongue (chorda tympani nerve), as well as paralysis of both upper and lower facial muscles.

Lesions between the geniculate ganglion and the point where the chorda tympani nerve leaves the facial nerve (6 mm above the stylomastoid fora-men), will cause loss of taste sensation in the anterior two-thirds of the tongue, as well as paralysis of the facial muscles, but lacrimation will still be present.

Lesions below the point where the chorda tympani nerve leaves the facial nerve will cause paralysis of the facial muscles, but both taste and lacrimation will be present. (Redrawn from an original drawing by Mr. Charles Keogh)

of the nose causes elevation of the upper lip and angle of the mouth (see Diamond and Frew 1979). The most important is the *blink reflex* (contraction of the palpebral orbicularis oculi evoked by tactile, visual, or acoustic stimuli). This reflex is the basis of the *glabellar tap sign* (p. 49 and p. 327). Tapping the forehead above the bridge of the nose evokes two contractions of both orbicularis oculi, one a transient contraction which can be recorded electri-cally but is invisible to the observer's eye as a rule and which is monosynaptic, the second a visible contraction of longer latency which is clearly polysynaptic. It is the latter component which habituates after repeated tapping in adults and older but not young children (Zametkin, Stevens, and Pittman 1979), suggest-ing that habituation reflects the maturity and integrity of dopami-nergic circuits in the brain. It is this late component which fails to habituate in parkinsonism so that blinking continues in time with the taps. The late component may be absent in coma (Lyon, Kimura, and McCormick 1972) but absence of both the early and the late components usually indicates a structural pontine lesion and is certainly seen in brain death (Mehta and Seshia 1976).

Facial paralysis

Facial paralysis may be due to:

1. A supranuclear lesion involving the corticospinal fibres concerned in voluntary facial movement.

2. A supranuclear lesion involving the fibres concerned in emotional movement of the face—mimic paralysis.

3. Nuclear and infranuclear lesions involving the lower motor neurones.

4. Primary degeneration or disorder of function of the facial muscles.

1. *Facial paralysis due to a supranuclear corticospinal lesion* is distinguished by the fact that movements of the lower face are affected more severely than those of the upper. There are no electrophysiological signs of denervation in the facial muscles.

2. Since there appears to be a pathway controlling emotional movement as distinct from voluntary movement of the opposite side of the face which originates in the frontal lobe and follows a different route from the corticospinal tract, a lesion of the latter tract above the internal capsule may paralyse voluntary movement of the lower face on the opposite side, leaving emotional movement, as in spontaneous smiling, intact. Very rarely a frontal or thalamic lesion may abolish contralateral emotional movement leaving voluntary movement unimpaired (*mimic paralysis*).

3. *Lesions involving the lower motor neurones* supplying the facial muscles, since they destroy the final common path, affect equally all forms of facial movement, and as a rule the upper and lower facial muscles are equally weakened. The symptoms and signs of facial paralysis due to lower motor-neurone lesions are described in the section dealing with Bell's paralysis. The facial lower motor neurones may be involved by a lesion:

(*a*) within the pons;
(*b*) within the posterior fossa, between the pons and the internal acoustic meatus;
(*c*) within the temporal bone;
(*d*) after emergence from the skull.

(*a*) *Pontine lesions.* Massive lesions involving the facial nucleus or the fibres of the facial nerve inevitably affect neighbouring structures as well. Facial paralysis is usually, therefore, associated with paralysis of the lateral rectus, or of conjugate ocular deviation to the same side, and often with paralysis of the ipsilateral jaw muscles. There may also be sensory loss due to involvement of the trigeminal nucleus and of the spinothalamic tract, or signs of a corticospinal lesion in the controlateral limbs. Acute and chronic degenerative lesions of the facial nuclei are likely to involve other bulbar motor nuclei. Pontine lesions causing facial paralysis include tumours, syringobulbia, vascular lesions, poliomyelitis, multiple sclerosis, and encephalomyelitis. Bilateral facial paralysis occasionally occurs as a congenital abnormality, probably due to a failure of development of the facial nuclei, and is usually then associated with congenital ocular palsies (Moebius' syndrome).

(*b*) *Within the posterior fossa* the proximity of the facial nerve to the nervus intermedius and the eighth nerve accounts for the fact that these nerves usually suffer together. Lesions may therefore cause deafness and loss of taste in the anterior two-thirds of the tongue, as well as facial paralysis. The commonest of such lesions are acoustic neuroma and other tumours in the region of the cerebellopontine angle such as meningioma, cholesteatoma, chordoma, and tumours of the glomus jugulare. In its extracerebral course, the facial, like other cranial nerves, may be damaged by polyneuritis cranialis (p. 528), granulomatous meningitis, sarcoidosis and nasopharyngeal or metastatic carcinoma, but is less often affected by these processes than the oculomotor nerves.

(*c*) *Within the temporal bone* the facial nerve may be involved in skull fracture or be involved in infections of the middle ear and mastoid. Facial paralysis may be the direct result of spread of infection to the facial canal, or may follow surgical operations on the ear, in which case the nerve may be merely contused or actually divided or exposed to invasion by the infecting organism. Delayed facial palsy developing within one or two weeks of a closed head injury appears to be due to a conduction defect in the nerve in its canal above the stylomastoid foramen and carries a prognosis less good than that of Bell's palsy (Puvanendran, Vitharana, and Wong 1977). Slow progressive facial palsy may be caused by an epidermoid within the temporal bone, and is then associated with deafness (Jefferson and Smalley 1938). Herpes zoster of the geniculate ganglion (p. 292) usually causes facial paralysis through secondary involvement of the motor fibres of the nerve (syndrome of Ramsay Hunt). Facial paralysis caused by a lesion within the middle ear is usually associated with loss of taste in the anterior two-thirds of the tongue, due to interruption of the fibres of the chorda tympani. Inflammation of the facial nerve within the stylomastoid foramen may be one cause of Bell's palsy. (see below).

(*d*) *After leaving the skull* the fibres of the facial nerve may be involved in inflammation from suppurating glands behind the angle of the jaw or be compressed by tumours or other lesions of the parotid gland. Various inflammatory and malignant processes sometimes cause unilateral or bilateral facial palsy, probably due to involvement of the nerve within the parotid. This may occur in uveoparotid fever (Heerfordt's syndrome), which is probably a form of sarcoidosis, in infective mononucleosis and in acute leukaemia.

Melkersson's syndrome is a name given to a condition of benign course and unknown aetiology in which recurrent episodes of facial oedema and unilateral or bilateral facial palsy occur in patients with deeply furrowed tongues.

The fibres of the facial nerve may also be compressed or divided, due to trauma to the face, as by obstetric forceps during delivery.

4. *Primary dysfunction of the facial muscles* is seen in myasthenia gravis in which the retractors of the angle of the mouth suffer earlier and more severely than the elevators and depressors of the lips, in the facioscapulohumeral type of muscular dystrophy, and in dystrophia mytonica. Facial weakness is rare in polymyositis, motor-neurone disease, and other forms of spinal muscular atrophy, but involvement of the orbicularis oculi is usual in ocular myopathy.

Bell's palsy (facial paralysis)

Definition. Facial paralysis of acute onset presumed to be due to non-suppurative inflammation (of unknown aetiology) of the facial nerve within its canal above the stylmastoid foramen.

Aetiology and pathology

The usual explanation given for Bell's palsy (named after Sir Charles Bell, 1774-1842) is that it is due to acute inflammation and oedema involving the nerve within its canal. The condition may occur at any time from infancy to old age, but in one series of cases of facial palsy in childhood (Manning and Adour 1972), 38 per cent were due to identifiable causes. It appears to be most common in young adults, and males are affected more frequently than females. An epidemiological survey carried out by Leibowitz (1969) suggested that small epidemics occur, suggesting an infective aetiology, but Adour and Wingerd (1974a) found no such evidence in a series of 419 cases.

Usually no predisposing cause can be found, but not uncommonly there is a history of exposure to chill, for example, riding in a vehicle next to an open window. In other cases the paralysis follows an acute upper respiratory-tract infection. While facial paralysis (often with ipsilateral deafness, facial numbness, and vesicles in the external meatus or on the soft palate) may occur in herpes zoster (the Ramsay Hunt syndrome), this is a comparatively rare cause. McCormick (1972) suggests that herpes simplex virus may be a common cause and Jamal and al-Husaini (1983) have implicated rubella infection, while in older patients with diabetes Korczyn (1971) postulated that it might be due to ischaemia; Abramsky, Webb, Teitelbaum, and Arnon (1975) advanced immunological evidence to suggest that the condition may be due to a lymphocyte-mediated hypersensitivity phenomenon. Adour and Doty (1973) adduced electronystagmographic findings to suggest that, even in idiopathic Bell's palsy, the fifth and eighth cranial nerves may sometimes be minimally involved, suggesting a polyneuropathy involving principally the seventh nerve.

Symptoms and signs

Bell's palsy is usually unilateral, rarely bilateral. The onset is sudden and often the patient awakens to find the face paralysed. He or his friends observe that his mouth is drawn to one side. There is frequently pain at the onset in the ear, in the mastoid region, or around the angle of the jaw.

There is paralysis of the muscles of expression (Fig. 2.12). The upper and lower facial muscles are usually equally affected and voluntary, emotional, and associated movements are involved. The eyebrow droops, and the wrinkles of the brow are smoothed out. Frowning and raising the eyebrow are impossible. Owing to paralysis of the orbicularis oculi the palpebral fissure is wider on the affected side and closure of the eye is impossible. When the patient attempts to close the eye, the globe rolls upwards and slightly inwards (Bell's phenomenon). Eversion of the lower lid (ectropism) impairs the absorption of tears, which tend to overflow the lower lid. The nasolabial furrow is smoothed out and the mouth drawn over to the sound side. The patient cannot retract the angle of the mouth or purse the lips, as in whistling. Owing to paralysis of the buccinator the cheek is puffed out in respiration, and food accumulates between the teeth and the cheek. Distortion of the mouth may cause the tongue to deviate to the sound side when protruded, thus giving a false impression of a hypoglossal lesion.

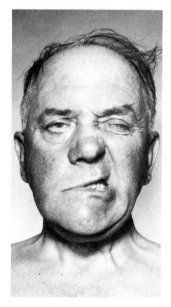

Fig. 2.12. An acute right-sided facial paralysis. The patient is trying to close his eyes and show his teeth. (Reproduced from Spillane 1975) by kind permission of the author and publisher.)

When the inflammatory process extends upwards to involve the nerve above the point at which the chorda tympani leaves it, there is loss of taste on the anterior two-thirds of the tongue, and when the branch to the stapedius is also involved the patient may complain of hyperacusis, an intensification of loud noises in the affected ear.

Diagnosis

Bell's palsy is distinguished from facial paralysis due to a pontine lesion by the presence in the latter case of signs of involvement of other pontine nuclei, especially the fifth and sixth, and sometimes of the long tracts. Lesions in the posterior fossa often involve the eighth nerve as well. A history of aural discharge and auroscopy make it easy to recognize facial paralysis secondary to otitis media. Unilateral facial palsy is sometimes an early symptom of multiple sclerosis, especially in young adults. A recurrent form associated with paroxysmal headache has been termed 'facioplegic migraine'. Electromyography and measurement of facial nerve conduction and/or excitability (see Fawcett and Barwick 1981) may assist in diagnosis but are of greater value in determining prognosis (see below).

Prognosis

More than 50 per cent of cases of Bell's palsy recover completely though this may take months (Taverner 1955). Factors associated with a poorer prognosis than average include hyperacusis, diminished lacrimation, an age greater than 60 years, diabetes mellitus, and hypertension (Adour and Wingerd 1974b; Adour, Bell, and Wingerd 1974). If at the end of three weeks from the onset there is some return of voluntary power in the face, recovery is likely to be rapid and will probably be complete in a few weeks. If within a few days after the onset electromyography shows that there are motor units under voluntary control in the facial muscles and if facial nerve conduction remains normal or only slightly slowed, then in all probability the lesion is mainly neurapraxial and recovery is likely to be rapid and complete. Measurement of minimal excitability values (MEV) in the affected nerve has proved especially useful (Devi, Challenor, Duarte, and Lovelace 1978), as has measurement of the amplitude of the maximal evoked motor response elicited by facial stimulation six or more days after the onset (Boongird and Vejjajiva 1978). If, however, paralysis is complete, if no motor units can be detected by needle electrode exploration of the facial musculature, and if within a few days the facial nerve is totally inexcitable, then the prognosis is much less good; spontaneous fibrillation potentials recorded from the muscle within two or three weeks indicate that at least some of the nerve fibres have undergone Wallerian degeneration.

In those cases in which recovery is incomplete, contracture often develops in the paralysed muscles and does much to improve the appearance of the face at rest, although the paralysis is evident when the patient smiles. When marked contracture develops, the nasolabial furrow may actually become deeper on the paralysed than on the normal side and the affected eyebrow is drawn downwards. Clonic facial spasm is an occasional sequel, but is not usually very severe. The syndrome of 'crocodile tears'—unilateral lacrimation on eating—occurs in a few cases. It is due to regenerating facial nerve fibres running from the geniculate ganglion through the greater petrosal nerve and the pterygopalatine ganglion to the lacrimal gland. Synkinetic movements due to aberrant motor regeneration can readily be assessed electrophysiologically and often an aberrant blink reflex appears on the affected side (Kimura, Rodnitzky, and Okawara 1975). Recurrent 'idiopathic' facial palsy is rare. It may occur first on one side and a year or two later on the other, and very occasionally develops simultaneously on the two sides.

Treatment

Robinson and Moss (1954) advocated the use of cortisone in the acute stage and Taverner, Cohen, and Hutchinson (1971) found that prednisone, 20 mg four times a day for 5 days followed by diminishing doses thereafter improved the prognosis and was superior to corticotrophin. In a prospective, randomized study of 259 cases, however, Wolf, Wagner, Davidson, and Forsythe (1978) found that only autonomic synkinesis was improved significantly by prednisone treatment. In their cases only 16 per cent of all the patients, whether in the treated or control groups, showed incomplete recovery which was mild in 14 percent and severe in only 2 per cent. Matthews (1982) provides a detailed review. It is sound treatment to try to prevent stretching of the paralysed muscles, which occurs when the mouth is drawn over to the sound side. Strips of adhesive strapping or transparent tape ('Sellotape' or 'Scotch Tape') applied above and below the mouth to counteract the pull of the muscles on the normal side (Pickerill and Pickerill 1945) are helpful.

Since Ballance and Duel (1932) first advocated decompression of the facial nerve in its canal, there have been many advocates of early operative treatment (Morris 1938, 1939) and more recently the operation has been recommended in cases presumed, on electrophysiological grounds, to carry a poor prognosis. However, a controlled trial (Mechelse, Goor, Huizing, Hammelburg, van Bolhuis, Staal, and Verjaal 1971) and Adour and Wingerd (1974b) have shown that the natural history of the condition is not favourably influenced by decompression in the second or third week after the onset.

After the acute stage, direct electrical stimulation of the facial muscles has had advocates but appears to predispose to the development of contracture and is not now widely used. When there is little or no recovery, facio-hypoglossal anastomosis, autografting of the facial nerve itself, and various plastic and cosmetic surgical procedures have been advocated but none is uniformly successful and most patients adjust to the residual deformity and weakness. Even after total resection of the parotid gland for malignant tumour, some facial movement may return after months or years due to misdirection into the facial nerve of regenerating axons from branches of the motor division of the trigeminus (Trojaborg and Siemssen 1972).

Clonic facial spasm (hemifacial spasm)

Definition. A disorder which occurs in both sexes but chiefly affects middle-aged or elderly women. There are frequent shock-like contractions of the facial muscles, limited to one side.

Aetiology and pathology

The condition is almost certainly the result of an irritative lesion at some point in the course of the nerve (Nielsen 1984a and b). It has been ascribed to a lesion of the geniculate ganglion or to a compressive lesion of the nerve (usually fibrosis of unknown aetiology) within its canal. Similar spasms, associated with synkinetic facial movements, may certainly develop after incomplete recovery from Bell's palsy (Auger 1979). Unquestionably in some cases the condition is due to compression of the trunk of the nerve by an aberrant artery shortly after it emerges from the brainstem but whether this accounts for the majority of cases is still uncertain (Maroon 1978).

Symptoms

Clonic facial spasm is much more common in women than in men and is rare before middle life. It usually begins in one orbicularis oculi as a fine intermittent twitching resembling the benign myokymia of the lower eyelid which occurs in normal individuals in states of fatigue and which is known as 'live flesh'. The spread of the spasm is extremely slow, but gradually the muscles of the lower face are involved, especially the retractors of the angle of the mouth. Finally strong spasms involve all the facial muscles on one side almost continuously. At this stage there is always slight weakness and wasting of the facial musculature. Taste may be lost over the anterior two-thirds of the tongue. Bilateral clonic facial spasm is less common: in such cases one side is usually affected after the other. The involuntary closure of both eyes then causes much more inconvenience. The condition may be associated with trigeminal neuralgia on the same or the opposite side.

Diagnosis

Clonic facial spasm must be distinguished from other facial involuntary movements (see below). A common movement, not truly involuntary, is tic or habit spasm, a brief compulsive movement, often bilateral, and usually seen in children and young adults. Blepharospasm, prolonged spasm of the orbicularis oculi, is usually seen in the elderly and, in this case also, the movements are bilateral and there is no twitching of lower facial muscles. However, it may be associated with choreic movements of the lips in cases of senile chorea while intermittent blepharospasm is a common 'hysterical' phenomenon and may sometimes be severe and disabling in patients of either sex with severe depression or anxiety. The involuntary movements of chorea and athetosis are also bilateral and are usually associated with similar movements in the limbs.

Prognosis

If untreated, clonic facial spasm is a slowly progressive disorder and spontaneous recovery does not occur. It may lead after many years to complete facial paralysis on the affected side, and the twitching then ceases.

Treatment

Drugs are of no lasting value although the condition is accentuated by tension and embarrassment so that chlordiazepoxide (*Librium*) in doses of 5-10 mg three times a day, or diazepam (*Valium*) 2-5 mg three times a day, are sometimes helpful. In the past the condition was sometimes treated by injection of the affected facial nerve behind the angle of the jaw with local anaesthetic, alcohol, or phenol, but the results were variable. Surgical decompression of the nerve in its canal also had its advocates but was rarely successful. More recently it has been shown that excellent results are achieved in many cases by exploration of the posterior fossa with decompression of the nerve trunk where it is being compressed by an aberrant artery (Maroon 1978; Fabinyi and Adams 1978; Kaye and Adams 1981; Fairholm, Wu, and Liu 1983).

Facial myokymia and other involuntary movements

Several other involuntary movements which may affect the face were mentioned above under the diagnosis of clonic facial spasm. Tardive dyskinesia (orofacial dyskinesia), which may result from phenothiazine administration, is described later under disorders of the basal ganglia, as are the facial movements of chorea; focal epilepsy (epilepsia partialis continua) can also involve the face (see *British Medical Journal* 1975). One unusual form of involuntary movement is *facial myokymia*, an irregular writhing or rippling movement occurring continuously, and usually only on one side of the face. It is most often a transient manifestation of multiple sclerosis (Matthews 1966) but is occasionally seen in polyneuropathy when it may be bilateral (Daube, Kelly, and Martin 1979); when it occurs in the Guillain–Barré syndrome (Wasserstrom and Starr 1977), limb myokymia (p. 557) may also be seen. In one case examined pathologically (Waybright, Gutmann, and Chou 1979), there was astroglial proliferation in the ipsilateral seventh-nerve nucleus with gliomatous change rostral to the nucleus suggesting that the latter was functionally deafferented.

References

Abramsky, O, Webb, C., Teitelbaum, D., and Arnon, R. (1975). Cellular immune response to peripheral nerve basic protein in idiopathic facial paralysis (Bell's palsy). *J. neurol. Sci.* **26**, 13.

Adour, K. K., Bell, D. N., and Wingerd, J. (1974). Bell palsy: dilemma of diabetes mellitus. *Arch. Otolaryngol.* **99**, 114.

—— and Doty, H. E. (1973). Electronystagmographic comparison of acute idiopathic and herpes zoster facial paralysis. *The Laryngoscope* **83**, 2029.

—— and Wingerd, J. (1974). Nonepidemic incidence of idiopathic facial paralysis: seasonal distribution of 419 cases in three years. *J. Am. med. Ass.* **227**, 653.

—— and —— (1974b). Idiopathic facial paralysis (Bell's palsy): factors affecting severity and outcome in 446 patients. *Neurology, Minneapolis* **24**, 1112.

Auger, R. G. (1979). Hemifacial spasm: clinical and electrophysiologic observations. *Neurology, Minneapolis* **29**, 1261.

Ballance, C. and Duel, A. B. (1932). Operative treatment of facial palsy by introduction of nerve grafts into fallopian canal and by other intratemporal methods. *Arch. Otolaryngol.* **15**, 1.

Boongird, P. and Vejjajiva, A. (1978). Electrophysiologic findings and prognosis in Bell's palsy. *Muscle & Nerve* **1**, 461.

British Medical Journal (1975). Involuntary facial movements. *Br. med. J.* **1**, 476.

Daube, J. R., Kelly, J. J., Jr., and Martin, R. A. (1979). Facial myokymia with polyradiculoneuropathy. *Neurology, Minneapolis* **29**, 662.

Devi, S. Challenor, Y., Duarte, N., and Lovelace, R. E. (1978). Prognostic value of minimal excitability of facial nerve in Bell's palsy. *J. Neurol. Neurosurg. Psychiat.* **41**, 649.

Diamond, C. and Frew, I. (1979). *The facial nerve.* Oxford University Press, Oxford.

Fabinyi, G. C. A. and Adams, C. B. T. (1978). Hemifacial spasm: treatment by posterior fossa surgery. *J. Neurol. Neurosurg. Psychiat.* **41**, 829.

Fairholm, D., Wu, J.-M., and Liu, K.-N. (1983). Hemifacial spasm; results of microvascular relocation. *Can. J. Neurol. Sci.* **10**, 187.

Fawcett, P. R. W. and Barwick, D. D. (1981). Studies in nerve conduction. In *Disorders of voluntary muscle*, 4th edn (ed. J. N. Walton) Chapter 27. Churchill Livingstone, Edinburgh.

Harris, W. (1926). *Neuritis and neuralgia.* Oxford University Press, London.

Jamal, G. A. and al-Husaini, A. (1983). Bell's palsy and infection with rubella virus. *J. Neurol. Neurosurg. Psychiat.* **46**, 678.

Jefferson, G. and Smalley, A. A. (1938). Progressive facial palsy produced by intratemporal epidermoids. *J. Laryng.* **53**, 417.

Kaye, A. H. and Adams, C. B. T. (1981). Hemifacial spasm; a long term follow-up of patients treated by posterior fossa surgery and facial nerve wrapping. *J. Neurol. Neurosurg. Psychiat.* **44**, 1100.

Kimura, J., Rodnitzky, R. L., and Okawara, S.-H. (1975). Electrophysiologic analysis of aberrant regeneration after facial nerve paralysis. *Neurology, Minneapolis* **25**, 989.

Korczyn, A. D. (1971). Bell's palsy and diabetes mellitus. *Lancet* **i**, 108.

Leibowitz, U. (1969). Epidemic incidence of Bell's palsy. *Brain* **92**, 109.

Lyon, L. W., Kimura, J., and McCormick, W. F. (1972). Orbicularis oculi reflex in coma: clinical, electrophysiological, and pathological correlations. *J. Neurol. Neurosurg. Psychiat.* **35**, 582.

McCormick, D. P. (1972). Herpes-simplex virus as cause of Bell's palsy. *Lancet* **i**, 937.

Manning, J. J. and Adour, K. K. (1972). Facial paralysis in children. *Pediatrics* **49**, 102.

Maroon, J. C. (1978). Hemifacial spasm: a vascular cause. *Arch. Neurol. Chicago* **35**, 481.

Matthews, W. B. (1966). Facial myokymia. *J. Neurol. Neurosurg. Psychiat.* **29**, 35.

—— (1982). Treatment of Bell's palsy. In *Recent advances in clinical neurology* (ed. W. B. Matthews and G. H. Glaser), Chapter 12, Vol. 3. Churchill-Livingstone, Edinburgh.

Mechelse, K., Goor, G., Huizing, E. H., Hammelburg, E.,van Bolhuis, A. H., Staal, A., and Verjall, A. (1971). Bell's palsy: prognostic criteria and evaluation of surgical decompression. *Lancet* **ii**, 57.

Mehta, A. J. and Seshia, S. S. (1976). Orbicularis oculi reflex in brain death. *J. Neurol. Neurosurg. Psychiat.* **39**, 784.

Morris, W. M. (1938). Surgical treatment of Bell's palsy. *Lancet* **i**, 429.

—— (1939). Surgical treatment of facial paralysis. *Lancet* **ii**, 558.

Nielsen, V. K. (1984). Pathophysiology of hemifacial spasm I and II. *Neurology, Cleveland* **34**, 418, 427.

Pickerill, H. S. and Pickerill, C. M. (1945). Early treatment of Bell's palsy. *Br. med. J.* **2**, 457.

Puvanendran, K. Vitharana, M., and Wong, P. K. (1977). Elctrodiagnostic study in delayed facial palsy after closed head injury. *J. Neurol. Neurosurg. Psychiat.* **40**, 351.

Robison, W. P. and Moss, B. F. (1954). Treatment of Bell's palsy with cortisone. *J. Am. med. Ass.* **154**, 142.

Spillane, J. D. and Spillane, J.A. (1982). *An atlas of clinical neurology* 3rd. edn. Oxford University Press, Oxford.

Taverner, D. (1955). Bell's palsy. A clinical and electromyographic study. *Brain* **78**, 209.

——, Cohen, S. B., and Hutchinson, B. C. (1971). Comparison of corticotrophin and prednisolone in treatment of idiopathic facial paralysis (Bell's palsy). *Br. med. J.*, **4**, 20.

Trojaborg, W. and Siemssen, S. O. (1972). Reinnervation after resection of the facial nerve. *Arch. Neurol. Chicago* **26**, 17.

Wasserstrom, W. R. and Starr, A. (1977). Facial myokymia in the Guillain-Barré syndrome. *Arch. Neurol. Chicago* **34**, 576.

Waybright, E. A., Gutmann, L., and Chou, S. M. (1979). Facial myokymia: pathological features. *Arch, Neurol. Chicago* **36**, 244.

Wolf, S. M. Wagner, J. H., Jr., Davidson, S., and Forsythe, A. (1978). Treatment of Bell palsy with prednisone: a prospective, randomized study. *Neurology, Minneapolis* **28**, 158.

Zametkin, A. J., Stevens, J. R., and Pittman, R. (1979). Ontogeny reflex. *Ann. Neurol.* **5**, 453.

The eighth or vestibulocochlear nerve

The eighth nerve contains two groups of fibres, those which supply the cochlea and are concerned in hearing, and those which supply the semicircular canals, the utricle and the saccule, and are concerned in postural and equilibratory functions. These two parts are described as the cochlear and vestibular nerves, respectively. They run together in the eighth nerve from the internal auditory meatus to its entry into the brainstem in the lateral aspect of the lower border of the pons, but differ in their peripheral distribution and their central connections. The eighth in its passage across the posterior fossa lies lateral to the seventh nerve, from which it is separated by the nervus intermedius.

Hearing

General considerations

While light (electromagnetic) waves can travel in a vacuum, sound waves are mechanically induced by vibrations which spread as pressure waves throughout the surrounding medium whether this is gaseous, liquid, or solid and are perceived by the ear, a specialized mechanoreceptor. Vibrations so recorded are modified in the conduction system (external auditory canal, tympanic membrane, ossicular system, and cochlear perilymph and endolymph) before reaching the auditory receptors, the hair cells of the organ of Corti, which are exquisitely sensitive, being responsive (at frequencies of maximum sensitivity—1000–2000 Hz) to displacements of as little as 10^{-10} cm.

However, the conduction system transmits some frequencies more efficiently than others. *Sound waves* travel in air with a velocity of 344 m/s at 20 °C. A simple sinusoidal wave gives rise to a *pure tone* (white noise) and its frequency (in Hz) determines its *pitch*, which is higher the greater the frequency; similarly there is a correlation between amplitude and loudness. Musical sounds produce *complex tones* consisting of a basic pure tone admixed with various harmonics which confer *quality* or *timbre* upon the sound, enabling one to recognize the distinctive sounds made by different instruments playing the same note. In addition, human experience is full of sounds of complex waveform which are disorganized and nonperiodic, simply called noises.

The *intensity* of sound, which is closely correlated with, but not identical to, *loudness* (a term which has psychological as well as physical connotations) is measured on a logarithmic scale in units known as bels (B) but for convenience the decibel (dB) is much more often used. Ten dB implies a 10-fold, 20dB a 100-fold increase in intensity.

Structure and function

Structure

The outer, middle, and internal ear are illustrated in Fig. 2.13. Sound passing via the *pinna* or *auricle* into the *external auditory canal* impinges on the tympanic membrane which transmits vibrations into the middle ear. The chain of *auditory ossicles* (malleus, incus, and stapes) in turn transmit the sound vibrations across the middle-ear cavity to the oval window of the cochlea where they are conveyed to the cochlear endolymph. This process is affected by the *tensor tympani muscle* (innervated by a branch from the motor trigeminus) which, being attached to the malleus and tympanic membrane, tenses the latter, and by the *stapedius* which joins the posterior wall of the middle ear to the head of the stapes; innervated by the facial nerve, this muscle can rock the stapes out of the oval window. The two muscles together increase tension in the ossicular chain, reducing energy transmission, and subserve a reflex protective function by protecting the ear against sound of exceptional intensity. In Bell's palsy, hyperacusis may be noted as the result of paralysis of the stapedius.

The structure of the inner ear is exceptionally complex (Figs. 2.14–2.16). The *bony labyrinth* contains fluid (*perilymph*) within which is the *membranous labyrinth* filled with *endolymph*.

The *organ of Corti*, the final cochlear sensory receptor organ, lies on the dorsal surface of the basilar membrane. The *rods or pillars of Corti* form a triangular arch enclosing the tunnel of Corti flanked by columns consisting of phalangeal (Deiters') cells and inner and outer *hair cells*. Projections from the phalangeal cells extend upwards between the hair cells and fuse to form the *reticular lamina or articular plate* (the roof of the organ), but even above this is a stiff, fibro-gelatinous plate (the *tectorial membrane*) which is hinged medially at the modiolar ridge. The sterocilia of the hair cells are attached to the undersurface of this membrane and therefore bend to and fro as the basilar membrane vibrates. *Soft columnar cells of Hensen and Claudius* cover the basilar membrane on either side of the hair cells. Up to 80 hairs or *sterocilia*, each about 1 μm in diameter, join the tips of each hair cell to the tectorial membrane; to-and-fro movement of these hairs generates potentials stimulating the cells of the *spiral ganglion*, which are the primary auditory neurones. Two types of nerve terminals can be identified in the base of the hair cells, clear endings which are afferent and convey the auditory impulse into the spiral ganglion, and granular terminals which are efferent, originating in the superior olivary nucleus and subserving the function of depressing hair-cell excitability.

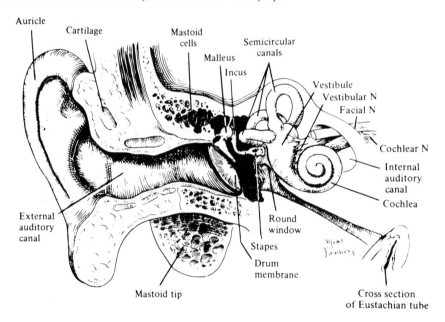

Fig. 2.13. The peripheral auditory apparatus. The cochlea is turned slightly to show its coils. The Eustachian tube runs forward as well as downward and inward. (Reproduced from Patton *et al.* (1976) and previously published in Davis and Silverman (1970), by kind permission of the authors and publishers.)

The three parts of the labyrinth are the *semicircular canals* (containing the *semicircular ducts*), the *vestibule* (containing the *utricle* and *saccule*), and the *cochlea* (containing the *cochlear duct* or *scala media*). Of these, the former two parts are concerned with balance and equilibrium (see below), the cochlear portion solely with hearing. The cochlea makes two and a half turns around its central pillar or *modiolus*, from which a bony shelf projects into the canal. Attached to the free edge of this shelf is the *basilar membrane*, joined to the lateral wall of the spiral ligament; below this membrane is the *scala tympani* filled with perilymph, above it the cochlear duct containing endolymph. *Reissner's membrane*, the delicate upper wall of the cochlear duct, separates its endolymph from the perilymph of the *scala vestibuli* which is continuous with that of the vestibule. The columnar cells which line the lateral wall of the cochlear duct form the *stria vascularis*; their activity controls the composition of the endolymph. At the apex of the cochlea, the scala tympani and scala vestibuli communicate through a tiny opening, the *helicotrema*; the scala tympani ends below at the round window, closed by a membrane separating it from the middle ear.

Function

Conduction. The external auditory canal acts like an organ pipe in adding resonance to sound entering it. The ossicular system, through a rocking action which gives a piston-like effect to the stapes in the oval window, effectively transmits pressure waves from a gaseous medium, through oscillation of the tympanic membrane, to a liquid medium (perilymph). These combined properties determine that sensitivity is most acute in the middle range of frequencies which predominate in human speech (400–3000 Hz). Air conduction can also occur through the round window, and the perilymph can also be made to vibrate by oscillations conducted through the bony skull (bone conduction). Bone conduction is much less sensitive than air conduction, a fact made use of in tuning fork tests; this function is utilized in various hearing aids.

Once oscillations conveyed to the oval window have induced pressure waves in the scala vestibuli perilymph, these, acting through Reissner's membrane, impinge on the basilar membrane, causing a shearing displacement of the hair-cell sterocilia. At the same time, pressure alters in the scala tympani perilymph with consequent bulging of the round window in and out of the middle ear. Outward movement of the stapes causes the organ of Corti to move upward and the hairs to bend laterally with consequent neuronal discharge which is then turned off by movement in the opposite direction.

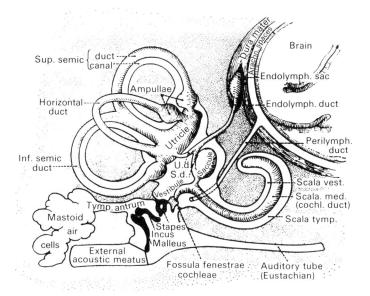

Fig. 2.14. The relationship of the osseous and membranous labyrinths. The former is filled with perilymph and at the vestibule communicates with the subarachnoid space via the perilymphatic duct. The membranous labyrinth floats in the perilymph and contains endolymph. Only part of the coiled cochlea is shown. Note that the cochlear duct (scala media) is part of the membranous system. It ends blindly at the cochlear apex and contains endolymph. The perilymph-filled scala vestibula communicates with the vestibule and, through the helicotrema, with the scala tympani, which ends at the round window. (Reproduced from Patton *et al.* (1976) and previously published in Bast and Anson (1949), by kind permission of the authors and publishers.)

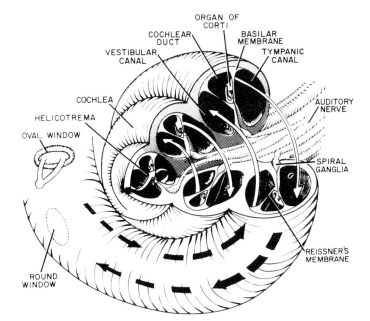

Fig. 2.15. The cochlea and the organ of Corti. Diagram of cochlea cut through to show the partition of the cavity by the basilar membrane and cochlear duct (scala media). Arrows show the pathway of transmission of pressure waves originating at the oval window. (Reproduced from Patton *et al.* (1976) and previously published in Curtis, Jacobson, and Marcus (1972), by kind permission of the authors and publishers.)

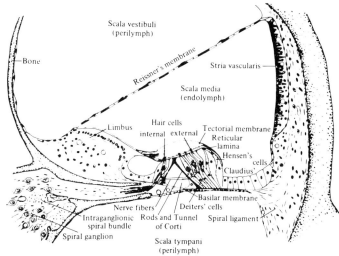

Fig. 2.16. The cochlear partition and the organ of Corti. (Reproduced from Patton *et al.* (1976) and previously published in Davis and Silverman (1970), by kind permission of the authors and publishers.)

Cochlear mechanisms. The auditory nerve fibres derived from the hair cells, because of their refractory period, have an upper frequency response of 1000 Hz, whereas the upper limit of the range of auditory perception and discrimination is about 20000 Hz. This discrepancy was explained by Helmholtz in the *place theory* of pitch perception, which concluded that the basilar membrane is differentially tuned at different points, thus allowing its different parts to respond to pressure waves of varying frequency. Subsequently, Békèsy showed that such waves in the perilymph produce propagated waves in the basilar membrane proceeding from the base towards the apex of the cochlea and that the amplitude of these waves at different points varied with the frequency of the sound wave. High-frequency waves reach maximal amplitude in the basal portion and die out before reaching the apex, while low frequencies produce minimal displacement at the base and much more towards the apex. Thus each frequency in the audible range has a point of maximal displacement of the membrane at which the relevant hair cells produce maximal rates of action potential discharge through which the pitch of the sound is recognized.

In 1930 Wever and Bray, while attempting to record electrical potentials from cat auditory nerve, recorded changes in potential closely analogous to the pure-tone sound-wave stimulus which they applied. Subsequently, it was shown that such potentials are *cochlear microphonics*, i.e. non-propagated hair-cell potentials generated by movement of the organ of Corti; these are best recorded from the round window but in man they can be picked up by electrodes applied behind the pinna above the mastoid process. Their amplitude is proportional to the intensity of the sound and gives an accurate indication of hair cell displacement. A positive *endocochlear potential* of about 80 mV is also generated by the cells of the stria vascularis, representing the potential difference between the endolymph and perilymph. This endocochlear potential combined with the *membrane potential* of the hair cells together produce a current which passes through the scala media and ultimately leaves the base of the hair cell to release a transmitter (as yet unidentified) which excites afferent neuronal endings. Movement of the membrane and consequently of the sterocilia of the hair cells causes variations in this leakage current which are responsible for the cochlear microphonic, the receptor potential of the ear.

The auditory nerve. The central processes of bipolar cells in the spiral ganglion form the cochlear nerve; the distal processes emerge and lose their myelin sheaths medial to the inner pillar of the organ of Corti. About 95 per cent of them innervate the inner hair cells, 20 fibres to a cell, while the remaining 5 per cent each innervate about 10 outer hair cells. Microelectrode recording from single afferent neurones in the auditory nerve has shown that most show random spontaneous resting discharges (about 100 spikes per second) even during absolute silence; these may be due to the leakage current from the hair cells mentioned above. When pure tones are applied to the ear, single fibres derived from different parts of Corti's organ each respond to a specific band of frequencies; it is assumed that the different tuning curves which can be plotted for each fibre indicate that they supply different groups of hair cells at various points on the basilar membrane.

Most of the granular, vesicular-containing efferent nerve endings are the terminals of neurones in the contralateral superior olivary nucleus in the brainstem; their fibres traverse the auditory nerve and spiral ganglion without synapsing to terminate either on the base of inner hair cells alongside afferent terminals or else on afferent fibres which innervate the outer cells. In addition, 20–25 per cent of efferent fibres arise from the ipsilateral olive and are largely distributed to inner hair cells. Like afferent fibres they show tuned behaviour and respond to auditory stimuli, having a threshold of about 40 dB. Stimulation of these fibres either blocks or reduces the neural response to auditory stimuli, but the cochlear microphonic is not reduced and is sometimes increased. It thus appears that this efferent system diminishes the masking effect of background noise, thus improving the signal-to-noise ratio.

Central auditory pathways. The afferent fibres of the auditory nerve synapse with secondary auditory neurones in the cochlear nuclei which lie dorsolaterally in the medulla just below the inferior cerebellar peduncle. In each there is one dorsal and two ventral nuclei, and the projection is organized tonotopically so that high frequencies are recorded dorsally, low frequencies ventrally. Pathways projecting centrally from these nuclei are exceptionally complex (Fig. 2.17). All fibres synapse in the inferior colliculus and again in the medial geniculate body, but their pathways are diverse. The fibres of the principal crossed pathway decussate in the trapezoid body and then enter the lateral lemniscus, with or without synapsing in the superior olive, while uncrossed fibres follow a similar route without crossing the midline. Most cells of the inferior colliculus project to the ipsilateral medial geniculate body, but some cross between the inferior colliculus to reach the contralateral medial geniculate. The final common path for auditory stimuli from the cells of the medial geniculate body is to the auditory (acoustic) cortex in the superior temporal gyrus. Multiple and complex tonotopic representation of the cochlea has been demonstrated in the lateral lemniscus, superior olive, inferior colliculus, medial geniculate body, and especially in the auditory cortex. This complex organization with multiple decussations explains why clinically overt disturbances of hearing rarely result from discrete lesions of the brainstem or auditory cortex.

Tests of auditory function

Damage to hair cells of the organ of Corti causes sensorineural deafness; lesions of the auditory cause nerve deafness. Lesions of the conducting mechanism in the middle ear give conductive deafness. Various tests are available to distinguish these clinically.

Weber's test. A vibrating tuning-fork (C=256) is applied to the forehead or vertex in the midline and the patient is asked whether the sound is heard in the midline or is localized in one ear. In normal individuals the sound appears to be in the midline. In conductive deafness it is usually localized in the affected ear, in nerve deafness in the normal ear. This is because in sensorineural or nerve deafness bone-conduction is reduced as well as air-conduction, whereas in conductive deafness air-conduction is reduced but bone-conduction is relatively enhanced.

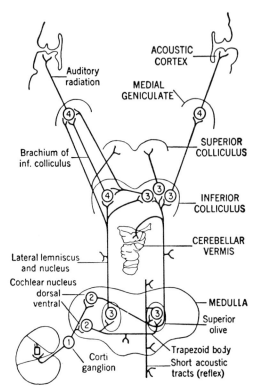

Fig. 2.17. Central auditory pathways. Numbers label first-, second-, third- and fourth-order neurones. (Reproduced from Patton *et al.* (1976) and previously published by Davis in Stevens (1951), by kind permission of the authors and publishers.)

Rinne's test. A vibrating tuning-fork is applied to the patient's mastoid process, the ear being occluded by the observer's finger. The patient is asked when he ceases to hear the sound, and the fork is then held at the acoustic meatus. In conductive deafness the sound cannot be heard by air-conduction after bone-conduction has ceased to transmit it. In sensorineural or nerve deafness, as in normal individuals, the reverse is the case. It is usual also to occlude the opposite ear during the test; even so, the results of Rinne's test may be misleading in unilateral nerve deafness when the sound of the tuning fork applied to the mastoid process of the deaf ear is heard in the opposite normal ear. A further distinction is that in sensorineural or nerve deafness loss of hearing is most marked for high-pitched tones, in conductive deafness for low-pitched tones.

Audiometry and other quantitative methods. Pure-tone audiometry, a quantitative method of testing hearing, should now be a routine procedure in all patients suspected of hearing loss. The threshold in decibels for the perception of pure tones of different frequencies is measured in each ear using both air- and bone-conduction, with the other ear masked. Characteristic patterns are then obtained for sensorineural or nerve deafness (of high and low frequencies or both), for conductive deafness and for mixed types. A 'peep-show' technique helps in the examination of young children (Dix and Hallpike 1952).

Loudness recruitment is a technique of particular value in detecting unilateral sensorineural deafness (due to cochlear end-organ disease, as in Ménière's syndrome). A pure tone of constant frequency is applied with increasing intensity (in decibels) to each ear alternately. In conductive deafness and in nerve deafness due to disease of the cochlear nerve central to the sensory end-organs, the ratio between the intensities required to produce sounds of equal loudness in both ears remains constant; in sensorineural deafness, however, with increasing intensity the sound eventually seems equally loud in both ears (Dix, Hallpike, and Hood 1948).

More refined tests have subsequently been introduced including the tone-decay test (Green 1963), Békèsy audiometry (Jerger 1960), measurement of the short increment sensitivity index (Jerger, Shedd, and Harford 1959), and speech audiometry (Johnson and House 1964; Hallpike 1976). Hood and Poole (1971) pointed out that the greatest social disability of the deaf is inability to hear and understand the spoken word; they showed that free-field speech audiometry is useful in distinguishing between conductive, cochlear, and retrocochlear hearing loss and in helping to correct cochlear deafness with hearing aids. Evoked-response audiometry, especially BAEPs (see below) has proved especially useful in detecting deafness in children (Doig 1972).

Auditory evoked potentials. The measurement of these potentials (see McCutchen and Iragui-Madoz 1979) is being used increasingly in diagnosis. When a click is delivered to the external auditory meatus, neurones in the internal ear, in the brainstem, and in the auditory and association areas of the cortex are activated sequentially and the electrical activity so generated can be recorded by means of sophisticated averaging techniques through electrodes applied over the mastoid process and vertex. At least seven components of the auditory evoked response have been identified of which five, occurring within the first 8 ms, are believed to originate from the auditory nerve and from brainstem nuclei (Stockard and Rossiter 1977). These short-latency components are known as the brainstem auditory evoked potentials (BAEP) and measurement of their interwave intervals, amplitude ratios, and responses to changing stimulus rates are being used increasingly as aids to the localization (and even identification) of brainstem lesions in adults and in children (Oh, Kuba, Soyer, Choi, Bonikowsski, and Vitek 1981; Hecox, Cone, and Blaw 1981). Intermediate-latency components occurring 8–50 ms after the stimulus and even less well-defined long-latency waves probably reflect activity in the auditory cortex and associated areas but have not proved as yet of much diagnostic value.

Lesions responsible for sensorineural and nerve deafness

The commonest causes of sensorineural deafness are Ménière's disease, damage by drugs or toxins (including streptomycin and its analogues–Cawthorne and Ranger 1957), and ageing (presbyacusis). Sudden unilateral (less often bilateral) deafness may be due to occlusion of the internal auditory artery, to virus infection (Rowson, Hincliffe, and Gamble 1975), or possibly to intracochlear membrane breaks (*The Lancet* 1977). The internal ear may also be involved in congenital syphilis, in congenital deaf-mutism, one form of which is associated with adenoma of the thyroid, and in otosclerosis. The many causes of hereditary deafness in man were reviewed by Konigsmark (1969). The vestibulocochlear nerve may be damaged within the petrous bone by spread of infection from the middle ear, by fractures of the skull, or by an intratemporal epidermoid, in both of which cases deafness may be associated with facial palsy, and it is sometimes compressed by bony hyperplasia of the internal auditory meatus in Paget's disease. In its passage across the posterior fossa the eighth nerve may be compressed by a tumour, such as an acoustic neuroma, or involved in an inflammatory lesion, e.g. meningovascular syphilis or other forms of granulomatous meningitis. Rare causes are avitaminosis, mumps, and polyneuritis cranialis, the deafness in both being bilateral. Deafness is a rare symptom of lesions within the central nervous system, though unilateral deafness may be caused by a pontine vascular lesion or tumour and by multiple sclerosis (Luxon 1980), and total bilateral deafness and loss of vestibular function may be associated with other signs of brainstem damage in head injury. Compression of the midbrain in the region of the inferior colliculi by tumours of the midbrain or pineal body may cause impairment of hearing. Clinical deafness does not result from lesions of the temporal lobe unless they are bilateral. Central deafness in childhood may be due to birth injury, perinatal anoxia, maternal rubella, or kernicterus. Cooper, Kay, Curry, Garside, and Roth (1974) showed that in elderly deaf patients there is an increased incidence of paranoid psychosis and to a lesser extent of affective illness (also see *British Medical Journal* 1977).

Tinnitus

Tinnitus is a sensation of noise caused by abnormal excitation of the acoustic apparatus or of its afferent paths or cortical areas. It may be continuous or intermittent, unilateral or bilateral. The noise may be high- or low- pitched and is variously described as hissing, whistling, or, in severe cases, as resembling that made by machinery. It may occur in time with the pulse. Apart from associated deafness, tinnitus when severe may interfere with hearing, and is most evident to the patient at night, when extraneous noises are few. Persistent tinnitus often leads to much distress in elderly people; it may be a manifestation of endogenous depression in such cases and can then be relieved by appropriate treatment. Tinnitus is often associated with conductive, sensorineural, nerve, or mixed deafness and sometimes with vertigo (Edwards 1973; Rudge 1982).

The causes of tinnitus are various. Wax in the external auditory meatus, Eustachian catarrh, and acute otitis media probably act by interfering with the conducting apparatus of the ear. The tinnitus produced by hemifacial spasm is attributed to associated spasm of the stapedius. In many cases it is probably due to ischaemia of the internal ear, and it may be produced by drugs, such as quinine, salicylates, streptomycin, and amyl nitrite, by acute labyrinthitis, arteriosclerosis, severe anaemia, aortic incompetence, and otosclerosis. Degeneration of Corti's organ is the commonest cause (*British Medical Journal* 1979). Abnormal sounds arising within the cranium may be conducted to the ear and so cause tinnitus. Thus a rhythmical bruit is sometimes heard by patients with carotico-cavernous fistula and intracranial aneurysm or arterial angioma. Irritation of the acoustic afferent paths may lead to tinnitus when the eighth nerve is compressed by tumour or involved in inflammatory processes. Tinnitus is rarely the result of a lesion of the central nervous system, but may occur in association with deafness after vascular or other lesions of the lateral pontine tegmentum. Noises heard as a result of irritative lesions of the temporal auditory cortex are usually more complex than those caused by irritation of the acoustic apparatus and its lower pathways. In this group fall auditory hallucinations comprising the aura of epileptic fits and those which sometimes occur as symptoms of temporal-lobe neoplasms or other lesions. Frazier and Rowe (1932) reported that tinnitus occurred in 25 per cent of their 51 verified cases of temporal-lobe tumour.

The treatment of tinnitus is often disappointing. Local lesions of the ear should receive appropriate treatment. Sedatives, tranquilizers, and nocturnal hypnotics have some palliative action and vasodilator drugs have been tried, usually with little benefit; when depression is severe, antidepressive drugs may be dramatically successful. There is some recent evidence that intravenous lignocaine (1–2 mg/kg, without adrenaline, well diluted, given over 3–4 min) may be helpful (Melding and Goodey 1979), as are carbamazepine (600–1000 mg daily) or phenytoin (up to 400 mg daily) (*British Medical Journal* 1979). In severe cases, in which tinnitus is intolerable, it may be justifiable to destroy the cochlea by ultrasound, but the patient must be informed that complete deafness in the ear thus treated will result and that tinnitus may persist in spite of the operation. Experimental work suggests that electrical stimulation of the cochlea may ultimately prove feasible and effective in some cases (*The Lancet* 1984).

The vestibular system

Structure and function

The vestibular portion of the eighth cranial nerve conveys impulses from the receptors of the vestibular labyrinth concerned with spatial orientation of the body into the central nervous system, where the information so derived is correlated with visual and proprioceptive inputs in order to control and modulate posture, balance and other motor activity.

Each vestibular labyrinth (Fig. 2.13–2.15) includes the three semicircular canals and the utricle and saccule, each of which contains a sensory epithelium containing receptor hair cells and supporting structures. At one end of each semicircular canal, there is a dilatation or *ampulla* containing the receptor organ or *crista ampullaris*; a gelatinous *cupula* covers the hair cells of this organ, each of which have numerous short sterocilia and a single longer kinocilium (Fig. 2.18) Movement of endolymph in the membranous labyrinth bends the cupula towards or away from the utricle; such a deflection bends the sterocilia towards the kinocilium and evokes increased discharge in afferent vestibular nerve fibres, while a deflection in the opposite direction reduces such neuronal firing. It is the extent of the angular deflection of the cupula which determines the frequency of firing in the vestibular neurones.

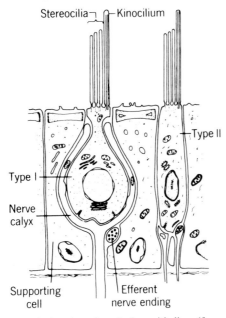

Fig. 2.18. Schematic drawing of vestibular epithelium (from electron micrographs), showing two types of hair cells. (Reproduced from Patton *et al.* (1976) and previously published in the second edn. of Brodal (1981), by kind permission of the authors and publishers.)

The three semicircular canals are arranged (Fig. 2.14) approximately at right angles to one another so that when the head is inclined 30° forwards from the erect position, the lateral canal is horizontal, a fact made use of in the caloric tests (see below). The relative position of the canals in relation to one another is such that any movement of the head in space evokes neuronal discharge which can be shown to be proportionate to the velocity of movement. The polarization of the sterocilia in relation to the kinocilia of respective groups of hair cells is such that vestibular nerve fibres derived from receptors in the horizontal canal are excited when endolymph moves towards the ampulla, whereas in the vertical canals excitation is induced by movement away from the ampulla.

In the utricle and saccule, the sensory epithelium is called the *macula*, which contains hair cells like those of the crista ampullaris but, in addition, crystals of calcium carbonate or *otoliths* lie in the gelatinous material overlying other hair cells. As these organs lie horizontally, movement of the upright head produces deflection of the hair-cell cilia but tilting of the head with the effect of gravity upon the otoliths causes deflections. Hence these organs, *static vestibular receptors* (or tonus elements), are not affected, like the semicircular canals, by velocity of head movement but by change of position of the head in relation to gravity.

The cell bodies of the vestibular neurones lie in *Scarpa's ganglion* in the internal auditory canal; most of their axons travel to the vestibular nuclei in the lateral pons and medulla, but a few pass through the nuclei without synapsing to enter the cerebellar flocculonodular lobe. There are medial, lateral (Deiters'), superior, and inferior vestibular nuclear groups which are connected with the spinal cord via the vestibulospinal tracts, with the third, fourth, and sixth cranial-nerve nuclei and proprioceptive pathways from the neck muscles via the medial longitudinal fasciculus, and with the cerebellum via the inferior cerebellar peduncle. Thus ocular deviation to the opposite side with nystagmus induced by stimulation of one horizontal semicircular canal is mediated via the medial longitudinal fasciculus as in the oculocephalic or vestibulo-ocular reflexes previously discussed.

Thus the function of the vestibular system is to assist the motor system in maintaining equilibrium by providing a continuing inflow of information into the nervous system relating to the effects of movement and of gravitational forces upon the body. If there is excessive output from the system, as after rapid rotation, or differing input from the two sides because of pathological processes, an illusion of movement or *vertigo* (see below) results. Such vertigo is nearly always accentuated by closing the eyes and lessened by opening them.

Examination of vestibular function

Tonic vestibular input on one side causes deviation of the eyes to the opposite side which is, however, quickly overcome by cerebral cortical mechanisms concerned with saccadic eye movements so that there is a rapid recoil. Thus a vestibular lesion may cause spontaneous *nystagmus* (p. 100) with a slow phase towards the opposite side and a rapid recoil. While the tonic vestibular component of the nystagmus is the slow phase, it is customary in clinical practice to describe the direction of nystagmus as being that of the quick phase, which is normally therefore *towards* the affected labyrinth. However, unlike the nystagmus which results from central brainstem lesions, that of labyrinthine origin is not altered by the direction of voluntary gaze.

In dysfunction of the semicircular canals or their peripheral neurones, the nystagmus is always accompanied by vertigo and is of limited duration because of central compensation. It nystagmus persists for more than a few weeks, it is usually due to changes in the central vestibular pathways. With central lesions subjective symptoms are less severe. Dix (1969) showed that nystagmus of peripheral origin is unidirectional and always conjugate; it is enhanced by eye closure or darkness (Korres 1978a), while central nystagmus may be multidirectional, dissociated in the two eyes, and unchanged or inhibited by eye closure (cessation of ocular fixation). The electronystagmographic recording of spontaneous nystagmus in light conditions, in darkness, and after eye closure has proved of value in the diagnosis of acoustic neuroma and of upper brainstem lesions (Korres 1978b).

Induced manifestations of vestibular dysfunction

Induced manifestations are shown by various clinical tests for vestibular function. Caloric tests and tests for positional and optokinetic nystagmus are necessary for diagnosis. Electronystagmography makes it possible to record details of the nystagmus (Hood 1977).

Caloric test. The caloric test of Fitzgerald and Hallpike is a method of demonstrating dysfunction of the canal and tonus elements of the vestibular system. The results remain remarkably constant regardless of repetition.

A moderate but effective thermal stimulus is applied to each labyrinth separately. The stimulus used is water at 7 °C below and 7 °C above body temperature. This produces equal and opposite horizontal nystagmus lasting approximately two minutes in the normal individual.

During the test the patient lies on a couch with his head raised 30 degrees from the horizontal. In this position the lateral semicircular canals are vertical, the position of maximal thermal sensitivity. The patient is asked to fix his gaze on a suitable spot throughout. Water at 30 °C is run into one ear continuously for 40 seconds, not less than 240 ml being used. In the normal subject, second-degree nystagmus away from the stimulated labyrinth occurs. The time is recorded in seconds from the beginning of irrigation to the point when nystagmus can no longer be seen with a good light at a distance of 25 cm. Irrigation at 30 °C is repeated in the other ear. Water at 44 °C is then used in each ear in turn, when the induced nystagmus is towards the irrigated side. Accuracy of temperature and duration of irrigation are essential. Experience in observing the end point and in interpreting the patterns is also necessary.

The caloric test is of great value in the diagnosis of organic lesions at all levels of the vestibular system. It may show suppression of activity on one side, canal paresis, or a directional preponderance of nystagmus, which means that nystagmus in one direction, from whichever canal it is obtained, is stronger and lasts longer than in the other direction, according to whether the canal or tonus elements of the vestibular system are affected. Combined responses showing directional preponderance and canal paresis frequently occur (Figs. 2.19–2.23).

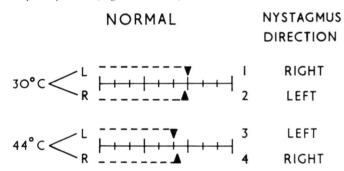

NORMAL   NYSTAGMUS DIRECTION

1 RIGHT
2 LEFT
3 LEFT
4 RIGHT

Fig. 2.19. Caloric responses: normal. (Reproduced from Fitzgerald and Hallpike (1942) by kind permission of the authors and editor.)

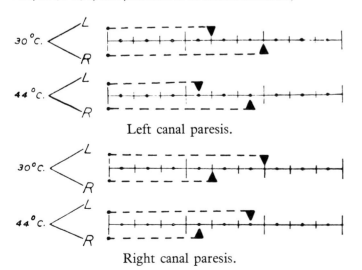

Left canal paresis.

Right canal paresis.

Fig. 2.20. Caloric responses: canal paresis. (Reproduced from Fitzgerald and Hallpike (1942) by kind permission of the authors and editor.)

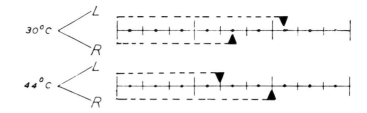

DIRECTIONAL PREPONDERANCE TO RIGHT.

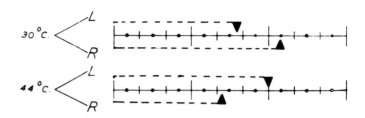

DIRECTIONAL PREPONDERANCE TO LEFT.

Fig. 2.21. Caloric responses: directional preponderance. (Reproduced from Fitzgerald and Hallpike (1942) by kind permission of the authors and editor.)

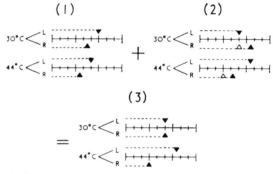

Fig. 2.22. Caloric responses: from a case of Ménière's disease of the right labyrinth. Combination of right-canal paresis (1) and directional preponderance to the left (2). (Reproduced from Hallpike (1965) by kind permission of the author and editor.)

In cerebral lesions involving the posterior temporal lobe, the cortical centre for the tonus pathway, marked directional preponderance of caloric nystagmus towards the side of the lesion is found (Carmichael, Dix, and Hallpike 1956).

In brainstem lesions, directional preponderance away from the lesion is found more often than canal paresis, which occurs when the lesion is at or above the level of the entry of the eighth nerve. Combined responses sometimes occur (Carmichael, Dix, and Hallpike 1965). Simple stimulation of one ear with a small quantity of ice-cold water is a useful rapid test of the responsiveness of pontine vestibular nuclei in comatose patients; absence of nystagmus implies a severe disturbance of brainstem function (p. 650).

In peripheral lesions the commonest abnormality is canal paresis, due to a lesion of the lateral semicircular canal or its peripheral neurones. Canal paresis is found in most patients with Ménière's disease, vestibular neuronitis, and acoustic neuroma. Combined lesions indicating a change in the utricle or its peripheral neurones as well as the lateral canal occur in 21 per cent of cases of Ménière's disease (Hallpike 1950). Directional preponderance of caloric nystagmus alone is found less often in peripheral disease. Various quantitative vestibulo-ocular test batteries involving the

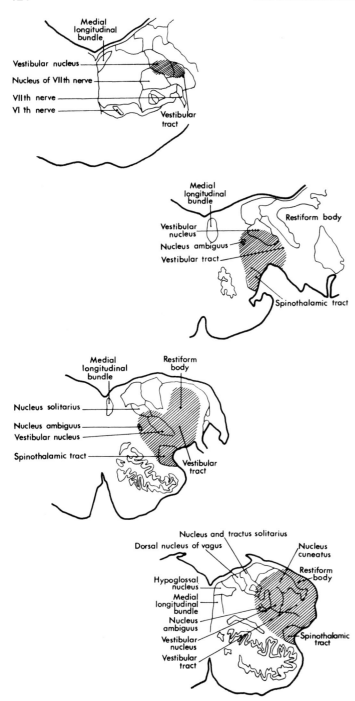

Fig. 2.23. Brainstem lesion: a case of lateral medullary syndrome with directional preponderance of the caloric responses to the left. (Reproduced from Carmichael, Dix, and Hallpike (1965) by kind permission of the authors and editor.)

recording of precise vestibular and ocular stimuli and responses such as caloric-induced nystagmus, smooth pursuit movement, optokinetic nystagmus, and rotational tests (involving sinusoidal acceleration) with digital computer analysis have been devised to improve diagnostic accuracy, especially in patients with suspected acoustic neuroma (Baloh, Konrad, Dirks, and Honrubia 1976).

Positional tests. Dix and Hallpike (1952) showed that nystagmus on sudden movement of the head in certain directions is produced by changes in the otolith organ of the utricle. The cause of this syndrome of benign positional vertigo or nystagmus (p. 126) is unknown.

Tests for otolith function cannot be confined to one ear, but there is a useful and simple test to elicit positional nystagmus (Barány's test-1921; Nylén 1939). The patient is seated on a couch. His head is held and he is briskly laid back to bring his head 30 degrees below the horizontal and rotated 30 to 40 degrees towards the observer (Fig. 2.24). In the normal subject no nystagmus or vertigo occur. In benign positional nystagmus, after a short, characteristic latent period, severe vertigo and rotary nystagmus towards the lowermost ear (the affected one) occur and last for several seconds. If the critical position is maintained, the nystagmus and vertigo gradually stop (Harrison and Ozahinoglu 1972). On returning to a sitting position a similar, though less severe, episode occurs. If the test is then repeated the phenomenon may not be seen, as adaptation occurs rapidly.

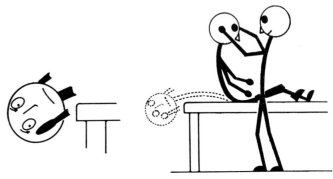

Fig. 2.24. The method of eliciting positional nystagmus. (Reproduced from Hallpike (1955) by kind permission of the author and editor.)

Positional nystagmus is sometimes seen in posterior fossa lesions and especially in patients with ependymomas or metastases (Cawthorne and Hinchcliffe 1961) in the fourth ventricle or in others with brainstem lesions of multiple sclerosis. In contrast to those with the benign syndrome, in these individuals nystagmus develops with a latent period, neither adapts nor fatigues, and is variable in direction depending upon how the head is moved; there is less severe subjective vertigo or even none at all (Dix 1969).

References

Baloh, R. W., Konrad, H. R., Dirks, D., and Honrubia, V. (1976). Cerebellar-pontine angle tumors: results of quantitative vestibulo-ocular testing. *Arch. Neurol., Chicago* **33**, 507.

Barany, R. (1921). Diagnose von Krankheitserscheinungen im Bereiche des Otolithenapparates. *Acta oto-laryngol.* **2**, 434.

Bast, R. and Anson, L. (1949). *The temporal bone and the ear.* Thomas, Springfield, Illinois.

British Medical Journal (1977). Deafness and mental health. *Br. med. J.* **1**, 191.

—— (1979). Treatment of tinnitus. *Br. med. J.* **1**, 1445.

Brodal, A. (1981). *Neurological anatomy in relation to clinical medicine*, 3rd. edn. Oxford University Press, Oxford.

Carmichael, E. A. Dix, M. R., and Hallpike, C. S. (1956). Pathology, symptomatology and diagnosis of organic affections of the eighth nerve system. *Brit. med. Bull.* **12**, 146.

——, ——, and —— (1965). Observations upon the neurological mechanism of directional preponderance of caloric nystagmus resulting from vascular lesion of the brainstem. *Brain* **88**, 51.

Cawthorne, T. E. and Hinchcliffe, R. (1961). Positional nystagmus of the central type as evidence of subtentorial metastases. *Brain* **84**, 415.

—— and Ranger, D. (1957). Toxic effect of streptomycin upon balance and hearing. *Br. med. J.* **1**, 1444.

Cooper, A. F., Kay, D. W. K., Curry, A. R., Garside, R. F., and Roth, M. (1974). Hearing loss in paranoid and affective psychoses of the elderly. *Lancet* **ii**, 851.

Curtis, B. A., Jacobson, S., and Marcus, E. M. (1972). *An introduction to the neurosciences.* Saunders, Philadelphia.

Davis, H. and Silverman, S. R. (1970). *Hearing and deafness.* Holt, Rinehart, and Winston, New York.

Dix, M. R. (1956). Loudness recruitment. *Br. med. Bull.* **12**, 119.

—— (1969). Modern tests of vestibular function, with special reference to their value in clinical practice. *Br. med. J.* **3**, 317.

—— and Hallpike, C. S. (1952). Further observations upon the diagnosis of deafness in young children. *Br. med. J.* **1**, 235.

——, ——, and Harrison, M. S. (1949). Some observations upon the otological effects of streptomycin intoxication. *Brain* **72**, 241.

——, ——, and Hood, J. D. (1948). Observations upon the loudness recruitment phenomenon, with especial reference to the differential diagnosis of disorders of the internal ear and VIII nerve. *Proc. R. Soc. Med.* **41**, 516.

Doig, J. A. (1972). Auditory and vestibular function and dysfunction. In *Scientific foundations of neurology* (ed. M. Critchley, J. L. O'Leary, and W. B. Jennett) Section V, Chapter 3. Heinemann, London.

Edwards, C. H. (1973). *Neurology of ear, nose, and throat diseases.* Butterworths, London.

Fitzgerald, G. and Hallpike, C. S. (1942). Studies in human vestibular function. **65**, 115.

Frazier, C. S. and Rowe, S. N. (1932). Certain observations upon the localization of 51 verified tumours of the temporal lobe. *Res. Publ. Ass. nerve. ment. Dis.* **13**, 251.

Green, D. S. (1963). Modified tone decay test (MTDT) as screening procedure for eighth nerve lesions. *Speech Hearing Dis.* **28**, 31.

Hallpike, C. S. (1950). In Discussion on the medical treatment of Ménière's disease. *Proc. Roy. Soc. Med.* **43**, 288.

—— (1955). Ménière's disease *Postgrad. med. J.* **31**, 330

—— (1965). Clinical otoneurology and its contributions to theory and practice. *Proc. R. Soc. Med.* **58**, 185.

—— (1967). Some types of ocular nystagmus and their neurological mechanisms. *Proc. R. Soc. Med.* **60**, 1043.

—— (1976). Sensori-neural deafness and derangements of the loudness function: their nature and clinical investigation. In *Handbook of sensory physiology* (ed. A. Iggo) Vol. V/3, Chapter 1. Springer Verlag, Berlin.

Harrison, M. S. and Ozsahinoglu, C. (1972). Positional vertigo: aetiology and clinical significance. *Brain* **95**, 369.

Hecox, K. E., Cone, B., and Blaw, M. E. (1981). Brainstem auditory evoked response in the diagnosis of pediatric neurologic disease. *Neurology, Minneapolis* **31**, 832.

Hood, J. D. (1977). Whither vestibular test? *Proc. R. Soc. Med.* **70**, 675.

—— and Poole, J. P. (1971). Speech audiometry in conductive and sensorineural hearing loss. *Sound* **5**, 30.

Jerger, J. F. (1960). Békèsy audiometry in analysis of auditory disorders. *J. speech Res.* **3**, 275.

——, Shedd, J. L., and Harford, E. (1959). On the detection of extremely small changes in sound intensity *Arch. Otolaryngol.* **69**, 200.

Johnson, E. W. and House, W. F. (1964). Auditory findings in 53 cases of acoustic neuroma. *Arch. Otolaryngol.* **80**, 667.

Konigsmark, B. W. (1969). Hereditary deafness in man. *New Engl. J. Med.* **281**, 713, 774, 827.

Korres, S. (1978a). Electronystagmographic criteria in neuro-otological diagnosis. 1. Peripheral lesions. *J. Neurol. Neurosurg. Psychiat.* **41**, 249.

——, (1978b). Electronystagmographic criteria in neuro-otological diagnosis. 2. Central nervous system lesions. *J. Neurol. Neurosurg. Psychiat.* **41**, 254.

The Lancet (1977). Sudden deafness. *Lancet* **ii**, 965.

The Lancet (1984). Tinnitus. *Lancet*, **i**, 543.

Luxon, L. M. (1980). Hearing loss in brainstem disorders. *J. Neurol. Neurosurg. Psychiat* **43**, 510.

McCutchen, C. B. and Iragui-Madoz, V. J. (1979). Evoked potentials. In *Current neurology* (ed. H. R. Tyler and D. M. Dawson) Vol. 2, Chapter 23. Houghton Mifflin, Boston.

Melding, P. S. and Goodey, R. J. (1979). The treatment of tinnitus with oral anticonvulsants. *J. Laryng. Otol.* **93**, 111.

Nylén, C. O. (1939). The otoneurological diagnosis of tumours of the brain. *Acta oto-laryngol* Suppl. 33.

Oh, S. J., Kuba, T., Soyer, A., Choi, I. S., Bonikowski, F. P., and Vitek, J. (1981). Lateralization of brainstem lesions by brainstem auditory evoked potentials. *Neurology, Minneapolis* **31**, 14.

Patton, H. D., Sundsten, J. W., Crill, W. E., and Swanson, P. D. (1976). *Introduction to basic neurology.* Saunders, Philadelphia.

Rowson, K. E. K., Hinchcliffe, R., and Gamble, D. R. (1975). A virological and epidemiological study of patients with acute hearing loss. *Lancet* **i**, 471.

Rudge, P. (1982). *Clinical neuro-otology.* Churchill-Livingstone, Edinburgh.

Stevens, H. (Ed.) (1951). *Handbook of experimental psychology.* John Wiley & Sons, New York.

Stockard, J. J. and Rossiter, V. S. (1977). Clinical and pathologic correlates of brainstem auditory response abnormalities. *Neurology, Minneapolis* **27**, 316.

Wever, E. G. and Bray, C. W. (1930). Present possibilities for auditory theory. *Psychol. Rev.* **37**, 365.

The nature of vertigo

Vertigo may be defined as an awareness of disordered orientation of the body in space. The derivation of the term implies a sense of rotation of the patient or of his surroundings, but this, though often present, is not invariable. As Brandt and Daroff (1980) have suggested, vertigo occurs with either physiological stimulation or pathological dysfunction of any of the three stabilizing sensory systems, vestibular, visual, and somatosensory; it has two principal forms:

1. The external world may appear to move, often in a rotatory fashion, but other forms of movement, such as oscillation, may be experienced.

2. The body itself may be felt to be moving, either in rotation or as a sensation of falling, or the movement may be referred to within the body, e.g. within the head.

3. The motor accompaniments of vertigo consist of involuntary movements of the whole body, such as falling, and disordered orientation of its parts, manifested in the eyes as nystagmus or rarely diplopia, and in the limbs as pass pointing, while visceral disturbances, such as pallor, sweating, alterations in the pulse rate and blood pressure, nausea, vomiting, and diarrhoea may be present. The maintenance of an appropriate position of the body in space depends in man upon several groups of afferent impulses, of which the following are the most important.

1. From the retinae are derived visual impulses which, in contributing to our perception of visual space, are intimately concerned in spatial orientation.

2. The labyrinth is a highly specialized spatial proprioceptor. The otoliths are mainly concerned in the orientation of the organism with reference to gravity, while the semicircular canals respond to movement and to angular momentum.

3. The proprioceptors of the joints and muscles of the neck are important in relating labyrinthine impulses, which convey information solely concerning the position of the head, to the attitude of the rest of the body.

4. The proprioceptors of the lower limbs and trunk are concerned with the position of the body in relation to such acts as sitting, standing, and walking.

The afferent impulses derived from these various sense organs are integrated by central mechanisms, of which the cerebellum, the vestibular nuclei, the medial longitudinal fasciculus, and the red nuclei are probably the most important, and which constitute reflex paths by which the position of the body is normally appropriately orientated. From these lower centres, impulses reach the cerebral cortex mainly in the temporal and parietal lobes and so influence voluntary movement. Vertigo may result from disordered function of the sensory end-organs, of the afferent paths, or of the central mechanisms concerned.

The causes of vertigo

It is clear from the anatomical and physiological considerations outlined above that vertigo may result from a disturbance of function at many different levels. We may therefore recognize: (1) psychogenic dizziness; (2) vertigo due to cortical disturbances; (3) vertigo of ocular origin; (4) vertigo of cerebellar origin; (5) vertigo due to brainstem lesions; (6) vertigo due to eighth-nerve lesions; and (7) aural vertigo. In many conditions it is difficult to define precisely the site of origin of the symptoms.

Psychogenic dizziness

In lay terminology, 'giddiness' is the term most often to be equated with genuine vertigo, while dizziness is used more often to identify less well-defined symptoms including vague feelings of instability, swimming in the head, feelings of faintness, and many more. Confusion results from the fact that some patients and doctors use these two terms as if they were interchangeable; analysis of these symptoms and differential diagnosis may be very difficult (Matthews 1975), and Drachman and Hart (1972) in an article on '. . . the dizzy patient' were clearly referring to vertigo. While some subjective sensations which cannot easily be distinguished from true vertigo may be one manifestation of hysteria, vague feelings of dizziness and instability, often with features of depersonalization, are common in patients with anxiety states or depressive illness and are prominent in those with panic attacks and hyperventilation.

Vertigo due to cortical disturbances

The aura of an epileptic attack may be a feeling of giddiness, as is not uncommon in minor epilepsy of temporal-lobe origin. Vertigo may also occur uncommonly in association with other localized temporal-lobe lesions.

Vertigo of ocular origin

Vertigo may occur in normal individuals in consequence of unusual visual perceptions. Giddiness at heights and on looking from the platform at a swiftly moving train are examples of this. Paralysis of one or more external ocular muscles is sometimes associated with vertigo. This is due to the spatial disorientation which is produced by false projection of the visual fields (see p. 96).

Vertigo of cerebellar origin

Vertigo may be slight or absent in spite of a massive lesion of the cerebellum, especially if this is limited to the lateral lobe. A cerebellar lesion is most likely to cause vertigo when it involves the flocculonodular lobe which is closely linked anatomically with the vestibular system. Thus severe vertigo may occur as a symptom of cerebellar infarction and it is invariable in those patients with primary intracerebral haemorrhage who remain conscious.

Vertigo due to brainstem lesions

Vascular or neoplastic lesions of the brainstem may cause vertigo if they involve vascular connections. Neoplasms in the fourth ventricle (ependymoma in young patients or metastases in the elderly) commonly produce vertigo induced by change in posture or sudden head movement. Streptomycin may damage the vestibular nuclei and cerebellum (Winston, Lewey, Parenteau, Marden, and Cramer 1948; Burns and Westlake 1949) but its principal toxic effect is upon the labyrinth itself (Cawthorne and Ranger 1957). Other drugs, such as barbiturates and anticonvulsants (e.g. phenytoin), produce giddiness, drowsiness, and ataxia through an action on central vestibular and cerebellar connections and a similar mechanism probably accounts for vertigo in metabolic disorders such as hypoglycaemia. A plaque of multiple sclerosis in the pons may cause severe vertigo with conspicuous nystagmus, vomiting, and prostration: so too may syringobulbia. Acute vertigo is a prominent presenting symptom of lateral medullary infarction due to vertebral or posterior inferior cerebellar artery occlusion; transient attacks due to brainstem ischaemia are common in basilar artery migraine, in patients with basilar aneurysm or brain stem angioma, and especially in vertebro-basilar insufficiency. Transitory ischaemia of the brainstem is the probable cause of vertigo evoked by head movement in patients with atheroma of the vertebral arteries, especially in the presence of cervical spondylosis.

Vestibular neuronitis and epidemic vertigo

Dix and Hallpike (1952) applied the term vestibular neuronitis to a disorder giving acute vertigo without deafness or tinnitus. Tests of cochlear function showed no abnormality: the caloric vestibular responses, however, were abnormal, often grossly so, on one or both sides. The onset was often associated with an infective illness and the prognosis was good. *Epidemic vertigo* produces a similar clinical picture occurring in epidemics, sometimes with symptoms of gastrointestinal or respiratory infection. It appears to be due to a mild viral encephalitis affecting the brainstem (Leishman 1955; Pedersen 1959). The onset is acute and prostrating; vertigo is precipitated by any movement of the head; the condition may last for days or even weeks and relapses have been described. Most cases of so-called acute labyrinthitis are probably of this type. However, Kohut, Waldorf, Haenel, and Thompson (1979) point out that a similar picture may result from minute perilymph leaks with fistulae at the round or oval window and that these may be corrected surgically. In such cases Hennebert's sign (subjective vertigo and nystagmus induced by pneumatic otoscopy) is usually positive (*The Lancet* 1979).

Vertigo due to lesions of the eighth nerve

Lesions of the vestibular nerve may cause giddiness, usually associated with deafness and tinnitus due to involvement of the cochlear nerve, but severe vertigo is uncommon. The commonest such lesion is an acoustic neuroma, but the nerve may also be compressed by abnormal vessels or involved in meningeal inflammation.

Other causes of aural vertigo

Mild vertigo can result from wax in the external auditory meatus or from blockage of the Eustachian tube. When inflammation due to acute or chronic otitis media invades the labyrinth, more severe vertigo results and Hennebert's fistula sign will be present. Sudden acute vertigo can result from occlusion of the internal auditory artery and is then associated with sudden unilateral deafness, and a similar syndrome of less abrupt onset may result from herpes zoster of the geniculate ganglion.

Other important causes include head injury, benign positional vertigo, the instability of motion sickness, and recurrent aural vertigo (benign, in childhood; and Ménière's syndrome or benign recurrent vertigo in adults).

Benign positional vertigo

Benign positional vertigo usually comes on relative acutely between the ages of 30 and 60. It is attributed to degeneration of the otolith apparatus, and is occasionally associated with middle-ear disease but is more often 'idiopathic'. Giddiness occurs on head movement and may be evoked by the test described on page 124. The condition is characterized by vertigo evoked by one specific movement of the head; it is often self-limiting and clears up spontaneously in a few months but occasionally persists for much longer. A similar syndrome in which any movement of the head (turning, or looking upwards or downwards) causes transient vertigo, presumed to be due to damage to the utricle, is a relatively frequent sequel of closed head injury (Harrison 1956; Cartlidge and Shaw 1981) and may take many months or even one or two years to resolve.

Ménière's disease

Definition. A condition giving recurrent attacks of severe vertigo often with vomiting and prostration, and usually associated with tinnitus and increasing deafness. The disorder runs a protracted course and the vertigo tends to disappear as the deafness increases (Ménière 1860–1).

Aetiology and pathology

Men suffer from Ménière's syndrome more often than women in a proportion of about 3 to 2. It is a disorder of middle age, especially late middle age, the average age of onset being 50, and more than one-third of all patients are first affected after the age of 60. Little is known about the aetiology. Pathological investigations by Hallpike and Cairns (1938) demonstrated a gross dilatation of the endolymph system of the internal ear. While it has been suggested that endolymphatic potassium which contaminates the perilymph after rupture of the cochlear membrane damages the organ of Corti, a primary abnormality of the endolymphatic sac has also been postulated and the cause of the hydrops of the labyrinth is still unknown (*The Lancet* 1981; Rudge 1982).

Symptoms

The usual history is that a patient, who has suffered from slowly progressive deafness and tinnitus in one or both ears for months or even years, suddenly becomes giddy. In some cases the giddiness develops so rapidly that the patient may fall; more often it takes a few minutes to become severe. In a severe attack the patient is literally prostrate, and there is an intense sensation of rotation of the surroundings, less often of the patient himself. Vomiting soon develops with severe nausea. Rarely there is also diarrhoea. The pulse may be rapid or slow, and the blood pressure raised or lowered, and there may be profuse sweating. Diplopia occurs rarely and in very severe cases fainting occurs. Deafness and tinnitus are sometimes intensified in the attack. The vertigo may last from half an hour to many hours, and then gradually subsides. On attempting to stand and walk, the patient is unsteady and staggers.

During the attack the patient usually lies on the sound side and shows rotary nystagmus, most evident on looking towards the affected ear. In the intervals between attacks, giddiness is occasionally brought on by sudden head movement and there may be a fine rotary nystagmus on extreme lateral fixation to either side. There may be some mild persistent ataxia. Deafness is usually unilateral, rarely bilateral. Both air- and bone-conduction are usually impaired and there is a selective loss of higher tones. Loudness recruitment is always present. The caloric test usually shows canal paresis in the affected ear. Directional preponderance is less frequent. Less often still, both are present.

Diagnosis

Aural vertigo is rarely confused with minor epilepsy, but when giddiness is a symptom of the latter condition the attacks last only a few seconds, consciousness is usually impaired or lost, and the giddiness disappears as rapidly as it develops. In Ménière's disease tinnitus and some hearing impairment are almost always present, and a lesion which impairs both cochlear and vestibular function must be situated either in the internal ear or in the eighth nerve. A lesion of the latter rarely gives severe vertigo and the ipsilateral corneal reflex is usually reduced or lost. When vertigo is due to lesions of the brainstem or cerebellum, hearing is usually unimpaired and other manifestations of these lesions are usually present.

Prognosis

The attacks recur at irregular intervals and with varying severity. Usually the intervals of freedom last only a few weeks; in rare cases the patient is free from attacks for years. The attacks tend to diminish in severity spontaneously, and finally to cease as deafness increases. Exceptionally, in the absence of radical treatment, the attacks continue for many years.

Treatment

During an attack the patient must rest lying perfectly still. An intramuscular injection of 50 mg of chlorpromazine will relieve the discomfort in severe cases. Dimenhydrinate 50 mg, promethazine 25 mg, thiethylperazine maleate 10 mg, or prochlorperazine 5 mg may be used regularly as vestibular sedatives. The patient should be warned about the risk of a sudden attack. If, after six months, there is no response to medical measures, and especially if the vertigo is severely incapacitating, surgical treatment should be considered. Labyrinthectomy once had a vogue but destroyed hearing totally in the affected ear and often caused troublesome ataxia in the elderly. Section of the vestibular nerve abolishes the vertigo while preserving the hearing and the tinnitus, but is a major neurosurgical operation. Ultrasonic irradiation can destroy vestibular function. Some reduction of hearing occurs in one-third of cases. Endolymphatic subarachnoid shunt has been used to correct the endolymphatic hydrops with occasional good results (House 1962). The operation of choice now appears to be decompression or cannulation of the endolymphatic sac (Booth 1980).

Benign recurrent vertigo

Slater (1979) and others (see *British Medical Journal* 1979) have drawn attention to a syndrome in which patients suffer repeated attacks of acute vertigo lasting from minutes to hours which are followed by a period in which positional nystagmus may be elicited. The attacks may occur once a day or as infrequently as once or twice a year. There is no associated deafness or tinnitus, audiometry and caloric tests are normal, but electronystragmography may suggest minor labyrinthine dysfunction. There is often a strong family history, as in familial paroxysmal nystagmus with vertigo and ataxia (White 1969), an association with migraine, and a tendency for the attacks to be precipitated by lack of sleep, stress, or alcohol. Prophylactic propranolol or pizotifen often controls the attacks.

Benign paroxysmal vertigo of childhood

This benign and self-limiting disorder gives severe but brief attacks of vertigo in children, usually below the age of three years. The episodes are distressing but generally resolve spontaneously within months or at the most a few years (Basser 1964; Koenigsberger, Chutorian, Gold, and Schvey 1970). The disorder is of labyrinthine origin but of unknown aetiology and is usually relieved substantially by treatment with dimenhydrinate.

References

Basser, L. S. (1964). Benign paroxysmal vertigo of childhood. *Brain* **87**, 141.

Booth, J. B. (1980). Ménière's disease: the selection and assessment of patients for surgery using electrocochleography. *Ann. R. Coll. Surg. Engl.* **62**, 415.

Brandt, T. and Daroff, R. B. (1980). The multisensory physiological and pathological vertigo syndromes. *Ann. Neurol.* **7**, 195.

British Medical Journal (1979). Benign recurrent vertigo. *Br. med. J.* **2**, 756.

Burns, P. A. and Westlake, R. E. (1949). In *Streptomycin* (ed. S. A. Waksman), p. 524. Williams & Wilkins, Baltimore.

Cairns, H. and Brain, W. R. (1933). Aural vertigo. Treatment by division of eighth nerve. *Lancet* i, 946.

Cartlidge, N. E. F. and Shaw, D. A. (1981). *Head injury*. Saunders, London.

Cawthorne, T. E., Fitzgerald, G., and Hallpike, C. S. (1942). Studies in human vestibular function: III. Observations on the clinical features of 'Ménière's disease with especial reference to the results of the caloric test. *Brain* **65**, 161.

—— and Ranger, D. (1957). Toxic effect of streptomycin upon balance and hearing. *Br. med. J.* **1**, 1444.

Dandy, W. E. (1933). Treatment of Ménière's disease by section of only the vestibular portion of the acoustic nerve. *Bull. Johns Hopkins Hosp.* **53**, 52.

Dix, M. R. and Hallpike, C. S. (1952). The pathology, symptomatology and diagnosis of certain disorders of the vestibular system. *Proc. R. Soc. Med.* **45**, 341.

Drachman, D. A. and Hart, C. W. (1972). An approach to the dizzy patient, *Neurology, Minneapolis* **22**, 323.

Hallpike, C. S. (1965). Clinical otoneurology and its contribution to theory and practice. *Proc. R. Soc. Med.* **58**, 185.
—— and Cairns, H. (1937–8). Observations on the pathology of Ménière's
syndrome. *Proc. R. Soc. Med.* **31**, 1317; also (1938) *J. Laryng.* **53**, 625.
Harrison, M. S. (1956). Notes on the clinical features and pathology of
post-concussional vertigo, with especial reference to positional nystagmus. *Brain* **79**, 474.
House, W. F. (1962). Subarachnoid shunt for drainage of endolymphatic
hydrops, a preliminary report. *Laryngoscope* **72**, 713.
Koenigsberger, M. R., Chutorian, A. M., Gold, A. P., and Schvey, M. S.
(1970). Benign paroxysmal vertigo of childhood. *Neurology, Minneapolis* **20**, 1108.
Kohut, R. I., Waldorf, R. A., Haenel, J. L., and Thompson, J. N. (1979).
Minute perilymph fistulas: vertigo and Hennebert's sign without hearing
loss. *Ann. Otol. Rhinol. Laryngol.* **88**, 153.
The Lancet (1979). Non-specific disturbances of balance. *Lancet* **ii**, 237.
—— (1981). Ménière's disease. *Lancet* **i**, 25.
Leishman, A. W. D. (1955). 'Epidemic vertigo' with oculomotor compli-
cation. *Lancet* **i**, 228.
Matthews, W. B. (1975). *Practical neurology*, 3rd edn. Blackwell, Oxford.
Pedersen, E. (1959). Epidemic vertigo. *Brain* **82**, 566.
Rudge, P. (1982). *Clinical neuro-otology*. Churchill-Livingstone, Edin-
burgh.
Slater, R. (1979). Benign recurrent vertigo. *J. Neurol. Neurosurg. Psy-
chiat.* **42**, 363.
White, J. C. (1969). Familial periodic nystagmus, vertigo, and ataxia.
Arch. Neurol., Chicago **20**, 276.
Winston, J., Lewey, F. H., Parenteau, A., Marden, P. A., and Cramer, F.
B. (1948). An experimental study of the toxic effects of streptomycin on
the vestibular apparatus of the cat. *Ann. Otol., St. Louis* **57**, 738.

The ninth or glossopharyngeal nerve

The glossopharyngeal nerve contains both sensory and motor
fibres. The sensory ganglion cells are situated in the inferior ganglion of the nerve. Their central processes mostly pass into the tractus solitarius and terminate in its nucleus. A few also enter the
dorsal nucleus of the vagus. The motor fibres originate partly in
the inferior salivary nucleus and partly in the nucleus ambiguus.
The nerve arises by a series of radicles from the posterior lateral
sulcus of the medulla between the fibres of origin of the vagus and
accessory nerves (Fig. 2.25). After crossing the posterior fossa it
emerges through the anterior compartment of the jugular foramen. In the neck it arches downwards and forwards between the
internal carotid artery and the internal jugular vein, and then
between the internal and external carotid arteries to the side of the
pharynx. Within the skull it gives off the tympanic nerve which
carries sensation from the tympanic cavity and joins the tympanic
plexus, from which the lesser petrosal nerve carries to the otic
ganglion fibres which excite salivary secretion. In the neck the
glossopharyngeal nerve gives a branch to the stylopharyngeus
muscle, its sole motor supply, and branches to the pharyngeal
mucous membrane. Its terminal branches supply the tonsil, the
lower border and posterior surface of the soft palate, and the posterior third of the tongue. The glossopharyngeal nerve is thus
motor to the stylopharyngeus and to the salivary glands, especially
the parotid gland. It supplies somatic sensibility to the posterior
third of the tongue, the tonsils, and the pharynx, and taste-fibres
to the same region. Isolated lesions of the glossopharyngeal nerve
are almost unknown. It is most often damaged along with the
vagus and accessory nerve at the jugular foramen (see below).

Glossopharyngeal neuralgia

Glossopharyngeal neuralgia resembles the much commoner trigeminal neuralgia. As in the latter, the pain occurs in brief attacks,
which may be of great severity. It usually begins in the side of the
throat and radiates down the side of the neck in front of the ear
and to the back of the lower jaw. Exceptionally, the pain begins
deep in the ear. Attacks are precipitated by swallowing or by pro-

truding the tongue, and the ear may be extremely sensitive to
touch.

Glossopharyngeal neuralgia is distinguished from trigeminal
neuralgia by the situation of the pain and its precipitation by swallowing. Pain of a similar distribution but of more continuous
character may result from neoplasms involving the tonsil and
pharynx, which must therefore be excluded. Rarely true glossopharyngeal neuralgia, like tic douloureux, may be symptomatic of
a posterior fossa neoplasm or of a nasopharyngeal cyst or bursa
(Tornwaldt's disease) (Stern and Hall 1972).

Carbamazepine (*Tegretol*) in doses of 200 mg three or four
times daily may completely control the pain. If it fails, interruption of the afferent fibres of the nerve may be necessary. Harris
successfully injected the nerve in the neck with alcohol but this is a
difficult procedure. To obtain permanent relief surgical avulsion
of the nerve may be needed; this can be performed in the neck
when the pain is predominantly pharyngeal, but should be carried
out intracranially in the posterior fossa when the deep part of the
ear is also the site of pain (Jefferson 1931). Chawla and Falconer
(1967) recommended intracranial section of the glosspharyngeal
nerve and of the upper two rootlets of the vagus as the operation
of choice. As in hemifacial spasm (p. 116), there is increasing evidence that the condition is often the result of compression of the
nerve trunk by an artery, when decompression alone may be successful. The artery in question may even be the vertebral (Brihaye, Perier, Smulders, and Franken 1956) which may have to be
tied back from the nerve.

References

Brihaye, J., Perier, O., Smulders, J., and Franken, L. (1956). Glossophar-
yngealneuralgia caused by compression of the nerve by an atheromatous
vertebral artery. *J. Neurosurg.* **13**, 299.
Chawla, J. C. and Falconer, M. S. (1967). Glossopharyngeal and vagal
neuralgia. *Br. med. J.* **3**, 529.
Dana, C. L. (1926). The story of the glossopharyngeal nerve and four cen-
turies of research concerning the cranial nerves of man. *Arch. Neurol.
Psychiat., Chicago* **15**, 675.
Dandy, W. E. (1927). Glossopharyngeal neuralgia (tic douloureux). *Arch.
Surg.* **15**, 198.
Fay, T. (1927–8). Observations and results from intracranial section of the
glossopharyngeus and vagus nerves in man. *J. Neurol. Psychopath.* **8**,
110.
Harris, W. (1926). *Neuritis and neuralgia*. Oxford University Press, Lon-
don.
Jefferson, G. (1931). Glossopharyngeal neuralgia. *Lancet* **ii**, 397.
Stern, L. Z. and Hall, S. W. (1972). Tornwaldt's disease. Onset as sympto-
matic (secondary) glosspharyngeal neuralgia. *Neurology, Minneapolis*
22, 1182.

The sense of taste

There are only four tastes: sweet, salt, bitter, and acid. All other
flavours are olfactory sensations. The acuity of taste, especially on
the anterior two-thirds on the tongue, varies considerably in normal individuals and tends to decline with increasing age (Brodal
1981). The sense of taste is tested with weak solutions or crystals
of sugar, common salt, quinine, and acetic acid or vinegar. The
patient keeps his tongue protruded and replies to questions by
nodding or shaking his head. It is convenient to have the names of
the four tastes written on cards, to which he can point. The protruded tongue is dried and substance is applied to the lateral border on one side. The patient is then asked to indicate what he
tastes. The anterior two-thirds and the posterior one-third of the
tongue must be tested separately but testing on the posterior third
is very difficult. Stimulation of the tongue with a galvanic current
applied by a naked copper electrode has also been used to examine taste (de Jong 1979) and Krarup (1958) designed a technique
of quantitative electrogustometry.

The taste fibres

Peripheral path

The fibres carrying taste impulses from the anterior two-thirds of the tongue pass through the lingual nerve to the chorda tympani, then into the facial nerve, and on to the geniculate ganglion which contains their ganglion cells. From the geniculate ganglion they pass to the pons by the nervus intermedius. Lesions of the third division of the trigeminus have been said to cause temporary impairment of taste on the anterior two-thirds of the tongue, possibly due not to interruption of taste fibres but to loss of background somatic sensation (Rowbotham 1939). Taste fibres from the posterior one-third of the tongue, from the pharynx, and from the lower border of the soft palate are carried by the glossopharyngeal nerve.

Central connections

The taste fibres after entering the pons pass into the tractus solitarius, the upper and middle part of which receives fibres from the nervus intermedius, and the lower part fibres from the glossopharyngeal. The fibres of the tractus solitarius terminate in a column of grey matter known as the nucleus of this tract, from which relay-neurones arise; these cross the midline and turn upwards in the tegmentum of the pons and medulla to form the gustatory lemniscus, which lies near the midline lateral to the medial longitudinal fasciculus. The gustatory lemniscus ascends to the VPM nucleus of the thalamus, from which taste fibres are further relayed to the cortical centre for taste at the foot of the postcentral gyrus.

Loss of taste

Loss of taste (ageusia) on the anterior two-thirds of the tongue may occur as a result of lesions of the chorda tympani or of the geniculate ganglion. There is no clear evidence as to whether or not it results from lesions of the nervus intermedius. Lesions of the glossopharyngeal nerve abolish taste on the posterior one-third of the tongue. Lesions of the tractus solitarius and its nucleus cause unilateral ageusia, while central pontine lesions may cause bilateral loss of taste from destruction of both gustatory leminsci (Harris 1926).

Cerebral lesions rarely impair taste though it is occasionally lost, together with the sense of smell, as a result of head injury. Sumner (1967) described 10 cases of post-traumatic ageusia, in 9 associated with anosmia. Rarely ageusia follows bilateral thalamotomy for parkinsonism.

Hallucinations of taste may occur along with those of smell as a result of an irritative lesion involving the uncus. Lesions in this region may also cause parageusia, a perversion of taste in which many substances have the same unpleasant flavour; this symptom occasionally develops without apparent cause in the elderly, causing troublesome anorexia; treatment rarely helps but antidepressive remedies are occasionally beneficial.

References

Brodal, A. (1981). *Neurological anatomy in relation to clinical medicine*, 3rd edn. Oxford University Press, Oxford.

Harris, W. (1926). *Neuritis and neuralgia*. Oxford University Press, London.

de Jong, R. N. (1979). *The neurological examination*, 4th edn. Hoeber, New York.

Krarup, B. (1958). Electro-gustometry; a method for clinical taste examination. *Acta oto-laryngol.* **49**, 294.

Rowbotham, G. F. (1939). Observations of the effect of trigeminal denervation. *Brain* **62**, 364.

Schwartz, H. G. and Weddell, G. (1938). Observations on the pathways transmitting the sensation of taste. *Brain* **61**, 99.

Sumner, D. (1967). Post-traumatic ageusia. *Brain* **90**, 187.

The tenth or vagus nerve

Central connections

The vagus nerve contains both sensory and motor fibres. The ganglion cells of the former are situated in the superior and inferior ganglia of the nerve. The cells of the superior are concerned with somatic sensation from part of the external ear and terminate in relation to the spinal tract of the trigeminal nerve and its nucleus. The cells of the inferior ganglion carry afferent impulses from the pharynx, larynx, trachea, oesophagus, and thoracic and abdominal viscera. Their central processes terminate in relation to the tractus solitarius and the dorsal nucleus of the vagus. The motor fibres are derived from two nuclei in the medulla. The dorsal nucleus, which is situated near the midline just beneath the floor of the fourth ventricle, sends fibres to the parasympathetic ganglia of the vagal plexuses to innervate the thoracic and abdominal viscera. The nucleus ambiguus is an elongated column of grey matter situated deep in the medulla between the dorsal accessory olive and the spinal nucleus of the trigeminus. Its fibres are distributed through the glossopharyngeal, vagus, and accessory nerves to the striated muscles of the palate, pharynx, and larynx.

Peripheral distribution

The vagus trunk

The vagus leaves the medulla by a series of radicles at the anterior margin of the inferior cerebellar peduncle and in series with the roots of the glossopharyngeal nerve above and the accessory below (Fig. 2.25). The roots form a single trunk, which leaves the skull through the jugular foramen, the same compartment as the accessory nerve. Within the neck it lies in the carotid sheath, behind the carotid arteries and the internal jugular vein. It enters the thorax behind the large veins, on the right side crossing over the subclavian artery, on the left lying between the left common carotid and subclavian arteries. In the thorax the relations of the two nerves differ. The right nerve passes downwards beside the brachiocephalic trunk and the trachea and behind the superior vena cava to the posterior surface of the lung root. The nerve passes downwards between the left common carotid and subclavian arteries and behind the left brachiocephalic vein and phrenic nerve. It crosses the aortic arch to reach the posterior surface of the root of the left lung. In the posterior mediastinum both nerves contribute to the pulmonary and oesophageal plexuses, and at the oesophageal opening of the diaphragm they enter the abdomen, the left nerve in front of the oesophagus and the right behind it, and terminate by supplying the stomach and other abdominal organs.

Branches. The superior ganglion of the vagus gives off a meningeal branch, which supplies the dura mater of the posterior fossa, and an auricular branch which carries somatic sensation from the back of the auricle and external auditory meatus. The inferior ganglion supplies a pharyngeal branch which combines with the pharyngeal branches of the glossopharyngeal and superior cervical ganglion of the sympathetic to form the pharyngeal plexus, to which it contributes motor fibres destined for the muscles of the pharynx and soft palate, except the stylopharyngeus and the tensor veli palatini. The superior laryngeal nerve arises from the inferior ganglion and has internal and external branches. The internal branch is the principal sensory nerve of the larynx. The external branch, after supplying fibres to the inferior pharyngeal constrictor, innervates the cricothyroid muscle.

Within the neck the vagus gives off cardiac branches, and the recurrent laryngeal nerves, which pursue different courses on the two sides. The right recurrent laryngeal arises at the root of the

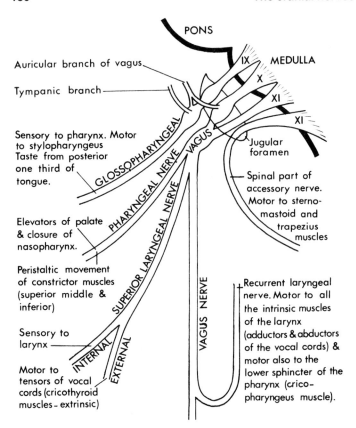

PONS

Auricular branch of vagus

Tympanic branch

IX MEDULLA

X

XI

XI

GLOSSOPHARYNGEAL

PHARYNGEAL NERVE

VAGUS

Sensory to pharynx. Motor
to stylopharyngeus
Taste from posterior
one third of
tongue.

Jugular
foramen

Spinal part of
accessory nerve.
Motor to sterno-
mastoid and
trapezius
muscles

Elevators of palate
& closure of
nasopharynx.

Peristaltic movement
of constrictor muscles
(superior middle &
inferior)

SUPERIOR LARYNGEAL NERVE

VAGUS NERVE

Sensory to
larynx

INTERNAL

EXTERNAL

Motor to
tensors of vocal
cords (cricothyroid
muscles – extrinsic)

Recurrent laryngeal
nerve. Motor to all
the intrinsic muscles
of the larynx
(adductors & abductors
of the vocal cords) &
motor also to the
lower sphincter of the
pharynx (crico-
pharyngeus muscle).

Fig. 2.25. The motor and sensory nerves supplying the pharynx and larynx, explaining the various patterns of paralysis commonly met with. (Redrawn from an original drawing by Mr. Charles Keogh.)

neck, where the vagus crosses the subclavian artery, around which it passes upwards and immediately behind the subclavian, the common carotid, and the thyroid gland. The left recurrent laryngeal leaves the vagus as it crosses the aortic arch, and after passing beneath the arch turns upwards in the superior mediastinum, between the trachea and the oesophagus, following the same course in the neck as the right nerve. The terminal branches of these nerves innervate all the laryngeal muscles (with the exception of the cricothroids, and some fibres of the transverse arytenoids), as well as the cricopharyngeus muscles which form the lower pharyngeal sphincter.

Symptoms and signs of lesions of the vagus

The pharynx and larynx

A unilateral lesion of the vagus paralyses on one side the muscles of the soft palate, the three constrictors of the pharynx, the intrinsic and extrinsic laryngeal muscles, and the lower pharyngeal sphincter, so that the patient has difficulty with saliva and nasopharyngeal secretions and in coughing, clearing the voice, and swallowing.

The pharynx functions as a muscular peristaltic tube in the second (involuntary) stage of deglutition. In its anterior wall are (*a*) the opening into the mouth and the back of the tongue, and (*b*) the opening into the larynx, and the thyroid and cricoid cartilages. Above is the nasopharyngeal sphincter, separating the pharynx from the nasal passages, and below is the cricopharyngeal sphincter, separating it from the oesophagus. During respiration the nasopharyngeal sphincter and the larynx remain open and the cricopharyngeal sphincter closes. When swallowing the nasopharyngeal sphincter and the larynx close, and the cricopharyngeal sphincter opens.

Paralysis of the palate

Motor fibres to the soft palate originate in the upper part of the nucleus ambiguus, leaving the vagus trunk at the inferior ganglion, just below the jugular foramen, in the pharyngeal nerve. Lesions of the vagus above the ganglion, or of the pharyngeal nerves, cause unilateral palatal paralysis. The tensors of the palate are supplied by the fifth nerve, and are unaffected by vagal lesions.

Unilateral palatal paralysis causes few symptoms, because of efficient compensation by the paired unparalysed muscles on the opposite side. Nevertheless there may be postnasal catarrh due to inefficient drainage of the nasopharynx, snoring, slight changes in phonation in singers, and ultimately slight changes in hearing because of inefficient function of the Eustachian tube on the same side. Unilateral paralysis is detected on examination by the fact that when the patient phonates, as in saying 'ah', the palate does not rise on the affected side, and the uvula is drawn over to the normal side.

Bilateral palatal paralysis causes regurgitation of food or fluid into the nose on swallowing, because the nasopharyngeal sphincter fails to close off the nasal passages. The voice has a nasal quality and there is altered pronunciation of those consonants which require the nasal passages to be occluded. This is most evident in the pronunciation of *b* and *g*, *rub* becoming *rum*, and *egg*, *eng*. There is often mouth-breathing and snoring at night, with difficulty in draining mucus from the nasal passages into the pharynx. The palate is immobile, and the palatal reflex is lost.

Causes of palatal paralysis include myasthenia gravis, polymyositis, and brainstem infarction. Bulbar poliomyelitis and diphtheritic polyneuropathy, once common, are now rare. Palatal myoclonus is associated with lesions of the olivodentate system (p. 349).

Paralysis of the pharynx

The motor fibres to the three paired pharyngeal constrictors, the muscles mainly responsible for propelling food into the oesophagus, originate in the middle of the nucleus ambiguus and leave the vagus trunk at the inferior ganglion. Lesions of these fibres cause pharyngeal paralysis. The palatal muscles (superior pharyngeal sphincter), the laryngeal muscles (laryngeal sphincter), and the cricopharyngeal muscles (lower pharygneal sphincter) are often involved at the same time. The pharyngeal wall droops on the affected side, and the pharyngeal reflex is present only on the other side. Frothy mucus collects above the opening of the oesophagus, indicating delay in pharyngeal emptying. This overflows into the larynx causing difficulty in clearing the voice, and coughing. Compensation by constrictor muscles on the unaffected side is often efficient, but the patient finds it easier to sleep on the affected side to prevent laryngeal irritation from mucus; there is always difficulty in clearing the throat and swallowing has to be deliberate.

Bilateral pharyngeal paralysis causes marked dysphagia and bilateral loss of the pharyngeal reflex. Soft pulpy foods are sometimes more readily swallowed than the usual solids and liquids. While dysphagia is a common consequence of bilateral upper motor-neurone dysfunction above the pons (as in pseudobulbar palsy) it may rarely be the consequence of a unilateral lesion involving either the precentral gyrus or more often the posterior part of the inferior frontal gyrus (Meadows 1973).

Paralysis of the larynx

Motor fibres to the larynx originate in the lowest part of the nucleus ambiguus; some probably leave the medulla with the accessory nerve, subsequently joining the vagus in the jugular foramen. Fibres destined for the cricothyroid muscle, a tensor of the vocal cords, leave the vagus by the superior laryngeal nerve and reach the muscle through its external branch. Those which innervate the abductors and adductors of the cords run in the recurrent laryngeal nerves. Abduction of the vocal cords occurs during inspiration, and they are adducted in phonation and coughing. Reflex adduction occurs in response to laryngeal irritation.

Supranuclear lesions
Little is known regarding the effects of supranuclear lesions. Hemiplegia does not impair movement of the vocal cords. Bilateral lesions involving the laryngeal centre in the cortex at the base of the percentral gyrus may do so; however, respiratory and reflex laryngeal movements are unaffected.

Nuclear and infranuclear lesions
The old terms adductor and abductor paralysis are misleading. The position of the vocal cords in varying forms of paralysis depends upon the site of the lesion, the extent to which different peripheral nerves are involved, and whether wasting of paralysed muscles has taken place. The ability of the unaffected laryngeal muscles to compensate for various forms of paralysis is remarkable.

The following varieties of laryngeal paralysis may occur.

Unilateral paralysis. (1) If the lesion affects the recurrent laryngeal nerve on one side only, there is unilateral paralysis of all laryngeal muscles except the tensors of the cords (cricothyroids) which are supplied by the external branch of the superior laryngeal. The lower sphincter of the pharynx (cricopharyngeus) is also paralysed on the same side. The appearance of the larynx when viewed through a laryngeal mirror (Fig. 2.26) shows a paralysed vocal cord lying near the midline, with the unparalysed cord coming across to meet it when the patient tries to say *E*. There is pooling of frothy mucus round the opening of the oesophagus on the same side with delay in pharyngeal emptying. As compensation is established, this tendency disappears. At first there is slight hoarseness of the voice and difficulty in swallowing fluids, but compensation by the paired unparalysed muscles is so efficient that the voice may appear normal, although it may tend to tire. Hence unilateral paralysis of the larynx often remains undiagnosed. Slight movement can be seen on the affected side, because the tensors of the paralysed cord are still functioning, and the paralysed arytenoid comes to lie just in front of the arytenoid on the unparalysed side. This is a useful diagnostic aid.

(2) If the lesion involves the superior laryngeal nerve as well as the recurrent laryngeal (that is between the nucleus ambiguus and the inferior ganglion of the vagus), there is total paralysis of one half of the larynx. The pharynx and palate on the same side are almost always paralysed as well, because of involvement of the pharyngeal branch of the vagus. The vocal cord on the affected side lies at rest slightly to one side of the midline, and the arytenoid cartilage on the same side appears to lie in front of its fellow. There is frothy mucus round the opening of the oesophagus. Cinematograph X-rays of patients swallowing opaque meals show that most of the meal passes down one piriform recess into the oesophagus. The cricopharyngeus closes firmly, shutting off the pharynx from the oesophagus, and oesophageal peristalsis continues to propel the food downwards. If the cricopharyngeus muscle is paralysed partly, or wholly, there is inefficient closure of this sphincter and some food regurgitates back into the pharynx. This accounts for the presence of frothy mucus in the lower pharynx in recurrent laryngeal nerve lesions.

Bilateral paralysis. This may be produced by bilateral lesions at any point between the nucleus ambiguus and the recurrent laryngeal nerves, but if the paralysis is complete the lesions must be above the inferior ganglion on both sides.

1. If the bilateral lesions are below the inferior ganglion, the motor fibres in the superior laryngeal nerve escape, and the main tensors of both cords are then intact and unopposed, because all the other muscles are paralysed. The cords are held close together, not more than 2 mm apart. Some apparent adduction

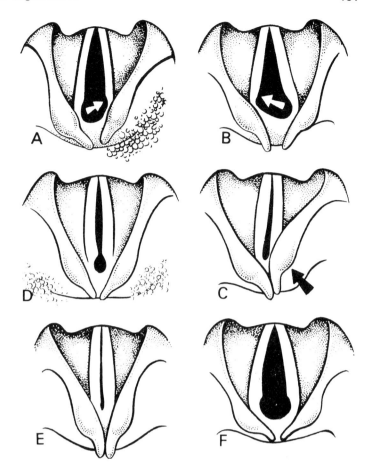

Fig. 2.26. Paralysis of the larynx (as seen through a laryngeal mirror). A: Paralysis of the left recurrent laryngeal nerve (neurofibroma). The paralysed arytenoid always lies slightly in front of the non-paralysed right arytenoid. Froth tends to collect round the opening of the oesophagus, owing to paralysis of the left cricopharyngeus muscle (lower sphincter of the pharynx, supplied by the same recurrent laryngeal nerve). On adduction the non-paralysed right vocal cord moves across to meet the paralysed left cord.) B: Paralysis of the right recurrent laryngeal nerve (thyroidectomy). There is no collected froth at the opening of the oesophagus because compensation is so good by the intact left paired cricopharyngeus muscle that it has been able to overcome the delay due to the paralysis of the right cricopharyngeus muscle. C: The same case showing closure of the larynx on adduction. The left non-paralysed cord now moves up to the paralysed cord, and the nonparalysed arytenoid now lies in front of the paralysed arytenoid. D: Paralysis of both vocal cords at the same time (thyroidectomy). The cords are held in adduction because their muscles are all paralysed except for the chief tensors of the cords, the cricothyroid muscles (supplied by the external branch of the superior laryngeal nerve). E: Normal closure of the vocal cords as seen in a laryngeal mirror. F: Normal abduction of the vocal cords as seen in a laryngeal mirror. (Redrawn from an original drawing by Mr Charles Keogh.)

can take place because the tensors are active, but abduction is impossible. There is pooling of mucus at the opening of the oesophagus indicating delay in pharyngeal emptying because the lower sphincter of the pharynx (cricopharyngeus) is paralysed. The voice is weak but remarkably clear; there is dyspnoea on exertion, and inspiratory stridor on deep inspiration (Fig. 2.27). Patients differ very greatly in their disabilities, some being able to do very little without stridor, breathlessness, and distress, while others manage very well except for breathlessness on exertion or distress during upper respiratory infections.

2. If there is complete bilateral laryngeal paralysis, the lesions must involve both superior laryngeal and both recurrent laryngeal nerves. The lesions are usually above the inferior ganglion of the vagus on both sides, or involve all four nerve trunks. Paralysis of

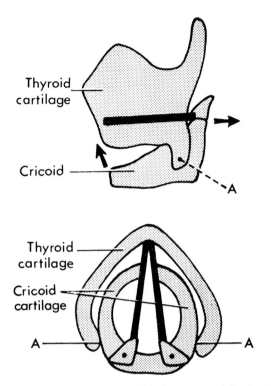

Thyroid cartilage

Cricoid

A

Thyroid cartilage

Cricoid cartilage

A ——————————— A

Fig. 2.27. Diagram of the mechanism of the larynx to explain why there is severe respiratory stridor when both recurrent laryngeal nerves are paralysed. The unopposed contraction of the non-paralysed cricothyroid muscles tilt the posterior border of the cricoid cartilage backwards, tensing the vocal cords and drawing them together. A–A shows the axis of tilt.

the palate and pharynx often accompanies complete bilateral laryngeal paralysis. The cords are immobile and lie to the midline in the so-called cadaveric position. The voice is weak but clear. The airway is adequate for most normal activity. There is, however, difficulty in clearing mucus, coughing is inefficient, and swallowing difficult, partly because there is overflow into the paralysed larynx, and partly because paralysis of the cricopharyngeus causes impaired pharyngeal emptying.

Speech in laryngeal paralysis

Some patients develop astonishingly good voices after complete removal of the larynx for carcinoma with permanent tracheostomy. With practice, air is sucked into the open oesophagus on deep inspiration, and expelled through folds in the pharynx. It is not suprising therefore that patients retain remarkably clear speech in all forms of vocal-cord paralysis, even though the voice is weak and hoarse.

Recovery in paralysis of the recurrent laryngeal nerves

Paralysis of the recurrent laryngeal nerves most often follows thyroid operations or results from poliomyelitis, aortic aneurysm, or from involvement of the left nerve in the mediastinum by lymph-node metastases from bronchial carcinoma or reticulosis. Occasionally paralysis of one nerve may take place without any apparent cause, even after exhaustive investigation; perhaps this rare event, which is also a rare, transient complication of treatment with vinca alkaloids (Whittaker and Griffith 1977), is comparable to Bell's palsy. Recovery from a recurrent laryngeal-nerve lesion, as after thyroid surgery, may occur either because the lesion was neurapraxial or through regeneration after division of axons if the epineurium remained in continuity. After prolonged laryngeal paralysis, muscular wasting may cause some subluxation of the cricoarytenoid joints. Indrawing of the arytenoid eminences and folds may then occur on forced inspiration.

Visceral function of the vagus

Little is known concerning the effects of high vagal lesions upon visceral function. In animals section of both vagi is usually fatal. In man tachycardia may follow bilateral lesions, as in subtentorial tumours, and in various forms of polyneuropathy. The parasympathetic function of the nerve is important in the regulation of cardiac and respiratory function and many abnormalities of cardiac rhythm and of respiration seen, for instance, in comatose patients (p. 649) are presumably mediated via this nerve. The trigeminal is afferent, the vagus efferent in the oculocardiac reflex (slowing of the heart rate induced by pressure upon the globe of the eye); in the carotid sinus reflex (p. 189) the glossopharyngeal nerve is afferent and the vagus efferent. The parasympathetic fibres are of course secretomotor to the acid-bearing area of the stomach and motor to the smooth muscle of the bowel wall. Surgical vagotomy has often been used to reduce acid secretion in patients with peptic ulcer and has been followed by a postvagotomy syndrome with abdominal discomfort and distension.

Lesions involving the vagus

Nuclear lesions

Lesions of the nucleus ambiguus may occur in lateral medullary infarction, syringobulbia, medullary tumour, motor-neurone disease, encephalitis, poliomyelitis, and rabies. Nuclear lesions usually cause an associated paralysis of the soft palate, pharynx, and larynx, though when the upper part of the nucleus only is affected the larynx escapes (palatopharyngeal paralysis: syndrome of Avellis).

Bilateral laryngeal paralysis may also be due to nuclear lesions, of which one cause is tabes. It is more often due to progressive bulbar palsy or cranial polyneuritis but is a rare manifestation of lead poisoning and botulism in which the nerve endings rather than the nuclei are involved.

Lesions in the posterior fossa

Lesions which involve the vagus between its emergence from the medulla and its exit from the skull in the jugular foramen almost invariably affect neighbouring cranial nerves, especially the ninth, eleventh, and twelfth. Such lesions include primary tumours (meningioma, glomus jugulare tumour) and metastases, and granulomatous inflammation involving the bone or meninges of the posterior fossa. The commonest combinations of cranial-nerve lesions in this region are glossopharyngeal, vagus, and accessory (the syndrome of the jugular foramen, and of Vernet); vagus and accessory (the syndrome of Schmidt); vagus, accessory, and hypoglossal (the syndrome of Hughlings Jackson).

Lesions of the trunk

Lesions of the trunk of the vagus above the origin of the superior laryngeal nerve cause unilateral anaesthesia of the larynx, with total paralysis of the ipsilateral vocal cord.

Lesions of the recurrent laryngeal nerve

Lesions of the recurrent laryngeal nerve do not affect sensation in the larynx. The left recurrent laryngeal nerve, owing to its longer course, is more vulnerable than the right. Within the thorax it may be compressed by aortic aneurysm, and rarely by the enlarged left atrium in mitral stenosis, or by neoplasm of the mediastinum or enlargement of mediastinal glands due to neoplastic metastases, lymphosarcoma, or Hodgkin's disease. In the neck both nerves are exposed to surgical trauma, to pressure from enlarged deep cervical glands, whether malignant or inflammatory, or from an enlarged thyroid, and may be involved in carcinoma of the oesophagus.

The superior laryngeal nerve

Lesions of this nerve are of little clinical importance; impairment of its sensory function does not give rise to symptoms. In the past its internal laryngeal branch was sometimes injected with alcohol for the relief of laryngeal pain due to tuberculosis or neoplasm. Kaeser and Richter (1965), however, reported four cases of isolated palsy of the nerve and pointed out that unilateral paralysis of the cricothyroid may give flabbiness of the corresponding vocal cord with impairment of the purity and strength of the voice. Strobsocopic examination of the vocal cords and electromyography of the cricothyroid were helpful in diagnosis; in two cases the palsy was due to trauma, in one to hypothermia, and in the other it followed thyroidectomy.

References

de Jong, R. N. (1979). *The neurologic examination*, 4th edn., Hoeber, New York.
Fay, T. (1927). Observations and results from intracranial section of the glossopharyngeus and vagus nerves in man. *J. Neurol. Psychopath.* **8**, 110.
Kaeser, H. E. and Richter, H. S. (1965). La paralysie isolée du muscle cricothyroïdien. *Rev. neurol.* **112**, 339
Meadows, J. C. (1973). Dysphagia in unilateral cerebral lesions. *J. Neurol. Neurosurg. Psychiat.* **36**, 853.
Schugt, H. P. (1926). Tuberculosis of the larynx. Treatment by surgical intervention in the superior and inferior laryngeal (recurrent) nerve. *Arch. Otolaryngol.* **4**, 479.
Taverner, D. (1969). The localisation of isolated cranial nerve lesions. In *Handbook of clinical neurology* (ed. P. J. Vinken and G. W. Bruyn) Vol. 2, Chapter 4. North-Holland, Amsterdam.
Terracol, J., Euzière, J., and Pagés, P. (1930). Les paralysies laryngées. *Rev. Oto-neuro-ophtal.* **8**, 241.
Whittaker, J. A. and Griffith, I. P. (1977). Recurrent laryngeal nerve paralysis in patients receiving vincristine and vinblastine. *Br. med. J.* **1**, 1251.

The eleventh or accessory nerve

Origin and distribution

The accessory is a purely motor nerve, which arises partly from the medulla and partly from the spinal cord. The cranial portion, or internal branch, is derived from cells in the lower part of the nucleus ambiguus. The spinal portion, or external branch, arises from cells in the lateral part of the anterior horn of spinal-cord grey matter, from the first cervical down to the fifth cervical segment. The cranial fibres emerge from the lateral aspect of the medulla below the roots of the vagus. The spinal fibres emerge from the lateral aspect of the cord between the ventral and dorsal roots. The spinal rootlets unite and then ascend in the spinal subdural space, posterior to the ligamentum denticulatum, to the foramen magnum, joining the cranial portion to form a single trunk, which leaves the skull though the jugular foramen with the vagus. In that foramen the cranial fibres join the vagus; their subsequent course to the pharynx and larynx has already been described. The spinal portion, or external branch, enters the neck between the internal carotid artery and the internal jugular vein. Passing downwards and laterally across the latter it descends beneath the steromastoid, which it then supplies. After crossing the posterior triangle, the nerve ends by entering the trapezius. In its course it communicates with branches of the second, third, and fourth cervical nerves.

Lesions of the accessory nerve

Nuclear lesions

Lesions of the nucleus ambiguus have been described in the section dealing with the vagus. The cells of origin of the spinal fibres may be attacked by poliomyelitis or degenerate in motor-neurone disease, or may be compressed in syringomyelia or by tumours involving the cervical spinal cord.

Lesions of the nerve trunk

Within the posterior fossa the nerve trunk may be damaged by tumours near the jugular foramen or involved in granulomatous meningitis or basal carcinoma, usually with the ninth, tenth, and twelfth nerves as described above. After leaving the skull, the nerve trunk may be compressed or involved in inflammation of upper deep cervical glands, or may be severed by penetrating wounds or in operations. When the lesion is deep to the steromastoid, both that muscle and the trapezius are paralysed; when it is in the posterior triangle, the sternomastoid escapes.

Lesions of the spinal branch

Unilateral lesions

Paralysis of one sternomastoid does not affect the position of the head at rest. The muscle is wasted and less prominent than its fellow. There is weakness of rotation of the head to the opposite side, and when the patient flexes the neck the chin is slightly turned to the paralysed side by the unopposed action of the normal muscle. A lesion of the accessory nerve paralyses only the upper fibres of trapezius. This part of the muscle is wasted and the normal curve formed on the back of the neck by its lateral border is flattened. The shoulder is lowered on the affected side, and the scapula rotates downwards and outwards, the lower angle being nearer the midline than the upper. There is also slight scapular winging, which disappears when serratus anterior is brought into action. There is weakness of elevation and retraction of the shoulder, and the patient cannot fully raise the arm above the head after it has been abducted by deltoid. It can still be raised in front of the body, however, through the action of the serratus anterior.

Bilateral lesions

Bilateral sternomastoid paralysis causes weakness of neck flexion, and the head tends to fall backwards when the patient is erect. Weakness of the sternomastoids is conspicuous in dystrophia myotonica. Paralysis of both trapezii causes weakness of neck extension and the head tends to fall forwards. This is most often seen in motor-neurone disease, polymyositis, and myasthenia gravis.

References

Seddon, H. (1976). *Surgical disorders of the peripheral nerves*, 2nd edn. Churchill Livingstone, London.
Strauss, W. L. and Howell, A. B. (1936). The spinal accessory nerve and its musculature. *Quart. Rev. Biol.* **11**, 387.
Sunderland, S. (1979). *Nerves and nerve injuries*, 2nd edn. Churchill-Livingstone, Edinburgh and London.

The twelfth or hypoglossal nerve

Origin and distribution

The hypoglossal nerve is the motor nerve of the tongue. Its fibres originate in the hypoglossal nucleus of the medulla, which represents an upward continuation of the anterior horn of spinal-cord grey matter. It is an elongated column, which in its upper part is subjacent to the floor of the fourth ventricle, near the midline, and below lies on the anterolateral aspect of the central canal. The nerve fibres pass forwards through the medulla to emerge from its ventral aspect between the olive and the pyramid. After a short course across the posterior fossa, the rootlets of the nerve unite in the hypoglossal canal through which it leaves the skull. In the neck the nerve passes downwards and forwards towards the hyoid bone, and then turns medially, passing forwards and downwards over the two carotid arteries, lying beneath the digastric and stylohyoid muscles. It then passes between the mylohyoid and hypoglossus muscles to reach the tongue.

The chief branch of the hypoglossal nerve, its descending branch, passes downwards in the anterior triangle to join the descending cervical nerve thus forming the ansa hypoglossi, from which branches are distributed to most of the infrahyoid muscles. A further branch supplies the thyrohyoid muscle but the fibres which leave the nerve by both the descending and the thyrohyoid branch are derived from the first and second cervical nerves.

Lesions of the hypoglossal nerve

A unilateral lesion of the hypoglossal nerve causes weakness and wasting of the muscles of the corresponding half of the tongue. The wasting throws the epithelium on the affected side into folds and, owing to the relative thickening of the epithelium, fur tends to accumulate on the paralysed side. The median raphe becomes concave towards the paralysed side and the tongue deviates to that side on protrusion (Fig. 2.28). Unilateral paralysis of the tongue does not impair articulation.

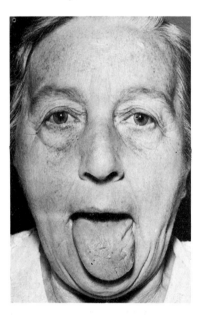

Fig. 2.28. Left hypoglossal-nerve palsy showing wrinkling and furrowing of the left side of the tongue and deviation to the left on protrusion. (Reproduced from Spillane (1975) by kind permission of the author.)

Bilateral lower motor-neurone lesions of the tongue cause marked wasting of both sides, associated, when the lesion is due to a progressive degeneration of the cells of the nuclei, with fasciculation. In severe cases, the tongue lies on the floor of the mouth and protrusion is impossible. Dysarthria and slight dysphagia are present. In dysarthia due to bilateral palsy of the tongue alone, the patient finds it difficult to pronounce *t* and *d*, and the anteriorly produced lingual vowels, *ĕ*, *ā*, *ī*, and *ē*. But bilateral paralysis is not usually an isolated phenomenon and dysphagia and dysarthria may therefore be due in part to paralysis of other muscles.

Unilateral lower motor-neurone lesions of the tongue may occur as a result of lesions involving the hypoglossal nucleus or the fibres of the nerve in their course through the medulla, as in acute poliomyelitis, syringobulbia, and thrombosis of median branches of the vertebral artery. In the last case one or both corticospinal tracts are usually also involved. Between the medulla and the hypoglossal canal the nerve roots may be compressed by a glomus tumour or meningioma or by a vertebral aneurysm or may be involved in granulomatous or carcinomatous meningitis. In such cases the glossopharyngeal, vagus, and accessory nerves often suffer in association with the hypoglossal (syndrome of Hughlings Jackson). Unilateral or, less often, bilateral atrophy and fasciculation of the tongue may also be due to congenital anomalies in the region of the foramen magnum (the Arnold–Chiari malformation, basilar impression of the skull). Unilateral paralysis has been speculatively ascribed to a periostitis of the hypoglossal canal analogous to the lesion thought to be responsible for Bell's facial paralysis. It is a rare sequel of head injury and has been reported as a rare sequel of central venous catheterisation (Whittet and Boscoe, 1984). In the neck the nerve may be injured in operations in this region, accidentally or intentionally, as in the operation of faciohypoglossal anastomosis. Hemiatrophy of the tongue may occur as part of the syndrome of facial hemiatrophy. It may also be caused by subluxation of the odontoid process or may follow retropharyngeal infection.

The commonest cause of a bilateral lower motor-neurone lesion of the tongue is involvement of the medullary nuclei in motor-neurone disease—progressive bulbar palsy. In such cases fasciculation is conspicuous as long as active degeneration is occurring.

There should be no difficulty in distinguishing upper from lower motor-neurone lesions involving the tongue. Bilateral upper motor-neurone paralysis occurs as a result of lesions involving both corticospinal tracts above the medulla and forms part of the syndrome known as pseudobulbar palsy. The commonest causes are double hemiplegia of vascular origin, diffuse cerebral ischaemia, multiple sclerosis, motor-neurone disease, and brainstem tumours. The tongue is somewhat smaller than normal owing to spasticicity but true wasting does not occur. Neighbouring muscles are also the site of spastic paralysis and the jaw-jerk is exaggerated.

References

de Jong, R. N. (1979). *The neurologic examination*, 4th edn. Hoeber, New York.

Goldenberg, N. A. and Sandler, J. G. (1931). Isolated paralysis of the hypoglossal nerve. *Rev. Oto-neuro-ophtal.* **9**, 429.

Spillane, J. D. (1975). *An atlas of clinical neurology*, 2nd edn. Oxford University Press.

Taverner, D. (1969). The localisation of isolated cranial nerve lesions. In *Handbook of clinical neurology* (ed. P. J. Vinken and G. W. Bruyn), Vol. 2, Chapter 4. North-Holland, Amsterdam.

Whittet, H. B. and Boscoe, M. J. (1984). Isolated palsy of the hypoglossal nerve after central venous catheterisation. *Br. med. J.* **i**, 1042.

3

Raised intracranial pressure, cerebral oedema, hydrocephalus, intracranial tumour, and headache

Raised intracranial pressure— pathophysiology

Many pathological processes may increase the intracranial pressure (ICP) but the most frequent are diffuse swelling of the brain (cerebral oedema), hydrocephalus, and intracranial space-occupying lesions, of which the commonest are tumours. The brain is unique among the viscera in being confined within a rigid box, the cranium. The total volume of the intracranial contents, namely the brain and its coverings, the blood vessels, and the blood and CSF is normally constant, so that an increase in any one of these can only occur at the expense of the others. However, the intracranial contents do not respond passively to changes in their volume or pressure but react in a number of complicated ways.

Since the late-nineteenth century it has been generally accepted that, as an intracranial mass lesion increases in size, there is initially a compensatory reduction in the intracranial CSF and blood volume, and only when this compensatory process is exhausted does the ICP increase. In this first or compensated stage, there is little change in the clinical condition of the patient but, in the second stage, as the compensatory process becomes increasingly ineffective, headache and drowsiness develop. The third stage of increasing intracranial pressure is characterized by increasing depression of consciousness, increased systemic arterial blood pressure (SAP), bradycardia, and irregular respiration, while in the fourth or terminal stage there is deep coma, a progressive fall in SAP and the pupils are fixed and dilated (Plum and Posner 1980).

The effects of mass lesions

General effects

The direct local effects of the increased mass of the brain, produced, say, by a tumour, play a comparatively small part initially, therefore, in raising intracranial pressure. Owing to the partial division of the cranial cavity into compartments by the falx and tentorium, the local rise of pressure is partly confined to the cranial compartment; this is in contrast to the increased pressure throughout the craniospinal axis which is usually produced by diffuse cerebral oedema, or to that which can be produced, for instance, in experimental animals by infusing saline into the lumbar subarachnoid space. Nevertheless, as compensation fails and the mass of the lesion increases, a volume/pressure curve can be derived, confirming the initial slight rise in ICP followed by an exponential increase as it grows larger. Recent work upon methods of *continuous monitoring of the ICP* (Richardson, Hide, and Eversden 1970; Lundberg 1972; Fishman 1980) has shown that there are at least three periodic waveforms superimposed upon base-line pressure, one due to the arterial pulse, one to respiration, and the other comprising slow waves of increased pressure ('X' waves) whose cause is still unknown. The higher the ICP, the greater the amplitude of the arterial pressure waves and the greater the increase in ICP produced by small increments in volume; by contrast, the respiratory and 'X' waves remain relatively constant in amplitude whether the ICP is normal or increased. However, as the mass of a focal lesion increases, the communication of the resultant increase in pressure to the whole of the subarachnoid space is reduced by the progressive herniation

of brain tissue from the compartment in which the mass lesion lies. The principal sites of such herniation are of the cingulate gyrus beneath the falx cerebri (*subfalcial herniation*), of the medial temporal lobe through the tentorial hiatus (*tentorial herniation*), or of the cerebellar tonsils into the foramen magnum (the *cerebellar pressure cone*). In these circumstances, pressure gradients develop between the various intracranial compartments, depending upon that in which the mass lesion lies. The effects of these lesions will be considered later.

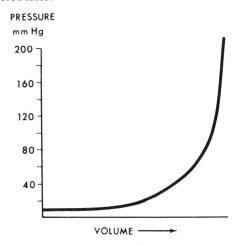

Fig. 3.1. Relationship between intracranial pressure and volume of space-occupying lesion. (Reproduced from Miller and Adams (1972) by kind permission of the authors, editors, and publisher.)

Thus an early effect of a mass lesion is to displace CSF from the cranial cavity and, if a lumbar puncture is performed, the pressure of the fluid in the lumbar subarachnoid space is increased. But, as previously stressed, this procedure carries grave risks in any tumour suspect as the removal of fluid with resultant reduced pressure in the lumbar theca may induce herniation. It must also be noted that mass lesions, depending upon their situation, can also obstruct the outflow of CSF from one lateral ventricle (due to pressure occlusion of one foramen of Monro), from the third ventricle (due to occlusion of the aqueduct), or less often from the fourth ventricle, giving rise to *hydrocephalus* with dilatation of one or more of the ventricles, thus causing an even greater increase in ICP.

The effect of ICP upon the *cerebral circulation* is also important. Compression of venous sinuses and cortical veins increases venous pressure, thus contributing to the rise in ICP, and is also one factor responsible for inducing cerebral oedema, often most severe in the neighbourhood of the tumour, an important complication of intracranial mass lesions. Pressure upon arteries may reduce blood flow focally or generally (if the rise in ICP is severe) and rarely infarction may result. An increase of ICP to over 30 mm Hg has been shown to reduce cerebral blood flow (CBF). Arterial hypertension then develops (the Cushing response—Fitch and McDowall 1977; Fitch, McDowall, Keaney, and Pickerodt 1977; Fishman 1980) partially in an attempt to compensate for the increased cerebral arterial resistance and to increase perfusion pressure. There may also be electrocardiographic (ECG) abnormalities such as prominent V waves, ST–T segment changes, notched T waves, and prolonged (or shortened) Q–T intervals (Jachuck, Ramani, Clark, and Kalbag 1975). The rise in SAP (and perhaps the ECG changes) are thought to result at least in part from medullary ischaemia due to stretching of perforating branches of the basilar artery induced in turn by downward brainstem displacement (Fitch *et al.* 1977). The situation may also be influenced by the cerebral vasodilatation induced by hypercapnia or hypoxia, which may in turn be a consequence of the respiratory irregularities induced by ICP, but these factors, like volatile anaesthetic agents, also increase ICP. Conversely, hyper-ventilation and consequent hypocapnia reduce it, as do hypothermia, hyperbaric oxygen, and some neuroleptic and analgesic drugs, especially the phenothiazines.

The effects of the *rigidity of the skull* must also be considered. That of the adult is rigid and unyielding but, as the ICP rises, an important consequence, at least in a radiological sense, is that downward pressure, sometimes of a dilated third ventricle, upon the sella turcica may cause initially decalcification and later erosion of the posterior clinoid processes. Sometimes the sella enlarges, giving rarely an empty-sella syndrome (Foley and Posner 1975), occasionally with clinical manifestations of hypopituitarism. In infants, non-union of the cranial sutures provides a partial safety-valve so that increased ICP (often due to hydrocephalus) leads to separation of the cranial sutures and the skull may yield a 'cracked-pot sound' on percussion. By contrast, premature union of the sutures (craniostenosis) causes a marked increase in ICP because skull growth is arrested while the brain is still increasing in size.

The *headache* associated with an increase in ICP, and especially that resulting from mass lesions, is mainly due to compression or distortion of the dura mater and of the pain-sensitive intracranial blood vessels. It is often paroxysmal, at first worse on waking, throbbing in character (due to the arterial pressure wave), and is accentuated by exertion, coughing, sneezing, vomiting, straining, or sudden changes in posture. The headache is often frontal or occipital or both and its distribution is of little localizing value, though it is occasionally unilateral, occurring upon the side upon which the mass lesion lies. Lesions in the posterior fossa often give suboccipital headache and, if there is associated neck stiffness or if pain is increased by attempted neck flexion, this may give warning of the presence of a cerebellar pressure cone.

The pathogenesis of *papilloedema* was considered on pp. 90–1. It develops more rapidly in patients with mass lesions in the posterior fossa because of their especial tendency to cause obstructive hydrocephalus and often appears late in patients with prefrontal lesions. Obstruction of CSF flow in the subarachnoid space and impaired absorption (demonstrated by RISA cisternography) both appear to be important factors in patients with tumours (Van Crevel 1979). It is sometimes worse on one side, but rarely unilateral except in the uncommon Foster Kennedy syndrome in which a subfrontal neoplasm (often a meningioma) on one side may compress the ipsilateral optic nerve giving optic atrophy on that side and papilloedema on the other.

The *vomiting* which often accompanies increased ICP often occurs in the mornings when the headache is at its height. It is generally attributed to compression or ischaemia of the vomiting centre in the medulla oblongata. Similarly, the *bradycardia* which is also common results from dysfunction in the cardiac centre but, in some patients with infratentorial lesions, tachycardia eventually develops. Similar effects upon the respiratory centre commonly give disorders of *respiration*. A sudden rise in ICP impairing consciousness (see Chapter 23) is often accompanied by slow and deep respiratory movements. Later breathing may become irregular (e.g. Cheyne–Stokes respiration) and periods of apnoea then alternate with others during which breathing waxes and wanes in amplitude. Central neurogenic hyperventilation or so-called

apneustic or ataxic breathing are less common effects of brainstem compression or distortion but, in terminal coma, breathing is often rapid or shallow. These abnormalities of respiratory rate and rhythm may be due to compression or distortion of the brainstem but more often to median raphe haemorrhages or infarcts in the midbrain and pons, resulting from tentorial herniation.

So-called '*false localizing signs*' may also arise as a consequence of a sustained rise in ICP. These include unilateral or bilateral sixth-nerve palsies due to compression of the trunks of one or both nerves as they cross the apex of the petrous temporal bone; bilateral extensor plantar responses or grasp reflexes resulting from ventricular dilatation in hydrocephalus; a third-nerve palsy or, more rarely, facial pain or sensory loss due to compression of the Gasserian ganglion in tentorial herniation; an ipsilateral extensor plantar response due to compression of the opposite cerebral peduncle against the free tentorial edge in tentorial herniation (Kernohan's sign); signs of cerebellar dysfunction rarely resulting from a massive frontal lesion and due to downward displacement of the brainstem; and bilateral fixed dilated pupils or defects of upward conjugate gaze due to a central cerebellar lesion displacing the midbrain upwards.

Subfalcial herniation
Herniation of the cingulate gyrus beneath the free edge of the falx cerebri can be identified radiologically, especially on angiography, and the ipsilateral lateral ventricle is often reduced in size, but usually there are no specific clinical features although there may be focal necrosis of the cingulate gyrus or extensive frontal infarction consequent upon compression of the pericallosal arteries.

Tentorial herniation
This most often develops as a consequence of lesions in the temporal lobe but may complicate any supratentorial mass lesion. As the herniated medial temporal lobe descends in the tentorial hiatus, the midbrain is pushed to the opposite side and downwards, the opposite cerebral peduncle is compressed against the free edge of the contralateral tentorium, the aqueduct is also compressed, and the ipsilateral third nerve is compressed against the tentorial edge, giving first a dilated fixed pupil and later other signs of a third-nerve palsy. There may be grooving of the uncus and hippocampal gyrus with focal necrosis or infarction.

If herniation increases, there is further downward displacement of the brainstem. The principal complications of this process are paresis or paralysis of upward conjugate gaze due to compression of the tectal plate; pressure upon one or both posterior cerebral arteries giving unilateral or bilateral occipital-lobe infarction with consequent hemianopia or cortical blindness; and most important of all, median raphe haemorrhages or infarction in the brainstem due sometimes to venous obstruction but more often to shearing effects upon perforating branches of the basilar artery, giving rise to irreversible coma due to necrosis of the reticular substance (Zülch, Mennel, and Zimmerman 1974; Plum and Posner 1980).

Tonsillar herniation (cerebellar pressure cone)
The principal effects of tonsillar herniation through the foramen magnum, which may complicate supratentorial, but more particularly infratentorial lesions, are first haemorrhagic infarction of the cerebellar tonsils themselves but more particularly, when there is associated downward displacement of the brainstem, compression of medullary structures with respiratory and/or cardiac arrest and death.

Infratentorial lesions
Infratentorial lesions, because of their effects upon the brainstem, aqueduct, and fourth ventricle, tend to cause obstructive hydrocephalus (see below) early in their course as well as tonsillar herniation. Medullary or cerebellar infarction may occur due to

compression of the medulla in the foramen magnum or distortion of the posterior inferior cerebellar arteries. Sometimes reversed tentorial herniation occurs with displacement of the brainstem and of the posterior fossa contents upwards, with infarction of the superior aspects of the cerebellar hemispheres due to compression of the superior cerebellar arteries; distortion of the hippocampal gyri due to upward pressure is rarely seen.

Cerebral oedema

Cerebral oedema accompanies many pathological processes involving the brain and is an important contributory factor in the resultant morbidity and mortality (Katzman, Clasen, and Klatz 1977). It plays a major role in head injury, stroke, and brain tumour, as well as cerebral infections, including brain abscess, encephalitis and meningitis, lead encephalopathy, hypoxia, hypo-osmolality, the disequilibrium syndromes associated with dialysis and diabetic keto-acidosis, and the various forms of obstructive hydrocephalus (Fishman 1980).

The terms, brain oedema and brain swelling, are synonymous, implying an increase in brain volume due to an increase in its water and sodium content. Oedema must be distinguished from engorgement due to an increase in the brain's blood volume due to venous obstruction or vasodilatation, though the latter, if prolonged, may lead to the former. When localized or mild and generalized, oedema produces few if any symptoms and signs but, if severe, it may cause major focal signs if it is localized, as it may be, say, to one cerebral hemisphere, while, if generalized, it can give rise to herniation as described above with medullary compression.

Fishman (1980) in a detailed review, classifies cerebral oedema into *vasogenic, cellular or cytotoxic* and *interstitial or hydrocephalic* subtypes. The vasogenic variety, associated with increased capillary permeability, is the commonest form observed in clinical practice, in conditions such as tumour, abscess, haemorrhage, infarction, contusion, lead encephalopathy, and purulent meningitis. The oedema is often localized around the primary lesion, producing focal symptoms and signs which are often due more to the oedema than to the primary lesion. Cellular or cytotoxic oedema, resembling that due to water intoxication in experimental animals, or that induced experimentally by triethyl tin (in which, however, there are also vacuoles and clefts in the cerebral white matter) is characterized by swelling of all the cellular elements of the brain (neurones, glia, and endothelial cells) with an associated reduction in extracellular fluid. This occurs in diffuse brain hypoxia, acute hypo-osmolality (in dilutional hyponatraemia, sodium depletion, or inappropriate ADH secretion) or in osmotic disequilibrium syndromes (as in haemodialysis or diabetic ketoacidosis). The clinical manifestations are usually less localized than in vasogenic oedema, including drowsiness leading to stupor or coma and sometimes convulsions. In ischaemic states a combination of vasogenic and cellular oedema, the latter coming first, is often seen. In Reye's syndrome the oedema is cellular and resembles that of triethyl tin intoxication. Interstitial or hydrocephalic oedema simply identifies the increased water content of the brain (largely extracellular) which is seen in hydrocephalus.

Recognition of the type of oedema has implications with respect to treatment. Thus high doses of glucocorticoids (dexamethasone, betamethasone) are of proven efficacy in most forms of vasogenic oedema but not in the cellular form (Fishman 1980) in which, however, osmotherapy with hypertonic mannitol or diuretics such as frusemide may be useful. While barbiturates appear to protect animals from the most severe effects of cerebral ischaemia, their role in the management of brain oedema is still uncertain (Marshall, Shapiro, and Smith 1979).

References

Fishman, R. A. (1980). *Cerebrospinal fluid in diseases of the nervous system*. Saunders, Philadelphia.

Fitch, W. and McDowall, D. G. (1977). Systemic vascular responses to increased intracranial pressure. 1. Effects of progressive epidural balloon expansion on intracranial pressure and systemic circulation. *J. Neurol. Neurosurg. Psychiat.* **40**. 833.

——, Keaney, N. P., and Pickerodt, V. W. A. (1977). Systemic vascular responses to increased intracranial pressure. 2. The 'Cushing' response in the presence of intracranial space-occupying lesions: systemic and cerebral haemodynamic studies in the dog and the baboon. *J. Neurol. Neurosurg. Psychiat.* **40**. 843.

Foley, K. M. and Posner, J. B. (1975). Does pseudotumor cerebri cause the empty sella syndrome? *Neurology, Minneapolis* **25**. 565.

Jachuck, S. J., Ramani, P. S., Clark, F., and Kalbag, R. M. (1975). Electrocardiographic abnormalities associated with raised intracranial pressure. *Br. med. J.* **1**. 242.

Katzman, R., Clasen, R., and Klatzo, I. (1977). Report of a Joint Committee for Stroke Resources. IV. Brain edema in stroke. *Stroke*. **8**. 509.

Lundberg, N. (1972). Monitoring of intracranial pressure. *Proc. R. Soc. Med.* **65**, 19.

Marshall, L. F., Shapiro, H. M., and Smith, R. W. (1979). Barbiturate treatment of intracranial hypertensive states in *Neural trauma* (ed. J. A. Popp, R. S. Bourke, L. R. Nelson, and H. K. Kimelberg) p. 347. Raven Press, New York.

Miller, D. and Adams, H. (1972). In *Scientific foundations of neurology* (ed. M. Critchley, J. L. O'Leary, and W. B. Jennett). Heinemann, London.

Plum, F. and Posner, J. B. (1980). *The diagnosis of stupor and coma*, 3rd edn. Blackwell, Oxford.

Richardson, A., Hide, T. A. H., and Eversden, I. D. (1970). Long-term continuous intracranial-pressure monitoring by means of a modified subdural pressure transducer. *Lancet* **ii**, 687.

Van Crevel, H. (1979). Papilloedema, CSF pressure, and CSF flow in cerebral tumours. *J. Neurol. Neurosurg. Psychiat.* **42**, 493.

Walton, J. N. (1981). Neurology (Section XII). In *Pathophysiology—the biological principles of disease* (ed. L. H. Smith, Jr. and O. Thier), *International textbook of medicine*. Saunders, Philadelphia.

Zülch, K. J., Mennel, H. D., and Zimmermann, V. (1974). Intracranial hypertension. In *Handbook of clinical neurology* (ed. P. J. Vinken and G. W. Bruyn) Vol. 16, Chapter 3. North-Holland, Amsterdam.

Hydrocephalus

Definition. An increase in the volume of the CSF within the skull.

Aetiology

Strictly, hydrocephalus means 'water on the brain' and this term has sometimes been used (*compensatory hydrocephalus* or '*hydrocephalus ex vacuo*') to embrace cases in which the amount of CSF within the cranial cavity is increased in order to compensate for cerebral atrophy, whatever its cause. Thus dilatation of the cerebral ventricles and an increased volume of CSF overlying the cortex and within the sulci is generally seen in patients with presenile or senile dementia solely as a consequence of loss of brain substance, but this finding is not now generally regarded as a form of hydrocephalus.

Hydrocephalus as now conventionally defined embraces those conditions in which there is at some stage an increased volume (and usually pressure) of CSF within the cranial cavity (sometimes called *hypertensive hydrocephalus*) due to: (1) increased formation of CSF; (2) obstruction to the flow of fluid at some point between the choroid plexuses of the lateral ventricles from which it is secreted and the arachnoidal villi in the sagittal sinus through which it is reabsorbed; and (3) impaired absorption of the fluid due to inflammation of the arachnoid (as in meningitis) or to thrombosis of the sagittal sinus.

Increased formation

Papilloedema and increased pressure were described in vitamin A deficient animals by Millen and Woollam (1958) who suggested that deficiency of this vitamin in infants, or in their mothers during pregnancy, might cause hydrocephalus. Whether this rare syndrome gives overproduction of CSF or deficient absorption due to squamous metaplasia of the arachnoid villi (Davson 1967) and whether it occurs in man remains undecided. The only clinical disorder in which hydrocephalus clearly results from increased production of fluid is that of choroid plexus papilloma (Guthkelch 1972); in such cases removal of the tumour is usually curative but occasionally, despite successful removal, hydrocephalus persists (McDonald 1969).

Obstructed circulation

Obstruction to the CSF circulation may occur at any point of its course. Within the ventricles the commonest cause is a neoplasm compressing one or both interventricular foramina or filling the third ventricle. The cerebral aqueduct may be obstructed by a tumour arising in the third ventricle, midbrain, or pineal body, or may be congenitally narrowed or even absent. Owing to its small calibre, slight swelling of its ependymal lining may lead to its obstruction, and cases have been reported in which hydrocephalus has been due to gliosis caused by ependymitis in this region. Aqueduct stenosis is a cause of infantile hydrocephalus and may give rise to increased intracranial pressure for the first time in adult life (McHugh 1964; Harrison, Robert, and Uttley 1974). The cause is unknown but the demonstration by Johnson, Johnson, and Edmonds (1967) and by Johnson and Johnson (1968) that aqueduct stenosis and hydrocephalus can be induced in suckling hamsters by inoculating mumps virus may be relevant. Restricted pulsatile flow of CSF during systole (White, Wilson, Carry, and Stevenson 1979) and associated congenital abnormalities (McMillan and Williams 1977) may also play a part.

Subtentorial tumours may obstruct the fourth ventricle. Its foramina may be blocked by a congenital septum (the Dandy–Walker syndrome), by adhesions following meningitis, or by displacement of the medulla into the foramen magnum by the pressure of a tumour. The Dandy–Walker syndrome may be due to atresia of the foramina of Magendie and Luschka or to dysplasia of the cerebellum developing early in fetal life, as the cerebellar vermis is often absent or vestigial in such cases (Benda 1954; Brodal and Hauglie-Hanssen 1959; Hart, Malamud, and Ellis 1972). The malformation may be accompanied by extra-axial leptomeningeal cysts in the posterior fossa (Haller, Wolpert, Rabe, and Hills 1971), while such cysts alone may give a similar clinical and radiological picture. Within the subarachnoid space, obstruction may again be due to tumour, to adhesions following trauma, inflammation, or haemorrhage, or to congenital abnormalities such as basilar impression or the Arnold-Chiari malformation.

The Arnold–Chiari malformation consists of congenital displacement of the cerebellar tonsils and of an elongated medulla oblongata downwards into the cervical canal. It prevents the egress of CSF from the fourth ventricle into the subarachnoid space; it is sometimes associated with lumbosacral spina bifida and with meningocele or meningomyelocele, but the Chiari type I anomaly consists of a simple ectasia of the cerebellar tonsils without any other primary malformation of the neuraxis. MacFarlane and Maloney (1957) found congenital narrowing of the cerebral aqueduct sufficient to cause hydrocephalus in 10 of 20 such cases. Gardner (1965) suggested that a Chiari malformation or, less often, the Dandy-Walker syndrome may result in dilatation of the central canal of the spinal cord early in life (hydromyelia) and that this, in turn, is the commonest mechanism producing syringomyelia. The observations of Appleby, Foster, Hankinson, and Hudgson (1968) and Barnett, Foster, and Hudgson (1974) support this view.

Impaired absorption

Absorption of fluid from the arachnoid villi may be restricted by a rise in the intracranial venous pressure, due to compression of

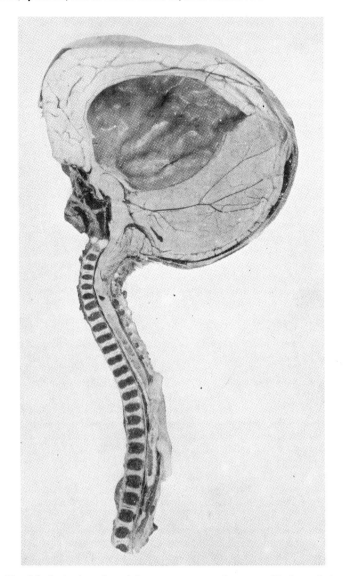

Fig. 3.2. Sagittal section of the nervous system in a case of hydrocephalus due to the Arnold–Chiari malformation. Note the abnormal cerebellum and the spina bifida. (By courtesy of the Photographic Department of the Hospital for Sick Children, Great Ormond Street, London.)

venous sinuses by an intracranial tumour, or impairment of venous drainage from the head by raised intrathoracic pressure in cases of intrathoracic neoplasm or pulmonary hypertension. Thrombosis of the superior sagittal sinus caused by extension of inflammation from the transverse sinus is one cause of the condition 'otitic hydrocephalus', in which symptoms of hydrocephalus complicate otitis media or mastoiditis (Symonds 1931, 1937), but most such patients are suffering from benign intracranial hypertension (p. 140). The arachnoid villi may also be obstructed by inflammatory, neoplastic, or leukaemic cells in infective or neoplastic meningitis.

Classification

Hypertensive hydrocephalus can be further subdivided into:

(a) *Obstructive hydrocephalus* (once called internal hydrocephalus), in which there is an obstruction to the circulation of the CSF, either within the ventricles or aqueduct or at the outlet from the fourth ventricle, which prevents free communication between the ventricles and the subarachnoid space, and

(b) *Communicating hydrocephalus* (once called external hydrocephalus), in which hydrocephalus is due either to disturbance in the formation and absorption of CSF, or to an obstruction to its circulation in the subarachnoid space itself. Hakim and Adams (1965) distinguished a form of communicating hydrocephalus, usually occurring in late life, which they called *low-pressure hydrocephalus* since although the cerebral ventricles are dilated the pressure within them at the time of measurement is either normal or only slightly raised (see below).

Laurence (1959) in 100 consecutive post-mortem examinations found that malformation alone was the cause in only 14 per cent of cases, but in association with infection or trauma it accounted for 46 per cent. Inflammatory reaction due to infection or haemorrhage without malformation accounted for another 50 per cent, the remaining 4 per cent being due to tumours. Thus malformation was present in 46 per cent and inflammation in 82 per cent. Cohen (1965), reviewing the radiological findings in Macnab's (1962) series of 200, found that 18 per cent were due to aqueduct block, 42 per cent to cistern block, and 40 per cent were associated with an Arnold-Chiari malformation (Fig. 3.2).

In the past, a distinction was often made between 'congenital' and 'acquired' hydrocephalus but this distinction is artificial. A congenital abnormality alone is the most likely cause of hydrocephalus developing before birth but congenital and acquired factors often both contribute to hydrocephalus in infancy. Nor do congenital factors cease to operate later since hydrocephalus developing in adult life may be the late result of aqueduct stenosis or Chiari malformation.

The commoner causes of hydrocephalus developing in the absence of congenital abnormality are meningeal adhesions following meningitis, arachnoiditis of obscure origin, thrombosis of intracranial venous sinuses, and intracranial tumour. Syphilitic meningitis or arachnoiditis following subarachnoid bleeding are rare causes. Obstruction within the third or fourth ventricle or in the subarachnoid space, is occasionally due to parasitic cysts.

Incidence

The incidence of all neural malformations, including hydrocephalus, has been shown to vary considerably between different countries, being much higher, for instance, in Scotland and Ireland than in Japan. In the United States, between 1959 and 1961, congenital malformations of the nervous system accounted for 94 deaths per 100 000 population in infants under one year of age, and 27 of these were due to hydrocephalus; the incidence was higher in the east, and especially the north-east, than elsewhere (Kurtzke, Goldberg, and Kurland 1973).

Pathology

Distension of the cerebral ventricles is the most conspicuous feature. When obstruction occurs in the aqueduct, only the lateral and third ventricles are distended. When the obstruction is more caudally situated, the aqueduct and fourth ventricle may also be enlarged. Ventricular distension causes thinning of the cerebral hemispheres, which in severe cases may be extreme and is associated with marked atrophy of the white matter and loss of cortical ganglion cells. The ventricular ependyma is normal, except in inflammatory cases, when a localized or diffuse ependymitis may be present. Meningeal adhesions indicate previous meningitis. Distension of the ventricles leads to pressure upon the calvarium, which becomes thin, especially over the cerebral gyri. Separation of the sutures occurs when hydrocephalus develops in early life, but is not seen as a rule after the age of 18. Compression of the base of the skull causes erosion of the clinoid processes and excavation of the sella turcica. The olfactory tracts and optic nerves are often atrophic.

Symptoms and signs

Infantile hydrocephalus
Englargement of the head is the most conspicuous sign in infantile hydrocephalus (Fig.3.3). It may occur before birth, but is often more evident during the first few weeks of life owing to the large head, prominent scalp veins, and turning down of the eyes ('rising sun sign'). In most cases it is slowly progressive and the head may attain a huge size, with a circumference of 75 cm or even more. The cranial sutures are widely separated and the anterior fontanelle is much enlarged. There is marked congestion of scalp veins. In extreme cases the head is translucent and yields a fluid thrill on percussion and an audible murmur on auscultation. Enlargement of the head occurs in all its diameters. The frontal region bulges forwards, and downward pressure upon the orbital plates causes the eyes to be protruded forwards and downwards. As the head becomes too heavy for the child to lift, gravity, acting upon it in the supine position, in time causes it to become relatively larger in the coronal than in the sagittal plane.

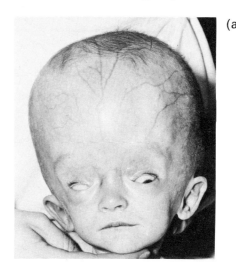

(a)

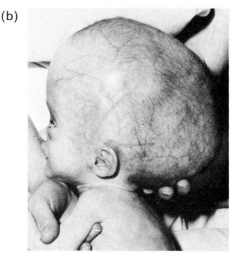

(b)

Fig. 3.3. (a) and (b). Gross enlargement of the head in an infant with obstructive hydrocephalus associated with a lumbar meningomyelocele and an Arnold–Chiari malformation. (Photographs kindly supplied by Mr L.P. Lassman.)

Owing to expansibility of the skull in infancy, symptoms of increased intracranial pressure are slight or absent. Hydrocephalic children seem little troubled by headache and rarely vomit. Convulsions are common. Bilateral anosmia may occur. Optic atrophy due to pressure upon the nerves is usually present, but in some cases there is papilloedema, and this may be superimposed upon optic atrophy. Papilloedema does not occur when the subarachnoid space is blocked. Visual acuity may be progressively reduced until the child becomes blind. Paralysis of other cranial nerves may occur, and squint is not uncommon. Nystagmus may be present. In the limbs there are usually weakness and incoordination, generally more marked in the lower than in the upper limbs. Spasticity with exaggeration of tendon reflexes is common in the lower limbs, though sometimes tendon reflexes are lost. The plantar reflexes are usually extensor. There is little or no disturbance of sensibility. The mental state varies in different cases. In severe cases there is usually dementia, but in milder cases this is slight or absent. Intelligence may be unimpaired even when ventricular dilatation is such that only 1 cm thickness of cerebral substance remains between the ventricles and the inner skull table. In milder cases there may be obesity and/or diabetes insipidus due to compression of the hypothalamus and pituitary, in more severe cases wasting. Cerebrospinal rhinorrhoea is a rare complication. An apparently unique hydrocephalic syndrome, the 'bobble-head doll syndrome' (Tomasoric, Nellhaus, and Moe 1975; Menkes 1980) is characterized by two to four oscillations of the head per minute with psychomotor retardation and results from obstructive lesions in or near the third ventricle or aqueduct.

Hydrocephalus after infancy

The clinical picture of hydrocephalus after infancy varies according to its cause. In obstructive hydrocephalus symptoms of increased intracranial pressure are conspicuous. Headache and vomiting are early symptoms and are often followed by the development of papilloedema. The headache is at first paroxysmal, but later becomes constant, and there are sometimes intense exacerbations characterized by severe headache radiating down the neck and associated with head retraction and even with opisthotonos, vomiting, and impairment of consciousness. Giddiness is a common symptom. Some mental deterioration usually occurs after a time, especially in later life, and hallucinations, delusions, and mood changes may occur. Convulsions are less common than in the infantile variety, and enlargement of the head does not occur after the age of 18. Before that age there is often slight separation of the cranial sutures, yielding a 'cracked-pot sound' on percussion and associated with venous congestion of the scalp. Cranial-nerve palsies may occur, especially paresis of the sixth and seventh nerves, and symptomatic trigeminal neuralgia or facial sensory loss have been reported (Maurice-Williams and Pilling 1977). Slight exophthalmos is not uncommon. Gross weakness of the limbs is absent, though clumsiness and slight incoordination are common. The tendon reflexes may be exaggerated or diminished. The plantar reflexes are often extensor. There is usually no sensory loss. Symptoms of hypopituitarism, obesity, and genital atrophy, are common in children and adolescents.

The pressure of CSF is generally increased at first but is often normal or may even be diminished late in the course of both communicating and obstructive hydrocephalus. In the syndrome of *'low-pressure hydrocephalus'* (Hakim and Adams 1965), fluctuating confusion, ataxia, and progressive dementia are the most prominent features; characteristically such patients often deteriorate strikingly following air encephalography which demonstrates marked dilatation of all the ventricles but no air diffuses over the cortex. The CT scan has proved helpful but the findings are not invariably conclusive, although it may show associated cortical atrophy, not revealed by air encephalography, in some such cases (Jacobs and Kinkel 1976); there is no apparent correlation between the presence or absence of such atrophy and postoperative ventricular size on the one hand or the clinical response to ventricular shunting (see below) on the other (*British Medical Journal* 1980). Large ventricles and small sulci shown on the CT scan, however, are suggestive of this condition, and continuous intracranial pressure monitoring, showing significant 'B' waves for at least two hours a day (Symon, Dorsch, and Stephens 1972; Crockard, Hanlon, Duda, and Mullan 1977), has been found helpful in identifying patients who may benefit from surgery. Thus, while the CSF pressure is usually normal or low, transient episodes of raised pressure occur in many cases. Serial psychometric tests are useful in assessing the response to treatment. The condition usually presents in middle or late life, sometimes with dementia alone (Crowell, Tew, and Mark 1973) or with the clinical picture of the parkinsonism–dementia complex (Sypert, Leffman, and Ojemann 1973) and 'drop' attacks are common (Botez, Ethier, Leveille, and Botez-Marquard 1977). Messert and Wannamaker (1974) suggested that cases selected for surgical treatment should have: (1) dementia, apraxia of gait, and incontinence; (2) a progressive course; (3) diagnostic air encephalography; and (4) definite evidence of block on RISA cisternography (Spoerri and Rösler 1966; Bannister, Gilford, and Kocen 1967; Harbert 1973). McCullough, Harbert, di Chiro, and Ommaya (1970) found a good correlation between ventricular stasis demonstrated by such RISA cisternograms on the one hand and clinical improvement after operation on the other. Measurement of the rate of clearance of intrathecal RISA into the plasma is also useful (Abbott and Alksne 1968). The cause of the communicating hydrocephalus in most such cases is unexplained though it may follow subarachnoid haemorrhage or develop many years after recovery from meningitis. Differential diagnosis from cerebral atrophy in presenile dementia is clearly important as shunting operations are of no value in the latter condition; however, no single method is absolutely reliable.

CSF changes and radiology

In most forms of obstructive and communicating hydrocephalus not due to tumour or meningeal inflammation, the CSF is normal in composition but Rogers and Dubowitz (1970) found that 5–HIAA (hydroxyindole acetic acid) was consistently raised in the ventricular CSF of 40 hydrocephalic children. Radiographs of the skull (Fig. 3.4) may show enlargement of the calvarium, with suture diastasis, thinning, and exaggeration of convolutional markings, but the latter finding alone may be normal and is an unreliable guide to raised intracranial pressure. Separation of the sutures may be present in children. The clinoid processes are often eroded and the sella turcica is deepened and expanded anteroposteriorly. Ventriculograms show enormous dilatation of the ventricular system (Fig. 3.4) and the sweep of the anterior cerebral arteries is increased in angiograms. Ventriculography with contrast medium may be needed to show the site of an obstruction. Isotope ventriculography or cisternography is not only useful in the diagnosis of communicating hydrocephalus but may also identify the site of leakage of CSF into the nasal cavity (CSF rhinorrhoea) which is an occasional complication of all forms of hydrocephalus.

Diagnosis

The diagnosis of infantile hydrocephalus is not usually difficult in view of the cranial enlargement. The rare condition of megalencephaly can be distinguished only by CT scan and ventriculography.

After infancy hydrocephalus often complicates the many conditions which cause increased intracranial pressure. Recognizing the hydrocephalus is usually simple. The discovery of its cause calls for the appropriate investigations of which radiographs and the CT scan are the most important. Spina bifida may suggest the presence of the Arnold–Chiari malformation. Brock, Bolton, and Scrimgeour (1974) and Wald, Brock, and Bonnar (1974) showed that estimation of the maternal plasma alpha-fetoprotein may be a reliable guide to the presence of fetal anencephaly or spina bifida and may allow early antenatal diagnosis and therapeutic abortion.

Benign intracranial hypertension

This term was used by Foley (1955) to describe a persistent rise of CSF pressure in the absence of a space-occupying lesion and with ventricles of normal or even reduced size. This syndrome, also called 'toxic hydrocephalus', occurs in two groups of patients. One

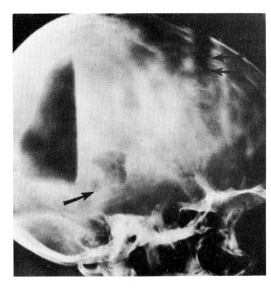

Fig. 3.4. A ventriculogram of a child with hydrocephalus due to aqueduct stenosis (single arrow) showing gross dilatation of the lateral ventricles. Note also the suture diastasis (double arrows)

consists predominantly of women, with a peak incidence in the fourth decade. The patient is often obese, and there is an association with pregnancy and miscarriage; in a smaller group, affecting the sexes equally, there is a previous history of middle-ear disease, non-specific infection, or mild head injury (Johnston and Paterson 1974*a*). In these cases the condition appears to be due to a diffuse cerebral oedema of unknown cause. Many pathogenetic mechanisms have been postulated to explain this brain swelling, including hypervitaminosis A (Feldman and Schlezinger 1970), the administration of tetracycline for the treatment of acne (Walters and Gubbay 1981), an abnormality of the cerebral microvasculature with increased water content of the brain (Raichle, Grubb, Phelps, Gado, and Caronna 1978), increased CSF production associated with an increase in circulating oestrone (Donaldson 1981), and increased CSF outflow resistance (Johnston and Paterson 1974*b*; Aisenberg and Rottenberg 1980). In a series of 34 cases reported by Boddie, Banna, and Bradley (1974), only 44 per cent showed small lateral ventricles and in many others the ventricular volume was increased radiologically. Nevertheless, the CT scan has shown that the ventricles are usually small (Reid, Matheson, and Teasdale 1980). In so-called 'otitic hydrocephalus', which is sometimes due to transverse or sagittal sinus thrombosis secondary to otitis, again the pressure of the fluid is raised but usually without ventricular enlargement. Papilloedema is constant, headache and vomiting are common though often not severe, and diplopia may occur. Symptoms and signs suggesting focal cerebral dysfunction are sometimes seen in the acute stage and transient paresis of one sixth or third cranial nerve is relatively common (McCammon, Kaufman, and Sears 1981). Despite their troublesome headache and high papilloedema, many affected patients seem surprisingly well. The condition, whether 'idiopathic' or 'otitic', is benign and if appropriately treated (see below) the prognosis is excellent on follow-up (Boddie *et al.* 1974; Bulens, de Vries, and van Crevel 1979) but in the acute stage papilloedema may constitute a serious threat to vision, and blindness or permanent central scotomas have been recorded.

Prognosis

Untreated infantile hydrocephalus is often fatal during the first few years of life, but Macnab (1966) showed that the average hydrocephalic alive at 3 months had a 26 per cent chance of reaching adult life without surgery, and if he survived to between 1 and 2 years he had a 50 per cent chance. Some who survive have mental retardation, epilepsy, or blindness. Laurence (1969) confirmed that, even in aqueduct stenosis, the hydrocephalic process often arrests spontaneously. In 41 per cent of 70 cases without spina bifida the IQ after 6 years was over 85, in 29 per cent below 50. There was a close relationship between IQ on the one hand and physical disability (e.g. spasticity and ataxia) and the severity of hydrocephalus on the other. In the past many children with the Arnold–Chiari malformation and myelomeningocele died from infection of the sac or hydrocephalus. The introduction of the Spitz-Holter valve has reduced the mortality of hydrocephalus with myelomeningocele to 30 per cent at the end of 2 years and that of uncomplicated hydrocephalus to less than 20 per cent. More recent figures (Milhorat 1972; Menkes 1980) suggest that two-thirds of cases treated surgically have an IQ of 75 or more. The prognosis of hydrocephalus after infancy depends upon its cause and how far this is amenable to treatment.

Treatment

Infantile hydrocephalus

In the past many operations, including excision of the choroid plexus, Torkildsen's ventriculo-cisternostomy, ventriculo-subdural, ventriculo-ureteric, and ventriculo-peritoneal drainage, were used with varying degrees of success, but there is now general agreement that the use of Spitz-Holter or Pudenz-Heyer or similar silastic valves inserted into one lateral ventricle with catheter drainage via a jugular vein into the cardiac atrium is the treatment of choice, even though there is a significant complication rate due to infection, thrombosis, and embolism (Nicholas, Kamal, and Epstein 1970; Noble, Lassman, Urquhart, and Aherne 1970). Colonization of the valves with *Staphylococcus albus* or diptheroids may be asymptomatic for some time. At least two-thirds of all shunts require revision because of infection or obstruction (Milhorat 1978; Menkes 1980). Hammon (1971) prefers ventriculo-peritoneal drainage, but this, too, carries a risk of serious complications (Davidson 1976). With increasing use of these methods, early closure of associated spina bifida sacs, with or without meningomyelocele, has become possible in the first few days and weeks of life, although the careful selection of cases, bearing in mind the prognosis of both the hydrocephalus and the spina bifida, is a matter for the expert and is still a controversial ethical problem (Lorber 1975). Neurological disability, including syringomyelia, resulting from the Arnold–Chiari malformation, may be alleviated in many cases by suboccipital decompression. In some neonatal cases with mild or moderate hydrocephalus and normal or slightly increased intracranial pressure, compressive head wrapping (Epstein, Hochwald, and Ransohoff 1973) seems helpful in promoting increased CSF absorption.

Hydrocephalus after infancy

The appropriate treatment of hydrocephalus after infancy depends upon its cause. When it is due to an intracranial tumour this must receive appropriate surgical treatment whenever possible. When there is a tumour in the third ventricle or midbrain or in some other area which is causing obstruction but cannot be removed or treated effectively by radiotherapy, temporary improvement may result from a shunting operation with insertion of a valve as in infancy, and a similar procedure may be dramatically successful in communicating 'low-pressure' hydrocephalus. While early reports were encouraging, with about two-thirds of all patients showing early intellectual as well as physical improvement, after three years less than half demonstrated continuing benefit (Greenberg, Shenkin, and Adam 1977) and Gustafson and Hagberg (1978) had a similar experience. In yet another series of patients only a third were improved (Hughes, Siegel, Coxe, Gado, Grubb, Coleman, and Berg 1978) and 50 per cent of a similar group of patients not operated upon failed to deteriorate over a three-year period; the surgical group also showed a high incidence of complications. Thus early optimism has not been borne out by long-term results; in some long-standing cases, there are irreversible neuropathological changes somewhat similar to those of Alzheimer's disease (Ball 1976).

In benign intracranial hypertension, treatment with high doses of steroids (dexamethasone or betamethasone 5 mg four times a day) is usually obligatory and rapidly reduces cerebral oedema and the threat to vision. In occasional cases with severe papilloedema and rapidly failing vision, surgical subtemporal decompression may still be needed as an emergency measure. Dehydrating agents such as diuretics (chlorthalidone, frusemide) may also be of some value (Jefferson and Clark 1976) but are now generally recognized to be inferior to steroid treatment in the acute phase. However, these remedies have been found useful for maintenance therapy in subacute cases.

References

Abbott, M. and Alksne, J. F. (1968). Transport of intrathecal I^{125} RISA to circulating plasma; a test for communicating hydrocephalus. *Neurology, Minneapolis* **18**, 870.

Aisenberg, R. M. and Rottenberg, D. A. (1980). The pathogenesis of pseudotumor cerebri: a mathematical analysis. *J. neurol. Sci.* **48**, 51.

Appleby, A., Foster, J. B., Hankinson, J., and Hudgson, P. (1968). The diagnosis and management of the Chiari anomalies in adult life. *Brain* **91**, 131.

Ball, M. J. (1976). Neurofibrillary tangles in the dementia of 'normal pressure' hydrocephalus. *Can. J. neurol. Sci.* **3**, 227.

Bannister, R., Gilford, E., and Kocen, R. (1967). Isotope encephalography in the diagnosis of dementia due to communicating hydrocephalus. *Lancet* ii, 1014.

Barnett, H. J., Foster, J. B., and Hudgson, P. (1974). *Syringomyelia*, Major problems in neurology. Vol. 1. Saunders, London.

Benda, C. E. (1954). The Dandy–Walker syndrome or the so-called atresia of the foramen Magendie. *J. Neuropath. exp. Neurol.* **13**, 14.

Boddie, H. G., Banna, M., and Bradley, W. G. (1974). 'Benign' intracranial hypertension—a survey of the clinical and radiological features, and long-term prognosis. *Brain* **97**, 313.

Botez, M. I., Ethier, R., Leveille, J., and Botez-Marquard, T. (1977). A syndrome of early recognition of occult hydrocephalus and cerebral atrophy. *Quart. J. Med.* **46**, 365.

British Medical Journal (1980). Cerebral atrophy or hydrocephalus? *Br. med. J.* **1**, 348.

Brock, D. J. H., Bolton, A. E., and Scrimgeour, J. B. (1974). Prenatal diagnosis of spina bifida and anencephaly through maternal plasma–alpha–fetoprotein measurement. *Lancet* i, 767.

Brodal, A. and Hauglie-Hanssen, E. (1959). Congenital hydrocephalus with defective development of the cerebellar vermis (Dandy–Walker syndrome). *J. Neurol. Neurosurg. Psychiat.* **22**, 99.

Bulens, C., de Vries, W. A. E. J., and Van Crevel, H. (1979). Benign intracranial hypertension: a retrospective and follow-up study. *J. neurol. Sci.* **40**, 147.

Cohen, S. J. (1965). See Macnab (1966).

Crockard, H. A., Hanlon, K., Duda, E. E., and Mullan, J. F. (1977). Hydrocephalus as a cause of dementia: evaluation by computerised tomography and intracranial pressure monitoring. *J. Neurol. Neurosurg. Psychiat.* **40**, 736.

Crowell, R. M., Tew, J. M., and Mark, V. H. (1973). Aggressive dementia associated with normal pressure hydrocephalus. Report of two unusual cases. *Neurology, Minneapolis* **23**, 461.

Dandy, W. E. (1918). Extirpation of the choroid plexus of the lateral ventricles in communicating hydrocephalus. *Ann. Surg.* **68**, 569.

Davidson, R. I. (1976). Peritoneal bypass in the treatment of hydrocephalus: historical review and abdominal complications. *J. Neurol. Neurosurg. Psychiat.* **39**, 640.

Davson, H. (1967). *The physiology of the cerebrospinal fluid.* Churchill, London.

Donaldson, J. O. (1981). Pathogenesis of pseudotumor cerebri syndromes. *Neurology, Minneapolis* **31**, 877.

Epstein, F., Hochwald, G. M., and Ransohoff, J. (1973). Neonatal hydrocephalus treated by compressive head wrapping. *Lancet.* i, 634.

Feldman, M. H. and Schlezinger, N. S. (1970). Benign intracranial hypertension associated with hypervitaminosis A. *Arch. Neurol. Chicago.* **22**, 1.

Foley, J. (1955). Benign forms of intracranial hypertension in 'toxic' and 'otitic' hydrocephalus. *Brain* **78**, 1.

Gardner, W. J. (1965). Hydrodynamic mechanism in syringomyelia: its relationship to myelocele. *J. Neurol. Neurosurg. Psychiat.* **28**, 247.

Globus, J. H. and Strauss, I. (1928). Subacute diffuse ependymitis, *Arch. Neurol. Psychiat. Chicago.* **19**, 623.

Greenberg, J. O., Shenkin, H. A., and Adam, R. (1977). Idiopathic normal pressure hydrocephalus—a report of 73 patients. *J. Neurol. Neurosurg. Psychiat.* **40**, 336.

Gustafson, L. and Hagberg, B. O. (1978). Recovery in hydrocephalic dementia after shunt operation. *J. Neurol. Neurosurg. Psychiat.* **41**, 940.

Guthkelch, A. N. (1972). High pressure hydrocephalus. In *Scientific foundations of neurology* (ed. M. Critchley, J. L. O'Leary and W. B. Jennett) Section VIII, Chapter 3. Heinemann, London.

Hakim, S. and Adams, R. D. (1965). The special clinical problem of symptomatic hydrocephalus with normal cerebrospinal fluid pressure. *J. neurol. Sci.* **2**, 307.

Haller, J. S., Wolpert, S. M., Rabe, E. F., and Hills, J. R. (1971). Cystic lesions of the posterior fossa in infants: a comparison of the clinical, radiological, and pathological findings in Dandy–Walker syndrome and extra-axial cysts. *Neurology, Minneapolis* **21**, 494.

Hammon, W. M. (1971). Evaluation and use of the ventriculo-peritoneal shunt in hydrocephalus. *J. Neurosurg.* **34**, 792.

Harbert, J. C. (1973). Radionuclide cisternography in adult hydrocephalus. *Proc. R. Soc. Med.* **66**, 827.

Harrison, M. J. G., Robert, C. M., and Uttley, D. (1974). Benign aqueduct stenosis in adults. *J. Neurol. Neurosurg. Psychiat.* **37**, 1322.

Hart, M. N., Malamud, N., and Ellis, W. G. (1972). The Dandy–Walker syndrome. A clinicopathological study based on 28 cases. *Neurology, Minneapolis* **22**, 771.

Hughes, C. P., Siegel, B. A., Coxe, W. S., Gado, M. H., Grubb, R. L., Coleman, R. E., and Berg, L. (1978). Adult idiopathic communicating hydrocephalus with and without shunting. *J. Neurol. Neurosurg. Psychiat.* **41**, 961.

Jacobs, L. and Kinkel, W. (1976). Computerized axial transverse tomography in normal pressure hydrocgphalus. *Neurology, Minneapolis.* **26**, 501.

Jefferson, A. and Clark, J. (1976). Treatment of benign intracranial hypertension by dehydrating agents with particular reference to the measurement of the blind spot area as a means of recording improvement. *J. Neurol. Neurosurg. Psychiat.* **39**, 627.

Johnson, R. T. and Johnson, K. P. (1968). Hydrocephalus following viral infection: the pathology of aqueductal stenosis developing after experimental mumps virus infection. *J. Neuropathol. exp. Neurol.* **27**, 591.

——, ——, and Edmonds, C. J. (1967). Virus-induced hydrocephalus: development of aqueductal stenosis in hamsters after mumps infection. *Science* **157**, 1066.

Johnston, I. and Paterson, A. (1974a). Benign intracranial hypertension. I. Diagnosis and prognosis. *Brain* **97**, 289.

—— and —— (1974b). Benign intracranial hypertension II. CSF pressure and circulation. *Brain* **97**, 301.

Kurtzke, J. F., Goldberg, I. D., and Kurland, L. T. (1973). The distribution of deaths from congenital malformations of the nervous system. *Neurology, Minneapolis* **23**, 483.

Laurence, K. M. (1959). The pathology of hydrocephalus. *Ann. R. Coll. Surg. Engl.* **24**, 388.

—— (1969). Neurological and intellectual sequelae of hydrocephalus. *Arch. Neurol., Chicago.* **20**, 73.

Lorber, J. (1975). Ethical problems in the management of myelomeningocele and hydrocephalus. *J. R. Coll. Phycns.* **10**, 47.

MacFarlane, A. and Maloney, A. F. J. (1957). The appearance of the aqueduct and its relationship to hydrocephalus in the Arnold–Chiari malformation. *Brain* **80**, 479.

Macnab, G. H. (1962). *see* Macnab, G. H. (1966).

Macnab, G. H. (1966). The development of the knowledge and treatment of hydrocephalus. In *Hydrocephalus and spina bifida*, p. 1. National Spastics Society. Heinemann, London.

Maurice-Williams, R. S. and Pilling, J. (1977). Trigeminal sensory symptoms associated with hydrocephalus. *J. Neurol. Neurosurg. Psychiat.* **40**, 641.

McCammon, A., Kaufman, H. H., and Sears, E. S. (1981). Transient oculomotor paralysis in pseudotumor cerebri. *Neurology, Minneapolis* **31**, 182.

McCullough, D. C., Harbert, J. C., di Chiro, G., and Ommaya, A. K. (1970). Prognostic criteria for cerebrospinal fluid shunting from isotope cisternography in communicating hydrocephalus. *Neurology, Minneapolis* **20**, 594.

McDonald, J. V. (1969). Persistent hydrocephalus following the removal of papillomas of the choroid plexus of the lateral ventricles. *J. Neurosurg.* **30**, 736.

McHugh, P. R. (1964). Occult hydrocephalus. *Quart. J. Med.* **33**, 297.

McMillan, J. J. and Williams, B. (1977). Aqueduct stenosis—case review and discussion. *J. Neurol. Neurosurg. Psychiat.* **40**, 521.

Menkes, J. H. (1980). *Textbook of child neurology*, 2nd edn. Lea and Febiger, Philadelphia.

Messert, B. and Wannamaker, B. B. (1974). Reappraisal of the adult occult hydrocephalus syndrome. *Neurology, Minneapolis.* **24**, 224.

Milhorat, T. H. (1972). *Hydrocephalus and the cerebrospinal fluid.* Williams and Wilkins, Baltimore.

—— (1978). Hydrocephalus. In *Paediatric neurosurgery.* F. A. Davis, Philadelphia.

Millen, J. W. and Woollam, D. H. M. (1958). *Vitamins and the cerebrospinal fluid. Ciba Foundation Symposium on the Cerebrospinal Fluid.* p. 168. Ciba Foundation, London.

Nicholas, J. L., Kamal, I. M., and Eckstein, H. B. (1970). Immediate shunt replacement in the treatment of bacterial colonisation of Holter valves. In *Studies in hydrocephalus and spina bifida, Develop. Med. Child Neurol. suppl.* **22**, p. 110.

Noble, T. C., Lassman, L. P., Urquhart, W., and Aherne, W. A. (1970). Thrombotic and embolic complications of ventriculo-atrial shunts. In *Studies in hydrocephalus and spina bifida, Develop. Med. Child Neurol.* suppl. 22, p. 114.

Raichle, M. E., Grubb, R. L., Phelps, M. E., Gado, M. H., and Caronna, J. J. (1978). Cerebral hemodynamics and metabolism in pseudotumor cerebri. *Ann. Neurol.* **4**, 104.

Reid, A. C., Matheson, M. S., and Teasdale, G. (1980). Volume of the ventricles in benign intracranial hypertension. *Lancet*, ii, 7.

Rogers, K. J. and Dubowitz, V. (1970). 5-Hydroxyindoles in hydrocephalus. A comparative study of cerebrospinal fluid and blood levels. *Develop. Med. Child Neurol.* **12**, 461.

Scarff, J. E. (1963). Treatment of hydrocephalus: an historical and critical review of methods and results. *J. Neurol. Neurosurg. Psychiat.* **26**, 1.

Spoerri, O. and Rösler, H. (1966). Isotope ventriculography with I^{131} and I^{125} in the evaluation of hydrocephalus. In *Hydrocephalus and spina bifida,* p. 88. National Spastics Society. Heinemann, London.

Symon, L., Dorsch, N. W. C., and Stephens, R. J. (1972). Pressure waves in so-called low-pressure hydrocephalus. *Lancet* ii, 1291.

Symonds, C. P. (1931). Otitic hydrocephalus. *Brain* **54**, 55.

—— (1937). Hydrocephalic and focal cerebral symptoms in relation to thrombophlebitis of the dural sinuses and cerebral veins. *Brain* **60**, 531.

Sypert, G. W., Leffman, H., and Ojemann, G. A. (1973). Occult normal pressure hydrocephalus manifested by Parkinsonism–dementia complex. *Neurology, Minneapolis* **23**, 234.

Tomasovic, J. A., Nellhaus, G., and Moe, P. G. (1975). The bobble-head doll syndrome: an early sign of hydrocephalus. *Neurology, Minneapolis* **19**, 533.

Wald, N. J., Brock, D. J. H., and Bonnar, J. (1974). Prenatal diagnosis of spina bifida and anencephaly by maternal serum-alpha-fetoprotein measurement: a controlled study. *Lancet* i 765.

Walters, B. N. J. and Gubbay, S. S. (1981). Tetracycline and benign intracranial hypertension: report of five cases. *Br. med. J.* **282**, 19.

White, D. N., Wilson, K. C., Curry, G. R., and Stevenson, R. J. (1979). The limitation of pulsatile flow through the aqueduct of Sylvius as a cause of hydrocephalus. *J. neurol. Sci.* **42**, 11.

Intracranial tumour

Definition. The term 'intracranial space-occupying lesion' is generally used to identify any lesion, whether vascular, neoplastic, or inflammatory in origin, which increases the volume of the intracranial contents and thus leads to a rise in the intracranial pressure. In the strictest sense the term 'intracranial tumour' should be reserved for neoplasms, whether benign or malignant, primary or secondary, but conventionally this inclusive term is often used to embrace lesions such as vascular malformations and granulomas of inflammatory origin (e.g. gumma and tuberculoma) as well as parasitic cysts, which are not neoplastic in the strict pathological sense.

Aetiology, incidence, and pathogenesis

Over 1 per cent of all deaths are due to intracranial tumours, which form about 10 per cent of all malignant neoplasms in man. Apart from those of inflammatory origin, the aetiology of these tumours is little undertood. In a minority of cases developmental abnormality plays an important part in causation, especially in the angiomas and angioblastomas, the ganglioneuromas, the cholesteatomas, and the craniopharyngiomas. Genetic factors are clearly important in the haemangioblastomas which are often familial, and in neurofibromatosis and tuberous sclerosis, both of which may be associated with intracranial growths; gliomas rarely occur in more than one member of a family (Russell and Rubinstein 1977). The causation of the gliomas is as obscure as that of neoplasms in general. It is uncertain whether the primitive character of the cells of which some gliomas are composed indicates that they are derived from embryonic cell rests or whether this is a cellular regression. While brain tumours have been induced in animals of various species by chemical means, using especially nitrosurea derivatives, or by virus infection (Bigner, Kredar, Thomas, Shaffer, Vick, Engel, and Day 1972), there is no convincing evidence that chemical carcinogens, viruses, or other environmental factors play a significant role in the pathogenesis of primary intracranial neoplasia in man, although the description of intracranial neoplasms of mesenchymal origin (especially reticulum-cell sarcoma) developing in patients after renal transplantation (Schneck and Penn 1971) suggests that iatrogenic immunosuppression may rarely play a part. There is little evidence that trauma is a predisposing factor, except, rarely, in the case of meningiomas which have been known to arise beneath the site of a previous head injury. Although particles resembling myxovirus have been identified in a patient with an intracranial hamartoma (Norris, Aguilar, and Harman 1972) and several viral strains (JC, SV40, BK, MMV) isolated from humans have induced glial neoplasms in animals, while the papovavirus JC has also been identified in a human subject with both multifocal leukoencephalopathy and multifocal glioblastomas, fluorescent antibody staining has failed to demonstrate T antigen, a virally coded nuclear antigen expressed in cells transformed by these viruses, in human gliomas (Spence 1979). Nevertheless, the possibility that some DNA viruses induce tumours in the human nervous system continues to arouse interest (Ibelgaufts 1982). There is also growing evidence to indicate that cell lines derived from human gliomas have surface antigens in common with one another but not with other normal human tissues or nonglial neoplasms (Spence 1979). An increased incidence of prior tuberculous infection in patients with gliomas has been adduced as evidence of defective immunity in such cases (Ward, Mattison, and Finn 1973) and there is evidence that many such tumours contain B lymphocytes which may be involved in host defence against the tumour (Sikora, Alderson, Phillips, and Watson 1982): the presence of lymphocytic infiltrates in such tumours may be associated with longer than average survival (Brooks, Markesbery, Gupta, and Roszman 1978). There is also growing evidence to indicate that the cells of human astrocytomas and other tumours may secrete various proteins and polypeptides, some of which may be neuroactive (McKeever, Quindlen, Banks, Williams, Kornblith, Laversen, Greenwood, and Smith 1981: McDermott, 1982).

An intracranial tumour may occur at any age, though, as will be seen later, certain types of glioma show a characteristic age incidence. The frequent occurrence of some forms of glioma in childhood (Gold and Gordis 1979a) accounts for the fact that the age incidence of intracranial tumours differs from that of most other malignant neoplasms, which are rare before middle life. Intracranial tumour generally affects the sexes equally and shows no significant variation in geographical incidence (Kurtzke 1969) except that tuberculomas and some forms of parasitic cyst are much commoner in under-developed countries. Cole (1978) found 27 previously unsuspected intracranial space-occupying lesions at autopsy in 200 patients dying in a mental hospital in South Africa. Barker, Weller, and Garfield (1976), in a detailed epidemiological survey in the Wessex region of England, found some evidence of geographical clustering of ependymomas, acoustic neuromas, and meningiomas, the latter being commoner in rural rather than urban areas. Gliomas had an average annual incidence of 3.94 per 100 000 population and seemed commoner in social classes 1 and 2 than in classes 4 and 5. Meningiomas (1.23 per 100 000, with a peak incidence of 2.48 per 100 000 at 60–69 years) were significantly commoner in females.

Pathology

Knowledge of the pathology of intracranial neoplasms has advanced greatly during the present century, following upon the work of Cajal, Hortega, and Cushing and his pupils, and is of considerable clinical importance. The different types of tumour, even the different varieties of glioma, often exhibit a characteristic age incidence and rate of growth and a predilection for certain parts of the brain. The clinician can now diagnose with increasing precision not only the presence and situation of an intracranial tumour, but also its precise pathological nature, and can form an accurate estimate of the prospects of its removal and of its probable malignancy. Modern techniques of investigation, including angiography, isotope encephalography, and CT scanning, often not only localize the tumour but give some indication of its pathological nature, and histological examination of biopsy specimens, where appropriate, often gives information of considerable value in determining treatment and prognosis.

In Cushing's (1932b) oft-quoted series of 2 023 intracranial tumours, about 43 per cent were gliomas, 18 per cent pituitary adenomas, 13 per cent meningiomas, 7 per cent sarcomas, and 4 per cent metastases, but since that time the proportion of metastases reported in all series has increased and that of sarcomas and pituitary adenomas has fallen. A representative recent series of 3 010 cases described by Courville (1967) gave the following percentage incidence:

Gliomas   41.5
Pituitary adenomas 3.4
Meningiomas   11.6
Acoustic neuromas 2.5
Congenital tumours 3.5
Metastases 23.7
Granulomatous tumours 2.5
Blood-vessel tumours 7.8
Sarcomas   0.3
Parasitic cysts 0.7
Miscellaneous lesions 2.2

There is now general agreement that gliomas constitute 40–45 per cent of all intracranial neoplasms, metastases about 20 per cent, meningiomas about 10 per cent, and acoustic neuromas and pituitary tumours not more than 5 per cent each. Figures derived from studies in India (Lalitha and Dastur 1980) are similar except that in that country acoustic neuromas are much commoner and metastases are less common.

Gliomas

The gliomas are tumours derived from glial cells but, unlike connective-tissue tumours elsewhere, they are of epiblastic origin. Their precise classification is still unsettled. Systematic examination of complete tumours reveals different types of cell in a single tumour. Moreover, tumours which are histologically identical may behave quite differently, e.g. the cerebral and cerebellar astrocytomas and the more and less rapidly growing oligodendrogliomas. Sometimes a glioma seems to arise diffusely, as in so-called 'gliomatosis cerebri', or from multiple centres at the same time. The diffusely infiltrating cells may be of the astrocytoma or glioblas-

toma series (Couch and Weiss 1974): sometimes diffuse meningeal gliomatosis may also occur (Yung, Horten, and Shapiro 1980). Kernohan, Mabon, Srien, and Adson (1949) recognized only five main groups of primary brain tumours, distinguishing within the group grades of malignancy. Though not universally accepted, their classification, based upon the characteristics of the predominant cell in the tumour in ascending grades of malignancy from 1 to 4, has been widely used. Thus the astrocytoma of Bailey and Cushing (1926) became their astrocytoma grade 1, the astroblastoma grade 2, and the glioblastoma multiforme an astrocytoma grade 3 or 4, depending upon the degree of malignancy. Similarly, the classical ependymoma became an ependymoma grade 1, the ependymoblastoma ependymoma grades 2–4, and the oligodendroglioma and oligodendroblastoma became oligodendrogliomas of grades 1–4. The classification of the medulloblastoma remained unchanged; the rare neurocytomas, ganglioneuromas, gangliocytomas, and gangliogliomas became the neuroastrocytoma grade 1, and the neuroblastoma, spongioneuroblastoma, and glioneuroblastoma were included in the neuroastrocytomas, grades 2–4. However, the World Health Organization has taken advice from 23 reference centres involving 300 pathologists from over 50 countries and has now devised an agreed classification of intracranial tumours including the gliomas (Table 3.1 and Barnard 1982) and the Kernohan classification has been discarded since anaplasia may be so localized a phenomenon that no prognostic value can be attached to the numerical grading of biopsies (Russell and Rubinstein 1977). This new histological classification, based upon the predominant cell type in the tumour, owes much to the pioneer work of Bailey and Cushing (1926). In this classification it is reasonable to regard the tumours of neuroepithelial tissue, including the neuronal tumours which also contain nerve-cell elements, loosely and collectively as gliomas. With the exception of the ependymoma and some pineal-cell tumours, these are all infiltrative neoplasms so that, unless they are very small, they cannot be removed surgically. Moreover, the fact that the glioma may leave nervous tissue which it infiltrates intact explains why a tumour may be much more extensive than would be supposed from the symptoms and physical signs. The most common gliomas are the astrocytomas, about 36 per cent, glioblastomas, about 34 per cent, and medulloblastomas, about 11 per cent.

Medulloblastoma. These are rapidly growing tumours which most often occur in the cerebellum in children, where they arise in the region of the roof of the fourth ventricle, but they are seen rarely in adults. They are composed of masses of rounded undifferentiated cells (Fig. 3.5) and often disseminate through the subarachnoid space both of the brain and of the spinal cord. Other gliomas similarly spread but much less often (Kepes, Striebinger, Brackett, and Kishore 1976); the medulloblastoma is also unique in that it may metastasize outside the cranial cavity giving secondary deposits especially in bone, particularly after partial operative removal or after a shunting operation carried out to relieve hydrocephalus. The medulloblastoma is one of the more malignant gliomas, but total or subtotal surgical removal followed by radiotherapy to the entire neuraxis gives a five-year survival rate of about 40 per cent and a 10-year rate of 20–30 per cent (Spence 1979).

Glioblastoma multiforme. This is an extremely malignant glioma arising in middle life and almost invariably found in the cerebral hemispheres. It infiltrates the brain extensively and often attains an enormous size. It is a reddish, highly vascular tumour, and often exhibits haemorrhages and areas of necrosis (Fig. 3.6). Microscopically it consists of relatively undifferentiated round or oval cells, together with spongioblastic and astroblastic forms; cellular polymorphism with frequent mitoses indicates its anaplastic character (Fig. 3.7). No form of treatment prolongs life for more than a few months, and the average survival is about 12 months.

Table 3.1. *Histological classification of tumours of the central nervous system**

I. **Tumours of Neuroepthelial Tissue**
  A. Astrocytic tumours
    1. Astrocytoma
      a. Fibrillary
      b. Protoplasmic
      c. Gemistocytic
    2. Pilocytic astrocytoma
    3. Subependymal giant-cell astrocytoma (ventricular tumour of tuberous sclerosis)
    4. Astroblastoma
    5. Anaplastic (malignant) astrocytoma
  B. Oligodendroglial tumours
    1. Oligodendroglioma
    2. Mixed oligo-astrocytoma
    3. Anaplastic (malignant) oligodendroglioma
  C. Ependymal and choroid plexus tumours
    1. Ependymoma
    Variants:
      a. Myxopapillary ependymoma
      b. Papillary ependymoma
      c. Subependymoma
    2. Anaplastic (malignant) ependymoma
    3. Choroid plexus papilloma
    4. Anaplastic (malignant) choroid plexus papilloma
  D. Pineal-cell tumours
    1. Pineocytoma (pinealocytoma)
    2. Pineoblastoma (pinealoblastoma)
  E. Neuronal tumours
    1. Gangliocytoma
    2. Ganglioglioma
    3. Ganglioneuroblastoma
    4. Anaplastic (malignant) gangliocytoma and ganglioglioma
    5. Neuroblastoma
  F. Poorly differentiated and embryonal tumours
    1. Glioblastoma
    Variants:
      a. Glioblastoma with sarcomatous component (mixed glioblastoma and sarcoma)
      b. Giant-cell glioblastoma
    2. Medulloblastoma
    Variants:
      a. Desmoplastic medulloblastoma
      b. Medullomyoblastoma
    3. Medulloepithelioma
    4. Primitive polar spongioblastoma
    5. Gliomatosis cerebri

II **Tumours of nerve sheath cells**
  A. Neurilemmoma (Schwannoma, neurinoma)
  B. Anaplastic (malignant) neurilemmoma (Schwannoma, neurinoma)
  C. Neurofibroma
  D. Anaplastic (malignant) neurofibroma (neurofibrosarcoma, neurogenic sarcoma)

III. **Tumours of meningeal and related tissues**
  A. Meningioma
    1. Meningotheliomatous (endotheliomatous, syncytial, arachnotheliomatous)
    2. Fibrous (fibroblastic)
    3. Transitional (mixed)
    4. Psammomatous
    5. Angiomatous
    6. Haemangioblastic
    7. Haemangiopericytic
    8. Papillary
    9. Anaplastic (malignant) meningioma
  B. Meningeal sarcomas
    1. Fibrosarcoma
    2. Polymorphic cell sarcoma
    3. Primary meningeal sarcomatosis
  C. Xanthomatous tumours
    1. Fibroxanthoma
    2. Xanthosarcoma (malignant fibroxanthoma)
  D. Primary melanotic tumours
    1. Melanoma
    2. Meningeal melanomatosis
  E. Others

IV. **Primary malignant lymphomas**

V. **Tumours of blood-vessel origin**
  A. Haemangioblastoma (capillary haemangioblastoma)
  B. Monstrocellular sarcoma

VI. **Germ-cell tumours**
  A. Germinoma
  B. Embryonal carcinoma
  C. Choriocarcinoma
  D. Teratoma

*Reproduced from Barnard (1982) by kind permission of the author and publisher.

Astrocytoma. These tumours have been divided into protoplasmic, fibrillary, pilocytic, and gemistocytic types (Russell and Rubinstein 1977) as well as the more malignant astroblastomas depending upon their predominant cellular constitution. They are usually white, infiltrating growths which may occur at any age, and in either the cerebral (Fig. 3.8) or the cerebellar hemispheres. They grow slowly, are relatively benign, and the average survival period after the first symptom is 67 months in the case of the former and 89 months in the case of the latter. The cerebellar astrocytoma of childhood is a particularly benign tumour. Microscopically (Fig. 3.9) they exhibit abundant astrocytes and, in the case of the fibrillary astrocytomas, a dense fibril network, and the tumour cells exhibit attachments to the blood vessels charac-teristic of the astrocyte. Astrocytomas are particularly liable to undergo cystic transformation. Gliomatous cysts, therefore, have on the whole a favourable prognosis, though cystic change is also fairly common in the glioblastomas.

The *astroblastoma* is somewhat less benign though not as malignant as the glioblastoma multiforme and usually occurs in the white matter of one cerebral hemisphere. Russell and Rubinstein (1959) identified the *polar spongioblastoma* as a relatively benign tumour of childhood or early adult life, occurring especially in the optic nerve and chiasm or brainstem, but this is now regarded as an astrocytoma of pilocytic type (Bernard 1982).

Less common gliomas are:

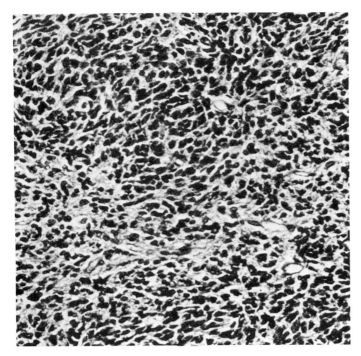

Fig. 3.5. Medulloblastoma, H & E × 160.

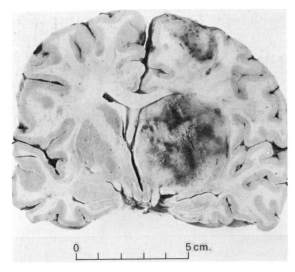

Fig. 3.6. Glioblastoma multiforme involving parietal cortex, centrum semiovale, and basal ganglia of the left cerebral hemisphere with oedema of the affected hemisphere and displacement of the ventricular system.

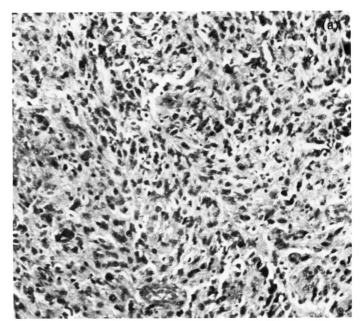

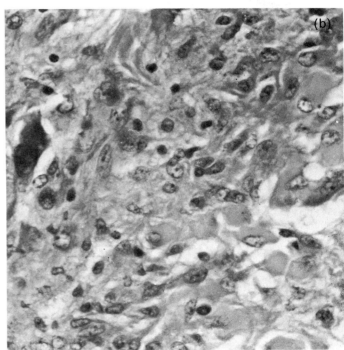

Fig. 3.7. Glioblastoma multiforme. (a) H & E, × 160; (b) H & E, × 400.

Oligodendroglioma. This is an uncommon, slowly growing, and usually relatively benign tumour occurring in the cerebral hemispheres in young adults. Oligodendrogliomas often calcify, giving a fine punctate or stippled pattern (Fig. 3.10) which, on a skull radiograph, may be virtually diagnostic; more malignant forms (oligodendroblastoma) are rare.

Ependymoma. This is a firm, whitish tumour, sometimes pedunculated, arising from the ependyma, frequently in the roof of the fourth ventricle and sometimes from the walls of the other ventricles or from the central canal of the spinal cord. Histologically it shows a characteristic 'rosette' formation (Fig. 3.11).

Neuroblastoma, ganglioglioma, gangliocytoma. These rare tumours all contain ganglion cells (Horten and Rubenstein 1976).

The neuroblastoma, ganglioneuroblastoma, and gangliocytoma are made up predominantly of neuroblasts (neuroastrocytoma grades 2–4), the ganglioglioma shows abnormal ganglion cells lying among proliferating astrocytes or astroblasts, and the gangliocytoma contains not only ganglion cells and astrocytes but also nerve fibres, usually unmyelinated (neuroastrocytoma grade 1). The ganglioneuroblastoma is more malignant, being made up of neuroblasts and primitive astrocytes.

Meningioma

These tumours (Fig. 3.12) were at one time thought to arise from the dura mater and hence were known as dural endotheliomas. It is now known, however, that, although many are attached to the dura, most arise from the arachnoid cells which penetrate the dura to form the arachnoid villi, projecting into the dural venous

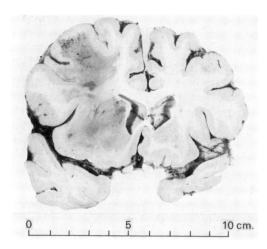

Fig. 3.8. An extensive astrocytoma of the right cerebral hemisphere.

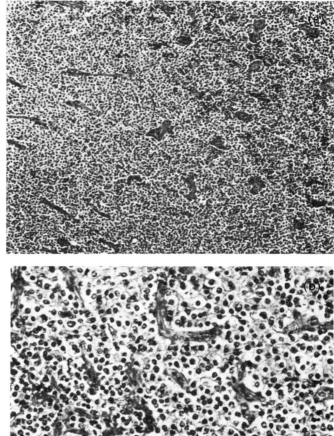

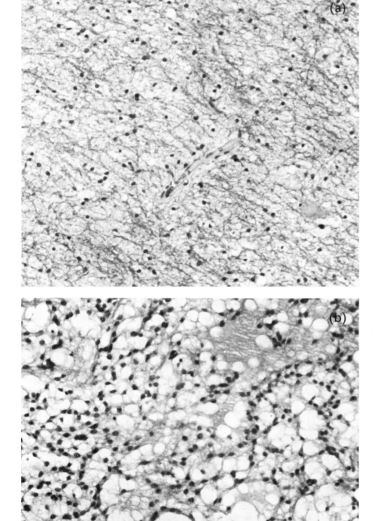

Fig. 3.9. Astrocytoma. (a) Fibrillary type, H & E, × 160; (b) protoplasmic microcystic type, H & E, × 160.

Fig. 3.10. Oligodendroglioma, H & E. Note the areas of calcification. (a) × 64; (b) × 160.

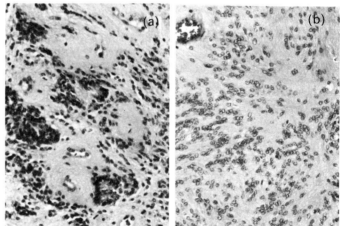

Fig. 3.11. (a) and (b) Two examples of fourth-ventricle ependymomas showing variations in the histological appearance, H & E, × 160.

sinuses. These cells are often present in columns or whorls (Fig. 3.13), and the tumour sometimes contains fibroglia together with collagen fibres and small calcified concretions known as psammoma bodies. Meningotheliomatous (syncytial), fibrous, transitional or mixed, psammomatous, angiomatous (highly vascular), and papillary types have been described (Barnard 1982). Haemorrhage into these tumours is closely correlated with their degree of vascularity (Helle and Conley 1980). The haemangioblastic variety (resembling the capillary haemangioblastoma) and the haemangiopericytic type (which resembles but can be differentiated from the very rare haemangiopericytoma—Choux, Christian, Tripier, Gambarelli, Hassoun, and Toga 1976) are more aggressive and more liable to recur following removal, while the anaplastic (malignant) variety may rarely develop as a primary tumour but more often represents sarcomatous change in a recurrent tumour.

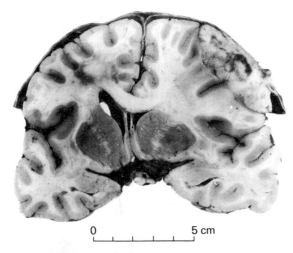

0   5 cm

Fig. 3.12. A left parietal meningioma.

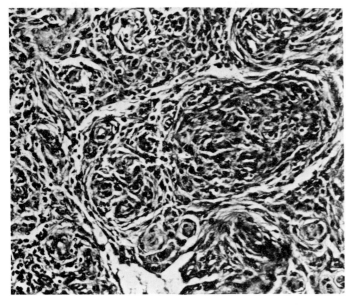

Fig. 3.13. A typical psammomatous meningioma, H & E, × 160.

Commonly the meningioma is a single, large, more or less irregularly lobulated growth, but less frequently it may form a flat plaque spreading over the inner surface of the dura ('meningioma en plaque'). A distinctive feature is the relationship of meningio-

mas to the bones of the skull. Though hyperostosis may occur as a reaction in the overlying bone without its having been invaded, these tumours invade bone in about 20 per cent of cases, resorption of bone and new bone formation occurring simultaneously. The outer table of the skull may then be rebuilt as a bony boss. Microscopically, meningioma cells fill the Haversian canals and spaces. New bone is laid down in spicules perpendicularly to the skull surface, the osteogenetic cells being derived from the outer layers of the dura or from the bone itself. Rarely a meningioma perforates the skull and infiltrates the extracranial tissues. The meningioma, which is of mesodermal origin, does not usually invade the brain but compresses it, and the resulting disturbance of cerebral function is usually much less marked in proportion to the size of the tumour than with the gliomas.

Since the meningiomas arise from cells of the arachnoid villi, they are often found in relation to the intracranial venous sinuses, and their sites of greatest predilection are the superior sagittal sinus—parasagittal meningiomas; the sphenoparietal sinus and middle meningeal vessels—meningiomas of the sphenoid ridge and the convexities; the olfactory groove of the ethmoid; and the circle of sinuses around the sella turcica—suprasellar meningiomas. They are uncommon below the tentorium but may arise from the tentorium itself or at the torcula. Occasionally they are found within the lateral ventricles. They are commoner in women than in men, especially in the spinal canal. Multiple meningiomas may occur in association with multiple neurofibromas (see p. 359) and a familial occurrence has been reported (Delleman, de Jong, and Bleeker 1978).

Reticuloses

Deposits of lymphoma, lymphosarcoma, and of leukaemic cells may, on occasion, develop in the cranial and spinal meninges, giving symptoms of cerebral or spinal compression (John and Nabarro 1955; Hutchinson, Leonard, Maudsley, and Yates 1958; Sohn, Valensi, and Miller 1967; Currie and Henson 1971; West, Graham-Pole, Hardisty, and Pike 1972; Spence 1979; Spillane, Kendall, and Moseley 1982). When deposits are solitary, the CT scan may suggest meningioma, when multiple, cerebral metastases (Spillane *et al.* 1982). Diffuse meningeal involvement may be difficult to differentiate from carcinomatous and meningeal gliomatosis (Ascherl, Hilal, and Brisman 1981). A solitary reticulum-cell sarcoma arising in the cranial bones or spinal column may similarly compress or invade nervous tissue. A reticulum cell sarcoma can also arise within the brain itself giving symptoms and signs of a focal cerebral lesion; alternatively such a neoplasm may arise diffusely throughout the cerebral substance ('microgliomatosis cerebri') (Schaumburg, Plank, and Adams 1972).

Acoustic neuroma

Acoustic neuromas are usually unilateral (Fig. 3.14). Rarely they are bilateral and are then usually, though not always, manifestations of generalized neurofibromatosis. Familial examples of bilateral acoustic neuroma have been reported. A solitary tumour consists of elongated cells like spindle fibroblasts with much collagen and reticulum, and exhibits marked palisading and parallelism of nuclei (Fig. 3.15). Some workers believe that these tumours arise from the perineurial or endoneurial connective tissue and that the fibroblast is their type cell. They have therefore been termed 'perineurial fibroblastomas'. Russell and Rubinstein (1977), however, regard them as Schwannomas, a view now widely accepted, but they are also called neurilemmomas or neurofibromas. Though the eighth cranial nerve is their commonest site, similar tumours may be found upon other cranial nerves, especially the optic and the trigeminal, upon spinal-nerve roots, usually the dorsal, and upon peripheral nerves.

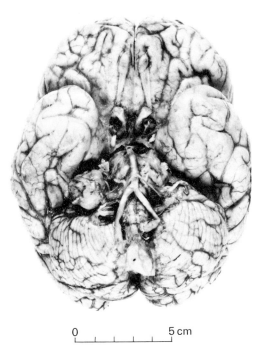

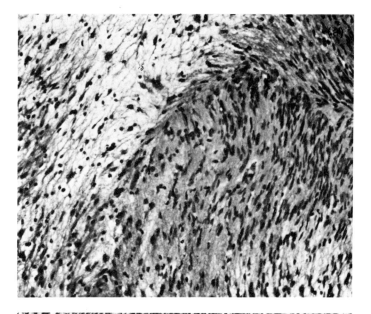

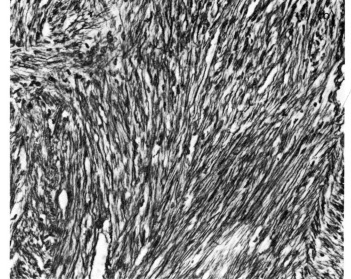

Fig. 3.14. A right-sided acoustic neuroma found at autopsy.

Blood-vessel tumours and malformations

The following are the commoner types:

1. The angiomatous malformations.
2. The cavernous haemangiomas.
3. The haemangioblastomas.
4. The Sturge–Weber syndrome.

The first two groups have sometimes been collectively described as blood-vessel hamartomas. However, the term hamartoma has also been applied to areas of ectopic neuronal and glial tissue, often encapsulated, and clearly of developmental origin, which are found within the brain substance or meninges. Thus some, but not all, hamartomas have a blood-vessel component.

1. *The angiomatous malformations*. These are congenital abnormalities of vascular development rather than true neoplasms. They may be divided into (*a*) telangiectases, (*b*) arteriovenous malformations.

(*a*) *Telangiectases*, or capillary angiomas, consist of greatly dilated capillaries. They may be associated with Osler's hereditary telangiectasia but are usually accidental post-mortem findings (often in the pons), though rupture has been known to cause death through haemorrhage (Becker, Townsend, Kramer, and Newton 1979).

(*b*) *Arteriovenous malformations*. These consist of a mass of enlarged and tortuous cortical vessels, supplied by one or more large arteries usually derived from the blood supply of one, but sometimes of both, hemispheres, and sometimes fed also from below the tentorium, and drained by one or more large veins. Sometimes there is also a contribution from the middle meningeal artery. These malformations are most frequently encountered in the field of the middle cerebral artery, but may involve the brain-stem (Logue and Monckton 1954). It appears that a single arteriovenous communication may be present initially but the consequential arterialization of draining veins leads to increasing size and tortuosity of the vessels involved so that these lesions increase steadily in size. They are rarely familial (Aberfeld and Rao 1981; also see p. 208).

Angiography has revealed that the angiomatous malformations

Fig. 3.15. An acoustic neuroma. (a) H & E, × 160, showing Antoni type A and B appearances, A to the right, B to the left; (b) reticulin, × 160, showing the close reticulin net in an Antoni type A area.

are commoner than used to be thought but even this technique sometimes fails to demonstrate angiomas which are subsequently revealed pathologically (Becker *et al.* 1979). Verified angiomas accounted in one series for 6.5 per cent of 200 cases of cerebral vascular disease. Increased vascularity of the scalp, with large and pulsating arteries, and hypertrophy of one or both carotids may be present, and even secondary cardiac hypertrophy may occur. A bruit is commonly heard over one or both carotid arteries in the neck and on the scalp overlying the angioma.

2. *The cavernous haemangiomas*. The cavernous haemangiomas are also congenital abnormalities rather than true neoplasms. They usually occur above the tentorium. They form a lobulated mass consisting of small and large spaces containing blood. Similar haemangiomas of vertebral bodies may cause vertebral collapse and spinal-cord compression (McAllister, Kendall, and Bull 1975).

3. *The haemangioblastomas*. The haemangioblastomas are tumours which, according to Cushing and Bailey (1928), are composed of angioblasts, the primitive cells which normally form the fetal blood vessels. They usually consist of vascular channels and

spaces with sparse intercapillary tissue containing swollen fat-laden endothelial cells (Fig. 3.16). They often form cysts in the surrounding nerve tissue, the cyst containing xanthochromic fluid which is an exudate from the tumour vessels. The cyst may be large and the tumour a small nodule in its wall; this must be excised if the cyst is not to refill. The haemangioblastomas are almost invariably subtentorial, but are rarely found above the tentorium. They are usually single, but there may be multiple growths in the cerebellum or in addition to a cerebellar lesion a tumour in the medulla or spinal cord. An important feature is the association with abnormalities elsewhere (Jeffreys 1975*a*). The most important of these, because the most easily observed, is a haemangioblastoma of the retina (von Hippel's disease). This is a small tumour usually situated in the periphery of the retina and supplied by an enlarged artery and vein. Secondary proliferative changes in, and rarely even detachment of, the retina may render it difficult to recognize. Other abnormalities which may coexist are haemangioblastoma of the spinal cord, cysts of the pancreas and kidneys, hypernephromas of the kidneys or the suprarenal glands. The coincidence of these abnormalities is known as Lindau's disease and is familial in about 20 per cent of cases. Polycythaemia may occur (Jeffreys 1975*b*) and malignant transformation and spread has been described following successful surgical removal (Mohan, Brownell, and Oppenheimer 1976).

4. *The Sturge–Weber syndrome.* In the fully developed form of this disorder, an extensive subcortical capillary malformation affects one hemisphere, particularly in the parieto-occipital region and is associated with a characteristic 'wavy' pattern of calcification which outlines the gyri and is visible radiologically after the third to fifth year of life. There is a 'port-wine' stain on the face on the affected side, often with an associated buphthalmos (ox eye), while most patients have a contralateral hemiparesis and epilepsy.

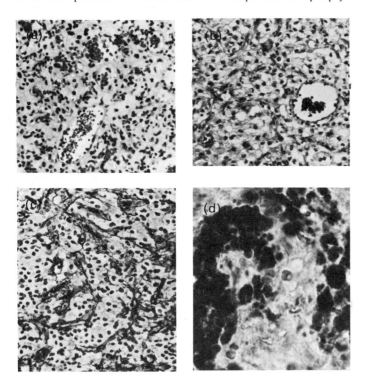

Fig. 3.16. Haemangioblastoma of cerebellum, showing fat-filled macrophages. (a) H & E, × 64; (b) H & E, × 160; (c) reticulin, × 160; (d) oil red O, × 400.

Craniopharyngioma

These tumours are also described as tumours of the craniopharyngeal, or Rathke's, pouch, adamantinomas, and hypophysial epidermoids. In order to understand their origin it is necessary briefly to review the development of the hypophysis (pituitary gland) in the embryo. The pituitary develops as a result of fusion of an evagination of the ectoderm of the stomadaeum with a process which extends downwards from the floor of the forebrain. The former loses its opening into the mouth cavity and becomes a closed sac from which are derived the anterior lobe and the pars intermedia. The process from the forebrain forms the posterior lobe and the infundibulum. The remnants of the craniopharyngeal pouch remain and, owing to rotation of the developing gland, come to lie anterior to the infundibulum and at the upper angle of the anterior lobe. They may also be found within the sella turcica itself.

Tumours arising from these embryonic relics show characteristics resulting from their origin. They contain cells resembling those of the embryonic buccal epithelium, including the ameloblasts of the embryonic enamel organ. Histologically, a cystic type lined by stratified squamous epithelium, an adamantinomatous type with fibrovascular cores, squamous and tall columnar cells (ameloblasts), and a much less common cyst of Rathke's cleft lined by ciliated columnar epithelium, sometimes containing goblet cells, are described (Bartlett 1971*a*, and *b*; Banna 1976; Hankinson and Banna 1976). Calcification within the cyst wall (Fig. 3.17) is common and ossification rarely occurs. These growths usually arise above the sellar diaphragm, and extend upwards into the third ventricle and hypothalamic region, but occasionally are seen within the sella itself.

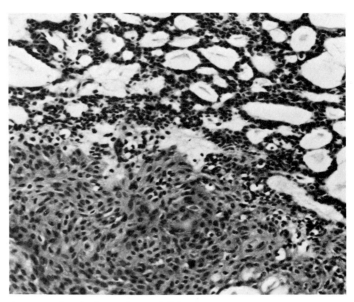

Fig. 3.17. Craniopharyngioma, H & E, × 160.

Tumours of the pituitary gland (hypophysis)

The cells of the anterior lobe of the pituitary are the alpha, eosinophil, or acidophil cells, which secrete growth hormone, luteinizing hormone, and prolactin; the beta or basophil cells, which secrete follicle-stimulating hormone, corticotrophin, and thyrotrophin, and the poorly staining chromophobe cells.

The common pituitary tumours are adenomas. The commonest is the chromophobe adenoma, composed of cells which sometimes show alveolar formation and resemble the chromophobe cells of the normal gland. The chromophil adenoma is composed of cells resembling the acidophil cells of the normal gland. It sometimes undergoes cystic degeneration. This tumour gives hyperpituitarism—gigantism if it develops before puberty and acromegaly in adults. The basophil adenoma is usually microscopic in size and only rarely causes pressure symptoms. It causes Cushing's syndrome. It has become increasingly evident, however, that relatively few pituitary tumours, and particularly the chromophobe adenomas, are made up of uniform cell types (Hankinson and Banna 1976), so that now these tumours are no longer classified according to histological staining characteristics but rather according to the clinical syndromes and typical hormonal changes which they produce (Gillespie and Mahaley 1981). Thus electron microscopic and immunofluorescent staining has enabled tumours to be classified according to the hormones they secrete. And careful hormonal studies have facilitated the recognition of very small pituitary tumours such as prolactin-secreting microadenomas, small growth-hormone-secreting or ACTH-secreting tumours. It was for long believed that Cushing's syndrome is usually due to hyperadrenalism but small adenomas involving basophil cells are now being found in the majority of such cases (Wilson, Tynell, and Fitzgerald 1979). Some of the larger growths made up largely of chromophobe cells also secrete prolactin (Franks, Nabarro, and Jacobs 1977) and have a particular tendency to undergo infarction or to bleed, giving the syndrome of pituitary apoplexy (Weiss, Apuzzo, Heiden, and Kurze 1976, and see p. 165).

The pituitary adenomas arise within the sella turcica, which they expand, and later may penetrate the sellar diaphragm and attain a considerable size, compressing structures at the base of the brain. Adenocarcinoma of the pituitary is a rare, rapidly growing tumour which gives rise to metastases. Metastases from extracranial neoplasms arising in the sella are rare and have most frequently been recorded in cases of carcinoma of the breast (Max, Deck, and Rottenberg 1981).

Osteoma and osteochondroma
Ivory osteomas may develop in the frontal or ethmoidal sinuses and are sometimes large enough to compress the frontal lobe. Osteochondroma of the base of the skull rarely gives neurological manifestations but can cause subarachnoid haemorrhage.

Cholesteatoma
The cholesteatoma, or cerebrospinal epidermoid, is a rare tumour of adult life. It affects males more frequently than females. It arises from fetal epithelial inclusions and is most often found in the subarachnoid cisterns at the base of the brain. Those arising below the tentorium, a common site, are situated either in the cerebellopontine angle or in the midline on the ventral aspect of the cerebellum, within the fourth ventricle or in the temporal bone. The naked-eye appearance of the tumour in the fresh state is highly characteristic. It is pearly white, smooth and glistening, firm but brittle. Microscopically a cholesteatoma is composed of several layers, of which the most characteristic—the stratum granulosum—consisting of several rows of large, finely granular cells, probably corresponds to the dermis. Rarely these tumours may leak keratin into the CSF causing degeneration of cranial nerves and the spinal cord (Tomlinson and Walton 1967).

Dermoid cysts
Posterior fossa dermoid cysts may occur in children but are uncommon.

Arachnoidal cysts
Arachnoidal cysts which contain CSF may enlarge progressively to compress the brain either above or below the tentorium, in both children and adults (Aicardi and Bauman 1975; Dyck and Gruskin 1977) and may mimic brain tumour. Diagnosis is usually possible by CT scanning.

Pinealoma
The commonest variety of tumour arising in the region of the pineal gland, and often erroneously called a pinealoma, is in fact a teratoma (Russell 1944; Russell and Rubinstein 1977) or a germinoma; these growths are commonest before the age of 30, being twice as common in males as in females. True pinealomas (pineo-cytoma or pineoblastoma) are much less common but are derived from pineal parenchymal cells (Herrick and Rubinstein 1979). Since these cells secrete melatonin and arginine vasotocin which probably affect ovarian maturation, this explains why sexual precocity sometimes results from such growths (Gillespie and Mahaley 1981).

Colloid cysts of the third ventricle
These are rounded cystic tumours measuring from 1 to 3 cm in diameter and arising from the paraphysis, ependyma, or choroid plexus. They are lined with ciliated epithelium and contain thick gelatinous material. Owing to their position they readily cause intermittent hydrocephalus.

Chordoma
These rare tumours, derived from primitive remnants of the notochord, arise either in the region of the clivus, causing cranial-nerve palsies and backward displacement of the pons, or in the body of the sacrum and sacral canal, causing a cauda equina syndrome.

Papilloma of the choroid plexus
Up to half of these benign vascular tumours occur in the fourth ventricle, about one-third in the lateral ventricles (usually left) and one-sixth in the third ventricle. Recurrent or chronic subarachnoid bleeding and communicating hydrocephalus may result. Malignant transformation sometimes occurs.

Glomus tumours
These tumours arise from the glomus jugulare and may invade the middle ear or the posterior fossa giving unilateral deafness and multiple palsies of lower cranial nerves; erosion of the skull base is often visible radiologically (Henson, Crawford, and Cavanaugh 1953; Siekert 1956). Sometimes the tumour invades the internal and middle ear and may be seen with the auriscope. Glomus intravagale tumours also occur but, like the histologically similar carotid body tumours, are usually extracranial. Though they are similar pathologically to other chromaffinomas, these neoplasms rarely, if ever, secrete noradrenaline.

Lipoma of the corpus callosum
This is a rare congenital condition which is sometimes asymptomatic but may present in childhood or adult life with epilepsy, hemiplegia, dementia, or headache (Wallace 1976; Gastaut, Regis, Gastaut, Yermenos, and Low 1980) or rarely with spontaneous periodic hypothermia (Summers, Young, Little, Stoner, Forbes, and Jones 1981). Plain radiographs may show a typical pattern of calcification and the CT scan is usually diagnostic.

Metastatic tumours
About 20–25 per cent of cerebral neoplasms are secondary to a primary growth elsewhere, usually in the lung, breast, stomach, prostate, kidney, or thyroid. In a recent series of 2 375 patients with cancer (Posner and Chernik 1978), 24 per cent had intracranial metastases, of which four-fifths were intradural and three-fifths intracerebral. There was leptomeningeal involvement in 3 per cent. Lung carcinomas accounted for about two-thirds, followed by breast, melanoma, leukaemia, and lymphoma in that order. More than half of the patients had multiple metastases; 72 per cent of melanomas and 34 per cent of bronchial carcinomas, but only 5 per cent of ovarian carcinomas spread to the brain, while prostatic carcinoma commonly gave extradural but very rarely intracerebral metastases. Leptomeningeal carcinomatosis is seen most often in leukaemia, melanoma, lymphoma, and breast carcinoma. In childhood the commonest tumours, other than the leukaemias and lymphomas, which spread to the brain are the neuroblastoma, embryonal rhabdomyosarcoma, Wilms' and Ewing's tumours, and osteogenic sarcoma (Vannucci and Baten

1974). Often the symptoms of the cerebral growth are more conspicuous than those of the primary. Metastases are often pinkish, rounded tumours, well defined from the oedematous surrounding brain tissue. Metastases in the fourth ventricle may give in middle or late life the same triad of symptoms (morning headache, morning vomiting, and postural vertigo) as is seen in younger patients with ependymomas in the same site. Leptomeningeal carcinomatosis or carcinomatosis of the meninges may rarely lead to subdural haematoma. More often many cranial nerves are compressed or infiltrated and multiple cranial-nerve palsies are accompanied by neck stiffness, headache, and confusion (Jacobs and Richland 1951; Olson, Chernik, and Posner 1974). The pituitary may be invaded and the tuber cinereum compressed, leading to metabolic and endocrine disorders. In such cases also metastatic deposits may also be present in the upper cervical lymph nodes. Secondary sarcoma of the brain is much rarer than secondary carcinoma. Malignant melanoma may metastasize rapidly to the brain and meninges (Gillespie and Mahaley 1981) and can produce subarachnoid haemorrhage.

Myeloma

Multiple myelomatosis frequently involves the cranial bones, giving multiple areas of osteolysis; it rarely involves the brain but extradural deposits from solitary or multiple myelomas may compress the spinal cord. Solitary myelomas have been described in the skull base or orbit (Gardner-Thorpe 1970) and in the substance of the brain (French 1947; Clarke 1954).

Tumours of infective origin

Tuberculoma. Tuberculoma of the brain is now much less frequent in Britain than a generation ago, when it was regarded as common, but it is seen largely in Asian immigrants (Loizou and Anderson 1982). It is still common in the Indian sub-continent. Cerebral tuberculomas are more often subtentorial than supratentorial and vary in size from small nodules up to large masses which may occupy more than one lobe of the brain. They are usually at some point subjacent to the pia mater. There is a yellow caseous centre surrounded by a pinkish-grey outer zone. Microscopically, cerebral tuberculomas show the features typical of tuberculous lesions. The caseous centre is surrounded by a zone containing giant cells and epithelioid cells and vessels showing endarteritis. Outside this area infiltration with compound granular corpuscles and fibrosis is conspicuous.

Gumma. Gumma of the brain is extremely rare. It is generally connected with the meninges, probably arising initially as a circumscribed patch of gummatous meningitis. Its pathology is described in the section on cerebral syphilis.

Parasitic cysts. Intracranial hydatid cysts are rare even in countries in which hydatid infection is common, the brain being infested in only 5 per cent of cases. They may be single or multiple. They sometimes occur outside the dura, and in one of Brain's patients, an extradural collection of hydatids eroded the frontal bone, and some cysts were extruded through the scalp. More often the cysts, which may reach the size of a hen's egg, develop within the cerebral hemispheres or within the ventricles. Cysticercus cellulosae and coenurus cerebralis cysts may cause symptoms of increased intracranial pressure. Either may occur in the ventricles or cause an adhesive arachnoditis in the posterior fossa. Cysticercus cellulosae may also behave as a space-occupying lesion in the cerebral hemisphere (Kuper, Mendelow, and Proctor 1958; see also p. 260). Rarely infestation of the brain with the ova of *Schistosoma japonicum* may cause tumour-like masses or areas of granulomatous change suggestive of multilocular abscess.

Mode of onset

The mode of onset of symptoms depends upon the nature and site of the tumour. It is often slower with astrocytomas, oligodendrog-

liomas, meningiomas, acoustic neuromas, and pituitary adenomas which may be present for years before the patient consults a doctor, and most rapid with glioblastoma multiforme and metastases. The commonest modes of onset are (1) progressive focal symptoms, e.g. focal epilepsy, monoplegia, hemiplegia, aphasia, cerebellar dysfunction, associated with symptoms of increased intracranial pressure; (2) symptoms of increased intracranial pressure alone; (3) progressive focal symptoms alone, e.g. visual failure, unilateral deafness, dementia; (4) generalized epileptic attacks preceding other symptoms by many years; both slowly-growing gliomas and meningiomas may cause epilepsy for as long as 20 years, before causing other symptoms; (5) rarely an apoplectiform onset with loss of consciousness, and perhaps hemiplegia.

Symptoms and signs of increased intracranial pressure

The manifestations of an intracranial tumour are conveniently divided into those attributable to increased intracranial pressure and those due to the local effects of the growth. It might be expected that focal symptoms would arise before a tumour was large enough to disturb the intracranial pressure. More often, however, the reverse is the case, and the symptoms often suggest the presence of a tumour which cannot be localized by physical examination alone. Headache, papilloedema, and vomiting are the classical triad of symptoms of increased intracranial pressure, but they are not found with equal frequency. In one series, headache was present in 88 per cent, papilloedema in 75 per cent, and vomiting in 65 per cent of cases of cerebral tumour. All three occurred together in only 60 per cent.

Headache. The headache of intracranial tumour is mainly due to compression or distortion of the dura and of the intracranial blood vessels. It is often paroxysmal, at least at first. It is usually described as a throbbing or a 'bursting' pain. It is generally worst in the early morning. Often the patient awakens with a headache which lasts from a few minutes to a few hours and then passes off, to recur next day. With gradual enlargement of the growth headaches become more prolonged and is ultimately continuous. It is generally intensified by activities which raise the intracranial pressure, such as exertion, excitement, coughing, sneezing, vomiting, stooping, coitus, or straining at stool. It may be influenced by posture, being worse when lying down, or lying on one side, and may be relieved by sitting up.

Owing to the diffuse increase in intracranial pressure in many cases of cerebral tumour, headache is of little localizing significance. Pain due to local pressure may be predominantly unilateral, on the side of the tumour, and occasionally gives tenderness of the skull on percussion in a limited area overlying it. In subtentorial tumours the headache may be mainly suboccipital at first, with some radiation down the back of the neck. In such cases neck flexion may increase the pain and this sign may warn of impending cerebellar herniation. As the intracranial pressure rises, the headache becomes diffuse, and hydrocephalus can give paroxysms of severe pain radiating down the neck, sometimes associated with head retraction. Pressure upon the trigeminal nerve may give unilateral pain, often in the distribution of the first division and associated with hyperpathia or analgesia over the same area.

Papilloedema. The pathogenesis and appearances of papilloedema are described on pages 90–1. Its incidence varies according to the situation of the tumour. It usually develops in tumours of the cerebellum, fourth ventricle, and temporal lobes, but is absent in many cases of pontine or subcortical tumour. It is usually late in developing in prefrontal tumours, and is often more severe with extracerebral than with intracerebral growths. Cerebellar tumours often cause papilloedema of the greatest severity. A slight asymmetry in the swelling of the two optic discs is not uncommon, but is of little localizing value. A tumour arising sufficiently near the optic canal to occlude the subarachnoid space of the optic nerve causes primary optic atrophy on the affected side and occasionally contralateral papilloedema results from the general effect of the tumour (the Foster Kennedy syndrome, often due to an olfactory-groove meningioma).

The changes in the visual fields due to papilloedema consist of enlargement of the blind spot with peripheral concentric constriction. Severe papilloedema may be present without impairment of visual acuity but transient episodes of unilateral or bilateral visual blurring or even blindness (obscurations of vision), sometimes precipitated by coughing, straining, or stooping, may warn of impending irreversible visual failure due to occlusion of one or both central retinal arteries.

Vomiting. Vomiting, when due to intracranial tumour, usually occurs in the early morning when headache is especially severe. Although sometimes, especially in children, there is little associated nausea, vomiting of cerebral origin is not always of precipitate or projectile type.

Epilepsy. While generalized epileptic seizures may occur in patients with hydrocephalus and increased intracranial pressure, in cases of intracranial tumour, epileptic fits are usually due to the direct effect of the neoplasm upon the surrounding or underlying brain. Schmidt and Wilder (1968), reviewing many published series, concluded that, in patients with epilepsy beginning over the age of 20, about 10 per cent are eventually shown to have intracranial tumours. Penfield, Erickson, and Tarlov (1940) found that about two-thirds of all patients with meningiomas or slowly growing astrocytomas and only about one-third of those with glioblastomas had fits at some stage. Such attacks are also commoner when the tumour involves the cortex rather than deeper structures (Marsden 1982). The incidence of tumour rises to about 30–40 per cent in patients with focal rather than generalized fits.

Vertigo. While many patients with increased intracranial pressure due to intracranial tumour complain of unsteadiness or dizziness, true vertigo is relatively uncommon, even in acoustic neuroma. However, severe vertigo induced by change in posture is an important manifestation of ependymomas or metastases in or near the fourth ventricle and vertigo is also a rare manifestation of temporal-lobe tumour.

Disturbances of pulse rate and blood pressure. An acute or subacute rise of intracranial pressure, as in intracranial haemorrhage or meningitis, often causes slowing of the pulse rate, usually to between 50 and 60 beats a minute. If pressure continues to increase the pulse later becomes extremely rapid. In either case it may be irregular. A gradual increase in intracranial pressure, as in intracranial tumour, does not usually cause bradycardia, but moderate tachycardia is not uncommon in cases of subtentorial tumour.

A rapid rise of intracranial pressure usually causes an increase in blood pressure. In intracranial haemorrhage this pressor effect may indicate that the bleeding is continuing and, in rapidly growing tumours or severe cerebral oedema, there may be a similar sustained rise. Rarely in patients with cerebellar tumours the hypertension is paroxysmal, mimicking the effects of a phaeochromocytoma (Cameron and Doig 1970). With slowly growing tumours, however, the blood pressure is more often normal or subnormal.

Respiratory rate. A gradual rise in intracranial pressure does not at first affect the respiratory rate. A rapid and sustained rise causing loss of consciousness usually leads at first to slow and deep respirations. Later the respiratory rate may become irregular, e.g. of the Cheyne–Stokes type, in which periods of apnoea alternate with a series of respirations which wax and wane in amplitude. In the terminal stages the respirations are rapid and shallow. These manifestations are due to compression or distortion of the brainstem, especially the medulla, where the respiratory centres lie. Central neurogenic hyperventilation (p. 649) is not uncommon in such cases and apneustic or ataxic breathing (Plum and Posner 1980) may each rarely occur. These abnormalities of respiratory rate and rhythm often result from the median-raphe haemorrhages or infarcts in the brainstem, which may result from tentorial herniation (p. 136); in such cases the patient usually lapses into irreversible coma. Hence these changes not only complicate posterior-fossa neoplasms which directly compress or distort the brainstem but also supratentorial lesions.

'Hypopituitarism.' Any chronic state of increased intracranial pressure with hydrocephalus may produce manifestations of 'hypopituitarism', such as adiposity and genital atrophy in some cases or loss of body hair and hypoadrenalism with hypothyroidism in others. This is due to downward pressure upon hypothalamic nuclei in the floor of the distended third ventricle, sometimes with erosion of the clinoid processes and diaphragma sellae and compression of the pituitary. These symptoms are most frequently seen in cases of cerebellar tumour in childhood. Radiography of the skull often shows erosion of the clinoid processes and enlargement of the sella turcica. These manifestations may lead to the erroneous diagnosis of a pituitary or suprasellar tumour.

Somnolence. Hypersomnia may occur in severe hydrocephalus and with tumours near the hypothalamus but true narcolepsy is virtually unknown.

Glycosuria. Glycosuria is occasionally encountered, sometimes with hyperglycaemia, more often with a normal blood-sugar and a lowered renal threshold.

Mental symptoms. Many varied mental symptoms are associated with increased intracranial pressure. If the pressure rises sufficiently, this leads to coma, and the more rapid the rise the more likely is this to occur. An acute or subacute rise insufficient to produce coma usually leads to a confusional state. Chronic hydrocephalus or frontal meningioma (Hunter, Blackwood, and Bull 1968) may lead to progressive dementia, with disintegration of intellect, emotional apathy, carelessness with regard to the person, and incontinence of urine and faeces. Less often, marked disturbances of mood are conspicuous, with episodes of excitement or euphoria, or of depression. In some cases impairment of memory and of concentration with irritability, may be the only mental symptoms. Such symptoms are most likely to occur when the tumour is situated in the frontal lobe or corpus callosum; but they can be produced by any tumour which increases the intracranial pressure. Thus any of the disturbances described can be produced by a cerebellar tumour; they are more likely to occur in the middle-aged and elderly than in younger patients.

False localizing signs

Collier first stressed the importance of signs, especially cranial-nerve palsies, produced by intracranial tumours in other ways than by direct compression. Since these may lead to errors in localization, he termed them 'false localizing signs'. A sixth-nerve palsy on one or both sides, or, less often, a third-nerve palsy, may be thus produced and have been variously attributed to stretching or compression of the nerves resulting from displacement of the cranial contents, e.g. tentorial herniation compressing one third nerve at the edge of the tentorium. Other false localizing signs include bilateral extensor plantar responses or bilateral grasp reflexes resulting from dysfunction of the cerebral hemispheres caused by distension of the ventricles in hydrocephalus; 'hypopituitarism' resulting from hydrocephalus, as already described; an extensor plantar response occurring on the same side as a tumour of one cerebral hemisphere produced by compression of the opposite cerebral peduncle against the tentorium (Kernohan's sign); cerebellar dysfunction due to tumours of the frontal lobe, and midbrain signs, especially fixed dilated pupils, produced by a tumour of the cerebellar vermis.

Examination of the head

Examination of the head may yield important information and should never be neglected. There may be visible enlargement when hydrocephalus develops before union of the cranial sutures. In such cases separation of the sutures may yield a 'cracked-pot sound' on percussion. Local tenderness of the skull may be present overlying the tumour. A bony boss may overlie a meningioma. Venous congestion of the scalp is not uncommon in increased intracranial pressure in children with marked separation of the sutures. Dilatation and tortuosity of scalp arteries are sometimes associated with a vascular intracranial tumour, especially a meningioma or an angioma. Such arterial congestion is usually confined to the side of the tumour and is often most evident in the superficial temporal artery. An audible bruit should be sought by auscultation. It is most often present over an arterial angioma, much less frequently over a highly vascular meningioma. However, cranial bruits are often heard in normal children, while bruits heard in the neck in adults and resulting from stenosis of major vessels (carotid, vertebral, subclavian) may be transmitted along temporal vessels so that auscultation of the neck is also essential. A bruit over the orbit is usually present,along with pulsating exophthalmos, in cases of carotico-cavernous fistula.

Facial naevus may be associated with the Sturge–Weber syndrome, retinal haemangioblastoma with cerebellar haemangioblastoma, and cutaneous pigmentation with neurofibromatosis, while unilateral exophthalmos may be due to a retro-orbital meningioma.

Management of the tumour suspect

In any patient in whom symptoms and/or physical signs suggest the possibility of an intracranial tumour, it is reasonable to begin by employing successively those investigations which are likely to give the maximum information with minimum risk to the patient and only subsequently to employ potentially hazardous investigations if the information necessary to localize and identify, or to exclude the presence of a neoplasm can be obtained in no other way. Thus radiography of the chest (to exclude, for instance, a bronchogenic carcinoma which may have metastasized to the brain) is invariably necessary, as are X-rays of the skull (see below). An echoencephalogram (p. 78) may confirm displacement of midline structures and may even be helpful in determining ventricular size and displacement, especially if the more sensitive B-scan is used (McKinney 1969) though the simpler A-scan can give useful information (Garg and Taylor 1968). An electroencephalogram (p. 76) may not only indicate a lesion in one cerebral hemisphere but may give some clue as to its situation; a negative recording, however, cannot exclude a tumour (Williams, Hicks, Herzberg, Williams, and Croft 1972). Unquestionably the greatest impact upon the diagnosis of intracranial tumour has resulted from the introduction of CT scanning (p. 80 and see below) and this technique is now the method of choice for imaging the brain and orbital contents (Anderson 1982), not only because it is non-invasive and safe but also because of its high diagnostic yield and its accuracy not only in localizing neoplasms within the skull but also in giving information which allows valid conclusions to be drawn about pathology in many cases (Oldendorf 1980, 1981). The diagnostic yield can be increased by combining the CT scan with isotope scanning in emission brain tomography (Ell, Deacon, Ducassou, and Brendel 1980), while positron emission tomography gives not only an image but also information about regional glycolysis and blood flow (Oldendorf 1981). It is now becoming evident (Doyle, Gore, Pennock, Bydder, Orr, Steiner, Young, Burl, Clow, Gilderdale, Bailes, and Walters 1981; Anderson 1982) that nuclear magnetic resonance (NMR scanning) is likely to become even more valuable. This technique makes use of non-ionizing radiofrequency photons which produce little or no image

from bone, and it already seems likely to be more accurate in consequence than CT scanning in demonstrating posterior fossa and parapituitary lesions. It will also give more information relating to chemical changes in nervous tissue while producing images of lesions, and is thus likely to contribute effectively to the diagnosis of cerebral and cerebellar degenerations, toxic, metabolic, and infective encephalopathies, meningitis, and multiple sclerosis as well as neoplasms. However, NMR is still being developed, and even the CT scan requires expensive instrumentation and skilled operators and is not universally available throughout the world, so that other diagnostic techniques may still be needed at least in some centres. The use of gamma-encephalography (p. 78) has declined sharply but may still be useful in demonstrating an increased uptake of isotope in a tumour (van Eck 1966; Boller, Patten, and Howes 1973; Penning, Front, Bechar, Go, and Rodermond 1973) or in multiple metastases. RISA cisternography (van Crevel 1979) is also of limited value in the diagnosis of supratentorial tumour.

Lumbar puncture is better avoided in the tumour suspect, certainly when symptoms and signs indicate raised intracranial pressure, because of the risk of tentorial or cerebellar herniation. In the past a rise in CSF pressure and in its protein content (pp. 65–71), was found useful, especially in cases of acoustic neuroma or meningioma; a substantial increase in CSF protein content was common in such cases with lesser rises in many patients with gliomas or intracranial metastases. Cytological examination of the fluid (Dyken 1975) is sometimes of value in detecting malignant cells, occasionally in patients with gliomas but more especially in carcinomatosis of the meninges, while the lactate dehydrogenase and glutamic oxalacetic transaminase activity of the fluid is sometimes increased in patients with cerebral metastases (Davies-Jones 1969). Lysozyme (Newman, Josephson, Cacatian, and Tsang 1974) and adenylate kinase (Ronquist, Frithz, Ericsson, and Hugosson 1977), absent from normal CSF, may each be found in the CSF of patients with primary or secondary malignant tumours, and CSF β-glucuronidase and carcinoembryonic antigen (Schold, Wasserstrom, Fleisher, Schwartz, and Posner 1980) are increased in cases of early meningeal carcinomatosis. It has also been found that after triparanol treatment of human CSF, a concentration of desmosterol (a precursor of cholesterol) of more than 0.1 μg ml indicates the presence of an intracranial tumour (Paoletti, Vandenheuvel, Fumagalli, and Paoletti 1969). Despite the value of these tests, the risks inherent in lumbar puncture mean that it is now used much less often in the tumour suspect than in the past. It should never be undertaken lightly and then only if evidence of raised pressure is lacking, if neurosurgical aid is immediately at hand, and if the information which it is likely to give cannot be obtained by less hazardous means.

For the same reasons, fractional pneumoencephalography (see below), which may demonstrate ventricular distortion or displacement produced by a neoplasm, is now employed much less often, though it still has a limited role when there is no evidence of raised pressure or of focal neurological signs, when there is no other reasonable means of excluding a tumour and when facilities are immediately available for neurosurgical exploration if a space-occupying lesion is demonstrated.

When no CT scan is possible, when there is evidence of raised intracranial pressure, and certainly when signs of a focal lesion are present, cerebral angiography is usually indicated, first because this may demonstrate hydrocephalus, or, in lesions of one cerebral hemisphere, it may show displacement of major vessels or a pathological tumour circulation. If no such localizing signs are found, or if the angiographic signs are those of hydrocephalus, the next step will usually be ventriculography (see below), either with air, or, on occasion, using contrast medium, especially when a neoplasm in one of the ventricles or in the brainstem or posterior fossa is suspected.

Accessory methods of investigation

Radiography. Some principles have already been outlined (pp. 79–80). In every suspected case of intracranial tumour lateral, anteroposterior, and posteroanterior views should be taken, and other positions, including basal views and Towne's view, are usually included in routine skull surveys (Bull 1951). Examination of the skull may reveal abnormalities in the bones, calcification in the tumour (Figs. 3.18–3.20), or displacement of the pineal body. Separation of the sutures may be seen when the intracranial pressure rises before the age at which these unite (Fig. 3.4, p. 141). Erosion of the posterior clinoid processes and erosion or decalcification of the dorsum sellae is a safer guide to the presence of raised intracranial pressure (see below) but decalcification in this area is also a common result of normal ageing processes. Local erosion of bone is most often seen in the skull overlying a meningioma. Around the eroded area new bone formation occurs, often in the form of spicules, perpendicular to the vault, and surrounding this there is frequently a network of deep vascular channels in the bone. The petrous temporal bone may be eroded by an acoustic neuroma which may lead to unilateral enlargement of the internal auditory meatus (Fig. 3.21). Bony changes in the region of the sella turcica are produced not only by tumours of the pituitary itself and those arising in its neighbourhood, but also by a general increase in the intracranial pressure (Fig. 3.22). Hypophysial tumours cause a uniform expansion of the sella with thinning of its walls (Fig. 3.23). The ballooned sella projects downwards and forwards into the sphenoidal sinuses, and upward pressure of the growth may erode the clinoid processes. Tumours arising outside the sella, but immediately above it, cause erosion of the clinoid processes and flattening of the sella, which is not, however, uniformly enlarged unless invaded by the tumour (Fig. 3.18); downward pressure of the floor of a distended third ventricle in hydrocephalus gives a very similar radiographic appearance.

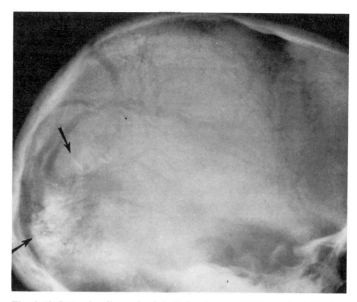

Fig. 3.19. Lateral radiograph of skull showing parallel lines of calcification in an occipital oligodendroglioma (arrows).

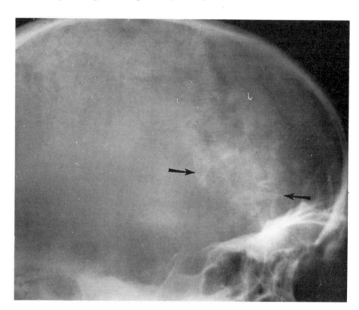

Fig. 3.20. Lateral radiograph of skull showing curvilinear calcification (arrows) in a frontal arteriovenous angioma.

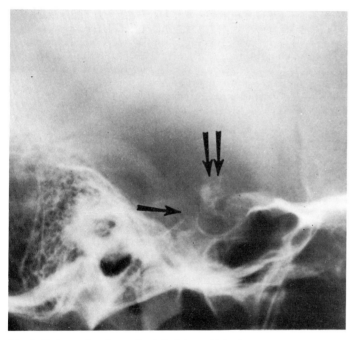

Fig. 3.18. Lateral radiograph of skull in a child with a suprasellar craniopharyngioma showing calcification (double arrows) and erosion of the tip of the dorsum sellae (single arrow).

Calcification is most often seen in craniopharyngiomas (Fig. 3.18)(in about 75 per cent of cases). They may exhibit on the X-ray film merely a few opaque flecks, or a mass the size of a hen's egg. Calcification may also occur in the angiomas (Fig. 3.20), sometimes with a characteristic convoluted appearance due to the deposit of calcium in the walls of the vessels composing the tumour but more often the pattern is nonspecific. Meningiomas also sometimes show calcified areas, and these may be encountered, though less often, in gliomas, especially oligodendrogliomas (Fig. 3.19), teratomas, tumours of the choroid plexuses, and tuberculomas. Chronic intracerebral haematomas, and, very rarely, subdural haematomas may also calcify. A typical form of calcification is also seen in the very rare lipoma of the corpus callosum, while bilateral calcification in the basal ganglia may be familial (Fahr's disease) or can occur in pseudohypoparathyroidism.

The pineal body is normally sufficiently calcified to be visible radiographically in 60 per cent of adults and is to be seen in the midline above and behind the sella turcica. It may be displaced to the opposite side by a neoplasm of one cerebral hemisphere. Calcification may also be seen in the normal choroid plexuses, in the petroclinoid ligaments, tuberculum sellae and falx cerebri, and even in the dura mater of the vault of the skull.

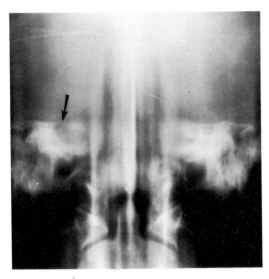

Fig. 3.21. Towne's view (tomogram) of skull showing gross erosion of the right internal auditory canal produced by an acoustic neuroma.

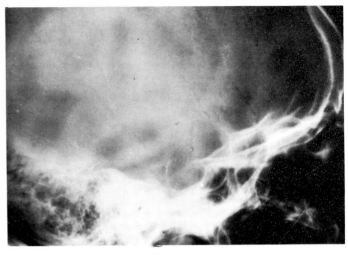

Fig. 3.23. Lateral radiograph of skull showing enlargement and thinning of the walls of the sella turcica due to a chromophobe adenoma of the pituitary.

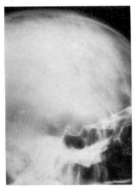 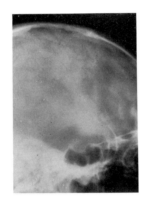

Fig. 3.22. On the left is a normal lateral radiograph of skull; on the right is a radiograph taken one year later of the same patient showing loss of the lamina dura of the dorsum sellae due to increased intracranial pressure.

Contrast methods

As stated above, the contrast methods in common use for the localization and identification of intracranial tumours are CT scanning, carotid and vertebral angiography, pneumoencephalography and ventriculography with air or contrast media (*Myodil, Metrizamide,* or *Conray*).

CT scanning. Many intracranial tumours are clearly identified by CT scanning but, with contrast enhancement following the intravenous injection of *Conray*, the diagnostic yield increases (Fig. 3.24). Thus meningiomas are usually revealed as homogeneous high-density lesions, enhancing uniformly, and acoustic neuromas are initially of low density but often enhance markedly. Slowly growing gliomas are often of low density and this is particularly so if they contain a cystic component; the actual tumour often has a speckled appearance (Weisberg, Nice, and Katz 1978). Glioblastomas show areas of alternating high and low density, while there is often evidence of a rim of oedema around tumours both of low and high malignancy, and this is particularly evident in relation to metastases (du Boulay 1978; Oldendorf 1980). Indeed some malignant tumours with a vascular periphery (Fig. 3.24(*c*)) may have a ring-like appearance on enhancement, resembling that of cerebral abscess (du Boulay 1978). In one early investigation of 366 cases of intracranial tumour (Ambrose, Gooding, and Richardson 1975), the diagnostic accuracy of CT scanning with enhancement was found to be 96 per cent and the introduction of

this diagnostic method has been shown to have transformed the management, for instance, of posterior-fossa tumours in childhood (Boltshauser, Hamalatha, Grant, and Till 1977).

Angiography. In carotid arteriography, the common carotid artery is injected with an iodine-containing contrast medium such as *Urografin* (60 per cent) or *Conray 80* (46 per cent). This technique is usually carried out by percutaneous injection under local or general anaesthesia; the internal carotid artery and its branches (the middle and anterior cerebral arteries and their radicals) are demonstrated and sometimes, but not often, one or both posterior communicating and posterior cerebral arteries may be filled. Vertebral angiography can also be performed by percutaneous puncture but complications are fewer if a catheter inserted into a limb artery such as the femoral or radial is used to inject contrast medium into one of the vertebral vessels. Aortic-arch angiography is particularly valuable in detecting lesions of the great vessels in the thorax and neck in patients with symptoms of cerebral vascular disease. It is less helpful in detecting intracranial tumours when it is necessary to demonstrate the fine detail of intracranial vessels. However, selective filling of the external carotid artery and its branches may be necessary in order to demonstrate tumours in the neck (e.g. carotid-body tumours) or others which are extracranial.

Fig. 3.24. (a) Meningioma, arising from the right sphenoidal wing, showing high-density well circumscribed mass, enhanced with Conray (right).

(b) Acoustic neuroma, right-sided, showing low-density mass, poorly circumscribed, distorting the brainstem, enhanced and well delineated with Conray (right).

(c) Glioma, left temporal, mainly cystic, showing low-density mass, but the margin of the cyst capsule is demonstrated by Conray (right). The low-density surrounding area is cerebral oedema.

(d) Glioma, left temporal, partly calcified, partly tumour. Showing irregular mixed-density mass in which the tumour component is enhanced in an irregular manner by Conray (right).

(e) Glioma, frontal midline, involving the corpus callosum with surrounding oedema on the right side, showing a moderately high-density mass surrounded by low-density area of oedema, slight enhancement with Conray (right).

(f) A solitary cerebral metastasis from carcinoma of the lung, right fronto-temporal, showing with Conray enhancement the tumour rim, the necrotic centre, surrounding oedema, and shift of midline structures (right).

(Reproduced from Bannister (1978) by kind permission of the author.)

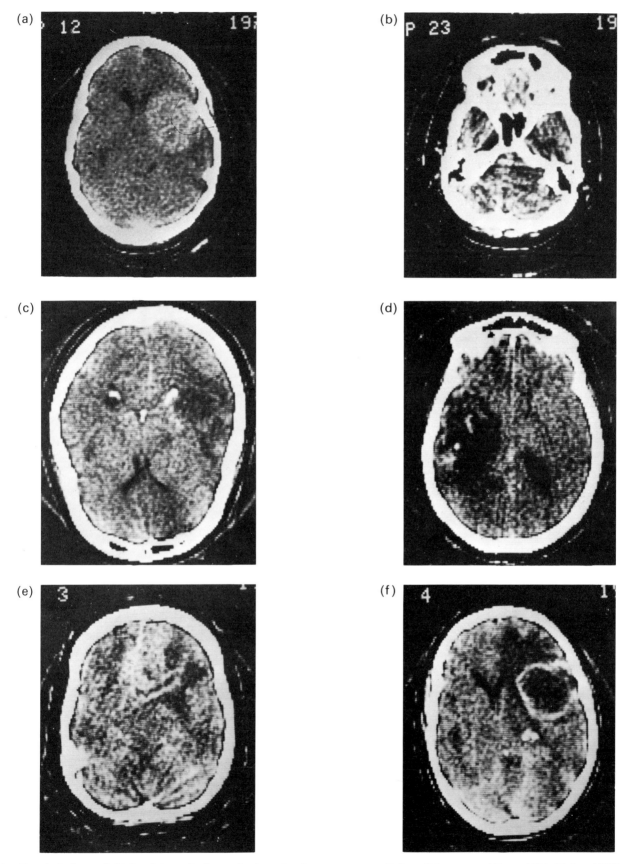

Subtraction techniques (which subtract the bony shadows leaving a clearer demonstration of the vessels) as well as image intensification or magnification using television are being used increasingly, but for details of technique the reader is referred to textbooks of neuroradiology (Newton and Potts 1974; Huber 1982). Normally at least three lateral, anteroposterior, and oblique views are taken at one-or two-second intervals to give early and late arterial and venous filling, but sometimes the demonstration of vascular lesions or of pathological tumour circulations requires much more frequent films (rapid serial angiography).

In cases of intracranial space-occupying lesion, displacement of arteries and/or veins may localize the lesion whether it be a tumour, an abscess, or a haemorrhage and an unusually wide 'sweep' of the anterior cerebral and pericallosal arteries around the corpus callosum may indicate ventricular dilatation due to hydrocephalus (Fig. 3.25). Some tumours show a characteristic pathological circulation. Astrocytomas tend to be relatively avascular (Fig. 3.26), glioblastomas and metastases often show tangles of small abnormal blood vessels (Figs. 3.27 and 3.28), arteriovenous angiomas contain greatly enlarged and tortuous arteries and veins (Fig. 3.29), and meningiomas often give a typical 'blush' in the venous phase of the angiogram owing to retention of contrast medium in the vessels of the tumour (Fig. 3.30), to quote only a few examples. Vertebral angiography may similarly be successful in demonstrating lesions in the posterior fossa, especially haemangioblastomas of the cerebellum (Fig. 3.31), and displacement of the basilar artery is a valuable sign of tumours lying in or in relation to the brainstem.

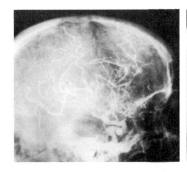
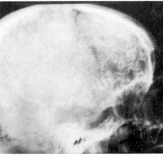

Fig. 3.27. A pathological circulation in a large frontal-lobe glioma.

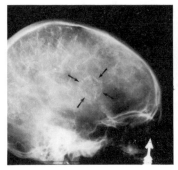
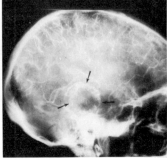

Fig. 3.28. Left carotid angiogram (left) showing a vascular metastasis in the fronto-parietal region (arrows). Right carotid arteriogram of the same patient (right) showing a similar lesion in the right temporal lobe.

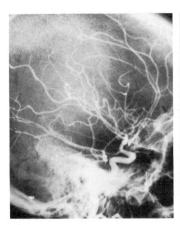
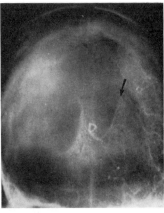

Fig. 3.25. Ventricular dilatation demonstrated by carotid angiography. On the left the anterior cerebral arteries are seen to take a wide sweep around the elevated corpus callosum. On the right, the thalamostriate vein (arrow) indicates the width of the lateral ventricle.

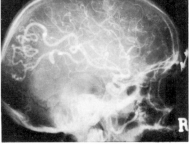
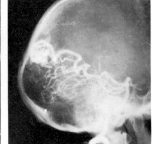

Fig. 3.29. An occipital arteriovenous angioma supplied by both the carotid (left) and vertebral (right) systems.

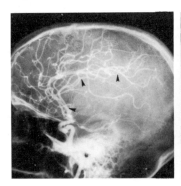
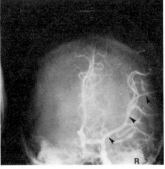

Fig. 3.26. Upward and inward displacement of the middle cerebral vessels produced by a temporal-lobe glioma (there is no pathological circulation).

Pneumoencephalography. Some contra-indications to pneumoencephalography were mentioned above; this technique is best avoided when there is reason to suspect that the intracranial pressure is raised or when there are strong grounds for suspecting the presence of a tumour in one cerebral hemisphere or in the posterior fossa. Nevertheless, if the CT scan or other investigations have given negative or equivocal findings or rarely when, for instance, it is necessary to define the upper limits of a tumour arising in the pituitary fossa, it may still be an appropriate examination in some

tumour suspects but should only be carried out in a specialized unit with neurosurgical aid immediately available. The method is still sometimes used to demonstrate cerebral atrophy in patients with presumed dementia or to confirm a diagnosis of communicating hydrocephalus but even in such cases it has been largely supplanted by the CT scan.

To perform a pneumoencephalogram (Robertson 1967), a lumbar puncture is performed with the patient sitting upright. After a few drops of CSF have been allowed to flow, sufficient only to determine that the needle is in position, 5 ml of air or oxygen is injected slowly and radiographs are taken as the bubble passes through the basal cisterns and fourth ventricle. Then 5 ml of CSF is removed, 10 ml of air is injected, and subsequently another 10 ml of fluid is withdrawn. The procedure is continued until 25–30 ml of air has been injected and adequate filling of the ventricular system has been obtained (Fig. 3.32). The procedure consistently produces severe headache and sometimes prostration and vomiting; the severity of these symptoms is usually in direct proportion to the amount of air injected. It is usual to give pethidine (demerol) or a similar analgesic both as a premedication and subsequently, and haloperidol or chlorpromazine may be required in

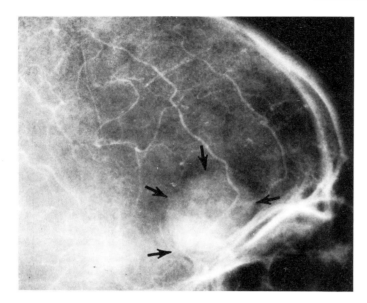

Fig. 3.30. A subfrontal meningioma showing a typical 'blush' (arrows) in the late arterial phase.

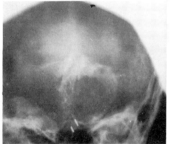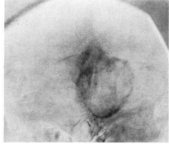

Fig. 3.31. A recurrent haemangioblastoma shown by vertebral angiography (left) to have a peripheral pathological circulation and an avascular centre; a subtraction print of the same angiogram is shown on the right.

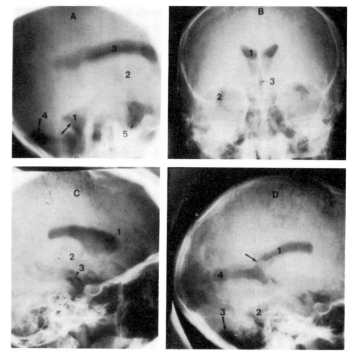

Fig. 3.32. A normal pneumoencephalogram.(A) Erect midline tomogram. 1. fourth ventricle, the choroid plexus is arrowed; 2. third ventricle; 3. lateral ventricle; 4. cisterna magna; 5. pre-pontine cistern. (B) Antero-posterior brow-up view. 1. Body of lateral ventricle; 2. temporal horn; 3. third ventricle. (C) Lateral brow-up view. 1. Frontal horn of lateral ventricle; 2. third ventricle; 3 temporal horn. (D) Lateral brow-down view. 1. Lateral ventricle (choroid plexus arrowed); 2. fourth ventricle; 3. cisterna magna; 4. occipital horn.

order to prevent or relieve vomiting. General anaesthesia is usually needed if the investigation is to be performed in children or restless or confused adults. The technique can help in defining the upper limits of a pituitary neoplasm (Fig. 3.33) and in demonstrating encroachment upon or distortion of the fourth ventricle produced by tumours such as brainstem gliomas, acoustic neuromas (Fig. 3.34), or other posterior-fossa lesions. Neoplasms of the cerebral hemispheres may be localized by signs of displacement of the lateral and/or third ventricles, but rarely is it possible to draw conclusions about the pathological character of the lesion except by inference according to its site.

Ventriculography. This technique requires shaving of the scalp and the insertion of bilateral posterior burr holes in the skull, after which air is injected into one lateral ventricle through a needle passed through a burr hole and then through brain tissue. The procedure is not without risk, first because the needle may pierce a vessel in its passage through the brain and secondly because the sudden release of pressure in one lateral ventricle may result in herniation of the opposite cerebral hemisphere beneath the falx cerebri. Immediate puncture of the opposite cerebral ventricle or operative decompression is then required. Hence the investigation is only performed when it is possible to proceed at once with any necessary neurosurgical operation.

Once air has been injected, the radiologist then manipulates the bubble throughout the cerebral ventricular system. As with pneumoencephalography, the method localizes neoplasms displacing

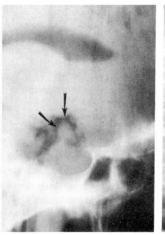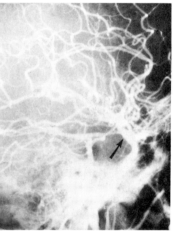

Fig. 3.33. Pneumoencephalogram (left) of the patient whose X-ray of skull is shown in Fig. 3.23. Air in the basal cisterns outlines a suprasellar extension of a chromophobe adenoma of the pituitary. Right carotid angiogram (right) shows deformity of the carotid siphon produced by the parasellar extension of the tumour.

or encroaching upon the lateral, third, or fourth ventricles (provided that the air will pass down the aqueduct) with considerable success (Figs. 3.35–3.38). The method is also valuable in demonstrating the site of obstruction (e.g. the aqueduct) in cases of hydrocephalus (Fig. 3.4, p. 141). Sometimes precise demonstration of the third or fourth ventricles requires injection of a contrast medium such as *Myodil* or *Conray* (Fig. 3.39). The latter technique should be used only when absolutely necessary as the injected material may act as a cerebral irritant unless it can be

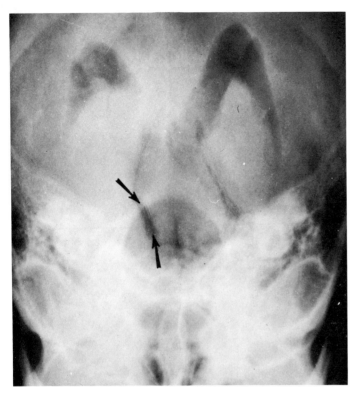

Fig. 3.34. Pneumoencephalogram of a case of acoustic neuroma showing displacement to the right of the cerebellopontine angle cistern (arrows).

made to pass downwards into the spinal theca at the conclusion of the examination and this is not always possible if the CSF pathways are obstructed.

Metrizamide cisternography. The introduction of the water-soluble contrast medium, metrizamide, now extensively used for myelography (Grainger and Lamb 1980), has been followed by the use of this substance in place of oily contrast media in outlining the cerebral ventricles (during ventriculography) and the basal cisterns (after injection by lumbar puncture). The method generally reduces the risk of subsequent arachnoiditis which is a complication of using oily contrast media, but sometimes precipitates attacks of epilepsy (Skalpe 1980) as well as headache. However it is particularly useful in demonstrating intrasellar and parasellar lesions (Hall 1980) as well as small acoustic neuromas in the internal auditory meati and other posterior-fossa tumours.

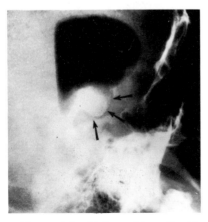

Fig. 3.35. A colloid cyst of the third ventricle outlined by ventriculography.

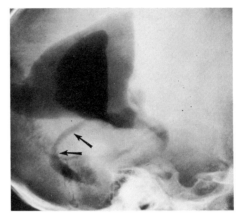

Fig. 3.36. A large ependymoma of the fourth ventricle demonstrated by ventriculography.

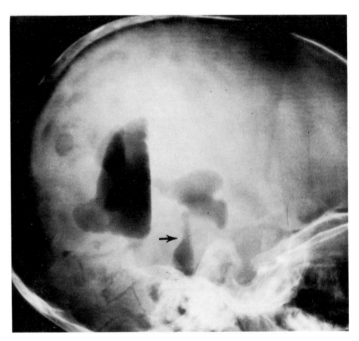

Fig. 3.37. A ventriculogram in a child with a medulloblastoma of the cerebellar vermis which is displacing the aqueduct and fourth ventricle forwards.

Focal symptoms

Frontal lobe
Prefrontal tumours. Prefrontal tumours are those confined to that part of the frontal lobe lying anterior to the precentral gyrus. Headache as a rule occurs early, but papilloedema and vomiting usually develop late and may be absent. As we have seen, mental symptoms may occur with a tumour in any situation, but there is evidence that they are more likely to occur when the tumour is in the corpus callosum or frontal lobe than when it is elsewhere. Moreover, in the absence of other localizing signs, the development of mental symptoms before signs of increased intracranial pressure favours a frontal localization (Botez 1974). The mental disturbance is a progressive dementia, with a defective grasp of situations and a failure of the synthetic function of thought. In more severe cases there is more severe intellectual decline and the patient becomes stupid, fails to appreciate the gravity of his illness, is careless of dress and appearance, and ultimately develops incontinence of urine and faeces without concern. Some patients are jocular and facetious and repeatedly make simple jokes or

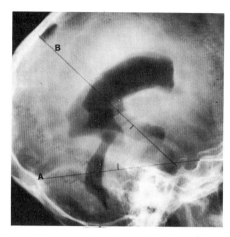

Fig. 3.38. A ventriculogram of a patient with a large glioma of the brain-stem.

A: Twining's line, the midpoint of which should normally lie in the fourth ventricle;

B: the Swedish line—the aqueduct should be at the junction of the anterior one-third and posterior two-thirds of the line. Both structures are displaced backwards and upwards.

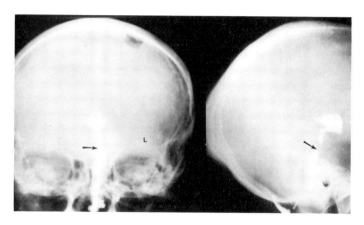

Fig. 3.39. Myodil ventriculogram of a patient with a cerebellar haem-angioblastoma. The aqueduct and fourth ventricle are displaced forwards and to the left. In the lateral view (right) contrast medium in the cisterna magna outlines the herniated cerebellar tonsils.

puns (Witzelsucht). Irritability of temper and depression are not uncommon.

Generalized convulsions occur in up to 50 per cent of cases. When the tumour lies inferiorly in the dominant hemisphere, the patient may experience an aura associated with speech. He may feel as if he wishes to speak but cannot do so, and may actually stammer before losing consciousness. There may be a sensation of something gripping the throat. When it is situated more superiorly, the motor element in the convulsion is likely to consist of turning of the head and eyes to the opposite side (adversive attacks) with complex clonic and tonic movements of the contralateral limbs.

Catatonia is a rare manifestation of organic brain disease, occurring more often in schizophrenia, but it has been described as an uncommon manifestation of frontal-lobe tumour. The patient becomes immobilized for some time in one attitude or may maintain indefinitely an attitude into which his limbs have been manipulated by the observer—waxy flexibility. Large frontal tumours sometimes cause considerable unsteadiness in walking with frequent falling, even without other evidence of paresis or reflex change. This ill-defined symptom has been thought to be an apraxia of gait, but is sometimes called 'frontal-lobe ataxia'.

Expressive aphasia (Broca's aphasia) may occur when the tumour involves the posterior part of the dominant inferior frontal gyrus.

The grasp reflex is an important sign, when present, as it is pathognomonic of a frontal-lobe lesion. It is most often seen in the opposite hand, but may be found only in the foot when the tumour lies in the upper part of the lobe.

A rare sign of a frontal-lobe lesion which must not be confused with the grasp reflex is tonic innervation or perseveration, which consists of a persistence of muscular contraction voluntarily initiated, with delay in relaxation. Tonic perseveration is usually most evident after finger flexion, but may occur after movements of other parts of the body on the side opposite to the lesion. Muscular relaxation is slow and may take several seconds.

Pressure upon neighbouring corticospinal fibres may lead to weakness of the opposite side of the body, usually most marked in the face and tongue. Pressure on the olfactory nerve, lying on the floor of the anterior fossa, may lead to anosmia on the side of the lesion. This most often occurs in the case of meningiomas arising from the olfactory groove. Such tumours extending backwards may compress the optic nerve, causing primary optic atrophy on the side of the lesion, while the rise of intracranial pressure causes papilloedema on the opposite side (the Foster Kennedy syndrome).

Precentral tumours. Precentral tumours are perhaps the easiest to localize because of the early development of symptoms of excitation and destruction of corticospinal fibres.

Corticospinal excitation finds expression in a focal convulsion, of which several forms are encountered. In a typical Jacksonian fit (Fig. 3.40) the convulsion begins with clonic movements, rarely with tonic spasm, in a limited area of the opposite side of the body, e.g. the thumb, and slowly spreads, involving other parts in the order in which they are represented in the precentral gyrus (see p.16). When the whole of one side of the body convulses the opposite side may become involved, and consciousness is then usually lost. Partial Jacksonian attacks may occur, restricted to a small part of one side of the body, without loss of consciousness. Such an attack may be continuous—'epilepsia partialis continua'. Jacksonian attacks can occur at long intervals, or very frequently, even up to several hundreds a day—serial Jacksonian epilepsy. When consciousness is not regained between successive attacks, the condition is described as Jacksonian status epilepticus.

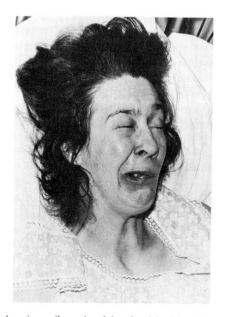

Fig. 3.40. Jacksonian epilepsy involving the right side of the face. (Photograph kindly provided by Dr J.D. Spillane.)

Motor weakness results from destruction or compression of corticospinal cells and fibres by the tumour, and exhibits a distribution corresponding to the representation of parts of the body in the precentral gyrus. Owing to the large surface area occupied by cortical motor cells, even a large tumour often causes weakness confined to one contralateral limb, that is, a monoplegia. With inferior tumours the weakness, often accompanied by apraxia, affects the face and tongue on the opposite side, and the thumb, which is represented in the adjacent area, may also be weak. If the tumour is at a higher level the thumb may escape, though the fingers and arm are affected, while a tumour mainly involving the medial aspect of the hemisphere is likely to cause a monoplegia involving only the foot or leg. The usual reflex changes associated with a corticospinal lesion are found and may be limited to the paretic part.

A tumour of the falx in the region of the paracentral lobule (a parasagittal meningioma) often produces weakness of both lower limbs, beginning in the feet, one usually being affected more than the other. Retention of urine may occur owing to compression of cortical centres where micturition is initiated. There may be an impairment of postural sensibility in the toes when the sensory area of the paracentral lobule is involved.

Jacksonian convulsions are usually associated with persisting weakness of the part of the body which is the focus of the fit, but after each convulsion there is often a temporary extension of this weakness to other parts (Todd's paralysis). Sensory loss is absent, unless the tumour extends to the postcentral gyrus.

Temporal lobe

The focal symptoms of temporal-lobe tumours are often slight, especially when the tumour is on the right. When it is anteriorly situated and involves the uncus, there is often a characteristic group of symptoms. This is the cortical centre for taste and smell, and the closely associated motor functions of licking, mastication, and swallowing are represented nearby. Tumours of the uncus may cause so-called uncinate fits characterized by an olfactory or gustatory aura often with certain motor accompaniments. The aura consists of an hallucination of taste or smell which is usually unpleasant but occasionally pleasant. It may be described as resembling paint, gas, acetylene, 'something burning', or even, as one patient put it, the monkey house at the zoo. There may also be 'butterflies in the stomach'. Involuntary licking, smacking the lips, or tasting movements often accompany the olfactory or gustatory aura and form the motor component of the uncinate fit.

Sometimes in association with such attacks other manifestations of temporal-lobe epilepsy (complex partial seizures—see p. 615) also occur as the epileptic discharge spreads more posteriorly. More often, and especially with small tumours of the medial temporal lobe (Cavanagh 1958), other symptoms including automatism, disordered consciousness, and perversions of memory and of the emotions characterize temporal-lobe attacks. The patient presents a dazed or dreamy appearance and usually stops what he is doing, but does not fall. He may have no recollection of the attack afterwards or may describe disturbances of memory, such as the *déjà vu* phenomenon, a feeling that everything that is happening has happened before like a recurrent dream, or he may in a short time relive in detail much of his past life. He may experience illusions relating to the external world or his own body. Objects may appear larger, smaller, or more distant than normal or unreal. There may be visual or auditory hallucinations. A sense of depersonalization or unreality (*jamais vu*) may occur. Emotional disturbances include fear (even 'panic attacks') and depression. Generalized convulsions sometimes occur, with or without a 'temporal-lobe' aura. Destruction in the region of the uncus gives impairment of taste and smell on the side of the lesion, though this is rarely noticed and does not as a rule proceed to complete loss. Rarely a hippocampal tumour in the dominant hemisphere may

produce transient global amnesia (Shuping, Toole, and Alexander 1980; and see p. 653).

Visual-field defects are found in about 50 per cent of temporal-lobe tumours. The lower fibres of the optic radiation are caught in their path around the tip of the inferior horn of the ventricle. The characteristic defect is thus a crossed upper quadrantic hemianopia, sometimes more extensive in the ipsilateral field. Although the cortical centre for hearing is situated in the posterior part of the lobe, temporal tumours do not cause complete deafness in either ear, though a unilateral lesion may give some bilateral impairment of hearing. Tumours in or near the auditory cortex may, however, cause tinnitus, while, if auditory association areas are involved, other crude auditory hallucinations or even organized hallucinations (e.g. voices or music) rarely occur. Lesions of the dominant temporal lobe may cause either nominal, receptive (Wernicke's), or conduction aphasia (see pp. 55–8). Most often the patient has difficulty in understanding spoken language and speaks in jargon with frequent paraphasia.

Commonly with larger lesions there is involvement of the lower cells and fibres of the corticospinal tract with contralateral facial weakness, perhaps with weakness of the arm and hand. Herniation of the medial temporal lobe through the tentorial hiatus can compress the trunk of the third nerve causing a fixed dilated pupil on the same side and sometimes ptosis, while compression of the trigeminal ganglion rarely causes loss of the ipsilateral corneal reflex.

Parietal lobe

The parietal lobe is the sensory area of the cerebral cortex. Sensory disturbances are therefore prominent symptoms of tumours of this region. Parts of the body are represented for recording sensation in the postcentral gyrus in a manner similar to their motor representation in the precentral gyrus. From below upwards we encounter in order the larynx and pharynx, the tongue, the buccal cavity, the face, neck, thumb, index, second, third, and fourth fingers, the hand, forearm, upper arm, shoulder, chest, abdomen, thigh, and leg. The areas of the foot and toes are situated at the superior border of the hemisphere, and on the medial aspect, in the paracentral lobule, lie those of the bladder, rectum, and genital organs (see p. 16).

Irritation of the postcentral gyrus causes sensory Jacksonian fits which consist usually of paraesthesiae, such as tingling or 'electric shocks', rarely of pain, and which begin in that part of the opposite side of the body corresponding to the focus of excitation. The paraesthesiae then spread to other parts in the order of their representation in the gyrus. Such sensory fits may occur alone, or be followed by a similar spreading motor discharge when excitation extends to the precentral gyrus, when the clonic convulsion often lags behind the advance of the paraesthesiae.

A destructive lesion of the postcentral gyrus gives sensory loss, corresponding in distribution to the extent of the cortical lesion. Sensory loss is of the cortical type, that is, it involves the spatial discriminative aspects of sensation, especially postural sensibility and tactile discrimination, while the crude appreciation of pain, heat, and cold is left intact. As a result, the patient may be unable to recognize objects placed in the affected hand—'stereoanaesthesia'.

Postcentral lesions lead also to hypotonia and wasting of the affected parts and to both static and kinetic ataxia. When the patient is at rest, there is often a conspicuous restlessness of the affected limb, sometimes amounting to 'pseudo-athetosis', and he may gesticulate exaggeratedly with the affected hand. There is likely to be considerable ataxia in the finger-nose test—'sensory ataxia'.

Parietal tumours reaching deep into the white matter may lead to 'thalamic over-reaction', an exaggerated response to unpleasant stimuli on the opposite side of the body, though this is usually slight. Involvement of fibres of the optic radiation causes a crossed homonymous visual-field defect; since the upper fibres are the more likely to be caught, the defect may be confined to the lower quadrant.

The posterior part of the parietal lobe constitutes a 'watershed' between the three great cortical sensory areas, the optic, acoustic, and somatic. A lesion of this area in the dominant hemisphere, therefore, commonly affects the comprehension of spoken and written speech (pp. 55–8). Lesions of the left angular gyrus usually cause alexia and agraphia with which may be associated finger-agnosia and acalculia. Lesions of the same area on the right side cause disturbance of awareness of the opposite side of the body and the opposite half of space. Such disturbances of the 'body image' in non-dominant parietal-lobe lesions may be associated with dressing apraxia. Other forms of apraxia and agnosia (see pp. 62–3) more often result from dominant parietal lesions.

Lesions of either parietal lobe occasionally cause contralateral tactile inattention; there is no evident sensory impairment when each side is examined independently, but when bilateral simultaneous stimuli are applied, those on the opposite side of the body from the lesion may be ignored.

Occipital lobe

Tumours of the occipital lobe are comparatively rare. Headache is an early symptom, and other signs of increased intracranial pressure are usually conspicuous. Epileptiform convulsions occur in many cases—50 per cent in one series. They may be preceded by a visual aura, such as flashes of light moving from one side towards the midline, but this is not constant. Such attacks may begin with turning of the eyes to the opposite side. Rarely, if the visual association areas are involved, formed visual hallucinations occur rather than the crude unformed hallucinations such as flashes of light which result from irritation of the striate cortex. The characteristic focal sign of an occipital tumour is a visual-field defect. This may be a crossed homonymous hemianopia extending to the fixation point, a crossed homonymous quadrantic defect, or a crescentic loss in the periphery of the opposite half-fields. Hemianopia may have been noticed by the patient owing to his colliding with people or objects on his blind side.

Lesions of the dominant occipital lobe may give visual-object agnosia as well as a field defect and rarely agnosia for colours. Prosopagnosia (inability to recognize faces) is a rare manifestation. If the lesion spreads more anteriorly to involve the posterior temporal lobe, jargon aphasia and/or auditory hallucinations may occur, while extension to the posterior parietal region may cause apraxia, dyslexia, acalculia, or even contralateral sensory loss or inattention (see above). Just as lesions of the parietal lobe may cause tactile inattention, those of the occipital lobe sometimes cause contralateral visual inattention; this may be defined by tachistoscopy (p. 87).

Corpus callosum

Tumours of the corpus callosum are more common than is generally realized. Bull (1967) pointed out that a quarter of all hemisphere astrocytomas show macroscopic or microscopic evidence invasion of the corpus callosum. Sometimes they yield a distinctive clinical picture but more often the presentation is non-specific. Mental symptoms are prominent and are often the first to be noticed. Probably they are more often found in cases of tumour here than when the growth is situated in any other part of the brain, including the frontal lobe. Apathy, drowsiness, and memory defect or dementia are the commonest disturbances, but many of the mental symptoms already described as occurring in cases of cerebral tumour may be present. General convulsions are common. Indeed, a combination of progressive dementia with major (or focal) attacks of epilepsy must always raise the possibility of a tumour in this position. Its situation in the midlin extending laterally into the central white matter on both sides

soon leads to damage to the corticospinal tracts. This is usually asymmetrical at first, leading to hemiplegia on one side, with on the other increased reflexes with little loss of power. Later, double hemiplegia may be found. Anteriorly placed tumours extending into the frontal lobes can cause a grasp reflex on one or both sides. Apraxia is present in a few cases. It may occur on the left side only, owing to interruption of fibres linking the left supramarginal gyrus with the right corticospinal tract. Tremor and choreiform movements sometimes occur and are probably due to involvement of the corpus striatum. Signs of increased intracranial pressure often develop late. The protein content of the CSF is often high.

Centrum semiovale and basal ganglia

The centrum semiovale consists mainly of corticospinal fibres converging on the internal capsule, and sensory fibres diverging from the latter to the cortical sensory areas. Tumours here may cause little increase in intracranial pressure, but usually cause motor or sensory symptoms early. Owing to the concentration of fibres near the internal capsule, the whole opposite side of the body is likely to be affected. Anteriorly placed tumours cause a progressive spastic hemiplegia. When the tumour is situated more posteriorly or in the thalamus, the presenting symptoms are sensory, all forms of sensation are usually impaired on the opposite side, and sensory ataxia is present. Very rarely, abrupt memory loss (Ziegler, Kaufman, and Marshall 1977) or dysphasia (if the lesion is in the dominant hemisphere) occurs in thalamic tumours; manifestations resembling those of degenerative disease of the basal ganglia are rare, although a craniopharyngioma extending into the basal ganglia has been thought to produce a parkinsonian syndrome (de Yébenes, Gervas, Iglesias, Mena, Martin del Rio, and Somoza 1981). Hemianopia may be added if the optic radiation is involved. Somnolence is not uncommon when the tumour invades the thalamic or subthalamic regions; and signs of pressure upon the upper part of the midbrain may be found, especially weakness of conjugate deviation upwards and inequality of the pupils. Involvement of the third ventricle by the tumour is followed rapidly by signs of increased intracranial pressure if these were not previously present (see McKissock and Paine 1958).

Third ventricle

The third ventricle may be the primary site of a tumour, e.g. a colloid cyst, or may be invaded by a tumour arising below, in the interpeduncular space, above, in the falx or corpus callosum, or laterally, in the basal ganglia. Extraventricular tumours usually yield ample evidence of their presence before invading the ventricle, but those arising in the ventricle are often difficult to localize. Astrocytomas arising in the wall of the ventricle are not uncommon in children (Stein 1972). Hydrocephalus may be acute, subacute, intermittent, or chronic. Severe paroxysmal headaches are common, and may be influenced by changes in head position. Headache and papilloedema are sometimes the only symptoms. Progressive dementia may occur, or coma may develop suddenly. Impairment of memory, including a Korsakow-like syndrome, may develop. In cases of colloid cyst in the ventricle (Fig. 3.35, p. 160), attacks of loss of consciousness without convulsive features, occurring often at the height of an attack of headache, are common, as are 'drop' attacks with transient weakness of the lower limbs and falling but without loss of the senses; occasionally episodes of paraesthesiae in the limbs also occur (Kelly 1951).

Somnolence, hyperglycaemia and glycosuria, obesity, sexual regression, and irregular pyrexia may be produced by downward pressure upon the tuber cinereum and pituitary while diabetes insipidus and/or cachexia may result from hypothalamic involvement. Lateral extension towards the internal capsule causes signs of corticospinal defect on one or both sides.

Midbrain

Tumours of the midbrain usually cause internal hydrocephalus early owing to obstruction of the aqueduct. Headache, papilloedema, and vomiting are therefore conspicuous. Owing to the presence here of the nuclei of the third and fourth cranial nerves and the supranuclear paths converging upon them, ocular abnormalities are prominent. Lesions of the upper midbrain usually cause paresis of conjugate ocular deviation upwards (Parinaud's syndrome, p. 98), and retraction of the upper lids may be associated with this. Lesions of the lower part cause paresis of conjugate ocular deviation downwards with which ptosis and paresis of convergence may be combined. Conjugate lateral movement of the eyes often escapes, at least in the early stages, though a lesion just above the pons can involve the decussating supranuclear fibres for lateral movement and so cause bilateral paralysis of lateral conjugate gaze. The pupils are often unequal and dilated. The reactions both to light and on convergence-accommodation may be lost, or the latter may be preserved when the former is lost. Asymmetrical nuclear ophthalmoplegia may occur.

The corticospinal tracts are usually involved on both sides, though one is often more severely affected than the other. The characteristic reflex changes are then present. Weakness and spasticity, slight in the early stages, progress until in some cases a condition of virtual decerebrate rigidity supervenes. 'Tonic' fits characterized by opisthotonos with extension of all four limbs and loss of consciousness may occur; less severe episodes (also seen sometimes in brainstem multiple sclerosis) give rigid extension of one or more limbs or other episodic postural changes in the limbs or trunk without loss of the senses. Tremor is common and nystagmus and ataxia result from injury to cerebellar connections. Sensory changes are due to damage to long ascending sensory paths. Extensive areas of analgesia and defects of postural sensibility may be encountered. Compression of the lateral lemniscus can lead to unilateral or bilateral deafness.

Pineal body

The symptoms of tumours of the pineal region are: (1) signs of increased intracranial pressure; (2) signs of pressure upon neighbouring parts of the brain; and (3) in exceptional cases hormonal disorders. As previously mentioned, most tumours arising in this region are teratomas or germinomas, and growths arising from pineal parenchymal cells (pineocytoma, pineoblastoma) are uncommon. Most pineoblastomas develop in the first decade of life and carry a poor prognosis (Gillespie and Mahaley 1981). Since the pineal body is situated between the splenium of the corpus callosum above and the superior colliculi below, growths here quickly cause hydrocephalus, owing to obstruction to the drainage of the third ventricle, and symptoms of compression of the upper midbrain. Signs of increased intracranial pressure therefore occur early and are associated with variable signs of a midbrain lesion as described above, namely, defective conjugate ocular deviation upwards, less often downwards and laterally; paresis of convergence; retraction or ptosis of the upper lids; inequality of the pupils, which are often dilated; reflex iridoplegia; bilateral signs of corticospinal lesion; nystagmus and ataxia; tremor and sensory loss, rarely including deafness.

Among the uncommon hormonal disturbances described in children (usually young boys) with pineocytomas have been abnormally rapid growth, sexual precocity, or alternatively pubertal delay. Whether these manifestations result from the excessive output of melatonin or arginine vasotocin from pineal cells or the suppression of such output is still uncertain (Gillespie and Mahaley 1981). The internal hydrocephalus caused by pineal tumour may lead to 'hypopituitarism', and obesity may then complicate the clinical picture.

The parasellar region (the region of the optic chiasm)

The small region at the base of the brain above the sella lying between the optic chiasm and the cerebral peduncles is the site of tumours arising in four principal situations, namely: (1) tumours of the pituitary (hypophysis); (2) craniopharyngiomas; (3) suprasellar meningiomas; and (4) gliomas of the optic chiasm.

Tumours of the pituitary gland. As already described, it has been conventional in the past to classify pituitary tumours into acidophil (chromophil), chromophobe, and basophilic adenomas according to the reaction of their constituent cells to eosin staining. Now, however, it is apparent that many such tumours contain mixed cellular components, that many are microadenomas not detectable radiologically but only by hormonal assay, and that over a third of all pituitary tumours secrete prolactin (Gillespie and Mahaley 1981). The manifestations of these tumours may be divided into: (1) endocrine disturbance; (2) pressure symptoms; and (3) radiological changes.

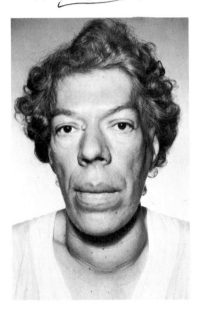

Fig. 3.41. The facial appearance of acromegaly. (Reproduced from Spillane (1975) by kind permission of the author.)

1. *Endocrine disturbances.* (*a*) *Growth hormone (GH)-secreting tumours.* In this tumour, the acidophil cells characteristic of the anterior lobe of the normal pituitary predominate, though chromophobe cells may also be present. When the tumour arises before growth has ceased, gigantism occurs; when, as more frequently happens, it begins during adult life, acromegaly is the result (Fig. 3.41). This is characterized by slow changes in the skin and subcutaneous tissues, bones, viscera, general metabolism, and sexual activity. The skin and subcutaneous tissues, especially of the fingers, lips, ears, and tongue, show fibrous hyperplasia, and paraesthesiae may occur in the fingers due to compression of the median nerve in the carpal tunnel. Overgrowth of the bones is most evident in the skull, face, mandible, and in the extremities. The calvarium is thickened and the bony ridges and points of attachment of muscles are increased in size. The zygomatic bones enlarge, and through overgrowth of the mandible the lower jaw becomes prognathous, and separation of the teeth occurs. The hands become broad and spade-like and hyperostoses may develop on the terminal phalanges ('tufting'). Similar changes occur in the feet, and the patient frequently notices that he requires a larger size in gloves and shoes. Kyphosis in the upper dorsal spine is common and hypertrophy of many of the viscera has been described.

Between 15 and 30 per cent of patients have overt diabetes mellitus, the glucose tolerance test is abnormal in 100 per cent, and 50 per cent die before 50 years of age from complications if untreated (Brodkey 1979). Usually the serum GH level is more than 10 ng/ml. Rarely such a tumour is associated with multiple endocrine adenomas elsewhere (Farhi, Dikman, Lawson, Cobin, and Zak

1976). Thyrotoxicosis and hypertrichosis may occur. Impairment of sexual function occurs in both gigantism and acromegaly, impotence in the male and relative or complete amenorrhoea in the female being the rule.

(*b*) *Chromophobe adenoma.* These tumours occur almost exclusively in adults and are three times as common as the GH-secreting tumours. While few such growths are exclusively composed of chromophobe cells and some secrete prolactin (see below), others corticotrophin, these tumours composed predominantly of chromophobe cells tend to be the largest growths originating in the sella, are often the least expressive in an endocrine sense, and are the most liable to cause chiasmal compression and/or pituitary apoplexy (see below). Their endocrine manifestations are usually those of hypopituitarism. The first symptom is usually depression of sexual function, with scanty menstruation, progressing to complete amenorrhoea in women and impotence in men. The skin becomes soft and pliable and there is often a loss of hair over the limbs and trunks (particularly in the axillae and pubic regions), and over the face in men. Moderate obesity often develops and hypoglycaemia may occur. The biochemical changes of hypothyroidism, hypo-adrenalism, and hypogonadism will be found. These symptoms may be present for many years before pressure symptoms develop.

(*c*) *Prolactinomas.* It is now apparent, following the introduction of a radioimmunoassay for prolactin, that the combination of amenorrhoea and galactorrhoea (the Forbes–Albright syndrome) in women is often due to the presence of a prolactin-secreting microadenoma in the pituitary gland. In men, impotence is the principal symptom but other manifestations of 'hypopituitarism' may occur. As the symptoms are more overt in women, they usually present with microadenomas, while men tend to have much larger tumours (Spark, Wills, O'Reilly, Ransil, and Bergland 1982). A microadenoma may coexist with an 'empty sella' demonstrated radiologically (Swanson 1979), but not all such tumours are small and many of the large growths classified in the past as chromophobe adenomas are now known to be prolactin-secreting. In patients with microadenomas the serum prolactin may be 75 ng/ml while in macroadenomas with suprasellar extension it may be 300 ng/ml.

(*d*) *Basophil adenoma.* The basophil adenoma rarely attains a sufficient size to cause pressure symptoms. It causes Cushing's disease due to hypersecretion of ACTH but a similar syndrome can result from adrenal tumours, hyperadrenalism, or ectopic ACTH-producing tumours in other organs. Serum ACTH measurement is, however, unreliable; secretion of this hormone by the pituitary may be suppressed (as indicated by plasma cortisol estimation) by 8 mg of dexamethasone, but not by 2 mg, and this test may help to identify Cushing's disease of pituitary origin, now believed to be much more common than that due to primary adrenal disease. The condition occurs three times as often in women as in men and its symptoms include painful, plethoric adiposity, 'moon-face' associated with purplish cutaneous striae, hirsutes, amenorrhoea, hyperglycaemia, hypertension, polycythaemia, osteoporosis, and myopathy. These symptoms are, of course, mimicked by the side-effects of corticosteroid drugs. Nelson's syndrome is a condition in which hyperpigmentation and myopathy may follow bilateral adrenalectomy for Cushing's disease and is due to an invasive ACTH-secreting tumour which commonly causes rapid sellar enlargement and visual field defects.

2. *Pressure symptoms.* Pressure symptoms may be entirely absent, particularly in the case of the microadenomas, which may for a long time produce only endocrine effects. Headache is usually an early symptom. In the early stages it is due to expansion of the sella and pressure upon the diaphragma sellae and is often described as a 'bursting' headache of bitemporal distribution. If later the tumour extends beyond the diaphragma, there may be a general increase in intracranial pressure. Vomiting is usually absent, except in the late stages. Since the optic chiasm lies above

the diaphragma sellae, visual-field defects are an important and early manifestation. Usually the tumour first compresses the decussating fibres of the chiasm, so that bitemporal hemianopia is the field defect most often found (see p. 88). This is as a rule asymmetrical, the defect beginning in the periphery of the upper temporal quadrant on one side, whence it extends towards the fixation point and then into the lower temporal quadrant. A similar change occurs either simultaneously or subsequently on the opposite side. Sometimes the defect begins as a scotoma on the temporal side of the fixation point. As the tumour grows, the nasal field of the eye first affected is involved so that the patient often passes through a stage of complete blindness in one eye with a temporal hemianopia on the opposite side. Later, if pressure is not relieved, the second eye also becomes blind. Less frequently one or other optic tract is compressed before the chiasm giving a homonymous hemianopia.

Compression of the optic chiasm causes optic atrophy, often more advanced in one eye than in the other. As the pressure at the same time obliterates the subarachnoid sheath of the optic nerves, papilloedema is rare. In the later stages, ocular palsies may be produced by compression of the third or sixth cranial nerves, trigeminal pain by pressure on the Gasserian ganglion, usually referred to the first division of the nerve and sometimes associated with analgesia. Rarely unilateral or bilateral ocular palsies without a visual-field defect may be the presenting symptom (Symonds 1962; Lopez, David, Gargano, and Post 1981). The title '*pituitary apoplexy*' has been given to the syndrome which may result from infarction in a chromophobe adenoma during a period of rapid growth (Conomy, Ferguson, Brodkey, and Mitsumoto 1975) or from actual bleeding into the tumour (Zervas and Medelson 1975; Mohanty, Tandon, Banerji, and Prakash 1977). This may give rise to intense headache, prostration, and even loss of consciousness with subarachnoid haemorrhage (Walton 1956); more often the tumour as it 'balloons' out of the sella causes compression of one third nerve and sometimes sudden blindness and optic atrophy (Jefferson and Rosenthal 1959).

Cerebral symptoms do not occur until the tumour has expanded beyond the sella, when compression of the cerebral peduncles or invasion of one hemisphere from below may lead to unilateral or bilateral signs of corticospinal-tract dysfunction; uncinate fits can result from compression of the uncus and pressure upon the frontal lobe may lead to marked mental deterioration, with or without abnormal emotional reactions. Somnolence, apathy, and confusion may be due to compression of the third ventricular floor and hypothalamus; such mental symptoms usually indicate a large extension.

3. *Radiographic appearances.* Pituitary macroadenomas cause a uniform expansion of the sella, with thinning of its walls and an upward extension may be demonstrated by the CT scan or by angiography or pneumoencephalography (Fig. 3.33, p. 159), but metrizamide cisternography is now generally preferred to the latter, though angiography may still be needed, especially to exclude suprasellar aneurysm. The single most sensitive radiological abnormality found in microadenomas is thinning of the lamina dura demonstrated by hypocycloidal polytomography (Gillespie and Mahaley 1981).

Craniopharygioma. The pathology of these tumours was described above. Since they depend upon developmental abnormalities, symptoms often appear early and in more than one-third of the cases the patient comes for treatment before the age of 15. Less often, however, they cause no symptoms until middle or late life. In a series of 85 cases Bartlett (1971 *a*) found that the sexes were equally affected: 30 were under the age of 15 when first seeking medical advice but the others were evenly distributed through the decades, the oldest being 71 years of age. In those under 15, 76 per cent presented with visual failure, 43 per cent with papilloedema, 40 per cent with growth disturbance; over that age, 74 per cent presented with visual symptoms, 32 per cent with dementia, and 32 per cent with pituitary failure, but only 5 per cent had papilloedema. These tumours usually arise above the sellar diaphragm, but exceptionally develop within the sella itself.

1. *Endocrine disturbances.* Since these growths arise between the floor of the third ventricle and the pituitary, often in childhood, they may produce many different disturbances of growth and metabolism, due to compression of the pituitary, hypothalamus or tuber cinereum. In Cushing's words, 'the patient may show extreme degrees of adiposity or emaciation, of polyuria or the reverse, of dwarfism, of sexual infantilism or of premature physical senility'. In the later stages the patient may be drowsy, and hyperpyrexia or diabetes may develop for the first time after surgery (Northfield 1957).

2. *Pressure symptoms.* Symptoms of increased intracranial pressure are much more conspicuous than with pituitary tumours. When the growth arises in childhood, the skull may be enlarged and the sutures separated. Headache and vomiting may be severe, and papilloedema is commoner than optic atrophy. The tumour may compress the optic nerves, chiasm, or tracts leading to corresponding field defects. The chiasm is compressed from above; hence the resulting bitemporal hemianopia usually begins in the lower quadrants. The frontal and temporal lobes and cerebral peduncles may also be compressed.

3. *Radiographic appearances.* These consist of: (i) general signs of increased intracranial pressure; (ii) erosion of the clinoid processes and flattening of the sella turcica, the result of downward pressure; and (iii) radiographic evidence of calcification within the tumour (Fig. 3.18, p. 155), which is present in about 75 per cent of cases and varies from faint, opaque flecks to a mass the size of a hen's egg, lying above the sella. Occasionally there is also calcification within the sella.

Suprasellar meningioma. Suprasellar meningiomas are tumours of adult life arising from the meninges covering the venous sinuses around the diaphragma sellae. Headache is not as a rule severe and endocrine symptoms are usually absent. The principal symptoms are visual and are due to compression of the optic nerve, chiasm, or tract, according to the position of the tumour. Optic atrophy is the rule and the visual-field defects may consist either of hemianopia of a central or paracentral scotoma. One eye is usually affected before the other and to a greater extent. Pressure upon the base of the brain may lead to uncinate attacks, general convulsions, and hemiparesis. Radiographs may show no abnormality, or the optic canal or clinoid processes may be eroded and the sella flattened, and there may be opacities due to calcification within the growth. Occasionally the tumour surrounds and may occlude one internal carotid artery. Extension upwards of metastases in the sella may have a similar effect (Scatliff and Bull 1965).

Glioma of the optic chiasm. This is a rare tumour which usually occurs in childhood, and may be associated with neurofibromatosis. Owing to its situation, visual deterioration usually draws attention to its presence before a marked rise of intracranial pressure occurs. Primary optic atrophy is the rule and the visual-field defects are often bizarre, depending upon the situation and extent of encroachment upon visual fibres. Proptosis may occur. Endocrine disturbances are absent. Radiographs usually show enlargement of one optic foramen (Fig. 3.42) and less often enlargement of the sella turcica forwards beneath the anterior clinoid processes (the J-shaped sella—see Cogan 1974). Gliomas in childhood tend to run a very slow course, often of many months or even years, before extending along the optic tracts into the midbrain. Rarely, if the diagnosis is made early it is possible to remove one eye and optic nerve before the chiasm is involved. Optic-nerve gliomas in adult life, however, are often aggressive, malignant and rapidly invasive, presenting with a picture like retrobulbar neuritis, giving total blindness within a few weeks and death in less than a year (Hoyt, Meshel, Lessell, Schatz, and Suckling 1973).

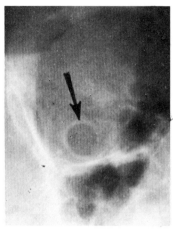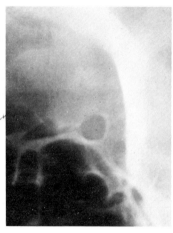

Fig. 3.42. Glioma of the right optic nerve. Radiographs show that the diameter of the right optic foramen (on the left) is 3 mm greater than the left (on the right).

Cerebellum

The cerebellum is a common site of tumour, especially in childhood. Medulloblastomas usually occur during the first decade of life. They arise in the midline in the region of the roof of the fourth ventricle. Astrocytomas, though they may occur either in the cerebrum or in the cerebellum, are common in the cerebellar hemispheres during childhood or early adult life, and are often cystic. Haemangioblastomas are almost exclusively cerebellar tumours, and are also usually cystic. The clinical effects differ according to whether the tumour is median or lateral.

Midline cerebellar tumours. In this group the history is usually short and the patient, generally a child, is likely to be brought for examination within a few weeks of the onset. Symptoms of increased intracranial pressure occur early, and often become severe. Headache, vomiting, and papilloedema are conspicuous, and in children hydrocephalus often leads to enlargement of the skull, with separation of the sutures. Signs of cerebellar dysfunction, to which the effects of ventricular dilatation may contribute (Maurice-Williams 1975), are usually most marked on standing and walking (truncal ataxia), and there may be little or no limb ataxia on examination. Giddiness is common, and there is usually unsteadiness on standing, especially with the eyes closed. The patient may sway or fall backwards or forwards. The gait is broad-based and unsteady, especially on turning and the patient cannot walk 'heel-to-toe'. Nystagmus is often absent, but there is often hypotonia which may be unequal on the two sides. Compression of the midbrain may lead to 'tonic fits', characterized by extension of all four limbs and opisthotonos, with loss of consciousness, and the pupils occasionally dilate and exhibit sluggish reactions, a misleading sign which may suggest a tumour of the third ventricle or pineal body. The other cranial nerves are often little affected, though weakness of one or both lateral recti and slight facial weakness may be found. There is as a rule little weakness of the limbs, though the plantar response may be extensor on one or both sides. The tendon reflexes are sometimes sluggish. Sensory loss is exceptional.

Tumours of the cerebellar hemisphere. As in the case of midline tumours, signs of increased intracranial pressure usually occur early, but a cystic haemangioblastoma can become large without causing conspicuous symptoms. In addition to suboccipital headache, early symptoms include clumsiness of the ipsilateral hand, a tendency to stagger to the side of the lesion, and giddiness on turning the head.

Nystagmus is usually marked and is most evident on conjugate lateral ocular deviation to the side of the lesion. The quick phase is directed towards the periphery and the slow phase towards the centre. It is usually confined to the plane in which the eyes are moved, but may occasionally be rotary. Other signs of cerebellar dysfunction are most marked in, and often confined to, the limbs on the side of the lesion. Hypotonia is usually conspicuous. The outstretched upper limb on the affected side tends to sway if unsupported. Ataxia is present on the affected side, being most evident in the upper limb during fine movements, as in the finger-nose test, and in the lower limb in walking. The gait is unsteady. The patient tends to walk on a wide base, to deviate to the affected side, and to fall to the affected side when standing with the feet together and the eyes closed. Rapid alternating movements are carried out in the affected limbs in an irregular, jerky manner. The shoulder on the affected side is sometimes held lower than the normal one, and there may be scoliosis concave towards the side of the lesion.

There is occasionally an abnormal attitude of the head, which is flexed to one side and rotated. Speech is usually little affected in cerebellar tumours, whether of the midline or lateral lobes. (For other signs of cerebellar lesions see p. 35.)

The cerebellar signs associated with a tumour of the cerebellum often seem disproportionately slight in relation to the size of the tumour. It is known that after cerebellar ablation a considerable recovery of function may occur; probably the slow growth of the tumour permits gradual compensation by other parts of the nervous system for the cerebellar lesion.

Neighbourhood symptoms are usually more conspicuous in patients with lateral cerebellar tumours than when the tumour is in the midline. Forward pressure may disturb the function of any of the cranial nerves from the fifth to the twelfth on the same side, the fifth, sixth, and seventh being most frequently affected. Pressure upon the ipsilateral half the pons and medulla may cause slight signs of corticospinal deficit on the opposite side of the body and occasionally sensory loss, especially impairment of postural sensibility, though this is rarely marked. Sometimes ipsilateral signs of corticospinal-tract dysfunction arise due to pressure of the contralateral crus cerebri against the free edge of the tentorium (the Kernohan–Woltman syndrome or Kernohan's sign).

Eighth nerve

Tumours of the eighth nerve (acoustic neuromas) may be either unilateral or bilateral. In the latter case they are usually manifestations of neurofibromatosis. They rarely cause symptoms before the third decade of life and most often during the fifth decade. They are tumours of slow growth, and focal signs commonly exist for years before those of increased intracranial pressure develop. The first symptoms are due to a disordered function of the eighth nerve; this feature is so constant that, if a tumour in the cerebello-pontine angle manifests itself in some other way, it is unlikely to be an acoustic neuroma. Tinnitus is usually the first symptom, followed by progressive deafness, though sometimes labyrinthine symptoms, for example giddiness, precede disturbances of hearing. Many patients, when first coming under observation, are completely deaf in the affected ear, having failed to notice unilateral hearing loss. Headache at first is usually occipital, but sometimes frontal, and may radiate from back to front through the mastoid region. In the late stages it becomes general and there may be attacks of severe occipital pain radiating down the spine, with retraction of the head and neck, respiratory embarassment, and, sometimes, loss of consciousness. Papilloedema and vomiting are comparatively late in developing. The patient may complain of paraesthesiae referred to the face on one or both sides, and attacks of hemifacial spasm may occur. Diplopia is not uncommon. Dysphagia occurs late.

On examination there are signs of dysfunction of the affected eighth nerve. Hearing is much reduced and may be completely lost. Tests of vestibular function usually show signs of a canal paresis. This usually occurs alone but sometimes in combination with a directional preponderance to the unaffected side (Carmichael, Dix, and Hallpike 1956).

Other signs result from pressure by the tumour upon neighbouring cranial nerves. There may be some facial weakness on the affected side, though this is often slight or absent. Sensory loss may occur in trigeminal distribution, but reduction or loss of the corneal reflex may be the only sign of involvement of this nerve. Nystagmus is almost invariable; if this sign is absent an acoustic neuroma is unlikely. Weakness of the lateral rectus may be present due to compression of the sixth nerve. The remaining cranial nerves are usually unaffected. Disturbance of function of the fifth, sixth, seventh, and eighth cranial nerves rarely occurs on the opposite side as well as on the side of the tumour. Compression of the ipsilateral cerebellar hemisphere can cause cerebellar signs on the side of the tumour. Signs of compression of the brainstem are not as a rule conspicuous, but crossed hemiparesis and hemianaesthesia may occur due to compression of long descending and ascending tracts, and weakness of conjugate ocular deviation to the side of the tumour, as a result of compression of the pons.

Atypical symptoms, occurring when the tumour arises more medially than usual, include acute hydrocephalus, causing rapid visual failure or slow mental deterioration, respectively, and paroxysmal disorders of consciousness, including epilepsy (Shephard and Wadia 1956). Radiographic examination may show erosion of the petrous portion of the temporal bone (Fig. 3.21, p. 156) or of the internal auditory meatus by the tumour. The size and situation of the tumour may be demonstrated by CT scan, ventriculography (Fig. 3.34, p. 160) or by metrizamide cisternography.

Pons and medulla

The commonest tumour of the brainstem is the pontine astrocytoma of childhood; less often these occur in adults. Owing to the close association in the pons and medulla of important cranial-nerve nuclei as well as of descending and ascending fibre tracts, tumours in this region soon produce localizing signs and symptoms (Barnett and Hyland 1952). Possibly for this reason signs of increased intracranial pressure are often slight when the patient first seeks advice. Vomiting is often absent, and papilloedema appears in under 50 per cent of cases. Headache, which at first is mainly occipital, and vertigo are common, and both may be intensified by head rotation. Diplopia due to a unilateral sixth-nerve palsy is usually the first focal symptom, a point of distinction from cerebellar medulloblastoma. At first the signs may point to a lesion on one side of the brainstem but they eventually become bilateral. Weakness of one or both lateral recti may be followed by paresis of conjugate ocular deviation, or the latter may occur alone. Crossed paralysis is usually seen at an early stage, the distribution of the weakness on the two sides of the body depending upon the level of the tumour. An acute hemiplegic onset in childhood has been described (Rothman and Olanow 1981). Sometimes there is weakness of jaw and facial muscles on one side and of the soft palate, tongue, and limbs on the other. Later bilateral paralysis of the bulbar muscles and limbs usually develops. Unilateral facial myokymia and contracture are rare manifestations of pontine glioma and have been observed in a case of pontine tuberculoma (Boghen, Filiatrault, and Descarries 1977). Sensory loss in trigeminal distribution with reduction of the corneal reflex is often present on one or both sides, and impairment of hearing may occur. Sensory loss on the limbs and trunk is variable. Analgesia and thermo-anaesthesia may occur without loss of postural sensibility or vice versa, or all forms of sensation may be affected. Sensory changes may be predominantly unilateral or bilateral. Nystagmus and some degree of limb ataxia are common due to involvement of central cerebellar connections. Paralysis of the ocular sympathetic on one or both sides is frequent, and medullary visceral functions may be disordered, leading to tachycardia or cardiac arrhythmia, alteration in respiratory rate and rhythm, hiccup, and glycosuria. The course of the illness is sometimes protracted, lasting for several years, as many of these tumours are very slow-growing (the condition which used to be called 'benign hypertrophy of the pons' is now known to be due to a slow-growing astrocytoma). 'Failure to thrive', like that seen in the so-called diencephalic syndrome of wasting in childhood, has been reported (Maroon and Albright 1977). Temporary remission of symptoms and signs is not infrequent (Sarkari and Bickerstaff 1969).

A chordoma arising between the pons and the clivus or a solitary plasmacytoma of the clivus (Gardner-Thorpe 1970) may give a similar picture to that of an intrinsic brainstem tumour with cranial-nerve palsies and long-tract signs. These tumours sometimes calcify and an area of calcification posterior to the clivus may be diagnostic. Arteriovenous angiomas of the brainstem can give a similar picture. CT scanning, vertebral angiography, metrizamide cisternography, or, where necessary venticulography (Fig. 3.38) are the methods of radiological investigation which are most useful in localizing tumours in or near the brainstem.

Fourth ventricle

Tumours arising in the fourth ventricle itself are usually ependymomas, though the fourth ventricle may be invaded by growths arising in the cerebellar vermis or pons. The characteristic symptom triad is headache, morning vomiting, and vertigo, with nystagmus increased or elicited by change in head position. In young patients ependymoma is the commonest cause but over the age of 50 the same syndrome may result from metastases in the fourth ventricle (usually from bronchial carcinoma). Headache is an early symptom, often with paroxysmal exacerbations and pain radiating to the neck and even to the shoulders and arms. Vomiting and papilloedema and other evidences of hydrocephalus usually develop rapidly. But headache and papilloedema may be absent: one patient had no symptoms except vomiting, for which he had had a laparotomy, and an ataxic gait. There is often some neck stiffness and truncal ataxia, but signs of cerebellar deficiency in the limbs may be slight or absent. Tonic fits may occur. Dysfunction of the cranial nerves is often slight, though there may be paresis of one or both lateral recti, and trismus has been noted. The tumour can affect the visceral centres of the medulla, causing attacks of tachycardia, dyspnoea and irregular respiration, hiccup, sweating, vasomotor disturbances, polyuria, and glycosuria. Sudden death may occur.

Rarely, the tumour grows out from the fourth ventricle to surround and compress the spinal cord at the level of the foramen magnum, producing analgesia and thermo-anaesthesia of the face and upper limbs, with signs of corticospinal involvement, and leading to a clinical picture closely resembling syringobulbia.

Foramen magnum and basal exit foramina

Tumours at or near the foramen magnum are often missed (*The Lancet* 1973). Many are meningiomas and they usually cause a clinical picture similar to that resulting from syringobulbia or basilar impression of the skull (p. 607) with signs of dysfunction of lower cranial nerves and of interference with long descending and ascending tracts. Severe impairment of position and joint sense in both hands and vertical nystagmus are signs which may point to a lesion in this neighbourhood.

The clinical manifestations of glomus tumours have already been mentioned (p. 151). Rarely a meningioma may develop near the jugular foramen giving unilateral paralysis of the ninth, tenth, and eleventh cranial nerves.

Basal meninges and skull base

Neoplastic infiltration of the basal meninges leads to a fairly distinctive clinical picture. This condition may be due to metastases from extracranial neoplasms, or to extension to the cranial cavity of a primary carcinoma of the naso-pharynx or of a paranasal sinus. It leads to progressive cranial-nerve palsies, which are usually unilateral but sometimes bilateral and asymmetrical. Often the neoplastic growth is wholly extradural, affecting particularly the third, fifth, and sixth cranial nerves as they emerge through their exit foramina, but sometimes the lower cranial nerves are selectively involved (tenth, eleventh, and twelfth). Radiographs of the skull base may demonstrate bony erosion (Fig. 3.43).

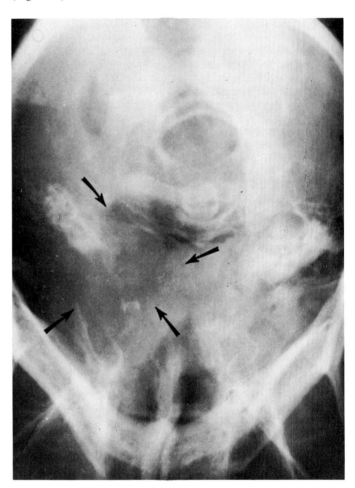

Fig. 3.43. Basal radiograph of skull demonstrating an ill-defined area of bony destruction (arrows) caused by a nasopharyngeal carcinoma. The foramina spinosum and ovale are completely destroyed on the left.

Greenberg, Deck, Vikram, Chu, and Posner (1981), in a report of 43 patients with metastases involving the bones of the base of the skull as distinct from the meninges, identified five clinical syndromes, *viz* orbital, parasellar, middle-fossa, jugular foramen, and occipital condyle. The orbital and parasellar syndromes were characterized by frontal headache, diplopia, and first-division trigeminal sensory loss. Proptosis occurred with the orbital but not the parasellar syndrome. The middle-fossa syndrome was characterized by facial pain or numbness, the jugular-foramen syndrome by hoarseness and dysphagia (ninth-, tenth-, and eleventh-nerve lesions) and the occipital-condyle syndrome by unilateral occipital pain and paresis of one side of the tongue.

In other instances, especially in the case of metastatic spread from extracranial visceral growths, the tumour is intradural, involving the arachnoid. Papilloedema may be present or absent. Invasion of the pituitary and tuber cinereum may cause polyuria, drowsiness, and other symptoms of hypothalamic disturbance. When the subarachnoid space is invaded, neck stiffness and pyrexia are present, the clinical picture then resembling that of tuberculous meningitis (carcinomatosis of the meninges). Neoplastic infiltration of the basal meninges may be associated with focal symptoms due to other metastases within the brain.

Gliomatosis cerebri
In this rare condition (p. 144), dementia and personality change are the commonest presenting feature but headache, papilloedema, fits, hemiparesis, ataxia, and brainstem signs may all occur (Couch and Weiss 1974); often angiography and air pictures give non-specific findings and diagnosis may ultimately depend upon brain biopsy.

Diagnosis
Other conditions may be confused with intracranial tumour, either because they increase the intracranial pressure or because they lead to a progressive cerebral lesion, or both. The following are the conditions most often mistaken for a growth.

Intracranial abscess
Usually, intracranial abscess is readily distinguished since its development is generally acute or subacute and a primary focus of infection is usually found either in the ears, sinuses, lungs, or elsewhere. Rarely, however, a chronic abscess may arise, its source of infection being latent or inapparent. In such cases clinical diagnosis from tumour may be impossible. A sudden or apoplectiform onset, the occurrence of a leucocytosis in the blood and of a slight CSF pleocytosis, and slight pyrexia are points in favour of abscess, but none of these is constant. The CT scan usually resolves the issue.

Arachnoidal cysts
Sometimes these cysts result from arachnoiditis after previous meningeal inflammation but most of those which mimic intracranial tumour are probably of developmental origin (Oliver 1958). They may occur between the hemispheres, in the cerebellopontine angle or at the base of the brain, where the optic chiasm may be involved. Preoperative diagnosis from tumour may be impossible without the CT scan which is often diagnostic.

Benign intracranial hypertension
The raised CSF pressure in this condition (p. 140) causes papilloedema, headache, and vomiting, but there are no progressive focal signs, the patients often seem surprisingly well (Foley 1955), and the ventricles are neither enlarged nor displaced; in fact they are usually small or normal in size.

Cerebral arterial disease
Cerebral softening due to vascular occlusion usually causes symptoms referable to a single lesion, though multiple lesions can occur. The onset of symptoms with a slight 'stroke' gives helpful evidence of their vascular origin, and support comes from evidence of vascular disease elsewhere. However, in some cases of cerebral infarction, particularly due to carotid occlusion, the evolution of symptoms is slow and diagnosis from tumour is difficult or impossible without contrast radiology. In malignant hypertension headache and papilloedema may coexist with signs of a focal cerebral lesion, but the blood pressure is high and typical retinal changes are present. Sometimes the diagnosis remains in doubt until investigation excludes a space-occupying lesion, but it must be remembered that in later life an intracranial tumour may coexist with arteriosclerosis and hypertension.

Neurosyphilis
Meningovascular neurosyphilis may be mistaken for tumour when headache and papilloedema coexist with signs of an intracranial lesion, while the dementia and convulsions of general paresis may suggest a tumour of the frontal lobe or corpus callosum. In both forms of neurosyphilis, however, reflex iridoplegia is usually present, and the V.D.R.L. reaction and other characteristic changes in the blood and CSF reveal the true nature of the disorder. Gumma of the brain is now extremely rare, and symptoms suggesting an intracranial tumour in a patient with a positive V.D.R.L. reaction must not be taken to indicate that the patient is suffering from such a lesion. Syphilis and cerebral tumour may occur in the same individual.

Epilepsy
Since epileptiform convulsions are a common symptom of intracranial tumour, differential diagnosis from other causes of epilepsy often arises. Constitutional epilepsy usually begins before the age of 25, though even in later life no cause may be found for fits even after prolonged observation. Convulsions beginning after this age always raise the possibility of tumour, though in late middle life and old age cerebral arteriosclerosis is probably the commonest cause. In idiopathic epilepsy headache is absent, except immediately after the fits, and there are no signs of a focal lesion. A focal onset or focal neurological signs in older patients with fits always raise the possibility of tumour and a CT scan should, where possible, be done in such cases.

Migraine
Headache, vomiting, visual hallucinations, and visual-field defects are common both to migraine and to tumours in the region of the occipital visual cortex, especially angioma. As a rule the field defects of migraine are transitory, lasting for one-half to one hour, but occasionally an exceptionally severe attack is followed by a permanent scotoma or hemianopia. Usually migraine begins at puberty, and there is often a family history. Signs of increased intracranial pressure are absent and there is no evidence of a progressive intracranial lesion. Visual-field defect associated with an occipital tumour is persistent. A bruit is sometimes heard over an angioma, and X-rays may show calcification or abnormal vascular markings in the skull. The CT scan and/or radiography are usually conclusive.

Retrobulbar neuritis
Acute bilateral retrobulbar neuritis may simulate intracranial tumour, because it causes disc swelling. It is distinguished, however, by the acute onset and by the fact that visual loss is disproportionately great compared with the disc oedema, which is usually slight. Headache is absent in retrobulbar neuritis, but pain in the eyes may be considerable, and they are often tender on pressure.

Leucodystrophy and demyelinating disease
Cerebral leucodystrophy or multiple sclerosis may simulate tumour when papilloedema is present. However, onset in early life, often with visual failure of subcortical origin, and the bilateral symptoms and signs should enable these conditions to be distinguished.

Chronic subdural haematoma
Since this is a slowly progressive space-occupying lesion, it may be indistinguishable from tumour in the absence of a history of trauma. The CT scan or angiography usually settle the diagnosis.

Encephalitis
Herpes simplex encephalitis (p. 280) may give a picture suggesting an acute temporal-lobe lesion but the apoplectiform onset is more likely to suggest abscess rather than tumour. Other forms of encephalitis and especially acute haemorrhagic leucoencephalitis sometimes give a 'pseudotumoural' picture of progressive hemiplegia in the early stages.

Aneurysm and other parasellar lesions

Large intracranial aneurysms may present as space-occupying lesions, especially when suprasellar in situation, but are readily recognized on angiography. It is also important to consider other parasellar lesions. In 102 patients with lesions in this region analysed by Thomas and Yoss (1970), 14 had tumours such as pituitary adenoma, craniopharyngioma, or meningioma, 13 other primary tumours (chondroma, plasmacytoma, lymphoma), 43 metastases, 19 aneurysms, and 13 inflammatory disorders such as herpes zoster, the 'Tolosa–Hunt syndrome', arachnoiditis, cranial arteritis, or Wegener's granulomatosis.

Hydrocephalus and dementia

Hydrocephalus of late onset, whether due to aqueduct stenosis giving symptoms first in adult life suggesting a posterior-fossa tumour, or to 'low-pressure hydrocephalus' which usually presents with dementia and ataxia, must be distinguished by appropriate radiological studies. Similar studies may be needed to exclude a corpus callosum glioma in some patients with dementia arising in the presenium.

Diagnosis of the nature of the tumour

Medulloblastoma

This is a rapidly growing, malignant tumour, usually found in or near the roof of the fourth ventricle in childhood. It should be suspected in children who present with symptoms of a midline cerebellar tumour and a history of a few weeks' or months' duration.

Glioblastoma multiforme

This is a malignant and rapidly growing tumour arising in middle life and usually found in the cerebral hemispheres. It should be suspected in middle-aged persons who have a short history of symptoms suggesting a tumour of one cerebral hemisphere. The CT scan is often diagnostic or gamma-encephalography shows enhanced radioactive uptake and angiography a pathological circulation.

Astrocytoma

The astrocytoma is a slowly growing tumour which may arise in the cerebral or cerebellar hemispheres or brainstem. When the history of an intracranial tumour in the cerebrum or cerebellum extends over several years, the growth is usually an astrocytoma or an oligodendroglioma but the latter is more liable to show calcification on plain X-rays than the former. Owing to its situation, the cerebellar astrocytoma is likely to bring the patient under observation sooner than one situated in the cerebral hemisphere. The CT scan is usually diagnostic but the gamma-encephalogram is less often positive than in more malignant growths and angiography often shows displacement of vessels only; as these growths are often avascular, a pathological circulation is relatively infrequent.

Meningioma

Meningiomas are predominently supratentorial tumours and exhibit certain sites of election which have already been described. They are rare before middle life and are commoner in females. There may be a very long history, e.g. of epilepsy for many years. Owing to their extracerebral origin they compress but do not invade the brain. The focal symptoms which they produce are less severe in relation to the size of the tumour than with gliomas, Meningiomas, therefore, often give a marked increase in intracranial pressure, with few if any signs of a focal lesion. Symptoms and signs may increase during pregnancy and remit after delivery (Bickerstaff, 1958; Michelsen and New 1969). Their proximity to the skull leads to erosion of bone, demonstrable on X-ray in up to 20 per cent of cases, and there may also be calcification within the tumour. The meningiomas are usually associated with increased vascularity, which may be extracranial as well as intracranial.

Radiographs may therefore show enlargement of the foramen spinosum in the base of the skull and the middle meningeal channels in the vault. The CT scan is usually diagnostic and angiography often demonstrates filling of the tumour from the meningeal circulation and vascular displacement; the typical 'blush' in the venous phase or other types of tumour circulation are seen in only about 50 per cent of cases (Banna and Appleby 1969).

Angioma

Since angiomas are of developmental origin, two-thirds cause symptoms below the age of 30. Epilepsy, intracerebral or subarachnoid haemorrhage, and hemiparesis are the commonest presenting symptoms. The diagnosis is confirmed by CT scan and angiography (Mackenzie 1953).

Haemangioblastoma

These tumours are almost exclusively cerebellar and are sometimes associated with haemangioblastoma of the retina and spinal cord, with cysts of the pancreas and kidneys and adrenals, or a hypernephroma. Only the first of these associated abnormalities, however, is likely to be identified clinically. As many of these tumours excrete erythropoietin, erythrocytosis is common (Jeffreys 1975 a, b) with haemoglobin levels often exceeding 16 g/100 ml; this is a valuable confirmatory sign. They occasionally cause paroxysmal hypertension mimicking the clinical picture of phaeochromocytoma (Cameron and Doig 1970). The CT scan is often diagnostic and vertebral angiography, using a subtraction technique, commonly shows a typical tumour circulation.

Tumours in the neighbourhood of the pituitary

Diagnosis of the nature of these tumours is described on pp. 164–6.

Acoustic neuroma

The clinical picture of this tumour, which usually arises in middle-aged persons, is distinctive, since the first symptoms are those of eighth- or fifth-nerve dysfunction on one side. A similar picture can result from a meningioma, cholesteatoma, or arachnoid cyst in the cerebellopontine angle.

Metastatic tumours

Metastatic tumours should be suspected in middle-aged or elderly individuals presenting with the history of a rapidly developing intracranial growth. In all such cases a thorough clinical and radiographic search for a primary neoplasm should be made. Often an intracranial metastasis gives rise to symptoms before the primary lesion, especially when this is in the lung, and sometimes the primary lesion is not discovered until autopsy.

Tuberculoma

Tuberculoma may occur at any age, but is most frequent in childhood and early adult life. It is now rare in Europe and the USA but is still common in India (Dastur and Desai 1965). These lesions are cortical or subcortical in the cerebral or cerebellar hemispheres and only rarely involve the brainstem. Remissions and relapses are somewhat characteristic, and the increase in intracranial pressure is often disproportionately slight. A pleocytosis may be found in the CSF. The presence of a tuberculous lesion elsewhere will afford some confirmatory evidence, but this is so common that it may coexist with a glioma.

Parasitic cysts

The possibility that the symptoms of an intracranial space-occupying lesion may be due to parasitic cyst should always be considered in a patient who has been exposed to the infestation. The presence of such cysts elsewhere in the body affords strong confirmatory evidence, and the CSF often shows a mononuclear pleocytosis.

The blood may show an eosinophilia. Complement fixation and flocculation tests, and Casoni's intradermal sensitization test may be of diagnostic value in suspected cases of hydatid infection.

Prognosis and treatment

The prognosis of intracranial tumour is influenced by the nature of the growth and its accessibility to the surgeon. In the absence of surgical interference almost all intracranial tumours increase in size, their rate of growth depending upon their nature. The resulting increase of intracranial pressure and destruction of brain tissue ultimately prove fatal. When papilloedema is severe, death may be preceded by blindness. The more malignant gliomas, such as medulloblastomas and glioblastomas, grow rapidly and usually prove fatal within one or two years, though temporary remission of symptoms and signs in medulloblastoma may follow radiotherapy and even the skeletal metastases of such tumours which can develop after partial operative removal or 'shunt' operations (p. 141) may remit temporarily after treatment with vincristine sulphate (Lassman, Pearce, Banna, and Jones 1969). The slowly growing astrocytomas may cause symptoms for many years before causing an overt increase in intracranial pressure (see Penman and Smith 1954). In a series of 184 brain tumours diagnosed in children over a 15 year period, Gold and Gordis (1979 *b*) found a 35 per cent five-year survival in 1960–4, improving to 49 per cent in 1970–4. Girls consistently did better than boys and those with supratentorial tumours showed a longer survival time than did those in whom the neoplasms lay beneath the tentorium.

Sudden death in cases of intracranial tumour is rare but can result from rapidly developing cerebral oedema and/or tentorial or cerebellar herniation. Increasingly severe headache, a unilateral dilated pupil, or increasing occipital pain and neck stiffness are important warning signs which may demand the urgent administration of high doses of steroids to reduce oedema, followed, where appropriate, by ventricular drainage or other neurosurgical measures.

Improvements in neurosurgical technique and anaesthesia, including the use of hypothermia when appropriate (Inglis and Turner 1957) and a careful choice of anaesthetic agents (Jennett, Barker, Fitch, and McDowell 1969) have greatly improved the outcome of surgical procedures in many patients. In a series of 766 patients subjected to surgery by Horrax (1954), the operative mortality was 13.2 per cent while almost 70 per cent engaged in useful activity for one to 20 years after operation. Even in cases of glioblastoma, partial removal of the tumour, creating an internal decompression, followed by the use of steroids (Lieberman, De Bran, Glass, Goodgold, Lux, Wise, and Ransohoff 1977) may improve the outcome, although attempted removal is less appropriate in tumours lying in relation to the motor and/or sensory cortex, in relation to the speech areas of the dominant hemisphere or in those which are deeply situated. In such cases, stereotaxic biopsy followed by implantation of ^{192}Ir and systemic chemotherapy (see below) has been shown to improve survival (Gillespie and Mahaley 1981). In slowly growing astrocytomas and oligodendrogliomas of the cerebral hemispheres, operative removal should not as a rule be attempted unless they lie in relatively silent areas, though exploration and biopsy may be necessary for diagnosis. By contrast, cerebellar astrocytomas can often be removed completely (see below), as can some haemangioblastomas. Most convexity meningiomas and pituitary adenomas can also be removed but operation upon basal and parasellar meningiomas may be much more hazardous because of encroachment upon major vessels or cranial nerves. Recurrence of meningiomas after apparent total removal is not infrequent and sometimes the recurrent growth becomes sarcomatous. Most colloid cysts of the third ventricle and other intraventricular tumours, such as choroid-plexus papillomas and ependymomas of the fourth ventricle, can also be removed and partial removal of clivus chordomas is also feasible, if hazardous. However, gliomas of the third ventricle and brainstem cannot be removed and the same is true of many pinealomas;

in such cases, if obstructive hydrocephalus develops, a 'shunt' operation may give at least temporary relief of symptoms. In some patients with craniopharyngiomas, a similar pallative operation is all that can be done, but, when the growth is relatively small, partial or even total removal is feasible and may lead to preservation of residual vision and prolonged remission of symptoms; even the drainage of an associated cyst or 'sump drainage' (Miles 1977) may also be beneficial, though a transient aseptic meningitis can result from the release of cholesterol into the subarachnoid space. Except in elderly patients with few focal signs and little evidence of raised pressure, all acoustic neuromas demand surgery but there is still some dispute among surgeons as whether total or intracapsular removal is to be preferred; the outcome in such cases is clearly related to the experience of the surgeon. There is also difference of opinion about the surgical treatment of arteriovenous angiomas; small or medium-sized malformations in relatively silent areas can be removed completely, even from the region of the basal ganglia (Garrido and Stein 1978); few surgeons are prepared to operate upon large angiomas but some advocate ligation or deliberate embolization of major feeding vessels. The rare intracranial gumma responds little if at all to antisyphilitic treatment but may demand surgical removal; the same principle applies to tuberculomas which should be removed if possible after prior treatment with antituberculous drugs which should be continued for some months after surgery in order to prevent meningitis. Surgery is of little or no value in the treatment of infiltrating basal neoplasms such as nasopharyngeal carcinoma and glomus tumours.

The introduction of steroid drugs to reduce intracranial pressure in such cases was a major advance; the usual initial treatment is with dexamethasone 5 mg every six hours. This remedy has now supplanted other dehydrating agents such as intravenous sucrose, rectal magnesium sulphate, and urea (Javid 1958). A dramatic reduction in brain oedema and in intracranial pressure usually results and operation is facilitated (*British Medical Journal* 1973). This treatment, followed by appropriate maintenance doses, may also produce prolonged remission of symptoms in many patients with intracranial metastases (Weinstein, Toy, Jaffe, and Goldberg 1973), and similar maintenance treatment may prolong and improve the quality of survival in some patients with other forms of intracranial tumour, including gliomas.

Radiotherapy has also been shown to be strikingly beneficial in patients with cerebral metastases from bronchial carcinoma (Deeley and Edwards 1968) and may even on occasions eradicate various metastatic lesions completely (Cairncross, Chernik, Kim, and Posner 1979). The results of irradiation in intracranial metastatic disease may be considerably improved by combining this method with surgical removal in some cases (Sharr and Garfield 1978) and also with high-dose steroids (Cairncross, Kim, and Posner 1980). Total craniospinal irradiation with a dose of 1800 cGy also plays an important part in the management of acute lymphoblastic leukaemia in childhood when the nervous system is involved (Nesbit, Sather, Robinson, Ortega, Littman, D'Angio, and Hammond 1981). The scope of radiotherapy in the treatment of other intracranial tumours is less clearly defined. Irradiation is indicated in most cases of medulloblastoma, in association with surgical treatment, and also plays a valuable role in patients with pontine glioma and nasopharyngeal carcinoma. It is commonly used in patients in whom only partial removal of ependymomas of the fourth ventricle or of cerebellar astrocytomas or haemangioblastomas has been possible, as well as in cases of pinealoma, glomus tumour, and chordoma.

The role of this treatment in gliomas of the cerebral hemisphere is less certain, though it is commonly used. Standard radiotherapy with 5000–6000 cGy seems undoubtedly to prolong life (Lieberman and Ransohoff 1979) and, even in glioblastomas, smaller-field and higher-dose irradiation can be of substantial benefit (Hochberg and Pruitt 1980) although doses of 7500 cGy or higher often carry a substantial risk of causing radiation necrosis of normal tissue. Fast-neutron and photon-beam irradiation are now being tested (Gillespie and Mahaley 1981) and the use of radio-sensitizers which increase the sensitivity of tumour cells, such as dianhydrogalactital, misonidazole, and hyperthermia, is also being studied. No firm rules can at present be laid down; the aim must be not just to prolong life but to be sure that the quality of survival is improved; there is little point in prolonging life only to prolong suffering. A similar dilemma relates to the use of chemotherapeutic agents such as vincristine and the various nitro-soureas which have been utilized systemically in patients with brain tumour. The agents most widely employed have been car-mustine (BCNU), lomustine (CCNU) and somustine (methyl CCNU) (Wilson, Gutin, Boldney, Crafts, Levin, and Enot 1976; Brisman, Housepian, Chang, Duffey, and Balis 1976; Vick, Khan-dekar, and Bigner 1977), of which carmustine, combined with sur-gery and radiotherapy, seems to be much the most successful (Gillespie and Mahaley 1981). It is also clear than the use of radiotherapy with intrathecal methotrexate is of considerable value in central-nervous-system leukaemia (*The Lancet* 1972) and in meningeal carcinomatosis (Theodore and Gendelman 1981). There have also been considerable advances in the treatment of pituitary tumours which until recently were almost invariably treated by surgery (via either the intracranial or transphenoidal routes) combined with radiotherapy and hormonal replacement therapy. However while hormonal therapy is often still needed to control the management of 'hypopituitarism' and surgery is still required in many cases, especially if visual failure threatens or in order to remove a microadenoma (Antunes, Housepian, Frantz, Holub, Hui, Carmel, and Quest 1977), there is now clear evidence that the dopamine agonist bromocriptine in an initial dose of 2.5 mg daily, increasing gradually to 5–10 mg six-hourly, is often remarkably successful in reducing the size of large pituitary tumours whether these secrete growth hormone (in acromegaly) or prolactin (Thorner, Chait, Aitken, Benker, Bloom, Mortimer, Sanders, Stuart Mason, and Besser 1975; McGregor Scanlon, Hall, and Hall 1979; Wass, Moult, Thorner, Dacie, Charlesworth, Jones, and Besser 1979; Wass, Williams, Charlesworth, Kinsley, Holliday, Doniach, Rees, McDonald, and Besser 1982). In Cush-ing's disease, interstitial irradiation of the pituitary using the local implantation of yttrium-90 rods, via the trans-sphenoidal route, seems to be more effective than conventional hypophysectomy, radiotherapy, and metyrapone (White, Doyle, Mashiter, and Jop-lin 1982).

It is therefore possible to conclude that some benign intracranial tumours can be removed completely and, provided irreversible damage to nervous structures has not occurred, in these cases the prognosis is excellent. Even in the case of malignant or inaccess-ible neoplasms, the judicious use of steroids, radiotherapy, chemotherapeutic agents, and surgery in appropriate cases may greatly improve the prognosis, but in many cases, especially those with slowly growing astrocytomas, excessively radical or mutilat-ing operations are contra-indicated. Every individual case must be treated on its merits in the light of experience and of new develop-ments in therapy.

References

Aberfeld, D. C. and Rao, K. R. (1981). Familial arteriovenous malforma-tion of the brain, *Neurology, Minneapolis* **31**, 184.

Aicardi, J. and Bauman, F. (1975). Supratentorial extracerebral cysts in infants and children. *J. Neurol. Neurosurg. Psychiat.* **38**, 57.

Alexander, G. L. and Norman, R. M. (1960). *The Sturge–Weber syn-drome*. John Wright, Bristol.

Ambrose, J., Gooding, M. R., and Richardson, A. E. (1975). An assess-ment of the accuracy of computerized transverse axial scanning (EMI scanner) in the diagnosis of intracranial tumour: a review of 366 patients. *Brain* **98**, 569.

Anderson, M. (1982). Nuclear magnetic resonance imaging and neur-ology. *Br. med. J.* **284**, 1359.

Antunes, J. L., Housepian, E. M., Frantz, A. G., Holub, D. A., Hui, R. M., Carmel, P. W., and Quest, D. O. (1977). Prolactin-secreting pitui-tary tumors. *Ann. Neurol.* **2**, 148.

Ascherl, G. F., Hilal, S. K., and Brisman, R. (1981). Computed tomogra-phy of disseminated meningeal and ependymal malignant neoplasms. *Neurology, Minneapolis.* **31**, 567.

Bailey, P. (1948). *Intracranial tumours*, 2nd edn. Thomas, Springfield, Illi-nois.

—— and Bucy, P. C. (1931). The origin and nature of meningeal tumors. *Am. J. Cancer* **15**, 15.

—— and Cushing, H. (1925). Medulloblastoma cerebelli, a common type of mid-cerebellar glioma of childhood. *Arch. Neurol. Psychiat., Chicago* **14**, 192.

—— and —— (1926). *A classification of the tumours of the glioma group*. Lippincott, Philadelphia.

Banna, M. (1976). Craniopharyngioma: based on 160 cases. *Br. J. Radiol.* **49**, 206.

—— and Appleby, A. (1969). Some observations on the angiography of supratentorial meningiomas. *Clin. Radiol.* **20**, 375.

Bannister, Sir Roger (Ed.) (1978). *Brain's clinical neurology*, 5th edn. Oxford University Press, Oxford.

Barker, D. J. P., Weller, R. O., and Garfield, J. S. (1976). Epidemiology of primary tumours of the brain and spinal cord: a regional survey in southern England. *J. Neurol. Neurosurg. Psychiat.* **39**, 290.

Barnard, R. O. (1982). The classification of tumours of the central nervous system. *Neuropath. appl. Neurobiol.* **8**, 1.

Barnett, H. J. and Hyland, H. H. (1952). Tumours involving the brain-stem. A study of 90 cases arising in the brain-stem, fourth ventricle, and pineal tissue. *Quart. J. Med.* **21**, 265.

Bartlett, J. R. (1971*a*). Craniopharyngiomas — a summary of 85 cases. *J. Neurol. Neurosurg. Psychiat.* **34**, 37.

—— (1971*b*). Craniopharyngiomas—an analysis of some aspects of symp-tomatology, radiology and histology. *Brain* **94**, 725.

Becker, D. H., Townsend, J. J., Kramer, R. A., and Newton, T. H. (1979). Occult cerebrovascular malformations: a series of 18 histologi-cally verified cases with negative angiography. *Brain* **102**, 249.

Bickerstaff, E. R., Small, J. M., and Guest, I. A. (1958). The relapsing course of certain meningiomas in relation to pregnancy and menstrua-tion. *J. Neurol. Neurosurg. Psychiat.* **21**, 89.

Bigner, D. D., Kvedar, J. P., Thomas, B. A., Shaffer, C., Vick, N. A., Engel, W. K., and Day, E. D. (1972). Factors influencing the cell type of brain tumors induced in dogs by Schmidt–Ruppin–Rous sarcoma virus. *J. Neuropathol. exp. Neurol.* **31**, 583.

Boghen, D., Filiatrault, R., and Descarries, L. (1977). Myokymia and facial contracture in brain stem tuberculoma: a clinicopathologic report. *Neurology, Minneapolis* **27**, 270.

Boller, F., Patten, D. H., and Howes, D. (1973). Correlation of brain-scan results with neuropathological findings. *Lancet* **i**, 1143.

Boltshauser, E., Hamalatha, H., Grant, D. N., and Till, K. (1977). Impact of computerised axial tomography on the management of poster-ior fossa tumours in childhood. *J. Neurol. Neurosurg. Psychiat.* **40**, 209.

Botez, M. (1974). Frontal lobe tumours. In *Handbook of clinical neur-ology* ed. P. J. Vinken and G. W. Bruyn, Vol. 17, Part II. North-Hol-land, Amsterdam.

Brady, J. I. and Rodriguez, F. (1961). Cerebellar hemangioblastoma and polycythemia. *Am. J. med. Sci.* **242**, 579.

Brisman, R., Housepian, E. M., Chang, C., Duffy, P., and Balis, E. (1976). Adjuvant nitrosurea therapy for glioblastoma. *Arch. Neurol., Chicago* **33**, 745.

British Medical Journal (1973). The swollen brain. *Br. med. J.* **3**, 463.

Brodkey, J. S. (1979). Hypersecreting pituitary tumors. In *Contemporary neurosurgery* (ed. G. T. Tindall and D. M. Long). Williams and Wil-kins, Baltimore.

Brooks, W. H., Markesbery, W. R., Gupta, G. D., and Roszman, T. L. (1978). Relationship of lymphocyte invasion and survival of brain tumour patients. *Ann. Neurol.* **4**, 219.

Bull, J. W. D. (1951). Diagnostic neuroradiology. In *Modern trends in neurology* (1st series) (ed. A. Fielding). Butterworths, London.

—— (1967). The corpus callosum. *Clin. Radiol.* **18**, 2.

—— and Marryat, J. (1965). Isotope encephalography: experience with 100 cases. *Br. med. J.* **1**, 473.

Cairncross, J.-G., Chernik, N. L., Kim, J. H., and Posner, J. B. (1979). Sterilization of cerebral metastases by radiation therapy. *Neurology, Minneapolis* **29**, 1195.

——, Kim, J.-H., and Posner, J. B. (1980). Radiation therapy for brain metastases. *Ann. Neurol.* **7**, 529.

Cairns, H. and Russell, D. S. (1931). Intracranial and spinal metastases in gliomas of the brain. *Brain* **54**, 377.

Cameron, S. J. and Doig, A. (1970). Cerebellar tumours presenting with clinical features of phaeochromocytoma. *Lancet* i, 492.

Carmichael, E. A., Dix, M. R., and Hallpike, C. S. (1956). Pathology, symptomatology and diagnosis of organic affections of the eighth nerve system. *Br. med. Bull.* **12**, 146.

Cavanagh, J. B. (1958). On certain small tumours encountered in the temporal lobe. *Brain* **81**, 389.

Choux, R., Christian, M. A., Tripier, M. F., Gambarelli, D., Hassoun, J., and Toga, M. (1976). Hémangiopéricytome cérébral: étude ultra-structurale d'un cas. *J. neurol. Sci.* **28**, 361.

Clarke, E. (1954). Cranial and intracranial myelomas. *Brain* **77**, 61.

Cogan, D. G. (1974). Tumours of the optic nerve. In *Handbook of clinical neurology* (ed. P. J. Vinken and G. W. Bruyn) Vol. 17, Part II.

Cole, G. (1978). Intracranial space-occupying masses in mental hospital patients: necropsy study. *J. Neurol. Neurosurg. Psychiat.* **41**, 730.

Conomy, J. P., Ferguson, J. H., Brodkey, J. S., and Mitsumoto, H. (1975). Spontaneous infarction in pituitary tumors: neurologic and therapeutic aspects. *Neurology, Minneapolis* **25**, 580.

Couch, J. R. and Weiss, S. A. (1974). Gliomatosis cerebri. Report of four cases and review of the literature. *Neurology, Minneapolis* **24**, 504.

Courville, C. B. (1967). Intracranial tumors. Notes upon a series of three thousand verified cases with some current observations pertaining to their mortality. *Bull. Los Angeles neurol. Soc.* **32**, (Suppl. no. 2).

Critchley, M. and Ferguson, F. R. (1928). The cerebrospinal epidermoids (cholesteatomata). *Brain* **51**, 334.

Currie, S. and Henson, R. A. (1971). Neurological syndromes in the reticuloses. *Brain* **94**, 307.

Cushing, H. (1912). *The pituitary body and its disorders.* Lippincott, Philadelphia.

—— (1917). *Tumors of the nervus acousticus and the syndrome of the cerebello–pontine angle.* Lippincott, Philadelphia.

—— (1930). The chiasmal syndrome of primary optic atrophy and bitemporal defects in adults with a normal sella turcica. *Arch. Ophthal., Chicago* **2**, 505, 707.

—— (1932a). The basophil adenomas of the pituitary body and their clinical manifestations (pituitary basophilism). *Bull. Johns Hopkins Hosp.* **1**, 137.

—— (1932b). *Intracranial tumors. Notes upon a series of two thousand verified cases with surgical-mortality percentages pertaining thereto.* Thomas, Springfield, Illinois.

—— and Bailey, P. (1928). *Tumors arising from the blood-vessels of the brain.* Thomas, Springfield, Illinois.

—— and Eisenhardt, L. (1938). *Meningiomas, their classification, regional behavior, life history, and surgical end results.* Thomas, Springfield, Illinois.

Dandy, W. E. (1928). Arteriovenous aneurysm of the brain and venous abnormalities and angiomas of the brain. *Arch. Surg.* **17**, 190, 715.

—— (1933). *Benign tumors in the third ventricle of the brain.* Bailliere, Tindall, and Cox, London.

Dastur, H. M. and Desai, A. D. (1965). A comparative study of brain tuberculomas and gliomas based upon 107 case records of each. *Brain.* **88**, 375.

Davies-Jones, G. A. B. (1969). Lactate dehydrogenase and glutamic oxalacetic transaminase of the cerebrospinal fluid in tumours of the central nervous system. *J. Neurol. Neurosurg. Psychiat.* **32**, 324.

Deeley, T. J. and Edwards, J. M. R. (1968). Radiotherapy in the management of cerebral secondaries from bronchial carcinoma. *Lancet* i, 1209.

Delleman, J. W., De Jong, J. G. Y., and Bleeker, G. M. (1978). Meningiomas in five members of a family over two generations, in one member simultaneously with acoustic neurinomas. *Neurology, Minneapolis* **28**, 567.

Doyle, F. H., Gore, J. C., Pennock, J. M., Bydder, G. M., Orr, J. S., Steiner, R. E., Young, I. R., Burl, M. Clow, H., Gilderdale, D. J., Bailes, D. R., and Walters, P. E. (1981). Imaging of the brain by nuclear magnetic resonance. *Lancet* ii, 53.

—— (1980). *Principles of X-ray diagnosis of the skull,* 2nd edn. Butterworths, London.

Du Boulay, G. H. (1978). The clinical application of computerised axial tomography (CT scanning). In *Recent advances in clinical neurology 2* (ed. W. B. Matthews and G. H. Glaser). Churchill-Livingstone, Edinburgh.

Dyck, P. and Gruskin, P. (1977). Supratentorial arachnoid cysts in adults: a discussion of two cases from a pathophysiologic and surgical perspective. *Arch. Neurol., Chicago* **34**, 276.

Dyken, P. R. (1975). Cerebrospinal fluid cytology: practical clinical usefulness. *Neurology, Minneapolis* **25**, 210.

Edwards, C. H. and Paterson, J. H. (1951). A review of the symptoms and signs of acoustic neurofibromata. *Brain* **74**, 144.

Ell, P. J., Deacon, J. M., Ducassou, D., and Brendel, A. (1980). Emission and transmission brain tomography. *Br. med. J.* **280**, 438.

Farhi, F., Dikman, S. H., Lawson, W., Cobin, R. H., and Zak, F. G. (1976). Paragangliomatosis associated with multiple endocrine adenomas. *Arch. Pathol. Lab. Med.* **100**, 495.

Fields, W. S. and Shankly, P. C. (1962). *The Biology and treatment of intracranial tumors.* Thomas, Springfield, Illinois.

Foley, J. (1955). Benign forms of intracranial hypertension. *Brain* **78**, 1.

Ford, R. and Ambrose, J. (1963). Echoencephalography. The measurement of the position of midline structures in the skull with high-frequency pulsed ultrasound. *Brain* **86**, 189.

Franks, S., Nabarro, J. D. N., and Jacobs, H. S. (1977). Prevalence and presentation of hyperprolactinaemia in patients with 'functionless' pituitary tumours. *Lancet* i, 778.

French, J. D. (1947). Plasmacytoma of hypothalamus: clinical–pathological report of case. *J. Neuropathol. exp. Neurol.* **6**, 265.

Gardner-Thorpe, C. (1970). Presumed plasmacytoma of clivus producing isolated hypoglossal nerve palsy. *Br. med. J.* **2**, 405.

Garg, A. G. and Taylor, A. R. (1968). A-scan echoencephalography in measurement of the cerebral ventricles. *J. Neurol. Neurosurg. Psychiat.* **31**, 245.

Garrido, E. and Stein, B. (1978). Removal of an arteriovenous malformation from the basal ganglion. *J. Neurol. Neurosurg. Psychiat.* **41**, 992.

Gastaut, H., Regis, H., Gastaut, J. L., Yermenos, E., and Low, M. D. (1980). Lipomas of the corpus callosum and epilepsy, *Neurology, Minneapolis* **30**, 132.

Gillespie, R. and Mahaley, M. S., Jr. (1981). Brain tumors: gliomas, pituitary tumors, pineal region tumors, and metastatic tumors. In *Current neurology* (ed. S. H. Appel) Chapter 15, Vol. 3. John Wiley, New York.

Gold, E. B. and Gordis, L. (1979a). Patterns of incidence of brain tumors in children. *Ann. Neurol.* **5**, 565.

—— and —— (1979b). Determinants of survival in children with brain tumors. *Ann. Neurol.* **5**, 569.

Grainger, R. G. and Lamb, J. T. (Eds.) (1980). *Myelographic techniques with metrizamide.* Nyegaard (UK), Birmingham.

Greenberg, H. S., Deck, M. D. F., Vikram, B., Chu, F. C. H., and Posner, J. B. (1981). Metastasis to the base of the skull: clinical findings in 43 patients. *Neurology, Minneapolis* **31**, 530

Hall, K. (1980). Metrizamide cisternography in sellar and parasellar lesions. In *Myelographic techniques with metrizamide* (ed. R. G. Grainger and J. T. Lamb). Nyegaard (UK), Birmingham.

Hankinson, J. and Banna, M. (1976). *Pituitary and parapituitary tumours.* Saunders, Eastbourne.

Helle, T. L. and Conley, F. K. (1980). Haemorrhage associated with meningioma: a case report and review of the literature. *J. Neurol. Neurosurg. Psychiat.* **43**, 725.

Henson, R. A., Crawford, J. V., and Cavanagh, J. B. (1953). Tumours of the glomus jugulare. *J. Neurol. Neurosurg. Psychiat.* **16**, 127.

Herrick, M. K. and Rubinstein, L. J. (1979). The cytological differentiating potential of pineal parenchymal neoplasms (true pinealomas). *Brain* **102**, 289.

Hochberg, F. H. and Pruitt, A. (1980). Assumptions in the radiotherapy of glioblastomas. *Neurology, Minneapolis* **30**, 907.

Horrax, G. (1924). Generalized cisternal arachnoiditis simulating cerebellar tumor. *Arch. Surg.* **9**, 95.

—— (1939). Meningiomas of the brain. *Arch. Neurol. Psychiat., Chicago* **41**, 140.

—— (1954). Benign (favourable) types of brain tumor. The end results (up to twenty years), with statistics of mortality and useful survival. *New Engl. J. Med.* **250**, 981.

—— and Bailey, P. (1925). Tumors of the pineal body, *Arch. Neurol. Psychiat., Chicago* **13**, 423.

Horten, B. C. and Rubenstein, L. J. (1976). Primary cerebral neuroblastoma. A clinicopathological study of 35 cases. *Brain* **99**, 735.

Hoyt, W. F., Meshel, L. G., Lessell, S., Schatz, N. J., and Suckling, R. D. (1973). Malignant optic glioma of adulthood. *Brain* **96**, 121.

Huber, P. (1982). *Krayenbühl and Yasargil's cerebral angiography* (2nd edn.). Thieme, Stuttgart.

Hunter, R., Blackwood, W., and Bull, J. W. D. (1968). Three cases of frontal meningiomas presenting psychiatrically. *Br. med. J.* **3**, 9.

Hutchinson, E. C., Leonard, B. J., Maudsley, C., and Yates, P. O. (1958). Neurological complications of the reticuloses. *Brain* **81**, 75.

Ibelgaufts, H. (1982). DNA viruses and brain tumours. *Trends Neurosci.* **5**, 16.

Inglis, J. M. and Turner, E. (1957). Use of hypothermia in nonvascular intracranial tumours. *Br. med. J.* **1**, 1335.

Ironside, R. and Guttmacher, M. (1929). The corpus callosum and its tumours. *Brain* **52**, 442.

Jacobs, L. L. and Richland, K. J. (1951). Carcinomatosis of the leptomeninges. Review of literature and report of four cases. *Bull. Los Angeles Neurol. Soc.* **16**, 335.

Javid, M. (1958). Urea—new use of an old agent. *Surg. Clin. N. Am.* **38**, 907.

Jefferson, M. and Rosenthal, F. D. (1959). Spontaneous necrosis in pituitary tumours (pituitary apoplexy). *Lancet* **i**, 61.

John, H. T. and Nabarro, J. D. N. (1955). Intracranial manifestations of malignant lymphoma. *Br. J. Cancer* **9**, 386.

Kelly, R. (1951). Colloid cysts of the third ventricle. *Brain* **74**, 23.

Kepes, J. J., Striebinger, C. M., Brackett, C. E., and Kishore, P. (1976). Gliomas (astrocytomas) of the brain-stem with spinal intra- and extra-dural metastases: report of three cases. *J. Neurol. Neurosurg. Psychiat.* **39**, 66.

Kernohan, J. W., Mabon, R. F., Svien, H. J., and Adson, A. W. (1949). A simplified classification of the gliomas. *Proc. Mayo Clin.* **24**, 71.

Kiloh, L. G., McComas, A. J., Osselton, J. W., and Upton, A. R. M. (1981). *Clinical electroencephalography*, 4th edn. Butterworths, London.

Kuper, S., Mendelow, H., and Proctor, N. S. F. (1958). Internal hydrocephalus caused by parasitic cysts. *Brain* **81**, 235.

Kurtzke, J. F. (1969). Geographic pathology of brain tumors. 1. Distribution of deaths from primary tumors. *Acta neurol. scand.* **45**, 540.

Lalitha, V. S. and Dastur, D. K. (1980). Neoplasms of the central nervous system—histological types in 2270 cases. *Ind. J. Cancer* **17**, 102.

The Lancet (1972). Treating the nervous system in acute leukaemia. *Lancet* **i**, 297.

—— (1973). Missed foramen-magnum tumours. *Lancet* **ii**, 1482.

Lassman, L. P., Pearce, G. W., Banna, M., and Jones, R. D. (1969). Vincristine sulphate in the treatment of skeletal metastases from cerebellar medulloblastoma, *J. Neurosurg.* **30**, 42.

Lieberman, A. and Ransohoff, J. (1979). Treatment of primary brain tumors. *Med. Clin. N. Am.* **63**, 835.

——, Le Brun, Y., Glass, P., Goodgold, A., Lux, W., Wise, A., and Ransohoff, J. (1977). Use of high dose corticosteroids in patients with inoperable brain tumours. *J. Neurol. Neurosurg. Psychiat.* **40**, 678.

Lindau, A. (1921). Studien über Kleinhirncysten. Bau, Pathogenese und Beziehungen zur Angiomatosis Retinae. *Acta pathol. microbiol. scand. Suppl.* **i**, 1.

Logue, V. and Monckton, G. (1954). Posterior fossa angiomas. *Brain* **77**, 252.

Loizou, L. A. and Anderson, M. (1982). Intracranial tuberculomas: correlation of computerized tomography with clinicopathological findings. *Quart. J. Med.* **51**, 104.

Lopez, R., David, N. J., Gargano, F., and Post, J. D. (1981). Bilateral sixth nerve palsies in a patient with massive pituitary adenoma. *Neurology, Minneapolis* **31**, 1137.

Mackenzie, I. (1953). The clinical presentation of the cerebral angiomas. *Brain* **76**, 184.

Maroon, J. C. and Albright, L. (1977). 'Failure to thrive' due to pontine glioma. *Arch. Neurol., Chicago* **34**, 295.

Marsden, C. D. and Reynolds, E. H. Neurology. In *A textbook of epilepsy* (ed. J. Laidlaw and A. Richens) 2nd edn., Chapter 4. Churchill-Livingstone, Edinburgh.

Maurice-Williams, R. S. (1975). Mechanism of production of gait unsteadiness by tumours in the posterior fossa. *J. Neurol. Neurosurg. Psychiat.* **38**, 143.

Max, M. B., Deck, M. D. F., and Rottenberg, S. A. (1981). Pituitary metastasis: incidence in cancer patients and clinical differentiation from pituitary adenoma. *Neurology, Minneapolis* **31**, 998.

Mayo Clinic (1976). *Clinical examinations in neurology*, 4th edn. Saunders, Philadelphia.

McAllister, V. L., Kendall, B. E., and Bull, J. W. D. (1975). Symptomatic vertebral angiomas. *Brain* **98**, 71.

McDermott, J. R., Smith, A. I., Biggins, J. A., Edwardson, J. A., and Griffiths, E. C. (1982). Mechanism of luteinizing hormone-releasing hormone degradation by subcellular fractions of rat hypothalamus and pituitary. *Regul. Peptides* **3**, 257.

McGregor, A. M., Scanlon, M. F., Hall, R., and Hall, K. (1979). Effects of bromocriptine on pituitary tumour size. *Br. med. J.* **2**, 700.

McKeever, P. E., Quindlen, E., Banks, M. A., Williams, U., Kornblith, P. L., Laversen, S., Greenwood, M. A., and Smith, B. (1981). Biosynthesized products of cultured neuroglial cells: selective release of proteins by cells from human astrocytomas. *Neurology, Minneapolis* **31**, 1445.

McKinney, W. M. (1969). Echoencephalography. In *Special techniques for neurological diagnosis* (ed. J. F. Toole), Contemporary Neurology Series, Chapter 3, no. 3. Davis, Philadelphia.

McKissock, W. and Paine, K. W. E. (1958). Primary tumours of the thalamus. *Brain* **81**, 41.

Michelsen, J. J. and New, P. E. J. (1969). Brain tumour and pregnancy. *J. Neurol. Neurosurg. Psychiat.* **32**, 305.

Miles, J. (1977). Sump drainage: a palliative manoeuvre for the treatment of craniopharyngioma. *J. Neurol. Neurosurg. Psychiat.* **40**, 120.

Mohan, J., Brownell, B., and Oppenheimer, D. R. (1976). Malignant spread of haemangioblastoma: report on two cases. *J. Neurol. Neurosurg. Psychiat.* **39**, 515.

Mohanty, S., Tandon, P. N., Banerji, A. K., and Prakash, B. (1977). Haemorrhage into pituitary adenomas. *J. Neurol. Neurosurg. Psychiat.* **40**, 987.

Mullan, S. (1962). Mortality of the surgical treatment of brain tumors. *J. Am. med. Ass.* **182**, 601.

Nesbitt, M. E., Jr., Sather, H. N., Robison, L. L., Ortega, J., Littman, P. S., D'Angio, G. J., and Hammond, G. D. (1981). Presymptomatic central nervous system therapy in previously untreated childhood acute lymphoblastic leukaemia: comparison of 1800 rad and 2400 rad. *Lancet* **i**, 461.

Newman, J., Josephson, A. S., Cacatian, A., and Tsang, A. (1974). Spinal-fluid lysozyme in the diagnosis of central-nervous-system tumours. *Lancet* **ii**, 756.

Newton, T. H. and Potts, D. G. (1974). *Radiology of the skull and brain*, Volume 2, Angiography. Mosby, St Louis.

Norris, F. H., Aguilar, M. J., and Harman, C. E. (1972). Virus-like particles in a case of vasculitis with brain tumor. *Arch. Neurol., Chicago* **26**, 212.

Northfield, D. W. C. (1957). Rathke-pouch tumours. *Brain* **80**, 293.

Oldendorf, W. H. (1980). *The quest for an image of brain*. Raven Press, New York.

—— (1981). Nuclear medicine in clinical neurology: an update. *Ann. Neurol.* **10**, 207.

Oliver, L. C. (1958). Primary arachnoid cysts: report of two cases. *Br. med. J.* **1**, 1147.

Olson, M. E., Chernik, N. L., and Posner, J. B. (1974). Infiltration of the leptomeninges by systemic cancer. A clinical and pathologic study, *Arch. Neurol., Chicago* **30**, 122.

Paoletti, P., Vandenheuvel, F. A., Fumagalli, R., and Paoletti, R. (1969). The sterol test for the diagnosis of human brain tumors. *Neurology, Minneapolis* **19**, 190.

Pendergrass, E. P., Schaeffer, J. P., and Hodes, J. P. (1956). *The head and neck in roentgen diagnosis*, 2nd edn. Blackwell, Oxford.

Penfield, W. (1931). A paper on classification of brain tumours and its practical application. *Br. med. J.* **1**, 337.

—— (1932). Tumours of the sheaths of the nervous system. *Arch. Neurol. Psychiat., Chicago* **27**, 1298.

——, Erickson, T. C., and Tarlov, I. (1940). Relation of intracranial tumours and symptomatic epilepsy. *Arch. Neurol. Psychiat., Chicago* **44**, 300.

Penman, J. and Smith, M. C. (1954). Intracranial gliomata. *Spec. Rep. Ser. med. Res. Coun., London* No. 285.

Penning, L., Front, D., Bechar, M., Go, K.G., and Rodermond, J. M. (1973). Factors governing the uptake of pertechnetate by human brain tumours—a scintigraphic study. *Brain* **96**, 225.

Plum, F. and Posner, J. B. (1980). *Diagnosis of stupor and coma*, 3rd edn. Davis, Philadelphia.

Posner, J. B. and Chernik, N. L. (1978). Intracranial metastases from systemic cancer. *Adv. Neurol.* **19**, 579.

Raimondi, A. J. (1966). Ultrastructure of brain tumours. In *Progress in neurological surgery* (ed. H. Krayenbuhl, P. E. Maspes, and W. H. Sweet). Karger, Basle.

Robertson, E. G. (1967). *Pneumoencephalography*, 2nd edn. Thomas, Springfield, Illinois.

Ronquist, G., Frithz, G., Ericsson, P., and Hugosson, R. (1977). Malignant brain tumours associated with adenylate kinase in cerebrospinal fluid. *Lancet* i, 1284.

Rothman, S. J. and Olanow, C. W. (1981). Brain stem glioma in childhood: acute hemiplegic onset. *Can. J. neurol. Sci.* **8**, 263.

Russell, D. S. (1944). The pinealoma: its relationship to teratoma. *J. Path. Bact.* **56**, 145.

—— and Cairns, H. (1930). Spinal metastases in a case of cerebral glioma of the type known as astrocytoma fibrillare. *J. Path. Bact.* **33**, 383.

—— and Rubenstein, L. J. (1959). *Pathology of tumours of the nervous system*. Edward Arnold, London.

—— and —— (1977). *Pathology of tumours of the nervous system*, 4th edn. Edward Arnold, London.

Sarkari, N. B. S. and Bickerstaff, E. R. (1969). Relapses and remissions in brain stem tumours. *Br. med. J.* **2**, 21.

Scatliff, J. H. and Bull, J. W. D. (1965). The radiological manifestations of suprasellar metastatic tissue. *Clin. Radiol.* **41**, 66.

Schaumburg, H. H., Plank, C. R., and Adams, R. D. (1972). The reticulum cell sarcoma—microglioma group of brain tumours. *Brain* **95**, 199.

Schmidt, R. P. and Wilder, B. J. (1968). *Epilepsy*, Contemporary Neurology Series, no. 2. Davis, Philadelphia.

Schneck, S. A. and Penn, I. (1971). De-novo brain tumours in renal-transplant recipients. *Lancet* i, 983.

Schold, S. C., Wasserstrom, W. R., Fleisher, M., Schwartz, M. K., and Posner, J. B. (1980). Cerebrospinal fluid biochemical markers of central nervous system metastases. *Ann. Neurol.* **8**, 597.

Sharr, M. M. and Garfield, J. S. (1978). Management of intracranial metastases. *Br. med. J.* **1**, 1535.

Shephard, R. H. and Wadia, N. H. (1956). Some observations on atypical features in acoustic neuroma. *Brain* **79**, 282.

Shuping, J. R., Toole, J. F., and Alexander, E., Jr. (1980). Transient global amnesia due to glioma in the dominant hemisphere. *Neurology, Minneapolis* **30**, 88.

Siekert, R. G. (1956). Neurologic manifestations of tumors of the glomus jugulare. *Arch. Neurol. Psychiat., Chicago* **76**, 1.

Sikora, K., Alderson, T., Phillips, J., and Watson, J. V. (1982). Human hybridomas from malignant gliomas. *Lancet* i, 11.

Skalpe, I. O. (1980). Early adverse effects of myelography. In *Myelographic techniques with metrizamide* (ed. R. G. Grainger and J. T. Lamb) Chapter 18. Nyegaard (UK), Birmingham.

Sohn, D., Valensi, Q., and Miller, S. P. (1967). Neurologic manifestations of Hodgkin's disease: intracerebral Hodgkin's granuloma. *Arch. Neurol., Chicago* **17**, 429.

Spark, R. F., Wills, C. A., O'Reilly, G., Ransil, B. J., and Bergland, R. (1982). Hyperprolactinaemia in males with and without pituitary macroadenomas. *Lancet* ii, 129.

Spence, A. M. (1979). Brain tumors: gliomas, meningiomas, lymphomas, and metastatic tumors. In *Current neurology* (ed. H. R. Tyler and D. M. Dawson) Chapter 17, Vol. 2. Houghton Mifflin, Boston.

Spencer, R. (1965). Scintiscanning in space-occupying lesions of the skull. *Br. J. Radiol.* **38**, 1.

Spillane, J. D. (1975). *An atlas of clinical neurology*, 2nd edn. Oxford University Press, Oxford.

Spillane, J. A. Kendall, B. E., and Moseley, I. F. (1982). Cerebral lymphoma: clinical radiological correlation. *J. Neurol. Neurosurg. Psychiat.* **45**, 199.

Stein, B. M., Fraser, R. A. R., and Tenner, M. S. (1972). Tumours of the third ventricle in children. *J. Neurol. Neurosurg. Psychiat.* **35**, 776.

Summers, G. D., Young, A. C., Little, R. A. Stoner, H. B., Forbes, W. S. T. C., and Jones, R. A. C. (1981). Spontaneous periodic hypothermia with lipoma of the corpus callosum. *J. Neurol. Neurosurg. Psychiat.* **44**, 1094.

Swanson, J. A. (1979). Coexistent empty sella and prolactin-secreting microadenoma. *Obstet. Gynecol.* **53**, 258.

Symonds, C. (1962). Ocular palsy as the presenting symptom of pituitary adenoma. *Bull. Johns Hopkins Hosp.* **111**, 72.

Taveras, J. M. and Wood, E. H. (1964). *Diagnostic neuroradiology*. Williams & Wilkins, Baltimore.

Theodore, W. H. and Gendelman, S. (1981). Meningeal carcinomatosis. *Arch. Neurol., Chicago* **38**, 696.

Thomas, J. E. and Yoss, R. E. (1970). The parasellar syndrome: problems in determining etiology. *Mayo Clin. Proc.* **45**, 617.

Thorner, M. O., Chait, A., Aitken, M., Benker, G., Bloom, S. R., Mortimer, C. H., Sanders, P., Stuart Mason, A., and Besser, G. M. (1975). Bromocriptine treatment of acromegaly. *Br. med. J.* **1**, 299.

Tomlinson, B. E. and Walton J. N. (1967). Granulomatous meningitis and diffuse parenchymatous degeneration of the nervous system due to an intracranial epidermoid cyst. *J. Neurol. Neurosrug. Psychiat.* **30**, 341.

Van Crevel, H. (1979). RIHSA cisternography in cerebral tumours. *Neuroradiology* **18**, 133.

Van Eck, J. H. M. (1966). Clinical value of isotope encephalography. *J. Neurol. Neurosurg. Psychiat.* **29**, 145.

Vannucci, R. C. and Baten, M. (1974). Cerebral metastatic disease in childhood. *Neurology, Minneapolis* **24**, 981.

Vick, N. A., Khandekar, J. D., and Bigner, D. D. (1977). Chemotherapy of brain tumors: the 'blood–brain barrier' is not a factor. *Arch. Neurol., Chicago* **34**, 523.

Wallace, D. (1976). Lipoma of the corpus callosum. *J. Neurol. Neurosurg. Psychiat.* **39**, 1179.

Walton, J. N. (1956). *Subarachnoid haemorrhage*. Livingstone, Edinburgh.

Ward, D. W., Mattison, M. L., and Finn, R. (1973). Association between previous tuberculous infection and cerebral glioma, *Br. med. J.* **1**, 83.

Wass, J. A. H., Moult, P. J. A., Thorner, M. O., Dacie, J. E., Charlesworth, M., Jones, A. E., and Besser, G. M. (1979). Reduction of pituitary-tumour size in patients with prolactinomas and acromegaly treated with bromocriptine with or without radiotherapy. *Lancet* ii, 66.

—— Williams, J., Charlesworth, M., Kingsley, D. P. E., Halliday, A. M., Doniach, I., Rees, L. H., McDonald, W. I., and Besser, G. M. (1982). Bromocriptine in management of large pituitary tumours. *Br. med. J.* **284**, 1908.

Weinstein, J. D., Toy. F. J., Jaffe, M. E., and Goldberg, H. I. (1973). The effect of dexamethasone on brain edema in patients with metastatic brain tumours. *Neurology, Minneapolis* **23**, 121.

Weisberg, L. A., Nice, C., and Katz, M. (1978). *Cerebral computed tomography: A text-atlas*. Saunders, Philadelphia.

Weiss, M. H. Apuzzo, M. L. J., Heiden, J. S., and Kurze, T. (1976). Pituitary apoplexy, therapeutic assessment. *Bull. Los Angeles Neurol. Soc.* **41**, 143.

West, R. J., Graham-Pole, J., Hardisty, R. M., and Pike, M. C. (1972). Factors in pathogenesis of central-nervous-system leukaemia. *Br. med. J.* **3**, 311.

White, M. C., Doyle, F. H., Mashiter, K., and Joplin, G. F. (1982). Successful treatment of Cushing's disease using yttrium-90 rods. *Br. med. J.* **285**, 280.

Williams, J. O., Hicks, E. P., Herzberg, L., Williams, N. E., and Croft, D. N. (1972). Overall value of brain scans and electroencephalograms in detecting neurosurgical lesions. *Lancet* ii, 642.

Wilson, C. B., Gutin, P., Boldrey, E. B., Crafts, D., Levin, V. A., and Enot, K. J. (1976). Single-agent chemotherapy of brain tumors: a five-year review. *Arch. Neurol., Chicago* **33**, 739.

——, Tynell, J. B., and Fitzgerald, P. (1979). Cushing's disease revisited. *Am. J. Surg.* **138**, 77.

de Yébenes, J. G., Gervas, J. J., Iglesias, J., Mena, M. A., Martin del Rio, R., and Somoza, E. (1982). Biochemical findings in a case of Parkinsonism secondary to brain tumor. *Ann. Neurol.* **11**, 313.

Yung, W. A., Horten, B. C., and Shapiro, W. R. (1980). Meningeal gliomatosis: a review of 12 cases. *Ann. Neurol.* **8**, 605.

Zervas, N. T. and Mendelson, G. (1975). Treatment of acute haemorrhage of pituitary tumours. *Lancet* , 604.

Ziegler, D. K., Kaufman, A., and Marshall, H. E. (1977). Abrupt memory loss associated with thalamic tumor. *Arch. Neurol, Chicago.* **34**, 545.

Zülch, K. J. (1965). *Brain tumors: their biology and pathology*. Heinemann, New York.

Headache

The investigation of a case of headache

Headache is a common symptom. Though frequently a trivial disorder, it is also at times a symptom of grave significance. Every patient with headache requires, therefore, careful consideration and sometimes thorough investigation. In taking the history, attention must be paid to the following points. How long has the patient suffered from headache? Is it increasing in severity? Is it constant or paroxysmal, and if paroxysmal what is the duration of the attacks, and do they occur at any special time of day? Are they precipitated by any circumstance or activity, and how, if at all, can they be relieved? What is the character of the headache and its situation? Is there associated tenderness of the scalp or skull, with visual disturbances, vomiting, or vertigo? Has there been a head injury? Are there symptoms of nasal obstruction or discharge, either from the nose or into the pharynx? Is the patient anxious, tense, or depressed?

Investigation of a case of headache involves a complete physical examination, special attention being paid to the ocular fundi, the nose and nasal air sinuses, the teeth, the blood pressure, and the urine. Radiography of the skull, including the nasal sinuses, of the cervical spine in cases of occipital headache, and other specialized neuroradiological investigations may be required in appropriate cases.

The mode of production of headache

All the tissues covering the cranium are sensitive to pain, especially the arteries but also the muscles and pericranium. The skull bone itself is insensitive. Within the cranium, the venous sinuses and their tributaries, the dura mater and the cerebral arteries, and the fifth, ninth, and tenth cranial nerves are the chief pain-sensitive structures.

The main factors causing headache (Lance 1981) are: (1) inflammation involving pain-sensitive structures of the head; (2) referred pain; (3) meningeal irritation; (4) traction on or dilatation of blood vessels; (5) pressure upon or distortion of pain-sensitive structures caused by tumours or other lesions; and (6) psychological causes, when the pain is often due to tension in muscles of the scalp and neck.

The causes of headache

Disease of the bones of the cranium

Osteitis of the cranial bones is an occasional cause. Usually it is secondary to suppuration in the middle ear or paranasal sinuses; syphilitic osteitis is now rare but Paget's disease (which is not truly an osteitis despite its name, osteitis deformans) is quite common. Headache due to these causes is of a burning, boring character and may be accompanied by tenderness of the skull, which often feels warmer than normal. Local or general thickening of the cranium is often present, and the radiological signs are characteristic. Metastases in skull bones, whether osteolytic (e.g. in bronchial or breast carcinoma) or osteosclerotic (as in carcinoma of the prostate) may also give similar headache, as may multiple myelomatosis.

Neuralgia

Pain in the head occurs in many neuralgic syndromes. Thus paroxysms of pain may radiate along the distribution of the supraorbital or infraorbital nerves. Sometimes the pain is due to local compression or irritation of the nerves in their respective bony canals, produced, for instance, by local scarring after injury or arising without evidence cause. In other cases, paroxysmal pain localized in this way may be the initial manifestation of trigeminal neuralgia (tic douloureux), but pain in the latter condition is commonest in the distribution of the second and third divisions of the trigeminus (p. 110). Attacks of neuralgia of undetermined cause occur also in the distribution of the auriculotemporal, posterior auricular, and occipital nerves, though auriculotemporal pain, like that in the distribution of the mandibular division of the fifth nerve, can be due to dental malocclusion with arthrosis of the temporomandibular joint (Costen's syndrome) and occipital pain can be a consequence of cervical spondylosis. Prolonged but paroxysmal attacks of severe boring pain in the eye ('ciliary neuralgia') or upper jaw

(sphenopalatine or Sluder's neuralgia) are variants of periodic migrainous neuralgia (p. 182), while constant upper jaw pain in the absence of signs of organic disease (atypical facial neuralgia) is often of psychogenic origin (pp. 111 and 665). Herpes zoster of the trigeminal ganglion sometimes causes severe and persistent neuralgic pain. After the acute stage the scars of the eruption remain visible, and there is usually cutaneous anaesthesia. Pain in the distribution of the trigeminal nerve may also be due to pressure upon it in its intracranial course by intracranial neoplasm or aneurysm, while its central fibres may be involved in a lesion within the medulla. Lateral medullary infarction (p. 196) and syringobulbia can in this way cause neuralgic pain over the face and scalp.

Referred pain

Lesions of many viscera cause pain referred to superficial tissues remote from the viscus involved, but innervated by the same segment of the nervous system (p. 47). Thus visceral disease in many situations can give pain in the head and localized hyperalgesia of the face or scalp. These symptoms may be produced by uncorrected visual refractive errors or latent squint, though this is not common (Waters 1970), by iritis, glaucoma, lesions of the middle ear, nasal sinuses, teeth including unerupted wisdom teeth, pharynx, and tongue, and also by disease of the intrathoracic and intra-abdominal viscera. The explanation of this reference of pain to the head from remote organs is that the trigeminal is the somatic sensory nerve corresponding to the vagus, by which so many viscera are innervated. Nasal obstruction, apart from sinusitis, is an occasional cause of persistent frontal headache. Occipital headache occurs often in cervical spondylosis.

Meningeal irritation

Meningeal irritation gives some of the most severe headaches. It is seen in the various forms of meningitis, or when non-infective irritant products such as extravasated blood come into contact with the meninges. The pain is constant, severe, and throbbing or 'bursting', and is usually associated with other signs of meningeal irritation, such as neck stiffness and Kernig's sign. Head movement increases discomfort and there is often photophobia and irritability.

Headaches of vascular origin

Paroxysmal throbbing or 'bursting' headaches may occur in patients with malignant hypertension, when the headache is less directly related to the height of the blood pressure than to distension of the cranial arteries (Wolff and Wolf 1948). Intracranial aneurysm is rarely large enough to increase the intracranial pressure before rupture. It may cause pain in the head, however, by compressing the trigeminal nerve. After rupture, subarachnoid haemorrhage causes headache through both increased intracranial pressure and meningeal irritation.

Changes in the calibre and permeability of cranial vessels probably account for the headaches which accompany or follow numerous toxic states such as severe infections, alcoholic overindulgence, general anaesthetics, uraemia, and diffuse cerebral inflammations—the various forms of encephalitis. In the 'hangover' headache, dehydration and reduced intracranial pressure play a part. Sudden prostrating headache simulating that of subarachnoid haemorrhage may occur in patients who eat cheese or broad beans or drink red wine while taking mono-amine oxidase inhibitor drugs, mainly tranylcypromine, for the treatment of depression; similar headache has been described after ingestion of nitrite in frankfurter sausages (Henderson and Raskin 1972) and all forms of vascular headache, including migraine (p. 177), may be accentuated or precipitated by alcohol. Similar 'vascular' headache has been described during orgasm (Lance 1976) and as a consequence of excessive coffee drinking (*British Medical Journal* 1977). Porter and Jankovic (1981) have identified as 'benign coital cephalalgia' a variety of headache coming on acutely during coitus which is relieved by propranolol prophylaxis and which they believe to be a migraine variant. Trigeminovascular sensory fibres and substance P may play a part in all vascular headaches (Moskowitz 1984).

Headache can also be caused by temporal or cranial arteritis; the scalp and the temporal arteries are usually tender (see p. 220).

Intracranial space-occupying lesions
The headache of intracranial neoplasm was described on p. 136.

Trauma
In severe head injury, headache is apt to be masked by impaired consciousness. It is a prominent symptom of concussion or cerebral contusion, and in the so-called post-concussional syndrome it may be paroxysmal, tends to be precipitated by noise, excitement, exertion, alcohol, and head movement, and is often associated with irritability, nervousness, and giddiness.

Lowered intracranial pressure
This may cause headache, as, for example, after lumbar puncture. The headache is throbbing and may be literally prostrating, being intensified by sitting or standing and relieved by lying flat or with the feet raised above the level of the head.

Cough headache
This is a distinctive, brief, but often severe 'bursting' kind of pain experienced after coughing, usually by a middle-aged man, who may clasp his head when he coughs in an attempt to relieve it. Its cause is obscure, but rarely it is a symptom of intracranial tumour. In most cases, however, it is benign and disappears spontaneously (Symonds 1956).

Psychogenic headache
Numerous abnormal cranial sensations are described by neurotic and psychotic patients. The commonest is a sense of pressure at the vertex, frequently encounted in anxiety states. One source of anxiety-headache is persistent contraction of the occipitofrontalis muscle. Such tension headaches are typically dull and aching in character and frontotemporal and/or occipital in distribution; they may be continuous but more often come on towards the end of the day, although in depressed patients the headache may be present on waking. Persistent 'neuralgic' pains associated with hyperaesthesia of the scalp and failing to respond to all analgesics may be encountered in hysteria as may bizarre headaches described in a florid manner ('like a nail being driven into the skull or an engine lifting off the top of the head'). Patients suffering from depression sometimes describe 'terrible pains in the head' of which they can give no more precise description (see also Chapter 23).

Treatment
Apart from palliative treatment with analgesics, which can safely be used in most cases, the treatment of headache is that of the causal disorder. Mild analgesics (aspirin, paracetamol) are safe in most cases; opiates and other drugs of addiction must be avoided, especially in cases of recurrent headache but also because drugs which depress respiratory function should not be used if the intracranial pressure is likely to be raised; nevertheless in severe headache due, for instance, to subarachnoid haemorrhage, pethidine or other similar powerful remedies may be needed. In a series of over 1000 cases of chronic headache, Lance, Curran, and Anthony (1965) found migraine (responding to ergot derivatives) and tension headaches (responding to tranquillizers) to be the most common varieties. Fitzpatrick and Hopkins (1981) found that, in a follow-up study of patients with headache not due to defined structural disease, many feared organic disease but few had overt psychiatric symptoms; most, save for some with long-standing migraine, improved over a period of one year.

References

British Medical Journal (1977). Headaches and coffee. *Br. med. J.* **2**, 284.
Dalessio, D. J. (1980). *Wolff's headache and other head pain*, 4th edn. Oxford University Press, New York.
Fitzpatrick, R. and Hopkins, A. (1981). Referrals to neurologists for headaches not due to structural disease. *J. Neurol. Neurosurg. Psychiat.* **44**, 1061.
Friedman, A. P. and Merritt, H. H. (1957). Treatment of headache. *J. Am. med. Ass.* **163**, 1111.
Henderson, W. R. and Raskin, N. H. (1972). 'Hot-dog' headache: individual susceptibility to nitrite. *Lancet* **ii**, 1162.
Kunkle, E. C. and Wolff, H. G. (1951). Headache. In *Modern trends in neurology* (ed. A. Feiling, 1st Series. Butterworths, London.
Lance, J. W. (1976). Headaches related to sexual activity. *J. Neurol. Neurosurg. Psychiat.* **39**, 1226.
—— (1978). *The mechanism and management of headache*, 3rd edn. Butterworths, London.
—— (1981). Headache. *Ann. Neurol.* **10**, 1.
—— Curran, D. A. and Anthony, M. (1965). Investigations into the mechanism and treatment of chronic headache. *Med. J. Aust.* **2**, 909.
Moskowitz, M. A. (1984). The neurobiology of vascular head pain. *Ann. Neurol.* **16**, 157.
Porter, M. and Jankovic, J. (1981). Benign coital cephalalgia: differential diagnosis and treatment. *Arch. Neurol., Chicago* **38**, 710.
Schumacher, G. A. and Wolff, H. G. (1941). Experimental studies in headache. *Arch. Neurol. Psychiat., Chicago* **45**, 199.
Symonds, C. (1956). Cough headache. *Brain* **79**, 557.
Waters, W. E. (1970). Headache and the eye; a community study. *Lancet* **ii**, i.
Wolff, H. G. and Wolf, S. (1948). *Pain*, p. 37. Thomas, Springfield, Illinois.

Migraine

Synonyms. Hemicrania; bilious attack; sick headache.

Definition. A paroxysmal disorder characterized in its fully developed form by visual and/or sensory phenomena in an aura associated with or followed by unilateral headache and vomiting. While this definition is satisfactory for 'classical' migraine, there are many patients who never experience an aura and in whom the headache is always bilateral; the single most characteristic and constant feature is that migraine is a paroxysmal disorder, i.e. the headaches occur in attacks, separated by intervals of freedom.

Aetiology, pathology, and incidence

Migraine has been known to medical science for nearly 2000 years. In the first century of the Christian era, Aretaeus of Cappadocia described it as heterocrania, and the term hemicrania, from which the word migraine was derived was introduced by Galen (A.D. 131–201). Among more modern studies, Liveing's (1873) is a classic.

The aetiology of migraine is complex. It is not a fatal disease and pathological observations in such cases are therefore scanty.

The intracranial disturbance of function
It has long been held that the most plausible hypothetical explanation of migraine is that it is due to arterial spasm, followed by dilatation, occurring within the distribution of the common carotid artery. During the scotomatous phase of an attack, focal EEG changes have been observed in the opposite cerebral cortex, consistent with cortical ischaemia (Engel, Ferris, and Romano 1945), and it has also been shown that amyl nitrite will temporarily abolish the scotoma (Schumacher and Wolff 1941). There is a generalized, rather than focal, reduction in cerebral blood flow during the aura (O'Brien 1971; Norris, Hachinski, and Cooper 1975; Hachinski, Olesen, Norris, Larsen, Enevoldsen, and Lassen 1977). Occlusion of retinal arteries has been observed during an attack (Graveson 1949), as has a persistent visual-field defect due to ischaemic papillopathy (McDonald and Sanders 1971) and cerebral infarction is not uncommon (*British Medical Journal* 1977;

Dorfman, Marshall, and Enzmann 1979). Confusion and agitation lasting from a few moments to hours may also occur during the aura in childhood (Ehyai and Fenichel 1978). It appears, therefore, that arterial spasm in the retina and/or the visual cortex is responsible for the subjective visual disturbances and other cortical symptoms at the onset of the attack, while subsequent vasodilatation causes the headache and is manifest in flushing of the face, congestion of the superficial temporal artery and of the conjunctiva and nasal mucosa on the side of the headache. Schumacher and Wolff showed that the headache is due to dilatation mainly of the extracerebral arteries of the dura and scalp and branches of the external carotid. The specific therapeutic effect of ergotamine tartrate is due to constriction of the branches of the artery. It is clear that the intracranial disturbance may be precipitated by more than one factor, and in susceptible individuals it is probable that more than one stimulus may cause an attack, though in different patients different causal factors predominate. Peatfield, Gawel, and Rose (1981) have pointed out that, in almost half of 111 patients, the symptoms of the aura which were presumably ischaemic occurred on the same side of the body as the headache, suggesting that ischaemia of one cerebral hemisphere was not necessarily followed by dilatation on the same side; they postulated that ischaemia and hyperaemia were both the result of a more generalized vasomotor disturbance. The CT scan has revealed evidence of cerebral oedema during attacks (Cala and Mastaglia 1976) and between attacks there may be unexpected evidence of cerebral atrophy and of cerebral infarction (Hungerford, du Boulay, and Zilkha 1976).

Ocular factors

Refractive errors and defective ocular muscle balance are often blamed for migraine, though with little justification. Attacks may, however, be precipitated by unusual visual stimuli, such as bright light.

Allergy

Sufferers from migraine are sometimes sensitive to one or more food proteins or other allergens, including pollen, chocolate, and tobacco, and may suffer from other allergic disorders.

Dietetic factors

While allergy may explain the precipitation of attacks by protein to which the patient is sensitive, other dietary factors may play a part. Thus the excessive consumption of animal fat or of alcohol may be followed by an attack; so, too, may missing a meal (Hockaday, Williamson, and Whitty 1971).

Psychological factors

Sufferers from migraine, though many are among the most intelligent and industrious members of the community, are not uncommonly of obsessional temperament, and attacks of migraine may be precipitated by mental fatigue or anxiety, or by other forms of stress. However, Waters (1971) found no evidence that individuals with migraine were more intelligent or of higher social class. Many women suffering frequent attacks at about the time of the menopause are depressed and treatment of the depression is then beneficial.

Endocrine and metabolic factors

On the whole there is little evidence that endocrine abnormality is important. The occurrence of 'menstrual migraine' has been quoted in favour of an ovarian disturbance. Water-retention occurs in some cases (Goldzieher 1941). Sicuteri, Testi, and Anselmi (1961) showed that the urinary excretion of 5-hydroxyindolacetic acid may be increased in severe attacks suggesting an intermittent release of 5-hydroxytryptamine (serotonin) into the circulation (Curzon, Theaker, and Phillips 1966). Injection of reserpine, 2.5 mg intramuscularly, was found to precipitate attacks in 9 out of 16 female subjects (Curzon, Barrie, and Wilkinson 1969), and similar observations were reported by Anthony, Hinterberger, and Lance (1969) who also found evidence to suggest that the catabolism of serotonin and norepinephrine is increased in the first 12 hours of an attack and postulated that an endogenous serotonin-releasing factor is present in the plasma during migraine headache. Adams, Orton, and Zilkha (1968) biopsied temporal arteries during attacks in six subjects and found that the tunica adventitia of the arteries in such patients has a marked capacity to bind noradrenaline. Abnormally high plasma cortisol levels (Ziegler, Hassanein, Kodanaz, and Meek 1979), increased concentrations of γ-aminobutyric acid (GABA) in the CSF (Welch, Chobi, Bartosh, Achar, and Meyer 1975), increased plasma total catecholamines and plasma noradrenaline (Hsu, Crisp, Kalucy, Koval, Chen, Carruthers, and Zilkha 1977), decreased platelet monamine–oxidase activity (Glover, Sandler, Grant, Rose, Orton, Wilkinson, and Stevens 1977), and diminished 5-hydroxytryptamine release from platelets (Damasio and Beck 1978; Hanington, Jones, Amess, and Wachowicz 1981), which may be due to a plasma factor (Pradalier and Launay 1982), have also been described. It has also been postulated that in such cases there is a disruption of the blood–brain barrier which renders the cerebral circulation vulnerable to circulating vasoactive substances (Harper, Mackenzie, McCulloch, and Pickard 1977) such as substance P and serotonin (Moskowitz, Reinhard, Romero, Melamed, and Pettibone 1979; Willoughby 1981).

Heredity

Hereditary predisposition is important, but not perhaps as important as previously believed (Waters 1971); nevertheless, migraine is often inherited as a dominant trait with incomplete penetrance. Various allergic disorders are common among relatives of migrainous subjects.

Association with epilepsy

Much stress has been laid by some writers on the association of migraine with epilepsy. Both are common and many have thought that the relationship is coincidental, but Basser (1969), in a study of 1800 cases, found the incidence of epilepsy in patients with migraine to be higher than in a control group. Occasionally a severe attack of migraine may terminate in an epileptic attack but loss of consciousness at the height of an attack is more often syncopal (Bickerstaff 1961b).

Age and sex

The age of onset is usually at or shortly after puberty, much less frequently in middle life or later, though an onset at about the menopause is not uncommon in women. Migraine is rare before puberty, but cyclical vomiting and travel-sickness are common in childhood in those who subsequently develop it. Women are slightly more subject than men and often suffer more severely.

Symptoms

The onset

Prodromal symptoms may be present or absent. The commonest are drowsiness, lassitude, hunger, and constipation or slight looseness of the bowels. Sometimes the subject feels exceptionally well before an attack. The onset may occur during the day, which is usually the case in migraine with a sensory aura. When headache is not preceded by such manifestations, the patient often awakens with it in the morning from a particularly heavy sleep.

Symptoms of cortical origin

Sensory symptoms, though not constant, are characteristic. Visual disturbances are commonest. These are usually homonymous in distribution, involving the corresponding halves of both visual fields. There may be a gradually developing hemianopia, sometimes preceded by positive symptoms such as flashes of light. The hemianopia can begin in the periphery of the field and spread towards the centre, or vice versa. A common onset is with a bright spot appearing near the centre. This gradually expands towards the periphery, the advancing edge exhibiting scintillating figures (*teichopsia*) which may be coloured and angular—*fortification spectra*. The spreading scintillation leaves behind it an area of blindness, so that when it reaches the periphery of the half-fields the patient is left with homonymous hemianopia. The spread of these symptoms lasts from 15 to 20 minutes, and the hemianopia then gradually fades away, the whole disturbance lasting about half an hour, though objects in the affected fields may appear less bright than normal for several hours. Many types of visual phenomena can occur. The symptoms may have a homonymous quadrantic distribution. Very rarely all peripheral vision is lost in both fields, leaving only a 'telescopic' central field of vision. Exceptionally also the hemianopia is bilateral giving temporary total blindness. In certain cases permanent visual-field defects (hemianopia or a quadrantic defect) may persist after a severe attack.

Paraesthesiae and numbness of parts of the body occur next in frequency. These symptoms occur in a 'cortical' distribution, involving the periphery of the limbs and the circumoral region. The upper limb is most often affected, tingling beginning in the fingers and gradually spreading up the limb, taking 15 or 20 minutes to do so. The lips, face, and tongue may be subsequently affected on one or both sides, or can be involved without the upper limb. The lower limb is rarely affected. Paraesthesiae usually develop shortly after the onset of the visual disturbances, but may occur without the latter as the first symptom. Less often they develop only after the headache has been present for several hours. Gustatory and auditory hallucinations have been reported, but are rare.

Weakness of a limb, usually the upper, or of half of the body may develop, usually following the paraesthesiae, and in very occasional cases recurrent attacks are each accompanied by transient hemiparesis ('*hemiplegic migraine*'). Sometimes this condition is sporadic, sometimes familial; the EEG in attacks may show slow waves over the hemisphere contralateral to the hemiplegia but the CT scan is usually normal (Gastaut, Yermenos, Bannefoy, and Cros 1981). Respiratory arrest in an attack leading to death has been described (Neligan, Harriman, and Pearce 1977). It also seems likely that some transient cerebral ischaemic attacks in older subjects for which no other cause can be found may be migrainous (Fisher 1980).

Aphasia, usually of expressive, less often receptive, type, may occur. In right-handed people, it may be associated with visual disturbances in the right half-fields and paraesthesiae on the right as well. There may be temporary disorientation in space.

Transitory diplopia may be experienced during an attack. Giddiness is not uncommon and there may be slight confusion. Loss of consciousness or even a fit rarely occur. When the symptoms of the aura suggest ischaemia in the distribution of the hind brain circulation, the condition has been called 'basilar artery migraine' (Bickerstaff 1961*a*; Swanson and Vick 1978).

It is often assumed that, in patients with a permanent visual-field defect, aphasia, ophthalmoplegia (see below), or motor weakness persisting after an attack, an intracranial vascular anomaly (e.g. aneurysm or angioma) will probably be present but an investigation of cases of 'complicated migraine' (Pearce and Foster 1965) showed that investigations designed to demonstrate such lesions are usually negative.

Headache

Headache is the most characteristic symptom of migraine and the one from which it derives its name. It may be the only manifestation of the disorder, or may follow the sensory symptoms des-

cribed. It usually begins as a boring pain in a localized area on one side, often in the temple, and gradually spreads till the whole of the affected side of the head is involved. Its boring or sharp, jabbing quality at the onset has been described as 'icepick-like pain' (Raskin and Schwartz 1980). Headache often but not invariably occurs on the side opposite to that to which the sensory symptoms are referred. Sometimes it extends to the whole head. It gradually increases in intensity and acquires a throbbing character, being intensified by stooping and by all forms of exertion. In milder cases it lasts for several hours but passes away if the patient can sleep, or after a night's rest. In more severe cases it persists for days.

Nausea is usually present during the stage of headache, and vomiting may or may not occur. In milder cases it seems to relieve the headache.

Vasomotor changes are often conspicuous (Appenzeller, Davison, and Marshall 1963; Dalessio 1980). The face is often pale and the extremities cold, until improvement begins, but congestion of the face, conjunctiva, and nasal mucosa may occur, often confined to the side of the headache. There may be subconjunctival haemorrhage or even bruising around the eyes. The superficial temporal artery on the affected side is congested and pulsates vigorously. There is often polyuria after the attack.

Electroencephalography

Dow and Whitty (1947) found a persistently abnormal EEG between the attacks in 30 of 51 patients examined and Slatter (1968) reported similar findings, with an unusual response to photic stimulation, but the appearances are non-specific.

Varieties of migraine

The commonest form is characterized by attacks of headache alone, or by headache and vomiting without other symptoms. Somewhat less often, visual or sensory disturbances precede the headache. Less often still, the visual or sensory symptoms, motor weakness, or aphasia occur without headache; in middle age, subjects who had classical migraine in earlier life sometimes experience an aura with associated malaise but without subsequent headache. Exceptionally vomiting may occur alone (one form of cyclical vomiting) or in association with abdominal pain ('migraine equivalents').

Ophthalmoplegic migraine

This term has been applied to recurrent attacks of headache associated with paralysis of one or more oculomotor nerves, often persisting for days or weeks after the attack and sometimes tending to become permanent. Although transitory diplopia is occasionally associated with true migraine, this diagnosis should be accepted with reserve when used to account for ocular palsies lasting more than an hour or two. Probably many such cases hitherto described had intracranial aneurysms. However, in a review of the ophthalmological complications of migraine, Pearce (1968) found that ophthalmoplegia, either isolated or recurrent, occurring in migrainous attacks often remained unexplained despite full investigation. A Horner's syndrome may develop after repeated attacks.

Hemiplegic and facioplegic migraine

Hemiplegic migraine was described above. Recurrent facial palsy in migraine attacks is very rare (Barraquer-Bordas, Peres-Serra, Grau-Veciana, and Saimon-Rabassa 1970). It is probably due to ischaemia of the nerve trunk or compression of it by a dilated artery as in ophthalmoplegic migraine.

Retinal migraine

Retinal vascular lesions in migraine are fortunately rare. Thrombosis of the central retinal artery and of single branches may occur

(Graveson 1949), and recurrent attacks of retinal ischaemia may lead to bilateral optic atrophy due to ischaemic papillopathy (McDonald and Sanders 1971). Retinal and vitreous haemorrhages may also occur.

Symptomatic migraine

A history of migraine is common in patients with intracranial aneurysm, especially upon the internal carotid or posterior communicating arteries, but whether the relationship is significant is dubious (Walton 1956). However, recurrent but increasing retro-orbital pain and ophthalmoplegia due to a supraclinoid aneurysm may simulate ophthalmoplegic migraine. Many patients with intracranial arteriovenous angiomas suffer attacks of headache indistinguishable from those of migraine; sometimes these occur consistently on the side of the head upon which the angioma lies (Mackenzie 1953).

Course and prognosis

The frequency of attacks varies considerably in different patients. Often they seem to possess a rhythm which is little influenced by extraneous factors. They may occur once a week, once a fortnight, or once a month, with great regularity. Attacks in which headache occurs alone are usually more frequent than those in which it is preceded by sensory symptoms. The latter usually recur at intervals of several months. Occasionally a patient has repeated frequent attacks, a condition which has been called status hemicranialis, by analogy with status epilepticus. Headache preceded by visual symptoms may occur more than once a day for several days. Attacks often tend to grow less frequent and severe as the patient grows older and to cease in late middle life. It is not uncommon for the character of the attack to change. For example, visual symptoms may cease or occur without headache.

Migraine does not shorten life, but frequent severe and uncontrolled attacks may be exhausting and debilitating. Depression is a common accompaniment in middle life, especially in women, and vigorous treatment of the latter may improve the migraine dramatically. In some such cases it is difficult to be sure when migrainous headache ends and tension headache begins and the patient may rarely be free from some form of pain in the head. In a few cases permanent hemianopia or other visual-field defects follow an exceptionally severe attack; then teichopsia may persist for weeks. Very rarely permanent aphasia and hemiplegia occur, but this should always suggest a structural lesion and a CT scan and angiography may then be indicated. Ultimately, on follow-up, there is a significantly higher incidence of hypertension and of cardiac infarction, but not of stroke, in sufferers from migraine (Leviton, Malvea, and Graham 1974).

Diagnosis

Migraine must be distinguished from similar symptoms resulting from organic brain disease. The early onset is an important point of distinction, since migraine usually begins at puberty whereas most organic conditions with which it may be confused are encountered in adult life. A tumour of the occipital lobe, especially an angioma, can give attacks of visual hallucinations associated with headache and vomiting. In these cases, however, careful perimetry usually shows a visual-field defect, persisting between the attacks, and increasing. Moreover, signs of increased intracranial pressure may ultimately develop, and there may be evidence of pressure upon neighbouring parts of the brain, and, in the case of an angioma, a cranial bruit.

Migraine is occasionally confused with epilepsy, since visual hallucinations may constitute the prodromal symptoms of both. In migraine, however, the progress of the attack is slow, in epilepsy it is rapid; and the usual retention of consciousness in the former helps to put the diagnosis beyond doubt.

When transitory attacks of paraesthesiae, weakness, and apha-sia occur in migraine without headache, diagnosis is more difficult. Such phenomena simulate cerebral ischaemia due to vascular lesions. In migraine, however, there is usually a history of previous attacks of headache, dating from an early age. The transitory ischaemic attacks of cerebral vascular disease occur chiefly in late middle and old age, and attacks of paraesthesiae in multiple sclerosis, usually lasting for several days or weeks, differ in distribution and duration from those of migraine, which last only half an hour or at the most a few hours. When headache occurs alone, it must be distinguished from that due to other causes: see pages 175–7.

Treatment

The sufferer from migraine should try to avoid both mental and physical fatigue as far as possible. Refractive errors, if present, should be corrected. Diet is sometimes important, but individual idiosyncrasies are marked. Articles of diet which seem occasionally to precipitate attacks, many of which contain vasoactive substances, include alcohol, eggs, chocolate, liver, pickled herring, cured meats (Dalessio 1980), and raw fruit, especially apples and oranges. While tyramine-containing foods (e.g. cheese and red wine) have been thought to be particularly important (Hanington 1967, 1969), Moffett, Swash, and Scott (1972), in a double-blind trial, did not find that tyramine consistently precipitated attacks. However, intravenous tyramine, given in successive doses of 0.5 mg until the systolic blood pressure rises by 30 mm Hg (the tyramine dose/pressor response test) has been found useful in identifying those patients who are likely to respond to treatment with the alpha-adrenergic blocking agent indoramin (Ghose, Coppen, and Carroll 1977).

Drug treatment can be divided into two categories, namely treatment of the attack and prophylaxis. While some attacks may be controlled by aspirin, paracetamol, or other simple analgesic tablets, the single most useful remedy is ergotamine tartrate which may be taken by mouth, sublingually, by suppository, by inhalation of a fine powder, or by intramuscular injection (0.5 mg). Useful commercial preparations in which ergotamine is combined with antihistamine or anti-emetic preparations include *Migril*, *Cafergot Q*, *Cafergot* suppositories, *Orgraine*, *Migraleve*, and *Medihaler ergotamine*. Buccal absorption of ergotamine seems to be no quicker than absorption from the stomach (Sutherland, Hooper, Eadie, and Tyrer 1974) and suppositories containing ergotamine, which had a vogue, are not demonstrably superior to oral medication. The prostaglandin inhibitor flufenamic acid (125 mg four to six times in an attack) has also been found helpful (Vardi, Rabey, Streifler, Schwartz, Lindner, and Zor 1976). Often trial and error is needed to find the most appropriate remedy in the individual patient. All such remedies must, however, be given early and preferably when the aura begins, if the attack is to be aborted. Vomiting is sometimes a troublesome side-effect. Some intelligent patients can be taught to inject themselves if oral medication fails.

In prophylaxis, antihistamine drugs such as prochlorperazine (*Stemetil*), 5 mg three times daily, are helpful in some mild cases and aspirin, 650 mg twice daily may also be effective (O'Neill and Mann 1978). A more powerful prophylactic remedy is dimethysergide (Curran and Lance 1964; Barrie, Fox, Weatherall, and Wilkinson 1968; Lance, Anthony, and Somerville 1970), given in a dosage of 1–3 mg three times daily. There is, however, a risk that retroperitoneal fibrosis may result from prolonged ingestion of this drug which should not therefore be given in a dose of more than 6 mg daily for more than three months at a time. Another powerful and effective serotonin antagonist without this dangerous side-effect is pizotifen, 1.5–3.0 mg daily, which can be continued over much longer periods. It is also clear that dihydroergotamine (1–2 mg three times daily) is also effective in prophylaxis; it can be continued for some months without significant risk of ergotism but must be used with caution in patients with coronary-artery disease and is contra-indicated in pregnancy. Propranolol, 160 mg daily, is also an effective prophylactic (Wideroe and Vigander 1974) as is clonidine (Zaimis and Hanington 1969) in a dose of 0.05 mg three times a day (Shafar, Tallett, and Knowlson 1972). Another remedy recently used with some success is opipramol 50 mg three times a day (Jacobs 1972). In the light of recent evidence implicating abnormalities of platelet formation, prostaglandin inhibitors other than aspirin such as dipyridamole (*The Lancet* 1982) have also been tried but with relatively little success and pizotifen or propranolol now seem the most popular remedies. In anxious and tense patients at any age, tranquillizing remedies such as trifluoperazine, 1 mg three times daily, or chlordiazepoxide, 5–10 mg three times daily, may be helpful, while, in the many women in the paramenopausal age group in whom frequent attacks of migraine and depression coexist, a similar tranquillizer along with amitriptyline, 25–50 mg three times daily, may be dramatically successful in reducing the frequency and severity of attacks. Amine-oxidase inhibitors such as phenelzine are better avoided except in cases resistant to other remedies (Anthony and Lance 1969). Interestingly, two careful studies (Couch, Ziegler, and Hassanein 1976; Couch and Hassanein 1979) have indicated that amitriptyline may be even more effective prophylactically in non-depressed patients of either sex than in those who are overtly depressed.

References

Adams, C. W. M., Orton, C. C., and Zilkha, K. J. (1968). Arterial catecholamine and enzyme histochemistry in migraine. *J. Neurol. Neurosurg. Psychiat.* **ii**, 237.

Adie, W. J. (1930). Permanent hemianopia in migraine and subarachnoid haemorrhage. *Lancet* **ii**, 237.

Anthony, M. and Lance, J. W. (1969). Monoamine oxidase inhibition in the treatment of migraine. *Arch. Neurol. Chicago* **21**, 263.

——, Hinterberger, H., and Lance, J. W. (1969). The possible relationship of serotonin to the migraine syndrome. *Res. clin. Stud. Headache* **2**, 29.

Appenzeller, O., Davison, K., and Marshall, J. (1963). Reflex vasomotor abnormalities in the hands of migrainous subjects. *J. Neurol. Neurosurg. Psychiat.* **26**, 447.

Barraquer-Bordas, L., Peres-Serra, J., Grau-Veciana, J. M., and Sagimon-Rabassa, E. (1970). Migraine prosoplégique familiale. *Acta neurol. belg.* **70**, 301.

Barrie, M. A., Fox, W. R., Weatherall, M., and Wilkinson, M. I. P. (1968). Analysis of symptoms of patients with headaches and their response to treatment with ergot derivatives. *Quart. J. Med.* **37**, 319.

Basser, L. (1969). The relation of migraine and epilepsy. *Brain* **92**, 285.

Bickerstaff, E. R. (1961a). Basilar artery migraine. *Lancet* **i**, 15.

—— (1961b). Impairment of consciousness in migraine. *Lancet* **ii**, 1057.

Bradshaw, P. and Parsons, M. (1965). Hemiplegic migraine. *Quart. J. Med.* **34**, 65.

British Medical Journal (1977). Migrainous cerebral infarction. *Brit. med. J.* **1**, 532.

Cala, L. A. and Mastaglia, F. L. (1976). Computerized axial tomography findings in a group of patients with migrainous headaches. *Proc. Aust. Ass. Neurol.* **13**, 35.

Couch, J. R. and Hassanein, R. S. (1979). Amitriptyline in migraine prophylaxis. *Arch. Neurol., Chicago* **36**, 695.

——, Ziegler, D. K., and Hassanein, R. S. (1976). Amitriptyline in the prophylaxis of migraine: effectiveness and relationship of antimigraine and antidepressant effects. *Neurology, Minneapolis* **26**, 121.

Curran, D. A. and Lance. J. W. (1964). Clinical trial of methysergide and other preparations in the management of migraine. *J. Neurol. Neurosurg. Psychiat.* **27**, 463.

Curzon, G., Barrie, M., and Wilkinson, M. I. P. (1969). Relationship between headache and amine changes after administration of reserpine to migrainous patients. *J. Neurol. Neurosurg. Psychiat.* **32**, 555.

——, Theaker, P., and Phillips, B. (1966). Excretion of 5-hydroxyindolyl acetic acid (5 HIAA) in migraine. *J. Neurol. Neurosurg. Psychiat.* **29**, 85.

Dalessio, D. J. (1962). On migraine headache, serotonin and serotonin antagonism. *J. Am. med. Ass.* **181**, 318.

—— (1980). *Wolff's headache and other head pain*, 4th edn. Oxford University Press, New York.

Damasio, H. and Beck, D. (1978). Migraine, thrombocytopenia, and serotonin metabolism. *Lancet* **i**, 240.

Dorfman, L. J., Marshall, W. H., and Enzmann, D. R. (1979). Cerebral infarction and migraine: clinical and radiologic correlations. *Neurology, Minneapolis* **29**, 317.

Dow, D. J. and Whitty, C. W. M. (1947). Electroencephalographic changes in migraine. *Lancet* **ii**, 52.

Ehyai, A. and Fenichel, H. M. (1978). The natural history of acute confusional migraine. *Arch. Neurol., Chicago* **35**, 368.

Engel, G. L., Ferris, E. B., Jr., and Romano, J. (1945). Focal encephalographic changes during scotomas of migraine, *Am. J. med. Sci.* **209**, 650.

Fisher, C. M. (1980). Late-life migraine accompaniments as a cause of unexplained transient ischemic attacks. *Can. J. neurol. Sci.* **7**, 9.

Friedman, A. P. (1963). The pathogenesis of migraine headache. *Bull. Los Angeles neurol. Soc.* **28**, 191.

——and Elkind, A. H. (1963). Methysergide in treatment of vascular headaches of migraine type. *J. Am. med. Ass.* **184**, 125.

Gastaut, J. L., Yermenos, E., Bonnefoy, M., and Cros, D. (1981). Familial hemiplegic migraine: EEG and CT scan study of two cases. *Ann. Neurol.* **10**, 392.

Ghose, K., Coppen, A., and Carroll, D. (1977). Intravenous tyramine response in migraine before and during treatment with indoramin. *Br. med. J.* **1**, 1191.

Glover, V., Sandler, M., Grant, E. Rose, F. C., Orton, D., Wilkinson, M., and Stevens, D. (1977). Transitory decrease in platelet monoamine-oxidase activity during migraine attacks. *Lancet* **i**, 391.

Goldzieher, M. A. (1941). Endocrine aspects of headaches. *J. lab. clin. Med.* **27**, 150.

Graveson, G. S. (1949). Retinal arterial occlusion in migraine. *Br. med. J.* **2**, 838.

Hachinski, V. C., Olesen, J., Norris, J. W., Larsen, B., Enevoldsen, E., and Lassen, N. A. (1977). Cerebral hemodynamics in migraine. *Can. J. neurol. Sci.* **4**, 245.

Hanington, E. (1967). Preliminary report on tyramine headache. *Br. med. J.* **2**, 550.

—— (1969. The effect of tyramine in inducing migrainous headache. In *Background to migraine, second migraine symposium, 1967* (ed. A. L. Cochrane) pp. 113–19. Heinemann, London.

——, Jones, R. J., Amess, J. A. L., and Wachowicz, B. (1981). Migraine: a platelet disorder. *Lancet* **ii**, 720.

Harper, A. M., MacKenzie, E. T., McCulloch, J., and Pickard, J. D. (1977). Migraine and the blood–brain barrier. *Lancet* **i**, 1034.

Hockaday, J. M., Williamson, D. H., and Whitty, C. W. M. (1971). Blood-glucose levels and fatty-acid metabolism in migraine related to fasting. *Lancet* **i**, 1153.

Hsu, L. K. G., Crisp, A. H., Kalucy, R. S., Koval, J., Chen, C. N., Carruthers, M., and Zilkha, K. J. (1977). Early morning migraine: nocturnal plasma levels of catecholamines, tryptophan, glucose, and free fatty acids and sleep encephalographs. *Lancet* **i**, 447.

Hungerford, G. D., Du Boulay, G. H., and Zilkha, K. J. (1976). Computerised axial tomography in patients with severe migraine: a preliminary report. *J. Neurol. Neurosurg. Psychiat.* **39**, 990.

Jacobs, H. (1972). A trial of opipramol in the treatment of migraine. *J. Neurol. Neurosurg. Psychiat.* **35**, 500.

Lance, J. W., Anthony, M., and Somerville, B. (1970). Comparative trial of serotonin antagonists in the management of migraine. *Br. med. J.* **2**, 327.

The Lancet (1982). Treatment of migraine. *Lancet* **i**, 1338.

Leviton, A., Malvea, B., and Graham, J. R. (1974). Vascular disease, mortality, and migraine in the parents of migraine patients. *Neurology, Minneapolis* **24**, 669.

Liveing, E. (1873). *On megrim, sick headache, and some allied disorders*. Churchill, London.

Mackenzie, I. (1953). The clinical presentation of the cerebral angiomas. *Brain* **76**, 184.

McDonald, W. I. and Sanders, M. D. (1971). Migraine complicated by ischaemic papillopathy. *Lancet* **ii**, 521.

Moffett, A., Swash, M., and Scott, D. F. (1972). Effect of tyramine in migraine: a double-blind study. *J. Neurol. Neurosurg. Psychiat.* **35**, 496.

Moskowitz, M. A., Reinhard, J. F., Jr., Romero, J., Melamed, E., and Pettibone, D. J. (1979). Neurotransmitters and the fifth cranial nerve: is there a relation to the headache phase of migraine? *Lancet* **ii**, 883.

Neligan, P., Harriman, D. G. F., and Pearce, J. (1977). Respiratory arrest in familial hemiplegic migraine: a clinical and neuropathological study. *Br. med. J.* **2**, 732.

Norris, J. W., Hachinski, V. C., and Cooper, P. W. (1975). Changes in cerebral blood flow during a migraine attack. *Br. med. J.* **2**, 676.

O'Brien, M. D. (1971). The relationship between aura symptoms and cerebral blood flow changes in the prodrome of migraine. *Proceedings of the International Headache Symposium*, Elsinore, Denmark, pp. 141–3.

O'Neill, B. P. and Mann. J. D. (1978). Aspirin prophylaxis in migraine. *Lancet* **ii**, 1179.

O'Sullivan, M. E. (1936). Termination of one thousand attacks of migraine with ergotamine tartrate. *J. Am. med. Ass.* **107**, 1208.

Pearce, J. (1968). The ophthalmological complications of migraine. *J. Neurol. Sci.* **6**, 73.

—— (1969). *Migraine*. Thomas, Springfield, Illinois.

—— and Foster, J. B. (1965). An investigation of complicated migraine. *Neurology, Minneapolis* **15**, 333.

Peatfield, R. C., Gawel, M. J., and Rose, F. C. (1981). Asymmetry of the aura and pain in migraine. *J. Neurol. Neurosurg. Psychiat.* **44**, 846.

Pradalier, A. and Launay, J. M. (1982). 5-Hydroxytryptamine uptake by platelets from migrainous patients. *Lancet* **i**, 862.

Raskin, N. H. and Schwartz, R. K. (1980). Icepick-like pain, *Neurology, Minneapolis* **30**, 203.

Schumacher, G. A. and Wolff, H. G. (1941). Experimental studies in headache. *Arch. Neurol. Psychiat., Chicago* **45**, 199.

Shafar, J., Tallett, E. R., and Knowlson, P. A. (1972). Evaluation of clonidine in prophylaxis of migraine: double-blind trial and follow-up. *Lancet* **i**, 403.

Sicuteri, F., Testi, A., and Anselmi, B. (1961). Biochemical investigations in headache; increase in the hydroxyindolacetic acid excretion during migraine attacks. *Int. Arch. Allergy.* **19**, 55.

Slatter, K. H. (1968). Some clinical and EEG findings in patients with migraine. *Brain* **91**, 85.

Sutherland, J. M., Hooper, W. D., Eadie, M. J., and Tyrer, J. H. (1974). Buccal absorption of ergotamine. *J. Neurol. Neurosurg. Psychiat.* **37**, 1116.

Swanson, J. W. and Vick, N. A. (1978). Basilar artery migraine: 12 patients, with an attack recorded electroencephalographically. *Neurology, Minneapolis* **28**, 782.

Vardi, Y., Rabey, I. M., Streifler, M., Schwartz, A., Lindner, H. R., and Zor, U. (1976). Migraine attacks: alleviation by an inhibitor of prostaglandin synthesis and action. *Neurology, Minneapolis* **26**, 447.

Walton, J. N. (1956). *Subarachnoid haemorrhage*. Livingstone, Edinburgh.

Waters, W. E. (1971). Migraine: intelligence, social class, and familial prevalence. *Br. med. J.* **2**, 77.

Welch, K. M. A., Chabi, E., Bartosh, K., Achar, V. S., and Meyer, J. S. (1975). Cerebrospinal fluid γ-aminobutyric acid levels in migraine. *Br. med. J.* **2**, 516.

Wideroe, T. E. and Vigander, T. (1974). Propranolol in the treatment of migraine. *Br. med. J.* **2**, 699.

Willoughby, J. O. (1981). The pathophysiology of vegetative symptoms in migraine. *Lancet* **ii**, 445.

Zaimis, E. and Hanington, E. (1969). A possible pharmacological approach to migraine. *Lancet* **ii**, 298.

Ziegler, D. K., Hassanein, R. S., Kodanaz, A., and Meek, J. C. (1979). Circadian rhythms of plasma cortisol in migraine. *J. Neurol. Neurosurg. Psychiat.* **42**, 741.

Periodic migrainous neuralgia

This term was applied by Harris (1926) to a highly distinctive type of headache involving chiefly the eye and frontal region on one side and characterized by its periodicity. Attacks may occur once or several times in 24 hours and last from one to several hours. The pain is intense, continuous and 'boring' or 'burning' in character; typically the attacks may awaken the patient from sleep in the early morning. They may also be precipitated by alcohol or vasodilator drugs (Ekbom 1970) and remission of anginal pain has been described in the attacks (Ekbom and Lindahl 1971). A bout tends to last for several weeks, after which the patient is free from symptoms for months or even one or two years when the headache recurs in the same way. Pearce (1980) has pointed out that in some patients once- or twice-daily attacks occur indefinitely without remission (chronic migrainous neuralgia) and Medina and Diamond (1981) have described another chronic non-remitting variant in which patients experience atypical localized headaches several times a day as well as short-lasting sharp pains of variable severity and location (multiple jabs). Lacrimation and nasal congestion on the affected side are apt to occur in the attacks. There are no abnormal physical signs, although a Horner's syndrome, either transient or permanent, sometimes develops on the affected side and has been attributed to damage to sympathetic fibres in the wall of the carotid artery resulting from recurrent dilatation of the vessel.

It now seems certain that the condition variously referred to as 'histamine headache' (Horton 1941) or 'cluster headache' (Wolff 1963) is the same as periodic migrainous neuralgia which probably also embraces the syndromes of ciliary neuralgia, vidian neuralgia, and sphenopalatine neuralgia described by the earlier neurologists. Symonds (1956) showed that ergotamine tartrate, 0.5 mg, given by subcutaneous injection once, twice, or even three times daily completely relieved the attacks. The injections are given for as long as may be necessary until the bout is over; this can only be determined by reducing or withdrawing treatment to see whether the attacks recur. Fortunately ergotism seems to be very rare in such cases. Balla and Walton (1964) found that in many cases ergotamine by mouth (*Migril*) was equally effective or, if this failed, dimethysergide, 1–2 mg three times daily. Dihydroergotamine (1–2 mg three times daily) is now one of the most favoured remedies. Probably oral medication should be tried before going on to treatment with injections. The fact that antagonists of histamine H1 and H2 are of no value in treatment (Russell 1979) makes it improbable that histamine is involved in the pathogenesis. However, there is increasing evidence to suggest that the prostaglandin inhibitor indomethacin may also be effective, as it is in 'benign exertional headache' (Diamond and Medina 1979).

References

Balla, J. I. and Walton, J. N. (1964). Periodic migrainous neuralgia. *Br. med. J.* **1**, 219.

Diamond, S. and Medina, J. L. (1979). Benign exertional headache: successful treatment with indomethacin. *Headache* **19**, 249.

Ekbom, K. (1970). *Studies on cluster headache*. Sundbyberg, Stockholm.

—— and Lindahl, J. (1971). Remission of angina pectoris during periods of cluster headache. *Headache* **11**, 57.

Harris, W. (1926). *Neuritis and neuralgia*. Oxford University Press, London.

Horton, B. T. (1941). Histamine cephalalgia. *J. Am. med. Ass.* **116**, 377.

Medina, J. L. and Diamond, S. (1981). Cluster headache variant: spectrum of a new headache syndrome. *Arch. Neurol., Chicago* **38**, 705.

Pearce, J. M. S. (1980). Chronic migrainous neuralgia: a variant of cluster headache. *Brain* **103**, 149.

Russell, D. (1979). Cluster headache: trial of a combined histamine H1 and H2 antagonist treatment. *J. Neurol. Neurosurg. Psychiat.* **42**, 668.

Symonds, C. (1956). A particular variety of headache. *Brain* **79**, 217.

Wolff, H. G. (1963). *Headache and other head pain*, 2nd edn. Oxford University Press, New York.

4

Disorders of the cerebral circulation

The cerebral arterial circulation

The intracranial blood supply is derived from the two internal carotid arteries and the two vertebral arteries which unite anteriorly to form the basilar artery. The circulus arteriosus cerebri (circle of Willis) which is situated at the base of the brain is formed by anastomoses between the internal carotid arteries, the basilar artery, and their branches. The basilar artery divides into the two posterior cerebrals, which are joined to the two internal carotids by the posterior communicating arteries. The internal carotids give off the two anterior cerebral arteries, which are united by the single anterior communicating artery, thus completing the circle.

Extracranial arterial disease, in the aorta and in the common and internal carotid and vertebral arteries in the neck, often accounts for symptoms of cerebrovascular insufficiency. Hence anomalies of the origin and formation of the arteries themselves, and of the circle of Willis, and the efficacy of collateral channels must all be considered in the pathogenesis of cerebral vascular disease. Among the commoner developmental anomalies are: marked inequality in the size of the two vertebral or posterior communicating arteries; hypoplasia or even absence of the anterior communicating artery and/or of the proximal portion of one anterior cerebral; an origin of one posterior cerebral artery from the carotid rather than the basilar; a persistent trigeminal artery joining the carotid to the basilar proximal to the cavernous sinus; an anomalous origin of one vertebral artery from the aorta or the carotid.

Many other rarer anomalies may occur but Hutchinson and Acheson (1975) concluded that all such abnormalities are of theoretical interest only unless occlusive vascular disease develops, when the collateral circulation may be affected (see p. 184).

The principal intracranial arteries and their areas of distribution (see Plates 1 and 2 and Sheldon 1981) are now described.

Arteries of the cerebral hemispheres

The internal carotid artery

The internal carotid artery after entering the cranium gives off small branches to the wall of the cavernous sinus, and to the third, fourth, fifth, and sixth cranial nerves, including the trigeminal ganglion, the pituitary, and the dura mater of the middle fossa. The next branch is the ophthalmic artery, from which the central artery of the retina is derived. The internal carotid next gives off the posterior communicating artery, which unites it with the posterior cerebral. The posterior communicating artery supplies the optic chiasm, pituitary, tuber cinereum, and hypothalamic region, the lower part of the anterior third of the posterior limb of the internal capsule, part of the lateral nucleus of the thalamus, the anterior third of the crus cerebri, and part of the midbrain, including the subthalamic nucleus and Forel's field. The anterior choroidal artery passes backwards and outwards from the internal carotid to enter the anterior extremity of the descending horn of the lateral ventricle, where it supplies the choroid plexus. It is distributed also to the optic tract, to the uncus, to the posterior two-thirds of the posterior limb of the internal capsule, and the origin of the optic radiation, to part of the lentiform nucleus, and some-

times to the anterior third of the crus cerebri, which is more often supplied by the posterior communicating; sometimes it also supplies the posterior two-thirds of the crus which is usually supplied by the posterior cerebral.

The anterior cerebral artery

The anterior cerebral artery passes forwards and medially from the internal carotid, turns round the genu of the corpus callosum, above which it runs backwards to terminate posteriorly, usually 2.5 cm anterior to the parieto-occipital sulcus. It gives off the following principal branches: (1) Basal branches, of which the most important is the recurrent branch (Heubner's artery). This branch enters the anterior perforated substance and supplies the anterior part of the caudate nucleus, the anterior one-third of the putamen, and the inferior half of the anterior limb of the internal capsule. (2) The anterior communicating artery, which is a short branch uniting the two anterior cerebrals and gives off no branches. (3) Branches to the frontal and parietal lobes including the pericallosal and callosomarginal branches. These supply the medial aspect of the hemisphere and the upper part of its lateral aspect extending outwards and downwards for 2 to 2.5 cm from the median edge throughout the length of the artery and also a corresponding area of the white matter of the frontal and parietal lobes, including the olfactory tract and lobe. The most important cortical branch of the anterior cerebral supplies the paracentral lobule, containing the leg area of the motor cortex. Other branches pass downwards to supply the genu, rostrum, and body of the corpus callosum.

The middle cerebral artery

The middle cerebral artery passes laterally from the internal carotid in the stem of the lateral sulcus to the surface of the insula, where it divides into its terminal cortical branches. When crossing the base of the brain it gives off its perforating striate branches. These supply part of the lentiform nucleus, the upper part of both anterior and posterior limbs of the internal capsule, and the horizontal part of the caudate nucleus behind the head. The cortical distribution of the middle cerebral artery is coterminous with that of the anterior cerebral as far back as the middle of the superior parietal lobule. It then extends to the edge of the median surface or is bounded by the territory of the posterior cerebral artery, passing downwards between the intraparietal sulcus and the occipital lobe to reach the middle of the inferior temporal or the lower border of the middle temporal gyrus. In about half of all cases the area of the middle cerebral artery extends to the occipital pole, or 1 cm anterior to it. It also supplies the tapetum of the corpus callosum and the white matter of the centrum semiovale corresponding to its cortical distribution. The cortical branches of the middle cerebral artery are the orbital, the frontal, which supply the inferior and middle frontal gyri, and are distributed to the precentral gyrus and the posterior part of the middle frontal gyrus; the parietal, which supply the postcentral gyrus and the adjacent superior parietal lobule; continuing in the direction of the main stem of the artery these also supply the inferior parietal lobule, part of the lateral surface of the occipital lobe, and the posterior temporal lobe; finally there are temporal branches, which supply the superior and middle temporal gyri.

The posterior cerebral artery

The two posterior cerebral arteries are the terminal branches of the basilar. They run backwards and upwards around the cerebral peduncles and beneath the splenium of the corpus callosum to the calcarine sulcus of the occipital lobe. Close to its origin the posterior cerebral artery gives off basal branches which supply the posterior part of the thalamus, including the pulvinar, the posterior two-thirds of the crus cerebri, and the red nucleus. Other branches pass around the brainstem to supply the colliculi and the geniculate bodies. The *posterior choroidal arteries*, of which there are usually two, supply some branches to the thalamus, brainstem, and third ventricle, and terminate in the choroid plexus of the third and lateral ventricles. There are four *cortical branches* of the posterior cerebral: the anterior temporal and posterior temporal, which supply especially the uncus; the calcarine, which passes along the calcarine sulcus and is distributed to the visual area of the cortex, and the parieto-occipital branch, which passes along the corresponding sulcus. The cortical area supplied by the posterior cerebral includes the medial surface of the temporal lobe, and of the occipital lobe as far forwards as the internal parieto-occipital sulcus, or to a point 2.5 cm anterior to this. The most anterior part of the temporal lobe, however, is supplied by the middle cerebral, and the anterior end of the uncus by the anterior choroidal artery. The cortical area of the posterior cerebral extends on to the outer surface for a distance of from 2 to 2.5 cm, being bounded here by the posterior limits of the anterior and middle cerebral arteries. Above, it usually extends anteriorly as far as the external parieto-occipital sulcus or in some cases to half-way along the superior parietal lobule; below, it supplies the medial aspect of the temporal lobe to within 2.5 cm of its tip.

Blood supply of internal capsule, basal ganglia, and optic radiation

The superior half of the anterior limb of the *internal capsule* is supplied by the middle cerebral artery, the inferior half by the anterior cerebral; the posterior limb is supplied as follows: the superior half by the middle cerebral, the anterior one-third of the inferior half by the posterior communicating, the posterior two-thirds by the anterior choroidal. The *thalamus* is supplied by vessels derived from the posterior cerebral, the posterior communicating, the anterior and posterior choroidal arteries, and the middle cerebral. The posterior half of the lateral nucleus is supplied by the middle and posterior cerebral arteries, the anterior half by the middle cerebral and posterior communicating arteries. The posterior half of the lateral nucleus is supplied by the lenticulo-optic, retromammillary, and thalamo-geniculate (the artery of the thalamic syndrome), the anterior half by the lenticulo-optic and thalamo-tuberal vessels. The oral one-third of the *caudate nucleus* and *putamen* is supplied by perforating branches of the anterior cerebral, the rest by striate branches of the middle cerebral. Most of the *globus pallidus* is supplied by the anterior choroidal. The *optic radiation* at its origin is supplied by the anterior choroidal artery: of the rest, the superior three-quarters is supplied by the middle cerebral and the inferior one-quarter by the posterior cerebral, unless the middle cerebral does not reach so far back, when the posterior cerebral supplies the whole.

Arteries of the brainstem

The arteries of the brainstem are mostly derived from the *basilar* and two *vertebral arteries*, though the upper midbrain receives in addition contributions from the posterior communicating artery, the anterior choroidal, and the posterior cerebral and its branches. The vertebral arteries enter a canal in the cervical spine at the level of the sixth cervical vertebra and then pass upwards to emerge at the level of the atlas and then form a loop before entering the foramen magnum. They fuse at the junction between the pons and the medulla to form the *basilar artery*, which terminates

at the upper border of the pons by dividing into the two posterior cerebrals. The arteries of the brainstem show considerable variations of distribution, but generally conform to the following scheme.

Paramedian arteries enter the brainstem near the midline anteriorly and supply a narrow zone extending from before backwards close to the midline. Short circumferential arteries supply an area, often wedge-shaped, on the lateral aspect, and long circumferential arteries are distributed to the posterior part and to the cerebellum.

The superior cerebellar artery is the highest branch derived from the basilar before its bifurcation. It passes outwards and backwards around the brainstem, giving small branches to the cerebral peduncle and the colliculi, and terminates by dividing to supply the upper surface of the vermis and of the lateral lobe of the cerebellum.

The anterior inferior cerebellar artery arises from the middle of the basilar and passes backwards to supply part of the pons, including the lateral tegmental region and the anterior part of the lower surface of the lateral lobes of the cerebellum. The *internal auditory artery* leaves the anterior inferior cerebellar artery, or less often the basilar or the vertebral, to accompany the cochlear part of the eighth nerve and enters the internal auditory meatus to supply the internal ear.

Throughout its length the basilar gives off small vessels to the anterior part of the pons. Its lowest lateral branch supplies a wedge-shaped area of the lateral aspect of the upper medulla corresponding to the area supplied by the posterior inferior cerebellar artery in the lower medulla.

The posterior inferior cerebellar artery is the largest branch of the vertebral. Its site of origin is variable, but it usually arises from this artery just below the lower border of the pons. It then passes outwards and backwards around the medulla, giving branches which supply a wedge-shaped area of the lateral aspect of the medulla, the base of which is on the surface, and the apex posterointernally, as well as the lower part of the inferior cerebellar peduncle. It also supplies the choroid plexus of the fourth ventricle. The main trunk divides into two terminal branches which supply the inferior vermis and the lower surface of the cerebellar hemisphere.

The vertebral artery, besides supplying the lateral medulla through the posterior inferior cerebellar, gives off branches to the paramedian region, a narrow zone adjacent to the middle line, including the pyramids of the medulla and extending backwards as far as the floor of the fourth ventricle. This paramedian area at the lowest medullary level is supplied by the *anterior spinal artery*, which arises by the fusion of branches from each vertebral artery.

The collateral channels

The experiments of McDonald and Potter (1951) showed that the internal carotid and vertebral arteries share the blood supply to their own half of the brain in such a way that there is normally no interchange of blood between them. Their respective streams meet in the posterior communicating artery at a 'dead point' at which the pressure of the two is equal, and do not mix there. If, however, both internal carotid or both vertebral arteries are occluded, blood crosses the middle line so that the area which would otherwise be deprived of blood is supplied by the contralateral fellow. Normally, the two streams from the vertebral arteries remain each on its own side of the basilar unmixed, like the Blue and White Nile for some miles below their union at Khartoum.

The circle of Willis is the principal collateral channel which helps to preserve circulation to the cerebral hemispheres if one of its principal feeding arteries is occluded (Sedzimir 1959; Gryspeerdt 1963). However, when there is occlusion of one internal carotid artery in the neck, important collateral channels may be

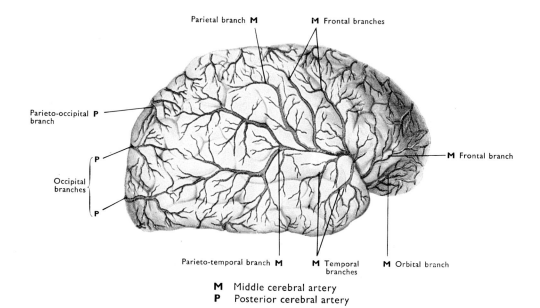

Parietal branch **M**   **M** Frontal branches

Parieto-occipital **P**
branch

P

Occipital
branches

P

M Frontal branch

Parieto-temporal branch **M**   **M** Temporal   **M** Orbital branch
branches

M   Middle cerebral artery
P   Posterior cerebral artery

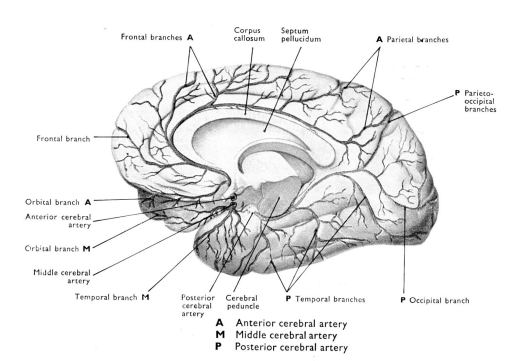

Frontal branches **A**   Corpus   Septum   **A** Parietal branches
callosum   pellucidum

P Parieto-
occipital
branches

Frontal branch

Orbital branch **A**
Anterior cerebral
artery
Orbital branch **M**
Middle cerebral
artery
Temporal branch **M**   Posterior   Cerebral   **P** Temporal branches   **P** Occipital branch
cerebral   peduncle
artery

A   Anterior cerebral artery
M   Middle cerebral artery
P   Posterior cerebral artery

Plate 1. (upper) Distribution of cerebral arteries on the supero-lateral surface of the right cerebral hemisphere. (lower) Distribution of cerebral arteries on the medial and tentorial surfaces of the right cerebral hemisphere.

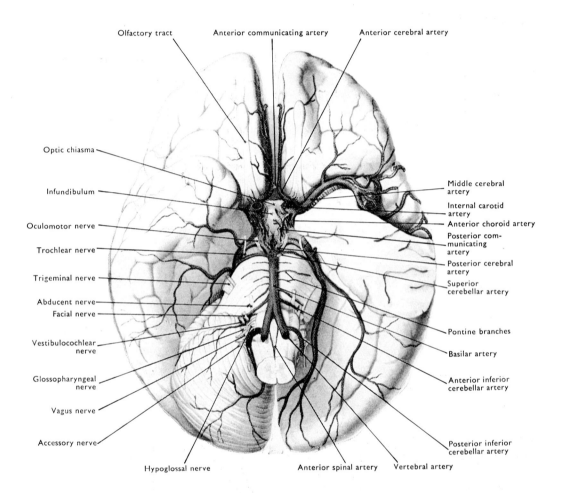

Olfactory tract

Anterior communicating artery

Anterior cerebral artery

Optic chiasma

Infundibulum

Oculomotor nerve

Trochlear nerve

Trigeminal nerve

Abducent nerve

Facial nerve

Vestibulocochlear nerve

Glossopharyngeal nerve

Vagus nerve

Accessory nerve

Hypoglossal nerve

Anterior spinal artery

Vertebral artery

Middle cerebral artery

Internal carotid artery

Anterior choroid artery

Posterior communicating artery

Posterior cerebral artery

Superior cerebellar artery

Pontine branches

Basilar artery

Anterior inferior cerebellar artery

Posterior inferior cerebellar artery

Plate 2. Arteries of the base of the brain.

established via the external carotid circulation with reverse flow through the ophthalmic artery. Less beneficial and indeed positively detrimental to the brain stem circulation is the reverse flow down one vertebral artery into the distal subclavian artery (subclavian steal) which may follow proximal occlusion of one subclavian artery. An external carotid 'steal' has also been described (Barnett, Wortzmann, Gladstone, and Lougheed 1970). In the cerebral cortex, areas of infarction due to occlusion of major arterial branches are limited by collateral flow through the profuse meningeal arterial anastomoses which exist at watershed areas between the anterior, middle, and posterior cerebral areas of supply (van der Eecken and Adams 1953; Gillilan 1959). However, perforating vessels which supply the internal capsule and basal ganglia are genuine end-arteries.

Cerebral blood flow and metabolism

While the extent and potency of the collateral channels is one important factor which limits the size of the area of infarction resulting from arterial occlusion, another important factor is the 'ability of the cerebral blood vessels to compensate rapidly for sudden changes in blood supply' (Hutchinson and Acheson 1975). These changes can be assessed by using the many methods now available to measure cerebral blood flow (CBF). Since Kety and Schmidt (1945) introduced the nitrous oxide method, many other techniques have been utilized. Cerebral 'transit time' can be measured by calculating the time taken for a radioactive bolus injected into the internal carotid artery to reappear in the jugular vein, but such measurements are of little diagnostic value. Similarly, the recording of circulation time, by injecting radioactive hippuran intravenously and recording gamma radiation over the intact skull (Rowan, Cross, Tedeschi, and Jennett 1970) is of little clinical value. An electromagnetic flow meter can be used to measure flow in the carotid artery (Hardesty, Brook, Tode, and Royster 1960; Meyer, Yoshida, and Sakamoto 1967; Welch, Spira, Knowles, and Lance 1974) but requires surgical exposure of the vessel. Gotoh, Meyer, and Tomita (1966) used hydrogen gas and measured hydrogen and other variables through electrodes inserted into the carotid artery and jugular vein, while Nylin, Silfverskiold, Lofstedt, Regnstione, and Hedlund (1960) injected radioactive erythrocytes and studied the dilution curve in the jugular bulb. Measurement of arteriovenous oxygen difference (Strandgaard, Olesen, Skinhøj, and Lassen 1973) allows multiple measurements over a short period. The non-invasive ^{15}oxygen inhalation technique is also useful (Lenzi, Jones, McKenzie, and Moss 1978). Techniques which have been more widely used, however, have generally made use of an inert gas such as ^{133}xenon or ^{85}krypton, either inhaled (Veall and Mallett 1965) or injected, dissolved in 5 ml of sterile saline, into the internal carotid artery through a catheter (Ingvar and Lassen 1962). With the latter technique it is possible, by using 16 or more scintillation crystals placed laterally over the head, to measure regional blood flow in different areas of the cerebral hemisphere (Skinhøj, Hø-edt-Rasmussen, Paulson, and Lassen 1970); calculations can also be applied to compare flow in the cortex and in the cerebral white matter (Rees, Bull, Ross Russell, Marshall, and Symon 1971). Using these methods it is possible to measure CBF in ml of blood per 100 g of brain per minute, a ratio (mean arterial BP/CBF) indicative of cerebral vascular resistance (CVR) and another indicating cerebral oxygen utilization (arteriovenous O_2 difference/CBF) ($CMRO_2$). It is also possible to use CT scanning after intravenous sodium isothalamate injection in order to measure cerebral blood volume (Ladurner, Zilkha, Iliff, du Boulay, and Marshall 1976; Zilkha, Ladurner, Iliff, du Boulay, and Marshall 1976).

Extensive studies using these techniques have shown first that the normal CBF is about 55 ml/100 g/min but diminishes with increasing age (Fazekas, Klein, and Finnerty 1955), especially in patients with hypertension, diabetes, and hyperlipidaemia (Naritomi, Meyer, Sakai, Yomaguchi, and Shaw 1979). The CBF is controlled by the perfusing pressure (which in normal subjects corresponds to the mean arterial blood pressure – MABP) and by the CVR; the ability of the brain to maintain CBF relatively constant despite variations in these parameters is known as autoregulation (Lassen 1966), a facility highly developed under normal conditions but which may be profoundly altered by cerebral vascular disease. Schmidt (1950) showed that cerebral vasomotor innervation plays little part in autoregulation, but Fog (1939) had previously shown that a rise in intravascular pressure caused constriction of pial arterioles and a fall caused dilatation. There is, however, evidence that one major factor which controls CVR in both man and animals is the CO_2 tension of the arterial blood (Kety and Schmidt 1948; Gotoh, Tazaki, and Meyer 1961; Harper and Bell 1963; Reivich 1964; Lassen 1968); inhalation of gas containing more than 3.5 per cent CO_2 causes a significant increase in CBF. Changes in O_2 tension tend to have the reverse effect in that inhalation of O_2 causes vasoconstriction and hypoxia tends to cause dilatation (Heyman, Patterson, and Whatley Duke 1952). A new dimension has been introduced since the development of positron-emission computed tomography (PET) which gives information about regional blood flow, relative perfusion and local cerebral oxygen and glucose utilization (Kuhl, Phelps, Kowell, Metter, Selin, and Winter 1980; Frackowiak, Lenzi, Jones, and Heather 1980; Mazziotta, Phelps, Miller, and Kuhl 1981; Phelps, Mazziotta, Kuhl, Nuwer, Packwood, Metter, and Engel 1981). Less expensive and not requiring, like the PET scan, access to a cyclotron, but potentially equally useful, is single-photon emission computed tomography (SPECT) after intravenous N-isopropyl-p-[^{123}I]-iodoamphetamine (Kuhl, Barrio, Huang, Selin, Ackermann, Lear, Wu, Lin, and Phelps 1982); this technique is still being validated. Another recent development in measuring regional CBF has been the use of emission computed tomography after inhalation of ^{133}xenon (Lassen, Henriksen, and Paulson 1981).

A vast literature has accumulated detailing studies of CBF in various forms of cerebral vascular disease. In patients with hypertension and cerebral atherosclerosis, earlier studies demonstrated consistent reductions in the over-all CBF, tending to be greater in patients with symptoms and signs of cerebral ischaemia (Scheinberg 1950; Alman and Fazekas 1957; Kempinsky, Boniface, Keating, and Morgan 1961). In patients with polycythaemia, there is a significant inverse relationship between CBF on the one hand and the haematocrit and blood viscosity on the other (Thomas, du Boulay, Marshall, Pearson, Ross Russell, Symon, Wetherley-Mein, and Zilkha 1977; Humphrey, du Boulay, Marshall, Pearson, Ross Russell, Symon, Wetherley-Mein, and Zilkha 1979). When angiography had demonstrated occlusion of a major vessel (internal carotid or middle cerebral) on one side, the total CBF was generally reduced more on the affected side of the head (McHenry 1966; O'Brien and Veall 1970) but in some cases, depending presumably upon the efficacy of the collateral circulation and the patency of small vessels, there was a general reduction of the CBF, even in the clinically uninvolved hemisphere. A similar unilateral reduction in CBF through the internal carotid circulation was reported in the prodromal phase of a migraine attack (O'Brien 1967; Skinhøj and Paulson 1969). The PET scan has clearly demonstrated localized areas of impaired perfusion and of glucose utilization in patients with stroke, especially in the affected cerebal hemisphere, and the SPECT method has given similar results (Kuhl *et al* 1980, 1982).

Not surprisingly in the light of the results described, many workers suggested that cerebral ischaemia should be treated by the inhalation of CO_2, and Hegedus and Shackleford (1965) recommended the inhalation of 5 per cent CO_2 in cases of unilateral carotid obstruction. However, Fazekas and Alman (1964) found that in 9 of 22 patients with occlusion of major vessels, inhaled CO_2 did not increase CBF and actually reduced $CMRO_2$;

they postulated that diseased small cerebral vessels were unresponsive.

Studies of regional blood flow (Høedt-Rasmussen 1967; Paulson, Skinhøj, Paulson, Ewald, Bjerram, Fahren-Krug, and Lassen 1970; Skinhøj et al 1970; Rees, Bull, Ross Russell, Marshall, and Symon 1970; Shah, Bull, du Boulay, Marshall, Ross Russell, and Symon 1972) clarified the position further. First, as Lassen (1966) showed, local hypoxia and tissue acidosis around an infarct may cause vasomotor vascular paralysis, vasodilatation, and loss of autoregulation which may in turn result in excessive blood flow around the periphery ('the luxury perfusion syndrome'). This phenomenon may cause venous engorgement (red venous blood) and even haemorrhage, thus extending the area of initial damage; inhaled CO_2 would be likely to increase flow into such areas and would thus be harmful. Høedt-Rasmussen et al (1967) and McHenry, Goldberg, Jaffe, Kenton, West, and Cooper (1972) showed that this process not only caused local tissue damage but also tended to divert blood away from an ischaemic focus ('intra-cerebral steal syndrome'). Fortunately such hyperaemic foci with loss of autoregulation usually perist for only two or three days, though occasionally they last much longer, and Rees et al (1970) found local areas of diminished CBF after transient cerebral ischaemic attacks for up to 90 days. In occasional cases autoregulation may be temporarily impaired over the entire affected hemisphere.

The importance of luxury perfusion and the 'intracerebral steal' phenomenon in relation to treatment was stressed by Paulson, Olesen, and Christensen (1972) who found that hypocapnia induced by hyperventilation (Raichle, Posner, and Plum 1970), often restored autoregulation in patients in whom it was lost. Hence, it appears that hyperventilation and hypocapnia do not cause cerebral ischaemic hypoxia in patients with cerebral ischaemia; on the contrary, they may increase local flow by producing vasoconstriction in the normal collateral channels, thus increasing the perfusing pressure to the ischaemic area (Hutchinson and Acheson 1975). However, there is also evidence that centres in the brainstem exercise a neurogenic controlling effect upon CBF and metabolism (Meyer, Teraura, Sakamoto, and Kondo 1971).

Blood flow in extracranial arteries

While angiography is the traditional method of identifying extra-cranial arterial stenoses which may influence the cerebral circulation in various ways, other techniques, such as computed tomography (Frisén, Kjällman, Lindberg and Svendsen 1979), oculoplethysmography, carotid phonoangiography (Ginsberg, Greenwood, and Goldberg 1979), and, more especially, directional Doppler ultrasonography (Müller 1972; Prichard, Martin, and Sherriff 1979; Hames, Humphries, Powell, and McLellan 1981), have proved useful, safe and atraumatic in identifying stenoses in the common carotid artery and its branches, including the internal carotid and ophthalmic arteries.

The blood–brain barrier

All vessels within the central nervous system are surrounded by a thin covering formed by astrocytic processes. The plasma in the vessels is separated from the nervous tissue by the endothelium of the capillaries and their basement membrane, outside which is the extracellular space of the nervous system. The blood–brain barrier consists of the endothelial lining cells, the basement membrane, and perivascular astrocytic processes. The intravenous injection of trypan blue gives staining only of the astrocytic processes and the dye does not reach the nervous parenchyma except where the barrier is incomplete, as in the pineal, pituitary, area postrema of the brainstem, choroid plexus, and locus caeruleus (Dempsey and Wislocki 1955; Brightman 1965). The restrictive permeability characteristics of capillaries in other parts of the brain are associated with a markedly increased content of mitochondria in their endothelial cells (Oldendorf, Cornford, and Brown 1977).

Injected large molecules (ferritin, horseradish peroxidase) cannot pass the tight junctions of these cells in either direction (Reese and Karnovsky 1968). However, gases, water, glucose, electrolytes, and amino acids diffuse freely across the blood–brain barrier into the intracellular space (glial cells and neurones) and into the extra-cellular space of the brain. Acute cerebral lesions, whether due to trauma, inflammation, or infarction, increase the permeability of the barrier and thus alter the extra- and intracellular concentrations of protein, water, and electrolytes (Millen and Hess 1958; Meyer 1958; Lassen and Ingvar 1963).

References

Alexander, L. (1942). The vascular supply of the striato-pallidum. *Res. Publ. Ass. nerv. ment. Dis.* **21**, 77.

Alman, R. W. and Fazekas, J. F. (1957). Disparity between low cerebral blood flow and clinical signs of cerebral ischaemia. *Neurology, Minneapolis* **7**, 555.

Atkinson, W. J. (1949). The anterior inferior cerebellar artery. *J. Neurol. Neurosurg. Psychiat.* **21**, 137.

Barnett, H. J. M., Wortzman, G., Gladstone, R. M., and Lougheed, W. M. (1970). Diversion and reversal of cerebral blood flow: external carotid artery 'steal'. *Neurology, Minneapolis* **20**, 1.

Brightman, M. W. (1965). The distribution within the brain of ferritin injected into the cerebrospinal fluid compartments. *Am. J. Anat.* **117**, 193.

Dempsey, E. W. and Wislocki, G. B. (1955). An electron microscopic study of the blood–brain barrier in the rat. *J. biophys. biochem. Cytol.* **1**, 245.

Fay, T. (1925). The cerebral vasculature. *J. Am. med. Ass.* **84**, 1727.

Fazekas, J. F. and Alman, W. R. (1964). Maximal dilatation of cerebral vessels. *Arch. Neurol., Chicago* **11**, 303.

——, Klein, J., and Finnerty, F. A. (1955). Influence of age and vascular disease on cerebral hemodynamics and metabolism. *Am. J. Med.* **18**, 477.

Fog, M. (1939). Reaction of pial arteries to increase in blood pressure. *Arch. Neurol. Psychiat., Chicago* **4**, 260.

Foix, C. (1925). Irrigation de la couche optique. *C.R. Soc. Biol., Paris* **92**, 55.

—— and Hillemand, P. (1925). Les artères de l'axe encéphalique jusqu'au diencéphale inclusivement. *Rev. Neurol., Paris* **32**, 705.

Frackowiaz, R. S. J., Lenzi, G. -L., Jones, T., and Heather, J. D. (1980). Quantitative measurement of regional cerebral blood flow and oxygen metabolism in man using O^{15} and positron emission tomography: theory, procedure, and normal values. *J. comput. assist. Tomogr.* **4**, 727.

Frisén, L. Kjällman, L., Lindberg, B., and Svendsen, P. (1979). Detection of extracranial carotid stenosis by computed tomography. *Lancet* i, 1319.

Gillilan, L. A. (1959). Significant superficial anastomosis in the arterial blood supply to the human brain. *J. comp. Neurol.* **112**, 55.

Ginsberg, M. D. Greenwood, S. A., and Goldberg, H. I. (1979). Noninvasive diagnosis of extracranial cerebrovascular disease: oculoplethys-mography–phonoangiography and directional Doppler ultrasonography. *Neurology, Minneapolis* s**29**, 623.

Gotoh, F. Meyer, J. S., and Tomita, M. (1966). Hydrogen method for determining cerebral blood flow in man. *Arch. Neurol., Chicago* **15**, 549.

——, Tazaki, Y., and Meyer, J. S. (1961). Transport of gases through brain and their extravascular vasomotor action. *Exp. Neurol.* **4**, 48.

Gryspeerdt, G. L. (1963). Angiographic studies of the blood flow in the circle of Willis: the value of various arterial compression tests. *Acta Radiol.* **1**, 298.

Hames, T. K., Humphries, K. N., Powell, T. V., and McLellan, D. L. (1981). Comparison of angiography with continuous wave Doppler ultrasound in the assessment of extracranial arterial disease. *J. Neurol. Neurosurg. Psychiat.* **44**, 661.

Hardesty, W. H., Brook, R., Toole, J. F., and Royster, H. P. (1960). Studies of carotid artery blood flow in man. *New Engl. J. Med.* **263**, 944.

Harper, A. M. and Bell, R. A. (1963). The effect of metabolic acidosis and alkalosis on the blood flow through the cerebral cortex. *J. Neurol. Neurosurg. Psychiat.* **26**, 341.

Hegedus, S. A. and Shackleford, R. T. (1965). Carbon dioxide and obstructed cerebral blood flow—correlation between cerebral blood flow crossfilling and neurological findings. *J. Am. med. Ass.* **191**, 279.

Heyman, A., Patterson, J. L., and Whatley Duke, T. (1952). Cerebral circulation and metabolism in sickle cell and other chronic anaemias with observations on the effects of oxygen inhalation. *J. clin. Invest.* **31**, 824.

Høedt-Rasmussen, K., Skinhøj, E., Paulson, O., Ewald, J., Bjerrum, J. K., Fahren-Krug, A., and Lassen, N. A. (1967). Regional cerebral blood flow in acute apoplexy. The 'luxury perfusion syndrome' of brain tissue. *Arch. Neurol., Chicago* **17**, 271.

Humphrey, P. R. D., du Boulay, G. H., Marshall, J., Pearson, T. C., Ross Russell, R. W., Symon, L., Wetherley-Mein, G., and Zilkha, E. (1979). Cerebral blood flow and viscosity in relative polycythaemia. *Lancet* **ii**, 873.

Hutchinson, E. C. and Acheson, E. J. (1975). *Strokes: Natural history, pathology and surgical treatment.* Saunders, London.

Ingvar, D. and Lassen, N. A. (1962). Regional blood flow of the cerebral cortex determined by Krypton[85]. *Acta physiol. scand.* **54**, 325.

Kempinsky, W. H., Boniface, W. R., Keating, J. B. A., and Morgan, P. P. (1961). Serial hemodynamic study of cerebral infarction in man. *Circulation Res.* **9**, 1051.

Kety, S. S. and Schmidt, C. F. (1945). The determination of cerebral blood flow in man by use of nitrous oxide in low concentrations. *Am. J. Physiol.* **143**, 53.

—— and —— (1948). Oxide method for the quantitative determination of cerebral blood flow in man. Theory, procedure and normal values. *J. clin. Invest.* **27**, 27, 476.

Kuhl, D. E., Barrio, J. R., Huang, S. -C., Selin, C., Ackermann, R. F., Lear, L. J., Wu, J. L., Lin, T. H., and Phelps, M. E. (1982). Quantifying local cerebral blood flow by N-isopropyl-p-[^{123}I]iodoamphetamine (IMP) tomography. *J. nuc. Med.* **23**, 196.

——, Phelps, M. E., Kowell, A. P., Metter, E. J., Selin, C., and Winter, J. (1980). Effects of stroke on local cerebral metabolism and perfusion: mapping by emission computed tomography of [18]FDG and [13]NH[3]. *Ann. Neurol.* **8**, 47.

Ladurner, G., Zilkha, E., Iliff, L. D., du Boulay, G. H., and Marshall, J. (1976). Measurement of regional cerebral blood volume by computerized axial tomography. *J. Neurol. Neurosurg. Psychiat.* **39**, 152.

Lassen, N. A. (1966). The luxury perfusion syndrome. *Lancet* **ii**, 1113.

—— (1968). Neurogenic control of cerebral blood flow. *Scand. J. clin. Lab. Invest.*, suppl. 102 VI: F.

—— and Ingvar, D. H. (1963). Regional cerebral blood flow measurements in man: a review. *Arch. Neurol., Chicago* **9**, 615.

——, Henriksen, L., and Paulson, O. B. (1981). Regional cerebral blood flow by radioxenon-133 inhalation and dynamic emission tomography. *Prog. Nucl. Med.* **7**, 110.

Lenzi, G. L., Jones, T., McKenzie, C. G., and Moss, S. (1978). Non-invasive regional study of chronic cerebrovascular disorders using the oxygen-15 inhalation technique. *J. Neurol. Neurosurg. Psychiat.* **41**, 11.

Mazziotta, J. C., Phelps, M. E., Miller, J., and Kuhl, D. E. (1981). Tomographic mapping of human cerebral metabolism: normal unstimulated state. *Neurology, Minneapolis* **31**, 503.

McDonald, D. A. and Potter, J. M. (1951). The distribution of blood to the brain. *J. Physiol., London* **114**, 356.

McHenry, L. C., Jr. (1966). Cerebral blood flow studies in cerebrovascular disease. *Arch. intern. Med.* **117**, 546.

——, Goldberg, H. I., Jaffe, M. E., Kenton, E. J., West, J. W., and Cooper, E. S. (1972). Regional cerebral blood flow: response to carbon dioxide inhalation in cerebrovascular disease. *Arch. Neurol, Chicago* **27**, 403.

Meyer, A. (1958). In *Neuropathology* (ed. J. G. Greenfield, W. Blackwood, W. H. McMenemey, A. Meyer and R. M. Norman), p. 230. Arnold, London.

Meyer, J. S., Yoshida, K., and Sakamoto, K. (1967). Autonomic control of cerebral blood flow measured by electromagnetic flowmeters. *Neurology, Minneapolis* **17**, 638.

——, Teraura, T., Sakamoto, K., and Kondo, A. (1971). Central neurogenic control of cerebral blood flow. *Neurology, Minneapolis* **21**, 247.

Millen, J. W. and Hess, A. (1958). The blood–brain barrier: an experimental study with vital dyes. *Brain* **81**, 248.

Müller, H. R. (1972). The diagnosis of internal carotid artery occlusion by directional Doppler sonography of the ophthalmic artery. *Neurology, Minneapolis* **22**, 816.

Naritomi, H., Meyer, J. S., Sakai, F., Yamaguchi, F., and Shaw, T. (1979). Effects of advancing age on regional cerebral blood flow: studies in normal subjects and subjects with risk factors for atherothrombotic stroke. *Arch. Neurol., Chicago* **36**, 410.

Nylin, G., Silfverskiold, B. P., Lofstedt, S., Regnstione, O., and Hed-

lund, S. (1960). Studies of cerebral blood flow in man using radioactive-labelled erythrocytes. *Brain* **83**, 293.

O'Brien, M. D. (1967). Cerebral-cortex-perfusion rates in migraine. *Lancet* **i**, 1036.

—— and Veall, N. (1970). The influence of carotid stenosis on cortex perfusion. *Research in Cerebral Circulaton, 3rd International Salzburg Conference* p. 165. Excerpta Medica, Amsterdam.

Oldendorf, W. H., Cornford, M. E., and Brown, W. J. (1977). The large apparent work capability of the blood–brain barrier: a study of the mitochondrial content of capillary endothelial cells in brain and other tissues of the rat. *Ann. Neurol.* **1**, 409.

Paulson, O. B., Lassen, N. A., and Skinhøj, E. (1970). Regional cerebral blood flow in apoplexy without arterial occlusion. *Neurology, Minneapolis* **20**, 125.

——, Olesen, J., and Christensen, M. S. (1972). Restoration of autoregulation of cerebral blood flow by hypocapnia. *Neurology, Minneapolis* **22**, 286.

Phelps, M. E., Mazziotta, J. C., Kuhl, D. E., Nuwer, M., Packwood, J., Metter, J., and Engel, J., Jr. (1981). Tomographic mapping of human cerebral metabolism: visual stimulation and deprivation. *Neurology, Minneapolis* **31**, 517.

Prichard, D. R., Martin, T. R. P., and Sherriff, S. B. (1979). Assessment of directional Doppler ultrasound techniques in the diagnosis of carotid artery disease. *J. Neurol. Neurosurg. Psychiat.* **42**, 563.

Raichle, M., Posner, J. B., and Plum, F. (1970). Cerebral blood flow during and after hyperventilation. *Arch. Neurol, Chicago* **23**, 394.

Rees, J. E., Bull, J. W. D., Ross Russell, R. W., Marshall, J., and Symon, L. (1970). Regional cerebral blood flow in transient ischaemic attacks. *Lancet,* **ii**, 1210.

——, ——, du Boulay, G. H., Marshall, J., Ross Russell, R. W., and Symon, L. (1971). The comparative analysis of isotope clearance curves in normal and ischaemic brain. *Stroke* **2**, 444.

Reese, T. S. and Karnovsky, M. J. (1968). Fine structural localisation of a blood–brain barrier to exogenous peroxidase. *J. Cell Biol.* **34**, 207.

Reivich, M. (1964). Arterial pCO_2 and cerebral hemodynamics. *Am. J. Physiol.* **206**, 25.

Rowan, J. O., Cross, J. N., Tedeschi, G. M., and Jennett, W. B. (1970). Limitations of circulation time in the diagnosis of intracranial disease. *J. Neurol. Neurosurg. Psychiat.* **33**, 739.

Scheinberg, P. (1950). Cerebral blood flow in vascular disease of the brain with observations on the effects of stellate ganglion block. *Am. J. Med.* **8**, 139.

Schmidt, C. F. (1950). *The cerebral circulation in health and disease.* Thomas, Springfield, Illinois.

Sedzimir, C. B. (1959). An angiographic test of collateral circulation, through the anterior segment of the circle of Willis. *J. Neurol. Neurosurg. Psychiat.* **22**, 64.

Shah, S., Bull, J. W. D., du Boulay, G. H., Marshall, J., Ross Russell, R. W., and Symon, L. (1972). A comparison of rapid serial angiography and isotope clearance measurements in cerebrovascular disease. *Br. J. Radiol.* **45**, 294.

Sheldon, J. J. (1981). Blood vessels of the scalp and brain. *Clinical Symposia.* CIBA Pharmaceutical Company, New Jersey.

Skinhøj, E. and Paulson, O. B. (1969). Regional blood flow in internal carotid distribution during migraine attack. *Br. med. J.* **3**, 569.

——, Høedt-Rasmussen, K., Paulson, O. B., and Lassen, N. A. (1970). Regional cerebral blood flow and its autoregulation in patients with transient focal cerebral ischemic attacks. *Neurology, Minneapolis* **20**, 485.

Strandgaard, S. Olesen, J., Skinhøj, E., and Lassen, N. A. (1973). Autoregulation of brain circulation in severe arterial hypertension. *Br. med. J.* **1**, 507.

Thomas, D. J., du Boulay, G. H., Marshall, J., Pearson, T. C., Ross Russell, R. W., Symon, L., Wetherley-Mein, G., and Zilkha, E. (1977). Cerebral blood-flow in polycythaemia. *Lancet* **ii**, 161.

van der Eecken, H. M. (1959). *The anastomoses between the leptomeningeal arteries of the brain.* Thomas, Springfield, Illinois.

—— and Adams, R. D. (1953). The anatomy and functional significance of the meningeal arterial anastomoses of the human brain. *J. Neuropath. exp. Neurol.* **12**, 132.

Veall, N. and Mallett, B. L. (1965). The partition of trace amounts of Xenon between human blood and brain tissues at 37 °C. *Phys. Med. Biol.* **10**, 375.

Welch, K. M. A., Spira, P. J., Knowles, L., and Lance, J. W. (1974). Effects of prostaglandins on the internal and external carotid blood flow in the monkey: possible relevance to cranial flow changes during migraine headache. *Neurology, Minneapolis* **24**, 705.

Zilkha, E., Ladurner, G., Iliff, D. L., du Boulay, G. H., and Marshall, J. (1976). Computer subtraction in regional cerebral blood-volume measurements using the EMI-scanner. *Br. J. Radiol.* **49**, 330.

Cerebral ischaemia

Cerebral ischaemia, or impairment of the blood supply to the brain, may be produced in many different ways. (1) Since, as we have seen, the cerebral blood flow is directly related to the blood pressure, a sudden fall of blood pressure from any cause may produce symptoms of cerebral ischaemia. The cause of this is discussed below. (2) The impaired supply may be the result of occlusion or stenosis of the cerebral arteries themselves due, for example, to atheroma or endarteritis. (3) A cerebral vessel may be obstructed by a substance carried into it from elsewhere by the circulation – cerebral embolism.

Complete circulatory arrest

The brain is very vulnerable to any interruption of its circulation. Irreversible dementia can follow severe blood loss in elderly subjects (Bedford 1956) and permanent cortical blindness has been a consequence of severe exsanguination resulting from haematemesis. Acute hypotension in the elderly is also an important cause of stroke (Mitchinson 1980). Loss of consciousness occurs within a few seconds after total interruption of the cerebral circulation as in cardiac arrest, and permanent damage (anoxic–ischaemic brain injury) is produced in about five to eight minutes (Plum 1973), though Meyer (1958) reported a case in which irreversible brain damage followed after one minute of cardiac and respiratory arrest. Irreversible anoxic–ischaemic cell changes occur in experimental animals within 15 minutes. Bell and Hodgson (1974), in a study of 284 patients resuscitated from cardiac arrest, found that only 19 per cent of comatose patients lived to be discharged from hospital compared with 54 per cent of non-comatose individuals. Snyder, Ramirez-Lassepas, and Lippert (1977) also found that the depth and duration of post-arrest coma, motor unresponsiveness, and absent oculocephalic responses were useful in predicting outcome, and many of those surviving after initial coma showed persisting neurological deficits. The EEG is of some value in predicting the prognosis (Pampiglione and Harden 1968). Brierley, Adams, Graham, and Simpson (1971) found neuropathological evidence of almost total neocortical death in two patients who survived for 5 months in coma. The effects of anoxia due, for instance, to carbon monoxide poisoning (p. 441) are similar, if less profound than those of total circulatory arrest. A vegetative state with restoration, after initial coma, of pupillary and caloric reflexes, with random roving eye movements but without purposive movements of the limbs implies severe bilateral cerebral hemisphere damage and carries a poor prognosis (Dougherty, Rawlinson, Levy, and Plum 1981).

Neurological complications of open-heart surgery

Cerebral ischaemic episodes may develop during open-heart surgery and vary in severity, sometimes simulating the effects of total cardiac arrest, sometimes those of diffuse cerebral anoxia (Gilman 1965; Javid, Tufo, Najafi, Dye, Hunter, and Julian 1969; *The Lancet* 1975; Sotaniemi 1980). Air or gas embolism due to the use of bubble oxygenators, which can be detected with Doppler ultrasonic flow detectors (Edmonds-Seal, Prys, Roberts, and Adams 1970) is sometimes the cause, but more often these complications are due to microembolic encephalopathy, the emboli consisting of blood products, platelets, or denatured plasma proteins as well as gas bubbles (Williams 1971; Brennan, Patterson, and Kessler

1971). Despite the use of a cerebral-function monitor during surgery and measurements of CSF creatine kinase and adenylate kinase activity (Aberg, Ronquist, Tydén, Åhlund, and Bergström 1982; *The Lancet* 1982) as indices of brain damage, the bypass procedure which is almost invariably required deactivates platelets, and there may be a case for using prostacyclin, a derivative of arachidonic acid, and/or barbiturates and a calcium-blocking agent such as flunarizine to protect the brain during operative procedures requiring cardiopulmonary bypass (*The Lancet* 1982). Similar complications, as well as many infective disorders of the nervous system, have complicated cardiac transplantation (Hotson and Pedley 1976).

Syncope

Definition. Syncope (fainting) is a brief and transitory loss of consciousness, due to impairment of the cerebral circulation, and usually occurring in the absence of organic brain disease. If the fall in cerebral perfusion is sufficiently prolonged, convulsions occur. Hence an isolated convulsion may sometimes be precipitated by circumstances which more usually cause syncope, but, in pathophysiological terms, syncope and epilepsy are quite distinct.

Aetiology

The essential feature of syncope is a temporary fall in cerebral perfusion below the level necessary to maintain consciousness. Apart from narrowing of the cerebral arteries, syncope is the result of low cardiac output, which may be produced in many ways, some of them complex.

Postural hypotension
Fainting occurs in a variety of circumstances which cause hypotension in the upright posture. Venous return to the heart is impaired because the blood accumulates in the veins in rapidly growing adolescents in hot rooms or in church, in young soldiers immobilized on parade, especially in hot weather, in patients getting up after long confinement to bed, in elderly men after emptying the bladder in the night (micturition syncope, *The Lancet* 1962), in those too rapidly assuming the erect posture after sympathectomy, spinal anaesthesia and high spinal-cord injuries, or while receiving hypotensive drugs, or in certain diseases, e.g. tabes, polyneuritis, and porphyria. In all these conditions, the reflex postural regulation of the blood pressure is inadequate. The reasons are often complex (Brigden, Howarth, and Sharpey-Schafer 1950). The pressor reflexes may be interrupted on their afferent side in tabes and polyneuritis, or centrally depressed by alcohol or other drugs, including phenothiazines, levodopa, and amine-oxidase inhibitors. Some patients show a lifelong tendency to faint (syncope proneness), a trait which may be familial (familial syncope); others may faint when sitting and eating a meal (prandial syncope), after a cold drink, a bowel movement, or during an episode of abdominal pain (when vagal stimulation—a true vasovagal attack—may be responsible) (Fisher 1979).

Chronic orthostatic hypotension (the Shy–Drager syndrome)
In this condition, which is often sporadic, but sometimes familial (Johnson, Lee, Oppenheimer, and Spalding 1966), the blood pressure falls as soon as the patient assumes the upright posture but there is no compensatory vasoconstriction of peripheral vessels or acceleration of the heart beat so that pallor, sweating, and tachycardia do not occur and there is abrupt loss of consciousness. Autopsy evidence (Shy and Drager 1960; Chokroverty, Barton, Katz, del Greco, and Sharp 1969; Hughes, Cartlidge, and Millac 1970; Roessman, van den Noort, and McFarland 1971; Thapedi, Ashenhurst, and Rozdilsky 1971; Bannister and Oppenheimer

1972) has revealed degeneration of the cells of the intermedio-lateral column of the spinal cord, confirming autonomic denervation, but the sympathetic ganglia are also abnormal (Petito and Black 1978), and pressor responses to vasoactive agents suggest 'denervation supersensitivity' (Polinsky, Kopin, Ebert, and Weise 1981). The condition has been described in association with the Holmes–Adie syndrome (Johnson, McLellan, and Love 1971). While orthostatic hypotension may be symptomatic of many neurological disorders (Martin, Travis, and van den Noort 1968) and while the primary autonomic failure is sometimes afferent and sometimes efferent (Love, Brown, Chinn, Johnson, Lever, Park, and Robertson 1971), in many cases of the chronic syndrome parkinsonian features, dysarthria, cerebellar ataxia, anhidrosis, impotence and incontinence, and amyotrophy develop in varying combinations and with variable severity, so that the condition is often called progressive multisystem degeneration and widespread degenerative changes are present in the central nervous system. Vocal-cord paralysis is not uncommon (Williams, Hanson, and Calne 1979; Bannister, Gibson, Michaels, and Oppenheimer 1981). In the early stages, attacks may be partially controlled by the use of drugs such as 9-α-fludrocortisone 0.1 mg twice daily with a high sodium intake to increase the blood volume. Levodopa alone may improve bradykinesia when present (de Lean and Deck 1976) but may also increase hypotension; when given with adrenergic drugs such as ephedrine or tranylcypromine it may be beneficial (Corder, Kanefsky, McDonald, Gray, and Redmond 1977). Infusions of angiotensin may cause greater hypertension and isoprenaline greater hypotension than in controls (Mathias, Matthews, and Spalding 1977) and pressor agents such as tyramine given with monoamine oxidase inhibitors are unpredictable (Davies, Bannister, and Sever 1978). Pindolol (in't Veld and Schalekamp 1981) has been found helpful by some but not by others (Davies, Bannister, Mathias, and Sever 1981) while indomethacin alone is unreliable but may be helpful with fludrocortisone (*The Lancet* 1981). Later the wearing of a G-suit may help but usually the disorder is progressive and ultimately fatal though the prognosis varies in individual cases.

Cough syncope

Cough syncope is precipitated by prolonged coughing, usually in middle-aged men with emphysema and chronic bronchitis. The changes in intrathoracic pressure produced by repeated coughing impede the venous return of blood to the heart. Treatment usually involves giving up smoking and other measures to prevent bouts of coughing. Another 'mechanical' mode of producing syncope by impairing venous return is by stretching with the arms extended and raised and the spine hyperextended—'stretch syncope'—which may occur in young people.

Swallow syncope

This rare disorder (Levin and Posner 1972), in which swallowing induces fainting, can be the result of demyelination in the vagus nerve and may be controlled by anticholinergic drugs.

Psychological causes

Syncope occurring as an immediate effect of sudden psychological shock is well known (Rook 1947). Hysteria is also a common cause of recurrent fainting in young girls. Here again there is often a fall of blood pressure due to complex factors but sometimes the attacks are very frequent, unaccompanied by pallor, sweating, or tachycardia, and may be difficult if not impossible to distinguish clinically from episodes of akinetic epilepsy except by collateral evidence of hysteria. Similar unexplained attacks resembling akinetic seizures can also occur in adults (Fisher 1979). McHenry, Fazekas, and Sullivan (1961) pointed out that hyperventilation, a common accompaniment of anxiety and hysteria, may also lead to cerebral ischaemia by producing hypocapnia. Fainting may also be a conditioned reaction to particular circumstances.

Physical shock

Many physical stimuli can cause syncope, and sometimes it is artificial to distinguish physical from psychological factors. Severe pain may precipitate loss of consciousness, but many stimuli causing little or no pain may also do so, such as venepuncture, cisternal and lumbar puncture, and pleural puncture ('pleural epilepsy').

Anaemia of sudden onset

Anaemia due to sudden severe haemorrhage may cause fainting, though an equally severe anaemia of gradual onset does not.

Polycythaemia vera

In polycythaemia vera the increased blood viscosity may predispose to cerebral infarction but many patients also experience episodes of cerebral or brainstem ischaemia similar to those of carotid or vertebro-basilar insufficiency (see below) (Silverstein, Gilbert, and Wasserman 1962). Others present with symptoms suggesting an intracranial space-occupying lesion (Kremer, Lambert, and Lawton 1972).

Cardiac disorder

Syncope may result from impaired cerebral perfusion resulting from low cardiac output caused by a disorder of the rate and rhythm of the heart in heart-block, auricular flutter, and paroxysmal tachycardia. Previously unrecognized episodes of cardiac dysrhythmia may be an important cause of episodes of transient cerebral ischaemia (McAllen and Marshall 1973) and may be detected by 24-hour electrocardiographic (ECG) monitoring (Luxon, Crowther, Harrison, and Coltart 1980). Syncope due to heart-block (the Stokes–Adams syndrome) is well recognized. The loss of consciousness is most likely to occur during the cardiac asystole which may develop in the transition between partial heart-block and complete block (Fairfax and Lambert 1976). The attacks may cease when the block is complete, but do not always do so. Many attacks may occur in a day, usually when the patient is at rest and not during physical effort. Typically loss of consciousness and pallor occur during asystole and flushing with a few myoclonic jerks of the extremities occur when the pulse returns and consciousness is quickly restored. These attacks rarely occur in patients with bundle-branch block. Low cardiac output may also be due to massive pulmonary embolism and mitral or aortic stenosis.

Carotid sinus syncope

The important role of the carotid sinus, the slight dilatation of the carotid in the region of the bifurcation, in controlling cardiac output was first pointed out by Hering, though previously the vagus had been held responsible for effects now known to originate in the sinus. A rise of pressure in the sinus causes a reflex fall in blood pressure and bradycardia, while a fall of pressure within it has the opposite effect. These reflex changes are mediated by the nerve to the sinus, a branch of the glossopharyngeal, and by medullary vasomotor centres. Disease in the neighbourhood of the sinus, or even hypersensitivity of its reflex, may cause syncopal attacks which can be reproduced by digital pressure on the sinus. Precipitation of attacks by spontaneous head movements is mentioned by Turner and Learmonth (1948).

Hutchinson and Stock (1960) reported 16 cases, all middle-aged or elderly males. Some had syncopal episodes alone, often with transient convulsive movements, but others experienced vertigo or other symptoms suggesting transient brainstem or cerebral ischaemia, presumably due to the effects of concomitant cerebral atheroma. Attacks were sometimes precipitated by head-turning. The diagnosis can be confirmed by recording the ECG during carotid sinus pressure when profound bradycardia and even transient asystole may occur (Reese, Green, and Elliott 1962).

The causes of carotid sinus attacks include lesions in its neighbourhood, such as scarring from tuberculous adenitis, atheroma of the artery, and rarely carotid-body tumour, but many cases are 'idiopathic'.

Cerebral atheroma

Cerebral ischaemia resulting from atheromatous narrowing of cerebral arteries is an unusual cause of syncope and is unlikely to cause such attacks unless the whole cerebral circulation is gravely impaired, or else the ischaemia specifically involves the central reticular formation. Faintness may then be induced particularly by turning the head or extending the neck, through impairment of the blood flow through one or other internal carotid or vertebral artery or both, independently of the carotid sinus reflex. Fainting attacks due to brainstem ischaemia rarely occur when occlusion of the left subclavian artery close to its origin results in retrograde flow of blood down the homolateral vertebral artery in order to supply the upper limb (the 'subclavian steal syndrome').

Symptoms

The onset of an attack of syncope may be sudden, but often takes a few seconds to develop. There may be prodromal symptoms such as coldness of the extremities, sweating, 'swimming' in the head, or blurred vision. The patient becomes cold and limp, and sinks to the ground, though the premonitory symptoms often enable him to sit or lie down first. Respiration is usually sighing, the pulse is generally slow, thin, and thready. The pupils may be dilated and react sluggishly to light; the corneal reflexes may be transiently lost and the tendon reflexes diminished. Muscular twitching and urinary incontinence occasionally occur, or, if the ischaemia is sufficiently prolonged, a general convulsion.

Electroencephalography

In syncope slow waves of high voltage develop in the EEG concurrently with the loss of consciousness (Hill and Driver 1962) and this may be followed by transient flattening of the EEG record (Gastaut and Fischer-Williams 1957).

Diagnosis

When syncope leads only to loss of consciousness, it must be distinguished from epilepsy. Syncope, being secondary to circulatory change, is usually more gradual in onset and cessation than an epileptic attack. Convulsive movements do not often occur, and the patient is limp rather than rigid, as in epilepsy. Syncopal convulsions, however, must be distinguished from epilepsy, while cardiac syncope due to arrhythmia may resemble fits (Schott, McLeod, and Jewitt 1977) and some faints are difficult to differentiate from akinetic seizures (Fisher 1979). Often the cause of the syncopal attacks is obvious. Syncope of carotid sinus origin can be reproduced by pressure on the sinus, but this is no longer effective after procaine has been injected into this region. In partial heart-block the diagnosis may be impossible without 24-hour ECG recording: in complete block the heart rate is usually from 26 to 30. Paroxysmal or focal epileptic discharges in the EEG are absent: if syncope can be induced, e.g. by ocular compression, the EEG changes are those described above.

Prognosis

A syncopal attack is rarely fatal and usually leaves no sequelae. However, prolonged and diffuse cerebral ischaemia which may, for example, occur during anaesthesia, particularly in the elderly, or severe recurrent faints, may lead to permanent anoxic brain damage. The prognosis is that of the causal condition.

Treatment

Little treatment is required for the ordinary faint, which is self-limiting. The patient should simply be laid flat. Any causal condition may, however, require treatment. Syncope of carotid sinus origin is best treated with anticholinergic drugs of which atropine, 0.5 mg two or three times daily or propantheline bromide, 15 mg three times a day, are usually the most successful. In intractable cases it may be justifiable to denervate the sinus surgically.

References

Aberg, T., Ronquist, G., Tydén, H., Åhlund, P., and Bergström, K. (1982). Release of adenylate kinase into cerebrospinal fluid during open-heart surgery and its relation to postoperative intellectual function. *Lancet* **i**, 1139.

Bannister, R. and Oppenheimer, D. R. (1972). Degenerative diseases of the nervous system associated with autonomic failure. *Brain* **95**, 457.

——, Gibson, W., Michaels, L., and Oppenheimer, D. R. (1981). Laryngeal abductor paralysis in multiple system atrophy: a report on three necropsied cases, with observations on the laryngeal muscles and the nuclei ambigui. *Brain* **104**, 351.

Bedford, P. D. (1956). Adverse cerebral effects following acute haemorrhage in elderly people. *Lancet* **ii**, 750.

Bell, J. A. and Hodgson, H. J. F. (1974). Coma after cardiac arrest. *Brain* **97**, 361.

Brennan, R. W., Patterson, R. H., and Kessler, J. (1971). Cerebral blood flow and metabolism during cardiopulmonary bypass: evidence of microembolic encephalopathy. *Neurology, Minneapolis* **21**, 665.

Brierley, J. B., Adams, J. H., Graham, D. I., and Simpson, J. A. (1971). Neocortical death after cardiac arrest: a clinical, neurophysiological, and neuropathological report of two cases. *Lancet* **ii**, 560.

Brigden, W., Howarth, S., and Sharpey-Schafer, E. P. (1950). Postural changes in the peripheral blood-flow of normal subjects with observations on vaso-vagal fainting reactions as a result of tilting, the lordotic posture, pregnancy and spinal anaesthesia. *Clin. Sci.* **60**, 79.

Chokroverty, S., Barron, K. D., Katz, F. H., del Greco, F., and Sharp, J. T. (1969). The syndrome of primary orthostatic hypotension. *Brain* **92**, 743.

Corder, C. N., Kanefsky, T. M., McDonald, R. H., Gray, J. L., and Redmond, D. P. (1977). Postural hypotension: adrenergic responsivity and levodopa therapy. *Neurology, Minneapolis* **27**, 921.

Davies, B., Bannister, R., Mathias, C., and Sever, P. (1981). Pindolol in postural hypotension: the case for caution. *Lancet* **ii**, 980.

——, ——, and Sever, P. (1978). Pressor amines and monoamine-oxidase inhibitors for treatment of postural hypotension in autonomic failure: limitations and hazards. *Lancet* **i**, 172.

de Lean, J. and Deck, J. H. N. (1976). Shy–Drager syndrome. Neuropathological correlation and response to levodopa therapy. *Can. J. neurol. Sci.* **3**, 167.

Dougherty, J. H., Jr., Rawlinson, D. G., Levy, D. E., and Plum, F. (1981). Hypoxic-ischemic brain injury and the vegetative state: clinical and neuropathologic correlation. *Neurology, Minneapolis* **31**, 991.

Edmonds-Seal, J., Prys Roberts, C., and Adams, A. P. (1970). Transcutaneous Doppler ultrasonic flow detectors for diagnosis of air embolism. *Proc. R. Soc. Med.* **63**, 831.

Fairfax, A. J. and Lambert, C. D. (1976). Neurological aspects of sino-atrial heart block. *J. Neurol. Neurosurg. Psychiat.* **39**, 576.

Fisher, C. M. (1979). Syncope of obscure nature. *Can. J. neurol. Sci* **6**, 7.

Gastaut, H. and Fischer-Williams, M. (1957). Electroencephalographic study of syncope. *Lancet* **ii**, 1018.

Gilman, S. (1965). Cerebral disorders after open-heart operations. *New Eng. J. Med.* **272**, 489.

Hill, D. and Driver, M. V. (1962). In *Recent advances in neurology and neuropsychiatry*, 7th edn. (ed. W. R. Brain), p. 219. Churchill, London.

Hohl, R. D., Frame, B., and Schatz, I. J. (1965). The Shy–Drager variant of idiopathic orthostatic hypotension. *Am. J. Med.* **39**, 134.

Hotson, J. R. and Pedley, T. A. (1976). The neurological complications of cardiac transplantation. *Brain* **99**, 673.

Hughes, R. C., Cartlidge, N. E. F., and Millac, P. (1970). Primary neurogenic orthostatic hypotension. *J. Neurol. Neurosurg. Psychiat.* **33**, 363.

Hutchinson, E. C. and Stock, J. P. P. (1960). The carotid-sinus syndrome. *Lancet* **ii**, 445.

In't Veld, A. J. M. and Schalekamp, M. A. D. H. (1981). Pindolol acts as beta-adrenoceptor agonist in orthostatic hypotension: therapeutic implications. *Clin Res.* **282**, 929.

Javid, H., Tufo, H. M., Najafi, H., Dye, W. S., Hunter, J. A., and Julian, O. C. (1969). Neurological abnormalities following open heart surgery. *J. thorac. cardiovasc. Surg.* **58**, 502.

Johnson, R. H., Lee, G. de J., Oppenheimer, W. R., and Spalding, J. M.

K. (1966). Autonomic failure due to intermedio-lateral column degeneration. *Quart. J. Med* **35**, 276.

——, McLellan, D. L., and Love, D. R. (1971). Orthostatic hypotension and the Holmes–Adie syndrome. *J. Neurol. Neurosurg. Psychiat.* **34**, 562.

Kremer, M., Lambert, C. D., and Lawton, N. (1972). Progressive neurological deficits in primary polycythaemia. *Br. med. J.* **3**, 216.

The Lancet (1962). Fainting on micturition. *Lancet* **ii**, 286.

—— (1975). Brain damage after open-heart surgery. *Lancet* **ii**, 399.

—— (1981). Management of orthostatic hypotension. *Lancet* **ii**, 963.

—— (1982). Brain damage after open-heart surgery. *Lancet* **i**, 1161.

Levin, B. and Posner, J. B. (1972). Swallow syncope. Report of a case and review of the literature. *Neurology, Minneapolis* **22**, 1086.

Love, D. R., Brown, J. J., Chinn, R. H., Johnson, R. H., Lever, A. F., Park, D. M., and Robertson, J. I. S. (1971). Plasma renin in idiopathic orthostatic hypotension: differential response in subjects with probable afferent and efferent autonomic failure. *Clin. Sci.,* **41**, 289.

Luxon, L. M., Crowther, A., Harrison, M. J. G., and Coltart, D. J. (1980). Controlled study of 24-hour ambulatory electrocardiographic monitoring in patients with transient neurological symptoms. *J. Neurol. Neurosurg. Psychiat.* **43**, 37.

Martin, J. B., Travis, R. H., and van den Noort, S. (1968). Centrally mediated orthostatic hypotension: report of cases. *Arch. Neurol, Chicago* **19**, 163.

Mathias, C. J., Matthews, W. B., and Spalding, J. M. K. (1977). Postural changes in plasma renin activity and responses to vasoactive drugs in a case of Shy–Drager syndrome. *J. Neurol. Neurosurg. Psychiat.* **40**, 138.

McAllen, P. M. and Marshall, J. (1973). Cardiac dysrhythmia and transient cerebral ischaemic attacks. *Lancet* **i**, 1212.

McHenry, L. C., Jr., Fazekas, J. F., and Sullivan, J. F. (1961). Cerebral haemodynamics of syncope. *Am. J. med. Sci.* **241**, 173.

Meyer, A. (1958). In *Neuropathology* (ed. J. G. Greenfield, W. Blackwood, W. H. McMenemey, A. Meyer, and R. M. Norman) p. 241. Arnold, London.

Mitchinson, M. J. (1980). The hypotensive stroke. *Lancet* **i**, 244.

Pampiglione, G. and Harden, A. (1968). Resuscitation after cardiocirculatory arrest. Prognostic evaluation of early electroencephalographic findings. *Lancet* **i**, 1261.

Petito, C. K. and Black, I. B. (1978). Ultrastructure and biochemistry of sympathetic ganglia in idiopathic orthostatic hypotension. *Ann. Neurol.* **4**, 6.

Plum, F. (1973). The clinical problem: how much anoxia-ischemia damages the brain? *Arch. Neurol, Chicago* **29**, 359.

Polinsky, R. J., Kopin, I. J., Ebert, M. H., and Weise, V. (1981). Pharmacologic distinction of different orthostatic hypotension syndromes. *Neurology, Minneapolis* **31**, 1.

Reese, C. L., Green, J. B., and Elliott, F. A. (1962). The cerebral form of carotid sinus syncope. *Neurology, Minneapolis* **12**, 492.

Roessmann, U., van den Noort, S., and McFarland, D. E. (1971). Idiopathic orthostatic hypotension. *Arch. Neurol, Chicago* **24**, 503.

Rook, A. F. (1947). Fainting and flying. *Quart. J. Med.* **40**, 181.

Schott, G. D., McLeod, A. A., and Jewitt, D. E. (1977). Cardiac arrhythmias that masquerade as epilepsy. *Br. med. J.* **1**, 1454.

Sharpey-Schafer, E. P. (1953). The mechanism of syncope after coughing *Br. med. J.* **2**, 860.

Shy, G. M. and Drager, G. A. (1960). A neurological syndrome associated with orthostatic hypotension. *Arch. Neurol., Chicago* **2**, 511.

Silverstein, A., Gilbert, H., and Wasserman, L. R. (1962). Hemiplegic complications of polycythaemia. *Ann. intern. Med.* **57**, 909.

Snyder, B. D., Ramirez-Lassepas, M., and Lippert, D. M. (1977). Neurologic status and prognosis after cardiopulmonary arrest: 1. A retrospective study. *Neurology, Minneapolis* **27**, 807.

Sotaniemi, K. (1980). Cerebral disorders in open-heart surgery patients: a neurological, electroencephalographic and neuropsychological follow-up study. *Acta Universitatis Ouluensis*, Series D, Med. No. 56, Neurol. No. 4.

Thapedi, I. M., Ashenhurst, E. M., and Rozdilsky, B. (1971). Shy–Drager syndrome: report of an autopsied case. *Neurology, Minneapolis* **21**, 26.

Turner, R. and Learmonth, J. R. (1948). Carotid-sinus syndrome. *Lancet* **ii**, 644.

Williams, A., Hanson, D., and Calne, D. B. (1979). Vocal cord paralysis in the Shy–Drager syndrome. *J. Neurol. Neurosurg. Psychiat.* **42**, 151.

Williams, I. M. (1971). Intravascular changes in the retina during open-heart surgery. *Lancet* **ii**, 688.

Classification of the cerebrovascular diseases

In 1958 an *ad hoc* committee of the National Advisory Council of the National Institute of Neurological Diseases and Blindness published a 'classification and outline of the cerebrovascular diseases', which remains a useful basis of classification today. This was revised and expanded in 1975 but the principal types of cerebrovascular disease may still be classified as follows.

Cerebral infarction
Transient cerebral ischaemia without infarction
Intracranial haemorrhage
Vascular malformations and developmental abnormalities
Inflammatory diseases of arteries
Vascular diseases without changes in the brain
Hypertensive encephalopathy
Dural sinus and cerebral venous thrombosis
Strokes of undetermined origin.

These broad diagnostic categories will in general be followed in the commentaries which follow. However, there is increasing evidence to indicate that diagnosis, however skilful, if based on clinical criteria alone, is often inaccurate and Capildeo, Haberman, and Rose (1977, 1978) have argued cogently in favour of using a revised classification based upon a cumulative numbering system which takes into account not only clinical but also investigative criteria and associated conditions; they have found this to be of much greater value than the traditional classification when considering management and prognosis.

The incidence and epidemiology of 'strokes'

Diagnostic information derived from epidemiological studies based upon death certificates must be treated with reserve (Hutchinson and Acheson 1975). Anderson and MacKay (1968) noted marked fluctuations in the incidence of recorded deaths due to cerebral thrombosis on the one hand and haemorrhage on the other between 1901 and 1961 but showed that in necropsy series the incidence had remained relatively constant. Statistics based upon hospital series are inaccurate as many elderly patients with strokes are not admitted to hospital. Whisnant, Fitzgibbon, Kurland, and Sayre (1971) in a survey of strokes in the population of Rochester, Minnesota, found that the incidence of all forms of cerebral vascular disease was 194 per 100 000 of the population per year, and infarction accounted for 146 per 100 000; cerebral haemorrhage accounted for less than 10 per cent of all strokes and subarachnoid haemorrhage for about 8 per cent. The incidence of cerebral haemorrhage seemed at first sight to be much higher in Japan (Johnson, Yano, and Katol 1967) but Kurtzke (1969) in a detailed multinational survey concluded that this was an artefact as autopsy evidence indicated that errors in diagnosis between haemorrhage and infarction may have varied from 10 per cent to as much as 40 per cent in different series. Capildeo *et al.* (1977, 1978), however, found that, in England and Wales in 1972–3, death certificates suggested that about 20 per cent of deaths were due to cerebral haemorrhage, 35 per cent to cerebral thrombosis, 24 per cent to acute but ill-defined cerebrovascular disease (CVD), 13 per cent to generalized ischaemic CVD, and about 5 per cent to subarachnoid haemorrhage. However, an analysis of the results recorded in the Harvard Co-operative Stroke Registry (Mohr, Caplan, Melski, Goldstein, Duncan, Kistler, Pessin, and Bleich 1978) which took into account investigative and post-mortem findings in a series of 694 patients admitted to hospital, showed that 53 per cent had cerebral thrombosis, 31 per cent embolism, 10 per cent intracerebral haemorrhage, and 6 per cent subarachnoid haemorrhage; about one-third of the patients with cerebral thrombosis had lacunar infarction. While ischaemic stroke and spontaneous intracerebral or subarachnoid haemorrhage are all uncommon in childhood, a survey at the Mayo Clinic gave an annual incidence rate of childhood strokes of 2.52 per 100 000 (Schoenberg, Mellinger, and Schoenberg 1978). So far unexplained is the evidence that the mortality of CVD is highest in the winter and spring and lowest in late summer (Haberman, Capildeo, and Rose 1981).

It is also clear that with an ageing population cerebrovascular disease imposes an increasingly heavy burden upon hospital and community services (Acheson and Fairbairn 1970). Though the prognosis of stroke may be somewhat better in females than in males (Marquardsen 1969), paradoxically mortality may be slightly higher in females (Eisenberg, Morrison, Sullivan, and Foote 1964); however, both morbidity and mortality are related linearly to age (Hutchinson and Acheson 1975). In England and Wales, however, the mortality from CVD (cerebral haemorrhage and thrombosis but not subarachnoid haemorrhage) has fallen, especially in females, while that from ischaemic heart disease has risen (Haberman, Capildeo, and Rose 1978; *The Lancet* 1978*a*). In neonates, cerebral infarction due to arterial occlusion is not unknown (Barmada, Moossy, and Shuman 1979). Cerebrovascular disease is ubiquitous in all races (Dalal, Shah, Aiyar, and Kikani 1968; Williams, Resch, and Loewenson 1969); evidence suggesting a higher incidence of cerebral haemorrhage in the American negro (Kane and Aronson 1969) is thought by some to be due to an artefact of reporting (Hutchinson and Acheson 1975) but the incidence of CVD overall in that ethnic group is higher than in Nigerians (Williams *et al.* 1969).

Cerebral infarction

Aetiology and pathology

The principal causes of cerebral infarction are atheroma, arterial hypertension, and cerebral embolism (p. 200) but rarer causes include direct trauma to the internal carotid artery in the neck (Hughes and Brownell 1968), as in attempted strangulation (Milligan and Anderson 1980), or to intracranial vessels in subarachnoid haemorrhage (Tomlinson 1959) and head injury (Blau and Richardson 1978), endarteritis due to meningovascular syphilis or other forms of meningitis (pp. 238 and 264), giant-cell arteritis, granulomatous arteritis, and other arteritides (pp. 219–21), collagen-vascular or connective-tissue disease (pp. 219–20), cerebral amyloid angiopathy (Mandybur 1979), fibromuscular hypoplasia of the internal carotid artery (Hartman, Yung, Bank, and Rosenblatt 1971; So, Toole, Dalal, and Moody 1981), spontaneous dissection of cervico-cerebral arteries (Fisher, Ojemann, and Roberson 1978), and ectasia of intracranial arteries (Yu, Moseley, Pullicino, and McDonald 1982). Acute hemiplegia in childhood (Solomon, Hilal, Gold, and Carter 1970) may be due to injury, infection, cardiac disease, or sickle-cell anaemia but most often results from occlusive vascular disease, sometimes due to atheroma or perhaps to inflamed cervical lymph nodes involving the internal carotid artery (Bickerstaff 1964). Disorders of the blood including anaemia, polycythaemia vera (Silverstein, Gilbert, and Wasserman 1962), thrombotic microangiopathy (p. 221), and hypercoagulability or intimal hyperplasia due to oral contraceptive medication (Inman and Vessey 1968; Schoenberg, Whisnant, Taylor, and Kempers 1970; Bickerstaff 1975; Irey, McAllister, and Henry 1978), or pregnancy and the puerperium (Cross, Castro, and Jennett 1968), also play an important role. Cerebral intravascular coagulation in diabetic ketoacidosis (Timperley, Preston, and Ward 1974) and the consequent ischaemia contribute to the morbidity of that condition. Occasionally, thrombosis in the carotid or vertebrobasilar system, even in young patients, occurs without demonstrable pathological cause (Graham and Adams 1972).

Atheroma (often called arteriosclerosis) is a process which affects primarily the arterial intima. Intimal thickening is followed by the deposition of cholesterol and often by calcification and ulceration, leading sometimes to breaching of the internal elastic lamina, ultimately with some encroachment upon the media of the vessel. Atheromatous lesions often occur as plaques, and thrombi may form on ulcerated areas; emboli arising from such plaques are sometimes made up of platelets or of cholesterol particles derived from breakdown of a disintegrating plaque. The aetiology of atheroma is still uncertain but hyperlipidaemia is one factor and it is often widespread in patients with diabetes and myxoedema. Atheroma is sometimes found in young children, and, while its incidence certainly increases with age, some elderly individuals show very little. It principally affects large- and medium-sized arteries.

While many patients with widespread atheroma are also hypertensive, arterial hypertension *per se* is more often associated with hypertrophy of the media of small arteries and arterioles, sometimes with associated intimal thickening (arteriolosclerosis). Miliary aneurysms are often found on such small vessels in the brain and retina in hypertensive subjects but may require special techniques of arterial injection at post-mortem or fluorescent retinal angiography during life for their demonstration. Thus atheroma is primarily a disorder of large vessels, while hypertension is associated with thickening of small arteries and arterioles with narrowing of their lumina, but the two often co-exist.

When nervous tissue is deprived of its blood supply for a few minutes due either to blockage of a vessel caused by thrombosis or embolism or when the flow through a narrowed but still patent artery falls below a critical level, nerve cells, fibres, and glial cells degenerate to give an area of infarction or softening. The area is subsequently invaded by activated microglial cells ('gitter' cells) and eventually a cystic cavity or glial scar remains. Infarcts may be small (a few millimetres in diameter) or large, and can be single or multiple, cortical or subcortical. Some are pale (anaemic), some haemorrhagic, and some mixed. Adams (1954) showed that many haemorrhagic infarcts are embolic and suggested that as an embolus impacts in a major vessel the initial infarct is pale, but if it then fragments and moves on, blood extravasates freely into the necrotic area. Lacunes are small trabeculated cavities often found in the deeper parts of the brains of hypertensive subjects (Fisher 1969) and, while there is some dispute about their pathogenesis (Hughes 1965), the view most widely accepted is that they result from small infarcts due to the occlusion of small perforating arteries. They may produce a number of specific and clearly-defined clinical syndromes (see below); while they can rarely if ever be demonstrated by angiography, they are often identified by high-resolution computerized tomography (Weisberg 1982).

If one excludes the rarer causes of cerebral infarction mentioned above, atheroma, hypertension, and/or embolism are usually responsible but intracranial arterial dissection is not uncommon (Farrell, Gilbert, and Kaufmann 1985). It is not always possible, even at post-mortem, to demonstrate an occluded vessel in such cases and infarction may occur when various haemodynamic factors combine with the effects of arterial narrowing to cause critical ischaemia of one or more parts of the brain. Factors which may contribute include anaemia, sudden hypotension due to blood loss, cardiac infarction, poorly controlled anaesthesia, syncope, cardiac arrhythmias, and transient narrowing or kinking of a major artery (as of the vertebral artery on turning the neck when there is severe cervical spondylosis) (Bauer, Sheehan, and Meyer 1961). However, the cross-sectional area of a stenosed carotid artery may have to be reduced to 10–15 per cent of normal to reduce blood flow significantly (Brice, Dowsett, and Lowe 1964).

'Moyamoya disease'

Takeuchi (1961) and Kudo (1968) were among the first to describe an unusual angiographic appearance in young Japanese patients in which the blood vessels supplying the cerebral hemispheres resembled the so-called 'rete mirabile' of lower animals; this appearance was entitled 'Moyamoya disease'. Children with this condition have sometimes presented with a choreiform syndrome, but affected adults of many ethnic backgrounds (Coakham, Duchen, and Scaravilli 1979) present more often with variable clinical features of cerebral ischaemia or of cerebral or subdural haemorrhage. In many Japanese reports, a developmental anomaly of the circle of Willis was postulated, but this angiographic appearance may be seen in adult non-Japanese patients following atherosclerotic occlusion of both internal carotid arteries (Poór and Gács 1974) and similar changes may be found in individuals with familial hypoplasia of these vessels (Austin and Stears 1971). The exact nature of the pathological process which accounts for the frequency of this finding in Japanese children, often in more than one family member (Kitahara, Ariga, Yamaura, Makino, and Maki 1979), is uncertain but it seems that this angiographic appearance results from the development of a collateral circulation following occlusion of major arteries of the circle of Willis.

The clinical features of 'strokes'

The term 'stroke' is now used colloquially and medically to identify all forms of cerebrovascular accident (CVA); some such attacks are called 'seizures' by the layman, but seizure in medical terminology is more often used to identify an attack of epilepsy. The classical term apoplexy may still be used for severe strokes (usually due to cerebral haemorrhage) which fell the patient, rendering him unconscious. A stroke or CVA can reasonably be defined (ad hoc Committee 1958) as a focal neurological disorder of abrupt development due to a pathological process in blood vessels.

Although the clinical varieties of stroke are numerous, depending upon the nature of the primary pathological abnormality and the vessel or vessels involved, a few general principles may reasonably be stated here, accepting that there is no certain means of distinguishing clinically between haemorrhage and infarction. In general, the onset of cerebral embolism is abrupt, hemiplegia, say, developing in a few seconds or minutes. Cerebral haemorrhage is often accompanied by headache at the onset, but loss of consciousness is usual with a neurological deficit which increases rapidly over 10–30 minutes; the condition may develop during exertion or in other circumstances which raise the blood pressure. The onset of non-embolic cerebral infarction (cerebral 'thrombosis') may be equally abrupt with headache if there is associated cerebral oedema; more often, however, the condition is noted on waking or soon after rising, or else weakness, say of one arm and leg, develops over about 30 minutes; less often the neurological deficit slowly extends over hours or days (stroke-in-evolution), presumably due to spreading vascular occlusion and an expanding infarct, when the picture may simulate that of an intracranial space-occupying lesion. In other cases the manifestations increase in a step-wise manner (a so-called 'stuttering' stroke). Sometimes an established stroke is preceded by warning symptoms in the form of transient ischaemic attacks (see below) or a series of 'little strokes'. When there is neck stiffness suggesting subarachnoid bleeding, this usually, but not invariably, indicates cerebral haemorrhage (a cerebellar infarct can cause neck stiffness at the onset). However, a massive infarct may cause loss of consciousness at the onset, while consciousness may be retained if a small, localized haemorrhage situated deeply does not reach the ventricles or subarachnoid space.

Before considering the specific clinical features associated with occlusion of the principal cerebral arteries and then describing the clinical effects of embolism and intracranial haemorrhage, it will now be convenient to consider the symptomatology of transient ischaemic attacks.

Transient cerebral ischaemic attacks

Transient cerebral ischaemic attacks are episodes indicating ischaemia of some part of one cerebral hemisphere or of the brainstem. They are defined as episodes of temporary and focal cerebral dysfunction of vascular origin leaving no persistent neurological deficit and lasting less than 24 hours (see Warlow 1982). The episodes may be isolated and infrequent or may occur many times in a day and tend to be consistent in their symptomatology in affected individuals, suggesting that the recurrent ischaemia consistently involves the same area of the brain. The clinical features and natural history of these episodes have been reviewed by Hutchinson and Acheson (1975), Toole, Yuson, Janeway, Johnston, Davis, Cordell, and Howard (1978), Warlow (1982), and others. By definition the attacks do not cause irreversible infarction of the affected brain substance, although in those attacks which last as long as 24 hours it seems possible that minute areas of permanent pathological change may persist. Conventionally, amaurosis fugax (p. 92) due to ischaemia of retina rather than brain is similarly defined, as it is usually due to microembolism in the carotid tree (Harrison and Marshall 1977), when attacks may be precipitated by bright light (Furlan, Whisnant, and Kearns 1979); however, it can, like other TIAs, be a complication of heart disease, such as rheumatic disease (Swash and Earl 1970) or atrial myxoma (DeSousa, Muller, Campbell, Batnitzky, and Rankin 1978).

The importance of atheroma in the carotid and vertebral arteries in the neck and/or in other major branches of the aortic arch in the pathogenesis of such attacks was stressed by Fisher and Cameron (1953) and by Yates and Hutchinson (1961) and has been amply confirmed (Toole, Janeway, Choi, Cordell, Davis, Johnston, and Miller 1975; Goldstein, Bolis, Fieschi, Gorini, and Millikan 1979). Attacks indicating ischaemia in the distribution of one carotid artery are often referred to as episodes of carotid insufficiency, those involving the brainstem as vertebro-basilar insufficiency.

Denny-Brown (1951) suggested that the attacks were often due to episodic hypotension, but Kendell and Marshall (1963) failed to reproduce them in affected individuals by lowering the blood pressure on a tilt table. Nevertheless, haemodynamic factors may play a part, especially in vertebro-basilar insufficiency (Naritomi, Sakai, and Meyer 1979). However, Millikan, Siekert, and Shick (1955), Fisher (1959) and Ross Russell (1961, 1963) showed that the attacks are usually due to recurrent microembolism arising from mural thrombi developing upon atheromatous plaques in major vessels in the neck and observed such emboli in the retinal arteries in some cases. That this is the commonest cause of such episodes which are often due to carotid or vertebral stenosis is now well-recognized and the emboli may consist of platelets (McBrien, Bradley, and Ashton 1963) or cholesterol (David, Klintworth, Friedberg, and Dillon 1963); the consistent symptomatology of the attacks seems to be due to the fact that blood flow in the major vessels is laminar so that emboli derived from the same thrombus or crumbling plaque ultimately reach the same peripheral intracranial branch. Sometimes the attacks may result, alternatively, from 'steal' phenomena (Ross Russell and Green 1971) (p. 196), or from episodes of cardiac arrhythmia (McAllen and Marshall 1973), or even from unruptured intracranial aneurysms (Fisher, Davidson, and Marcus 1980; Stewart, Samson, Diehl, Hinton, and Ditmore 1980). A bruit in the neck may be a useful indication of arterial stenosis but the absence of such a bruit does not exclude a surgically treatable stenosis and four-vessel angiography carried out by aortic-arch catheterization is usually indicated and is relatively safe in such cases (Marshall 1971). Negative arteriography does not necessarily imply a good prognosis (Toole and Yson, 1977). There is also recent evidence (de Bono and Warlow 1981; Warlow 1982) that haemodynamically insignificant cardiac valvular lesions, including mitral-valve leaflet prolapse and also previous cardiac infarction, may be a commoner cause of TIAs than is generally realized. Hence, echocardiography may be necessary when angiography is negative.

The incidence of such episodes has been estimated at between 0.3 and 1.3 per 1 000 individuals in the population per year. Various studies (Baker, Ramseyer, and Schwartz 1968; Whisnant, Matsumoto, and Elveback 1973a; Toole et al. 1975; Hutchinson and Acheson 1975; Whisnant, Cartlidge, and Elveback 1978; Warlow 1982) have estimated the incidence of subsequent stroke in such cases at between 2 and 62 per cent, occurring from 12 to 30 months after the onset; occasionally the episodes first develop after a stroke (Barnett 1978) but this is uncommon. The attacks cease spontaneously in about 50 per cent of cases within 1–3 years; the prognosis is worse in hypertensive patients and in many under 65 than in those who are older, a fact which underlines the importance of investigating younger patients who present in this way. However, under the age of 50 when there is no evidence of vascular disease, the outlook is better (Marshall 1982).

Syndromes of the cerebral arteries

Obstruction of a cerebral artery gives a clinical picture which depends upon loss of function of the parts of the brain supplied by the vessel. This is influenced by the point at which the obstruction occurs, since blockage at the origin of a vessel may impair the function of a larger region than is the case when the block lies more distally or involves only a single branch. However, as already mentioned, occlusion of a small perforating artery may have more profound and permanent effects (as these are end-arteries) than may proximal occlusion of a major trunk as the latter can be compensated for by meningeal arterial anastomoses. Variations in the clinical picture also relate to variability in the distribution of the arteries. Because of the importance of the collateral circulation, obstruction of either the vertebral or the internal carotid artery may intensify symptoms due to obstruction of the other (Hutchinson and Yates 1956).

The internal carotid artery
Angiography (Fig. 4.1) has taught us much about the symptoms of occlusion of the internal carotid artery. There may be no symptoms. At the other extreme, the hemiplegia may be complete almost at its onset—the 'completed stroke'. Progressive obliteration of the lumen by atheroma may cause TIAs, giving aphasia, confusion, or contralateral paraesthesiae or weakness, or ultimately 'stuttering hemiplegia' terminating in a persistent hemiplegia. Internal carotid-artery stenosis (*The Lancet* 1981; Parkin, Kendall, Marshall, and McDonald 1982) is the commonest cause of amaurosis fugax, though this may rarely result from stenosis of the external carotid when this vessel and its branches are fulfilling an anastomotic role after internal carotid-artery occlusion (Burnbaum, Selhorst, Harbison, and Brush 1977). TIAs may continue over a prolonged period without a stroke occurring, even after total occlusion of the artery, when microemboli are presumed to originate from the distal end of the thrombus (Barnett, Peerless, and Kaufmann 1978). Finally, a stroke may develop slowly over hours or a day or two—the 'stroke-in-evolution'. Unilateral frontal headache can occur with any of these. The manifestations of complete occlusion depend upon the adequacy of the collateral circulation through the circle of Willis and external carotid artery, and may include contralateral homonymous hemianopia, hemiplegia, and loss of spatial and discriminative sensibility on the opposite side of the body, and, when the lesion is of the dominant hemisphere, aphasia, either receptive, expressive, or global. The internal carotid pulse may be diminished or lost but in the neck it may be difficult to distinguish from that of the external carotid artery and palpation with a finger in the lateral wall of the pharynx

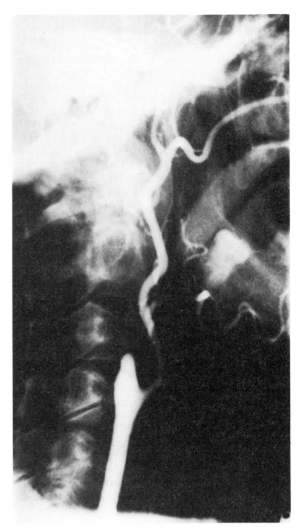

Fig. 4.1. Left carotid arteriogram demonstrating stenosis at the origin of the internal carotid artery. (Reproduced from Walton (1966) by kind permission of the publisher.)

behind the tonsillar fossa is a safer guide. Dissection of the artery in the neck can cause Horner's syndrome and ipsilateral head and neck pain (West, Davies, and Kelly 1976). When the internal carotid artery is occluded, facial and orbital pulses may be accentuated (Fisher 1970a) and there may be a haemodynamic bruit over the contralateral internal carotid (Fisher 1957). A bruit on the side of the lesion is a useful clue to the presence of stenosis at or near the origin of the vessel, a lesion often associated with transient ischaemic attacks (Fig. 4.1) but Ziegler, Zileli, Dick, and Sebaugh (1971) found stenosis in the absence of a bruit in 73 per cent of cases and a bruit without stenosis in 10 per cent. Carotid stenosis or occlusion rarely results from giant-cell arteritis (Cull 1979), while both fibromuscular hyperplasia of the arterial wall (Corrin, Sandok, and Houser 1981) and a kinked carotid artery (*British Medical Journal* 1977a) may cause TIAs and mimic stenosis. Thermography of the supraorbital region indicating increased flow through supraorbital branches of the external carotid artery was found by some workers to be a useful guide to internal carotid-artery occlusion but is now outmoded, as is ophthalmodynamometry (Heyman, Karp, and Bloor 1957; Mawdsley, Samuel, Sumerling, and Young 1968). Carotid arterography is the most reliable diagnostic method in confirming the diagnosis of atheromatous stenosis (Croft, Ellam, and Harrison 1980) but the ultrasonic Doppler method (Blackwell, Merory, Toole, and McKinney 1977; Lakeman, Sherriff, and Martin 1981) is now very reliable in skilled hands and can also be used to assess ophthalmic artery flow after total carotid occlusion (Kaneda, Irino, Watanabe, Kadota, and Taneda 1979); it is possibly the best non-invasive technique (Ackerman 1979). Occlusion of the ophthalmic branch of the internal carotid, if it extends into the central retinal artery, may give unilateral blindness; however, total occlusion is more often related to hypertension and total carotid occlusion, branch occlusion in the retina to TIAs and stenosis (Wilson, Warlow, and Russell 1979). A perforating branch of the posterior communicating usually supplies the subthalamic nucleus (body of Luys) and an infarct here, seen usually in the elderly, generally gives contralateral hemiballismus. Thrombosis of the anterior choroidal artery is rare but may give contralateral hemiplegia and hemianalgesia; it is more often asymptomatic (Toole and Patel 1974).

The anterior cerebral artery

This long vessel may be occluded at several different points with varying clinical effects. The following are the most important.

Occlusion at its origin, proximal to Heubner's artery. This causes hemiplegia on the opposite side together with sensory loss of cortical type in the paralysed lower limb. When the lesion is on the dominant side there is also expressive aphasia, and apraxia on the left, non-paralysed side, due to interruption in the corpus callosum of fibres running from the left supramarginal gyrus to the right precentral gyrus. A disorder of language has also been reported as a rare consequence of occlusion of the artery to the non-dominant hemisphere, supplying the supplementary motor area (Brust, Plank, Burke, Guobadia, and Healton 1982).

Occlusion of Heubner's artery. Since this artery supplies part of the frontal lobe, together with the anterior limb of the internal capsule, its occlusion leads to paralysis of the face, tongue, and upper limb on the opposite side, movements at the proximal joints of the limb being more affected than those at the distal. When the lesion is on the left side, there is often expressive aphasia.

Occlusion distal to Heubner's branch. This leads to contralateral hemiplegia, weakness being most marked in the lower limb. In addition, there is often forced grasping and groping in the affected limb.

Occlusion of the paracentral artery. This is the branch of the artery which supplies the paracentral lobule. The result of this lesion is a crural spastic monoplegia on the opposite side, with or without sensory loss of cortical type in the affected lower limb. Angiography may demonstrate obstruction of the main anterior cerebral artery.

Occlusion of both anterior cerebral arteries. This syndrome which may follow operation upon aneurysms of the anterior communicating artery, is characterized by profound dementia and apathy with variable long-tract signs and often incontinence. Bilateral grasp reflexes may be present and in severe cases the clinical picture resembles that of 'akinetic mutism' (Freemon 1971).

The middle cerebral artery

Obstruction of the middle cerebral artery at its origin (Fig. 4.2) causes hemiplegia with sensory loss on the opposite side. Lhermitte, Gautier, Derouesné, and Guiraud (1968) suggested that embolism is the commonest cause but thrombosis is not uncommon. The weakness is most marked in the face, tongue, and upper limb. When the lesion involves the dominant hemisphere, Broca's aphasia and/or Wernicke's aphasia may occur. Eslinger and Damasio (1981) found that Broca's and/or conduction aphasia was commoner in younger subjects, Wernicke's or global aphasia in the older, suggesting that the cortical distribution of the artery may change with age. Obstruction of the frontal branch which supplies the inferior frontal gyrus causes severe Broca's aphasia with little or no weakness, except possibly of the face and tongue on the

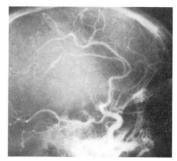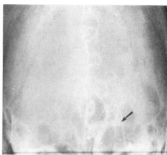

Fig. 4.2. Left carotid arteriogram (lateral view on right, anteroposterior view on left) showing total occlusion of the trunk of the middle cerebral artery close to its origin.

opposite side. Obstruction of the main artery distal to this branch causes hemiplegia of the opposite side, weakness being most marked in the upper limb, but there may be little or no speech abnormality. Obstruction of parietal and temporal branches, when the lesion is on the left, causes marked aphasia of the conduction type, with disturbance of comprehension of heard and written speech, and sometimes Wernicke's aphasia. In addition, there may be a contralateral homonymous visual-field defect (Lascelles and Burrows 1965). Occlusion of the right (non-dominant) middle cerebral can cause acute confusional states (Mesulam, Waxman, Geschwind, and Sabin 1976), while bilateral occlusion may give infarction of both opercula; the posterior opercular syndrome is characterized by pure word deafness, the bilateral anterior syndrome by facio-pharyngo-glosso-masticatory diplegia (the Foux–Chavany–Marie syndrome) (Mariani, Spinnler, Sterzi, and Vallar 1980). Occlusion of small perforating branches has been thought by Fisher (1979) to cause small infarcts in the internal capsule giving rise to lacunes which may be associated either with a 'pure sensory stroke' (contralateral hemianaesthesia) or a 'pure motor hemiplegia' (without sensory loss), though the latter syndrome can also result from pontine infarction (Fisher, Mohr, and Adams 1974). Stenosis of the middle cerebral can cause TIAs (Hinton, Mohr, Ackerman, Adair, and Fisher 1979).

The posterior cerebral artery

This artery supplies the visual cortex of the occipital lobe. Its occlusion, therefore, causes contralateral homonymous hemianopia, sometimes with 'macular sparing' (p. 88). Ischaemia of the left occipital lobe may cause visual agnosia. If the obstruction is proximal to the supply to the thalamus, the thalamic syndrome may develop. The thalamo-perforating stalk arises from the junction of the basilar and the proximal part of the posterior cerebral artery. Bilateral occlusion of this vessel can cause vertical oculomotor apraxia and memory loss (Mills and Swanson 1978), while unilateral occlusion in the dominant hemisphere can cause transcortical aphasia (McFarling, Rothi, and Heilman 1982). The 'top of the basilar syndrome' (Caplan 1980), which usually occurs when an embolus impacts at the termination of the basilar artery where both posterior cerebral arteries originate, can give bilateral cortical blindness (see below) but, in incomplete occlusion, rostral brainstem infarction can give disorders of vertical gaze and of convergence, atypical skew deviation of the eyes, small, poorly reacting pupils, and various ocular and behavioural features (including amnesia) due to bilateral temporal-lobe infarction.

The basilar and vertebral arteries

Complete occlusion of the main trunk of the basilar artery is usually rapidly fatal. It leads to impairment of consciousness, small fixed pupils, pseudobulbar palsy, and quadriplegia, but sensation may escape (Kubik and Adams 1946; Biemond 1951). Incomplete obstruction in the vertebro-basilar system, however, is much commoner and may lead to many transitory or permanent disorders of brainstem function, including deafness, vertigo, drop-attacks, ophthalmoplegia, ataxia, nystagmus, and bilateral dysaesthesiae over the body and bilateral corticospinal-tract signs (vertebro-basilar insufficiency). Symonds and Mackenzie (1957) suggest that bilateral loss of vision from cerebral infarction is due to embolism or thrombosis in the basilar at or close to its bifurcation. Thrombi in this region may also cause occlusion of the posterior thalamo-subthalamic paramedian artery, giving bilateral infarction of periventricular grey matter around the posterior part of the third ventricle and of the upper midbrain and part of the thalamus; clinically akinetic mutism is the usual consequence (Segarra 1970) ('*the syndrome of the mesencephalic artery*'). This clinical state (see p. 645) must be distinguished from the so-called '*locked-in syndrome*' (Kemper and Romanul 1967) which results from massive pontine infarction, again often due to basilar-artery occlusion; in this condition, the patient, though tetraparetic and mute, is alert and able to signal by means of voluntary eye movement. Small lacunar infarcts in the pons due to occlusion of single perforating branches of the basilar (Fisher and Caplan 1971) have been noted to cause either '*a pure motor hemiplegia*' or the so-called '*dysarthria–clumsy hand syndrome*' (Fisher 1967).

Many eponymous syndromes of brainstem infarction due to occlusion of branches (especially perforating branches) of the vertebral and basilar arteries have been described and were reviewed by Minderhoud (1971). Most are now included in the syndrome of vertebro-basilar insufficiency (Williams and Wilson 1962). Some, however, occur with sufficient frequency to deserve separate identification. These are Weber's syndrome, Claude's syndrome, Benedikt's syndrome, the Millard–Gubler syndrome, Foville's syndrome, and, most consistent of all, the lateral medullary syndrome of Wallenberg (see below).

Weber's syndrome (a unilateral third-nerve palsy and contralateral hemiplegia) and *Claude's syndrome* (a unilateral third-nerve palsy with ipsilateral tremor and contralateral hemiplegia) usually result from infarction of one cerebral peduncle and (in Claude's syndrome) one red nucleus, supplied by a branch of the posterior cerebral artery. *Benedikt's syndrome*, due to a midbrain lesion involving the third-nerve nucleus and red nucleus, consists of a third-nerve palsy on one side with contralateral tremor and hyperaesthesia. The *Millard–Gubler syndrome* (unilateral sixth- and seventh-nerve palsy and contralateral hemiparesis) and the *Foville syndrome* (unilateral facial palsy with paralysis of conjugate gaze to the affected side and a contralateral hemiplegia) result from pontine infarction due to occlusion of perforating branches of the basilar. *Occlusion of the internal auditory artery* is another uncommon but identifiable syndrome giving acute severe vertigo, with unilateral deafness and tinnitus (Millikan, Siekert, and Whisnant 1959). Much less common are the syndromes of *Avellis* (ninth- and tenth-nerve palsy with contralateral hemiparesis and hemianaesthesia), *Babinski-Nageotte* (ataxia, Horner's syndrome, and contralateral hemiparesis), *Schmidt* (ninth-, tenth-, and eleventh-nerve palsies with contralateral hemiparesis), and *Hughlings Jackson* (eleventh- and twelfth-nerve palsies and contralateral hemiplegia). Minderhoud (1971) found that most patients with brainstem infarction did not present with any of these so-called classical syndromes.

Occlusion of the *superior cerebellar artery* causes ipsilateral ataxia sometimes with choreiform movements, and occasionally contralateral hemianalgesia. Massive cerebellar infarction may cause oedema sufficient to give brainstem compression and a clinical picture simulating a posterior-fossa tumour (Lehrich, Winkler, and Ojemann 1970). The CT scan can be helpful in demonstrating a small localized infarct and in such cases the outlook is usually good, the only residua within four weeks being ipsilateral-limb ataxia (Scotti, Spinnler, Sterzi, and Vallar 1980), but, when there is progressive impairment of consciousness with signs of brainstem compression and the scan shows a large expanding lesion, surgical removal of infarcted cerebellum may be required (Woodhurst 1980).

Within recent years it has been noted that occlusion of the first part of one subclavian artery can produce a syndrome in which exercise of the affected arm induces retrograde flow of blood down the ipsilateral vertebral artery in order to supply the arm, thus effectively 'stealing' blood from the brainstem. In this '*subclavian steal syndrome*' (Mannock, Suter, and Hume 1961; North, Fields, de Bakey, and Crawford 1962; Patel and Toole 1965), there is often a bruit over the affected subclavian artery and the pulse and blood pressure in the affected arm are reduced when compared with the normal side. Symptoms of vertebro-basilar insufficiency (vertigo, transient bilateral blindness, syncope, and even olfactory hallucinations (Cameron and Wright 1964)) may occur spontaneously or on exercising the affected arm. Similar symptoms may occur when one vertebral artery is occluded in the neck (Fisher 1970*b*).

The *lateral medullary syndrome of Wallenberg* has usually been attributed to occlusion of one posterior inferior cerebellar artery. It is probably more often due to thrombosis of one vertebral artery. Left-sided vertebral occlusion is usually atheromatous; right-sided occlusion in women is often associated with oral contraceptives (Ask-Upmark and Bickerstaff 1976). In either case there is a typical clinical picture resulting from infarction of a wedge-shaped area of the lateral aspect of the medulla and the inferior surface of the cerebellum. The onset is associated with severe vertigo, and hiccup and vomiting may occur. There is often dysphagia and sometimes pain or paraesthesiae, like a feeling of hot water running over the face, may be referred to the trigeminal area on the affected side. There is some ipsilateral cerebellar ataxiat, with nysagmus, hypotonia, and incoordination. Ipsilateral paralysis of the soft palate, pharynx, and vocal cord is due to involvement of the nucleus ambiguus. Horner's syndrome—myosis, enophthalmos, and ptosis—is present on the affected side. Usually analgesia and thermo-anaesthesia are present on the face on the same side as the lesion and on the contralateral trunk and limbs. This is due, respectively, to involvement of the spinal tract and nucleus of the trigeminal nerve and of the spinothalamic tract. The sensory loss on the face may be confined to the first, or to the first and second, divisions of the nerve, as these regions are represented in the lower part of the spinal nucleus, which may alone be supplied by the posterior inferior cerebellar artery. Persistent neuralgic pain in the face on the side of the lesion, and sometimes in the contralateral limbs and trunk, as well as dysphagia are common and troublesome sequelae.

Lacunar infarction

When small arteries or arterioles already thickened as a result of hypertension are occluded by thrombus or by emboli from larger atherosclerotic vessels, this may cause areas of microinfarction which ultimately lead to small slit-like cavities known as lacunes (see p. 192 and Toole and Patel 1974). Some affected vessels show lipohyalinosis (Fisher 1979). In severe hypertension, multiple lacunes (a lacunar state) may be found in putamen, pons, thalamus, caudate, internal capsule, and cerebral or cerebellar white matter and may be responsible for the clinical syndrome often attributed to diffuse cerebral atherosclerosis, and especially pseudobulbar palsy (see below).

However, we owe to Fisher (1965, 1967, 1978) the identification of four specific clinical syndromes each of which may be associated with a single lacunar infarct. These are:

1. Hemiparesis with ataxia in the same limbs, involving the leg more than the arm, due to a lacune in the contralateral internal capsule.

2. Pure motor hemiplegia, when the lacune can be either in the opposite side of the pons or internal capsule. This can rarely result, however, from a discrete cortical lesion (Chokroverty,

Rubino, and Haller 1977) or from one in the medullary pyramid (Ropper, Fisher, and Kleinman 1979), when the face is spared.

3. The 'dysarthria–clumsy hand syndrome' due to a pontine lacune, giving the acute onset of dysarthria, slight dysphagia, central facial weakness, deviation of the tongue to the affected side, and clumsiness and ataxia in the hand on the side of the lesion.

4. A pure sensory stroke with unilateral sensory loss for all modalities of sensation due to a lacune in the contralateral posterolateral thalamic nucleus. Rarely a similar clinical syndrome can result from a slit haemorrhage in the posterior limb of the internal capsule close to the thalamus (Groothuis, Duncan, and Fisher 1977).

In fact, Fisher (1982) has recently pointed out that some 21 clinical syndromes in all have been attributed to lacunar strokes, but of these the four listed above were by far the commonest.

Diffuse cerebral atherosclerosis

Many cases of progressive dementia previously attributed to cerebral atherosclerosis were undoubtedly due to other forms of diffuse degenerative brain disease such as presenile dementia. Nevertheless, repeated episodes of cerebral infarction with multiple areas of softening, sometimes unilateral but more often bilateral, can undoubtedly cause progressive impairment of memory and intellectual function, often accompanied by epileptic attacks, variable signs of focal brain damage, and ultimately an irreversible dementia with incontinence (multi-infarct dementia) (Tomlinson, Blessed, and Roth 1968; Harrison, Thomas, du Boulay, and Marshall 1979; Ladurner, Iliff, and Lechner 1982). When this syndrome results primarily from atheroma (large-vessel disease), deterioration often occurs in a step-like manner, in that each stroke leaves more evidence of mental and physical deterioration. Depending upon the parts of brain involved, dysarthria, aphasia, apraxia, hemiparesis, and other focal symptoms and signs may occur. Bilateral frontal-lobe infarction may cause severe apraxia of gait, bilateral grasp reflexes, dementia, and incontinence. In such cases, deterioration often follows general anaesthesia.

The syndrome of pseudobulbar palsy (spastic dysarthria, brisk jaw and snout reflexes, and pathological emotional lability with inappropriate laughter and crying) can be a late consequence of multiple bilateral infarcts as described above, but is more often seen in a slowly progressive syndrome, often without clinical evidence of actual minor strokes, which results from multiple small areas of softening (a lacunar state as defined above) occurring deep within the hemispheres and resulting from small-vessel disease associated with severe hypertension. This syndrome has sometimes been called 'atherosclerotic parkinsonism' as the patients show a slow, shuffling gait (marche à petits pas), usually with bilateral spasticity and rigidity of the limbs and extensor plantar responses; some degree of dementia is usual but facial masking and other stigmata of parkinsonism are absent.

Accessory investigations

The CSF is usually normal except after an acute infarct, when the protein may be raised up to 1.0–2.0 g/l for two or three weeks, and the fluid may be xanthochromic at first. There may also be a pleocytosis including a moderate excess of polymorphonuclear cells. Polymorphs are found more often in cases of intracranial haemorrhage and in haemorrhagic infarction than in patients with ischaemic infarcts (Sörnäs, Östland, and Müller 1972). The ECG is often abnormal but the abnormality is more often due to concomitant myocardial damage and hypertension than to any central effect caused by the cerebral infarct (Tomkin, Coe, and Marshall 1968). The serum uric acid and serum triglycerides are often raised in patients with strokes (Pearce and Aziz 1969, 1970). Moderate increases in serum and CSF creatine kinase, aldolase, and lactic dehydrogenase occur but are less striking than those found in patients with intracranial haemorrhage (Wolintz, Jacobs, Chris-

toff, Solomon, and Chernik 1969). Norepinephrine and other catecholamines are also raised in the serum and CSF of patients with strokes, but again the rise is substantially greater in haemorrhage than infarction (Meyer, Stoica, Pascu, Shimazu, and Hartmann 1973). EEG changes are too variable and imprecise to be of diagnostic value.

Gamma-encephalography is of limited help, in that a focal abnormality due to an infarct usually improves with time, while that due to a tumour usually becomes worse. The CT scan has proved very successful in localizing and identifying sizeable infarcts (Kinkel and Jacobs 1976), especially after contrast enhancement (Masdeu, Azar-Kia, and Rubino 1977; Tubman, Ethier, Melançon, Bèlanger, and Taylor 1981); sometimes it will even identify a lacunar infarct (Rosenberg and Koller 1981). However, it is not usually helpful in patients with transient ischaemic attacks (British Medical Journal 1978a). The value of Doppler ultrasound in identifying arterial stenosis in the neck has already been discussed (p. 194). This and other non-invasive techniques have been reviewed by Kappert (1982). By far the greatest information, however, is likely to be derived from cerebral angiography which often reveals evidence of arterial occlusion or stenosis not previously diagnosed accurately on clinical grounds (Bull, Marshall, and Shaw 1960; Acheson, Boyd, Hugh, and Hutchinson 1969; Weibel and Fields 1969; Caplan and Rosenbaum 1975; Thiele, Young, Chikos, Hirsch, and Strandness 1980). Aortic-arch catheterization is necessary to demonstrate the major vessels in the neck, but direct injection of the common carotid arteries is still the best method of revealing the detail of the intracranial vessels, especially if magnification and subtraction techniques are used. While the risks are low in skilled hands, the examination should never be undertaken lightly, and much depends upon the age and condition of the patient and the information which is sought. The risks of precipitating further infarction are greater in older patients, possibly in hypertensive and diabetic subjects, but above all in those with diffuse arterial disease and multiple stenoses, the very group in whom the investigation is most informative (Faught, Trader, and Hanna 1979). Digital subtraction angiography using intravenous contrast is a major advance (Schneidau 1984). Angiography is indicated in young patients with strokes but should be employed more sparingly in the elderly. Its purpose is first to exclude a tumour, aneurysm, or angioma whose effects may be mimicking those of an infarct, secondly to exclude an intracranial haematoma, thirdly to demonstrate an arterial stenosis or occlusion which may be amenable to surgical or other treatment, and fourthly to give evidence relating to the collateral circulation if a vessel is occluded.

Diagnosis

Cerebral atheroma usually presents in one of four ways: (1) as a focal lesion of sudden onset; (2) as a focal lesion of insidious onset; (3) with remittent and recurrent symptoms; and (4) with diffuse and progressive symptoms.

1. A focal lesion of sudden onset, leading, for example, to hemiplegia, may be due to atheromatous occlusion of a large artery. This may be simulated by cerebral haemorrhage due to hypertension, or from a ruptured aneurysm or angioma invading the brain substance. Coma is more likely, and, if present, to be deeper in cerebral haemorrhage than in infarction, unless the internal carotid artery is occluded. Severe hypertension favours haemorrhage. The CSF can be helpful as it is likely to contain some red cells, as well as a raised protein, immediately after a cerebral haemorrhage, and, if the haemorrhage has reached the subarachnoid space, the blood will be visible to the naked eye. Clinical evidence of a cardiac lesion may suggest that the infarct is embolic. When there is doubt as to whether a focal lesion is ischaemic or haemorrhagic the question may be settled by a CT scan and/or angiography, but, even with these aids, misdiagnosis is still common (Norris and Hachinski 1982).

An intracranial tumour rarely causes sudden focal symptoms; when it does this is generally due to oedema and papilloedema is often present. Transient hemiplegia of sudden onset may occur in migraine, when diagnosis rests upon its association with other symptoms of migraine and rapid recovery without residua. General paresis is a rare cause of sudden hemiplegia. Very rarely a single lesion will develop sufficiently suddenly in multiple sclerosis to suggest a vascular lesion. Dissecting aneurysm of the aorta rarely causes sudden cerebral ischaemia. Infarction may be diffuse and is accompanied by chest pain, and, usually, hypotension.

The diagnosis of arterial occlusion or stenosis due to atheroma as the cause of infarction rests upon the age of the patient, the presence of atheroma elsewhere, particularly in retinal arteries, a bruit, if present, the absence of other forms of vascular disease, and in some cases upon the presence of another predisposing disorder, e.g. diabetes or myxoedema. Syphilitic endarteritis is associated with characteristic changes in the CSF and blood. Tuberculous endarteritis is a sequal of tuberculous meningitis. The rarer causes of arterial disease, such as polyarteritis nodosa and giant-cell (temporal) arteritis can be diagnosed only through their systemic manifestations.

2. *Focal lesions of insidious onset.* Ischaemic brain disease, especially atheroma of one internal carotid artery, may cause a progressive focal lesion of gradual onset which it may be difficult to distinguish from a neoplasm. Conversely, a glioma in an elderly atheromatous subject sometimes progresses so rapidly, and with so little evidence of increased intracranial pressure, that it closely simulates an infarct. A third condition which may deserve consideration is a chronic subdural haematoma. In such cases diagnosis may require a CT scan or angiogram.

3. *Lesions producing remittent and recurrent symptoms.* Cerebral atheroma may lead to recurrent episodes of disordered brain function within the territory of a single artery (transient ischaemic attacks), or successive lesions involving different parts of the brain. These syndromes are unlikely to be confused with any other condition, but occasionally sensory Jacksonian epilepsy due to a glioma simulates the former, while multiple metastases may produce symptoms resembling those of multiple infarcts. Recurrent epileptic attacks may be the sole manifestation of previous asymptomatic infarction, and other causes of epilepsy of late onset must then be excluded. The rare 'pulseless disease' (Takayasu's disease) (p. 221) may also cause intermittent cerebral ischaemia.

4. *Lesions producing diffuse and progressive symtoms.* Failing intellectual powers and impairment of memory, characteristic of diffuse atheromatosis of smaller cerebral vessels (multi-infarct dementia), may simulate dementia due to any other cause (see p. 657). General paresis is distinguished by appropriate serological and other tests. In the absence of symptoms of increased intracranial pressure, it may be difficult to exclude an intracranial tumour as the cause of dementia of insidious onset. The CT scan is then helpful as may be isotope encephalography and pneumoencephalography in establishing the diagnosis of presenile dementia. 'Atherosclerotic parkinsonism' must be distinguished from paralysis agitans (see p. 329) and other rare degenerative cerebral diseases of the second half of life may also simulate cerebral atherosclerosis.

Prognosis

The prognosis of cerebral ischaemia due to atheroma depends upon several factors, chief among which are the age of the patient, the adequacy of the collateral circulation, the extent and degree of the arterial disease, the condition of the circulation as a whole, and the presence or absence of associated disorders, such as diabetes, renal disease, etc.

It may be difficult to assess the prognosis of a focal ischaemic lesion during the first two or three days after the onset. When it lies within the territory of the internal carotid artery, the greater the extent of the area of cerebral damage the worse the outlook. Unconsciousness, and the association of sensory loss and hemiplegia are bad prognostic signs. A small focal lesion in any part of the brain, however, is usually less serious than a large infarct. An elderly patient may live for years after a small focal lesion, even causing hemiplegia, with no recurrence. Adams and Merrett (1961) studied a series of 736 hemiplegics. Their figures showed that expectation of life after a stroke is greatly shortened, being less than half the normal for people of the same age. They divided their patients into those who recovered in that they became fully independent or were able to walk, though handicapped by a useless arm, and those who failed to improve appreciably after three months of intensive treatment. In the latter group a patient's chance of being able to get about and look after himself was shown to be little better than that of becoming a relatively helpless invalid. Age, however, did not in itself preclude good recovery nor did a lesion of the dominant hemisphere. Adams and Hurwitz (1963) analysed the associated defects of cerebral function held to be responsible for a failure to respond to treatment. These included defects of comprehension and various forms of apraxia and agnosia.

In a detailed survey based upon their personal experience and a thorough review of the literature, Hutchinson and Acheson (1975) found an immediate mortality of 30 per cent in cases of stroke in the first month. Long-term mortality at five years was 35–45 per cent; between 25 and 50 per cent of patients suffered recurrent strokes. Mortality and long-term prognosis were adversely influenced by hypertension; this was the single most important adverse factor to emerge from a careful analysis, although an abnormal ECG was also significantly associated with a tendency to have a second or subsequent stroke. However, they found only minimal evidence that the artery involved influenced prognosis; those with episodes involving the vertebro-basilar system did marginally better than those in whom the first stroke occurred in the internal-carotid territory. More recent analyses of various risk factors (Goldstein *et al.* 1979) and of their influence upon prognosis (Barnett 1980) have reached similar conclusions. Furlan, Whisnant, and Baker (1980) found a five-year survival rate of 77 per cent (compared with 85 per cent in a matched normal population) and a stroke recurrence rate of 3 per cent per year over the age of 35 years in patients with proven carotid artery occlusion who had little or no neurological deficit.

The clinical picture of diffuse cerebral ischaemia is insidiously progressive with or without exacerbations over several years. In the terminal stage the patient is bedridden, with variable dementia, with or without hemiplegia, pseudobulbar palsy, 'arteriosclerotic parkinsonism', or similar physical concomitants. Death occurs either in coma from further infarction, from intercurrent disease, or from cardiac infarction (Baker *et al.* 1968).

Treatment

When a patient is comatose or semicomatose as the result of an ischaemic stroke, the usual measures necessary in managing the unconscious patient are required (p. 650). It has been suggested that in severe strokes in which the infarct has caused oedema of the affected hemisphere, treatment with steroids (dexamethasone 5 mg four times daily), as employed in cerebral oedema due to any cause (p. 137), may reduce mortality and improve the prognosis (Patten, Mendell, Bruun, Curtin, and Carter 1972). Others (Meyer, Charney, Rivera, and Mathew 1971) suggested, again in severe cases, that intravenous (1.2 g per kg body weight) or oral (1.5g per kg) glycerol might have a similar effect. However, carefully controlled blind trials using glycerol (Larsson, Marinovich, and Barber 1976) and high-dose steroids, either alone or in combination with low-molecular-weight dextran (Matthews, Oxbury, Grainger, and Greenhall 1976; Kaste, Fogelholm, and Waltimo 1976; *British Medical Journal* 1977*b*) have failed to show significant benefit. And while barbiturates may lessen the immediate effects of hypoxia or ischaemia upon the brain (*The Lancet* 1980), there is no evidence that these drugs are likely to be helpful in stroke. Many antispasmodic, vasodilator, and other vasoactive drugs have been used extensively in the past, not only in acute stroke but also in patients with diffuse cerebral arterial disease. While some such remedies may increase regional cerebral blood flow (McHenry, Jaffe, West, Cooper, Kenton, Kawamura, Oshiro, and Goldberg 1972), there is no sound evidence that they are of any clinical value (Barnett 1980).

The role of anticoagulant therapy in cerebral ischaemic disorders has been a source of controversy for many years (Marshall and Shaw 1959; Hill, Marshall, and Shaw 1960; Carter 1964; Whisnant, Matsumoto, and Elveback 1973*b*; Toole and Patel 1974; Marshall 1976; Brust 1977; Barnett 1980). It is now generally agreed that these drugs are of no value in the treatment of a completed stroke, and although some workers still use them in cases of 'stroke-in-evolution', in an attempt to restrict extension of the thrombus and of the infarct, in such cases, too, their use has been largely abandoned. The principal risk, even after full investigation, is still that of mistaking a small haemorrhage or haemorrhagic infarct for an ischaemic infarct as it is only in the latter type of lesion that these drugs would be likely to be successful. However, there is still fair agreement that anticoagulant therapy, given for at least six months and more often for two years or more, is effective in many cases of TIA, both in abolishing the attacks and in preventing a completed stroke (Millikan 1971; Whisnant *et al.* 1973*b*; Toole and Patel 1974). Hence this treatment is still sometimes given to patients with TIAs in whom an arterial stenosis inaccessible to surgery has been demonstrated or in whom no evident cause has been found; in such cases the treatment is only likely to be successful if microemboli of platelets and not cholesterol are causing the attacks. Heparin is not appropriate for long-term treatment; the drugs most often used are phenindione or warfarin, and the dose must be regulated in order to reduce the prothrombin to about 10 per cent of normal.

It has become evident that platelet aggregation is increased especially in younger patients with stroke (Couch and Hassanein 1976; Dougherty, Levy, and Weksler 1977), and, in consequence, aspirin, dipyridamole, sulphinpyrazone, pentoxifylline, and other drugs which reduce such aggregation have been tried both in the treatment of TIAs and in an effort to prevent ischaemic stroke (Fields, Lemak, Frankowski, and Hardy 1977, 1978; Canadian Cooperative Study Group 1978; *British Medical Journal* 1978*b*; *The Lancet* 1978*b*; Hallam, Goldman, and Fryers 1981; Herskovits, Vazquez, Famulari, Smud, Tamaroff, Fraiman, Gonzalez, Vila, and Matera 1981). Aspirin, 600 mg daily, is certainly effective in amaurosis fugax (Harrison, Marshall, Meadows, and Russell 1971). While much of the evidence is conflicting, there seems little doubt that aspirin, 1300 mg daily is at least as effective and probably more so than the other antiplatelet drugs, certainly in men, less certainly in women, in controlling TIAs and in preventing subsequent stroke.

When there is hypercholesterolaemia, clofibrate is likely to be of theoretical benefit but does not give clinical improvement; similarly, hypotensive drugs do not seem to help in the immediate management of the acute stroke, although the potential risk of increasing ischaemia by sudden blood pressure reduction has probably been overestimated, and, if the pressure is reduced gradually, the CVR is reduced and the CBF rises (Meyer, Sawada, Kitamura, and Toyda 1968). Clearly, however, the effective control of hypertension substantially improves the prognosis in stroke survivors (Carter 1970; Beevers, Fairman, Hamilton, and Harpur 1973; Hutchinson and Acheson 1975).

Within recent years, operations upon the large arteries in the neck have been carried out increasingly, sometimes in an effort to reduce the effects of a completed stroke, but much more often in order to relieve TIAs. Without doubt surgical disobliteration of the occluded segment of the affected subclavian artery will abolish the symptoms of the 'subclavian steal' syndrome, and carotid endarterectomy, first performed by Rob and Eastcott (Eastcott, Pickering, and Rob 1954) in a case of recurring amaurosis fugax and contralateral hemiparesis, has been widely used in treating stenosis of the internal carotid artery, especially where there is a circumscribed atheromatous plaque close to the bifurcation (Edwards, Gordon, and Rob 1960; Edwards and Gordon 1962; Dickinson, Hankinson, and Marshall 1964; Morris 1968; Sundt, Sandok, and Whisnant 1975). However, few controlled series have been reported, and those which have, have not shown the results of surgical treatment to be immeasurably superior to those achieved by other methods (Fields, Maslenikov, Meyer, Hass, Remington, and MacDonald 1970; *The Lancet* 1974). A recently reported randomized trial of carotid endarterectomy showed that the operation significantly reduced the frequency of TIAs in the relevant vascular territory (Shaw, Venables, Cartlidge, Bates, and Dickinson 1984). However, that same study and many others (Barnett, Plum, and Walton 1984) have demonstrated that in many centres the post-operative morbidity and mortality is unacceptably high, sufficiently so to cast doubt upon whether the operation, the third most frequently performed in the United States in 1983 (Plum *et al.* 1984) is justified except in a few highly specialized centres dealing with large numbers of cases where the morbidity and mortality has been shown to be acceptable. However, in skilled hands, the mortality and morbidity of endarterectomy is small and the removal of accessible stenotic lesions in patients with frequent TIAs is probably sensible though each case must be considered individually in the light of the patient's age, general condition, and clinical presentation. Another exciting development has been the introduction of the technique of extracranial-intracranial (ECIC) anastomosis in which one superficial temporal artery is anastomosed through a trephine hole in the skull to the trunk of the middle cerebral. This operation is particularly valuable in patients with intracranial stenosis or proximal occlusion of the internal carotid or middle cerebral arteries and may be strikingly beneficial (Murray 1978; Samson, White, and Clark 1977; Lee, Ausman, Geiger, Latchaw, Klassen, Chou, and Resch 1979). An international randomized controlled study of its effects is in progress (Barnett 1980).

Finally, the invaluable role of physiotherapy, occupational therapy, and other methods of rehabilitation must be stressed (Hurwitz and Adams 1972). Exercise, re-education, the provision, where appropriate, of walking aids, toe-raising springs or calipers, and other appliances, adaptation to the home and domestic environment, speech therapy in the aphasic, anticonvulsant drugs in the management of post-hemiplegic epilepsy, antibiotics for the management of complications, attention to diet and vitamin intake in the confused elderly subject, and instruction of relatives and home-helps; all these and many more are invaluable. Treatment in a specialized unit and well-organized out-patient physiotherapy and occupational therapy after discharge from hospital improves the outcome (Garraway, Akhtar, Hockey, and Prescott 1980*a, b*; Smith, Goldenberg, Ashburn, Kinsella, Sheikh, Brennan, Meade, Zutshi, Perry, and Reeback 1981). Special attention should be paid to shoulder pain and immobility in the hemiplegic patient (Brocklehurst, Andrews, Richards, and Laycock 1978). The risk of deep venous thrombosis in the legs and of consequent pulmonary embolism (Warlow, Ogston, and Douglas 1976) should also be recognized. The treatment of aphasia and apraxia or agnosia (*British Medical Journal* 1978*c*) may require special skills, but even in these cases, as in those who are paralysed, untrained volunteer helpers can play a valuable role (Meikle, Wechsler, Tupper, Benenson, Butler, Mulhall, and Stern 1979). With appropriate and intensive treatment, many patients with strokes, of whatever age, can resume a useful life in society despite residual disability. Many problems may require to be resolved relating to employment, driving of motor vehicles, hostel or hospital residential care, and the like, but can only be determined in the light of the patient's progress and the doctor's experience of similar cases.

Cerebral embolism

Aetiology and pathology

Embolism of an intracranial artery is a complication of many disorders which allow thrombi, or, less frequently, other material, such as cholesterol derived from an atheromatous plaque, air, or fat, to enter the circulation in such a way that it can reach the brain. The nearest sources of thrombus are the internal carotid, vertebral, and common carotid arteries. In rare cases of thrombosis of the right subclavian artery due to pressure by a cervical rib, the thrombus extends into the right common carotid and a detached portion is carried to the brain (Symonds 1927). A clot may come also from an aneurysm of the innominate artery or of the aorta or from mural thrombosis on an atheromatous ulcer in this vessel; cholesterol emboli may be dislodged during cardiac surgery (Price and Harris 1970). A vegetation may become detached from the aortic or mitral valves in bacterial endocarditis. The left ventricle may be the source of an embolus, following coronary thrombosis, when a clot forms on the endocardium over the infarcted area or when aneurysm of the ventricle results (McAllen and Marshall 1977); the risk of stroke is greater with larger myocardial infarcts (Thompson and Robinson 1978). In auricular fibrillation, whether due to mitral stenosis or to some other cause, a clot may form in the atrium and may become wholly or partially detached spontaneously (Wolf, Dawber, Thomas, and Kannel 1978) or following the restoration of the normal cardiac rhythm by drugs or other means. This may also occur in auricular flutter or after mitral valvulotomy and microemboli often form during cardiopulmonary bypass (Brennan, Patterson, and Kessler 1971). Even in cases of rheumatic heart disease without endocarditis, transient visual obscurations presumed to be due to microembolism, perhaps from small thrombi on a roughened valve, have been described (Swash and Earl 1970) and embolism may also result from 'mute' juvenile endocarditis (Reske-Nielsen, Svendsen, and Søgaard 1965). An important but rare cause of cerebral embolism, usually occurring in young women, is atrial myxoma (Maroon and Campbell 1969; Price, Harris, New, and Cantu 1970; Schwarz, Schwartzman, and Joyner 1972; Yufe, Karpati, and Carpenter 1976; Roeltgen, Weimer, and Patterson 1981); in such cases a cardiac murmur which varies with time and with changing body position, is a useful sign. It is important to be aware of this possibility as many myxomas can be removed surgically. Episodes of cerebral embolism of undetermined origin have also been described in young women taking oral contraceptives (Enzell and Lindemalm 1973). The importance of prolapse of one or more leaflets of the mitral valve with associated vegetations as a cause of strokes and, less often, of TIAs in young people, has been recognized increasingly (Barnett, Jones, Boughner, and Kostuk 1976; Wilson, Keeling, Malcolm, Russell, and Webb-Peploe 1977; Kostuk, Boughner, Barnett, and Silver 1977); this condition and other intracardiac sources of emboli may be recognized by means of two-dimensional echocardiography (Donaldson, Emanuel, and Earl 1981).

The source of the thrombus is rarely in the lung, when thrombosis of a pulmonary vein occurs. Infected emboli from the lungs cause cerebral abscess complicating pulmonary infection, and tumour cells may pass in the same way from lung to brain. The lung capillaries constitute a filter which protects the arterial circulation from emboli of any size derived from the systemic veins. Fat globules, however, may pass through the pulmonary circulation and so reach the brain after fracture of one of the long bones (Larson 1968; Boutros and Henry 1982). An atrial septal defect short-circuits the pulmonary capillary filter and provides a route by which emboli from the systemic veins can in very exceptional circumstances reach the brain—*paradoxical embolism*.

The arteries of the left side of the brain are embolized more often than those of the right, and the left middle cerebral is the vessel most often affected. The point at which the embolus lodges depends upon its size. A large clot may be arrested in the internal carotid. A small one may pass to a cortical branch of one of the main arteries. Following impaction of an embolus, a thrombus usually forms in the vessel and may spread distally or, less frequently, proximally, and the area of brain deprived of blood supply is infarcted. If an embolus impacts and then moves on, arterial blood may then enter the infarcted area; thus embolism is the commonest cause of haemorrhagic infarction (Adams 1954). When the embolus is infected, meningitis or cerebral abscess may subsequently develop, or, when the infection is of low virulence, embolism may be followed by infective softening of the vessel wall and aneurysm formation. Such mycotic aneurysms may rupture into the subarachnoid space or into the brain (see pp. 207–14).

Symptoms

The onset of the symptoms of cerebral embolism is usually very sudden, as lodgement of the embolus occurs more rapidly than either cerebral haemorrhage or thrombosis. However, cases of less sudden onset, resembling that of 'stroke-in-evolution', have been described (Fisher and Pearlman 1967). Loss of consciousness is not very common. A convulsion may occur at the onset, and there is sometimes headache. The nature of the focal symptoms depends upon the vessel in which the embolus is impacted (see p. 194). After the onset there may be a gradual increase in the severity of the symptoms due to the development of oedema or the proximal extension of thrombosis. On the other hand, symptoms may diminish in severity if the embolus becomes dislodged and passes on peripherally.

Fat embolism. Fat embolism causes symptoms after a latent interval lasting from hours to days following the injury. Restlessness, tachycardia, precordial pain, and dyspnoea are the symptoms of fat embolism of the lungs, and, when the fat reaches the brain, insomnia, disorientation, and delirium occur, passing into stupor or coma, with signs of cortical irritation or paralysis. The patient is usually pyrexial, petechial haemorrhages may be present, especially on the chest and neck, and fat may be found in the urine.

Air embolism. Gas bubbles (of nitrogen) may appear in the arterial circulation of the central nervous system in decompression sickness or Caisson disease (p. 442) but, in addition, air can enter the circulation accidentally during cardiac surgery, during venous or arterial catheterization, or in the course of diagnostic procedures involving air insufflation into joints, the mediastinum, or the perirenal space to quote only a few examples. The condition can be fatal but, if the amount of air is relatively small, focal or generalized epileptic attacks, focal neurological signs, or failure to awake from anaesthesia are the commonest presentations (Menkin and Schwartzman 1977). Patients who survive usually show few residua.

Diagnosis

Differential diagnosis is as in thrombotic infarction.

Prognosis

The immediate mortality of cerebral embolism is 7–10 per cent. There is always a risk that embolism of other organs may occur and the prognosis of the condition causing the embolism must also be considered. As shock passes off and the oedema of the infarcted area diminishes, the symptoms decline in severity, and the patient is finally left with such disabilities as result from destruction of the region of the brain supplied by the obstructed artery. Epilepsy is a common sequel.

Treatment

Hypotension, if present, should be treated. Wright and McDevitt (1954) stressed the prophylactic value of anticoagulants for patients with heart disease who are liable to embolism. Treatment of the cerebral lesion is the same as that of cerebral infarction from any cause. Carter (1957) also found anticoagulants of value (see p. 199) but they should not be used when the embolus is due to infective endocarditis. Adams, Merrett, Hutchinson, and Pollock (1974) in a long-term follow-up of cases of mitral stenosis over 20 years showed conclusively that long-term anticoagulant therapy greatly reduces the risks of recurrent cerebral embolism; Koller (1982) and Furlan, Cavalier, Hobbs, Weinstein, and Modie (1982) reached a similar conclusion.

When the source of emboli can be identified with confidence and when the causal condition can be eradicated, appropriate treatment (often surgical) is indicated when the patient's condition permits. Phenoxybenzamine 1 mg per kg body weight intravenously or other vasodilator drugs have been recommended in the acute stage but are of doubtful value. Intravenous low-molecular-weight dextran and surface cooling (hypothermia) have been recommended in cases of fat embolism, combined with assisted positive pressure respiration when necessary (Larson 1968).

References

(Cerebral atheromatosis; syndromes of the cerebral arteries; cerebral embolism.)

Achar, V. S., Coe, R. P. K., and Marshall, J. (1966). Echoencephalography in the differential diagnosis of cerebral haemorrhage and infarction. *Lancet* i, 161.

Acheson, J., Boyd, W. N., Hugh, A. E., and Hutchinson, E. C. (1969). Cerebral angiography in ischemic cerebrovascular disease. *Arch. Neurol.*, *Chicago* **20**, 527.

Acheson, R. M. and Fairbairn, A. S. (1970). Burden of cerebrovascular disease in the Oxford area in 1963 and 1964. *Br. med. J.* **2**, 621.

Ackerman, R. H. (1979). A perspective on noninvasive diagnosis of carotid disease. *Neurology, Minneapolis* **29**, 615.

Adams, G. F. and Hurwitz, L. J. (1963). Mental barriers to recovery from strokes. *Lancet* ii, 533.

—— and Merrett, J. W. (1961). Prognosis and survival in the aftermath of hemiplegia. *Br. med. J.* **1**, 309.

——, ——, Hutchinson, W. M., and Pollock, A. M. (1974). Cerebral embolism and mitral stenosis: survival with and without anticoagulants. *J. Neurol. Neurosurg. Psychiat.* **37**, 378.

Adams, R. D. (1954). Mechanisms of apoplexy as determined by clinical and pathological correlations. *J. Neuropath. exp. Neurol.* **13**, 1.

Ad Hoc Committee, National Advisory Council of the National Institute of Neurological Diseases and Blindness (1958). *Neurology, Minneapolis* **8**, (supplement).

Ad Hoc Committee, National Advisory Council of the National Institute of Neurological and Communicative Disorders and Stroke (1975). A classification and outline of cerebrovascular diseases II. *Stroke* **6**, 565.

Anderson, A. G., Lockhart, R. D., and Souter, W. C. (1931). Lateral syndrome of the medulla. *Brain* **54**, 460.

Anderson, T. W. and MacKay, J. S. (1968). A critical reappraisal of the epidemiology of cerebrovascular disease. *Lancet* i, 1137.

Ask-Upmark, E. and Bickerstaff, E. R. (1976). Vertebral artery occlusion and oral contraceptives. *Br. med. J.* **1**, 487.

Austin, J. H. and Stears, J. C. (1971). Familial hypoplasia of both internal carotid arteries. *Arch. Neurol, Chicago* **24**, 1.

Baker, R. N., Ramseyer, J. C., and Schwartz, W. (1968). Prognosis in patients with transient cerebral ischemic attacks. *Neurology, Minneapolis* **18**, 1157.

Barmada, M. A. Moossy, J., and Shuman, R. M. (1979). Cerebral infarcts with arterial occlusion in neonates. *Ann. Neurol.* **6**, 495.

Barnett, H. J. M. (1978). Delayed cerebral ischemic episodes distal to occlusion of major cerebral arteries. *Neurology, Minneapolis* **28**, 769.

—— (1980). Progress towards stroke prevention: Robert Wartenberg Lecture. *Neurology, Minneapolis* **30**, 1212.

——, Jones, M. W., Boughner, D. R., and Kostuk, W. J. (1976). Cerebral

ischemic events associated with prolapsing mitral valve. *Arch. Neurol.*, *Chicago* **33**, 777.

——, Peerless, S. J., and Kaufmann, J. C. E. (1978). 'Stump' of internal carotid artery—a source for further cerebral embolic ischemia. *Stroke* **9**, 448.

——, Plum, F., and Walton, J. N. (1984). Carotid endarterectomy—an expression of concern. *Stroke* **15**, 941.

Bauer, R. B., Sheehan, S., and Meyer, J. S. (1961). Arteriographic study of cerebrovascular disease. II. Cerebral symptoms due to kinking, tortuosity and compression of carotid and vertebral arteries in the neck. *Arch. Neurol.*, *Chicago* **4**, 119.

Beevers, D. G., Fairman, M. J., Hamilton, M., and Harpur, J. E. (1973). Antihypertensive treatment and the course of established cerebral vascular disease. *Lancet* i, 1407.

Bickerstaff, E. R. (1964). Aetiology of acute hemiplegia in childhood. *Br. med. J.* **2**, 82.

—— (1975). *Neurological complications of oral contraceptives*. Oxford University Press, Oxford.

Biemond, A. (1951). Thrombosis of the basilar artery and vascularization of the brain stem. *Brain* **74**, 300.

Blackwell, E., Merory, J., Toole, J. F., and McKinney, W. (1977). Doppler ultrasound scanning of the carotid bifurcation. *Arch. Neurol.*, *Chicaco* **34**, 145.

Blau, A. and Richardson, J. C. (1978). Strokes and head injury. *Can. J. neurol Sci.* **5**, 263.

Boutros, A. R. and Henry, C. E. (1982). Electrocerebral silence associated with adequate spontaneous ventilation in a case of fat embolism: a clinical and medicolegal dilemma. *Arch. Neurol.*, *Chicago* **39**, 314.

Brennan, R. W., Patterson, R. H., Jr., and Kessler, J. (1971). Cerebral blood flow and metabolism during cardiopulmonary bypass: evidence of microembolic encephalopathy. *Neurology, Minneapolis* **21**, 665.

Brice, J. G., Dowsett, D. J., and Lowe, R. D. (1964). Haemodynamic effects of carotid artery stenosis. *Br. med. J.* **2**, 1363.

British Medical Journal (1977a). Kinked carotid arteries. *Br. med. J.* **1**, 1177.

—— (1977b). Treatment of acute cerebral infarction. *Br. med. J.* **1**, 1.

—— (1978a). Investigating stroke. *Br. med. J.* **1**, 1503.

—— (1978b). Preventing stroke. *Br. med. J.* **2**, 454.

—— (1978c). Non-paralytic motor dysfunction after strokes. *Br. med. J.* **1**, 1165.

Brocklehurst, J. C., Andrews, K., Richards, B., and Laycock, P. J. (1978). How much physical therapy for patients with stroke? *Br. med. J.* **1**, 1307.

Brust, J. C. M. (1977). Transient ischemic attacks: natural history and anticoagulation. *Neurology, Minneapolis* **27**, 701.

——, Plank, C., Burke, A., Guobadia, M. M. I., and Healton, E. B. (1982). Language disorder in a right-hander after occlusion of the right anterior cerebral artery. *Neurology, Minneapolis* **32**, 492.

Bull, J. W. D., Marshall, J., and Shaw, D. A. (1960). Cerebral angiography in the diagnosis of the acute stroke. *Lancet* i, 562.

Burnbaum, M. D., Selhorst, J. B., Harbison, J. W., and Brush, J. J. (1977). Amaurosis fugax from disease of the external carotid artery. *Arch. Neurol.*, *Chicago* **34**, 532.

Cameron, W. J. and Wright, I. S. (1964). Subclavian steal syndrome with olfactory hallucinations. *Ann. intern. Med.* **61**, 128.

Canadian Cooperative Study Group (1978). A randomized trial of aspirin and sulfinpyrazone in threatened stroke. *New Engl. J. Med.* **299**, 53.

Capildeo, R., Haberman, S., and Rose, F. C. (1977). New classification of stroke: preliminary communication. *Br. med. J.* **2**, 1578.

——, ——, and —— (1978). The definition and classification of stroke. *Quart. J. Med.* **47**, 177.

Caplan, L. R. (1980). 'Top of the basilar' syndrome. *Neurology, Minneapolis* **30**, 72.

—— and Rosenbaum, A. E. (1975). Role of cerebral angiography in vertebrobasilar occlusive disease. *J. Neurol. Neurosurg. Psychiat.* **38**, 601.

Carter, A. B. (1957). The immediate treatment of cerebral embolism. *Quart. J. Med.* **26**, 335.

—— (1964). *Cerebral infarction*. Pergamon Press, Oxford.

—— (1970). Hypotensive therapy in stroke survivors. *Lancet* i, 485.

Chokroverty, S., Rubino, F. A., and Haller, C. (1977). Pure motor hemiplegia due to cerebral cortical infarction. *Arch. Neurol.*, *Chicago* **34**, 93.

Coakham, H. B., Duchen, L. W., and Scaravilli, F. (1979). Moya-Moya disease: clinical and pathological report of a case with associated myopathy. *J. Neurol. Neurosurg. Psychiat.* **42**, 289.

Corrin, L. S., Sandok, B. A., and Houser, O. W. (1981). Cerebral ischemic events in patients with carotid artery fibromuscular dysplasia. *Arch. Neurol., Chicago* **38**, 616.

Couch, J. R. and Hassanein, R. S. (1976). Platelet aggregation, stroke, and transient ischemic attack in middle-aged and elderly patients. *Neurology, Minneapolis* **26**, 888.

Critchley, M. (1929). Arteriosclerotic parkinsonism. *Brain* **52**, 23.

Croft, R. J. Ellam, L. D., and Harrison, M. J. G. (1980). Accuracy of carotid angiography in the assessment of atheroma of the internal carotid artery. *Lancet* **i**, 997.

Cross, J. N. Castro, P. O., and Jennett, W. B. (1968). Cerebral strokes associated with pregnancy and the puerperium. *Br. med. J.* **3**, 214.

Cull, R. E. (1979). Internal carotid artery occlusion caused by giant cell arteritis. *J. Neurol. Neurosurg. Psychiat.* **42**, 1066.

Dalal, P. M. Shah, P. M., Aiyar, R. R., and Kikani, B. J. (1968). Cerebrovascular diseases in West Central India. A report on angiographic findings from a prospective study. *Br. med. J.* **3**, 769.

David, N. J., Klintworth, G. K., Friedberg, S. J., and Dillon, M. (1963). Fatal atheromatous cerebral embolism associated with bright plaques in the retinal arterioles. *Neurology, Minneapolis* **13**, 709.

Davison, C., Goodhart, S. P., and Savitsky, N. (1935). The syndrome of the superior cerebellar artery and its branches. *Arch. Neurol. Psychiat., Chicago* **33**, 1143.

de Bono, D. P. and Warlow, C. P. (1981). Potential sources of emboli in patients with presumed transient cerebral or retinal ischaemia. *Lancet* **i**, 343.

Denny-Brown, D. (1951). The treatment of recurrent cerebrovascular symptoms and the question of 'vasospasm'. *Med. Clin. N. Am.* **35**, 1457.

—— (1960). Recurrent cerebro-vascular episodes. *Arch. Neurol., Chicago* **2**, 194.

DeSousa, A. L., Muller, J., Campbell, R. L., Batnitzky, S., and Rankin, L. (1978). Atrial myxoma: a review of the neurological complications, metastases and recurrences. *J. Neurol. Neurosurg. Psychiat.* **41**, 1119.

Dickinson, P. H., Hankinson, J., and Marshall, M. (1964). Internal carotid artery stenosis. *Br. J. Surg.* **51**, 703.

Donaldson, R. M. Emanuel, R. W., and Earl, C. J. (1981). The role of two-dimensional echocardiography in the detection of potentially embolic intracardiac masses in patients with cerebral ischaemia. *J. Neurol. Neurosurg. Psychiat.* **44**, 803.

Dougherty, J. H., Jr., Levy, D. E., and Weksler, B. B. (1977). Platelet activation in acute cerebral ischaemia. Serial measurements of platelet function in cerebrovascular disease. *Lancet* **i**, 821.

Eastcott, H. H. G., Pickering, G. W., and Rob, C. G. (1954). Reconstruction of internal carotid artery in a patient with intermittent attacks of hemiplegia. *Lancet* **ii**, 994.

Edwards, C. H. and Gordon, N. S. (1962). Surgical treatment of narrowing of the internal carotid artery. *Br. med. J.* **1**, 1289.

——, ——, and Rob, C. G. (1960). The surgical treatment of internal carotid artery occlusion. *Quart. J. Med.* **29**, 67.

Eisenberg, H., Morrison, J. T., Sullivan, P., and Foote, F. M. (1964). Cerebrovascular accidents. *J. Am. med. Ass.* **189**, 883.

Enzell, K. and Lindemalm, G. (1973). Cryptogenic cerebral embolism in women taking oral contraceptives. *Br. med. J.* **4**, 507.

Eslinger, P. J. and Damasio, A. R. (1981). Age and type of aphasia in patients with stroke. *J. Neurol. Neurosurg. Psychiat.* **44**, 377.

Farrell, M.A., Gilbert, J. J., and Kaufmann, J. C. E. (1985). Fatal intracranial arterial dissection. *J. Neurol. Neurosurg. Psychiat.* **48**, 111.

Faught, E., Trader, S. D., and Hann, G. R. (1979). Cerebral complications of angiography for transient ischemia and stroke: prediction of risk. *Neurology, Minneapolis* **29**, 4.

Fields, W. S., Lemak, N. A., Frankowski, R. F., and Hardy, R. J. (1977). Controlled trial of aspirin in cerebral ischemia. *Stroke* **8**, 301.

——, ——, ——, and —— (1978). Controlled trial of aspirin in cerebral ischemia. Part II: Surgical group. *Stroke* **9**, 309.

——, Maslenikov, V., Meyer, J. S., Hass, W. K., Remington, R. D., and Macdonald, M. (1970). Joint study of extracranial arterial occlusion. *J. Am. med. Ass.* **211**, 1993.

Fisher, C. M. (1957). Cranial bruit associated with occlusion of the internal carotid artery. *Neurology, Minneapolis* **7**, 299.

—— (1959). Observations of the fundus oculi in transient monocular blindness. *Neurology, Minneapolis* **9**, 333.

—— (1965). Pure sensory stroke involving face, arm and leg. *Neurology, Minneapolis* **15**, 76.

—— (1967). A lacunar stroke: the dysarthria–clumsy hand syndrome. *Neurology, Minneapolis* **17**, 614.

—— (1969). The arterial lesions underlying lacunes. *Acta neuropath.* **12**, 1.

—— (1970a). Facial pulses in internal carotid artery occlusion. *Neurology, Minneapolis* **20**, 476.

—— (1970b). Occlusion of the vertebral arteries causing transient basilar symptoms. *Arch. Neurol, Chicago* **22**, 13.

—— (1978). Thalamic pure sensory stroke: a pathologic study. *Neurology, Minneapolis* **28**, 1141.

—— (1979). Capsular infarcts: the underlying vascular lesions. *Arch. Neurol, Chicago* **36**, 65.

—— (1982). Lacunar strokes and infarcts: a review. *Neurology, Minneapolis* **32**, 871.

—— and Cameron, D. G. (1953). Case report: concerning cerebral vasospasm. *Neurology, Minneapolis* **3**, 468.

—— and Caplan, L. R. (1971). Basilar artery branch occlusion: a cause of pontine infarction. *Neurology, Minneapolis* **21**, 900.

—— and Pearlman, A. (1967). The nonsudden onset of cerebral embolism. *Neurology, Minneapolis* **17**, 1025.

——, Mohr, J. P., and Adams, R. D. (1974). In *Harrison's principles of internal medicine*, 7th ed., (ed. M. M. Wintrobe, G. W. Thorn, R. D. Adams, E. Braunwald, K. J. Isselbacher, and R. D. Petersdorf) p. 1749. Blakiston, New York.

——, Ojemann, R. G., and Robertson, G. H. (1978). Spontaneous dissection of cervico-cerebral arteries. *Can. J. neurol. Sci.* **5**, 9.

Fisher, M., Davidson, R. I., and Marcus, E. M. (1980). Transient focal cerebral ischemia as a presenting manifestation of unruptured cerebral aneurysms. *Ann. Neurol.* **8**, 367.

Freemon, F. R. (1971). Akinetic mutism and bilateral anterior cerebral artery occlusion. *J. Neurol. Neurosurg. Psychiat.* **34**, 693.

Furlan, A. J., Cavalier, S. J., Hobbs, R. E., Weinstein, M. A., and Modie, M. T. (1982). Hemorrhage and anticoagulation after nonseptic embolic brain infarction. *Neurology, Minneapolis* **32**, 280.

——, Whisnant, J. P., and Baker, H. L., Jr., (1980). Long-term prognosis after carotid artery occlusion. *Neurology, Minneapolis* **30**, 986.

——, ——, and Kearns, T. P. (1979). Unilateral visual loss in bright light: an unusual symptom of carotid artery occlusive disease. *Arch. Neurol., Chicago* **36**, 675.

Garraway, W. M., Akhtar, A. J., Hockey, L., and Prescott, R. J. (1980a). Management of acute stroke in the elderly: follow-up of a controlled trial. *Br. med. J.* **281**, 827.

——, Prescott, R. J., and Hockey, L. (1980b). Management of acute stroke in the elderly: preliminary results of a controlled trial. *Br. med. J.* **280**, 1040.

Goldstein, M., Bolis, L., Fieschi, C., Gorini, S., and Millikan, C. H. (Eds.) (1979). *Cerebrovascular disorders and stroke*, Advances in Neurology, Vol. 25. Raven Press, New York.

Graham, D. I. and Adams, H. (1972). 'Idiopathic' thrombosis in the vertebrobasilar artery system in young men. *Br. med. J.* **1**, 26.

Groothuis, D. R., Duncan, G. W., and Fisher, C. M. (1977). The human thalamocortical sensory path in the internal capsule: evidence from a small capsular hemorrhage causing a pure sensory stroke. *Ann. Neurol.* **2**, 328.

Gunning, A. G., Pickering, G. W., Robb-Smith, A. H. T., and Russell, R. (1964). Mural thrombosis of the internal carotid artery and subsequent embolism. *Quart. J. Med.* **33**, 155.

Haberman, S., Capildeo, R., and Rose, F. C. (1978). The changing mortality of cerebrovascular disease. *Quart. J. Med.* **47**, 71.

——, ——, and —— (1981). The seasonal variation in mortality from cerebrovascular disease. *J. neurol. Sci.* **52**, 25.

Hallam, J., Goldman, L., and Fryers, G. R. (eds.) (1981). *Aspirin Symposium 1980*, International Congress and Symposium Series, Number 39. Royal Society of Medicine, London.

Harrison, M. J. G. and Marshall, J. (1977). Evidence of silent cerebral embolism in patients with amaurosis fugax. *J. Neurol. Neurosurg. Psychiat.* **40**, 651.

——, ——, Meadows, J. C., and Russell, R. W. R. (1971). Effect of aspirin in amaurosis fugax. *Lancet* **ii**, 743.

——, Thomas, D. J., du Boulay, G. H., and Marshall, J. (1979). Multi-infarct dementia. *J. neurol. Sci.* **40**, 97.

Hartman, J. D., Young, I., Bank, A. A., and Rosenblatt, S. A. (1971). Fibromuscular hyperplasia of internal carotid arteries. Stroke in a young adult complicated by oral contraceptives. *Arch. Neurol., Chicago* **25**, 295.

Herskovits, E., Vazquez, A., Famulari, A., Smud, R., Tamaroff, L., Fraiman, H., Gonzalez, A. M., Vila, J., and Matera, V. (1981). Randomised trial of pentoxifylline versus acetylsalicylic acid plus dipyridamole in preventing transient ischaemic attacks. *Lancet* **i**, 966.

Heyman, A., Karp, H. R., and Bloor, B. M. (1957). Determination of retinal artery pressure in diagnosis of carotid artery occlusion. *Neurology, Minneapolis* **7**, 97.

Hill, A. B., Marshall, J., and Shaw, D. A. (1960). A controlled clinical trial of long-term anticoagulant therapy in cerebro-vascular disease. *Quart. J. Med.* **29**, 597.

Hinton, R. C., Mohr, J. P., Ackerman, R. H., Adair, L. B., and Fisher, C. M. (1979). Symptomatic middle cerebral artery stenosis. *Ann. Neurol.* **5**, 152.

Hughes, J. T. and Brownell, B. (1968). Traumatic thrombosis of the internal carotid artery in the neck. *J. Neurol. Neurosurg. Psychiat.* **31**, 307.

Hughes, W. (1965). Origin of lacunes. *Lancet* **ii**, 19.

Humphrey, J. G. and Newton, T. H. (1960). Internal carotid occlusion in young adults. *Brain* **83**, 565.

Hurwitz, L. J. and Adams, G. F. (1972). Rehabilitation of hemiplegia: indices of assessment and prognosis. *Br. med. J.* **1**, 94.

Hutchinson, E. C. and Acheson, E. J. (1975). *Strokes: natural history, pathology and surgical treatment.* Saunders, London.

—— and Yates, P. O. (1956). The cervical portion of the vertebral artery: a clinico-pathological study. *Brain* **79**, 319.

Inman, W. H. W. and Vessey, M. P. (1968). Investigation of deaths from pulmonary, coronary, and cerebral thrombosis and embolism in women of child-bearing age. *Br. med. J.* **2**, 193.

Irey, N. S., McAllister, H. A., and Henry, J. M. (1978). Oral contraceptives and stroke in young women: a clinicopathologic correlation. *Neurology, Minneapolis* **28**, 1216.

Johnson, K. G., Yano, K., and Kato, H. (1967). Cerebral vascular disease in Hiroshima, Japan. *J. Chron. Dis.* **20**, 545.

Kane, W. C. and Aronson, S. M. (1969). Cerebrovascular disease in an autopsy population. I. Influence of age, ethnic background, sex, and cardiomegaly upon frequency of cerebral hemorrhage. *Arch. Neurol., Chicago* **20**, 514.

Kaneda, H., Irino, T., Watanabe, M., Kadota, E., and Taneda, M. (1979). Semiquantitative evaluation of ophthalmic collateral flow in carotid artery occlusion: ultrasonic Doppler study. *J. Neurol. Neurosurg. Psychiat.* **42**, 1133.

Kappert, A. (1982). New noninvasive methods of investigating cerebrovascular insufficiency. *Triangle* **21**, 1.

Kaste, M., Fogelholm, R., and Waltimo, O. (1976). Combined dexamethasone and low-molecular-weight dextran in acute brain infarction: double-blind study. *Br. med. J.* **2**, 1409.

Kemper, T. L. and Romanul, F. C. A. (1967). State resembling akinetic mutism in basilar artery thrombosis. *Neurology, Minneapolis* **17**, 74.

Kendell, R. E. and Marshall, J. (1963). Role of hypotension in the genesis of transient focal cerebral ischaemic attacks. *Br. med. J.* **2**, 344.

Kinkel, W. R. and Jacobs, L. (1976). Computerized axial transverse tomography in cerebrovascular disease. *Neurology, Minneapolis* **26**, 924.

Kitahara, T., Ariga, N., Yamaura, A., Makino, H., and Maki, Y. (1979). Familial occurrence of Moya-Moya disease: report of three Japanese families. *J. Neurol. Neurosurg. Psychiat.* **42**, 208.

Koller, R. L. (1982). Recurrent embolic cerebral infarction and anticoagulation. *Neurology, Minneapolis* **32**, 283.

Kostuk, W. J., Boughner, D. R., Barnett, H. J. M., and Silver, M. D. (1977). Strokes: a complication of mitral-leaflet prolapse? *Lancet* **ii**, 313.

Kubik, C. S. and Adams, R. D. (1946). Occlusion of the basilar artery—a clinical and pathological study. *Brain* **69**, 73.

Kudo, T. (1968). Spontaneous occlusion of the circle of Willis. A disease apparently confined to Japanese. *Neurology, Minneapolis* **18**, 485.

Kurtzke, J. F. (1969). *Epidemiology of cerebrovascular disease.* Springer-Verlag, Berlin, Heidelberg, New York.

Ladurner, G., Iliff, L. D., and Lechner, H. (1982). Clinical factors associated with dementia in ischaemic stroke. *J. Neurol. Neurosurg. Psychiat.* **45**, 97.

Lakeman, M. J., Sherriff, S. B., and Martin, T. R. P. (1981). A prospective study of the accuracy of Doppler ultrasound in detecting carotid artery disease. *J. Neurol. Neurosurg. Psychiat.* **44**, 657.

The Lancet (1974). Carotid endarterectomy and T.I.A.s. *Lancet* **i**, 51.

—— (1978a). Cerebral infarction and myocardial infarction: a similar aetiology? *Lancet* **i**, 1239.

—— (1978b). Aspirin and stroke prevention. *Lancet* **ii**, 245.

—— (1980). Barbiturate therapy in cerebral ischaemia. *Lancet* **i**, 965.

—— (1981). Carotid stenosis. *Lancet* **i**, 535.

Larson, A. G. (1968). Treatment of cerebral fat-embolism with phenoxybenzamine and surface cooling. *Lancet* **ii**, 250.

Larsson, O., Marinovich, N., and Barber, K. (1976). Double-blind trial of glycerol therapy in early stroke. *Lancet* **i**, 832.

Lascelles, R. G. and Burrows, E. H. (1965). Occlusion of the middle cerebral artery. *Brain* **88**, 85.

Lee, M. C., Ausman, J. I., Geiger, J. D., Latchaw, R. E., Klassen, A. C., Chou, S. N., and Resch, J. A. (1979). Superficial temporal to middle cerebral artery anastomosis: clinical outcome in patients with ischemia or infarction in internal carotid artery distribution. *Arch. Neurol., Chicago* **36**, 1.

Lehrich, J. R., Winkler, G. D., and Ojemann, R. G. (1970). Cerebellar infarction with brain stem compression: diagnosis and surgical treatment. *Arch. Neurol., Chicago* **22**, 490.

Lhermitte, F., Gautier, J. C., Derouesné, C., and Guiraud, B. (1968). Ischemic accidents in the middle cerebral artery territory: a study of the causes in 122 cases. *Arch. Neurol., Chicago* **19**, 248.

Mandybur, T. I. (1979). Cerebral amyloid angiopathy: possible relationship to rheumatoid vasculitis. *Neurology, Minneapolis* **29**, 1336.

Mannock, J. A., Suter, L. G., and Hume, D. M. (1961). The 'subclavian steal' syndrome. *J. Am. med. Ass.* **182**, 254.

Mariani, C., Spinnler, H., Sterzi, R., and Vallar, G. (1980). Bilateral perisylvian softenings: bilateral anterior opercular syndrome (Foix–Chavany–Marie syndrome). *J. Neurol.* **223**, 269.

Maroon, J. C. and Campbell, R. L. (1969). Atrial myxoma: a treatable cause of stroke. *J. Neurol. Neurosurg. Psychiat.* **32**, 129.

Marquardsen, J. (1969). The natural history of acute cerebrovascular disease. A retrospective study of 769 patients. *Acta neurol. scand.* suppl. **38**.

Marshall, J. (1971). Angiography in the investigation of ischaemic episodes in the territory of the internal carotid artery. *Lancet* **i**, 719.

—— (1976). *The management of cerebrovascular disease*, 3rd edn. Blackwell, Oxford.

—— (1982). The cause and prognosis of strokes in people under 50 years. *J. neurol. Sci.* **53**, 473.

—— and Shaw, D. A. (1959). Anticoagulant therapy in cerebrovascular disease. *Proc. R. Soc. Med.* **52**, 547.

Masdeu, J. C., Azar-Kia, B., and Rubino, F. A. (1977). Evaluation of recent cerebral infarction by computerized tomography. *Arch. Neurol., Chicago* **34**, 417.

Matthews, W. B., Oxbury, J. M., Grainger, K. M. R., and Greenhall, R. C. D. (1976). A blind controlled trial of dextran 40 in the treatment of ischaemic stroke. *Brain* **99**, 193.

Mawdsley, C., Samuel, E., Sumerling, M. D., and Young, G. B. (1968). Thermography in occlusive cerebrovascular diseases. *Br. med. J.* **3**, 521.

McAllen, P. M. and Marshall, J. (1973). Cardiac dysrhythmia and transient cerebral ischaemic attacks. *Lancet* **i**, 1212.

—— and —— (1977). Cerebrovascular incidents after myocardial infarction. *J. Neurol. Neurosurg. Psychiat.* **40**, 951.

McBrien, D. J., Bradley, R. D., and Ashton, W. (1963). The nature of retinal emboli in stenosis of the internal carotid artery. *Lancet* **i**, 697.

McFarling, D., Rothi, L. J., and Heilman, K. M. (1982). Transcortical aphasia from ischaemic infarcts of the thalamus: a report of two cases. *J. Neurol. Neurosurg. Psychiat.* **45**, 107.

McHenry, L. C., Jaffe, M. E., West, J. W., Cooper, E. S., Kenton, E. J., Kawamura, J., Oshiro, T., and Goldberg, H. I. (1972). Regional cerebral blood flow and cardiovascular effects of hexobendine in stroke patients. *Neurology, Minneapolis* **22**, 217.

Meikle, M., Wechsler, E., Tupper, A., Benenson, M., Butler, J., Mulhall, D., and Stern, G. (1979). Comparative trial of volunteer and professional treatments of dysphasia after stroke. *Br. med. J.* **2**, 87.

Menkin, M. and Schwartzman, R. J. (1977). Cerebral air embolism: report of five cases and review of the literature. *Arch. Neurol, Chicago* **34**, 168.

Mesulam, M.-M., Waxman, S. G., Geschwind, N., and Sabin, T. D. (1976). Acute confusional states with right middle cerebral artery infarctions. *J. Neurol. Neurosurg. Psychiat.* **39**, 84.

Meyer, J. S., Charney, J. Z., Rivera, V. M., and Mathew, N. T. (1971). Treatment with glycerol of cerebral oedema due to acute cerebral infarction. *Lancet* **ii**, 993.

——, Sawada, T., Kitamura, A., and Toyoda, M. (1968). Cerebral blood flow after control of hypertension in stroke. *Neurology, Minneapolis* **18**, 772.

——, Stoica, E., Pascu, I., Shimazu, K., and Hartmann, A. (1973). Catecholamine concentrations in CSF and plasma of patients with cerebral infarction and haemorrhage. *Brain* **96**, 277.

Milligan, N. and Anderson, M. (1980). Conjugal disharmony: a hitherto unrecognised cause of strokes. *Br. med. J.* **281**, 421.

Millikan, C. H. (1971). Reassessment of anticoagulant therapy in various types of occlusive cerebral vascular disease. *Stroke* **2**, 201.

——, Siekert, R. G., and Shick, R. N. (1955). Studies in cerebrovascular disease. III. Use of anticoagulant drugs in treatment of insufficiency or thrombosis within basilar arterial system. *Mayo Clin. Proc.* **30**, 116. V. Use of anticoagulant drugs in treatment of intermittent insufficiency of internal carotid system. *Mayo Clin. Proc.* **30**, 578.

——, ——, and Whisnant, J. P. (1959). The syndrome of occlusion of the labyrinthine division of the internal auditory artery. *Trans. Am. neurol. Ass.* **84**, 11.

Mills, R. P. and Swanson, P. D. (1978). Vertical oculomotor apraxia and memory loss. *Ann. Neurol.* **4**, 149.

Minderhoud, J. M. (1971). Diagnostic significance of symptomatology in brain stem ischaemic infarction. *Eur. Neurol.* **5**, 343.

Mohr, J. P., Caplan, L. R., Melski, J. W., Goldstein, R. J., Duncan, G. W., Kistler, J. P., Pessin, M. S., and Bleich, H. L. (1978). The Harvard Cooperative Stroke Registry: a prospective registry. *Neurology, Minneapolis* **28**, 754.

Morris, W. R. (1968). Long-term results of carotid artery surgery. A report of 65 cases. *Guy's Hosp. Rep.* **117**, 225.

Murray, P. J. (1978). Microvascular anastomosis for cerebral ischemia in 19 patients: a preliminary report. *Can. J. neurol. Sci.* **5**, 21.

Naritomi, H., Sakai, F., and Meyer, J. S. (1979). Pathogenesis of transient ischemic attacks within the vertebrobasilar arterial system. *Arch. Neurol., Chicago* **36**, 121.

Norris, J. W. and Hachinski, V. C. (1982). Misdiagnosis of stroke. *Lancet* **i**, 328.

North, R. R., Fields, W. S., de Bakey, M. E., and Crawford, E. S. (1962). Brachiobasilar insufficiency syndrome. *Neurology, Minneapolis* **12**, 810.

Parkin, P. J., Kendall, B. E., Marshall, J., and McDonald, W. I. (1982). Amaurosis fugax: some aspects of management. *J. Neurol. Neurosurg. Psychiat.* **45**, 1.

Patel, A. and Toole, J. F. (1965). Subclavian steal syndrome—reversal of cephalic blood flow. *Medicine* **44**, 289.

Patten, B. M., Mendell, J., Bruun, B., Curtin, W., and Carter, S. (1972). Double-blind study of the effects of dexamethasone on acute stroke. *Neurology, Minneapolis* **22**, 377.

Pearce, J. and Aziz, H. (1969). Uric acid and plasma lipids in cerebrovascular disease. Part 1: Prevalence of hyperuricaemia. *Br. med. J.* **4**, 78.

—— and —— (1970). Uric acid and serum lipids in cerebrovascular disease. Part 2: Uric acid–plasma lipid correlations, *J. Neurol. Neurosurg. Psychiat.* **33**, 88.

Poór, G. and Gács, G. (1974). The so-called 'Moyamoya disease'. *J. Neurol. Neurosurg. Psychiat.* **37**, 370.

Price, D. L. and Harris, J. (1970). Cholesterol emboli in cerebral arteries as a complication of retrograde aortic perfusion during cardiac surgery. *Neurology, Minneapolis* **20**, 1209.

——, ——, New, P. F. J., and Cantu, R. (1970). Cardiac myxoma: a clinicopathologic and angiographic study. *Arch. Neurol., Chicago* **23**, 558.

Reske-Nielsen, E., Svendsen, K., and Søgaard, H. (1965). Cerebral emboli as a result of 'mute' juvenile endocarditis. *Acta path. microbiol. scand* **63**, 321.

Roeltgen, D. P., Weimer, G. R., and Patterson, L. F. (1981). Delayed neurologic complications of left atrial myxoma. *Neurology, Minneapolis* **31**, 8.

Ropper, A. H., Fisher, C. M., and Kleinman, G. M. (1979). Pyramidal infarction in the medulla: a cause of pure motor hemiplegia sparing the face. *Neurology, Minneapolis* **29**, 91.

Rosenberg, N. L. and Koller, R. (1981). Computerized tomography and pure sensory stroke. *Neurology, Minneapolis* **31**, 217.

Russell, R. W. R. (1961). Observations on the retinal blood vessels in monocular blindness. *Lancet* **ii**, 1422.

—— (1963). Atheromatous retinal embolism. *Lancet* **ii**, 1354.

—— and Green, M. (1971). Mechanisms of transient cerebral ischaemia. *Br. med. J.* **1**, 646.

Samson, D., Watts, C., and Clark, K. (1977). Cerebral revascularization for transient ischemic attacks. *Neurology, Minneapolis* **27**, 767.

Schneidau, A. (1984). Digital subtraction angiography in ischaemic cerebrovascular disease. *Brit. J. hosp. Med.* **30**, 176.

Schoenberg, B. S., Mellinger, J. F., and Schoenberg, D. G. (1978). Cerebrovascular disease in infants and children: a study of incidence, clinical features, and survival. *Neurology, Minneapolis* **28**, 763.

——, Whisnant, J. P., Taylor, W. F., and Kempers, R D. (1970). Strokes in women of childbearing age: a population study. *Neurology, Minneapolis* **20**, 181.

Schwarz, G. A. Schwartzman, R. J., and Joyner, C. R. (1972). Atrial myxoma: cause of embolic stroke. *Neurology, Minneapolis* **22**, 1112.

Scotti, G., Spinnler, H., Sterzi, R., and Vallar, G. (1980). Cerebellar softening. *Ann. Neurol.* **8**, 133.

Segarra, J. M. (1970). Cerebral vascular disease and behavior. I. The syndrome of the mesencephalic artery (basilar artery bifurcation). *Arch. Neurol., Chicago* **22**, 408.

Shaw, D. A., Venables, G. S., Cartlidge, N. E. F., Bates, D., and Dickinson, P. H. (1984). Carotid endarterectomy in patients with transient cerebral ischaemia. *J. neurol. Sci.* **64**, 45.

Silverstein, A., Gilbert, H., and Wasserman, L. R. (1962). Hemiplegic complications of polycythaemia. *Ann. intern. Med.* **57**, 909.

Smith, D. S., Goldenberg, E., Ashburn, A., Kinsella, G., Sheikh, K., Brennan, P. J., Meade, T. W., Zutshi, D. W., Perry, J. D., and Reeback, J. W. (1981). Remedial therapy after stroke: a randomised controlled trial. *Br. med. J.* **282**, 517.

So, E. L., Toole, J. F., Dalal, P., and Moody, D. M. (1981). Cephalic fibromuscular dysplasia in 32 patients: clinical findings and radiologic features. *Arch. Neurol., Chicago* **38**, 619.

Solomon, G. E., Hilal, S. K., Gold, A. P., and Carter, S. (1970). Natural history of acute hemiplegia of childhood. *Brain* **93**, 107.

Sörnäs, R., Östlund, H., and Müller, R. (1972). Cerebrospinal fluid cytology after stroke. *Arch. Neurol., Chicago* **26**, 489.

Stewart, R. M., Samson, D., Diehl, J., Hinton, R., and Ditmore, Q. M. (1980). Unruptured cerebral aneurysms presenting as recurrent transient neurologic deficits. *Neurology, Minneapolis* **30**, 47.

Sundt, T. M., Jr., Sandok, B. A., and Whisnant, J. P. (1975). Carotid endarterectomy: complications and preoperative assessment of risk. *Mayo Clin. Proc.* **50**, 301.

Swash, M. and Earl, C. J. (1970). Transient visual obscurations in chronic rheumatic heart-disease. *Lancet* **ii**, 323.

Symonds, C. P. (1927). Cervical rib: thrombosis of subclavian artery. Contralateral hemiplegia of sudden onset, probably embolic. *Proc. R. Soc. Med.* **20**, 1244.

—— and Mackenzie, I. (1957). Bilateral loss of vision from cerebral infarction. *Brain* **80**, 415.

Takeuchi, K. (1961). Occlusive diseases of the carotid artery. Recent advances. *Res. nerv. Syst.* **5**, 511.

Thiele, B. L., Young, J. V., Chikos, P. M. Hirsch, J. H., and Strandness, D. E., Jr. (1980). Correlation of arteriographic findings and symptoms in cerebrovascular disease. *Neurology, Minneapolis* **30**, 1041.

Thompson, P. L. and Robinson, J. S. (1978). Stroke after acute myocardial infarction: relation to infarct size. *Br. med. J.* **2**, 457.

Timperley, W. R., Preston, F. E., and Ward, J. D. (1974). Cerebral intravascular coagulation in diabetic ketoacidosis. *Lancet* **i**, 952.

Tomkin, G., Coe, R. P. K., and Marshall, J. (1968). Electrocardiographic abnormalities in patients presenting with strokes. *J. Neurol. Neurosurg. Psychiat.* **31**, 250.

Tomlinson, B. E. (1959). Brain changes in ruptured intracranial aneurysms. *J. Clin. Pathol.* **12**, 391.

——, Blessed, G., and Roth, M. (1968). Observations on the brains of non-demented old people. *J. neurol. Sci.* **7**, 331.

Toole, J. F. and Patel, A. N. (1974). *Cerebrovascular disorders*, 2nd edn. McGraw-Hill, New York.

—— and Tucker, S. H. (1960). Influence of head position upon cerebral circulation. *Arch. Neurol., Chicaco* **2**, 616.

—— and Yuson, C. P. (1977). Transient ischemic attacks with normal arteriograms: serious or benign prognosis? *Ann. Neurol.* **1**, 100.

——, Janeway, R., Choi, K., Cordell, R., Davis, C., Johnston, F., and Miller, H. S. (1975). Transient ischemic attacks: a prospective study of 225 patients. *Neurology, Minneapolis* **28**, 746.

Tubman, D. E., Ethier, R., Melançon, D., Bèlanger, G., and Taylor, S. (1981). The computerized tomographic assessment of brain infarcts. *Can. J. neurol Sci.* **8**, 121.

Walton, J. N. (1966). *Essentials of neurology*, 2nd edn. Pitman Publishing Co. Ltd., London.

Warlow, C. P. (1982). Transient ischaemic attacks. In *Recent advances in neurology—3* (ed. W. B. Matthews and G. H. Glaser). Churchill-Livingstone, Edinburgh.

——, Ogston, D., and Douglas, A. S. (1976). Deep venous thrombosis of the legs after strokes. Part I—Incidence and predisposing factors. Part II—Natural history. *Br. med. J.* **1**, 1178, 1181.

Weibel, J. and Fields, W. S. (1969). *Atlas of arteriography in occlusive cerebrovascular disease.* Saunders, Philadelphia.

Weisberg, L. A. (1982). Lacunar infarcts: clinical and computed tomographic correlations. *Arch. Neurol., Chicago* **39**, 37.

West, T. E. T., Davies, R. J., and Kelly, R. E. (1976). Horner's syndrome and headache due to carotid artery disease. *Br. med. J.* **1**, 818.

Whisnant, J. P., Cartlidge, N. E. F., and Elveback, L. R. (1978). Carotid and vertebral-basilar transient ischemic attacks: effect of anticoagulants, hypertension, and cardiac disorders on survival and stroke occurrence—a population study. *Ann. Neurol.* **3**, 107, 1978.

——, Fitzgibbon, J. P., Kurland, L. T., and Sayre, G. P. (1971). Natural history of stroke in Rochester, Minnesota, 1945 through 1954. *Stroke* **2**, 11.

——, Matsumoto, N., and Elveback, L. R. (1973a). Transient cerebral ischaemic attacks in a community, Rochester, Minnesota, 1955 through 1969. *Mayo Clin. Proc.* **48**, 194.

——, ——, and —— (1973b). The effect of anticoagulant therapy on the prognosis of patients with transient cerebral ischemic attacks in a community, Rochester, Minnesota, 1955 through 1969. *Mayo Clin. Proc.* **48**, 844.

Williams, A. O., Resch, J. A., and Loewenson, R. B. (1969). Cerebral atherosclerosis—a comparative autopsy study between Nigerian Negroes and American Negroes and Caucasians. *Neurology, Minneapolis* **19**, 205.

Williams, D. and Wilson, T. G. (1962). The diagnosis of the major and minor syndromes of basilar insufficiency. *Brain* **85**, 741.

Wilson, L. A., Keeling, P. W. N., Malcolm, A. D., Russell, R. W. R., and Webb-Peploe, M. M. (1977). Visual complications of mitral leaflet prolapse. *Br. med. J.* **2**, 86.

——, Warlow, C. P., and Russell, R. W. R. (1979). Cardiovascular disease in patients with retinal arterial occlusion. *Lancet* **i**, 292.

Wolf, P. A., Dawber, T. R., Thomas, H. E., Jr., and Kannel, W. B. (1978). Epidemiologic assessment of chronic atrial fibrillation and risk of stroke: The Framingham Study. *Neurology, Minneapolis* **28**, 973.

Wolintz, A. H., Jacobs, L. D., Christoff, N., Solomon, M., and Chernik, N. (1969). Serum and cerebrospinal fluid enzymes in cerebrovascular disease: creatine phosphokinase, aldolase, and lactic dehydrogenase. *Arch. Neurol., Chicago* **20**, 54.

Woodhurst, W. B. (1980). Cerebellar infarction—review of recent experiences. *Can. J. neurol. Sci.* **7**, 97.

Wright, I. S. and McDevitt, E. (1954). Cerebral vascular diseases. *Ann. intern. Med.* **41**, 682.

Yates, P. O. and Hutchinson, E. C. (1961). Cerebral infarction: the role of stenosis of the extracranial vessels. *Spec. Rep. Ser. med. Res. Coun. (Lond.),* No. 300. HMSO, London.

Yu, Y. L., Moseley, I. F., Pullicino, P., and McDonald, W. I. (1982). The clinical picture of ectasia of the intracerebral arteries. *J. Neurol. Neurosurg. Psychiat.* **45**, 29.

Yufe, R., Karpati, G., and Carpenter, S. (1976). Cardiac myxoma: a diagnostic challenge for the neurologist. *Neurology, Minneapolis* **26**, 1060.

Ziegler, D. K., Zileli, T., Dick, A., and Sebaugh, J. L. (1971). Correlation of bruits over the carotid artery with angiographically demonstrated lesions. *Neurology, Minneapolis* **21**, 860.

Hypertensive encephalopathy

Definition. An acute and largely reversible disorder of cerebral function occuring in association with severe arterial hypertension, usually in association with malignant hypertension, less often with acute or chronic nephritis or eclampsia. The cardinal symptoms are headache and drowsiness, sometimes with nausea and vomiting, focal neurological symptoms and signs, and/or epileptic fits.

Aetiology and pathology

The term hypertensive encephalopathy was first used by Oppenheimer and Fishbery (1928) to identify a constellation of cerebral symptoms occurring in severely hypertensive individuals. Byrom (1954) suggested that it was due to acute constriction of cerebral arterioles caused by a sudden rise in intravascular pressure, but more recent evidence indicates that it is more probably consequent upon failure of the normal autoregulatory vasoconstriction of cerebral arterioles which usually accompanies a given rise in blood pressure (*British Medical Journal* 1979). Chester, Agamanolis, Banker, and Victor (1978) found in the brains of fatal cases fibrinoid necrosis of arteriolar walls, thrombosis in arterioles and capillaries, multiple microinfarcts, and petechial haemorrhages involving much of the brain but most severe in the brainstem. Cerebral oedema, previously thought to be a common finding in such cases, was uncommon even in patients with papilloedema and increased CSF pressure, but similar vascular changes were found in the eyes, kidneys, and other organs. Attacks have been described following the ingestion of tyramine-containing foods such as cheese in patients taking aminoxidase inhibitors for the treatment of depression and may also occur in paroxysms of hypertension in cases of phaeochromocytoma (see Toole and Patel 1974).

The age incidence of hypertensive encephalopathy is that of the causal disorders. Acute nephritis is commonest in childhood, adolescence, and early adult life; chronic nephritis in the second and third decade; eclampsia during the early child-bearing period; and malignant hypertension in the thirties and forties, though it may occur in childhood or late middle age.

Symptoms and signs

The onset of symptoms is usually subacute, the patient complaining of headaches of increasing severity, which are often associated with vomiting. Epileptic convulsions are common and may be followed either by confusion or coma. Drowsiness and impairment of memory and intellect suggestive of dementia or even at times of psychosis are common (Healton, Brust, Feinfeld, and Thomson 1982). Impairment of vision, or even complete blindness, may occur. This is often cortical in origin, and during recovery of vision one homonymous pair of visual half-fields may recover before the other. Other focal disturbances include aphasia and hemiparesis. Irreversible blindness and paraplegia due to infarction of the optic nerves and spinal cord has been described in severe childhood hypertension (Hulse, Taylor, and Dillon 1979).

Arterial hypertension is present in every case, and a sudden rise in an already high blood pressure frequently heralds the encephalopathy. The retinae usually show bilateral papilloedema and the exudative changes of hypertensive retinopathy. Cervical rigidity, tachycardia, and fever sometimes occur. Jellinek, Painter, Prineas, and Ross Russell (1964) noted that transient blindness of cortical type was common and that during this stage the EEG often showed diffuse slow activity, loss or impairment of the alpha rhythm, and absence of the normal 'following' response to photic stimulation. The pressure of the CSF is usually increased but its composition is generally normal.

Diagnosis

Hypertensive encephalopathy must be distinguished from uraemia, cerebral vascular lesions such as haemorrhage and infarction, and intracranial tumour. In uraemia convulsive phenomena consist usually of myoclonic twitches rather than of epileptiform attacks and amaurosis is rare. Cerebral vascular lesions do not usually produce such a diffuse picture of cerebral disturbance and their manifestations do not resolve rapidly as the blood pressure is lowered. On the other hand, severe encephalopathy can lead to infarction (Healton *et al.* 1982). The diagnosis from intracranial tumour may be difficult in the presence of papilloedema, since a tumour may develop in a patient who also has hypertension. When a CT scan is inconclusive, other contrast studies may be needed to exclude neoplasm or benign intracranial hypertension, but the symptoms of hypertensive encephalopathy are usually so transient that this is rarely necessary. Urinalysis, estimations of the blood urea, and serial blood pressure recording usually support the diagnosis, and other tests of renal function may be needed to determine whether the primary cause is renal disease.

Prognosis

Alarming though the symptoms are, the outlook in hypertensive encephalopathy is on the whole good with respect to the neurological manifestations unless the episode is severe and prolonged and leads to infarction or other irreversible pathological changes; however, the ultimate outcome depends upon the underlying cause. Most patients recover from encephalopathy complicating acute nephritis and from eclampsia. Even in malignant hypertension the patient usually recovers from an attack if hypertension is vigorously treated. Severe and frequent convulsions are a bad sign. Recovery from visual disturbance, aphasia, and other focal symptoms is usually complete in a few days.

Treatment

Hypotensive drugs may bring an attack of encephalopathy to an end, and usually produce dramatic relief within hours. However, it is important that the blood pressure should be lowered slowly over hours or days, since if it is reduced too rapidly at a time when cerebrovascular autoregulation is impaired, severe ischaemia or even extensive infarction can occur (Ledingham and Rajagopalan 1979). Toole and Patel (1974) recommended treatment with pentolinium (20–200 mg/l) given by slow intravenous infusion with constant monitoring of the blood pressure, preferably in an intensive care unit. Many now prefer sodium nitroprusside (0.5–10 μg/kg/min) given by infusion pump with similar monitoring; an appropriate beta-blocking drug should be started, with oral hydrallazine and a potent diuretic, at the same time (*British Medical Journal* 1979). If the convulsions prove intractable, phenytoin or intravenous diazepam are indicated. The treatment appropriate to the causal condition will also be required.

References

British Medical Journal (1979). Hypertensive encephalopathy *Br. med. J.* **2**, 1387.

Byrom, F. B. (1954). The pathogenesis of hypertensive encephalopathy. *Lancet* **i**, 201.

Chester, E. M., Agamanolis, D. P., Banker, B. Q., and Victor, M. (1978). Hypertensive encephalopathy: a clinicopathologic study of 20 cases. *Neurology, Minneapolis* **28**, 928.

Finnerty, F. A. (1972). Hypertensive encephalopathy. *Am. J. Med.* **52**, 672.

Healton, E. B., Brust, J. C., Feinfeld, D. A., and Thomson, G. E. (1982). Hypertensive encephalopathy and the neurologic manifestations of malignant hypertension. *Neurology, Minneapolis* **32**, 127.

Hulse, J. A., Taylor, D. S. I., and Dillon, M. J. (1979). Blindness and paraplegia in severe childhood hypertension. *Lancet* **ii**, 553.

Jellinek, E. H., Painter, M., Prineas, J., and Ross Russell, R. (1964). Hypertensive encephalopathy with cortical disorders of vision. *Quart. J. Med.* **33**, 239.

Kung, P. C., Lee, J. C., and Bakay, L. (1968). Electron microscopic study of experimental acute hypertensive encephalopathy. *Acta neuropath., Berlin* **10**, 263.

The Lancet (1965). Pressor attacks during treatment with monoamine-oxidase inhibitors. *Lancet* **i**, 945.

Ledingham, J. G. G. and Rajagopalan, B. (1979). Cerebral complications in the treatment of accelerated hypertension. *Quart. J. Med.* **48**, 25.

Oppenheimer, B. S. and Fishberg, A. M. (1928). Hypertensive encephalopathy. *Arch. intern. Med.* **41**, 264.

Skinhøj, E. and Strandgaard, S. (1973). Pathogenesis of hypertensive encephalopathy. *Lancet* **i**, 461.

Toole, J. F. and Patel, A. N. (1974). *Cerebrovascular disorders*, 2nd edn. McGraw-Hill, New York.

Intracranial aneurysm

Definition. A localized dilatation of an intracranial artery which may cause symptoms either through localized pressure upon neighbouring structures, especially cranial nerves, or by sudden rupture leading to subarachnoid haemorrhage.

Aneurysm of congenital origin

'Berry' or so-called 'congenital' aneurysms

Pathology

A congenital abnormality is an important factor in the aetiology of intracranial aneurysm. 'Congenital' aneurysms appear to arise, as Turnbull (1914–15) and Forbus (1930) showed, at a point where there is a deficiency in the media at the junction of the components of the circle of Willis, at a bifurcation of one of the cerebral arteries, or where a vestigial vessel is present in association with a congenital anomaly of the circle. However, a medial defect alone is not sufficient to cause aneurysmal formation and there must also be an acquired lesion which breaches the internal elastic lamina at the same point, as the latter alone will withstand more than twice the highest recorded arterial blood pressure. This acquired lesion is usually atheroma; this explains why, despite the ubiquity of congenital medial defects in cerebral arteries, aneurysms usually appear and produce their clinical effects in middle life (Carmichael 1950; Walton 1956). These aneurysms may be single or multiple, as many as 13 having been present in the same individual (Zacks 1978); they are sometimes discovered fortuitously at autopsy or when angiography is performed for other reasons (Zacks, Russell, and Miller 1980). They are most frequently found on the internal carotid artery, on the middle cerebral, and at the junction of the anterior communicating with the anterior cerebral arteries, but may occur on any cerebral artery. Only about 10 per cent are in the posterior fossa. They range in size from smaller than a pin's head to 30 mm or more in diameter (Fig. 4.3). 'Congenital' intracranial aneurysms have occurred in more than one member of the same family (Beumont 1968; Bannerman, Ingall, and Graf 1970; Acosta-Rua 1978) and subarachnoid haemorrhage resulting from the rupture of almost identical aneurysms has been reported in identical twins (Fairburn 1973). They may be found at any age, even in infancy (Thompson and Pribram 1969), but more than half first cause symptoms between the ages of 40 and 55 (Fearnsides 1916) (Fig. 4.7, p. 209), and they occur almost equally in the two sexes with perhaps a slight predominance in females. Sooner or later most aneurysms, except the largest, rupture, and the extravasated blood passes into the subarachnoid space and sometimes into the substance of the brain, even reaching the ventricles. Rupture into the subdural space (Clarke and Walton 1953) and even through the dura has been observed. Subarachnoid haemorrhage accounts for about 6–8 per cent of all cases of cerebral vascular disease, and occurs about as often as intracerebral haemorrhage.

The pathological effects of rupture of an aneurysm were studied by Tomlinson (1959) and Crompton (1964a, b), who stressed the frequency of cerebral infarction and of damage to the hypothalamus (Crompton 1963). Aneurysms are often found in normotensive subjects, though a rise of blood pressure in later life may well be responsible, if not for the formation of the aneurysm, at least for its rupture.

Other congenital vascular abnormalities, such as congenital heart disease, aneurysms or defects of the media of abdominal arteries leading to intraperitoneal haemorrhage, coarctation of the aorta, and cutaneous naevi, have occasionally been observed in patients with intracranial aneurysm and these may also co-exist with an intracranial angioma. Intracranial aneurysms are also common in patients with renal polycystic disease.

Symptoms

The symptoms of congenital intracranial aneurysm differ according to whether the patient is observed: (1) before rupture; (2) immediately after rupture; or (3) after recovery from the immediate effects of rupture.

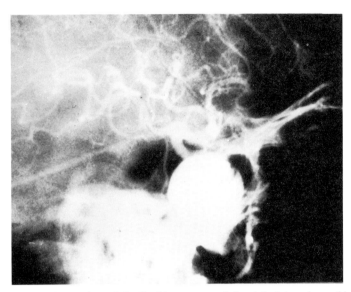

Fig. 4.3. A very large infraclinoid aneurysm of the right internal carotid artery shown by angiography to be within the cavernous sinus.

Symptoms before rupture of the aneurysm

It is often impossible to diagnose an intracranial aneurysm before it ruptures as it may be too small to produce symptoms by compressing structures in its vicinity. However, if such symptoms occur, it is frequently possible to make a correct diagnosis. Unless the aneurysm is very large (Bull 1969), symptoms of increased intracranial pressure do not occur. Some 25 per cent of patients suffer from recurrent headaches—about half from typical migraine. The diagnosis of aneurysm rests upon evidence of focal pressure fairly sharply localized and only slowly, if at all, progressive. The nature of such focal symptoms depends upon the situation of the aneurysm. Those placed anteriorly in the circle of Willis may compress the optic nerve, leading to unilateral impairment of vision, which may vary in severity with transient unilateral visual obscurations, superficially resembling amaurosis fugax. In such cases optic atrophy and rarely slight papilloedema may be found in the affected eye and exophthalmos may be present. Hemianopia may result from compression of one optic tract, or the chiasm may be compressed (Jefferson 1937, 1938; Peiris and Ross Russell 1980). Paralysis of the third, fourth, or sixth cranial nerves may occur with or without exophthalmos and pain, sometimes of sudden onset, often with anaesthesia in the cutaneous area supplied by the first (and less often the second) divisions of the trigeminal nerve. This is the characteristic picture which may result from an aneurysm of the internal carotid artery within the cavernous sinus (Fig. 4.3) (an infraclinoid aneurysm) (Barr, Blackwood, and Meadows 1971) and, if sudden expansion occurs, there is pain behind the eye. Aneurysms situated on the cortical course of the middle cerebral artery occasionally cause monoplegia or hemiplegia either through direct pressure if they are very large or through ischaemia in the distribution of their parent vessel, and this is the main situation in which an aneurysm is likely to cause convulsions. These aneurysms may also present with TIAs (p. 193). Aneurysm of the posterior part of the circle of Willis, for example the posterior communicating artery, usually causes paralysis of the third nerve and possibly hemianopia due to compression of the optic tract. An isolated third-nerve palsy is not infrequently produced by pressure from an enlarging aneurysm of the internal carotid artery above the cavernous sinus (Sengupta, Gryspeerdt, and Hankinson 1976) (a supraclinoid aneurysm—Fig. 4.4). Aneurysms in this situation rarely cause Raeder's paratrigeminal syndrome (ocular sympathetic paralysis as in Horner's

syndrome but without anhidrosis and with fifth-nerve sensory loss) (Law and Nelson 1968) or even hypopituitarism if the sella is invaded (Cartlidge and Shaw 1972). Aneurysm of the posterior cerebral artery may cause crossed hemianopia, owing to coincident thrombosis of the vessel. Aneurysm of the basilar artery (Fig. 4.5) usually causes conspicuous localizing signs early. There is often a crossed hemiplegia with paresis of some of the cranial nerves originating from the pons on one side, and of the limbs on the opposite side. Very rarely such a lesion may cause paroxysmal hypertension simulating the effects of a phaeochromocytoma (Emanuele, Dorsch, Scarff, and Lawrence 1981). A somewhat similar picture may be produced by an aneurysm of the vertebral artery which is, however, less common; aneurysms on the vertebro-basilar system can produce effects either through direct pressure or by causing ischaemia in the distribution of small arterial branches. Those of the cerebellar arteries (Fig. 4.6) rarely give localizing signs.

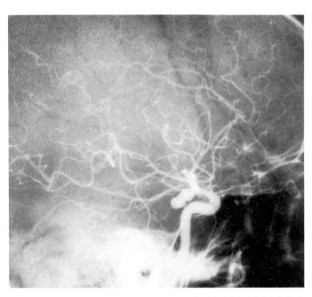

Fig. 4.4. A supraclinoid aneurysm arising at the junction of the right internal carotid and posterior communicating arteries.

Thus, while large or expanding intracranial aneurysms, and particularly those at the base of the brain (Bull 1969), may produce localizing signs due to compression of the brain, brainstem, or cranial nerves, many are asymptomatic prior to rupture. Unruptured aneurysms may develop intramural calcification which is seen on skull radiographs and some can be identified by CT scans (Weir, Miller, and Russell 1977), but angiography is necessary for diagnosis and localization (Bull 1962). Surgical treatment of large aneurysms is often difficult and may be unrewarding (see p. 212). Rupture of an aneurysm is the commonest cause of subarachnoid haemorrhage (pp. 208–12).

Embolic intracranial aneurysm

Embolic or 'mycotic' aneurysms are rare. They arise following impaction in a cerebral vessel of an embolus, bearing organisms of low virulence and are the result of infective softening of the vessel wall. More virulent organisms usually cause cerebral abscess or meningitis. The embolus usually lodges in a cortical branch of one or other middle cerebral artery, the right and left being involved with equal frequency. Less often the main trunk of the middle cerebral or the anterior cerebral artery is affected. Embolic aneurysms elsewhere in the intracranial circulation are rare. Subacute bacterial endocarditis is the commonest cause, but these

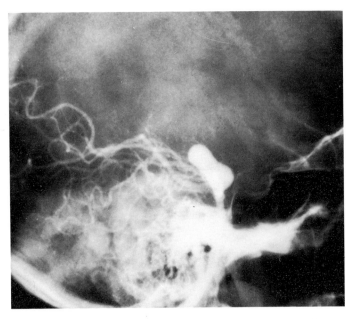

Fig. 4.5. A large aneurysm at the bifurcation of the basilar artery demonstrated by vertebral angiography.

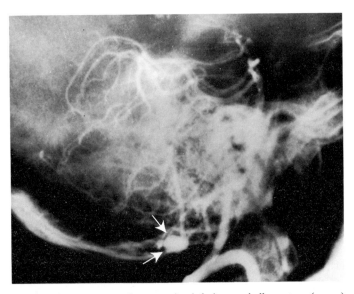

Fig. 4.6. An aneurysm of a posterior inferior cerebellar artery (arrow) shown by vertebral angiography.

aneurysms rarely result from other chronic forms of septicaemia and pyaemia, including brucellosis. Usually, the aneurysm subsequently ruptures as would a 'berry' aneurysm giving subarachnoid haemorrhage.

The initial impaction of the embolus will often have caused a 'stroke'. The signs of subacute bacterial endocarditis or of some other pyaemic source are usually evident and emboli may occur elsewhere in the body. Treatment of rupture is the same as in subarachnoid haemorrhage due to rupture of a 'berry' aneurysm but the underlying infective condition will also need treatment.

Carotico-cavernous-sinus aneurysm or fistula

Arteriovenous aneurysm produced by rupture of the internal carotid artery into the cavernous sinus may arise spontaneously or can follow head injury with or without skull fracture. Hamby (1966)

thinks that 'the majority of spontaneous fistulas develop as a result of rupture of pre-existing aneurysms'. However, some cases follow cranial trauma and in others angiography fails to reveal any predisposing cause for arterial rupture. The resulting clinical picture is distinctive, consisting of unilateral pulsating exophthalmos, with oedema of the eyelids, conjunctivae, and cornea, and sometimes papilloedema. There is a loud systolic murmur, audible to the patient and to the examiner on auscultation over the eye and temporal region, and suppressible by compression of the ipsilateral carotid artery. There is usually complete or partial ophthalmoplegia of the affected eye. The other eye may become involved, as blood at arterial pressure is carried by the circular sinus to the opposite cavernous sinus. Common carotid ligation is the method of treatment usually employed and, though not without risk is generally successful. Some few fistulae heal spontaneously.

Other causes of intracranial aneurysm

Other causes of intracranial aneurysms are extremely rare, though examples due to polyarteritis nodosa, to atheroma, and to syphilis have been described. An atheromatous aneurysm is usually a fusiform dilatation of the internal carotid or basilar artery. The characteristic syphilitic change in the small elastic and muscular arteries, such as the intracranial vessels, is an obliterative endarteritis; this explains the rarity of syphilitic intracranial aneurysm. Most verified syphilitic aneurysms have been situated upon the basilar artery; in these cases, which are now very rare, the usual treatment for syphilis is required.

Arteriovenous angioma

The pathology of these malformations was discussed in the previous chapter (pp. 149 and 170) where it was noted that these lesions commonly present with recurrent headache resembling migraine, epilepsy, or subarachnoid haemorrhage. Rarely they may be large enough to cause fatal haemorrhage or infarction in childhood (Takashima and Becker 1980), while in adult life they infrequently produce focal manifestations such as extrapyramidal manifestations (Lobo-Antunes, Yahr, and Hilal 1974); dementia, once thought to be a result of relative ischaemia due to shunting of arterial blood into the venous circulation, is, in fact, rare (Waltimo and Putkonen 1974). Lesions in the brainstem often produce a progressive but fluctuating clinical course resembling that of multiple sclerosis (Stahl, Johnson, and Malamud 1980), while those in the spinal cord may behave similarly though they also often cause spinal subarachnoid haemorrhage (Caroscio, Brannan, Budabin, Huang, and Yahr 1980). While angiography remains the single most useful diagnostic method (Stein and Wolpert 1980), some small malformations are angiographically occult (Bell, Kendall, and Symon 1978) and the CT scan with enhancement is often helpful (Leblanc and Ethier 1981).

Subarachnoid haemorrhage

Aetiology

Subarachnoid haemorrhage may occur as the result of any condition in which there is rupture of one or more blood vessels so placed that the extravasated blood reaches the subarachnoid space. The bleeding may be arterial, capillary, or venous, and its site of origin single or multiple. Head injury, including birth injury, may thus cause subarachnoid bleeding. Capillary damage leading to haemorrhage may occur in exceptionally acute forms of encephalitis or encephalopathy, and subarachnoid haemorrhage is rarely a symptom of haemorrhagic diseases or of intravascular coagulation (Heron, Hutchinson, Boyd, and Aber 1974) and may complicate anticoagulant therapy. Rarely it may be the result of septic or aseptic venous sinus thrombosis or of an intracranial tumour (angioblastic meningioma, glioma, pituitary adenoma, intracranial metastases—particularly of malignant melanoma; Walton 1956). Choroid plexus papilloma is another rare cause (Ernsting 1955). It has also been described as a result of an acute hypertensive reaction following the ingestion of cheese in a patient receiving tranylcypromine, one of the amine-oxidase inhibitor drugs (Espir and Mitchell 1963). It has been reported in so-called Moyamoya disease in Chinese patients, secondary to carotid occlusion (Lee and Cheung 1973). Intracerebral haemorrhage, due to vascular degeneration associated with high blood pressure, may reach the subarachnoid space either by rupture into the ventricular system or, more rarely, to the surface of the brain, while that due to aneurysm or angioma beginning in the subarachnoid space may also invade the brain. The chief causes of intracranial subarachnoid haemorrhage are intracranial aneurysm (see p. 206) and angioma (see p. 208), the former being nine or ten times as common as the latter. In a series of 3042 cases Richardson (1969) found an aneurysm in 1571, an angioma in 142, a primary intracerebral, cerebellar, or brainstem haemorrhage in 725, and 604 were unexplained. In a small proportion of cases no cause can be found even at autopsy; it is thought that in most such cases a tiny aneurysm may have been present but was destroyed by the force of the bleeding (Hayward 1977). Spontaneous spinal subarachnoid haemorrhage usually results from an angioma of the spinal cord (Henson and Croft 1956) or less often from a tumour such as a neurofibroma or an ependymoma of the filum terminale (Walton 1956; Nassar and Correll 1968).

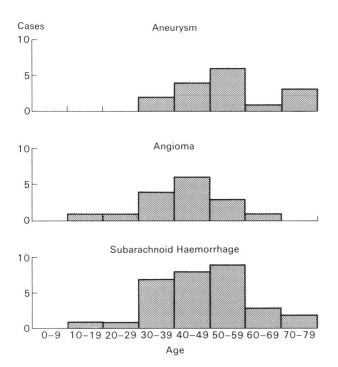

Fig. 4.7. Subarachnoid haemorrhage, angioma and aneurysm age incidence

Subarachnoid haemorrhage was found in 15 per cent of 200 patients suffering from cerebral vascular disease seen by Brain: its age incidence, and that of its two principal causes, is shown in Fig. 4.7. Females are affected slightly more than males, and about 50 per cent of the patients are normotensive. Cigarette smoking appears significantly to increase the risk of suffering such a haemorrhage in both sexes (Bell and Symon 1979), especially in patients with aneurysms (Taha, Ball, and Illingworth 1982). The incidence of the condition appears to have remained constant at 11 cases per year per 100 000 population in Rochester, Minnesota (Phillips, Whisnant, O'Fallon, and Sundt 1980).

In addition to blood in the subarachnoid space, secondary haemorrhages may occur in the brainstem, and spasm of the artery on which the aneurysm lies may lead to infarction of the part of the brain which it supplies. Infarction may also result from compression, tearing, or distortion of arteries resulting from subarachnoid haematoma formation within sulci (Tomlinson 1959) or from spasm of other intracranial arteries (Millikan 1975; Richardson 1976).

Symptoms and signs

When subarachnoid haemorrhage is due to head injury, acute encephalitis or encephalopathy, or extension of an intracerebral haemorrhage, it usually constitutes a minor part of the total clinical picture. When it is caused by an aneurysm or an angioma, it is usually the most prominent and sometimes the sole manifestation. The following account will therefore be limited to such cases.

The symptoms and signs of subarachnoid haemorrhage may be divided into: (1) those due to rapidly increasing intracranial pressure with meningeal irritation; (2) focal symptoms; (3) changes in the CSF; and (4) radiographic evidence.

1. The intensity of the symptoms of *increasing intracranial pressure* varies according to the rapidity and extent of the haemorrhage. The onset or ictus may occur during physical exertion but also during sleep and it seems likely that effort or a rise in blood pressure may simply precipitate bleeding from an aneurysm or angioma which was about to rupture spontaneously (Walton 1956). Loss of consciousness occurs rapidly when bleeding is substantial. Vomiting is common at the onset; convulsions occasionally occur. When coma is deep, the breathing is usually irregular and the pulse slow. The patient may present a picture of profound shock with generalized flaccidity and there may be no cervical rigidity. In less severe case the patient may not lose consciousness completely, but passes into a semi-stuporose state, lying in an attitude of general flexion, resenting interference, and being confused and irritable when roused. Headache is severe, and the presence of blood in the subarachnoid space produces signs of meningeal irritation, such as neck stiffness and Kernig's sign. Moderate pyrexia is common at this stage. Minor leakage of blood may, however, give only mild headache with little or no neck stiffness at first and is then difficult to detect clinically; however, one or more such episodes may occasionally presage a more severe haemorrhage.

Changes are often found in the ocular fundi. Papilloedema is sometimes present, though usually slight. Small scattered retinal haemorrhages are sometimes seen but a brick-red subhyaloid haemorrhage extending outwards from the disc margin, though uncommon, is more characteristic. This has been attributed to the passage of blood from the subarachnoid space of the optic nerves into the eye, but it is now evident that these haemorrhages occur as a result of acute compression of the central vein of the retina caused by the blood in the optic sheaths.

Other signs of subarachnoid haemorrhage include occasional diminution or loss of the tendon reflexes, and of the abdominal reflexes, and extensor plantar responses in the absence of paralysis. Albuminuria and glycosuria may occur while hyperpyrexia and severe transient arterial hypertension may result from damage to hypothalamic centres. Adipsia and hypothermia have been described (Spiro and Jenkins 1971) as well as other disturbances of hypothalamic-pituitary-adrenal function (Jenkins, Buckell, Carter, and Westlake 1969), and a delay and/or deficiency of thromboplastin generation has been reported (Uttley and Buckell 1968). A fall in CSF pH, presumed to be due to an increase in CSF lactic acid, is associated with a poor prognosis and there is often evidence of salt and water depletion (Sambrook, Hutchinson, and Aber 1973*a*, *b*). Changes in the ECG are common, including peaking of the P and T waves, a short PR interval, a long Q-Tc and tall U waves, and have been shown to be associated with increased urinary catecholamine excretion; excess catecholamine production may also be associated with the arterial spasm often found in subarachnoid haemorrhage (Cruickshank, Neil-Dwyer, and Brice 1974). Myocardial lesions found in such cases at autopsy have been attributed, like hypothalamic lesions, to increased sympathetic activity (Doshi and Neil-Dwyer 1977) and it has been suggested that these complications might be prevented by adrenergic blockade (*British Medical Journal* 1981; Walter, Neil-Dwyer, and Cruickshank 1982). The blood leucocyte count is often raised and a persistent rise in the WBCs to above 10 000/mm³ is associated with a less good prognosis (Neil-Dwyer and Cruickshank 1974).

2. *Focal symptoms and signs* are due to compression of neighbouring cranial nerves by blood clot or to invasion of brain substance by the haemorrhage or to infarction. Visual-field defects may occur as a result of compression of the optic nerves, chiasm, or tracts. The third, fourth, and sixth cranial nerves are likely to be compressed if an aneurysm is near the cavernous sinus. Haemorrhage from an aneurysm at the junction of the anterior cerebral and anterior communicating arteries is apt to invade the frontal lobe and may cause mental impairment, incontinence or, less commonly, urinary retention (Andrew 1966), hemiparesis, and, if on the left side, expressive aphasia. Leakage from an aneurysm on the cortical course of the middle cerebral may cause epileptiform convulsions, and a monoplegia; and rupture of an aneurysm on the cortical course of the posterior cerebral may cause a crossed homonymous hemianopia as a result of haemorrhage into the substance of the occipital lobe or thrombosis of the artery. Leakage from an aneurysm of the basilar artery may lead to quadriplegia or to one of the various forms of 'crossed paralysis'; and neck stiffness is likely to be particularly severe when the haemorrhage comes from an aneurysm in the posterior fossa.

Haemorrhage from an intracranial angioma may pass into the neighbouring brain tissue, or into the subarachnoid space, or both. Subarachnoid haemorrhage seems more likely to arise from a small cortical angioma which has given rise to no other symptoms than from the massive malformations which extend widely and deeply into the white matter. Herpes zoster is an occasional sequel of subarachnoid bleeding.

Spinal subarachnoid haemorrhage usually begins with pain in the back and lower limbs and sphincter disturbances, with rigidity of the spine and Kernig's sign. Later there may be flaccid weakness of the lower limbs with sensory loss and loss of reflexes, depending upon the degree of damage to the cord and/or cauda equina which results. Extension of the haemorrhage to the cerebral subarachnoid space causes headache, cervical rigidity, and other symptoms of intracranial bleeding.

3. *The cerebrospinal fluid.* Subarachnoid haemorrhage causes characteristic changes in the CSF, the pressure of which is raised at first. In the first week or more red cells are present, and the supernatant fluid exhibits a yellow coloration which persists for from two to three weeks. The faint coloration which appears within 4–6 hours is due to oxyhaemoglobin, while bilirubin first appears within 36–48 hours (Barrows, Hunter, and Banker 1955; Roost, Pimstone, Diamond, and Schmid 1972). The protein con-

tent of the fluid is raised, though rarely above 1.0 g/l. Irrigation of the meninges by the extravasated blood leads to a pleocytosis consisting usually of mononuclear cells, though rarely polymorphs may be present when the substance of the brain has been invaded. In some cases the colloidal gold curve is 'paretic' in type after a severe haemorrhage. Red cells may disappear from the fluid within a few days but may persist, with xanthochromia, depending upon the severity of the haemorrhage, for as long as 4–6 weeks (Walton 1956). Metabolic acidosis in the fluid due to presence of red cells (Shannon, Shore, and Kazemi 1972; Sambrook *et al* 1973*a*) may cause systemic respiratory alkalosis and altered consciousness. There is evidence that an as yet unidentified substance (which may contribute to arterial spasm and thus to infarction) is present in the fluid after subarachnoid bleeding (Boullin, Mohan, and Grahame-Smith 1976; Hunt, du Boulay, Blaso, Forster, and Boullin 1979).

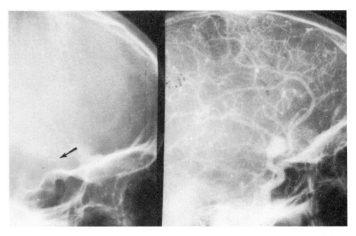

Fig. 4.8. A lateral radiograph of skull (left) showing curvilinear calcification in the wall of an aneurysm of one middle cerebral artery later demonstrated by angiography (on the right).

4. *Radiology.* Plain X-rays rarely show evidence of the source of a subarachnoid haemorrhage, though there may be X-ray signs of an angioma (see p. 79) or very rarely an aneurysm may show calcification in its wall (Fig. 4.8). Angiography is usually obligatory in such cases unless the patient's level of consciousness, age, general condition, or neurological status would make surgery impracticable even if the causal lesion were demonstrated. Martindale and Garfield (1978) have suggested that full investigation is rarely justified after the age of 59 years, but this view is not generally accepted and each patient must be assessed individually. Except in the comatose patient, therefore, bilateral carotid arteriography should be performed as soon as possible after the ictus and if this fails to demonstrate an aneurysm or angioma, vertebral angiography is then indicated. Even if an aneurysm on one carotid tree is shown, it is still wise to visualize the vertebrobasilar system, depending upon the condition of the patient, as many individuals have multiple aneurysms. When multiple lesions are shown, the presence of arterial spasm may be a valuable guide in indicating which has bled, but this is not always possible and the EEG, though relatively imprecise, may help (Binnie, Margerison, and McCaul 1969). Even with improved radiological techniques, including the use of oblique views, magnification, and image intensification, in about 20 per cent of cases no causal lesion is demonstrated though some of these later prove to have aneurysms at autopsy (Richardson 1969). The CT scan is often useful in demonstrating focal collections of blood over the brain surface which may give a clue to the location of the bleeding point and in estimating the amount of blood in the basal CSF cisterns as this can be correlated with outcome (Bell,

Kendall, and Symon 1980); the noninvasive measurement of vasospasm by measuring regional cerebral blood flow with the ^{133}xenon inhalation technique has also been found useful in planning management and in assessing prognosis (Yamamoto, Meyer, Naritomi, Sakai, Yamaguchi, and Shaw 1979). Spinalcord angiography (Djindjian, Merland, Djindjian, and Stoeter 1981), the whole-body CT scan and myelography are most useful in the diagnosis of spinal-cord lesions causing haemorrhage.

Diagnosis

The essence of the clinical picture of subarachnoid haemorrhage is the acute or subacute onset of symptoms of meningeal irritation associated with the presence of blood in the CSF demonstrated by lumbar puncture. To this extent the diagnosis is usually easy. Meningitis rarely comes on so acutely, and is readily distinguished by examination of the fluid. A lumbar puncture, again, usually enables subarachnoid haemorrhage to be distinguished from other conditions causing coma. But the presence of subarachnoid haemorrhage having been established, it is still necessary to decide its origin. Subarachnoid bleeding is occasionally found in exceptionally acute forms of encephalitis, but in such cases the blood is present only in small amounts, and there is evidence of diffuse disease of the nervous system. Traumatic subarachnoid haemorrhage is usually easily recognized through the history. Intracerebral haemorrhage, due to vascular degeneration associated with hypertension, may reach the subarachnoid space either by rupture into the ventricular system, or, more rarely, to the surface of the brain. Such patients usually exhibit hemiplegia, which is less common in subarachnoid haemorrhage from intracranial aneurysm, and hypertension and arterial degeneration which are not necessarily associated with it. When, however, an aneurysm bleeds both into the subarachnoid space and into the substance of one hemisphere, the clinical picture may be indistinguishable from that of a primary intracerebral haemorrhage which has ruptured into the ventricle. In such a case angiography will often settle the diagnosis by demonstrating the presence, or absence, of an aneurysm. Rupture of a mycotic aneurysm may give a clinical picture indistinguishable from that which occurs when a 'berry' aneurysm has caused the haemorrhage. The former, however, is usually associated with subacute bacterial endocarditis, and its embolic origin is often indicated by the sudden development of hemiplegia some time before. An angioma is a much less common cause of subarachnoid haemorrhage than an aneurysm; there may be a cranial bruit and angiography will again be diagnostic. The possibility of the rarer causes mentioned on pages 208–9 should also be considered. Finally, in 10–20 per cent of all cases, the source of the haemorrhage is not found, however thorough the investigation.

Prognosis

The prognosis of subarachnoid haemorrhage depends upon many factors such as the size and site of the bleeding, whether it can be found and treated surgically, the age of the patient, and the condition of the cardiovascular system, especially the presence or absence of hypertension and cerebral atherosclerosis.

In an analysis of 312 personal cases not treated surgically, Walton (1956) found a mortality of 45 per cent in the first 8 weeks; about 15 per cent of patients died within the first 48 hours, 15 per cent within 7–14 days as a result of the initial haemorrhage, and 15 per cent from recurrent bleeding with a peak incidence in the second week. About 20 per cent of those who survived for 8 weeks died later of recurrent bleeding, half within the first 6 months; of the survivors most were able to pursue some useful activity but about a third were disabled by hemiplegia, epilepsy, headache, or severe neurotic symptoms and fear of recurrence. A more recent survey of 364 patients not treated surgically (Winn, Richardson, and Jane 1977; Winn, Richardson, O'Brien,

and Jane 1978) gave similar results with a rebleeding rate after six months in the survivors of 3.5 per cent per year over the first decade and an enhanced mortality of 67 per cent in recurrent haemorrhage. In general the immediate prognosis of angiomal bleeding is better than that of aneurysmal rupture as many angiomas tend to bleed little and often, except for small angiomas in children which may cause a fatal intracerebral haematoma (Henderson and Gomez 1967). Sahs *et al.* (1969), in a national cooperative study in the USA, found that the prognosis was adversely influenced by increasing age, hypertension, the presence of hemiplegia or other focal neurological signs indicating bleeding into the brain or concomitant infarction, and loss of consciousnesss. They and Alvord, Loeser, Bailey, and Copass (1972) found that a method of clinical grading of cases was useful in predicting outcome; thus patients in coma or semicoma consistently did worse, as did those subjected to angiography or surgery too early when vasospasm was often severe and widespread (Weir, Rothberg, Grace, and Davis 1975). Thus it is generally unwise to operate upon a comatose patient except in order to remove an intracerebral haematoma and the time of operation must be carefully judged in each case; if the aneurysm is accessible it is often best to operate (see below) at about 7–10 days when vasospasm is diminishing and if possible before the period when the risk of recurrent bleeding is at its peak. There is no doubt that surgical treatment improves prognosis and lessens the risk of recurrent bleeding (Kaste and Troupp 1978).

A rare complication of chronic or recurrent subarachnoid bleeding is superficial haemosiderosis of the nervous system causing deafness, dementia, cerebellar ataxia, and other progressive neurological signs (Tomlinson and Walton 1964; Hughes and Oppenheimer 1967).

Treatment

In treating subarachnoid haemorrhage it is necessary first to relieve headache with appropriate analgesics such as pethidine (demerol) 100 mg by mouth or injection as required, and often combined with phenothiazine drugs such as chlorpromazine 50 mg or haloperidol 1–2 mg, which have the effect of sedating the patient while at the same time reducing body temperature, transient hypertension, and cerebral metabolism. Unconscious patients should be treated in the usual way antibiotics are often needed to prevent respiratory infection, catheterization may be required, and the airway must be kept patent, but it is rarely, if ever, justifiable to begin assisted respiration if spontaneous breathing ceases as this usually implies irreversible brainstem damage. Induced hypotension and/or hypothermia had a vogue but are no longer widely employed because of the risk of infarction (Walton 1956). However, it has been suggested that epsilonaminocaproic acid (EACA) (0.1 g/kg body weight by mouth or intravenous infusion every four hours) may reduce the risk of recurrent bleeding by inhibiting fibrinolysis (*Today's Drugs* 1967); tranexamic acid (AMCA) (15–20 mg/kg four hourly in an intravenous infusion) seems to be even more effective (Andersson, Nilsson, Nilehn, Hedner, Granstrand, and Melander 1965; Melander, Gliniecki, Granstrand, and Hanshoff 1965; Tovi, Nilsson, and Thulin 1972). Chandra (1978) found in a double-blind trial that AMCA 6 g daily reduced mortality and rebleeding, while Chowdhary, Carey, and Hussein (1979) found that EACA was particularly useful in reducing early recurrent haemorrhage. In yet further trials, Chowdhary and Sayed (1981) concluded that EACA and tranexamic acid were equally effective, but the results achieved by Ramirez-Lassepas (1981) and Ameen and Illingworth (1981) were less conclusive and there was a suggestion that ischaemic infarction might possibly be increased by the use of these remedies. Furthermore EACA produces rarely a severe necrotizing myopathy (Mastaglia and Argov 1981); nevertheless, this drug and AMCA are widely used in preparing patients for surgery or in patients deemed unsuitable for surgical treatment. Surviving patients, depending upon their disability, often require speech therapy, physiotherapy, and occupational therapy; epilepsy will require appropriate anticonvulsant drugs.

Although it has proved difficult to compare directly the results of surgical treatment of ruptured aneurysms with those of conservative management (Walton 1956; McKissock and Paine 1959), a vast literature has accumulated which indicates without reasonable doubt that, whereas surgical treatment carries an appreciable mortality and morbidity, the prognosis of the condition is considerably improved by the judicious use of operative treatment (Kaste and Troupp 1978). Carotid ligation or temporary clamping of the vessel (Atkinson 1975) is often employed in the management of aneurysms on the internal carotid artery (McKissock and Walsh 1956) but in the acute phase it carries a considerable risk of infarction and may not prevent further bleeding (McKissock, Richardson, and Walsh 1960; Sahs, Perret, Locksley, and Nishioka 1969). Nevertheless, in selected cases unsuitable for intracranial attack, it is still of value provided the cerebral blood flow is monitored before and during the operation (Jennett, Miller, and Harper 1976); the risk of post-operative epilepsy is much less after this procedure than after intracranial operation (Cabral, King, and Scott 1976). Cerebral blood flow studies are also useful in predicting outcome after surgery (Merory, Thomas, Humphrey, du Boulay, Marshall, Ross Russell, Symon, and Zilkha 1980); those patients without a significant post-operative rise in CBF do less well.

The intracranial operation most commonly employed is clipping of the neck of the aneurysm (Paterson 1968) or trapping of it between two clips when the parent vessel can safely be ligated; the use of the operating microscope and of techniques of microneurosurgery (Adams, Loach, and O'Laoire 1976) has greatly improved the results, as have advances in neuroanaesthesia, including the use of controlled hypothermia. Even giant aneurysms can often be treated successfully by various techniques including the induction of intramural thrombosis, aneurysmorrhaphy, or even excision followed by anastomosis of the parent vessel (Hosobuchi 1979). Many other surgical techniques have been used including investment of the aneurysm with plastic (Dutton 1959). The results are somewhat better in aneurysms on the internal carotid and middle cerebral arteries (McKissock, Richardson, and Walsh 1962) than in those in the region of the anterior communicating (Fig. 4.9), and some aneurysms on the vertebral, basilar, and cerebellar vessels can be treated successfully (Dimsdale and Logue 1959; Drake 1968); however, satisfactory results have also been reported with anterior communicating aneurysms (Logue 1956; Sengupta 1975).

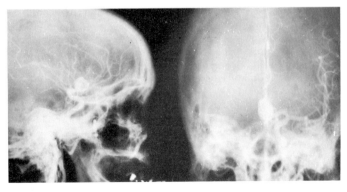

Fig. 4.9. An aneurysm of the anterior communicating artery.

Some arteriovenous angiomas can be removed, if small and situated in comparatively 'silent' areas of the brain (Paterson and McKissock 1956); very rarely these lesions may resolve sponta-

neously (Levine, Misko, Seres, and Snodgrass 1973), presumably due to thrombosis. With improving neurosurgical technique, some larger angiomas may now be excised; ligation of major feeding vessels is less successful and radiotherapy ineffective. Therapeutic embolization with silicone spheres, Gelfoam fragments, or rapidly solidifying liquids (Kendall and Moseley 1977) has also proved successful, especially in preparing the patient for subsequent surgical excision (Stein and Wolpert 1980).

References

Acosta-Rua, G. J. (1978). Familial incidence of ruptured intracranial aneurysms. *Arch. Neurol, Chicago* **35**, 675.

Adams, C. B. T., Loach, A. B., and O'Laoire, S. A. (1976). Intracranial aneurysms: analysis of results of microneurosurgery. *Br. med. J.* **2**, 607.

Alvord, F. C., Loeser, J. D., Bailey, W. L., and Copass, M. K. (1972). Subarachnoid haemorrhage due to ruptured aneurysms. A simple method of estimating prognosis. *Arch. Neurol., Chicaco* **27**, 273.

Ameen, A. A. and Illingworth, R. (1981). Anti-fibrinolytic treatment in the pre-operative management of subarachnoid haemorrhage caused by ruptured intracranial aneurysm. *J. Neurol. Neurosurg. Psychiat.* **44**, 220.

Andersson, L., Nilsson, I. M., Nilehn, J. E., Hedner, U., Granstrand, B., and Melander, B. (1965). Experimental and clinical studies on AMCA, the antifibrinolytically active isomer of p-aminomethyl cyclohexane carboxylic acid. *Scand. J. Haematol.* **2**, 230.

Andrew, J., Nathan, P. W., and Spanos, N. C. (1966). Disturbances of micturition and defaecation due to aneurysms of anterior communicating or anterior cerebral arteries. *J. Neurosurg.* **24**, 1.

Atkinson, W. J. (1975). New approach to management of intracranial aneurysms. *Lancet* **i**, 5.

Bannerman, R. M., Ingall, G. B., and Graf, C. J. (1970). The familial occurrence of intracranial aneurysms. *Neurology, Minneapolis* **20**, 283.

Barr, H. W. K., Blackwood, W., and Meadows, S. P. (1971). Intracavernous carotid aneurysms. A clinical-pathological report. *Brain* **94**, 607.

Barrows, L., Hunter, T., and Banker, B. (1955). The nature and clinical significance of pigments in cerebrospinal fluid. *Brain* **78**, 59.

Bell, B. A. and Symon, L. (1979). Smoking and subarachnoid haemorrhage. *Br. med. J.* **1**, 577.

——, Kendall, B. E., and Symon, L. (1978). Angiographically occult arteriovenous malformations of the brain. *J. Neurol. Neurosurg. Psychiat.* **41**, 1057.

——, ——, and —— (1980). Computed tomography in aneurysmal subarachnoid haemorrhage. *J. Neurol. Neurosurg. Psychiat.* **43**, 522.

Beumont, P. J. V. (1968). The familial occurrence of berry aneurysm. *J. Neurol. Neurosurg. Psychiat.* **31**, 399.

Binnie, C. D., Margerison, J. H., and McCaul, I.R. (1969). Electroencephalographic localization of ruptured intracranial aneurysms. *Brain* **92**, 679.

Boullin, D. J., Mohan, J., and Grahame-Smith, D. G. (1976). Evidence for the presence of a vasoactive substance (possibly involved in the aetiology of cerebral arterial spasm) in cerebrospinal fluid from patients with subarachnoid haemorrhage. *J. Neurol. Neurosurg. Psychiat.* **39**, 756.

British Medical Journal (1981). Subarachnoid haemorrhage. *Br. med. J.* **283**, 1347.

Bull, J. W. D. (1962). Contribution of radiology to the study of intracranial aneurysms. *Br. med. J.* **2**, 1701.

—— (1969). Massive aneurysms at the base of the brain. *Brain* **92**, 535.

Cabral, R. J., King, T. T., and Scott, D. F. (1976). Epilepsy after two different neurosurgical approaches to the treatment of ruptured intracranial aneurysm. *J. Neurol. Neurosurg. Psychiat.* **39**, 1052.

Carmichael, R. (1950). The pathogenesis of non-inflammatory cerebral aneurysms. *J. Path. Bact.* **62**, 1.

Caroscio, J. T., Brannan, T., Budabin, M., Huang, Y. P., and Yahr, M. D. (1980). Subarachnoid hemorrhage secondary to spinal arteriovenous malformation and aneurysm: report of a case and review of the literature. *Arch. Neurol, Chicago* **37**, 101.

Cartlidge, N. E. F. and Shaw, D. A. (1972). Intrasellar aneurysm with subarachnoid hemorrhage and hypopituitarism: case report. *J. Neurosurg.* **36**, 640.

Chandra, B. (1978). Treatment of subarachnoid hemorrhage from ruptured intracranial aneurysm with tranexamic acid: a double-blind clinical trial. *Ann. Neurol.* **3**, 502.

Chowdhary, U. M. and Sayed, K. (1981). Comparative clinical trial of epsilon amino-caproic acid and tranexamic acid in the prevention of early recurrence of subarachnoid haemorrhage. *J. Neurol. Neurosurg. Psychiat.* **44**, 810.

——, Carey, P. C., and Hussein, M. M. (1979). Prevention of early recurrence of spontaneous subarachnoid haemorrhage by ε-aminocaproic acid. *Lancet* **9**, 741.

Clarke, E. and Walton, J. N. (1953). Subdural haematoma complicating intracranial aneurysm and angioma. *Brain* **76**, 378.

Crompton, M. R. (1963). Hypothalamic lesions after rupture of cerebral aneurysms. *Brain* **86**, 301.

—— (1964a). Cerebral infarction following the rupture of cerebral berry aneurysms. *Brain* **87**, 263.

—— (1964b). The pathogenesis of cerebral infarction following the rupture of cerebral berry aneurysms. *Brain* **87**, 491.

Cruickshank, J. M., Neil-Dwyer, G., and Brice, J. (1974). Electrocardiographic changes and their prognostic significance in subarachnoid haemorrhage. *J. Neurol. Neurosurg. Psychiat.* **37**, 755.

Dandy, W. E. (1944). *Intracranial arterial aneurysms.* Comstock Publishing Company, Ithaca, New York.

Dimsdale, H. and Logue, V. (1959). Ruptured posterior fossa aneurysms and their surgical treatment. *J. Neurol. Neurosurg. Psychiat.* **22**, 202.

Djindjian, R., Merland, J.-J., Djindjian, M., and Stoeter, P. (1981). *Angiography of spinal column and spinal cord tumors.* Georg Thieme, Stuttgart.

Doshi, R. and Neil-Dwyer, G. (1977). Hypothalamic and myocardial lesions after subarachnoid haemorrhage. *J. Neurol. Neurosurg. Psychiat.* **40**, 821.

Drake, C. G. (1968). The surgical treatment of aneurysms of the basilar artery. *J. Neurosurg.* **29**, 436.

Dutton, J. (1959). Acrylic investment of intracranial aneurysms. *Br. med. J.* **2**, 597.

Emanuele, M. A., Dorsch, T. R., Scraff, T. B., and Lawrence, A. M. (1981). Basilar artery aneurysm simulating pheochromocytoma. *Neurology, Minneapolis* **31**, 1560.

Ernsting, J. (1955). Choroid plexus papilloma causing spontaneous subarachnoid haemorrhage. *J. Neurol. Neurosurg. Psychiat.* **18**, 134.

Espir, M. L. E. and Mitchell, L. (1963). Tranylcypromine and intracranial haemorrhage. *Lancet* **ii**, 639.

Fairburn, B. (1973). 'Twin' intracranial aneurysms causing subarachnoid haemorrhage in identical twins. *Br. med. J.* **1**, 210.

Falconer, M. A. (1951). The surgical treatment of bleeding intracranial aneurysms. *J. Neurol. Neurosurg. Psychiat.* **14**, 153.

Fearnsides, E. G. (1916). Intracranial aneurysms. *Brain* **39**, 224.

Forbus, W. D. (1930). On the origin of miliary aneurysms of the superficial cerebral arteries. *Bull. Johns Hopkins Hosp.* **47**, 239.

Hamby, W. B. (1966). *Carotid-cavernous fistula.* Thomas, Springfield, Illinois.

Hayward, R. D. (1977). Subarachnoid haemorrhage of unknown aetiology. *J. Neurol. Neurosurg. Psychiat.* **40**, 926.

Henderson, W. R. and Gomez, R. de R. L. (1967). Natural history of cerebral angiomas. *Br. med. J.* **4**, 571.

Henson, R. A. and Croft, P. B. (1956). Spontaneous spinal subarachnoid haemorrhage. *Quart. J. Med.* **25**, 53.

Heron, J. R., Hutchinson, E. C., Boyd, W. N., and Aber, G. M. (1974). Pregnancy, subarachnoid haemorrhage, and the intravascular coagulation syndrome. *J. Neurol. Neurosurg. Psychiat.* **37**, 521.

Hosobuchi, Y. (1979). Direct surgical treatment of giant intracranial aneurysms. *J. Neurosurg.* **51**, 743.

Hughes, J. T. and Oppenheimer, D. R. (1967). Superficial siderosis of the central nervous system: a report on nine cases with autopsy. *Acta neuropath., Berlin* **13**, 56.

Hunt, T. M., du Boulay, G. H., Blaso, W. P., Forster, D. M. C., and Boullin, D. J. (1979). Relationship between presence of vasoconstrictor activity in cerebrospinal fluid and time after subarachnoid haemorrhage from rupture of cerebral arterial aneurysms. *J. Neurol. Neurosurg. Psychiat.* **42**, 625.

Jefferson, G. (1937). Compression of the chiasma, optic nerves and optic tracts by intracranial aneurysms. *Brain* **60**, 444.

—— (1938). On the saccular aneurysms of the internal carotid artery in the cavernous sinus. *Br. J. Surg.* **26**, 267.

Jenkins, J. S., Buckell, M., Carter, A. B., and Westlake, S. (1969).

Hypothalamic–pituitary–adrenal function after subarachnoid haemorrhage. *Br. med. J.* **4**, 707.

Jennett, W. B., Miller, J. D., and Harper, A. M. (1976). *Effect of carotid artery surgery on cerebral blood-flow.* Excerpta Medica, Amsterdam.

Kaste, M. and Troupp, H. (1978). Subarachnoid haemorrhage: long-term follow-up results of late surgical versus conservative treatment. *Br. med. J.* **1**, 1310.

Kendall, B. and Moseley, I. (1977). Therapeutic embolisation of the external carotid arterial tree. *J. Neurol. Neurosurg. Psychiat.* **40**, 937.

Law, W. R. and Nelson, E. R. (1968). Internal carotid aneurysm as a cause of Raeder's paratrigeminal syndrome. *Neurology, Minneapolis* **18**, 43.

Leblanc, R. and Ethier, R. (1981). The computerized tomographic appearance of angiographically occult arteriovenous malformations of the brain. *Can. J. neurol. Sci.* **8**, 7.

Lee, M. L. K. and Cheung, E. M. T. (1973). Moyamoya disease as a cause of subarachnoid haemorrhage in Chinese. *Brain* **96**, 623.

Levine, J., Misko, J. C., Seres, J. L., and Snodgrass, R. G. (1973). Spontaneous angiographic disappearance of a cerebral arteriovenous malformation: third reported case. *Arch. Neurol., Chicago* **28**, 195.

Lobo-Antunes, J., Yahr, M. D., and Hilal, S. K. (1974). Extrapyramidal dysfunction with cerebral arteriovenous malformations. *J. Neurol. Neurosurg. Psychiat.* **37**, 259.

Logue, V. (1956). Surgery in spontaneous subarachnoid haemorrhage. Operative treatment of aneurysms on the anterior cerebral and anterior communicating artery. *Br. med. J.* **1**, 473.

Martindale, B. V. and Garfield, J. (1978). Subarachnoid haemorrhage above the age of 59: are intracranial investigations justified? *Br. med. J.* **1**, 465.

Mastaglia, F. L. and Argov, Z. (1981). Drug-induced neuromuscular disorders in man. In *Disorders of voluntary muscle*, 4th edn. (ed. J. N. Walton). Chapter 25. Churchill Livingstone, Edinburgh.

McKissock, W. and Paine, K. W. E. (1959). Subarachnoid haemorrhage. *Brain* **82**, 356.

——, Richardson, A., and Walsh, L. (1960). Posterior communicating aneurysms. *Lancet* **ii**, 1203.

——, ——, and —— (1962). Middle cerebral aneurysms. *Lancet* **ii**, 417.

—— and Walsh, L. (1956). Subarachnoid haemorrhage due to intracranial aneurysms: results of treatment of 249 verified cases. *Br. med. J.* **2**, 559.

Melander, B., Gliniecki, G., Granstrand, B., and Hanshoff, G. (1965). Biochemistry and toxicology of Amikapron, the antifibrinolytically active isomer of AMCHA (a comparative study with ε-aminocaproic acid). *Acta pharmacol. toxicol.* **22**, 340.

Merory, J., Thomas, D. J., Humphrey, P. R. D., du Boulay, G. H., Marshall, J., Ross Russell, R. W., Symon, L., and Zilkha, E. (1980). Cerebral blood flow after surgery for recent subarachnoid haemorrhage. *J. Neurol. Neurosurg. Psychiat.* **43**, 214.

Millikan, C. H. (1975). Cerebral vasospasm and ruptured intracranial aneurysm. *Arch. Neurol., Chicago* **32**, 433.

Nassar, S. I. and Correll, J. W. (1968). Subarachnoid hemorrhage due to spinal cord tumors. *Neurology, Minneapolis* **18**, 87.

Neil-Dwyer, G. and Cruickshank, J. (1974). The blood leucocyte count and its prognostic significance in subarachnoid haemorrhage. *Brain* **97**, 79.

Paterson, A. (1968). Direct surgery in the treatment of posterior communicating aneurysms. *Lancet* **ii**, 808.

Peiris, J. B. and Ross Russell, R. W. (1980). Giant aneurysms of the carotid system presenting as visual field defect. *J. Neurol. Neurosurg. Psychiat.* **43**, 1053.

Phillips, L. H., Whisnant, J. P., O'Fallon, W. M., and Sundt, T. M. (1980). The unchanging pattern of subarachnoid hemorrhage in a community. *Neurology, Minneapolis* **30**, 1034.

Ramirez-Lassepas, M. (1981). Antifibrinolytic therapy in subarachnoid hemorrhage caused by ruptured intracranial aneurysm. *Neurology, Minneapolis* **31**, 316.

Richardson, A. (1969). Subarachnoid haemorrhage. *Br. med. J.* **4**, 89.

Richardson, J. T. E. (1976). Arterial spasm and recovery from subarachnoid haemorrhage. *J. Neurol. Neurosurg. Psychiat.* **39**, 1134.

Riddoch, G. and Goulden, C. (1925). On the relationship between subarachnoid and intraocular haemorrhage. *Br. J. Ophthal.* **9**, 209.

Roost, K. T., Pimstone, N. R., Diamond, I., and Schmid, R. (1972). The formation of cerebrospinal fluid xanthochromia after subarachnoid haemorrhage. Enzymatic conversion of hemoglobin to bilirubin by the arachnoid and choroid plexus. *Neurology, Minneapolis* **22**, 973.

Sahs, A. L., Perret, G. E., Locksley, H. B., and Nishioka, H. (1969). *Intracranial aneurysms and subarachnoid hemorrhage. A co-operative study*, p. 296. Lippincott, Philadelphia.

Sambrook, M. A., Hutchinson, E. C., and Aber, G. M. (1973*a*). Metabolic studies in subarachnoid haemorrhage and strokes. I. Serial changes in acid-base values in blood and cerebrospinal fluid. *Brain* **96**, 171.

——, ——, and —— (1973*b*). Metabolic studies in subarachnoid haemorrhage and strokes. II. Serial changes in cerebrospinal fluid and plasma urea, electrolytes and osmolality. *Brain* **96**, 191.

Sengupta, R. P. (1975). Quality of survival following direct surgery of anterior communicating aneurysms. *J. Neurosurg.* **43**, 58.

——, Gryspeerdt, G. L., and Hankinson, J. (1976). Carotid-ophthalmic aneurysms. *J. Neurol. Neurosurg. Psychiat* **39**, 837.

Shannon, D. C., Shore, N., and Kazemi, H. (1972). Acid–base balance in hemorrhagic cerebrospinal fluid. *Neurology, Minneapolis* **22**, 585.

Spiro, S. G. and Jenkins, J. S. (1971). Adipsia and hypothermia after subarachnoid haemorrhage. *Br. med. J.* **3**, 411.

Stahl, S. M., Johnson, K. P., and Malamud, N. (1980). The clinical and pathological spectrum of brainstem vascular malformations: long-term course simulates multiple sclerosis. *Arch. Neurol, Chicago* **37**, 25.

Stein, B. M. and Wolpert, S. M. (1980). Arteriovenous malformations of the brain: current concepts and treatment. *Arch. Neurol, Chicago* **37**, 1, 69.

Symonds, C. P. (1924–5). Spontaneous subarachnoid haemorrhage. *Quart. J. Med.* **18**, 93.

Taha, A., Ball, K. P., and Illingworth, R. D. (1982). Smoking and subarachnoid haemorrhage. *J. R. Soc. Med.* **75**, 332.

Takashima, S. and Becker, L. E. (1980). Neuropathology of cerebral arteriovenous malformations in children. *J. Neurol. Neurosurg. Psychiat.* **43**, 380.

Thompson, R. A. and Pribram, H. F. W. (1969). Infantile cerebral aneurysm associated with ophthalmoplegia and quadriparesis. *Neurology, Minneapolis* **19**, 785.

Today's Drugs (1967). Epsilon aminocaproic acid. *Br. med. J.* **4**, 725.

Tomlinson, B. E. (1959). Brain changes in ruptured intracranial aneurysm. *J. clin. Pathol.* **12**, 391.

—— and Walton, J. N. (1964). Superficial haemosiderosis of the central nervous system. *J. Neurol. Neurosurg. Psychiat.* **27**, 332.

Tovi, D., Nilsson, I. M., and Thulin, C. A. (1972). Fibrinolysis and subarachnoid haemorrhage. Inhibitory effect of tranexamic acid. *Acta neurol. scand.* **48**, 393.

Turnbull, H. M. (1914–15). Alterations in arterial structure, and their relation to syphilis. *Quart. J. Med.* **8**, 201.

Uttley, A. H. C. and Buckell, M. (1968). Biochemical changes after spontaneous subarachnoid haemorrhage. Coagulation and lysis with special reference to recurrent haemorrhage. *J. Neurol. Neurosurg. Psychiat.* **31**, 621.

Walter, P., Neil-Dwyer, G., and Cruickshank, J. M. (1982). Beneficial effects of adrenergic blockade in patients with subarachnoid haemorrhage. *Br. med. J.* **284**, 1661.

Waltimo, O. and Putkonen, A.-R. (1974). Intellectual performance of patients with intracranial arteriovenous malformations. *Brain* **97**, 511.

Walton, J. N. (1956). *Subarachnoid haemorrhage*. Livingstone, Edinburgh.

Wechsler, I. S., Gross, S. W., and Cohen, I. (1951). Arteriography and carotid artery ligation in intracranial aneurysm and vascular malformation. *J. Neurol. Neurosurg. Psychiat.* **14**, 25.

Weir, B., Miller, J., and Russell, D. (1977). Intracranial aneurysms: a clinical, angiographic and computerized tomographic study. *Can. J. neurol. Sci.* **4**, 99.

——, Rothberg, C., Grace, M., and Davis, F. (1975). Relative prognostic significance of vasospasm following subarachnoid hemorrhage. *Can. J. neurol. Sci.* **2**, 109.

Winn, H. R., Richardson, A. E., and Jane, J. A. (1977). The long-term prognosis in untreated cerebral aneurysms: I. The incidence of late hemorrhage in cerebral aneurysm: a 10-year evaluation of 364 patients. *Ann. Neurol.* **1**, 358.

——, ——, O'Brien, W., and Jane, J. A. (1978). The long-term prognosis in untreated cerebral aneurysms: II. Late morbidity and mortality. *Ann. Neurol.* **4**, 418.

Yamamoto, M., Meyer, J., Naritomi, H., Sakai, F., Yamaguchi, F., and

Shaw, T. (1979). Noninvasive measurement of cerebral vasospasm in patients with subarachnoid hemorrhage. *J. neurol. Sci.* **43**, 301.

Zacks, D. J. (1978). Multiple intracranial aneurysms. *Am. J. Roentgenol* **130**, 180.

——, Russell, D. B., and Miller, J. D. R. (1980). Fortuitously discovered intracranial aneurysms. *Arch. Neurol., Chicago* **37**, 39.

Cerebral haemorrhage

Aetiology and pathology

Intracranial haemorrhage may be venous, capillary, or arterial. Bleeding from ruptured veins traversing the subdural space is the usual cause of subdural haematoma (p. 231) which generally follows trauma to the head, though it sometimes develops spontaneously, especially in patients with liver disease or in those receiving anticoagulants. We are concerned here with haemorrhage into the brain substance; bleeding from venous sources is rare but may occur in pyaemia (Alpers and Gaskill 1944) or in venous sinus thrombosis (p. 223). Capillary or petechial haemorrhages are found in toxic and infective conditions, such as acute encephalitis, septicaemia, severe anaemia, leukaemia, and thrombocytopenic purpura. Acute brain purpura due to anaphylaxis or to other acute hypersensitivity reactions is similar. In such cases, however, the haemorrhages are small and focal and of little clinical relevance. Even in hereditary haemorrhagic telangiectasia, intracerebral haemorrhage is rare, other than from an associated arteriovenous angioma (Adams, Subbiah, and Bosch 1977). Haemorrhage may occur into a cerebral tumour, for example a glioma; bleeding from an angioma is common, either into the substance of the brain or into the subarachnoid space. Severe trauma, especially if it involves fracture of the skull or penetration of the brain by a missile, may also cause haemorrhage. In 108 cases of cerebral haemorrhage Richardson and Einhorn (1963) found that 77 were due to hypertension, 10 were unexplained, 7 were due to neoplasms, 6 to blood disease, 3 to arteritis, 2 to anticoagulants, and 3 resulted from other miscellaneous causes.

Arterial haemorrhage may be extradural, rarely subdural, subarachnoid, or intracerebral. The first three are usually traumatic (Chapter 5). The commonest cause of intracerebral arterial haemorrhage is rupture of an atheromatous artery in a hypertensive individual. The rise in blood pressure is usually due to essential hypertension, much less frequently to chronic nephritis or polycystic kidney. As already mentioned, hypertension causes medial hypertrophy in small arteries and arterioles. The hypertrophied media degenerates and along with atheroma of the intima produces a thickened but brittle vessel. Miliary aneurysms are often present on the small intracerebral vessels in arteriosclerosis, and Ross Russell (1963) showed that they are much commoner in hypertensive than in normotensive subjects.

There are thus two factors in the causation of arterial cerebral haemorrhage, the degeneration of the vessel and the raised blood pressure. The former in the absence of the latter is more likely to cause thrombosis rather than haemorrhage, while haemorrhage does not necessarily occur even when the blood pressure is very high, unless the vessel wall is fragile; even so, the ultimate cause of rupture is not yet fully understood (Ojemann and Mohr 1976). As in subarachnoid haemorrhage, spontaneous bleeding into the brain substance may also result from angiomal rupture and from rare causes such as bleeding diseases (haemophilia, Christmas disease, thrombocytopenic purpura, thrombotic microangiopathy, etc), leukaemia, collagen disease, and septic embolism. Lobar haemorrhages (localized to the frontal, temporal, parietal, or occipital lobes), unlike the more common putaminal and thalamic haemorrhages, are more likely to be due to these causes or to anticoagulant therapy than to hypertension (Ropper and Davis 1980).

Most cases of cerebral haemorrhage occur in middle or late life. Freytag (1968) found that 11 per cent of her cases were under 40 years of age, 36 per cent over 60. It is comparatively rare in younger hypertensives and thrombosis with infarction is commoner in extreme old age. Males are more frequently affected than females. A familial incidence is common (Marshall 1973). There is evidence, however, that its overall incidence is declining while its age incidence is increasing (Furlan, Whisnant, and Elveback 1979).

While cerebral haemorrhage may occur in any situation, Freytag (1968) in a study of 393 cases found that 42 per cent were in the region of the internal capsule and corpus striatum (putaminal haemorrhage), 16 per cent in the pons, 15 per cent in the thalamus, 12 per cent in the cerebellum, and 10 per cent in the cerebral white matter. Seventy-five per cent ruptured into the ventricles, 15 per cent through the cortex into the subarachnoid space, and 6 per cent into the subdural space. Secondary haemorrhages were found in the midbrain and pons in 54 per cent of cases with supratentorial haematomas.

After a large intracerebral haemorrhage, the affected hemisphere is enlarged and the gyri are flattened. The site of haemorrhage is occupied by a red clot and the surrounding tissues are compressed and often oedematous. Later the clot is absorbed and is replaced by a neuroglial scar or by a cavity containing yellow serous fluid. During absorption of the clot, gliosis occurs in the walls of the cavity with phagocytosis of destroyed neural tissue by compound granular corpuscles. Multiple haemorrhages sometimes occur.

Symptoms and signs

The onset of cerebral haemorrhage is always sudden, but the patient may be known to be hypertensive and there may have been premonitory symptoms, such as transitory speech disturbances or attacks of weakness of a limb. The actual rupture of the vessel may be precipitated by mental excitement or physical effort, or may occur during sleep. Usually the patient complains of sudden severe headache and may vomit. He becomes dazed, and in all but the mildest cases loses consciousness in a few minutes. Convulsions may occur at the onset, but are exceptional. The physical signs depend upon the situation and size of the haemorrhage.

Haemorrhage in the region of the corpus striatum and internal capsule

The patient is usually unconscious, but the depth of coma depends upon the size of the haemorrhage and the extent of pressure upon or of secondary haemorrhage into the brainstem. The advent of CT scanning, however, has allowed the accurate diagnosis and localization of many small non-fatal haemorrhages in this region which do not cause loss of consciousness and which would previously have remained undiagnosed (Hier, Davis, Richardson, and Mohr 1977). In unconscious patients, the pulse rate is generally slow—50 to 60—and the pulse full and bounding. The respirations are deep and stertorous, and the respiratory rate may be either slow, increased, or irregular, for example Cheyne–Stokes respiration. An unconscious patient is unable to swallow. The head is usually rotated and the eyes deviated towards the side of the lesion, due to paralysis of rotation of the head and of conjugate deviation of the eyes to the opposite side and the consequent unbalanced action of the undamaged cerebral hemisphere. The fundi usually show retinal arteriosclerosis, but the discs are usually normal, though slight paiplloedema is not uncommon. The pupils may be unequal, but react to light unless the patient is deeply comatose. A divergent squint is common, and the eyes often exhibit irregular, jerky movements. The corneal reflexes are often lost when coma is profound. A capsular haemorrhage causes contralateral hemiplegia, but voluntary movement cannot be tested in the comatose patient and hence it is necessary to use indirect methods of demonstrating paralysis.

Flattening of the nasolabial furrow may be evident on the paralysed side, and the cheek is often distended more on the paralysed than on the normal side during expiration. If the patient is not deeply comatose, he may also be seen to move the limbs spontaneously on the normal but not on the paralysed side. Spasticity takes two or three weeks to develop in the paralysed limbs; before this the limbs are flaccid, and this flaccidity is a most valuable sign of hemiplegia in a comatose patient. The arm and leg if lifted up fall to the bed limply, whereas even in deep coma the normal arm and leg subside more gradually. Painful stimuli may be used to demonstrate paralysis. Pricking with a pin in a semicomatose patient usually causes contraction of facial muscles and withdrawal of the limb which is pricked. These movements do not occur on the paralysed side. Their absence, however, may also be due to hemianalgesia. This may often be demonstrated by the fact that reflex facial grimacing occurs when the patient is pricked on the normal side of the body, but not when he is pricked on the analgesic side. The tendon reflexes are variable. They may be much diminished or abolished on the paralysed side; sometimes they are exaggerated. The plantar reflex on the affected side is extensor; on the other side it may be flexor or extensor. The abdominal reflexes are often lost on both sides in coma. Retention or incontinence of urine and faeces is the rule as long as the patient is unconscious.

Thalamic haemorrhage
Like a capsular or putaminal haemorrhage, a thalamic haemorrhage also gives hemiplegia due to pressure on the internal capsule but, in addition, the sensory deficit is usually prominent. There may be transient hemianopia and aphasia if the dominant hemisphere is involved (Ciemins 1970). Extension medially or into the subthalamus may cause paralysis of vertical gaze, occasionally skew deviation with downward displacement of the contralateral eye, ipsilateral ptosis and miosis, and even hemiballismus; mutism has been described in non-dominant thalamic lesions.

Lobar haemorrhage
Haemorrhage largely restricted to the white matter of one lobe of the brain (Ropper and Davis 1980) can produce distinctive clinical features. Occipital haemorrhage usually gives pain around the ipsilateral eye and dense hemianopia; haemorrhage into the dominant temporal lobe pain in the region of the ear with fluent dysphasia and an incomplete contralateral hemianopia; frontal haemorrhage severe weakness of the contralateral arm and minimal face and leg weakness with frontal headache; and parietal haemorrhage ipsilateral anterior temporal headache and a contralateral hemisensory deficit.

Pontine haemorrhage
If the patient is seen soon after the ictus, the signs may be those of a unilateral lesion of the pons, with, say, facial paralysis on the side of the lesion and flaccid paralysis of the limbs on the opposite side. Owing to paralysis of conjugate ocular deviation and of rotation of the head to the side of the lesion, the patient often lies with his head and eyes turned towards the side of the paralysed limbs. Even when the signs at the outset are those of a unilateral lesion of the pons, extension of the haemorrhage may involve the opposite side, or the signs may be bilateral from the beginning. When both sides of the pons are thus affected, there is paralysis of the face and limbs on both sides, with bilateral extensor plantar reflexes and sometimes decerebrate rigidity. Marked contraction of the pupils, 'pinpoint pupils', the result of bilateral destruction of ocular sympathetic fibres, is also characteristic. Moreover, destruction of the pons divides fibres coming from the heat-regulating centres in the hypothalamus, and the

patient becomes poikilothermic so that hyperpyrexia is common. Absence of nystagmus induced by cold water injected into one or both auditory meati is useful in distinguishing the condition from cerebral haemorrhage. Caplan and Goodwin (1982) have pointed out that lateral tegmental brainstem haemorrhages, which can be diagnosed with the CT scan, sometimes remain localized to that area or may spread to the dorsal basis pontis. They usually produce an ipsilateral palsy of conjugate gaze, ipsilateral internuclear ophthalmoplegia, small reacting pupils with a smaller pupil on the side of the lesion, cerebellar ataxia which is usually worse on the same side, and contralateral hemiplegia and sensory loss.

Haemorrhage into the ventricles

A putaminal haemorrhage sometimes bursts into the lateral ventricle. It may then be difficult to differentiate ventricular from pontine haemorrhage. After ventricular haemorrhage, coma deepens and signs of corticospinal-tract dysfunction are usually present on both sides of the body. The upper limbs often adopt a posture of rigid extension. The temperature frequently exhibits a terminal rise, also seen in pontine haemorrhage.

Neonatal intraventricular haemorrhage

Intracranial haemorrhage is a major cause of death and an important cause of handicap in low-birthweight infants. Subdural haemorrhage has become rare with improved obstetric care, transient subarachnoid haemorrhage is relatively common but of little importance clinically, and cerebellar haemorrhage is rare, occurring only in the small premature infant (Volpe 1979). The commonest and most important conditions are periventricular subependymal and intraventricular haemorrhage from the capillaries of the subependymal germinal matrix, usually occurring in the region of the head of the caudate nucleus, invariably in premature, immature neonates, and often in association with hyaline-membrane disease (*The Lancet* 1976, 1980; Ahmann, Lazzara, Dykes, Brann, and Schwartz 1980). The CT scan is diagnostic, the mortality rate is 25–30 per cent despite intensive care, and hydrocephalus, which may resolve spontaneously but may require shunt surgery, is the major complication.

Cerebellar haemorrhage

Cerebellar haemorrhage is usually sudden, and in many cases consciousness is lost sooner or later, but in one series of 56 patients, two-thirds were responsive on admission to hospital (Ott *et al.* 1974). Occipital headache and vomiting are common at the onset. Only a few patients show localizing signs: in many others, the clinical picture suggests a cerebrovascular accident without clear evidence as to its site (McKissock *et al.* 1960). Repeated vomiting and intense vertigo at the onset in a conscious patient who is ataxic and complains of headache but may have no classical 'cerebellar signs' should always suggest this diagnosis as a possibility. Ocular signs such as paralysis of conjugate gaze to the side of the lesion, a sixth-nerve palsy, or 'skew deviation' are seen in some cases. A similar picture may result from small cerebellar angiomas in children (Erenberg, Robin, and Shulman 1972). If the haemorrhage is not evacuated, coma due to brainstem compression supervenes. Without surgery the prognosis is poor; evacuation of the haematoma may lead to complete recovery especially when undertaken in a conscious patient (Freeman *et al.* 1973; Brennan and Bergland 1977).

Investigations

Lumbar puncture is not without risk in cases of cerebral haemorrhage because of the risk of cerebellar or tentorial herniation with consequent increased brainstem compression and/or secondary haemorrhage. The CT scan, if available, may make it unnecessary. Nevertheless, in selected cases it is still of diagnostic value. *The CSF* after cerebral haemorrhage is under increased pressure and its protein content may be somewhat raised. The

presence of blood visible to the naked eye in the fluid indicates usually that the haemorrhage has ruptured into the ventricular system, less frequently that it has come to the surface of the brain and ruptured into the subarachnoid space. Even when no blood can be seen with the naked eye, red cells may be seen microscopically. There is often a slight leucocytosis, the sedimentation rate is raised, and glycosuria and/or albuminuria are common. Hypertension and signs of cardiovascular disease are usually present.

Whereas in the past angiography was often thought necessary in younger conscious patients and ventriculography was commonly used when cerebellar haemorrhage was suspected (Norris, Eisen, and Branch 1969), the CT scan (Wiggins, Moody, Toole, Laster, and Ball 1978) is so successful in identifying and localizing haematomas and in demonstrating significant subarachnoid bleeding that other contrast methods are less often required. However, although the location of the haematoma can often be used with confidence to distinguish primary intracerebral haemorrhage from aneurysmal rupture (Hayward and O'Reilly 1976), angiography may still be wise when there is a possibility that the bleeding could be of aneurysmal origin.

Diagnosis

In most cases an intracerebral haemorrhage leads to impairment or loss of consciousness, usually very rapidly, sometimes more gradually. It must then be distinguished from other conditions causing coma (see p. 648). Important diagnostic points are the association of impaired consciousness with the physical signs of a focal cerebral lesion of acute or subacute onset, other evidence of cardiovascular disease, particularly hypertension and atheroma, and the presence of blood, visible either microscopically or macroscopically, in the CSF.

A cerebral vascular lesion having been diagnosed, it is necessary to decide whether it is haemorrhagic or ischaemic. Ischaemic lesions are either embolic, or due to atheroma, hypotension, ischaemic anoxia, polycythaemia, or arteritis, with or without thrombosis. An embolic lesion usually comes on suddenly with a clinical picture indicating obstruction of a particular artery and the source of the embolus is often evident. Ischaemic infarction due to atheroma is usually more gradual than haemorrhage. There may have been previous recurrent episodes with complete or partial recovery, or the onset is insidious over a period of 24 to 48 hours. Exceptionally, however, it is as sudden as haemorrhage. Unconsciousness is less common and when it occurs usually less profound. The blood pressure is less often raised, and there may be evidence of pre-existing associated disease, such as diabetes.

The CSF is often helpful. The presence of red blood cells is more suggestive of haemorrhage, while after infarction the fluid is more often free from red cells but may contain a raised protein.

Primary subarachnoid haemorrhage is distinguished from intracerebral haemorrhage by the prominent signs of meningeal irritation, i.e. neck stiffness and Kernig's sign, and the lack of signs of a focal cerebral lesion. It may, however, be impossible to distinguish clinically between an intracerebral haemorrhage reaching the ventricles or subarachnoid space, and a subarachnoid bleed from an aneurysm or angioma invading one cerebral hemisphere. However, the CT scan and, when necessary, angiography will usually be decisive.

An intracranial tumour rarely simulates a cerebral vascular lesion unless it is itself the site of bleeding or causes rapidly developing oedema. Such a lesion may be difficult to recognize if there have been no preceding symptoms of increased intracranial pressure. However, the CT scan will again be diagnostic. The 'congestive attacks' of general paresis or hemiplegia due to meningovascular syphilis may simulate a cerebral haemorrhage closely owing to the rapid onset of hemiplegia with loss of consciousness, but are now rare.

Prognosis

The immediate problem in a case of cerebral haemorrhage is whether or not the haemorrhage will prove fatal. Death may occur from medullary compression or brainstem haemorrhage as a result of continued bleeding. Even if the bleeding stops, the destruction of brain tissue and rise of intracranial pressure may cause coma so prolonged that the patient dies of exhaustion or from intercurrent infection, such as pneumonia. When haemorrhage continues, death may occur rapidly, though rarely in less than a few hours, usually during the first two days. The patient may, however, linger in a comatose state for a week or more. If the haemorrhage continues, there is progressive deepening of the coma, indicated by inability to rouse a formerly responsive patient, and loss of the corneal, pupillary, oculocephalic, and caloric reflexes; the pulse becomes rapid and irregular; the respiratory rate is often irregular and finally becomes rapid and shallow, and both the temperature and the blood pressure tend to rise.

Bilateral paralysis of the limbs is a sign of bad prognostic import, because it usually indicates either ventricular or pontine haemorrhage, both of which are often fatal. Visibly bloodstained CSF usually means a ventricular haemorrhage. If the patient shows no signs of recovery from coma 48 hours after the ictus, the chances of recovery are poor, even though the haemorrhage may have stopped. McKissock, Richardson, and Taylor (1961) in a series of 180 cases had an over-all mortality of 51 per cent and it was about twice as high in men as in women. Freytag (1968) found that almost all patients with pontine haemorrhage died within 24 hours, while the immediate mortality of haemorrhage in the cerebral white matter was 48 per cent. However, since the CT scan has allowed the accurate diagnosis of many smaller haemorrhages which must previously have gone undiagnosed, it is evident that many such patients survive, some with minimal deficit, even after pontine haemorrhage (Payne, Maravilla, Levinstone, Heuter, and Tindall 1978); Hier, Davis, Richardson, and Mohr (1977) found a mortality rate of only 37 per cent in putaminal haemorrhage.

When the patient recovers consciousness, he is naturally anxious to know whether he will have a permanent disability. This depends upon the situation of the haemorrhage, and the extent of the resulting destruction of brain tissue. Neural shock and oedema of surrounding areas usually cause a more severe initial depression of function than is actually due to the destructive effect of the lesion. Some improvement may therefore be expected in most cases.

Haemorrhage in the region of the posterior part of the inferior frontal gyrus on the left side may cause for a time total expressive aphasia, but considerable recovery of speech usually occurs in time, and improvement may continue for up to two years. The speech defect which follows a capsular haemorrhage is more often dysarthria and usually improves rapidly. Frontal-lobe haemorrhage can leave residual impairment of memory and concentration, irritability, and emotional lability. Damage to the corticospinal tract by a haemorrhage in the region of the internal capsule causes contralateral spastic hemiplegia as previously described (see p. 33). Some return of power always occurs in the lower limb, so that the patient is likely to be able to walk. If the upper limb shows returning power at the end of a month after the onset, a considerable degree of recovery of movement at the larger joints will probably occur in it. If, however, there is no improvement after three months, the paralysis is likely to be permanent. When the posterior part of the capsule is involved, sensory loss and homonymous hemianopia on the side opposite to the lesion may be added to the paralysis and are usually perma-

nent. Pain on the paralysed side may occur after a capsular or thalamic haemorrhage, and it is likely to be persistent. Involuntary movements sometimes follow cerebral haemorrhage, but only when limb paralysis is incomplete. They usually appear several weeks or months after the onset, with the return of voluntary power, and are always more marked in the upper than in the lower limbs. Action tremor (p. 323) is common; less often there is static tremor of the parkinsonian type and athetosis is also sometimes seen. All these movements tend to be persistent, though some improvement may occur, especially in the tremor. They are probably due to involvement of the corpus striatum. Choreiform movements or even frank hemiballismus may follow haemorrhage in the region of the subthalamic nucleus. Although cerebral haemorrhage is often fatal, improvement and even recovery may take place. Trophic changes often develop in the paralysed limbs and post-hemiplegic epilepsy is not uncommon.

Treatment

Continuing cerebral haemorrhage causes death from brainstem compression or secondary haemorrhage in this region. The objects of treatment are, therefore, to stop the haemorrhage and to reduce the intracranial pressure. Steroids may be helpful as in all cases of raised intracranial pressure (pp. 137 and 142).

Surgical evacuation of the clot is a rational procedure but is rarely practicable or beneficial, save in cerebellar haemorrhage. It should, however, be considered when cerebral haemorrhage occurs before middle life, in view of the possibility of haemorrhage from a small angioma which may be demonstrable by angiography (Small, Holmes, and Connolly 1953) or, in conscious patients in good condition, with accessible haematomas shown by CT scanning. McKissock, Richardson, and Walsh (1959) compared surgical and conservative treatment in a series of 244 cases of primary intracerebral haemorrhage. They concluded that no group of patients fared better with operation than with conservative treatment. However, there is no doubt that surgical evacuation of an intracerebellar haematoma in cases of primary cerebellar haemorrhage often saves life and lessens morbidity (McKissock, Richardson, and Walsh 1960; Ott, Kase, Ojemann, and Mohr 1974; Freeman, Onofrio, Okazaki, and Dinapoli 1973; Brennan and Bergland 1977). Hypotensive therapy appears to be of no value in the acute stage.

The usual treatment of the unconscious patient should be carried out. After recovery from the immediate effects of the haemorrhage, the principles of rehabilitation are the same as in cerebral infarction (p. 199).

References

Adams, H. P., Jr., Subbiah, B., and Bosch, E. P. (1977). Neurologic aspects of hereditary hemorrhagic telangiectasia. *Arch. Neurol, Chicago* **34**, 101.

Ahmann, P. A., Lazzara, A., Dykes, F. D., Brann, A. W., Jr., and Schwartz, J. F. (1980). Intraventricular hemorrhage in the high-risk preterm infant: incidence and outcome. *Ann. Neurol.* **7**, 118.

Alpers, B. J. and Gaskill, H. S. (1944). The pathological characteristics of embolic or metastatic encephalitis. *J. Neuropath. exp. Neurol.* **3**, 210.

Brennan, R. W. and Bergland, R. M. (1977). Acute cerebellar hemorrhage: analysis of clinical findings and outcome in 12 cases. *Neurology, Minneapolis* **27**, 527.

Caplan, L. R. and Goodwin, J. A. (1982). Lateral tegmental brainstem hemorrhages. *Neurology, Minneapolis* **32**, 252.

Ciemins, V. A. (1970). Localized thalamic hemorrhage: a cause of aphasia. *Neurology, Minneapolis* **20**, 776.

Erenberg, G., Rubin, R., and Shulman, K. (1972). Cerebellar haematomas caused by angiomas in children. *J. Neurol. Neurosurg. Psychiat.* **35**, 304.

Fields, W. S. (1961). *Pathogenesis and treatment of cerebrovascular disease*. Thomas, Springfield, Illinois.

Freeman, R. E., Onofrio, B. M., Okazaki, H., and Dinapoli, R. P.

(1973). Spontaneous intracerebellar hemorrhage: diagnosis and surgical treatment. *Neurology, Minneapolis* 23, 84.

Freytag, E. (1968). Fatal hypertensive intracerebral haematomas: a survey of the pathological anatomy of 393 cases. *J. Neurol. Neurosurg. Psychiat.* 31, 616.

Furlan, A. J., Whisnant, J. P., and Elveback, L. R. (1979). The decreasing incidence of primary intracerebral hemorrhage: a population study. *Ann. Neurol.* 5, 367.

Hayward, R. D. and O'Reilly, G. V. A. (1976). Intracerebral haemorrhage: accuracy of computerised transverse axial scanning in predicting the underlying aetiology. *Lancet* i, 1.

Hier, D. B., Davis, K. R., Richardson, E. P., Jr., and Mohr, J. P. (1977). Hypertensive putaminal hemorrhage. *Ann. Neurol.* 1, 152.

The Lancet (1976). Neonatal cerebral intraventricular haemorrhage. *Lancet* ii, 1341.

—— (1980). Towards the prevention of intraventricular haemorrhage. *Lancet* i, 236.

Marshall, J. (1973). Familial incidence of cerebral hemorrhage. *Stroke* 4, 38.

McKissock, W., Richardson, A., and Taylor, J. (1961). Primary intracerebellar haemorrhage. *Lancet* ii, 221.

——, ——, and Walsh, L. (1959). Primary intracerebral haemorrhage: results of surgical treatment in 244 consecutive cases. *Lancet* ii, 683.

——, ——, and —— (1960). Spontaneous cerebellar haemorrhage. *Brain* 83. 1.

Norris, J. W., Eisen, A. A., and Branch, C. L. (1969). Problems in cerebellar haemorrhage and infarction. *Neurology, Minneapolis* 19, 1043.

Ojemann, R. G. and Mohr, J. P. (1976). Hypertensive brain hemorrhage. In *Clinical neurosurgery* (ed. W. Mosberg), Vol. 23, p. 220. Congress of Neurological Surgeons, London.

Ott, K. M., Kase, C. S., Ojemann, R. G., and Mohr, J. P. (1974). Cerebellar hemorrhage: diagnosis and treatment. *Arch. Neurol., Chicago* 31, 160.

Payne, H. A., Maravilla, K. R., Levinstone, A., Heuter, J., and Tindall, R. S. A. (1978). Recovery from primary pontine hemorrhage. *Ann. Neurol.* 4, 557.

Richardson, J. C. and Einhorn, R. W. (1963). In *Clinical neurosurgery* (ed. W. Mosberg), p. 114. Congress of Neurological Surgeons, London.

Riishede, J. (1957). Cerebral apoplexy. *Acta psychiat., Copenhagen* 32, Suppl. 118.

Ropper, A. H. and Davis, K. R. (1980). Lobar cerebral hemorrhages: acute clinical syndromes in 26 cases. *Ann. Neurol.* 8, 141.

Russell, R. W. Ross (1963) Observations on intracranial aneurysms. *Brain* 86, 425.

Small, J. M., Holmes, J. M., and Connolly, R. C. (1953). The prognosis and role of surgery in spontaneous intracranial haemorrhage. *Br. med. J.* 2, 1072.

Toole, J. F. and Patel, A. N. (1974). *Cerebrovascular disorders*, 2nd edn. McGraw-Hill, New York.

Volpe, J. J. (1979). Intracranial hemorrhage in the newborn: current understanding and dilemmas. *Neurology, Minneapolis* 29, 632.

Wiggins, W. S., Moody, D. M., Toole, J. F., Laster, D. W., and Ball, M. R. (1978). Clinical and computerized tomographic study of hypertensive intracerebral hemorrhage. *Arch. Neurol., Chicago* 35, 832.

Other degenerative vasculopathies

Binswanger's disease (chronic progressive subcortical encephalopathy)

Binswanger (1894) described eight patients in whom the pathological changes were confined to the white matter of the cerebral hemispheres with virtually total sparing of the cortex. He called the condition encephalitis subcorticalis chronica progressiva, but in 1962 Olszewski postulated a vascular cause for the condition and coined the title subcortical arteriosclerotic encephalopathy. Caplan and Schoene (1978) stressed the almost invariable association with progressive dementia and hydrocephalus as well as the invariable hypertension and diffuse thickening of small vessels, the widespread gliosis of cerebral white matter, and the multiple lacunar infarcts; many of their patients had pseudobulbar palsy. De Reuck, Crevits, de Coster, Sieben, and Vander Eecken

(1980) also found multiple lacunes and areas of white-matter softening, especially in periventricular watershed areas, but felt that the condition is simply one form of multi-infarct dementia in which arteriosclerosis involves particularly small perforating arteries. Loizou, Kendall, and Marshall (1981) have described a characteristic pattern of low white-matter attenuation with linear capsular infarcts demonstrated by the CT scan which may allow diagnosis during life. Possibly many patients with 'diffuse cerebral atherosclerosis' show such changes (p. 197).

Köhlmeier–Degos disease (malignant atrophic papulosis)

This condition is associated with a disseminated occlusive vasculopathy (McFarland, Wood, Drowns, and Meneses 1978) and also a coagulopathy (Dastur, Singhal, and Shroff 1981). Patients present as a rule with pathognomonic papular skin lesions due to microinfarcts, followed by abdominal pain, bowel perforation, peritonitis, and death. In very occasional cases, gastrointestinal symptoms are absent and the manifestations may then be neurological with headache, paraesthesiae, unilateral or bilateral paresis or paralysis, and other features resulting from progressive, multiple, haemorrhagic infarction.

Ehlers–Danlos syndrome

This rare disorder of connective tissue of autosomal dominant inheritance is characterized by cutaneous fragility and hyperelasticity, excessive joint mobility and a bleeding tendency. Because the internal elastic laminae of arteries are also abnormal, many patients die from subarachnoid haemorrhage due to aneurysmal rupture; multiple aneurysms are common (Rubinstein and Cohen 1964). Arterial dissection and carotico-cavernous fistula are also well-recognized complications (Schoolmand and Kepes 1967).

Pseudoxanthoma elasticum

This condition, of autosomal recessive inheritance, causes degeneration and calcification of elastic tissue giving cutaneous lesions, retinal angioid streaks, and vascular lesions in many bodily organs. In the nervous system (Messis and Budzilovich 1970), cerebral ischaemia, infarction or haemorrhage, and aneurysmal rupture have all been described.

Familial cerebral amyloid angiopathy

This rare disorder of dominant inheritance is a microangiopathy with amyloid deposition in the walls of small cerebral arteries and arterioles and gives rise to recurrent cerebral haemorrhage and/or haemorrhagic infarction (Wattendorff, Bots, Went, and Endtz 1982; Griffiths, Mortimer, Oppenheimer, and Spalding 1982).

Idiopathic regressing arteriopathy

This title was given to a condition seen by Mokri, Houser, and Sundt (1977) in relatively young patients, who developed nonatheromatous occlusive cervicocephalic arterial disease causing vascular stenosis or occlusion which later resolved spontaneously. As yet, pathological evidence about the nature of this disorder is lacking.

Radiation-induced cerebrovascular disease

The effects of radiation on the nervous system will be considered later (p. 422). However, there is no doubt that radiation-related carotid arteritis in the neck following treatment of cancer of the neck may cause a stroke in the adult (Conomy and Kellermeyer 1974), while in childhood, neonatal irradiation of an orbital haemangioma was followed six years later by cerebral ischaemia associated with stenosis of the internal carotid and occlusion of the anterior and middle cerebral arteries (Wright and Bresnan 1976).

References

Binswanger, O. (1984). Die abgrenzung der allgemeinen progressiven paralyse. *Berliner Klin. Wschr.* **31**, 1103, 1137, 1180.

Caplan, L. R. and Schoene, W. C. (1978). Clinical features of subcortical arteriosclerotic encephalopathy (Binswanger disease). *Neurology, Minneapolis* **28**, 1206.

Conomy, J. P. and Kellermeyer, R. (1974). Delayed cerebrovascular consequences of therapeutic radiation: a clinico-pathologic study of stroke due to radiation-related cervical carotid arteritis. *Neurology, Minneapolis* **24**, 394.

Dastur, D. K., Singhal, B. S., and Shroff, H. J. (1981). CNS involvement in malignant atrophic papulosis (Köhlmeier–Degos disease): vasculopathy and coagulopathy. *J. Neurol. Neurosurg. Psychait.* **44**, 156.

de Reuck, J., Crevits, L., de Coster, W., Sieben, G., and Vander Eecken, H. (1980). Pathogenesis of Binswanger chronic progressive subcortical encephalopathy. *Neurology, Minneapolis* **30**, 920.

Griffiths, R. A., Mortimer, T. F., Oppenheimer, D. R., and Spalding, J. M. K. (1982). Congophilic angiopathy of the brain: a clinical and pathological report of two siblings. *J. Neurol. Neurosurg. Psychiat.* **45**, 396.

Loizou, L. A., Kendall, B. E., and Marshall, J. (1981). Subcortical arteriosclerotic encephalopathy: a clinical and radiological investigation. *J. Neurol. Neurosurg. Psychiat.* **44**, 294.

McFarland, H. R., Wood, W. G., Drowns, B. V., and Meneses, A. C. O. (1978). Papulosis atrophicans maligna (Köhlmeier–Degos disease): a disseminated occlusive vasculopathy. *Ann. Neurol.* **3**, 388.

Messis, C. P. and Budzilovich, G. N. (1970). Pseudoxanthoma elasticum. report of an autopsied case with cerebral involvement. *Neurology, Minneapolis* **20**, 703.

Mokri, B., House, O. W., and Sundt, T. M., Jr. (1977). Idiopathic regressing arteriopathy. *Ann. Neurol.* **2**, 466.

Olszewski, J. (1962). Subcortical arteriosclerotic encephalopathy. *World Neurol.* **3**, 359.

Rubinstein, M. K. and Cohen, N. H. (1964). Ehlers–Danlos syndrome associated with multiple intracranial aneurysms. *Neurology, Minneapolis* **14**, 125.

Schoolman, A. and Kepes, J. J. (1967). Bilateral spontaneous carotid-cavernous fistulae in Ehlers–Danlos syndrome. Case report. *J. Neurosurg.* **26**, 82.

Wattendorff, A. R., Bots, G. T. A. M., Went, L. N., and Endtz, L. J. (1982). Familial cerebral amyloid angiopathy presenting as recurrent cerebral haemorrhage. *J. neurol. Sci.* **55**, 121.

Wright, T. L. and Bresnan, M. J. (1976). Radiation-induced cerebrovascular disease in children. *Neurology, Minneapolis* **26**, 540.

Vascular diseases without changes in the brain and strokes of undetermined aetiology

These categories of cerebral vascular disease were included by the Ad Hoc Committee of NINDB (1958) (see p. 191) in their classification simply in order to indicate that the pathologist may find evidence of extensive atherosclerosis and/or arteriolosclerosis at autopsy in patients without symptoms of cerebral ischaemia and without pathological evidence of disease in the cerebral parenchyma. Similarly it is evident that despite extensive clinical and pathological study it may still be impossible, using techniques at present available, to determine the cause of certain strokes.

Reference

Ad Hoc Committee National Advisory Council of the National Institute of Neurological Diseases and Blindness (NINDB) (1958). A classification and outline of cerebrovascular disease. *Neurology, Minneapolis* **8**, Supplement.

Inflammatory diseases of intracranial arteries

Polyarteritis nodosa (periarteritis nodosa)

This disorder is characterized by multiple arterial focal lesions which begin with necrosis of the media and the internal elastic lamina, followed by extension of the inflammation to the adventitia, and periarteritis. Proliferation of the intima produces gradual narrowing of the lumen of the vessels. Secondary aneurysm formation is exceptional. The nervous system is said to be involved in between 8 and 40 per cent of cases; and lesions may occur in the meninges, cerebral cortex, medulla, spinal cord, and peripheral nerves (due to occlusion of vasa nervorum). The disease is commoner in men than women, by a ratio of 4:1, and usually begins between the ages of 20 and 40 years (Ford and Seikert 1965). Wegener's granulomatosis, which is histologically similar but which involves electively the upper respiratory tract and kidneys, may give similar neurological complications.

Cerebral lesions may lead to headache, convulsions, hemiplegia, psychosis, dementia, and coma. Pupillary changes may be present. The symptoms of involvement of the peripheral or cranial nerves are often those of multiple neuropathy ('mononeuritis multiplex') rather than symmetrical polyneuritis. Pain and muscular weakness may develop over a few hours. Tenderness of the nerve trunks and muscles with muscular wasting and weakness, loss of reflexes, and sensory loss are irregularly distributed according to the distribution of the spinal roots and peripheral nerves affected. Isolated cranial-nerve palsies may also occur or syndromes suggesting infarction of the brain or spinal cord when a large vessel is occluded; vascular rupture causing haemorrhage is rare. The spinal fluid may be under increased pressure with xanthochromia and polymorphonuclear pleocytosis.

Changes are often present in the ocular fundi. There may be choroidal exudates in the form of perivascular hillocks resembling choroidal tubercles. Detachment of the retina may occur, and in the later stages hypertensive retinopathy.

The general symptoms include fever and loss of weight, and focal visceral symptoms depending upon the situation of the lesions, which involve especially the kidneys, heart, liver, and gastrointestinal tract. The spleen may be enlarged, and radiographically the lungs may show a characteristic infiltration. There is often a leucocytosis in the blood and occasionally eosinophilia. Asthma is common. Hypertension and albuminuria usually occur in the later stages. The ESR is usually greatly raised. Muscle infarcts may occur and a biopsy may show the characteristic vascular lesion. Many patients improve when treated with steroid drugs, a few recover after long-term treatment, and in some the disease appears to become 'burnt-out', but there is still an appreciable mortality.

References

Ford, R. G. and Seikert, R. G. (1965). Central nervous system manifestations of periarteritis nodosa. *Neurology, Minneapolis* **15**, 114.

Kernohan, J. W. and Woltman, H. W. (1938). Periarteritis nodosa. A clinico-pathologic study with special reference to the nervous system. *Arch. Neurol. Psychiat., Chicago* **39**, 665.

Systemic lupus erythematosus

Symptoms and signs of cerebral ischaemia have been reported as an uncommon manifestation of systemic lupus erythematosus; the manifestations are often those of a restricted brainstem stroke but cerebral-hemisphere lesions, often resulting from small areas of perisulcal softening, occasionally occur and focal spinal-cord lesions have also been described (Johnson and Richardson 1968; Berry 1971). The clinical manifestations of cerebral involvement are diverse, including not only manifestations of focal ischaemia, sometimes giving TIAs, at other times a more typical single stroke (Haas 1982), but also epileptiform seizures, cranial-nerve palsies, chorea, and arachnoiditis in some cases (Glaser 1952; *British Medical Journal* 1975). Optic neuritis has also been described (Hackett, Martinez, Larson, and Paddison 1974) and a progressive spinal-cord syndrome resembling multiple sclerosis (Fulford, Catterall, Delhanty, Doniach, and Kremer 1972), while symmetrical sensorimotor polyneuropathy is also relatively common. Kurland, Hauser, Ferguson, and Holley (1969) reviewed the relative incidence of systemic lupus and of other collagen or connective-tissue diseases which may involve the nervous system.

References

Berry, R. G. (1971). Lupus erythematosus. In *Pathology of the nervous system* (ed. J. Minckler), Vol. 2, pp. 1482–8. McGraw-Hill, New York.
British Medical Journal (1975). Cerebral lupus. *Br. med. J.* **1**, 537.
Fulford, K. W. M., Catterall, R. D., Delhanty, J. J., Doniach, D., and Kremer, M. (1972). A collagen disorder of the nervous system presenting as multiple sclerosis. *Brain* **95**, 373.
Glaser, G. H. (1952). Lesions of the central nervous system in disseminated lupus erythematosus. *Arch. Neurol. Psychiat., Chicago* **67**, 745.
Haas, L. F. (1982). Stroke as an early manifestation of systemic lupus erythematosus. *J. Neurol. Neurosurg. Psychiat.* **45**, 554.
Hackett, E. R., Martinez, R. D., Larson, P. F., and Paddison, R. M. (1974). Optic neuritis in systemic lupus erythematosus. *Arch. Neurol. Psychiat., Chicago* **31**, 9.
Johnson, R. T. and Richardson, E. P. (1968). The neurological manifestations of systemic lupus erythematosus. *Medicine, Baltimore* **47**, 337.
Kurland, L. T., Hauser, W. A., Ferguson, R. H., and Holley, K. E. (1969). Epidemiologic features of diffuse connective tissue disorders in Rochester, Minn., 1951 through 1967, with special reference to systemic lupus erythematosus. *Mayo Clin. Proc.* **44**, 649.

Buerger's disease

It has been suggested in the past that thromboangiitis obliterans may sometimes involve cerebral vessels, but it is now generally agreed, on the basis of pathological evidence, that most cases so diagnosed have resulted either from atheroma or from granulomatous arteritis (Fisher 1957; Bruetsch 1971; Hutchinson and Acheson 1975).

References

Bruetsch, W. L. (1971). Cerebral thromboangiitis obliterans. In *Pathology of the nervous system* (ed. J. Minckler), Vol. 2, Chapter XVII, Section 108. McGraw-Hill, New York.
Fisher, C. M. (1957). Cerebral thromboangiitis obliterans. *Medicine, Baltimore* **36**, 169.
Hutchinson, E. C. and Acheson, E. J. (1975). *Strokes: natural history, pathology, and surgical treatment.* Saunders, London.

Temporal (giant-cell) arteritis

The disorder originally described as temporal, or cranial arteritis is now recognized to be a generalized vascular disease which attacks elderly patients, being rare before the age of 60 years. The pathological features are those of subacute inflammation, spreading by the vasa vasorum to the media of the arteries and longitudinally along the vessels in contrast to the lesion in polyarteritis nodosa. The intima becomes hypertrophied, and thrombosis is a common sequel. Giant cells are often found, and the disorder is also called giant-cell arteritis. The characteristic path-

ological changes may be found in many large and small vessels (Crompton 1959), including the aorta and the retinal arteries. Biopsy of an affected portion of a superficial temporal artery may confirm the diagnosis.

The characteristic symptoms and signs are anorexia, loss of weight, joint and muscle pains, fever and sweating, painful arterial thrombosis, and severe headache. Sometimes diffuse muscular pain is the presenting symptom, and there is a clear association with polymyalgia rheumatica (p. 566). Trismus, dysphagia, and peripheral neuropathy are rare manifestations. The superficial temporal arteries are intensely tender during the acute stage and may become thrombosed through part or the whole of their length. Papilloedema may occur, and unilateral or bilateral loss of vision is common. Indeed, in 80 personal cases Meadows (1966) found that unilateral or bilateral blindness due to central retinal artery occlusion occurred in over half and diplopia in 15 per cent. Sudden unilateral blindness in an elderly patient, even when other evidence of arteritis is unobtrusive, should always raise the possibility of this condition and an ESR (this is almost invariably raised in the untreated case) is the single most useful investigation. Only very exceptionally is the ESR normal in a histologically proven case (Kansu, Corbett, Savino, and Schatz 1977). Treatment with steroid drugs (prednisone 30–40 mg daily in the first instance) is mandatory as this may be the only means of preserving remaining vision. The disease usually burns itself out in 1–2 years when treatment can gradually be withdrawn. Cerebral symptoms due to involvement of the carotid and vertebral arteries are occasionally seen and brainstem strokes are not uncommon, though intracranial vessels are rarely involved (Wilkinson and Russell 1972).

References

Cooke, W. T., Cloake, P. C. P., Govan, A. D. T., and Colbeck, J C. (1946). Temporal arteritis: a generalized vascular disease. *Quart. J. Med* **15**, 47.
Crompton, M. R. (1959). The visual changes in temporal (giant-cell) arteritis. Report of a case with autopsy findings. *Brain* **82**, 377.
Kansu, T., Corbett, J. J., Savino, P., and Schatz, N. J. (1977). Giant cell arteritis with normal sedimentation rate. *Arch. Neurol., Chicago* **34**, 624.
Meadows, S. P. (1966). Temporal or giant-cell arteritis. *Proc. R. Soc. Med.* **59**, 329.
Wilkinson, I. M. S. and Russell, R. W. R. (1972). Arteries of the head and neck in giant cell arteritis. A pathological study to show the pattern of arterial involvement. *Arch. Neurol., Chicago* **27**, 378.

Granulomatous angiitis

Within recent years several cases have been described in adults of all ages and both sexes of a disorder presenting with symptoms of focal or generalized cerebral dysfunction, epileptic seizures, and evidence of spinal-cord involvement which may precede cerebral symptoms and in which a diffuse granulomatous angiitis of small intracerebral and meningeal arteries has been discovered at autopsy. The pathological changes, with giant cells in the inflammatory lesions in the affected vessels, resemble in some degree those of sarcoidosis and in other respects those of temporal arteritis, with which condition earlier cases of this disorder were confused (McCormick and Neuburger 1958); however, as mentioned above, the latter condition affects mainly larger extracranial vessels. The CSF is usually under increased pressure and contains an excess of protein and lymphocytes; the aetiology of the disorder is unknown; most cases have proved fatal within months or exceptionally a few years, but in rare instances where cerebral biopsy has established the diagnosis, steroid treatment has been found helpful (Kolodny, Rebelz, Caviness, and Richardson 1968; Nurick, Blackwood, and Mair 1972).

References

Kolodny, E. H., Rebeiz, J. J., Caviness, V. S., and Richardson, E. P. (1968). Granulomatous angiitis of the central nervous system. *Arch. Neurol.*, *Chicago* **19**, 510.

McCormick, H. M. and Neubuerger, K. T. (1958). Giant-cell arteritis involving small meningeal and intracerebral vessels. *J. Neuropath. exp. Neurol.* **17**, 471.

Nurick, S., Blackwood, W., and Mair, W. G. P. (1972). Giant cell granulomatous angiitis of the central nervous system. *Brain* **95**, 133.

Other forms of cerebral arteritis

A necrotizing form of cerebral arteritis is now well recognized to occur in young adult drug addicts, especially in those addicted to amphetamines (Citron, Halpern, McCarron, Lundberg, McCormick, Pincus, Tatter, and Haverback 1970) and can cause manifestations of cerebral ischaemia, infarction, or even intracerebral or subarachnoid haemorrhage (Edwards 1977). A granulomatous angiitis causing segmental stenosis of intracranial arteries and giving rise to cerebral infarction has also been described as a complication of ophthalmic herpes zoster (MacKenzie, Forbes, and Karnes 1981).

References

Citron, B. P., Halpern, M., McCarron, M., Lundberg, G. D., McCormick, R., Pincus, I. J., Tatter, D., and Haverback, B. J. (1970). Necrotizing angiitis associated with drug abuse. *New Engl. J. Med.* **283**, 1003.

Edwards, K. R. (1977). Hemorrhagic complications of cerebral arteritis. *Arch. Neurol.*, *Chicago* **34**, 549.

MacKenzie, R. A., Forbes, G. S., and Karnes, W. E. (1981). Angiographic findings in herpes zoster arteritis. *Ann. Neurol.* **10**, 458.

Pulseless disease

Episodes of cerebral ischaemia or infarction in patients with absent or reduced pulses, especially in the upper limbs, have been recognized for many years to occur in young Japanese women with that form of obliterative arteritis of the brachiocephalic branches of the aortic arch first described by Takayasu (1908) and often now called Takayasu's disease. This condition, though rare, has been described in racial groups other than the Japanese, but in Western countries 'pulseless disease' more often results from atherosclerotic occlusion of major vessels, though it has been described in systemic lupus erythematosus (Lessof and Glynn 1959). In true Takayasu's disease the illness runs a subacute course with fever, arthralgia, anaemia, a raised ESR, and sometimes haemoptysis and pleural effusion. The main arterial trunks in the neck are often tender and multiple bruits can usually be heard. Steroids and immunosuppressive drugs seem to be effective (Riehl and Brown 1965; *British Medical Journal* 1977).

References

British Medical Journal (1977). Takayasu's arteritis. *Br. med. J.* **1**, 667.

Lessor, M. H. and Glynn, L. E. (1959). The pulseless syndrome. *Lancet* **i**, 799.

Riehl, J. L. and Brown, W. J. (1965). Takayasu's arteritis: an autoimmune disease. *Arch. Neurol.*, *Chicago* **12**, 92.

Takayasu, M. (1908). A case with peculiar changes of the central retinal vessels. *Acta Soc. ophthal. Jap.* **12**, 554.

Disseminated intravascular coagulation

Disseminated intravascular coagulation (DIC) is a process characterized by the activation of the coagulation system with the for-

mation of either soluble or insoluble fibrin. Clotting factors and platelets are consumed and there is secondary activation of fibrinolysis (Davies-Jones, Preston, and Timperley 1980; Preston 1982). There are many precipitating causes including trauma, surgical operations, infections, disorders of the immune system, neoplasia, diabetes, and pregnancy (Heron, Hutchinson, Boyd, and Aber 1974); the condition has been thought to arise occasionally in patients with primary cerebral lesions due to the release of thromboplastin from damaged brain tissue (Preston, Malia, Sworn, Timperley, and Blackburn 1974). It usually gives rise to widespread thrombosis causing ischaemia or infarction of many tissues and organs, including the brain. The clinical manifestations are commonly those of involvement of the respiratory or renal systems but, when the brain is involved, a variety of focal neurological manifestations and even coma may be seen. Confusion, delirium, seizures, dysphasia, and variable pareses are all common (Davies-Jones *et al* 1980; Schwartzmann and Hill 1982). The CT scan may show multiple areas of softening; the platelet count is invariably low and tests for the presence of soluble fibrin monomer usually confirm the diagnosis.

Thrombotic thrombocytopenic purpura

This is one relatively specific variety of DIC, sometimes called thrombotic microangiopathy (Symmers 1952, 1956), in which thrombocytopenia, haemolytic anaemia, and neurological manifestations including stupor or coma, mental changes, variable pareses, dysphasia, convulsions, ataxia, and visual-field defects as well as cranial-nerve palsies and, rarely, spinal-cord symptoms may also be seen (Davies-Jones *et al.* 1980). Pyrexia, petechial haemorrhages, arthralgia, and gastrointestinal bleeding are all common. Pathologically, many small cerebral vessels are blocked with platelet thrombi. There is a close relationship with systemic L.E. and many workers consider that so-called acute haemorrhagic leucoencephalitis is usually due to this cause. Steroid drugs combined with splenectomy have sometimes been helpful, but not invariably, and more spectacular improvement has followed plasma exchange, but generally the prognosis is very poor.

References

Davies-Jones, G. A. B., Preston, F. E., and Timperley, W. R. (1980). *Neurological complications in clinical haematology*, p. 193. Blackwell, Oxford.

Heron, J. R., Hutchinson, E. C., Boyd, W. N., and Aber, G. M. (1974). Pregnancy, subarachnoid haemorrhage, and the intravascular coagulation syndrome. *J. Neurol. Neurosurg. Psychiat.* **37**, 521.

Preston, F. E. (1982). Disseminated intravascular coagulation. *Br. J. hosp. Med.* **28**, 129.

——, Malia, R. G., Sworn, M. J., Timperley, W. R., and Blackburn, E. K. (1974). Disseminated intravascular coagulation as a consequence of cerebral damage. *J. Neurol. Neurosurg. Psychiat.* **37**, 241.

Schwartzmann, R. J. and Hill, J. B. (1982). Neurologic complications of disseminated intravascular coagulation. *Neurology*, *Minneapolis* **32**, 791.

Symmers, W. St. C. (1952). Thrombotic microangiopathic haemolytic anaemias (thrombotic microangiopathy). *Br. med. J.* **2**, 897.

—— (1956). Thrombotic microangiopathy (thrombotic thrombocytopenic purpura) associated with acute haemorrhagic leucoencephalitis and sensitivity to oxophenarsine. *Brain* **79**, 511.

The cerebral venous circulation

The venous sinuses

The intracranial sinuses (Fig. 4.10) are spaces lying between layers of the dura mater and are lined with endothelium. They receive blood from the veins of the brain and directly or indirectly drain into the internal jugular vein. They communicate with the meningeal veins, and by emissary veins with those of the scalp.

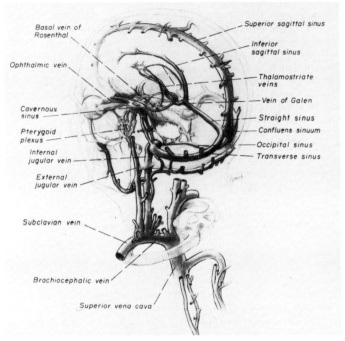

Fig. 4.10 The cerebral venous system. (Reproduced from Toole and Patel (1974) by kind permission of the authors and publisher.)

The following sinuses are unpaired:

The superior sagittal sinus. The superior sagittal sinus begins anteriorly at the crista galli where it communicates through the foramen caecum with the nasal veins, and passes upwards, backwards, and finally downwards at the convex upper margin of the falx. It ends at the level of the internal occipital protuberance by turning, usually to the right, into the right transverse sinus. Occasionally it turns into the left transverse sinus. It has a terminal dilatation—the confluence of the sinuses—from which a communication passes to the junction of the straight sinus and left transverse sinus. The superior sagittal sinus receives the superior group of superficial cerebral veins and thus drains the upper part of the cerebral hemispheres.

The inferior sagittal sinus. The inferior sagittal sinus lies in the free lower border of the falx for its posterior two-thirds and terminates posteriorly by joining the great cerebral vein to form the straight sinus, which passes between layers of the dura along the line of junction of the falx with the tentorium. Posteriorly it turns to the left at the level of the internal occipital protuberance to become the left transverse sinus.

The following sinuses are paired:

The transverse sinuses. The transverse sinuses arise posteriorly, the right from the superior sagittal sinus, the left from the straight sinus, and pass laterally and forwards in the attached border of the tentorium, lying in a groove in the occipital bone. Each then turns downwards on the inner surface of the mastoid process and leaves the skull by the jugular foramen, to enter the internal jugular vein.

The cavernous sinuses. The cavernous sinuses lie one on either side of the body of the sphenoid. They begin anteriorly at the inner end of the superior orbital fissure, where they receive the ophthalmic veins, and terminate posteriorly at the apex of the petrous temporal bone by dividing into the superior and inferior petrosal sinuses. In the lateral wall of the cavernous sinus

lie the internal carotid artery with its sympathetic plexus, the third and fourth nerves, and first and second divisions of the fifth nerve, and the sixth nerve.

The petrosal sinuses. The superior petrosal sinuses run in the posterior margin of the tentorium to join the transverse sinuses while the inferior sinuses pass through the jugular foramina to enter the internal jugular vein.

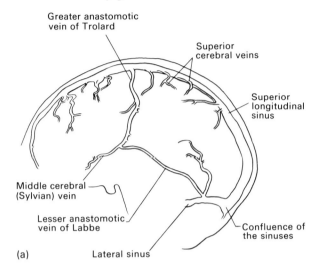

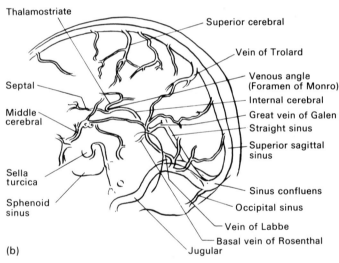

Fig. 4.11. Diagrams drawn from the venous phase of an angiogram, showing the more important veins. (a) The superficial veins. (b) The deep venous system. (Reproduced from Toole and Patel (1974) by kind permission of the authors and publisher.)

The cerebral veins. The venous sinuses receive as tributaries the cerebral veins (Fig. 4.11). The superficial cerebral veins are divided into two groups—the superior, including the veins of Trolard (which usually follow the Rolandic fissure), which run upwards to the superior sagittal sinus and drain the upper halves of the hemispheres, and the inferior, including the vein of Labbé, which drain the lower halves of the hemispheres and run downwards to join the venous sinuses of the base. The most important of the deep cerebral veins is the great cerebral vein of Galen, which, having received contributions from the septal and thalamostriate veins via the internal cerebral vein and the basal veins of Rosenthal, thus drains the choroid plexuses of the third and lateral ventricles and the basal ganglia, and terminates by joining the inferior sagittal sinus to form the straight sinus. Much new information about the cerebral venous system, identifying specific veins not previously named in anatomical texts, has been derived in recent years from angiographic studies (Newton and Potts 1974; Toole and Patel 1974). Displacement of these structures is valuable in the angiographic localization of intracranial tumours. Thus, for example, the 'venous angle' at the foramen of Monro, formed by the junction of the thalamostriate and internal cerebral veins, may be distorted by frontal tumours, a wide sweep of the thalamostriate veins is seen in hydrocephalus, and lateral displacement of the internal cerebral vein, seen in anteroposterior projections, indicates a mass lesion of one cerebral hemisphere.

The diploic veins. The venous channels in the bones of the skull, the diploic veins, drain either into the venous sinuses or into the superficial veins of the scalp.

Thrombosis of the intracranial venous sinuses and veins

Aetiology

Thrombosis of the intracranial venous sinuses may result from the extension of infection from neighbouring structures or from direct injury. Sometimes it occurs in the absence of any evident local cause (Averback 1978). These two varieties of sinus thrombosis are rather unsatisfactorily distinguished as 'secondary' and 'primary', respectively.

'Primary' sinus thrombosis is uncommon and is most often seen at the extremes of life, especially during the first year. It occurs in wasted, debilitated infants, especially as a complication of congenital heart disease or gastrointestinal infections, and later in life in individuals suffering from severe anaemia (including sickle-cell disease and haemolytic anaemia), exhausting infections such as enteric fever, or emaciating diseases such as carcinoma, tuberculosis, and ulcerative colitis. It has also been described as a complication of oral contraceptive medication (Bickerstaff 1975), of polycythaemia vera (Melamed, Rachmilewitz, Reches, and Lavy 1976), and in pregnancy and the puerperium (Carroll, Leak, and Leel 1966). The principal predisposing factors of 'primary' sinus thrombosis appear to be anaemia, increased coagulability of the blood, low blood pressure, cachexia, and dehydration. It may form part of the picture of thrombophlebitis migrans.

'Secondary' sinus thrombosis may follow direct injury to a sinus through fracture of the skull or a surgical operation, or puncture of the superior sagittal sinus in infancy for therapeutic purposes. Infection may spread to the sinuses from an area of osteitis of one of the cranial bones. The transverse sinus may thus become infected from mastoiditis, or through the jugular vein from the fauces. Infection may spread from the transverse to the superior sagittal sinus. The latter and the cavernous sinus may be directly infected from frontal sinusitis or from infection in other nasal sinuses. Owing to the comparatively free communication between the intracranial venous sinuses and the superficial veins of the face and scalp, cutaneous sepsis may also cause sinus thrombosis. The cavernous sinus is especially liable to become infected from pyogenic infections in the region of the upper lip.

Though sinus thrombosis may be the only manifestation of infection, it may also be associated with extradural or subdural abscess, intracerebral abscess, or localized or diffuse leptomeningitis.

Pathology

The affected sinus contains a reddish clot, which eventually becomes paler and adherent to the sinus wall. In sinus thrombophlebitis due to pyogenic organisms, the clot may become purulent. It may extend into tributary veins or into other sinuses. The internal jugular vein is often involved by extension from the transverse sinus. The area of brain drained by the affected sinus shows congestive oedema and sometimes haemorrhagic venous infarction, while the development of a collateral venous circulation causes congestion of neighbouring veins. Obstruction of a large sinus, such as the superior sagittal, may so impede the absorption of CSF that hydrocephalus results. Involvement of the Galenic vein may cause softening in the central areas of the brain. Extension of infection from the sinus may cause localized or diffuse leptomeningitis or intracerebral abscess, while the liberation of organisms or of fragments of infected clot into the general circulation may lead to pyaemia and pyaemic abscesses, especially in the lungs. The pathology of the condition, as well as its clinical features, were reviewed by Kalbag and Woolf (1967).

Symptoms and signs

The clinical features in intracranial venous sinus thrombosis consist of: those of the predisposing condition; those of obstruction to the venous drainage of tissues adjacent to the sinus; in the case of infective thrombophlebitis, those of extension of the infection to neighbouring structures and of its dissemination in the blood stream; and in some cases hydrocephalus due to defective absorption of CSF. Predisposing conditions have already been mentioned. The manifestations of obstructed venous drainage differ according to the sinus affected.

Thrombosis of the cavernous sinus
Pain is often severe and is felt in the eye and forehead on the affected side sometimes with hyperpathia over the cutaneous distribution of the ophthalmic division of the trigeminal nerve. There is marked oedema of the eyelids, the cornea, and the root of the nose, with exophthalmos due to congestion of orbital veins. Papilloedema is sometimes present, but the optic disc may be normal and vision is usually unimpaired. Since the third, fourth, and sixth cranial nerves lie in the lateral wall of the sinus, ocular palsies are usually present and there may be complete internal and external ophthalmoplegia. Cavernous sinus thrombosis is usually unilateral at the outset, but the process can readily extend through the circular sinus to the cavernous sinus on the opposite side when the signs become bilateral.

Thrombosis of the transverse sinus
Thrombosis of the transverse sinus is almost always due to extension of infection from the mastoid. The patient complains of headache and of pain in the ear, which may be intensified by moving the head. Vomiting may occur. Venous congestion is common in the region of the mastoid process and extension of phlebitis to the jugular vein causes tenderness in the neck. Rarely, the vein is palpable as a tender cord. Papilloedema is sometimes present, but is usually slight and may be confined to the eye on the affected side. Focal cerebral symptoms include convulsions and contralateral hemiparesis. Aphasia may be present when the left transverse sinus is affected.

Thrombosis of the superior sagittal sinus
Thrombosis of the superior sagittal sinus usually leads to increased intracranial pressure. The earliest symptoms are headache, vomiting, delirium, and in some cases convulsions. Rarely there is congestion of the scalp and external nasal veins, and in infants the fontanelle is tense. Papilloedema is common but not invariable. Since the superior sagittal sinus receives the superior cortical veins which drain the upper half of the hemispheres, and since the lower limbs are represented in the areas of the precentral gyrus nearest the vertex, thrombosis of this sinus may cause symptoms of bilateral corticospinal lesions, which are most marked in, and may be confined to, the lower limbs. Focal symptoms may be unilateral, e.g. Jacksonian epilepsy and hemiplegia, or even absent. Subarachnoid haemorrhage has been described (Walton 1956). The symptoms may be mainly or exclusively

those of hydrocephalus, as in so-called 'otitic hydrocephalus' (see p. 141).

Thrombosis of other sinuses

Thrombophlebitis may spread from the transverse sinus to the superior petrosal sinus and so reach cerebral veins draining the lower part of the precentral gyrus, causing faciobrachial monoplegia. Thrombophlebitis of the inferior petrosal sinus may cause Gradenigo's syndrome (Symonds 1944) or may involve the posterior group of cranial nerves.

Thrombophlebitis in pregnancy

According to Carroll *et al.* (1966) the presenting symptoms in order of frequency are severe headache, convulsions, speech disturbances, and drowsiness and confusion.

The CSF

The fluid is usually under increased pressure, but may be otherwise normal. In thrombosis of the superior sagittal sinus, however, red blood cells are often present in considerable numbers, with a corresponding rise in the protein content, and even a xanthochromic fluid. A slight excess of leucocytes, usually both polymorphonuclear and mononuclear, is not uncommon and indicates a localized extension of the infection to the neighbouring leptomeninges. When one transverse sinus is filled with clot, the pressure of the CSF may fail to show the normal rise when the jugular vein on the affected side is compressed alone (the Tobey–Ayer test), but the sinus may be infected without being obstructed.

Other investigations

Carotid angiography, especially the appearances in the venous phase, is the definitive investigation and frequently demonstrates occlusion of, or filling defects in, the affected sinus or sinuses (Fig. 4.12). The CT scan is helpful, though the appearances, often indicating simply cerebral oedema, are relatively non-specific (Kingsley, Kendall, and Moseley 1978).

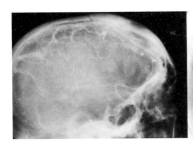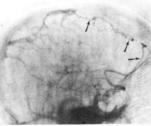

Fig. 4.12. Occlusion of the superior sagittal sinus in the frontal region demonstrated by carotid angiography (on the left). A subtraction film (on the right) shows the anastomotic venous arcade (arrows).

General symptoms

Infective sinus thrombosis often gives the general symptoms of septicaemia. The patient is extremely ill, with a swinging temperature and rapid pulse, and rigors are common. Detachment of fragments of clot with resulting pulmonary embolism occurs most often in transverse sinus thrombosis with extension to the jugular vein. This event is indicated by sudden pain in the chest, with dyspnoea and sometimes haemoptysis, followed by signs of pulmonary consolidation and often a pleural rub. A lung abscess may follow. The commonest intracranial extension of the infection is to the leptomeninges, often resulting in diffuse meningitis, characterized by an increase in the severity of the headache, neck stiffness, Kernig's sign and other typical symptoms, together with a marked polymorphonuclear pleocytosis with or without organ-

isms in the CSF. In many cases, however, thrombophlebitis of cranial sinuses develops insidiously, or after the acute phase of the infection has passed.

Diagnosis

Cavernous sinus thrombosis is occasionally confused with other lesions in the neighbourhood of the superior orbital fissure. Similar local symptoms may be produced by carotico-cavernous fistula due to trauma or aneurysmal rupture (p. 208). Pulsation is present in the eye and a bruit is audible to the patient and often to the observer. Symptoms of infection are absent. The symptoms of retro-orbital or orbital tumour are of gradual onset and unassociated with evidence of infection. Unilateral exophthalmos due to Graves' disease, mucocele of the ethmoid sinus, orbital myositis or pseudotumour (*British Medical Journal* 1974) occasionally cause diagnostic difficulty, as may the syndrome of painful ophthalmoplegia (p. 108).

Thrombosis of the superior sagittal sinus, when it occurs in infancy, may be difficult to distinguish from other causes of hydrocephalus, which it often produces. In adults selective paralysis of the lower limbs, when present, is the most useful distinctive feature.

Transverse sinus thrombosis may be difficult to distinguish from other intracranial complications of mastoiditis, especially extradural, subdural, and intracerebral abscess, with any of which it may coexist. Radiological evidence, and especially the CT scan, will then be helpful. However, surgical exploration through the ear is still sometimes necessary under antibiotic cover.

Prognosis

Antibiotic treatment has transformed the prognosis of infective thrombophlebitis, and recovery is now usual even from cavernous sinus thrombosis which was formerly often fatal. The outlook is also good in transverse sinus thrombosis treated by aural surgery combined with antibiotic treatment. Hydrocephalus due to thrombosis of the superior sagittal sinus also resolves eventually as a rule, and cranial-nerve palsies usually recover. Some permanent loss of function is likely after extensive cortical venous thrombosis which may be followed by epilepsy as a late sequel. The mortality rate in thrombophlebitis of pregnancy is 33 per cent and 19 per cent of the survivors are left with permanent neurological deficits (Carroll *et al.* 1966).

Treatment

When sinus thrombosis is infective in origin, the source of infection must be treated with appropriate antibiotics. Ligature of the jugular vein, once commonly used in transverse sinus thrombosis, is now outdated. The value of anticoagulants is controversial because of the risk of haemorrhage: they are most likely to be useful if given in cases of primary thrombophlebitis before venous infarction has occurred but are now rarely used. Intravenous infusion of low-molecular-weight dextran is sometimes employed. Meningitis requires appropriate treatment. Otherwise treatment is symptomatic; dexamethasone in high dosage (p. 142) is useful in reducing cerebral oedema, especially when there are symptoms and signs of hydrocephalus.

References

(The cerebral venous circulation, thrombosis of the intracranial venous sinuses and veins.)

Averback, P. (1978). Primary cerebral venous thrombosis in young adults: the diverse manifestations of an underrecognized disease. *Ann. Neurol.* **3**, 81.

Bailey, O. T. and Hass, G. M. (1937). Dural sinus thrombosis in early life. *Brain* **60**, 293.

Bickerstaff, E. R. (1975). *Neurological complications of oral contraceptives*. Oxford University Press, Oxford.

British Medical Journal (1974). Pseudotumours of the orbit. *Br. med. J.* **2**, 5.

Carroll, J. D., Leak, D.and Lee, H. A. (1966). Cerebral thrombophlebitis in pregnancy and the puerperium. *Quart. J. Med.* **35**, 347.

Davies-Jones, G. A. B., Preston, F. E., and Timperley, W. R. (1980). *Neurological complications in clinical haematology.* Blackwell, Oxford.

Holmes, G. and Sargent, P. (1915). Injuries of the superior longitudinal sinus. *Br. med. J.* **2**, 493.

Kalbag, R. M. and Woolf, A. L. (1967). *Cerebral venous thrombosis.* Oxford University Press, London.

Kingsley, D. P. E., Kendall, B. E., and Moseley, I. F. (1978). Superior sagittal sinus thrombosis: an evaluation of the changes demonstrated on computed tomography. *J. Neurol. Neurosurg. Psychiat.* **41**, 1065.

Martin, J. P. and Sheehan, H. L. (1941). Primary thrombosis of cerebral veins (following childbirth). *Br. med. J.* **1**, 349.

Melamed, E., Rachmilewitz, E. A., Reches, A., and Lavy, S. (1976). Aseptic cavernous sinus thrombosis after internal carotid arterial occlusion in polycythaemia vera. *J. Neurol. Neurosurg. Psychiat.* **39**, 320.

Newton, T. H. and Potts, D. F. (1974). *Radiology of the skull and brain,* Vol. 2 (Angiography). Mosby, St. Louis.

Symonds, C. P. (1937). Hydrocephalic and focal cerebral symptoms in relation to thrombophlebitis of the dural sinuses and cerebral veins. *Brain* **60**, 531.

—— (1944). Venous thrombosis in the central nervous system. *Proc. R. Soc. Med.* **37**, 387.

Toole, J. F. and Patel, A. N. (1974). *Cerebrovascular disorders,* 2nd edn. McGraw-Hill, New York.

Walton, J. N. (1956). *Subarachnoid haemorrhage.* Livingstone, Edinburgh.

Weill, G. (1929). De la thrombo-phlébite du sinus caverneux. *Rev. Oto-neuro-ophthal.* **7**, 737.

5

Head injury

Non-penetrating injuries of the brain

Aetiology

In recent years head injuries have occurred with increasing frequency, owing to the high speed of modern life. In civil life most are due to direct violence resulting from motor and industrial accidents. Less frequently they are produced by indirect violence after falls on the feet or buttocks. Sporting injuries are not infrequent. Penetrating wounds of the brain are comparatively rare except in the missile injuries associated with war or civil unrest. Sewing needles inserted through a fontanelle have been used for attempted infanticide in some countries (Abbassioun, Ameli, and Morshed 1979). There is no direct parallelism between the severity of an injury to the skull and the extent to which the brain is damaged. Though severe skull fractures are often associated with severe cerebral injury, the brain may be extensively damaged without fracture and, on the other hand, fracture may occur without severe damage to the brain. Compound fractures, especially those involving the base and extending into the nasopharynx, nasal air sinuses, middle ear, and mastoid, assume additional importance, being liable to cause infection of intracranial contents giving meningitis or intracranial abscess. Apart from this risk, however, the crucial question after head injury is the state of the brain rather than that of the skull, and this alone will be considered here. For the physics of brain injury, and the characteristics of fractures of the skull and their treatment, see Gurdjian and Webster (1958), Rowbotham (1964), and Feiring (1974). For a discussion of epidemiology, see Field (1976) and Cartlidge and Shaw (1981). Accident is now the commonest cause of death under 45 years in developed countries; a million patients attend British hospitals each year with head injury, even more in relation to population in the USA, Australia, West Germany, and France; there are 7 000 deaths a year in Britain and 1 500 patients leave hospital with permanent brain damage (Jennett 1980), Injuries due to assault, to falls from bicycles in children (Cartlidge and Shaw 1981) and to falls in steeplechase jockeys (Foster, Leiguarda, and Tilley 1976) appear to be increasing.

Pathology

The factors operating upon the brain in head injury are multiple and complex, and their results often equally so. As Gurdjian, Lissner, Hodgson, and Patrick (1966) put it, 'compression, acceleration, and deceleration may occur during the traumatic episode. Tissues are injured by compression, tension, and shear. All of these modes of injury may occur simultaneously or in succession in the same accident.' These factors and their effects on the brain were described and discussed by Greenfield and Russell (1963) and by Tomlinson (1964). These processes, of which shearing forces may well be the most important, may give widespread microscopic lesions throughout the brain and brainstem (Oppenheimer 1968), microglial clusters (Clark 1974), and ischaemic or haemorrhagic lesions of the anterior hypothalamus (Crompton 1971). Ommaya and Gennarelli (1974) suggested that rotational and accelerative forces produce a graded centripetal progression of diffuse cortical–subcortical disconnection phenomena maximal at the periphery and enhanced at junctions between grey and white matter. Studies of cerebral blood flow and angiography have shown that after severe closed head injury there is widespread vascular spasm and slowing of the cerebral circulation (Macpherson and Graham 1973) but these changes do not invariably correlate with the pathological finding of widespread ischaemic lesions which were found in 55 per cent of a series

of fatal cases (Graham and Adams 1971). Unexplained haemorrhages in spinal posterior root ganglia may also be found (Spicer and Strich 1967). The persistent vegetative state (see below) can be associated with widespread axonal and diffuse degeneration of central white matter, but also with diffuse cortical and/or brainstem damage (Jennett and Plum 1972). Localized intracranial haematomata can occur without skull fracture at all ages from childhood to late life (Galbraith and Smith 1976) and the picture may be complicated by disseminated intravascular coagulation (Vecht, Sibinga, and Minderhoud 1975). Pathological examination of the brains of fatal cases has been helpful in identifying primary and secondary changes, thus helping to determine which avoidable factors in management may have contributed to death (Adams, Graham, Scott, Parker, and Doyle 1980; *British Medical Journal* 1981).

Concussion

Concussion was defined by Trotter as 'a condition of widespread paralysis of the functions of the brain which comes on as an immediate consequence of a blow on the head, has a strong tendency to spontaneous recovery, and is not necessarily associated with any gross organic change in the brain substance'. He stressed the reversibility of the process and suggested that concussion is a reversible impairment of consciousness of comparatively brief duration. It is now clear, however, that this cannot occur without some damage to nerve cells and fibres and it is now doubtful if any pathophysiological distinction can be drawn between concussion as just defined and more prolonged states of unconsciousness resulting from head injury (Symonds 1962). We know that consciousness depends upon the integrity of the ascending reticular alerting formation, and there is evidence that 'this system can be reversibly blocked by acceleration concussion' (Ward 1966). But even if concussion is associated with actual physical damage to nerve cells and fibres, in mild cases recovery is complete and there are no detectable sequelae, though the effects of a second injury may be cumulative (Gronwall and Wrightson 1975). The brainstem, attached above to the massive cerebral hemispheres and passing through an opening in the tentorium may well be especially vulnerable to brief displacements of cranial contents. This fact led to the view that head injuries producing a decerebrate state or prolonged unconsciousness probably resulted from primary brainstem injury (Maciver, Lassman, Thomson, and McLeod 1958a, b), but it is now clear that brainstem injury does not exist in isolation but is only one aspect of diffuse brain damage (Mitchell and Adams 1973; Ommaya and Gennarelli 1974). Nevertheless, acute pontine syndromes with retention of consciousness do sometimes occur (Turazzi and Bricolo 1977).

Cerebral contusion

The term cerebral contusion has traditionally been used to identify bruising of the brain, or a diffuse state more severe than concussion characterized by diffuse nerve-cell and axonal damage, multiple punctate haemorrhages, and oedema. As indicated above, it is doubtful whether it is now useful to distinguish this condition from concussion, as the pathological changes in the two conditions are similar, differing only in degree and depending upon the severity of the injury. Larger areas of haemorrhage are sometimes found, either in the cortex beneath the site of the blow, or in the contralateral hemisphere where the brain has been driven forcibly against the interior of the skull vault (*contre-coup* injury). Superficial haemorrhages are often found in one or both frontal, temporal, or occipital poles (Fig. 5.1) and may sometimes occur even after relatively minor injury, especially in the elderly. Diffuse degeneration of white matter is an important sequel of severe injury (Strich 1956; Tomlinson 1964).

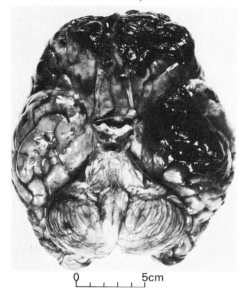

Fig. 5.1. The brain in a case of fatal closed head injury showing extensive areas of superficial haemorrhage over both frontal poles and in the left temporal region.

Hydrocephalus
The cerebral oedema which usually accompanies severe head injury generally causes a substantial rise in intracranial pressure (Johnston, Johnston, and Jennett 1970) with an accompanying increase in the pressure of the CSF in the ventricles and lumbar theca but arachnoidal adhesions may subsequently form resulting in disturbances of CSF formation and flow and even communicating hydrocephalus; rarely rupture of the arachnoid allows CSF to enter the subdural space, producing a subdural hygroma.

Cerebral laceration
'Cerebral laceration' is the term used when a contusion is sufficiently severe to cause a visible breach in the continuity of the brain substance. This may occur either beneath the site of the blow or by *contre-coup* on the opposite side.

Intracranial haemorrhage
Traumatic intracranial haemorrhage may be either intracerebral, subarachnoid, subdural, or extradural. An intracerebral haematoma may develop immediately after the injury but is rarely delayed, giving symptoms after an asymptomatic interval of hours or days, especially in older patients (Baratham and Dennyson 1972). Bleeding into the subarachnoid space is generally associated with cortical contusion. Acute subdural haemorrhage is usually the result of a severe laceration, which may either involve the surface of the hemisphere or cause a large cavity filled with blood within its substance. Less often it is due to rupture of venous tributaries of the superior sagittal sinus or to laceration of a venous sinus. Chronic subdural haematoma (p. 231) usually develops after a latent interval following minor trauma but sometimes arises spontaneously. Extradural haemorrhage is almost invariably the result of tearing of the middle meningeal artery or one of its branches due to a fracture of the skull vault crossing the groove in which it lies.

Symptoms and signs

Concussion and contusion
After a slight injury the patient may be merely dazed or unconscious for a few seconds only, but his higher mental functions may

subsequently be impaired for a period of several hours, during which he may carry out complicated activities automatically, afterwards remembering nothing of these events. This is the period of *post-traumatic amnesia* (Russell 1971) which is best measured from the injury to the time when continuous awareness is restored. This loss of memory may also extend to incidents which occurred before the accident, and is then known as *retrograde amnesia*. For example, a patient sustaining a head injury in an aeroplane crash may remember nothing that happened after he left the ground; or one injured in a motor accident may forget the incidents of a long drive (see p. 653); retrograde amnesia does not occur without post-traumatic amnesia (Yarnell and Lynch 1970; Wolpaw 1971). A simple quantitative questionnaire and test involving the naming and recall of people and common objects has been shown to give an accurate indication of the duration of post-traumatic amnesia (Fortuny, Briggs, Newcombe, Ratcliff, and Thomas 1980). In cases of more severe injury, unconsciousness is more prolonged, and in addition the patient often shows signs of brainstem dysfunction. The pupils may be dilated and may fail to react to light, and the cutaneous and tendon reflexes may be lost, the musculature being flaccid; in severe cases a decerebrate or decorticate state is present. The blood pressure is low and the pulse slow, or, in some cases, rapid and feeble, or imperceptible. Respiration may stop or may be shallow and sighing. Death may occur in severe cases from medullary paralysis. Many methods of assessing the severity of head injury have been introduced. The Ommaya scale assesses levels of impairment of consciousness on a five-point scale and the now widely used Glasgow Coma Scale (Jennett 1976; Jennett and Teasdale 1977; Table 5.1) depends upon the hierarchical scoring of responses to appropriate stimuli in three separate areas of function—eye-opening, limb movement, and verbal response (see Cartlidge and Shaw 1981).

Table 5.1. *Glasgow coma scale**

Eye-opening	Spontaneous
	To speech
	To pain
	None
Motor response	Obedience to commands
	Localization of pain
	Withdrawal
	Flexion to pain
	Extension to pain
	None
Verbal response	Orientated
	Confused conversation
	Inappropriate words
	Incomprehensible sounds
	None

In each category, responses to appropriate stimuli are graded from the highest to the lowest.
*Reproduced from Cartlidge and Shaw (1981) by kind permission of the authors and publishers.

Recovery is manifest first in an improvement of visceral function; the volume of the pulse increases, respiration becomes deeper, pupillary, brainstem, and other reflexes return, the eyes are opened on command, and voluntary semi-purposive movements appear. Vomiting is common at this stage. On recovering consciousness the patient may be delirious, restless, and irritable, and almost always complains of headache. In cases of mild concussion, however, these symptoms, with the possible exception of headache, usually disappear within a few days, though even after mild injury, the post-concussional syndrome (see below) may develop, especially in a compensation setting.

Traumatic encephalopathy

Focal brain damage may occur in the absence of clinical manifestations of concussion or contusion, especially when a localized blow causes a depressed fracture of the skull, when consciousness is often retained (Miller and Jennett 1968); the severity of the underlying damage to the brain may be dependent upon whether or not the dura is penetrated. In such cases, infection, haemorrhage, and focal neurological symptoms and signs are the most important complications. In moderate or severe closed head injury, with or without linear skull fracture, however, consciousness is usually lost immediately. In the most severe cases, the depth of coma steadily increases, and the patient dies from medullary paralysis within a few hours. In less severe cases the patient passes into a state of stupor or confusion. He is usually drowsy and presents the picture long known as 'cerebral irritation', but better described as traumatic delirium, lying in a flexed attitude, resenting interference, confused and disorientated when roused, and at times noisy and violent. This may last for days or even weeks with a corresponding duration of post-traumatic amnesia, and in favourable cases gradually passes away. Or the patient may remain stuporose (persistent vegetative state—Jennett and Plum 1972) for many months. Symptoms of a focal lesion of the brain are usually absent, but focal convulsions, hemiparesis, or aphasia (Heilman, Safran, and Geschwind 1971; Levin, Grossman, and Kelly 1976) may follow a contusion involving the cortex; injury to the basal ganglia may cause mutism and extrapyramidal syndromes, and damage to the midbrain may cause quadriplegia, tonic convulsions, and in less severe cases ocular palsies, diplopia, and nystagmus; other cranial-nerve palsies may be present (see below); and diabetes insipidus and disorders of hypothalamic function (Byrne 1951) are rare complications.

The post-concussional syndrome

Though a patient may recover rapidly and completely from a cerebral contusion, persistent disabling symptoms are common. The three cardinal late symptoms are headache, giddiness, and mental disturbances, which usually develop out of the symptoms of the acute stage. Headache tends to be severe and occurs in paroxysms which may last several hours, often against a background of continuous pain. It is brought on or exacerbated by stooping, sneezing, physical exertion, noise and excitement. The giddiness is not always a sense of rotation, but a feeling of instability, though true vertigo and staggering on sudden head movement are common. Post-traumatic vertigo induced by change of posture is probably due to damage to the utricle and saccule of the internal ear and is accompanied by nystagmus which can be recorded in the electronystagmogram (Cartlidge and Shaw 1981). Residual spastic pareses, and occasionally a parkinsonian syndrome after severe injury may be permanent but vertigo and nystagmus usually resolve in up to three years.

The commonest mental symptoms are inability to concentrate, fatigability and impairment of memory, together with nervousness and anxiety, and intolerance of alcohol. All grades are encountered between the common milder cases and the less frequent more severe examples. In the latter the patient passes from the initial stupor into a stage of profound disorientation and confusion with defects of perception and disorganization of speech, and then sometimes into a stage resembling Korsakow's psychosis with gross defects of memory for recent events and sometimes confabulation (Friedman and Brenner 1945). The final picture depends on many factors, especially the psychological constitution of the patient. Residual intellectual impairment is common: severe dementia is uncommon but not as rare as has been suggested (Fahy, Irving, and Millac 1967). Moods of excitement or depression are not infrequent in cyclothymic individuals while, after severe head injury with prolonged unconsciousness, paranoid and other psychotic manifestations have been reported (Fahy et al. 1967)

There has been considerable dispute as to whether the so-called post-concussional or post-traumatic syndrome as described above, when occurring in a setting which may involve financial compensation (e.g. in industrial or road accidents) is largely an organic disorder or an 'accident neurosis' (Miller 1961). Unquestionably headache, giddiness, impaired concentration, and the other symptoms described above occurring after moderate or severe head injury are the result of organic brain damage and may take between one and three years to recover, if indeed they ever do so (Cartlidge and Shaw 1981). These symptoms tend to be directly proportional in severity and duration to the duration of the post-traumatic amnesia (Steadman and Graham 1970) but may sometimes occur after relatively minor head injury (Gronwall and Wrightson 1974). However, neurotic and hysterical manifestations may cloud the clinical picture, especially when prolonged disability follows minor or even trivial injury and even frank malingering may be difficult to recognize (Miller and Cartlidge 1971). Considerable experience is necessary in the assessment of such cases; detailed psychometric testing may be needed but reliable objective measures are few and it may only be possible to talk of 'the balance of probabilities'. Foster (1976) has reviewed the medico-legal aspects. Gronwall and Wrightson (1981) found no clear correlation between tests of memory and information-processing on the one hand and the duration of post-traumatic amnesia on the other, though Brooks (1976) had found a correlation between the latter and memory defects as demonstrated on the Wechsler scale.

'Punch-drunkenness' is a chronic traumatic encephalopathy which may occur in professional boxers. It leads to deterioration of the personality, impairment of memory, dysarthria, tremor, parkinsonian features, and ataxia (Critchley 1957; Neubuerger, Sinton, and Denst 1959; Royal College of Physicians 1969; *The Lancet* 1973). Pneumoencephalography in such cases often shows not only cortical atrophy but absence or cavitation of the septum pellucidum (Harvey and Davis 1974). Even in young amateur boxers acute intracranial haemorrhage may occur (Cruikshank, Higgens, and Gray 1980). CT scans performed after a knock-out in professional boxers commonly reveal unexpected cerebral atrophy (Casson, Sham, Campbell, Tarlau, and Didomenico 1982). A chronic traumatic encephalopathy comparable to that found in boxers can occur in steeplechase jockeys after repeated head injury (Foster et al. 1976).

Acute traumatic cerebral compression

Cerebral compression leads to progressively deepening coma, indicated by the failure of the patient to respond to stimuli which previously roused him, and by loss of corneal reflexes. Deepening coma is of special importance when it follows a lucid interval after concussion. Ocular symptoms are important, the pupil on the side of the haemorrhage being first contracted and later dilated and failing to react to light, the same sequence of events subsequently occurring on the opposite side (Hutchinson pupil). These signs are due to tentorial herniation with pressure upon the trunk of one or both third cranial nerves. Papilloedema is usually absent, though the optic discs and fundi may show venous congestion. These signs must always raise the possibility of an extradural haematoma which is a neurosurgical emergency, but similar signs result from an acute subdural haematoma, an intracerebral haemorrhage, or even severe unilateral cerebral oedema associated with contusion or laceration, a fact which underlines the importance of CT scanning and skilled neurosurgical assessment and management of such cases. Symptoms and signs of a progressive lesion of the affected hemisphere, focal convulsions, or a flaccid hemiparesis are more likely to be due to an intracerebral lesion but rarely occur in extradural haemorrhage. Medullary symptoms are prominent, especially in the later stages. The pulse at first is slow and full, later rapid, thready, and irregular. The blood pressure may be subnormal or may rise steadily. The respirations are at first slow and deep, later irregular, e.g. of the Cheyne–Stokes type, and finally rapid and shallow.

Cranial-nerve palsies

Cranial-nerve palsies may be due to injury of the brainstem or of the nerves, either in their intracranial or in their extracranial course. Bilateral anosmia (p. 83) is a common complication due to tearing of olfactory nerve filaments as they pass through the cribriform plate of the ethmoid; ageusia (p. 129) is much less common. Contusion of the midbrain may leave permanent paresis of ocular movement, usually in the vertical plane, either unilaterally or bilaterally, resulting in diplopia and often associated with nystagmus. Intracranial injuries of the nerves are usually the result of fracture of the base of the skull. After the olfactory, the seventh is the nerve most frequently affected and then the eighth, sixth, second, third, and fourth in this order (Sherren 1908). Facial palsy may first appear several days after injury (Puvanendran, Vitharana, and Wong 1977a, b). The facial nerve, or its branches, and branches of the trigeminal may be divided or contused as a result of wounds of the face. Permanent diplopia can result from oculo-orbital displacement (Whitaker and Schaffer 1977). Traumatic cranial-nerve palsies are sometimes permanent, but recovery occurs when intracranial or extracranial nerve trunks have been contused rather than divided. Cartlidge and Shaw (1981) found that, while anosmia, unilateral blindness, or deafness were often permanent, delayed facial palsy or other cranial-nerve injuries usually recovered.

Cerebrospinal fluid

Examination of the CSF may yield information of value, but lumbar puncture is not without risk because of the risk of herniation of swollen brain. It should not be performed, therefore, unless absolutely necessary for diagnostic purposes. It is rarely needed in the acute stage if the CT scan and angiography are available, but may be necessary to exclude meningitis. Blood is present in the fluid immediately after the accident in most cases of cerebral contusion. The number of red cells present is not always proportionate to the severity of the injury; the protein content of the fluid is proportionate to the number of red cells. The supernatant fluid is xanthochromic. The red cells tend to disappear in four or five days, but the xanthochromia may remain for two or three weeks.

Electroencephalography

Suppression of the normal frequencies, widespread slow waves, and outbursts of high-voltage 2 to 3 Hz waves are seen in the acute stage. In the chronic post-traumatic state, generalized low-voltage 2 to 7 Hz waves, often seen in one or both temporal regions, are the rule and the disturbance is on the whole proportional to the severity of the injury (Williams 1941 a, b). However, the EEG may be surprisingly normal after severe brain injury and is disappointing in predicting which patients will and which will not develop post-traumatic epilepsy (Walton, Barwick, and Longley 1964).

Radiography

Radiography in the acute stage may show an unsuspected fracture of the skull, which often proves of greater medico-legal than clinical importance. Echo-encephalography and angiography were often used in the past to detect intracranial haematomata but have been largely supplanted by CT scanning which generally gives much more precise diagnostic information (Ambrose, Gooding, and Uttley 1976; Kalbag 1981). This investigation, like air encephalography (which often revealed evidence of ventricular dilatation or cortical atrophy in up to 80 per cent of severe cases) may also show, in the presence of an extensive cortical scar, a diverticulum from one cerebral ventricle (traumatic porencephaly). Enlargement of the Sylvian aqueduct may indicate midbrain damage (Boller, Albert, Le May, and Kertesz, 1972). Communicating hydrocephalus due to meningeal adhesions is an occasional late complication. Isotope encephalography (p. 78) may be needed to identify sites of CSF leakage following skull fracture.

Other investigations

Inspection and palpation of the scalp and skull form part of the routine examination of cases of head injury, the presence of haematomas being noted and the bones carefully examined for depressed fracture. Bleeding from the nasopharynx and ears in the absence of external injury is an important sign of fracture of the skull base, and inquiry should always be made as to the discharge of watery CSF, which may be recognized by its sugar content. The urinary output should be measured because of the risk of renal failure (Taylor 1957). As profound disturbances of hydration and acid-base balance readily occur in patients with head injury, and as pulmonary complications leading to cerebral anoxia are also common (Maciver, Frew, and Matheson 1958 a), regular monitoring of the blood urea and serum electrolytes and of the blood gases (oxygen and carbon dioxide) is necessary in the unconscious patient. The regular monitoring of intracranial pressure via an extradural transducer inserted surgically is needed in some cases and studies of the ventilatory response to rising CO_2, using a rebreathing method, are sometimes useful in assessing the severity of brain damage (North and Jennett 1976). Measurement of serum levels of myelin basic protein (Thomas, Palfreyman, and Ratcliffe 1978) also appears to be of some value in this respect and in predicting outcome.

Diagnosis

Although in most cases the injury to the head is clearly the cause of the patient's symptoms, it is necessary to bear in mind the possibility that a pre-existing illness, such as a stroke or intoxication with alcohol or other drugs, may have led to an accident in which the head has been injured, in which case the symptoms may not be due to the injury. When this source of confusion is eliminated, it is necessary to determine the nature of the brain injury. If after a head injury the patient remains unconscious for more than a few minutes, or if after recovery of consciousness he remains confused or exhibits other symptoms of cerebral dysfunction, it is reasonable to conclude that he has suffered concussion or cerebral contusion. The symptoms which distinguish acute traumatic cerebral compression from cerebral contusion were described above. The occurrence of cerebral fat embolism in a patient also suffering from a head injury may give rise to difficulty. The existence of a latent interval, pulmonary symptoms and signs, and cutaneous haemorrhages may enable the correct diagnosis to be made. The onset of meningitis is to be suspected, in a patient with known traumatic subarachnoid haemorrhage, when the patient develops increasing cervical rigidity and pyrexia, and is confirmed by the presence of a polymorphonuclear pleocytosis, with or without pyogenic organisms, in the CSF.

When confusion and drowsiness increase in severity, the possibility of intracranial haemorrhage or increasing oedema must be considered. When these are present, the symptoms tend to get worse, whereas in concussion or contusion the early symptoms tend to improve. Progressive symptoms in the later stages may suggest chronic subdural haematoma and render further investigation advisable.

Prognosis

Concussion is rarely fatal and, when the patient survives the immediate effects of the injury, is followed by complete recovery within a few weeks or months, provided it is not severe or complicated by contusion or more serious injuries. The post-concussional syndrome has been discussed above.

Traumatic encephalopathy, when severe, may prove fatal, usually within a few hours, from medullary paralysis. However, in Lewin's (1966 *a*) series of 7 000 patients with non-missile injuries admitted to hospital, the mortality rate was only 48 per cent. After severe injury some patients remain comatose for days or weeks and subsequently die from respiratory infection or other complications, but with modern nursing and medical care this is relatively uncommon and many enter, after a few weeks, a 'persistent vegetative state' (Jennett and Plum 1972), showing periods of apparent wakefulness, random eye movements, and primitive postural and reflex motor activity. Most remain in this state for months or even years but a few ultimately regain limited speech and volitional motor activity though all have severe residual intellectual and neurological deficits. Among the factors which have been shown to have an adverse influence upon prognosis are age (children often recover remarkably from severe injuries), decerebrate rigidity or extensor spasms, prolonged coma, hypertension, a low arterial $p(CO_2)$, a high respiratory minute volume, and a temperature persistently above 39 °C. (Vapalahti and Troupp 1971; Overgaard, Christensen, Huid-Hansen, Haase, Land, Heim, Pedersen, and Tweed 1973). In comatose patients, careful neurological examination with particular attention being paid to caloric, oculocephalic, and other brainstem reflexes and to the respiratory pattern may give valuable prognostic clues (Plum and Posner 1980). Jennett and Bond (1975) devised a useful five-point scale (the Glasgow outcome scale) for assessing the ultimate outcome, namely: (1) death; (2) persistent vegetative state; (3) severe disability (conscious but disabled); (4) moderate disability (disabled but independent); (5) good recovery. Miller and Stern (1965) reviewed the condition of 100 consecutive cases of severe head injury at a mean interval of 11 years. Eight patients had died, 21 out of 25 with spastic pareses showed unexpectedly good recovery, 19 had developed epilepsy, and 16 had persisting psychiatric symptoms, of whom 10 had dementia. Of 479 severe cases reviewed by Lewin, Marshall, and Roberts (1979), 4 per cent were totally disabled and 14 per cent severely so, but 49 per cent had recovered. Of 64 patients who were unconscious for a month or more, 40 had survived between three and 25 years after injury. While the value of the Glasgow outcome scale has been confirmed in the UK and in the Netherlands (Jennett, Teasdale, Braakman, Minderhoud, and Knill-Jones 1976; Jennett, Snoele, Bond, and Brooks 1981), more complex numerical scales for grading neurological and neuropsychological data in the early stages may be of even greater predictive value (Yen, Bourke, Nelson, and Popp 1978; Eson, Yen, and Bourke 1978). In minor head injuries with concussion, positive neurological manifestations observed 24 hours after injury correlate well with residual symptomatology at six months (Rutherford, Merrett, and McDonald 1977); emotional sequelae are generally greater in those with significant neuropsychological deficits in the early stages (Dikmen and Reitan 1977) and even after severe injury social recovery may be remarkably good (Oddy, Humphrey, and Uttley 1978). In a consecutive series of 372 cases admitted to hospital in Newcastle upon Tyne (Cartlidge and Shaw 1981), there were remarkably few severe head injuries with disabling sequelae; and anxiety and depression, post-traumatic headache, and dizziness were all common but generally improved; cognitive and memory defects showed most improve-

ment in the first six months but some patients showed lasting personality change. True malingering was rare.

Acute traumatic cerebral compression is fatal in many cases, the outlook being worse in acute subdural haemorrhage (which usually implies severe underlying cortical damage) than in extradural or intracerebral haematoma, provided surgical treatment is undertaken early. After successful evacuation of a clot, many patients recover completely but others are left with some disability.

Prophylactic chemotherapy has much reduced the incidence of meningitis, and lessened its dangers if it occurs. Late results of head injury, which include aphasia, persisting symptoms of injuries to the hypothalamus and midbrain (such as diplopia and diabetes insipidus), cranial-nerve palsies, intracranial aerocele, cerebrospinal rhinorrhoea, subdural haematoma, and traumatic epilepsy, are described elsewhere.

Treatment

The usual treatment of the unconscious patient should be carried out (see p. 650). If there is respiratory embarrassment, this should be treated by suction or tracheostomy. Oxygen should be administered by nasal tube or tracheostomy catheter. Hypothermia should be used if necessary to control pyrexia and may be useful in other severe cases. Hyperosmolarity of the blood may require intravenous fluid and other disorders of acid–base balance will require appropriate treatment. Convulsions, if severe, may need to be controlled by intravenous diazepam or thiopentone. Traumatic cerebral oedema responds well to steroids such as dexamethasone (see p. 171). Avoidable factors which contribute to death and morbidity include delay in treatment of an intracranial haematoma, poorly controlled epilepsy, meningitis, hypoxia, and hypotension (Rose, Valtonen, and Jennett 1977; *The Lancet* 1978 *a, b*). Prophylactic antibiotics should be given in all comatose patients and in severe cases the routine administration of sodium valproate or phenytoin has been shown to reduce the incidence of early and late post-traumatic epilepsy (see *The Lancet* 1980).

For details of surgical treatment the reader is referred to neurosurgical texts (Rowbotham 1964; Northfield 1973). The most important principles are first, to maintain an adequate airway and pulmonary ventilation from the outset, secondly, to reduce cerebral oedema and thus the intracranial pressure, and thirdly, to be prepared to operate immediately when an expanding intracranial haematoma is present.

The broad outlines of rehabilitation are now well defined; they were well set out by Jefferson (1942), Cairns (1942), Symonds (1942) and Lewis (1942) and have been reviewed by Tobis, Lowenthal, and Maringer (1957), Trethowan (1970), and Feiring (1974). It is essential to ascertain and take into account the personality of the patient before the accident. Explanation of symptoms and reassurance play an important part as soon as consciousness is regained. The patient should get out of bed as soon as he feels able to do so. After getting up, activity is increased, beginning with walking, games, and light exercises, and going on to more strenuous exercises. Supervised occupation should begin as early as possible and occupational therapy should gradually merge into therapeutic occupation. Throughout convalescence the patient's mental attitude must be kept constantly in mind. Psychological tests are of value for discovering specific disabilities, but the patient's emotional attitude to his difficulties is of equal importance, and explanation and encouragement are necessary throughout. Miller (1980) has shown that, in the acquisition of psychomotor skills, severely head injured patients have very poor starting levels compared with controls but may nevertheless learn rapidly and quickly close the gap. In cases uncomplicated by focal lesions, absence from work may last from six weeks to many months according to the severity of the injury. Persistent disabilities may make it impossible for patients to return to their pre-accident occupations. Special disabilities, especially speech disturbances, require prolonged treatment by experts.

Traumatic pneumocephalus and CSF rhinorrhoea

Synonym. Intracranial aerocele.

Definition. The presence of air within the skull as a result of head injury.

Aetiology and pathology

Trauma is the commonest cause of air within the skull; this is usually due to a fracture of the skull affording communication between an air-containing cranial cavity and the interior of the cranium. It may occur as the result of a fracture involving the frontal, ethmoidal, or sphenoidal sinuses or mastoid air cells or rarely follows operation on a nasal sinus. Occasionally, however, air enters the skull as a result of erosion of bone from within, for example by intracranial tumour, abscess, or hydrocephalus. Within the cranial cavity the collection of air may be external to the brain. Both subdural and subarachnoid collections have been described, but as the arachnoid is often torn, they are difficult to differentiate. The air sometimes penetrates one cerebral hemisphere, in which it becomes encysted.

Symptoms and signs

Cerebrospinal rhinorrhoea, a discharge of CSF from the nose, is usually an accompaniment of traumatic pneumocephalus. It may, however, occur when the base of the skull is eroded from within by intracranial tumour, abscess, or internal hydrocephalus. The volume of the discharge is variable: it may be small or profuse. The discharge is usually influenced by change of posture and may occur, for example, only when the patient sits up and leans forward. It often affords relief from headache. The presence of sugar in the fluid can be demonstrated by appropriate tests and is a useful diagnostic point. Air within the skull may occasionally be demonstrated by means of a tympanitic note on percussion, more frequently by a succussion splash audible to the patient and to the observer on shaking the patient's head. This sign implies the presence of both air and fluid within the same part of the cranial cavity.

Air within the skull may lead to focal symptoms, especially when it has invaded one cerebral hemisphere. They may include confusion, convulsions, aphasia, hemiparesis, and a grasp reflex. They tend to fluctuate in severity and may be relieved by an attack of CSF rhinorrhoea. Symptoms of increased intracranial pressure, for example headache and papilloedema, may also be present. In severe cases coma may develop.

X-ray examination of the skull is the most valuable single method of diagnosis, the situation of the air being exactly demonstrated. When fluid is also present within the cavity, it may be demarcated from the air by a horizontal line which varies in position in relation to gravity.

Diagnosis

Diagnosis offers little difficulty. All cases of serious head injury should be X-rayed and the air is then demonstrated. Isotope encephalography is valuable in localizing the point of leakage in CSF rhinorrhoea (p. 78).

Prognosis

Two factors influence the prognosis: the risks of a focal lesion of the brain associated with increased intracranial pressure and the risks of meningitis due to infection entering the skull through the opening in the bone.

Air in the ventricles and in the subarachnoid space is normally absorbed in from 10 to 14 days. It is doubtful, however, whether absorption occurs when the air is encysted by brain tissue. The risk of infection is high and, in most cases of head injury with CSF rhinorrhoea, meningitis supervenes in the absence of prophylactic antibiotic therapy and/or operative interference.

Treatment

In order to diminish the risks both of further entry of air and/or meningeal infection, the patient should be advised to avoid forcibly blowing his nose. Prophylactic chemotherapy should be employed. In Lewin's view 'operative repair is the treatment of choice for all cases of paranasal sinus fracture with cerebral fluid rhinorrhoea, whether this is of early or late onset, of brief or long duration' (Lewin 1966 *b*).

Subdural haematoma

Definition. An encysted collection of blood between the dura mater and the arachnoid, sometimes traumatic, but also occurring in the absence of obvious injury.

Pathology

Acute subdural haematoma is common in fatal cases of head injury: an extensive but thin layer of haemorrhage may raise the intracranial pressure enough to cause herniation of the uncus, or midbrain haemorrhages.

In chronic subdural haematoma, blood slowly accumulates in the subdural space. It is usually the result of a minor head injury causing rupture of veins which traverse the subdural space In most cases the collection of blood, which may become large, lies over the frontal and parietal lobes, and in some cases there are bilateral haematomas. Subdural bleeding in the posterior fossa is rare. The blood is encysted between an outer wall consisting of a layer of highly vascularized granulation tissue slightly adherent to the dura ('the membrane'), and a thinner, inner wall of fibrous tissue with a single layer of mesothelium on the side next to the arachnoid. It is mostly fluid, though a coagulum may be present. Subdural hygroma is a collection of CSF, which eventually becomes xanthochromic, and is indistinguishable (except by the CT scan) before operation from a subdural haematoma.

Aetiology

Males are affected more often than females in the ratio of three to one. Subdural haematoma may occur at any age. It is sometimes seen in infancy, when it has been attributed to birth injury but is sometimes due to postnatal trauma (Yashon, Jane, White, and Sugar 1968) as in the 'battered baby syndrome'. Subdural effusions may, however, develop as a complication of meningitis in infancy (Rabe, Flynn, and Dodge 1968). In adult life it is commonest in the elderly, usually resulting from trauma which may be trivial. Wintzen (1980) reviewed 212 cases of which the majority had a history of trauma but about 25 per cent did not. Of the 50 cases without such a history, eight showed an acute onset with severe symptoms within six hours, 42 were subacute or chronic. The condition is also an uncommon complication of aneurysmal rupture, especially recurrent bleeding, when the aneurysm may rupture directly into the subdural space (Golden, Odom, and Woodhall 1953; Clarke and Walton 1953). It may also follow air encephalography (Robinson 1957) or whiplash injury to the neck (Ommaya and Yarnell 1969) and has been reported during haemodialysis (Leonard, Weil, and Scribner 1969). Other causes include chronic alcoholism, liver disease, neurosyphilis, streptococcal infections, blood diseases such as scurvy and thrombocytopenic purpura, treatment with anticoagulants, and carcinoma of the dura; in such cases there is rarely any history of injury.

Symptoms and signs

The symptoms of subdural haematoma may follow an injury immediately. Alternatively there is a latent interval lasting weeks or months, less often more than a year, rarely of many years. During the latent interval the patient may be free from symptoms or may feel vaguely unwell (Scheinberg and Scheinberg 1964). After this interval, there is a gradual onset of headache, drowsiness, and often confusion: epilepsy is rare. The symptoms may fluctuate in severity but headache is often severe, paroxysmal, and induced by bending or coughing. Signs of focal cerebral dysfunction may be lacking or slight, even with a large haematoma. However, Luxon and Harrison (1979), in a retrospective study of 194 cases, found that epilepsy, aphasia, hemianopia, and dense hemiplegia were all found from time to time. Papilloedema is often absent. Pupillary dilatation and other features of a third-nerve palsy due to tentorial herniation may develop on the side of the haematoma.

In infants the onset occurs during the first year. Enlargement of the head may be the first abnormality to be noticed, but convulsions, irritability, and vomiting are common and pyrexia may be present (Till 1968). The head is enlarged, with a bulging anterior fontanelle and often separation of the sutures. The veins of the scalp are often dilated. Papilloedema and retinal and subhyaloid haemorrhages are usually present, sometimes leading to optic atrophy. The symptoms are therefore those of increased intracranial pressure with cortical irritation, and limb paralysis is usually absent. The CSF may be blood-stained or xanthochromic with increased protein, and is rarely normal. The diagnosis is established by subdural puncture, carried out at the lateral margin of the anterior fontanelle, xanthochromic or blood-stained fluid being withdrawn from the subdural space.

Diagnosis

The diagnosis of subdural haematoma offers little difficulty when there is a clear history of recent head injury. Without this the clinical picture may simulate that of intracranial tumour, especially when papilloedema is present. The fluctuating character of the drowsiness and confusion, however, may suggest the true diagnosis. In an elderly patient with a history of head injury, it may be difficult to distinguish subdural haematoma from a cerebral vascular accident. Luxon and Harrison (1979) found that the clinical presentation could mimic those of tumour, dementia, stroke, or subarachnoid haemorrhage. Chronic alcoholism may lead to confusion and drowsiness, and, since it is a predisposing cause of subdural haematoma and can also cause accidents which involve head injury, may give rise to difficulties in diagnosis. The CSF is often normal, but the protein may be increased, and the fluid may be xanthochromic. The pressure is usually raised but may be subnormal. There is rarely a pleocytosis. Spectrophotometry of the fluid (Kjellin and Steiner 1974) can be helpful. The CT scan is usually diagnostic but the diagnosis is confirmed unexpectedly at angiography in some cases (Luxon and Harrison 1979); this shows a characteristic displacement of arteries, with an avascular area beneath the skull vault (Fig. 5.2). Calcification is occasionally observed radiographically in a haematoma of very long standing, and Bull (1951) showed that the floor of the middle fossa may be excavated.

Prognosis

The prognosis of subacute or chronic subdural haematoma is good, provided the diagnosis is made sufficiently early for operation to be performed before the patient's condition has deteriorated seriously. Complete recovery is then the rule. In other cases, however, the patient fails to respond to evacuation. Echlin, Sordillo, and Garvey (1956) reported a mortality rate of 39 per cent in 300 cases. McKissock, Richardson, and Bloom (1960), dividing their cases into acute, subacute, and chronic, had a mortality rate of 57 per cent in the acute, 24 per cent in the subacute, and 6 per

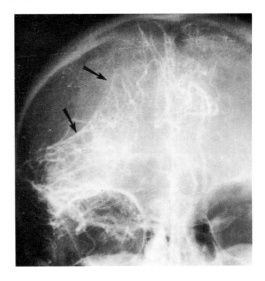

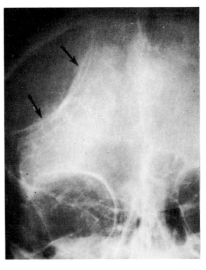

Fig. 5.2. A right-sided chronic subdural haematoma demonstrated by carotid angiography; arterial phase on the left, capillary phase on the right.

cent in the chronic group. The poor prognosis in acute cases applies not only to those following immediately after head injury when there is usually severe damage to the underlying brain, but also to those in which the condition develops apparently spontaneously (Wintzen 1980). In subacute or chronic cases the outlook worsens with increasing age, but operation is almost always justified.

Treatment

Treatment consists of surgical evacuation of the blood clot. Occasionally in chronic cases, craniotomy and removal of the membrane is required. Among others, Bender and Christoff (1974) advised non-surgical treatment, but this view has received little acceptance.

Post-traumatic epilepsy

Aetiology and pathology

Much early knowledge of the factors influencing the development of epilepsy after head injury was derived from studies of cases of gunshot wound of the head. Such injuries are not strictly comparable with most head injuries of civil life, since they include many more penetrating wounds and fewer cases of simple concussion and fracture of the skull base.

The incidence of epilepsy after penetrating wounds was assessed at 45 per cent by Russell and Whitty (1952), but Caveness (1966) suggested that with dural penetration it was 40 per cent, without it 20 per cent, and it is more frequent with posterior frontal and parietal injuries than with those at other sites (Watson 1947; Cartlidge and Shaw 1981). The incidence in 500 closed head injuries in soldiers was 6 per cent (Phillips 1954). Probably about 5 per cent represents the average incidence in civil life (Jennett 1975).

The latent period between the injury and the onset of fits is variable. In a few cases fits occur immediately after the injury, or in the first week (early post-traumatic epilepsy) (Jennett 1969), and status epilepticus has been described after relatively minor injury in childhood (Grand 1974). These usually cease and, if convulsions subsequently develop, they do so only after an interval of freedom (late post-traumatic epilepsy). There is some evidence (Whitty 1947; Jennett 1975; Cartlidge and Shaw 1981) that early attacks predispose to late ones. Apart from these early attacks, attacks may develop within a month or two of the injury or may be delayed for many years. A patient of Brain's, with a retained metallic foreign body, had his first attack 27 years after being wounded. The commonest time of onset is between six and 12 months after the injury, but figures vary. Jennett (1965) found that half the patients had their first attack within a year of the injury but, both in missile wounds (Adeloye and Odeku 1971) and in closed head injury, there is a substantial, though declining, subsequent risk which can be calculated by actuarial methods (Jennett, Teather, and Bennie 1973). However, the majority who become epileptic do so within two years (Miller and Stern 1965). Feeney and Walker (1979) have devised a mathematical method of predicting whether or not epilepsy is likely to occur, based upon the numerical assessment of various risk factors.

The severity of the injury is one important factor. Foerster and Penfield (1930) stressed the part played by scar tissue in aetiology; epilepsy is most likely to occur when vascularized scar tissue unites the surface of the brain to the dura, a process most likely to occur when the dura has been penetrated. Jennett (1965) found that, except in children, late epilepsy was rare with a duration of post-traumatic amnesia of less than 24 hours. Epilepsy following trivial head injury in adult life is rare (except in the elderly), but certainly occurs in childhood (Small and Woolf 1957). A family history is sometimes present, so inherited predisposition probably plays a part in aetiology in some cases.

Symptoms and signs

Attacks may be focal or generalized. Focal attacks often occur immediately after the injury. Their character and the nature of the aura, if any, depends upon the situation of the lesion. Even when early attacks are focal, there is a tendency for subsequent episodes to be major or, if minor, of the 'temporal lobe' type (pp. 614–15). The CT scan or air encephalography may be of diagnostic value, since air may fail to reach the area of cortex adherent to the dura and there may be a 'traction diverticulum', the lateral ventricle being drawn towards the lesion by atrophy of the white matter and by the scar. But in most cases there are no abnormal neurological signs and the scar is not detectable radiologically. The EEG may be normal between attacks (Walter 1938; Walton et al. 1964; Jennett and van de Sande 1975).

Diagnosis

For the diagnosis of epilepsy see page 619. Post-traumatic syncope and hysterical 'faints' can give rise to especial difficulty, especially in a setting involving financial compensation. Eye-witness descriptions of the attacks may be particularly important. The traumatic origin of genuine epilepsy can usually be established only when there is a history of injury, and this should be sought,

since the patient may not realize its importance if the attacks do not begin until several years later. A previous head injury may not necessarily be the cause of the attacks, but its aetiological significance is reinforced if the fits have a focal onset, if there are persistent signs of a focal cerebral lesion, and if the radiographic abnormalities already described are present.

Prognosis

The factors which influence the prognosis of 'idiopathic' epilepsy apply equally to post-traumatic cases, but when a gross focal lesion of the brain is present the prognosis as to recovery is worse than in epilepsy not so complicated. The attacks ceased in one-third of Ashcroft's cases. The prognosis is best when they begin within two weeks of the injury, worst when the latent interval is over two years. The life expectancy of patients with post-traumatic epilepsy is slightly reduced (Walker, Leuchs, Lechtape-Grüter, Caveness, and Kretschman 1971).

Treatment

Patients with post-traumatic epilepsy should receive anticonvulsant drugs as in cases of idiopathic epilepsy. Only very rarely, when drugs fail to control the attacks, should operation be considered. Foerster and Penfield (1930) and Penfield and Erickson (1941) claimed good results in selected cases. If operation is to be successful, the presence of a focal cerebral lesion must be established by the methods already described, ad it should be possible to find electrocorticographic abnormalities on the exposed cortex in the affected area. Treatment consists in a free excision of the scar tissue (Rasmussen and Gossman 1963). Improvements in drug treatment have meant that very few cases now require surgery.

References

Abbassioun, K., Ameli, N. O., and Morshed, A. A. (1979). Intracranial sewing needles: review of 13 cases. *J. Neurol. Neurosurg. Psychiat.* **42**, 1046.

Adams, J. H., Graham, D. I., Scoot, G., Parker, L. S., and Doyle, D. (1980). Brain damage in fatal non-missile head injury. *J. clin. Pathol.* **33**, 1132.

Adeloye, A. and Odeku, E. L. (1971). Epilepsy after missile wounds of the head. *J. Neurol. Neurosurg. Psychiat.* **34**, 98.

Ambrose, J., Gooding, M. R., and Uttley, D. (1976). E.M.I. scan in the management of head injuries. *Lancet* **i**, 847.

Ashcroft, P. B. (1941). Traumatic epilepsy after gunshot wounds of the head. *Br. med. J.* **1**, 739.

Baratham, G. and Dennyson, W. G. (1972). Delayed traumatic intracerebral haemorrhage. *J. Neurol. Neurosurg. Psychiat.* **35**, 698.

Bender, M. B. and Christoff, N. (1974). Nonsurgical treatment of subdural haematomas. *Arch. Neurol., Chicago* **31**, 73.

Boller, F. C., Albert, M. L., LeMay, M., and Kertesz, A. (1972). Enlargement of the Sylvian aqueduct: a sequel of head injuries. *J. Neurol. Neurosurg. Psychiat.* **35**, 463.

British Medical Journal (1981). Pathologists and head injuries. *Br. med. J.* **282**, 1344.

Brooks, D. N. (1976). Wechsler memory scale performance and its relationship to brain damage after severe closed head injury. *J. Neurol. Neurosurg. Psychiat.* **39**, 593.

Bull, J. W. D. (1951). Diagnostic radiology. In *Modern trends in neurology*, 1st series (ed. A. Feiling) Chapter 8. Butterworths, London.

Byrne, E. A. J. (1951). Post-traumatic disturbance of hypothalmic function. *Br. med. J.* **1**, 850.

Cairns, H. (1937). Injuries of the frontal and cthmoidal sinuses with special reference to cerebrospinal rhinorrhoea and aerocele. *J. Laryng.* **52**, 589.

—— (1941–2). Rehabilitation after injuries to the central nervous system. *Proc. R. Soc. Med.* **35**, 299.

Cartlidge, N. E. F. and Shaw, D. A. (1981). *Head injury*. Saunders, London.

Casson, I. R., Sham, R., Campbell, E. A., Tarlau, M., and Didomenico, A. (1982). Neurological and CT evaluation of knocked-out boxers. *J. Neurol. Neurosurg. Psychiat.* **45**, 170.

Caveness, W. F. (1966). Post traumatic sequelae. In *Head injury*, (ed. W. F. Caveness and A. E. Walker) p. 209. Lippincott, Philadelphia.

Clark, J. M. (1974). Distribution of microglial clusters in the brain after head injury. *J. Neurol. Neurosurg. Psychiat.* **37**, 463.

Clarke, E and Walton, J. N. (1953). Subdural haematoma complicating intracranial aneurysm and angioma. *Brain* **76**, 378.

Critchley, M. (1957). Medical aspects of boxing. *Br. med. J.* **1**, 357.

Crompton, M. R. (1971). Hypothalamic lesions following closed head injury. *Brain* **94**, 165.

Cruikshank, J. K., Higgens, C. S., and Gray, J. R. (1980). Two cases of acute intracranial haemorrhage in young amateur boxers. *Lancet* i, 626.

Dandy, W. E. (1925). Pneumocephalus (intracranial pneumatocele or aerocele). *Arch. Surg.* **12**, 949.

Denny-Brown, D. and Russell, W. R. (1941). Experimental cerebral concussion. *Brain* **64**, 93.

Dikmen, S. and Reitan, R. M. (1977). Emotional sequelae of head injury, *Ann. Neurol.* **2**, 492.

Echlin, F. A., Sordillo, S. V. R., and Garvey, T. Q. (1956). Acute, subacute and chronic subdural haematoma. *J. Am. med. Ass.* **161**, 1345.

Eson, M. E., Yen, J. K., and Bourke, R. S. (1978). Assessment of recovery from serious head injury. *J. Neurol. Neurosurg. Psychiat.* **41**, 1036.

Fahy, T. J., Irving, M. H., and Millac, P. (1967). Severe head injuries. *Lancet* ii, 475.

Feeney, D. M. and Walker, A. E. (1979). The prediction of posttraumatic epilepsy: a mathematical approach. *Arch. Neurol. Chicago* **36**, 8.

Feiring, E. H. (1974). *Brock's injuries of the brain and spinal cord and their coverings*, 5th edn. Springer, New York.

Field, J. H. (1976). *Epidemiology of head injuries in England and Wales*. HMSO, London.

Foerster, O. and Penfield, W. (1930). The structural basis of traumatic epilepsy and results of radical operation. *Brain* **53**, 99.

Fortuny, L. A. I., Briggs, M., Newcombe, F., Ratcliff, G., and Thomas, C. (1980). Measuring the duration of post traumatic amnesia. *J. Neurol. Neurosurg. Psychiat.* **43**, 377.

Foster, J. B. (1976). Medico-legal aspects of head injury. In *Handbook of clinical neurology* (ed. P. J. Vinken and G. W. Bruyn) Vol. 24, Part II, Chapter 39. North-Holland, Amsterdam.

——, Leiguarda, R., and Tilley, P. J. B. (1976). Brain damage in National Hunt jockeys. *Lancet* i, 981.

Friedman, A. P. and Brenner, C. (1945). Amnestic-confabulatory syndrome (Korsakoff psychosis) following head injury. *Am. J. Psychiat.* **102**, 61.

Galbraith, S. and Smith, J. (1976). Acute traumatic intracranial haematoma without skull fracture. *Lancet* i, 501.

Golden, J., Odom, G. L., and Woodhall, B. (1953). Subdural haematoma following subarachnoid hemorrhage. *Arch. Neurol. Psychiat., Chicago* **69**, 486.

Graham, D. I. and Adams, J. H. (1971). Ischaemic brain damage in fatal head injuries. *Lancet* i, 265.

Grand, W. (1974). The significance of post-traumatic status epilepticus in childhood. *J. Neurol. Neurosurg. Psychiat.* **37**, 178.

Greenfield, J. G. and Russell, D. S. (1963). Traumatic lesions of the central and peripheral nervous systems. In *Greenfield's neuropathology* (ed. W. Blackwood, W. H. McMenemey, A. Meyer, R. M. Norman and D. S. Russell) 2nd edn., p. 441. Arnold, London.

Gronwall, D. and Wrightson, P. (1974). Delayed recovery of intellectual function after minor head injury. *Lancet* ii, 605.

—— and —— (1975). Cumulative effect of concussion. *Lancet* ii, 995.

—— and —— (1981. Memory and information processing capacity after closed head injury. *J. Neurol. Neurosurg. Psychiat.* **44**, 889.

Gurdjian, E. S. and Webster, J. E. (1958). *Head injuries*. Little Brown, Boston.

——, Lissner, H. R., Hodgson, V. R., and Patrick, L. M. (1966). Mechanism of head injury. In *Clinical neurosurgery*, p. 112. Congress of Neurological Surgeons, Baltimore, Maryland.

Harvey, P. K. P. and Davis, J. N. (1974). Traumatic encephalopathy in a young boxer. *Lancet* ii, 928.

Heilman, K. M., Safran, A., and Geschwind, N. (1971). Closed head trauma and aphasia. *J. Neurol. Neurosurg. Psychiat.* **34**, 365.

Jefferson, G. (1941–2). Rehabilitation after injuries to the central nervous system. *Proc. R. Soc. Med.* **35**, 295.

Jennett, B. (1965). Predicting epilepsy after blunt head injury. *Br. med. J.* **1**, 1215.

—— (1969). Early traumatic epilepsy: definition and identity. *Lancet* i, 1023.

—— (1975). *Epilepsy after non missile head injuries*, 2nd edn. Heinemann, London.

—— (1980). Research in brain trauma. *Trends Neurosci.* **3**, 10.

—— and Bond, M. (1975). Assessment of outcome after severe brain damage: a practical scale. *Lancet* i, 480.

—— and Plum, F. (1972). Persistent vegetative state after brain damage: a syndrome in search of a name. *Lancet* i, 734.

—— and Teasdale, G. (1977). Aspects of coma after severe head injury. *Lancet* i, 878.

—— and Van de Sande, J. (1975). EEG prediction of post-traumatic epilepsy. *Epilepsia* **16**, 251.

——, Snoek, J., Bond, M. R., and Brooks, N. (1981). Disability after severe head injury: observations on the use of the Glasgow Outcome Scale. *J. Neurol. Neurosurg. Psychiat.* **44**, 285.

—— Teasdale, G., Braakman, R., Minderhoud, J., and Knill-Jones, R. (1976). Predicting outcome in individual patients after severe head injury. *Lancet* i, 1031.

——, Teather, D., and Bennie, S. (1973). Epilepsy after head injury. Residual risk after varying fit-free intervals since injury. *Lancet* ii, 652.

Johnston, I. H., Johnston, J. A., and Jennett, B. (1970). Intracranial-pressure changes following head injury. *Lancet* ii, 433.

Kalbag, R. M. (1981). Management of head injuries. In *Head injury* (ed. N. E. F. Cartlidge and D. A. Shaw) Chapter 13. Saunders, London.

Kjellin, K. G. and Steiner, L. (1974). Spectrophotometry of cerebrospinal fluid in subacute and chronic subdural haematomas. *J. Neurol. Neurosurg. Psychiat.* **37**, 1121.

The Lancet (1973). Boxing brains. *Lancet* ii, 1064.

—— (1978 a). Preventing secondary brain damage after head injury. *Lancet* ii, 1189.

—— (1978 b). Head injuries—from accident department to necropsy room. *Lancet* i 589.

—— (1980). Epilepsy after head trauma and fitness to drive. *Lancet* i, 401.

Leonard, C. D., Weil, E., and Scribner, B. H. (1969). Subdural haematomas in patients undergoing haemodialysis. *Lancet* ii, 239.

Levin, H. S., Grossman, R. G., and Kelly, P. J. (1976). Aphasic disorder in patients with closed head injury. *J. Neurol. Neurosurg. Psychiat.* **39**, 1062.

Lewin, W. (1966 a). Nonsurgical treatment of patients with head injuries. In *Clinical neurosurgery*, p 75. Congress of Neurological Surgeons, Baltimore, Maryland.

—— (1966 b). Cerebrospinal fluid rhinorrhea in nonmissile head injuries. in *Clinical Neurosurgery*, p. 237. Congress of Neurological Surgeons, Baltimore, Maryland.

——, Marshall, T. F. de C., and Roberts, A. H. (1979). Long-term outcome after severe head injury. *Br. med. J.* **2**, 1533.

Lewis, A. (1941–2). Differential diagnosis and treatment of post-contusional states. *Proc. R. Soc. Med.* **35**, 607.

Luxon, L. M. and Harrison, M. J. G. (1979). Chronic subdural haematoma. *Quart. J. Med.* **48**, 43.

Maciver, I. N., Frew, I. J. C., and Matheson, J. G. (1958 a). The role of respiratory insufficiency in the mortality of severe head injuries. *Lancet* i, 390.

——, Lassman, L. P., Thomson, C. W., and McLeod, I. (1958 b). Treatment of severe head injuries. *Lancet* ii, 544.

Macpherson, P and Graham, D. I. (1973). Arterial spasm and slowing of the cerebral circulation in the ischaemia of head injury. *J. Neurol. Neurosurg. Psychiat.* **36**, 1069.

McKissock, W., Richardson, A., and Bloom, W. H. (1960). Subdural haematoma. *Lancet* i, 1365.

McLaurin, R. M. (1966). Metabolic changes accompanying head injury. In *Clinical neurosurgery*, p. 143. Congress of Neurological Surgeons, Baltimore, Maryland.

Miller E. (1980). The training characteristics of severely head-injured patients: a preliminary study. *J. Neurol. Neurosurg. Psychiat.* **43**, 525.

Miller, H. (1961). Accident neurosis. *Br. med. J.* **1**, 919, 992.

—— and Cartlidge, N. (1972). Simulation and malingering after injuries to the brain and spinal cord. *Lancet* i, 580.

—— and Stern, G. (1965). The long-term prognosis of severe head injury. *Lancet* i, 225.

Miller, J. D. and Jennett, W. B. (1968). Complications of depressed skull fracture. *Lancet* ii, 991.

Mitchell, D. E. and Adams, J. H. (1973). Primary focal impact damage to the brainstem in blunt head injuries. Does it exist? *Lancet* ii, 215.

Neubuerger, K. T., Sinton, D. W., and Denst, J. (1959). Cerebral atrophy associated with boxing. *Arch. Neurol. Psychiat., Chicago* **81**, 403.

North, J. B. and Jennett, S. (1976). Response of ventilation and of intracranial pressure during rebreathing of carbon dioxide in patients with acute brain damage. *Brain*, **99**, 169.

Northfield, D. W. C. (1973). *The surgery of the central nervous system*. Blackwell, Oxford.

Oddy, M., Humphrey, M., and Uttley, D. (1978). Subjective impairment and social recovery after closed head injury. *J. Neurol. Neurosurg. Psychiat.* **41**, 611.

Ommaya, A. K. and Gennarelli, T. A. (1974). Cerebral concussion and traumatic unconsciousness. *Brain* **97**, 633.

—— and Yarnell, P. (1969). Subdural haematoma after whiplash injury. *Lancet ii*, 237.

Oppenheimer, D. R. (1968). Microscopic lesions in the brain following head injury. *J. Neurol. Neurosurg. Psychiat.* **31**, 229.

Overgaard, J., Christensen, S., Hvid-Hansen, O., Haase, J., Land, A. M., Heim, O., Pedersen, K. K., and Tweed, W. A. (1973). Prognosis after head injury based on early clinical examination. *Lancet ii*, 631.

Penfield, W. and Erickson, T. C. (1941). *Epilepsy and cerebral localization*. Thomas, Springfield, Illinois.

Phillips, G. (1954). Traumatic epilepsy after closed head injury. *J. Neurol. Neurosurg. Psychiat.* **17**, 1.

Plum, F. and Posner, J. B. (1980). *The diagnosis of stupor and coma*, 3rd edn. Davis, Philadelphia.

Puvanendran, K., Vitharana, M., and Wong, P. K. (1977 *a*). Delayed facial palsy after head injury. *J. Neurol. Neurosurg. Psychiat.* **49**, 342.

——, ——, and —— (1977 *b*). Electrodiagnostic study in delayed facial palsy after closed head injury. *J. Neurol. Neurosurg. Psychiat.* **40**, 351.

Rabe, E. F., Flynn, R. E., and Dodge, P. R. (1968). Subdural collections of fluid in infants and children: a study of 62 patients with special reference to factors influencing prognosis and the efficacy of various forms of therapy. *Neurology, Minneapolis* **18**, 559.

Rand, C. W. (1930). Traumatic pneumocephalus. *Arch. Surg.* **20**, 935.

Rasmussen, T. and Gossman, H. (1963). Epilepsy due to gross destructive brain lesions: results of surgical therapy, *Neurology, Minneapolis* **13**, 659.

Robinson, R. G. (1957). Subdural haematoma in an adult after air encephalography. *J. Neurol. Neurosurg. Psychiat.* **20**, 131.

Rose, J., Valtonen, S., and Jennett, B. (1977). Avoidable factors contributing to death after head injury. *Br. med. J.* **2**, 615.

Rowbotham, G. F. (1964). *Acute injuries of the head*, 4th edn. Livingstone, Edinburgh.

Royal College of Physicians (1969). *Report on the medical aspects of boxing*. London.

Russell, W. R. (1947). The anatomy of traumatic epilepsy. *Brain* **70**, 225.

—— (1971). *The traumatic amnesias*. Oxford University Press, London.

—— and Whitty, C. W. M. (1952). Studies in traumatic epilepsy: 1. Factors influencing the incidence of epilepsy after brain wounds. *J. Neurol. Neurosurg. Psychiat.* **15**, 93.

Rutherford, W. H., Merrett, J. D., and McDonald, J. R. (1977). Sequelae of concussion caused by minor head injuries, *Lancet i*, 1.

Scheinberg, S. C. and Scheinberg, L. (1964). Early description of chronic subdural hematoma: etiology, symptomatology and treatment. *J. Neurosurg.* **21**, 445.

Sherren, J. (1908). *Injuries of nerves and their treatment*. Nisbet, London.

Sherwood, D. (1930). Chronic subdural hematoma in infants. *Am. J. Dis. Childh.* **39**, 980.

Small, J. M. and Woolf, A. L. (1957). Fatal damage to the brain by epileptic convulsions after a trivial injury to the head. *J. Neurol. Neurosurg. Psychiat.* **20**, 293.

Spicer, E. J. F. and Strich, S. J. (1967). Haemorrhages in posterior-root ganglia in patients dying from head injuries. *Lancet ii*, 1389.

Steadman, J. H. and Graham, J. G. (1970). Head injuries: an analysis and follow-up study. *Proc. R. Soc. Med.* **63**, 23.

Strich, S. J. (1956). Diffuse degeneration of the cerebral white matter in severe dementia following head injury. *J. Neurol. Psychiat.* **19**, 163.

Symonds, C. P. (1941–2). Rehabilitation after injuries to the central nervous system. *Proc R. Soc. Med.* **35**, 601.

—— (1960). Concussion and contusion of the brain and their sequelae. In *Injuries of the brain and spinal cord* (ed. S. Brock), p. 69. Springer, New York.

—— (1962). Concussion and its sequelae. *Lancet i*, 1.

Taylor, W. H. (1957). Management of acute renal failure following surgical operation and head injury. *Lancet ii*, 703.

Thomas, D. G. T., Palfreyman, J. W., and Ratcliffe, J. G. (1978). Serum-myelin-basic-protein assay in diagnosis and prognosis of patients with head injury. *Lancet i* 113.

Till, K. (1968). Subdural haematoma and effusion in infancy, *Br. med. J.* **3**, 400.

Tobis, J. S., Lowenthal, M., and Maringer, S. (1957). Evaluation and management of the brain-damaged patient. *J. Am. Med. Ass.* **165**, 2035.

Tomlinson, B. E. (1964). Pathology. In *Acute injuries of the head*, 4th edn. (ed. G. F. Rowbotham) Chapter V. Livingstone, Edinburgh.

Trethowan, W. H. (1970). Rehabilitation of the brain injured: the psychiatric angle. *Proc. R. Soc. Med.* **63**, 32.

Turazzi, S. and Bricolo, A. (1977). Acute pontine syndromes following head injury. *Lancet ii*, 62.

Vapalahti, M. and Troupp, H. (1971). Prognosis for patients with severe brain injuries. *Br. med. J.* **3**, 404.

Vecht, C. J., Sibinga, C. T. S., and Minderhoud, J. M. (1975). Disseminated intravascular coagulation and head injury. *J. Neurol. Neurosurg. Psychiat.* **38**, 567.

Walker, A. E., Leuchs, H. K., Lechtape-Grüter, H., Caveness, W. F., and Kretschman, C. (1971). Life expectancy of head injured men with and without epilepsy. *Arch. Neurol., Chicago* **24**, 95.

Walter, W. G. (1938). The technique and applications of electroencephalography. *J. Neurol. Psychiat., N.S.* **1**, 359.

Walton, J. N., Barwick, D. D., and Longley, B. P. (1964). The electroencephalogram in brain injury. In *Acute injuries of the head*, 4th edn (ed. G. F. Rowbotham) Chapter XIV. Livingstone, Edinburgh.

Ward, A. A. (1966). The physiology of concussion, In *Clinical neurosurgery*, p. 95. Congress of Neurological Surgeons, Baltimore, Maryland.

Watson, C. W. (1947). The incidence of epilepsy following craniocerebral injury. *Res. Publ. Ass. nerv. ment. Dis.* **26**, 516.

Whitaker, L. A. and Schaffer, D. B. (1977). Severe traumatic oculo-orbital displacement. *Plastic reconstructive surg.* **59**, 352.

Whitty, C. W. M. (1947). Early traumatic epilepsy. *Brain* **70**, 416.

Williams, D. (1941 *a*). The EEG in acute head injuries. *J. Neurol. Psychiat., N.S.* **4**, 107.

—— D. (1941 *b*). The EEG in chronic post-traumatic states. *J. Neurol. Psychiat., N.S.* **4**, 131.

Wintzen, A. R. (1980). The clinical course of subdural haematoma: a retrospective study of aetiological, chronological and pathological features in 212 patients and a proposed classification. *Brain* **103**, 855.

Wolpaw, J. R. (1971). The aetiology of retrograde amnesia. *Lancet ii*, 356.

Yarnell, P. R. and Lynch, S. (1970). Retrograde memory immediately after concussion. *Lancet i*, 863.

Yashon, D., Jane, J. A., White, R. J., and Sugar, O. (1969). Traumatic subdural hematoma of infancy: long-term follow-up of 92 patients. *Arch. Neurol., Chicago* **18**, 370.

Yen, J. K., Bourke, R. S., Nelson, L. R., and Popp, A. J. (1978). Numerical grading of clinical neurological status after serious head injury. *J. Neurol. Neurosurg. Psychiat.* **41**, 1125.

Intracranial birth injuries

Aetiology and pathology

Normal labour involves considerable compression of the fetal head and probably in many cases slight intracranial damage, as is indicated by the presence of red blood cells in the CSF in some normal new-born infants. It is not surprising, therefore, that serious intracranial injury may result from excessive or otherwise abnormal compression due to abnormal presentations or contracted pelvis or difficult forceps delivery. The most serious intracranial birth injuries are tears of the dura involving rupture of important venous sinuses with consequent haemorrhage. As Holland (1922 *a, b*) showed, a major aetiological factor is excessive longitudinal stress leading to abnormal tension on the falx, which is anchored posteroinferiorly to the tentorium; as a result the tentorium may be torn or the internal cerebral vein ruptured. Large basal haemorrhages occur in such cases. In Holland's series of 167 fresh fetuses, the tentorium was torn in 81 (48 per cent) and the falx in 5. Subdural haemorrhages occurred in all but 6. Overriding of the parietal bones may lead to rupture of the superior sagittal sinus or of one or more

of its venous tributaries, with the production of a supracortical subdural haemorrhage, which is usually confined to, or predominates
upon, one side. Abnormal longitudinal stress is most likely to occur
in breech presentations, which are, therefore, especially hazardous. In such presentations, moreover, the thorax may be subjected
to considerable compression, thus leading to intracranial venous
congestion, oedema, and petechial haemorrhages. Those types of
major birth injury which usually occur in the full-term infant have
become progressively less common with improvements in obstetric
care (Menkes 1980). However, as these have decreased, intraventricular haemorrhage in the premature neonate (p. 351) which is
associated with perinatal hypoxia, respiratory distress, and hyaline-membrane disease has increased (Ellison and Farina 1980).
The route of delivery of the infant has little if any influence upon
the occurrence of these haemorrhages (Leviton, Gilles, and Strassfeld 1977). Measurement at birth of the Apgar score (Apgar 1953;
The Lancet 1982), which measures heart rate, breathing, reflex irritability, muscle tone, and colour, each on a three-point scale, has
proved to be a useful method of assessing the severity of the
infant's condition and of predicting subsequent disability.

The borderline between brain damage resulting from direct
trauma to the head during delivery and that which may result from
perinatal hypoxia, acidosis, hypoglycaemia, and cerebral ischaemia due to vascular distortion and compression (Norman, Urich,
and McMenemey 1957; Norman 1963; Courville 1971) is indistinct. Whereas traumatic haemorrhage *per se* is also rarely the
direct cause of cerebral palsy in the usual sense of spastic diplegia
(Ingram 1964), there can be little doubt that most of the syndromes of cerebral palsy (see Chapter 13) result from a combination of the factors referred to above, often identified by the
inclusive term 'perinatal trauma', though various cerebral malformations also play a part (Menkes 1980). Among the consequent
pathological changes are ulegyria (atrophic sclerosis of gyri), porencephaly, cystic degeneration of the central white matter (Benda
1952), periventricular encephalomalacia, especially in premature
infants (Banker and Larroche 1962), communicating hydrocephalus, and *état marbré* of the corpus striatum. Localized damage to
the cerebellum is sometimes seen (Courville 1971).

Symptoms

After a severe intracranial haemorrhage the child may be stillborn. If born alive it may show 'white asphyxia' due to medullary
paralysis. If it recovers from this, it may be cyanosed, breathing
slowly and irregularly. The pulse may be slow or thin and rapid.
The child cries feebly and is difficult to feed. Generalized rigidity
with head retraction is common, and local or general convulsions
may occur. A supracortical haemorrhage often causes hemiplegia.
Papilloedema and retinal haemorrhages may be present, and in
some cases exophthalmos, inequality of the pupils, squint, and
nystagmus occur. The fontanelles may be bulging and non-pulsat-
ing. The CSF is likely to be blood-stained and under increased
pressure, and in subdural haemorrhage, it may be possible to withdraw blood by subdural puncture at the lateral angle of the anterior fontanelle. Sometimes the signs of injury are absent at birth
but develop gradually in the course of the first four or five days.

Diagnosis

There is usually little doubt about the diagnosis, though the effects

of hypoxia, hypercarbia, acidosis, and hypoglycaemia, which may
occur in various combinations, giving cerebral oedema (Menkes
1980) may be similar, but in these disorders the CSF contains only
a few red cells and sometimes a raised protein. A high CSF bilirubin is a useful indication of intracranial haemorrhage (Menkes
1980). The CT scan is usually diagnostic.

Prognosis

In most cases in which the symptoms are sufficiently severe to
enable an intracranial birth injury to be diagnosed, death occurs,
if not before or immediately after birth, within three or four days.
Infants who survive may suffer from infantile hemiplegia, epilepsy, mental handicap, or hydrocephalus. The various forms of
cerebral palsy are considered on pages 351–6.

Treatment

Maintenance of an adequate airway, oxygen, the treatment of respiratory infection, the correction of metabolic abnormalities, steroids to reduce cerebral oedema, and the provision of adequate
fluid and nutrition are all important. A subdural haematoma may
require surgical evacuation.

References

Apgar, V. (1953). A proposal for a new method of evaluation of the newborn infant. *Current Res. Anaesth. Analges.* **32**, 260.
Banker, B. Q. and Larroche, J. C. (1962). Periventricular leukomalacia of
infancy. *Arch. Neurol., Chicago* **7**, 386.
Benda, C. E. (1952). *Developmental disorders of mentation and cerebral
palsies.* Grune and Stratton, New York.
Byers, R. K. (1920). Late effects of obstetrical injuries at various levels of
the nervous system. *New Engl. J. Med.* **203**, 507.
Christensen, E. and Melchior, J. (1967). *Cerebral palsy, a clinical and
neuropathological study*, Clinics in Developmental Medicine, No. 25.
Heinemann, London.
Courville, C. B. (1971). *Birth and brain damage.* Courville, Pasadena.
Ellison, P. H. and Farina, M. A. (1980). Progressive central nervous system deterioration: a complication of advanced chronic lung disease of
prematurity. *Ann. Neurol.* **8**, 43.
Holland, E. (1922a). *The causation of foetal death*, Ministry of Health
Reports, No. 7. HMSO, London.
—— (1922b). Cranial stress in the foetus during labour and on the effects
of excessive stress on the intracranial contents; with an analysis of
eighty-one cases of torn tentorium cerebelli and subdural cerebral hae-
morrhage. *J. Obstet. Gynaec. Br. Emp* **29**, 549.
Ingram, T. T. S. 81964). *Paediatric aspects of cerebral palsy.* Livingstone,
Edinburgh.
The Lancet (1982). The value of the Apgar score. *Lancet* i, 139.
Leviton A., Gilles, F., and Strassfeld, R. (1977). The influence of route
of delivery and hyaline membranes on the risk of neonatal intracranial
hemorrhages. *Ann. Neurol.* **2**, 451.
Menkes, J. H. (1980). *Textbook of child neurology*, 2nd edn. Lea and
Febiger, Philadelphia.
Munro, D. (1930). Symptomatology and immediate treatment of cranial
and intracranial injury in the new-born. *New Engl. J. Med.* **103**, 502.
Norman, R. M. (1963). Cerebral birth injury. In *Greenfield's neuropatho-
logy*, 2nd edn (ed. W. Blackwood, W. H. McMenemey, A. Meyer, R.
M. Norman, and D. S. Russell) p. 382. Arnold, London.
——, Urich, H., and McMenemey, W. H. (1957). Vascular mechanisms of
birth injury. *Brain* **80**, 49.
Schwartz, P. (1965). Parturitional injury of the newborn as a cause of men-
tal deficiency. In *Medical aspects of mental retardation* (ed. C. H.
Carter) Chapter 6, Thomas, Springfield, Illinois.

6

Diseases of the meninges

The anatomy of the meninges

The brain and spinal cord are covered by three membranes or meninges named, from without inwards, the dura mater, the arachnoid, and the pia mater.

The *dura mater* is thick and fibrous and serves as the internal periosteum of the skull bones, to which it is closely applied. The inner surface is covered with a layer of endothelial cells. Sheaths of dura extend outwards for a short distance as a covering for the cranial nerves as they pass through their respective foramina. Certain folds of the dura, or septa, partially separate the cranial cavity into compartments. These are the falx cerebri, the tentorium, the falx cerebelli, and the diaphragma sellae. The falx cerebri descends from the cranial vault in the midline lying between the cerebral hemispheres in the longitudinal fissure. It is attached anteriorly to the crista galli and posteriorly to the tentorium. At its superior attached border it splits into two layers to contain the superior sagittal sinus, and its lower free border splits similarly to contain the inferior sagittal sinus. The tentorium cerebelli separates the posterior and middle fossae of the skull, its free border surrounding the midbrain, while its attached border is fixed to the occipital and parietal bones and to the superior border of the petrous temporal bone. The posterior part of its attached border splits to enclose the transverse sinus, and the anterior part similarly encloses the superior petrosal sinus. The falx cerebelli lies in the midline between the tentorium and the internal occipital protuberance, to both of which it is attached, and its free border separates the cerebellar hemispheres posteriorly. The diaphragma sellae forms a roof to the sella turcica and contains an opening, through which passes the infundibulum.

The *pia mater* is a delicate membrane lined with endothelial cells, which intimately clothes the surface of the brain, dipping into the sulci.

The *arachnoid* is a similar membrane, lying between the dura and the pia and bridging over the sulci. The space between the arachnoid and the pia, known as the subarachnoid space, contains the CSF. Its expansions are known as the subarachnoid cisterns. The cerebellomedullary cistern (the cisterna magna) lies between the inferior surface of the cerebellum and the posterior surface of the medulla. The cisterna pontis, continuous with this, lies anterior to the pons and continues upwards into the cisterna interpeduncularis. This in turn continues forwards into a cistern lying in front of the optic chiasm—the cisterna chiasmatis. The subarachnoid space and its continuations into the brain substance—the perivascular spaces—have been described in the section on the CSF (p. 64). Between the dura mater and the arachnoid lies a potential space, the subdural space. The spinal meninges are described in the section on the spinal cord (p. 390).

The dura mater is sometimes called the pachymeninx, the arachnoid and the pia mater the leptomeninges. Inflammation of the dura has been called pachymeningitis, but this term is now rarely used; inflammation of the pia and arachnoid is sometimes called leptomeningitis, but more often simply meningitis.

Tumours of the meninges

See Intracranial Tumour, page 143.

Calcification of the falx

Calcification of the falx may be found incidentally in routine radiographs of the skull. It is best seen in postero-anterior radiographs as a well-defined linear opacity in the midline. It is much less evident in lateral views, in which it appears as scattered opaque flecks, most evident just above the crista galli and extending backwards for a variable distance. It is of no pathological significance: the same is true of the patchy dural calcification less often seen in the diaphragma sellae and in the dura of the skull vault.

Pachymeningitis

This term is now outmoded but syphilitic pachymeningitis was once common (p. 264). Suppuration between the dura and the skull (extradural abscess) is usually due to cranial osteitis; subdural abscess (p. 251) usually complicates paranasal sinusitis. Subdural haematoma was once identified by the obsolete term pachymeningitis interna haemorrhagica.

Acute leptomeningitis (meningitis)

Definition. Acute inflammation of the leptomeninges.

Aetiology

Infection may reach the meninges by the following routes.

1. *Direct spread from without.* This may occur as a result of skull fracture with either penetrating wounds of the cranial vault or fractures of the base, when organisms may spread to the meninges from the nasopharynx. In the latter case the fracture may be unsuspected until meningitis develops. Other external sources of meningitis are osteitis of cranial bones, especially mastoiditis, infection of the nasal air sinuses, especially the frontal sinus, and of the soft tissues of the scalp, and thrombophlebitis of the intracranial venous sinuses. Organisms are introduced rarely by lumbar puncture.

2. *Direct spread from within* may occur when the meninges are breached by a brain abscess or in tuberculous meningitis due to a cerebral tuberculoma.

3. *Infection through the blood stream.* In such cases meningitis follows bacteraemia. It may be the only or the principal manifestation, as in so-called 'primary' pneumococcal meningitis, meningococcal meningitis, and acute lymphocytic meningitis, or the meningeal infection may be secondary to focal infection elsewhere as, for example, in pneumonia, empyema, osteomyelitis, erysipelas, typhoid fever, etc., in which case the bacteraemia may or may not be associated with endocarditis due to the infecting organism. Tuberculous meningitis may thus be a manifestation of miliary tuberculosis.

4. *Meningitis complicating encephalitis and myelitis.* Meningeal inflammation often plays a subordinate role in encephalitis or myelitis. Poliomyelitis is one example of such a meningo-encephalomyelitis, and meningeal inflammation occurs similarly in other viral encephalitides. In such cases meningeal symptoms may be either prominent or slight, but the CSF yields evidence of meningeal involvement.

5. *Other forms of meningitis.* Subarachnoid haemorrhage excites an inflammatory reaction in the meninges, though organisms are absent. Aseptic meningitis may also result from the release of other irritative substances (e.g. air, cholesterol, keratin, spinal anaesthetics) into the subarachnoid space. The term 'serous meningitis' has no precise meaning and is outmoded. 'Meningism' occurs as a complication of acute infections, especially in childhood. Symptoms of meningeal irritation are associated with a rise in CSF pressure, often due to cerebral oedema.

Meningitis arising in, and at first limited to, the spinal canal (spinal meningitis) is rare; it may result from vertebral osteitis but has been described in tuberculosis (Wadia and Dastur 1969; Dastur and Wadia 1969) and is a rare consequence of staphylococcal infection.

The organisms commonly responsible for meningitis are the *Neisseria meningitidis, Diplococcus pneumoniae, Haemophilus influenzae, Listeria monocytogenes* (particularly in neonates), streptococcus, staphylococcus, *Escherichia coli, Citrobacter diversus* (Levy and Saunders 1981), *Eikenella corrodens* (Brill, Pearlstein, Kaplan, and Mancall 1982), all of which cause pyogenic meningitis; the *Mycobacterium tuberculosis*; and various viruses which cause 'lymphocytic meningitis'. Other organisms less frequently the cause of meningitis are *Salmonella typhosa, Bacillus anthracis, Brucella abortus, Pseudomonas aeruginosa,* leptospira, *Mycoplasma pneumoniae* (Decaux, Szyper, Ectors, Cornil, and Franken 1980), various parasites, and yeasts such as *Cryptococcus neoformans (Torula histolytica).* Mixed infections may occur; since antibiotic usage in minor infection has become common, community-acquired purulent meningitis of unknown aetiology (Geiseler, Nelson, and Levin 1981), without identification of the causal organism, has become more common but usually carries a good prognosis.

Acute pyogenic meningitis

Pathology

Whatever the causative organism, the pathological changes in acute pyogenic meningitis are similar in all cases. Whether the organism reaches the meninges by direct spread or through the blood stream, inflammation usually spreads rapidly through the whole subarachnoid space of the brain and spinal cord. The space between the pia and the arachnoid becomes filled with purulent exudate, which may cover the whole cortex or is occasionally confined to the sulci. In cranial osteitis and cerebral abscess the pus may be most evident near the source of the infection. The cortical veins are congested, and the gyri are often flattened due to oedema and hydrocephalus. Microscopically the meninges show inflammatory-cell infiltration which in the early stages consists wholly of neutrophils, though in the later stages lymphocytes and plasma cells are present (Fig. 6.1). In acute cases the brain shows little change except for perivascular inflammatory-cell infiltration in the cortex. In pneumococcal meningitis, greenish-yellow pus is particularly evident over the vertex and at the base of the brain. Indolent meningitis due to staphylococcus albus has been described in cases of hydrocephalus treated by shunting procedures (Holt 1969). If a purulent infection becomes subacute, due to inadequate treatment, or in meningitis due to *H. influenzae*, which often runs a subacute course, especially in children, there may be diffuse degeneration and even sometimes necrosis with glial proliferation in the superficial areas of the cerebral and cerebellar cortex and spinal cord (toxic encephalomyelopathy) and in the cranial nerves (especially the second and eighth, giving visual loss and/or deafness, but sometimes also in the third, fourth, sixth, and seventh). Similar changes may occur in the hypothalamus and corpora mammillaria, with perivascular cellular infiltration around subependymal veins, and thrombosis of subarachnoid veins and

even of the venous sinuses (Adams and Kubik 1947); subdural empyema is a rare complication. Hydrocephalus results in part from inflammatory adhesions in the basal cisterns and foramina of the fourth ventricle, in part from impairment of absorption of CSF due to blockage of arachnoidal villi. In tuberculous and other granulomatous meningitides, and occasionally in pyogenic meningitis (Smith, Norman, and Urich 1957), there may also be endarteritis of the circle of Willis and its branches, giving cerebral ischaemia or infarction.

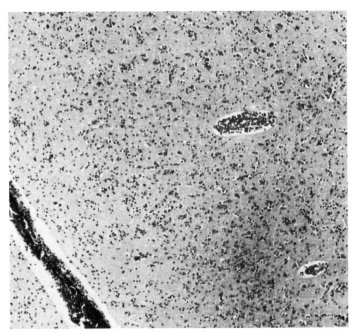

Fig. 6.1. Suppurative meningitis; a dense collection of inflammatory cells is present in the subarachnoid space and there is a superficial encephalitis with cellular infiltration of the cortex, especially around venules and capillaries. H & E, × 64.

Symptoms and signs

All forms of acute meningitis, whatever their cause, have certain symptoms in common. The onset may be fulminating, acute, or, less commonly, insidious. Headache, increasing in severity, is usually the first symptom.

General symptoms of infection are usually conspicuous. Fever is the rule, though the pyrexia varies. The temperature is usually between 37.8 °C and 38.9 °C though hyperpyrexia may occur, especially terminally. The pulse rate is also variable. It is sometimes slow in the early stages, for example between 50 and 60, but always rises as the illness progresses and at the end is usually very rapid and often irregular. The respiratory rate is usually slightly increased, and various forms of irregular respiration, especially Cheyne–Stokes breathing, may occur. Headache is prominent and usually very severe, possessing a 'bursting' character. It may be diffuse or mainly frontal, and usually radiates down the neck and into the back, sometimes being associated with pain in the spine radiating to the limbs, especially the lower. Vomiting may occur, especially in the early stages. Convulsions are common in children, especially in influenzal meningitis (Menkes 1980) but rare in adults. The patient tends to lie in an attitude of general flexion, curled up under the bed-clothes and resenting interference. There may be a high-pitched 'meningeal' cry in infants.

Signs of meningeal irritation

Cervical rigidity. Cervical rigidity (neck stiffness) is present at an early stage in almost every case. It is elicited by the observer placing his hand beneath the patient's occiput and endeavouring to flex the head so as to bring the chin towards the chest. In a normal individual this is accomplished with ease and without pain. In meningitis there is resistance due to spasm of the extensor muscles of the neck, and an attempt to overcome this causes pain.

Head retraction. Head retraction is an extreme degree of cervical rigidity brought about by spasm of extensor muscles. Flexion of the neck causes a rise in the tension of the CSF in the cisterna magna. When the meninges are inflamed this is painful; neck stiffness and head retraction represent reflex protective spasm. Cervical rigidity is usually associated with some rigidity of the lower spine.

Kernig's and Brudzinski's signs. To elicit Kernig's sign one knee is extended with the hip fully flexed; when positive there is pain and spasm of the hamstrings. Brudzinski's sign consists first of spontaneous flexion of the knees and hips on attempted neck flexion and secondly spontaneous flexion of one leg when the other is flexed passively These signs result from the presence of inflammatory exudate around the roots in the lumbar theca; they are often present in subarachnoid haemorrhage.

Other signs

The mental state of the patient varies according to the stage and progress of the disease. Delirium is common in the early stages, but often, as the disease progresses, gives place to drowsiness and stupor, which is followed by coma. Photophobia is also common. The fundi may be normal or may show venous congestion or, sometimes, papilloedema. The pupils are often unequal and may react sluggishly; they tend to be dilated and fixed. Ptosis is common as are squint and diplopia. Any of the ocular muscles may be paralysed, most frequently one or both lateral recti. Facial paresis is not rare. Dysphagia may also occur in the later stages. Muscular power in the limbs is usually preserved, though slight incoordination and tremor are common and there is often marked hypotonia. Diffuse flaccid paralysis is a terminal event. The tendon reflexes are usually sluggish and often soon lost; the abdominal reflexes also disappear early; the plantar reflexes are usually flexor at first, though later one or both may become extensor. Sensory loss is rare. True paralysis of sphincter control occurs only late, but stupor or coma may lead to retention or incontinence of urine early in the illness. *Tache cérébrale* is often elicitable (p. 241), but is not pathognomonic.

Meningitis localized for a time to one hemisphere may cause Jacksonian convulsions, hemiparesis, and even hemianopia. The toxic encephalomyelopathy referred to above, and/or hydrocephalus and cranial-nerve involvement may give rise to dementia, amnesia, epilepsy, paresis of the limbs, ataxia, blindness and deafness, paraplegia, and many other complications depending upon the site of maximal pathological change, but with the increasingly effective control of meningitis with antibiotics these late complications are becoming much less common. Nevertheless, cerebral herniation remains an important and potentially fatal complication, especially in infants and children (Horwitz, Boxerbaum, and O'Bell 1980). Persistent pyrexia, and increased intracranial pressure, along with vomiting, convulsions, and focal neurological signs present 72 hours after the start of treatment in infants should make one suspect the presence of a subdural effusion (Rabe, Flynn, and Dodge 1968; Menkes 1980).

The cerebrospinal fluid

The CSF is under increased pressure. Its appearance depends upon the number of leucocytes present, and ranges from slight turbidity to frank purulence. When it is turbid the deposit is yellow, and when macroscopic pus is present the supernatant fluid is often xanthochromic. The spontaneous formation of a fine coagulum is not uncommon. The cells are predominantly polymorphonuclear and may be present in very large numbers, amounting to many thousands per mm³. Often there are a few large mononuclear cells. The protein is increased, and in frankly purulent fluids may reach a high level—5.0 g/l or more. A reduction in chloride is usually secondary to vomiting and is of no diagnostic value. Glucose rapidly disappears from the fluid, or is at least greatly reduced and lactate rises reciprocally (Fishman 1980). IgA and IgG levels in the fluid are increased in all forms of meningitis, less so in the viral varieties, but in purulent meningitis the most striking increase occurs in IgM, a finding which may be used for diagnostic purposes (Smith, Bannister, and O'Shea 1973). Lactic dehydrogenase (Beaty and Oppenheimer 1968), aminotransferase (GOT) (Belsy 1969), and creatine kinase (Katz and Liebman 1970) may all be raised in the fluid, as may acid phosphatase and betaglucuronidase, especially in chronic meningitis (Shuttleworth and Allen 1968). Many amino acids are increased in the fluid (Corston, McGale, Stonier, Hutchinson, and Aber 1979). Organisms may be demonstrated in the films or on culture. Meningococci may be difficult to find and to culture but other cocci and *H. influenzae* may be present in profusion, unless the patient has been treated with antibiotics. Specific bacterial antigens can be sought using the technique of countercurrent immunoelectrophoresis (CIE test) with commercially available antisera against common meningeal pathogens (see Fishman 1980); however, the sensitivity of the test is limited because of the small concentration of bacteria in some patients. Nevertheless, in pneumococcal meningitis, the identification of pneumococcal polysaccharide antigen is very reliable (Tugwell, Greenwood, and Warrell 1976). The limulus lysate test can also be used for the detection of specific bacterial endotoxin and is especially useful in meningitis due to gram-negative bacteria. Tubercle bacilli should be sought, using the Ziehl–Neilsen stain, on centrifuged deposits of CSF (p. 239). Special methods are needed to isolate or culture viruses and yeasts.

Electrolyte and other metabolic disturbances

About 6 per cent of patients show hyponatraemia, sometimes with inappropriate secretion of antidiuretic hormone, giving hypervolaemia, oliguria, and symptoms of water intoxication (restlessness, irritability, and convulsions) requiring restriction of water intake and the administration of sodium. Persistent depression of CSF glucose levels probably indicates a persistent defect in the membrane transport of glucose or increased glycolysis in adjacent cerebral tissue (Fishman 1980) and this abnormality of cerebral carbohydrate metabolism, especially notable in pneumococcal meningitis (Tugwell *et al.* 1976) is an important cause of morbidity and mortality.

Diagnosis

Acute pyogenic meningitis must be distinguished from: (1) general infections with toxaemia, especially when headache is a prominent symptom; (2) meningism; (3) acute cerebral infections, including encephalitis and intracranial abscess; (4) subarachnoid haemorrhage; (5) other forms of meningitis and meningeal irritation.

1. *Acute general infections* which most often simulate meningitis are influenza, pneumonia, typhoid fever, and various viral infections. These are distinguished by the characteristic local and general symptoms of the infection and by the absence of signs of meningeal irritation, especially neck stiffness and Kernig's sign. However, acute infections may lead to meningism or may be complicated by meningitis, and in either case signs of meningeal irritation will be present. When diagnosis is in doubt, therefore, lumbar puncture should be performed.

2. *Meningism* is a state of meningeal irritation complicating acute infections. It is usually observed in the acute specific fevers and pneumonia in childhood, but may occur in adults with typhoid fever (Osuntokun, Bademosi, Ogunremi, and Wright 1972). Neck stiffness and Kernig's sign are present, but the CSF, though under increased pressure, is normal in composition.

3. Symptoms of meningeal irritation are usually present in *acute meningoencephalomyelitis* in childhood and in *acute disseminated encephalomyelitis* complicating the specific fevers, are almost constant in the early stages of *poliomyelitis*, and are not uncommon in all forms of *encephalitis*. The diagnosis of these disorders is based upon signs of involvement of the nervous system, especially the grey matter of the midbrain in meningo-encephalitis and of the corticospinal tracts in the various forms of acute disseminated encephalomyelitis. In acute poliomyelitis the stage of meningeal irritation precedes that of paralysis. In meningo-encephalitis and acute disseminated encephalomyelitis the CSF usually shows a modest mononuclear pleocytosis. In acute poliomyelitis the fluid contains an excess of cells, which in the first few days are both polymorphonuclear cells and lymphocytes. After the first week lymphocytes alone are found. This lymphocytic pleocytosis differentiates the condition from acute pyogenic leptomeningitis, and the normal glucose content from tuberculous meningitis. *Intracranial abscess* may simulate meningitis when it gives rise to neck stiffness, but this is not usually severe unless meningitis coexists. In cases of abscess the CSF usually contains an excess of cells, though not often more than 100 per mm^3, the majority being lymphocytes. The protein may be disproportionately increased. The sugar content of the fluid is normal and organisms are absent.

4. *Subarachnoid haemorrhage*, since it gives meningeal irritation, closely simulates meningitis. Its onset, however, is usually more rapid, and the true diagnosis is readily established by the demonstration of blood in the CSF.

5. *Other forms of meningitis.* Localized aseptic meningitis may occur as a complication of pyogenic infection close to the meninges, especially in mastoiditis, subdural abscess, and intracranial thrombophlebitis. In such cases the CSF is usually under increased pressure and shows a slight excess of cells, which may be either polymorphonuclear, mononuclear, or mixed. Organisms are absent. *Virus meningitis* should be suspected in cases of meningitis of acute onset running a benign course, in which no focal source of infection can be detected, in which there is a lymphocytic pleocytosis in the fluid and organisms cannot be demonstrated on repeated examination by ordinary methods. *Tuberculous meningitis* usually develops much more insidiously than the pyogenic variety, and symptoms of meningeal irritation, for example neck stiffness and Kernig's sign, are often slight and sometimes absent. The CSF contains an excess of cells, consisting usually of polymorphonuclear and mononuclear cells in varying proportions. The glucose content is diminished, usually to 0.1—0.4 g/l. Tubercle bacilli may be demonstrable in fluid or on culture, and there is usually evidence of tuberculous infection elsewhere. *Syphilitic meningitis* is occasionally sufficient acute to cause confusion. In such cases the CSF contains an excess of cells which are usually mononuclear, but in acute cases polymorphonuclear cells may also be present. The VDRL or other appropriate reactions are usually positive in the fluid and also in the blood. A subacute or chronic meningitis with an excess of cells in the CSF may also be due, for example, to *brucellosis, cysticercosis*, infection with *Cryptococcus neoformans*, *Behçet's disease, sarcoidosis, carcinomatosis of the meninges*, or *Mollaret's meningitis*.

Prognosis

The prognosis of acute pyogenic meningitis depends upon the nature of the invading organism, the number of organisms present in the CSF, the possibility of removing the source of infection, and the effectiveness of treatment. The introduction of the sulphonamides, of penicillin and streptomycin and other newer antibiotics revolutionized the prognosis of many forms of meningitis. Previously pneumococcal meningitis was almost invariably fatal and streptococcal meningitis was fatal in more than 90 per cent of cases. With early diagnosis, a recovery rate of 90 per cent or over may be expected in cases of 'primary' pneumococcal meningitis

and meningitis due to *H. influenzae* in developed countries but even comparatively recently the mortality of pneumococcal meningitis was up to 50 per cent (Baird, Whittle, and Greenwood 1976; Tugwell *et al.* 1976). Menkes (1979) has suggested that the use of intravenous glucose infusions in addition to antibiotic treatment is likely to improve the outcome. In meningitis complicating surgical conditions the mortality rate is still between 10 and 20 per cent. In uncomplicated meningococcal meningitis treated early the mortality rate is now usually under five per cent but may be much higher in infancy. Early and effective treatment should lead to recovery without residual symptoms. In any form of pyogenic meningitis treated late or inadequately, permanent damage may lead to dementia, epilepsy, deafness, blindness, or spastic weakness.

Treatment
See page 244.

Special features of meningococcal meningitis

Aetiology

Neisseria meningitidis is usually obtainable from the nasopharynx of both patients and 'carriers', and in the early stages of the infection can often be isolated from the blood. Meningococcal meningitis occurs both in epidemics and sporadically. It occurs worldwide and in the tropics; it is especially prevalent in the 'meningitis belt' of central Africa (Artenstein 1978). Since antibiotics came to be widely used for minor infections, epidemics have become much less frequent in temperate zones and developed countries. Group A organisms were once the commonest but have been superseded by Groups B and C which are less sensitive to sulphonamides. Sporadic cases occur at any time of year but epidemics are commonest in the spring.

The disease, although infectious, is only slightly so, and it is exceptional for multiple cases to occur in a single household or for the infection to spread in hospital. It is spread by droplet infection, mainly through 'carriers'. These are usually individuals who have been in contact with a patient and who usually harbour the organism in the nasopharynx for only two or three weeks. Such 'carriers', who greatly outnumber overt cases, may infect others without themselves developing the disease, or after a period of apparently good health may develop meningitis. An important cause of epidemics is overcrowding, and the disease is thus especially prevalent among school-children, and soldiers who are crowded together. Both sexes are affected equally, and the age of greatest susceptibility is from infancy to 10 years, the highest incidence being in the first year of life. It is rare after the age of 40. The incubation period varies from one to seven days and is usually about four days; during this period the organisms spread from the nasopharynx to the meninges via the blood stream.

Pathology

The pathology of meningitis is described on page 238. Some of the toxic changes in the brain found in severe cases are probably due to meningococcal endotoxin in the CSF (Ducker and Simmons 1968) while endotoxaemia may give increased peripheral vascular resistance, decreased visceral perfusion, and other manifestations of shock (Lillehei, Longerbeam, Bloch, and Manax 1964). Myocarditis and intravascular coagulation are serious complications in severe cases (Artenstein 1978). In the 'adrenal type', there is haemorrhage in both adrenals.

Symptoms and signs

Several clinical types of infection are recognized, viz.: (1) the average meningitic type; (2) the fulminating cerebral type; (3) the adrenal type; and (4) ameningitic meningococcal septicaemia. The symptoms of the average meningitic type are described on page 238.

The skin
Several types of rash may occur, the most typical being a purpuric eruption in the form of petechiae, which are purple at first, fading to a brownish colour, and do not disappear on pressure. They are especially liable to occur in areas subjected to pressure. The purpuric patches may be larger, even up to 2 cm in diameter in very severe cases. The purpuric eruption may appear during the first 24 hours and, if present, develops before the third day. It is seen in about one-third of all cases. A maculopapular rash is present less frequently, usually appearing before the fourth day, first on the trunk and later on surfaces of the thighs and forearms. Erythematous rashes can occur at any stage and facial herpes febrilis is common.

The blood
A well-marked polymorphonuclear leucocytosis occurs in the blood. Meningococci can sometimes be cultured from the blood in the early stages, but rarely after the signs of meningitis have appeared, unless chronic meningococcal septicaemia develops, as it does rarely. In acute septicaemia, the petechiae (as described above) may be due to small bacterial emboli; rarely there is extensive bruising with intravascular coagulation (Margaretten and McAdams 1958).

The cerebrospinal fluid
The changes are those of pyogenic meningitis (see p. 239). Meningococci can sometimes be demonstrated but are often difficult to find. If present, they are best found in smears made from centrifuged deposit. Most are intracellular, lying within polymorphonuclear leucocytes; many extracellular meningococci are believed to indicate a severe infection. If meningococci are not demonstrable on the first day, they may nevertheless be cultured. Meningococcal polysaccharide antigen is often, but not invariably, detectable by counter-immunoelectrophoresis and in many cases the limulus lysate test will detect meningococcal endotoxin.

It may be necessary to examine ventricular or cisternal fluid if hydrocephalus develops or if, in spite of improvement in the lumbar CSF, symptoms of infection persist. In infants showing such a picture, subdural tap is indicated (pp. 67 and 232).

Other manifestations
Slight cardiac dilatation may occur as a result of toxaemia, but true myocarditis and/or pericarditis may occur (see below). Catarrhal inflammation of the upper respiratory tract is also common. Rapid flushing of the skin in response to a light scratch (*tache cérébrale*), is often present, but is not pathognomonic.

Complications of meningococcal origin
The symptoms already described are those attributable to the meningitis and the bacteraemia which precedes it. Neurological complications of all forms of meningitis, including hydrocephalus, deafness and blindness, toxic encephalomyelopathy, and paraparcsis, have already been described. They were once relatively common sequelae of meningococcal meningitis but have become rare since effective chemotherapy and antibiotic treatment were introduced.

The eye. Conjunctivitis is fairly common. More severe ocular lesions, such as keratitis or panophthalmitis, are fortunately rare (Williams and Geddes 1970).

The heart. Fibrinopurulent pericarditis is a rare complication in severe cases but myocarditis is commonly found at autopsy in fatal cases (Hardman and Earle 1969). Bacterial endocarditis is rare.

Arthritis. This used to occur in from 10 to 15 per cent of cases in epidemics but is now much less common. Purulent arthritis was once the rule, but aseptic joint effusions are now seen more often. The knee- and shoulder-joints are most frequently affected, but almost any joint may be involved.

Genito-urinary system. Albuminuria is common. Rarely a focal nephritis develops, often with haematuria, presumably due to septicaemia and bacterial embolism. Epididymitis and orchitis are rare.

Non-meningococcal complications
Though bronchopneumonia may rarely result from the meningococcus, it is more often due to a secondary infection. Infection of the urinary tract may occur, especially when frequent catheterization is needed.

Other clinical types
In the *fulminating cerebral type*, presumably due to severe meningococcal septicaemia and endotoxaemia, the onset is sudden and the patient rapidly becomes comatose. Death may occur in a few hours without signs of meningeal irritation and with a clear CSF. In less acute cases there is slight neck stiffness and the fluid is turbid and contains meningococci.

In the *adrenal type*—the Waterhouse–Friderichsen syndrome—the characteristic features are grave hypotension and cyanosis (circulatory collapse), with biochemical changes characteristic of acute adrenal failure. There is a petechial rash with larger purpuric elements. The affected patients (usually children) are often alert and signs of meningitis are usually absent as the condition is due to septicaemia.

Chronic posterior basic meningitis. This chronic form of meningococcal meningitis occurring in infants, usually between the ages of 4 months and 2–3 years was once relatively common, due either to failure to recognize the nature of the initial infection, or to inadequate treatment; it is now rare. Head retraction is usually well marked, often with opisthotonos, and hydrocephalus soon develops.

Chronic meningococcaemia. While acute meningococcal septicaemia usually gives the more explosive clinical features described above, chronic septicaemia may give mild recurrent fever, fleeting maculopapular rashes, joint pains and swelling, and meningococci may be cultured from the blood. Spontaneous recovery may occur but a few patients ultimately develop meningitis.

Prophylaxis
Since meningococcal meningitis is spread chiefly by droplet infection from carriers, measures should be taken to ensure adequate ventilation and to avoid overcrowding in institutions and communities exposed to infection. Detection of carriers by swabbing the nasopharynx is impracticable on a large scale but may be of value in communities in which infection has occurred. A carrier should be isolated from children and young persons. Sulphadiazine was found by Kuhns, Nelson, Feldman, and Kuhn (1943) to protect individuals exposed to infection, but unfortunately most organisms of Group C are resistant to sulphadiazine so that this drug has been abandoned and antibiotics have generally been unsuccessful when used prophylactically (Artenstein 1978). The administration of penicillin to high-risk individuals as soon as they show any evidence of infection is now recommended. Mass vaccination with polyvalent vaccine containing Groups A and C polysaccharide antigen in Nigeria was shown to reduce dramatically the incidence of the disease and there were no untoward reactions (Mohammed and Zaruba 1981); it was suggested that a sustained programme of vaccination in the 'meningitis belt' may well eradicate the disease.

Listerial meningitis

Diffuse infection with *Listeria monocytogenes* may be found in aborted, premature, and stillborn children or in neonates dying soon after birth. Listerosis is also a common cause of pyogenic meningitis occurring within the first four weeks of life and cannot be differentiated from other forms of pyogenic meningitis except by culture of the organism, which is, however, readily mistaken for a diphtheroid bacillus. Listerial meningitis has also been reported rarely in adults, particularly in elderly subjects with debilitating diseases (Ford, Herzberg, and Ford 1968; Heck 1978). The organism is very sensitive to penicillin and to sulphonamides, chloramphenicol and erythromycin, so that prompt recognition of the condition in neonates is important, as is treatment of genital listerosis in the pregnant female, as treatment may prevent infection of the fetus.

The other organism which commonly causes neonatal meningitis is *E. coli*.

Tuberculous meningitis

Aetiology

Tuberculous meningitis may be a consequence of miliary tuberculosis, especially in children. Rich and McCordock (1933) and MacGregor and Green (1937), however, showed that in most cases the infection spreads to the meninges from a haematogenous caseous focus in the brain in contact with either the subarachnoid space or the ventricles. In children the condition is most often a consequence of primary or miliary tuberculosis, but in adults it usually develops in those with known tuberculosis elsewhere, especially in the lung. In Lincoln's (1947) series 50 per cent of patients were known sufferers from tuberculosis and 57 per cent had tuberculous contacts. While about a quarter of all cases used to be due to the bovine bacillus (MacGregor and Green 1937), most now result from the human organism. Once a disease mainly of childhood, it is now seen at any age and is equally frequent in adults. The pattern of tuberculous infection of the nervous system has changed (Kocen and Parsons 1970): thus some patients with symptoms of meningitis may show no pleocytosis in the spinal fluid, at least initially; others may show a transient aseptic meningitis which recovers spontaneously, despite culture of *M. tuberculosis* from the fluid (Emond and McKendrick 1973). Some, especially after BCG inoculation, present a clinical picture of a mild meningitic illness strongly suggesting benign lymphocytic meningitis, and others present with symptoms and signs of chronic spinal meningitis with evidence of spinal-cord compression but with, at least initially, no evidence of intracranial spread (Wadia and Dastur 1969; Dastur and Wadia 1969; Kocen and Parsons; Tandon 1978). Meningitis may also develop in patients with those intracranial tuberculomas which initially give symptoms of an intracranial space-occupying lesion.

Pathology

In acute cases, macroscopically, the brain is usually pale and the gyri are flattened. A yellowish gelatinous exudate is found matting together the meninges at the base and extending along the lateral sulci. Miliary tubercles may be visible on the meninges, being most conspicuous along the vessels, especially the middle cerebral artery and its branches. In many cases, however, careful sectioning of the brain is needed in order to demonstrate the causal focus. Microscopically the tubercles consist of collections of round cells, chiefly mononuclear (Fig. 6.2), often with central caseation. Giant cells are rare. Hydrocephalus, toxic encephalomyelopathy, involvement of cranial nerves, endarteritis (Fig. 6.2*b*) with consequent cerebral infarction (Smith and Daniel 1947), and other complications of subacute or chronic meningitis (p. 238) are especially common in tuberculous meningitis.

Symptoms and signs

The onset of symptoms is insidious, and there is almost always a prodromal phase of vague ill health. In children lassitude, anorexia, loss of weight, and intermittent vomiting are prominent. In adults symptoms of a confusional state may precede those of meningitis. This prodromal phase usually lasts two or three weeks, and is followed by symptoms of meningeal irritation. The pulse, previously rapid, becomes slow and irregular. Fever, if previously absent, usually now appears but the temperature, which is often markedly variable, does not usually rise much above 38.9 °C. Headache and vomiting appear and convulsions may occur. The patient becomes drowsy and at times delirious, but lucid intervals, even up to a late stage of the illness, are characteristic. Signs of meningeal irritation are usually less than in pyogenic meningitis. There is usually slight neck stiffness, but this may be absent and actual head retraction is rare. Kernig's sign is usually present. The patient frequently lies in a flexed attitude, resenting interference, and in the early stages often exhibits photophobia. Children sometimes utter what has been called a 'meningeal cry', a high-pitched scream.

Papilloedema is inconstant and when present develops only in the late stages. Choroidal tubercles are present in up to 20 per cent of patients and are visible ophthalmoscopically as ill-defined rounded or oval yellowish bodies about half the size of the disc. The pupils are usually contracted at first, but later become dilated and fixed. In subacute, chronic, or inadequately treated cases, involvement of cranial nerves may give ptosis, diplopia, facial weakness, deafness, or dysphagia. Endarteritis leading to cerebral infarction may give hemiplegia, while if hydrocephalus and diffuse arachnoiditis develop, there may be paresis and spasticity of all four limbs with extensor rigidity or even opisthotonos. Often in the early stages the tendon reflexes in the lower limbs are depressed but later are often increased and the plantars extensor. Retention of urine may be followed by incontinence of urine, less often of faeces. The *tache cérébrale* is common. In the uncommon localized spinal form, back pain and rigidity and progressive paraparesis with early urinary retention are usual; girdle or root pains are frequent (Tandon 1978).

Tuberculous lesions are usually found outside the nervous system. In one series radiography of the chest showed miliary dissemination in the lungs in 27 per cent, and enlarged hilar glands or active primary complex in 25 per cent; 13 per cent showed other lesions in lung, skin, or bone. The Mantoux text is positive in 85 per cent of cases (Lincoln 1947; Lincoln and Sewell 1963).

The cerebrospinal fluid

The CSF is under increased pressure. It is generally clear, but a fine 'cobweb' clot frequently forms on standing. There is an increase in cells, usually to about p. 100/mm^3 but varying from 10 to 1 000. These may all be mononuclear or a mixture of mononuclear and polymorphonuclear, the former predominating. There is a moderate increase in the protein, up to about 1.0–4.0 g/l but increasing to 10 g/l or more in the presence of severe arachnoidal adhesions or in the spinal form. The chloride content of the fluid is usually much reduced, but this is simply a result of the vomiting which occurs in most cases. There is a diminution in the glucose content, usually to below 0.5 g/l, and Lange's gold curve is meningitic. The frequency with which tubercle bacilli are found in the fluid varies in the hands of different workers. Some report that they are almost invariably demonstrable: others find them less often. Consequently, though their presence clinches the diagnosis, their absence is less significant. The organism should be cultured

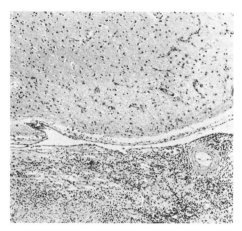

Fig. 6.2 Tuberculous meningitis.

(a) Lymphoid and epithelioid cells in the meninges with neuronal loss and gliosis in the cotex. H & E, × 64.

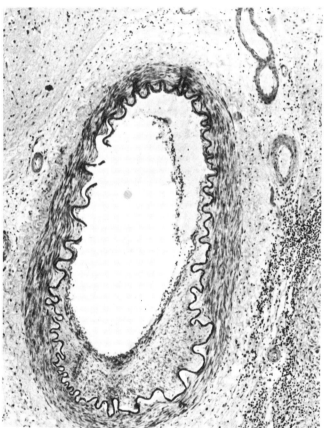

(b) Endarteritis in tuberculous meningitis. H & E, × 64.

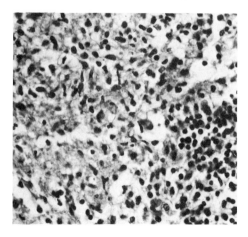

(c) Collections of lymphoid and epithelioid cells in the subarachnoid space. H & E, × 400.

and its sensitivity to streptomycin tested; guinea-pig inoculation should be used in doubtful cases.

The bromide test, in which serum and CSF bromide concentrations are measured after oral bromide administration or a single intravenous dose of 2–4 g in 10 ml of sterile water, has been found useful, as in tuberculous meningitis the CSF: serum ratio approaches unity, while in normal individuals it is about 1:3 (Taylor, Smith, and Hunter 1954). The test is often also positive in sarcoidosis and meningeal carcinomatosis and is now little used. A rapid latex particle agglutination test which detects *M. tuberculosis* plasma membrane antigen is both quick and accurate (Krambovitis, McIllmurray, Lock, Hendrickse, and Holzel 1984).

Diagnosis

Since effective treatment is now available, early diagnosis is vital. The general diagnosis of meningitis was discussed on page 239. Owing to the importance of examination of the CSF, lumbar puncture should be carried out without delay in any doubtful case, especially in any patient known to be tuberculous who develops symptoms or signs of meningitis. Sometimes when there is no such evidence, a CT scan may first be wise to exclude a space-occupying lesion. If a patient with meningitis has a mononuclear pleocytosis in the CSF with a glucose content below 0.5 g/l, if no malignant cells are detected by cytological examination of a centrifuged deposit, and if there is no evidence of syphilis, sarcoid, or fungal infection, it may be wise to treat him for tuberculous meningitis even though no mycobacteria are discoverable initially (even if the latex test is negative).

Prognosis

Before the introduction of streptomycin and other antituberculous drugs, tuberculous meningitis was almost invariably fatal in from 1 to 4 weeks after the onset, though recovery was very occasionally reported after tubercle bacilli had been demonstrated in the CSF and still occurs in the transient aseptic meningitis which has been occasionally reported as a consequence of tuberculosis (Emond and McKendrick 1973).

It is still too early to be certain what proportion of patients can be cured by modern treatment. Recoveries have been claimed in between 10 and 50 per cent of cases in different centres. Cairns and Taylor (1949) reported a fatality rate of 20 out of 49 patients, but a review by Miller, Seal, and Taylor (1963) showed that, whereas up to 1952 a mortality of about 30 per cent was usual, the introduction of isoniazid transformed the situation so that the mortality in Western countries fell to less than 10 per cent and recurrence after adequate treatment became rare. However, in developing countries even in the last decade, a mortality rate of between 30 and 55 per cent (see Tandon 1978) was still the rule, while in the West, especially in childhood, the outlook has continued to improve (Miller 1982). As would be expected, the earlier the patient is treated the better the prognosis and, if he is already comatose when first seen, the outlook is almost hopeless. Otherwise, the treated disease may run one of several courses, though the reasons for these variations are unclear. In cases which are ultimately fatal the patient may show no response to treatment, deteriorating rapidly and dying within the period expected of untreated cases, or show slow progressive deterioration with no period of improvement. Others show a short initial period of improvement, followed by progressive deterioration; others again improve for so long that they seem to be recovering and then relapse and progressively deteriorate. Those who survive show an equal variability. Some improve uninterruptedly from the beginning; others only after an initial stationary or fluctuating period. Some recover in spite of a relapse, and some after a long period of deterioration remain stationary with evidence of gross cerebral lesions. Broadly, among patients treated early the mortality-rate should be under 10 per cent and of those who survive 70 per cent should be free from sequelae.

The treatment of meningitis

The choice of drug

The appropriate treatment of meningitis depends upon the isolation of the organism and tests of its sensitivity to the available chemotherapeutic and antibiotic agents. The treatment of meningitis is a field in which, owing to the rapidity of new developments, techniques change rapidly. This is particularly evident in the management of tuberculous meningitis, where new developments quickly render older methods out of date. All that can be done in a textbook, therefore, is to provide an up-to-date summary of the methods which, at the time of writing, are generally regarded as best. Valuable reviews are given by Garrod, Lambert, and O'Grady (1980), Menkes (1980) and Bell (1981) who point out that the policy of administering immediately 10 000 units (6 mg) of benzylpenicillin in 10 ml saline intrathecally as soon as turbid fluid is found on lumbar puncture has much to commend it. Until a bacteriological diagnosis is made, ampicillin, 105 mg/kg body weight per day, is the most satisfactory initial systemic treatment.

The fundamental principles involved are that the infecting organism shall be sensitive to the agent used, and that this shall be used in such a way as to reach the organism in sufficient strength. The application of these principles will be considered in relation to particular varieties of meningitis.

Pyogenic meningitis

Many authorities believe that by giving massive systemic doses of antibiotics most cases of pyogenic meningitis, especially in meningococcal infection, can be satisfactorily treated without intrathecal injections. Nevertheless there are cases, especially those of pneumococcal infection or of infection with gram-negative organisms (*The Lancet* 1976), in which the response to a combination of intrathecal and systemic therapy is more rapid than that of systemic therapy alone. Hence many authorities still believe that it is wise to use both routes of administration at least initially in severe infections.

When a tentative diagnosis of meningitis has been made, no treatment should be given until a lumbar puncture has been performed, since the administration of antibiotics at that stage may make it impossible to identify the causal organism. If the fluid is turbid it may be assumed that the meningitis is pyogenic. Ten ml in two consecutive portions of 5 ml each should be removed for examination and culture. Testing the sensitivity of the organism takes time and valuable time may be lost if treatment is delayed until this has been reported upon. Hence in all cases of pyogenic meningitis it is wise to begin treatment at once with an intrathecal injection of benzylpenicillin (penicillin G) at the initial puncture, once CSF has been obtained. The dose for an adult is 10 000 units (6 mg) mixed with 10 ml of saline or of the patient's CSF, that for a child being calculated in proportion to its weight; 600 mg of penicillin G should also be given intramuscularly. If the infection proves to be pneumococcal, treatment should be continued with 4-hourly intramuscular injections of 1.2 g of penicillin G in an adult. Some authorities still recommend daily intrathecal injections of 10 000 units (6 mg) until the infection is well under control (usually in about one week) but others now regard these as unnecessary and rely on systemic treatment (see below). It is, however, important to note that multiple resistant pneumococci (*Steptococcus pneumoniae*), insensitive to penicillin and chloramphenicol, are now emerging (Radetsky, Istre, Johansen, Parmalee, Lauer, Wiesenthal, and Glade 1981) but may be sensitive to rifampicin. Streptococcal and staphylococcal infections should be treated similarly, but substituting ampicillin, or another drug, for penicillin should the organism be penicillin-resistant.

While recommendations relating to the use of chemotherapeutic agents and antibiotics in case of meningitis change rapidly from year to year, and while no simple guide can be comprehensive, taking account of all eventualities in the light of varying sensitivity of organisms to different remedies, Table 6.1 (Menkes 1980) presents the current position clearly, and useful reviews are also given by Garrod *et al.* (1980), Bell (1981), and Davidson and Lenman (1981). Sulphadiazine, once the drug of choice in meningococcal infections and in influenzal and *E. coli* meningitis, has now been largely discarded in favour of the antibiotics.

Table 6.1. *Choice of antibiotic in meningitis**

Organism	Conventional therapy
Bacteroides fragilis	Clindamycin, chloramphenicol, metronidazole
Bacteroides, other	Penicillin G
Clostridium	Penicillin G
Corynebacterium	Penicillin G, erythromycin
Streprococcus pneumoniae	Penicillin G
Enterobacter	Gentamicin, carbenicillin
Escherichia coli	Ampicillin, gentamicin, or kanamycin
Hemophilus influenzae	Ampicillin or chloramphenicol
Klebsiella	Gentamicin or kanamycin
Listeria monocytogenes	Ampicillin, gentamicin, or kanamycin
Neisseria meningitidis	Penicillin G
Neisseria gonorrhoeae	Penicillin G
Proteus mirabilis (indole negative)	Ampicillin
Proteus morganii (indole positive)	Gentamicin, kanamycin, or carbenicillin
Pseudomonas	Gentamicin, colistin, polymyxin, or carbenicillin
Salmonella	Ampicillin, gentamicin, or chloramphenicol
Staphylococci—penicillinase negative	Penicillin G
Staphylococci—penicillinase positive	Methicillin
Streptococci	Penicillin G
Unknown	Ampicillin, gentamicin, or kanamycin; methicillin if question of staphylococcal infection

*From Menkes (1980), p. 285.

Ampicillin is normally given by mouth in a dose of 250 mg 6-hourly to an adult, 125 mg 6-hourly to a child, but can also be given by intravenous injection in a dose of 200–400 mg/kg body weight in children. It is particularly recommended for infections with *H. influenzae*, *Streptococcus viridans*, and enterococci. Methicillin (100–200 mg/kg daily in four to six divided doses in a child or 1 g four times daily in an adult) or erythromycin (250–500 mg four times daily in an adult) are recommended for staphylococcal infections with penicillinase-producing organisms. Gentamicin is a wide-spectrum antibiotic, effective in most coccal infections, including those with methicillin-resistant staphylococci, but also of particular value in infections with *Enterobacter*, *Bacteroides*, *B. proteus*, *E. coli*, and *Pseudomonas*; the dose is 0.8–1.2 mg/kg daily in two to four equally divided doses in childhood and 60–80 mg 8-hourly in adults. Kanamycin is another antibiotic of value in infections with *Enterobacter*, *B.proteus*, and *E. coli*, but also with *Klebsiella*; the dose is 5–15 mg/kg intramuscularly in divided daily doses in children, 250–500 mg 6-hourly by mouth in adults. Both gentamicin and kanamycin must be used cautiously if there is evidence of impaired renal function and both may cause labyrinthine damage if high blood levels are maintained for more than a week.

Polymyxin B (1.5–2.5 mg/kg daily in four equally divided doses), colistin (2.5–5.0 mg/kg), or carbenicillin (400–600 mg/kg) are especially recommended for pseudomonas infections but may occasionally be useful in other infections; streptomycin, once widely used in infection with *H. influenzae*, *E. coli*, and *Pseudomonas*, is now used as a rule only in tuberculous meningitis. Chloramphenicol, too (75–100 mg/kg daily in children, 250 mg four times daily in adults), is less often used in meningitis because of the risk of bone-marrow suppression, unless the organism responsible is not sensitive to any other available antibiotic. Bell (1981) has tabulated in detail precise dosage required of these and other antibiotics given systemically and intrathecally in neonates and young infants. Other agents sometimes used rarely are clindamycin (adult dose 150–300 mg 6-hourly) and lincomycin (500 mg 6-hourly), especially in the treatment of penicillin-resistant staphylococcal infections and when *Bacteroides fragilis* is the infective agent; but these remedies carry a serious risk of causing pseudomembranous colitis. Vancomycin (500 mg every 6 hours) can be useful in enterococcal infections. Metronidazole (400 mg 8-hourly in adults) is effective against anaerobic bacteria such as *Bacteroides fragilis* and against protozoa. *Citrobacter* infection may require moxalactam (Levy and Saunders 1981). Most of the remedies listed can also be given, if need be, by intramuscular injection; the reader is referred to the manufacturer's instructions for details.

The question as to whether intrathecal as well as systemic treatment is necessary was mentioned above. While penicillin and some other antibiotics mentioned above only cross the normal blood-brain barrier in very small amounts, all cross the inflamed meninges in adequate concentration to deal with meningeal infections. Nevertheless it seems that meningitis is often controlled more rapidly if intrathecal therapy is given. In meningococcal meningitis, a single intrathecal injection followed by systemic treatment will usually suffice, but in other infections it is still the practice in some centres to give an intrathecal injection daily or every other day for the first one or two weeks, depending upon the condition of the patient, until the infection is under control. Among drugs which can be given intrathecally are penicillin G, 10 000 units (6 mg), streptomycin, 5–10 mg, polymyxin, 2 mg in children, 5 mg in adults, ampicillin, 3–5 mg for children, 10–20 mg for adults, methicillin, 3–5 mg for children, 10 mg for adults, amikacin, 1–3 mg in children, 10 mg in adults, erythromycin, 3–10 mg in the child, 20 mg in the adult, and gentamicin, 1 mg; all should be given well diluted in 10 ml of saline or CSF. Systemic antibiotic therapy should be given for about one week after the fluid has become sterile and relatively free from cells and after all clinical evidence of infection has subsided.

In all cases of pyogenic meningitis other than meningococcal, a careful search should be made for a source of infection, especially in the ears or paranasal sinuses, and the possibility of a coexistent intracranial abscess should be borne in mind.

Tuberculous meningitis

Each introduction of a new antibiotic effective against the tubercle bacillus has been followed by an improvement in the recovery rate from tuberculous meningitis. Routine treatment consists of the systemic administration of isoniazid and streptomycin in the following doses for an adult: isoniazid, 100 mg thrice daily by mouth, and streptomycin, 1 g daily by intramuscular injection. PAS is also often given in a dosage of 18–20 g daily. The doses in childhood are isoniazid, 20 mg/kg, streptomycin 20 mg/kg, and PAS 200 mg/kg daily. When the causal organism is resistant to isoniazid or streptomycin, rifampicin (10 mg/kg daily in the adult as a single morning dose) with ethambutol (25 mg/kg daily) should be given instead, but the latter drug is better avoided in children. Even after clinical recovery treatment should probably be continued for six to 12 months. As in pyogenic infections, some workers believe that tuberculous meningitis can be adequately treated without intrathecal injections. This is true in some cases, but there still appears to be a place for such injections, particularly in severely ill patients or in those who are not otherwise responding well. The intrathecal dose of streptomycin is from 20 to 50 mg daily or every

other day for 10 injections. The routine administration of steroid drugs (e.g. prednisone, 40 mg daily at first and later 30 mg or 20 mg daily) during the first few weeks probably helps to reduce complications such as adhesive arachnoiditis and communicating hydrocephalus and is now recommended by most authorities. When a rise in CSF protein and a fall in its pressure suggests that a spinal subarachnoid block is developing, an intrathecal dose of 10–25 mg of hydrocortisone, repeated daily if necessary for a week, is often valuable. Pyridoxine in doses of 40 mg daily should be given to prevent the development of isoniazid neuropathy, and anticonvulsants are often given prophylactically for several weeks. Now that more drug-resistant strains of tubercle bacilli are emerging, newer remedies such as ethionamide, pyrazinamide, or cycloserine may be needed in some cases. The development of hydrocephalus calls for surgical intervention and rarely for the administration of streptomycin into the ventricles.

The main index of a good response to treatment is the disappearance of tubercle bacilli from the CSF. In favourable cases these usually disappear within the first two weeks. Of the chemical constituents the glucose level is the most useful but is of little help after streptomycin has been given intrathecally. The protein content may rise considerably after such treatment, and a high protein with a falling cell count has been regarded as a good sign, though both ultimately fall. A high cell count, mainly polymorphonuclear, may be a reaction to the streptomycin.

A relapse is indicated by gradual or sudden deterioration in the condition of a patient who has previously been making good progress. Fever, vomiting, increase in headache, irritability, and apathy are the chief symptoms, while the CSF is likely to show a fall in glucose content, a rising cell count, and a reappearance of the organism in films or cultures. This calls for further intrathecal treatment. The development of resistance to streptomycin by the organism during treatment is fortunately rare. Details of treatment and of prognosis are given by Miller *et al.* (1963) and Menkes (1980).

Toxic effects of streptomycin include vertigo, which is often transitory, and possibly an ataxic gait in the convalescent, which also usually disappears after re-education. Deafness is a more serious complication, since when it occurs it is usually permanent. After an illness involving many weeks in bed, convalescence is necessarily prolonged, and the after-care is that of any form of chronic tuberculosis.

General measures

Good nursing is of the utmost importance and in severe cases the long illness, often with relapses, and the need for repeated lumbar punctures, make heavy demands upon the skill and patience of the nurses. Nasal or parenteral feeding and the administration of dextrose saline by intravenous drip is often required with particular attention to correction of electrolyte imbalance. An indwelling catheter is often needed for a time. Sedatives will usually be needed to control restlessness and in some cases convulsions. Ounsted (1951) stressed the dangers of status epilepticus. In childhood especially prophylactic anticonvulsant therapy with sodium phenytoin 50 mg twice daily is often wise. Repeated convulsions may require intravenous diazepam as given in the treatment of status epilepticus (p. 625).

References

Adams, R. D. and Kubik, C. (1947). The effects of influenzal meningitis on the nervous system. *NY State J. Med.* **47**, 2676.

Artenstein, M. S. (1978). Meningococcal meningitis. In *Handbook of clinical neurology* (ed. P. J. Vinken and G. W. Bruyn) Vol. 33, Chapter 2. North-Holland, Amsterdam.

Ashby, M. and Grant, H. (1955). Tuberculous meningitis treated with cortisone. *Lancet i*, 65.

Baird, D. R., Whittle, H. C., and Greenwood, B. M. (1976). Mortality from pneumococcal meningitis. *Lancet* **ii**, 1344.

Banks, H. S. (1948). Meningococcosis. *Lancet* **ii**, 635.

—— and McCartney, J. E. (1943). Meningococcal adrenal syndromes and lesions. *Lancet* **i**, 771.

Beaty, H. N. and Oppenheimer, S. (1968). Cerebrospinal fluid lactic dehydrogenase and its isoenzymes in infections of the central nervous system. *New Engl. J. Med.* **279**, 1197.

Bell, W. E. (1981). Treatment of bacterial infections of the central nervous system. *Ann. Neurol.* **9**, 313.

Belsy, M. A. (1969). CSF glutamic oxaloacetic transaminase in acute bacterial meningitis. *Am. J. Dis. Child.* **117**, 288.

Bhagwati, S. N. (1971). Ventriculo-atrial shunt in tuberculous meningitis with hydrocephalus. *J. Neurosurg.* **35**, 309.

Brill, C. B., Pearlstein, L. S., Kaplan, J. M., and Mancall, E. L. (1982). CNS infections caused by *Eikenella corrodens*. *Arch. Neurol., Chicago* **39**, 431.

Cairns, H., Smith, H. V., and Vollum, R. L. (1950). Tuberculous meningitis. *J. Am. med. Ass.* **144**, 92.

—— and Taylor, M. (1949). Streptomycin in tuberculous meningitis. *Lancet* **i**, 148.

Corston, R. N., McGale, E. H. F., Stonier, C., Hutchinson, E. C., and Aber, G. M. (1979). Abnormalities of cerebrospinal fluid amino-acids in purulent meningitis. *J. Neurol. Neurosurg. Psychiat.* **42**, 881.

Dastur, D. K. and Wadia, N. H. (1969). Spinal meningitides with radiculo-myelopathy. Part 2: Pathology and pathogenesis. *J. neurol. Sci.* **8**, 261.

Davidson, D. L. W. and Lenman, J. A. R. (1981). *Neurological therapeutics*. Pitman Medical, London.

Decaux, G., Szyper, M., Ectors, M., Cornil, A., and Franken, L. (1980). Central nervous system complications of mycoplasma pneumoniae. *J. Neurol. Neurosurg. Psychiat.* **43**, 883.

Drury, M. I., O'Lochlainn, S., and Sweeney, E. (1968). Complications of tuberculous meningitis. *Br. med. J.* **1**, 842.

Ducker, T. B. and Simmons, R. L. (1968). The pathogenesis of meningitis. Systemic effects of meningococcal endotoxin within the cerebrospinal fluid. *Arch. Neurol., Chicago* **18**, 123.

Emond, R. T. D. and McKendrick, G. D. W. (1973). Tuberculosis as a cause of transient aseptic meningitis. *Lancet* **ii**, 234.

Fishman, R. A. (1980). *Cerebrospinal fluid in diseases of the nervous system*. Saunders, Philadelphia.

Ford, P. M., Herzberg, L., and Ford, S. E. (1968). Listeria monoctyogenes: six cases affecting the central nervous system. *Quart. J. Med.* **37**, 281.

Freiman, I. and Geefhuysen, J. (1970). Evaluation of intrathecal therapy with streptomycin and hydrocortisone in tuberculous meningitis. *J. Pediat,* **76**, 895.

Garrod, L. P., Lambert, H. P., and O'Grady, F. (1980). *Antibiotic and chemotherapy*, 5th edn. Churchill-Livingstone, Edinburgh.

Geiseler, P. J., Nelson, K. E., and Levin, S. (1981). Community-acquired purulent meningitis of unknown etiology: a continuing problem. *Arch. Neurol., Chicago* **38**, 749.

Harding, J. W. and Brunton, G. B. (1972). *Listeria monocytogenes* meningitis in neonates. *Lancet* **ii**, 484.

Hardman, J. M. and Earle, K. M. (1969). Myocarditis in 200 fatal meningococcal infections. *Arch. Pathol.* **87**, 318.

Heck, A. F. (1978). Listeria monocytogenes. In *Handbook of clinical neurology* (ed. P. J. Vinken and G. W. Bruyn), Vol. 33. Chapter 7, North-Holland, Amsterdam.

Hoeprich, P. D. (1958). Infection due to *Listeria monocytogenes*. *Medicine, Baltimore* **37**, 142.

Holt, R. (1969). The classification of staphylococci from colonized ventriculo-atrial shunts. *J. clin. Pathol.* **22**, 475.

Horwitz, S. J., Boxerbaum, B., and O'Bell, J. (1980). Cerebral herniation in bacterial meningitis in childhood. *Ann. Neurol.* **7**, 524.

Illingworth, R. S. and Wright, T. (1948). Tubercles of the choroid. *Br. med. J.,* **2**,365.

Katz, R. M. and Liebman, W. (1970). Creatine phosphokinase activity in central nervous system disorders and infections. *Am. J. Dis. Child.* **120**, 543.

Kocen, R. S. and Parsons, M. (1970). Neurological complications of tuberculosis: some unusual manifestations. *Quart. J. Med.* **39**, 17.

Krambovitis, E., McIllmurray, M. B., Lock, P. E., Hendrickse, W., and Holzel, H. (1984). Rapid diagnosis of tuberculous meningitis by latex particle agglutination. *Lancet* **ii**, 1229.

Kuhns, D. M., Nelson, C. T., Feldman, H. A., and Kuhn, L. R. (1943). The prophylactic value of sulfadiazine in the control of meningococcic meningitis. *J. Am. med. Ass.* **123**, 335.

The Lancet (1976). Intrathecal antibiotics in purulent meningitis. *Lancet* **ii**, 1068.

Levy, R. L. and Saunders, R. L. (1981). *Citrobacter* meningitis and cerebral abscess in early infancy: cure by moxalactam. *Neurology, Minneapolis* **31**, 1575.

Lillehei, R. C., Longerbeam, J. K., Block, J. H., and Manax, W. G. (1964). The modern treatment of shock based on physiologic principles. *Clin. Pharmacol. Ther.*, 63.

Lincoln, E. M. (1947). Tuberculous meningitis in children, with special reference to serous meningitis. *Am. Rev. Tuberculosis* **56**, 75.

—— and Sewell, E. M. (1963). *Tuberculosis in children*. McGraw-Hill, New York.

Lorber, J. (1960). Treatment of tuberculous meningitis. *Br. med. J.* **1**, 1309.

MacGregor, A. R. and Green, C. A. (1937). Tuberculosis of the central nervous system, with special reference to tuberculous meningitis. *J. Path. Bact.* **45**, 613.

Margaretten, W. and McAdams, A. J. (1958). An appraisal of fulminant meningococcemia with reference to the Schwartzman phenomenon. *Am. J. Med.* **25**, 868.

McKendrick, G. D. W. (1954*a*). Pyogenic meningitis. *Lancet* **ii**, 510.

—— (1954*b*). Pneumococcal meningitis. *Lancet* **ii**, 512.

Menkes, J. H. (1980). *Textbook of child neurology*, 2nd edn. Lea and Febiger, Philadelphia.

Menkes, J. J. (1979). Improving the long-term outlook in bacterial meningitis. *Lancet* **ii**, 559.

Miller, F. J. W. (1982). *Tuberculosis in childhood*. Churchill-Livingstone, Edinburgh.

——, Seal, R. M. E., and Taylor, M. D. (1963). *Tuberculosis in children*. Churchill, London.

Mohammed, I. and Zaruba, K. 81981). Control of epidemic meningococcal meningitis by mass vaccination. *Lancet* **ii**, 80.

Osuntokun, B. O., Bademosi, O., Ogunremi, K., and Wright, S. G. (1972). Neuropsychiatric manifestations of typhoid fever in 959 patients. *Arch. Neurol., Chicago* **27**, 7.

Ounsted, C. (1951). Significance of convulsions in children with purulent meningitis. *Lancet* **i**, 1245.

Rabe, E. F., Flynn, R. E., and Dodge, P. R. (1968). Subdural collections of fluid in infants and children: a study of 62 patients with special reference to factors influencing prognosis and the efficacy of various forms of therapy. *Neurology, Minneapolis* **18**, 559.

Radetsky, M. S., Istre, G. R., Johansen, T. L., Parmalee, S. W., Lauer, B. A., Wiesenthal, A. M., and Glode, M. P. (1981). Multiply resistant pneumococcus causing meningitis: its epidemiology within a day-care centre. *Lancet* **ii**, 771.

Rich, A. R. and McCordock, H. A. (1933). The pathogenesis of tuberculous meningitis. *Bull. Johns Hopk. Hosp.* **52**, 5.

Shuttleworth, E. C. and Allen, N. (1968). Early differentiation of chronic meningitis by enzyme assay. *Neurology, Minneapolis* **18**, 534.

Smellie, J. M. (1954). The treatment of tuberculous meningitis without intrathecal therapy. *Lancet* **ii**, 1091.

Smith, H., Bannister, B., and O'Shea, M. J. (1973). Cerebrospinal-fluid immunoglubulins in meningitis. *Lancet* **ii**, 591.

Smith, H. V. and Daniel, P. (1947). Some clinical and pathological aspects of tuberculosis of the central nervous system. *Tubercle, London* **28**, 64.

—— and Vollum, R. L. (1950). Effects of intrathecal tuberculin and streptomycin in tuberculous meningitis. *Lancet* **ii**, 275.

——, Norman, R. M., and Urich, H. (1957). The late sequelae of pneumococcal meningitis. *J. Neurol. Neurosurg. Psychiat.* **20**, 250.

Tandon, P. N. (1978). Tuberculous meningitis. In *Handbook of clinical neurology* (ed. P. J. Vinken and G. W. Bruyn), Vol. 33, Chapter 12. North-Holland, Amsterdam.

Taylor, L. M., Smith, H. V., and Hunter, G. (1954). The blood–cerebrospinal fluid barrier to bromide in the diagnosis of tuberculous meningitis. *Lancet* **i**, 700.

Tugwell, P., Greenwood, B. M., and Warrell, D. A. (1976). Pneumococcal meningitis: a clinical and laboratory study. *Quart. J. Med.* **45**, 583.

Wadia, N. H. and Dastur, D. K. (1969). Spinal meningitides with radiculo-myelopathy. Part 1: Clinical and radiological features. *J. neurol. Sci.* **8**, 239.

Williams, D. N. and Geddes, A. M. (1970). Meningococcal meningitis complicated by pericarditis, panophthalmitis, and arthritis, *Br. med. J.* **2**, 93.

Leptospiral meningitis

Infection with either *Leptospira icterohaemorrhagica* or *Leptospira canicola* may present solely or mainly as meningitis. *L. icterohaemorrhagica* is excreted in the urine of infected rats and is transmitted to humans who come in contact with material contaminated by this urine. Fish-workers, coal-miners, sewer-workers, and farm-labourers are exposed to the risk of infection by their occupations. The other chief source is accidental immersion or bathing in contaminated water, and the meningitic form of Weil's disease is particularly likely to follow infection while bathing (Buzzard and Wylie 1947). *L. canicola* is transmitted to man from dogs, in which it may cause diarrhoea, but which may harbour the organism while remaining apparently in normal health.

The clinical picture of the meningeal form of both diseases is similar. The usual manifestations of meningitis may be severe. Symptoms and signs of involvement of the cerebral hemispheres or brainstem rarely occur (Alston and Broom 1958). The fundi are often congested and there may be papilloedema. The CSF is under increased pressure and contains many cells. In Weil's disease neutrophils predominate at the outset, later giving place to lymphocytes, while in canicola fever a lymphocytosis is characteristic. The number of cells ranges from 50 to over 1 000 per mm^3 and the protein content of the fluid may be normal or as high as 4.0 g/l.

Though in either disease meningitis may be associated with the typical general symptoms, these may be absent. The most distinctive sign outside the nervous system appears to be ciliary congestion. In canicola fever there may be a morbilliform rash and the spleen may be enlarged. In Weil's disease jaundice may be absent, and there may be no haemorrhages or severe renal damage.

The clinical picture may thus be that of so-called acute aseptic meningitis, and the only clues pointing to the cause may be the ciliary congestion, the occupation of the patient, or a history of recent immersion. The diagnosis is confirmed by a rising serum-agglutination titre to the infecting organism and by the demonstration by appropriate techniques of leptospirae in the blood, urine, or conjunctival secretion.

When the clinical picture is purely or predominantly meningeal, the prognosis is good and complete recovery is the rule, but leptospiral encephalitis is less benign (Menkes 1980). Penicillin is often given systemically, but its value is doubtful.

References

Alston, J. M. and Broom, J. C. (1958). *Leptospirosis in man and animals*. Livingstone, Edinburgh.

Buzzard, E. M. and Wylie, J. A. H. (1947). Meningitis leptospirosa. *Lancet* ii, 417.

Edwards, G. A. and Domm, B. M. (1960). Human leptospirosis. *Medicine, Baltimore* 39, 117.

Laurent, L. J. M., Norris, T. St. M., Starks, J. M., Broom, J. C., and Alston, J. M. (1948). Four cases of leptospira canicola infection in England. *Lancet* ii, 48.

Mackay-Dick, J. and Watts, R. W. E. (1949). Canicola fever in Germany. *Lancet* i, 907.

Menkes, J. H. (1980). *Textbook of child neurology*, 2nd edn. Lea and Febiger, Philadelphia.

Weetch, R. S., Kolquhoun, J., and Broom, J. D. (1949). Fatal human case of canicola fever. *Lancet* i, 906.

Acute lymphocytic choriomeningitis and acute aseptic meningitis

(See page 288)

Mollaret's meningitis

Mollaret (1944, 1952) and Bruyn and Straathof (1961) described a clinical syndrome characterized by recurrent febrile episodes of about two to four days' duration accompanied by headache, neck stiffness, and myalgia. The CSF showed a mononuclear pleocytosis, often with large, fragile endothelial cells present in the attack. The aetiology of the condition is unknown although Kinnman, Kam-Hansen, Link, and Norby (1979) demonstrated a defect in the regulatory function of T lymphocytes, and Steel, Dix, and Baringer (1982) isolated herpes simplex virus type 1 from a patient with the condition. Mora and Gimeno (1980) reported a patient with recurrent episodes occurring over 22 months, uninfluenced by antibiotics but apparently cured by colchicine.

References

Bruyn, G. W. and Straathof, L. J. A. (1961). La méningite endothélioleucocytaire multirécurrente bénigne de Mollaret, *Presse Méd.* **69**, 1741.

Kinnman, J., Kam-Hansen, S., Link, H., and Norrby, E. (1979). Studies on the humoral and cell-mediated immune response in a patient with Mollaret's meningitis. *J. neurol. Sci.* **43**, 265.

Mollaret, P. (1944). La méningite endothélio-leukocytaire multirécurrente bénigne: syndrome nouveau ou maladie nouvelle? *Rev. Neurol.* **72**, 57.

—— (1952). Benign recurrent pleocytic meningitis and its presumed causative virus. *J. nerv. ment. dis.* **116**, 1072.

Mora, J. S. and Gimeno, A. (1980). Mollaret meningitis: report of a case with recovery after colchicine. *Ann. Neurol.* **8** 631.

Steel, J. G., Dix, R. D., and Baringer, J. R. (1982). Isolation of herpes simplex virus type 1 in recurrent (Mollaret) meningitis. *Ann. Neurol.* **11**, 17.

Brucellosis

Any of the three organisms *Brucella melitensis*, *Brucella abortus*, and *Brucella suis*, may directly or indirectly affect the nervous system. There are many recorded cases of meningo-encephalitis due to these organisms. To the naked eye, the rare fatal cases show greyish-white 'tubercles' in the meninges; histologically these consist of hyalinized connective tissue infiltrated with chronic inflammatory cells, with, in places, necrosis. The meninges themselves are invaded by lymphocytes, plasma cells, and a few neutrophils. Although vigorous campaigns of eradication have resulted in the disappearance of the disease from many countries, notably in Scandinavia, *abortus* infection is still prevalent, though diminishing in incidence, in Britain and the USA (Sahs 1978).

The clinical picture is often one of a subacute or chronic meningitis, or there may be symptoms of increased intracranial pressure suggesting a tumour, or the picture may be that of focal encephalitis. Epilepsy, aphasia, confusion or dementia, and spastic weakness of the limbs have all been observed. Myelitis is rare, polyneuritis uncommon. The CSF contains an excess of mononuclear cells, usually below 100 per mm^3. The protein is raised as a rule, but is sometimes disproportionately high, and the fluid may be xanthochromic. In one reported case it was blood-stained, owing to rupture of a mycotic aneurysm.

Headache, fatigability, irritability, and toxic confusional states may occur as toxic symptoms without direct involvement of the nervous system. Brucellosis may lead to spondylitis, and neurological symptoms may be secondary to this, lumbar spondylitis, for example, causing sciatica.

The clinical picture of meningeal irritation associated with lymphocytosis in the CSF may lead to confusion with tuberculous meningitis or meningitis due to *Cryptococcus neoformans*. Diagnosis rests upon the appropriate serological tests for brucellosis, reinforced by the isolation of the organism, which may be obtained from the CSF. These organisms are largely resistant to antibiotics but tetracycline is the drug of choice (Spink 1981); some strains are sensitive to gentamicin or kanamycin.

References

Dalrymple-Champneys, W. (1960). *Brucella infection and undulant fever in man*. Oxford University Press, London.
Harris, H. J. (1950). *Brucellosis (undulant fever)*. Hoeber, New York.
Huddleson, I. F. (1943). *Brucellosis in man and animals*. The Commonwealth Fund, New York.
Sahs, A. L. (1978). Brucellosis (Malta fever; undulant fever). In *Handbook of clinical neurology* (ed. P. J. Vinken and G. W. Bruyn) Vol. 33. Chapter 15, North-Holland, Amsterdam.
Spink, W. W. (1981). Brucella. In *Medical microbiology and infectious disease* (ed. A. I. Braude), Chapter 34. Saunders, Philadelphia.

Meningitis due to *Cryptococcus neoformans* (*Torula histolytica*)

Cryptococcus neoformans, also known as *Torula histolytica*, is a fungus consisting of a round or oval body surrounded by a thick polysaccharide capsule. It appears to be of world-wide distribution, but most cases of infection are seen in the southern United States and in Australia (Edwards, Sutherland, and Tyrer 1970). It is also found in Great Britain. Its usual portal of entry appears to be the lung where it forms lesions not unlike those of pulmonary tuberculosis, but these rarely cavitate. The brain, however, is the most important site of infection. There it causes irregular granulomatous thickening of the meninges which are infiltrated with lymphocytes and occasional plasma cells. Multinucleated giant cells are also present. Capsulated cryptococci are scattered throughout the meninges. To the naked eye the brain shows a diffuse or more localized opacity of the meninges with flattening of gyri and other evidence of increased intracranial pressure. Other organs, including the kidneys, spleen, and lymph nodes may be involved. The histological changes in lymph nodes have been likened to those of Hodgkin's disease but Hodgkin's disease may predispose to true infection with the cryptococcus as may carcinomatosis and other debilitating diseases.

Clinically there is an insidious onset of symptoms with a history varying from weeks to years, but usually measured in months. Symptoms of meningitis are usually present, including neck stiffness and Kernig's sign, but papilloedema and signs of a focal cerebral lesion may suggest an intracranial tumour. The CT scan may demonstrate hydrocephalus but sometimes shows low-density areas which enhance with contrast medium, indicating intracerebral torulomas (Weenink and Bruyn 1978; de Wytt, Dickson, and Holt 1982). The CSF is very variable. It may be clear with only a small excess of cells and protein, or may contain many cells, usually lymphocytes and occasionally neutrophils, with or without a high protein. A paretic colloidal gold curve is characteristic. A latex agglutination test is also available. Cryptococci may be present in the fluid or may be cultured on Sabouraud's medium; special stains are required to stain the capsule. The condition must be distinguished from other forms of subacute or chronic meningitis, sarcoidosis, intracranial tumour, and carcinomatosis of the meninges. The presence of a characteristic pulmonary lesion may be helpful, with fever and hepatosplenomegaly, but these features are rare. Spinal arachnoiditis giving signs of cord compression has been described (Davidson 1968).

Amphotericin B given intravenously in a dosage of 0.25 mg, increasing to 1.0 mg/kg body weight daily by slow infusion, is an effective treatment but may be toxic, giving renal damage. The same drug given intrathecally is also effective (McIntyre 1967). Steroids, given with amphotericin B, may have an adjuvant value; given alone they cause exacerbation of the condition and have been used as a provocative diagnostic test, since after giving prednisone, 30 mg daily for 48 hours, the cryptococcus may be found

for the first time in the CSF. 5-fluorocytosine, 100–200 mg per kg body weight, given by mouth for 6–8 weeks, may be more effective than amphotericin B and is usually less toxic (Watkins, Gardner-Medwin, Ingham, and Murray 1969). Miconazole 400–800 mg intravenously two or three times daily and 20 mg intrathecally each day may prove still better than amphotericin and flucytosine combined (de Wytt *et al.* 1982); the mortality with amphotericin alone in de Wytt's series was 43 per cent, with flucytosine added 13 per cent, and with miconazole 0 per cent.

References

Butler, W. T., Alling, D. W., Spickard, A., and Utz, J. (1964). Diagnostic and prognostic value of clinical and laboratory findings in cryptococcal meningitis. *New Engl. J. Med.* **270**, 59.
Davidson, S. (1968). Cryptococcal spinal arachnoiditis. *J. Neurol. Neurosurg. Psychiat.* **31**, 76.
de Wytt, C. N., Dickson, P. L., and Holt, G. W. (1982). Cryptococcal meningitis: a review of 32 years experience. *J. neurol. Sci.* **53**, 283.
Edwards, V. E., Sutherland, J. M., and Tyrer, J. H. (1970). Cryptococcosis of the central nervous system: epidemiological, clinical, and therapeutic features. *J. Neurol. Neurosurg. Psychiat.* **33**, 415.
Greenfield, J. G. (1958). In *Neuropathology* (ed. J. G. Greenfield, W. Blackwood, W. H. McMenemey, A. Meyer, and R. M. Norman), p. 149. Arnold, London.
McIntyre, H. B. (1967). Cryptococcal meningitis. A case successfully treated by cisternal administration of amphotericin B with a review of recent literature. *Bull. Los Angeles neurol. Soc.* **32**, 213.
Rose, F. C., Grant, C., and Jeanes, A. L. (1958). Torulosis of the central nervous system in Britain. *Brain* **81**, 542.
Watkins, J. S., Gardner-Medwin, D., Ingham, H. R., and Murray, I. G. (1969). Two cases of cryptococcal meningitis, one treated with 5-fluorocytosine. *Br. med. J.* **3**, 29.
Weenink, H. R. and Bruyn, G. W. (1978). Cryptococcosis of the nervous system. In *Handbook of clinical neurology* (ed. P. J. Vinken and G. W. Bruyn), Vol. 35, Chapter 22. North-Holland, Amsterdam.

Actinomycosis

While the commonest site of human infection with *Actinomyces* is the mouth and jaw, the nervous system may rarely be involved with the formation of a multiloculated brain abscess (see Chapter 7) due to haematogenous spread from a pulmonary focus; meningitis does not occur as a primary event but only very rarely due to rupture of an abscess into the ventricles or subarachnoid space (Causey 1978).

Reference

Causey, W. A. (1978). Actinomycosis. In *Handbook of clinical neurology* (ed. P. J. Vinken and G. W. Bruyn) Vol. 35, Chapter 17. North-Holland, Amsterdam.

Coccidiomycosis

This fungal infection occurs in semi-arid areas of the southwestern United States and in Central and South America. It is acquired by inhaling arthrospores of *Coccidioides immitis* from contaminated soils. Most infections are self-limiting; sometimes the lungs alone are involved but occasionally there is similar or haematogenous spread which may lead to multiple small intracerebral granulomas and subacute or chronic meningitis. The CSF findings are similar to those of cryptococcosis: spherules may be identified in the CSF, the fungus may be cultured from sputum or lymph nodes (rarely CSF), and there is a specific coccidioidin skin test indicative of prior infection. Amphotericin B is effective in this condition, too (Goldstein and Lawrence 1978).

Reference

Goldstein, E. and Lawrence, R. M. (1978). Coccidioidomycosis of the central nervous system. In *Handbook of clinical neurology* (ed. P. J. Vinken and G. W. Bruyn), Vol. 35, Chapter 21. North-Holland, Amsterdam.

Amoebic meningoencephalitis

Primary amoebic meningoencephalitis, due to the amoebae *Naegleria* and *Hartmannella*, acquired by bathing in infected water, has been reported to cause either a mild meningitic illness or a fatal meningoencephalitis in children in Australia (Fowler and Carter 1965), the United States (Duma, Ferrell, Nelson, and Jones 1969), and in Great Britain (Symmers 1969); amphotericin B appears to be an effective treatment (Apley, Clarke, Roome, Sandry, Saygi, Silk, and Warhurst 1970).

References

Apley, J., Clarke, S. K. R., Roome, A. P. C. H., Sandry, S. A., Saygi, G., Silk, B., and Warhurst, D. C. (1970). Primary amoebic meningo-encephalitis in Britain. *Br. med. J.* **1**, 596.

Duma, R. J., Ferrell, H. W., Nelson, E. C., and Jones, M. M. (1969). Primary amebic meningoencephalitis. *New Engl. J. Med.* **281**, 1315.

Fowler, M. and Carter, R. F. (1965). Acute pyogenic meningitis probably due to *Acanthamoeba*: a preliminary report. *Br. med. J.* **2**, 740.

Symmers, W. St. C. (1969). Primary amoebic meningoencephalitis in Britain. *Br. med. J.* , 449.

Other rare fungal infections

Other rare fungal infections include aspergillosis (multiple brain abscesses and vascular thrombosis—see Beal, O'Carroll, Kleinman, and Grossman 1982), blastomycosis and cephalosporium infection (both giving meningitis), mucormycosis (thrombosis of cerebral and meningeal arteries), and nocardiosis (meningitis, multiple abscesses) (see Menkes 1980). Most of these also respond to amphotericin B.

References

Beal, M. F., O'Carroll. P., Kleinman, G. M., and Grossman, R. I. (1982). Aspergillosis of the nervous system. *Neurology, Minneapolis* **32**, 473.

Menkes, J. H. (1980). *Textbook of child neurology*, 2nd edn. Lea and Febiger, Philadelphia.

7

Suppurative encephalitis: intracranial abscess

Pathology

Intracranial abscess may be: (1) extradural; (2) subdural; (3) subarachnoid; or (4) intracerebral. (1) Extradural abscess is secondary to osteitis of a cranial bone. The infection passes through the bone, but as its further advance is arrested by the dura, the accumulating pus strips off the dura. (2) In subdural abscess the pus lies between dura and arachnoid. (3) Subarachnoid abscess is a rare form in which the pus is confined to the subarachnoid space and spreads along the brain surface. (4) Intracerebral abscess may follow the spread of infection from the surface of the brain, or may be haematogenous. In the former case it usually, but not necessarily, has a track communicating with the surface. Intracerebral abscesses are usually single, but may be multilocular, or, less commonly, multiple. The developing intracerebral abscess passes through three stages. The first is focal acute inflammation without pus formation. In the second stage pus appears (suppurative encephalitis), but the abscess is not well defined from surrounding tissue. In the third stage a definite wall is formed, and the abscess is localized (Fig. 7.1). Its encapsulation depends upon various factors, of which the resistance of the patient to the organism is one of the most important. In some rapidly fatal cases the condition remains one of a spreading suppurative encephalitis.

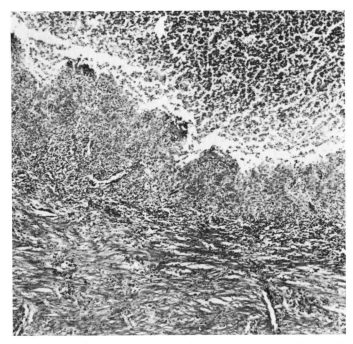

Fig. 7.1. The wall of a chronic pyogenic cerebral abscess with pus cells above, a line of granulation tissue in the centre and the fibroglial capsule below. Mallory's PTAH, × 40.

Abscesses of otitic origin are usually found in the middle or posterior part of the temporal lobe or in the cerebellum, the former situation being about twice as common as the latter. An otitic cerebellar abscess usually occupies the anterosuperior part of the lateral lobe and is adherent to the posterior part of the petrous bone (Pennybacker 1948). Much more rarely such abscesses occur in the pons, frontal, or parietal lobes. In otitic cases the brain may

become infected as a result of: (1) purulent thrombosis of the transverse sinus; (2) osteomyelitis of the petrous temporal bone; or (3) by spread along the adventitia of perforating blood vessels (Evans 1931). The anterior frontal lobe is the usual site of abscess following frontal sinusitis. Haematogenous abscesses occur in any situation, but are usually above the tentorium. The left hemisphere is more often affected than the right, and most often the abscess lies in the area supplied by the middle cerebral artery and rather superficially.

Microscopically an intracerebral abscess consists of an inner layer of pus cells, surrounded by a layer of granulation tissue containing new blood vessels and hyperplastic fibrous tissue. Outside this is a layer of glial reaction, mainly cellular in the early stages, mainly fibrous later. Fat-granule cells, plasma cells, and neutrophil leucocytes are plentiful, especially in the middle layer. There is an inflammatory reaction in the overlying meninges, and in extradural and subdural abscess granulation tissue is present on the dural surface.

Aetiology

The causes of intracranial abscess in approximate order of frequency are: (1) infection of the middle ear or nasal sinuses; (2) pyaemia or bacteraemia; (3) metastasis from intrathoracic suppuration; and (4) head injury. Of Evans's (1931) 194 cases, 121 were due to infection in the ear or paranasal sinuses, 24 to pyaemia, 22 to pulmonary suppuration; even today up to 40 per cent of cases in adults, but even more in children (Nestadt, Lowry, and Turner 1960), result from ear or sinus infection, but in about 20 per cent the source of infection may never be traced (Pennybacker and Sellors 1948; Beller, Sahar, and Praiss 1973). In a review of 172 cases, McClelland, Craig, and Crockard (1978) found that the incidence had fallen from five to three per million over three decades and the condition was three times as common in males as in females; 29 per cent of abscesses were in the temporal lobe, 25 per cent frontal, 10 per cent parietal, 6 per cent cerebellar, 3 per cent occipital, 7 per cent subdural or thalamic, and 20 per cent multiple. Chronic ear disease was still the commonest cause. Hence:

1. Infection of the middle ear is from four to nine times as common a cause as is sinus infection; the frontal sinus is most often involved, the sphenoidal sinus next.

2. Pyaemia is now rare, following widespread use of antibiotics, but a cerebral abscess may still arise as a consequence of acute infective endocarditis; it is rare in subacute bacterial endocarditis in view of the low virulence of the infecting organism. Unsuspected bacteraemia in acute osteomyelitis and in other pyogenic infections including simple cutaneous sepsis is sometimes the cause.

3. When intracranial abscess is secondary to infection elsewhere, the thorax is often the source, and many cases complicate bronchiectasis, empyema, or lung abscess. Rarely the primary abscess is elsewhere, as in the liver. There is a clear association between cerebral abscess and cyanotic congenital heart disease (Maronde 1950; Campbell 1957; Nestadt et al. 1960; Matson and Salem 1961). Single or multiple abscesses may also develop in the immunosuppressed patient, as after cardiac transplantation (Britt, Enzmann, and Remington 1981), when the organisms may be aspergillus, toxoplasma, candida, klebsiella, cryptococcus, coccidioides, listeria, mucor, or rhizopus.

4. Fracture of the skull is liable to cause abscess when an injury

leads to free communication between the body surface and the brain, especially when fragments of bone, clothing, or a missile penetrate the latter. Pencil-tip injuries penetrating the orbital roof or temporal bone may, for example, have this effect in children (Foy and Sharr 1980); in adults compound depressed skull fracture with a dural tear is the commonest cause.

Any of the common pyogenic organisms may cause intracranial abscess, the commonest in the past being *Staphylococcus aureus*, streptococci, and pneumococci, or organisms of the *E. coli* group. More recently, Louvois, Gortval, and Hurley (1977) and Ingham, Selkon, and Roxby (1977), while identifying such organisms in many cases, also noted an increasing incidence of mixed infections with aerobic and obligate anaerobic bacteria including *bacteroides fragilis* and less often organisms such as proteus, klebsiella, or haemophilus. The causal agent may also be a streptothrix, as in actinomycotic abscess, and amoebic abscess sometimes occurs. In certain parts of South-east Asia, chronic cerebral abscess due to paragonimiasis is relatively common and may be associated with recurrent episodes of low-grade meningitis (Oh 1969).

Symptoms and signs

Mode of onset
The history may be of greater diagnostic importance than the physical signs, which are often slight at the stage when treatment is most likely to be effective.

When abscess follows skull fracture it usually develops soon after the injury, though when a missile penetrates the brain there may be a latent interval of days or weeks. These cases, however, offer little difficulty. The history is particularly important when abscess is secondary to otitis media. In some such cases the onset is acute or subacute. After an exacerbation of pre-existing otitis, or a temporary suppression of aural discharge, or operation on the ear, the patient rapidly develops headache, vomiting, and delirium. In other cases there is a 'latent interval' of weeks or even months before the *signs* of abscess appear. The existence of *symptoms* during this period may suggest that all is not well. There may be fluctuating headache, loss of appetite and weight, occasional unexplained pyrexia, and a change in temperament leading to lassitude, depression, and irritability.

Abscess of haematogenous origin may develop insidiously, in which case, unless the primary infective focus is discovered, it may be clinically indistinguishable from an intracranial tumour. It is rare, since the virtual disappearance of pyaemia, to obtain a history of an acute episode due to impaction of an infected embolus in the brain. Even so, in very occasional cases there may be a history of sudden headache with impairment of consciousness, and weakness of a limb, followed by remission of symptoms for weeks or months before those of the abscess develop.

The symptoms of intracranial abscess may be conveniently divided into: (1) general symptoms of infection; (2) symptoms of increased intracranial pressure; (3) focal symptoms; and (4) changes in the CSF.

General symptoms
The severity of the general symptoms is usually proportionate to the acuteness of the abscess, and is thus most marked in cases of acute suppurative encephalitis. In acute cases irregular pyrexia is the rule; in chronic cases the temperature may be intermittently raised but not invariably. In both there may be a neutrophil leucocytosis in the blood.

Symptoms and signs of increased intracranial pressure
Headache is usually present. In chronic abscess it is often paroxysmal, being increased by stooping and exertion, and presenting the other features of headache due to increased intracranial pressure. In more acute cases it is persistent and severe. Papilloedema is a late sign and is often absent or slight. When present it is sometimes more marked on the side of the lesion. Bradycardia is common, but is not constant, and when it occurs usually indicates a rapid increase in the severity of the condition. In severe cases delirium, somnolence, stupor, and coma develop. Exceptionally signs of increased intracranial pressure are slight or lacking, even when a large abscess is present.

Focal symptoms
Extradural abscess. This is difficult to diagnose because, unless the abscess is large, focal symptoms are absent, except for headache radiating from the ear or from the infected sinus towards the vertex. Increasing local headache with tenderness and/or oedema of the scalp in the region of the infected ear or sinus when surgical drainage seems adequate are suspicious signs.

Subdural abscess or empyema. This condition is usually a complication of frontal sinusitis but rarely complicates sphenoidal sinusitis, otitis media, or meningitis. A layer of pus forms in the subdural space over one frontal lobe (or rarely over the temporal lobe). The clinical manifestations usually consist of high fever, fits (either focal or generalized) and a rapidly-developing hemiplegia, with aphasia if the major hemisphere is involved (Farmer and Wise 1973). Early surgical evacuation of the pus and irrigation of the subdural space with a weak solution of an appropriate antibiotic is imperative; thrombosis of cortical veins is an important complication which can lead to substantial residual disability even if appropriate treatment is given.

Intracerebral abscess. 1. *Temporal lobe abscess.* An abscess in this position, if situated on the left side in a right-handed individual, can cause aphasia, often of the nominal or amnestic type. A patient who can name familiar objects accurately often hesitates or misnames less familiar articles. Abscess on either side may produce a visual-field defect. This is usually a homonymous upper quadrantic defect on the opposite side due to involvement of the lower fibres of the optic radiation. Damage to the corticospinal tract is usually slight, and weakness is most marked in the face and tongue. The opposite plantar reflex may be extensor. Oculomotor paralyses may result from pressure upon the third or sixth cranial nerves.

2. *Cerebellar abscess.* Headache in cerebellar abscess (Shaw and Russell 1975) is often predominantly suboccipital. It may radiate down the neck and be associated with neck stiffness. The head may be flexed to the side of the lesion or retracted. Signs of cerebellar dysfunction vary in severity and may be slight. The most important are: phasic nystagmus, most marked on looking to the side of the lesion; and hypotonia and incoordination in the limbs on the affected side, with an inability to carry out rapid alternating movements with the upper limb on the affected side as well as on the normal side. Pressure upon the brainstem may occur, leading to compression of cranial nerves, especially the sixth and seventh, on the side of the abscess, and slight signs of corticospinal defect on the opposite side. Pass-pointing outwards with the affected hand and a tendency to deviate or fall to the side of the lesion when walking are seen in some cases.

3. *Frontal abscess.* Headache, drowsiness, apathy, and impairment of memory and attention are usually conspicuous, but focal signs are often lacking. A large abscess with oedema may cause aphasia or hemiparesis. Unilateral anosmia and slight exophthalmos may be present.

4. *Abscesses in other situations.* The focal symptoms depend upon the position of the abscess, and usually resemble those of tumour in the same situation. Chronic abscess of the brainstem (Russell and Shaw 1977), though uncommon, may give features closely resembling those of pontine glioma and may even give the clinical picture of the 'locked-in syndrome' (Murphy, Brenton, Aschenbrener, and Van Gilder 1979).

Subarachnoid abscess. This rather rare condition may be suspected when the signs suggest abscess of otitic origin, though none of the clinical pictures described above is present. Convulsions may occur with a superficial abscess over a cerebral hemisphere. When the signs suggest involvement of the cerebellum but no abscess is evident in the cerebellum itself, a superficial abscess in the cerebellopontine angle may be present.

The cerebrospinal fluid

Examination of the CSF may be of great diagnostic value, but lumbar puncture may be dangerous because of the risk of tentorial or cerebellar herniation and is better avoided in favour of a CT scan if an abscess is strongly suspected (Garfield 1969). While an abscess remains localized, the fluid is clear. Its pressure may be increased. There is usually an excess of cells, though not often more than 100 per mm^3, the majority being lymphocytes, the remainder neutrophils: the protein is somewhat raised, often to 2.0 g/l. There is usually no diminution in the sugar content, and organisms are absent. If meningitis develops, the changes are those of pyogenic meningitis (p. 239).

Other methods of investigation

The EEG may yield valuable evidence as to the site of an abscess, demonstrating a striking focus of high-amplitude slow delta activity. Echoencephalography may indicate displacement of the midline as in intracranial tumour. Isotope encephalography, too, may accurately locate an abscess (Planiol 1963). Angiography has been shown to locate the lesion in 90 per cent of cases and to suggest its character in 61 per cent (Beller *et al* 1973), but the CT scan has virtually supplanted all of these methods in view of its diagnostic precision, with a false negative rate of less than one per cent (Shaw and Russell 1977), and ventriculography, once thought to be needed in many cases (Garfield 1969), is now rarely, if ever, necessary. Once an abscess has been diagnosed and localized, if aspiration is preferred to excision, contrast medium may be injected into the cavity (Fig. 7.2) in order to observe its subsequent shrinkage.

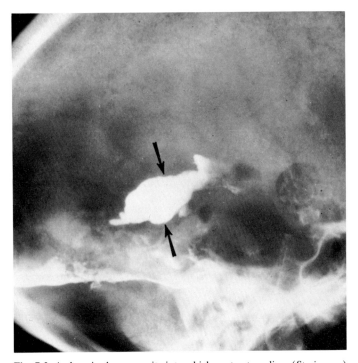

Fig. 7.2. A chronic abscess cavity into which contrast medium (*Steripaque*) has been injected; some of the medium has leaked out into the subarachnoid space.

Diagnosis

Intracranial abscess is occasionally found without an evident source of infection when it may be exposed at operation for a supposed intracranial tumour. Diagnosis of such cases from tumour is difficult and often impossible. Pyrexia, leucocytosis, and pleocytosis in the CSF, however, may suggest the correct diagnosis, as may the CT scan. When the causal infective focus is obvious, abscess must be distinguished from other pyogenic intracranial complications. Meningitis, which may coexist with abscess, is distinguishable by signs of meningeal irritation, cervical rigidity, Kernig's sign, and the changes in the CSF already described. Transverse sinus thrombosis causes few cerebral symptoms, though it can cause papilloedema, more marked on the affected side, and slight signs of contralateral corticospinal weakness. The signs of pyaemia are usually conspicuous with swinging temperature and rigors. A useful but inconstant sign may be demonstrated in some such cases by Queckenstedt's test. The rise of CSF pressure may be slight or absent when the jugular vein on the affected side is compressed alone, because the blocked transverse sinus prevents communication of the raised jugular pressure to the cranial cavity. Acute vestibular neuronitis or spread of suppuration to the labyrinth may be confused with cerebellar abscess. In the former vertigo is more, and headache less, intense than in the latter. Hypotonia favours a cerebellar lesion. Papilloedema and changes in the CSF indicate that the infection has spread beyond the internal ear.

Prognosis

Very rarely an intracranial abscess becomes quiescent and is found accidentally at post-mortem, surrounded by a layer of gliosis. Recovery by spontaneous drainage through the ear or nose may also occur. These occurrences, however, are too exceptional to have any bearing upon prognosis, which is almost uniformly fatal in the absence of antibiotic and surgical treatment. While vigorous antibiotic treatment with serial CT scans may show resolution of some abscesses without surgery (Berg, Franklin, Cuneo, Boldrey, and Strimling 1978), most authorities still regard surgery as being necessary in the average case. Spreading encephalitis, rupture of the abscess into the ventricular system, meningitis, and sinus thrombosis are the usual terminations. Even after surgical drainage or excision these complications may occur, and the mortality rate is high. In 1969 Garfield found it to be 40 per cent and even in 1977 Jefferson and Keogh found an overall mortality of 28 per cent in a personal series of 49 cases, while predicting that the rate should fall to around 10 per cent with modern antibiotic therapy and improved neurosurgical techniques. In fact Alderson, Strong, Ingham, and Selkon (1981) found in 90 cases treated in Newcastle that in three consecutive five-year periods the rate fell from 42 to 21 and finally to 9.7 per cent. Thoracogenic and otitic cerebellar abscesses are the most serious. Epilepsy is an important sequel, occurring in between 50 and 72 per cent of cases (Jooma, Pennybacker, and Tutton 1951; Legg, Gupta, and Scott 1973), usually within 12 months.

Treatment

The treatment of choice is, first, systemic wide-spectrum antibiotic therapy, say with gentamicin and ampicillin, followed by the introduction of metronidazole (especially in otogenic abscess) and of other appropriate antibiotics once the organism or organisms have been identified (*British Medical Journal* 1977; *The Lancet* 1978) and then either surgical excision or drainage. Excision has the lowest mortality (Jooma *et al* 1951) but is not always practicable and much depends upon the situation of the lesion. In the early stages, dexamethasone may be useful in reducing cerebral oedema, provided antibiotic cover is adequate, and the widespread use of steroids may have contributed to the observed reduction in mortality (Alderson *et al*, 1981).

References

Alderson, D., Strong, A. J., Ingham, H. R., and Selkon, J. B. (1981). Fifteen-year review of the mortality of brain abscess. *Neurosurgery*, **8**, 1.

Beller, A. J., Sahar, A., and Praiss, I. (1973). Brain abscess: review of 89 cases over a period of 30 years. *J. Neurol. Neurosurg. Psychiat.* **36**, 757.

Berg, B., Franklin, G., Cuneo, R., Boldrey, E., and Strimling, B. (1978). Nonsurgical cure of brain abscess: early diagnosis and follow-up with computerized tomography. *Ann. Neurol.* **3**, 474.

British Medical Journal (1977). Treatment of cerebral abscesses. *Br. med. J.* **2**, 978.

Britt, R. H., Enzmann, D. R., and Remington, J. S. (1981). Intracranial infection in cardiac transplant recipients. *Ann. Neurol.* **9**, 107.

Campbell, M. (1957). Cerebral abscess in cyanotic congenital heart disease. *Lancet* **i**, 111.

Evans, W. (1931). The pathology and aetiology of brain abscess. *Lancet*, **i**, 1231 and 1289.

Farmer, T. W. and Wise, G. R. (1973). Subdural empyema in infants, children and adults. *Neurology, Minneapolis* **23**, 254.

Foy, P. and Sharr, M. (1980). Cerebral abscesses in children after pencil-tip injuries. *Lancet* **ii**, 662.

Garfield, J. (1969). Management of supratentorial intracranial abscess: a review of 200 cases. *Br. med. J.* **2**, 7.

Ingham, H. R., Selkon, J. B., and Roxby, C. M. (1977). Bacteriological study of otogenic cerebral abscesses: chemotherapeutic role of metronidazole. *Br. med. J.* **2**, 991.

Jefferson, A. A. and Keogh, A. J. (1977). Intracranial abscesses: a review of treated patients over 20 years. *Quart. J. Med.* **46**, 389.

Jooma, O. V., Pennybacker, J., and Tutton, G. K. (1951). Brain abscess, aspiration, drainage or excision?, *J. Neurol. Psychiat.* **14**, 308.

The Lancet (1978). Chemotherapy of brain abscess. *Lancet* **ii**, 1081.

Legg, N. J., Gupta, P. C., and Scott, D. F. (1973). Epilepsy following cerebral abscess—a clinical and EEG study of 70 patients. *Brain* **96**, 259.

Louvois, J. de, Gortval, P., and Hurley, R. (1977). Bacteriology of abscesses of the central nervous system: a multicentre prospective study. *Br. med. J.* **2**, 981.

Maronde, R. F. (1950). Brain abscess and congenital heart disease. *Ann. intern. Med.* **33**, 602.

Matson, D. D. and Salem, M. (1961). Brain abscess in congenital heart disease. *Pediatrics* **27**, 772.

McClelland, C. J., Craig, B. F., and Crockard, H. A. (1978). Brain abscesses in Northern Ireland: a 30 year community review. *J. Neurol. Neurosurg. Psychiat.* **41**, 1043.

Murphy, M. J., Brenton, D. W., Aschenbrener, C. A., and Van Gilder, J. C. (1979). Locked-in syndrome caused by a solitary pontine abscess. *J. Neurol. Neurosurg. Psychiat.* **42**, 1062.

Nestadt, A., Lowry, R. B., and Turner, E. (1960). Diagnosis of brain abscess in infants and children. *Lancet* **ii**, 449.

Oh, S. J. (1969). Cerebral paragonimiasis. *J. neurol. Sci.* **8**, 27.

Pennybacker, J. (1948). Cerebellar abscess. *J. Neurol. Neurosurg. Psychiat.* **11**, 1.

—— and Sellors, T. H. (1948). Treatment of thoracogenic brain abscess. *Lancet* **ii**, 90.

Planiol, T. (1963). La gamma-encéphalographie. *Rev. Prat., Paris* **13**, 3625.

Russell, J. A. and Shaw, M. D. M. (1977). Cerebellar abscess. *J. Neurol. Neurosurg. Psychiat.* **38**, 429.

—— and —— (1977). Value of computed tomography in the diagnosis of intracranial abscess. *J. Neurol. Neurosurg. Psychiat.* **40**, 214.

8

Nervous complications of miscellaneous infections

Acute toxic encephalopathy

Definition. An acute cerebral disturbance occurring chiefly in children, sometimes in small epidemics; it is characterized pathologically by toxic changes in the nervous system and clinically by delirium or coma and convulsions, variable pareses of the limbs, and symptoms of meningeal irritation.

Pathology

The changes in the nervous system distinguish this disorder both from viral encephalitis and from post-infective encephalomyelitis. Pathologically there is acute degeneration of the ganglion cells with hyperaemia and conspicuous oedema, and focal collections of glial cells and round cells. 'Acute brain purpura', in which multiple punctate haemorrhages in perivascular distribution are conspicuous, may be an intense variety of this disorder if not due to thrombotic microangiopathy or disseminated intravascular coagulation.

Aetiology

The pathological changes are thought to be due to a toxaemia with variable effects upon nerve cells and the blood vessels, giving different combinations of neural degeneration, oedema, and haemorrhage. In some cases the source of the toxaemia is an acute, systemic infection and it can occur in children with burns (Warlow and Hinton 1969). However, burn encephalopathy, which occurred in 5 per cent of 287 children suffering from burns (Mohnot, Snead, and Benton 1982), and in which hypocalcaemia is common, probably results from a series of complex metabolic, haematological, and haemodynamic abnormalities. The 'idiopathic' variety of encephalopathy resembles that which may follow pertussis and rabies vaccination (pp. 301–2). In other cases the cause is unknown, especially in the small epidemics which sometimes attack young children during the summer months. It is uncommon in infancy, most cases occurring between the ages of two and 10 years.

Symptoms

The onset of the illness is usually acute and may be fulminating. It is sometimes preceded by sore throat or gastrointestinal disturbance. Severe headache, vomiting, and convulsions are common and the latter are occasionally unilateral. The child is usually delirious, but may later pass into coma. There is usually high fever. Meningeal symptoms are often conspicuous. Aphasia, monoplegia, hemiplegia or double hemiplegia, optic neuritis, and trismus may all occur and facial paresis is frequently present. The tendon reflexes are usually exaggerated, and the plantar reflexes extensor on one or both sides, Retention and incontinence of urine are common when consciousness is clouded. The CSF is usually normal in composition though under increased pressure. Haematuria or albuminuria may occur rarely and a purpuric rash has been described.

Diagnosis

The fact that the CSF is usually normal in composition distinguishes acute toxic encephalopathy from the various forms of meningitis, encephalitis, and poliomyelitis. Lead encephalopathy must also be excluded.

Prognosis

The prognosis varies in different groups of reported cases. In some epidemics almost all the affected individuals died. In others almost all recovered. The condition accounted for 6 per cent of all infants and children coming to autopsy at the Massachusetts General Hospital in one decade (Lyon, Dodge, and Adams 1961). In fatal cases death usually occurs within two or three days of the onset, coma having supervened within a few hours. In those who survive, the dangers are persistent mental handicap, aphasia, hemiplegia, or epilepsy. Sometimes the patient recovers in a few days. In other cases improvement is slower but recovery may still be surprisingly complete.

Treatment

Treatment is symptomatic. Anticonvulsant drugs may be required to control the convulsions. Cerebral oedema may be treated by dexamethasone, 2–5 mg three times daily in the acute stage, depending upon the age of the patient.

Reye's syndrome

This condition, also called acute toxic encephalopathy with fatty degeneration of the viscera, is a disorder of childhood in which a toxic encephalopathy as described above is associated with hypoglycaemia and with fatty degeneration of the liver giving symptoms and signs of hepatic dysfunction; similar degenerative changes have been described in the kidney (Reye, Morgan, and Baral 1963). Typically, the condition develops in a child who is apparently recovering from an acute viral illness or exanthem and who then develops intractable vomiting followed by increasing drowsiness, leading to coma, often with convulsions (*The Lancet* 1982). The mortality is as high as 85 per cent; hyperkalaemia, hyperpnoea, and haematemesis are unfavourable signs, but if the patient survives two or three days, recovery may be complete. While the condition has been described in association with various viral infections (Jenkins, Dvorak, and Patrick 1976) and has been attributed to chemical toxins (Glasgow and Ferris 1968), the aetiology is unknown. An association with type I vaccine-like poliovirus has been reported (Brunberg and Bell 1974) and the condition has also followed influenza A infection (Harrington and Draper 1981). There is now clear evidence of diffuse mitochondrial damage in brain, liver, and kidney in such cases (de Vivo 1978); an inability to metabolize salicylate has been postulated as an aetiological factor of importance (Partin, Partin, Schubert, and Hammond 1982) and many affected children have been treated with aspirin. The serum prolactin is also greatly raised in comatose patients (Newman, Faraj, Caplan, Ali, Camp, and Ahmann 1979). Treatment must be directed to controlling cerebral oedema and manifestations of hepatic dysfunction, including a rising blood ammonia (Menkes 1980). The clearance of organic acidaemia is also important (Trauner, Sweetman, Holm, Kulovich, and Nyhan 1977) and Trauner (1980), in summarizing a treatment regimen, has stressed the importance of controlling temperature and of using hypertonic solutions to reduce oedema, neomycin enemas to reduce blood ammonia, and barbiturate-induced coma to reduce intracranial pressure in severe cases.

References

British Medical Journal (1973). Clinical diagnosis of Reye's syndrome. *Br. med. J.* **3** 308.

Brunberg, J. A. and Bell, W. E. (1974). Reye syndrome. An association with type I vaccine-like poliovirus. *Arch. Neurol.*, *Chicago* **30**, 304.

De Vivo, D. C. (1978). Reye syndrome: a metabolic response to an acute mitochondrial insult? *Neurology, Minneapolis* **28**, 105.

Glasgow, H. F. T. and Ferris, J. A. J. 81968). Encephalopathy and visceral fatty infiltration of probable toxic aetiology. *Lancet* **i**, 451.

Harrington, M. and Draper, I. T. (1981). Post-influenzal encephalitis and Reye's syndrome. *J. Neurol. Neurosurg. Psychiat.* **44**, 649.

Jenkins, R., Dvorak, A., and Patrick, J. (1967). Encephalopathy and fatty degeneration of the viscera associated with chickenpox. *Pediatrics* **39**, 769.

The Lancet (1982). Reye's syndrome—epidemiological considerations. *Lancet* **i**, 941.

Lyon, G., Dodge, P. R., and Adams, R. D. (1961). The acute encephalopathies of obscure origin in infants and children. *Brain* **84**, 680.

Menkes, J. H. (1980). *Textbook of child neurology*, 2nd edn. Lea and Febiger, Philadelphia.

Mohnot, D., Snead, O. C., and Benton, J. W. (1982). Burn encephalopathy in children. *Ann. Neurol.* **12**, 42.

Newman, S. L. Faraj, B. A., Caplan, D. B., Ali, F. M., Camp, V. M., and Ahmann, P. A. (1979). Prolactin and the encephalopathy of Reye's syndrome. *Lancet* **ii**, 1097.

Partin, J. S., Partin, J. C., Schubert, W. K., and Hammond, J. G. (1982). Serum salicylate concentrations in Reye's disease: a study of 130 biopsy-proven cases. *Lancet* **i**, 191.

Reye, R. D., Morgan, G., and Baral, J. (1963). Encephalopathy and fatty degeneration of the viscera. A disease entity in childhood. *Lancet* **ii**, 749.

Trauner, D. A. (1980). Treatment of Reye syndrome. *Ann. Neurol.* **7**, 2.

——, Sweetman, L., Holm, J., Kulovich, S., and Nyhan, W. L.(1977). Biochemical correlates of illness and recovery in Reye's syndrome. *Ann. Neurol.* **2**, 238.

Warlow, C. P. and Hinton, P. (1969). Early neurological disturbances following relatively minor burns in children. *Lancet* **ii**, 978.

Scarlet fever

Nervous complications of scarlet fever are rare. The pathological changes in most cases have been those of acute haemorrhagic encephalitis (Ferraro 1944). Meningism is not uncommon, symptoms of meningeal irritation coexisting with a normal CSF. True meningitis occurs less frequently and is usually secondary to otitis or other complications. Cerebral abscess may occur without otitis. Hemiplegia was once the commonest complications, resulting from vascular occlusion; Rolleston collected 66 cases from the literature. Hypertensive encephalopathy due to acute nephritis has been described and chorea is a not uncommon sequel. Hemiplegia of vascular origin is usually permanent, but symptoms due to hypertensive encephalopathy disappear if the patient recovers.

References

Ferraro, A. (1944). Allergic brain changes in post-scarlatinal encephalitis. *J. Neuropath. Exp. Neurol.* 3, 239.

Forbers, J. G. (1926). Post-scarlatinal meningitis. *Lancet* **ii**, 1207.

Miller, H. G., Stanton, J. B., and Gibbons, J. L. (1956). Para-infectious encephalomyelitis and related syndromes. *Quart. J. Med.* **25, 427.**

Neal, J. B. and Jones, A. (1972). Streptococcic meningitis following scarlet fever recovery. *Arch. Pediat.* 44, 395.

Neurath, R. (1912). Die Rolle des Scharlachs in der Ätiologie der Nervenkrankheiten. *Ergebn. inn. Med. Kinderheilk.* 9, 103.

Rolleston, J. D. (1927–8). Hemiplegia following scarlet fever. *Proc. R. Soc. Med.* **21**, 213.

Toomey, J. A., Dembo, L. H., and McConnell, G. (1923). Acute hemorrhagic encephalitis: report of a case following scarlet fever. *Am. J. Dis. Child.* **25**, 98.

Whooping cough

Some neurological complications of pertussis are due to focal vascular lesions, especially small haemorrhages. Askin and Zimmerman (1929) reported a case of encephalitis with focal collections of inflammatory cells. Convulsions are not uncommon especially in young children. Though they may sometimes by due to encephalitis, in other cases the changes are those of an encephalopathy, possibly resulting from the mechanical effects of venous congestion due to repeated coughing. Focal symptoms, which include aphasia, unilateral or bilateral hemiplegia, blindness, and deafness, are probably the result of focal haemorrhage or softening. Severe and repeated convulsions may be fatal. Neurological complications are becoming less frequent but in the past, of the group with focal lesions, approximately one-fifth died, two-fifths were incapacitated by residual symptoms, and two-fifths recovered.

An encephalopathy has been described as a sequel to pertussis inoculation, usually occurring within two to three days after the injection (Byers and Moll 1948; Berg 1958; Ström 1960). The reaction is an acute, monophasic, allergic, demyelinating process, involving fewer than 1 in 100000 of those inoculated (Fenichel 1982). Convulsions leading to coma are common; most patients survive and some recover but many are left with permanent mental retardation, variable signs of diffuse brain damage, and recurrent seizures.

References

Askin, J. A. and Zimmerman, H. M. (1929). Encephalitis accompanying whooping-cough: clinical history and report of postmortem examination. *Am. J. Dis. Child.* **38**, 97.

Berg, J. M. (1958). Neurological complications of pertussis immunization. *Br. med. J.* **2**, 24.

Byers, R. K. and Moll, F. C. (1948). Encephalopathies following prophylactic pertussis vaccine. *Pediatrics* **1**, 437.

Dubois, R., Ley, R. A., and Dagnelie, J. (1932). Protocoles anatomo-cliniques de huit cas de complications nerveuses de la coqueluche. *J. Neurol., Brux.* **32**, 645.

Ellison, J. B. (1934). Whooping-cough eclampsia. *Lancet* **i**, 227.

Fenichel, G. M. (1982). Neurological complications of immunization. *Ann. Neurol.* **12**, 119.

Miller, H. G., Stanton, J. B., and Gibbons, J. L. (1956). Para-infectious encephalomyelitis and related syndromes. *Quart. J. Med.* **25**, 427.

Ström, J. (1960). Is universal vaccination against pertussis always justified? *Br. med. J.* **2**, 1184.

Typhoid fever

Mental symptoms are common, the commonest being acute toxic confusional states during the febrile period and post-typhoid psychosis or amnesia; psychotic reactions of schizophrenic type may be particularly common in the African (Osuntokun, Bademosi, Ogunremi, and Wright 1972). Meningeal symptoms are usually due to meningism, the CSF being normal. Much more rarely true typhoid meningitis occurs (p. 238). Suppurative meningitis may also result from infection with other pyogenic organisms, with or without the *Salmonella typhi*. The nervous parenchyma is less often involved than the meninges, but focal symptoms, especially hemiplegia, with or without aphasia, convulsions, myoclonus, or parkinsonian features, may occur (Osuntokun *et al.* 1972; Keusch 1981). Optic neuritis is rare. Cerebral abscess may occur either by extension from otitis media or by metastasis from a focus of pyogenic infection elsewhere. Such abscesses are usually due to a secondary invader, but are rarely caused by the *S. typhi*. Occasionally spinal symptoms predominate, yielding a picture of transverse myelitis. Polyneuritis is a rare sequel, predominantly involving the feet and causing tenderness of the soles. Similar complications may occur in paratyphoid fever, but much less frequently than in typhoid.

Meningitis and cerebral abscess in typhoid fever were once very serious complications which usually terminated fatally, but the use of chloramphenicol has greatly improved the prognosis. Focal lesions do not threaten life to the same extent, but frequently cause permanent disability, e.g. hemiplegia.

References

Keusch, G. T. (1981). Typhoid fever. In *Medical microbiology and infectious diseases* (ed. A. I. Braude), Chapter 179, p. 1399. Vol. II in *International textbook of medicine*. Saunders, Philadelphia.

Laroche, G. and Peju, G. (1920). Méningite typhique bénigne au cours d'une septicémie typhique à rechute. *Bull. Soc. méd. Hôp., Paris* **44**, 150.

Osuntokun, B. O., Bademosi, O., Ogunremi, K., and Wright, S. G. (1972). Neuropsychiatric manifestations of typhoid fever in 959 patients. *Arch. Neurol., Chicago* **27**, 7.

Typhus fever

The classical or European epidemic form of typhus fever is transmitted to man through the body-louse; the murine type is endemic all over the world and is passed on by rat fleas; Brill's disease is the name given to a form of recurrent typhus often seen in the past in European immigrants to the USA, but now very rare (Woodward 1959; Brezina 1981).

Nervous symptoms are common and there is abundant evidence that they are usually due to infection of the nervous system by the causative organism. Histologically microscopic nodules in the walls of very small blood vessels—typhus nodules—have frequently been found in the nervous system, and consist of perivascular collections of glial, endothelial, and other mononuclear cells. Thrombosis frequently occurs in the affected vessel. *Rickettsia prowazeki*, the causal organism, has been seen in the vascular endothelium and sometimes in the typhus nodules.

Headache, delirium, and insomnia, which are common during the initial febrile stage, are probably toxic in origin and do not necessarily indicate invasion of the nervous system. Focal symptoms indicative of the latter usually occur during the last few days of the febrile period or a few days afterwards. Meningeal symptoms are common, and any part of the nervous system may be involved (Herman 1949). Cerebral symptoms often indicate multiple lesions, a disseminated encephalitis, but hemiplegia is also common. Acute cerebellar ataxia occurs in a few cases, and multiple bulbar foci may occur, leading to dysphagia and dysarthria. Lesions are sometimes confined to the spinal cord, giving the clinical picture of myelitis. The cranial and peripheral nerves frequently suffer. Optic neuritis may occur. Facial paralysis is particularly common, and deafness may develop. In the peripheral nerves the symptoms may be those of a focal mononeuritis, associated with pain and tenderness, or of a polyneuritis.

Changes are frequently found in the CSF, which is sometimes xanthochromic and may show a lymphocytosis. The protein content of the fluid is usually slightly raised and this may persist for from two to eight months after the acute stage. Severe nervous symptoms naturally add to the gravity of the prognosis but in patients who survive, these symptoms usually recover.

Other Rickettsial infections

Q fever and trench fever are both due to rickettsiae but do not as a rule give neurological manifestations. However, in tick-borne Rocky mountain spotted fever (or Colorado fever) which is due to the *Rickettsia rickettsii* and which is similar to many other rickettsial illnesses seen in other parts of the world (e.g. Kenya fever, Brazilian spotted fever), neurological complications similar to those of typhus are quite common (Miller and Price 1972; Bisno

1981). In this condition, now the commonest rickettsial infection seen in the United States (Menkes 1980), meningoencephalitis with myoclonus, tremors, choreoathetosis, focal motor seizures, variable pareses of the limbs and cranial nerves, as well as papilloedema, have all been reported, usually developing in four to eight days. The same is true of scrub typhus (Tsutsugamushi disease) (Ripley 1946; Brezina 1981) in which the ulcerated lesion on the skin where bitten by the mite may give a useful clue to the diagnosis.

References

Bisno, A. L. (1981). Rocky Mountain spotted fever. In *Medical microbiology and infectious diseases*, (ed. A. I. Braude), Chapter 189, p. 1458. Vol. II in *International textbook of medicine*. Saunders, Philadelphia.

Brezina, R. (1981). Epidemic (louse-borne) typhus, and endemic (murine) typhus. In *Medical microbiology and infectious diseases* (ed. A. I. Braude), Chapters 186 and 187, pp. 1441 and 1446. Vol. II. in *International textbook of medicine*. Saunders, Philadelphia.

Herman, E. (1949). Neurological syndromes in typhus fever. *J. Nerv. ment. Dis.* **109**, 25.

Menkes, J. H. (1980). *Textbook of child neurology*, 2nd edn. Lea and Febiger, Philadelphia.

Miller, J. Q. and Price, T. R. (1972). The nervous system in Rocky mountain spotted fever. *Neurology, Minneapolis* **22**, 561.

Ripley, H. S. (1946). Neuropsychiatric observations on Tsutsugamushi fever (scrub typhus). *Arch. Neurol. Psychiat., Chicago* **56**, 42.

Woodward, T. E. (1959). Rickettsial diseases in the United States, *Med. Clin. N. Am.* **43**, 1507.

Malaria

Acute nervous symptoms in malaria, or cerebral malaria, occur chiefly in infections with the malignant tertian parasite in blackwater fever, and are due to sporulation of the parasite in the cerebral capillaries. Sections of brain show macroscopically a smoky grey appearance with oedema, hyperaemia, and punctate haemorrhages. Histologically, there is more or less complete blockage of capillaries with parasitized red cells, leading to thrombosis, oedema, and petechial haemorrhages. The leptomeninges show perivascular infiltration with small, round cells. Malarial nodules (granulomas) have been observed and consist of a central capillary filled with parasitized red cells and surrounded by a perivascular necrotic area, with glial proliferation (Thompson and Annecke 1926).

Acute cerebral malaria is characterized by hyperpyrexia and rapidly evolving coma, with or without prior convulsions. Symptoms of meningeal irritation may occur, especially in children. The prognosis is always grave. Focal manifestations include hemiplegia, aphasia, and cerebellar ataxia, which are usually transitory. Paraplegia has been described. Optic neuritis and retinal haemorrhages are often seen, and complete external ophthalmoplegia may occur. In the acute stage, the response to dexamethasone has been thought to be dramatic (Woodruff and Dickinson 1968), but a more recent trial by White and Warrell (1982) showed that steroids were positively detrimental and that treatment rests upon the administration of intravenous quinine given in a dose of 10 mg/kg by infusion over four hours, every eight hours (*The Lancet* 1982; *British Medical Journal* 1982).

Chronic nervous symptoms in malaria are probably toxic in origin and are usually due to neuropathy. Trigeminal neuralgia, facial palsy, mononeuropathy, and polyneuropathy may all occur.

References

British Medical Journal (1982). Dexamethasone deleterious in cerebral malaria. *Br. med. J.* **284**, 1588.

The Lancet (1982). Corticosteroids for cerebral malaria. *Lancet* **i**, 840.

Manson-Bahr, P. E. C. and Apted, F.I.C. (eds.) (1982). *Manson's tropical diseases*, 18th edn. Baillière Tindall, London.

Thompson, J. G. and Annecke, S. (1926). Pathology of the central nervous system in malignant tertian malaria. *J. trop. Med. Hyg.* **29**, 343.

White, N. J. and Warrell, D. A. (1982). Managing cerebral malaria. *Br. med. J.* **285**, 439.

Woodruff, A. W. and Dickinson, C. J. (1968). Use of dexamethasone in cerebral malaria. *Br. med. J.* **3**, 31.

Trypanosomiasis

African trypanosomiasis is transmitted to man by the bite of the tsetse fly. After an incubation period of about two weeks a local erythematous nodule may form at the site of the bite and this is followed by insomnia, impaired concentration, formication, and deep muscular aching. The parasites may not enter the central nervous system for several years; the onset may then be explosive with convulsions, coma, and death within a few days but more often there is a chronic fluctuating illness characterized by progressive drowsiness, apathy, dysarthria, and involuntary movements ('sleeping sickness'). The condition is usually fatal within a few months. The serum IgM is greatly raised. The CSF shows a mononuclear pleocytosis and a rise in protein. Tryparsamide, suramin sodium, or melarsoprol by intravenous injection or pentamidine intramuscularly may be effective in treatment of such cases (Barrett-Connor 1981).

South American trypanosomiasis (Chagas's disease) is acquired as a result of a bite from an affected bug. Meningo-encephalitis may occur, particularly in childhood but severe cardiomyopathy and/or diffuse myositis with swelling of the face (pseudomyxoedema) is more common in the adult although central nervous system involvement may result in convulsions and paralysis. Nitrofurazone analogues such as nifurtimox may be an effective treatment (Lumsden 1981).

References

Barrett-Connor, E. (1981). African sleeping sickness. In *Medical microbiology and infectious diseases* (ed. A. I. Braude), Chapter 163, p. 1287. Vol. II in *International textbook of medicine*. Saunders, Philadelphia.

Bogaert, L. Van and Vansen, P. (1957). Contribution à l'étude de la neurologie et neuropathologie de la trypanosomiase humaine. *Ann. Soc. Belge med. Trop.* **37**, 380.

Chagas, C. (1922). Descoberta do tripanozomia cruzi e verificação da Tripanozomiase americana. *Mem. Inst. Oswaldo Cruz* **15**, 67.

Lumsden, W. H. R. (1981). Trypanosomiasis. In *Medical microbiology and infectious diseases* (ed. A. I. Braude) Chapter 196, p. 1492. Vol. II in *International textbook of medicine. Saunders. Philadelphia.*

Manson-Bahr, P. E. C. and Apted, F. I. C. (Eds.) (1982). *Manson's tropical diseases*, 18th edn. Baillière Tindall, London.

Influenza

Nervous symptoms are frequently attributed to influenza, but the diagnosis is usually speculative. Small epidemics of encephalitis and polyneuritis have been observed to coincide with epidemics of influenza. Proof, however, is lacking that these forms of encephalitis are actually due to the influenza virus, since a precedent febrile illness, when it occurs, may well be due to invasion by another organism which is responsible for the nervous symptoms. Alternatively, influenza may be one of the many specific and non-specific infections which may be followed by a post-infective encephalitis or myelitis, or both, due to an allergic or hypersensitivity phenomenon. Thus, during certain influenza epidemics, especially the pandemic of 1957, cases of acute, sometimes fulminating, encephalomyelitis occurred (McConkey and Daws 1958; Flewett and Hoult, 1958; Thiruvengadam 1959). In the most acute cases

the pathology was that of an acute haemorrhagic encephalomyelitis, and it seems likely that these were cases of acute disseminated encephalomyelitis (see p. 304) complicating influenza. Several severe cases of acute encephalitis also occurred during an epidemic in Finland in 1979/80 (Sulkava, Rissanen, and Phyala 1981) and were shown to be associated with influenza A (H3N2) infections; all recovered completely. Other neurological manifestations affecting predominantly the spinal cord and roots such as transverse myelopathy have been described by Wells (1971). Influenza A virus may certainly cause a fatal encephalitis in mice (Bell, Narang, and Field 1971); the fact that the virus has been isolated from the brain in human subjects is not incompatible with the hypersensitivity theory and it is still uncertain whether this is the cause of neurological complications or whether they are due to a direct effect of the virus itself. Influenzal myositis (p. 563) may also occur.

References

Bell, T. M., Narang, H. K., and Field, E. J. (1971). Influenzal encephalitis in mice. A histopathological and electron microscopical study. *Arch. ges. Virusfors.* **34**, 157.

Dunbar, J. M., Jamieson, W. M., Langlands, H. M., and Smith, G. H. (1958). Encephalitis and influenza. *Br. med. J.* **1**, 913.

Flewett, T. H. and Hoult, J. G. (1958). Influenzal encephalopathy and post-influenzal encephalitis. *Lancet* **i**, 11.

Greenfield, J. G. (1930). Acute disseminated encephalomyelitis as a sequel to 'influenza'. *J. Path. Bact.* **33**, 453.

McConkey, B. and Daws, R. A. (1958). Neurological disorders associated with Asian influenza. *Lancet* **ii**, 15.

Sulkava, R., Rissanen, A., and Phyala, R. (1981). Post-influenzal encephalitis during the influenza A outbreak in 1979/1980. *J. Neurol. Neurosurg. Psychiat.* **44**, 161.

Thiruvengadam, K. V. (1959). Disseminated encephalomyelitis after influenza. *Br. med. J.* **2**, 1233.

Wells, C. E. C. (1971). Neurological complications of so-called 'influenza': a winter study in south-east Wales. *Br. med. J.* **i**, 369.

Infective hepatitis

Serious nervous complications of infective hepatitis and serum hepatitis (types A and B) are uncommon, though mild cerebral, meningeal, and neuritic symptoms have been seen in some epidemics. Brain saw one case with unilateral convulsions and hemiplegia, and other with myelitis and neuritis. Byrne and Taylor (1945) reported five cases, one with myelitis. The nervous symptoms usually develop four or five days before the jaundice appears. Jaundice, however, may coexist with nervous symptoms in other diseases—with meningitis in leptospirosis, and with encephalitis in St. Louis and equine encephalomyelitis, while the influenza virus may cause hepatitis (Kapila, Kaul, Kupur, Kalayanam, and Banerjee 1958). The rare focal lesions of the nervous system in infective hepatitis must be distinguished from those of encephalopathy due to acute hepatic failure in fulminant hepatitis (see p. 451).

References

Byrne, E. A. J. and Taylor, G. F. (1945). An outbreak of jaundice with signs in the nervous system. *Br. med. J.* **1**, 477.

Kapila, C. C., Kaul, S., Kapur, S. C., Kalayanam, T. S., and Banerjee, D. (1958). Neurological and hepatic disorders associated with influenza. *Br. med. J.* **2**, 1311.

Newman, J. L. (1942). Infective hepatitis: the history of an outbreak in the Lavant valley. *Br. med. J.* **1**, 61.

Walshe, J. M. (1951). Observations on the symptomatology and pathogenesis of hepatic coma. *Quart. J. Med.* **20**, 421.

Infectious mononucleosis

Nervous complications of infectious mononucleosis are not uncommon. The clinical picture may be meningitic, encephalitic, myelitic, or polyneuritic. Anosmia, optic neuritis, ophthalmoplegia, facial palsy, and acute cerebellar ataxia (Lascelles, Longson, Johnson, and Chiang 1973) have been described. Poliomyelitis may be simulated, or the Guillain-Barré syndrome. The CSF may contain an excess of lymphocytes.

Dolgopol and Husson (1949) reported a fatal case with respiratory paralysis. There was selective degeneration of the nerve cells of the third and fourth cranial nerves, of the cerebellar Purkinje cells, and of the ventral portion of the inferior reticular nucleus, together with recent haemorrhages in the grey matter of the spinal cord. In the polyneuritic cases mononuclear cell infiltration of the spinal roots and nerves has been described. Gautier-Smith (1965) pointed to the occurrence of mononeuritis (of cranial of peripheral nerves) in some cases and gave reasons for supposing that in some cases there is direct viral invasion of the central nervous system; however, in some patients with encephalomyelitis the aetiology of the nervous manifestations may be allergic. When the general symptoms and blood changes are typical no difficulty in diagnosis arises, but the nervous symptoms may come first, and the diagnosis may then depend upon the positive heterophile antibody test. Antibodies to the causal Epstein–Barr virus may be discovered in both the serum and CSF (Lascelles *et al* 1973).

References

Dolgopol, V. B. and Husson, G. S. (1949). Infectious mononucleosis with neurologic complications. *Arch. intern. Med.* **83**, 179.

Gautier-Smith, P. C. (1965). Neurological complications of glandular fever (infectious mononucleosis). *Brain* **88**, 323.

Lascelles, R. G. Longson, M., Johnson, P. J., and Chiang, A. (1973). Infectious mononucleosis presenting as acute cerebellar syndrome. *Lancet* **ii**, 707.

Sarcoidosis

Lesions of Boeck's sarcoidosis may involve any level of the nervous system and the muscles (see Colover 1948; Jefferson 1957; and Matthews 1965). The meninges or peripheral nerves may be infiltrated with endothelioid cells, giant cells, lymphocytes, plasma cells, and mononuclear leucocytes. Associated with the meningo-encephalitis there may be tumour-like masses in the dura mater. Adhesive arachnoiditis can cause hydrocephalus and the hypothalamus may be involved. This may cause amenorrhoea, galactorrhoea, and uterine–ovarian atrophy (the Chiari–Frommel syndrome) (Brust, Rhee, Plank, Newmark, Felton, and Lewis 1977). Dementia simulating Alzheimer's disease has also been described (Cordingley, Navarro, Brust, and Healton). The eyes may suffer in various ways. There may be papilloedema, optic neuropathy (Gudeman, Selhorst, Susac, and Waybright 1982), or retinal lesions, uveitis, or even exophthalmos while paresis of the third or sixth nerves is not uncommon. Facial paralysis on one or both sides, with or without loss of taste, is common, and the glossopharyngeal and vagus nerves may also suffer. The limbs may be the site of polyneuritis or of a focal mononeuritis. An affected peripheral nerve may be palpably thickened. The characteristic lesions of sarcoidosis are likely to be found elsewhere in the body, e.g. the lymph nodes, liver, and spleen and phalanges. The combination of iridocyclitis with parotitis and polyneuritis was the first neurological manifestation to be recognized. Crompton and MacDermot (1961) reported three cases of sarcoidosis confined to muscle, presenting with progressive muscular wasting and weakness (sarcoid myopathy). The condition tends to run an indolent course, sometimes with relapses and remissions (James and

Sharma 1967; Wells 1967), but many cases are ultimately fatal (Douglas and Maloney 1973). Temporary or sustained remission is often produced by large doses of steroids although maintenance therapy of as much as 30-40 mg of prednisone daily may have to be given, sometimes for several years.

References

Brust, J. C. M., Rhee, R. S., Plank, C. R., Newmark, M., Felton, C. P., and Lewis, L. D. (1977). Sarcoidosis, galactorrhea, and amenorrhea: 2 autopsy cases, 1 with Chiari–Frommel syndrome. *Ann. Neurol.* **2**, 130.

Colover, J. (1948). Sarcoidosis with involvement of the nervous system. *Brain* **71**, 451.

Cordingley, G., Navarro, C., Brust, J. C. M., and Healton, E. B. (1981). Sarcoidosis presenting as senile dementia. *Neurology, Minneapolis* **31**, 1148.

Crompton, M. R. and MacDermot, V. (1961). Sarcoidosis associated with progressive muscular wasting and weakness. *Brain* **84**, 62.

Douglas, A. C. and Maloney, A. F. J. 81973). Sarcoidosis of the central nervous system. *J. Neurol. Neurosurg. Psychiat.* **36**, 1024.

Garcin, R. (1960). Les atteintes neurologiques et musculaires dans la maladie de Besnier–Boeck–Schaumann. *Psychiat. Neurol. Neurochir., Amsterdam* **63**, 285.

Gudeman, S. K., Selhorst, J. B., Susac, J. O., and Waybright, E. A. (1982). Sarcoid optic neuropathy. *Neurology, Minneapolis* **32**, 597.

James, D. G. and Sharma, O. P. (1967). Neurosarcoidosis. *Proc. R. Soc. Med.* **60**, 1169.

Jefferson, M. (1957). Sarcoidosis of the nervous system. *Brain* **80**, 540.

Matthews, W. B. (1965). Sarcoidosis of the nervous system. *J. Neurol. Neurosurg. Psychiat.* **28**, 23.

Wells, C. E. C. (1967). The natural history of neurosarcoidosis. *Proc. R. Soc. Med.* **60**, 1172.

Mycoplasma infection

Infection with *Mycoplasma pneumoniae*, which usually causes primary atypical pneumonia, has been reported to cause polymyositis, transverse myelitis, ascending polyneuritis, bilateral optic neuritis, and hearing loss, perhaps as a postinfective allergic response to the primary infection (Rothstein and Kenny 1979).

Reference

Rothstein, T. L. and Kenny, G. E. (1979). Cranial neuropathy, myeloradiculopathy, and myositis: complications of Mycoplasma pneumoniae infection. *Arch. Neurol., Chicago.* **36**, 476.

Toxoplasmosis

Toxoplasmosis is the result of infection with *Toxoplasma gondii*, an obligate intracellular protozoon found in animals, birds, and reptiles and conveyed to man from domestic animals, rats, or mice. It is a crescentic organism 2 to 4μm wide and 4 to 7μm long, which is found intracellularly and extracellularly in the central nervous system, retina, heart muscle, kidneys, and endocrine glands. Pathologically it leads to disseminated encephalomyelitis with areas of yellow necrotic softening of the cerebral cortex and a contiguous leptomeningitis (Sabin, 1941; Cowen, Wolf, and Paige 1942; Remington, Jacobs, and Kaufman 1960). Miliary granulomata are found. The spinal cord may also show softening and necrosis (Wyllie and Fisher 1950).

Campbell and Clifton (1950) recognized the following clinical types—congenital infantile, acquired infantile, acquired adult, and latent. In the congenital infantile type the cerebral symptoms are present at or soon after birth. Microcephaly occurs in 13 per cent, hydrocephalus in about 28 per cent of affected infants (Remington and McLeod 1981). The fundi show characteristic choroidoretinitis and there may be mental retardation, epilepsy, hemiplegia, or diplegia. In the acquired forms the patient often complains of headache and vomiting and joint pains, and may exhibit a rash and fever. Choroidoretinitis is less common than in the congenital form, but papilloedema, glaucoma, or optic atrophy may be present together with nerve deafness and the symptoms of a meningo-encephalitis. The spleen may be enlarged and the blood may show eosinophilia. Toxoplasmic polymyositis has been described (Rowland and Greer 1961). The cells and protein in the CSF are usually increased and it may be possible to isolate the organism from the fluid. In the serum, the Sabin–Feldman dye test, the indirect fluorescent antibody (IFA) test, and indirect haemagglutination (HIA) test are usually diagnostic. Calcification is often observed in the brain radiologically in the form of multiple subcortical flakes and linear or granular areas in the basal ganglia (Sutton 1951). Pyrimethamine, sulphadiazine, and spiramycin are the most effective drugs in treatment.

References

Campbell, A. M. G. and Clifton, F. (1950). Adult toxoplasmosis in one family. *Brain* **73**, 281.

Cowen, D., Wolf, A., and Paige, B. H. (1942). Toxoplasmic encephalomyelitis. *Arch. Neurol. Psychiat., Chicago* **48**, 689.

Remington, J. S., Jacobs, L., and Kaufman, H. E. (1960). Toxoplasmosis in the adult. *New Engl. J. Med.* **262**, 180.

—— and McLeod, R. (1981). Toxoplasmosis. In *Medical microbiology and infectious diseases* (ed. A. I. Braude) Chapter 248, p. 1816. Vol. II in *International textbook of medicine*. Saunders, Philadelphia.

Rowland, L. P. and Greer, M. (1961). Toxoplasmic polymyositis. *Neurology, Minneapolis* **11**, 367.

Sabin, A. B. (1941). Toxoplasmic encephalitis in children. *J. Am. med. Ass.* **116**, 801.

Sutton, D. (1951). Intracranial calcification in toxoplasmosis. *Br. J. Radiol.* **24, 31**.

Wyllie, W. G. and Fisher, H. J. W. (1950). Congenital toxoplasmosis *Quart. J. Med.* N.S. **19**, 57.

Benign myalgic encephalomyelitis

(Epidemic neuromyasthenia)

Benign myalgic encephalomyelitis is the term applied to a puzzling disorder which has occurred often in small epidemics, especially in institutions, and has been recognized recently in many parts of the world. An epidemic in the Royal Free Hospital, London, some years ago led to its being sometimes called the Royal Free Disease. Its puzzling features are the severity of the symptoms in relation to the slightness of the physical signs, its selective incidence upon females, and the absence of any evidence as to its cause (Dillon, Marshall, Dudgeon, and Steigman 1974). Its mode of spread in institutions is unknown. Sporadic cases undoubtedly occur.

The onset is usually that of a febrile illness, sometimes with throat, upper gastrointestinal, respiratory or gastrointestinal symptoms, and often a generalized lymphadenopathy. Jaundice is occasionally seen. In many cases there is no evidence of involvement of the nervous system and the patient recovers completely in a few days. When the nervous system is involved—in 10 out of 48 cases in an outbreak in Newcastle (Pool, Walton, Brewis, Uldall, Wright, and Gardner 1961)—psychological disturbances are prominent, particularly depression, disturbances of sleep, and reactions commonly described as hysterical. The limbs are prominently affected with flaccid weakness, muscle pain and tenderness, and paraesthesiae, 'hyperaesthesia', or relative analgesia of irregular distribution. The tendon jerks may be normal, but are sometimes slightly exaggerated or slightly depressed. The plantar reflexes are usually flexor, but rarely extensor. Cranial-nerve palsies are sometimes observed, but are rare. A characteristic feature of the muscular weakness is the jerkily intermittent muscular contraction, confirmed by electromyography (see below). Objective sensory changes are uncommon.

The CSF is usually normal, the only abnormality found on laboratory investigation being that of occasional abnormal lymphocytes in the blood. Changes which are believed to be characteristic have been found on electromyography, in particular some grouping of motor-unit activity with brief silent intervals between groups of two or three action potentials.

The disease is never fatal and thus its pathology is unknown. Major persistent disability is rare. A striking feature is the tendency for relapses to occur during the months, and in some cases even years, after the initial illness. Many neurologists believe that its regular occurrence in closed communities (such as colleges and nurse-training schools) indicate that it is due to a 'mass' hysterical reaction in a community afflicted by an epidemic due to various benign non-neurotropic viruses. Others, however, are confident that it is organic and possibly due to an autoimmune response to viral infection, especially with Coxsackie viruses (Behan and Behan 1982); these workers have recommended treatment with plasmapheresis and immunoglobulin G. As Pool *et al.* say, 'the condition should be borne in mind in any patient suffering from a relapsing illness characterized by muscular weakness and by emotional lability'.

References

Acheson, E. D. (1959). The clinical syndrome variously called benign myalgic encephalomyelitis, Iceland disease and epidemic neuromyasthenia. *Am. J. Med.* **26**, 569–95.

Behan, P. O. and Behan, W. M. H. (1982). Immunotherapy in myalgic encephalomyelitis. *J. Neuroimmunol.* Suppl. 1, 52.

Dillon, M. J., Marshall, W. C., Dudgeon, J. A., and Steigman, A. J. (1974). Epidemic neuromyasthenia: outbreak among nurses at a children's hospital. *Br. med. J.* **1**, 301.

Fields, W. S. and Blattner, R. J. (1958). *Viral encephalitis*. Thomas, Springfield, Illinois.

Medical Staff of the Royal Hospital (1957). An outbreak of encephalomyelitis in the Royal Free Hospital Group, London, in 1955. *Br. med. J.* **2**, 895.

Pool, J. H., Walton, J. N., Brewis, E. G., Uldall, P. R., Wright, A. E., and Gardner, P. S. (1961). Benign myalgic encephalomyelitis in Newcastle upon Tyne. *Lancet* **i**, 733.

Behçet's disease

Behçet's disease is an obscure disorder characterized by ulceration of the mouth and genitalia usually with iridocyclitis, which runs a remittent course characteristically with attacks recurring three or four times a year.

The nervous system may also be involved, the typical lesions being those of disseminated encephalomyelitis with low-grade perivascular inflammatory exudates in the meninges and cortex, but more particularly in the white matter, foci of softening in relation to the blood vessels, and extensive and patchy areas of cortical infarction. The lesions may be widespread, but show a predilection for the upper brainstem. Evans, Pallis, and Spillane (1957) claimed to have isolated a virus, but it is now generally accepted that the condition is due to allergy or hypersensitivity and not to specific infection (McMenemey and Laurence 1957; Kawakita, Nishimura, Satoh, and Shibata 1967; Alema 1978). The relationship of Behçet's syndrome to Reiter's disease is unknown, but in Reiter's disease, too, ocular lesions may be associated with meningoencephalitis or with radiculoneuropathy (Oates and Hancock 1959).

When the nervous system is involved headache is a common symptom. Progressive dementia, parkinsonian features, ophthalmoplegia leading to diplopia, and spastic weakness of the limbs have all been observed. Intracranial venous sinus thrombosis may lead to papilloedema (Pamir, Kansu, Erbengi, and Zileli 1981). During an active phase the CSF contains an excess of cells, usually lymphocytes. They rarely number more than a hundred per mm^3, but occasionally much larger numbers have been observed with many neutrophils. Aphthous ulceration of the mouth and ulceration of the vagina or scrotum are characteristic. The iritis may lead to hypopyon, and other ocular lesions include conjunctivitis, keratitis, retinitis, retrobulbar neuritis, retinal haemorrhage, and thrombophlebitis. Permanent blindness may occur. Thrombophlebitis of small or large veins elsewhere is said to occur in 25 per cent of cases. Remissions may occur, but the mortality rate varies from about 21 per cent in Japan to almost 50 per cent in Western countries (Kawakita *et al* 1967).

Diagnostic difficulty is likely to arise only if the mouth and skin lesions are small or overlooked. Then the neurological manifestations may be confused with tuberculous meningitis, but in Behçet's syndrome the CSF sugar is normal (Wadia and Williams 1957). Alternatively the subacute development of spastic limb weakness may suggest multiple sclerosis, but the cell count in the CSF is likely to be considerably larger than is commonly found in that disease. There is increasing evidence to suggest that long-term treatment with steroid drugs may be effective; benefit has also been claimed from repeated plasmapheresis (Pamir *et al.* 1981).

References

Alema, G. (1978). Behçet's disease. In *Handbook of clinical neurology* (ed. P. J. Vinken and G. W. Bruyn) Vol. 34, Chapter 24, p. 475. North-Holland, Amsterdam.

Evans, A. D., Pallis, C. A., and Spillane, J. D. (1957). Involvement of the nervous system in Behçet's syndrome. *Lancet* ii, 349.

Kawakita, H., Nishimura, M., Satoh, Y., and Shibata, N. (1967). Neurological aspects of Behçet's disease: a case report and clinico-pathological review of the literature in Japan. *J. neurol. Sci.* 5, 417.

McMenemey, W. H. and Laurence, B. J. (1957). Encephalomyelopathy in Behçet's disease. *Lancet* ii, 353.

Oates, J. K. and Hancock, J. A. H. (1959). Neurological symptoms and lesions occurring in the course of Reiter's disease. *Am. J. med. Sci.* 238, 79.

Pallis, C. A. and Fudge, B. J. (1956). The neurological complications of Behçet's syndrome. *Arch. Neurol. Psychiat., Chicago* 75, 1.

Pamir, M. N., Kansu, T., Erbengi, A., and Zileli, T. (1981). Papilloedema in Behçet's syndrome. *Arch. Neurol., Chicago* 38, 643.

Wadia, N. and Williams, E. (1957). Behçet's syndrome with neurological complications. *Brain* 80, 59.

(For neurological sequelae and complications of prophylactic inoculation and of childhood exanthemata, mumps, and some other common viral infections, see Chapters 10 and 11. For bacterial infections such as tetanus and botulism which produce their neurological effects through exotoxin production, see Chapter 15 and for nervous complications of diphtheria, see Chapter 17.)

Metazoal infections

Taenia solium (cysticercosis)

Cysticercosis is the infestation of man with the encysted larval stage of the human tapeworm, *Taenia solium*, resulting from the ingestion of the ova. The embryos are carried to all parts of the body, and may invade the nervous system and the muscles. Many cases seen in Great Britain resulted from infection of British soldiers serving in India. Dixon and Lipscomb (1961) found the incidence of clinical cysticercosis to be between 1.2 and 2.0 per thousand men serving in that country. The incidence of the condition has increased in the south-western United States, especially in immigrants from Central or South America (Grisolia and Wiederholt 1982; McCormick, Zee, and Heiden 1982).

In man, the cysts grow for a time, but the larvae die, and the cysts then tend to calcify. This happens more often in the muscles than in the brain. In the brain, the cysts usually measure about 1 cm in diameter, and are found in the subarachnoid space, in the cerebral cortex, and to a lesser extent in the white matter. A race-mose form is encountered particularly in the fourth ventricle and basal cisterns, giving a cluster of grape-like cystic bodies with thin, perhaps translucent, walls containing colourless fluid.

The incubation period between infection and the development of symptoms varies from less than one year to 30 years, the average interval being about five years. In Dixon and Lipscomb's series, 91.8 per cent of patients had focal or generalized seizures and other neurological symptoms were relatively rare, mental disorder occurring in 8.7 per cent, intracranial hypertension in 6.4 per cent, focal nervous lesions of the brain in 2.7 per cent, and of the spinal cord in 0.2 per cent. Intracranial hypertension may result from hydrocephalus caused by the racemose type, while occasional patients demonstrate the characteristic triad of occipital headache, postural vertigo, and morning vomiting which can result from lesions in the fourth ventricle (Bickerstaff, Small, and Woolf 1956; Kuper, Mendelow, and Proctor 1958). In a recent series reported by Grisolia and Wiederholt (1982), intracranial hypertension was commoner than epilepsy, but McCormick *et al.* (1982) found the reverse.

Exceptionally, the clinical picture is that of a subacute meningoencephalitis or recurrent lymphocytic meningitis. In chronic cases, there may be a moderate excess of protein and a lymphocytic pleocytosis in the fluid and an indirect haemagglutination titre may be positive in both serum and CSF.

Subcuticular nodules are found in approximately half of all cases, and exceptionally a nodule is seen in the eye or in the tongue. The muscular lesions are usually asymptomatic but hypertrophic myopathy has been reported (Pallis and Lewis 1981) and, in many cases, calcified cysts can be demonstrated by X-ray. Calcification of intracranial cysts occurs in only about one-third of all cases, and then very rarely less than 10 years after infection. The CT scan was positive in two-thirds of a series of 127 cases (McCormick *et al*, 1982). Biopsy of a subcuticular nodule may be helpful in diagnosis (see Mehringer 1983).

A fatal outcome is uncommon, usually being due to status epilepticus or intracranial hypertension. Epilepsy should be treated along the usual lines: this often controls or abolishes the attacks. Intracranial hypertension calls for surgical shunting and possibly resection of intraventricular cysts. High-dose dexamethasone may also be helpful in the acute stage.

Multiceps multiceps (coenures cerebralis)

In some countries, especially South Africa, *Multiceps multiceps* is the common tapeworm of dogs, and human infection may lead to the presence of cysts in the ventricles or in the posterior fossa, the clinical picture being predominantly that of intracranial hypertension.

References

Bickerstaff, E. R., Small, J. M., and Woolf, A. L. (1956). Cysticercosis of the posterior fossa. *Brain* 79, 622.

Dixon, H. B. F. and Lipscomb, F. M. (1961). Cysticercosis: an analysis and follow-up of 450 cases. *Spec. Rep. Ser. med. Res. Counc. London*, No. 299.

Grisolia, J. S. and Wiederholt, W. C. (1982). CNS cysticercosis. *Arch. Neurol., Chicago* 39, 540.

Kuper, S., Mendelow, H., and Proctor, N.S. F. (1958). Internal hydrocephalus caused by parasitic cysts. *Brain* 81, 235.

McCormick, G. W., Zee, C.-S., and Heiden, J. (1982). Cysticercosis cerebri: review of 127 cases. *Arch. Neurol., Chicago* 39, 534.

Mehringer, M. C. (Ed.) (1983). Symposium on cysticercosis. *Bull. Clin. Neurosci.* 48, 1.

Pallis, C. and Lewis, P. D. (1981). Involvement of human muscle by parasites. In *Disorders of voluntary muscle* (ed. J. N. Walton). Chapter 15, Part II. Churchill-Livingstone, Edinburgh.

Pawlowski, Z. S. (1981). Cestodiasis. In *Medical microbiology and infectious diseases* (ed. A. I. Braude) Chapter 133, p. 1087. Vol. II in *International textbook of medicine*. Saunders, Philadelphia.

Toxocara infection

In children in frequent contact with dogs or cats or who eat dirt (pica), a syndrome of recurrent wheezy bronchitis or pneumonitis may be accompanied by fleeting urticarial rashes and convulsions. The condition is due to ingestion of the larvae of the dog round-worm *Toxocara canis* or *Toxocara cati* which may produce a widespread granulomatous reaction in liver, lungs, skeletal muscle, and brain. Focal epilepsy in an adult has been reported (Brain and Allan 1964), as have ataxia, coma, hemiparesis, and the Guillain-Barré syndrome (Huntley 1981), and uveitis or endophthalmitis may occur (Ashton 1960). There is often a striking eosinophilia and a skin test may be diagnostic (Duguid 1961). Diethylcarbamazine is probably an effective treatment.

References

Ashton, N. (1960). Larval granulomatosis of the retina due to *Toxocara*. *Br. J. Ophthal.* **44**, 129.

Brain, W. R. and Allan, B. (1964). Encephalitis due to infection with Toxocara cania. *Lancet* **i**, 1355.

Duguid, I.M. (1961). Chronic endophthalmitis due to *Toxocara*. *Br. J. Ophthal.* **45**, 705, 589.

Huntley, C. C. (1981). Visceral larva migrans. In *Medical microbiology and infectious diseases* (ed. A. I. Braude) Chapter 250, p. 1837. Vol. II in *International textbook of medicine*. Saunders, Philadelphia.

Trichinosis

This condition develops in man following the ingestion of pork infected with *Trichinella spiralis*. Usually the condition gives rise to fever, periorbital oedema, and widespread muscle pain due to myositis (Gross and Ochoa 1979), but the central nervous system is involved in between 10 and 24 per cent of cases (Kramer and Aita 1972). In the brain larvae become impacted in cerebral capillaries giving petechial haemorrhages, perivascular cellular infiltration, and/or granulomatous nodules. The clinical manifestations include confusion, delirium, and focal neurological signs such as hemiparesis (Gould 1945; Dalessio and Wolff 1961); unilateral lateral rectus palsy has been described (Kramer and Aita 1972). Treatment with steroids and thiabendazole 2 g daily is recommended.

References

Dalessio, D. and Wolff, H. G. (1961). Trichinella spiralis infection of the central nervous system. *Arch. Neurol., Chicago* **4**, 407.

Gould, S. E. (1945). *Trichinosis*. Thomas, Springfield, Illinois.

Gross, B. and Ochoa, J. (1979). Trichinosis: clinical report and histochemistry of muscle. *Muscle & Nerve* **2**, 394.

Kramer, M. D. and Aita, J. F. (1972). Trichinosis with central nervous system involvement. *Neurology, Minneapolis* **22**, 485.

Schistosomiasis (bilharzia)

This condition, which is common in the Middle East and Orient, is due to bathing in infested water. The ova of the trematodes may be deposited in the bladder wall, giving haematuria, and in the lungs. Involvement of the nervous system is comparatively uncommon, but *S. japonicum* shows a predilection for the cerebral hemispheres (Blankfein and Chirico 1965), *S. haematobium* and *S. mansoni* for the spinal cord (Bird 1964). Cerebral involvement may give oedema and papilloedema, headache, convulsions, and focal neurological signs; when the spinal cord is involved the signs are generally those of an incomplete transverse myelopathy. The CSF may show an increase in both cells and protein. Skin and complement fixation tests and/or rectal biopsy and eosinophilia are helpful in diagnosis. Metriphonate is effective against *S. haematobium* only, oxamniquine against *S. mansoni* only, and praziquantel against all human schistosomal species (Webbe 1981).

References

Bird, A. V. (1964). Acute spinal schistosomiasis. *Neurology, Minneapolis* **14**, 647.

Blankfein, R. J. and Chirico, A. M. (1965). Cerebral schistosomiasis. *Neurology, Minneapolis* **15**, 957.

Webbe, G. (1981). Schistosomiasis: some advances. *Br. med. J.* **283**, 1104.

Echinococcosis (hydatid cysts)

Rarely, and especially in sheep-rearing countries, man becomes the intermediate host of the *Erchinococcus granulosus*. Hydatid cysts are most common in the liver and lungs but rarely occur in the brain (Araná-Iniguez and San Julian 1955; Pawlowski 1981) where they are usually single and present as space-occupying lesions; even more rarely they are found in the spine, giving spinal-cord compression (Malloch 1965).

References

Araná-Iniguez, R. and San Julian, J. (1955). Hydatid cysts of the brain. *J. Neurosurg.* **12**, 323.

Malloch, J. D. (1965). Hydatid disease of the spine. *Br. med. J.* **1**, 633.

Pawlowski, Z. S. (1981). Cestodiasis. In *Medical microbiology and infectious diseases* (ed. A. I. Braude) Chapter 133, p. 1087. Vol. II in *International textbook of medicine*. Saunders, Philadelphia.

Gnathostoma and angiostrongylus infection

Human infection by *Gnathostoma spinigerum* is usually characterized by painless migratory cutaneous swellings, but in Thailand cases of eosinophilic meningoencephalomyelitis due to this infection have been described causing either a subacute meningoencephalitis, often with cranial-nerve palsies, or an acute painful myelitis with paraparesis (Punyagupta, Juttijudata, Bunnag, and Comer 1968*a*; Punyagupta, Limtrakul, Vichipanthu, Karnchanachetanee, and Nye, 1968*b*). However, the commonest cause of eosinophilic meningitis is infection with *Angiostrongylus cantonensis*, usually acquired by ingesting raw snails or poorly cooked crustaceans (Kuberski and Wallace 1979); rarely the condition is fatal but most patients recover completely without specific treatment.

References

Kuberski, T. and Wallace, G. D. (1979). Clinical manifestations of eosinophilic meningitis due to *Angiostrongylus cantonensis*. *Neurology, Minneapolis* **29**, 1566.

Punyagupta, S., Juttijudata, P., Bunnag, T., and Comer, D. S. (1968*a*). Two fatal cases of eosinophilic myeloencephalitis: a newly recognized disease caused by *Gnathostoma spinigerum*. *Trans. R. Soc. trop. Med. Hyg.* **62**, 801.

——, Limtrakul, C., Vichipanthu, P., Karnchanachetanee, C., and Nye, S. W. (1968*b*). Radiculomyeloencephalitis associated with eosinophilic pleocytosis. *Am. J. trop. Med. Hyg.* **17**, 551.

Whipple's disease

The cause of this condition, which usually gives progressive weight loss, malabsorption, and polyarthritis, is unknown. The intestinal wall and lymphatics are infiltrated by macrophages filled with glycoprotein. Neurological complications associated with subependymal granulomatous lesions containing the characteristic sickleform particle-containing (SPC) cells have been described in about 6 per cent of cases (Tengström and Werner 1966). Trigeminal neuralgia, myoclonus, and ophthalmoplegia were the clinical features in a case shown at autopsy to have a nodular encephalitis (Stoupel, Monseu, Pardoe, Heimann, and Martin 1969). Diagnosis depends upon finding periodic acid–Schiff (PAS)-positive macrophages in the tissues involved, and when neurological manifestations are present, PAS-positive cells may be found in the

CSF. Ultrastructural studies confirm that these cells contain membrane-bound bacilliform bodies. Remission may follow treatment with penicillin G and tetracycline (Kirsner and Shorter 1980). Very rarely the disease process appears to be totally confined to the nervous system (Halperin, Landis, and Kleinman 1982).

References

Halperin, J. J., Landis, D. M. D., and Kleinman, G. M. (1982). Whipple disease of the nervous system. *Neurology, Minneapolis* **32**, 612.

Kirsner, J. B. and Shorter, R. G. (Eds.)(1980). *Inflammatory bowel disease*. Lea and Febiger, Philadelphia.

Stoupel, N., Monseu, G., Pardoe, A., Heimann, R., and Martin, J. J. (1969). Encephalitis with myoclonus in Whipple's disease. *J. Neurol. Neurosurg. Psychiat.* **32**, 338.

Tengström, B. and Werner, I. (1966). Whipple's disease. A report of two cases and a review of the literature. *Acta Soc. Med. Upsalien.* **71**, 237.

9

Syphilis of the nervous system

Aetiology

Syphilis has become less common and less dangerous as a result of modern treatment. The Registrar General's Annual Statistical Review shows that in England and Wales the mortality from general paresis declined by 94 per cent between 1916 and 1954 and that from tabes dorsalis by 86.2 per cent. Headache and palsies were attributed to syphilis in the Middle Ages, but little was known about neurosyphilis before the nineteenth century. Bayle described general paralysis in 1822, though the term was first used by Delaye in 1824, and the first adequate account of tabes was given by Romberg in 1846, and amplified by Duchenne and Charcot. Argyll Robertson described the pupillary abnormalities which bear his name in 1869. Fournier, also in 1869, described congenital syphilis. The discovery of the causal organism, in the spirochaete *Treponema pallidum*, by Schaudinn and Hoffmann in 1903 and the elaboration of the Bordet–Wassermann reaction (1901–7) were other important landmarks. The serological diagnosis of syphilis depends on the demonstration of antibodies, either the non-specific, non-treponemal globulin complex called reagin or else specific treponemal antibodies, in the patient's serum (see Storm-Mathisen 1978). Of the reagin tests, the Wasserman complement-fixation test is now outmoded, having been largely replaced by the VDRL flocculation test. The treponemal immobilization (TPI) test, the first of the specific reactions, has now been largely supplanted by the very sensitive fluorescent treponemal antibody absorption (FTA–ABS) test.

Although the earliest manifestation of acquired syphilitic infection is the primary chancre, spirochaetes may reach the blood and be present in the spleen within 10 days of infection and before the chancre appears. In the secondary stage spirochaetes may reach the nervous system in many infected persons, though they may not then give rise to symptoms. The secondary stage is usually followed by a latent period, but even within a year, often within two or three years, symptoms of the tertiary stage may develop. Latent syphilis (an asymptomatic patient, not previously treated for syphilis, who shows no clinical abnormality but has a positive serological test for syphilis or gives birth to a child with congenital syphilis) may, however, last for several years. Asymptomatic neurosyphilis is a term often applied to such patients who show no neurological abnormality but in whom the CSF shows a pleocytosis or a positive VDRL test.

On clinical grounds a distinction has long been drawn between two types of neurosyphilis, one of which has been known as tertiary meningovascular or cerebrospinal syphilis, the other, which comprises tabes and general paresis, being distinguished as quaternary or parenchymatous neurosyphilis. In meningovascular or cerebrospinal syphilis symptoms may occur within a few years of infection, tend to be focal, and on the whole respond well to treatment. Tabes and general paresis, on the other hand, exhibit a longer latent interval, are characterized by diffuse or systematized pathological changes, and are less influenced by treatment. In cerebrospinal or meningovascular syphilis the essential changes affect blood vessels and mesoblastic tissues and the parenchyma of the nervous system suffers secondarily, while in tabes and general paresis there is invasion of the nervous tissue itself by spirochaetes in addition.

Clinical neurosyphilis occurs in only a few—about 10 per cent—of persons infected with the *Treponema pallidum*. In patients with untreated asymptomatic neurosyphilis, the cumulative probability of progression to clinical neurosyphilis is about 20 per cent in the first 10 years and increases with the passage of time, being greatest in those with substantial CSF pleocytosis and elevation of protein (Holmes 1974). There is no evidence that any single strain of *T. pallidum* is specifically neurotropic. However, in populations more recently exposed to syphilitic infection, acute secondary and tertiary manifestations of the infection (meningoencephalitis, meningovascular manifestations, and gumma) are commoner, whereas in those communities long exposed to the disease, such as the North American Indian, parenchymatous disease occurs more frequently. The predicted rise in the number of cases of neurosyphilis resulting from untreated infections in the Second World War did not materialize, possibly due to the widespread use of antibiotics in treating other infections. However, there is also evidence that mild modified neurosyphilis still occurs and may go unrecognized because of its minimal symptoms and signs (*British Medical Journal* 1978; Luxon, Lees, and Greenwood 1979; Hooshmand 1981). Traviesa, Prystowsky, Nelson, and Johnson (1978) examined the CSF in untreated or inadequately treated asymptomatic patients in whom the FTA–ABS test was positive in the serum; they found minor neurological signs in a few patients, and very few showed increases in cells, protein, or IgG or a positive VDRL test, but the TPI and FTA–ABS tests were positive in a much larger number. Hence these, rather than the reagin tests, may be a sensitive index of nervous-system involvement.

Secondary syphilis

Pathology

Spirochaetes may reach the nervous system during the primary stage and there may be a lymphocytosis in the CSF in up to 9 per cent of cases; Cutler, Bauer, Price, and Schwimmer (1954) found positive serological reactions in 1.5 per cent. In the secondary stage abnormalities such as pleocytosis or a raised protein, which may be transitory, have been found in the fluid in from 36 to 80 per cent of cases in different series. Cutler *et al.* (1954) found serological abnormalities in CSF in 6 per cent. The changes in the nervous system are those of a lymphocytic meningitis.

Symptoms and signs

There may be no symptoms referable to the nervous system in spite of slight abnormalities in the CSF, or the symptoms may be simply the headache and pains in the back and limbs commonly associated with the secondary stage. An acute meningitic illness occurs in 1-2 per cent of cases with headache, neck stiffness, and a marked CSF pleocytosis; meningoencephalitis is rare but may occur if the untreated condition remits spontaneously with a subsequent relapse. While fever, malaise, anorexia, skin eruptions including condylomata, lymphadenopathy, uveitis, hepatitis, and nephritis may all be seen, when meningoencephalitis does occur, the headache, papilloedema, convulsions, and confusion or coma which can result may be similar to the manifestations of tertiary meningovascular syphilis. Paresis of vertical gaze, presumably due to mesencephalitis, has been reported in the secondary stage (Page, Lean, and Sanders 1982).

The cerebrospinal fluid

In patients in the secondary stage who show no symptoms of nervous-system involvement the changes are usually slight, consisting of a slight increase in the number of mononuclear cells or of protein or both. The VDRL and FTA–ABS reactions may be negative in the fluid and positive or negative in the blood, according to whether the patient has received treatment. Patients with nervous symptoms show more marked changes which are usually proportional to their severity. When there is clinical evidence of meningitis, the pressure of the fluid is usually raised and the cell content is increased to as many as 1000 per mm^3. The cells are usually mononuclear, but in some acute cases neutrophils may also be found. CSF gamma globulin, especially the IgM and IgG fractions, are increased and the serological reactions are usually positive in the fluid.

For Diagnosis, Prognosis, and Treatment, see page 266.

Tertiary meningovascular syphilis

Cerebral syphilis

Pathology

The principal pathological changes in tertiary syphilis of the brain are first subacute meningitis, secondly vascular and perivascular inflammation involving large- and medium-sized arteries, and thirdly gumma formation. *Cranial pachymeningitis* is usually secondary to syphilitic cranial osteitis; though often described in the past, it is now rare. *Subacute leptomeningitis* is comparatively common in the basal meninges and over the convexity of the hemispheres; the changes are granulomatous, frequently involving cranial nerves and giving adhesive arachnoiditis, often with communicating hydrocephalus, and rarely arachnoid cyst formation.

The principal arterial lesion is an *obliterative endarteritis*; the vessel may be occluded either by intimal thickening or consequent thrombosis, with cerebral infarction or even infarction of cranial nerves due to involvement of vasa nervorum. The walls of the affected vessels are infiltrated with lymphocytes and plasma cells and there is perivascular fibrosis.

A gumma is a syphilitic granuloma, often with central necrosis which may be around a small vessel, surrounded by mononuclear and epithelioid cells, occasional giant cells, and an outer layer of fibroblasts and connective tissue. *T. pallidum* is only rarely isolated from gummas and from the inflamed blood vessels and meninges. Gummas may be small and multiple or large and single, up to several cm in diameter. Though they are commonest in skin, bone, and abdominal viscera, they may occur in the dura and meninges though they, like all tertiary manifestations, are now rare in Western countries.

Symptoms and signs

Meningovascular syphilis may cause symptoms within a few months of infection or at any time subsequently. In most cases, however, symptoms develop between 5 and 10 years after infection. Frequently symptoms of both cerebral and spinal syphilis are present in the same patient and may even coexist with evidence of parenchymatous disease.

Asymptomatic neurosyphilis

In some patients abnormalities are found in the CSF though the nervous system is clinically normal. This is known as asymptomatic neurosyphilis.

Cranial pachymeningitis

This rare condition may give no symptoms other than headache, but if the dura is adherent to the cortical meninges there may be focal convulsions and paresis of the limbs.

Cerebral leptomeningitis

The symptoms may be relatively diffuse or sharply focal, for example, limited to one cranial nerve. When the lesions are diffuse, the onset is usually insidious. Headache is often severe, with nocturnal exacerbations, and papilloedema may occur. Confusion and impairment of memory are common. The patient becomes inefficient, often anxious and nervous and may be thought to be neurotic. In more severe cases there is apathy and dementia, or a Korsakow syndrome. Aphasia may be present, and loss of sphincter control is common. The patient may finally pass into a state of semi-stupor. When the meninges over the convexity of the cerebral hemispheres are involved, focal or generalized convulsions may occur. Paresis and incoordination of the limbs on one or both sides are common. Basal meningitis often involves the chiasm and may thus give optic atrophy or visual-field defects. Hypothalamic involvement may cause obesity, diabetes insipidus, transient glycosuria, or somnolence. Hydrocephalus occasionally occurs. Reflex iridoplegia is usual and single or multiple cranial-nerve palsies, often unilateral, are common, the nerves being involved in inflammation in the subarachnoid space. The third nerve is most often affected, painless third-nerve palsy of rapid onset being a common isolated symptom. The paralysis of the intrinsic and extrinsic ocular muscles supplied by the nerve may be incomplete. Next in frequency the sixth, seventh, and fifth cranial nerves are liable to be attacked. Thus facial paralysis clinically indistinguishable from Bell's palsy is rarely seen. When the fifth nerve suffers, sensory disturbances are more common than motor weakness. Neuralgic pain in the distribution of one or more of its branches may be associated with either hyperpathia or analgesia, and sometimes with ophthalmic herpes zoster or neuropathic keratitis. Lesions of the eighth nerve can cause vertigo and deafness. The medullary nerves may also be involved, the twelfth suffering more often than the tenth and eleventh, but any of the three may be affected either alone or in combination with the others.

Cerebral endarteritis

Any cerebral artery may be involved. Before occlusion is complete there are frequently premonitory motor or sensory symptoms due to ischaemia. Finally, thrombosis gives symptoms of infarction which are described elsewhere (p. 192). The middle cerebral artery or its branches and the posterior cerebral are most frequently affected, but the anterior cerebral or the vertebrobasilar system may be involved.

Hemiplegia is the commonest effect and may result from occlusion of the middle cerebral artery itself or of one of its basal branches supplying the internal capsule. Its onset is rapid and associated with headache, but not often with loss of consciousness. It is rarely bilateral. Once a common cause of hemiplegia in young adults, syphilis is now rarely responsible; atheromatous occlusion of the internal carotid is much commoner. Parkinsonian features rarely occur in syphilitic mesencephalitis.

Cerebral gumma

Small gummatous lesions may be found in the meninges in syphilitic meningitis but a large gumma gives the symptoms of an intracranial tumour, usually situated subcortically in one cerebral hemisphere. The syphilitic origin of the tumour can only be inferred from a history of infection, signs of syphilis elsewhere and positive serological reactions in the blood and/or CSF. Cerebral gumma is now rare, however, whereas intracranial neoplasm and syphilitic infection are both common, and may be present in the same individual. A positive VDRL reaction, therefore, must not be interpreted as indicating that a space-occupying lesion within the skull is necessarily, or even probably, a gumma.

The cerebrospinal fluid

In meningovascular syphilis the VDRL reaction is positive in the blood in 60 or 70 per cent of cases. The TPI and FTA–ABS tests are even more specific, a positive result invariably being indicative of syphilitic infection. The pressure of the CSF may be either normal or increased. There is usually an excess of cells ranging between 20 and 100 per mm^3. The cells are mononuclear. The protein content of the fluid is usually increase to between 0.5 and 1.5 g/l. An increase in gamma-globulin (IgG and IgM) is almost invariable. In cases of luetic cerebral thrombosis, the VDRL reaction may be positive in the blood and negative in the fluid. Lange's colloidal gold test yields either a 'paretic' curve, e.g. 5543211000, or a 'luetic' curve—1345421000.

Diagnosis

Cerebral syphilis is protean its manifestations. Fortunately, serological tests come to the aid of clinical observations. It is rare that the VDRL reaction is negative in the CSF in active cerebral syphilis, and still more rare to find the reaction negative in both the CSF and the blood. Any suspicion of syphilis should, therefore, lead to the examination of both and to the performance of the more specific FTA–ABS test.

Mental changes associated with cerebral syphilis must be distinguished from other mental disorders and in their milder forms from neurosis. A clue to their nature is usually afforded by the presence of neurological signs, especially in the pupillary reactions.

When meningovascular syphilis causes papilloedema, it may be confused with intracranial tumour. Focal symptoms of subacute onset in syphilis, however, are relatively uncommon (except in the rare gumma) and, if they are present, the possibility of a tumour should not be too readily dismissed, even if the VDRL reaction is positive, since it is not very rare for a tumour to develop in a patient with syphilis.

Cerebral thrombosis of syphilitic origin usually occurs at an earlier age than that due to atheroma, but otherwise it can be distinguished from the latter only when a history of infection or other signs of syphilis are present, or, in their absence, by serological tests.

Meningovascular syphilis, as it often causes multiple cerebral lesions, may be confused with encephalitis, other forms of granulomatous meningitis, and multiple sclerosis. In encephalitis, impairment of consciousness is often more profound and pupillary changes are uncommon; nevertheless diagnosis ultimately rests upon serological tests in blood and CSF. These too are important in distinguishing meningovascular syphilis from sarcoidosis, carcinomatosis of the meninges, and cryptococcosis, all of which may give a clinical picture of subacute meningitis with multiple cranial-nerve palsies. In multiple sclerosis the pupillary reflexes are rarely affected, while nystagmus and ataxia in the absence of sensory loss are rare in syphilis. In multiple sclerosis the tendon jerks are exaggerated; in cerebral syphilis they are more often diminished or lost.

Prognosis

The prognosis is on the whole good, and excellent results are usually obtained with energetic treatment. When severe mental symptoms have occurred, however, despite marked improvement, the patient may have some residual impairment of memory, intellectual capacity, or emotional stability. The results of vascular occlusion are permanent, and though some improvement is usual as in all cases of cerebral infarction, variable permanent disability persists, while the hemianopia resulting from posterior cerebral thrombosis remains unaltered. Relapses are not uncommon, especially in patients who abandon treatment. They are unlikely in those who are thoroughly treated and kept under regular observation.

Treatment

See page 266.

Spinal syphilis

Pathology

The lesions of meningovascular syphilis have already been described.

Spinal pachymeningitis

Syphilitic inflammation of the spinal dura mater may follow syphilitic osteitis of the spine or may occur independently but is now very rare. The cervical region is usually involved—pachymeningitis cervicalis hypertrophica—the dura mater is thickened and adherent to the arachnoid and pia. The vessels and nerve roots entering and leaving the cord are involved; the cord becomes ischaemic and may contain a central cavity. Compression of long tracts is followed by ascending and descending degeneration.

Meningomyelitis

As in cerebral syphilis the meninges and blood vessels are both involved, though often unequally. When meningitis predominates, degenerative changes in the cord itself may be superficial. When the vessels also suffer severely, lesions of the cord substance are more extensive. Though the lesions are chronic, thrombosis of a major vessel may lead to an acute or subacute transverse lesion of the cord ('Erb's syphilitic spastic paraplegia'). In such cases the leptomeninges are adherent to the cord, which is visibly softened. Microscopically the vessels show endarteritis and perivascular cellular infiltration, and the meninges are also infiltrated. Within the cord there is degeneration of both myelin sheaths and axons. Ganglion cells exhibit chromatolysis, and there is ascending and descending degeneration. Syphilitic myelitis usually involves the dorsal region and, though the leptomeninges may be extensively infiltrated, the area of softening is usually limited to two or three segments.

Spinal endarteritis

As in the brain, endarteritis of a spinal artery or of its branches may cause thrombosis leading to a circumscribed area of softening within the cord, corresponding to the area of supply of the obstructed vessel.

Radiculitis

The spinal roots may be involved in syphilitic meningeal inflammation.

Symptoms and signs

Cervical pachymeningitis

The earliest symptom is pain due to compression of spinal nerves; it radiates round the neck, shoulders, and down the upper limbs. The pain is followed by atrophy of muscles supplied by the affected roots. Finally, compression and ischaemia of the cord lead to progressive spastic paraplegia with sensory loss below the level of the lesion.

Meningomyelitis

Myelitis is frequently an early symptom and may occur within three to five years of infection. The dorsal region of the cord is usually affected but when the cervical region is involved, and the course is subacute, pain in the neck and upper limbs may be followed by amyotrophy and sensory loss in the upper extremities due to root involvement. When sensory loss is slight or absent, the combination of lower motor-neurone involvement in the upper limbs and upper motor-neurone signs in the lower (syphilitic amyotrophy) may mimic that of motor-neurone disease (amyotrophic lateral sclerosis). Motor symptoms due to a dorsal lesion are generally preceded by pain in the back and in girdle distribution. Weakness of the lower limbs develops between a few days and several weeks after the onset of pain. In some cases complete flaccid paraplegia develops rapidly, with retention of urine and impairment or loss of all forms of sensibility below the level of the lesion. Sometimes the onset is more gradual and the functions of the cord are less severely affected. In such cases the patient develops spastic paraplegia-in-extension; bladder control is less severely impaired and sensory loss may be slight ('Erb's syphilitic spastic paraplegia'). In flaccid paraplegia the reflexes in the lower limbs are at first lost; extensor plantar responses soon appear, however, and as spinal shock passes off, severe flexor spasms usually develop.

Spinal endarteritis

Endarteritis and arterial thrombosis play an important part in syphilitic myelitis. Exceptionally thrombosis of anterior or posterior spinal arteries comparable with luetic cerebral thrombosis occurs. Rarely the picture of complete anterior spinal artery occlusion is seen (p. 423). When a lateral branch of the artery is occluded, there is a sudden onset of weakness, followed by wasting of muscles innervated by the affected spinal segment. The spinothalamic tract on the same side is often affected, giving hemianalgesia and hemi-thermo-anaesthesia on the opposite side of the body, with an upper level a few segments below that involved in the lesion. When thrombosis of one posterior spinal artery occurs, this usually affects only a few segments. All forms of sensibility are then impaired in the corresponding cutaneous segments owing to destruction of the posterior horn of grey matter. The posterior columns and the corticospinal tract on the same side are also infarcted so that position and joint sense and vibration sense are lost below the level of the lesion on the same side, with spastic paralysis below the lesion also on the same side.

Radiculitis

Syphilitic radiculitis usually affects dorsal roots causing pain and hyperpathia or analgesia in the corresponding segments. Herpes zoster is a common complication. When ventral roots are also affected, weakness and wasting develop in the muscles they supply.

The cerebrospinal fluid

In spinal syphilis the changes in the CSF are generally the same as those found in cerebral syphilis (p. 265). In a subacute condition, such as meningomyelitis, there is often a considerable excess of protein and of mononuclear cells; in this condition and in syphilitic pachymeningitis meningeal adhesions may obstruct the subarachnoid space giving spinal block (p. 67). Rarely, in vascular lesions of the spinal cord, the spinal fluid is normal, but the VDRL and FTA–ABS reactions are usually positive in the blood.

Diagnosis

Spinal syphilis must be differentiated from other conditions causing paraplegia or spinal-root lesions, especially spinal tumour, cervical spondylosis, motor-neurone disease, and multiple sclerosis. The diagnosis is not difficult when a history of infection is obtainable. Signs of cerebral syphilis, especially irregular pupils and impairment of their light reaction are often present and characteristic changes, especially a positive VDRL reaction, are found in the CSF. Nevertheless, myelography may still be necessary to exclude cord compression.

Prognosis

Spinal syphilis may respond well to treatment, the determining factor being the extent to which irreparable damage has been done to the spinal cord. Even when myelitis has led to complete paraplegia, improvement can occur as shock passes off and oedema disappears. Complete recovery, however, is not to be expected and this is especially the case after cord infarction. In amyotrophy the progress of the muscular wasting is sometimes arrested and slight improvement may occur, but much of the disability will be permanent. Root pains can usually be relieved, but are occasionally intractable.

Treatment of meningovascular syphilis

Before treatment is begun, the serum VDRL and FTA–ABS reactions should be examined and the CSF should be examined for comparison with future findings. The object of treatment is the destruction of all the spirochaetes in the body. Before penicillin this could not be accomplished with certainty with bismuth, iodine, and the arsenobenzene derivatives, alone or in combination, but penicillin can achieve a complete cure.

Penicillin

Experience showed that the smaller doses of penicillin at first given were inadequate and the dose now employed is 600 mg of benzylpenicillin (penicillin G) or procaine penicillin daily. Dattner, Kaufman, and Thomas (1947) gave an intramuscular injection every 3 hours, Nicol and Whelen (1947) only once a day. Most workers are now agreed that a single daily injection of 600 mg of penicillin G for 20 days is all that is required (Storm-Mathison 1976; Hooshmand 1981). However, occasional untoward allergic reactions to penicillin occur (Beerman, Nicholas, Schamberg, and Greenberg 1962) and chloramphenicol and chlortetracycline are also effective. Erythromycin, 500 mg four times daily for 10-15 days, is probably the drug of choice in patients known to be allergic to penicillin (Thomas 1964; Brown 1971; Holmes 1974; Muster 1981).

The routine of treatment

Penicillin is the foundation of treatment. To diminish the risk of Herxheimer reactions some authorities have advised beginning with small doses of penicillin, then gradually increasing but it is now agreed that this is no longer necessary. After the initial course no other treatment should be necessary for 6 months, when the blood and CSF VDRL and FTA–ABS reactions are re-examined. The first favourable change in the fluid is a fall in the cell count, the protein falls next, sometimes after an initial rise, and changes in the immunoglobulins and VDRL and FTA–ABS reactions come last. If the fluid shows improvement at the end of 6 months and the patient's clinical condition is satisfactory, he can safely be left without treatment for a further 6 months, when the blood and CSF are examined again; continuing evidence of activity in the fluid is an indication for a further course of treatment. If, however, the abnormality of the fluid is much less, the serological reactions should be examined every 6 months and the CSF once a year. The primary objectives are the relief of symptoms and arrest of the progress of the disease. The latter is only achieved when the CSF is normal, with negative serological reactions, and the reactions in the blood are also negative. When this has taken place the patient should be examined clinically and the blood examined once a year for 5 years, but it is unnecessary to examine the CSF again unless fresh symptoms appear. Sometimes, however, patients in whom the clinical course of the disease appears to be arrested continue to show positive reactions in the blood or fluid or both. If, in spite of several courses of treatment given over two or three years, the patient remains 'VDRL-fast' and his clinical condition is satisfactory, further treatment is not advisable.

General paresis

Synonyms. Dementia paralytica; general paralysis of the insane (G.P.I.).

Aetiology

General paresis was recognized as a clinical entity about 100 years ago, though, as its name implies, it was at first regarded as a form of paralysis supervening in persons who had already become insane. In the later nineteenth century its relationship to syphilitic infection was established, though syphilis was then regarded as predisposing to general paresis rather than as actually causing it. Noguchi first demonstrated in 1911 the presence of spirochaetes in the brains of sufferers from general paresis.

As McIntosh and Fildes (1914) showed, the effects of tertiary meningovascular syphilis upon the nervous system are secondary to granulomatous inflammatory changes in blood vessels and meninges, while in general paresis the spirochaetes actually invade the substance of the brain and spinal cord and themselves attack neurones. As previously mentioned, populations and races long exposed to syphilis (North America and Europe) are more liable to develop quaternary neurosyphilis (general paresis and tabes) while those which acquired the infection more recently (e.g. in many tropical countries) tend to develop the more florid secondary and tertiary manifestations (gummas and meningovascular syphilis).

General paresis affects about five out of 12 sufferers from neurosyphilis. Males are more liable to it than females in the proportions of four to one. It usually develops 10–15 years after infection, though the interval may be much shorter, and exceptionally it is 30 years or longer. It is rare, however, for the incubation period to be more than 20 years. The first symptoms usually appear between the ages of 40 and 50 but a congenital form occurs rarely (see p. 272).

Pathology

Macroscopically the brain is shrunken, the gyri being usually well defined, and the cerebral atrophy is usually confined to the anterior two-thirds of the hemispheres. The pia-arachnoid is usually somewhat opaque and the walls of the ventricles show granular ependymitis. A true communicating hydrocephalus occurs rarely, but may cause unexpected clinical deterioration (Giménez-Roldán, Benito, and Martin 1979).

Microscopic changes are predominantly cortical involving meninges, blood vessels, and neurones. The leptomeninges are diffusely infiltrated with lymphocytes and plasma cells. Similar cells occupy the perivascular spaces in the cerebral cortex, and there is often evidence of new capillary formation. The cortical ganglion cells show variable degrees of degeneration, going on to complete disappearance. These changes are most marked in the molecular layer and the layers of small- and medium-sized pyramidal cells. The deeper layers, including the large pyramidal cells, show less severe changes. Demyelination of cortical and subcortical fibres is also seen, often in focal distribution. There is widespread gliosis, often with giant astrocytes and activated microglial cells.

These cortical changes are diffuse, but the frontal and temporal regions suffer most severely. Similar changes may be found in the basal ganglia and cerebellar cortex. There is no relationship between the severity of the cortical degeneration and the degree of infiltration of the overlying leptomeninges. Spirochaetes are demonstrable in about 50 per cent of cases, especially in the frontal region, and are sometimes found in ganglion cells. In the 'Lissauer type' of general paresis, localized cortical atrophy, a 'spongy state' and patchy demyelination of the white matter are found. The pathological changes of tabes may coexist with general paresis (taboparesis). Aortitis is often present.

Symptoms

Mental symptoms

The earliest symptoms are usually mental and are often so slight as to be apparent only to those who known the patient well. It is thus important to obtain a history from a relative or friend. The earliest change is usually impaired intellectual efficiency. The patient is less effective in his work. He loses the power to concentrate, and his memory becomes unreliable. His inefficiency is often apparent to others but not to himself, though exceptionally anxiety is prominent and may lead to a mistaken diagnosis of neurosis. As the condition progresses, the patient's behaviour becomes more abnormal, he becomes careless about dress and personal appearance, and about money, and may lose large sums in extravagance or in ill-judged speculations. Alcoholic excess and sexual aberrations are common. These are symptoms of dementia see (p. 657), and this form is sometimes described as the 'simple dementing type'.

The type of disorder, however, doubtless depends upon the patient's premorbid personality, and thus other clinical pictures occur. The grandiose form, though often regarded as typical, is less common than simple dementia. These patients are euphoric, and develop delusions in which they figure as exceptional persons endowed with superhuman strength, immense wealth, or other magnificent attributes. They readily act on these delusions, and may order large quantities of goods or write cheques for huge sums, and see no discrepancy between their imaginary attributes and their debilitated and unfortunate actual condition. Occasionally, in this stage, affected individuals have been known to produce unusual works of art of exceptional quality (Fraser 1981). Other emotional states may dominate the picture, leading to depressed, agitated, and maniacal, types. Sometimes the condition resembles Korsakow's syndrome. As the patient deteriorates however, the symptoms of dementia become more prominent; in the terminal stage the sufferer, bedridden, incontinent, and dirty, leads virtually a vegetative existence.

Speech suffers both in its receptive and expressive functions. Difficulty in naming objects is common. Echolalia may occur.

Physical symptoms and signs

Epileptic attacks occur in about 50 per cent of cases. They may take the form of focal seizures, without loss of consciousness; generalized attacks, in which consciousness is lost; or minor seizures, in which brief impairment or loss of consciousness occurs without a convulsion. Status epilepticus is rarely seen.

Apoplectiform episodes, so-called 'congestive attacks', were once common but are now rare. The resulting symptoms, of which hemiplegia is the commonest, but which may include aphasia, apraxia, and hemianopia, are always transitory and the associated loss of consciousness is usually brief. Recovery is often complete in a week or two.

Although physical abnormalities are usually present when the patient first seeks advice, physical signs may be absent even when mental changes are conspicuous. The expression is often vacant or fatuous, less often mask-like. The pupils are usually contracted and irregular and react sluggishly to light. Typical Argyll Robertson pupils are common. Optic atrophy is not uncommon, but is rarely severe enough to cause marked loss of visual acuity.

Voluntary power becomes progressively impaired, and weakness is usually associated with tremor, most conspicuous on voluntary movement, and best seen in the facial muscles, especially the lips and the tongue and in the outstretched fingers. Slow slurred speech is characteristic. In addition, incoordination usually develops later, rendering the gait unsteady and movements of the upper limbs ataxic.

Owing to bilateral degeneration of the corticospinal tracts, the tendon reflexes are usually exaggerated, the abdominal reflexes diminished or lost, and the plantar reflexes extensor. When tabes is associated with general paresis—'taboparesis'—the tendon reflexes are lost. Except in taboparesis, when the sensory changes typical of tabes are present, sensation is unimpaired. Loss of sphincter control is common at a comparatively early stage, but is the result of the cerebral changes.

The cerebrospinal fluid

The CSF shows changes of great diagnostic importance. The pressure is normal or slightly increased. There is usually an excess of mononuclear cells, rarely exceeding 100 per mm^3. The protein content is also increased and usually lies between 0.5 and 1.0 g/l. There is usually a marked increase of globulin and of the total more than 25 per cent may be found to be gamma-globulin with a considerable increase in IgG and IgM. Lange's colloidal gold curve is of the paretic type, e.g. 5554311000 or even 5555555444. The VDRL reaction is positive in the CSF in 100 per cent of cases, and in the blood in from 90 to 100 per cent. The TPI and FTA–ABS tests are even more specific, being invariably positive in the fluid in the untreated case.

Diagnosis

The constancy of serological abnormalities in the blood and CSF in general paresis is of the utmost diagnostic importance, as it frequently confirms a diagnosis which on clinical grounds alone might be doubtful.

The mental symptoms in the early stage may simulate neurosis or manic-depressive psychosis. Neither condition, however, is associated with signs of organic nervous disease.

General paresis must be distinguished from the presenile and senile dementias and from arteriosclerotic (multi-infarct) dementia in which tremor, spasticity, and extensor plantar responses may be present. In such cases the diagnosis is made only after examination of the blood and CSF. Alcoholic dementia— 'alcoholic pseudoparesis'—may simulate general paresis and is again distinguishable only by serological tests.

It is often difficult to distinguish general paresis from meningovascular syphilis when the latter condition causes severe mental changes, since the VDRL reactions and FTA–ABS may be positive in both blood and CSF in both conditions.

Prognosis

Before the introduction of malarial treatment general paresis was invariably fatal, and it was exceptional for a patient to survive more than three years. Exceptionally the disease ran a rapid course and was fatal within a year. Remissions, however, occurred spontaneously in from 10 to 20 per cent of cases. Malarial treatment greatly improved the outlook, but penicillin is much more effective (Hahn, Webster, Weickhardt, Thomas, Timberlake, Solomon, Stokes, Heyman, Gammon, Gleeson, Curtis, and Cutler 1958). Arrest can usually be achieved, hence the earlier the diagnosis is made and treatment is begun, the better the outlook. Nevertheless, complete cure is unusual and in a series of 100 cases followed up for 10 years after initial treatment, 31 per cent developed new neurological manifestations (Wilner and Brody 1968).

Treatment

Penicillin

Penicillin is the treatment of choice, or other antibiotics, as in meningovascular syphilis (p. 266).

Malarial therapy

The introduction of malaria treatment by Wagner-Jauregg in 1917 was a great advance. The parasite of benign tertian malaria (*P. vivax*) was generally employed (Rudolf 1927; Meagher 1929), being inoculated by the bite of an infected mosquito or by injection of infected donor blood. Though malarial and/or other types of fever therapy were still used until about 20 years ago, this method is no longer necessary if adequate antibiotic therapy is given.

Tabes dorsalis

Synonym. Locomotor ataxia

Aetiology

Tabes was first recognized by Romberg and Duchenne. Its association with syphilis was first suspected by Fournier, and was established by the introduction of the Wassermann reaction and the discovery of spirochaetes in the brain and spinal cord of affected individuals by Noguchi, Marinesco, and Minea. Tabes, like general paresis, differs from tertiary syphilis with respect to the parenchymatous nature of the spinal lesions and the unsatisfactory response of advanced cases to treatment.

As in general paresis, it is not uncommon to find that tabetic patients deny having had primary or secondary syphilis. These signs of infection may, therefore, have passed unnoticed. Tabes affects males much more frequently than females in a ratio of at least 4 to 1, and affects 3 out of 12 cases of neurosyphilis. Although trauma has sometimes been blamed for precipitating the onset it seems likely that the relationship is fortuitous. Tabetic symptoms usually appear between 8 and 12 years after infection. Exceptionally they may develop within 3 years, or be delayed for 20 years or longer. The age of onset is usually between 35 and 50 years.

Pathology

Macroscopically there is atrophy of the dorsal spinal roots, especially in the lower thoracic and lumbosacral regions. The posterior columns of the spinal cord are flat or even sunken; hence the name tabes dorsalis or dorsal wasting. On section the posterior columns appear grey and translucent, in contrast to the normal appearance of the remaining white matter.

Microscopically the primary lesion is degeneration of the central processes of the dorsal-root ganglion cells, which themselves are usually little affected. Since the only exogenous fibres which follow a long course within the cord lie in the posterior columns, these degenerate selectively and their demyelination is conspicuous when stained by myelin stains (Fig. 9.1). The endogenous fibres in the commissural zone, that part of the posterior columns lying just posterior to the grey commissure, usually escape. Since the lower thoracic and lumbosacral roots are first attacked and their fibres entering the posterior columns move towards the midline as they ascend, the fasciculus gracilis suffers earlier than the fasciculus cuneatus in the cervical region. In early cases the intraspinal portion of the posterior roots may be infiltrated with lymphocytes and plasma cells (Merritt 1946); later there is secondary gliosis in the posterior columns and the overlying pia mater is thickened. Exceptionally degeneration of anterior horn cells occurs in certain segments, with atrophy of the fibres of the corresponding ventral roots.

Many theories have been proposed to explain the selective degenerative lesions of tabes. Obersteiner and Redlich (1894–5) believed that it was due to compression of the dorsal root fibres by meningeal constriction at the point where they pass through the pia mater and this view is still generally favoured.

Optic atrophy is common, the degeneration of the nerve fibres being either primary or secondary to granulomatous syphilitic inflammation of the interstitial tissues (see p. 264). The Argyll Robertson pupil has been variously explained (see p. 104). Sensory fibres of the cranial nerves, especially the trigeminal and glossopharyngeal, like those of the dorsal roots, may be involved as they approach the brain-stem, and degeneration has also been des-

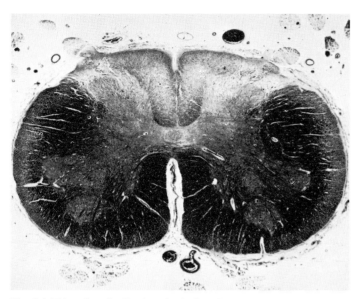

Fig. 9.1. Tabes dorsalis. Section of spinal cord.

cribed in the sympathetic fibres. The pathological changes of men-ingovascular syphilis rarely coexist with those of tabes, and lesions of general paresis may also be found ('taboparesis').

Tabes is an important cause of trophic arthropathy—Charcot's joints. Destruction of cartilage and erosion of the epiphyses occur and are often associated with the development of osteophytic out-growths. There is an increased volume of synovial fluid, and sub-luxation of an affected joint is not uncommon. Trauma frequently contributes to the development of arthropathy. Syphilitic aortitis is a common complication.

Symptoms and signs

The principal symptoms of tabes are readily explained by the degeneration of the afferent fibres of the dorsal roots. Pain and paraesthesiae result from irritation of the affected sensory fibres. Sensory loss, i.e. analgesia and impairment of postural sensibility and vibration sense, are due to interruption of many such fibres. Sensory ataxia is due in part to impaired appreciation of position and joint sense. Diminution and loss of the tendon reflexes are due to interruption of their reflex arcs on the afferent side. Impo-tence and sphincter disturbances are the result of loss of afferent impulses concerned in sexual function and in evacuation of the bladder and rectum.

Mode of onset
The onset of tabes is usually insidious but exceptionally it is rapid and rarely a patient can become grossly ataxic within three months. Usually sensory symptoms, especially pain, precede ataxia by months or years (the pre-ataxic stage), but ataxia may develop early. Frequently the early symptoms are so slight that the patient does not seek advice until a more serious symptom deve-lops. Hence the symptom which brings him to the doctor may be pain, ataxia, vomiting, impotence, disorder of micturition, failing vision, diplopia, or even arthropathy.

Sensory symptoms and signs
Pain is the commonest early symptom and usually takes the form of 'lightning pains'. These pains, which are stabbing in character, occur in brief paroxysms in the lower limbs and may be very severe. As a rule they do not radiate longitudinally, but are loca-lized to one spot, where the patient feels as if a sharp object were being driven into the limb. Each attack lasts only a few seconds, but attacks can recur repeatedly in the same place, or may shift from place to place in the limb. A fresh attack may be precipitated

by a change in the weather or by intercurrent illness. Hyperpathia is common with vasodilatation of the skin in the area to which the pains are referred, and in severe cases ecchymosis may occur. Similar severe paroxysmal pains may occur in the upper limbs or in the distribution of the trigeminal nerve. Other forms of pain may be felt, such as burning or tearing pains in the feet, sciatica, or a constricting pain around the chest or abdomen —'root pains' or 'girdle pains'.

Paraesthesiae are common, especially in the lower limbs. The patient may complain that the feet feel numb or cold, and a sensa-tion as of walking on wool is a common complaint. The skin of the trunk and lower limbs is often hypersensitive to touch and to heat and cold. The patient may recognize that some parts of the body are anaesthetic. Thus he may be unable to feel the chair upon which he sits, and may notice that he is unaware when his bladder is full, and that he cannot feel the act of defaecation.

Objective sensory changes
The forms of sensation first impaired are usually those mediated by the posterior columns. Appreciation of vibration suffers early, and usually before recognition of posture and passive movement. As a rule the lower limbs are affected before the upper, though exceptionally the upper limbs suffer first—so-called 'cervical tabes'.

Painful sensibility is also impaired early, deep tissues becoming insensitive before the skin. Squeezing of muscles and of the tendo calcaneus evokes no pain, and testicular sensation is often lost. The appreciation of painful cutaneous sensation is usually lost first on the side of the nose, the ulnar border of the arm and forearm, the trunk between the nipples and the costal margin, the outer border of the leg and dorsum and sole of the foot, and the perianal region. In these areas, even when pin-prick is appreciated as pain-ful, there is often a long delay of up to several seconds, between the application of the stimulus and its perception. Cutaneous sen-sibility to light touch, heat, and cold is usually unimpaired at first, but finally there may be loss of all forms of sensibility over much of the body.

Ataxia
Sensory ataxia usually begins in the lower limbs with slight unsteadiness in walking and turning. Since the patient is able to some extent to compensate by means of vision for the deficit, his ataxia is worse in the dark or when he closes his eyes, whence arises the characteristic symptom of falling into the wash-basin when the eyes are closed in washing the face. As the ataxia increases, movements of the lower limbs become increasingly incoordinate. The patient walks on a wide base; the feet are lifted too high and brought down to the ground too violently. Walking becomes difficult without a stick, and finally he can only walk when supported.

In the early stages ataxia of the lower limbs is best demonstrated by asking the patient to stand with the toes and heels together and the eyes closed, noting whether he sways—Romberg's test—or by asking him to walk along a line placing one heel in front of the opposite toe.

In severe cases ataxia of the trunk muscles may cause the patient to be unable to sit up in bed without support. Ataxia of the upper limbs is manifest in the clumsy fine movements of the fingers. The defective maintenance of posture can be demon-strated in the outstretched fingers by asking the patient to close his eyes. When their posture is no longer controlled by vision they either droop or wander in space ('pseudoathetosis').

Muscle tone
Partial deafferentation leads to diffuse muscular hypotonia.

The reflexes of the limbs and trunk

Degeneration of afferent fibres of the reflex arc leads to depression of tendon reflexes and ultimately to their disappearance. The ankle-jerks are thus affected before the knee jerks. The tendon-jerks of the upper limbs are usually diminished early but are finally lost only after those of the lower limbs have disappeared. The plantar reflexes usually remain elicitable and are flexor, except in taboparesis, when they are extensor. The abdominal reflexes are also obtainable as a rule.

Sphincter disturbances

Disturbances in bladder control may occur early when sacral roots are involved. When lumbar roots suffer first, ataxia of the lower limbs may precede bladder symptoms. The patient may complain either of difficulty of micturition or of incontinence. The bladder is large and atonic; catheterization often reveals the presence of substantial residual urine, and complete retention may occur. Urinary-tract infection develops sooner or later, and ascending pyelonephritis may develop. Constipation is the rule, but faecal incontinence can occur, especially when the patient is unaware of the act of defaecation. Impotence is sometimes an early symptom but is not invariable.

Ocular symptoms and signs

Pupillary abnormalities are present in more than 90 per cent of patients at some time in the course of the disease. The pupils are usually contracted and often irregular. Exceptionally they are moderately or even widely dilated, especially in congenital neurosyphilis. Occasionally one is moderately dilated and the other contracted. The reaction to light is at first impaired and later lost, while that on accommodation-convergence is retained. The iris is pale and atrophic. The complete Argyll Robertson pupil (p. 104), however, often appears late, and in the early stages it is commoner to find that the light reaction is present but reduced in amplitude, exhibits a long latent period, and is ill-sustained. The reflex is often brisker in one eye than in the other, and the consensual reaction may be brisker than the direct. Rarely the pupil dilates in response to light. The contracted pupil fails to dilate in response to a scratch upon the skin of the neck; both the myosis and loss of this ciliospinal reflex are due to degeneration of oculosympathetic fibres. Moderate ptosis, also due to oculosympathetic paralysis, is common, and compensatory contraction of the frontalis muscle contributes to the characteristic facies. Diplopia occurs in about 20 per cent of cases; in the early stages it is often transitory, but permanent paralysis of the third or sixth nerve develops rarely.

Optic atrophy is of the 'primary' variety (see p. 93). The optic disc is small and pale, the physiological cup is preserved, and the lamina cribrosa is often visible. The atrophy is often slight and non-progressive, with little or no subjective impairment of visual acuity, being discovered only on routine examination. When, however, the patient complains of failing vision it is more likely to progress and to terminate in blindness. Usually there is a peripheral constriction of the visual fields; less often there is a central scotoma.

Other cranial nerves

Pain and analgesia in trigeminal distribution have already been described. Loss of smell and taste occasionally occur. Degeneration of the eighth nerve may give deafness, and involvement of vestibular fibres vertigo. Exceptionally, degeneration of part of the nucleus ambiguus causes bilateral laryngeal-abductor paralysis, and paralysis of the accessory and hypoglossal nerves is occasionally observed.

Trophic changes

Arthropathies—Charcot's joints—are common; symptoms not infrequently appear after injury. The onset of the joint change is frequently rapid, with considerable swelling and increase in the synovial fluid. The skin may seem hot, but pain is almost invariably absent. Later, osteophytes frequently develop, the joint becomes much enlarged, and considerable disorganization with subluxation may occur. Radiographs show marked erosion of the joint surfaces with formation of new bone at the articular margins or from the adjacent shaft (Fig. 9.2). The knee is most frequently affected, and after that the hip. The shoulder, tarsal joints, elbow, ankle, small joints of the fingers and toes and spine are involved in approximately this order of frequency. The long bones are brittle, and fractures can occur after slight trauma.

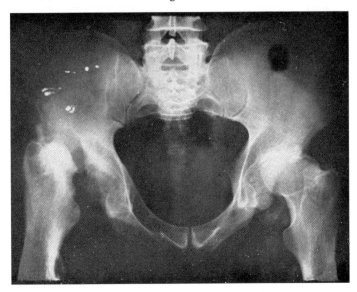

Fig. 9.2. Radiograph of bilateral Charcot hips in a tabetic patient. Note the opacities due to bismuth injections in the right buttock.

The commonest trophic change in the skin is the perforating ulcer, usually seen under the pad of the great toe or at other pressure-points on the sole (Fig. 9.3). The first stage is epithelial thickening resembling a corn, and, either spontaneously or following attempts to cut it away, an indolent ulcer develops. Sometimes a sinus extends down the underlying bone, and bony disorganization and deformity may then result. Other trophic changes include bruising, loss of hair, and even occasionally of the teeth. Symptomatic herpes zoster may occur.

Tabetic crises

Paroxysmal painful disorders of function of various viscera occur in tabes, and are called crises. The gastric crisis is the commonest. It is characterized by attacks of epigastric pain with severe vomiting, and can last from a few hours to several days. Laryngeal crises are attacks of dyspnoea with cough and both inspiratory and expiratory stridor, and are associated with vocal-cord paresis. Rectal crises, characterized by tenesmus, and vesical crises, with pain in the bladder or penis and strangury, may also occur, and renal and other crises have been described. The feature common to most such crises seems to be increased motility of a hollow viscus, presumably due to autonomic dysfunction.

The cerebrospinal fluid

The pressure is normal and there is usually an excess of cells, which are mononuclear and do not often exceed 70 per mm^3. The total protein is normal or slightly increased. The gamma-globulin is raised in 90 per cent of cases. The colloidal gold curve is usually of the 'luetic' type. The VDRL and FTA–ABS reactions are positive in both blood and CSF in 65 per cent of cases, positive in the fluid alone in 10 per cent, in the blood alone in 5 per cent, and negative in both in 20 per cent. The test is positive in the fluid in about 60 per cent of all cases but is almost invariably positive in

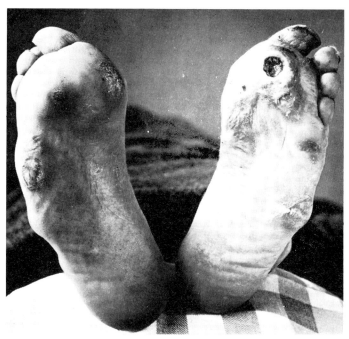

Fig. 9.3. Perforating ulcers in tabes dorsalis.

the blood (Duperrat and Cayol 1962). The VDRL and FTA–ABS reactions may be negative in the fluid in spite of an excess of cells, protein, and globulin, and a negative reaction in both blood and fluid or even a completely normal fluid is rarely found in a patient with progressive disease.

Complications

Symptoms of meningovascular syphilis, including muscular wasting, can coexist with those of tabes, but this is unusual. A tabetic patient may, after some years, develop general paresis, or some symptoms of tabes may be present in an individual who presents with symptoms of the latter disorder. Psychotic reactions, often with paranoia, have also been described in cases of tabes. Syphilitic aortitis is often present, but is often asymptomatic. However, even after the successful treatment of neurosyphilis, cardiovascular manifestations, and particularly signs of aortitis, can appear several years later.

Diagnosis

When the patient is frankly ataxic, diagnosis usually presents little difficulty, for the typical physical signs are then well developed, and the matter is clinched by investigation of the blood and CSF. In multiple sclerosis ataxia is usually associated with spasticity, exaggerated tendon reflexes, and extensor plantar responses. Friedreich's ataxia resembles tabes in the association of lower-limb ataxia with diminution or loss of tendon reflexes, but begins at an early age and is differentiated clinically by the presence of nystagmus, dysarthria, extensor plantar responses, scoliosis, and pes cavus. Polyneuropathy may simulate tabes when there is ataxia of the lower limbs. In alcoholic neuropathy the pupillary reactions may be sluggish, the tendon reflexes diminished or lost, pains occur in the limbs, and there is impairment of postural sensibility. In this condition, however, weakness of distal-limb muscles is also conspicuous and wrist- and foot-drop are often present, while the deep tissues, especially the muscles, are tender on pressure and not, as in tabes, analgesic. However, some patients with diabetic polyneuropathy also experience pain in the limbs and on examination show pupillary changes, areflexia, and peripheral impairment of pain sensation ('diabetic pseudotabes'); the coincidental association of tabes dorsalis may then have to be excluded

by serological tests and motor-nerve conduction velocity measurements, which are usually abnormal in diabetic neuropathy and normal in tabes. Argyll Robertson pupils have been described in peroneal muscular atrophy (Charcot–Marie–Tooth disease), but in this condition the peripheral amyotrophy is diagnostic.

When ataxia is absent the prominence of other symptoms may lead to an error in diagnosis; for example, pains in the limbs may be attributed to arthritis, root pains in the trunk to visceral lesions, gastric crises to ulceration of the stomach or duodenum, disturbances of the vesical sphincter to prostatism or other bladder lesions, arthropathy to arthritis, facial pain to trigeminal neuralgia, and optic atrophy to toxic amblyopia. These mistakes can be avoided only by systematic neurological examination, special stress being laid upon the pupillary reflexes and upon diminution, absence, or inequality of lower-limb tendon reflexes. In doubtful cases the blood and CSF should be examined. It must always be borne in mind that tabes may coexist with other disorders. All patients suspected of gastric crisis should have a barium meal and/or gastroscopy, as the failure to diagnose peptic ulcer in a tabetic may be more serious for the patient than to mistake a gastric crisis for such a lesion.

Prognosis

Tabes is very variable in its rate of progress and in the extent to which it responds to treatment. A rapidly progressive course leading to ataxia in a few months is rare. Usually the pre-ataxic stage lasts from 2 to 5 years. In some cases overt ataxia never develops and there are a few abortive cases with Argyll Robertson pupils and absent knee- and ankle-jerks, but no symptoms. The rate of progression can be roughly assessed from the duration of the pre-ataxic stage. The longer this is, the slower will be the subsequent deterioration. The response to treatment is equally variable. Sometimes considerable improvement occurs and the disorder seems arrested. Other patients go downhill rapidly or slowly in spite of treatment. Optic atrophy is not necessarily progressive, but when the patient complains of failing vision it often leads to blindness. Early treatment is likely to arrest the condition in about 50 per cent of cases. Gastric crises often respond, and perforating ulcers which are not too far advanced can usually be induced to heal. No improvement can be expected in the arthropathy. Sphincter control often improves, and impotence, though often permanent, is not necessarily so. In fatal cases death usually occurs from intercurrent infection, or from cardiovascular complications.

Treatment

General treatment

Special attention to the bladder and bowels, to the treatment of secondary infections, and the care of the feet is needed.

Antisyphilitic treatment should be given as indicated for meningovascular syphilis (p. 266). Various appliances, including walking sticks, supporting bandages for neuropathic joints, and even spinal corsets, are sometimes needed.

Treatment of special symptoms

Pain. Tabetic pains are often relieved by simple analgesics; when lightning pains are more severe and frequent, systemic steroids (Moore 1953) or intrathecal prednisone (Bertini 1958) have been recommended, but the most successful drug seems to be carbamazepine (*Tegretol*) given in a dosage of 400–800 mg daily (Ekbom 1972).

Ataxia. Limb coordination may be improved by suitable re-educational exercises.

The bladder. Precipitancy of micturition may be relieved by propantheline, 15mg three times daily, or similar remedies. The atonic bladder should not be treated surgically unless renal function is impaired or there is urinary infection which has failed to respond to chemotherapy. The choice will then lie between suprapubic cystostomy, and transurethral division of the internal sphincter. Catheterization and cystometrography may be needed with measurement of the residual urine. The patient should be instructed to pass urine at four-hourly intervals whether he feels the need to micturate or not. Even when the bladder has become overdistended it is probably best treated in this way, with the addition of appropriate drugs such as carbamylcholine. Surgical intervention should be postponed as long as possible.

Crises. A gastric crisis can frequently be cut short by an injection of pethidine hydrochloride, 100 mg but this, and other potentially addictive drugs should be avoided unless absolutely essential. In severe recurrent cases benefit has followed section of lower thoracic spinal dorsal roots, and very rarely bilateral upper cervical cordotomy may be necessary.

Perforating ulcer. Tabetic patients should wear well-fitting shoes and should be warned against cutting their own corns, as a perforating ulcer may follow a slight injury. Regular attention from a skilled chiropodist is recommended. When an ulcer has developed, antibiotic and protective dressings may promote healing.

Arthropathy. The objective is to relieve the strain on the damaged joint. The knee or ankle may be supported by a firm elastic support. Spinal arthropathy necessitates a leather corset or spinal brace. When there is much fluid in the joint, this may be aspirated. Excision of an arthropathic joint or the insertion of prostheses should not be attempted, since the results are uniformly unsatisfactory.

Optic atrophy. No treatment other than penicillin or other appropriate antibiotics is of any value; surgical decompression of the optic nerves is ineffective (Bruetsch 1948).

Congenital neurosyphilis

Active neurosyphilis used to occur in from 8 to 10 per cent of congenitally syphilitic children, males being affected slightly more often than females (Jeans and Cooke 1930). Neither in its pathological nor in its clinical features does congenital neurosyphilis differ in any essential respects from the acquired form save for the fact that fixed dilated pupils rather than those of typical Argyll Robertson type are more common in the congenital variety. Both meningovascular and parenchymatous neurosyphilis occur. Intrauterine infection with the spirochaete may lead to actual developmental arrest so that the cerebral hemispheres are unusually small. Gross loss of Purkinje cells with gliosis of the cerebellar cortex are characteristic of juvenile general paresis.

Symptoms and signs

The meningovascular form is commoner than the parenchymatous. Both mental handicap (Schachter 1959) and convulsions are common. Mild communicating hydrocephalus is relatively common. The pupils are often large, irregular, and unequal and the reaction to light is sluggish or absent. Optic atrophy is often present; it may be secondary to choroidoretinitis or to involvement of the optic nerves or chiasm in basal syphilitic meningitis, or may be parenchymatous in congenital general paresis or tabes. Facial weakness is common, as is deafness, due in most cases to a lesion of the eighth nerve within the temporal bone and not in its intracranial course. Destruction of corticospinal fibres may lead to diplegia or hemiplegia and moderate infantilism is not uncommon. Hypersomnia and diabetes insipidus are rare manifestations.

Parenchymatous neurosyphilis is rare. Stewart (1933) estimated that general paresis occurred in 1 per cent of congenital syphilitics. Symptoms usually develop during the first half of the second decade of life. They are similar to those of the acquired form, though the mental symptoms are usually less florid and are those of acquired dementia. Grandiose delusions, if present, are puerile in type; for example, a boy stated that he owned all the sweet shops in the country. The course of the disorder is usually slower than in the adult, and the untreated patient may live for 10 or more years.

Congenital tabes usually develops somewhat later than congenital general paresis, and may not appear until early adult life but taboparesis can occur in adolescence (Joffe, Black, and Floyd 1968). Optic atrophy is common in both, and in both the pupils are often widely dilated and fixed.

The blood VDRL and FTA–ABS reactions are usually positive and the TPI test is always so when congenital neurosyphilis is progressive, but the VDRL test is sometimes negative in latent or arrested cases. The CSF usually shows the changes associated with the acquired disorders.

Diagnosis

The diagnosis is usually easy when it is considered, as other signs of congenital syphilis are usually present, and is confirmed by serological studies in the child and its parents. However, juvenile general paresis or taboparesis, when presenting with fits, dementia, and akinetic mutism, with or without areflexia and sphincter disturbance, may be mistaken for encephalitis or polyradiculitis.

Prognosis

The response to treatment is disappointing in patients first seen because of nervous symptoms, especially in congenital general paresis and tabes. Hence it is important that the CSF should be examined in all congenitally syphilitic children at an early age, in order to detect neurosyphilis.

Treatment

Treatment should be carried out on the same lines as for acquired syphilis.

References

Adams, R. D. and Merritt, H. H. (1944). Meningeal and vascular syphilis of the spinal cord. *Medicine, Baltimore* **23**, 181.

Beerman, H., Nicholas, L., Schamberg, I. L., and Greenberg, M. S. (1962). Syphilis: review of the recent literature, 1960–1. *Arch. intern. Med.* **109**, 323.

Bertini, F. (1958). Terapia cortisonica a scopo antalgico nella tabe dorsale. *Gazz. med. ital.* **117**, 417.

Bogaert, L. van and Verbrugge, J. (1928). The pathogenesis and the surgical treatment of gastric crisis of tabes: neuroramisectomy. *Surg. Gynec. Obstet.* **47**, 543.

British Medical Journal (1978). Modified neurosyphilis. *Br. med. J.* **2**, 647.

Brown, W. J. (1971). Status and control of syphilis in the United States. *J. infect. Dis.* **124**, 428.

Breutsch, W. L. (1948). Surgical treatment of syphilitic primary atrophy of the optic nerves (syphilitic optochiasmatic arachnoiditis). *Arch. Ophthal.* **38**, 735.

Clark, E. G. and Danbolt, N. (1964). The Oslo study of the natural course of untreated syphilis. *Med. Clin. N. Amer.* **48**, 613.

Curtis, A. C., Kruse, W. T., and Norton, D.H. (1950). Neurosyphilis. IV. Post-treatment evaluation 4–5 years following penicillin and penicillin plus malaria. *Am. J. Syph.* **24**, 554.

Cutler, J. C., Bauer, T. J., Price, E. V., and Schwimmer, B. H. (1954). Comparison of spinal fluid findings among syphilitic and nonsyphilitic individuals. *Am. J. Syph.* **38**, 447.

Dattner, B. (1948*a*). Neurosyphilis and the latest methods of treatment. *Med. Clin. N. Amer.* **32**, 707.

—— (1948*b*). Treatment of neurosyphilis with penicillin alone. *Amer. J. Syph.* **32**, 399.

——, Kaufman, S. S., and Thomas, E. W. (1947). Penicillin in treatment of neurosyphilis. *Arch. Neurol. Psychiat. Chigago* **58**, 426.

Duperrat, B. and Cayol, J. (1962). Le test de Nelson dans les tabès. *Bull. Soc. Méd. Paris.* **113**, 556.

Ekbom, K. (1972). Carbamazepine in the treatment of tabetic lightning pains. *Arch. Neurol. Chicago* **26**, 374.

Foix, C., Crusem, L., and Nacht, S. (1926). Sur l'anatomo-pathologie de la syphilis médullaire en général et en particulier des paraplégies syphilitiques progressives. *Ann. Méd.* **20**, 81.

Fraser, I. (1981). General paralysis of the insane. *Br. med. J.* **283, 1631.**

Gillespie, E. J. and Brown, B. C. (1964). New laboratory methods in the diagnosis of syphilis and other treponematoses. *Med. Clin. N. Amer.* **48**, 731.

Giménez-Roldán, S., Benito, C., and Martin, M. (1979). Dementia para-lytica: deterioration from communicating hydrocephalus. *J. Neurol. Neurosurg. Psychiat.* **42**, 501.

Goldman, D. (1945). Treatment of neurosyphilis with penicillin. *J. Am. med. Ass.* **128**, 274.

Hahn, R. D. (1951). The treatment of neurosyphilis with penicillin and with penicillin plus malaria. *Am. J. Syph.* **35**, 433.

——, Cutler, J. C., Curtis, A. C., Gammon, G., Heyman, A., Johnwick, E., Stokes, J. H., Solomon, H., Thomas, E., Timberlake, W., Webster, B., and Gleeson, G. (1956). Penicillin treatment of asymptomatic central nervous system syphilis, I and II. *Arch. Derm.* **74**, 355, 367.

——, Webster, B., Weickhard, G., Thomas, E., Timberlake, W., Solomon, H., Stokes, J. H., Heyman, A., Gammon, G., Gleeson, G. A., Curtis, A. C., and Cutler, J. C. (1958). The results of treatment in 1,086 general paralytics the majority of whom were followed for more than five years. *J. chron. Dis.* **7**, 209.

Hassin, G. B. (1929). Tabes dorsalis. *Arch. Neurol. Psychiat., Chicago* **21**, 311.

Hoff, H. and Kauders, O. (1926). Über die Malariabehandlung der Tabes dorsalis. *Z. ges. Neurol. Psychiat.* **104**, 306.

Holmes, K. K. (1974). Syphilis. In *Harrison's Principles of Internal Medicine*, 7th edn. (ed. M. M. Wintrobe, G. W. Thorn, R. D. Adams, E. Braunwald, K. J. Isselbacher, and R. G. Petersdorf) Chapter 159, p. 876. McGraw Hill, New York.

Hooshmand, H. (1981). Nerosyphilis. In *Medical microbiology and infectious diseases* (ed. A. I. Braude) Chapter 161, p. 1274. Vol. II in *International textbook of medicine*. Saunders, Philadelphia.

Huriez, C., Agache, P., and Soullart, F. (1963). Panorama actuel des syphilis viscérales. *Vie méd.* **44**, 369.

Jauregg, W. (1929). La malariathérapie de la paralysie générale et des affections syphilitiques du systéme. *Rev. neurol.* **36**, 889.

Jeans, P. C. and Coke, J. V. (1930). Prepubescent syphilis. *Clin. Pediatr.* **xviii**, 9.26 New York.

Joffe, R., Black, M. M., and Floyd, M. (1968). Changing clinical picture of neurosyphilis: report of seven unusual cases. *Br. Med.J.* **1**, 211.

Kenney, J. A. and Curtis, A. C. (1953). The treatment of syphilitic optic atrophy by penicillin with and without therapeutic malaria. *Am. J. Syph.* **37**, 449.

Léri, A. (1925). Sur certaines pseudo-scléroses latérales amyotrophiques syphilitiques. *Rev. neurol.* **32**, 827.

Lhermitte, J. (1933). La syphilis diencéphalique et les syndromes végetatifs qu'elle conditionne—étude clinique. *Ann. Méd.* **33**, 272.

Luxon, L., Lees, A. J., and Greenwood, R. J. (1979). Neurosyphilis today. *Lancet* **i**, 90.

Martin, J. P. (1948). Treatment of neurosyphilis with penicillin *Br. med. J.* **1**, 922.

McIntosh, J. and Fildes, P. (1914). The demonstration of *Spirochaeta pallida* in chronic parenchymatous encephalitis (dementia paralytica). *Brain* **37**, 401.

Meagher, E. T. (1929). *General paralysis and its treatment by induced malaria*. Board of Control, London.

Merritt, H. H., Adams, R. D., and Solomon, H. C. (1946). *Neurosyphilis*. Oxford University Press, New York.

—— and Moore, M. (1935). Acute syphilitic meningitis. *Medicine, Baltimore* **14**, 119.

Montgomery, C. H. and Knox, J. M. (1959). Antibiotics other than penicillin in the treatment of syphilis. *New Engl. J. Med.* **261**, 277.

Moore, J. E. (1932). The syphilitic optic atrophies. *Medicine, Baltimore* **11**, 263.

—— (1953). The effect of adronocortical hormones on the lightning pains and visceral crises of tabes dorsalis. *Am. J. Syph.* **37**, 226.

Moritz, A. R. (1928). Tabische Arthropathie. *Virchows Arch. path. Anat.* **267**, 746.

Musher, D. M. (1981). Syphilis of the genital tract. In *Medical microbiology and infectious diseases* (ed. A. I. Braude) Chapter 150, p. 1210. Vol. II in *International textbook of medicine*. Saunders, Philadelphia.

Nageotte, J. (1894). La lésion primitive du tabes. *Bull. Soc. Anat. de Paris* **69**, 808.

Nelson, R. A. and Duncan, L. (1945). Acute syphilitic meningitis treated with penicillin *Am. J. Syph.* **29**, 141.

Nicol, W. D. and Whelen, M. (1947). Penicillin in the treatment of neurosyphilis. *Proc. R. Soc. Med.* **40**, 684.

Nielsen, A. and Idsoe, O. (1962) *Evaluation of the fluorescent treponemal antibody test (FTA)* WHO Monograph No. 102.

Obersteiner, H. and Redlich, E. (1894-5). Ueber das Wesen und Pathogenese der tabischen Hinterstrangs Degeneration. *Arbeiten aus dem Hirnanatomischen Institut* **2**, 158, and **3**. 192.

Page, N. G. R., Lean, J. S., and Sanders, M. D. (1982). Vertical supra-nuclear gaze palsy with secondary syphilis. *J. Neurol. Neurosurg. Psychiat.* **45**, 86.

Richter, H. (1921). Zur Histogenese der Tabes. *Z. ges. Neurol. Psychiat.* **67**, 1.

Rimbaud, P. (1958). Le traitement des syphilis sérologiques asymptomtiques. *Sem. méd. Paris* **34**, 1209.

Rose, A. S. and Carmen, L. R. (1951). Clinical follow-up studies of 130 cases of long-standing paretic neurosyphilis treated with penicillin. *Am. J. Syph.* **35**, 278.

Rudolf, G. de M. (1927). *Therapeutic malaria*. Oxford University Press, London.

Spitzer, H. (1926). Zur Pathogenese der tabes dorsalis. *Arb. neurol. Inst. Univ. Wien* **28**, 227.

Stewart, R. M. (1933). Juvenile types of general paralysis. *J. ment. Sci.* **79**, 602.

Storm-Mathisen, A. (1978). Syphilis. In *Handbook of clinical neurology* (ed. P. J. Vinken and G. W. Bruyn) Vol. 33, Chapter 17, p. 337. North-Holland, Amsterdam.

Thomas, E. W. (1964). Some aspects of neurosyphilis. *Med. Clin. N. Amer.* **48**, 699.

Traviesa, D. C., Prystowsky, S. D., Nelson, B. J., and Johnson, K. P. (1978). Cerbrospinal fluid findings in asymptomatic patients with reactive serum fluorescent treponemal absorption tests. *Ann. Neurol.* **4**, 524.

Wilkinson, A. E. (1963). The fluorescent treponemal antibody test in the serological diagnosis of syphilis. *Proc. roy. Soc. Med.* **56**, 478.

Wilner, E. and Brody, J. A. (1968). Prognosis of general paresis after treatment. *Lancet* **ii**, 1370.

Wilson, S. A. K. and Cobb, S. (1924–5). Mesencephalitis syphilitica *J. Neurol. Psychopath.* **5**, 44.

10

Virus infections of the nervous system

General considerations

The nature of viruses

The term 'neurotropic virus' was formerly used to describe minute terable pathogenic agents which attack the nervous system. The first such virus, the causal organism of rabies, was discovered by Pasteur in 1884, and poliomyelitis was shown to be due to a virus in 1909. More recently, organisms responsible for many other nervous diseases, both in man and in animals, have been found to be viruses, and it has become apparent that the former distinction drawn between neurotropic and non-neurotropic viruses according to whether or not the nervous system is the primary or secondary site of attack is largely artificial (Harter 1973). Nevertheless, various neural cells do display selective vulnerability to various viral infections (Johnson 1980). Most viruses which attack the nervous system first multiply in other organs; invasion of the nervous system results from haematogenous spread or retrograde dissemination along nerve fibres after endocytosis at axonal terminals (Blinzinger and Anzil 1974).

Viruses have been classified according to their nucleic acid content, size, sensitivity to lipid solvents, morphology, and method of development in cells. They can be defined as 'entities whose genomes are elements of nucleic acid that replicate inside living cells using the cellular synthetic machinery and causing the synthesis of specialized elements that can transfer the viral genome to other cells' (Luria, Darnell, Baltimore and Campbell 1978). Definition is no longer dependent upon size, lack of a cell wall, or morphology; but each specific virus contains only one species of nucleic acid, and organisms which contain both DNA and RNA such as the agents of psittacosis, lymphogranuloma venereum, and trachoma, even though they cannot replicate outside living cells, are now called *Chlamydia*—not so complex as a bacterium and not so simple as a virus (Johnson 1982). If the virus contains DNA, it is usually, but not always, double-stranded,like herpes simplex, if RNA it is usually, but not always, single-stranded like poliovirus. DNA virus replication is like that of any cellular organism and these viruses act by transcription to messenger RNA and then translation to polypeptides and protein. RNA virus replication may be direct, by the formation of a complementary RNA strand, or indirect, by reverse transcription to a DNA provirus template from which identical RNA strands are then transcribed; RNA viruses act directly as messenger RNA (Legg 1975). Viruses of virtually every known animal group have caused neurological illnesses in animals or man (see Table 10.1). Their names sometimes reflect the diseases (e.g. rabies, mumps) or the pathological changes (e.g. encephalitis) they produce, sometimes their cytopathic effects (foamy viruses), their ultrastructural appearances (e.g. arenaviruses), the anatomical site of most frequent isolation (e.g. enterovirus, adenovirus) or the geographical site of first recovery (e.g. Coxsackie) (Johnson 1982). Their effects vary depending upon the nature of the virus, the human or experimental conditions relating to infection, and various complex immunological responses. They can produce neoplastic transformation (as in Burkitt's lymphoma in man and brain tumours in various animals), various developmental abnormalities if infection is prenatal or neonatal, including microcephaly, cerebellar hypoplasia, and aqueduct stenosis with hydrocephalus (Johnson 1968; Raine and Fields 1973), as well as the more typical acute inflammatory changes normally associated with viral infections. Most viruses seem to be obligatory intracellular parasites and damage the nervous system by attacking ganglion cells or, sometimes, glial cells; some show an affinity for specific cells or areas of the nervous system, so that poliovirus attacks principally motor neurones, herpes simplex virus the temporal and frontal lobes, and some myxoviruses attack ependymal cells (Harter 1973). Pathologically they produce chromatolysis followed by necrosis and neuronophagia, microglial proliferation, perivascular cellular infiltration, meningeal inflammation, and often inclusion bodies in nerve or glial cells in various combinations.

Most epidemic forms of viral encephalomyelitis are due to picornaviruses (enteroviruses) or togaviruses; the latter multiply in mosquitoes or ticks before infecting man (see Table 10.1). Neurological disease due to viruses of other groups usually occurs sporadically as part of a disorder first involving primarily other organs or systems. Thus it has long been known that the neurological complications of mumps are due to invasion of the nervous system by the causal virus; however, it has been thought that encephalomyelitis complicating other childhood exanthemata (e.g. measles) or following smallpox vaccination is due to an allergic or hypersensitivity reaction of the nervous system so that these disorders have been classified traditionally with the demyelinating diseases, as in this volume (Chapter 11). However, the isolation of measles virus from the brain of a patient with measles encephalitis (ter Meulen, Müller, Käckell, Katz, and Meyermann 1972) has suggested that some such cases may provide to be due to viral invasion rather than hypersensitivity.

Much interest has been aroused of late by the concept of 'slow virus' infections. Thus it is now evident that subacute sclerosing panencephalitis is due to the persistence of measles virus in the brain for many years after the initial infection. Kuru, a progressive and fatal disorder of the nervous system seen in the eastern highlands of New Guinea, is due to an unidentified transmissible agent, presumably viral, which shows some affinities with those responsible for subacute spongiform encephalopathy (Creutzfeldt–Jakob disease) and for scrapie, a disease of sheep; all three disorders have a long incubation period after initial inoculation. Progressive multifocal leukoencephalopathy (due to polyoma virus) and cytomegalic inclusion body disease are other slow virus infections. However, the hope that other chronic progressive neurological disorders such as multiple sclerosis or motor-neurone disease would prove to be due to specific viruses has not been fulfilled (Johnson 1982).

Viral infections can be diagnosed by a variety of serological tests involving complement fixation, haemagglutination-inhibition, or antibody neutralization reactions, or by the inoculation of blood, nasopharyngeal exudates, faeces, or CSF into animals or tissue culture systems. If a viral agent is isolated, final identification depends upon neutralization of specific antiserum. Immunofluorescent techniques for the identification of specific antibodies can be applied to brain biopsy sections or to cells isolated from the fluid (Dayan and Stokes 1973; Lindemann, Müller, Versteeg, Bots, and Peters 1974; Legg 1975); 'immune electron microscopy', counter-immunoelectrophoresis, and radioimmunoassay after labelling specific viral antibody with ^{125}I have all been shown to be of some value, but the enzyme-linked immunosorbent assay (ELISA), in which an enzyme such as alkaline phosphatase is used as the immunoglobulin marker in place of the radioactive isotope, is much more specific and sensitive and is becoming the method of choice (Johnson 1982).

Table 10.1. *Viral infections of the nervous system**

	Some representative viruses causing neurological disease in man and animals
RNA viruses	
Paramyxovirus	
Paramyxovirus	Parainfluenza virus
	Mumps virus
Morbillivirus	Measles virus
Rhabdovirus	
Lyssavirus	Rabies virus
Bunyavirus	California encephalitis virus
	Rift Valley fever virus
Reovirus	
Orbivirus	Colorado tick fever virus
Togavirus	
Alphavirus (formerly group A arboviruses)	Eastern Encephalitis virus
	Western encephalitis virus
	Venezuelan equine encephalitis virus
Rubivirus	Rubella virus
Flavivirus (formerly group B arboviruses)	St Louis encephalitis virus
	Japanese encephalitis virus
	Murray Valley encephalitis virus
	Tick-borne encephalitis virus
	Louping-ill
	Yellow fever virus
	Dengue viruses
Picornavirus	
Enterovirus	Polioviruses
	Coxsackie viruses A and B
	Echoviruses
Cardiovirus	Encephalomyocarditis virus
Arenavirus	Lymphocytic choriomeningitis
DNA viruses	
Herpes viruses	Herpes simplex, types 1 and 2
	Varicella-zoster
	Cytomegalovirus
	Epstein–Barr virus (infectious mononucleosis)
Papova virus	Polyoma virus (progressive multifocal leucoencephalopathy)
Poxvirus	Vaccinia
	Variola
Retrovirus	AIDS
Unidentified presumed viral illnesses	Encephalitis lethargica
	Kuru
	Creutzfeldt–Jakob disease
	Scrapie

* Modified from Johnson (1982)

References

Blinzinger, K and Anzil, A. P. (1974). Neural route of infection in viral diseases of the central nervous system *Lancet* ii, 1374.

Dayan, A. D. and Stokes, M. I. (1973). Rapid diagnosis of encephalitis by immunofluorescent examination of cerebrospinal fluid cells. *Lancet* i, 177.

Fields, W. S. and Blattner, R. J. (1958). *Viral encephalitis*. Thomas, Springfield, Illinois.

Harter, D. (1973). Viral infections. In *A textbook of neurology* (ed. H. H. Merritt) 5th edn. Lea and Febiger, New York.

Johnson, R. T. (1968). Mumps virus encephalitis in the hamster: studies of the inflammatory response and noncytopathic infection of neurons *J. Neuropath. exp. Neurol.* **27**, 80.

—— (1980). Selective vulnerability of neural cells to viral infections. *Brain* **103**, 447.

—— (1982). *Viral infections of the nervous system*. Raven Press, New York.

Legg, N. (1975). How viruses affect the nervous system. In *Modern trends in neurology—6* (ed. D. Williams). Butterworths, London.

Lindemann, J., Müller, W. K., Versteeg, J., Bots, G. T. A. M., and Peters, A. C. B. (1974). Rapid diagnosis of meningoencephalitis, encephalitis. *Neurology, Minneapolis* **24**, 143.

Luria, S. E., Darnell, J. E., Baltimore, D., and Campbell, A. (1978). *General virology*, 3rd edn. John Wiley, New York.

Miller, J. D. and Ross, C. A. C. (1968). Encephalitis: a four-year survey. *Lancet* i, 1121.

Raine, C. S. and Fields, B. N. (1973). Neurotropic viruses and the developing brain. *NY State J. Med.* **73**, 1169.

ter Meulen, V., Müller, D., Käckell, Y., Katz, M., and Meyermann, R. (1972). Isolation of infectious measles virus in measles encephalitis. *Lancet* ii, 1172.

Epidemic encephalitis lethargica

Synonyms. Epidemic encephalitis, type A; 'sleepy sickness'.

Definition. An epidemic disease probably due to a virus with an acute, subacute, or insidious onset and in most cases a chronic course, characterized pathologically by inflammatory and degenerative changes, especially in the midbrain grey matter, and clinically in the acute stage by disturbance of the sleep rhythm, lethargy, and pupillary abnormalities, and in the chronic stage by a parkinsonian syndrome.

Aetiology

Encephalitis lethargica was first described by von Economo in May 1917, and about the same time by Cruchet, Moutier, and Calmette. It seems to have first appeared in 1915, though some authorities believe that previous epidemics can be recognized in medical historical texts. During the next decade widespread epidemics occurred, but now an illness with the characteristic clinical features is virtually unknown. It affected the sexes equally and no age was exempt, though it was commonest in early adult life. There was a seasonal incidence, most cases occurring in the first quarter of the year. Numerous attempts to isolate a causative organism failed, but there is little doubt that it was a virus. Outbreaks of epidemic hiccup sometimes coincided with epidemics of encephalitis lethargica, and it is possible that both were due to the same agent.

Pathology

Macroscopic changes in the nervous system were slight, consisting, in the acute stage, of congestion, oedema, and sometimes petechial haemorrhages. Microscopically (Figs. 10.1 and 10.2) the smaller vessels showed perivascular cuffs of inflammatory cells, chiefly lymphocytes and plasma cells. In addition the brain was diffusely infiltrated with mononuclear cells, and the neurones themselves showed degenerative changes. In the acute stage the principal changes were in the grey matter of the upper midbrain, the oculomotor nuclei, and the substantia nigra. The basal ganglia, pons, and medulla were affected next in frequency. The spinal cord was sometimes affected. In the chronic stage also degenerative changes were diffuse. The substantia nigra usually suffered severely, but the grey matter of the cerebral cortex and basal ganglia was also involved.

Symptoms and signs

When it first appeared this was an acute disease, often with a fulminating onset. After several years the acute stage became less severe and the chronic one more prominent. It is now doubtful if acute cases ever occur, and post-encephalitic parkinsonism is gradually disappearing. Many authorities believe that the disease has died out, although sporadic cases showing some of its features are rarely seen. Espir and Spalding (1956) reported three possible cases occurring in British soldiers serving in Western Germany and Rail,

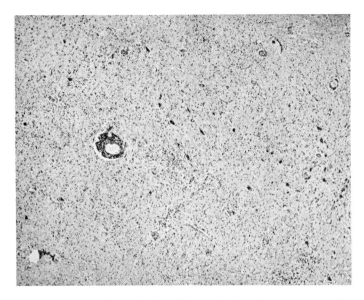

Fig. 10.1. Encephalitis lethargica. Substantia nigra showing perivascular and diffuse inflammatory infiltration. H & E, × 36.

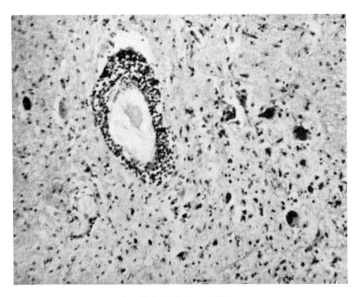

Fig. 10.2. The same as Fig. 10.1. H & E, × 145.

Scholtz, and Swash (1981) reported another eight possible cases; other sporadic reports continue to appear of small numbers of cases, often observed during influenza epidemics (*The Lancet* 1981). Bojinov (1971) described 11 cases of an encephalitis causing an acute parkinsonian syndrome in patients from 4 to 33 years of age. The illness developed acutely with symptoms reaching maximum severity in one to three weeks; four patients died and autopsy revealed bilateral inflammatory necrosis of the substantia nigra, but the other seven improved, four recovering completely. In most patients there was a mild lymphocytic pleocytosis in the CSF but attempts to isolate a causal virus and serological tests were all negative. Parkinsonian syndromes have also been reported as the immediate consequence of infections with Western, St. Louis, Japanese, and Coxsackie viruses but these have not given rise to oculogyric crises, nor have they developed after the long latent period so characteristic of post-encephalitic parkinsonism (Johnson 1982).

Symptoms of the acute stage

The onset was sudden or gradual. In early epidemics it was often fulminant with headache, vertigo, delirium, convulsions, and severe pain in the trunk or limbs. Later the onset became more gradual. The three most constant symptoms of the acute stage were headache, disturbance of sleep rhythm, and visual abnormalities, such as diplopia. The characteristic disturbance of sleep rhythm was severe lethargy by day with insomnia or restlessness at night. The patient could always be roused except when lethargy passed into coma. Delirium and fever occurred only in the more severe cases.

Visual disturbances were common; papilloedema and optic atrophy were rare but the pupils were often irregular and unequal. The reaction on accommodation was more often lost than that to light. Ptosis was frequent as was external ophthalmoplegia, the sixth nerve being most often affected. Nuclear and supranuclear ophthalmoplegias were less common, but all forms of conjugate ocular palsy were seen.

Facial weakness was common and usually transitory, as were vertigo and nystagmus due to damage to vestibular nuclei. Bulbar symptoms, aphasia, and hemiplegia were rare, though slight corticospinal tract damage with unilateral or bilateral extensor plantar responses was common.

Extrapyramidal disturbances typical of the chronic stage could also appear in the acute. A parkinsonian facies was often seen, but the muscles were usually hypotonic. Rigidity, when present, was catatonic: true parkinsonian rigidity was never seen in the acute stage. Choreiform movements were often found between 1916 and 1922, as was myoclonus, including hiccup. More often myoclonic jerks at any frequency from 10 to 80 contractions a minute occurred in the abdominal muscles but sometimes synchronous, painful myoclonus affected several limbs and the trunk. Static or intention tremor sometimes occurred; sensory loss was rare but a unilateral thalamic syndrome was reported. Signs of cerebellar or spinal-cord dysfunction were also rare but a transverse myelitic form was described, as was polyneuropathy. The tendon reflexes were often diminished in the acute stage. There was usually no sphincter disturbance until the patient became comatose.

Signs of meningeal irritation were rare and the CSF was usually normal, though a slight excess of lymphocytes and a modest increase in protein and globulin was sometimes found.

After the acute stage the disease sometimes became arrested or persisted as a chronic and slowly progressive disorder. The chronic progressive form of the disease could follow an acute attack, or develop insidiously, without being preceded by acute symptoms. It seems probable that in these cases the infection persisted in a chronic form as in other 'slow virus' infections.

Symptoms and signs of the chronic stage

Parkinsonism. This is described in Chapter 12, pages 325–336.

Sleep disturbances. Lethargy and/or insomnia frequently outlasted the acute attack.

Mental symptoms. Though dementia was reported in only 27 per cent of cases, if less severe degrees of mental impairment were included, this figure would have been much higher. In adults, nervousness, fatigability, inability to concentrate, anxiety, and depression often persisted for long periods. Behaviour disorders were common in children, who often became restless and unstable with abnormalities ranging from mere naughtiness to stealing, cruelty, acts of violence, and sexual offences.

Ocular abnormalities. Gross persistent abnormalities, such as nystagmus, squint, and diplopia, were rare, but the patient often complained of blurred vision, due to defective muscle balance or weakness of accommodation with accompanying pupillary abnormalities. Oculogyric crises, one of the most striking sequelae, are described in the section on parkinsonism.

Involuntary movements. (1) Choreiform movements were common in acute but rare in chronic cases. (2) Slow, regular, rhythmical movements of large amplitude, involving the limbs and trunk were common. Other involuntary movements included: (3) myoclonus; (4) tremor; (5) dyskinesias of the jaw, lips, tongue, and palate; and (6) torticollis.

Respiratory disturbances. In chronic cases, disorders of respiratory rate and rhythm were common.

Metabolic and endocrine disorders. Metabolic and endocrine disorders due to hypothalamic involvement were rare but included obesity, genital atrophy, diabetes insipidus, and hyperthyroidism.

Convulsions. Epileptiform convulsions were an uncommon sequel.

Diagnosis

Encephalitis lethargica was distinguished from other forms of encephalitis and from poliomyelitis and acute multiple sclerosis by the characteristic disturbance of sleep rhythm, the prominence of ocular symptoms, and the rarity of convulsions and paralysis; and from meningitis by the absence of neck stiffness and Kernig's sign and often of a CSF pleocytosis.

Prognosis

When it first made its appearance, epidemic encephalitis lethargica was an acute illness. Today, if it occurs at all, the acute stage may pass unnoticed. The mean death-rate in one large series of over 2000 cases was 38.2 per cent. Most patients who died in the acute stage did so in the first month, and 14 days was the commonest length of a fatal attack. The mortality rate in the acute stage was highest in the first year of life and after the age of 70, and lowest between 20 and 30.

Complete recovery occurred in only about 25 per cent of cases. The remainder who survived were more or less severely disabled, most being unable to carry on their usual occupations. Even after apparent recovery from an acute attack, the patient could suffer from relapses at intervals of a year or two before passing into the chronic stage; this could occur 20 years or more after the acute attack.

The prognosis of parkinsonism is described in Chapter 12, page 330.

Treatment

The Matheson Commission reported upon 75 methods of treating encephalitis lethargica, none of which influenced its course. All treatment was therefore symptomatic. Treatment in the chronic stage was also disappointing but modern remedies may ameliorate post-encephalitic parkinsonism (p. 332).

References

Bojinov, S. (1971). Encephalitis with acute Parkinsonian syndrome and bilateral inflammatory necrosis of the substantia nigra. *J. neurol. Sci.* **12**, 383.

Eaves, E. C. and Croll, M. M. (1930). The pituitary and hypothalamic region in chronic epidemic encephalitis. *Brain* **53**, 56.

Ebaugh, F. G. (1923). Neuropsychiatric sequelae of acute epidemic encephalitis in children. *Am. J. Dis. Child.* **25**, 89.

Espir, M. L. E. and Spalding, J. M. K. (1956). Three recent cases of encephalitis lethargica. *Br. med. J.* **1**, 1142.

Hall, A. J. and Yates, A. G. (1926). Clinical report. Report of sub-committee on the Sheffield outbreak of epidemic encephalitis in 1924. *Spec. Rep. Ser. med. Res. Coun., Lond.* No. 108, p. 29.

Holt, W. L., Jnr. (1937). Epidemic encephalitis. A follow-up study of two hundred and sixty-six cases. *Arch. Neurol. Psychiat. Chicago* **38**, 1135.

Johnson, R. T. (1982). *Viral infections of the nervous system.* Raven Press, New York.

The Lancet (1981). Encephalitis lethargica. *Lancet* **ii**, 1396.

Levaditi, C. (1929). Etiology of epidemic encephalitis, its relation to herpes, epidemic poliomyelitis, and post-vaccinal encephalopathy. *Arch. Neurol. Psychiat., Chicago* **22**, 767.

Matheson Commission (1929). *Epidemic encephalitis. Report of a survey by the Matheson Commission.* New York.

—— (1932). *Second report by the Matheson Commission.* New York.

Parsons, A. C. (1928). Report of an enquiry into the after-histories of persons attacked by encephalitis lethargica. *Min. Hlth. Rep. publ. Hlth,* No. 49, London.

Rail, D., Scholtz, C. and Swash, M. (1981). Post-encephalitic parkinsonism in current experience. *J. Neurol. Neurosurg. Psychiat.* **44**, 670.

Reimold, W. (1925). Über die myoklonische Form der Encephalitis. *Z. ges. Neurol. Psychiat.* **95**, 21.

Riser, M. and Meriel, P. (1931). Les 'séquelles' neurologiques de l'encéphalite épidémique. *Rev. Oto-neuro-ophtal.* **9**, 297, 323.

Turner, W. A. and Critchley, M. (1927–28). The prognosis and the late results of post-encephalitic respiratory disorders. *J. Neurol. Psychopath.* **8**, 191.

von Economo, C. (transl. K. O. Newman) (1931). *Encephalitis Lethargica; its sequelae and treatment.* Oxford University Press, London.

Epidemic encephalitis: Japanese type B, St. Louis type, and Murray Valley type

Definition. These varieties of epidemic encephalitis, one occurring in Japan and other Asian countries, another in the United States, and the third in Australia, have been shown to be due to togaviruses which are distinct because there is no cross-immunity between them, but the epidemiology, pathology, and clinical features of the three diseases are so similar that they can conveniently be considered together.

Aetiology

These diseases are all caused by viruses which measure 40–70 nm in diameter. They used to be called arboviruses (meaning arthropod-borne) but this title is no longer accepted taxonomically as it embraces most of the togaviruses, some reoviruses, and the bunyaviruses (Table 10.1). However, it is still useful biologically when taken simply to mean that large groups of viruses which undergo biological transmission via arthropods (Johnson 1982). Of this large group of arboviruses, relatively few are encephalitogenic. The natural reservoir of these viruses is mammals or birds, and the virus is usually transmitted to man by the bite of a mosquito or tick. The St. Louis virus is found in wild birds in the Western USA but more often in *Culex* mosquitoes breeding on stagnant water with high organic content, in the urban Midwest. Urban epidemics of encephalitis occur in drought years because of poor drainage, while rural epidemics are more often associated with high rainfall (Johnson 1982).

Japanese encephalitis type B is caused by a virus which was first transmitted to monkeys by Hayashi. Kawamura and his colleagues transmitted the virus to mice and monkeys (Inada 1937 *a* and *b*), and showed that it was immunologically distinct from the virus of the St. Louis epidemic which was also transmitted to monkeys and mice by Muckenfuss, Armstrong, and McCordock (1933) and Webster and Fite (1935). Russian autumnal encephalitis is now generally regarded as identical with Japanese type B encephalitis while the Murray Valley type (Australian X disease) which occurs in Australia and New Guinea is clinically indistinguishable from the Japanese variety and is due to a very similar but nevertheless distinctive virus. Also closely related are the so-called Far Eastern tick-borne encephalitis complex (formerly Russian spring-summer encephalitis), West Nile encephalitis, and louping-ill (which is the only disease of this group to occur in Great Britain (Webb, Connolly, Kane, O'Reilly, and Simpson 1968) and in which the reservoir of infection is in the sheep).

Epidemiology

Eight epidemics of encephalitis occurred in Japan in various summers between 1871 and 1919, since when outbreaks have occurred every few years, and in 1935 there were 5000 cases. A St. Louis epidemic occurred in 1933 when there were over 1000 cases in the neighbourhood during the late summer. There were smaller outbreaks in other cities in the United States, including one in Toledo in 1934. In 1975 a further epidemic with over 2000 documented cases occurred in the American Midwest. Multiple cases in the same family were not common. The incubation period was usually between 9 and 14 days. There was a marked susceptibility of the elderly, and a relatively small incidence in children; children are more commonly affected by the Japanese and Murray Valley types. In rural areas the usual cycle of transmission is from bird to mosquito to man, but in urban districts it is more often from man to mosquito to man (Johnson 1982). It has been shown that mosquitoes may infect patients with the viruses of St. Louis and Western equine encephalitis at the same time (Hammon 1941).

Pathology

The pathological picture in the three diseases is virtually identical except that Japanese observers described areas of softening in the brain which were not observed in the American epidemics, and in the Japanese B and Murray Valley types selective damage to Purkinje cells is seen. All levels of the nervous system may be affected, and severe inflammation is always found in the brainstem, the basal ganglia, and the white matter of the hemispheres. The inflammatory changes are diffuse, involving the basal pons, the entire medulla, the cortex and white matter of the cerebellum, the basal ganglia, and also the cerebral cortex (Löwenberg and Zbinden 1936; Robertson 1952). There is neuronal degeneration, diffuse microglial and macroglial proliferation, and perivascular cuffing (Reyes, Gardner, Poland, and Monath 1981). Intranuclear inclusion bodies have been found in the renal tubular epithelium.

Symptoms

Several workers classify cases as: (1) abortive; (2) mild; and (3) severe; including fulminating cases. Abortive cases, with fever, headache, malaise, and recovery in a few days are occasionally seen in epidemics but are uncommon. The onset of the disease is usually acute with fever, 40–40.6 °C, headache and neck stiffness, and within a few hours many patients develop mental confusion and tremor of the lips, tongue, and hands. Rigidity may involve the upper limbs or the whole body. Drowsiness is common but the patient may be hyperexcitable. In severe cases coma develops early. The optic discs are usually normal as are the pupils and their reactions. Nystagmus, facial palsy, monoparesis, and spastic tetraparesis are not infrequent. Opsoclonus and myoclonus may occur, as may dysuria, and up to 25 per cent of patients show inappropriate secretion of antidiuretic hormone.

The CSF is usually clear and under increased pressure. There is an excess of cells, usually between 50 and 500 per mm^3, predominantly lymphocytes. The globulin content is increased but the sugar is normal. The blood usually shows a polymorphonuclear leucocytosis.

Diagnosis

Clinical diagnosis depends mainly upon recognition of an encephalitic illness in an endemic area after exposure to an insect vector. Laboratory diagnosis depends upon the recognition of complement-fixing and neutralizing antibodies which appear at about the seventh day (MacCallum 1967; Hannoun, Shiraki, and Osetowska 1970). The ELISA test (p. 274) may well prove to be specific.

Prognosis

In the St. Louis epidemic the mortality rate was 20 per cent, but in the 1975 US epidemic it was 8.5 per cent (Johnson 1982). In the Japanese and Murray Valley epidemics it has been much higher, usually 50 to 60 per cent. The mortality rate increases after the age of 50. In favourable cases recovery is often rapid and complete. Many patients in the St. Louis epidemic had apparently recovered completely in from 10 to 14 days, but the disease sometimes ran a protracted course with residual emotional instability and tremors, especially in the elderly. A study by Bredeck, Broun, Hempelmann, McFadden, and Spector (1938) of survivors of the 1933 St. Louis epidemic showed that 66 per cent had made a complete recovery and only 6.3 per cent were physically unfit for work. Finley (1958) made similar observations in a follow-up of 350 cases.

Prophylaxis and treatment

Prophylaxis consists of measures to eliminate insect vectors. Attempts to prepare specific protective vaccines have to date been unsuccessful. No specific treatment is known, and it is therefore purely symptomatic.

References

Beckmann, J. W. (1935). Neurologic aspects of the epidemic of encephalitis in St. Louis. *Arch. Neurol. Psychiat.*, *Chicago* 33, 732.

Bredeck, J. F., Broun, G. O., Hempelmann, T. C., McFadden, J. F., and Spector, H. I. (1938). Follow-up studies of the 1933 St. Louis epidemic of encephalitis. *J. Am. med. Assoc.* 111, 15.

Finley, K. H. (1958). In *Viral encephalitis* (ed. W. S. Fields and R. J. Blattner). Thomas, Springfield, Illinois.

Hammon, W. M. (1941). Encephalitis in Yakima valley: mixed St. Louis and Western equine types. *J. Am. med. Ass.* 117, 161.

Hannoun, C., Shirak, H., and Osetowska, E. (1970). Encephalitides due to arboviruses. In *Clinical virology* (ed. R. Debré and T. Celers). Saunders, Philadelphia.

Inada, R. (1937). Recherches sur l'encéphalite épidémique du Japon. *Presse méd.* 45, 99.

—— (1937). Du mode d'infection dans l'encéphalite épidémique. *Presse méd.* 45, 386.

Johnson, R. T. (1982). *Viral infections of the nervous system*. Raven Press, New York.

Kawakita, Y. (1939). Cultivation *in vitro* of the virus of Japanese encephalitis. *Jap. J. exp. Med.* 17, 211.

Löwenberg, K. and Zbinden, T. (1936). Epidemic encephalitis (St. Louis type) in Toledo, Ohio. *Arch. Neurol. Psychiat. Chicago.* 36, 1155.

Muckenfuss, R. S., Armstrong, C., and McCordock, H. A. (1933). Encephalitis: studies on experimental transmission. *Publ. Hlth Rep., Washington* 48, 1341.

Reyes, M. G., Gardner, J. J., Poland, J. D., and Monath, T. P. (1981). St. Louis encephalitis. Quantitative histologic and immunofluorescent studies. *Arch. Neurol., Chicago* 38, 329.

Robertson, E. G. (1952). Murray Valley encephalitis: pathological aspects. *Med. J. Aust.* i, 107.

—— and McLorinan, H. (1952). Murray Valley encephalitis: clinical aspects. *Med. J. Aust.* i, 103.

Webb, H. E., Connolly, J. H., Kane, F. F., O'Reilly, K. J., and Simpson, D. I. H. (1968). Laboratory infections with louping-ill with associated encephalitis. *Lancet* ii, 255.

Webster, L. T. and Fite, G. L. (1935). Experimental studies on encephalitis. *J. exp. Med.* 61, 103.

Wolstenholme, G. E. W. and Cameron, M. P. (1960). *Virus meningoencephalitis*. Ciba Foundation Study Group No. 7, London.

Eastern and Western (equine) encephalomyelitis

These forms of encephalomyelitis have been known in the United States for many years. In 1931 a virus was first identified as the cause of an outbreak among mules in California (hence 'equine'), and a few years later a virus was isolated from an epizootic occurring in the Eastern states. These viruses, though similar, are immunologically distinct, and are known as the Western and Eastern strains; like those responsible for the disorders considered above and like those of Venezuelan equine encephalitis they belong to the togavirus group. Numerous cases of human infection have been observed, and in 1941 an epidemic of infection with the Western virus affected at least 1700 persons in Minnesota and North Dakota with 150 deaths. It has been shown that various species of bird constitute a reservoir of infection, that a wood-tick also harbours the virus, and that mosquitoes transmit it to man (Johnson 1982). The term 'equine' has been discarded since the horse or mule is, like man, a 'dead-end host' (Johnson 1982) and is not the reservoir from which man acquires the infection.

Pathological changes differ somewhat in the two forms. In the Western type the vessels of the nervous system are always much congested, and petechial haemorrhages are common. Both neutrophil and mononuclear inflammatory cells are present in the perivascular spaces and as focal or diffuse infiltrations. Small, discrete patches of demyelination are scattered irregularly throughout the brain. The nervous parenchyma appears to suffer secondarily. The spinal cord may also be involved, mainly in the central grey matter. The meninges show little change as a rule.

In the Eastern variety, on the other hand, there is widespread involvement of nerve cells, ranging from early nuclear changes to complete disappearance. Polymorphonuclear infiltration of the brain is conspicuous and there is an inflammatory infiltration of the meninges, lymphocytes predominating.

The clinical features of the two diseases also differ. In the Western form the onset is sudden, with generalized headache, nausea, elevation of temperature, and lethargy. However, there is a very high ratio of inapparent to overt infections. Focal signs of nervous involvement are usually absent, but in overt cases there are stiffness of the neck, muscular weakness, and diminution of tendon reflexes. The CSF shows a moderate, predominantly mononuclear, pleocytosis. The mortality rate is very low. Most patients make a complete recovery in a week or two, but mental defect, epilepsy, and spastic palsies have been observed as sequelae, especially in infants after perinatal infection and in young children (Finley 1958; Aguilar, Calanchini, and Finley 1968). These features may be due to the effect of the virus upon cerebral development (Raine and Fields 1973).

In the Eastern form, which chiefly attacks children and in which there are many fewer inapparent infections, the onset is very abrupt with severe general symptoms; lethargy soon appears, passing into stupor or coma. Cervical rigidity and Kernig's sign are present. Aphasia, diplopia, and paralyses indicate damage to the brain. The spinal fluid contains many cells, often more than 1000 per mm^3, and polymorphonuclears may predominate. There is a mortality rate of 60 per cent, and severe sequelae are common in those who survive.

Prophylaxis is directed to the destruction of mosquitoes and protection from their bites. Treatment is symptomatic.

References

Aguilar, M. J., Calanchini, P. R., and Finley, K. H. (1968). Perinatal arbovirus encephalitis and its sequelae. In *Infections of the nervous system* (ed. H. M. Zimmerman) Vol. 1, Chapter 13. Baltimore.

Baker, A. B. and Noran, H. H. (1942). Western variety of equine encephalitis in man. *Arch. Neurol. Psychiat. Chicago* **47**, 565.

David, W. A. (1940). A study of birds as hosts for the virus of Eastern equine encephalomyelitis. *Am. J. Hyg.* **32**, 45.

Finley, K. H. (1958). In *Viral encephalitis* (ed. W. S. Fields and R. J. Blattner). Thomas, Springfield, Illinois.

Fothergill, N. D., Dingle, J. H., Farber, S., and Connerley, M. L. (1938). Human encephalitis caused by the virus of the Eastern variety of equine encephalomyelitis. *New Engl. J. Med.* **219**, 411.

Hammon, W. H. (1941). Encephalitis in Yamika Valley: mixed St. Louis and Western equine types. *J. Am. med. Ass.* **117**, 161.

Johnson, R. T. (1982). *Viral infections of the nervous system.* Raven Press, New York.

Raine, C. S. and Fields, B. N. (1973). Neurotropic viruses and the developing brain. *NY State J. Med.* **73**, 1169.

Syverton, J. T. and Berry, G. P. (1941). Hereditary transmission of the Western type of equine encephalitis by the wood tick, Dermacentor Andersoni Stiles. *J. exp. Med.* **73**, 507.

Other forms of viral encephalitis

Other arthropod-borne forms of encephalitis have recently been reviewed by Johnson (1982). In the Venezuelan form, which usually gives a mild and transient influenza-like illness with recovery in a few days and which occurs not only in South America but also in the southern United States, the horse is in fact the reservoir from which man is infected via the mosquito; immunization of horses can control epidemics (*The Lancet* 1973). Also benign is the illness resulting from the California arthropod-borne bunyavirus of which the commonest strain is the la Crosse which does not have an avian reservoir but is transmitted by a woodland treehole mosquito from small forest mammals. The illness is commonest in children, paradoxically in the eastern USA rather than in California; it often gives an aseptic meningitis, much less often a severe encephalitis, but the mortality rate is very low. Irritability and other behavioural sequelae persist in some cases. Colorado tick fever virus usually produces a benign febrile illness with headache and myalgia but rarely it causes aseptic meningtitis and very rarely indeed stupor, coma, and convulsions.

References

Johnson, R. T. (1982). *Viral infections of the nervous system.* Raven Press, New York.

The Lancet (1973). Venezuelan encephalitis. *Lancet* **i**, 29.

Subacute sclerosing panencephalitis

First described by Dawson (1933) and subsequently by van Bogaert (1945), who called the condition subacute sclerosing leuco-encephalitis, this condition later became known as subacute inclusion body encephalitis as Dawson (1933), Brain, Greenfield, and Russell (1948), Greenfield (1950), Foley and Williams (1953), and many others found characteristic acidophilic intranuclear and cytoplasmic inclusion bodies within affected neurones and glial cells. The distinctive pathological changes are first widespread neuronal degeneration with associated inflammatory changes, and secondly extensive gliosis. Connolly, Allan, Hurwitz, and Millar (1967) found that antibody titres to measles virus rose in the serum during the course of the illness, while Dayan, Gostling, Greaves, Stevens, and Woodhouse (1967) and Lennette, Magoffin, and Freeman (1968) found paramyxovirus-like particles in the brain of the affected patients and Saunders, Knowles, Chambers, Caspary, Gardner-Medwin, and Walker (1969) found lymphocyte transformation in response to measles antigen in such a case. Subsequently Horta-Barbosa, Fuccillo, London, Jabbour, Zeman, and Sever (1969) isolated measles virus from brain-cell cultures in two cases and it is now agreed that the condition is due to the long persistence of this virus in the brain after an attack of measles (Brody, Detels, and Sever 1972; Detels, Brody, McNew, and Edgar 1973) though there are still many complex and unanswered virological and immunological problems to be resolved (Legg 1975; Johnson 1982).

In Israel SSPE was found to be commoner in the poor and in rural areas, but there is no convincing evidence of genetic susceptibility (Soffer, Rannon, Alter, Kahana, and Feldman 1976). The report of a case in which the condition followed natural measles after the prior administration of immune globulin (Rammohan, McFarland, and McFarlin 1982) raises the question as to whether viral persistence could be the result of antibody transfer during viral infection. The condition has also developed very rarely as a sequel to vaccination with attentuated measles vaccine (Johnson

1982). It is now evident that a similar clinical picture can rarely be due to the rubella virus (Townsend, Baringer, Wolinsky, Mala-mud, Mednick, Panitch, Scott, Oshiro, and Cremer 1975; Weil, Itabashi, Cremer, Oshiro, Lennette, and Carnay 1975). As in measles SSPE, this condition may follow many years after child-hood German measles (Wolinsky, Berg, and Maitland 1976; Townsend, Walinsky, and Baringer 1976) and should be con-sidered as a possibility in adolescents presenting with progressive dementia and pyramidal and cerebellar dysfunction.

The disease runs a slowly progressive course of from 2 to 18 months in which three stages can be recognized. First the mood changes and there is some intellectual deterioration, sometimes accompanied by epileptic attacks or more often by recurrent myoc-lonic jerking. This is followed by progressive dementia leading to akinetic mutism often with complex involuntary movements. The third stage is one of decortication. The CSF may show mild pleocy-tosis, a rise in protein, a paretic colloidal gold curve with increased IgB, and characteristic EEG changes are found in the form of com-plex generalized slow-wave complexes, recurring repetitively and often in time with the myoclonic jerks and separated by intervals of comparative electrical silence in the record (Cobb and Hill 1950). Synthesis of oligoclonal IgG and measles antibody activity within the central nervous system were shown by Link, Panelius, and Salmi (1973) and Mehta, Tetley and Thormer (1975) demonstrated measles-specific IgG in the serum. Measles-virus specific IgM and IgC responses in both serum and CSF can be identified by radioim-munoassay (Kiessling, Hall, Yung, and ter Meulen 1977); the brain tissue of such patients lacks detectable M protein (Hall and Chop-pin 1981), a finding which could be related to individual susceptibi-lity to the disease or to an attenuated immune response to M protein resulting from the disease (Johnson 1982). The disease has been reproduced in dogs (Notermans, Tijl, Willems, and Slooff 1973), hamsters (Lehrich, Katz, Rorke, Barbonti-Brodano, and Koprowski 1970; Raine, Bynington, and Johnson 1974), and the ferret (Mehta *et al.* 1975) by inoculation of brain material from human subjects.

The disease usually terminates fatally, but may become arrested and occasional cases of prolonged spontaneous improvement or even recovery have been reported (Pearce and Barwick 1964; Cobb and Morgan-Hughes 1968; Risk, Haddad, and Chemali 1978). No treatment is known to be of value. Amantadine hydro-chloride has been found to be unsuccessful by Haslam, McQuillen, and Clark (1969), but Robertson, Clark, and Markesbery (1980) have claimed that this drug may promote remission in some cases, and Huttenlocher and Mattson (1979) and Dyken, Swift, and Dur-ant (1982) have had even more encouraging results when using iso-prinosine (inosiplex) over a period of several years. Partly purified human leucocyte interferon appeared recently to have been of no benefit in three cases (Behan 1981).

Herpes simplex encephalitis

It is well known that herpes simplex virus may occasionally cause an acute and fatal illness in neonates with encephalitic and multiple necrotic lesions in brain, liver, kidneys, adrenals, and other organs (Legg 1975). The virus implicated is usually herpes simplex type II which is often found in the female genital tract (Pettay, Leinikki, Donner, and Lapinleimu 1972) but occasionally a similar illness is due to the type I strain which is responsible for oral and labial herpes.

For many years occasional cases of acute necrotizing encephalitis have been reported in adults (Greenfield 1950; Crawford and Robinson 1957) and some such cases have been called limbic ence-phalitis because of selective and severe damage to the temporal lobes and often to other parts of the limbic system. However, some cases of so-called limbic encephalitis (Brierley, Corsellis, Hierons, and Nevin 1960), especially when occurring in association with car-

cinoma (Corsellis, Goldberg, and Norton 1968), have run a chronic course with severe and persistent loss of recent memory or severe dementia. Nevertheless, it is now clear that most cases of acute necrotizing encephalitis with necrosis of one or both temporal lobes are due to herpes simplex virus Type I. The illness is usually explosive with coma, hyperpyrexia, convulsions, and often hemi-paresis with other features suggesting a temporal-lobe lesion. Often intracerebral haemorrhage or cerebral abscess is suspected and angiography may suggest a space-occupying lesion. The EEG sometimes shows periodic sharp-wave discharges (Upton and Gumpert 1970) but the changes are not pathognomonic (Illis and Taylor 1972; Ch'ien, Boehm, Robinson, Liu, and Frenkel 1977). Diagnosis may be confirmed by serological tests or by the identifi-cation of specific antibodies in the CSF (Koshiniemi and Vaheri 1982) and, especially in childhood, the combination of EEG find-ings with areas of low attenuation in the temporal lobe on CT scan-ning may be virtually diagnostic (Schauseil-Zipf, Harden, Hoare, Lyen, Lingam, Marshall, and Pampiglione 1982); the EEG is less helpful, the CT scan equally so, in adults (Dutt and Johnston 1982). However, periodic EEG complexes may also be found in encephalitis due to infective mononucleosis (Greenberg, Weinkle, and Aminoff 1982). It has been suggested that the temporal-lobe localization is due to spread of virus along fifth-nerve fibres which innervate the middle fossa meninges (Davis and Johnson 1979). For rapid confirmation brain biopsy followed by identification of the virus by immunofluorescence (Johnson 1964), culture (John-son, Rosenthal, and Lerner 1972), or electron microscopy (Har-land, Adams, and McSeveney 1967; Joncas, Berthiaume, McLaughlin, and Granger-Julien 1976) is more reliable. The mor-tality rate is high but more patients have recovered following the use of dexamethasone 5 mg four times daily to reduce oedema, and surgical decompression. The role of antiviral agents such as idoxur-idine (80–200 mg/kg body weight daily by intravenous infusion) (Meyer, Bauer, Rivera-Olmes, Nolan, and Lerner 1970; Illis and Merry 1972) and cytosine arabinoside (Sarubbi, Sparling, and Gle-zen 1973) is controversial; some have found them of value (Mar-shall 1967), others have not and have reported unacceptable toxic side-effects (Johnson *et al.* 1972; Joncas *et al.* 1976). Vidarabine (adenine arabinoside) has been more successful (Taber, Green-berg, Perez, and Couch 1977) and acyclovir, a safe and more ideal drug (Johnson 1982) is now clearly the treatment of choice (Camp-bell, Klapper, and Longson 1982; Sköldenberg *et al.* 1984). In patients who recover, variable defects of memory and focal neuro-logical signs may persist (Rennick, Nolan, Bauer, and Lerner 1973; Hierons, Janota, and Corsellis 1978), but a few recover comple-tely. Rarely a similar clinical picture may be due to Coxsackie B5 virus infection (Heathfield, Pilsworth, Wall, and Corsellis 1967), while it has also been reported that milder subacute encephalitic illnesses and even chronic limbic encephalitis may on occasion be due to herpes simplex (Corsellis, Janota, and Hierons 1975).

References

Behan, P. O. (1981). Interferon in treatment of subacute sclerosing pan-encephalitis. *Lancet* i, 1059.

Brain, W. R., Greenfield, J. G., and Russell, D. (1948). Subacute inclusion encephalitis (Dawson type). *Brain* **71**, 365.

Brierley, J. B., Corsellis, J. A. N., Hierons, R., and Nevin, S. (1960). Subacute encephalitis of later adult life, mainly affecting the limbic areas. *Brain* **83**, 357.

Brody, J. A., Detels, R., and Sever, J. L. (1972). Measles-antibody titres in sibships of patients with subacute sclerosing panencephalitis and con-trols. *Lancet* i, 177.

Campbell, M., Klapper, P. E., and Longson, M. (1982). Acyclovir in herpes encephalitis. *Lancet* i, 38.

Ch'ien, L. T., Boehm, R. M., Robinson, H., Liu, C., and Frenkel, L. D. (1977). Characteristic early electroencephalographic changes in herpes simplex encephalitis. *Arch. Neurol., Chicago* **34**, 361.

Cobb, W. A. and Hill, D. (1950). Electroencephalogram in subacute pro-gressive encephalitis. *Brain* **73**, 392.

—— and Morgan-Hughes, J. A. (1968). Non-fatal subacute sclerosing leu-coencephalitis. *J. Neurol. Neurosurg. Psychiat.* **31**, 115.

Connolly, J. H., Allen, I. V., Hurwitz, L. J., and Millar, J. H. D. (1967). Measles-virus antibody and antigen in subacute sclerosing panencephali-tis. *Lancet* **i**, 532.

Corsellis, J. A. N., Goldberg, G. J., and Norton, A. R. (1968). 'Limbic encephalitis' and its association with carcinoma. *Brain* **91**, 481.

——, Janota, I., and Hierons, R. (1975). A clinicopathological study of long-standing cases of limbic encephalitis. Paper presented to the Associ-ation of British Neurologists.

Crawford, A. R. and Robinson, F. L. J. (1957). Necrotizing encephalitis. *Brain* **80**, 209.

Davis, L. E. and Johnson, R. T. (1979). An explanation for the localization of herpes simplex encephalitis? *Ann. Neurol.* **5**, 2.

Dawson, J. R. (1933). Cellular inclusions in cerebral lesions of lethargic encephalitis. *Am. J. Path.* **9**, 7.

Dayan, A. D., Gostling, J. V. T., Greaves, J. L., Stevens, D. W., and Woodhouse, M. A. (1967). Evidence of a pseudomyxovirus in the brain in subacute sclerosing leucoencephalitis. *Lancet* **i**, 980.

Detels, R., Brody, J. A., McNew, J., and Edgar, A. H. (1973). Further epidemiological studies of subacute sclerosing panencephalitis. *Lancet* **ii**, 11.

Dutt, M. K. and Johnston, I. D. A. (1982). Computed tomography and EEG in herpes simplex encephalitis: their value in diagnosis and progno-sis. *Arch. Neurol., Chicago* **39**, 99.

Dyken, P. R., Swift, A., and Durant, R. H. (1982). Long-term follow-up of patients with subacute sclerosing panencephalitis treated with inosiplex. *Ann. Neurol.* **11**, 359.

Foley, J. and Williams, D. (1953). Inclusion encephalitis and its relation to subacute sclerosing leuco-encephalitis. *Quart. J. Med.* **22**, 157.

Gostling, J. V. T. (1967). Herpetic encephalitis. *Proc. R. Soc. Med.* **60**, 693.

Greenberg, D. A., Weinkle, D. J., and Aminoff, M. J. (1982). Periodic EEG complexes in infectious mononucleosis encephalitis. *J. Neurol. Neurosurg. Psychiat.* **45**, 648.

Greenfield, J. G. (1950). Encephalitis and encephalomyelitis in England and Wales during the last decade. *Brain* **73**, 141.

Hall, W. W. and Choppin, P. W. (1981). Measles virus proteins in the brain tissue of patients with subacute sclerosing panencephalitis: absence of M protein. *New Engl. J. Med.* **304**, 1152.

Harland, W. A., Adams, J. H., and McSeveney, D. (1967). Herpes-sim-plex particles in acute necrotizing encephalitis. *Lancet* **ii**, 581.

Haslam, R. H. A., McQuillen, M. P., and Clark, D. B. (1969). Amanta-dine therapy in subacute sclerosing panencephalitis: a preliminary report. *Neurology, Minneapolis* **19**, 1080.

Heathfield, K. W. G., Pilsworth, R., Wall, B. J., and Corsellis, J. A. N. (1967). Coxsackie B5 infections in Essex, 1965, with particular reference to the nervous system. *Quart. J. Med.* **36**, 579.

Hierons, R., Janota, I., and Corsellis, J. A. N. (1978). The late effects of necrotizing encephalitis of the temporal lobes and limbic areas: a clinico-pathological study of 10 cases. *Psych. Med.* **8**, 21.

Horta-Barbosa, L., Fuccillo, D. A., London, W. T., Jabbour, J. T., Zeman, W., and Sever, J. L. (1969). Isolation of measles virus from brain cell cultures of two patients with subacute sclerosing panencephalitis. *Proc. Soc. exp. Biol. Med.* **132**, 272.

Huttenlocher, P. R. and Mattson, R. H. (1979). Isoprinosine in subacute sclerosing panencephalitis. *Neurology, Minneapolis* **29**, 763.

Illis, L. S. and Merry, R. T. G. (1972). Treatment of herpes simplex ence-phalitis. *J. R. Coll. Phycns. Lond.* **7**, 34.

—— and Taylor, F. M. (1972). The electroencephalogram in herpes-sim-plex encephalitis. *Lancet* **i**, 718.

Johnson, K. P., Rosenthal, M. S., and Lerner, P. I. (1972). Herpes simplex encephalitis. The course in five virologically proven cases. *Arch. Neurol., Chicago* **27**, 103.

Johnson, R. T. (1964). The pathogenesis of herpes virus encephalitis. I: Virus pathways to the nervous system of suckling mice demonstrated by fluorescent antibody stain. *J. exp. Med.* **119**, 343.

—— (1982). *Viral infections of the nervous system.* Raven Press, New York.

Joncas, J. H., Berthiaume, L., McLaughlin, B., and Granger-Julien, M. (1976). Herpes encephalitis: rapid diagnosis and treatment with antiviral drugs. *J. neurol. Sci.* **23**, 203.

Kiessling, W. R., Hall, W. W., Yung, L. L., and ter Meulen, V. (1977). Measles-virus-specific immunoglobulin-M response in subacute scleros-ing panencephalitis. *Lancet* **i**, 324.

Koskiniemi, M. L. and Vaheri, A. (1982). Diagnostic value of cerebro-spinal fluid antibodies in herpes simplex virus encephalitis. *J. Neurol. Neurosurg. Psychiat.* **45**, 239.

The Lancet (1972). What's new in SSPE? *Lancet* **ii**, 263.

Legg, N. (1975). How viruses affect the nervous system. In *Modern trends in neurology—6* (ed. D. Williams). Butterworth, London.

Lehrich, J. R., Katz, M., Rorke, L. B., Barbanti-Brodano, G., and Koprowski, H. (1970). Subacute sclerosing panencephalitis: encephalitis in hamsters produced by viral agents isolated from human brain cells. *Arch. Neurol., Chicago* **23**, 97.

Lennette, E. H., Magoffin, R. L., and Freeman, J. N. (1968). Immunologi-cal evidence of measles virus as an etiologic agent in subacute sclerosing panencephalitis. *Neurology, Minneapolis* **18**, 21.

Link, H., Panelius, M., and Salmi, A. A. (1973). Immunoglobulins and measles antibodies in subacute sclerosing panencephalitis. Demon-stration of synthesis of oligoclonal IgG with measles antibody activity within the central nervous system. *Arch. Neurol., Chicago* **28**, 23.

Marshall, W. J. S. (1967). Herpes simplex encephalitis treated with idoxuri-dine and external decompression. *Lancet* **ii**, 579.

Mehta, P. D., Tetley, A. J., and Thormar, H. (1975). Measles antibodies and immunoglobulins in sera from patients with subacute sclerosing panence-phalitis (SSPE) and from an infected ferret. *J. neurol. Sci.* **26**, 283.

Meyer, J. S., Bauer, R. B., Rivera-Olmos, V. M., Nolan, D. C., and Lerner, A. M. (1970). Herpesvirus hominis encephalitis. Neurological manifestations and use of idoxuridine. *Arch. Neurol., Chicago* **23**, 438.

Notemans, S. L. H., Tijl, W. F. J., Willems, F. T. C., and Slooff, J. L. (1973). Experimentally induced subacute sclerosing panencephalitis in young dogs. *Neurology, Minneapolis* **23**, 543.

Pearce, J. M. S. and Barwick, D. D. (1964). Recovery from presumed subacute inclusion-body encephalitis. *Br. med. J.* **2**, 611.

Pettay, O., Leinikki, P., Donner, M., and Lapinleimu, K. (1972). Herpes simplex virus infection in the newborn. *Arch. Dis. Childh.* **47**, 97.

Raine, C. S., Byington, D. P., and Johnson, K. P. (1974). Experimental subacute sclerosing panencephalitis in the hamster: ultrastructure of the chronic disease. *Lab. Invest.* **31**, 355.

Rammohan, K. W., McFarland, H. F., and McFarlin, D. E. (1982). Sub-acute sclerosing panencephalitis after passive immunization and natural measles infection: role of antibody in persistence of measles virus. *Neur-ology, Minneapolis* **32**, 390.

Rennick, P. M., Nolan, D. C., Bauer, R. B., and Lerner, A. M. (1973). Neuropsychologic and neurologic follow-up after herpesvirus hominis encephalitis. *Neurology, Minneapolis* **23**, 42.

Risk, W. S., Haddad, F. S., and Chemali, R. (1978). Substantial spon-taneous long-term improvement in subacute sclerosing panencephalitis: six cases from the Middle East and a review of the literature. *Arch. Neurol., Chicago* **35**, 494.

Robertson, W. C., Clark, D. B., and Markesbery, W. R. (1980). Review of 38 cases of subacute sclerosing panencephalitis: effect of amantadine on the natural course of the disease. *Ann. Neurol.* **8**, 422.

Sarubbi, F. A., Sparling, P. F., and Glezen, W. P. (1973). Herpesvirus hominis encephalitis. Virus isolation from brain biopsy in seven patients and results of therapy. *Arch. Neurol., Chicago* **29**, 268.

Saunders, M., Knowles, M., Chambers, M. E., Caspary, E. A., Gardner-Medwin, D., and Walker, P. (1969). Cellular and humoral responses to measles in subacute sclerosing panencephalitis. *Lancet* **i**, 72.

Schauseil-Zipf, U., Harden, A., Hoare, R. D., Lyen, K. R., Lingam, S., Marshall, W. C., and Pampiglione, G. (1982). Early diagnosis of herpes simplex encephalitis in childhood. *Eur. J. Pediatr.* **138**, 154.

Sköldenberg, B., Alestig, K., and others (1984). Acyclovir versus vidara-bine in herpes simplex encephalitis. *Lancet* **ii**, 707.

Soffer, D., Rannon, L., Alter, M., Kahana, E., and Feldman, S. (1976). Subacute sclerosing panencephalitis: an epidemiologic study in Israel. *Am. J. Epidemiol.* **103**, 67.

Taber, L. H., Greenberg, S. B., Perez, F. I., and Couch, R. B. (1977). Herpes simplex encephalitis treated with vidarabine (adenine arabino-side). *Arch. Neurol., Chicago* **34**, 608.

Townsend, J. J., Baringer, J. R., Wolinsky, J. S., Malamud, N., Mednick, J. P., Panitch, H. S., Scott, R. A. T., Oshiro, L. S., and Cremer, N. E. (1975). Progressive rubella panencephalitis: late onset after congenital rubella. *New Engl. J. Med.* **292**, 990.

——, Wolinsky, J. S., and Baringer, J. R. (1976). The neuropathology of progressive rubella panencephalitis of late onset. *Brain* **99**, 81.

Upton, A. and Gumpert, J. (1970). Electroencephalography in diagnosis of herpes-simplex encephalitis. *Lancet* **i**, 650.

van Bogaert, L. (1945). Une leuco-encéphalite sclérosante subaigue. *J. Neurol. Neurosurg. Psychiat.* **8**, 101.

Weil, M. L., Itabashi, H., Cremer, N. E., Oshiro, L. S., Lennette, E. H., and Carnay, L. (1975). Chronic progressive panencephalitis due to rubella virus simulating SSPE. *New Engl. J. Med.* **292**, 994.

Wolinsky, J. S., Berg, B. O., and Maitland, C. J. (1976). Progressive rubella panencephalitis. *Arch. Neurol., Chicago* **33**, 722.

Poliomyelitis

Synonyms. Infantile paralysis; Heine–Medin disease.

Definition. An acute infective disease due to a virus with a predilection for the anterior horn cells of the spinal cord and the motor nuclei of the brainstem, destruction of which causes muscular paralysis and atrophy.

Pathology

In the acute stage naked-eye examination often reveals parenchymatous degeneration of the liver and kidneys, and general enlargement of lymphoid tissue. The spinal cord is congested, soft, and oedematous, and minute haemorrhages may be visible in the grey matter.

Histologically the changes in the nervous system are usually most marked in the grey matter of the spinal cord and medulla. The basal ganglia and cerebral cortex are little affected. In the cord the changes consist of degeneration of the anterior horn cells and an inflammatory reaction with small haemorrhages in the grey matter. The anterior horn cells show changes varying from slight chromatolysis to complete destruction with neuronophagia. The inflammatory reaction consists of perivascular cuffing, mainly with lymphocyes but with a smaller number of neutrophils, and diffuse infiltration of the grey matter with similar cells and cells of neuroglial origin (Fig. 10.3). The white matter may also show some perivascular infiltration. The meninges share in the inflammatory reaction, also showing infiltration with lymphocytes.

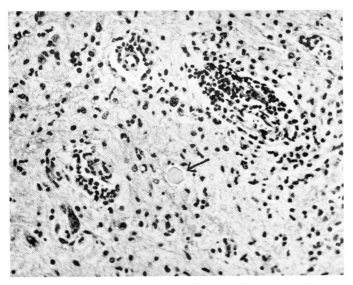

Fig. 10.3. Poliomyelitis. Anterior horn showing inflammatory infiltration and advanced chromatolysis of neurone (arrow). H & E, × 215.

Cortical lesions are similar but more focal, and inflammatory changes have been found in spinal dorsal roots and in peripheral nerves. Rarely the brunt of the infection falls upon the brainstem (polioencephalitis). Focal necroses are found in the liver, and inflammatory hyperplasia of lymphoid tissue. The virus has been demonstrated in the pharyngeal wall, the small and large intestines, and mesenteric lymph nodes, as well as in the nervous system.

Recovery from the acute stage is by restoration of ganglion cells

which have not been too severely damaged. Others disappear completely, and sections therefore show a paucity of cells in the anterior horns in the affected regions with secondary degeneration in corresponding ventral roots and peripheral nerves. The affected muscles show varying degrees of neurogenic atrophy with a relative increase of connective tissue and fat.

Aetiology

Our knowledge of the causative organism of poliomyelitis dates from the observation of Landsteiner and Popper in 1909 that the disease could be transmitted to monkeys, and it has since been shown to be an enterovirus. Detailed reviews of the virology and epidemiology have been given by Russell (1956), Drouhet, Debré and Celers (1970), and Johnson (1982). Three strains of virus have been isolated, known as 'Brunhilde' (Type 1), 'Lansing' (Type 2), and 'Leon' (Type 3). The virus was first grown in tissue culture by Enders, Weller, and Robbins (1949). It is a spherical particle measuring 30 nm in diameter. The virus can be obtained from the nasopharyngeal mucosa of patients in the acute stage, healthy contacts, and convalescents, and also from stools. Monkeys can be successfully inoculated by direct intracerebral injection or by injection subcutaneously, intraperitoneally, into lymph nodes, or into a nerve trunk, but the usual route of infection in man is from the alimentary tract, and it has been suggested that the virus reaches the nervous system by way of the autonomic nerves (Howe and Bodian 1941 *a*, *b*, 1942). Fairbrother and Hurst (1930) showed that the virus can travel along axis cylinders both in the peripheral nerves and in the central nervous system. However, spread by the blood or lymph system is also common (Horstmann 1952; Bodian 1952) and the pharynx is a common portal of entry, especially from the raw tonsillar bed after tonsillectomy (Aycock and Luther 1929). There is also good evidence that physical exertion during the stage of incubation may predispose to paralysis, particularly of those muscles which have been most used and paralysis may also develop in a limb which has been traumatized, as by an injection. For these reasons prophylactic inoculations and tonsillectomy are generally abandoned during an epidemic and physical exercise is unwise in unprotected individuals who have been exposed to infection (Russell 1956). The virus is highly resistant to chemical agents, but sensitive to heat and to desiccation. It can readily be cultured in HeLa cells or monkey kidney cells, and a series of specific serological tests, including complement-fixing and antibody neutralization methods are available. Specific monoclonal antibodies against the various strains have now been produced (Ferguson, Yi-Hua, Minor, Magrath, Spitz, and Schild 1982). Coxsackie A7 virus may produce a clinical illness indistinguishable from paralytic poliomyelitis.

Epidemiology

In Great Britain and the United States poliomyelitis now occurs only sporadically, but considerable epidemics occurred in the past. Wickman (1909) found that spread of the disease could often be traced to a healthy individual who had been in contact with a paralytic case but never himself developed it. Such healthy carriers and abortive cases, in which recovery occurs before the paralytic stage is reached, greatly outnumber paralytic cases and are probably mainly responsible for spread of the infection, though it can certainly be acquired from a paralytic case. Most members of a household have probably been infected by the time a paralytic case appears, though multiple paralytic cases in a household occur in less than 10 per cent of infected families. For every person with symptoms there may be 10 to 100 infected individuals with no obvious illness. Infectivity is probably greatest in the viraemic phase. Some strains of virus have seemed much more virulent than others, as shown by the high incidence of paralysis and fatality in British and American troops in India and in the Philippines in

1944–5. Type I virus is generally more virulent than Types II and III. Genetically determined susceptibility has also been postulated but remains unproven (Wyatt 1975 *a*, *b*). The virus has been demonstrated in the pharyngeal secretions and faeces of patients, in sewage, and in flies. Personal contact and the faecal contamination of food appear to be the principal modes of transmission.

The seasonal incidence in late summer and early autumn may be explained by these facts. Infants under the age of 1 year are rarely attacked. In a country where hygiene is poor most sufferers are between the ages of 2 and 4 years. After the age of 5 susceptibility rapidly diminishes, and after 25 the disease is rare. During and after the Second World War in the USA and in Great Britain the age incidence rose steadily. In Massachusetts in 1907, 7 per cent of those affected were over 15, in 1945, 25 per cent; and cases in adults became commoner (Horstmann 1948). The incidence in adult white immigrants to South Africa was shown to be much higher than in the South African born population of all races (Dean and Malk 1967). Males suffer somewhat more often than females. The incubation period appears to be usually from 7 to 14 days, but may be as long as 5 weeks.

The last 30 years has seen a dramatic decline in the incidence of the disease in all countries in which campaigns of prophylactic inoculation have been carried out using first injections of the Salk (Salk 1960) and British vaccines and subsequently the Sabin type oral attenuated live vaccine (Sabin 1959). While very occasional cases of paralytic poliomyelitis have been shown to follow oral vaccination, there is at present no justification for the view that it would be wise to return to using the injected killed vaccines (*The Lancet* 1977; *British Medical Journal*, 1978). Monoclonal antibodies (Ferguson *et al.* 1982) can accurately distinguish natural infections from those due to oral vaccination. It seems probable that the disease will eventually be totally controlled. However, other enteroviruses are now causing polio-like syndromes in vaccinated populations (Johnson 1982).

Symptoms

There are four possible ways in which a person may react to infection. (1) Exposure to the virus may lead to the development of immunity without any symptoms of illness. This is subclinical or inapparent infection. (2) In some patients the symptoms in the phase of viraemia are those of a mild general infection not involving the nervous system. These are abortive cases. (3) Many patients, in some epidemics as many as 75 per cent, develop fever, headache, malaise, and often meningism, and show an excess of cells in the CSF yet never develop paralysis. These are called meningitic or non-paralytic cases. (4) Only in a minority does the infection run its full course and cause paralysis.

Pre-paralytic or non-paralytic cases
In the pre-paralytic stage two phases can often be recognized. The first symptoms are fever, malaise, headache, drowsiness or insomnia, sweating, flushing, faucial congestion, and often gastro-intestinal disturbances such as anorexia, vomiting, and diarrhoea. This phase, the 'minor illness', which lasts one or two days, is followed by temporary improvement with remission of fever for 48 hours or may merge into the second phase, 'the major illness', in which headache is more severe and associated with pain in the back and limbs, sometimes with muscle tenderness. The symptoms closely resemble those of other forms of viral meningitis.

Delirium may occur and neck stiffness and Kernig's sign may be found. In the absence of such signs the 'spinal sign' is of occasional diagnostic value; attempted passive flexion of the spine is prevented by pain. Convulsions may occur in infants in either of the first two phases. In non-paralytic cases the patient recovers after exhibiting in mild or more severe form either or both of the phases of the pre-paralytic stage.

The cerebrospinal fluid
In the second phase the CSF shows changes of mild meningitis. The pressure is increased and there is an excess of cells, usually 50 to 250 mm³. At first both neutrophils and lymphocytes are present, but after the first week lymphocytes alone are found. The protein and globulin show a moderate increase, but the glucose content of the fluid is normal. During the second week the protein may rise to between 100 and 200 mg.

Paralytic cases

Spinal form. The onset of paralysis, often ushered in by muscular fasciculation, usually follows rapidly upon the pre-paralytic stage, with considerable pain in the limbs and tenderness of the muscles on pressure. Exceptionally the pre-paralytic phase may last for a week or even two. The paralysis may be widespread or localized. In severe cases the muscles of the neck, trunk, and all four limbs may be paralysed. When paralysis is less extensive, its asymmetry and patchy character are conspicuous features; some muscles may be severely affected on one side of the body and escape on the other. Usually paralysis reaches its maximum within 24 hours, but less often it is progressive. In the ascending form it gradually spreads upwards from the legs, and endangers life through respiratory paralysis. A descending form also occurs. Sometimes the infection seems to smoulder on and fresh weakness appears a week or more after the onset. The lower limbs are more often affected than the upper. Movement of the intercostals and the diaphragm must be observed carefully. A useful test for early respiratory paralysis is to ask the patient to count aloud without taking a breath; if he cannot count beyond 12 to 15, there is serious respiratory insufficiency and appropriate measurements of forced expiratory volume should be carried out in order to confirm the probability that assisted respiration will be needed urgently.

Fortunately only a proportion of the muscles affected at the outset remain permanently paralysed. The disease produces temporary loss of function in many anterior horn cells which ultimately recover. Improvement usually begins at the end of the first week after the onset of paralysis. Like other causes of lower motor-neurone paralysis, poliomyelitis leads to wasting of, and loss of cutaneous and tendon reflexes subserved by, the affected muscles. Complete paralysis of the muscles around a joint may result in subluxation. When opposing muscle groups are unequally affected, contractures develop in the stronger muscles. In the upper limb this most often happens at the shoulder after deltoid paralysis; in the lower limb, in the calf muscles, after paralysis of the peronei and anterior tibial group. Talipes equinovarus results from contracture of the calf. Asymmetrical palsy of spinal muscles causes scoliosis. The affected limbs are blue and cold, often with oedema or chilblains. Fasciculation may continue for years in partially paralysed muscles. Bone growth is retarded in the paralysed limbs (Ring 1957, 1958), and the bones show atrophy and rarefaction radiographically (Walton and Warrick 1954).

Rarely inflammation extends to the white matter of the lateral columns of the cord. Involvement of the spinothalamic tracts then gives impaired appreciation of pain, heat, and cold, and damage to the corticospinal tracts spastic paralysis. Except in such unusual cases sphincter disturbance is rare and sensory loss absent.

Brain stem form (polioencephalitis). In a few cases the brunt of the infection falls upon the brainstem, leading to facial, pharyngeal, laryngeal, lingual, or rarely ocular paralysis. Vertigo and nystagmus may occur and there is grave danger of involvement of the cardiac and respiratory centres.

Diagnosis

Diagnosis is rarely possible in the abortive or pre-paralytic stages, except in an epidemic. Even then suspicion cannot be confirmed until changes in the CSF indicate that the nervous system is invaded. In sporadic cases the disease has then to be distinguished from other causes of meningitis. In the acute pyogenic forms the glucose content of the CSF is reduced, and the cells are exclusively neutrophils. Mumps meningitis, also lymphocytic, is not likely to cause confusion if parotitis is present. Tuberculous meningitis may be difficult to distinguish but its onset is usually more gradual. Diagnosis, however, rests upon the examination of the CSF, which in both may contain an excess of cells, both neutrophils and lymphocytes, and an excess of protein. In poliomyelitis the sugar content is normal; in tuberculous meningitis the sugar is invariably diminished. Tubercle bacilli, if present, are, of course, conclusive.

The spinal form in the paralytic stage is usually easy to diagnose. When pain and tenderness are severe, it may be confused with acute rheumatism and acute osteomyelitis. In these, however, the tenderness is more localized and is in or near a joint. Moreover, the tendon reflexes are not lost as in poliomyelitis. A curious and, as yet unexplained, poliomyelitis-like syndrome has been reported to follow acute asthmatic attacks in childhood (Hopkins 1974; Wheeler and Ochoa 1980; The Lancet 1980). This syndrome of 'post-asthmatic pseudo-polio' can only be distinguished by the association with asthma and the lack of any rise in antibody titres against poliovirus.

In adults poliomyelitis must be distinguished from acute transverse myelitis and from the Guillain–Barré syndrome, but in the former condition flaccid paralysis of the legs is associated with extensor plantar reflexes, sensory loss, and loss of sphincter control, and in the latter weakness is usually proximal and asymmetrical and the CSF shows an increase in protein but rarely any pleocytosis.

When the patient is seen years after the acute attack the muscular wasting may suggest motor-neurone disease, syringomyelia, or myopathy. The fact that the wasting is not usually progressive, however, excludes these alternatives. The absence of fasciculation helps to distinguish it from the first named, and the absence of sensory loss from the second, while the wasting is usually too patchy and asymmetrical to simulate myopathy.

The bulbar form must be distinguished from other forms of encephalitis. In encephalitis complicating the exanthemata and vaccination, the primary cause is usually obvious, and the long tracts, both motor and sensory, are usually involved. Diagnosis from other viral encephalitides will usually depend upon serological and antibody tests and virus isolation.

Prognosis

The mortality has varied in different epidemics from under 5 per cent to over 25 per cent. The cause of death is usually respiratory paralysis due to direct involvement of the respiratory centre in the bulbar form or to ascending paralysis involving the intercostals and diaphragm; mortality has been much lower since the introduction of refined methods of assisted respiration.

When the progress of the paralysis has ceased, it is safe to predict that considerable recovery will occur (Russell and Fischer-Williams 1954). Favourable indications are the presence of voluntary movement, of reflex responsiveness, and of muscular contraction evoked by nerve stimulation three weeks after the onset of the paralysis. Improvement once begun may be expected to continue for at least a year and sometimes for even longer. The nature and extent of the residual disability will depend upon the distribution of the paralysis; disability often increases to the extent of impairing mobility and employability solely through the superimposition of the effects of ageing (Jennekens, Tomlinson, and Walton 1971; Anderson, Levine, and Gellert 1972; Hayward and Seaton 1979). Late-onset respiratory failure is also an uncommon sequel, often accentuated by kyphoscoliosis and sometimes heralded by prolonged alveolar hypoventilation (Lane, Hazleman, and Nichols 1974). Second attacks, though very rare, are well authenticated but are usually due to a different strain of virus.

Motor-neurone disease is thought to be a rare sequel of acute anterior poliomyelitis, which it may follow after many years, the progressive wasting usually beginning in the region originally affected (Campbell, Williams, and Pearce 1969). Others feel that this is not true motor-neurone disease but simply the result of superimposed ageing processes as discussed above (Johnson 1982).

Treatment

General management
Immediate and complete rest should be insisted on in every suspected case, however mild, since physical activity in the pre-paralytic stage increases the risk of severe paralysis (Russell 1949, 1955).

Three categories of paralytic case must be distinguished because in each the treatment needed is different. These are: (1) the patient with neither respiratory nor bulbar paralysis; (2) the patient with respiratory paralysis with or without bulbar paralysis; and (3) the patient with bulbar paralysis.

The treatment of a patient without respiratory and bulbar paralysis
Aspirin in doses of 300–600 mg or other analgesics and sedatives, such as diazepam, will be required for the relief of pain and restlessness. Gentle passive movements are the only form of physical treatment permissible at this stage. Antibiotics are of no value except as prophylactics against pneumonia in patients with respiratory paralysis, and immune globulin is also valueless at this stage.

The course of the disease after the onset of paralysis can be divided into: (1) An acute stage, in which pain and tenderness of the muscles persist. This usually lasts for three or four weeks. (2) A convalescent stage, during which improvement in muscular power continues. This may last from six months to two years. (3) A chronic stage in those left with permanent paralysis after maximum recovery has occurred.

The principal object in the acute stage is to prevent stretching of the paralysed muscles and contracture of their antagonists. Damage may be done in a few days which it will take months to repair. The patient should be nursed on a firm bed and the limbs kept in the positions in which the paralysed muscles are relaxed (but not stretched) by means of sandbags and pillows.

During the convalescent stage prolonged bed rest is necessary only in severe cases, contractures being prevented by suitable splints if necessary. Passive movements should be carried out from the beginning. Except when the trunk muscles are severely paralysed, the patient should as soon as possible be allowed to stand several times daily, but paralysis of spinal muscles requires suitable spinal supports if severe spinal deformity is to be prevented. Active exercises are of great importance. They may need to be assisted or carried out in baths or in a sling-suspension apparatus. The affected parts should be put through a full range of movement at least once, and if possible twice, a day. Adequate instrumental support for the spine and limbs may be required and both the physiotherapist and occupational therapist play an important role (Taylor 1955). In the later stages contractures and deformities may require tenotomy or other surgical treatment, but these can usually be avoided by adequate care during the acute stage.

In the chronic stage when oedema, cyanosis, and chilblains are troublesome in the feet, lumbar sympathectomy may improve the circulation.

Treatment of respiratory paralysis (with or without bulbar paralysis)
A patient with respiratory paralysis must be treated by some method of artificial respiration which may be needed for weeks, for months or occasionally indefinitely. As Beaver (1962) pointed out, the proper handling of respiratory failure is now so rewarding that it must be instituted as soon as respiratory insufficiency threatens. This is the case when the $p(CO_2)$ and $p(O_2)$ can be kept within nor-

mal limits only by excessive effort which soon becomes exhausting. It was customary in the past when respiratory paralysis was not accompanied by pharyngeal paralysis, so that the patient could swallow his own secretions, to use either a cuirass or cabinet respirator. The cuirass applies external positive and negative pressure directly to the chest wall (Kelleher, Wilson, Russell, and Stott 1952) while the cabinet, in which the entire patient other than the head is enclosed, works by applying negative pressure to the chest so that air is sucked into the lungs. The use of these respirators, once widely employed with excellent results, requires considerable skill (Bourdillon, Davies-Jones, Stott, and Taylor 1950; Russell 1956). Now they have been largely abandoned in favour of intermittent positive pressure respiration (IPPR) applied either through a nasal or oral endotracheal tube through which the lungs are inflated (when respiratory paralysis is unlikely to last more than two or three days at the most) or through a cuffed tube inserted via a tracheostomy (Lassen 1953; Spalding, and Russell 1954; Beaver 1962). Occasionally, when respiratory insufficiency is slight, and the patient can survive the hours of sleep without becoming dangerously hypoxic or hypercapnic, intermittent diurnal inflation of the lungs via a Bird type respirator with the nose occluded, via a mouthpiece held between the closed lips, is sufficient. Sometimes even simpler devices suffice (Lane, Hazleman, and Nichols 1974). Whenever possible, assisted ventilation, if likely to be prolonged, should be carried out under expert supervision in an intensive care unit with regular monitoring of the blood gases in order to avoid under- or over-ventilation.

The great advantage of IPPR is that if pharyngeal (bulbar) paralysis is also present, the cuffed intratracheal tube effectively prevents the passage of pharyngeal secretions into the lungs and also prevents the inhalation of food and vomit. Infection is an important complication requiring appropriate antibiotics; pulmonary collapse may necessitate bronchoscopy and suction; acute dilatation of the stomach, once a common accompaniment of respiratory failure, is rare now that gastric intubation is routine. Patients on artificial respiration also require the usual care of the skin, bladder (often including catheterization), and bowels.

Treatment of bulbar paralysis alone

Russell (1956) and Lassen (1956) did much to clarify the treatment of bulbar paralysis in poliomyelitis. When this occurs without respiratory paralysis the danger to the patient arises from his inability to prevent fluids, or pharyngeal secretions, from being sucked into the lungs with inspiration. Vomiting, for example, may be followed by fatal inhalation. Dysphagia also leads to difficulty in feeding. A proper posture of the patient is all-important. He should be nursed in the semi-prone position, being turned from one side to the other every few hours, while the foot of the bed is raised to make an angle of 15 degrees with the horizontal. This posture should be relaxed for nursing or other purposes only for short periods under close supervision. Tracheostomy in such cases is rarely necessary except in the presence of bilateral abductor paralysis of the vocal cords. A mechanical sucker is required to remove pharyngeal secretions. After about 24 hours of starvation, feeding should be carried out by an oesophageal catheter, preferably passed through the nose.

Prophylaxis

Since the nasopharyngeal secretions, the urine, and the faeces of the patient may contain the virus, barrier nursing is wise. Virus is present in the stools 3 weeks after the onset in 50 per cent of patients and 5–6 weeks after the onset in 25 per cent. Isolation should be continued for at least 6 weeks.

During an epidemic, residential schools should not be closed. Closure of a school will not necessarily modify the spread of the disease among those already exposed to it, and there is a risk that such a course might disseminate the infection among younger and therefore more susceptible children. Children in an affected household should be isolated from other children for three weeks after

isolation of the patient. Modern immunization is so successful in halting epidemics that measures which were once traditional (e.g. the closure of swimming baths) are no longer needed. Operations on the ear, nose, and throat and inoculations should not be carried out during an epidemic, and dental extractions should be avoided if possible.

The protective value of the Salk vaccine was well established between 1950 and 1960. Three doses, giving 90 per cent protection, were given as a routine, and a fourth was often added later in special circumstances. Immunity induced by injection did not prevent colonization of the gut by wild virus; hence an immune person could still be a carrier. On the other hand, attenuated live vaccine, given orally, by multiplying in the gut blocked the entry of wild virus (Koprowski 1960). Its capacity to confer immunity is now well established and the Sabin vaccine, given as one or two drops on a sugar lump, appears to confer almost total immunity for three years or more. In the United States it was customary to give Type I vaccine first followed by a combination of Types II and III 6–8 weeks later, but tritypic vaccine is preferred in Great Britain and the latter type should certainly be used in an epidemic or after exposure to a paralytic case in an endemic area. In children and young adults 'booster' doses at regular intervals are recommended.

References

Anderson, A. D., Levine, S. A., and Gellert, H. (1972). Loss of ambulatory ability in patients with old anterior poliomyelitis. *Lancet* ii, 1061.

Aycock, W. L. and Luther, E. H. (1929). The occurrence of poliomyelitis following tonsillectomy. *New Engl. J. Med.* **200**, 164.

Beaver, R. (1962). The management of respiratory failure. In *Modern trends in neurology* (ed. D. Williams), Vol. 3. Butterworth, London.

Bodian, D. (1952). A reconsideration of the pathogenesis of poliomyelitis. *Am. J. Hyg.* **55**, 414.

Bourdillon, R. B., Davies-Jones, E., Stott, F. D., and Taylor, L. M. (1950). Respiratory studies in paralytic poliomyelitis. *Br. med. J.* **2**, 539.

British Medical Journal (978). Poliomyelitis vaccines: killed or live? *Br. med. J.* **2**, 845.

Campbell, A. M. G., Williams, E. R., and Pearce, J. (1969). Late motor neuron degeneration following poliomyelitis. *Neurology, Minneapolis* **19**, 1101.

Cox, H. R., Cabasso, V. J., Markham, F. S., Moses, M. J., Mayer, A. W., Roca-Garcia, M., and Ruegsegger, J. M. (1959). Immunological response to trivalent and oral poliomyelitis vaccine. *Br. med. J.* **2**, 591.

Dane, D. S., Dick, G. W. A., McAlister, J. J., and Nelson, R. T. (1960). Epidemic control of poliomyelitis with inactive virus vaccines. *Lancet* i, 835.

Dean, G. and Malk, M. (1967). Poliomyelitis among white immigrants to South Africa. *S.A. med. J.* **41**, 294.

Droughet, V., Debré, R., and Celers, J. (1970). Laboratory diagnosis of enterovirus infections. Poliomyelitis: pathophysiology, and Poliomyelitis: prophylaxis. In *Clinical virology* (ed. R. Debré and J. Celers). Saunders, Philadelphia.

Enders, J. F., Weller, T. H., and Robbins, F. C. (1949). Cultivation of the Lansing strain of poliomyelitis virus in tissue culture. *Science* **109**, 85.

Fairbrother, R. W. and Hurse, E. W. (1930). The pathogenesis of, and propagation of the virus in, experimental poliomyelitis. *J. Path. Bact.* **33**, 17.

Ferguson, M., Yi-Hua, Q., Minor, P. D., Magrath, D. I., Spitz, M., and Schild, G. C. (1982). Monoclonal antibodies specific for the Sabin vaccine strain of poliovirus 3. *Lancet* ii, 122.

Hale, J. H., Doraisingham, M., Kanagaratnam, K., Leong, K. W., and Monteiro, E. S. (1959). Large scale use of Sabin type 2 attenuated poliomyelitis vaccine in Singapore during a type I poliomyelitis epidemic. *Br. med. J.* **1**, 1541.

Hayward, M. and Seaton, D. (1979). Late sequelae of paralytic poliomyelitis: a clinical and electromyographic study. *J. Neurol. Neurosurg. Psychiat.* **42**, 117.

Hopkins, I. J. (1974). A new syndrome: poliomyelitis-like illness associated with acute asthma in childhood. *Aust. Paediatr. J.* **10**, 273.

Horstman, D. M. (1948). Problems in the epidemiology of poliomyelitis. *Lancet* i, 273.

—— (1952). Poliomyelitis virus in blood of orally infected monkeys and chimpanzees. *Proc. Soc. exp. Biol. (NY)* **79**, 417.

Howe, H. A. and Bodian, D. (1941*a*). The pathology of early, arrested and nonparalytic poliomyelitis. *Bull. Johns Hopk. Hosp.* **69**, 135.

—— and —— (1941*b*). Poliomyelitis in the chimpanzee: a clinical-pathological study. *Bull. Johns Hopk. Hosp.* **69**, 149.

—— and —— (1942). *Neural mechanisms in poliomyelitis.* Hoeber, New York.

Hurse, E. W. (1930). A further contribution to the pathogenesis of experimental poliomyelitis: inoculation into the sciatic nerve. *J. Path. Bact.* **33**, 1133.

Hurst, E. W. (1932). Further observations on the pathogenesis of experimental poliomyelitis: intrathecal inoculation of the virus. *J. Path. Bact.* **35**, 41.

Jennekens, F. G. I., Tomlinson, B. E., and Walton, J. N. (1971). Histochemical aspects of five limb muscles in old age: an autopsy study. *J. neurol. Sci.* **14**, 259.

Johnson, R. T. (1982). *Viral infections of the nervous system.* Raven Press, New York.

Kelleher, W. H., Wilson, A. B. K., Russell, W. R., and Stott, F. D. (1952). Notes on cuirass respirators. *Br. med. J.* **2**, 413.

Koprowski, H. (1960). Historical aspects of the development of live virus vaccine in poliomyelitis. *Br. med. J.* **2**, 85.

Kramer, S. D., Hoskwith, B., and Grossman, L. H. (1939). Detection of virus poliomyelitis in nose and throat and gastro-intestinal tract of human beings and monkeys. *J. exp. Med.* **59**, 49.

The Lancet (1977). Poliomyelitis vaccines. *Lancet* **ii**, 21.

—— (1980). Post-asthmatic pseudo-polio in children. *Lancet* **i**, 860.

Lane, D. J., Hazleman, B., and Nichols, P. J. R. (1974). Late onset respiratory failure in patients with previous poliomyelitis. *Quart. J. Med.* **43**, 551.

Lassen, H. C. A. (1953). A preliminary report on the 1952 epidemic of poliomyelitis in Copenhagen. *Lancet* **i**, 37.

—— (1956). *Management of life-threatening poliomyelitis.* Livingstone, Edinburgh and London.

Paul, J. R., Trask, J. W., Bishop, M. B., Melnick, J. L., and Casey, A. E. (1941). The detection of poliomyelitis virus in flies. *Science* **94**, 395.

Ring, P. A. (1957). Shortening and paralysis in poliomyelitis. *Lancet* **ii**, 980.

—— (1958). Prognosis of limb inequality following paralytic poliomyelitis. *Lancet* **ii**, 1306.

Russell, W. R. (1949. Paralytic poliomyelitis. *Br. med. J.* **1**, 465.

—— (1956). *Poliomyelitis.* 2nd edn. Arnold, Bristol.

—— and Fischer-Williams, M. (1954). Recovery of muscular strength after poliomyelitis. *Lancet* **i**, 330.

Sabin, A. B. (1959). Present position of immunization against poliomyelitis with live virus vaccines. *Br. med. J.* **1**, 663.

Salk, J. E. (1960). Persistence of immunity after administration of formalin-treated poliovirus vaccine. *Lancet* **ii**, 715.

Seddon, H. J. (1947). The early treatment of poliomyelitis. *Br. med. J.* **2**, 319.

Smith, A. C., Spalding, J. M. K., and Russell, W. R. (1954). Artificial respiration by intermittent positive pressure in poliomyelitis and other diseases. *Lancet* **i**, 939.

Taylor, R. A. R. (1955). *Poliomyelitis and polioencephalitis..* Butterworths, London.

Trask, J. D., Vignec, A. J., and Paul J. R. (1938). Poliomyelitis virus in human stools. *J. Am. med. Ass.* **111**, 6.

Walton, J. N. and Warrick, C. K. (1954). Osseous changes in myopathy. *Br. J. Radiol.* **27**, 1.

Wheeler, S. D. and Ochoa, J. (1980). Poliomyelitis-like syndrome associated with asthma: a case report and review of the literature. *Arch. Neurol., Chicago* **37**, 52.

Wickman, I. (1909). *Beitrage zur Kenntnis der Heine-Medinschen Krankheit.* Berlin.

World Health Organization Expert Committee on Poliomyelitis, First Report (1954). *Wld Hlth Org. techn. Rep. Ser.*, No. 81.

Wyatt, H. V. (1975*a*). Is poliomyelitis a genetically-determined disease? I: a genetic model. *Med. Hypothesis* **1**, 23.

—— (1975*b*). Is poliomyelitis a genetically-determined disease? II: A critical examination of the epidemiological data. *Med. Hypothesis* **1**, 35.

Rabies

Synonym. Hydrophobia.

Definition. An infection of the nervous system due to a virus communicated to man by the bite of an infected animal. The resulting encephalitis, which is almost always fatal, is distinguished by the characteristic pharyngeal spasm evoked by the attempt to drink.

Aetiology

Rabies is due to a rhabdovirus (*Lyssavirus*) of the RNA type, about 60–80 nm in diameter. It is commonly found in mucus-secreting glands (such as the salivary glands), but its most devastating effects are upon the central nervous system. It is communicated to man by the bite of an infected animal which carries the virus in its saliva. Most cases of human infection are due to dog bites, though bites of jackals, cats, bats, and wolves are occasionally responsible. The bites of rabid horses and cattle hardly ever communicate the disease. An epidemic in Trinidad was attributed to vampire bats which were believed to carry the infection from cattle to man. The virus of rabies has been isolated from a fatal case occurring in a human epidemic of encephalitis in Japan. The risk of infection is influenced by the severity of the bite and is much diminished when the individual is bitten through clothes, which to some extent free the animal's teeth from saliva. The virus, having entered the body, is transmitted only along nerve trunks, moving in both directions. The condition has been transmitted by corneal transplant (Baer, Shaddock, Houff, Harrison, and Gardner 1982).

Pathology

The pathological changes in the nervous system are in part those usually associated with virus infection. Severe degenerative changes are found in the ganglion cells of the brain, cord, and sympathetic ganglia. The small vessels are narrowed with swollen endothelial cells, and marked perivascular round-cell infiltration. The neuronal degeneration is more diffuse than the inflammatory reaction, and the ganglion cells of the cortex may be extensively affected. There is considerable microglial reaction with collections of inflammatory and glial cells known as Babes' nodes. The Negri body is diagnostic; it is an acidophil inclusion body contained within the cytoplasm or protoplasmic processes of neurones, especially those of the hippocampus, but it is seen less often in the cortical pyramidal cells, the cerebellar Purkinje cells, and ganglion cells elsewhere. Negri bodies are not constantly present in human rabies nor in experimental infection in animals.

The pathological changes resulting from complications of rabies vaccination are different (see p. 301).

Symptoms and signs

Rabies in animals

The first symptoms of rabies in the dog are a change in behaviour with perversion of appetite. The animal will gnaw and swallow paper, sticks, earth, and other unusual substances. This is followed by excitement, in which it will snap at and bite other animals. There is a free flow of saliva, and the bark often becomes high-pitched. After one or two days paralysis develops, first in the hind limbs and spreading to the forelimbs and jaw. Muscular spasms may occur affecting the whole body. Emaciation is marked and death is almost invariable. In other animals, especially rodents and herbivora, the stage of excitement does not occur, and symptoms are paralytic from the beginning; this paralytic form occurs rarely in dogs.

Rabies in man

The incubation period in man depends upon the distance of the infected lesion from the central nervous system. When the bite is on the head it is about 27 days, when on the arm 32 days, when on the leg 64 days, but these periods vary widely. During the incubation period there are no symptoms. Local pain in the bitten limb is often the first symptom. The first general symptom is depression, often with apprehension, and disturbed sleep. The next is pharyngeal spasm brought on by an attempt to drink and rapidly extending to involve both the ordinary and the accessory muscles of respiration, and later all the muscles of the body, often with opisthotonos. When this stage is at its height not only any attempt to drink but the sound and even the thought of water will bring on the spasm, which may also be excited by other stimuli, even a current of air. Salivation is excessive, and vomiting is common. A horror of water develops and hallucinations may appear. The human patient does not develop the impulse to bite characteristic of the rabid dog. Later the symptoms of excitement and the spasm diminish and may give place to terminal paralysis. Fever is usual and terminal hyperpyrexia may occur. Death may occur during the spasmodic stage from respiratory or cardiac failure, or the patient may die paralysed and in coma.

Rarely spasms and mental excitement are absent and the symptoms are paralytic from the beginning, as in some animals. An epidemic of paralytic rabies occurred in Trinidad in 1931. In such cases the clinical picture is one of ascending paralysis with loss of sphincter control. The upper limbs may or may not be affected and sensory loss is inconstant. Finally, bulbar paralysis leads to dysphagia, and death occurs from respiratory paralysis.

Diagnosis

The diagnosis is usually easy on account of the history of the bite and the distinctive pharyngeal spasm. The condition must be distinguished from tetanus, the incubation period of which is shorter. Symptoms of tetanus unmodified by the injection of anti-serum usually begin within 14 days of the injury and almost invariably within 3 weeks. Trismus is an early symptom and pharyngeal spasm is usually absent.

Hysteria may simulate hydrophobia in a patient who has been bitten by a dog thought to be rabid. In hysteria, however, true pharyngeal spasm does not occur and the condition is usually amenable to drugs and suggestion.

The paralytic form of rabies should offer no diagnostic difficulty when there is a history of a bite, but when the mode of infection is obscure, the diagnosis was often established in the past only by means of animal inoculation. More recently, it has been shown that the diagnosis may be confirmed by finding specific fluorescence in corneal impression smears, skin or brain biopsies, or by detecting fluorescent antibody in serum (*British Medical Journal* 1975; Johnson 1982).

Prognosis

The risk of contracting rabies is estimated at about 5 per cent of individuals bitten by animals supposed to be rabid. Adequate prophylactic treatment reduces this incidence to about 1.5 per cent. The mortality rate is almost 100 per cent, but very occasional patients treated with curarization and assisted ventilation have recovered (Hattwick, Weis, Stechschulte, Baer, and Gregg 1972; Porras, Barboza, Fuenzalida, Adaros, Oviedo de Diaz, and Furst 1976).

Prophylaxis and treatment

The prophylactic treatment of rabies introduced first by Pasteur is still used, though it has been modified in various ways. It consists of successive doses of a vaccine derived from animals which have been infected with the virus. The vaccine may consist of living or dead virus from the cord or brain of infected animals and may be given alone or combined with antiserum. The Semple vaccine prepared from rabbit brain is still used. A vaccine free from brain tissue and prepared in duck embryo was introduced in the United States and is given in a course of 14 daily injections to an individual exposed to infection. The indications for vaccine treatment were given in the report of the WHO Committee (1966). The administration should be begun as early as possible after the bite. The long incubation period permits the development of acquired immunity after infection. The prophylactic vaccine treatment of rabies is thus analogous to the vaccination of individuals after exposure to smallpox. The risk of producing acute or subacute demyelinating encephalomyelitis as a complication (p. 301) should be borne in mind and treatment is interrupted if this is suspected. Though complications have been most frequent following the use of vaccines prepared in brain or spinal-cord tissue (Gibbs, Carpenter, and Spies 1961), a case of transverse myelitis following the use of duck embryo vaccine has been described (Prussin and Katabi 1964) and other neurological complications have been reported, including an illness resembling the Guillain-Barré syndrome (Ozer, Finnigan, Petzold, Spitter, Emmons, and Rothenberg 1973). The Flury vaccine made from living but attenuated virus is successful in protecting animals (Koprowski and Cox 1948) but has not been thought safe enough for use in man; hyper-immune gamma-globulin given to confer temporary passive immunity is often given with vaccine but only gives short-term protection. Newer vaccines have now been developed; the inactivated vaccine grown in the human diploid cell strain WI–38 (Wicktor, Fernandez, and Koprowski 1964) is now the safest and most effective yet produced and is being progressively refined (Wiktor, Plotkin, and Grella 1973). It has been shown to be safe, acceptable, and effective (Aoki, Tyrrell, Hill, and Turner 1975; Johnson 1982). The bite itself should be treated, though cauterization has little influence in preventing the development of the disease. When rabies has developed, treatment is purely symptomatic, its principal object being to diminish the spasms. Total paralysis with curare and assisted respiration may be the only hope.

References

Aoki, F. Y., Tyrrell, D. A. J., Hill, L. E., and Turner, G. S. (1975). Immunogenicity and acceptability of a human diploid-cell culture rabies vaccine in volunteers. *Lancet* **i**, 660.

Baer, G. M., Shaddock, J. H., Houff, S. A., Harrison, A. K., and Gardner, J. J. (1982). Human rabies transmitted by corneal transplant. *Arch. Neurol., Chicago* **39**, 103.

Baltazard, M. (1970). Rabies. In *Clinical virology*. (ed. R. Debré and J. Celers). Saunders, Philadelphia.

British Medical Journal (1975). Diagnosis and management of human rabies. *Br. med. J.* **3**, 721.

Gibbs, F. A., Gibbs, E. L., Carpenter, P. R., and Spies, H. W. (1961). Comparison of rabies vaccines grown on duck embryo and on nervous tissue. *New Engl. J. Med.* **265**, 1002.

Hattwick, A. W., Weis, T. T., Stechschulte, J., Baer, G. M., and Gregg, M. B. (1972). Recovery from rabies; a case report. *Ann. intern. Med.* **76**, 931.

Hurst, E. W. and Pawan, J. L. (1931). An outbreak of rabies in Trinidad without history of bites and with the symptoms of acute ascending myelitis. *Lancet* **ii**, 622.

—— and —— (1932). A further account of the Trinidad outbreak of acute rabies myelitis. Histology of the experimental disease. *J. Path. Bact.* **35**, 301.

Johnson, R. T. (1982). *Viral infections of the nervous system*. Raven Press, New York.

Knutt, R. E. (1929). Acute ascending paralysis and myelitis due to the virus of rabies. *J. Am. med. Ass.* **93**, 754.

Koprowski, H. and Cox, H. R. (1948). Studies in chick embryo adapted rabies virus. *J. Immunol.* **60**, 533.

Mozer, H. N., Finnigan, F. B., Petzold, H., Spitter, L. E., Emmons, R. W., and Rothenberg, B. (1973). Myelopathy after duck embryo rabies vaccine. *J. Am. med. Ass.* **224**, 1605.

Porras, C., Barboza, J. J., Fuenzalida, E., Adaros, H. L., Oviedo de Diaz, A. M., and Furst, J. (1976). Recovery from rabies in man. *Ann. intern. Med.* **85**, 44.

Prussin, G. and Katab, G. (1964). Dorsolumbar myelitis following antirabies vaccination with duck embryo vaccine. *Ann. intern. Med.* **60**, 114.

Viets, H. R. (1926). A case of hydrophobia with Negri bodies in the brain. *Arch. Neurol. Psychiat., Chicago* **15**, 735.

Wiktor, T. J., Fernandes, M. V., and Koprowski, H. (1964). Cultivation of rabies virus in human diploid cell strain WI–38. *J. Immunol.* **93**, 353.

——, Plotkin, S. A., and Grella, D. W. (1973). Human cell culture rabies vaccine. Antibody response in man. *J. Am. med. Ass.* **224**, 1170.

World Health Organization Expert Committee on Rabies (1966). *Wld Hlth Org. techn. Rep. Ser.*, No. 321.

Virus meningitis

Synonyms. Acute benign lymphocytic meningitis; epidemic serous meningitis; acute aseptic meningitis.

Aetiology

There is no absolute distinction between encephalitis and meningitis, as is evident from the term meningo-encephalitis. Nevertheless, many virus infections can produce the clinical picture of an acute meningitis with a pleocytosis in the CSF, and little or no evidence of involvement of the substance of the nervous system. These agents include those of acute lymphocytic choriomeningitis, mumps, infectious mononucleosis, some of the Coxsackie and Echo viruses, poliomyelitis, louping-ill, and the *Chlamydia* of psittacosis.

Recent observations suggest that benign lymphocytic meningitis accounts for about 50 per cent of all cases of infectious meningitis seen in hospital. Mumps is a common cause in Britain, being found in 26 per cent of a series of cases in Glasgow in which Echo 9 virus accounted for 61 per cent and other enteroviruses for 13 per cent; lymphocytic choriomeningitis was uncommon (Grist 1967). Oligoelonal IgG and less often IgM is usually demonstrable in such patients but there is no evidence of association with any HLA antigen (Frydén and Link 1979; Frydén, Möller, and Link 1979).

Acute lymphocytic choriomeningitis

The disorder occurs sporadically and also in small epidemics. Children are usually affected, but it may also occur in adults. Armstrong and Lillie (1934), Findlay, Alcock, and Stern (1936), and others showed that it is caused by a virus now classified as an arenavirus; it has been recovered from the CSF of patients and transmitted to mice and monkeys. Mice are subject to the disease in the wild state and may be the source of the human disease, which has been encountered in Europe, North America, New Zealand, and Malaya. Hamsters may also be a reservoir of human infection (Johnson 1982).

Pathology

Animals infected experimentally show intense lymphocytic infiltration of the leptomeninges, the ventricular ependyma, and the choroid plexuses. Viets and Warren (1937) reported similar changes in a fatal case together with degeneration of cerebral neurones with cytoplasmic inclusion bodies in the midbrain. Perivascular lymphocytic infiltration was seen in both the brain and the spinal cord. Fatal cases of bulbar paralysis, ascending paralysis, and acute meningoencephalitis due to this virus have been reported by Adair, Gould, and Smadel (1953) and Warkel, Rinaldi, Bancroft, Cardiff, Holmes, and Wilsnack (1973).

Symptoms and signs

The onset is acute, and symptoms of meningeal irritation usually develop rapidly but there may be prodromal manifestations of a general infection followed by a remission before nervous symptoms occur. The symptoms are those of any acute meningitis (see p. 237). Papilloedema may occur, and squint and nystagmus are common. Apart from the occasional occurrence of facial paralysis, the other cranial nerves are normal. Paraplegia and retention of urine have been described, but symptoms of encephalomyelitis are rare. There is usually high fever at the onset, and the temperature falls by lysis in about a week. Pneumonitis—'atypical pneumonia'—may occur (Smadel, Green, Paltauf, and Gonzales 1942), and indeed a general infection without meningitis may be the commonest form of the disease (Farmer and Janeway 1942).

The CSF is under increased pressure and may be clear or turbid. The protein is increased and a 'cobweb clot' has occurred in some cases. There is an excess of cells ranging from 50 to 1500 per mm^3. These may be mainly mononuclear from the onset, but in a few cases neutrophils predominate at the beginning, giving place to mononuclear cells during the first week. The sugar of the fluid is usually little, if at all, depressed. The pleocytosis in the CSF is often remarkably persistent, and mononuclear cells may be present for many weeks after the disappearance of symptoms, when the patient is apparently in normal health.

Diagnosis

For the diagnosis of meningitis see page 239.

Acute lymphocytic choriomeningitis is most likely to be confused with tuberculous meningitis, and since inability to find tubercle bacilli in the CSF cannot exclude the latter, the two conditions may be difficult to distinguish. A low sugar content in the fluid, however, is against the benign disorder. A bromide partition test using bromine–82 was shown to be of some value (Crook, Duncan, Gutteridge, and Pallis 1960) in identifying the abnormal serum/CSF bromide ratio which suggests tuberculous meningitis. The acute onset of symptoms in lymphocytic choriomeningitis is the single criterion most useful in distinguishing acute viral meningitis of all types from the tuberculous form, but, except sometimes on the basis of associated clinical or haematological findings, it is not possible to distinguish lymphocytic choriomeningitis from the meningitides resulting from mumps, mononucleosis, herpes simplex Type I, poliomyelitis, Echo virus, and Coxsackie virus infections. Serum antibodies do not usually appear for about two weeks but CSF antibodies may be detected earlier, as may specific immunofluorescence in cells isolated from the fluid or a positive ELISA test (see Johnson 1982). In mumps, Echo virus and Coxsackie infections, the virus may be cultured from the CSF within two or three days, sufficiently early to influence management (*The Lancet* 1982).

Prognosis

The prognosis is good and complete recovery is the rule, though rare fatal cases have been reported (Warkel *et al.* 1973). Relapses occasionally occur. Paraplegia, however, may be permanent and diffuse arachnoiditis has been described as a rare sequel.

Treatment

Treatment is purely symptomatic; appropriate analgesics should be given for the relief of headache; chemotherapy is of no value.

References

Adair, C. V., Gould, R. L., and Smadel, J. E. (1953). Aseptic meningitis: a disease of diverse etiology. *Ann. intern. Med.* **39**, 675.

Armstrong, C. and Lillie, R. D. (1934). Experimental lymphocytic choriomeningitis of monkeys and mice. *Publ. Hlth Rep., Washington* **49**, 1019.

Crook, A., Duncan, H., Gutteridge, B., and Pallis, C. (1960). Use of ^{82}Br in differential diagnosis of lymphocytic meningitis. *Br. med. J.* **i**, 704.

Farmer, T. W. and Janeway, C. A. (1942). Infections with the virus of lymphocytic choriomeningitis. *Medicine, Baltimore* **21**, 1.

Findlay, G. M., Alcock, N. S., and Stern, R. O. (1936). The virus aetiology of one form of lymphocytic meningitis. *Lancet* **i**, 650.

Frydén, A. and Link, H. (1979). Predominance of oligoclonal IgG type λ in CSF in aseptic meningitis. *Arch. Neurol., Chicago* **36**, 478.

——, Möller, E., and Link, H. (1979). No association between oligoclonal immunoglobulins in cerebrospinal fluid and HLA antigens in acute aseptic meningitis. *Neurology, Minneapolis* **29**, 1422.

Grist, N. R. (1967). Acute viral infections of the nervous system. *Proc. R. Soc. Med.* **60**, 696.

Johnson, R. T. (1982). *Viral infections of the nervous system*. Raven Press, New York.

The Lancet (1982). Viral cultures from cerebrospinal fluid. *Lancet* **ii**, 250.

MacCallum, F. O. and Findlay, G. M. (1939). Lymphocytic choriomeningitis. Isolation of the virus from the nasopharynx. *Lancet* **i**, 1370.

Smadel, J. E., Green, R. H., Paltauf, R. M., and Gonzales, T. A. (1942). Lymphocytic choriomeningitis: two human fatalities following an unusual febrile illness. *Proc. Soc. exp. Biol., NY* **49**, 683.

Viets, H. R. and Warren, S. (1937). Acute lymphocytic meningitis. *J. Am. med. Ass.* **108**, 357.

Warkel, R. L., Rinaldi, C. F., Bancroft, W. H., Cardiff, R. D., Holmes, G. E., and Wilsnack, R. E. (1973). Fatal acute meningoencephalitis due to lymphocytic choriomeningitis virus. *Neurology, Minneapolis* **23**, 198.

Nervous complications of mumps

Aetiology

Gordon (1927) showed that mumps is due to a virus with neurotropic propensities. He produced meningitis in monkeys by the intracerebral injection of a filtrate of the saliva of patients suffering from mumps. The commonest nervous complication is meningitis, and in such cases the mumps paramyxovirus has been recovered from the CSF. While many other neurological manifestations including hemiplegia, quadriplegia, blindness, and deafness have been described, encephalomyelitis is much less common, occurring in 9 of a series of 64 cases with neurological involvement (Levitt, Rich, Kinde, Lewis, Gates, and Bond 1979); the remaining 55 patients had meningitis alone. However, a recent case (Vaheri, Julkunen, and Koskiniemi 1982) has suggested that occasionally this virus can produce chronic encephalomyelitis. The observation of Johnson, Johnson, and Edmonds (1967) that inoculation of the virus into suckling hamsters produced hydrocephalus and aqueduct stenosis may eventually prove to be of importance in relation to the aetiology of similar lesions in man.

Pathology

Mumps meningitis is rarely fatal; in encephalomyelitis the pathological changes are those of any viral encephalomyelitis with meningeal infiltration with inflammatory cells and perivascular demyelination and cellular infiltration within the nervous parenchyma (Miller *et al.* 1956; Bistrian, Phillips, and Kaye 1972).

Symptoms and signs

Nervous symptoms may occur at the onset or during the first stage of the disease, but usually develop somewhat later, in the adult male just before orchitis appear. They may occur without parotitis but with orchitis or may be the sole manifestation. The symptoms are usually those of acute meningitis, but encephalomyelitis may occur and in rare cases aphasia and hemiplegia or paraplegia have been described. Optic neuritis and optic atrophy are rare complications. Deafness, either unilateral or bilateral, is commoner.

A few cases of polyneuritis associated with mumps have been recorded, usually developing 2 or 3 weeks after the onset of the primary symptom. In many reported cases there has been flaccid paralysis of all four limbs, and in some cases cranial-nerve paralyses have occurred, most often facial paralysis. Isolated facial palsy occurs rarely.

The CSF usually shows a marked lymphocytosis. This is often present in mumps in the absence of any meningeal symptoms and may also occur in contacts who never develop other symptoms of the disease.

Diagnosis

The parotitis usually renders the diagnosis easy. In cases of lymphocytic meningitis for which no cause is apparent, inquiry should always be made whether symptoms of parotitis or orchitis have been present, as this may not have been mentioned spontaneously.

Tests for complement-fixing antibodies in paired sera (Enders and Cohen 1942; Kane, Cohen and Levens 1945) or CSF may confirm the diagnosis and occasionally the virus can be isolated from the fluid (Bistrian, Phillips, and Kaye 1972). Immunoprecipitation may also demonstrate specific antibodies against mump-virus envelope glycoprotein (Vaheri *et al.* 1982).

Prognosis

Recovery from mumps meningitis is the rule, but the condition is rarely fatal. Patients with polyneuritis usually recover, though slowly or incompletely. The mortality rate of encephalomyelitis is about 20 per cent (Russell and Donald 1958).

Treatment

Treatment is purely symptomatic. Specific mumps immune globulin may be used to protect susceptible adolescents and adults during an epidemic and active immunization with a vaccine may confer temporary immunity.

References

Bistrian, B., Phillips, C. A., and Kaye, I. S. (1972). Fatal mumps meningoencephalitis. *J. Am. med. Ass.* **222**, 478.

Collens, W. S. and Rabinowitz, M. A. (1928). Mumps polyneuritis; quadriplegia with bilateral facial paralysis. *Arch. intern. Med.* **41**, 61.

Enders, J. F. and Cohen, S. (1942). Detection of antibodies by complement-fixation in sera of man and monkey convalescent from mumps. *Proc. Soc. exp. Biol.* **1**, 180.

Finklestein, H. (1938). Meningo-encephalitis in mumps. *J. Am. med. Ass.* **111**, 17.

Gordon, M. H. (1927). Experimental production of the meningo-encephalitis of mumps. *Lancet* **i**, 652.

Grist, N. R. (1967). Acute viral infections of the nervous system. *Proc. R. Soc. Med.* **60**, 696.

Harris, W. and Bethell, H. (1938). Meningo-encephalitis and orchitis as the only symptoms of mumps. *Lancet* **ii**, 422.

Johnson, R. T., Johnson, K. P., and Edmonds, C. J. (1967). Virus-induced hydrocephalus: development of aqueductal stenosis in hamsters after mumps infection. *Science* **157**, 1066.

Kane, L. W., Cohen, S., and Levens, J. H. (1945). Immunity in mumps. *J. exp. Med.* **81**, 93.

Lennette, E. H., Caplan, G. E., and Magoffin, R. L. (1960). Mumps virus infection simulating paralytic poliomyelitis. *Pediatrics* **25**, 788.

Levitt, L. P., Rich, T. A., Kindie, S. W., Lewis, A. L., Gates, E. H., and Bond, J. O. (1970). Central nervous system mumps: a review of 64 cases. *Neurology, Minneapolis* **20**, 829.

Miller, H. G., Stanton, J. B., and Gibbons, J. L. (1956). Para-infectious encephalomyelitis and related syndromes. *Q. J. med.* **25**, 427.

Russell, R. R. and Donald, J. C. (1958). The neurological complications of mumps. *Br. med. J.* **ii**, 27.

Vaheri, A., Julkunen, I., and Koskiniemi, M. L. (1982). Chronic encephalomyelitis with specific increase in intrathecal mumps antibodies. *Lancet* **ii**, 685.

The Coxsackie viruses

Following the isolation in Coxsackie, New York, of a virus which could produce paralysis in mice, the term Coxsackie or C. viruses has been applied to a group which now includes a number of enteroviruses. In infant mice some strains attack the muscles, and some the nervous system also. In man the chief clinical manifestations so far recognized are: (1) Aseptic meningitis. The CSF does not usually contain more than 100 cells per mm^3, and the percentage of neutrophils ranges from 10 to 50. The febrile period lasts on an average five days, and recovery is usually complete. However, it is now evident that the Coxsackie A7 virus, which closely resembles that of poliomyelitis, may on occasion cause paralysis which is similar to but generally less severe than that of poliomyelitis. This infection can occur in individuals immunized against poliomyelitis. In a series of hospital cases diagnosed neurologically over an eight-year period, paralysis was found in 70 per cent of poliovirus infections and in 19 per cent of Coxsackie A7 virus infections (Grist, Bell, and Assaud 1978). (2) Encephalomyelitis. Coxsackie virus of type B3 and B5 was cultured from throat swabs or faeces obtained from 10 patients suffering from encephalitis in Essex in 1965; one patient had a fatal necrotizing encephalitis and the B5 virus was isolated from her CSF (Heathfield, Pilsworth, Wall, and Corsellis 1967). Coxsackie A9 virus has also been shown to produce focal encephalitis causing acute infantile hemiplegia and porencephaly (Chalhub, Devivo, Siegel, Gado, and Feigin 1977). (3) Epidemic myalgia or pleurodynia. It is now established that Bornholm disease is usually caused by Coxsackie B5 virus and some patients also have pericarditis (Heathfield *et al.* 1967). Epidemic myalgia and acute aseptic meningitis may both occur in the same patient. (4) Herpangina. This is a febrile illness with pharyngitis characterized by vesicular or ulcerative lesions. Vomiting and abdominal pain may be present. (5) Encephalomyocarditis of the new-born (see Johnson 1982). Typically all enterovirus infections occur predominantly between July and October in the Northern Hemisphere.

Diagnosis depends upon the isolation of one of the Coxsackie viruses from the faeces, from oropharyngeal swabs, or from CSF, and the appearance of, or an increase in, neutralizing antibodies against the virus in the patient's serum at appropriate intervals.

C. virus has often been recovered from the faeces of patients suffering from poliomyelitis, but there is no evidence that either virus influences the patient's reaction to the other.

No specific treatment is known.

References

Chalhub, E. C., Devivo, D. C., Siegel, B. A., Gado, M. H., and Feigin, R. D. (1977). Coxsackie A9 focal encephalitis associated with acute infantile hemiplegia and porencephaly. *Neurology, Minneapolis* **27**, 574.

Giunchi, G. (1960). Clinical aspects of Coxsackie viruses. In *Virus meningo-encephalitis* (ed. G. E. W. Wolstenholme and M. P. Cameron). P. 37. Ciba Foundation, London.

Grist, N. R., Bell, E. J., and Assaad, F. (1978). Enteroviruses in human disease. *Prog. Med. Virol.* **24**, 114.

Heathfield, K. W. G., Pilsworth, R., Wall, B. J., and Corsellis, J. A. N. (1967). Coxsackie B5 infections in Essex, 1965, with particular reference to the nervous system. *Quart. J. Med.* **36**, 579.

Hummelen, K., Kirk, D., and Ostapick, M. (1954). Aseptic meningitis caused by Coxsackie virus and isolation of virus from cerebrospinal fluid. *J. Am. med. Ass.* **156**, 676.

Johnson, R. T. (1982). *Viral infections of the nervous system.* Raven Press, New York.

The Echo viruses

There are at least 28 distinct antigenic types of the Echo virus (enteric cytopathic human orphan). They infect the gastrointestinal tract and are excreted mainly in the stools. They cause a febrile illness, sometimes with a rash. Some types cause an acute aseptic meningitis and some encephalitis (Johnson 1982); it has been suggested that they can cause a poliomyelitis-like illness but it now seems more probable that in such cases paralysis may be caused by a concomitant infection with poliovirus or Coxsackie A7 virus, as enterovirus infections are commonly multiple. In the meningitic cases there may be more than 500 cells per mm^3, usually mainly mononuclear, in the CSF. The virus may be isolated from the fluid or stools. Antibodies may be present in the blood.

References

Grist, N. R. (1961). Echo viruses. In *Virus meningo-encephalitis* (ed. G. E. W. Wolstenholme and M. P. Cameron), p. 17. Ciba Foundation, London.

Johnson, R. T. (1982). *Viral infections of the nervous system.* Raven Press, New York.

Kahlmeter, O. (1961). Clinical aspects of Echo viruses. In *Virus meningo-*

encephalitis. (ed. G. E. W. Wolstenholme and M. P. Cameron), p. 24. Ciba Foundation, London.

Acute haemorrhagic conjunctivitis (AHC)

This virus, closely related to the Coxsackie and Echo viruses, usually causes acute haemorrhagic conjunctivitis but has been shown in epidemics in India to cause a radiculomyelopathy in some cases (Wadia, Irani, and Katrak 1972; Bharucha and Mondkar 1972); inoculation of the virus into monkeys caused an inflammatory myelopathy (Kono, Uchida, Sasagana, Akao, Kodama, Mukoyama, and Fujiwara 1973). It is now known that the virus concerned is enterovirus 70 (EV70) and in a recent epidemic in the Americas (see *The Lancet* 1982) the conjunctivitis, usually in men, much less often in women and children, was followed after about two weeks in many patients by acute, hypotonic, areflexic proximal paralysis in the lower limbs. Isolated cranial-nerve palsies (notably of the facial nerve) are also seen.

References

Bharucha, E. P. and Mondkar, V. P. (1972). Neurological complications of a new conjunctivitis. *Lancet* **ii**, 970.

Kono, R., Uchida, N., Sasagawa, A., Akao, Y., Kodama, H., Mukoyama, J., and Fujiwara, T. (1973). Neurovirulence of acute-haemorrhagic-conjunctivitis virus in monkeys. *Lancet* **i**, 61.

The Lancet (1982). Neurovirulence of enterovirus 70. *Lancet* **i**, 373.

Wadia, N. H., Irani, P. F., and Katrak, S. M. (1972). Neurological complications of a new conjunctivitis. *Lancet* **ii**, 970.

Other miscellaneous viral CNS infections

The neurological complications of influenza, including influenza A encephalitis (Kennard and Swash 1981), and of infectious mononucleosis were described in Chapter 8. Post-infective encephalomyelitis following measles and other exanthemata will be considered in Chapter 11, but it should be noted that a true encephalitis due to measles virus, distinct both from SSPE and from post-infectious encephalitis, has been reported during the treatment of acute lymphoblastic leukaemia with immunosuppressive agents (*British Medical Journal* 1976) and immunosuppressive remedies have been noted to activate many other viruses including herpes simplex, zoster, cytomegalovirus, and adenoviruses (see Johnson, 1982). Epilepsia partialis continua has been reported in such cases of measles encephalitis (Aicardi, Goutieres, Arsenio-Nunes, and Lebon 1977) and there is considerable evidence to suggest that this clinical syndrome is commonly due to focal viral encephalitis (Johnson 1982). Spinal myoclonus (Hopkins and Michael 1974), subacute myoclonic spinal neuronitis (Campbell and Garland 1956), and progressive encephalomyelitis with rigidity (Howell, Lees, and Toghill 1979) are other somewhat ill-defined clinical syndromes which have been attributed to viral infection but in which no specific organism has been identified. A viral aetiology has also been postulated, so far without proof, in Mollaret's meningitis, Behçet's disease, and in the Vogt–Koyanagi–Harada syndrome of uveoparotid fever with encephalitis.

References

Aicardi, J., Goutieres, F., Arsenio-Nunes, M., and Lebon, P. (1977). Acute measles encephalitis in children with immunosuppression. *Pediatrics* **59**, 232.

British Medical Journal (1976). Measles encephalitis during immunosuppressive treatment. *Br. med. J.* **i**, 1552.

Campbell, A. M. G. and Garland, H. (1956). Subacute myoclonic spinal neuronitis. *J. Neurol. Neurosurg. Psychiat.* **19**, 268.

Hopkins, A. P. and Michael, W. F. (1974). Spinal myoclonus. *J. Neurol. Neurosurg. Psychiat.* **37**, 1112.

Howell, D. A., Lees, A. J., and Toghill, P. G. (1979). Spinal internuncial neurones in progressive encephalomyelitis with rigidity. *J. Neurol. Neurosurg. Psychiat.* **42**, 773.

Johnson, R. T. (1982). *Viral infections of the nervous system*, Raven Press, New York.

Kennard, C. and Swash, M. (1981). Acute viral encephalitis: its diagnosis and outcome. *Brain* **104**, 129.

Herpes zoster

Synonym. Shingles.

Definition. An acute infection involving primarily the first sensory neurone and the corresponding area of skin.

Pathology

The pathological changes in the nervous system are those of acute inflammation involving the first sensory neurone. The dorsal root ganglia and the corresponding sensory ganglia of the cranial nerves are the commonest sites, but the posterior horn of grey matter of the spinal cord, the dorsal roots and the peripheral nerves may also be involved. One or more successive metameric segments may be affected, but it is very rare for the lesion to be bilateral. The microscopic changes in the acute stage consist of haemorrhages and infiltration with mononuclear and occasional neutrophil leucocytes, especially in the form of perivascular cuffs, and degenerative changes in the nerve cells. Fibrosis and secondary degeneration follow in severe cases. Inflammatory changes are present in the neighbouring leptomeninges. In fatal cases of zoster meningo-encephalitis, neuronal chromatolysis, and perivascular infiltration are found at all levels of the nervous system up to the cerebral cortex (Biggart and Fisher 1938). Focal areas of necrosis may also be found with Type A intranuclear inclusion bodies in oligodendroglial cells and the causal virus has been isolated from and identified by electron microscopy in, such lesions (McCormick, Rodnitzky, Schochet, and McKee 1969). The cutaneous lesions show inflammatory infiltration of the epidermis and dermis, with vesicle formation produced by serous exudation beneath the stratum corneum. Acidophil nuclear inclusion bodies have been described in the cells of the vesicle epithelium. Angiitis may occur (see below).

Aetiology

The contagiousness of the infection is well established. It is now clear that the same DNA virus causes zoster and varicella (chickenpox) so that it is known as varicella-zoster (VZ) virus. Either may give rise to the other in contacts, though varicella follows exposure to zoster more frequently than the reverse. While varicella occurs in epidemics especially in winter and spring, zoster does not do so either by year or season (Johnson 1982). It has been suggested that herpes zoster may be due to reactivation of varicella virus which is latent in the tissues (Gajdusek 1965). The VZ virus is serologically distinct from that of herpes simplex but resembles it closely under the electron microscope (Kaplan 1969; McCormick *et al.* 1969); it is circular and between 196 and 218 nm in size (Nagler and Rake 1948; Farrant and O'Connor 1949).

Zoster may occur without any evident predisposing cause, or as a complication of some other disease or toxic state, especially when this causes damage to the first sensory neurone. These two groups are distinguished as 'idiopathic' and 'symptomatic' zoster, but the evidence indicates that both are due to the same virus. 'Symptomatic' zoster may be precipitated by intoxication with various poisons, and may occur in the course of infections such as pneumonia and tuberculosis or toxic states such as uraemia. It may complicate any lesion of the dorsal roots and can therefore follow fracture-dislocation of the spine, secondary carcinoma of the vertebral column, meningococcal and other forms of meningitis, subarachnoid hae-morrhage, prolapsed disc, and spinal tumour. It occasionally follows quite a slight injury.

Zoster may occur at any age, but is rare in infancy and more frequent in the second half of life than in the first. It is most often seen in patients over 50 and about half of those who live to 85 years of age will have had an attack (Johnson 1982).

The incubation period is from 7 to 24 days, and is usually about a fortnight.

Symptoms and signs

General symptoms

The eruption is often preceded by malaise, anorexia, and sometimes by fever, and there is enlargement of the lymph nodes draining the affected area of skin. The general symptoms are usually slight but may be severe in the aged.

Zoster of the limbs and trunk

The first local symptom is usually pain in the segment or segments involved; it is burning or shooting in character and is often associated with hyperpathia in the area of skin supplied by the affected roots. Three or four days after the onset of pain the eruption appears as a series of localized papules which develop into vesicles grouped together upon an erythematous base (Fig. 10.4). The eruption also has a segmental distribution. After a few days the eruption fades, the vesicles drying into crusts which separate, leaving small permanent scars. The skin in the affected area usually becomes partially or completely analgesic, though pain may persist, the association of pain with sensory loss being sometimes described as anaesthesia dolorosa. Thermal and postural sensibility may also be impaired. Pain may persist for weeks or months or indefinitely, and this 'post-herpetic neuralgia' is the more likely to occur the older the patient. Severe itching is sometimes a troublesome sequel.

Segmental complications of zoster

In addition to involving the first sensory neurone and the skin, zoster may cause a disturbance of function of other structures innervated by the spinal segment affected. Muscular wasting of segmental distribution is more common than generally realized (Weiss, Streifler, and Weiser 1975) and is probably due to extension of the infection from the posterior to the anterior horn of grey matter in the spinal cord. Such wasting is easily overlooked when intercostal muscles are involved, zoster being commonest in the dorsal roots (Fig. 10.4), but is more readily identified when the infection involves cervical or lumbar roots giving weakness in the upper or lower limb. These palsies may be permanent but often recover slowly over several months. Visceral manifestations of zoster may also occur. Arthritis is rare; it has been described in the joints of the hand and wrist complicating zoster involving the upper limb. There is severe pain and peri-articular swelling with limitation of movement, which is likely to be permanent. Radiographically the bones are rarefied. Other visceral manifestations of zoster include zoster of the pleura, and urinary bladder, and symptoms resembling those of duodenal ulceration.

Ophthalmic zoster

When the zoster virus invades the trigeminal ganglion, the eruption appears in some part of the cutaneous distribution of the trigeminal nerve, being usually confined to one division. When the ophthalmic division is involved, vesicles usually appear on the forehead but the cornea may be attacked, usually only when the eruption also appears on the part of the nose supplied by the nasociliary branch, as Jonathan Hutchinson pointed out. The corneal lesion takes the form of small, round infiltrations in the more superficial layers of the substantia propria. Often there is severe swelling of the conjunctiva and eyelids. Other orbital structures may be involved, rarely giving optic neuritis, followed by atrophy and

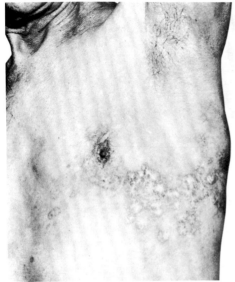

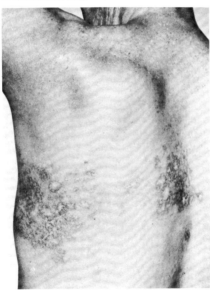

Fig. 10.4. Focal scarring and pigmentation due to herpes zoster in the mid-dorsal region on the left side (kindly provided by Dr J.D.Spillane).

blindness. Oculomotor paralyses may occur, the third nerve being more often affected than the fourth and sixth. Contralateral hemiparesis due to middle cerebral arteritis is an uncommon complication (Reshef, Greenberg, and Jankovic 1985). Trigeminal zoster, like zoster elsewhere, may be either idiopathic or symptomatic. In the latter case it may follow any intracranial lesion of the fifth nerve, including alcohol injection of the ganglion.

Geniculate zoster

Zoster of the geniculate ganglion was the explanation proposed by Ramsay Hunt (1915) for cases in which the vesicles are found in the auricle and less often on the anterior pillar of the fauces. There is pain in the ear and mastoid region radiating to the anterior pillar of the fauces and to the vertex. There may be a serosanguineous discharge from the ear. Taste may be lost on the anterior two-thirds of the tongue on the same side, the region innervated by the geniculate ganglion through the chorda tympani. Almost invariably the infection spreads to the trunk of the facial nerve leading to facial paralysis or clonic facial spasm. The eighth nerve may be involved, with resultant deafness or vestibular dysfunction and facial sensory loss on the same side is not uncommon. Some workers have

doubted whether the geniculate ganglion is always involved (Denny-Brown, Adams, and Fitzgerald 1944; O'Neill 1945) and have suggested that the seat of infection in such cases is more often the brainstem but in a typical case examined at autopsy there were unequivocal pathological changes in the geniculate ganglion (Aleksic, Budzilovich, and Lieberman 1973).

Meningitis, encephalitis, myelitis, and polyneuritis

Some degree of meningeal inflammation is the rule in zoster and is indicated by an excess of mononuclear cells and a raised protein content in the CSF. Less frequently clinical signs of meningitis are observed, headache and cervical rigidity complicating zoster of the trigeminal ganglion, and pain in the lower limbs and Kernig's sign being associated with dorsal or lumbar zoster. Extension of the infection to the cerebral substance or the spinal-cord white matter is less common. Nevertheless, zoster encephalitis and myelitis have been observed and necrosis of the cord resembling subacute necrotizing myelopathy was found in a fatal case (Rose, Brett, and Burston 1964). A Guillain–Barré syndrome has also been described (Gardner-Thorpe, Foster, and Barwick 1976). When the cord is involved, myoclonus, intractable hiccup, and spastic monoparesis or paraparesis may all occur.

Generalized zoster

Besides the segmental eruption, the patient may exhibit scattered vesicles. These may be few in number—'aberrant vesicles'— or a widespread eruption resembling varicella. Usually the generalized rash appears within three or four days of the onset, but the interval may be longer.

Diagnosis

The diagnosis of herpes zoster offers little difficulty, as in no other condition is there a vesicular eruption associated with pain and hyperpathia in segmental distribution. Herpes febrilis (simplex) is less painful, is usually situated in proximity to a mucous membrane, is often bilateral, and leaves neither residual pain nor scarring. Post-herpetic neuralgia is distinguished from other types of root pain by the history of the eruption, the scars of which can usually be found. Diagnosis is difficult in the pre-eruptive stage, but the possibility of zoster should be suggested by root pains of sudden onset accompanied by fever and malaise. Varicella-zoster antigen may be demonstrated in cells in the CSF when the diagnosis is in doubt (Peters, Versteeg, Bots, Lindeman, and Smeets 1979).

Prognosis

Most sufferers from zoster recover without residual symptoms, except for cutaneous scarring. One attack may confer permanent immunity but second or repeated attacks sometimes occur especially in the symptomatic form. Severe secondary infection of the vesicles is a rare complication. Zoster of the cornea may be followed by corneal ulceration, and the occurrence of optic atrophy has already been mentioned. Recovery from facial paralysis following geniculate zoster is often complete, less commonly incomplete (Heathfield and Mee 1978). Segmental muscular weakness due to anterior horn-cell involvement (Thomas and Howard 1972; Weiss, Streifler, and Weiser 1975) usually recovers in a few months but various focal neurological signs, including spastic paresis, may persist after encephalomyelitis. The most troublesome sequel of zoster is persistent intractable pain, which may endure for years in elderly patients.

Treatment

In most cases treatment is simple. Dusting powder and a dry dressing are all that are needed for the cutaneous eruption. Powerful analgesics are usually required. Dihydrocodeine or paracetamol may be sufficient in some cases but more often stronger remedies such as pethidine are required in the acute stage, particularly in ophthalmic cases. Amantadine hydrochloride had no significant effect in a double-blind trial carried out in general practice (Galbraith 1973). However, vidarabine produced rapid improvement in a case of zoster myelitis (Corston, Logsdail, and Godwin-Austen 1981) and acyclovir produced rapid healing of skin lesions and rapid relief of pain in a controlled trial (Peterslund, Seyer-Hansen, Ipsen, Esmann, Schonheyder, and Juhl 1981). Steroids are of no proven value. Persistent post-herpetic pain is a very troublesome complication, especially in the elderly. In severe cases analgesics are almost useless. It makes life a burden and may lead the patient to the verge of suicide. Morphine is contra-indicated owing to the risk of addiction and carbamazepine (*Tegretol*) is only rarely helpful. Irradiation of the spinal cord and nerve roots or of the trigeminal ganglion has been tried and is occasionally successful but rarely has a lasting effect. Surgical division of sensory nerves or roots and alcohol or phenol injection of the Gasserian ganglion have also been advocated but relief is often temporary. The local application for up to 20 minutes three times a day of an electrical vibrator to the painful area (Russell, Espir, and Morganstern 1957) or repeated freezing of the skin segment involved with an ethyl chloride spray (Taverner 1960), if continued for several weeks or months, may give lasting relief. Sometimes self-administered electrical cutaneous stimulation is even more successful (Nathan and Wall 1974). Often dihydrocodeine and chlorpromazine three or four times daily must be given for as long as the local treatment is continued. The accompanying depression which is often present in severe cases must also be treated with aminoxidase inhibitors or with amitriptyline, imipramine, or related remedies in appropriate dosage. Frequently it is best to admit the patient to hospital initially to teach him to use the vibrator, cooling spray, or stimulator, depending upon which is the more effective in the individual case.

References

Aleksic, S. N., Budzilovich, G. N., and Lieberman, A. N. (1973). Herpes zoster oticus and facial paralysis (Ramsay-Hunt syndrome): clinicopathologic study and review of literature. *J. neurol. Sci.* **20**, 149.

Biggart, J. H. and Fisher, J. A. (1938). Meningo-encephalitis complicating herpes zoster. *Lancet* **ii**, 944.

Brain, W. R. (1931). Zoster, varicella and encephalitis. *Br. med. J.* **1**, 81.

Chauffard, A. and Rendu, H. (1907). Méningite zonateuse tardive dans un cas de zona ophthalmique. *Bull. Soc. méd. Hôp. Paris* **24**, 141.

Corston, R. N., Logsdail, S., and Godwin-Austen, R. B. (1981). Herpes-zoster myelitis treated successfully with vidarabine. *Br. med. J.* **283**, 698.

Denny-Brown, D., Adams, R. D., and Fitzgerald, P. J. (1944). Pathologic features of herpes zoster: a note on 'geniculate herpes'. *Arch. Neurol. Psychiat., Chicago* **51**, 216.

Farrant, J. L. and O'Connor, J. L. (1949). Elementary bodies of varicella and herpes zoster. *Nature, London* **163**, 260.

Gajdusek, D. C. (1965). In *Slow and latent and temperate virus infections*, N.I.N.D.B. Monograph No. 2, p. 3. Bethesda, Maryland.

Galbraith, A. W. (1973). Treatment of acute herpes zoster with amantadine hydrochloride (Symmctrcl). *Br. med. J.* **4**, 693.

Gardner-Thorpe, C., Foster, J. B., and Barwick, D. D. (1976). Unusual manifestations of herpes zoster: a clinical and electrophysiological study. *J. neurol. Sci.* **28**, 427.

Heathfield, K. W. G. and Mee, A. S. (1978). Prognosis of the Ramsay Hunt syndrome. *Br. med. J.* **1**, 343.

Hunt, J. R. (1915) The sensory field of the facial nerve: a further contribution to the symptomatology of the geniculate ganglion. *Brain* **38**, 418.

Johnson, R. T. (1982). *Viral infections of the nervous system.* Raven Press, New York.

Lidsky, M. D., Klass, D. W., McKenzie, B. F., and Goldstein, N. P. (1962). Herpes zoster encephalitis. Case report with electroencephalographic and cerebrospinal fluid studies. *Ann. intern. Med.* **56**, 779.

McCormick, W. F., Rodnitzky, R. L., Schochet, S. S., and McKee, A. P. (1969). Varicella-zoster encephalomyelitis: a morphologic and virologic study. *Arch. Neurol., Chicago* **21**, 559.

Nagler, F. P. O. and Rake, G. (1948). The use of the electron microscope in the diagnosis of variola, vaccinia and varicella. *J. Bact.* **55**, 45.

Nathan, P. W. and Wall, P. D. (1974). Treatment of post-herpetic neuralgia by prolonged electric stimulation. *Br. med. J.* **3**, 645.

O'Neill, H. (1945). Herpes zoster auris ('geniculate' ganglionitis). *Arch. Otolaryng.* **42**, 309.

Peters, A. C. B., Versteeg, J. Bots, G. T. A. M., Lindeman, J., and Smeets, R. E. H. (1979). Nervous system complications of herpes zoster: immunofluorescent demonstration of varicella-zoster antigen in CSF cells. *J. Neurol. Neurosurg. Psychiat.* **42**, 452.

Peterslund, N. A., Seyer-Hansen, K., Ipsen, J., Esmann, V., Schonheyder, H., and Juhl, H. (1981). Acyclovir in herpes zoster. *Lancet* **ii**, 827.

Reshef, E., Greenberg, S.B., and Jankovic, J. (1985). Herpes zoster ophthalmicus followed by contralateral hemiparesis. *J. Neurol. Neurosurg. Psychiat.* **48**, 122.

Rose, F. C., Brett, E. M., and Burston, J. (1964). Zoster encephalomyelitis. *Arch. Neurol., Chicago* **11**, 155.

Russell, W. R., Espir, M. L. E., and Morganstern, F. S. (1957). Treatment of post-herpetic neuralgia. *Lancet* **i**, 242.

Schiff, C. I. and Brain, W. R. (1930). Acute meningo-encephalitis associated with herpes zoster. *Lancet* **ii**, 70.

Taverner, D. (1960). Alleviation of post-herpetic neuralgia. *Lancet* **ii**, 671.

Thomas, J. E. and Howard, F. M. (1972). Segmental zoster paresis—a disease profile. *Neurology, Minneapolis* **22**, 459.

Weiss, S., Streifler, M., and Weiser, H. J. (1975). Motor lesions in herpes zoster. Incidence and special features. *Eur. Neurol.* **13**, 332.

Cytomegalovirus infection

Cytomegalovirus is ubiquitous; the factors causing an infection which gives rise to clinical manifestations are unclear. The virus has an affinity for the subependymal cells lining the cerebral ventricles and, as infection of the fetus usually occurs in the third trimester of pregnancy, there is failure of brain growth with periventricular and intracerebral calcification (see Menkes 1980). Intranuclear inclusion bodies are found in neurones and endothelial cells.

The typical clinical manifestations include persistent neonatal jaundice, hepatosplenomegaly, anaemia, and thrombocytopenia. Neurologically, microcephaly and microgyria and, less often, hydrocephalus and other cerebral malformations occur. Variable ocular abnormalities include chorioretinitis, retinal calcification, cataract, and optic atrophy (Hanshaw 1971). It has been suggested that mental retardation may be the result of less overt chronic infection (Stern, Elek, Booth, and Fleck 1969). The virus can also cause rare cases of meningitis and/or encephalitis in adults, and an association, as yet somewhat dubious, with the Guillain-Barré syndrome has been postulated (Johnson 1982).

References

Hanshaw, J. B. (1971). Congenital cytomegalovirus infection: a fifteen year perspective. *J. infect. Dis.* **123**, 555.

Johnson, R. T. (1982). *Viral infections of the nervous system.* Raven Press, New York.

Menkes, J. H. (1980). *Textbook of child neurology*, 2nd edn. Lea and Febiger, Philadelphia.

Stern, H., Elek, S. D., Booth, J. C., and Fleck, D. G. (1969). Microbial causes of mental retardation. The role of prenatal infections with cytomegalovirus, rubella virus, and toxoplasma. *Lancet* **ii**, 443.

Progressive multifocal leucoencephalopathy

This condition, due to papovavirus, occurring usually in association with reticulosis, is considered on page 485.

Congenital rubella

An acute encephalitis rarely occurs during the course of rubella (see p. 304) and, as indicated previously, this virus can produce a clinical picture like that of subacute sclerosing panencephalitis (p. 280). However, Gregg (1941) showed that maternal rubella was sometimes responsible for congenital cataract and it is now evident that many developmental anomalies may result from fetal infection, being more severe the earlier in pregnancy the maternal infection occurs. The commonest abnormalities are deafness, heart disease, and cataract, but chorioretinitis, mental retardation of varying severity, epilepsy, and spasticity have all been recorded, as have various cerebral malformations, and spina bifida (Menkes 1980).

References

Gregg, N. (1941). Congenital cataract following German measles in the mother. *Trans. ophthal. Soc. Aust.* **3**, 35.

Menkes, J. H. (1980). *Textbook of child neurology*, 2nd edn. Lea and Febiger, Philadelphia.

Infectious mononucleosis

For the neurological complications of this disorder, due to infection with the Epstein–Barr virus, see page 258.

Acquired immune deficiency syndrome (AIDS)

Since 1979 much interest has centred upon the appearance of an infective syndrome carrying a high mortality, reported first in homosexual males in the USA but now known not to be confined to homosexuals or to the male sex. Many cases of this acquired cellular immune deficiency, sometimes associated with Kaposi's sarcoma, have subsequently been reported from the USA, from Europe, and from many other parts of the world (Waterson 1983). The condition is now known to be due to lymphocylopathic retrovirus variously known as human T-lymphotropic virus type III, lymphadenopathy—associated virus or AIDS—associated retrovirus (ARV). Full-blown AIDS is the late result of severe T helper cell immunodeficiency (see Cooper *et al.* 1985). Many patients present with a pneumonia due to *Pneumocystis carinii* or with fever, lymphadenopathy, loss of weight and diarrhoea, or with opportunistic infections of various kinds. Many neurological complications have been reported including cerebral abscesses due to *Toxoplasma gondii*, progressive multifocal leukoencephalopathy, cryptococcal meningitis, candidal meningitis, subacute encephalitis possibly due to cytomegalovirus, or diffuse lymphoma with meningeal involvement (Snider, Simpson, Nielsen, Gold, Metroka, and Posner 1983).

References

Cooper, D. A., Maclean, P., Finlayson, R., Michelmore, H. M., Gold, J., Donovan, B., Barnes, T. G., Brooke, P., and Penny, R. (1985). Acute AIDS retrovirus infection. *Lancet* **i**, 537.

Snider, W. D., Simpson, D. M., Nielsen, S., Gold, J. W. M., Metroka, C. E. and Posner, J. B. (1983). Neurological complications of acquired immune deficiency syndrome: analysis of 50 patients. *Ann. Neurol.* **14**, 403.

Waterson, A. P. (1983). Acquired immune deficiency syndrome. *Br.Med.J.* **286**, 743.

'Slow virus' infections

Kuru, scrapie, and Creutzfeldt–Jakob disease

Kuru, a progressive and fatal disease of the nervous system which occurs in the Fore people of the Eastern highlands of New Guinea,

has been shown to be due to a transmissible agent, presumably viral, though no virus has yet been identified. Commoner in young women, but also seen in male adults and rarely in children, the condition is characterized by difficulty in walking, tremulous legs, headache, and pains in the legs in some cases and by disorders of mood, frequent dementia, and sometimes hyperreflexia. The condition is usually fatal within 6 to 24 months (Hornabrook 1968); transmission from subject to subject has been thought to be due to cannibalism (it was customary for members of the family to eat the brain of the deceased as a mark of respect). The incubation period of the disease has been shown, following transmission to the chimpanzee by inoculation of brain material from affected subjects, to be a minimum of one and often several years (Beck, Daniel, Asher, Gajdusek, and Gibbs 1973; Gajdusek 1973; *The Lancet* 1974). The histological changes in affected brains, showing spongiform change with loss of ganglion cells and fibrillary astrocytosis, closely resemble those of scrapie, a disorder of sheep also believed to be of viral origin, and also with a long incubation period (Hadlow 1959; Alper 1972). The pathological changes of Creutzfeldt–Jakob disease or subacute spongiform encephalopathy of man (p. 379) are also similar and this condition, too, has been transmitted to the chimpanzee and to New World monkeys, again with a very long incubation period (Gibbs, Gajdusek, Asher, Alpers, Beck, Daniel, and Matthews 1968; Roos, Gajdusek, and Gibbs 1973). The condition has been transmitted from one human subject to another by corneal tranplantation, by neurosurgical procedures, and possibly by direct contact (Will and Matthews 1982). Virus-like particles and nucleoprotein-type filaments have been demonstrated by electron microscopy in brain tissue from two patients (Vernon, Horta-Barbosa, Fuccillo, Sever, Baringer, and Birnbaum 1970) but as yet the causal virus of this condition, too, has not been isolated.

References

Alper, T. (1972). The nature of the scrapie agent. *J. clin. Path., London* **25**, suppl. 154.

Beck, E., Daniel, P. M. Asher, D. M., Gajdusek, D. C., and Gibbs, C. J. (1973). Experimental kuru in the chimpanzee: a neuropathological study. *Brain* **96**, 441.

Gajdusek, D. C. (1973). Kuru and Creutzfeldt–Jakob disease. Experimental models of noninflammatory degenerative slow virus disease of the central nervous system. *Ann. clin. Res.* **5**, 254.

Gibbs, C. J., Gajdusek, D. C., Asher, D. M., Alpers, M. P., Beck, E., Daniel, P. M., and Matthews, W. B. (1968). Creutzfeldt–Jakob disease (spongiform encephalopathy): transmission to the chimpanzee. *Science, NY* **161**, 388.

Hadlow, W. J. (1959). Scrapie and kuru. *Lancet* **ii**, 289.

Hornabrook, R. W. (1968). Kuru—a subacute cerebellar degeneration. The natural history and clinical features. *Brain* **91**, 53.

The Lancet (1974). Kuru, Creutzfeldt–Jakob, and scrapie. *Lancet* **ii**, 1551.

Roos, R., Gajdusek, D. C., and Gibbs, C. J. (1973). The clinical characteristics of transmissible Creutzfeldt–Jakob disease. *Brain* **96**, 1.

Snider, W. D., Simpson, D. M., Nielsen, S., Gold, J. W. M., Metroka, C. E., and Posner, J. B. (1983). Neurological complications of acquired immune deficiency syndrome: analysis of 50 patients. *Ann. Neurol.* **14**, 403.

Vernon, M. L., Horta-Barbosa, L., Fuccillo, D. A., Sever, J. L., Baringer, J. R., and Birnbaum, G. (1970). Virus-like particles and nucleoprotein-type filaments in brain tissue from two patients with Creutzfeldt–Jakob disease. *Lancet* **i**, 964.

Waterson, A. P. (1983). Acquired immune deficiency syndrome. *Br. med. J.* **286**, 743.

Will, R. G. and Matthews, W. B. (1982). Evidence for case-to-case transmission of Creutzfeldt–Jakob disease. *J. Neurol. Neurosurg. Psychiat.* **45**, 235.

11

Neuroimmunology and the demyelinating diseases of the nervous system

The foundations of neuroimmunology

It will be convenient at this point to consider some recent developments in knowledge concerning normal and abnormal immune responses in the nervous and neuromuscular systems, not least because these have thrown light upon the pathogenesis of many neurological and neuromuscular disorders, notably many of those classified as demyelinating in type. These comments are, however, relevant to many other diseases in which disordered autoimmunity plays an important role, including the vasculitides (Chapter 4), some nervous complications of specific infections (Chapter 8), many viral infections (Chapter 10), paraneoplastic syndromes (Chapter 17), some forms of polyneuropathy (Chapter 18), myasthenia gravis, and some inflammatory diseases of muscle (Chapter 19).

Johnson (1982) has drawn attention to Panum's observation in 1846 that a single attack of measles often confers lifelong immunity. This observation documented two salient features of immune responses, namely their specificity and their memory. The specificity of such responses, it is now known, is conferred by surface configurations or receptors on cells of the immune system and by the active or variable ends of antibody molecules, while specialized lymphocytes confer memory; how the latter is preserved over many decades is still a mystery.

The next major development was Pasteur's recognition in the 1880s of the encephalomyelitis which could be induced in the rabbit by vaccination with rabies virus; an even more fundamental discovery was the production of experimental allergic encephalomyelitis by Rivers, Sprunt, and Berry (1933) followed later by the experimental induction of an allergic neuritis by Waksman and Adams (1955) and that of an allergic myositis by Dawkins (1965). It later became clear that man possesses many complex and heterogeneous immune systems which help the body to dispose of dangerous infectious agents, to protect against re-infection, and to monitor and attempt to destroy, for example, neoplastic cells that are identified as non-self. When these responses are harmful to the host they are called allergic or hypersensitivity reactions, but if they develop against a host's own antigens they are called autoimmune responses (Behan and Currie 1978; Aarli and Tönder 1980). Whether or not these are humoral or cell-mediated, or both, they demonstrate specificity and memory.

Modern immunology (see Humphrey 1982) dates from about 1960 when the general structure of antibodies was discovered and the fact that lymphocytes are the cells responsible for their production and for cellular immunity was established. While a central theme of immunology is the study of the properties and functions of lymphocytes and their products, it is also concerned with the behaviour of monocytes, macrophages, and granulocytes including mast cells. It also takes account of the activities of the complement system. Because antibodies are useful in identifying, isolating, and quantifying substances which are otherwise difficult to discern or assay, the production of antibodies, and especially those which are monoclonal with uniform combining sites specific for a single determinant on a molecule, has become a major industry in biological laboratories. These are used in immunofluorescent techniques, radioimmunoassay, and other diagnostic methods because of their specificity. An adult human has some 2×10^{12} lymphocytes which originate in adult life from haemopoietic stem cells concentrated in bone marrow. Their progeny develop in two lines, one of which migrates to the thymus in which they differentiate, emerging as thymus-dependent or T lymphocytes which subsequently undergo further maturation in peripheral lymphoid tissues. The other line also undergoes several maturation steps solely in peripheral tissues; these are the B lymphocytes. Both develop surface receptors; those on B lymphocytes are immunoglobulins similar to the antibodies which they secrete when suitably stimulated. The structure of receptor molecules on T lymphocytes is still unknown but they interact best with molecules associated with others controlled by the major histocompatibility complex (MHC) locus.

Neurological and neuromuscular disorders associated with disordered immunity

In the late-1940s and early-1950s, acute haemorrhagic leucoencephalitis and so-called brain purpura were regarded as the archetypes of allergic disease of the nervous system, and the post-infective and post-vaccinal encephalomyelitides were widely held to be due to some unknown allergic response. By analogy, the same was thought likely to be true of multiple sclerosis (MS), and although there were some who thought that the Guillain-Barré syndrome was genuinely an infective polyneuritis, the view that it was due to allergy was gaining ground. At about that time Walton and Adams (1958) and others suggested that polymyositis was almost certainly an autoimmune disease and the astute clinical observations of Simpson (1960) first gave credence to the view that this was also true of myasthenia gravis.

While there is now evidence that many encephalitides once thought to be post-infective or autoimmune may after all be due to, or associated with, direct viral invasion of the nervous system (Johnson 1982), the early concepts implicating disordered immunity in the diseases mentioned above have been amply confirmed by recent research. And while in some rare diseases of the nervous system, such as ataxia telangiectasia, and even myotonic dystrophy, some unusual and at times unexpected immunological defects have been defined, it has become apparent that the response of the host, sometimes to a specific infective agent and on other occasions to as yet undefined pathogens, has played a major role in modifying the disease process and consequentially the clinical features and course of such illnesses as neurosyphilis, subacute sclerosing panencephalitis, multifocal leucoencephalopathy, slow virus infections such as kuru and Creutzfeldt–Jakob disease, sarcoidosis, and some non-metastatic complications of malignant disease. Conversely, the acquired immune deficiency syndrome, itself clearly due to an infective agent (p. 294) may render the nervous system vulnerable to a variety of opportunistic infections. The new techniques of modern neuroimmunology have cast light upon some previously unexplained mysteries in each of these disorders.

Immunoregulation

Three major concepts have become central to an understanding of immunoregulation (Weiner and Hauser 1982a, b; Waksman 1983): these are immunoregulatory T cells, idiotype–antiidiotype networks, and immune response genes. It is also important to recall that each lymphocyte and its progeny stem from individual ancestors which bear unique membrane receptors capable of binding a specific antigen. When a lymphocyte is exposed to that antigen, whatever its nature, it divides or undergoes clonal expansion. Normally clones reactive against the host's own antigens probably exist but are not operational; when regulatory mechanisms break down and these autoreactive clones proliferate, autoimmune disorders may result.

Immunoregulatory T cells

Different subsets of regulatory T cells are identified through the surface glycoproteins which they possess and which serve as phenotypic markers for the functional properties of the cell. They consist of suppressor and helper (or inducer) cells (Fig. 11.1). These cells regulate both humoral immunity (B cell production of antibody) and cellular immune responses. Other effector cells including macrophages, neutrophil leucocytes, and mast cells are influenced by these immunoregulatory T cells and their products. Monoclonal antibodies selectively recognize T lymphocyte subpopulations. In man, approximately 65 per cent of peripheral blood lymphocytes are T cells; the remainder are B cells, monocytes, or cells without T or B cell markers (null cells).

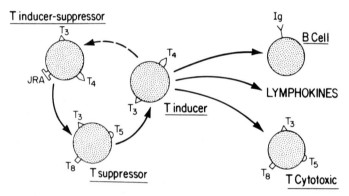

Fig. 11.1. The immunoregulatory T cell network in human beings. Intracting networks of T cells regulate the immune response and can be identified on the basis of surface glycoproteins, which serve as phenotypic markers for the functional properties of the cell. For example, T inducer cells, which bear T_4 and T_3 markers, induce B cells, which have immunoglobulin (Ig) on their surface, to produce immunoglubulin. B cells without T inducer cells will not produce immunoglobulin when stimulated. If sufficient T suppressor cells (which bear T_3, T_5, and T_8 markers) are added to B cells and T inducer cells, the production of antibody by B cells is shut off. T inducer cells also produce lymphokines, soluble substances that amplify the immune response and induce T cytotoxic cells. Although T suppressor and T cytotoxic cells have different functional properties, surface markers have yet to be found that distinguish between these cells. A subgroup of T inducer cells possess the 'JRA' marker (a surface structure reactive with serum from patients with juvenile rheumatoid arthritis). These cells are believed to be inducers of suppressor cells. Based on murine studies, a cell that induces the inducer–suppressor cell (represented by the dotted line) may exist, though it has yet to be described in humans. In summary, all T cells possess the T_3 marker, inducer cells possess the T_4 marker, and suppressor/cytotoxic cells possess the T_5 and T_8 markers. (Reproduced from Weiner and Hauser (1982) by kind permission of the authors, editor, and publisher.)

Idiotypes and the network hypothesis

The network theory states that the library of different receptors, whether on T or B lymphocytes, is likely to contain some that can recognize each different and unique receptor site on other receptor molecules. The name given to such a unique receptor site is an idiotype. In an initial random state, the concentration of any one idiotype is too low to stimulate lymphocytes bearing the corresponding antiidiotype, but when its concentration is increased following stimulation by an antigen, it can stimulate B cells to secrete

antiidiotype. Alternatively, it may stimulate T cells which act on cells expressing antiidiotype, either to help or more usually to shut them off (Humphrey 1982). In turn, the antiidiotype molecules stimulate other lymphocytes which express anti-antiidiotypes (Fig. 11.2) and an infinite network of interactions is potentially established; this will not only regulate the initial response to antigen but will leave the whole balance altered. It seems that it is the idiotype with which specific suppressor T cells react on helper T cells or B cells, and that the way in which specific T cells stimulate B cells to secrete, also involves reacting with the idiotype. Many experimental systems are now being used to study idiotype–antiidiotype interactions. For example, antiidiotypic antibodies against oligoclonal immunoglobulin G (IgG) from the CSF of patients with MS have been made in an attempt to determine the antigenic specificity of the immunoglobulin.

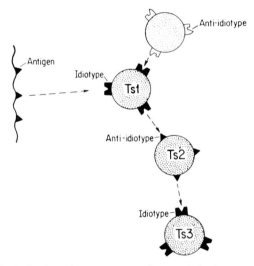

Fig. 11.2. Activation of a suppressor-cell network in the mouse. Antigen binds to specific receptors (idiotypes) on the surface of some T cells. These cells, the first-order cells of the suppressor network, are termed Ts1. Ts1 products then react with a second population of cells, Ts2, that possess complementary (antiidiotypic) receptors, or receptors which bind the idiotype. This population in turn reacts with a third subset of cells, Ts3, with anti-antiidiotypic (or idiotypic) receptors. Ts3 appears to represent the active cell that mediates suppression. Note that while the antiidiotype may be antigenically similar to the initial antigen, this is not always the case. (Reproduced from Weiner and Hauser (1982) by kind permission of the authors, editor, and publisher.)

Immune response genes

Most antigens elicit a complex network of functionally distinct T cells that regulate B cells and each other, and idiotypic–antiidiotypic reactions act within this network. But immune regulation also involves immune response genes, i.e. those which code for antigens within the major histocompatibility complex (MHC). In animals these gene products probably act in part by determining the way in which macrophages present antigens to T cells, thus influencing whether or not T cells will respond and whether the responding cells will be helper or suppressor. And the gene products may also determine the ultimate T cell repertoire while T cells are maturing in the thymus, so that susceptibility to autoimmune disorders may be strongly influenced by them. The human MHC contains four major loci, HLA-A, B, C, and D. Susceptibility to certain diseases is associated with particular haplotypes, the strongest association being that between HLA-B27 and ankylosing spondylitis. The D locus seems to be specifically involved in the regulation of suppressor and helper T cell networks, and in neurology multiple sclerosis appears to be associated with HLA-DR2 and myasthenia gravis with HLA-B8, though even these associations have been questioned. Attempts made to identify similar associations in other autoimmune diseases of the nervous and neuromuscular systems have as yet been inconclusive.

It is, however, of some interest that abnormalities of immuno-regulatory T cells have been observed in various human disease states such as lupus erythematosus, juvenile rheumatoid arthritis, haemolytic anaemia, and many more. In relation to nervous disease, however, there is clearly decreased suppression in MS (Weiner and Hauser 1982) but not in myasthenia gravis or the Guillain-Barré syndrome, while increased suppression occurs in lepromatous leprosy, cytomegalovirus infection, and sarcoid.

Immunoregulation in neurological disease

One can apply to each of the major autoimmune disorders of the nervous system the questions posed by Weiner and Hauser (1982) in asking first what is the antigen, secondly what is the mechanism of immune damage, and thirdly what triggers the autoimmune response, to see how current knowledge has been extended by modern neuroimmunology.

Multiple sclerosis (MS)

While we know that myelin basic protein (MBP) is the encephalitogenic determinant which can produce experimental allergic encephalomyelitis (EAE) and optic neuritis (EON) in animals (Wisniewski and Bloom 1975; Wisniewski and Keith 1977; Traugott, Stone, and Raine 1979), there is no convincing evidence that this antigen plays a major role in the pathogenesis of MS. While there is also some evidence to suggest that there may be a surface antigen on the CNS oligodendrocytes which is important in EAE and in this disease (Lisak, Saida, Kennedy, Saida, Silberberg, and Leibowitz 1980), no such antigen or antigens have yet been defined, nor is there any evidence that myelin-associated glycoprotein plays a major role. However, lymphocyte sensitivity to MBP has been demonstrated in chronic progressive MS (Brinkman, Nillesen, Hommes, Lamers, de Pauw, and Delmotte 1982). That oligoclonal IgG is locally produced within the CNS in this disease seems well established (Tourtellotte and Ma 1978) but we do not know what stimulates its production. Similarly, there is no information available at present as to what causes the suppressor-cell loss in this disease (Antel, Arnason, and Medof 1979), and while exposure to several viruses, including measles and canine distemper, has been thought by some to play an important part in pathogenesis (see below), this view remains somewhat speculative. Hence, not just one but several enigmas persist.

Myasthenia gravis

Here at least we are on safer ground in relation to antigen identification, but recent work has clearly shown that AChR is not a single antigen but contains multiple determinants (Lisak and Barchi 1982). That the immune damage is antibody-mediated is clear in the light of mother-to-child transmission of neonatal myasthenia, and experimental transfer of the disease through a serum IgG fraction. But in looking at what triggers the immune response, we are on much less certain ground. Certainly there is no evidence that any specific virus or group of viruses play a role, and various significant associations, as with thyroid disease, remain to be fully explained. Nevertheless, evidence is growing to suggest (Lisak and Barchi 1982) that AChR-specific helper cells are generated in the thymus and migrate to the periphery where they promote anti-AChR antibody synthesis. In this disease we seem to be much closer to a full understanding of the nature of the process than in MS.

Guillain–Barré syndrome

Clearly the antigen must be a component of peripheral nerve, but we still do not know which of the three major proteins (P0, P1, and P2), if indeed it is any of these, is responsible. Probably P1 equates with MBP, while P2 is most effective in inducing experimental allergic neuritis in animals. That cell-mediated immunity plays an important role is clear and there is histological and ultra-structural evidence that activated macrophages strip myelin from the affected nerves. Perhaps this is T cell-induced but there is also good evidence that immune complexes play a role, as experimental demyelination of peripheral nerve may be induced by serum derived from patients with this disease (see Chapter 19). When one looks at factors which potentially trigger the response, the situation is more complex since in different cases a myriad of viruses have been implicated, including the Epstein–Barr agent, cytomegalovirus, Echo, Coxsackie, varicella, mumps, and many more. The occurrence of the condition after surgical operation is well substantiated and an association with lymphoma has been described, as has one with mycoplasma infection. There seems little doubt that the precipitants may be multifactorial, but how they produce their effect remains to be determined.

Polymyositis

It should be noted (Chapter 19) that there may be significant differences, not only clinically but also immunologically, between certain cases of childhood polymyositis and dermatomyositis on the one hand and the superficially similar clinical disorder occurring in adults on the other. While the evidence that the condition is autoimmune seems incontrovertible, the nature of the antigen remains undefined. Certainly it is not just myosin of skeletal muscle, though it seems that Z band protein may be of importance. No clear-cut association with any HLA haplotype has been defined, but the disease has been described in association with C2 deficiency (Dawkins, Garlepp, and McDonald 1982). Several workers have demonstrated cytotoxicity upon muscle in culture of killer T cells derived from patients with the disease (Mastaglia and Walton 1982) but others have failed to substantiate these findings. However, in some negative studies it appears that the patients being examined were under treatment with prednisone at the time. Cambridge and Stern (1981) and Isenberg and Cambridge (1982) have used a sensitive assay of specific *in vitro* muscle-cell cytotoxicity using radio-labelled carnitine which is only taken up by muscle cells in the culture; their findings support the concept of cell-mediated myotoxicity in this disease, and Rowe, Isenberg, McDougall, and Beverley (1981) have demonstrated large numbers of T lymphocytes in the infiltrates found in muscle biopsy sections in many polymyositis patients. That circulating immune complexes also play an important part in many cases is, however, evident (Behan, Barkas, and Behan 1982), and Walker, Mastaglia, and Roberts (1982) have found serum C3 and C4 complement to be increased in many patients. Thus, while cell-mediated immune responses appear predominant, disordered humoral immunity is clearly also of considerable importance. There is also convincing evidence that viral particles in skeletal muscle may be a significant precipitating factor. How associated malignant disease plays a role, as it undoubtedly does in patients with dermatomyositis over middle age, is still uncertain.

References

Aarli, J. A. and Tönder, O. (1980). *Immunological aspects of neurological diseases.* Karger, Basle.

Antel, J. P., Arnason, B. G. W., and Medof, M. E. (1979). Suppressor cell function in multiple sclerosis: correlation with clinical disease activity. *Ann. Neurol.* **5**, 338.

Behan, P. O. and Currie, S. (1978). *Clinical neuroimmunology.* Saunders, London.

Behan, W. M. H., Barkas, T., and Behan, P. O. (1982). Detection of immune complexes in polymyositis. *Acta neurol. scand.* **65**, 320.

Brinkman, C. J. J., Nillesen, W. M., Hommes, O. R., Lamers, K. J. B., de Pauw, B. E. J., and Delmotte, P. (1982). Cell-mediated immunity in multiple sclerosis as determined by sensitivity of different lymphocyte populations to various brain tissue antigens. *Ann. Neurol.* **11**, 450.

Cambridge, G. and Stern, C. M. (1981). The uptake of tritium-labelled carnitine by monolayer cultures of human fetal muscle and its potential as a label in cytotoxicity studies. *Clin. Exp. Immunol.* **43**, 211.

Dawkins, R. L. (1965). Experimental myositis associated with hypersensitivity to muscle. *J. Path. Bact.* **90**, 6l9.

——, Garlepp, M., and McDonald, B. (1982). Immunopathology of muscle. In *Skeletal muscle pathology,* (ed. F. L. Mastaglia and J. N. Walton) Chapter 15. Churchill Livingstone, Edinburgh.

Humphrey, J. H. (1982).The value of immunological concepts in medicine. *J. R. Coll. Physns., London.* **16**, 141.

Isenberg, D. and Cambridge, G. (1982). Polymyositis. *Hosp. Update* **8**, 639.

Johnson, R. T. (1982). *Viral infections of the nervous system.* Raven Press, New York.

Lisak, R. P. and Barchi, R. L. (1982). *Myasthenia gravis.* Saunders, Philadelphia.

——, Saida, T., Kennedy, P. G. E., Saida, K., Silberberg D. H., and Leibowitz, S. (1980). EAE, EAN, and galactocerebroside sera bind to oligodendrocytes and Schwann cells. *J. neurol. Sci.* **48**, 287.

Mastaglia, F. L. and Walton J. N. (1982). Inflammatory myopathies. In *Sketetal muscle pathology* (ed. F. L. Mastaglia and J. N. Walton), Chapter 11. Churchill Livingstone, Edinburgh.

Panum, P. L. (1940). *Observations made during the epidemic of measles on the Faroe Islands in the year 1846.* American Public Health Association, Delta Omega Society, New York.

Rivers, T. M., Sprunt, D. H., and Berry, G. P. (1933). Observations on attempts to produce acute disseminated encephalomyelitis in monkeys. *J. exp. Med.* **58**, 39.

Rowe, D., Isenberg, D., McDougall, J., and Beverley, P. C. L. (1981). Characterization of polymyositis infiltrates using monoclonal antibodies to human leucocyte antigens. *Clin. exp. Immunol.* **45**, 290.

Simpson, J. A. (1960). Myasthenia gravis: a new hypothesis. *Scot. med. J.* **5**, 419.

Tourtellotte, W. W. and Ma, B. I. (1978). Multiple sclerosis: the blood–brain–barrrier and the measurement of de novo central nervous system IgG synthesis. *Neurology, Minneapolis.* **28**, 76.

Traugott, U., Stone, S. H., and Raine, C. S. (1979). Chronic relapsing experimental allergic encephalomyelitis. *J. neurol. Sci.* **41**, 17.

Waksman, B. H. and Adams, R. D. (1955). Allergic neuritis. An experimental disease of rabbits induced by the injection of peripheral nervous tissue and adjuvants. *J. exp. Med.* **102**, 213.

Walker, G. L., Mastaglia, F. L., and Roberts, D. F. (1982). A search for genetic influence in idiopathic inflammatory myopathy. *Acta neurol. scand.* **66**, 432.

Waksman, B. H. (1983). Immunity and the nervous system: basic tenets. *Ann. Neurol.* **13**, 587.

Walton, J. N. and Adams, R. D. (1958). *Polymyositis.* Livingstone, Edinburgh.

Weiner, H. L. and Hauser, S. L. (1982). Neuroimmunology I: immunoregulation in neurological disease. *Ann. Neurol.* **11**, 437.

——, —— (1982). Neuroimmunology II: antigenic specificity of the nervous system. *Ann. Neurol.* **12**, 499.

Wisniewski, H. M. and Bloom, B. R. (1975). Experimental allergic optic neuritis (EAON) in the rabbit: a new model to study primary demyelinating diseases. *J. neurol. Sci.* **24**, 257.

—— and Keith, A. B. (1977). Chronic relapsing experimental allergic encephalomyelitis: an experimental model of multiple sclerosis. *Ann. Neurol.* **1**, 144.

Classification of the demyelinating diseases

Large and important group of diseases of the nervous system possess, as a common pathological feature, foci in which the myelin sheaths of the nerve fibres are destroyed. These foci, mainly situated in the white matter, vary in size, shape, and distribution and also in the acuteness of the pathological process of which they are the result, but they are sufficiently similar in the different diseases to justify the appelation, *demyelinating diseases of the nervous system.* However, the axis cylinders often suffer in varying degree as well as their myelin sheaths and it is not certain that myelin destruction is always the primary change: it may be part of a more diffuse process. Moreover, as Lumsden (1961) pointed out, 'we mostly use the word 'myelin' for a complex structural unit consisting of a formed sheath of myelin with satellite nutrient cells'. Not

only does it not follow, but it is very unlikely, that destruction of myelin is always the result of the same process. Myelin has been the subject of much study (see Pette, Westphal, Burdzy, and Kallos 1969; Field, Bell, and Carnegie 1972; Adams 1972; Lumsden 1972; Wisniewski 1977; Davison and Cuzner 1977). Much new information has been derived from studies involving the electron microscope and tissue culture of myelin, from biochemical studies of its composition (Eylar 1971; Martenson, Deibler and Kies 1971; Adams 1972; Thompson 1977), from complex immunological investigations of demyelinating processes in animals and man (see Rowland 1971; Lumsden 1972; Lassmann and Wisniewski 1979a, b; Weiner and Hauser 1982), and from virological studies (Dal Canto and Rabinowitz 1982); these investigations will, where necessary, be considered in commenting upon individual disease entities within his group.

Apart from the fact that all but the most acute forms of demyelinating disease are sometimes familial, and that some follow acute infections, especially the exanthemata such as measles and smallpox or vaccination, the aetiology of most of the demyelinating disorders remains obscure, though many seem to be due to a complex interrelationship of genetic, infective, immunological, and biochemical mechanisms. An aetiological classification is therefore impossible.

Any attempt to classify these conditions upon a pathological basis raises the difficulty that although many pathological varieties have been distinguished, they overlap with one another. A purely clinical classification is equally unsatisfactory in that it fails to accommodate transitional forms with features of two clinical varieties which can usually be clearly distinguished. The best available classification is clinico-pathological, based upon the recognition that clinical and pathological features can often be closely correlated. Such a classification must be provisional and qualified by the recognition of transitional forms. Increased knowledge may well show that clinico-pathological distinctions do not correspond to aetiological differences, being simply an expression of differences in the acuteness of the process, which may be influenced by the patient's genetic constitution, his age, the nature of the precipitating factors, and also by immunological mechanisms. There is growing evidence to indicate that some such diseases are precipitated by viral or other infections and, as many now believe, that post-infectious encephalomyelitis may be due to actual viral invasion of the nervous system; others take the view that the primary pathological process is autoimmune, whether lymphocyte-mediated or humoral, and that any virus present acts merely as the trigger which initiates the process. It has also become clear that many disorders traditionally embraced by the term diffuse sclerosis are due to specific metabolic defects which influence the formation or lipid composition of myelin and that they should be considered to be dysmyelinating disorders or so-called leukodystrophies (see pp. 320 and 460), i.e. disorders of myelin formation or composition rather than demyelinating diseases in the traditional sense. The confusion which has arisen in relation to Schilder's disease and through the use of 'diffuse sclerosis' to identify demyelinating as well as dysmyelinating disorders will be considered later in this chapter. It is uncertain, therefore, when a demyelinating disorder affects the brain and spinal cord, whether encephalitis or encephalopathy, myelitis or myelopathy is the more appropriate term. Encephalitis and myelitis are employed here as being less cumbersome and better known. Table 11.1 gives a convenient clinico-pathological classification.

Demyelination may also be produced in man and animals by many drugs, toxic agents, and viruses. Thus it was an occasional complication of the arsphenamine treatment of syphilis and in animals it may result from cyanide intoxication (Adams 1972) when it shows some resemblance to the demyelination which is a feature of the pathological changes in the nervous system in human vitamin B_{12} deficiency. Demyelination may also be produced experimentally by diphtheria toxin (Weller 1965; Hallpike and Adams

Table 11.1. *The demyelinating diseases*

Variety	Synonyms	Incidence	Distribution of lesions	Course
Acute disseminated enchephalomyelitis following acute infections, e.g. measles, chickenpox, smallpox, and following vaccination against smallpox and rabies	Acute perivascular myelinoclasis	Sporadic, very rarely familial: usually in children or adolescents	Patchy in brain and spinal cord, tending especially to a perivenous distribution; rarely in optic nerves	Acute or subacute and self-limited
Acute haemorrhagic leuco-encephalitis	Acute necrotizing haemorrhagic leuco-encephalopathy	Sporadic, in all age groups	Patchy in white matter of brain, generally perivascular	Explosive, often fatal within 24–48 hours
Disseminated myelitis with optic neuritis	Neuromyelitis optica Ophthalmoneuromyelitis (Devic's disease)	Sporadic (once reported in twins), any age from childhood onwards	Massive in optic nerves and chiasm and spinal cord which may undergo softening and cavitation	Acute or subacute in onset; sometimes self-limited, sometimes relapsing and progressive
Multiple sclerosis	Insular sclerosis Disseminated sclerosis	Sporadic, occasionally familial; usually in the first half of adult life	Patchy in brain, optic nerves, and spinal cord, the lesions being multiple and successive	Progressive, ranging from acute to extremely chronic with a conspicuous tendency to remissions and relapses
'Diffuse sclerosis'	Encephalitis periaxialis diffusa (Schilder's disease)* Centrolobar sclerosis. Progressive degenerative subcortical encephalopathy Concentric demyelination (Baló's disease).	Sporadic, usually in infancy and adolescence, less often in adult life	Diffuse and massive, usually symmetrical, cerebral much more than spinal	Acute, subacute, and chronic, steadily progressive or intermittent
Central pontine myelinolysis	No synonyms at present	Sporadic, usually in alcoholic or malnourished patients or in those with chronic liver disease	Central in pons	Subacute, progressive

*It now seems likely that X-linked recessive adrenoleucodystrophy, once equated with Schilder's disease, is a dysmyelinating disorder as are the other leucodystrophies (Chapter 13).

1969) but in human diphtheria this change is usually confined to the peripheral nerves. Similarly, demyelination due to organophosphorus compounds (Cavanagh 1954, 1963) is due to a 'dying-back' degeneration of the axon, again particularly in peripheral nerves, with secondary demyelination. In the brain, secondary demyelination can result from oedema, trauma, vascular disease, or hypercapnic hypoxia (Cuzner, Davison, and Thompson 1981). Vascular damage due to circulating immune complexes has been suggested as another cause (Reik 1980), while it has been suggested that glial changes in areas of demyelination may rarely lead to neoplastic transformation (Anderson, Hughes, Jefferson, Smith, and Waterhouse 1980).Naturally occurring dysmyelinating disorders of animals, including swayback disease of sheep due to copper deficiency (Innes and Shearer 1940; Howell, Davison, and Oxberry 1964) are known to be different from any naturally occur-

ring demyelinating disease which occurs in man though there is a possible indirect analogy with Menkes' kinky hair disease (Chapter 13), but not with other leucodystrophies. However, as already seen, several close analogies can be drawn between EAE and human encephalomyelitis. The analogy between relapsing EAE and MS is less clear-cut, just as the experimental forms of demyelination produced by viruses and/or various chemicals differ in certain important respects from those seen in MS (see Allen 1981). Certainly the view that subacute fat embolism is responsible for MS (James 1982) has won few adherents. The pathophysiology of remission in this disease, however (McDonald 1974) continues to excite interest and it has been suggested (Dalakas, Wright, and Prineas 1980) that this may be due to an astrocytic lesion with inflammation and oedema causing conduction block without actual demyelination.

References

Adams, C. W. M. (1972). *Research on multiple sclerosis*. Thomas, Springfield, Illinois.

Allen, I. V. (1981). The pathology of multiple sclerosis – fact, fiction and hypothesis. *Neuropath. appl. Neurobiol.* **7**, 169.

Anderson, M., Hughes, B.,Jefferson, M., Smith, W. T., and Waterhouse, J. A. H. (1980). Gliomatous transformation and demyelinating diseases. *Brain* **103**, 603.

Cavanagh, J. B. (1954). The toxic effects of triorthocresyl phosphate on the nervous system—an experimental study in hens. *J. Neurol. Neurosurg. Psychiat.* **17**, 163.

—— (1963). Organo-phosphorus neurotoxicity, a model 'dying-back' process comparable to certain human neurological disorders. *Guy's Hosp. Rep.* **112**, 303.

Cuzner, M. L., Davison, A. N., and Thompson, R. H. S. (1981). The demyelinating diseases of the central nervous system. In *The molecular basis of neuropathology* (ed. A. N. Davison and R. H. S. Thompson), Chapter 15. Arnold, London.

Dalakas, M., Wright, R. G., and Prineas, J. W. (1980). Nature of the reversible white matter lesion in multiple sclerosis: effects of acute inflammation on myelinated tissue studied in the rabbit eye. *Brain*, **103**, 515.

Dal Canto, M. C. and Rabinowitz, S. G. (1982). Experimental models of virus-induced demyelination of the central nervous system. *Ann. Neurol.* **11**, 109.

Davison, A. N. and Cuzner, M. L. (1977). Immunochemistry and biochemistry of myelin. *Br. med. Bull.* **33**, 60.

Eylar, E. H. (1971). Basic Al protein of myelin: relationship to experimental allergic encephalomyelitis. In *Immunological disorders of the nervous system* (A.R.N.M.D. Vol. XLIX) (ed. L. P. Rowland) p. 50. Williams and Wilkins, Baltimore.

Field, E. J., Bell, T. M., and Carnegie, P. R. (1972). *Multiple sclerosis: progress in research*. North Holland, Amsterdam.

Finean, J. B. (1961). Electron microscopy of the myelin. *Proc. R. Soc. Med.* **54**, 19.

Hallpike, J. F. and Adams, C. W. M. (1969). Proteolysis and myelin breakdown: a review of recent histochemical and biochemical studies. *Histochem. J.* **1**, 559.

Howell, J. McC., Davison, A. N., and Oxberry, J. (1964). Biochemical and neuropathological changes in swayback. *Res. vet. Sci.* **5**, 376.

Innes, J. R. M. and Shearer, G. D. (1940). Swayback, a demyelinating disease of lambs with affinities to Schilder's encephalitis in man. *J. comp. Neurol.* **53**, 1.

James, P. B. (1982). Evidence for subacute fat embolism as the cause of multiple sclerosis. *Lancet* **i**, 380.

Lassmann, H. and Wisniewski, H. M. (1979*a*). Chronic relapsing experimental allergic encephalomyelitis: clinicopathological comparison with multiple sclerosis. *Arch. Neurol. Chicago.* **36**, 490.

—— and —— (1979*b*). Chronic relapsing experimental allergic encephalomyelitis: morphological sequence of myelin degradation. *Brain Res.* **169**, 357.

Lumsden, C. E. (1961). Consideration of multiple sclerosis in relation to the autoimmunity process. *Proc. R. Soc. Med.* **54**, 11.

—— (1972). The clinical pathology of multiple sclerosis. In *Multiple sclerosis: a reappraisal* (ed. D. McAlpine, C. E. Lumsden, and E. D. Acheson) Part III, p. 311. Churchill-Livingstone, Edinburgh.

McDonald, W. I. (1974). Pathophysiology of multiple sclerosis. *Brain* **97**, 179.

Martenson, R. E., Deibler, G. E., and Kies, M. W. (1971). Microheterogeneity and species-related differences among myelin basic proteins. In *Immunological Disorders of the Nervous System* (A.R.N.M.D., vol XLIX) (ed. L. P. Rowland) p. 76. Williams and Wilkins, Baltimore.

Pette, E., Westphal, O., Burdzy, K., and Kallos, P. (1969). *Pathogenesis and etiology of demyelinating diseases*. Karger, Basle.

Reik, L. (1980). Disseminated vasculomyelinopathy: an immune complex disease. *Ann. Neurol.* **7**, 291.

Rowland, L. P. (Ed.) (1971). *Immunological disorders of the nervous system* (A.R.N.M.D., vol. XLIX). Williams and Wilkins, Baltimore.

Thompson, E. J. (1977). Laboratory diagnosis of multiple sclerosis: immunological and biochemical aspects. *Br. med. Bull.* **33**, 28.

Weiner, H. L. and Hauser, S. L. (1982). Neuroimmunology I: immunoregulation in neurological disease. *Ann Neurol.* **11**, 437.

Weller, R. O. (1965). Diphtheritic neuropathy in the chicken: an electron-microscopic study. *J. Path. Bact.* **89**, 591.

Wisniewski, H. M. (1977). Immunopathology of demyelination in autoimmune diseases and virus infections. *Br. med. Bull.* **33**, 54.

Wright, G. P. (1961). The metabolism of myelin. *Proc. R. Soc. Med.* **54**, 26.

Acute disseminated encephalomyelitis

Synonym. Acute perivascular myelinoclasis.

Definition. An acute disorder characterized by demyelination of the nervous system, usually in perivascular distribution, and by symptoms of damage to the brain and spinal cord, especially in the white matter, following infection with the virus of one of the exanthemata, such as measles, German measles, smallpox, mumps, or chickenpox, or vaccination against smallpox or rabies, banal infection, or occurring spontaneously.

Pathology

Naked-eye changes consist merely of congestion and oedema of the nervous system. Microscopically (Fig. 11.3) there is marked perivascular infiltration of the brain and spinal cord with lymphocytes and plasma cells both within the perivascular spaces and still more conspicuously at a greater distance from the vessels. In the white matter the most striking feature is the presence of zones of demyelination around the vessels, especially the veins. Activated microglial cells and fat-laden macrophages are common in the demyelinated areas and oligodendroglial cells are often pyknotic but the neurones usually remain intact, unlike the usual findings in viral encephalomyelitis (Adams and Kubik 1952; De Vries 1960). The most intense changes are often found in cerebral white matter and/or in the lumbosacral regions of the spinal cord, and in the pons. In the midbrain the substantia nigra is the structure most affected. Inflammatory changes may be present throughout the whole length of the nervous system. Meningeal infiltration is relatively slight. Herkenrath (1935) reported a case of recovery from post-vaccinal encephalitis followed by death from another cause 18 months later. The nervous system showed only a few fat-laden macrophages in the perivascular spaces of the cerebellum, pons, medulla, and spinal cord. It was inferred that perivascular demyelination is capable of complete reversal resulting in clinical and anatomical recovery.

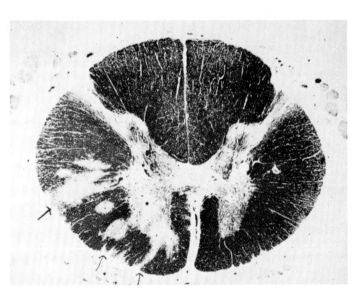

Fig. 11.3. Spinal cord in post-vaccinal encephalomyelitis. The arrows indicate patches of demyelination. (By courtesy of Dr Urich.)

Aetiology

It has been suggested that this form of encephalomyelitis may be due to direct viral invasion of the brain by the agent which causes the exanthem; Shaffer, Rake, and Hodes (1942) and Adams (1968) either isolated measles virus or identified cytoplasmic and nuclear inclusion bodies suggestive of viral infection from the brains of patients with measles encephalitis. However, as stated above, the pathological picture of this condition differs in many respects from that usually associated with viral encephalomyelitis, and although many viruses, including that of canine distemper (Allen 1981; Dal Canto and Rabinowitz 1982) can produce experimental primary demyelination in animals, this is not true of the vaccinia and rabies agents, for example. Demyelination is also seen in 'slow virus infections' such as SSPE and is characterized by phospholipid breakdown and increased lysosomal hydrolase activity like that found in MS, but the accompanying pathological changes are quite different from those of MS (Cuzner, Davison, and Thompson 1981).

Glanzmann (1927), van Bogaert (1933), and Finley (1937, 1938) were among the first to suggest that post-infectious encephalomyelitis might be due to an allergic response on the part of the nervous system to a variety of different infective agents, and this concept that the condition is due to hypersensitivity of the nervous system to viral multiplication or to the products of viral injury is now generally accepted. Since Rivers and Schwentker (1935) showed that experimental allergic encephalomyelitis (EAE) could be induced in animals by the injection of brain emulsion with Freund's adjuvant, much work has been done upon the animal model of the human disease and a chronic relapsing form has been produced (Lassmann and Wisniewski 1979 a, b).Both the acute and the chronic experimental disorder may be suppressed by steroids, antilymphocytic serum, immunosuppressive agents, and by COP 1, a synthetic polypeptide (Traugott, Stone, and Raine 1979; Keith, Arnon, Teitelbaum, Caspary, and Wisniewski 1979), and there is evidence of both lymphocyte-mediated hypersensitivity (to MBP) (Eggers and Hibbard 1981) and circulating humoral antibodies (Kristensson, Wisniewski, and Bornstein 1976) in animals with the disease. The fact that a similar disorder may occur in man after the inoculation of antirabic vaccine prepared in animal brain or spinal cord supports the analogy between the experimental disorder in animals and the naturally occurring human disease.

References

Adams, J. M. (1968). Clinical pathology of measles encephalitis and sequelae. *Neurology, Minneapolis.* **18**, 2.

Adams, R. D. and Kubik, C. S. (1952). The morbid anatomy of the demyelinative diseases. *Am. J. Med.* **12**, 510.

Allen, I. V. (1981). The pathology of multiple sclerosis—fact, fiction and hypothesis. *Neuropath. appl. Neurobiol.* **7**, 169.

Cuzner, M. L., Davison, A. N., and Thompson, R. H. S. (1981). The demyelinating diseases of the central nervous system. In *The molecular basis of neuropathology* (ed. A. N. Davison and R. H. S. Thompson) Chapter 15. Arnold, London.

Dal Canto, M. C. and Rabinowitz, S. G. (1982). Experimental models of virus-induced demyelination of the central nervous system. *Ann. Neurol.* **11**, 109.

—— Wisniewski, H. M., Johnson, A. B., Brostoff, S. W., and Raine, C. S. (1975). Vesicular disruption of myelin in autoimmune demyelination. *J. neurol. Sci.* **24**, 313.

De Vries, E.(1960). *Postvaccinal perivenous encephalitis.* Elsevier, Amsterdam.

Eggers, A. E. and Hibbard, C. A. (1981). Direct cell-mediated cytotoxicity in experimental allergic encephalomyelitis. *J. neurol. Sci.* **49**, 109.

Finley, H. K. (1937). Perivenous changes in acute encephalitis associated with vaccination, variola and measles. *Arch. Neurol. Psychiat., Chicago.* **37**, 505.

—— (1938). Pathogenesis of encephalitis occurring with vaccination, variola and measles. *Arch. Neurol. Psychiat., Chicago.* **39**, 1047.

Glanzmann, E. (1927). Die nervösen komplikationen der Varizellen, Variola under Vakzine. *Schweiz med. Wschr.* **8**, 145.

Herkenrath, B. (1935). Pathologisch-anatomisch gesicherte Ausheilung eines Falles von Encephalitis post vaccinationem. *Z. ges. Neurol. Psychiat.* **152**, 293.

Kabat, E. A., Wolf, A., and Bezer, A. E. (1947). The rapid production of a demyelinating encephalomyelitis in Rhesus monkeys by injection of heterologous and homologous brain tissue with adjuvants. *J. exp. Med.* **85**, 117.

Keith, A. B., Arnon, R., Teitelbaum, D. Caspary, E. A., and Wisniewski, H. M. (1979). The effect of Cop 1, a synthetic polypeptide, on chronic relapsing experimental allergic encephalomyelitis in guinea pigs. *J. neurol. Sci.* **42**, 41.

Kies, M. W. and Alvord, E. C., Jr. (1959). *Allergic encephalomyelitis.* Thomas, Springfield, Illinois.

Kristensson, K., Wisniewski, H. M., and Bornstein, M. B. (1976). About demyelinating properties of humoral antibodies in experimental allergic encephalomyelitis: in vivo and in vitro studies. *Acta neuropath, Berlin.* **36**, 307.

Lassmann, H. and Wisniewski, H. M. (1979*a*). Chronic relapsing experimental allergic encephalomyelitis: clinicopathological comparison with multiple sclerosis. *Arch. Neurol., Chicago.***36**, 490.

—— and —— (1979*b*), Chronic relapsing experimental allergic encephalomyelitis: morphological sequence of myelin degradation. *Brain Res.* **169**, 357.

Raunch, H. C. and Griffin, J. (1969). Passive transfer studies in experimental allergic encephalomyelitis. In *Pathogenesis and etiology of demyelinating diseases.* ed. E. Pette, O. Westphal, K. Burdzy, and P. Kallos, p. 387. Karger, Basle.

Rivers, T. M. and Schwentker, F. F. (1935). Encephalomyelitis accompanied by myelin destruction experimentally produced in monkeys. *J. exp. Med.* **61**, 689.

Shaffer, M. F., Rake, G., and Hodes, H. L. (1942). Isolation of virus from a patient with fatal encephalitis complicating measles. *Am. J. Dis. Child.* **64**, 815.

Traugott, U., Stone, S. H., and Raine, C. S. (1979). Chronic relapsing experimental allergic encephalomyelitis. *J. neurol. Sci.* **41**, 17.

van Bogaert, L. (1933). Les manifestations nerveuses au cours des maladies eruptives. *Rev. neurol., Paris.* **40**, 150.

Wisniewski, H. M. (1975). Morphogenesis of the demyelinating process. In *Multiple sclerosis research* (ed. A. N. Davison, J. H. Humphrey, L. A. Liversedge, W. I. McDonald, and J. S. Porterfield) p. 132. HMSO, London.

Encephalomyelitis following vaccination against rabies

It is now established that the nervous complications of antirabic inoculation, whose incidence varies from 1 in 1000 to 1 in 4000 persons treated with vaccines prepared in animal brain or spinal cord, are due to sensitization to the central nervous tissue contained in the vaccine and are therefore comparable with EAE (see above). The pathological changes are those of acute disseminated encephalomyelitis (Uchimura and Shiraki 1957). The clinical picture may be encephalitic, myelitic, or polyradiculitic. A clinical picture resembling that of the Guillain-Barré syndrome has been described (Adaros and Held 1971). Retrobulbar neuritis, either unilateral or bilateral, may also occur. The death rate in the encephalitic and myelitic types of case is about 30 per cent. The incidence of these complications has been reduced by using vaccines grown in duck embryos or tissue culture (p. 287). Lumsden (1961) found that the pathological changes in nine fatal cases were in certain respects different from those of MS on the one hand and from acute 'spontaneous' disseminated encephalomyelitis on the other.

References

Adaros, H. L. and Held, J. R. (1971). Guillain-Barré syndrome associated with immunization against rabies: epidemiological aspects. In *Immunological disorders of the nervous system* (A. R. N. M. D. vol. XLIX) (ed. L. P. Rowland), p. 178. Baltimore.

Bassoe, P. and Grinker, R. R. (1930). Human rabies and rabies vaccine encephalomyelitis. *Arch. Neurol. Psychiat., Chicago.* **23**, 1138.

Johnson, R. T. (1982). *Viral infections of the nervous system.* Raven Press, New York.

Lumsden, C. E. (1961). The pathology and pathogenesis of multiple sclerosis. In *Scientific aspects of neurology* (ed. H. Garland). Livingstone, Edinburgh.

Uchimura, I. and Shiraki, H. (1957). A contribution to the classification and the pathogenesis of demyelinating encephalomyelitis. *J. Neuropath. exp. Neurol.* **16**, 139.

Post-vaccinal encephalomyelitis and encephalopathy

Aetiology

See page 298.

Pathology

See page 300 and Fig. 11.3.

Epidemiology

Nervous complications, such as hemiplegia,had been known to follow vaccination since 1860, but seemed to be isolated occurrences until 1922, when epidemics of post-vaccinal encephalomyelitis began to occur. Ninety-three cases were reported in England between 1922 and 1927, and 124 cases had been observed in Holland prior to the latter date. Cases were also observed elsewhere in Europe and the United States, though they were much rarer than in the countries mentioned. In Holland it was estimated that one case occurred in about 5000 persons vaccinated. It followed primary vaccination much more frequently than revaccination, the incidence in Holland being approximately one case in 300 primary vaccinations and one in 50 000 revaccinations. Johnson (1982) gives the incidence as between 1:63 and 1:200 000 vaccinations. It is practically unknown in infants vaccinated under the age of 1 year and most cases have occurred in children of school age. Though no age is exempt, it is rare after 30. Both sexes are affected equally.

The condition has occurred in epidemics coinciding with an increase in the number of persons vaccinated owing to the prevalence of smallpox. In an English outbreak of 1923 the 51 cases reported were distributed across the country. In the 1962 epidemic of smallpox in South Wales, Spillane and Wells (1964) recorded that of 800 000 individuals vaccinated, some 39 individuals (24 primary vaccinations, 15 revaccinations) suffered neurological complications. There were 11 cases of post-vaccinal encephalomyelitis, 3 of encephalopathy (convulsions and focal neurological signs in infants), 7 cases of meningism, 3 of epilepsy, 6 with focal lesions of brain or cord, 5 with polyneuritis, and 2 with brachial neuritis, while 2 patients with myasthenia gravis relapsed. De Vries (1965) also stressed the importance of encephalopathy as a cause of convulsions and coma in infancy, following either vaccination or other infections and pointed out that the pathological changes are non-inflammatory and thus different from those of encephalomyelitis. There is no evidence of spread of encephalomyelitis by contagion, but it has been noticed that there are often proportionately more cases in small communities and rural areas than in large towns. On several occasions two members of the same family who had been vaccinated at the same time both developed encephalomyelitis. The source of vaccine lymph is not of any aetiological significance but Johnson (1982) points out that there is evidence of vaccinia virus replication in the brain in many cases.

Symptoms and signs

Incubation period

In most cases the symptoms of encephalomyelitis develop between the tenth and the twelfth days after vaccination, though the onset has occurred as early as the second day or as late as the twenty-fifth. When the disorder follows revaccination the incubation period is often less than when it occurs after primary vaccination.

The clinical picture

The onset is usually rapid with headache, vomiting, drowsiness, fever,and in some cases convulsions. When fully developed, the clinical picture is one of meningeal irritation associated with widespread disturbance of function of the brain and spinal cord. In severe cases drowsiness passes into stupor and coma. Cervical rigidity and Kernig's sign are often present. The fundi are usually normal, but transient papilloedema is occasionally observed. The incidence of ocular abnormalities is variable. In some cases impairment of pupillary reflexes and ocular palsies have been noted. Trismus has frequently been described, and more than one case has been mistaken for tetanus in consequence. Flaccid paralysis of the limbs often develops, associated with loss of tendon reflexes and extensor plantar responses. Retention or incontinence of urine and faeces is the rule in severe cases. Sensory loss is inconstant,but may be marked when the spinal cord is severely affected. The CSF may be normal, though under increased pressure, but more often an excess of mononuclear cells and of protein is found. The cutaneous site of vaccination shows the usual inflammatory changes corresponding to the stage at which the patient is seen. Not uncommonly there is a severe local reaction, and occasionally a generalized vaccinial rash is observed.

Diagnosis

Diagnosis is rarely difficult, since there is a history of recent vaccination and the skin lesions are still visible. Otherwise, the clinical picture cannot be distinguished from other forms of acute disseminated encephalomyelitis or encephalopathy occurring spontaneously or complicating exanthemata. The severe involvement of the nervous parenchyma indicated by flaccid paralysis distinguishes the condition from meningitis, while the signs of meningeal irritation and the subsequent occurrence of convulsions, trismus, and paralysis of the limbs, together with the inconstancy of ocular abnormalities, distinguish it from encephalitis lethargica. Unlike the findings in poliomyelitis, the paralysis is upper rather than lower motor-neurone in type, there is usually associated sensory loss and sphincter involvement, and the plantar responses are generally extensor. Post-vaccinal encephalopathy is similar to that which may follow pertussis inoculation (p. 255).

Prognosis

The mortality rate has ranged from 10 to 30 per cent and rarely even 50 per cent in different epidemics. In most fatal cases the patient dies in coma from medullary paralysis within a few days. Less frequently death is due to bronchopneumonia or urinary infection. If recovery occurs, it is usually remarkably complete and residual symptoms are exceptional (Johnson 1982). Rarely, however, there is some persistent weakness or sensory loss or, in the case of young children, mental retardation.

Prophylaxis

With the object of preventing post-vaccinal encephalomyelitis as far as possible, the British Ministry of Health recommended in 1929 and again in 1956 that 'as long as the smallpox prevalent in this country retains it present mild character, it is not generally expedient to press for the vaccination of persons of these ages who have not previously been vaccinated, unless they have been in personal contact with a case of smallpox or directly exposed to smallpox infection'. With the virtual disappearance of smallpox throughout the world, routine vaccination has now been abandoned in practically all countries, as recommended by Brown (1971), and this illness has also disappeared in consequence.

Treatment

See page 305.

References

Bastiaanse, F. S. van B. (1925). Encéphalite consécutive à la vaccination antivariolique. *Bull. Acad. Méd., Paris.* **94**, 815.

Brown, G. C. (1971). Is routine smallpox vaccination necessary in the United States? *Am. J. Epidemiol.* **93**, 221.

de Vries, E. (1965). The acute encephalopathic reaction in infants. *Psychiat. Neurol. Neurochir. Amsterdam.* **68**, 85.

Johnson, R. T. (1982). *Viral infections of the nervous system.* Raven Press, New York.

Ministry of Health. *Reports of the committee on vaccination.* London, 1928 and 1930.

Perdrau, J. R. (1928). The histology of post-vaccinal encephalitis. *J. Path. Bact.* **31**, 17.

Spillane, J. D. and Wells, C. E. C. (1964). The neurology of Jennerian vaccination. *Brain* **87**, 1.

Turnbull, H. M. and McIntosh, J. (1926). Encephalomyelitis following vaccination. *Br. J. exp. Path.* **7**, 181.

Wiersma, D. (1929). Remarks on the etiology of encephalitis after vaccination. *Acta psychiat. Kbh.* **4**, 75.

Encephalomyelitis complicating smallpox

The occurrence of nervous symptoms in smallpox has been known for many years, but is rare, having been observed in only about 2.5 per 1000 cases. Troup and Hurst (1930) and McIntosh and Scarff (1928) showed that the pathological changes in the nervous system are indistinguishable from those of post-vaccinal encephalomyelitis. In some cases bulbar symptoms, especially dysarthria, are prominent and may be accompanied by paralysis of the limbs. In other cases paraplegia occurs, with or without sphincter disturbances and impairment of sensibility. Mental changes are sometimes present. Complete recovery is usual but the patient may die during the acute attack or subsequently from complications of paraplegia.

References

Marsden, J. P. and Hurst, E. W. (1932). Acute perivascular myelinoclasis ('acute disseminated encephalomyelitis')in smallpox. *Brain* **55**, 181.

McIntosh, J. and Scarff, R. W. (1927-8). The histology of some virus infections of the central nervous system. *Proc. R. Soc. Med.* **21**, 705.

Troup, A. G. and Hurst, E. W. (1930). Disseminated encephalomyelitis following smallpox. *Lancet* **i**, 566.

Encephalomyelitis complicating measles

According to Miller, Stanton, and Gibbons (1956) neurological complications occur in less than 1 in 1000 cases: 95 per cent are encephalitic or encephalomyelitic, less than 3 per cent myelitic, and less than 2 per cent polyradiculitic. The pathological picture ranges from congestion, perivascular infiltration, and occasional haemorrhages in the more acute cases to typical perivenous demyelination in the later stages (also see Behan and Currie 1978; Johnson 1982).

Symptoms and signs

Nervous complications of measles have been known for over a century, but appear to have become more common. The onset of symptoms is usually 4 to 6 days after the onset of the illness when the fever has fallen and the rash is fading. Tyler (1957) reviewed the literature and distinguished several clinical types. Acute disseminated encephalomyelitis may not account for all the nervous complications of measles. Johnson (1982) points out that viral-induced encephalopathy, a non-inflammatory disorder, may complicate measles and the other exanthemata and differs in its effects from encephalomyelitis. This encephalopathy resembles in many respects that which may complicate pertussis inoculation (Griffith 1978; Fenichel 1982; and see p. 255). It is also clear that encephalomyelitis is a rare complication of vaccination with live attenuated measles vaccine. The following are the commonest clinical presentations.

1. The symptoms may be relatively mild and transient and the clinical picture resembles 'meningism' or encephalopathy. In such cases headache, stupor, signs of meningeal irritation, and sometimes convulsions occur, but signs of focal lesions of the nervous parenchyma are absent.

2. Multiple focal or diffuse lesions of the nervous system may occur, involving the cerebral cortex, basal ganglia, brainstem, cerebellum, optic nerves, and spinal cord in various combinations.

3. There may be a single focal cerebral lesion, hemiplegia and aphasia being the commonest manifestations.

4. The symptoms may be predominantly those of cerebellar dysfunction.

5. The spinal cord may be mainly affected, the clinical picture being an acute ascending paralysis leading to paraplegia, with or without concurrent involvement of the brain. Neuromyelitis optica may be simulated.

6. Other nervous symptoms are rare, the clinical picture of polyradiculitis being the most important. The CSF may be normal in cases of encephalopathy but in encephalomyelitis usually shows a moderate increase in lymphocytes and protein.

7. It is now clear that subacute sclerosing panencephalitis is a late but rare sequel of measles infection (p. 279).

Diagnosis

The diagnosis is usually easy, since the measles rash is generally present when the symptoms develop. If the measles attack has passed unnoticed, the disorder cannot be distinguished from other forms of acute disseminated encephalomyelitis.

Prognosis

The mortality rate is 10 to 25 per cent in different series, and probably about 50 per cent are left with residual symptoms, of which the most important are hemiplegia, ataxia, mental handicap or change of personality, often with hyperkinesis and perceptual defects (Meyers and Byers 1952), and epilepsy. Coma and convulsions are bad prognostic signs.

Treatment

See page 305.

References

Behan, P. O. and Currie, S. (1978). *Clinical neuroimmunology.* Saunders, London.

Fenichel, G. M. (1982). Neurological complications of immunization. *Ann. Neurol.* **12**, 119.

Ferraro, A. and Scheffer, I. H. (1931). Encephalitis and encephalomyelitis in measles. *Arch. Neurol. Psychiat., Chicago.* **25**, 748.

Ford, F. R. (1928). The nervous complications of measles with a summary of the literature and publication of 12 additional case reports. *Bull. Johns Hopk. Hosp.* **43**, 140.

Greenfield, J. G. (1929). The pathology of measles encephalomyelitis. *Brain* **52**, 171.

Griffith, A. H. (1978). Reactions after pertussis vaccine: a manufacturer's experiences and difficulties since 1964. *Br. med. J.* **1**, 809.

Johnson, R. T. (1982). *Viral infections of the nervous system.* Raven Press, New York.

Malamud, N. (1937). Encephalomyelitis complicating measles. *Arch. Neurol. Psychiat., Chicago.* **38**, 1025.

Miller, H. G., Stanton, J. B., and Gibbons, J. L. (1956). Parainfectious encephalomyelitis and related syndromes. *Quart. J. Med.* **25**, 427.

Tyler, H. R. (1957). Neurological complications of rubeola (measles). *Medicine, Baltimore.* **36**, 147.

Encephalomyelitis complicating rubella

Encephalomyelitis is a rare complication of rubella, occurring in between 1 in 5000 and 1 in 20000 cases (Sherman, Michaels, and Kenny 1965; Johnson 1982). The clinical and pathological features are similar to those of measles encephalomyelitis; contrary to the common view, the illness tends to be more acute and severe than in either measles or varicella with a mortality of about 20 per cent. Coma and convulsions are common, and cerebellar involvement (Cantwell 1957), myelitis, and polyradiculitis have been reported but recovery is usually rapid and complete in surviving cases within two weeks (Margolis, Wilson, and Top 1943). As in measles, a late, progressive panencephalitis resulting from rubella virus has been described (p. 280).

References

Cantwell, R. J. (1957). Rubella encephalitis. *Br. med. J.* **2,** 1471.

Johnson,, R. T. (1982). *Viral infections of the nervous system.* Raven Press, New York.

Margolis, F. J., Wilson, J. L., and Top, F. H. (1943). Post-rubella encephalomyelitis. *J. Pediat.* **23,** 158.

Merritt, H. H. and Koskoff, Y. D. (1936). Encephalomyelitis following German measles. *Am. J. med. Sci.* **191,** 690.

Miller, H. G., Stanton, J. B., and Gibbons, J. L. (1956). Para-infectious encephalomyelitis and related syndromes. *Quart. J. Med.* **25,** 427.

Sherman, F. E., Michaels, R. H., and Kenny, F. M. (1965). Acute encephalopathy (encephalitis) complicating rubella. *J. Am. med. Ass.* **192,** 675.

Encephalomyelitis complicating chickenpox

Encephalitis and/or myelitis are rare complications of chickenpox (varicella).

Pathology

Owing to the relatively benign nature of this disorder there have been few opportunities of studying its pathology. The pathological picture is similar to that found in measles encephalomyelitis though van Bogaert (1933) found foci of demyelination in the cerebral hemisphere of one case resembling early plaques of multiple sclerosis and Miget (1933) was impressed by the meningeal inflammation.

Symptoms and signs

Symptoms of involvement of the nervous system develop in such cases between the fifth and the twentieth day after the appearance of the rash, usually during the first half of the second week. Encephalitis is said to occur in 90 per cent of cases, myelitis in 3 per cent, and polyradiculitis in 7 per cent (Miller, Stanton, and Gibbons 1956). However, Johnson (1982) points out that not all neurological complications in this illness are due to encephalomyelitis, since acute toxic encephalopathy and Reye's syndrome (p. 254) also occur, while the common acute cerebellar ataxia (see below) may not be of inflammatory origin either. When encephalitis does occur, the onset is acute with fever, headache, vomiting, and giddiness, and sometimes delirium. Coma and convulsions are less common than in other forms of post-infectious encephalomyelitis, occurring only in about 3 per cent of cases. The disturbance may be mainly meningeal, mainly cerebral, or mainly spinal but about 50 per cent of cases present with what seems to be an almost 'pure' cerebellar ataxia. In these cases, incoordination is the commonest symptom, occurring with or without involuntary movements. The ataxia is often so gross as to render the child incapable of walking. Tremor and choreic or choreo-athetoid movements sometimes occur. Signs of corticospinal-tract lesions may be present, but diplegia and hemiplegia are rare. Ophthalmoplegia has been observed. The meningeal form resembles any viral meningitis. The spinal form usually produces the picture of a dorsal transverse myelitis. The CSF may be normal, or may show an excess of protein and cells, usually mononuclear.

Diagnosis

The cause of the nervous symptoms is evident when the diagnosis of chickenpox has already been made. If, however, this has passed unnoticed, the encephalomyelitis cannot be distinguished from other forms of acute disseminated encephalomyelitis, except that cerebellar ataxia is peculiarly frequent (Boughton 1966).

Prognosis

The prognosis is good, both as to life and as to recovery of function. The mortality rate in encephalitic cases is less than 10 per cent and sequelae are rare in those who survive.

Treatment

See page 305.

References

Boughton, C. R. (1966). Neurological complications of varicella. *Med. J. Aust.* **2,** 444.

Brain, W. R. (1931). Zoster, varicella, and encephalitis. *Br. med. J.* **1,** 81.

Gordon, M. B. (1924). Acute hemorrhagic nephritis and acute hemorrhagic encephalitis following varicella *Am. J. Dis. Child.* **28,** 589.

Johnson, R. T. (1982). *Viral infections of the nervous system.* Raven Press, New York.

Krabbe, K. H. (1925). Varicella myelitis. *Brain.* **48,** 535.

Miget, A. (1933). Les complications nerveuses de la varicelle. *Médecine* **14,** 137.

Miller, H. G., Stanton, J. B., and Gibbons, J. L. (1956). Para-infectious encephalomyelitis and related syndromes. *Quart. J. Med.* **25,** 4271.

van Bogaert, L. (1933). Les manifestations nerveuses au cours des maladies eruptives. *Rev. neurol.* **1,** 150.

Zimmermann, H. M. and Yannet, H. (1931). Nonsuppurative encephalomyelitis accompanying chickenpox. *Arch. Neurol. Psychiat., Chicago.* **26,** 322.

Spontaneous acute disseminated encephalomyelitis and acute cerebellar ataxia

A form of acute disseminated encephalomyelitis clinically and pathologically identical with that which follows the above-mentioned exanthems may occur spontaneously or as a complication of a febrile illess of an 'influenzal' type. The condition can present as encephalitis, as an ascending transverse myelitis (p. 420) or as a combination of the two. Acute disseminated encephalomyelitis appears to represent a non-specific allergic reaction of the nervous system to various antigens, chiefly of bacterial or virus origin. Thus the 'spontaneous' form of the disease may be a reaction to a banal infection (as with influenza or *mycoplasma*), or may rarely follow an inoculation, the administration of antiserum, or even an adverse drug reaction (Behan and Currie 1978; Johnson 1982).

Symptoms and signs

The symptoms and signs of spontaneous acute disseminated encephalomyelitis are indistinguishable from those of the post-exanthematous varieties described above. However, *acute cerebellar ataxia of infancy and childhood* is a distinctive syndrome, occurring usually in infants between 1 and 2 years of age and often following a non-specific infective illness (Weiss and Carter 1959). As Menkes (1980) points out, the acute onset of cerebellar ataxia in childhood can be due to many causes but in this distinctive syndrome which is characterized by severe truncal ataxia, nystagmus in most cases, and often by tremor of the head, trunk, and limbs (Brumlik and Means 1969), there may be evidence of ECHO, Coxsackie, or even poliovirus infection, but most cases seem to be the result of an autoimmune response similar to that which occurs in other forms of encephalomyelitis. Ataxia may be so severe that the child cannot sit unsupported, and speech is often affected; the condition may last for two or more months, even though mildly affected children may recover in one or two weeks, and relapses may follow recurrent respiratory infection. Recovery is often complete but in up to a third of cases there is residual ataxia, dysarthria, and even mental retardation. The relationship between this condition and the so-called subacute myoclonic encephalopathy of infants described by Kinsbourne (1962)and by Dyken and Kolar (1968) in which bizarre random eye movements (opsoclonus) and coarse irregular jerking movements of the extremities are also accompanied by variable ataxia is uncertain but the rapid response to treatment with ACTH in many of the latter cases suggests that the aetiology and pathogenesis are probably similar. The CSF may be normal but sometimes shows a modest lymphocytic pleocytosis and an increased protein count, particularly of immunoglobulins.

Diagnosis

The diagnosis of encephalomyelitis rests upon the occurrence of a febrile illness with evidence of subacute lesions of the white matter of the brain or spinal cord or both, usually in multiple foci, and with or without signs of meningeal irritation (see also p. 302). The main difficulty lies in distinguishing the condition from acute multiple sclerosis.

McAlpine, Lumsden, and Acheson (1972) pointed out that whereas in the acute stage distinction between the two conditions may be impossible on clinical grounds, an acute attack of encephalomyelitis or myelitis may resolve completely and subsequently the patient may remain free from relapse for many years. Pette (1928) first suggested that no clinical or pathological distinction could be made between the two conditions and this 'unitary' theory was later supported by Ferraro (1958) and Miller and Schapira (1959).

Van Bogaert (1950) pointed out that some cases of acute encephalomyelitis are in every respect similar to those which occur after specific infectious fevers; others run a course typical of MS, while others recover and remain well. The encephalitic form is particularly common in children and young adults and may affect principally the cerebral hemispheres, brainstem, or cerebellum, while the myelitic form may occur at any age (McAlpine *et al.* 1972). After the acute stage has subsided, if the patient has residual physical signs, diagnosis from MS may be difficult or impossible. It must be based upon the history of the onset and the development of symptoms in the acute stage and the absence of any extension of the physical signs after the first few weeks of the illness. Normal visual evoked responses (see p. 87) may also be helpful.

Prognosis

Although fresh lesions may occur within two or three weeks of the onset, acute disseminated encephalomyelitis is usually a self-limiting disease, and relapses are uncommon. Miller and Evans (1953) pointed out that recurrences do rarely occur, especially when the disorder follows a non-specific minor infection in which the development of lasting immunity is known to be exceptional, and in which repeated antigenic insults furnish a possible pathogenetic mechanism. In all acute demyelinating disorders a substantial degree of recovery of function can be expected, but if the initial disorder is severe some residual disability is likely, and this may be added to if recurrences occur. In general, however, when relapses do occur, a diagnosis of MS should be seriously entertained.

Treatment

When hyperpyrexia occurs in such cases, cooling may be necessary. In comatose patients, tube-feeding, parenteral fluids, careful nursing care, and even tracheostomy with or without assisted respiration may be required. Miller (1953) and Miller and Gibbons (1953) recommended corticotrophin (ACTH), 80 units daily, in the acute phase and it is now generally agreed that this drug is beneficial in limiting the spread of the inflammatory process, in promoting clinical remission, and in reducing sequelae, although no controlled trials have been done. Most now prefer prednisone with or without immunosuppressive agents such as azathioprine (Behan and Currie 1978). In cases of encephalopathy in childhood, dexamethasone in appropriate dosage depending upon age may be preferred in order to reduce cerebral oedema in the acute stage. Appropriate antibiotics are often needed to control secondary infections and anticonvulsants may also be required in selected cases to control convulsions.

References

Behan, P. O. and Currie, S. (1978). *Clinical neuroimmunology*. Saunders, Philadelphia.
Brumlik, J. and Means, E. D. (1969). Tremorine-tremor, shivering and acute cerebellar ataxia in the adult and child—a comparative study. *Brain* **92**, 157.
Ferraro, A. (1958). Studies on multiple sclerosis. *J. Neuropath.* **17**, 278.
Johnson, R. T. (1982). *Viral infections of the nervous system*. Raven Press, New York.
Kinsbourne, M. (1962). Myoclonic encephalopathy of infants. *J. Neurol. Neurosurg. Psychiat.* **25**, 71.
McAlpine, D., Lumsden, C. E., and Acheson, E. D. (1972). *Multiple sclerosis: a reappraisal*, 2nd edn. Livingstone, Edinburgh.
Menkes, J. H. (1980).*Textbook of child neurology*. 2nd edn. Lea and Febiger, Philadelphia.
Miller, H. G. (1953). Acute disseminated encephalomyelitis treated with ACTH. *Br. med. J.* **1**,177.
—— and Evans. M. J. (1953). Prognosis in acute disseminated encephalomyelitis; with a note on neuromyelitis optica. *Quart. J. Med.* N. S. **22**, 347.
—— and Gibbons, J. L. (1953). Acute disseminated encephalomyelitis and acute multiple sclerosis; results of treatment with ACTH *Br. med. J.* **2**, 1345.
—— and Schapira, K. (1959). Aetiological aspects of multiple sclerosis. *Br. med. J.* **1**, 737.
Pette, H. (1928). Klinische und anatomische Studien über die Pathogenese der multiplen Sklerose. *Dtsch. med. Wschr.* **84, g22061.**
van Bogaert, L. (1950). Post-infectious encephalomyelitis and multiple sclerosis. *J. Neuropathol.* **9**, 219.
Weiss, S. and Carter, S. (1959). Course and prognosis of acute cerebellar ataxia in children. *Neurology, Minneapolis* **9**, 711.

Acute haemorrhagic leuco-encephalitis

Acute haemorrhagic leuco-encephalitis (also called acute necrotizing haemorrhagic leucoencephalopathy) was first described by Hurst (1941) and subsequently by Henson and Russell in 1942. It is characterized pathologically by macroscopic oedema of the brain with numerous minute haemorrhages and microscopically by severe damage to the vessel walls, perivascular necrosis, perivascular and focal demyelination, intense polymorphonuclear exudation, and microglial reaction. Clinically there is a febrile illness characterized by headache, vomiting, deepening stupor with or without hemiparesis, and a leucocytosis in the blood. Hurst suggested, and Greenfield (1950) accepted, the view that the haemorrhagic lesions and the non-haemorrhagic areas of necrosis or demyelination represent different degrees of injury by a single noxious agent, and Russell (1955) agreed that acute haemorrhagic leuco-encephalitis is simply a hyperacute and explosive form of acute disseminated encephalomyelitis. This view is now widely held (Johnson 1982); nevertheless, the condition is explosive and may occur as a complication of 'septic shock' in gram-negative septicaemia, when it resembles a generalized Schwartzman reaction, and may be associated with disseminated intravascular coagulation, with widespread complement activation (Graham, Behan, and More 1979).

References

Graham, D. I., Behan, P. O., and More, I. A. R. (1979). Brain damage complicating septic shock. Acute haemorrhagic leucoencephalitis as a complication of the generalised Schwartzman reaction. *J. Neurol. Neurosurg. Psychiat.* **42,** 19.

Greenfield, J. G. (1950). Encephalitis and encephalomyelitis in England and Wales during the last decade. *Brain.* **73,** 141.

Henson, R. A. and Russell, D. S. (1942). Acute haemorrhagic leuco-encephalitis. *J. Path. Bact.* **54,** 227.

Hurst, E. W. (1941). Acute haemorrhagic leuco-encephalitis, a previously undefined entity. *Med. J. Aust.* **2,** 1.

Johnson, R. T. (1982. *Viral infections of the nervous system.* Raven Press, New York.

Russell, D. S. (1955). The nosological unity of acute haemorrhagic leucoencephalitis and acute disseminated encephalomyelitis. *Brain* **78,** 369.

Disseminated myelitis with optic neuritis

Synonyms. Acute disseminated myelitis; diffuse myelitis with optic neuritis; neuromyelitis optica; ophthalmoneuromyelitis; Devic's disease.

Definition. A form of subacute encephalomyelitis characterized by massive demyelination of the optic nerves and spinal cord, sometimes running a self-limited and sometimes a progressive course.

Pathology

Both the optic nerves and spinal cord show massive demyelination. This is extensive in the optic nerve and chiasm, but in the spinal cord may be limited to a few segments, usually in the lower cervical and upper dorsal region, or it may be more diffuse, extending through the greater part of the cord. In severe cases cavitation may occur. Marked perivascular infiltration is not only present in the demyelinated areas but may be found throughout the nervous system. The infiltrating cells are principally mononuclear, but polymorphonuclear cells may also be present. In the demyelinated areas there is a great multiplication of vessels surrounded by many fat-granule cells and also neuroglial cells, though with little formation of new neuroglial fibres. To the naked eye the affected areas are swollen, congested, and softened.

Aetiology

The cause of Devic's disease is unknown. It is rare and affects both sexes at all ages from 12 to 60 years. McAlpine (1938) reported its occurrence in identical twins. While the condition was once regarded as an independent clinical and pathological entity, McAlpine, Lumsden, and Acheson (1972) point to the growing body of opinion which favours the view that it is simply a form of multiple sclerosis (MS). Even in Japan where it is very common, Okinaka, McAlpine, Miyagawa, Suwa, Kuroiwa, Shiraki, Araki, and Kurland (1960) have reached a similar conclusion. Nevertheless, Scott (1961, 1967), who followed up cases seen in Edinburgh between 1937 and 1949, found that despite clear evidence of bilateral optic-nerve involvement and variable signs of spinal-cord disease, none of his patients had developed episodes of subsequent neurological illness to suggest recurring demyelination as would have been expected in MS and in general the ultimate prognosis was good. This clinical syndrome rarely results from systemic lupus erythematosus (April and Vansonnenberg 1976).

Symptoms and signs

Stansbury (1949) and Scott (1952) pointed out that the illness often begins with a sore throat, cold, or other febrile illness. Either the ocular or the spinal lesion may develop first, separated by days or weeks, or both may occur simultaneously. Usually one eye is first affected, to be followed by the other after an interval varying from a few hours to several weeks. Rarely the onset of the myelitis intervenes between the affection of the two eyes.

The ocular lesion may be a true optic neuritis or a retrobulbar neuritis, depending upon whether it is situated sufficiently anteriorly to involve the optic discs. In the former case papilloedema is present, though the swelling is usually slight; in the latter the discs are normal. The characteristic field defect is a bilateral central scotoma. In severe cases blindness may be complete or almost so. Homonymous field defects have been described. The two eyes are often unequally affected. Pain in the eyes is often severe and is accentuated by moving them and by pressure upon the globes.

The spinal-cord lesion, which may be heralded by severe pain in the back and limbs, leads to the usual features of transverse myelitis, with paralysis of upper motor-neurone type and loss of sensation below the level of the lesion and of sphincter control.

The CSF may show no abnormality or there may be an increase of protein and globulin and an excess of cells, usually mononuclear, though occasionally neutrophils have been described. There is usually an increase in oligoclonal immunoglobulins.

Probably the disorder may abort after the development of optic neuritis and before the spinal symptoms appear and the reverse may also occur, so that some cases of acute bilateral optic neuritis without other symptoms, and also some cases of acute transverse meylitis without optic neuritis, may belong to this group.

Diagnosis

The presence of bilateral optic neuritis before symptoms of the spinal-cord lesion appear, may suggest a diagnosis of intracranial tumour. The disc swelling is, however, slight in proportion to the severity of the loss of vision and the characteristic field defect is bilateral central scotomas, in contrast to the peripheral constriction of the fields associated with papilloedema. Moreover, in cases of optic neuritis, headache, and vomiting are absent, though pain in the eyes may be severe.

Prognosis

The mortality rate was once about 50 per cent, death occurring either from respiratory paralysis, or from infection complicating paraplegia. If the patient survived, recovery was often remarkably complete. Cases occurring in the last 30 years have seemed less severe and assisted respiration has greatly improved the outcome. Complete blindness may be followed by considerable recovery of vision, though some degree of optic atrophy is likely to persist. Similarly, the functions of the spinal cord may be largely, if not completely, restored. Recovery, once achieved, may be permanent, but progressive and relapsing cases occur.These underline the close relationship of the disorder to MS.

Treatment

Corticotrophin (ACTH) 80 units daily at first, with subsequent reduction to 40 units daily, continuing until progressive clinical improvement is manifest, and giving thereafter smaller maintenance doses for several weeks, or prednisone in standard dosage are now generally recommended. The usual measures for the care of the skin and urinary and intestinal tracts, which are required in paraplegia, will be necessary and assisted respiration may be required in severe cases with ascending paralysis.

References

April, R. S. and Vansonnenberg, E. (1976). A case of neuromyelitis optica (Devic's syndrome) in systemic lupus erythematosus: clinicopathologic report and review of the literature. *Neurology, Minneapolis* **26,** 1066.

Hassin, G. B. (1937). Neuroptic myelitis versus multiple sclerosis. *Arch. Neurol. Psychiat., Chicago* **37,** 1083.

Holmes, G. (1927). Discussion on diffuse myelitis associated with optic neuritis. *Brain.* **50,** 702.

Kuroiwa, Y., Shibasaki, H., Tabira, T., and Itoyama, Y. (1982). Clinical picture of multiple sclerosis in Asia. In *Multiple sclerosis East and West* (ed. Y. Kuroiwa and L. T. Kurland). P. 31. Kyushu University Press, Kyushu.

McAlpine, D. (1938). Familial neuromyelitis optica: its occurrence in identical twins. *Brain* **61,** 430.

——, Lumsden, C. E., and Acheson, E. D. (1972). *Multiple sclerosis: a reappraisal,* 2nd edn. Livingstone, Edinburgh.

Okinaka, S., McAlpine, D., Miyagawa, K., Suwa, N., Kuroiwa, Y., Shiraki, H., Araki, S., and Kurland, L. T. (1960). Multiple sclerosis in Northern and Southern Japan. *Wld Neurol.* **1,** 22.

Scott, G. I. (1952). Neuromyelitis optica. *Am. J. Ophthal.* **35,** 755.

—— (1961). Ophthalmic aspects of demyelinating diseases. *Proc. R. Soc. Med.* **54,** 38.

—— (1967). Optic disc oedema. *Trans. ophthal. Soc. UK* **87,** 733.

Stansbury, F. C. (1949). Neuromyelitis optica (Devic's disease). *Arch. Ophthal., Chicago* **42,** 292, 465.

Multiple sclerosis (MS)

Synonyms. Disseminated sclerosis; insular sclerosis.

Definition. A disease of unknown aetiology characterized pathologically by the widespread occurrence in the nervous system of patches of demyelination followed by gliosis. In many cases the early manifestations are followed by improvement or even apparent complete clinical recovery, so that remissions and relapses are a striking feature of the disorder, the course of which may extend over many years. The early symptoms are often those of focal lesions of the nervous system, while the later clinical picture is often one of progressive dissemination tending to produce the classical features of ataxic paraplegia.

Pathology

The first pathological accounts of the disease were given by Cruveilhier in 1835 and Carswell in 1838. The pathological 'unit' in MS is a circumscribed lesion beginning with destruction of the myelin sheaths of the nerve fibres and to a much lesser extent of the axis cylinders, and ending with the formation of a 'sclerotic plaque' (Fig. 11.4). These plaques occur predominantly in the white matter of the brain and spinal cord. They are sometimes found in the grey matter of the cerebral cortex and in cranial or spinal-nerve roots, rarely in the grey matter of the spinal cord (Allen 1981). Many writers have stressed their perivascular distribution, and Putnam (1937) emphasized their relationship to cerebral venules, but Dow and Berglund (1942) found many exceptions to this. The optic nerves and chiasm, the periventricular regions, and the subpial region of the spinal cord are favourite sites. In an extensive review, Lumsden (1970) confirmed that there is no evidence to indicate that venous thrombosis plays any part in pathogenesis, but immunofluorescent studies (Lumsden 1971) showed that immunoglobulins and complement accumulate in areas of active demyelination. Since then much work has been done on the disordered immunological processes found in this disease. There is evidence that the inflammatory cells present in MS plaques are mainly T lymphocytes but some B cells, macrophages, and plasma cells may also be found (Prineas and Connell 1978; Prineas and Wright 1978; Nyland, Mörk, and Matre 1982). Many immunoglobulin-containing cells are found in the plaques (Esiri 1977, 1980) and the brains of such patients contain bound IgG (Mehta, Frisch, Thormar, Tourtellotte, and Wisniewski 1981). There is also good evidence to indicate that circulating immune complexes (Tachovsky, Lisak, Koprowski, Theofilopoulos, and

Dixon 1976; Goust, Chenais, Carnes, Hames, Fudenberg, and Hogan 1978) and circulating T cells sensitized to myelin basic protein (MBP) are of importance (Colby, Sheremata, Bain, and Eylar 1977; Symington, Mackay, Whittingham, White, and Buckley 1978; Fraser, Haire, Millar, and McCrea 1979; Traugott, Scheinberg, and Raine 1979; Turner, Cuzner, Davison, and Rudge 1980) and similar cells may be found in the CSF (Kam-Hansen 1980). There is also evidence that IgG is manufactured by B cells in MS plaques (Tourtellotte and Ma 1978; Esiri 1980) and that some of this enters the CSF-producing oligoclonal bands (Roström 1981); high lymphokine activity may also be found in the fluid (Meyer-Rienecker, Jenssen, and Werner 1979). It has also been shown that the autologous mixed lymphocytic reaction (MLR) is significantly increased in active MS (Birnbaum and Kotilinek 1981) and that activity of the disease can be correlated with changes in T-cell subsets (Hauser, Bresnan, Reinherz, and Weiner 1982), and with reduced suppressor-cell function (Antel, Arnason, and Medof 1979). That these immunological abnormalities may be related to infection with several viruses now seems clear (see below). Biochemical changes in myelin and the activation of proteolytic enzymes, as previously discussed, seem to be secondary to the immunological abnormalities and not primary (Davison and Cuzner 1977).

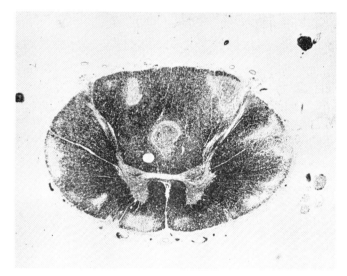

Fig. 11.4. Multiple sclerosis: spinal cord, T9.

To the naked eye the sclerotic plaque appears slightly sunken, greyish, and more translucent than normal nervous tissue. The myelin of the nerve sheaths degenerates and undergoes phagocytosis, and the axis cylinders may show diffuse or irregular swellings. There is marked reactive gliosis and in late plaques the myelin has been removed; the axis cylinders are reduced in number, some of those persisting are abnormal, and there is a thick condensation of the glial meshwork. Ultrastructural studies of plaques have confirmed inflammatory-cell infiltration and phagocytosis of myelin. Mechanisms of remyelination, which may account for remission of symptoms, and the role of the oligodendroglia in this process have been reviewed by McDonald (1974*a, b*). A claim that there may be histological changes in the jejunum in MS patients has been disproved (Jones, Pallis, and Peters 1979; Bateson, Hopwood, and MacGillivray 1979).

There has been much dispute in the past as to whether there is any pathological distinction between the lesions of acute disseminated encephalomyelitis on the one hand and those of MS on the other. Lumsden (1970, 1972) and Lassmann and Wisniewski (1979) hold the view that the primary pathological process is identical in the two disorders but point out that in the chronic lesion of MS the appearances are such that it is impossible to determine what may have been the primary process. Massive and widespread demyelination may well be the end-result of several processes of varying aetiology and acute disseminated encephalomyelitis, Devic's disease, MS, the concentric demyelination of Baló and certain cases previously diagnosed as Schilder's disease (see below) may represent the differing end-stages of what is, in the first instance, the same essential pathological change.

Aetiology

General considerations

The aetiology of MS is still unknown. The gliosis was once thought to be the primary process, hence the word 'sclerosis', but it is now clear that the glial scar is simply the end-result of the initial inflammatory and demyelinating process. Theories suggesting that the disease might be due to infection with a spirochaete or a rickettsial agent, to venular thrombosis, to the ingestion of heavy metals such as copper, or to excessive dietary fat have now been largely abandoned and the isolation of a specific virus claimed by Margulis, Soloviev, and Shubladze (1946) was never confirmed. Epidemiological studies (see below) have given some support to the possibility that the condition could prove to be due to a 'slow virus' infection, while experimental work on recurrent rather than monophasic encephalomyelitis induced by EF and adjuvant (see Wisniewski 1975) as well as much clinical, immunological, and genetic evidence suggests that the disease is due to disordered immunity.

Many groups of workers have now reported the finding of significantly increased levels of measles antibodies in the serum and CSF of MS cases, and measles-specific immunoglobulin was identified in CSF samples (Dowling, Kim, Murray, and Cook 1968; Salmi, Panelius, Halonen, Rinne, and Pettinen 1972; Norrby, Link, and Olsson 1974). In other cases, however, raised levels of antibodies to viruses as diverse as RSV virus, herpes simplex, mumps, varicella, and adenovirus were found (Ross, Lenman, and Melville 1969; Sever, Kurtzke, Alter, Schumacher, Gilkeson, Ellenberg, and Brody 1971), and McDermott, Field, and Caspary (1974) pointed out that EF and measles virus have similar antigenic determinants. An association postulated on epidemiological grounds between MS on the one hand and enterovirus infections such as poliomyelitis on the other (Poskanzer, Schapira, and Miller 1963b) was not supported by virological studies. Subsequently, however, evidence implicating vaccinia as well as measles virus and possibly mumps and rubella has accumulated, based upon studies of serum and CSF antibodies, virus-specific IgG in serum and CSF, and lymphoblastic transformation (Miyamoto, Walker, Ginsberg, Burks, McIntosh, and Kempe 1976; Symington and Mackay 1978; Weiner, Cherry, and McIntosh 1978; McFarland and McFarlin 1979; Arnadottir, Reunanen, Meurman, Salmi, Panelius, and Halonen 1979; Walker and Cook 1979; Vartdal, Vandvik, and Norrby 1980; Röströ, Link, Laurenzi, Kam-Hansen, Norrby, and Wahen 1981; Tobler, Johnson, and Buehring 1982). It has also been suggested that herpes simplex virus type 2 (HSV−2) may play a part in persons lacking HSV−1 immunity (Martin 1981). It must, however, be noted that HLA determinants (see below) may influence antibody titres (Poskanzer, Sever, Terasaki, Prenney, Sheridan, and Park 1980a). Much interest has also been aroused by a possible relationship between canine distemper, other canine viruses, and dog ownership on the one hand and MS on the other (Cook and Dowling 1977; Cook, Dowling, and Russell 1979) and this had been thought by Cook and Dowling to be a possible factor responsible for post-war 'epidemics' of MS in the Faroe Islands and in Iceland (Nathanson, Palsson, and Gudmundsson 1978; Kurtzke and Hyllested 1979; Kurtzke, Gudmundsson, and Bergmann 1982). However, much recent evidence has failed to confirm any association with distemper or other canine viruses (Kurtzke and Priester 1979;

Appel, Glickman, Raine, and Tourtellotte 1981; Read, Nassim, Smith, Patterson, and Warlow 1982).

Many claims have been made that a virus has been isolated from the brains of MS patients (Nemo, Brody, and Waters 1974; Carp, Licursi, Merz, and Merz 1972; Carp, Merz, and Licursi 1975; Melnick, Seidel, Inoue, and Nishibe 1982); paramyxovirus-like agents have been identified by electron microscopy (Narang and Field 1973; Raine, Powers, and Suzuki 1974), while ter Meulen, Koprowski, Iwasaki, Käckell, and Müller (1972) isolated an infective agent resembling parainfluenza virus from MS brain tissue cultured *in vitro*, and Mitchell, Porterfield, Micheletti, Lange, Goswami, Taylor, Jacobs, Hockley, and Salsbury (1978) isolated an infectious agent from bone marrow. Nevertheless the consensus view (see *The Lancet* 1981) is that no single agent is responsible but that both genetic (see below) and environmental factors are involved. The environmental agent is probably infective and the infection may be acquired in early life (Millar 1971; Leibowitz and Alter 1973; more than one exposure may be involved (Poskanzer, Walker, Prenney, and Sheridan 1981).

The role of inherited predisposition

Multiple cases of MS sometimes occur in the same family. In most instances two sibs are affected. Affection of two successive generations is less common but conjugal cases rarely occur (Schapira, Poskanzer, and Miller 1963) and the disease has been reported in the daughter of parents each of whom had MS (Gilbert 1971). Twin studies (Bobowick, Kurtzke, Brody, Hrubec, and Gillespie 1978; Williams, Eldridge, McFarland, Houff, Krebs, and McFarlin 1980) have demonstrated a 25–50 per cent concordance for clinical MS in monozygotic twins and a much lower concordance (15 per cent) in the dizygotic. The fact that clinically normal twins may show CSF IgG abnormalities raises the possibility that subclinical MS may be present in some such individuals (Williams *et al.* 1980).

McAlpine, Lumsden, and Acheson (1972) concluded that the risk that MS will develop in a first-degree relative is about 15 times as great as in the general population. No definite pattern of inheritance emerges but much interest has been aroused by histocompatibility antigen studies. In Caucasoids and in Iran (Lotfi, Nikbin, Derakhshan, Aghai, and Ala 1978) there is a weak association with HLA−A3 and −B7 and a stronger association with the related antigens DW2 and DR2 (Paty, Mervart, Campling, Rand, and Stiller 1974; Lehrich and Arnason 1976; Olsson, Möller, and Link 1976; Eldridge, McFarland, Sever, Sadowsky, and Krebs 1978; Stendahl-Brodin, Link, Möller, and Norrby 1979; Visscher, Myers, Ellison, Malmgren, Detels, Lucia, Madden, Sever, Park, and Coulson 1979; *The Lancet* 1971; Engell, Raun, Thomsen, and Plutz 1982). In Arab populations there is a weak association with DR4 and with the B-lymphocyte alloantigen BT 102 (Kurdi, Ayesh, Abdallat, Maayta, McDonald, Compston, and Batchelor 1977). Madigand, Oger, Fauchet, Sabouraud, and Genetet (1982) suggest that HLA profiles may indicate two forms of the disease and that certain haplotypes (B12, B35, DR1, DR7) could be protective. Ebers, Paty, Stiller, Nelson, Seland, and Larsen (1982), from studies of sib pairs, conclude that there is no single MS susceptibility gene linked to HLA. Roberts and co-workers (Roberts, Papiha, and Poskanzer 1979a; Roberts, Roberts, and Poskanzer 1979b and Poskanzer, Terasaki, Prenney, Sheridan, and Park 1980b) found no clear-cut association with HLA in the Orkney and Shetland islands and concluded that multifactorial genetic involvement in the disease is probable.

Precipitating factors

Many events may immediately precede the onset of the illness and have been regarded as precipitating factors though their mode of operation is unknown. They include influenza and other respiratory infections, the specific fevers, superficial sepsis, surgical operations, and the extraction of teeth. Doubt has been cast on the danger of surgical operations (Miller 1961) but relapses have followed vaccination against smallpox (Miller, Cendrowski, and Schapira 1967), and Currier, Martin, and Woolsey (1974) found a significantly increased incidence of infectious illness, trauma, and surgical operation before the age of 20 years in 60 MS patients when compared with matched control subjects. A more recent study (Currier and Eldridge 1982) defined similar risk factors in a national study of 51 twin pairs, as between affected and unaffected twins. Cigarette smoking has no obvious aetiological influence (Simpson, Newell, and Schapira 1966) but may temporarily worsen symptoms (McAlpine *et al.* 1972). Millar, Allison, Cheeseman, and Merrett (1959) believed that pregnancy did not influence the relapse rate but Schapira, Poskanzer, Newell, and Miller (1966) showed that relapses were particularly common in the 3 months after delivery. Relapse has also occurred after emotional stress, as an allergic reaction to various drugs, including penicillin, after insect bites, blood transfusion, and as a result of exertion, fatigue, or exposure to high or low temperature (McAlpine *et al.* 1972). In Switzerland, Wüthrich, and Rieder (1970) showed that most relapses occurred in winter and spring. McAlpine and Compston (1952) obtained a history of physical injury preceding the onset of symptoms by less than 3 months in 14.4 per cent of cases, but in only 5.2 per cent of controls, and a relation between the site of the injury and that of the first symptom has been postulated (Miller 1964). Trauma has thus been thought to precipitate the onset of the disease or a relapse but in a careful study Bamford, Sibley, Thies, Laguna, Smith, and Clark (1981) found no such association.

Distribution, age, and sex

MS is most prevalent in Northern Europe and Switzerland. It is less common in North America and in Japan, in South Africa, and in tropical counties but is seen world-wide and in all races (Ames and Louw 1977; Ben Hamida 1977; Kuroiwa, Hung, Landsborough, Park, Singhal, Soemargo, Vejjajiva, and Shibasaki 1977; Chopra, Radhakrishnan, Sawhney, Pal, and Banerjee 1980; Baum and Rothschild 1981). A vast literature has now accumulated upon the incidence and prevalence of the disease, based upon careful population surveys carried out in many parts of the world and this was reviewed in detail by Acheson (1972). In general the crude prevalence rate rises the further one moves north or south from the equator. Figures vary from 10 per 100 000 in New Orleans and 14 per 100 000 in rural Western Australia to 33 per 100 000 in Hobart, Tasmania, 41 per 100 000 in Boston, Massachusetts, 50 per 100 000 in Northumberland, and Durham, England, and about 80 per 100 000 in south-eastern Norway. The prevalence in northern Canada is 129 per 100 000 (Shepherd and Downie 1980) but that in the Orkneys (309) and Shetland (184 per 100 000) islands is the highest in the world (Poskanzer, Prenney, Sheridan, and Kondy 1980c). However, there are many examples of a relatively high prevalence rate in isolated populations in low-risk areas and vice versa (Rinne, Panelius, Kivalo, Hokkanen, and Meurman 1968; McCall, Brereton, Dawson, Millingen, Sutherland, and Acheson 1968; Panelius 1969; Kurtzke 1975a, b;1980a; Granieri and Rosati 1982). There is also evidence that the clinical picture of the disease may be changing in some low-risk areas (Kuroiwa and Shibasaki 1973; Shibasaki and Kuroiwa 1973). In particular, the incidence of bilateral optic-nerve involvement and of neuromyelitis optica in Japan, though still much higher than in Britain, is declining (Shibasaki, McDonald, and Kuroiwa 1981). Much work has also been done upon the incidence and prevalence of the disease in migrant populations (Leibowitz, Kahana, and Alter 1969; Kurtzke, Kurland, and Goldberg 1971; Leibowitz and Alter 1973; Dean, McLoughlin, Brady, Adelstein, and Tallett-Williams 1976; Alter, Kahana, and Loewenson 1979; Kurtzke and Bui-Quoc-Huong 1980) and in general this supports the view that migrants retain the risk associated with their mother country, a finding suggesting that, as Millar (1971) proposed, the environmental factor of aetiological importance may be acquired in childhood. Acheson

(1972) concluded that the disease is neither one of affluence nor one associated with malnutrition or atmospheric pollution. It is associated with particular localities rather than race and whatever agent or agents cause it are not freely transportable to other countries. In his view no particular factors other than latitude characterize low-risk and high-risk areas but Leibowitz and Alter (1973) suggest that hygiene and sanitation may be important. The postwar epidemics in the Faroe islands and in Iceland coincided with occupation by British troops (Kurtzke, 1980b) but the significance of this association is unclear. HLA studies in different populations have failed to explain the unusual geographical distribution of the disease. The disease principally attacks young adults. In two-thirds of all cases it begins between 20 and 40, rather more often in the third than the fourth decade. Its occurrence below the age of 10 is rare, but it is occasionally seen in children between the ages of 12 and 15. In recent years the proportion of patients in whom the disease begins after 50 has increased, but onset after 60 is very uncommon. In most published series males have been affected more often than females, but the disease often begins earlier and runs a more rapid course in females (Acheson 1972).

Symptoms and signs

The clinical picture

The disease produces a very varied clinical picture. In the early stages it is often that of a single acute focal lesion which remits or becomes quiescent. As time goes on, the cumulative effects of earlier lesions produce a persistent background of incapacity upon which fresh disabilities due to new lesions are superimposed. Thus, in the early stages there are usually long and often remarkably complete remissions, while later the patient's condition fluctuates only to the extent that fresh lesions temporarily regress. However, some severe cases beginning in early adult life and more indolent chronic cases of onset in middle life run a progressive course from the outset, without remission.

Mode of onset

The disease usually begins with the rapid development, within a few hours or a day or two, of symptoms of a single focal lesion of white matter. Much less often symptoms appear insidiously. In a series of 100 consecutive patients the first symptom noticed was as follows:

Weakness or loss of control over limbs	No.
Involving both lower limbs	18
Involving one lower limb	14
Involving one upper limb	9
Involving one upper and one lower limb	7
Involving all four limbs	2
	—
	50

Visual symptoms	
'Blindness' in one eye	16
Double vision	8
'Dimness' of vision	4
Homonymous field defect	1
	—
	29

Sensory symptoms	
Numbness and other painless paraesthesiae	11

Miscellaneous symptoms	
Vertigo	2
Tremor	2
Multiple symptoms	2
Ptosis	1
Loss of taste	1
Epilepsy	1
Impotence	1
	—
	10

Thus weakness of one or both lower limbs is the first symptom in about one-third of all cases, and a disturbance of vision in almost one-third more. Sensory symptoms which cause no disability are often forgotten and probably occur more frequently than in 11 per cent. Patients who are carefully questioned when first seeking advice often describe symptoms of multiple small lesions occurring within a period of a few weeks. Weakness of the lower limbs is the commonest presenting symptom in patients in whom the disease develops insidiously, and in those in whom it begins after the age of 35.

Rarely the onset is fulminating, with an acute encephalitic, myelitic, or encephalomyelitic picture (see p. 312).

Motor symptoms

Motor weakness. Loss of power in the lower limbs is first manifest as fatigability or a feeling of heaviness, and later as spastic paraparesis; often patients with early spastic weakness complain of aching in the legs on exertion. Sometimes sudden weakness of one upper limb occurs, often associated with loss of postural sensibility in the fingers, the 'useless hand' of Oppenheim. Facial weakness and hemiplegia occur occasionally. Monoparesis of one lower limb occurs occasionally but even when the patient complains that only one leg is weak, signs of corticospinal-tract dysfunction are often bilateral, if worse in the affected leg.

Muscular wasting is very rare owing to the infrequency of involvement of the anterior horn cells, but very occasional cases with amyotrophy, often in the small hand muscles, are seen.

Incoordination. This is common. In the upper limbs it may take the form of *intention tremor*, a tremor occurring only on voluntary movement and increasing in intensity the greater the accuracy demanded. In touching the nose with the finger the tremor increases in amplitude as the finger approaches the target. The same phenomenon is seen when the patient is asked to touch his own nose and the observer's finger alternately or to lift a glass of water to the lips. Ataxia may, however, occur without intention tremor. In exceptionally severe cases cerebellar ataxia is so severe that the wild 'flinging' movements of the limbs which occur on attempted volitional activity make it virtually impossible for the patient to use the limbs at all. In the lower limbs incoordination is revealed by an ataxic gait and an abnormal heel-knee test. Tremor of the head is common in the late stages if cerebellar involvement is prominent.

Dysarthria and aphasia. Dysarthria may be due either to spastic weakness or to ataxia of the muscles of articulation or to a combination of the two. In the early stages speech is often slurred and later may become explosive and almost unintelligible. The 'syllabic' or 'scanning' speech, sometimes regarded as typical, is exceptional and only occurs when cerebellar ataxia is severe. Transitory aphasia is rare (Olmos-Lau, Ginsberg, and Geller 1977).

Sensory symptoms

Paraesthesiae occur at some stage of the disease in most cases, often in the form of numbness and tingling over one side of the face or one upper or both lower limbs. Impairment of position and joint sense and of finer sensibility due to a lesion in the posterior columns of the spinal cord is often accompanied by sensations of apparent swelling of the limb and by feelings suggested that tight strings or bandages have been applied to the trunk or extremities. When there is a plaque in the posterior columns of the cervical cord, a sensation resembling an electric shock may radiate down the back and limbs on flexing the neck ('Lhermitte's sign'). Pain is uncommon except in spastic limbs with flexor spasms, but typical

trigeminal neuralgia, sometimes bilateral, is occasionally encountered. Objective sensory loss is present in at least 50 per cent of cases. Defects of postural sensibility and of appreciation of vibration are the commonest abnormalities, but sensory loss suggesting trigeminal neuropathy occasionally occurs. Occult trigeminal-nerve involvement may be detectable electrophysiologically (Eisen, Paty, Purves, and Hoirch 1981). Inability to recognize objects placed in the hand may result from a plaque in the fasciculus cuneatus in the cervical region. There may be a sharply defined upper level of sensory loss on the trunk suggesting myelitis or spinal tumour and unilateral loss of pain and temperature sensation, often with contralateral spastic paresis (a partial Brown–Séquard syndrome) is another uncommon presentation. Sensory symptoms may be effectively localized and monitored by measurement of somatosensory evoked responses (Namerow 1970, and see below).

Visual symptoms

Acute unilateral retrobulbar neuritis is one of the most important early symptoms. It occurs most often between the ages of 20 and 30. The vision of one eye becomes misty and in 24 or 48 hours is reduced to a perception of hand movement or of light only. The eye is painful on movement and tender on pressure, and there is a central scotoma larger for red and green than for white. The optic disc is usually normal in appearance during the acute stage, but if the lesion is near the disc papillitis may occur, though swelling is usually slight. In a few weeks vision improves, but the residual damage to the nerve manifests itself in some degree of optic atrophy with pallor of the disc, especially in its temporal half and often a persistent though smaller central scotoma (Patterson and Heron 1980). Enlargement of such a scotoma after exertion or a hot bath (p. 91) is well recognized (see McAlpine 1972), and has been thought to be due to the effects of temperature upon axonal conduction (Davis 1970). Sensitive tests of visual acuity and of contrast sensitivity often give abnormal findings (Regan, Raymond, Ginsburg, and Murray 1981). Permanent blindness is very rare but progressive visual failure has been reported (Ormerod and McDonald 1984). Simultaneous retrobulbar or optic neuritis in both eyes is uncommon in MS but undoubtedly occurs. The lesions of the optic nerves may be so insidious as to produce the characteristic temporal pallor of the disc, which is found in over 50 per cent of cases, without the patient's being aware of any impairment of vision. The measurement of the shape and latency of pattern-evoked, averaged, visual responses Halliday, McDonald, and Mushin 1973; Asselman, Chadwick, and Marsden 1975) and the assessment of delayed conduction in visual pathways using the Pulfrich pendulum (Rushton 1975) may detect visual lesions which are unsuspected clinically and are thus of considerable diagnostic value, say, in patients with undiagnosed spastic paraparesis (see below). Lesions of the optic chiasm and optic tracts are uncommon, but when they occur cause distinctive defects of the visual fields.

Nystagmus. This is present in about 70 per cent of cases. It is usually absent on central fixation and appears on conjugate deviation laterally. The slow phase is towards the central fixation point and the quick phase away from it. A rotary element is sometimes present, especially on vertical fixation. Nystagmus on central fixation is rare in MS but pendular nystagmus and oscillopsia have been described (Aschoff, Conrad, and Kornhuber 1974). Nystagmus may be evoked or accentuated by heating the patient (Jestico and Ellis 1976).

Ocular movement disorders. Paralysis of conjugate ocular deviation may occur as the result of a plaque in the midbrain or pons, but is uncommon: paresis of single ocular muscles occurs in about

6 per cent of cases; but diplopia without objective ocular palsy is commoner (34 per cent of cases). Dissociation of lateral conjugate deviation may occur, the adducting eye being less completely deviated than the abducting. When this occurs (Harris' sign, a form of 'internuclear ophthalmoplegia') nystagmus is often apparent only in the abducting eye (so-called 'ataxic' nystagmus); the lesion lies in the medial longitudinal fasciculus. The sign is almost pathognomonic of MS and is commoner in this disease than other forms of internuclear ophthalmoplegia (p. 98) Ptosis is rare, retraction of the upper lids slightly commoner. Subclinical eye-movement disorders (Solingen, Baloh, Myers, and Ellison 1977; Mastaglia, Black, and Collins 1979) may also be identified by recordings of saccadic and smooth-pursuit eye movements.

Pupillary abnormalities. The pupillary reactions are usually normal. Loss of the reaction to light with preservation of that to accommodation is very rarely observed and is more often unilateral than in syphilis. Total internal ophthalmoplegia may occur. Paresis of the ocular sympathetic leading to ptosis, enopthalmos, and miosis may be seen as the result of a brainstem lesion.

Auditory and vestibular symptoms

Cortical deafness is a rare manifestation (Tabira, Tsuji, Nagashima, Nakajima, and Kuroiwa 1981), but vertigo is a common and early symptom, usually beginning with a mild sense of instability. Sometimes severe vertigo with vomiting and coarse nystagmus occurs in attacks lasting for several days, but is usually accompanied by other signs indicating the presence of a pontine plaque involving vestibular nuclei and other contiguous structures.

Paroxysmal symptoms

Paroxysmal symptoms occurring in MS include focal or generalized epileptiform attacks which occur in about 2 per cent of cases (McAlpine 1972), tonic seizures (brief and often painful episodes in which the limbs on one side adopt a posture reminiscent of tetany and which are often precipitated by movement or sensory stimulation) (Matthews 1958; Shibasaki and Kuroiwa 1974), paroxysmal dysarthria and ataxia (Osterman and Westerberg 1975), and sensory symptoms, pain or paresis of very brief duration (Twomey and Espir 1980). Matthews (1975) suggested that these attacks may be due to lateral spread of axonal excitation within demyelinated plaques.

Mental symptoms

Some reduction in the intellectual capacity of the patient is not uncommon, but emotional changes are more frequent. A sense of mental and physical well-being (euphoria) is well known. On the other hand, depression and irritability are sometimes conspicuous (Whitlock and Siskind 1980). Some disinhibition and emotional lability, leading to involuntary laughter and tears, is common, especially in the later stages. Delusional states are uncommon but dementia occurs relatively frequently, especially in the later stages. Kahana, Leibowitz, and Alter (1971) found that cerebral manifestations (hemiparesis, hemianopia, aphasia, convulsions, and/or dementia) occurred in 10 per cent of their cases at the onset and in 34 per cent at some stage of the illness.

Reflex changes

As corticospinal-tract involvement is very common, the tendon reflexes are usually exaggerated in paretic limbs and generalized hyperreflexia with clonus as well as flexor or extensor spasms (p. 391) are frequently seen, especially in advanced cases. Occasionally spasticity is so great that the reflexes are difficult to elicit; loss of reflexes is uncommon but is occasionally seen, especially when sensory lesions are severe with interruption of the reflex arc. The abdominal reflexes are absent in at least two-thirds of all cases and may be lost at an early stage, and extensor plantar responses occur in from 80 to 90 per cent of cases in the later stages.

Other symptoms and signs

Sphincter control is frequently impaired. In the early stages urgency or precipitancy of micturition is common (Jameson 1982). Later, retention or reflex evacuation of both urine and faeces may occur. Occasionally acute retention of urine is the first symptom; impotence is common and sweating is often impaired (Cartlidge 1972). Some patients show other evidence of autonomic dysfunction specifically involving the cardiovascular system (Senaratine, Carroll, Warren, and Kappagoda 1984). There is no consistent endocrine abnormality (Teasdale, Smith, Wilkinson, Latner, and Miller 1967).

Pyrexia may develop during acute exacerbations which are consequently described by the patient as having begun with an attack of 'influenza'. Headache sometimes occurs and indeed the clinical picture rarely mimics that of cerebral tumour (Sagar, Warlow, Sheldon, and Esiri 1982).

Cerebrospinal fluid

Some abnormality is found in the CSF in most cases. An excess of mononuclear cells is found in about 10 per cent. T and B lymphocytes can be identified in the fluid in such cases (Allen, Sheremata, Cosgrove, Osterlaud, and Shea 1976) and the percentage of T cells rises in relapses but their activity is depressed (Kam-Hansen 1979). Those mononuclear cells which have a surface receptor for the Fc portion of IgG, also fall during an exacerbation, at which time the concentration of immune complexes in the fluid is also reduced (Coyle, Brooks, Hirsch, Cohen, O'Donnell, Johnson, and Wolinsky 1980). A paretic colloidal gold curve was regarded in the past as a characteristic change. The total protein is often normal or only moderately raised (Fishman 1980) but it was shown many years ago, using crude paper electrophoretic and zinc sulphate precipitation techniques (Kabat, Moore, and Landow 1942; Prineas, Teasdale, Latner, and Miller 1966) that the proportion of gamma globulin is raised. Much more specific is the estimation of immunoglobulins by electrophoresis or immunoelectrophoresis (Kolar and Zeman 1967; Kolar, Ross, and Herman 1970; Link and Müller 1971; Fischer-Williams and Roberts 1971; Olsson and Link 1973) or by electroimmunodiffusion (Schneck and Claman 1969). The IgG is increased to more than 14 per cent of the total CSF protein in most patients with MS, and IgA, various complements, tranferrin (Olsson and Link 1973), and IgM (Williams, Mingioli, McFarland, Tourtellotte, and McFarlin 1978) may also be raised. There is, in fact, a reduction in CSF C9 complement suggesting consumption during relapse, due to the formation of membrane attack complexes (Morgan, Campbell, and Compston 1984). As previously mentioned, most of the IgG appears to be manufactured in the central nervous system but abnormalities in serum immunoglobulins are sometimes found (Kolar *et al.* 1970). Agarose and polyacrylamide gel electrophoresis with immunofixation have demonstrated oligoclonal bands in the CSF in over 90 per cent of cases, almost invariably for IgG but sometimes for IgA and IgM (Vandvik, Natvig, and Wiger 1976; Link and Laurenzi 1979; Thompson, Kaufmann, Shortman, Rudge, and McDonald 1979), but immunoelectrophoresis and isoelectric focusing (Hosein and Johnson 1981) may also demonstrate abnormalities not revealed as an increase in IgG or as oligoclonal gammopathy (Kolar, Rice, Jones, Defalque, and Kincaid 1980). The CSF protein serine residue is also increased (Poser, Sylwester, Ho, and Alpert 1975) and α_1-antitrypsin activity is reduced (Price and Cuzner 1979), but the finding of an increased concentration of the P1 fragment of MBP, using radioimmunoassay (Whitaker 1977; Jacque, Delassalle, Rancurel, Raoul, Lesourd, and LeGrand 1982) seems even more sensitive. CSF esterase, peptidase, and proteinase activity has been shown to be greatly increased, particularly in acute cases. While these tests have added precision to diagnosis, none is yet absolutely specific for MS, as similar abnormalities may occur in other in nervous diseases associated with an altered immune response, including some forms of meningitis and encephalitis.

Other diagnostic tests

Since the recognition of unsuspected lesions in the visual pathways has been made possible by techniques of visual evoked response (VER) recording (p. 87), methods have been considerably refined (Regan, Milner, and Heron 1976; Matthews, Small, Small, and Pountney 1977; Collins, Black, and Mastaglia 1978; Bodis-Wollner, Hendley, Mylin, and Thornton 1979; Mastaglia and Carroll 1982); this technique, together with quantitative perimetry (Ellenberger and Ziegler 1977), can detect clinically silent lesions in the optic nerves or more posteriorly in about 70 per cent of patients with MS in whom clinically the disease seems to be confined, for example, to the spinal cord (*The Lancet* 1982). The recording of auditory (Robinson and Rudge 1977) and of somato-sensory evoked potentials (Matthews and Small 1979; Eisen and Nudleman 1979; Ganes 1980) may also reveal unsuspected abnormalities in about 50 per cent. In some patients there is also electro-physiological evidence of abnormalities in sensory peripheral nerves (Hopf and Eysholdt 1978) and in the neuromuscular system (Weir, Hansen, and Ballantyne 1979, 1980) but, unlike evoked potential recording, these changes have not proved to be of diagnostic value. The erythrocyte-UFA (E-UFA) mobility test, which measures the mobility of erythrocytes before and after the addition of linoleic acid and which has been claimed to be a virtually specific diagnostic test for the disease (Field, Joyce, and Smith 1977), has not been found to be of value by many other workers (Cuypers and Reddemann 1980).

Much interest has been aroused by reports that the CT scan may successfully demonstrate focal areas of cerebral demyelination, shown as foci of reduced density, in patients with MS (Cala and Mastaglia 1976; Warren, Ball, Paty, and Banna 1976; Cala, Mastaglia, and Black 1978; Lane, Carroll, and Pedley 1978) and that the plaques may show contrast enhancement (Sears, Tindall, and Zarnow 1978; Lebow, Anderson, Mastri, and Larson 1978; Harding, Radue, and Whiteley 1978). It is now evident that nuclear magnetic resonance (NMR) tomography (Young, Hall, Pallis, Legg, Bydder, and Steiner 1981; Mastaglia and Cala 1982) is likely to be even more successful.

Symptom complexes

The variability of the clinical picture justifies the recognition of 'forms' of the disease due to predominant involvement of different parts of the nervous system.

1. The classical triad of Charcot, namely nystagmus, intention tremor, and scanning speech, is comparatively rare, and occurs in under 10 per cent of cases, being accompanied usually by severe ataxia (*the cerebellar form*).

2. The *generalized form*, common in younger patients, is characterized by temporal pallor of the optic discs, nystagmus, slight intention tremor, ataxia, weakness and spasticity of the lower limbs, and defective sphincter control.

3. Onset with *ocular symptoms*. Retrobulbar neuritis or transient diplopia may be the only symptom without subsequent relapse until many years later.

4. *The sensory form*. In some patients recurrent episodes of paraesthesiae with loss of postural sensibility in one or more limbs indicating a plaque in the posterior column of the cord may occur and often resolves after a few days or weeks only to recur months or years later in some other part. This form often runs a benign course with long intervals between relapses before signs of corticospinal-tract involvement appear. Isolated unilateral facial sensory loss (trigeminal neuropathy) occasionally occurs.

5. *The cerebral form*. An onset with hemiplegia, hemianopia, aphasia, or epileptiform convulsions is uncommon and may simulate cerebral tumour; remission in a few weeks or months is usual but subsequently dementia often develops.

6. *Spinal forms*. (a) *Progressive spastic paraplegia* may occur with few if any other physical signs, especially in middle-aged patients. (b) *Unilateral spinal lesions* occur chiefly in the cervical cord. The posterior and lateral columns are usually involved. A partial Brown-Séquard syndrome developing in a young person is not uncommon and usually remits within a few months. (c) *Sacral form*. A plaque in the conus medullaris may lead to incontinence of urine and faeces, impotence, and anaesthesia in the region of the sacral cutaneous supply.

7. *The brainstem form*. Apart from transient diplopia, mentioned above, which may be due to involvement of a single oculomotor nerve or alternatively may be of internuclear type, transient unilateral facial palsy, an acute episode of vertigo resembling vestibular neuronitis, and various other syndromes due to combined lesions of cranial nerves and long tracts are seen (see below).

8. *Acute multiple sclerosis*. Rarely the illness is of very acute onset, with clinical manifestations of any of the above syndromes. A fatal termination within a few months is very rare. In such acute cases fever may be present. Headache, vomiting, vertigo, and delirium may all occur in severe cases. The symptoms may be predominantly cerebral, predominantly spinal, or both brain and cord may be diffusely affected. The affection may extend to hitherto unaffected parts of the nervous system after days or even weeks. The symptoms of the cerebral type include mental changes, convulsions, aphasia, hemiplegia, hemianopia, nystagmus, vertigo, and ataxia of the upper limbs. However, aphasia and hemianopia are signs of exceptional rarity. Optic neuritis may occur bilaterally. Cranial-nerve palsies involving other than the ocular, trigeminal, and facial nerves are comparatively uncommon. Symptoms of meningeal irritation are rare. In the spinal type, simulating 'transverse myelitis', pains in the back and limbs in girdle distribution are not uncommon. Total paraplegia, sensory loss, and sphincter paralysis develop in the more severe cases of this type. The tendon reflexes may be exaggerated, but are often diminished or lost in the acute stage of 'spinal shock' and the plantars are usually extensor. The spinal cord may be swollen, simulating intramedullary tumour (Feasby, Paty, Ebers, and Fox 1981).

Diagnosis

MS must be distinguished from the various forms of *diffuse sclerosis*, which often occur in childhood, are usually steadily progressive, and by destroying symmetrically the white matter of the cerebral hemispheres lead to blindness, spastic tetraplegia, and dementia.

In *neuromyelitis optica* the symptoms of retrobulbar neuritis are associated with those of transverse myelitis, both developing rapidly. Acute bilateral retrobulbar neuritis can occur without myelitis but, except in Japan, it is uncommon for both eyes to be affected simultaneously and concurrently with spinal-cord involvement in MS. Nevertheless, most authorities now regard neuromyelitis optica as simply being one mode of presentation of MS (McAlpine *et al.* 1972).

Meningovascular syphilis. MS is distinguished from meningovascular syphilis by the rarity of pupillary changes and of diminished reflexes in the former and by the markedly dissimilar CSF changes. Nystagmus and signs of cerebellar dysfunction are very rare in neurosyphilis.

Tabes may be superficially simulated by the ataxic gait of MS, but in the latter there is usually spasticity, exaggerated tendon jerks, and extensor plantar reflexes, while the pupillary reflexes are normal.

Friedreich's ataxia causes, as in many cases of MS, nystagmus, absent abdominal reflexes, ataxia of the lower limbs, loss of postural sensibility, and extensor plantar responses. In this disease, however, the ankle-jerks, and later the knee-jerks, are lost or diminished, there is scoliosis, and pes cavus, and the frequent onset in childhood, slow progressive course, and occurrence of multiple cases in one family are distinctive.

Other familial ataxias. Some forms of familial ataxia have been described which are virtually indistinguishable from MS, e.g. the family described by Ferguson and Critchley (1929). Differential points, however, are the familial incidence, the steadily progressive course, and certain manifestations, e.g. marked ocular palsies, extrapyramidal signs, and extensive sensory loss, which are unusual in MS.

Subacute combined degeneration may lead to confusion as a cause of 'ataxic paraplegia'. It usually begins, however, later in life than do most cases of MS, paraesthesiae appear early and persist, the tendon reflexes in the lower limbs are often lost, and gastric achylia, megalocytic anaemia, and a low serum B_{12} activity are distinctive features.

Spinal tumour. MS may closely simulate spinal tumour when it gives rise to progressive spastic paraplegia, with or without sensory loss up to a segmental level, and without evident physical signs above this level. VER recording may be helpful. In any case of doubt spinal CT scanning and/or myelography will be needed.

Cervical spondylosis with myelopathy may lead to ataxia, weakness of the upper limbs and spastic paraplegia, and so be confused with MS. Plain X-rays of the cervical spine and myelography may help, but the two conditions are so common that they often coexist. Here again, evoked-potential recording as well as CSF IgG estimation may give the answer.

Other spinal lesions. The neurological complications of Behçet's disease (p. 259) may give a picture similar to MS, especially if mucosal lesions in the mouth and genitalia are unobtrusive. An arteriovenous angioma of the cord and subacute necrotic myelitis can also give similar symptoms and signs but CSF examination and myelography and/or CT scanning or spinal angiography are usually diagnostic.

Hysteria is often confused with MS but a thorough examination of the nervous system usually clarifies the position. Such early symptoms as giddiness, paraesthesiae, and paresis may, however, be unaccompanied by convincing signs at first and it is not rare for a patient to develop hysterical symptoms in addition to those of MS. An hysterical overlay present in the early stages often therefore causes difficulty in initial diagnosis.

Prognosis

The extremely variable course renders prognosis difficult. The disease in its acute form may terminate fatally in three months or less, or the patient may still be able to work 50 years after the onset. When retrobulbar neuritis is the first symptom the next may not follow for many years. Among Brain's patients there were remissions of 13, 15, 17, and 19 years after such an attack of retrobulbar neuritis, and of 20 and 25 years after another symptom, before the disease recurred. Hutchinson (1976) found a probability of 78 per cent that a patient with retrobulbar neuritis would develop MS within 15 years. Factors thought to increase this probability have included an onset in the winter, an association with HLA BT 101, and recurrent attacks (Compston, Batchelor, Earl, and McDonald 1978; Cohen, Lessell, and Wolf 1979). It is conceivable that a remission may last a lifetime and the patient recovers permanently from his first attack (McAlpine *et al.* 1972). McAlpine and Compston (1952) found the average number of fresh 'attacks' of all types to be about 0. 4 per year for patients of both sexes. It was often said in the past that the disease is generally fatal within 5 to 25 years of the onset but there is now convincing evidence (*British Medical Journal* 1980*a*) that many patients survive much longer, not simply due to the more effective treatment of intercurrent infection with antibiotics and of bedsores and other complications. Certainly patients presenting in early adult life with progressive ataxic paraparesis or signs of multiple lesions and especially those with severe cerebellar ataxia have a much worse prognosis than average (Leibowitz *et al.* 1969). Even so, unexpectedly complete remission may occur and Kurtzke, Beebe, Nagler, Auth, Kurland, and Nefzger (1973) found that most patients recovered from an initial severe episode, especially if the manifestations were predominantly sensory; prolonged but milder relapses recovered less completely. Kurtzke, Beebe, Nagler, Nefzger, Auth, and Kurland (1970) found that 69 per cent of male patients lived more than 25, and 50 per cent more than 35 years after the onset. Stendahl-Brodin and Link (1980) found a positive correlation between a benign course and a low-grade humoral immune response in the CSF. Confavreux, Aimard, and Devic (1980) found that there was a poorer prognosis in cases of late onset, in those with a short interval between the first two relapses, and with an early onset of the progressive phase, and the findings of Detels, Clark, Valdiviezo, Visscher, Malmgren, and Dudley (1982) were similar save that in their series the outlook was more unfavourable in males of all ages. Confavreux *et al.* (1980) estimated that 50 per cent of patients can expect to be moderately disabled but still walking in six years, severely disabled and unable to walk in 18 years, and dead in 30 years.

This evidence that the disease often runs a benign course and that some patients remain mobile and relatively unrestricted in their activity for 20 years or more and survive to a normal age does not, however, detract from the fact that in many severe cases the patient is confined to a wheelchair for many years or even, in the end, to bed. The terminal stages may be very distressing. Graphic accounts have been given by sufferers, such as W.N.P. Barbellion, in *The diary of a disappointed man* and *Enjoying life* and by Gould (1982). Ataxia, weakness, and spasticity confine the patient to bed and prevent him or her from carrying out the simplest actions. Swallowing becomes difficult and speech almost unintelligible. Urinary infection or pneumonia finally releases the sufferer. In rare cases the last event is an acute exacerbation of the disease itself, taking the form of an acute myelitis or encephalomyelitis.

Treatment

General measures

The management of the patient requires tact and judgement. Because of the public image of MS as a progressive and incurable disease, it may be best in an early attack to use terms such as 'neuritis' to identify it, but when the disease enters upon a progressive course or if the patient asks 'Am I suffering from MS?' it is unjustifiable to withhold the diagnosis. Every effort should be made to keep the patient at his usual occupation as long as possible. The attachment of weights to an affected limb may lessen distressing intention tremor (Hewer, Cooper, and Morgan 1972) and isoniazid has been found helpful in four such cases (Sabra, Hallett, Sudarsky, and Mullally 1982); when such tremor is very severe it may be abolished by stereotaxic ventrolateral thalamotomy but relief is often temporary and the procedure may cause confusion or hasten the progression of incipient dementia. In later stages encouragement and suggestion, and vigorous physiotherapy including active and passive movements and re-educational walking exercises may long postpone the bedridden state. Even though pregnancy may not influence the relapse rate it may accelerate deterioration in a moderately advanced case, so that contraceptive advice or even sterilization may be indicated. Spasticity may be relieved by drugs such as diazepam, 2-5 mg, dantrolene sodium 50-75 mg, or baclofen (5 mg initially, increasing to 15 mg), each given three or four times daily, while in selected cases intrathecal phenol or hypertonic saline injections are useful for the relief of flexor spasms. Electrical stimulation of the spinal dorsal columns, either percutaneously or using implanted epidural electrodes, has been thought greatly to lessen disability (Cook and Weinstein 1973; Illis, Oygar, Sedgewick, and Subbahi Awadalla 1976; Illis, Sedgewick, and Tallis 1980) but others have found the procedure ineffective (Rosen and Barsoum 1979; Hawkes, Wyke, Desmond,

Bultitude, and Kanegaonkar 1980: Read, Matthews, and Higson 1980; *British Medical Journal* 1980b). Carbamazepine, 200 mg three times daily or other anticonvulsant drugs usually control paroxysmal symptoms such as tonic fits (Espir and Millac 1970). Propantheline, 15 mg two or three times daily, may control urgency of micturition. Calipers and other mechanical aids are of value in appropriate cases and the advice of an occupational therapist may be of great benefit. In the late stages the skin, bladder, and rectum will require attention, as in paraplegia from any cause. In such patients investigation will often reveal residual urine and impaired renal efficiency.

Specific treatment

Assessment of the effects of treatment upon the disease is difficult in a condition like MS which remits and relapses spontaneously, and which is so variable in its clinical course. The number, duration, and severity of relapses occurring in a given period is one helpful guide. Various scales or scores of disability assessment have been designed (see Kurtzke 1955, 1970; McAlpine *et al.* 1972) and Schumacher (1974) has defined the minimal acceptable criteria for assessing the effects of treatment while Brown, Beebe, Kurtzke, Loewenson, Silberberg, and Tourtellotte (1979) have laid down comprehensive guidelines for clinical trials. Claims of benefit with intrathecal tuberculin (Smith, Espir, Whitty, and Russell 1957) or with a low-fat diet (Swank 1955, 1970) have not been substantiated. However, there is some evidence that ACTH given in a dosage of 80 units daily for a week, every other day for 2 weeks and then twice weekly for 3 weeks may reduce the severity and duration of a relapse (Rose, Kuzma, Kutzke, Namerow, Sibley, and Tourtellotte 1970; McAlpine *et al.* 1972) though long-term treatment with prednisone or ACTH is ineffective despite the occasional occurrence of patients who are apparently steroid-dependent (Miller, Newell, and Ridley 1961; Boman, Hokkanen, Jarho, and Kivalo 1966; Millar, Vas, Noronha, Liversedge, and Rawson 1967; Millar, Rahman, Vas, Noronha, Liversedge, and Swinburn 1970). Early investigations with immunosuppressive agents (Neumann and Ziegler 1972) showed that 6-mercaptopurine or methotrexate alone are of no value; antilymphocyte globulin (ALG) has been found effective in some hands (Seland, McPherson, Grace, Lamoureux, and Blain 1974) but not in others (MacFayden, Reeve, Bratty, and Thomas 1973; Kastrukoff, McLean, and McPherson 1978), while the place of intensive immunosuppression with thoracic-duct drainage, ALG, azathioprine, and prednisone (Brendel, Seifert, and Lob 1972; Ring, Seifert, Lob, Coulin, Angstwurm, Frick, Brass, Mertin, Backmund, and Brendel 1974) is still uncertain. Mertin and co-workers (Mertin, Knight, Rudge, Thompson, and Healy 1980; Mertin, Rudge, Kremer, Healey, Knight, Compston, Batchelor, Thompson, Halliday, Denman, and Medawar 1982) found that vigorous immunosuppression reduced the relapse rate, especially in females and in those who were HLA-A3 positive, while Patzold, Hecker, and Pocklington (1982) have claimed significant benefit from long-term treatment with azathioprine in a dose of 2 mg/kg/day. Desensitization therapy with MBP has been proposed by Alvord, Shaw, Hruby, and Kies (1979), and Bornstein, Miller, Teitelbaum, Arnon, and Sela (1982) have treated 12 patents, apparently with benefit, with the synthetic polypeptide COP 1 which suppresses EAE in experimental animals. It has also been suggested that transfer factor (Fog, Pedersen, Raun, Kam-Hansen, Mellerup, Platz, Ryder, Jakobsen, and Grob 1978; Basten, McLeod, Pollard, Walsh, Stewart, Garrick, Frith, and Van de Brink 1980) may retard the progress of the disease, as may intrathecal interferon (Jacobs, O'Malley, Freeman, Murawski, and Ekes 1982), but plasmapheresis, recommended by Dau, Petajan, Johnson, Panitch, and Bornstein (1980), has been found ineffective by others (Tindall, Walker, Ehle, Near, Rollins, and Becker 1982). ACTH in relapses and azathioprine for long-term treatment seem at present to be the treatments of choice, but the position is continually changing. There is no scientific evidence to support the use of a gluten-free diet, despite the publicity given to remission in one severe case on such a diet, and there is no convincing evidence to support the use of linoleic acid supplements either (Millar, Zilkha, Langman, Wright, Payling Smith, Belin, and Thompson 1973; Bates, Fawcett, Shaw, and Weightman 1978).

References

Acheson, E. D. (1972). The epidemiology of multiple sclerosis. In *Multiple sclerosis: a reappraisal* (ed. D. McAlpine, C. E. Lumsden, and E. D. Acheson) 2nd edn. Part I, p. 3. Churchill-Livingstone, Edinburgh.

Allen, I. V. (1981). The pathology of multiple sclerosis—fact, fiction and hypothesis. *Neuropath. appl. Neurobiol.* **7**, 169

Allen, J. C., Sheremata, W., Cosgrove, J. B. R., Osterland, K., and Shea, M. (1976). Cerebrospinal fluid T and B lymphocyte kinetics related to exacerbations of multiple sclerosis. *Neurology, Minneapolis* **26**, 579.

Allison, R. S. (1950). Survival in disseminated sclerosis. *Brain* **73**, 103.

Alter, M., Kahana, E., and Loewenson, R. (1978). Migration and risk of multiple sclerosis. *Neurology, Minneapolis* **28**, 1089.

Alvord, E. C., Shaw, C. M., Hruby, S., and Kies, M. W. (1979). Has myelin basis protein received a fair trial in the treatment of multiple sclerosis? *Ann. Neurol.* **6**, 461.

Ames, F. R. and Louw, S. (1977). Multiple sclerosis in coloured South Africans. *J. Neurol. Neurosurg. Psychiat.* **40**, 729.

Antel, J. P., Arnason, B. W., and Medof, M. E. (1979). Suppressor cell function in multiple sclerosis: correlation with clinical disease activity. *Ann. Neurol.* **5**, 338

Appel, M. J., Glickman, L. T., Raine, C. S., and Tourtellotte, W. W. (1981). Canine viruses and multiple sclerosis. *Neurology, Minneapolis* **31**, 944.

Arnadottir, T., Reunanen, M., Meurman, O., Salmi, A., Panelius, M., and Halonen, P. (1979). Measles and rubella virus antibodies in patients with multiple sclerosis: a longitudinal study of serum and CSF specimens by radioimmunassay. *Arch. Neurol., Chicago* **36**, 261.

Arnason, B. G. W., Fuller, T. C., Lehrich, J. R., and Wray, S. H. (1974). Histocompatability types and measles antibodies in multiple sclerosis and optic neuritis. *J. neurol. Sci.* **22**, 419.

Aschoff, J. C., Conrad, B., and Kornhuber, H. H. (1974). Acquired pendular nystagmus with oscillopsia in multiple sclerosis: a sign of cerebellar nuclei disease. *J. Neurol. Neurosurg. Psychiat.* **37**, 570.

Asselman, P., Chadwick, D. W., and Marsden, C. D. (1975). Visual evoked responses in the diagnosis and management of patients suspected of multiple sclerosis. *Brain* **98**, 261.

Bamford, C. R., Sibley, W. A., Thies, C., Laguna, J. F., Smith, M. S., and Clark, K. (1981). Trauma as an etiologic and aggravating factor in multiple sclerosis. *Neurology, Minneapolis* **31**, 1229.

Basten, A., McLeod, J. G., Pollard, J. D., Walsh, J. C., Stewart, G. J., Garrick, R., Frith, J. A., and Van der Brink, C. M. (1980). Transfer factor in treatment of multiple sclerosis. *Lancet* ii, 931.

Bates, D., Fawcett, P. R. W., Shaw, D. A., and Weightman, D. (1978). Polyunsaturated fatty acids in treatment of acute remitting multiple sclerosis. *Br. med. J.* **2**, 1390.

Bateson, M. C., Hopwood, D., and MacGillivray, J. B. (1979). Jejunal morphology in multiple sclerosis. *Lancet* i, 1108.

Baum, H. M. and Rothschild, B. B. (1981). The incidence and prevalence of reported multiple sclerosis. *Ann. Neurol.* **10**, 420.

Ben Hamida, M. (1977). La sclérose en plaques en Tunisie: étude clinique de 100 observations. *Rev. Neurol., Paris* **133**, 109.

Birnbaum, G. and Kotilinek, L. (1981). Autologous lymphocyte proliferation in multiple sclerosis and the effect of intravenous ACTH. *Ann. Neurol.* **9**, 439.

Bobowick, A. R., Kurtzke, J. F., Brody, J. A., Hrubec, Z., and Gillespie, M. (1978). Twin study of multiple sclerosis: an epidemiologic inquiry. *Neurology, Minneapolis* **28**, 978.

Bodis-Wollner, I., Hendley, C. D., Mylin, L. H., and Thornton, J. (1979). Visual evoked potentials and the visuogram in multiple sclerosis. *Ann. Neurol.* **5**, 40.

Boman, K., Hokkanen, E., Jarho, L., and Kivalo, E. (1966). Double-blind study of the effect of corticotropin treatment in multiple sclerosis. *Ann. Med. Int. Fenn.* **55**, 71.

Bornstein, M. B., Miller, A. I., Teitelbaum, D., Arnon, R., and Sela, M. (1982). Multiple sclerosis: trial of a synthetic polypeptide. *Ann. Neurol.* **11**, 317.

Brendel, W., Seifert, J., and Lob, G. (1972). Effect of 'maximum immune suppression' with thoracic duct drainage, ALG, azathioprine and cortisone in some neurological disorders. *Proc. R. Soc. Med.* **65**, 531.

British Medical Journal (1972). Benign forms of multiple sclerosis. *Br. med. J.* **1**, 392.

—— (1980a). The prognosis of multiple sclerosis. *Br. med. J.* **281**, 824.

—— (1980b). Dorsal column stimulation in multiple sclerosis. *Br. med. J.* **280**, 1287.

Brown, J. R., Beebe, G. W., Kurtzke, J. F., Loewenson, R. B., Silberberg, D. H., and Tourtellotte, W. W. (1979). The design of clinical studies to assess therapeutic efficacy in multiple sclerosis. *Neurology, Minneapolis* **29**, 3.

Cala, L. A. and Mastaglia, F. L. (1976). Computerized axial tomography in multiple sclerosis. *Lancet* i, 689.

—— and Black, J. L. (1978). Computerized tomography of brain and optic nerve in multiple sclerosis: observations in 100 patients, including serial studies in 16. *J. neurol. Sci.* **36**, 411.

Carp, R. I., Licursi, P. A., and Merz, G. S. (1972). Decreased percentages of polymorphonuclear neutrophils in mouse peripheral blood after inoculation with material from multiple sclerosis patients. *J. exp. Med.* **136**, 618.

——, Merz, G. S., and Licursi, P. C. (1975). A non-cytopathic infectious agent associated with multiple sclerosis material. *Neurology, Minneapolis* **25**, 492.

Cartlidge, N. E. F. (1972). Autonomic function in multiple sclerosis. *Brain* **95**, 661.

Chopra, J. S., Radhakrishnan, K., Sawhney, B. B., Pal, S. R., and Banerjee, A. K. (1980). Multiple sclerosis in North-West India. *Acta neurol. scand.* **62**, 312.

Cohen, M. M., Lossell, S., and Wolf, P. A. (1979). A prospective study of the risk of developing multiple sclerosis in uncomplicated optic neuritis. *Neurology, Minneapolis* **29**, 208.

Colby, S. P., Sheremata, W., Bain, B., and Eylar, E. H. (1977). Cellular hypersensitivity in attacks of multiple sclerosis. 1. A comparative study of migration inhibitory factor production and lymphoblastic transformation in response to myelin basic protein in multiple sclerosis. *Neurology, Minneapolis* **27**, 132.

Collins, D. W. K., Black, J. L., and Mastaglia, F. L. (1978). Pattern-reversal visual evoked potential: method of analysis and results in multiple sclerosis. *J. neurol. Sci.* **36**, 83.

Compston, D. A. S., Batchelor, J. R., Earl, C. J., and McDonald, W. I. (1978). Factors influencing the risk of multiple sclerosis developing in patients with optic neuritis. *Brain* **101**, 495.

Confavreux, C., Aimard, G., and Devic, M. (1980). Course and prognosis of multiple sclerosis assessed by the computerized data processing of 349 patients. *Brain* **103**, 281.

Cook, A. W. and Weinstein, S. P. (1973). Chronic dorsal column stimulation in multiple sclerosis: preliminary report. *NY State J. Med.* **73**, 2826.

Cook, S. D. and Dowling, P. C. (1977). A possible association between house pets and multiple sclerosis. *Lancet* i, 980.

——, ——, and Russell, W. C. (1979). Neutralizing antibodies to canine distemper and measles virus in multiple sclerosis. *J. neurol. Sci.* **41**, 61.

Coyle, P. K., Brooks, B. R., Hirsch, R. L., Cohen, S. R., O'Donnell, P., Johnson, R. T., and Wolinsky, J. S. (1980). Cerebrospinal-fluid lymphocyte populations and immune complexes in active multiple sclerosis. *Lancet* ii, 229.

Currier, R. D. and Eldridge, R. (1982). Possible risk factors in multiple sclerosis as found in a national twin study. *Arch. Neurol., Chicago* **39**, 140.

——, Martin, E. A., and Woolsey, P. C. (1974). Prior events in multiple sclerosis. *Neurology, Minneapolis* **24**, 748.

Cuypers, J. and Reddemann, H. (1980). Evaluation of the erythrocyte-UFA mobility test for the diagnosis of multiple sclerosis. *J. Neurol. Neurosurg. Psychiat.* **43**, 995.

Dau, P. C., Petajan, J. H., Johnson, K. P., Panitch, H. S., and Bornstein, M. B. (1980). Plasmapheresis in multiple sclerosis: preliminary findings. *Neurology, Minneapolis* **30**, 1023.

Davis, F. A. (1970). Axonal conduction studies based on some considerations of temperature effects in multiple sclerosis. *Electroenceph. clin. Neurophysiol.* **28** 281.

Davison, A. N. and Cuzner, M. L. (1977). Immunochemistry and biochemistry of myelin. *Br. med. Bull.* **33**, 60.

Dawson, J. W. (1916). The histology of disseminated sclerosis. *Trans. R. Soc., Edinburgh* **50**, 517.

Dean, G., McLoughlin, H., Brady, R., Adelstein, A. M., and Tallett-Williams, J. (1976). Multiple sclerosis among immigrants in Greater London. *Br. med. J.* **1**, 861.

Detels, R., Clark, V. A., Valdiviezo, N. L., Visscher, B. R., Malmgren, R. M., and Dudley, J. P. (1982). Factors associated with a rapid course of multiple sclerosis. *Arch. Neurol., Chicago* **39**, 337.

Dow, R. S. and Berglund, G. (1942). Vascular pattern of lesions of disseminated sclerosis. *Arch. Neurol. Psychiat., Chicago* **47**, 1.

Dowling, P. C., Kim, S. U., Murray, M. R., and Cook, S. D. (1968). Serum 19s and 7s demyelinating antibodies in multiple sclerosis. *J. Immunol*, **101**, 1101.

Dubois-Dalcq, M., Schumacher, G., and Sever, J. L. (1973). Acute multiple sclerosis: electron-microscopic evidence for and against a viral agent in the plaques. *Lancet,* **ii**, 1408.

Ebers, G. C., Paty, D. W., Stiller, C. R., Nelson, R. F., Seland, T. P., and Larsen, B. (1982). HLA-typing in multiple sclerosis sibling pairs. *Lancet* ii, 88.

Einstein, E. R., Csejtey, J., Dalal, K. B., Adams, C. W. M., Bayliss, O. B., and Hallpike, J. (1972). Proteolytic activity and basic protein loss in and around multiple sclerosis plaques: combined biochemical and histochemical observations. *J. Neurochem.* **19**, 653.

Eisen, A. and Nudleman, K. (1979). Cord to cortex conduction in multiple sclerosis. *Neurology, Minneapolis* **29**, 189.

——, Paty, D., Purves, S., and Hoirch, M. (1981). Occult fifth nerve dysfunction in multiple sclerosis. *Can. J. neurol. Sci.* **8**, 221.

Eldridge, R., McFarland, H., Sever, J., Sadowsky, D., and Krebs, H. (1978). Familial multiple sclerosis: clinical, histocompatibility, and viral serological studies. *Ann. Neurol.* **3**, 72.

Ellenberger, C. and Ziegler, S. B. (1977). Visual evoked potentials and quantitative perimetry in multiple sclerosis. *Ann. Neurol.* **1**, 561.

Engell, T., Raun, N. E., Thomsen, M., and Platz, P. (1982). HLA and heterogeneity of multiple sclerosis. *Neurology, Minneapolis* **32**, 1043.

Esiri, M. M. (1977). Immunoglobulin-containing cells in multiple sclerosis plaques. *Lancet* ii, 478.

—— (1980). Multiple sclerosis: a quantitative and qualitative study of immunoglobulin-containing cells in the central nervous system. *Neuropath. appl. Neurobiol.* **6**, 9.

Espir, M. L. E. and Millac, P. (1970). Treatment of paroxysmal disorders in multiple sclerosis with carbamazepine (Tegretol). *J. Neurol. Neurosurg. Psychiat.* **33**, 528.

Feasby, T. E., Paty, D. W., Ebers, G. C., and Fox, A. J. (1981). Spinal cord swelling in multiple sclerosis. *Can. J. neurol. Sci.* **8**, 151.

Ferguson, F. R. and Critchley, M. (1929). A clinical study of an heredo-familial disease resembling disseminated sclerosis. *Brain* **52**, 203.

Field. E. J., Joyce, G., and Smith, B. M. (1977). Erythrocyte-UFA (EUFA) mobility test for multiple sclerosis: implications for pathogenesis and handling of the disease. *J. Neurol.* **214**, 113.

Fischer-Williams, M. and Roberts, R. C. 81971). Cerebrospinal fluid proteins and serum immunoglobulins. Occurrence in multiple sclerosis and other neurological diseases: comparative measurement of γ-globulin and the IgG class. *Arch. Neurol., Chicago* **25**, 526.

Fishman, R. A. (1980). *Cerebrospinal fluid in diseases of the nervous system.*. Saunders, Philadelphia.

Fog, T., Pedersen, L., Raun, N. E., Kam-Hansen, S., Mellerup, E., Platz, P., Ryder, L. P., Jakobsen, B. K., and Grob, P. (1978). Long-term transfer-factor treatment for multiple sclerosis. *Lancet* i, 851.

Fraser, K. B., Haire, M., Millar, J. H. D., and McCrea, S. (1979). Increased tendency to spontaneous in-vitro lymphocyte transformation in clinically active multiple sclerosis. *Lancet* ii, 715.

Ganes, T. (1980). Somatosensory evoked responses and central afferent conduction times in patients with multiple sclerosis. *J. Neurol. Neurosurg. Psychiat.* **43**, 948.

Gilbert, G. J. (1971). Multiple sclerosis in the child of conjugal multiple sclerosis patients. *Neurology, Minneapolis* **21**, 1169.

Gould, J. (1982). Disabilities and how to live with them: multiple sclerosis. *Lancet* ii, 1208.

Goust, J. M., Chenais, F., Carnes, J. E., Hames, C. G., Fudenberg, H. H., and Hogan, E. L. (1978). Abnormal T cell subpopulations and circulating immune complexes in the Guillain–Barré syndrome and multiple sclerosis. *Neurology, Minneapolis* **28**, 421.

Granieri, E. and Rosati, G. (1982). Italy: a medium or high-risk area for multiple sclerosis? An epidemiologic study in Barbagia, Sardinia, southern Italy. *Neurology, Minneapolis* **32**, 466.

Greenfield, J. G. and King, L. S. (1936). Histopathology of the cerebral lesions in disseminated sclerosis. *Brain* **59**, 445.

Halliday, A. M., McDonald, W. I., and Mushin, J. (1973). Visual evoked responses in diagnosis of multiple sclerosis. *Br. med. J.* **4**, 661.

Harding, A. E., Radue, E. W., and Whiteley, A. M. (1978). Contrast-enhanced lesions on computerised tomography in multiple sclerosis. *J. Neurol. Neurosurg. Psychiat.* **41**, 754.

Hauser, S. L., Bresnan, M. J., Reinherz, E. L., and Weiner, H. L. (1982). Childhood multiple sclerosis: clinical features and demonstration of changes in T cell subsets with disease activity. *Ann. Neurol.* **11**, 463.

Hawkes, C. H., Wyke, M., Desmond, A., Bultitude, M. I., and Kanegaonkar, G. S. (1980). Stimulation of dorsal column in multiple sclerosis. *Br. med. J.* **280**, 889.

Hewer, R. L., Cooper, R., and Morgan, M. H. (1972). An investigation into the value of treating intention tremor by weighting the affected limb. *Brain* **95**, 579.

Hopf, H. C. and Eysholdt, M. (1978). Impaired refractory periods of peripheral sensory nerves in multiple sclerosis. *Ann. Neurol.* **4**, 499.

Hosein, Z. Z. and Johnson, K. P. (1981). Isoelectric focusing of cerebrospinal fluid proteins in the diagnosis of multiple sclerosis. *Neurology, Minneapolis* **31**, 70.

Hutchinson, W. M. (1976). Acute optic neuritis and the prognosis for multiple sclerosis. *J. Neurol. Neurosurg. Psychiat.* **39**, 283.

Illis, L. S., Oygar, A. E., Sedgwick, E. M., and Sabbahi Awadalla, M. A. (1976). Dorsal-column stimulation in the rehabilitation of patients with multiple sclerosis. *Lancet* **i**, 1383.

——, Sedgwick, E. M., and Tallis, R. C. (1980). Spinal cord stimulation in multiple sclerosis: clinical results. *J. Neurol. Neurosurg. Psychiat.* **43**, 1.

Jacobs, L., O'Malley, J., Freeman, A., Murawski, J., and Ekes, R. (1982). Intrathecal interferon in multiple sclerosis. *Arch. Neurol., Chicago* **39**, 609.

Jacque, C., Delassalle, A., Rancurel, G., Raoul, M., Lesourd, B., and Legrand, J. -C. (1982). Myelin basic protein in CSF and blood: relationship between its presence and the occurrence of a destructive process in the brains of encephalitic patients. *Arch. Neurol., Chicago* **39**, 557.

Jameson, R. M. (1982). The bladder in multiple sclerosis. *J. R. Soc. Med.* **75**, 75.

Jestico, J. V. and Ellis, P. D. M. 81976). Changes in nystagmus on raising body temperature in clinically suspected and proven multiple sclerosis. *Br. med. J.* **2**, 970.

Jones, P. E., Pallis, C., and Peters, T. J. (1979). Morphological and biochemical findings in jejunal biopsies from patients with multiple sclerosis. *J. Neurol. Neurosurg. Psychiat.* **42**, 402.

Kabat, E. A., Moore, D. H., and Landow, H. (1942). An electrophoretic study of the protein components of cerebrospinal fluid and their relationship to the serum proteins. *J. clin. Invest.* **21**, 571.

Kahana, E., Leibowitz, U., and Alter, M. (1971). Cerebral multiple sclerosis. *Neurology, Minneapolis* **21**, 1179.

Kam-Hansen, S. 81979). Reduced number of active cells in cerebrospinal fluid in multiple sclerosis. *Neurology, Minneapolis* **29**, 897.

—— (1980). Distribution and function of lymphocytes from the cerebrospinal fluid in patients with multiple sclerosis. *Acta neurol. scand.* **62**, suppl. 75.

Kastrukoff, L.F., McLean, D. R., and McPherson, T. A. (1978). Multiple sclerosis treated with antithymocyte globulin—a five year follow-up. *Can. J. neurol. Sci.* **5**, 175.

Kolar, O. J., Rice, P. H., Jones, F. H., Defalque, R. J., and Kincaid, J. (1980). Cerebrospinal fluid immunoelectrophoresis in multiple sclerosis. *J. neurol. Sci.* **47**, 221.

——, Ross, A. T., and Herman, J. T. (1970). Serum and cerebrospinal fluid immunoglobulins in multiple sclerosis. *Neurology, Minneapolis* **20**, 1052.

—— and Zeman, W. (1967). Immunoelectrophoretic changes of serum IgG during subacute inflammatory and demyelinating diseases of the central nervous system. *Z. Immunitätsforsch.* **134**, 267.

Kurdi, A., Ayesh, I., Abdallat, A., Maayta, U., McDonald, W. I., Compston, D. A. S., and Batchelor, J. R. (1977). Different B lymphocyte alloantigens associated with multiple sclerosis in Arabs and north Europeans. *Lancet* **i**, 1123.

Kuroiwa, Y., Hung, T. -P., Landsborough, D., Park, C. S., Singhal, B. S., Soemargo, S., Vejjajiva, A., and Shibasaki, H. (1977). Multiple sclerosis in Asia. *Neurology, Minneapolis* **27**, 188.

—— and Shibasaki, H. (1973). Clinical studies of multiple sclerosis in Japan. 1. A current appraisal of 83 cases. *Neurology, Minneapolis* **23**, 611.

Kurtzke, J. F. (1955). A new scale for evaluating disability in multiple sclerosis. *Neurology, Minneapolis* **5**, 580.

—— (1970). Neurologic impairment in multiple sclerosis and the disability status scale. *Acta neurol. scand.* **46**, 493.

—— (1972). Multiple sclerosis death rates from underlying cause and total deaths. *Acta neurol. scand.* **48**, 148.

—— (1975a). A reassessment of the distribution of multiple sclerosis—Part One. *Acta neurol. scand.* **51**, 110.

—— (1975b). A reassessment of the distribution of multiple sclerosis—Part Two. *Acta neurol. scand.* **51**, 137.

—— (1980a). Geographic distribution of multiple sclerosis: an update reference to Europe and the Mediterranean region. *Acta neurol. scand.* **62**, 65.

—— (1980b). Epidemiologic contributions to multiple sclerosis: an overview. *Neurology, Minneapolis* **30**, 61.

—— Beebe, G. W., Nagler, B., Auth, T. L., Kurland, L. T., and Nefzger, M. D. (1973). Studies on the natural history of multiple sclerosis. 7. Correlates of clinical change in an early bout. *Acta neurol. scand.* **49**, 379.

——, ——, ——, Nefzger, M. D., Auth, T. L., and Kurland, L. T. (1970). Studies on the natural history of multiple sclerosis. V. Long-term survival in young men. *Arch. Neurol., Chicago* **22**, 215.

—— and Bui-Quoc-Huong (1980). Multiple sclerosis in a migrant population: 2. Half-Orientals immigrating in childhood. *Ann. Neurol.* **8**, 256.

——, Gudmundsson, K. R., and Bergmann, S. (1982). Multiple sclerosis in Iceland: 1. Evidence of a postwar epidemic. *Neurology, Minneapolis* **32**, 143.

—— and Hyllested, K. (1979). Multiple sclerosis in the Faroe Islands: 1. Clinical and epidemiological features. *Ann. Neurol.* **5**, 6.

——, Kurland, L. T., and Goldberg, I. D. (1971). Mortality and migration in multiple sclerosis. *Neurology, Minneapolis* **21**, 1186.

—— and Priester, W. A. (1979). Dogs, distemper, and multiple sclerosis in the United States. *Acta neurol. scand.* **60**, 312.

Lampert, F. and Lampert, P. (1975). Multiple sclerosis: morphologic evidence of intranuclear paramyxovirus or altered chromatin fibers? *Arch. Neurol., Chicago* **32**, 425.

The Lancet (1981). The aetiology of multiple sclerosis. *Lancet* **i**, 1347.

—— (1982). Evoked potentials in multiple sclerosis. *Lancet* **i**, 1445.

Lane, B., Carroll, B. A., and Pedley, T. A. (1978). Computerized cranial tomography in cerebral diseases of white matter. *Neurology, Minneapolis* **28**, 534.

Lassmann, H. and Wisniewski, H. M. 81979). Chronic relapsing experimental allergic encephalomyelitis: clinicopathological comparison with multiple sclerosis. *Arch. Neurol., Chicago* **36**, 490.

Lebow, S., Anderson, D. C., Mastri, A., and Larson, D. (1978). Acute multiple sclerosis with contrast-enhancing plaques. *Arch. Neurol. Chicago* **35**, 435.

Lehrich, J. R. and Arnason, B. G. W. (1976). Histocompatibility types and viral antibodies. *Arch. Neurol., Chicago* **33**, 404.

——, ——, Fuller, T. C., and Wray, S. H. (1974). Parainfluenza, histocompatibility, and multiple sclerosis. Association of parainfluenza antibodies and histocompatibility types in MS and optic neuritis. *Arch. Neurol., Chicago* **30**, 327.

Leibowitz, U. and Alter, M. (1973). *Multiple sclerosis: clues to its cause.* Elsevier, Amsterdam.

——, Kahana, E., and Alter, M. (1969). Multiple sclerosis in immigrant and native populations of Israel. *Lancet* **ii**, 1323.

Link, H. and Laurenzi, M. A. (1979). Immunoglobulin class and light chain type of oligoclonal bands in CSF in multiple sclerosis determined by agarose gel electrophoresis and immunofixation. *Ann. Neurol.* **6**, 107.

—— and Müller, R. (1971). Immunoglobulins in multiple sclerosis and infections of the nervous system. *Arch. Neurol., Chicago* **25**, 326.

Lofti, J., Nikbin, B., Derakhshan, I., Aghai, Z., and Ala, F. (1978). Histocompatibility antigens (HLA) in multiple sclerosis in Iran. *J. Neurol. Neurosurg. Psychiat.* **41**, 699.

Lumsden, C. E. (1970). The neuropathology of multiple sclerosis. In *Handbook of clinical neurology* (ed. P. J. Vinken and G. W. Bruyn) Volume 9, p. 217. North-Holland, Amsterdam.

—— (1971). The immunogenesis of the multiple sclerosis plaque. *Brain Res.* **28**, 365.

—— (1972). The clinical pathology of multiple sclerosis. In *Multiple sclerosis: a reappraisal* (ed. D. McAlpine, C. E. Lumsden and E. D. Acheson) 2nd ed. p. 311. Churchill-Livingstone, Edinburgh.

MacFadyen, D. J., Reeve, C. E., Bratty, P. J. A., and Thomas, J. W. (1973). Failure of antilymphocytic globulin therapy in chronic progressive multiple sclerosis. *Neurology, Minneapolis* **23**, 592.

Madigand, M., Oger, J. J. -F., Fauchet, R., Sabouraud, O., and Genetet, B. (1982). HLA profiles in multiple sclerosis suggest two forms of disease and the existence of protective haplotypes. *J. neurol. Sci.* **53**, 519.

Mandelbrote, B. M., Stanier, M. W., Thompson, R. H. S., and Thruston, M. N. (1948). Studies on copper metabolism in demyelinating diseases of the nervous system. *Brain* **71**, 212.

Margulis, M. S., Soloviev, V. D., and Shubladze, A. K. (1946). Aetiology and pathogenesis of acute sporadic encephalomyelitis and multiple sclerosis. *J. Neurol. Neurosurg. Psychiat.* **9**, 63.

Martin, J. R. (1981). Herpes simplex virus types 1 and 2 and multiple sclerosis. *Lancet* **ii**, 777.

Mastaglia, F. L., Black, J. L., and Collins, D. W. K. (1979). Quantitative studies of saccadic and pursuit eye movements in multiple sclerosis. *Brain* **102**, 817.

—— and Cala, L. A. (1982). Nuclear magnetic resonance imaging (NMR) and computerised tomography (CT) in multiple sclerosis. *Lancet* **i**, 850.

—— and Carroll, W. M. (1982). Evoked potentials in neurological diagnosis. *Br. med. J.* **285**, 1678.

Matthews, W. B. (1958). Tonic seizures in disseminated sclerosis. *Brain* **81**, 193.

—— (1975). Paroxysmal symptoms in multiple sclerosis. *J. Neurol. Neurosurg. Psychiat.* **38**, 617.

—— and Small, D. G. (1979). Serial recording of visual and somatosensory evoked potentials in multiple sclerosis. *J. neurol. Sci.* **40**, 11.

——, ——, Small, M., and Pountney, E. (1977). Pattern reversal evoked visual potential in the diagnosis of multiple sclerosis. *J. Neurol. Neurosurg. Psychiat.* **40**, 1009.

McAlpine, D. (1931). Acute disseminated encephalomyelitis: its sequelae and its relationship to disseminated sclerosis. *Lancet* **i**, 846.

—— (1972). Clinical studies . In *Multiple sclerosis: a reappraisal* (ed. D. McAlpine, C. E. Lumsden, and E. D. Acheson) 2nd edn. Part II, p. 82. Churchill-Livingstone, Edinburgh.

—— and Compston, N. (1952). Some aspects of the natural history of disseminated sclerosis. *Quart. J. Med.* **21**, 135.

——, Lumsden, C. E., and Acheson, E. D. (Eds.) (1972). *Multiple sclerosis: a reappraisal*, 2nd edn. Churchill-Livingstone, Edinburgh.

McCall, M. G., Brereton, T. le G., Dawson, A., Millingen, K., Sutherland, J. M., and Acheson, E. D. (1968). Frequency of multiple sclerosis in three Australian cities—Perth, Newcastle, and Hobart. *J. Neurol. Neurosurg. Psychiat.* **31**, 1.

McDermott, J. R., Field, E. J., and Caspary, E. A. (1974). Relation of measles virus to encephalitogenic factor with reference to the aetiopathogenesis of multiple sclerosis. *J. Neurol. Neurosurg. Psychiat.* **37**, 282.

McDonald, W. I. (1974a). Pathophysiology in multiple sclerosis. *Brain* **97**, 179.

—— (1974b). Remyelination in relation to clinical lesions of the central nervous system. *Br. med. Bull.* **30**, 186.

McFarland, H. F. and McFarlin, D. E. (1979). Cellular immune response to measles, mumps, and vaccinia viruses in multiple sclerosis. *Ann. Neurol.* **6**, 101.

Mehta, P. D., Frisch, S., Thormar, H., Tourtellotte, W. W., and Wisniewski, H. M. (1981). Bound antibody in multiple sclerosis brains. *J. neurol. Sci.* **49**, 91.

Melnick, J. L., Seidel, E., Inoue, Y. K., and Nishibe, Y. (1982). Isolation of virus from the spinal fluid of three patients with multiple sclerosis and one with amyotrophic lateral sclerosis. *Lancet* **i**, 830.

Mertin, J., Knight, S. C., Rudge, P., Thompson, E. J., and Healy, M. J. R. (1980). Double-blind, controlled trial of immunosuppression in the treatment of multiple sclerosis. *Lancet* **ii**, 949.

——, Rudge, P., Kremer, M., Healey, M. J. R., Knight, S. C., Compston, A., Batchelor, J. R., Thompson, E. J., Halliday, A. M., Denman, M., and Medawar, P. B. (1982). Double-blind controlled trial of immunosuppression in the treatment of multiple sclerosis: final report. *Lancet* **ii**, 351.

Meyer-Rienecker, H. J., Jenssen, H. L., and Werner, H. (1979). Aspects of cellular immunity in multiple sclerosis: antigen-reactivity of lymphocytes and lymphokine activity. *J. neurol. Sci.* **42**, 173.

Millar, J. H. D. (1971). *Multiple sclerosis: a disease acquired in childhood*, Thomas, Springfield, Illinois.

——, Allison, R. S., Cheeseman, E. A., and Merrett, J. D. (1959). Pregnancy as a factor influencing relapse in disseminated sclerosis. *Brain* **82**, 417.

——, Rahman, R., Vas, C. J., Noronha, M. J., Liversedge, L. A., and Swinburn, W. R. (1970). Effect of withdrawal of corticotrophin in patients on long-term treatment for multiple sclerosis. *Lancet* **i**, 700.

——, Vas, C. J., Noronha, M. J., Liversedge, L. A., and Rawson, M. D. (1967). Long-term treatment of multiple sclerosis with corticotrophin. *Lancet* **ii**, 429.

——, Zilkha, K. J., Langman, M. J. S., Wright, H., Payling Smith, A. D., Belin, J., and Thompson, R. H. S. (1973). Double-blind trial of linoleate supplementation of the diet in multiple sclerosis. *Br. med. J.*, **1**, 765.

Miller, H. (1961). Aetiological factors in disseminated sclerosis. *Proc. R. Soc. Med.* **54**, 7.

—— (1964). Trauma and multiple sclerosis. *Lancet* **i**, 848.

——, Cendrowski, W., and Schapira, K. (1967). Multiple sclerosis and vaccination. *Br. med. J.* **2**, 210.

——, Newell, D. J., and Ridley, A. (1961). Multiple sclerosis. Trials of maintenance treatment with prednisolone and soluble aspirin. *Lancet* **i**, 127.

—— and Schapira, K. (1959). Aetiological aspects of multiple sclerosis. *Br. med. J.* **1**, 737, 811.

Mitchell, D. N., Porterfield, J. S., Micheletti, R., Lange, L. S., Goswami, K. K. A., Taylor, P., Jacobs, J. P., Hockley, D. J., and Salsbury, A. J. (1978). Isolation of an infectious agent from bone-marrow of patients with multiple sclerosis. *Lancet* **ii**, 387.

Miyamoto, H., Walker, J. E., Ginsberg, A. H., Burks, J. S., McIntosh, K., and Kempe, H. (1976). Antibodies to vaccinia and measles viruses in multiple sclerosis patients. *Arch. Neurol., Chicago* **33**, 414.

Morgan, B. P., Campbell, A. K., and Compston, D. A. S. (1984). Terminal component of complement (C9) in cerebrospinal fluid of patients with multiple sclerosis. *Lancet* **ii**, 251.

Namerow, N. S. (1970). Somatosensory recovery functions in multiple sclerosis patients. *Neurology, Minneapolis* **20**, 813.

Narang, H. K. and Field, E. J. (1973). Paramyxovirus like tubules in multiple sclerosis biopsy material. *Acta neuropath., Berlin* **25**, 281.

Nathanson, N., Palsson, P. A., and Gudmundsson, G. (1978). Multiple sclerosis and canine distemper in Iceland. *Lancet* **ii**, 1127.

Nemo, G. J., Brody, J. A., and Waters, D. J. (1974). Serological responses of multiple-sclerosis patients and controls to a virus isolated from a multiple-sclerosis case. *Lancet* **ii**, 1044.

Neumann, J. W. and Ziegler, D. K. (1972). Therapeutic trial of immunosuppressive agents in multiple sclerosis. *Neurology, Minneapolis* **22**, 1268.

Norrby, E., Link, H., and Olsson, J. -E. (1974). Measles virus antibodies in multiple sclerosis: comparison of antibody titers in cerebrospinal fluid and serum. *Arch. Neurol., Chicago* **30**, 285.

Nyland, H., Mörk, S., and Matre, R. (1982). In-situ characterization of mononuclear cell infiltrates in lesions of multiple sclerosis. *Neuropath, appl. Neurobiol,* **8**, 403.

Olmos-Lau, N., Ginsberg, M. D., and Geller, J. B. (1977). Aphasia in multiple sclerosis. *Neurology, Minneapolis* **27**, 623.

Olsson, J. -E. and Link, H. (1973). Immunoglobulin abnormalities in multiple sclerosis: relation to clinical parameters. *Arch. Neurol., Chicago* **28**, 392.

——, Möller, E., and Link, H. (1976). HLA haplotypes in families with high frequency of multiple sclerosis. *Arch. Neurol., Chicago* **33**, 808.

Ormerod, I. E. C. and McDonald, W. I. (1984). Multiple sclerosis presenting with progressive visual failure. *J. Neurol. Neurosurg. Psychiat* **47**, 943.

Osterman, P. O. and Westerberg, C. -E. (1975). Paroxysmal attacks in multiple sclerosis. *Brain* **98**, 189.

Panelius, M. (1969). Studies on epidemiological, clinical and etiological aspects of multiple sclerosis. *Acta neurol. scand.* **45**, suppl. 39.

Patterson, V. H. and Heron, J. R. (1980). Visual field abnormalities in multiple sclerosis. *J. Neurol. Neurosurg. Psychiat.* **43**, 205.

Paty, D. W., Mervart, H., Campling, B., Rand, C. G., and Stiller, C. R. (1974). HL-A frequencies in patients with multiple sclerosis. *Can. J. neurol. Sci.* **1**, 211.

Patzold, U., Hecker, H., and Pocklington, P. (1982). Azathioprine in treatment of multiple sclerosis: final results of a 4.5-year controlled study of its effectiveness covering 115 patients. *J. neurol. Sci.* **54**, 377.

Percy, A. K., Nobrega, F. T., Okazaki, H., Glattre, E., and Kurland, L. T. (1971). Multiple sclerosis in Rochester, Minnesota—a 60-year appraisal. *Arch. Neurol., Chicago* **25**, 105.

Poser, C. M., Sylwester, D. L., Ho, B., and Alpert, A. (1975). Amino acid residues of serum and CSF protein in multiple sclerosis: clinical application of statistical discriminant analysis. *Arch. Neurol., Chicago* **32**, 308.

Poskanzer, D. C., Miller, H., and Schapira, K. (1963). Epidemiology of multiple sclerosis in the counties of Northumberland and Durham. *J. Neurol. Neurosurg. Psychiat.* **26**, 368.

——, Prenney, L. B., Sheridan, J. L., and Kondy, J. Y. (1980c). Multiple sclerosis in the Orkney and Shetland Islands. I: Epidemiology, clinical factors, and methodology. *J. Epidemiol. Community Hlth* **34**, 229.

——, Schapira, K., and Miller, H. (1963b). Multiple sclerosis and poliomyelitis. *Lancet* **ii**, 917.

——, Sever, J. L. Terasaki, P. I., Prenney, L. B., Sheridan, J. L., and Park, M. S. (1980a). Multiple sclerosis in the Orkney and Shetland Islands. V: The effect on viral titres of histocompatibility determinants. *J. Epidemiol. Community Hlth.* **34**, 265.

——, Terasaki, P. I., Prenney, L. B., Sheridan, J. L., and Park, M. S. (1980b). Multiple sclerosis in the Orkney and Shetland Islands. III: Histocompatibility determinants. *J. Epidemiol. Community Hlth.* **34**, 253.

——, Walker, A. M., Prenney, L. B., and Sheridan, J. L. (1981). The etiology of multiple sclerosis: temporal-spatial clustering indicating two environmental exposures before onset. *Neurology, Minneapolis* **31**, 708.

Price, P. and Cuzner, M. L. (1979). Proteinase inhibitors in cerebrospinal fluid in multiple sclerosis. *J. neurol. Sci.* **42**, 251.

Prineas, J. W. and Connell, F. (1978). The fine structure of chronically active multiple sclerosis plaques. *Neurology, Minneapolis* **28**, 68.

——, Teasdale, G., Latner, A. L., and Miller, H. (1966). Spinal fluid gamma-globulin and multiple sclerosis. *Br. med. J.* **2**, 922.

—— and Wright, R. G. (1978). Macrophages, lymphocytes, and plasma cells in the perivascular compartment in chronic multiple sclerosis. *Lab. Invest.* **38**, 409.

Putnam, T. J. (1937). Evidence of vascular occlusion in multiple sclerosis and 'encephalomyelitis'. *Arch. Neurol. Psychiat., Chicago* **37**, 1298.

Raine, C. S., Powers, J. M., and Suzuki, K. (1974). Acute multiple sclerosis. Confirmation of 'paramyxovirus-like' intranuclear inclusions. *Arch. Neurol., Chicago* **30**, 39.

Read, D. J., Matthews, W. B., and Higson, R. H. (1980). The effect of spinal cord stimulation on function in patients with multiple sclerosis. *Brain* **103**, 803.

——, Nassim, D., Smith, P., Patterson, C., and Warlow, C. (1982). Multiple sclerosis and dog ownership: a case-control investigation. *J. neurol.Sci.* **55**, 359.

Regan, D., Milner, B. A., and Heron, J. R. (1976). Delayed visual perception and delayed visual evoked potentials in the spinal form of multiple sclerosis and in retrobulbar neuritis. *Brain* **99**, 43

——, Raymond, J., Ginsburg, A. P., and Murray, T. J. (1981). Contrast sensitivity, visual acuity and the discrimination of Snellen letters in multiple sclerosis. *Brain* **104**, 333.

Ring, J., Seifert, J., Lob, G., Coulin, K., Angstwurm, H., Frick, E., Brass, B., Mertin, J., Backmund, H., and Brendel, W. (1974). Intensive immunosuppression in the treatment of multiple sclerosis. *Lancet* **ii**, 1093.

Rinne, U. K., Panelius, M., Kivalo, E., Hokkanen, E., and Meurman, T. (1968). Multiple sclerosis in Finland: further studies on its distribution and prevalence. *Acta neurol. scand.* **44**, 631.

Roberts, D. F., Papiha, S. S., and Poskanzer, D. C. (1979a). Polymorphisms and multiple sclerosis in Orkney. *J. Epidemiol. Community Hlth.* **33**, 236.

——, Roberts, M. J., and Poskanzer, D. C. (1979b). Genetic analysis of multiple sclerosis in Orkney. *J. Epidemiol. Community Hlth.* **33**, 229.

Robinson, K. and Rudge. P. 81977). Abnormalities of the auditory evoked potentials in patients with multiple sclerosis. *Brain* **100**, 19.

Rose, A. S., Kuzma, J. W., Kurtzke, J. F., Namerow, N. S., Sibley, W. A., and Tourtellotte, W. W. (1970). Cooperative study in the evaluation of therapy in multiple sclerosis: ACTH vs. placebo. *Neurology, Minneapolis* **20** (5), Part 2.

Rosen, J. A. and Barsoum, A. H. (1979). Failure of chronic dorsal column stimulation in multiple sclerosis. *Ann. Neurol.* **6**, 66.

Ross, C. A. C., Lenman, J. A. R., and Melville, I. D. (1969). Virus antibody levels in multiple sclerosis. *Br. med. J.* **3**, 512.

Rostrôm, B. (1981). Specificity of antibodies in oligoclonal bands in patients with multiple sclerosis and cerebrovascular disease. *Acta neurol. scand.* **63**, suppl. 86.

——, Link, H., Laurenzi, M. A., Kam-Hansen, S., Norrby, E., and Wahren, B. (1981). Viral antibody activity of oligoclonal and polyclonal immunoglobulins synthesized within the central nervous system in multiple sclerosis. *Ann. Neurol.* **9**, 569.

Rushton, D. (1975). Use of the Pulfrich pendulum for detecting abnormal delay in the visual pathway in multiple sclerosis. *Brain* **98**, 283.

Sabra, A. F., Hallett, M., Sudarsky, L., and Mullally, W. (1982). Treatment of action tremor in multiple sclerosis with isoniazid. *Neurology, Minneapolis* **32**, 912.

Sagar, H. J., Warlow, C. P., Sheldon, P. W. E., and Esiri, M. M. (1982). Multiple sclerosis with clinical and radiological features of cerebral tumour. *J. Neurol. Neurosurg. Psychiat.* **45**, 802.

Salmi, A. A., Panelius, M., Halonen, P., Rinne, U. K., and Penttinen, K. (1972). Measles virus antibody in cerebrospinal fluids from patients with multiple sclerosis. *Br. med. J.* **1**, 477.

Schapira, K., Poskanzer, D. C., and Miller, H. (1963). Familial and conjugal multiple sclerosis. *Brain* **86**, 315.

——, ——, Newell, D. J., and Miller, H. (1966). Marriage, pregnancy and multiple sclerosis. *Brain* **89**, 419.

Schneck, S. A. and Claman, H. N. (1969). CSF immunoglobulins in multiple sclerosis and other diseases: measurement by electroimmunodiffusion. *Arch, Neurol., Chicago* **20**, 132.

Schumacher, G. A. (1974). Critique of experimental trials of therapy in multiple sclerosis. *Neurology, Minneapolis* **24**, 1010.

Sears, E. S., Tindall, R. S. A., and Zarnow, H. (1978). Active multiple sclerosis: enhanced computerized tomographic imaging of lesions and the effect of corticosteroids. *Arch. Neurol., Chicago* **35**, 426.

Seland, T. P., McPherson, T. A., Grace, M., Lamoureux, G., and Blain, J. G. (1974). Evaluation of antithymocyte globulin in acute relapses of multiple sclerosis. *Neurology, Minneapolis* **24**, 34.

Senaratne, M. P. J., Carroll, D., Warren, K. C., and Kappagoda, T. (1984). Evidence for cardiovascular autonomic nerve dysfunction in multiple sclerosis. *J. Neurol. Neurosurg. Psychiat.* **47**, 947.

Sever, J. L., Kurtzke, J. F., Alter, M., Schumacher, G., Gilkeson, M. R., Ellenberg, J. H., and Brody, J. A. (1971). Virus antibodies and multiple sclerosis. *Arch. Neurol., Chicago* **24**, 489.

Shepherd, D. I. and Downie, A. W. (1980). A further prevalence study of multiple sclerosis in north–east Scotland. *J. Neurol. Neurosurg. Psychiat.* **43**, 310.

Shibasaki, H. and Kuroiwa, Y. (1973). Clinical studies of multiple sclerosis in Japan. II. Are its clinical characteristics changing? *Neurology, Minneapolis* **23**, 618.

—— and —— (1974). Painful tonic seizure in multiple sclerosis. *Arch. Neurol., Chicago* **30**, 47.

——, McDonald, W. I., and Kuroiwa, Y. (1981). Racial modification of clinical picture of multiple sclerosis: comparison between British and Japanese patients. *J. neurol. Sci.* **49**, 253.

Simpson, C. A., Newell, D. J., and Schapira, K. (1966). Smoking and multiple sclerosis. *Neurology, Minneapolis* **16**, 1041.

Smith, H. V., Espir, M. L. E., Whitty, C. W. M., and Russell, W. R. (1957). Abnormal immunological reactions in disseminated sclerosis. *J. Neurol. Psychiat.* **20**, 1.

Solingen, L. D., Baloh, R. W., Myers, L., and Ellison, G. (1977). Subclinical eye movement disorders in patients with multiple sclerosis. *Neurology, Minneapolis* **27**, 614.

Stendahl-Brodin, L. and Link, H. (1980). Relation between benign course of multiple sclerosis and low-grade humoral immune response in cerebrospinal fluid. *J. Neurol. Neurosurg. Psychiat.* **43**, 102.

——, ——, Möller, E., and Norrby, E. (1979). Genetic basis of multiple sclerosis: HLA antigens, disease progression, and oligoclonal IgG in CSF. *Acta neurol. scand.* **59**, 297.

Swank, R. L. (1955). Treatment of multiple sclerosis with low fat diet. *Arch. Neurol. Psychiat., Chicago* **73**, 631.

—— (1970). Multiple sclerosis: twenty years on low fat diet. *Arch. Neurol., Chicago* **23**, 460.

Symington, G. R. and Mackay, I. R. (1978). Cell-mediated immunity to measles virus in multiple sclerosis: correlation with disability. *Neurology, Minneapolis* **28**, 109

Symington, G. R., Mackay, I. R., Whittingham, S., White, J., and Buckley, J. D. (1978). A 'profile' of immune responsiveness in multiple sclerosis. *Clin. exp. Immunol.* **31**, 141.

Tabira, T., Tsuji, S., Nagashima, T., Nakajima, T., and Kuroiwa, Y. (1981). Cortical deafness in multiple sclerosis. *J. Neurol. Neurosurg. Psychiat.* **44**, 433.

Tachovsky, T. G., Lisak, R. P., Koprowski, H., Theofilopoulos, A. N., and Dixon, F. J. (1976). Circulating immune complexes in multiple sclerosis and other neurological diseases. *Lancet* **ii**, 997.

Teasdale, G. M., Smith, P. A., Wilkinson, R., Latner, A. L., and Miller, H. (1967). Endocrine activity in multiple sclerosis. *Lancet* **i**, 64.

Ter Meulen, V., Koprowski, H., Iwasaki, Y., Käckell, Y. M., and Müller, D. (1972). Fusion of cultured multiple-sclerosis brain cells with indicator cells: presence of nucleocapsids and virions and isolation of parainfluenza-type virus. *Lancet* **ii**, 1.

Thompson E. J., Kaufmann, P., Shortman, R. C., Rudge, P., and McDonald, W. I. (1979). Oligoclonal immunoglobulins and plasma cells in spinal fluid of patients with multiple sclerosis. *Br. med. J.* **i**, 16.

Tindall, R. S. A., Walker, J. E., Ehle, A. L., Near, L., Rollins, J., and Becker, D. (1982). Plasmapheresis in multiple sclerosis: prospective trial of pheresis and immunosuppression versus immunosuppression alone. *Neurology, Minneapolis* **32**, 739.

Tobler, T. H., Johnson, K. P., and Buehring, G. C. (1982). Measles- or mumps virus-infected cells forming rosettes with lymphocytes from patients with multiple sclerosis. *Arch. Neurol., Chicago* **39**, 565.

Tourtellotte, W. W. and Ma, B. I. (1978). Multiple sclerosis: the blood-brain-barrier and the measurement of de novo central nervous system IgG synthesis. *Neurology, Minneapolis* **28**, 76.

Traugott, U., Scheinberg, L. C., and Raine, C. S. (1979). Multiple sclerosis: circulating antigen-reactive lymphocytes. *Ann. Neurol.* **6**, 425.

Turner, A., Cuzner, M. L., Davison, A. N., and Rudge, P. (1980). On the role of sensitised T-lymphocytes in the pathogenesis of multiple sclerosis. *J. Neurol. Neurosurg. Psychiat.* **43**, 305.

Twomey, J. A. and Espir, M. L. E. (1980). Paroxysmal symptoms as the first manifestations of multiple sclerosis. *J. Neurol. Neurosurg. Psychiat.* **43**, 296.

Vandvik, B., Natvig, J. B., and Wiger, D. (1976). IgGl subclass restriction of oligoclonal IgG from cerebrospinal fluids and brain extracts in patients with multiple sclerosis and subacute encephalitides. *Scand. J. Immunol.* **5**, 427.

Vartdal, F., Vandvik, B., and Norrby, E. (1980). Viral and bacterial antibody responses in multiple sclerosis. *Ann. Neurol.* **8**, 248.

Visscher, B. R., Myers, L. W., Ellison, G. W., Malmgren, R. M., Detels, R., Lucia, M. V., Madden, D. L., Sever, J. L., Park, M. S., and Coulson, A. H. (1979). HLA types and immunity in multiple sclerosis. *Neurology, Minneapolis* **29**, 1561.

Walker, J. E. and Cook, J. D. (1979). Lymphoblastic transformation in response to viral antigens in multiple sclerosis. *Neurology, Minneapolis* **29**, 1341.

Warren, K. G., Ball, M. J., Paty, D. W., and Banna, M. (1976). Computer tomography in disseminated sclerosis. *Can. J. neurol. Sci.* **3**, 211.

Weiner, H. L., Cherry, J., and McIntosh, K. (1978). Decreased lymphocyte transformation to vaccinia virus in multiple sclerosis. *Neurology, Minneapolis* **28**, 415.

Weir, A., Hansen, S., and Ballantyne, J. P. (1979). Single fibre electromyographic jitter in multiple sclerosis. *J. Neurol. Neurosurg. Psychiat.* **42**, 1146.

——, ——, and —— , (1980). Motor unit potential abnormalities in multiple sclerosis: further evidence for a peripheral nervous system defect. *J. Neurol. Neurosurg. Psychiat.* **43**, 999.

Whitaker, J. N. (1977). Myelin encephalitogenic protein fragments in cerebrospinal fluid of persons with multiple sclerosis. *Neurology, Minneapolis* **27**, 911.

Whitlock, F. A. and Siskind, M. M. (1980). Depression as a major symptom of multiple sclerosis. *J. Neurol. Neurosurg. Psychiat.* **43**, 861.

Williams, A., Eldridge, R., McFarland, H., Houff, S., Krebs, H., and McFarlin, D. (1980). Multiple sclerosis in twins. *Neurology, Minneapolis* **30**, 1139.

——, Mingioli, E. S., McFarland, H. F., Tourtellotte, W. W., and McFarlin, D. E. (1978). Increased CSF IgM in multiple sclerosis. *Neurology, Minneapolis* **28**, 996.

Wisniewski, H. M. (1975). Morphogenesis of the demyelinating process. In *Multiple sclerosis research* (ed. A. N. Davison, J. H. Humphrey, L. A. Liversedge, W. I. McDonald, and J. S. Porterfield). HMSO. London.

Young, I. R., Hall, A. S., Pallis, C. A., Legg, N. J., Bydder, G. M., and Steiner, R. E. (1981). Nuclear magnetic resonance imaging of the brain in multiple sclerosis. *Lancet* **ii**, 1063.

Wüthrich, R. and Rieder, H. P. (1970). The seasonal incidence of multiple sclerosis in Switzerland. *Europ. Neurol.* **3**, 257.

Central pontine myelinolysis

In 1959 Adams, Victor, and Mancall described four patients in whom autopsy studies revealed a single sharply outlined focus of myelin destruction in the rostral part of the pons, involving all fibre tracts indiscriminately but largely sparing nerve fibres and axis cylinders. The process seemed to begin centrally and to spread centrifugally. In two of their patients the clinical picture was one of a rapidly evolving flaccid paraplegia with facial and tongue weakness, dysphagia, and anarthria; the clinical picture in the other two cases was less dramatic. Three of the patients were alcoholics, the other was severely malnourished. While the condition is provisionally classified at present as a demyelinating disease, it seems evident that it is of metabolic or nutritional origin. It has subsequently been described in association with Wernicke's encephalopathy, cirrhosis of the liver, and Wilson's disease (Goebel and Herman-Ben Zur 1972) in leukaemia (Rosman, Kakulas, and Richardson 1966), and as a complication of uraemia and haemodialysis (Tyler 1965). Three affected children were all found to be suffering from severe liver disease which is a common association (Valsamis, Peress, and Wright 1971). Ultrastructural studies support the view that the condition is due to a toxic-metabolic process (Powers and McKeever 1976), possibly affecting the oligodendroglia specifically (Tomlinson, Pievides, and Bradley 1976). Prolonged hyponatraemia now seems to be the cause in most if not all cases and the condition can be recognized before death with the CT scan (Telfer and Miller 1979; Satran and Griggs 1981).

References

Adams, R. D., Victor, M., and Mancall, E. L. (1959). Central pontine myelinolysis. *Arch. Neurol. Psychiat., Chicago* **81**, 154.

Goebel, H. H. and Herman-Ben Zur, P. (1972). Central pontine myelinolysis—a clinical and pathological study of 10 cases. *Brain* **95**, 495.

Powers, J. M. and McKeever, P. E. (1976). Central pontine myelinolysis: an ultrastructural and elemental study. *J. neurol. Sci.* **29**, 65.

Rosman, N. P., Kakulas, B. A., and Richardson, E. P., (1966). Central pontine myelinolysis in a child with leukemia. *Arch. Neurol., Chicago* **14**, 273.

Satran, R. and Griggs, R. C. (1981). Metabolic encephalopathy. In *Current neurology* (ed. S. H. Appel), Vol. 3, p. 23. John Wiley, New York.

Telfer, R. B. and Miller, E. M. (1979). Central pontine myelinolysis following hyponatremia, demonstrated by computerized tomography. *Ann. Neurol.* **6**, 455.

Tomlinson, B. E., Pierides, A. M., and Bradley, W. G. (1976). Central pontine myelinolysis. *Quart J. Med.* **45**, 373.

Tyler, H. R. (1965). Neurological complications of dialysis, transplantation, and other forms of treatment in chronic uremia. *Neurology, Minneapolis* **15**, 1081.

Valsamis, M. P., Peress, N. S., and Wright, L. D. (1971). Central pontine myelinolysis in childhood. *Arch. Neurol., Chicago* **25**, 307.

Diffuse sclerosis (Schilder's disease)

Classification, definition, pathology, and aetiology

As Poser (1973) and Menkes (1980) have pointed out, the term 'diffuse cerebral sclerosis' has long been used to identify a heterogeneous group of diseases of cerebral white matter, many of which are now known to be dysmyelinating disorders or leucodystrophies which are genetically determined disorders of myelin formation and metabolism (see p. 298). Thus of the diseases classified by Greenfield (1958) under this title, familial sudanophilic diffuse sclerosis, Pelizaeus–Merzbacher disease, Krabbe's diffuse sclerosis (globoid body disease) and metachromatic leucodystrophy, to name but a few of the many disorders recognized , are all leucodystrophies and are considered on pages 452–61. Binswanger's subcortical encephalopathy is now known to be an uncommon consequence of diffuse cerebral arteriosclerosis and Baló's concentric sclerosis (Baló 1928) is now regarded as but one pathological manifestation of severe MS.

In 1912 Schilder described, under the title of 'encephalitis periaxalia diffusa', a brain in which there was extensive demyelination, particularly in the posterior parts of both cerebral hemispheres with relative sparing of axons and comparative preservation of the cortex and of subcortical U fibres. Subsequently in 1924 he described another case in which the areas of demyelination were sharply demarcated; there was extensive glial proliferation and massive infiltration of lipid-laden phagocytes with some inflammatory cells. It is now accepted that such a disorder, though rare, may indeed occur sporadically in childhood and the term 'Schilder's disease' can reasonably be retained provided it is recognized that very many cases so diagnosed in the past, when male, were suffering from adrenoleukodystrophy (see below) and others from various other forms of leukodystrophy. Poser and van Bogaert (1956) and Poser (1973) identified two varieties which they called myelinoclastic diffuse sclerosis; they distinguished between the severe and diffuse variety in which most of the central white matter is demyelinated and transitional diffuse sclerosis in which there are extensive areas of demyelination as well as smaller plaques resembling those of MS. They point out that transitional diffuse sclerosis, like MS, usually occurs in early adult life, the more severe and diffuse variety, corresponding to Schilder's original description, being commoner in childhood. Even in severe childhood cases, occasional complete recovery is seen (Ellison and Barron 1979). Many authors now believe that Schilder's disease is probably no more than an exceptionally severe and generalized variety of MS occurring in early life.

Pathologically, Schilder's diffuse sclerosis is characterized macroscopically by the conversion of the white matter of the posterior parts of both cerebral hemispheres into translucent, greyish, gelatinous areas. The subcortical U fibres are spared less often than in the leucodystrophies, though the cortex is usually intact; on the other hand, the axons are generally spared whereas in leucodystrophy they are usually damaged early, while inflammatory-cell infiltration is common in Schilder's disease, and rare in leucodystrophy. We know as little about the aetiology of the disease as we do about MS; the CSF changes in such cases are similar to those found in MS.

Symptoms and signs

The condition usually begins in a previously healthy child between the ages of 5 and 12 years with intellectual impairment and a gait disorder. The onset is sometimes rapid, sometimes insidious. Headache and giddiness may occur, but fever is exceptional. Visual impairment is often an early symptom, but may be preceded by mental deterioration, epileptic attacks, aphasia, or weakness and incoordination of the limbs. Visual failure is usually due to destruction of the optic radiations. When one occipital lobe is first involved, the first field defect is contralateral homonymous hemianopia, the remaining halves of the visual fields being subsequently gradually lost as the opposite occipital lobe is involved. More often both sides are involved symmetrically. In either case the end-result is blindness. Less often visual impairment is due to bilateral retrobulbar neuritis with bilateral central scotomas. In such cases disc swelling is occasional in the acute stage and is followed by optic atrophy. Acute widespread demyelination may cause cerebral oedema, raised intracranial pressure, and papilloedema. Unless the optic nerves are involved the pupillary reactions are normal. Diplopia is not uncommon and is usually due to lateral rectus paralysis. Third-nerve palsy occurs much less frequently. Nystagmus is common. Loss of smell and taste, deafness, and tinnitus have been described.

Progressive spastic weakness of the extremities gradually develops. One side of the body may be affected before the other, but a spastic tetraplegia is the final state. Sensory loss of cortical type is not uncommon with loss of postural sensibility, appreciation of passive movement, and tactile discrimination, but capsular involvement may also give analgesia involving one or both halves of the body. Aphasia may occur, but later tends to be masked by spastic dysarthria, and dysphagia due to pseudobulbar palsy often supervenes. The mental changes are those of a progressive dementia. Epileptic attacks, which may be either generalized or Jacksonian, may occur at any stage.

Diagnosis

In a typical case the early onset of blindness with progressive dementia and spastic paralysis constitute a distinctive clinical picture. When symptoms are for a time predominantly unilateral and especially when papilloedema occurs, intracranial tumour may be simulated. The EEG is of considerable value in diagnosis from SSPE and the various lipidoses; it usually shows only diffuse slow activity in no way comparable to the recurrent bizarre complexes of SSPE or the irregular spike and wave discharges often seen in Tay–Sachs disease, for example. The CT scan is very helpful, demonstrating extensive areas of attenuation in the white matter of both cerebral hemispheres. Diagnosis from the leucodystrophies may, however, be difficult if not impossible, especially if the family history is negative. In Krabbe's diffuse sclerosis the CSF is usually much more abnormal, while slowing of motor nerve conduction is common due to peripheral-nerve involvement; the latter is also true in cases of metachromatic leucodystrophy in which metachromatic granules may be detected in the urine and aryl-sulphatase estimation in leucocyte suspensions may be diagnostic (p. 460). In the final analysis, however, diagnosis from some of the familial leucodystrophies is sometimes dependent upon brain biopsy, a procedure which may rarely be justified in some cases of progressive dementia and paralysis in childhood, if only to determine the prognosis and to give informed genetic counselling.

Prognosis

The disease is almost invariably progressive and usually terminates fatally, although exceptionally temporary remissions occur and, very rarely, arrest or recovery (Ellison and Barron 1979). It may run an acute course, leading to death within one or two months. Few patients survive more than three years after the onset but rarely life may be prolonged for several years.

Treatment

The cause of the disease being unknown, treatment is empirical and none is known to arrest its course. Steroids and/or immunosuppressive drugs appear to be of no value. The usual anticonvulsants should be used to control convulsions.

Adrenoleucodystrophy (Addison–Schilder's disease)

This X-linked recessive disorder, manifest in males and transmitted by clinically unaffected carrier females, gives a clinical picture indistinguishable from that of Schilder's disease as described above (Siemerling and Creutzfeldt 1923) save for the fact that the affected patients also show adrenal atrophy; some but not all develop the typical endocrinological and biochemical manifestations of Addison's disease. In some cases (adrenomyeloneuropathy) the brunt of the disease falls upon the spinal cord and peripheral nerves (Vercruyssen, Martin, and Mercelis 1982), and in others the condition can present as X-linked Addison's disease without any evidence of nervous system involvement (O'Neill, Moser, and Saxena 1982). Estimation of the plasma ACTH, which is usually raised, may be helpful in diagnosis (Rees 1975) but adrenal biopsy is usually diagnostic, as ultrastructural studies of adrenal sections show membrane-like cytoplasmic inclusions which may also be found in brain tissue (Schaumburg, Power, Suzuki, and Raine 1974; Schaumburg, Powers, Raine, Suzuki, and Richardson 1975). The diagnosis may also be made by examining ultrastructurally nerve twigs found in skin or conjunctival biopsies (Martin, Ceuterick, and Libert 1980) which show typical curved clefts and leaflets in Schwann cells. Recording the auditory-evoked brainstem responses may help in the diagnosis of the carrier state (Moloney and Masterson 1982). The condition appears to be due to a disorder of very long-chain fatty-acid metabolism (O'Neill *et al.* 1982). Moser, Moser, Singh, and O'Neill (1984) have reviewed the biochemistry, diagnosis, and therapy of the condition in 303 cases: even bone marrow transplantation was of no benefit.

References

Baló, J. (1928). Encephalitis periaxalis concentrica. *Arch. Neurol. Psychiat., Chicago* **19**, 242.

Bielschowsky, M. and Henneberg, R. (1928). Über familiäre diffuse Sklerose. (Leukodystrophia Cerebri Progressiva Hereditaria). *J. Psychiat. Neurol.* **36**, 131.

Collier, J. and Greenfield, J. G. (1924). The encephalitis periaxalis of Schilder. *Brain* **47**, 489.

Ellison, P. H. and Barron, K. D. (1979). Clinical recovery from Schilder disease. *Neurology, Minneapolis* **29**, 244.

Ferraro, A. (1937). Primary demyelinating processes of the central nervous system. *Arch. Neurol. Psychiat., Chicago* **37**, 1100.

Greenfield, J. G. (1958). Demyelinating diseases. In *Neuropathology*, 1st edn. (ed. J. G. Greenfield, W. Blackwood, W. H. McMenemey, A. Meyer, and R. M. Norman). Chapter 11. Arnold, London.

—— and Norman, R. M. (1965). Demyelinating diseases. In *Greenfield's neuropathology*, 2nd edn. (ed. W. Blackwood, W. H. McMenemey, A. Meyer, R. M. Norman, and D. S. Russell). Chapter 11. Arnold, London.

Martin, J. J., Ceuterick, C., and Libert, J. (1980). Skin and conjunctival nerve biopsies in adrenoleukodystophy and its variants. *Ann. Neurol.* **8**, 291.

Menkes, J. H. (1980). *Textbook of child neurology*, 2nd edn. Lea and Febiger, Philadelphia.

Moloney, J. B. M. and Masterson, J. G. (1982). Detection of adrenoleucodystrophy carriers by means of evoked potentials. *Lancet* **ii**, 852.

Moser, H. W., Moser, A. E., Singh, I., and O'Neill, B. P. (1984). Adrenoleucodystrophy: survey of 303 cases: biochemistry, diagnosis and therapy. *Ann. Neurol.* **16**, 628.

O'Neill, B. P., Moser, H. W., and Saxena, K. M. (1982). Familial X-linked Addison disease as an expression of adrenoleukodystrophy (ALD): elevated C_{26} fatty acids in cultured skin fibroblasts. *Neurology, Minneapolis* **32**, 543.

Poser, C. M. (1973). Diseases of the myelin sheath. In *A textbook of neurology* (ed. H. H. Merritt). Lea and Febiger, Philadelphia.

—— and Van Bogaert, L. (1956). Natural history and evolution of the concept of Schilder's diffuse sclerosis. *Acta Psychiat. Neurol. Scand.* **31**, 285.

Rees, L. H., Grant, D. B., and Wilson, J. (1975). Plasma corticotrophin levels in Addison-Schilder's disease. *Br. med. J.* **3**, 201.

Schaumburg, H. H., Powers, J. M., Raines, C. S., Suzuki, K., and Richardson, E. P., Jr. (1975). Adrenoleukodystophy. *Arch. Neurol., Chicago* **32**, 577.

——, ——, Suzuki, K., and Raine, C. S. (1974). Adrenoleukodystrophy (sex-linked Schilder disease). *Arch. Neurol., Chicago* **31**, 210.

Schilder, P. (1912). Zur Kenntnis der sogenannten diffusen Sklerose. *Z. ges. Neurol. Psychiat.* **10**, 1.

Siemerling, E. and Creutzfeldt, H. G. (1923). Bronzenkrankheit und sklerosierende Encephalomyelitis. *Arch. Psychiat. Nervenkr.* **68**, 217.

—— (1924). Die Encephalitis periaxalis diffusa. *Arch. Psychiat. Nervenkr.* **71**, 327.

Stewart, T. G., Greenfield, J. G., and Blandy, M. A. (1927). Encephalitis periaxalis diffusa. Report of three cases with pathological examinations. *Brain* **50**, 1.

Symonds, C. P. (1928). A contribution to the clinical study of Schilder's encephalitis. *Brain* **51**, 24.

Vercruyssen, A., Martin, J. J., and Mercelis, R. (1982). Neurophysiological studies in adrenomyeloneuropathy: a report on five cases. *J. neurol. Sci.* **56**, 327.

12

Extrapyramidal syndromes

The basal ganglia

The anatomy of the basal ganglia and brief comments upon their function were given on pp. 17–18. More detailed reviews of their anatomy, physiology, and pathophysiology may be found in Brodal (1981), Lance and McLeod (1981), Burke and Fahn (1981), and Marsden (1981, 1982).

Disorders of the basal ganglia and their interpretation

Studies of the pathophysiology (to be considered below) of diseases of the basal ganglia have long been recognized to be difficult because the yield of clinical neuropathological techniques has been limited and the pathological substrate, for example, of conditions such as torsion dystonia remains poorly defined. However, new developments in neuropharmacology (Marsden 1982) have cast considerable light upon many of these disorders and it will therefore be useful to consider first their general symptomatology and what little is known about clinicopathological and pathophysiological correlations. Marsden points out that these diseases usually present with movement disorders, either poverty of movement with rigidity (akinetic-rigid syndromes) or abnormal and excessive involuntary movements (dyskinesias) (Table 12.1). A more comprehensive classification of the extrapyramidal disorders has been prepared by the World Federation of Neurology (Research Group on Extrapyramidal Disease 1981).

Table 12.1. *Classification of movement disorders**

Akinetic-rigid syndromes	Dyskinesias
Parkinson's disease	Tremor
Post-encephalitic parkinsonism	Benign essential tremor
Drug-induced parkinsonism	Cerebellar tremor
Multiple system atrophy	Chorea
Shy–Drager syndrome	Huntington's disease
Striatonigral degeneration	Rheumatic chorea
Olivopontocerebellar degeneration	Benign hereditary chorea
Progressive supranuclear palsy	Myoclonus
	Epileptic myoclonus
Wilson's disease	Symptomatic myoclonus:
	post-anoxic
Hallervorden–Spatz disease	cerebellar degeneration
	Essential myoclonus
Pallido-pyramidal degenerations	(see Chapter 22)
	Tics
	Gilles de la Tourette syndrome
Symptomatic parkinsonism	Torsion dystonia
Multi-infarct dementia	Hereditary dystonia
Alzheimer's disease	Symptomatic dystonia
Head injury	Paroxysmal dystonia
Manganese intoxication	Spasmodic torticollis
Anoxia	

*Modified from Marsden (1982) with permission.

Symptoms and signs of striatal and other extra-pyramidal disorders

In considering the manifestations of striatal disorder, it is important to note that these are in a sense artificial abstractions from a larger whole. This is so first, because one specific symptom tends to merge into others, however clear-cut it may be in an individual patient. Thus, there are intermediate forms between chorea and athetosis and between athetosis and dystonia, while parkinsonian rigidity tends to merge into other forms of hypertonia. Hence a particular symptom may be regarded as part of a spectrum rather than as an isolated entity. Second, although in some patients a symptom of striatal disease may remain virtually unchanged for years, in many others, who suffer from a progressive disorder, the clinical picture itself changes with time, moving as it were along the spectrum from one group of symptoms to another.

Athetosis
Athetosis means instability of posture, and is a term applied to a disturbance of both posture and motor control resulting in involuntary movements. It may be unilateral or bilateral. In the upper limb, when, for example, the arm is outstretched, there is a typical alternation between two postures. The first gives exaggerated flexion of the wrist and hyperextension of the fingers, particularly at the metacarpophalangeal joints, the forearm tending to be pronated. This is apt to change into a posture of flexion of the fingers, often with the thumb flexed beneath the other digits, and the wrist flexed and somewhat supinated. The change from extension to flexion tends to occur successively in one digit after another. Athetotic movements are less marked in the lower limb, where the picture is usually one of plantar flexion of the ankle and dorsiflexion of the great toe. Voluntary movement is impeded, and, in the upper limb particularly, wild excursions may occur at shoulder and elbow when it is attempted. The lips, jaw, and tongue are involved, particularly when athetosis is bilateral, leading to facial grimaces and dysarthria.

Chorea
There is no sharp distinction between athetosis and chorea. Typical chorea, however, consists of continuous involuntary movements involving the face, tongue and limbs, chiefly in their distal joints, and even trunk and respiratory muscles. Choreic movements are rapid and are sometimes described as 'pseudo-purposive'. Thus they resemble fragmentary and disordered forms of emotional and voluntary movement, continually interrupted, and never proceeding to completion. As in athetosis, voluntary movement is grossly disturbed in severe chorea by the involuntary movements. Associated movements are exaggerated. When a choreic patient is asked to clench his fists, his whole body participates in movements which are an exaggerated and disorganized form of those associated movements which normally accompany muscular effort. The disorganization consists of loss of reciprocal relaxation with incoordination of the synergic muscular contractions necessary for orderly movement. Chorea is also characterized by hypotonia and impaired ability to maintain a posture. Many patients have a combination of the largely peripheral and relatively rapid movements of chorea with the slower, more proximal writhing movements of athetosis and are then said to show choreo-athetosis.

Hemiballismus

Hemiballismus is an uncommon form of involuntary movement related to chorea. It is limited to one side of the body, and differs from chorea chiefly in the greater involvement of proximal joints and a prominent tendency to rotation of the limbs. The wild 'flinging' and continuous character of the movement in severe cases may produce virtual exhaustion of the patient and excoriation of skin due to repeated trauma to the affected limbs.

Dystonia

Whereas in one direction athetosis merges into chorea, in another it merges into dystonia. Dystonia is the term applied to the persistent maintenance of a posture by exaggerated muscle tone, the posture not usually being one intermidiate between flexion and extension as in parkinsonism, but an extreme degree of one or the other, usually extension in the lower limb and either extension or flexion in the upper limb. Dystonia often begins with exaggerated plantar-flexion and inversion of the foot, or hyperextension of the fingers. In extreme cases, as Denny-Brown (1962) points out, the extremity becomes set in one of the postures of athetosis. The facial muscles and tongue may be involved. The disorder may be unilateral or bilateral, and the asymmetrical distribution of the hypertonia may lead to torsion of the trunk and torticollis. Many authorities believe that *spasmodic torticollis* is a fractional variety of torsion dystonia.

Rigidity

Rigidity of the muscles is characteristic of parkinsonism. It is often described as being of plastic type and is characterized by a relatively constant resistance to passive stretching of the muscles, a resistance which is approximately equal in the flexors and extensors. It is usually evident in the flexors of the wrist and fingers, and pronators of the forearm. Denny-Brown pointed out that this plastic rigidity can be made to disappear if the limb is completely supported and the patient instructed to relax. In such a state of relaxation unimpeded passive movement is possible in either direction at any joint within a small range of 5 to 10 degrees. Movement of larger range, however, immediately evokes contraction in the stretched muscle, demonstrating that the rigidity is due to a stretch reflex. Denny-Brown stated that 'the plastic quality of parkinsonian rigidity, that distinguishes it from spasticity, is due to a tendency of motor units recruited into a contraction by stretching, to drop out again one by one as others are recruited. When a spastic muscle is stretched more and more motor units respond, and resistance to stretch mounts to a peak. At this point many units suddenly cease responding, and resistance to further stretch melts away ('lengthening reaction'). In plastic rigidity the lengthening reaction affects one motor unit after another from the beginning of stretch, so that resistance to stretch remains approximately constant. So-called 'cog-wheel rigidity' is often thought to be due to a combination of rigidity and tremor, resistance to passive movement waxing and waning with phases of contraction and relaxation of the muscle produced by the tremor. However, Lance, Schwab and Peterson (1963) pointed out that cog-wheel rigidity may be found in patients without resting tremor and suggested that it may be due to an exaggerated physiological tremor which has a different frequency from the resting tremor of parkinsonism.

Tremor

Tremor is a rhythmical alternating contraction of opposing muscle groups (Yahr 1972). It is commonly associated with rigidity in parkinsonism, but may occur independently. The typical tremor of parkinsonism is present at rest (resting or static tremor) and abolished by movement but may also persist to some extent during such movement. Postural or action tremor, present with the arms outstretched or throughout the entire range of movement, may be due to anxiety, thyrotoxicosis, drug intoxication, or many other causes but is also characteristic of so-called *benign or essential tremor*. Tremor which increases towards the end of movement as the limb approaches a target (intention tremor or kinetic tremor, sometimes erroneously called action tremor) is characteristic of disease of cerebellar connections in the brainstem, less often of the cerebellum itself.

The relationship of symptoms to lesions of the basal ganglia

The precise correlation of specific clinical manifestations with pathological changes in individual nuclei of the basal ganglia is difficult. There are, however, certain well-established correlations but these fill in only part of the picture.

Athetosis

Pathological evidence suggests that the lesion responsible for athetosis is situated in the outer segment of the putamen as in the *état marbré* responsible for congenital double athetosis.

Chorea

Probably past experimental work has not sufficiently distinguished between chorea and hemiballismus. True chorea seems to result from a lesion of the corpus striatum involving particularly the caudate nucleus. Hemiballismus is almost always due to damage to the opposite subthalamic nucleus or to lesions which isolate it from the globus pallidus (Martin 1957).

Dystonia

The close relationship between dystonia and athetosis has already been noted, and the causative lesions may be in a similar situation. The putamen can be involved in both, but in dystonia the thalamus and cerebral cortex may possibly be involved as well; however the neuropathology of dystonia is still very poorly defined.

Parkinsonian tremor and rigidity

These manifestations are closely related both clinically and physiologically, and it is not yet possible to distinguish their pathological bases. Parkinsonism was once attributed to lesions of the globus pallidus, but the importance of the substantia nigra, which suffers severely in encephalitis lethargica, was subsequently stressed (Greenfield 1958). Pakkenberg and Brody (1965) found a significant reduction in the number of melanin-containing neurones in this structure in patients with parkinsonism when compared with controls. Alvord (1958) and others stressed the finding of Lewy bodies (eosinophilic inclusions) in the nigral neurones of patients with paralysis agitans and the same cells often show Alzheimer's neurofibrillary change in post-encephalitic cases. And low doses of MPTP (1-methyl-4-phenyl-1, 2, 3, 6-tetrahydropyridine) selectively destroy these neurones giving parkinsonian responsive to levodopa (see Williams 1984; Langston 1985). Degeneration of cells in the locus ceruleus (Forno 1982) is also common. Neurofibrillary tangles, granulovacuolar bodies, and 'rod-like' structures are common in the Guam parkinsonism-dementia complex (Hirano, Dembitzer, Kurland and Zimmerman 1968; Brody, Hirano and Scott 1971) but not in idiopathic cases. It is now agreed that the principal pathological abnormalities in parkinsonism lie in the zona compacta of the substantia nigra, the locus ceruleus, and in the ascending nigrostriatal pathway (Stern 1966; Calne 1970; Yahr 1972; Forno 1982; Marsden 1982).

Massive lesions of the basal ganglia

Important light is thrown upon the functions of the corpus striatum by the clinical pictures which result from massive bilateral lesions of the putamen and caudate nucleus on the one hand, and of the globus pallidus on the other. Denny-Brown (1962) noted that the characteristic effect of the former lesion is muscular rigidity with the upper limbs in flexion and the lower in extension, particularly evident when the patient is lifted from the ground. The effect of symmetrical necrosis of the globus pallidus, commonly due to carbon monoxide poisoning, is an akinetic mute state with generalized rigidity of all four limbs in a semi-flexed attitude. However, bilateral lesions of the substantia nigra produced experimentally in monkeys caused hypokinesia and immobility which was enhanced by further lesions in the globus pallidus, but neither rigidity nor tremor developed (Stern 1966); by contrast, Denny-Brown (1962) found that bilateral pallidal lesions *did* produce plastic rigidity.

The pathophysiology of disease of the basal ganglia

As Lance and McLeod (1981) point out, the action of the extrapyramidal system on spinal motor neurones is largely mediated through reticulospinal pathways. The extrapyramidal system is made up of a succession of relatively short neurones which descend from the cortex through relay nuclei, often as multiple paths in parallel. At each relay the flow of caudally directed impulses is regulated by neurones which project rostrally from areas such as the subthalamic nucleus, substantia nigra, and midbrain reticular formation providing a feedback control mechanism. There is a cortico-cortical current passing through the basal ganglia which regulates the cortical control of voluntary movement by a process of graded inhibition which assists in its smooth control. Sensory input is also important and Denny-Brown (1962) suggested that many symptoms of lesions of the corpus striatum are due to abnormalities of the righting reflexes since in many extrapyramidal syndromes the posture of the patient and his involuntary movements can be modified by changing the position of the body in space. Martin (1967) also stressed abnormalities of postural reflexes, indicating in particular the way in which a patient with Parkinson's disease who cannot initiate the act of walking (akinesia) can be made to walk if he leans forward, thus moving the centre of gravity of his body, an act which may initiate the walking reflex. He believed that the globus pallidus controlled this 'starter function'.

Much work has also been done upon the role of the basal ganglia in controlling the activity of the alpha and gamma motor neurones and it has been suggested that there is a disorder of gamma innervation in Parkinson's disease. However, study of the Jendrassik manoeuvre (reinforcement of tendon reflexes) and of the H-reflex (the electrical analogue of the ankle jerk) in such patients has given somewhat conflicting results relating to muscle spindle activity (Gassel and Diamantopoulos 1964; Yap 1967; Calne 1970; McLeod and Walsh 1972; McLellan 1973). It is, however, known that 'long-loop' reflexes (Lance and McLeod 1981; Burke and Fahn 1981) are greatly enhanced (up to five times the normal amplitude) in parkinsonian rigidity. Muscle stretch evokes three reflex responses, M1, M2, and M3, the first of which, M1, is of short latency (20 ms) and corresponds to the monosynaptic tendon jerk; M2 with a latency of 50–70 ms (too short to be a voluntary response) is often called Marsden's automatic response (Marsden, Merton, Morton, Adam and Hallett 1978); and the third or late M3 response has a latency of 120 ms (the 'functional stretch reflex'). It is now agreed that the basal ganglia are concerned with controlling the balance of alpha and gamma motor-neurone activity and that in parkinsonism there are two components responsible for rigidity; there is an enhancement of tonic stretch reflexes which depends upon both the alpha and gamma systems, and in addition there is, in advanced cases, a progressive flexion dystonia (responsible for the stooped posture) which results from increasing alpha neurone activity and which may ultimately become irreversible (Lance and McLeod 1981). How the balance of reticulospinal activity is altered so as to increase activity in static fusimotor and alpha motor neurones is, however, unknown. Neurophysiological studies have also confirmed that the typical static tremor of parkinsonism is different in frequency from

the action tremor which is seen in some cases and which is an exaggeration of physiological tremor; it is the latter, rather than the former, when superimposed on rigidity, which accounts for the cog-wheel phenomenon. Akinesia seems due in part to a disorder of postural reflexes (Martin 1967) and in part to flexion dystonia involving particularly the lower limbs (Andrews 1973).

It is now agreed that the globus pallidus is the final efferent-cell station in the basal ganglia and that its activity is regulated by an input from the cortex, caudate nucleus, putamen, substantia nigra, and subthalamic nucleus. The involuntary movements which result from diffuse partial lesions of the putamen and globus pallidus are due to impaired control of various reflexes and of the incoming impulses which normally modify them; thus in a sense they are release phenomena, due to loss of normal inhibitory activity. Lesions of the putamen usually release the movements of athetosis, those of the caudate chorea, in which, in contrast to parkinsonism, associated movements are increased, while motor-neurone excitability and the tonic stretch reflexes are often diminished. The subthalamic nucleus seems to be concerned with stabilization of the limbs on the opposite side of the body in relation to their resting posture and voluntary movement, so that a lesion of this structure leads to the violent uncontrolled movements of hemiballismus. As already mentioned, the patho-anatomical substrate of torsion dystonia is still undefined but in this disorder which gives fixed alterations in posture, tonic stretch reflexes and alpha motor-neurone activity are markedly enhanced.

Each extrapyramidal syndrome may thus be due to disturbance of the delicate physiological balance which normally exists in this intricate system. The fact that lesions produced surgically in the globus pallidus or ventrolateral nucleus of the thalamus may abolish contralateral tremor and reduce rigidity in parkinsonism (Cooper 1961) and that the same operation may be beneficial in abolishing hemiballismus or the intention tremor of cerebellar disease, while it is less effective in dystonia, chorea, and torticollis and almost totally ineffective in athetosis, is still difficult to explain. Probably the lesion blocks the main efferent pathway from the globus pallidus which passes rostrally via the ventro-lateral thalamic nucleus. Why interruption of this output leaves the patient with little or no disability remains unanswered.

Some unsolved patho-physiological problems are becoming more easily understood as a result of recent neuropharmacological research. It is now known (Marsden 1982, and Fig. 12.1) that dopamine is the neurotransmitter in the nigrostriatal pathway and also in certain mesolimbic and mesocortical systems, while cortico-striatal pathways utilize glutamate and striatonigral neurones γ-aminobutyric acid (GABA) as their transmitters. Thalamostriate neurones, by contrast, are cholinergic; pathways from the midbrain raphe nuclei to the striatum utilize serotonin and there are also peptidergic strionigral and striopallidal pathways which contain substance P and metenkephalin. Cholecystokinin may indeed coexist with dopamine in the same neuronal system. Ehringer and Hornykiewicz (1960) first showed that the concentration of dopamine was reduced in the basal ganglia of patients with parkinsonism. Reserpine and the phenothiazines which may produce drug-induced parkinsonism, act by depleting dopamine stores in the basal ganglia through inhibition of dopamine-stimulated adenylate cyclase activity (Calne, Chase and Barbeau 1975). By giving levodopa, a precursor of dopamine, or dopamine agonists such as bromocriptine, dopamine stores can generally be repleted with amelioration of many symptoms of parkinsonism (p. 332). On the other hand, important side effects of levodopa therapy include troublesome involuntary movements which may resemble chorea or athetosis; similarly, phenothiazine derivatives are known on occasion to produce facial dyskinetic movements and/or postural changes resembling those of dystonia. There is also convincing evidence, reviewed fully by Calne (1970, 1971), that cholinergic activation in thalamostriate neurones aggravates the symptoms of parkinsonism, a fact which probably explains the

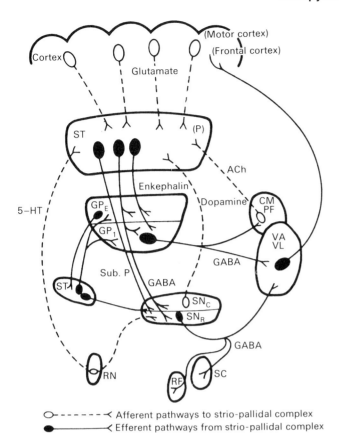

○------< Afferent pathways to strio-pallidal complex
●——< Efferent pathways from strio-pallidal complex

Fig. 12.1. Neurotransmitter anatomy of basal ganglia. ST = striatum (caudate nucleus and putamen (P)); GP$_E$ = globus pallidus externa; GP$_I$ = globus pallidus interna; SN$_C$ = substantia nigra compacta; SN$_R$ = substantia nigra reticulata; ST = subthalamus; RN = raphe nuclei; SC = superior colliculus; RF = reticular formation; CM = centremedian; PF = parafascicular nucleus; VA = nucleus ventralis anterior of the thalamus; VL = nucleus ventralis lateralis of thalamus. Gluta = glutamate; GABA = γ-aminobutyric acid; Sub. P = substance P; DA = dopamine; 5HT = serotonin; ACh = acetylcholine. (Reproduced from Marsden (1982) by kind permission of the author, editor, and publisher.)

beneficial effect of anticholinergic drugs in this disease. It is thus probable that many symptoms of disease in the basal ganglia are due to an imbalance in the relative activities of cholinergic and dopaminergic neurones and their receptors. Much can be learned of these mechanisms by studying the concentration of metabolites of dopamine such as homovanillic acid (HVA) and of other catecholamines in the CSF and in the urine.

References

Abbé-Fessard, D., Guiot, G., Lamarre, Y., and Arfel, G. (1966). Activation of thalamocortical projections related to tremorogenic processes. In *The thalamus* (ed. D. O. Purpura, and M. D. Yahr). Columbia University Press, New York.

Alvord, E. C., Jr., (1958). Pathology of Parkinsonism. In *Pathogenesis and treatment of Parkinsonism* (ed. W. S. Fields), Thomas, Springfield, Illinois.

Andrews, C. J. (1973). The influence of dystonia on the response to long-term L-dopa therapy. *J. Neurol. Neurosurg. Psychiat.* **36**, 630.

Borit, A., Rubinstein, L. J., and Urich, H. (1975). The striatonigral degenerations—putaminal pigments and nosology. *Brain* **98**, 101.

Brodal, A. (1981). *Neurological anatomy in relation to clinical medicine*, 3rd edn. Oxford University Press, London.

Brody, J. A. Hirano, A., and Scott, R. M. (1971). Recent neuropathologic observations in amyotrophic lateral sclerosis and parkinsonism-dementia of Guam. *Neurology, Minneapolis* **21**, 528.

Burke, R. E. and Fahn, S. (1981). Movement disorders. In *Current neurology* (ed. S. H. Appel) Vol. 3, p. 92. John Wiley, New York.

Calne, D. B. (1970). *Parkinsonism: Physiology, pharmacology and treatment*. Arnold, London.

—— (1971). Parkinsonism—physiology and pharmacology. *Br. med. J.* **3**, 693.

——, Chase, T. N., and Barbeau, A. (1975). *Dopaminergic mechanisms* Advances in Neurology, Vol. 9. Raven Press, New York.

Cooper, I. S. (1961). *Parkinsonism. Its medical and surgical therapy.* Thomas, Springfield, Illinois.

Denny-Brown, D. (1962). *The basal ganglia and their relation to disorders of movement.* Oxford University Press, Oxford.

Ehringer, H. and Hornykiewicz, O. (1960). Verteilung von Noradrenalin und Dopamin (3-hydroxytyramin) im Gehirn des Menschen und ihr Verhalten bei Erkrankungen des extrapyramidalen Systems. *Klin. Wschr.* **38**, 1236.

Forno, L. S. (1982). Pathology of Parkinson's disease. In *Movement disorders* (ed. C. D. Marsden and S. Fahn). p. 25. Butterworths, London.

Gassel, M. M. and Diamantopoulos, E. (1964). The Jendrassik maneuver. I. The pattern of reinforcement of monosynaptic reflexes in normal subjects and patients with spasticity or rigidity. *Neurology, Minneapolis* **14**, 555.

Greenfield, J. G. (1958). In *Neuropathology* (ed. J. G. Greenfield, W. Blackwood, W. H. McMenemey, A. Meyer, and R. M. Norman) p. 530. Arnold, London.

Hirano, A., Dembitzer, H. M., Kurland, L. T., and Zimmerman, H. M. (1968). The fine structure of some intraganglionic alterations: neurofibrillary tangles, granulovacuolar bodies and 'rod-like' structures as seen in Guam amyotrophic lateral sclerosis and Parkinsonism-dementia complex. *J. Neuropath. exp. Neurol.* **27**, 167.

Hornykiewicz, O. (1963). Die topische Lokalisation und das Verhallen von Noradrenaline und Dopamin im der Substantia der normallen und Parkinson Kranken Menschen. *Wien. Klin. Wschr.* **75**, 309.

Lance, J. W. and McLeod, J. G. (1981). *A physiological approach to clinical neurology*, 3rd edn. Butterworth, London.

——, Schwab, R. S., and Peterson, E. A. (1963). Action tremor and the cogwheel phenomenon in Parkinson's disease. *Brain* **86**, 95.

Langston, J. W. (1985). MPTP and Parkinson's disease. *Trends Neurosci.* **8**, 79.

Marsden, C. D. (1981). Extrapyramidal diseases. In *The molecular basis of neuropathology* (ed. A. N. Davison and R. H. S. Thompson) p. 345. Arnold, London.

—— (1982). Basal ganglia disease. *Lancet* **ii**, 1141.

——, Merton, P. A., Morton, H. B., Adam, J. E. R., and Hallett, M. (1978). Automatic and voluntary responses to muscle stretch in man. In *Progress in human neurophysiology* (ed. J. E. Desmedt), Vol. 4, p. 167. Karger, Basle.

Martin, J. P. (1957). Hemichorea (hemiballismus) without lesions in the corpus Luysii. *Brain* **80**, 1.

—— (1967). *The basal ganglia and posture*. Pitman, London.

McLellan, D. L. (1973). Dynamic spindle reflexes and the rigidity of Parkinsonism. *J. Neurol. Neurosurg. Psychiat.* **36**, 342.

McLeod, J. G. and Walsh, J. C. (1972). H reflex studies in patients with Parkinson's disease. *J. Neurol. Neurosurg. Psychiat.* **35**, 77.

Mettler, F. A. (1968). Anatomy of the basal ganglia. In *Diseases of the basal ganglia* (ed. P. J. Vinken and G. W. Bruyn), Handbook of clinical neurology, Vol. 6, p. 1. North Holland, Amsterdam.

Pakkenberg, H. and Brody, H. (1965). The number of nerve cells in the substantia nigra in paralysis agitans. *Acta Neuropath., Berlin* **5**, 320.

Research Group on Extrapyramidal Disease (1981). Classification of extrapyramidal disorders. *J. neurol. Sci.* **51**, 311.

Stern, G. (1966). The effects of lesions in the substantia nigra. *Brain* **89**, 449.

Watkins, E. S. (1972). The basal ganglia. In *Scientific foundations of neurology* (ed. M. Critchley, J. L. O'Leary, and B. Jennett). p. 75. Heinemann, London.

Williams, A. (1984). MPTP parkinsonism. *Br. med. J.* **2**, 1401.

Yahr, M. D. (1972), Involuntary movements. *In Scientific foundations of neurology.* (ed. M. Critchley, J. L. O'Leary, and B. Jennett). p. 83, Heinemann, London.

Yap, C.-B. (1967). Spinal segmental and long-loop reflexes and spinal motorneurone excitability in spasticity and rigidity. *Brain* **90**, 887.

The parkinsonian syndrome

Definition. The parkinsonian syndrome, named after James Parkinson, who first described paralysis agitans in 1817, is a disturbance of motor function characterized chiefly by slowing of emotional and voluntary movement, akinesia, muscular rigidity, and tremor. Parkinsonism may be produced by several different pathological processes involving the substantia nigra and its efferent pathways.

Aetiology and pathology

Jakob and Ramsay Hunt considered that loss of large ganglion cells of the corpus striatum was the cause of parkinsonism, but, as mentioned above (p. 323), it is now clear that the substantia nigra is the principal site of pathological change (Earle 1968; Lewis 1971; Forno 1982).

The histological changes depend upon the cause. Greenfield and Bosanquet (1953) and Greenfield (1958) reviewed the pathology of idiopathic (paralysis agitans) and post-encephalitic parkinsonism, with special reference to the substantia nigra and the locus ceruleus. They described five types of cell change: (1) saccular distension with lipochrome granules; (2) vacuolation; and (3) binucleated cells—all changes found in post-encephalitic parkinsonism; (4) Lewy's spherical concentric hyaline inclusions, found in idiopathic parkinsonism (Fig. 12.2); and (5) neurofibrillary tangles, found in post-encephalitic cases and in the parkinsonism-dementia complex. These changes are not affected by prior treatment with levodopa (Yahr, Wolf, Antunes, Miyoshi, and Duffy 1972). Den Hartog Jager (1969) suggested that the Lewy bodies contain sphingomyelin and postulated a disorder of lipid storage in this disease. However, Issidorides, Mytilineou, Whetsell, and Yahr (1978) found spherical cytoplasmic bodies in neurones of the substantia nigra and locus ceruleus containing a protein rich in free basic amino groups, and similar changes were found in the core of the Lewy bodies; they felt that these findings indicated a disorder of protein synthesis.

As Marsden (1982) has pointed out, at least 80–85 per cent of nigral neurones must be lost and the striatum must be depleted of 80 per cent of its dopamine content before symptoms of Parkinson's disease appear. The nigral dopaminergic neurones which remain intact increase their activity in a compensatory manner and there is also postsynaptic compensation in that striatal dopamine receptors also increase in the early stages of the disease (postsynaptic receptor supersensitivity induced by denervation). Some asymptomatic individuals may be found at autopsy to have Lewy bodies and probably represent preclinical cases in whom these compensatory mechanisms have been fully effective; eventually compensation breaks down and symptoms appear.

Other biochemical changes include: lesser degrees of dopamine deficiency in mesolimbic and mesocortical dopamine systems (Javoy-Agid and Agid 1980); alterations in [³H] spiperone binding in caudate, substantia nigra, and frontal cortex, indicating a loss of dopamine receptor sites (Quik, Spokes, Mackay, and Bannister 1979), especially those of D2 type (Burke and Fahn 1981); a moderate reduction of noradrenaline in the nucleus accumbens (Hornykiewicz 1982); reduced glutamic acid decarboxylase (GAD) activity, a marker of GABA activity, and met-enkephalin (Diamond and Borison 1978) in the substantia nigra; and reduced cortical choline acetyl transferase (ChAT) activity, similar to that found in Alzheimer's disease, especially in patients who become demented (Hakim and Mathieson 1979).

Despite increasing knowledge of the biochemical pathology of the disease, however, the primary cause of the degenerative process of paralysis agitans is unknown; while the condition may be precipitated by alcoholism, this is uncommon (Carlen, Lee, Jacob, and Livshits 1981); it is presumed that in post-encephalitic parkinsonism, the causal virus (which was never isolated) damaged the neuronal systems involved. The view that the idiopathic disorder may also be a sequel of subclinical lethargic encephalitis (Poskanzer, Schwab, and Fraser 1969; Brown and Knox 1972) is not generally accepted and there is no convincing evidence that any other virus is responsible (Burke and Fahn 1981). Drug-induced parkinsonism due to dopamine antagonists such as reserpine,

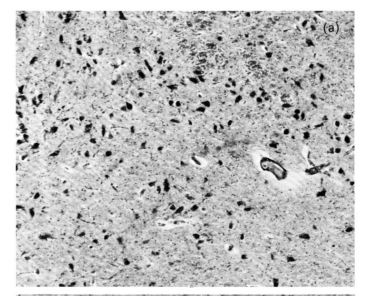

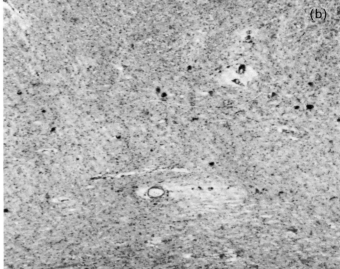

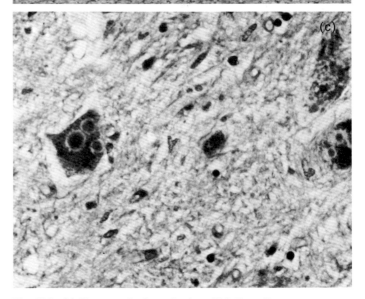

Fig. 12.2. (a) The normal substantia nigra, H & E, × 40.
(b) The substantia nigra in idiopathic parkinsonism, H & E, × 40.
(c) Lewy bodies in the substantia nigra, H & E, × 400. (Illustrations kindly provided by Professor B.E. Tomlinson.)

haloperidol, tetrabenazine, and other phenothiazines is common (Ayd 1961; Calne 1970) but usually resolves when the offending drug is withdrawn.

So-called arteriosclerotic parkinsonism or the parkinsonian syndrome in multi-infarct dementia (Table 12.1) differs from Parkinson's disease in several essential respects (see p. 330); clinical features resembling those of parkinsonism may also result from manganese intoxication, carbon monoxide poisoning, severe head injury, and the 'punch-drunk syndrome' of professional boxers. Rarely, too, parkinsonism may be symptomatic of brain tumour (de Yébenes, Gervas, Iglesias, Mena, Martin del Rio, and Somoza 1982). Parkinsonian features are also seen in various other degenerative diseases of the basal ganglia including progressive bulbar palsy, corticostriatonigral degeneration, progressive supranuclear palsy, progressive multisystem degeneration (the Shy–Drager syndrome), and the parkinsonism-dementia complex which occurs on the island of Guam, but each of these disorders is distinct from Parkinson's disease in the usual sense of the term.

The idiopathic disease occurs more often in more than one member of a family than can be accounted for by chance, and families suggesting dominant inheritance with incomplete penetrance have been described (Pratt 1967; Kondo, Kurland, and Schull 1973). Rarely, the familial disorder is associated with axonal peripheral neuropathy (Byrne, Thomas, and Zilkha 1982). Polygenic inheritance of the disease, possibly related to an inherited deficiency of tyrosine hydroxylase, has been postulated (Martin, Young, and Anderson 1973). In a rare fatal familial syndrome characterized by depression, parkinsonism, and alveolar hypoventilation (Purdy, Hahn, Barnett, Bratty, Ahmad, Lloyd, McGeer, and Perry 1979), degeneration of the nigrostriatal dopaminergic system is accompanied by low taurine concentrations in fasting plasma and CSF and by reduced tyrosine hydroxylase in the brain. There is some evidence that malignant disease occurs more often in patients with parkinsonism than in a control population (Pritchard and Netsky 1973). A prevalence rate of between 1 in 200 (Yahr 1967) and 1 in 1 000 (Brewis, Poskanzer, Rolland, and Miller 1966) has been reported; there is no convincing evidence of any specific racial or geographical incidence. The condition is slightly more common in males than females (Calne 1970) and the commonest age of onset is in the fifth and sixth decades with death occurring in from 1 to 33 years with a mean of 9 years after the development of symptoms, in the pre-levodopa era (Hoehn and Yahr 1967). Levodopa treatment has increased life expectancy by between 1.3 and 1.5 times (Diamond and Markham 1979; Burke and Fahn 1981). A very rare juvenile form, often familial, has been described, beginning in adolescence (Hunt 1917; Martin et al. 1973) often with dystonic features and diurnal fluctuation of symptoms (Sunohara, Mano, Ando and Satoyoshi 1985).

Symptoms and signs

A general description of the symptoms of the parkinsonian syndrome will first be given, and the distinctive features of the various forms will then be considered separately.

Facies and attitude

The parkinsonian facies is characteristic. The palpebral fissures may be wider than normal, and blinking is infrequent. The eyes have a staring appearance, due partly to these features and partly to the fact that spontaneous ocular movements are reduced. The *glabellar tap reflex* fails to habituate; thus in normal persons, tapping on the glabella produces blinking which ceases after the first few taps, whereas in many patients with parkinsonism the blinking continues in time with the taps for as long as the stimulus is applied. Electrophysiological studies have shown that this reflex has two components of different latency (see Kugelberg 1952; Rushworth 1962; and page 113) and the abnormal reflex of parkinsonism may be modified by treatment (Klawans and Goodwin 1969; Penders and Delwaide 1971). The facial muscles exhibit an

unnatural immobility. The attitude of the limbs and trunk is one of moderate flexion with a typical 'stoop' (Fig. 12.3). The spine is usually somewhat flexed, but is occasionally extended. There is little rotatory movement of the cervical spine. The limbs are moderately flexed and adducted, but the wrist is usually slightly extended. The fingers are flexed at the metacarpophalangeal, and extended or only slightly flexed at the interphalangeal joints, and adducted. The thumb is usually adducted, and extended at the metacarpo- and interphalangeal joints.

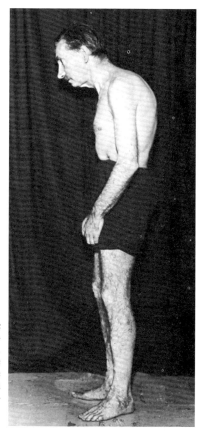

Fig. 12.3. The characteristic posture of severe paralysis agitans (idiopathic parkinsonism). Note the typical stoop and the flexion of the arms at the elbows. (Reproduced from Spillane (1975) by kind permission of the author.)

Ocular manifestations

Visual evoked potential studies have shown increased latency in over two-thirds of affected individuals (Bodis-Wollner and Yahr, 1978) and may improve with levodopa therapy. Slowing of saccadic ocular movements, suggesting that bradykinesia (see below) affects ocular as well as other muscles, is also a common finding (Shibasaki, Tsuji, and Kuroiwa 1979).

Disorders of movement (akinesia and bradykinesia)

Voluntary movement shows some reduction in power, but more striking are the difficulty in initiating movement (akinesia) and the slowness with which it is performed (bradykinesia). In many cases, signs may initially be present on one side of the body and not on the other ('hemiplegic' parkinsonism; Gilbert 1976). In general, movements carried out by small muscles suffer most. Hence the patient shows weakness of some ocular movements, especially convergence; of facial movements, associated with tremor of the eyelids on eye closure; and of movements concerned in mastication, deglutition, and articulation. The speech in severe cases is slurred, quiet, and monotonous, owing to defective pronunciation of consonants and lack of variation in pitch (Critchley 1981). Rarely palilalia occurs and occasionally in severe cases phonation and articulation are so impaired that the patient is virtually mute (Nakano, Zubick, and Tyler 1973). Movements of the hands are also markedly affected, with resulting clumsiness and inability to perform fine movements, such as those used in needlework, dealing cards, and taking money from a pocket. Characteristically the range of movement, as in opposition of the thumb and individual fingers, is greatly reduced. There is often a close correlation between slowness of movement and slowness of mental processes (Mortimer, Pirozzolo, Hansch, and Webster 1982). Micrographia is common; the writing becomes progressively smaller and may trail away to nothing. Certain associated and synergic movements suffer conspicuously. Swinging of the arms in walking is diminished and later lost, and synergic extension of the wrist, normally associated with flexion of the fingers, is also impaired. Various methods of analysing the movement defects, using 'tracking tasks' and recording devices have been designed in order to assess the abnormality quantitatively (Calne 1970; Angel, Alston, and Higgins 1970). Thoracic expansion in inspiration is reduced, but contraction of the diaphragm may be increased in compensation. Emotional movements of the face are also reduced in amplitude, slow in developing, and unduly protracted.

Muscular rigidity

Rigidity does not always develop *pari passu* with the disorders of movement just described, which often precede it. It differs from the hypertonia associated with corticospinal lesions in being present to an equal extent in opposing muscle-groups, for example, the flexors and extensors of the elbow; it is uniform throughout the whole range of movement at a joint. Sometimes the rigidity is interrupted when tested by passive movement, the muscles yielding to stretch in a series of jerks ('cog-wheel rigidity') while sometimes it is smooth and of the so-called 'plastic' or 'lead-pipe' variety. Parkinsonian rigidity, like other parkinsonian symptoms, is often unequal on the two sides of the body. Nevertheless, full passive movement is usually possible at all joints. Occasionally, however, in the post-encephalitic type, contractures occur which limit such movement, most often in the hands and the feet. The fingers may be so strongly flexed that a pad may be needed to prevent the nails being driven into the palm. Similar flexor deformity of the toes may occur, and talipes equinovarus may be produced.

Gait

The parkinsonian gait is in part at least the outcome of the patient's attitude and rigidity. It is usually slow, shuffling, and composed of small steps (*marche à petits pas*). The patient is often unable to stop quickly when pushed forwards or backwards—propulsion and retropulsion. When propulsion occurs spontaneously in walking, the patient shows a 'festinant' gait, hurrying with small steps in a bent attitude as if trying to catch up his centre of gravity. Often there is difficulty in beginning to walk and his feet seem to 'freeze' to the floor (akinesia); there may also be great difficulty in getting out of a chair. Often the patient seems to 'mark time' on one spot and then takes a few short, shuffling steps before beginning to walk more normally. If he looks down at a line on the floor in front of him, or leans forward slightly on to a frame-type walking aid (Martin 1967) the walking reflex may be initiated so that he then walks without difficulty. A striking feature is the frequent ability of the patient to carry out rapid movements requiring considerable exertion better than slower and less energetic movements. Thus a patient who can walk only very slowly may be able to run quite fast. This phenomenon has been called 'kinesia paradoxa'.

Tremor

Tremor is the characteristic involuntary movement of parkinsonism. Tremor, rigidity, akinesia, and bradykinesia are, however, largely independent variables. Tremor may be the first symptom, as it often is in paralysis agitans, and may precede rigidity by months or years. An onset with unilateral tremor often implies a benign course, especially in cases of early onset, i.e. at less than 40 years of age (Scott, Brady, Schwab, and Cooper 1970; Scott and

Brody 1971); it usually begins in one hand and arm, later involves the leg, and may not spread to the other side of the body for many months or years. In post-encephalitic parkinsonism rigidity more often precedes tremor. The head is involved late, if at all.

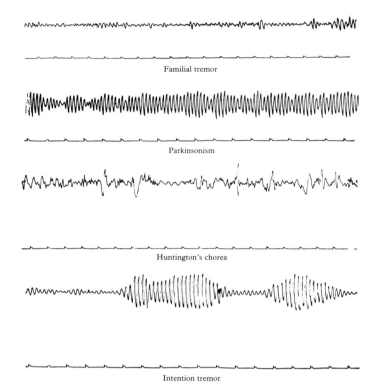

Familial tremor

Parkinsonism

Huntington's chorea

Intention tremor

Fig. 12.4. Recordings of four different types of tremor. The intervals on the time marker are one second. (By courtesy of Professor John Marshall.)

The tremor consists of rhythmic alternating movements of opposing muscle-groups (Fig. 12.4). In the upper limb the hand is most affected. Movements of the fingers occur at the metacarpophalangeal joints and may be combined with movements of the thumb—the 'pill-rolling movement'. Movements at the wrist may be flexion and extension, lateral displacement, or pronation and supination. Often the tremor shifts from one group of muscles to another while the patient is under observation. Little movement usually occurs at joints above the wrist. In the lower limb, tremor is most marked at the ankle, at which flexion and extension occur. Either flexion and extension or a rotatory tremor of the head may occur. When mandibular muscles are involved, rhythmical opening and closure of the mouth are seen, and the tongue is sometimes involved.

The frequency of the tremor is 4–8 Hz, being slower in paralysis agitans than in post-encephalitic parkinsonism. It is present when the patient is at rest ('static tremor'), and is often temporarily or wholly suppressed when the limb is moved voluntarily. Action tremor, which is not uncommon (p. 323), is more rapid with a frequency of 7–12 Hz (Teräväinen and Calne 1980; Lance and McLeod 1981). Tremor can often be inhibited for a time by conscious effort, but is liable to break from this control with increased intensity. It is increased by emotion and almost always disappears during sleep.

Akithisia

This is a form of intolerable restlessness and associated discomfort, requiring continual changes of position, occasionally seen in parkinsonism.

Sensory symptoms

There is no loss of sensibility in parkinsonism. Pain, however, is common, especially in the later stages, when most patients complain of cramp-like pains in the limbs and spine due to rigidity and to the changes induced in the joints and ligaments by the abnormal posture. Even in early cases, aching discomfort in the affected limbs is occasionally the presenting symptom, especially when rigidity is unilateral.

The reflexes

Parkinsonism does not always produce changes in the reflexes, though rigidity may render the tendon-jerks difficult to elicit and reduced in amplitude. However, in the early stages tendon-jerks may actually be increased in limbs showing early rigidity and in 'hemiplegic' parkinsonism this may give diagnostic difficulty. The plantar reflexes are flexor in uncomplicated paralysis agitans, but one or both may be extensor in post-encephalitic parkinsonism or when there is associated cervical spondylosis leading to myelopathy. Extensor plantar responses are common in so-called arteriosclerotic 'parkinsonism' and in the parkinsonism-dementia complex; they are also seen in various forms of degenerative disease which show parkinsonian features, including some types of presenile dementia, cortico-striatonigral degeneration, and sometimes in progressive multisystem degeneration. Hence the finding of such responses should always cast doubt upon the diagnosis of idiopathic paralysis agitans.

Changes in the H-reflex excitability curve and in 'long-loop reflexes' have been reported in such cases (see p. 324).

Autonomic symptoms

Autonomic dysfunction accounts for certain symptoms which often cause much discomfort. Flushing of the skin may occur accompanied by uncomfortable sensations of heat and sometimes sweating. These symptoms may be limited to, or more marked upon, one side of the body; cutaneous sebum excretion is increased (Burton and Shuster 1970). Oedema and cyanosis of a limb are rare. Parkinsonian patients usually tolerate cold much better than heat; this fact, combined with their immobility, renders them particularly liable to suffer episodes of hypothermia, particularly if confined to bed in an unheated room in cold weather. Excessive salivation is also seen in many cases. There is usually a gradual loss of weight.

The resting blood pressure is often low (Aminoff and Wilcox 1972) and many patients also show orthostatic hypotension with an abnormal fall of pressure on tilting (Gross, Bannister, and Godwin-Austen 1972; Rajpat and Rozdilsky 1976). In post-encephalitic cases particularly, but to a lesser extent in paralysis agitans, the resting respiratory rate may be increased with fewer variations in amplitude than in normal subjects (Kim 1968). Retention of urine is relatively common, but is often due to the effects of treatment with anticholinergic drugs rather than to the disease itself.

Mental state

Parkinsonism is not necessarily accompanied by any mental change, and the sufferer's intellectual capacity and emotional reactions may continue unimpaired behind the mask in which his features become fixed. However, it has long been known that disorders of personality and mood and dementia are common sequelae of encephalitis lethargica. Depression, which may respond to appropriate drugs, is also a very common accompaniment of paralysis agitans, occurring in up to 90 per cent of cases (Mindham 1970; Mayeux, Stern, Rosen, and Leventhal 1981). Psychotic episodes have often been attributed to the effects of treatment but are now known to occur spontaneously and there is growing evidence to indicate that progressive dementia occurs in idiopathic parkinsonism much more frequently than has been appreciated in the past (Loranger, Goodell, McDowell, Lee, and Sweet 1972;

British Medical Journal 1973*a*, Pirozzolo, Hansch, Mortimer, Webster, and Kuskowski 1982; Brown and Marsden 1984) and is often associated with progressive cerebral atrophy (Selby 1968; Schneider, Fischer, Jacobi, Becker, and Hacker 1979) which is readily demonstrated by CT scanning (Becker, Schneider, Hacker, and Fischer, 1979). Pathologically the changes in the brain are usually those of Alzheimer's disease (Marsden 1982).

Forms of parkinsonism

Paralysis agitans

Synonyms. Parkinson's disease; shaking palsy.

Pathology and aetiology
See page 326.

Symptoms and signs

Tremor is often the first symptom, beginning either unilaterally or bilaterally, but in many other patients stiffness and slowness of movement, sometimes beginning on one side, are the presenting features. Often, slight facial immobility, a stoop, early fatigue, and slowness of movement are thought by the patient and his family to be due simply to ageing and the early manifestations of the illness may go unrecognized for months or years. As rigidity and akinesia increase, difficulty in getting out of a chair, bed, or bath or even in turning over in bed develop and in severe cases the patient is ultimately immobile and bed-ridden.

Prognosis

The disease is always progressive, though cases differ considerably in the rate of progress. Symptoms may be confined to one limb for months or years, and the spread to other limbs when it occurs may be slow or fairly rapid. When tremor in one upper limb is the only manifestation of the disease for several years, the outlook is very much better than the average. It is worse when the condition begins with akinesia and progressive rigidity leading to immobility, but even helpless patients may survive for many years. There is growing evidence that levodopa therapy favourably influences the natural history (Stern, McDowell, Miller, and Robinson (1972) and, with carbidopa or its analogues, it greatly increases longevity (Diamond and Markham 1979). The average duration of the disease before levodopa was about 10 years, but it was not uncommon for patients to live considerably longer (Hoehn and Yahr 1967). Death occurs usually from complications such as pneumonia, vascular disease, or neoplasia (Calne 1970). Occasionally there is a terminal stage of lethargy passing into coma.

Parkinsonism following encephalitis lethargica

Pathology and aetiology
See pages 275 and 326.

Symptoms

It was common to observe some parkinsonian symptoms in the acute attack of encephalitis and often parkinsonism developed insidiously during the succeeding 12 months. The interval, however, was sometimes as long as 20 years; or no history of an acute attack was obtainable. Since the greatest incidence of the disease was in early adult life, for 20 years after the epidemic of the 1920s most cases of encephalitic parkinsonism occurred before the age of 40. Subsequently many cases beginning as late as 60 years of age appeared. With the virtual disappearance of encephalitis lethargica this form of the disease is gradually disappearing.

Stiffness, slowness of movement, and weakness usually preceded tremor. These symptoms were usually more marked upon, and often confined to, one side of the body. Sometimes they involved only one upper limb, or one upper limb and the same side of the face. Rigidity was usually more conspicuous than tremor throughout the course of the illness. The pupillary reactions to accommodation or to light or to both were often impaired, and apathy, depression, or dementia conspicuous. There was often an excess of sebaceous secretion over the face, and of saliva which characteristically dripped from the open mouth.

Oculogyric crises

Spasm of conjugate ocular muscles was a common complication of post-encephalitic parkinsonism, but is now rare. Attacks last from a few seconds to hours. The eyes usually deviate upwards, with lids retracted, less often laterally, and rarely downwards or obliquely. There may be associated spasmodic deviation of the head in the same direction and occasionally the patient falls over backwards. Sometimes the eyes become fixed when the gaze is directed forwards, or in a position of convergence. During the attack the patient's attempts to move the eyes in other directions result in only a feeble, jerky displacement from the position of spasmodic deviation.

Other symptoms

Other symptoms such as torticollis or other dystonic attitudes of the trunk and limbs were occasionally seen. Bizarre contractures of the extremities were not uncommon in severe post-encephalitic cases but are rare in paralysis agitans.

Prognosis

In most cases parkinsonism following soon after encephalitis was progressive and ran a much shorter course than paralysis agitans. Occasionally, the disorder became arrested and this happened most often when symptoms were predominantly unilateral. In severe cases the patient became quite incapacitated within a year of the onset of symptoms, but chronic cases were usually milder and the disorder often reached a stationary phase. Progressive amyotrophy resembling motor-neurone disease is an occasional late sequel (Greenfield and Matthews 1954). Death is due to pneumonia, vascular disease, or general cachexia terminating in coma.

Arteriosclerotic 'parkinsonism'

Clinical features resembling those of parkinsonism may develop in the course of cerebral arteriosclerosis, but the resulting clinical picture is not only very variable in itself but is generally complicated by other symptoms of vascular disease. Thus there are usually accompanying signs of pseudobulbar palsy, corticospinal lesions, and multi-infarct dementia, or of a lesion of the midbrain.

Some cases are due to atheroma with low or normal blood pressure, and are, therefore, found in late middle life or old age. However, some patients with severe hypertension and with consequent multiple small lacunar softenings in the cerebral hemispheres and brainstem may develop a slow shuffling gait, facial immobility, emotional lability (pathological over-emotionalism) with rigidity of the limbs, hyperreflexia, and extensor plantar responses. They often develop other signs of pseudobulbar palsy and dementia. The condition often develops later than does paralysis agitans, though in severely hypertensive patients it may occur earlier in life. The onset is usually insidious, but sometimes follows a 'stroke'; and a series of mild 'strokes' may each be followed by an increase in the severity of the symptoms.

Of the manifestations which resemble those of parkinsonism, the bodily attitude, slowness of movement, and the festinant gait are the commonest, while facial immobility and tremor are rare.

The rigidity is often atypical, being variable in degree and predominating in the flexors of the elbows and the extensors of the knees. Catatonia is not uncommon. Probably the signs are in part due to lesions at a higher level than the corpus striatum, interrupting corticostriate fibres.

The course of the disorder is more rapid than that of paralysis agitans. It shows little or no response to treatment with levodopa and other remedies (Godwin-Austen, Bergmann, and Frears 1971; Parkes, Marsden, Rees, Curzon, Kantamaneni, Knill-Jones, Akbar, Das, and Kataria 1974). When the blood pressure is high, a fatal cerebral haemorrhage may occur. Progressive dementia, dysphagia, and eventual incontinence render nursing difficult, and the patient succumbs in a few years.

The diagnosis of parkinsonism

The parkinsonian syndrome must be distinguished from other conditions which simulate it. Since the most striking manifestations are tremor and rigidity, parkinsonism is most likely to be confused with conditions causing one or other of these symptoms.

Other causes of tremor

Senile tremor. Tremor in old age differs from parkinsonian tremor in being finer and more rapid, like exaggerated physiological tremor. At first it is absent when the limbs are at rest and occurs only on voluntary movement ('action' tremor). Later it appears during rest. It is most marked in the upper limbs, but more often affects the head than parkinsonian tremor. The rhythmical to-and-fro 'titubating' movements of the head are characteristic. It is not associated with muscular weakness or rigidity and probably represents benign tremor of late onset.

Benign or 'essential' familial tremor. This is a form of tremor which may occur in several members of the same family, often in successive generations (Critchley 1949; Larsson and Sjögren 1960; Critchley 1972). It may begin in childhood, when it may be associated with 'shuddering attacks' (Vanasse, Bédard, and Andermann 1976), and usually develops during the first 25 years of life. It may be fine and rapid or slower and coarser, is usually absent at rest in the early stages, and tends to be increased by voluntary movement and emotion. It is thus an action tremor; senile tremor (see above) may be regarded as a similar disorder of sporadic occurrence in late life. It may be generalized or involve especially the hands, lips, and tongue. As a rule it worsens slightly throughout life and no other neurological signs appear. In rare instances paralysis agitans has been observed in a member of a family afflicted with familial tremor. A curious feature of benign familial tremor is that it is almost specifically, though temporarily, relieved by ethyl alcohol (Growdon, Shahani, and Young 1975). Propranolol (Morgan, Hewer, and Cooper 1973; Sweet, Blumberg, Lee, and McDowell 1974; Rajput, Jamieson, Hirsch, and Quraishi 1975) and/or diazepam may also reduce the tremor, and controlled trials with various β-adrenoreceptor antagonists such as propranolol, sotalol, atenolol, and pindolol have shown that it is those against β_2 adrenoreceptors which are successful and not β_1 antagonists (Teräväinen, Fogelholm, and Larsen 1976; Teräväinen, Larsen, and Fogelholm 1977; Jefferson, Jenner, and Marsden 1979a; *The Lancet* 1979; Dietrichson and Espen 1981); a satisfactory blood level of propranolol is usually achieved with daily doses of 120–240 mg (Jefferson, Jenner, and Marsden 1979b), but Sørensen, Paulson, Steiness, and Jansen (1981) did not find measurement of blood levels helpful. Treatment with primidone in doses up to 750 mg daily may be even more effective in some cases (O'Brien, Upton, and Toseland 1981; Chakrabarti and Pearce 1981). In severe cases stereotaxic surgery is very rarely necessary.

Hysterical tremor. Two forms of hysterical tremor are encountered: a fine tremor, localized to one limb or generalized, and resembling the shaking of extreme fear, and a coarse, irregular shaking, intensified by voluntary movement. In common with other hysterical symptoms, hysterical tremor is characterized by its irregularity, variability from time to time, and by a tendency to diminish when the patient's attention is distracted and to increase when attention is directed to the affected part. The tremor of acute anxiety is similar but less florid and variable.

Tremor in hyperthyroidism. This is a fine, rapid action tremor seen best in the outstretched arms and sometimes more marked on one side than the other. The associated exophthalmos, thyroid enlargement, tachycardia, and flushed and sweating skin usually render diagnosis easy.

Toxic tremor. Tremor may be a sign of intoxication with or withdrawal of various poisons or drugs, especially mercury, cocaine, and alcohol. The tremor of cocaine addiction and chronic alcoholism is fine and of action type. That of chronic poisoning and delirium tremens and that due to withdrawal of barbiturates or other drugs is somewhat coarser, but does not have the rhythmical character of static parkinsonian tremor. The 'flapping' or 'wing-beating' tremor (asterixis) of chronic liver disease is also distinctive. In all these cases the cause is usually evident.

Multiple sclerosis. In multiple sclerosis with cerebellar involvement intention tremor is common. It is absent when the limb is at rest and develops only during voluntary movement, increasing as the limb approaches its objective. In this respect it is the opposite of parkinsonian tremor, which is present at rest and diminishes on movement. Static tremor is rare in multiple sclerosis, but may be seen rarely in the head. In this disease there are usually nystagmus and signs of corticospinal dysfunction, which, apart from the character of the tremor, distinguish it from parkinsonism.

Hereditary ataxia
Intention tremor similar to that observed in multiple sclerosis is sometimes a feature of inherited cerebellar degeneration. Static tremor, closely resembling that of parkinsonism, is seen in olivo-ponto-cerebellar degeneration in which, however, the associated features of dementia, cerebellar ataxia, and corticospinal-tract degeneration are distinctive.

General paresis. Tremor affecting especially the face, tongue, and hands is an early symptom of general paresis. This is a fine tremor, increased by voluntary movement. The mental changes, Argyll Robertson pupils, signs of corticospinal tract lesions, and positive serological reactions in blood and CSF distinguish the condition from parkinsonism.

The parkinsonism-dementia complex
This is a degenerative disease of unknown aetiology, thought by some to be genetically determined and by others to be due to unidentified environmental factors in genetically susceptible individuals (Hoffman, Robbins, Gibbs, Gajdusek, Garruto, and Terasaki 1977), which occurs only in the Chamorro people of Guam and the Mariana islands. Most affected patients develop bradykinesia, rigidity, and tremor but progressive dementia also occurs and few patients survive formore than a few years. Some also develop signs of amyotrophic lateral sclerosis (motor-neurone disease) (Hirano, Malamud, and Kurland 1961; Hirano, Malamud, and Elizan 1966; Brody and Chen 1969). A somewhat similar disorder has been reported in the Australian aborigine (Kiloh, Lethlean, Morgan, Cawte, and Harris 1980). The pathological changes differ from those of paralysis agitans; the rigidity and tremor may improve with levodopa (Schnur, Chase, and Brody 1971) but the dementia does not. Cases which are similar clinically but which occur sporadically in other countries may be due to low-pressure hydrocephalus (Botez, Bertrand, Léveillé, and Marchand 1977) or more often to the common association of paralysis agitans and Alzheimer's disease.

Corticostriatonigral degeneration
This familial and progressive disorder is indistinguishable from paralysis agitans in its early stages except that it usually produces severe akinesia and rigidity but little if any tremor; dementia may rarely develop and pathological changes in the putamen and globus pallidus are much more severe than in idiopathic parkinsonism (Adams, van Bogaert, and vander Eecken 1964; Takei and Mirra 1973). Similar clinical and pathological features are often seen in advanced cases of so-called progressive multisystem degeneration (the Shy–Drager syndrome, see page 188), in which, however, severe orthostatic hypotension and/or cerebellar ataxia are more often the presenting features.

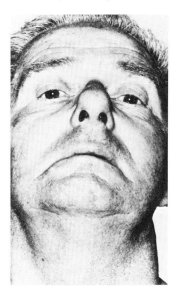
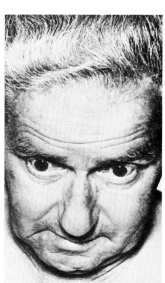

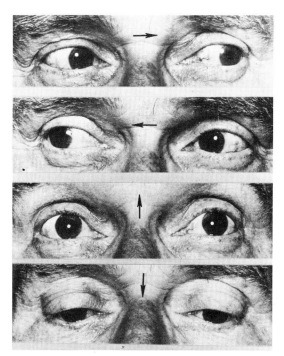

Fig. 12.5. Progressive supranuclear palsy. (Kindly provided by Dr J.D. Spillane.)

(a) Even on head flexion there is no reflex upward movement of the eyes. Note the parkinsonian features.

(b) Voluntary upward gaze is totally lost but lateral and downward gaze is retained.

Progressive supranuclear palsy

This rare condition (Steele, Richardson, and Olszewski 1964; Behrman, Carroll, Janota, and Matthews 1969; Kurihara, Landau, and Torack 1974; also see p. 99) is characterized by progressive paralysis of upward vertical gaze (Fig. 12.5), paroxysmal dysequilibrium, progressive parkinsonian features, and sometimes increasing dementia. The neck muscles become rigid and retrocollis is sometimes seen as is corticospinal-tract involvement. All patients show 'square-wave jerks' giving defective ocular fixation (Troost and Daroff 1977). Many show evidence of cortical atrophy on CT scanning (Perkin, Lees, Stern, and Kocen 1978; Haldeman, Goldman, Hyde, and Pribram 1981) and Alzheimer-type neuropathological changes. While these patients show little if any response to drugs normally of benefit in parkinsonism, they may show some response to serotonin inhibitors such as methysergide (Rafal and Grimm 1981).

Other causes of rigidity

Hysterical rigidity. In such cases the degree of the rigidity is proportional to the observer's efforts to move the limb. In parkinsonism the rigidity is, by contrast, a definite quantum which always yields to the exercise of slightly greater force.

Spasticity due to corticospinal-tract lesions. This is distinguished by the selective distribution of the rigidity to certain muscle groups, usually the flexors in the upper and the extensors in the lower limbs. Moreover, it is usually maximal at the beginning of passive movement and diminishes as the movement proceeds. Parkinsonian rigidity is uniform both in its distribution and throughout the angle of joint movement. In spastic paraplegia the plantar reflexes are extensor, whereas they are flexor in uncomplicated parkinsonism.

Arthritis and arthropathy. Rigidity due to joint disease occasionally simulates parkinsonism, especially when vertebral joints are affected as in ankylosing spondylitis. The flexion of the spine and immobility of the head may at first glance be deceptive. Pain in such cases, however, is usually severe at some stage, and it is easy to demonstrate that the rigidity is bony and not muscular in origin.

Treatment

The sufferer from parkinsonism should be encouraged to lead an active life as long as possible. Passive movements are valuable for their temporary effect in diminishing rigidity, but more as a means of postponing the development of contractures. Re-educational walking exercises under the supervision of a skilled physiotherapist are often helpful. A walking-stick is invaluable in many cases and in patients with severe akinesia a frame walking aid which encourages the patient to lean forwards and to initiate those walking reflexes which are impaired by the disease process is of great benefit. Chairs with seats which can be electrically or mechanically elevated and many other appliances may be needed. For many years the only drugs available to diminish rigidity were those of the belladonna group, which also reduced salivation and sweating. Traditional remedies such as hyoscine hydrobromide, belladonna, and stramonium were later supplanted by synthetic antispasmodic drugs, which are still useful in some cases despite the much greater benefit obtained with dopamine precursors and agonists (see below).

The most useful are benzhexol (*Artane*), beginning with 2 mg two or three times a day, or orphenadrine hydrochloride (*Disipal*), 50–100 mg up to three times a day. It may be necessary to try several preparations, since the drug which suits one patient may not suit another. Benztropine (*Cogentin*), 1–2 mg at night, and methixene (*Tremonil*), 5–10 mg three times a day, may be a little more successful than other remedies in controlling tremor but no such drug is really effective. All of these may produce dryness of the mouth, constipation, and blurring of vision. The latter

may be helped by adding pilocarpine eye-drops. Glaucoma may be a serious complication (Friedman and Neumann 1972). Confusion is an even more important side-effect, particularly in elderly patients and may be accompanied by disturbing visual and auditory hallucinations. Retention of urine may also occur. Such side-effects may even necessitate withdrawal of all drugs in a few cases but some patients are best treated by a combination of two such drugs. The improvement produced by anticholinergic remedies is limited; not more than 80 per cent of patients show up to 30 per cent improvement (Duvoisin 1965; Calne 1970). Amphetamine was once used for oculogyric crises and depression and may give limited improvement in parkinsonism (Parkes *et al* 1974) but has been supplanted in treating depression by tricyclic antidepressant drugs such as imipramine and its derivatives (Calne 1970). Beta-adrenergic blocking remedies such as propranolol and nadolol improve tremor (Owen and Marsden 1965; Foster *et al.* 1984). When the patient becomes bed-ridden much care is needed to prevent the development of bed-sores and to maintain nutrition.

An important addition to the therapeutic armamentarium, first used in 1969, was amantadine hydrochloride, originally used as an antiviral agent. The drug is certainly beneficial (Butzer, Silver, and Sahs 1975); the usual dose is 100 mg twice daily and it is still given in some cases of mild and early parkinsonism. It is believed to act by blocking the presynaptic uptake of dopamine, thereby prolonging its effective half-life (Grelak, Clark, and Stump 1970). It improves akinesia and rigidity, and tremor to a lesser extent, but is significantly less effective than levodopa (Hunter, Stern, Laurence, and Armitage 1970) though it may have an adjuvant effect when combined with the latter (Godwin-Austen, Frears, Bergmann, Parkes, and Knill-Jones 1970; Schwab, Poskanzer, England, and Young 1972; Cox, Danta, Schnieden, and Yuill 1973; Bauer and McHenry 1974).

The most major advance of the last 25 years was the introduction into treatment of levodopa and a vast literature upon its use has now accumulated. Its effects may be monitored by estimating homovanillic acid and its other metabolites in the CSF (Curzon, Godwin-Austen, Tomlinson, and Kantamaneni 1970). Examination of brains at autopsy has confirmed that levodopa significantly increases cerebral dopamine (Rinne and Sonninen 1973). When levodopa alone was used, without peripheral decarboxylase inhibitors (see below), it was usual to begin treatment with 250 mg levodopa daily or twice daily, increasing by 250–500 mg daily every three or four days until the maximum tolerated dosage was reached. Side-effects such as nausea and vomiting were often troublesome but could be controlled by cyclizine or similar remedies. The most troublesome side-effect was the development of involuntary movements which often included features of chorea, athetosis, and dystonia as well as bizarre foot-paddling and facial dyskinetic movements which are difficult to classify (Mones, Elizan, and Siegel 1971) but may resemble those of Meige's syndrome of blepharospasm—oromandibular dystonia (Weiner and Nausieda 1982). These movements usually cease or lessen when the dose is reduced and may be reduced by deanol in a dosage of 100 mg three times daily (Miller 1974) or by oxiperomide, 15 mg daily (Bédard, Parkes, and Marsden 1978). The dose of levodopa, when given alone, which could be tolerated by individual patients varied from 1 g to 8 g daily. It could not be given with most amine oxidase inhibitors or with pyridoxine, which inhibits its effects. It was usually combined with anticholinergic remedies and/or amantadine for maximum therapeutic effect and sudden withdrawal of anticholinergic drugs sometimes produced rapid deterioration (Hughes, Polgar, Weightman, and Walton 1971; Horrocks, Vicary, Rees, Parkes, and Marsden 1973). The drug was effective in paralysis agitans and in post-encephalitic parkinsonism (Cotzias, van Woert, and Schifter 1967; Yahr, Duvoisin, Schear, Barrett, and Hoen 1969; Duvoisin, Lobo-Antunes, and Yahr 1972); it was of limited benefit in the parkinsonism–dementia complex and corticostriatonigral degeneration but not in the Shy–Drager syndrome. In supranuclear palsy it temporarily modified the parkinsonian manifestations (Mendell, Chase, and Engell 1970; Klawans and Ringel 1971) but not other features. It improved akinesia and rigidity most but also improved tremor and oculogyric crises (Klawans and Erlich 1970) and had a marked alerting effect (Marsh, Markham, and Ansel 1971) but did not improve dementia and the disease often progressed despite partial control of its clinical manifestations (Hunter, Laurence, Shaw, and Stern 1973). Occasional cases showed a remarkable lack of response for reasons which are difficult to determine (*British Medical Journal* 1973b) and there was sometimes progressive deterioration after long-term treatment with episodes of severe akinesia and an 'on-off' effect (Markham 1972) with marked variation in the patient's condition from one part of the day to another, often related to the timing of the medication, the so-called long-term levodopa syndrome (Barbeau 1972). This may be due to increasing receptor hypersensitivity.

Despite these problems, as well as that of 'peak-dose' dyskinesia (Shaw, Lees, and Stern 1980) in which involuntary movements are at their most troublesome 60–90 minutes after a dose of levodopa, there is no doubt that since levodopa was introduced, the mortality rate and long-rate morbidity in patients suffering from parkinsonism has declined (Joseph, Chassan, and Koch 1978). Responsiveness to treatment may be partially restored after a 'drug holiday' of as little as five to seven days (Weiner, Koller, Perlik, Nausieda, and Klawans 1980). Lesser, Fahn, Snider, Cote, Isgreen, and Barrett (1979) suggested that because of the 'wearing-off' and 'on-off' effects, levodopa should be withheld in mild cases until the patient's condition is significantly impaired by his disease, but Markham and Diamond (1981) have shown that withholding treatment in the earlier stages confers no long-term benefit. Selegeline, a selective monoamine-oxidase B inhibitor, in a dose of 5–10 mg daily, has been shown to prolong the therapeutic effect of levodopa and to reduce 'on-off' disability and end-of-dose akinesia (Lees, Shaw, Kohout, Stern, Elsworth, Sandler, and Youdim 1977; Schachter, Marsden, Parkes, Jenner, and Testa 1980). Sodium valproate, a GABA inhibitor, is of no value in this respect (Nutt, Williams, Plotkin, Eng, Ziegler, and Calne 1979), but naloxone, an opiate antagonist, has also been found to reduce the 'on-off' effect and levodopa-induced dyskinesia (Trabucchi, Bassi, and Frattola 1982); as it must be given intravenously, it is unlikely to find general favour.

Much of the above section has been written in the past tense, since levodopa is now rarely, if ever, given alone, but is almost invariably combined with a decarboxylase inhibitor which reduces the peripheral degradation of dopamine, thus making more available in the brain (Calne, Reid, Vakil, Rao, Petrie, Pallis, Gawler, Thomas, and Hilson 1971; Marsden, Barry, Parkes, and Zilkha 1973; Mars 1973; Yahr 1973). The usual preparations are of levodopa with L-α-methyldopa-hydrazine (carbidopa) combined in a 10:1 ratio (*Sinemet*) or levodopa with benserazide in a 4:1 ratio (*Madopar*). Both combinations have been found to be effective and significantly to reduce side-effects such as involuntary movements. Some patients find greater benefit and fewer side-effects with one remedy, some with the other, but several controlled trials (e.g. Diamond, Markham, and Treciokas 1978) have found both to be equally effective. Levodopa must be withdrawn as one or other of these remedies is gradually introduced. For example, one tablet of *Sinemet* 110 or one of *Madopar* 125 has a similar therapeutic effect to one 500-mg dose of levodopa alone. One or other of these preparations is now generally regarded as the initial treatment of choice in Parkinson's disease. Other remedies (amantadine, anticholinergic drugs), if being given, can be continued during the changeover.

Another major advance has been the introduction of dopamine agonists which stimulate the production of endogenous dopamine. Of these, the most widely used has been bromocriptine in a dosage of 15–75 mg daily given either alone or in combination with levodopa and carbidopa or benserazide (Calne, Teychenne, Claveria, Eastman, Greenacre, and Petrie 1974; Calne, Plotkin, Williams, Nutt, Neophytides, and Teychenne 1978; Parkes, Debono, and Marsden 1976; Rascol, Guiraud, Montastruc, David, and Clanet 1979; Pearce and Pearce 1978). When given in combination with domperidone, a peripheral dopamine blocking agent, nausea and vomiting, a troublesome side-effect, is largely overcome (Agid, Pollak, Bonnet, Signoret, and Lhermitte 1979; Quinn, Illas, Lhermitte, and Agid 1981). This drug is about as effective as levodopa but appears to have little advantage over the latter in long-term treatment (Lees, Haddad, Shaw, Kohout, and Stern 1978), though there is some evidence that low-dose treatment (5–20 mg daily) may be effective without inducing an on-off effect or dyskinesia (Teychenne, Bergsrud, Racy, Elton, and Vern 1982). Generally, bromocriptine is now reserved for patients who do poorly with *Sinemet* or *Madopar* or deteriorate after initial benefit. Another class of remedies which may prove to be of benefit are the semisynthetic ergolines, lisuride, and pergolide (Parkes, Schachter, Marsden, Smith, and Wilson 1981; Lieberman, Goldstein, Leibowitz, Neophytides, Gopinathan, Walker, and Pact 1981a; Lieberman, Goldstein, Leibowitz, Neophytides, Kupersmith, Pact, and Kleinberg 1981b; Gopinathan, Teräväinen, Dambrosia, Ward, Sanes, Stuart, Evarts, and Calne 1981), which are powerful dopamine agonists and can, like bromocriptine, be given with levodopa but may produce troublesome drowsiness.

Surgery

The operations of pallidectomy and ventrolateral thalamotomy, or both combined, had a considerable vogue in the treatment of parkinsonism after Cooper (1953) showed that infarction of the globus pallidus resulting from anterior choroidal artery ligation improved contralateral rigidity and tremor. In general, surgery gave best results in idiopathic parkinsonism with unilateral symptoms in a patient under the age of 65. Severe akinesia, generalized cerebral atheroma, dementia, and severe hypertension were contra-indications (Cooper 1961; Gillingham, Watson, Donaldson, and Naughton 1960). Various stereotaxic techniques were used by different neurosurgeons; chemopallidectomy (injection of alcohol) was largely supplanted by methods involving thermocoagulation or freezing (cryothalamotomy). It became evident that tremor could be greatly reduced or abolished and rigidity reduced but akinesia, speech disturbance, and salivation were uninfluenced. Bilateral operations carried out simultaneously, or with an interval of a few months between the two procedures, were commonly done, even in patients of 70 years or older who were in good general condition, but confusion and permanent intellectual impairment were more common after bilateral procedures. Surgical treatment was only one component of the treatment in such cases and did not supplant the use of appropriate drugs (Hankinson 1960; Cooper 1965; Selby 1967). The number of operations performed has fallen dramatically since the introduction of levodopa, but surgery still has a limited place if severe tremor is poorly controlled by drugs.

References

Adams, R. D., van Bogaert, L., and Vander Eecken, H. (1964). Striato-nigral degeneration. *J. Neuropath. exp. Neurol.* **23**, 584.

Agid, Y., Pollak, P., Bonnet, A. M., Signoret, J. L., and Lhermitte, F. (1979). Bromocriptine associated with a peripheral dopamine blocking agent in treatment of Parkinson's disease. *Lancet* **i**, 570.

Aminoff, M. J. and Wilcox, C. S. (1972). Control of blood pressure in Parkinsonism. *Proc. R. Soc. Med.* **65**, 944.

Angel, R. W., Alston, W., and Higgins, J. R. (1970). Control of movement in Parkinson's disease. *Brain* **93**, 1.

Ayd, F. J., Jr. (1961). A survey of drug-induced extrapyramidal reactions. *J. Am. med. Ass.* **175**, 1054.

Barbeau, A. (1972). Long-term appraisal of levodopa therapy, *Neurology, Minneapolis* **22**, 22.

——, Campanella, G., Butterworth, R. F., and Yamada, K. (1975).

Uptake and efflux of ^{14}C-dopamine in platelets: evidence for a generalized defect in Parkinson's disease. *Neurology, Minneapolis* **25**, 1.

Bauer, R. B. and McHenry, J. T. (1974). Comparison of amantadine, placebo, and levodopa in Parkinson's disease. *Neurology, Minneapolis* **24**, 715.

Becker, H., Schneider, E., Hacker, H., and Fischer, P. -A. (1979). Cerebral atrophy in Parkinson's disease—represented in C. T. *Arch. Psychiat. Nervenkr.* **227**, 81.

Bédard, P., Parkes, J. D., and Marsden, C. D. (1978). Effect of new dopamine-blocking agent (oxiperomides) on drug-induced dyskinesias in Parkinson's disease and spontaneous dyskinesias. *Br. med. J.* **1**, 954.

Behrman, S., Carroll, J. D., Janota, I., and Matthews, W. B. (1969). Progressive supranuclear palsy. *Brain* **92**, 663.

Bodis-Wollner, I. and Yahr, M. D. (1978). Measurements of visual evoked potentials in Parkinson's disease. *Brain* **101**, 661.

Botez, M. I., Bertrand, G., Léveillé, J., and Marchand, L. (1977). Parkinsonism-dementia complex, hydrocephalus and Paget's disease. *Can. J. neurol. Sci.* **4**, 139.

Brewis, M., Poskanzer, D. C., Rolland, C., and Miller, H. (1966). Neurological disease in an English city. *Acta neurol. scand.* **24**, Supp. 42.

British Medical Journal (1973a). Mental symptoms and Parkinsonism. *Br. med. J.* **2**, 67.

——, (1973b). Failure to respond to levodopa. *Br. med. J.* **4**, 314.

Brody, J. A. and Chen, K. -M. (1969). Changing epidemiologic patterns of amyotrophic lateral sclerosis and Parkinsonism-dementia in Guam. In *Motor neuron diseases* (ed. F. H. Norris and L. T. Kurland), p.61. Grune and Stratton, New York.

Brown, E. L. and Knox, E. G. (1972). Epidemiological approach to Parkinson's disease. *Lancet* i, 974.

Brown, R. G. and Marsden, C. D. (1984). How common is dementia in Parkinson's disease? *Lancet* ii, 1262.

Burke, R. E. and Fahn, S. (1981). Movement disorders. In *Current neurology* (ed. S. H. Appel), Vol. 3, p. 92. John Wiley, New York.

Burton, J. L. and Shuster, S. (1970). Effect of L-dopa on seborrhoea of Parkinsonism. *Lancet* ii, 19.

Butzer, J. F., Silver, D. E., and Sahs, A. L. (1975). Amantadine in Parkinson's disease: a double-blind, placebo-controlled, crossover study with long-term follow-up. *Neurology, Minneapolis* **25**, 603.

Byrne, E., Thomas, P. K., and Zilkha, K. J. (1982). Familial extrapyramidal disease with peripheral neuropathy. *J. Neurol. Neurosurg. Psychiat.* **45**, 372.

Calne, D. B. (1970). *Parkinsonism: physiology, pharmacology and treatment.* Arnold, London.

——, Plotkin, C., Williams, A. C., Nutt, J. G., Neophytides, A., and Teychenne, P. F. (1978). Long-term treatment of Parkinsonism with bromocriptine. *Lancet* i, 735.

——, Reid, J. L., Vakil, S. D., Rao, S., Petrie, A., Pallis, C. A., Gawler, J., Thomas, P. K., and Hilson, A. (1971). Idiopathic Parkinsonism treated with an extracerebral decarboxylase inhibitor in combination with levodopa, *Br. med. J.* **3**, 729.

——, Teychenne, P. F., Claveria, L. E., Eastman, R., Greenacre, J. K., and Petrie, A. (1974). Bromocriptine in Parkinsonism. *Br. med. J.* **4**, 442.

Carlen, P. L., Lee, M. A., Jacob, M., and Livshits, O. (1981). Parkinsonism provoked by alcoholism. *Ann. Neurol.* **9**, 84.

Chakrabarti, A. and Pearce, J. M. S. (1981). Essential tremor: response to primidone. *J. Neurol. Neurosurg. Psychiat.* **44**, 650.

Cooper, I. E. (1953). Anterior choroidal artery ligation for involuntary movements. *Science* **118**, 193.

—— (1961). *Parkinsonism, its medical and surgical treatment.* Thomas, Springfield, Illinois.

—— (1965). The surgical treatment of Parkinsonism. *Ann. Rev. Med.* **16**, 309.

Cotzias, G. C., Van Woert, M. H., and Schiffer, L. M. (1967). Aromatic amino acids and modification of Parkinsonism. *New Engl. J. Med.* **276**, 374.

Cox, B., Danta, G., Schnieden, H., and Yuill, G. M. (1973). Interactions of L-dopa and amantadine in patients with Parkinsonism. *J. Neurol. Neurosurg. Psychiat.* **36**, 354.

Critchley, E. (1972). Clinical manifestations of essential tremor. *J. Neurol. Neurosurg. Psychiat.* **35**, 365.

—— (1981). Speech disorders of Parkinsonism: a review. *J. Neurol. Neurosurg. Psychiat.* **44**, 751.

Critchley, M. (1929). Arteriosclerotic Parkinsonism. *Brain* **52**, 23.

—— (1949). Observations on essential (heredofamilial) tremor. *Brain* **72**, 113.

Curzon, G., Godwin-Austen, R. B., Tomlinson, E. G., and Kantamaneni, B. D. (1970). The cerebrospinal fluid homovanillic acid concentration in patients with Parkinsonism treated with L-dopa. *J. Neurol. Neurosurg. Psychiat.* **33**, 1.

Den Hartog Jager, W. A. (1969). Sphingomyelin in Lewy inclusion bodies in Parkinson's disease. *Arch. Neurol., Chicago* **21**, 615.

Denny-Brown, D. (1962). *The basal ganglia and their relation to disorders of movement.* Oxford University Press, Oxford.

de Yébenes, J. G., Gervas, J. J., Iglesias, J., Mena, M. A., Martin del Rio, R., and Somoza, E. (1982). Biochemical findings in a case of Parkinsonism secondary to brain tumor. *Ann. Neurol.* **11**, 313.

Diamond, B. I. and Borison, R. L. (1978). Enkephalins and nigrostriatal function. *Neurology, Minneapolis* **28**, 1085.

Diamond, S. G. and Markham, C. H. (1979). Mortality of Parkinson patients treated with Sinemet. In *Advances in neurology* (ed. L. J. Poirier, T. L. Sourkes, and P. J. Bédard) Vol. 24, p. 489. Raven Press, New York.

——, ——, and Treciokas, L. J. (1978). A double-blind comparison of levodopa, Madopar, and Sinemet in Parkinson disease. *Ann. Neurol.* **3**, 267.

Dietrichson, P. and Espen, E. (1981). Effects of timolol and atenolol on benign essential tremor: placebo-controlled studies based on quantitative tremor recording. *J. Neurol. Neurosurg. Psychiat.* **44**, 677.

Duvoisin, R. C. (1965). A review of drug therapy in Parkinsonism. *Bull. NY Acad. Sci.* **41**, 898.

——, Lobo-Antunes, J., and Yahr, M. D. (1972). Response of patients with postencephalitic Parkinsonism to levodopa. *J. Neurol. Neurosurg. Psychiat.* **35**, 487.

Earle, K. M. (1968). Studies on Parkinson's disease including X-ray fluorescent spectroscopy of formalin fixed brain tissue. *J. Neuropath. exp. Neurol.* **27**, 1.

Forno, L. S. (1982). Pathology of Parkinson's disease. In *Movement disorders* (ed. C. D. Marsden and S. Fahn), p. 25. Butterworths, London.

Foster, N. L., Newman, R. P., LeWitt, P. A. Gillespie, M. M., Larsen, T. A., and Chase, T. N. (1984). Peripheral beta-adrenergic blockade treatment of parkinsonian tremor. *Ann. Neurol.* **16**, 505.

Friedman, Z. and Neumann, E. (1972). Benzhexol-induced blindness in Parkinson's disease. *Br. med. J.* **1**, 605.

Gilbert, G. J. (1976). A pseudohemiparetic form of Parkinson's disease. *Lancet* ii, 442.

Gillingham, F. J., Watson, W. S., Donaldson, A. A., and Naughton, J. A. L. (1960). The surgical treatment of Parkinsonism. *Br. med. J.* **2**, 1395.

Godwin-Austen, R. B., Bergmann, S., and Frears, C. (1971). Effect of age and arteriosclerosis on the response of Parkinsonian patients to levodopa. *Br. med. J.* **4**, 522.

——, Frears, C., Bergmann, S., Parkes, J. D., and Knill-Jones, R. P. (1970). Combined treatment of Parkinsonism with L-dopa and amantadine. *Lancet* ii, 383.

Gopinathan, G., Teräväinen, H., Dambrosia, J. M., Ward, C. D., Sanes, J. N., Stuart, W. K., Evarts, E. V., and Calne, D. B. (1981). Lisuride in parkinsonism. *Neurology, Minneapolis* **31**, 371.

Greenfield, J. G. (1958). In *Neuropathology* (ed. J. G. Greenfield, W. H. McMenemey, A. Meyer, and R. M. Norman), p. 530. Arnold, London.

—— and Bosanquet, F. D. (1953). The brain-stem lesions in Parkinsonism. *J. Neurol. Neurosurg. Psychiat.* **16**, 213.

—— and Matthews, W. B. (1954). Post-encephalitic Parkinsonism with amyotrophy. *J. Neurol. Neurosurg. Psychiat.* **17**, 50.

Grelak, R. P., Clark, R., and Stump, J. M. (1970). Amantadine–dopamine interaction: possible mode of action in Parkinsonism. *Science* **169**, 203.

Gross, M., Bannister, R., and Godwin-Austen, R. B. (1972). Orthostatic hypotension in Parkinson's disease. *Lancet* i, 174.

Growdon, J. H., Shahani, B. T., and Young, R. R. (1975). The effect of alcohol on essential tremor. *Neurology, Minneapolis* **25**, 259.

Hakim, A. M. and Mathieson, G. (1979). Dementia in Parkinson disease: a neuropathologic study. *Neurology, Minneapolis* **29**, 1209.

Haldeman, S., Goldman, J. W., Hyde, J., and Pribram, H. F. W. (1981). Progressive supranuclear palsy, computed tomography, and response to antiparkinsonian drugs. *Neurology, Minneapolis* **31**, 442.

Hall, A. J. (1931). Chronic epidemic encephalitis, with special reference to the ocular attacks. *Br. med. J.* **2**, 833.

Hankinson, J. (1960). The surgical treatment of Parkinson's disease. *Postgrad. med. J.* **36**, 242.

Hirano, A., Malamud, N., and Elizan, T. S. (1966). Amyotrophic lateral sclerosis and parkinsonism-dementia complex in Guam. *Arch. Neurol., Chicago* **15**, 35.

——, ——, and Kurland, L. T. (1961). Parkinsonism–dementia complex—

an endemic disease on the island of Guam, II. Pathological features. *Brain* **84**, 662.

Hoehn, M. M. and Yahr, M. D. (1967). Parkinsonism: onset, progression, and mortality. *Neurology, Minneapolis* **17**, 427.

Hoffman, P. M., Robbins, D. S., Gibbs, C. J., Gajdusek, D. C., Garruto, R. M., and Terasaki, P. I. (1977). Histocompatibility antigens in amyotrophic lateral sclerosis and Parkinsonism–dementia on Guam. *Lancet* **ii**, 717.

Hornykiewicz, O. (1982). Brain neurotransmitter changes in Parkinson's disease. In *Movement disorders* (ed. C. D. Marsden and S. Fahn). Butterworths, London.

Horrocks, P. M., Vicary, D. J., Rees, J. E., Parkes, J. D., and Marsden, C. D. (1973). Anticholinergic withdrawal and benzhexol treatment in Parkinson's disease. *J. Neurol. Neurosurg. Psychiat* **36**, 936.

Hughes, R. C., Polgar, J. G., Weightman, D., and Walton, J. N. (1971). Levodopa in Parkinsonism: the effects of withdrawal of anticholinergic drugs. *Br. med. J.* **2**, 487.

Hunt, J. R. (1917). Progressive atrophy of the globus pallidus. *Brain* **40**, 58.

Hunter, K. R., Laurence, D. R., Shaw, K. M., and Stern, G. M. (1973). Sustained levodopa therapy in Parkinsonism. *Lancet* **ii**, 929.

Hunter, K. M., Stern, G. M., Laurence, D. R., and Armitage, P. (1970). Amantadine in Parkinsonism *Lancet* **i**, 1127.

Issidorides, M. R., Mytilineou, C., Whetsell, W. O., and Yahr, M. D. (1978). Protein-rich cytoplasmic bodies of substantia nigra and locus ceruleus. *Arch. Neurol., Chicago* **35**, 633.

Javoy-Agid, F. and Agid, Y. (1980). Is the mesocortical dopaminergic system involved in Parkinson's disease? *Neurology, Minneapolis* **30**, 1326.

Jefferson, D., Jenner, P., and Marsden, C. D. (1979*a*). β-adrenoreceptor antagonists in essential tremor. *J. Neurol. Neurosurg. Psychiat.* **42**, 904.

——, ——, and —— (1979*b*). Relationship between plasma propranolol concentration and relief of essential tremor. *J. Neurol. Neurosurg. Psychiat.* **42**, 831.

Joseph, C., Chassan, J. B., and Koch, M.-L. (1978). Levodopa in Parkinson disease: a long-term appraisal of mortality. *Ann. Neurol.* **3**, 116.

Kiloh, L. G., Lethlean, A. K., Morgan, G., Cawte, J. E., and Harris, M. (1980). An endemic neurological disorder in tribal Australian aborigines. *J. Neurol. Neurosurg. Psychiat.* **43**, 661.

Kim, R. (1968). The chronic residual respiratory disorder in post-encephalitic Parkinsonism. *J. Neurol. Neurosurg. Psychiat.* **31**, 393.

—— and Goodwin, J. A. (1969). Reversal of the glabellar reflex in Parkinsonism by L-dopa. *J. Neurol. Neurosurg. Psychiat.* **32**, 423.

—— and Ringel, S. P. (1971). Observations on the efficacy of L-dopa in progressive supranuclear palsy. *Eur. Neurol.* **5**, 115.

Kondo, K., Kurland, L. T., and Schull, W. J. (1973). Parkinson's disease. Genetic analysis and evidence of a multifactorial etiology. *Mayo Clin. Proc.* **48**, 465.

Kugelberg, E. (1952). Facial reflexes. *Brain* **75**, 385.

Kurihara, T., Landau, W. M., and Torack, R. M. (1974). Progressive supranuclear palsy with action myoclonus, seizures. *Neurology, Minneapolis* **24**, 219.

Kurland, L. T. (1958). In *The pathology and treatment of Parkinsonism* (ed. W. S. Fields) p. 5. Thomas, Springfield, Illinois.

Lance, J. W. and McLeod, J. G. (1981). *A physiological approach to clinical neurology.* Butterworth, London.

The Lancet (1979). Beta-blockers in essential tremor. *Lancet* **ii**, 1280.

Larsson, T. and Sjögren, T. (1960). Essential tremor. *Acta psychiat., (Kbh)* **36**, Suppl. 144.

Lees, A. J., Haddad, S., Shaw, K. M., Kohout, L. J., and Stern, G. M. (1978). Bromocriptine in Parkinsonism: a long-term study. *Arch. Neurol., Chicago* **35**, 503.

——, Shaw, K. M., Kohout, L. J., Stern, G. M., Elsworth, J. D., Sandler, M., and Youdim, M. B. H. (1977). Deprenyl in Parkinson's disease. *Lancet* **ii**, 791.

Lesser, R. P., Fahn, S., Snider, S. R., Cote, L. J., Isgreen, W. P., and Barrett, R. E. (1979). Analysis of the clinical problems in parkinsonism and the complications of long-term levodopa therapy. *Neurology, Minneapolis* **29**, 1253.

Lewis, P. D. (1971). Parkinsonism—neuropathology. *Br. med. J.* **3**, 690.

Lieberman, A., Goldstein, M., Leibowitz, M., Neophytides, A., Gopinathan, G., Walker, R., and Pact, V. (1981*a*). Lisuride combined with levodopa in advanced Parkinson disease. *Neurology, Minneapolis* **31**, 1466.

——, ——, ——, ——, Kupersmith, M., Pact, V., and Kleinberg, D. (1981*b*). Treatment of advanced Parkinson disease with pergolide. *Neurology, Minneapolis* **31**, 675.

Loranger, A. W., Goodell, H., McDowell, F. H., Lee, J. E., and Sweet, R. D. (1972). Intellectual impairment in Parkinson's syndrome. *Brain* **95**, 405.

Markham, C. H. (1972). Thirty months' trial of levodopa in Parkinson's disease. *Neurology, Minneapolis* **22**, 17.

—— and Diamond, S. G. (1981). Evidence to support early levodopa therapy in Parkinson disease. *Neurology, Minneapolis* **31**, 125.

Mars, H. (1973). Modification of levodopa effect by systemic decarboxylase inhibition. *Arch. Neurol., Chicago* **28**, 91.

Marsden, C. D. (1982). Basal ganglia disease. *Lancet* **ii**, 1141.

——, Barry, P. E., Parkes, J. D., and Zilkha, K. J. (1973). Treatment of Parkinson's disease with levodopa combined with L-alpha-methyldopahydrazine, an inhibitor of extracerebral dopa decarboxylase. *J. Neurol. Neurosurg. Psychiat.* **36**, 10.

Marsh, G. G., Markham, C. H., and Ansel, R. (1971). Levodopa's awakening effect on patients with Parkinsonism. *J. Neurol. Neurosurg. Psychiat.* **34**, 209.

Martin, J. P. (1967). *The basal ganglia and posture.* Butterworths, London.

Martin, W. E., Resch, J. A., and Baker, A. B. (1971). Juvenile Parkinsonism. *Arch. Neurol., Chicago* **25**, 494.

——, Young, W. I., and Anderson, V. E. (1973). Parkinson's disease: a genetic study. *Brain* **96**, 495.

Mayeux, R., Stern, Y., Rosen, J., and Leventhal, J. (1981). Depression, intellectual impairment, and Parkinson disease. *Neurology, Minneapolis* **31**, 645.

Mendell, J. R., Chase, T. N., and Engel, W. K. (1970). Modification by L-dopa of a case of progressive supranuclear palsy. *Lancet* **i**, 593.

Miller, E. (1974).Deanol in the treatment of levodopa-induced dyskinesias. *Neurology, Minneapolis* **24**, 116.

Mindham, R. H. S. (1970). Psychiatric symptoms in Parkinsonism. *J. Neurol. Neurosurg. Psychiat.* **33**, 188.

Mones, R. J., Elizan, T. S., and Siegel, G. J. (1971). Analysis of L-dopa induced dyskinesias in 51 patients with Parkinsonism. *J. Neurol. Neurosurg. Psychiat.* **34**, 668.

Morgan, M. H., Hewer, R. L., and Cooper, R. (1973). Effect of the beta adrenergic blocking agent propranolol on essential tremor. *J. Neurol. Neurosurg. Psychiat.* **36**, 618.

Mortimer, J. A., Pirozzolo, F. J., Hansch, E. C., and Webster, D. D. (1982). Relationship of motor symptoms to intellectual deficits in Parkinson disease. *Neurology, Minneapolis* **32**, 133.

Nakano, K. K., Zubick, H., and Tyler, H. R. (1973). Speech defects of parkinsonian patients. Effects of levodopa therapy on speech intelligibility. *Neurology, Minneapolis* **23**, 865.

Nutt, J., Williams, A., Plotkin, C., Eng, N., Ziegler, M., and Calne, D. B. (1979). Treatment of Parkinson's disease with sodium valproate: clinical, pharmacological, and biochemical observations. *Can. J. neurol. Sci.* **6**, 337.

O'Brien, M. D., Upton, A. R., and Toseland, P. A. (1981). Benign familial tremor treated with primidone. *Br. med. J.* **282**, 178.

Owen, D. A. L. and Marsden, C. D. (1965). Effect of adrenergic β-blockade on Parkinsonian tremor. *Lancet* **ii**, 1259.

Parkes, J. D., Debono, A. G., and Marsden, C. D. (1976). Bromocriptine in Parkinsonism: long-term treatment, dose response, and comparison with levodopa. *J. Neurol. Neurosurg. Psychiat.* **39**, 1101.

——, Marsden, C. D., Rees, J. E., Curzon, G., Kantamaneni, B. D, Knill-Jones, R., Akbar, A., Das, S., and Kataria, M. (1974). Parkinson's disease, cerebral arteriosclerosis, and senile dementia. *Quart. J. Med.* **43**, 49.

——, Schachter, M., Marsden, C. D., Smith, B., and Wilson, A. (1981). Lisuride in Parkinsonism. *Ann. Neurol.* **9**, 48.

Pearce, I. and Pearce, J. M. S. (1978). Bromocriptine in Parkinsonism. *Br. med. J.* **1**, 1402.

Penders, C. A. and Delwaide, P. J. (1971). Blink reflex studies in patients with Parkinsonism before and during therapy. *J. Neurol. Neurosurg. Psychiat.* **34**, 674.

Perkin, G. D., Lees, A. J., Stern, G. M., and Kocen, R. S. (1978). Problems in the diagnosis of progressive supranuclear palsy (Steele–Richardson–Olszewski syndrome). *Can. J. neurol. Sci.* **5**, 167.

Pirozzolo, F. J., Hansch, E. C., Mortimer, J. A., Webster, D. D., and Kuskowski, M. A. (1982). Dementia in Parkinson disease: a neuropsychological analysis. *Brain and Cognition* **1**, 71.

Pollock, M. and Hornabrook, R. W. (1966). The prevalence, natural history and dementia of Parkinson's disease. *Brain* **89**, 429.

Poskanzer, D. C., Schwab, R. S., and Fraser, D. W. (1969). In *Third sym-*

posium on Parkinson's disease (ed. F. J. Gillingham and I. M. L. Donaldson). Livingstone, Edinburgh.

Pratt, R. T. C. (1967). *The genetics of neurological disorders.* Oxford University Press, London.

Pritchard, P. B. and Netsky, M. G. (1973). Prevalence of neoplasms and causes of death in paralysis agitans: a necropsy study. *Neurology, Minneapolis* **23**, 215.

Purdy, A., Hahn, A., Barnett, H. J. M., Bratty, P., Ahmad, D., Lloyd, K. G., McGeer, E. G., and Perry, T. L. (1979). Familial fatal Parkinsonism with alveolar hypoventilation and mental depression. *Ann. Neurol.* **6**, 523.

Quik, M., Spokes, E. G., Mackay, A. V. P., and Bannister, R. (1979). Alterations in [³H] spiperone binding in human caudate nucleus, substantia nigra and frontal cortex in the Shy–Drager syndrome and Parkinson's disease. *J. neurol. Sci* **43**, 429.

Quinn, N., Illas, A., Lhermitte, F., and Agid, Y. (1981). Bromocriptine and domperidone in the treatment of Parkinson disease. *Neurology, Minneapolis* **31**, 662.

Rafal, R. D. and Grimm, R. J. (1981). Progressive supranuclear palsy: functional analysis of the response to methysergide and antiparkinsonian agents. *Neurology, Minneapolis* **31**, 1507.

Rajput, A. H., Jamieson, H., Hirsh, S., and Quraishi, A. (1975). Relative efficacy of alcohol and propranolol in action tremor. *Can. J. neurol. Sci.* **2**, 31.

—— and Rozdilsky, B. (1976). Dysautonomia in Parkinsonism: a clinico-pathological study. *J. Neurol. Neurosurg. Psychiat.* **39**, 1092.

Rascol, A., Guiraud, B., Montastruc, J. L., David, J., and Clanet, M. (1979). Long-term treatment of Parkinson's disease with bromocriptine. *J. Neurol. Neurosurg. Psychiat.* **42**, 143.

Rinne, U. K. and Sonninen, V. (1973). Brain catecholamines and their metabolites in Parkinsonian patients. Treatment with levodopa alone or combined with a decarboxylase inhibitor. *Arch. Neurol., Chicago* **28**, 107.

Rushworth, G. (1962). Observations on blink reflexes. *J. Neurol. Neurosurg. Psychiat.* **25**, 93.

Schachter, M., Marsden, C. D., Parkes, J. D., Jenner, P., and Testa, B. (1980). Deprenyl in the mangement of response fluctuations in patients with Parkinson's disease on levodopa. *J. Neurol. Neurosurg. Psychiat.* **43**, 1016.

Schneider, E., Fischer, P. -A. Jacobi, P., Becker, H., and Hacker, H. (1979). The significance of cerebral atrophy for the symptomatology of Parkinson's disease. *J. neurol. Sci.* **42**, 187.

Schnur, J. A., Chase, T. N., and Brody, J. A. (1971). Parkinsonism-dementia of Guam: treatment with L-dopa. *Neurology, Minneapolis* **21**, 1236.

Schwab, R. S., Poskanzer, D. C., England, A. C., and Young, R. R. (1972). Amantadine in Parkinson's disease. Review of more than two years' experience. *J. Am. med. Ass.* **222**, 792.

Scott, R. M. and Brody, J. A. (1971). Benign early onset of Parkinson's disease: a syndrome distinct from classic postencephalitic parkinsonism. *Neurology, Minneapolis* **21**, 366.

——, ——, Schwab, R. S., and Cooper, I.S. (1970). Progression of unilateral tremor and rigidity in Parkinson's disease. *Neurology, Minneapolis* **20**, 710.

Selby, G. (1967). Stereotactic surgery for the relief of Parkinson's disease. *Quart. J. Med.* **49**, 283.

Shibasaki, H., Tsuji, S., and Kuroiwa, Y. (1979). Oculomotor abnormalities in Parkinson's disease. *Arch. Neurol., Chicago* **36**, 360.

Sørensen, P. S., Paulson, O. B., Steiness, E., and Jansen, E. C. (1981). Essential tremor treated with propranolol: lack of correlation between clinical effect and plasma propranolol levels. *Ann. Neurol.* **9**, 53.

Spillane, J. D. (1975). *An atlas of clinical neurology,* 2nd edn. Oxford University Press, Oxford.

Steele, J. C., Richardson, J. C., and Olszewski, J. (1964). Progressive supranuclear palsy. *Arch. Neurol., Chicago* **10**, 333.

Stern, P. H., McDowell, F., Miller, J. M., and Robinson, M. B. (1972). Levodopa therapy effects on natural history of Parkinsonism. *Arch. Neurol., Chicago* **27**, 481.

Sunohara, N., Mano, Y., Ando, K., and Satoyoshi, E. (1985). Idiopathic dystonia-parkinsonism with marked diurnal fluctuation of symptoms. *Ann. Neurol.* **17**, 39.

Sweet, R. D., Blumberg, J., Lee, J. E., and McDowell, F. H. (1974). Propranolol treatment of essential tremor. *Neurology, Minneapolis* **24**, 64.

Takei, Y. and Mirra, S. S. (1973). Striatonigral degeneration: a form of multiple system atrophy with clinical Parkinsonism. In *Progress in neuropathology* (ed. H. M. Zimmerman), Vol. II, p. 217. Raven Press, New York.

Terävainen, H. and Calne, D. (1980). Action tremor in Parkinson's disease. *J. Neurol. Neurosurg. Psychiat.* **43**, 257.

——, Fogelholm, R., and Larsen, A. (1976). Effect of propranolol on essential tremor. *Neurology, Minneapolis* **26**, 27.

——, Larsen, A., and Fogelholm, R. (1977). Comparison between the effects of pindolol and propranolol on essential tremor. *Neurology, Minneapolis* **27**, 439.

Teychenne, P. F., Bergsrud, D., Racy, A., Elton, R. L., and Vern, B. (1982). Bromocriptine: low-dose therapy in Parkinson disease. *Neurology, Minneapolis* **32**, 577.

Trabucchi, M., Bassi, S., and Frattola, L. (1982). Effect of naloxone on the 'on-off' syndrome in patients receiving long-term levodopa therapy. *Arch. Neurol., Chicago* **39**, 120.

Troost, B. T. and Daroff, R. B. (1977). The ocular motor defects in progressive supranuclear palsy. *Ann. Neurol.* **2**, 397.

Vanasse, M., Bédard, P., and Andermann, F. (1976). Shuddering attacks in children: an early clinical manifestation of essential tremor. *Neurology, Minneapolis* **26**, 1027.

Weiner, W. J., Koller, W. C., Perlik, S., Nausieda, P. A., and Klawans, H. L. (1980). Drug holiday and management of Parkinson disease. *Neurology, Minneapolis* **30**, 1257.

—— and Nausieda, P. A. (1982). Meige's syndrome during long-term dopaminergic therapy in Parkinson's disease. *Arch. Neurol., Chicago* **39**, 451.

Yahr, M. D. (1973). *The treatment of parkinsonism—the role of dopa decarboxylase inhibitors,* Advances in Neurology, Vol. 2. Raven Press, New York.

——, Duvoisin, R. C., Schear, M. J., Barrett, R. E., and Hoehn, M. M. (1969). Treatment of Parkinsonism with levodopa. *Arch. Neurol., Chicago* **21**, 343.

——, Wolf, A., Antunes, J.-L., Miyoshi, K., and Duffy, P. (1972). Autopsy findings in parkinsonism following treatment with levodopa. *Neurology, Minneapolis* **22**, 56.

Wilson's disease

Synonyms. Tetanoid chorea (Gowers); pseudosclerosis (Westphal); progressive lenticular degeneration; hepatolenticular degeneration.

Definition. A progressive disease, usually of early life, due to an autosomal recessive gene and characterized by a disorder of copper metabolism leading to degeneration of certain parts of the brain, especially the corpus striatum, and cirrhosis of the liver, and clinically by increasing muscular rigidity, tremor, and progressive dementia. Although pseudosclerosis, first investigated by Alzheimer, Westphal, and others between 1883 and 1898, and progressive lenticular degeneration, described by Wilson in 1912, were once thought to be different diseases, they are now considered to be identical and are included under the title Wilson's disease.

Pathology

The pathological changes in the brain consist of degeneration of ganglion cells with conspicuous glial proliferation, but without evidence of inflammation or vascular abnormality. Macroscopically the most striking abnormality is softening and cavitation of both lentiform nuclei. In other cases the nucleus is shrunken and only occasionally is its naked-eye appearance normal. Microscopically, Alzheimer's type 2 cells are present, especially in the putamen. The caudate nucleus is usually similarly affected though to a lesser extent, but the globus pallidus is less often involved. Pericapillary concretions staining heavily for copper are often found, especially in the putamen. The so-called Opalski cell (see Greenfield 1958), a large, rounded cell with a large nucleus and a finely granular or foamy cytoplam which stains a light rose colour with Nissl stains is thought to be specific for Wilson's disease. These cells, thought to be of glial origin, are rare in the striatum and are most often seen in thalamus, globus pallidus, and substantia nigra. Similar changes are often present in other parts of the brain; for example, in the cerebral cortex, the thalamus, the red nucleus, and the cerebellum. Spongy degeneration of cortical grey matter, often seen in such cases, with Alzheimer type 2 glia, is comparable to that found in acquired hepatocerebral degeneration in patients with chronic portal-systemic encephalopathy (Finlayson and Superville 1981). The copper in the basal ganglia and cortex is sequestered in lysosomes which are more than normally sensitive to rupture (see Menkes 1980).

In the liver the changes are those of a multilobular cirrhosis with no distinctive characteristics save for a reddish, brown, or even greenish colour due to the presence of copper; splenomegaly is common. The typical Kayser–Fleischer ring around the edge of the cornea is also due to copper deposition.

Aetiology

The condition is clearly one of autosomal recessive inheritance with a gene frequency of about 1 in 1000 of the population (Bearn 1957). It is usually first manifest clinically between 10 and 25 years of age with a slightly earlier age of onset in female subjects (Strickland, Frommer, Leu, Pollard, Sherlock, and Cumings 1973); it appears to be ubiquitous in all races, having been reported from India (Dastur, Manghani, and Wadia 1968) and Taiwan (Strickland *et al.* 1973), and many cases have been described in the United Kingdom and in the USA. Rarely, the condition can first give rise to symptoms in middle life (Czlonkowska and Rodo 1981). Glazebrook (1945) and Cumings (1948) showed that the concentration of copper in brain and liver was greatly increased in such cases and it was later shown that caeruloplasmin, the copper-carrying protein of the plasma, is reduced to 10 per cent of normal values; Walshe (1967) suggested that a failure to synthesize this protein is the fundamental genetic abnormality. However, in occasionally well-authenticated cases, the serum caeruloplasmin has been found normal (see below). Ingested copper is deposited in the tissues and excreted in increased quantities in the urine. The whole body turnover of ^{64}Cu or ^{67}Cu is prolonged, with a greatly reduced release from liver in affected subjects (O'Reilly, Strickland, Weber, Beckner, and Shipley 1971a; O'Reilly, Weber, Oswald, and Shipley 1971b) and in gene carriers (O'Reilly, Weber, Pollycove, and Shipley 1970). The plasma iron and transferrin are also low (O'Reilly, Pollycove, and Bank 1968) and there is an increased urinary output of amino acids (Matthews, Milne, and Bell 1952; Denny-Brown 1953). A very rare disorder with neurological manifestations similar to those of Wilson's disease has been found to be associated with low concentrations of copper in plasma, urine, and liver, but increased amounts in the lower bowel, and a defect of mucosal transport has been postulated (Godwin-Austen, Robinson, Evans, and Lascelles 1978).

Symptoms and signs

Nervous manifestations

In some cases choreiform movements of the face and hands or flapping tremor are the first symptoms. These movements may occur when the limbs are apparently at rest and yet are abolished by complete relaxation or support. They are increased by voluntary movement. Athetoid and writhing movements of the trunk and limbs have also been seen. In many cases, dysarthria (see below) is the first manifestation. In general, plastic rigidity followed by tremor or athetoid movements is common in younger patients while tremor precedes rigidity in those in whom the onset is over the age of 20.

Rigidity in its distribution and character resembles that of parkinsonism. The limbs become fixed, usually in flexion, and contractures ultimately develop, but in younger patients the terminal state is one of bilateral hemiplegic dystonia.

Voluntary movement is impaired, and articulation and deglutition are early and severely affected. Speech may become unintelligible or the patient may even become totally anarthric. The facies exhibits, as in Parkinsonism, a vacant, expressionless appearance, or a vacuous smile. Loss of emotional control is usual, and involuntary laughing and crying may occur. There seems always to be some mental deterioration amounting to mild dementia. There is no consistent change in the tendon-jerks or the abdominal reflexes, though muscular rigidity may render them difficult to elicit. The plantar reflexes are flexor and there is no disturbance of sensibility.

Corneal pigmentation (the Kayser–Fleischer ring)

Corneal pigmentation, as first observed by Kayser and Fleischer, is a sign of great diagnostic value. It may be invisible in daylight and is best seen with the slit lamp which shows that it is present in virtually all cases. It consists of a zone of golden-brown granular pigmentation about 2 mm in diameter on the posterior surface of the cornea towards the limbus, and may be present before any nervous symptoms have developed.

Symptoms of cirrhosis of the liver

Although these may be inconspicuous, they sometimes prove fatal before any nervous symptoms develop. In the early stages pyrexial attacks, with slight jaundice, may occur; later the liver may enlarge, and ascites, haematemesis, and other symptoms of portal obstruction may appear.

Renal lesions

Apart from aminoaciduria (Uzman and Denny-Brown 1948), especially of threonine and cystine, patients with Wilson's disease sometimes have glycosuria, increased urinary phosphate excretion, low urate excretion, proteinuria, a reduced glomerular filtration rate, and evidence of tubular damage produced by the copper. Spontaneous pseudofractures and osteomalacia and osteochondritis have been described (see Bearn 1957).

Biochemical changes

Biochemical tests of value include a low serum copper (normal 86–112 μg per 100 ml) and copper oxidase, a low caeruloplasmin in the blood (normal 27–38 mg per 100 ml), and a high urinary copper (normal 24-hour excretion 0–26 μg), especially if this is increased after treatment with BAL or penicillamine. Patients do not incorporate ^{64}Cu or ^{67}Cu normally with caeruloplasmin (Matthews 1954) and radiocopper turnover may be abnormal in clinically normal heterozygotes. The fact that metallothionein–copper binding is abnormally tight could provide a unifying explanation for the biochemical abnormalities (see Menkes 1980). Measurement of copper levels in liver-biopsy specimens using neutron activation analysis may give figures more than five times normal in Wilson's disease but the copper is also much increased in samples from patients with long-standing biliary obstruction, as in biliary cirrhosis (Smallwood, Williams, Rosenoer, and Sherlock 1968).

Radiology

The CT scan may show areas of reduced density in the lenticular nuclei (Ropper, Hatten, and Davis 1979) or in the thalamocapsular area, but the usual findings are those of ventricular dilatation and cortical and brainstem atrophy with hypodense areas in the basal ganglia in about 45 per cent of cases, improving after treatment (Williams and Walshe 1981).

Diagnosis

There are few disorders with which Wilson's disease can be confused. No other disease is characterized by the familial occurrence of tremor and rigidity with liver damage in the second decade of life. Corneal pigmentation and symptoms of cirrhosis of the liver, when present, are pathognomonic. Sporadic cases may simulate other disorders in which the corpus striatum is damaged. Double athetosis is usually congenital. Symptoms are therefore present from an early age, and some improvement may occur. Neurological manifestations of acquired liver disease (p. 451) usually develop much later in life and are non-familial, but juvenile cirrhosis (Lygren 1959) occasionally gives diagnostic difficulty.

Other rare familial degenerative disorders of the corpus striatum, without liver damage, cause progressive rigidity, spasmodic laughing, dysarthria, and dementia beginning in childhood, e.g. Hallervorden–Spatz disease and progressive pallidal degeneration.

When Wilson's disease is suspected in one member of a family, all the sibs should be examined for nervous abnormalities, cirrhosis of the liver, corneal pigmentation, and biochemical change. Any symptoms, if present, will not only make it possible to anticipate the development of the disorder in other family members but will support the diagnosis in the patient already affected.

Prognosis

The course of the disease may be acute, subacute, or chronic, but it is invariably fatal if not treated. In the shortest illness on record death occurred five weeks after the onset of symptoms. Before effective treatment became available 50 per cent of patients died in from 1 to 6 years though a few survived very much longer (Hall 1921). The prognosis has been transformed by treatment with D-penicillamine, and many patients survive to a normal age with little or no disability provided treatment is started early before irreversible brain or liver damage has occurred. However, about 25 per cent of children with the mixed hepatocerebral picture when first seen continue to deteriorate despite treatment (Menkes 1980).

Treatment

Cumings (1951) and Denny-Brown (1953) showed that substantial improvement could follow the use of dimercaprol (BAL) and another chelating agent, calcium versenate, was subsequently tried with some success. Oral potassium sulphide was also given to reduce the absorption of copper. However, the introduction of D-penicillamine in 1956 by Walshe transformed the prognosis. The drug is given in a daily dosage of 1.0–2.0 g, with an average dose of 1.5 g (Richmond, Rosenoer, Tompsett, Draper, and Simpson 1964; Goldstein, Tauxe, McCall, Randall, and Gross 1971; Strickland *et al.* 1973). If given early enough, many affected subjects grow and develop normally and may remain symptom-free for as long as maintenance treatment is continued. Unfortunately, toxic side-effects of penicillamine have emerged in recent years, of which nephropathy leading to the nephrotic syndrome and thrombocytopenia are the most troublesome (Walshe 1969). In such cases there may be no alternative to withdrawal of treatment; fortunately, triethyl tetramine given in a dosage of 1.2 g daily, is an effective alternative treatment (Walshe 1973, 1982). Rarely, when liver disease is exceptionally severe, liver transplantation may be successful (Starzl, Giles, Lilly, Takagi, Martineau, Schroter, Halgrimson, Penn, and Putnam 1971).

References

Bearn, A. G. (1957). Wilson's disease. An inborn error of metabolism with multiple manifestations. *Am. J. Med.* **22**, 747.

Bickel, H., Neale, F. C., and Hall, G. (1957). A clinical and biochemical study of hepatolenticular degeneration (Wilson's disease). *Quart. J. Med.* **26**, 527.

Cumings, J. N. (1948). The copper and iron content in the brain and liver in the normal and in hepatolenticular degeneration. *Brain* **71**, 410.

—— (1951). The effects of B.A.L. in hepatolenticular degeneration. *Brain* **74**, 10.

Czlonkowska, A. and Rodo, M. (1981). Late onset of Wilson's disease: report of a family. *Arch. Neurol.*, *Chicago* **38**, 729.

Dastur, D. K., Manghani, D. K., and Wadia, N. H. (1968). Wilson's disease in India. I. Geographic, genetic, and clinical aspects in 16 families. *Neurology*, *Minneapolis* **18**, 21.

Denny-Brown, D. (1953). Abnormal copper metabolism and hepatolenticular degeneration. *Res. Publ. Ass. nerv. ment. Dis.* **32**, 190.

Finlayson, M. H. and Superville, B. (1981). Distribution of cerebral lesions in acquired hepatocerebral degeneration. *Brain* **104**, 79.

Glazebrook, A. J. (1945). Wilson's disease. *Edinburgh med. J.* **52**, 83.

Godwin-Austen, R. B., Robinson, A., Evans, K., and Lascelles, P. T. (1978). An unusual neurological disorder of copper metabolism clinically resembling Wilson's disease but biochemically a distinct entity. *J. neurol. Sci.* **39**, 85.

Goldstein, N. P., Tauxe, W. N., McCall, J. T., Randall, R. V., and Gross, J. B. (1971). Wilson's disease (hepatolenticular degeneration). Treatment with penicillamine and changes in hepatic trapping of radioactive copper. *Arch. Neurol.*, *Chicago* **24**, 391.

Greenfield, J. G. (1958). Hepatolenticular degeneration, in *Neuropathology* (ed. J. G. Greenfield, W. Blackwood, W. H. McMenemey, A. Meyer, and R. M. Norman) Chapter 4. Arnold, London.

Hall, H. C. (1921). *La dégénérescence hépato-lenticulaire*. Paris.

Lygren, T. (1959). Hepatolenticular degeneration (Wilson's disease) and juvenile cirrhosis in the same family. *Lancet* **i**, 275.

Matthews, W. B. (1954). The absorption and excretion of radiocopper in hepatolenticular degeneration (Wilson's disease). *J. Neurol. Neurosurg. Psychiat.* **17**, 242.

——, Milne, M. D., and Bell, M. (1952). The metabolic disorder in hepatolenticular degeneration. *Quart. J. Med.* **21**, 425.

Menkes, J. H. (1980). *Text book of child neurology*, 2nd edn. Lea and Febiger, Philadelphia.

O'Reilly, S., Pollycove, M., and Bank, W. J. (1968). Iron metabolism in Wilson's disease. Kinetic studies with iron[59]. *Neurology*, *Minneapolis* **18**, 634.

——, Strickland, G. T., Weber, P. M., Beckner, W. M., and Shipley, L. (1971*a*). Abnormalities of the physiology of copper in Wilson's disease. I. The whole-body turnover of copper. *Arch. Neurol.*, *Chicago* **24**, 385.

——, Weber, P. M., Oswald, M., and Shipley, L. (1971*b*). Abnormalities of the physiology of copper in Wilson's disease. III. The excretion of copper. *Arch. Neurol.*, *Chicago* **25**, 28.

——, ——, Pollycove, M., and Shipley, L. (1970). Detection of the carrier of Wilson's disease. *Neurology*, *Minneapolis* **20**, 1133.

Richmond, J., Rosenoer, V. M., Tompsett, S. L., Draper, I., and Simpson, J. A. (1964). Hepato-lenticular degeneration (Wilson's disease) treated by penicillamine. *Brain* **82**, 619.

Ropper, A. H., Hatten, H. P., and Davis, K. R. (1979). Computed tomography in Wilson disease: report of 2 cases. *Ann. Neurol.* **5**, 102.

Smallwood, R. A., Williams, H. A., Rosenoer, V. M., and Sherlock, S. (1968). Liver-copper levels in liver disease. Studies using neutron activation analysis. *Lancet* **ii**, 1310.

Starzi, T. E., Giles, G., Lilly, J. R., Takagi, H., Martineau, G., Schroter, G., Halgrimson, C. G., Penn, I., and Putnam, C. W. (1971). Indications for orthotopic liver transplantation: with particular reference to hepatomas, biliary atresia, cirrhosis, Wilson's disease and serum hepatitis. *Transplantation Proc.* **3**, 308.

Strickland, G. T., Frommer, D., Leu, M.-L., Pollard, R., Sherlock, S., and Cumings, J. N. (1973). Wilson's disease in the United Kingdom and Taiwan. I. General characteristics of 142 cases and prognosis. II. A genetic analysis of 88 cases. *Quart. J. Med.* **42**, 619.

Uzman, L. and Denny-Brown, D. (1948). Amino-aciduria in hepatolenticular degeneration (Wilson's disease). *Am. J. med. Sci.* **215**, 599.

Walshe, J. M. (1956). Penicillamine: a new oral therapy for Wilson's disease. *Am. J. Med.* **21**, 487.

—— (1967). The physiology of copper in man and its relation to Wilson's disease. *Brain* **90**, 149.

—— (1969). Management of penicillamine nephropathy in Wilson's disease: a new chelating agent. *Lancet* **ii**, 1401.

—— (1973). Copper chelation in patients with Wilson's disease. A comparison of penicillamine and triethylene tetramine dihydrochloride. *Quart. J. Med.* **42**, 441.

—— (1982). Treatment of Wilson's disease with trientine (triethylene tetramine) dihydrochloride. *Lancet* **i**, 643.

Williams, F. J. B. and Walshe, J. M. (1981). Wilson's disease. An analysis of the cranial computerized tomographic appearances found in 60 patients and the changes in response to treatment with chelating agents. *Brain* **104**, 735.

Wilson, S. A. K. (1911–12). Progressive lenticular degeneration: a familial nervous disease associated with cirrhosis of the liver. *Brain* **34**, 295.

Hallervorden–Spatz disease and infantile neuroaxonal dystrophy

The rare familial disorder first described by Hallervorden and Spatz in 1922 presents in childhood or adolescence as a progressive, predominantly extrapyramidal disorder running a protracted course of several years but usually terminating fatally. Clinically the affected children usually show choreoathetosis and progressive dystonia (Yanagisawa, Shiraki, Minakawa, and Narabayashi 1966); dementia, dysarthria, fits, and signs of corticospinal-tract involvement sometimes but not invariably develop. Pathologically the brains of affected individuals show degeneration of neurones in the globus pallidus and substantia nigra with many rounded hyaline bodies or spheroids and mineral pigment deposits often containing iron. Dooling, Schoene, and Richardson (1974) treated two cases with chelating agents without effect but thought that levodopa produced some improvement. In agreeing that the condition is a primary axonal dystrophy of unknown cause, however, Menkes (1980) concludes that no specific defect of iron metabolism has been demonstrated and that no effective treatment is available. In 1952 Seitelberger reported a disorder of similar clinical presentation (see p. 468) in which hyaline swelling and eventuall breakdown of nerve cells were demonstrated in the cerebellum, basal ganglia, and brainstem and which he called neuroaxonal dystrophy; the pallidum showed spheroids, spongy degeneration, and deposits of pseudocalcium. Defendini, Markesbery, Mastri, and Duffy (1973) drew attention to the presence of Lewy-type inclusions in nerve cells in some cases and pointed out that the two disorders were difficult if not impossible to distinguish both clinically and pathologically.

References

Defendini, R., Markesbery, W. R., Mastri, A. R., and Duffy, P. E. (1973). Hallervorden–Spatz disease and infantile neuro-axonal dystrophy. Ultrastructural observations, anatomical pathology and nosology. *J. neurol. Sci.* **20**, 7.

Dooling, E. C., Schoene, W. C., and Richardson E. P. (1974). Hallervordern–Spatz syndrome. *Arch. Neurol.*, *Chicago* **30**, 70.

Hallervorden, J. and Spatz, H. (1922). Eigenartige Erkrankung im extrapyramidalen System mit besonderer Beteiligung des Globus Pallidus und der Substantia Nigra. *Z. ges. Neurol. Psychiat.* **79**, 254.

Menkes, J. H. (1980). *Textbook of child neurology*, 2nd edn. Lea and Febiger, Philadelphia.

Seitelberger, F. (1952). Eine unbekannte Form von infantiler Lipoid-Speicher-Krankheit des Gehirns. In *Proceedings of the 1st International Congress of Neuropathology*, Vol. 3, p. 323. Turin.

Yanagisawa, N., Shiraki, H., Minakawa, M., and Narabayashi, H. (1966). Clinicopathological and histochemical studies of Hallervorden-Spatz disease with torsion dystonia, with special reference to diagnostic criteria of the disease from the clinico-pathological viewpoint. *Progress in Brain Research* **21B**, 373.

Neuronal intranuclear inclusion disease

This rare condition, which has been reported in identical twins (Haltia, Somer, Palo, and Johnson 1984) was characterized in these two patients by slurred speech, nystagmus and oculogyral spasms starting at 11 years of age. Subsequently rage attacks, extrapyramidal and lower motor neurone dysfunction increased, with death at 21 years of age. At post-mortem there was severe loss of nigral and craniospinal motor neurones and many nerve cells contained round, eosinophilic, autofluorescent inclusion bodies, 3–10 μm in diameter, shown ultrastructurally to contain masses of proteinaceous filaments (Palo, Haltia, Carpenter, Karpati, and Mushynski 1984).

References

Haltia, M., Somer, H., Palo, J., and Johnson, W. G. (1984). Neuronal intranuclear inclusion disease in identical twins. *Ann. neurol.* **15**, 316.

Palo, J., Haltia, M., Carpenter, S., Karpati, G., and Mushynski, W. (1984). Neurofilament subunit-related proteins in intranuclear inclusion body disease. *Ann. neurol.* **15**, 322.

Torsion dystonia

Synonym. Dystonia musculorum deformans (Oppenheim).

Definition. A syndrome characterized by involuntary movements producing torsion of the limbs and the vertebral column, which may occur as a symptom of more than one pathological state.

Aetiology and pathology

Torsion dystonia is a rare syndrome first described by Schwalbe in 1908 in three sibs. Mendel in 1919 collected 30 cases from the literature. Symptomatic dystonia may occur in many neurological disorders including cerebral palsy, infantile hemiplegia, Wilson's disease, Hallervorden–Spatz disease, and intoxication with phenothiazines and other drugs (Zeman and Whitlock 1968) and in such cases the pathology is that of the primary disorder. Dystonia may not develop for many years after the initial cerebral insult, whether this is perinatal axonia, head injury, or infarction (Burke, Fahn, and Gold 1980). Idiopathic torsion dystonia, however, may be inherited as an autosomal recessive trait in Ashkenazic Jews and as an autosomal dominant disorder in some non-Jewish populations; many cases are sporadic. However, Korczyn, Kahana, Zilber, Streifler, Carasso, and Alter (1980) found autosomal dominant inheritance with incomplete penetrance to be relatively common in Israeli Jews. In Japan (Segawa, Hosaka, Miyagawa, Nomura, and Imai 1976) but also in Australia (Ouvrier 1978), familial progressive dystonia has been found sometimes to show a remarkable diurnal variation in the severity of symptoms. In the idiopathic disorder extensive neuropathological studies have failed to demonstrate any consistent abnormalities in the basal ganglia or elsewhere (Zeman and Dyken 1967; Zeman 1970). However, Wooten, Eldridge, Axelrod, and Stern (1973) and Ebstein, Freedman, Lieberman, Goldstein, and Pasternack (1974) found elevated serum dopamine-beta-hydroxylase levels in such cases, whether of dominant or recessive inheritance, and the disorder may prove to be due to a biochemical abnormality involving central dopaminergic systems. Tabaddor, Wolfson, and Sharpless (1978) reported low concentrations of homovanillic acid in ventricular CSF in adult-onset cases suggesting diminished dopaminergic activity. While manganese intoxication may induce dystonia and dementia (Banta and Markesbery 1977), there is no evidence that heavy metals play a part in the aetiology of the idiopathic syndrome and a postulated abnormality of melanin metabolism (Korein 1981) remains unsubstantiated as yet. In a review of 42 cases, Marsden and Harrison (1974) pointed out that a childhood onset is usually associated with a progressive course leading to severe disability, while in cases first developing in adult life it is much more benign and symptoms often remain localized indefinitely.

Symptoms and signs

In severe familial cases the onset usually occurs in childhood or adolescence, and the abnormality is frequently first noticed when the patient walks. The disorder often begins with spasmodic plantar-flexion of one foot, rendering it impossible to place the heel on the ground. The resultant bizarre gait, when first observed in an otherwise healthy child, is often misconstrued as being hysterical. The involuntary movements in the upper limbs consist of rotation or torsion round the long axes and are associated with similar torsion movements of the vertebral column, especially in the lumbar

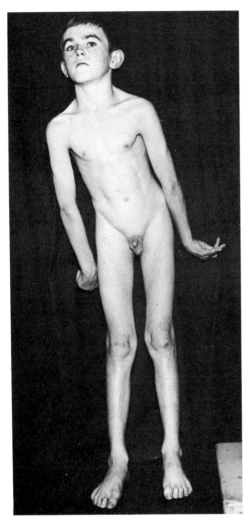

Fig. 12.6. A case of torsion dystonia; note the abnormal posture of the head, neck, trunk, and upper limbs. (Reproduced from Spillane (1975) by kind permission of the author.)

region (Fig. 12.6). Lordosis and scoliosis are common and are conspicuous when the patient walks, but tend to disappear when he lies down. Other forms of involuntary movement, such as tremor and occasional myoclonus, have been described. Muscular tone is variable, being exaggerated during spasms which may be very painful, and sometimes diminished in the intervals between them. Signs of corticospinal-tract dysfunction are absent. There is no muscular wasting except as a result of cachexia in the terminal stages. The reflexes are normal, and sensibility is unimpaired. The intellect is unimpaired and speech and swallowing are usually unaffected until the later stages though 'whispering dysphonia' (Parker 1985) may occur.

Diagnosis

Torsion dystonia must be distinguished especially from athetosis and chorea. In athetosis the movements, which are of a slow, writhing character, involve the peripheral parts of the limbs, rather than the proximal as in dystonia. Double athetosis, moreover, is usually congenital, and hence the movements develop at an earlier age also. Choreic movements involve the peripheral parts of the limbs. In chorea, however, rotational movements of the limbs and trunk do occur, but are quicker and briefer than those of dystonia. Dystonic movements may develop in the affected limbs after some years in occasional cases of infantile hemiplegia. Hysteria may cause bizarre involuntary movements; these

movements, however, rarely involve the trunk and the proximal parts of the limbs, and in hysteria the emotional attitude of the patient to the disorder and the presence of other manifestations usually settle the diagnosis.

Electromyography may be helpful (Yanagisawa and Goto 1971), demonstrating tonic non-reciprocal involuntary activity in agonists and antagonists and regular or irregular grouping of action potentials appearing synchronously in many muscles.

Prognosis

In symptomatic dystonia due to Wilson's disease, cerebral palsy, infantile hemiplegia, and other disorders the prognosis is that of the underlying disease. In very occasional idiopathic cases spontaneous recovery has been described. In the 'idiopathic' disorder the condition may remain static or localized to one limb or other part of the body for many years, especially when the onset is in adult life but in most childhood cases there is slow progressive deterioration and death eventually results from the combined effects of cachexia and respiratory or urinary infection.

Treatment

Rest and physiotherapy are of little value but various drugs may be helpful. Levodopa (Barbeau 1970; Chase 1970) alone or with haloperidol (Mandell 1970) has been recommended but seems of little long-term benefit. Other remedies recommended have included diazepam alone, up to 30 mg daily (Ziegler 1981), or combined with isoniazid, pyridoxine, and L-glutamine (Korein, Lieberman, Kupersmith, and Levidou 1981), carbamazepine with levodopa (Garg 1982), bromocriptine (Stahl and Berger 1981), lithium (Marti-Masso, Obeso, Carrera, Astudillo, and Martinez Lage 1982) and tetrabenazine with benzhexol (Marsden, Marion, and Quinn 1984), but the multiplicity of remedies used testifies to their relative inefficacy. Cooper (1970) and others reported improvement following bilateral ventrolateral thalamotomy, a procedure still worth considering in severe cases, although the results of such stereotaxic operations have been variable and unpredictable.

References

Banta, R. G. and Markesbery, W. R. (1977). Elevated manganese levels associated with dementia and extrapyramidal signs. *Neurology, Minneapolis* **27**, 213.

Barbeau, A. (1970). Rationale for the use of L-dopa in the torsion dystonias. *Neurology, Minneapolis* **20**, 96.

Burke, R. E., Fahn, S., and Gold, A. P. (1980). Delayed onset dystonia in patients with 'static' encephalopathy. *J. Neurol. Neurosurg. Psychiat.* **43**, 789.

Chase, T. N. (1970). Biochemical and pharmacologic studies of dystonia. *Neurology, Minneapolis* **20**, 122.

Cooper, I. S. (1970). Neurosurgical treatment of dystonia. *Neurology, Minneapolis* **20**, 133.

Ebstein, R. P., Freedman, L. S., Lieberman, A., Goldstein, M., and Pasternack, B. (1974). A familial study of serum dopamine-β-hydroxylase levels in torsion dystonia. *Neurology, Minneapolis* **24**, 684.

Garg, B. P. (1982). Dystonia musculorum deformans: implications of therapeutic response to levodopa and carbamazepine. *Arch. Neurol., Chicago* **39**, 376.

Korczyn, A. D., Kahana, E., Zilber, N., Streifler, M., Carasso, R., and Alter, M. (1980). Torsion dystonia in Israel. *Ann. Neurol.* **8**, 387.

Korein, J. (1981). Iris pigmentation (melanin) in idiopathic dystonic syndromes including torticollis. *Ann. Neurol.* **10**, 53.

——, Lieberman, A., Kupersmith, M., and Levidow, L. (1981). Effect of L-glutamine and isoniazid on torticollis and segmental dystonia. *Ann. Neurol.* **10**, 247.

Larsson, T. and Sjögren, T. (1966). Dystonia musculorum deformans. A genetic and population study of 121 cases. *Acta neurol. scand.* **42**, Suppl. 17.

Mandell, S. (1970). The treatment of dystonia with L-dopa and haloperidol. *Neurology, Minneapolis* **20**, 103.

Marsden, C. D. and Harrison, M. J. G. (1974). Idiopathic torsion dystonia (dystonia musculorum deformans). A review of forty-two patients. *Brain* **97**, 793.

——, Marion, M.-H. and Quinn, N. (1984). The treatment of severe dystonia in children and adults. *J. Neurol. Neurosurg. Psychiat.* **47**, 1166.

Marti-Masso, J. R., Obeso, J. A., Carrera, N., Astudillo, W., and Martinez Lage, J. M. (1982). Lithium therapy in torsion dystonia. *Ann. Neurol.* **11**, 106.

Mendel, K. (1919). Torsiondystonie. *Mschr. Psychiat. Neurol.* **46**, 309.

Ouvrier, R. A. (1978). Progressive dystonia with marked diurnal fluctuation. *Ann. Neurol.* **4**, 412.

Parker, N. (1985). Hereditary whispering dysphonia. *J. Neurol. Neurosurg. Psychiat.* **48**, 218.

Segawa, M., Hosaka, A., Miyagawa, F., Nomura, Y., and Imai, H. (1976). Hereditary progressive dystonia with marked diurnal fluctuation. In *Advances in neurology*, (ed. R. Eldridge and S. Fahn) Vol. 14, p. 215. Raven Press, New York.

Spillane, J. D. (1975). *An atlas of clinical neurology*, 2nd edn. Oxford University Press, Oxford.

Stahl, S. M. and Berger, P. A. (1981). Bromocriptine in dystonia. *Lancet* **ii**, 745.

Tabaddor, K., Wolfson, L. I., and Sharpless, N. S. (1978). Diminished ventricular fluid dopamine metabolites in adult-onset dystonia. *Neurology, Minneapolis* **28**, 1254.

Wooten, G. F., Eldridge, R., Axelrod, J., and Stern, R. S. (1973). Elevated plasma dopamine-β-hydroxylase activity in autosomal dominant torsion dystonia. *New Engl. J. Med.* **288**, 284.

Yanagisawa, N. and Goto, A. (1971). Dystonia musculorum deformans. Analysis with electromyography. *J. neurol. Sci.* **13**, 39.

Zeman, W. (1970). Pathology of the torsion dystonias (dystonia musculorum deformans). *Neurology, Minneapolis* **20**, 79.

—— and Dyken, P. (1967). Dystonia musculorum deformans. Clinical, genetic and pathoanatomical studies. *Psychiat. Neurol. Neurochir., Amsterdam* **70**, 77.

—— and Whitlock, C. C. (1968). Symptomatic dystonias. In *Handbook of clinical neurology* (ed. P. J. Vinken and G. W. Bruyn), Vol. 6, p. 544. North-Holland, Amsterdam.

Ziegler, D. K. (1981). Prolonged relief of dystonic movements with diazepam. *Neurology, Minneapolis* **31**, 1457.

Spasmodic torticollis

Synonym. Wry neck.

Definition. A disorder characterized by spasmodic rotation of the head, brought about by clonic or tonic contraction of the cervical muscles; it is usually a symptom of organic disease of the nervous system but is rarely hysterical. Torticollis of organic origin is probably a fragmentary form of torsion spasm. Retrocollis and antecollis are similar disorders, in which the neck is extended or flexed.

Aetiology and pathology

In the past, confusion as to the nature of torticollis arose from a failure to distinguish the uncommon hysterical torticollis from the commoner variety due to organic disease. The hysterical syndrome is a form of tic and the nature of the symptoms in such cases is proved by their response to treatment of the primary emotional disorder. However, there are now ample grounds for regarding most cases as being due to a restricted segmental form of dystonia (Lal 1979). It may occur as a sequel to encephalitis lethargica, with or without parkinsonism, or as a part of other extrapyramidal syndromes. Since torticollis as an isolated symptom is not fatal, pathological evidence is scanty. Foerster (1933) reported a case in which bilateral focal lesions of the corpus striatum were present, but Tarlov (1970) was unable to find any significant abnormality in an extensive study of the brain of a typical case. In a detailed review, Lal (1979) noted that focal lesions induced experimentally in the ascending dopaminergic fibres from the midbrain tegmentum in animals may produce abnormal neck postures, while in man, various neuroleptic agents such as metoclopramide which block dopamine receptors may cause drug-induced torticollis. However, no specific neurotransmitter abnormality has yet been identified in idiopathic cases and there is no evidence of vestibular dysfunction (Matthews, Beasley, Parry-Jones, and Garland 1978). Both sexes are affected, and the onset is usually during adult life. The disorder may be familial.

Symptoms and signs

The onset is usually insidious but may be sudden. The rotation of the head is brought about by contraction of the cervical muscles, and though both the superficial and deep neck muscles are involved, the contraction is evident to the observer only in the sternomastoid, trapezius, and splenius. The precise posture of the head varies in different cases. Contraction of the sternomastoid alone causes rotation to the opposite side, with flexion of the neck to the side of the contracted muscle. Rotation, however, may occur without lateral flexion, or the head may be flexed to the side to which it is rotated, when contraction of the sternomastoid on one side is associated with contraction of the contralateral splenius and trapezius. The muscles involved hypertrophy. The condition may be predominantly tonic, leading to a sustained posture, or may consist of repeated clonic jerks. It may be possible to modify the abnormal posture by altering the position of the patient in relation to gravity. There may or may not be resistance to passive movement of the head in the direction opposite to the abnormal position. In a few cases torticollis is associated with paralysis of rotation to the opposite side. There may be spasm of the facial muscles and platysma on the side to which the head is rotated, or spasmodic torsion movements of one upper limb. The patient not infrequently finds that he can inhibit the torticollis by exerting slight pressure with his finger upon the jaw on the side to which the head is rotated (counterpressure, see Stejskal 1980), and the movement ceases during sleep. Pain may occur in the cervical muscles. The reflexes and sensation are normal. Long-continued torticollis may cause cervical spondylosis.

Retrocollis is due to a bilateral contraction of the splenius and trapezius; antecollis, due to spasmodic contraction of neck flexors, is very rare.

Diagnosis

The distinction between hysterical and organic torticollis may be difficult, but most cases are now recognised as organic. Hysteria should be suspected when the symptom resembles a tic and develops suddenly after mental stress, and also when it can be controlled by relaxation and suggestion, though these measures can also produce some improvement in the organic disorder. Kjellin and Stibler (1974) claimed that alkaline end-fractions found in isoelectric focusing of samples of CSF helped to distinguish organic from hysterical cases but this observation has not been confirmed.

Spasmodic torticollis is distinguished by the age of onset from congenital torticollis due either to fibrosis of one sternomastoid following a haematoma in the muscle, or to a congenital hemi-vertebra. It is also necessary to exclude as causes of torticollis localized myositis, caries of the cervical spine, and adenitis of the cervical lymph nodes.

Prognosis

Torticollis is almost always intractable, but in the rare hysterical cases improvement and even cure may be effected by psychotherapy, abreaction, or hypnosis. Radical surgical treatment using radiculectomy and neurectomy has given good results in some cases, though the spasm may recur after operation. Generally, the outlook is poor (Matthews *et al.* 1978) though spontaneous remission rarely occurs.

Treatment

Hysterical torticollis should be treated by psychotherapy or abreaction along the same lines as other hysterical symptoms (Paterson 1945). Sedative and tranquillizing drugs such as chlordiazepoxide (*Librium*), 10 mg three or four times daily, or diazepam (*Valium*), 2–5 mg three times a day, are of limited value, even in some organic cases. In the latter, benefit has been claimed from treatment with amantadine and haloperidol (Gilbert 1972) and from bromocriptine (see *The Lancet* 1978). Tetrabenazine, too, is occasionally dramatically successful but its effect is usually only temporary and then at the expense of an unacceptable degree of drug-induced parkinsonism. Brudny, Grynbaum, and Korein (1974) claimed benefit from teaching patients volitional control with the aid of a feedback display of the electromyogram. Levodopa is of no value (Ansari, Webster, and Manning 1972).

Several surgical operations have been recommended. Finney and Hughson (1925) divided the accessory and upper cervical nerves, while Dandy (1930) combined division of the accessory nerves with interruption of the upper three cervical sensory and motor roots within the spinal canal, and Foerster performed intra-dural section of both the ventral and dorsal roots of the upper three cervical segments.

Sorensen and Hamby (1966) reviewed the results obtained in 71 cases treated surgically and found that patients subjected to anterior cervical rhizotomy and subarachnoid section of the spinal accessory nerve did best. However, this operation rarely has disastrous consequences as in a case where delayed brainstem ischaemia led to tetraplegia (Adams 1984). In intractable cases simultaneous bilateral lesions produced in ventrolateral thalamic nuclei by stereotaxic methods may be beneficial but the results of this treatment are variable (Cooper 1965).

References

Adams, C. B. T. (1984). Vascular catastrophe following the Dandy McKenzie operation for spasmodic torticollis. *J. Neurol. Neurosurg. Psychiat.* **47**, 990.

Ansari, K. A., Webster, D., and Manning, N. (1972). Spasmodic torticollis and L-dopa. Results of therapeutic trial in six patients. *Neurology, Minneapolis* **22**, 670.

Brudny, J., Grynbaum, B. B., and Korein, J. (1974). Spasmodic torticollis: treatment by feedback display of the EMG. *Arch. Phys. Med. Rehabil.* **55**, 403.

Cooper, I. S. (1965). Clinical and physiologic implications of thalamic surgery for disorders of sensory communication, pt. 2 (Intention tremor, dystonia, Wilson's disease and torticollis). *J. neurol. Sci.* **2**, 520.

Dandy, W. E. (1930). An operation for the treatment of spasmodic torticollis. *Arch. Surg.* **20**, 1021.

Finney, J. M. T. and Hugheson, W. (1925). Spasmodic torticollis. *Ann. Surg.* **81**, 255.

Foerster, O. (1933). Mobile spasm of the neck muscles and its pathological basis. *J. comp. Neurol.* **58**, 725.

Gilbert, G. J. (1972). The medical treatment of spasmodic torticollis. *Arch. Neurol., Chicago* **27**, 503.

Kjellin, K. G. and Stibler, H. (1974). Protein pattern of cerebrospinal fluid in spasmodic torticollis. *J. Neurol. Neurosurg. Psychiat.* **37**, 1128.

Lal, S. (1979). Pathophysiology and pharmacotherapy of spasmodic torticollis: a review. *Can. J. neurol. Sci.* **6**, 427.

The Lancet (1978). Spasmodic torticollis. *Lancet* **ii**, 301.

Matthews, W. B., Beasley, P., Parry-Jones, W., and Garland, G. (1978). Spasmodic torticollis: a combined clinical study. *J. Neurol. Neurosurg. Psychiat.* **41**, 485.

Paterson, M. (1945). Spasmodic torticollis: results of psychotherapy in 21 cases. *Lancet* **ii**, 556.

Sorensen, B. F. and Hamby, W. B. (1966). Spasmodic torticollis. Results in surgically-treated patients. *Neurology, Minneapolis* **16**, 867.

Stejskal, L. (1980). Counterpressure in torticollis. *J. neurol. Sci.* **48**, 9.

Tarlov, E. (1970). On the problem of the pathology of spasmodic torticollis in man. *J. Neurol. Neurosurg. Psychiat.* **33**, 457.

Athetosis

Definition. Athetosis, or 'mobile spasm', is the term applied to a form of involuntary movement which in some respects resembles chorea, as is recognized by the use of the term 'choreo-athetosis' to describe an intermediate condition. Athetoid movements, however, are slower, coarser, and more writhing than those of chorea. Athetosis is due to a variety of pathological states which damage the basal ganglia.

Aetiology and pathology

There is considerable evidence that the lesion causing athetosis is usually situated in the putamen. Bilateral athetosis is occasionally familial (see below). Athetosis is one of the many involuntary movements which may be induced by the use of drugs such as levodopa or the phenothiazines (Lader 1970; Singer and Cheng 1971).

Bilateral athetosis

Bilateral athetosis may be congenital and due to cerebral palsy, when it may be due to the état marbré of the corpus striatum described by Oppenheim and Vogt (1911). Rarely it may develop during adolescence as a progressive disorder terminating in generalized rigidity, as a result of degeneration of the corpus striatum described by C. and O. Vogt (1919) as état dysmyélinique. The common pathological factor, according to Denny-Brown (1946), the état marbré or status marmoratus, is a disorder of glial formation leading to hypermyelination, involving to a varying extent the cortex, basal ganglia, and other structures; it usually underlies double athetosis, and some cases of congenital diplegia. Glutaric acidaemia, a rare inborn metabolic error, gives rise to psychomotor retardation, recurrent metabolic acidosis, and choreoathetosis with tetraparesis (Leibel, Shih, Goodman, Bauman, McCabe, Zwendling, Bergman, and Costello 1980). Athetosis may rarely occur as a symptom of Wilson's disease, or may follow kernicterus; cases developing in adult life are usually due to drugs. Paroxysmal kinesigenic choreoathetosis, a disorder in which choreoathetotic, ballistic, and dystonic movements of the extremities occur in brief paroxysmal episodes precipitated by voluntary movement (Kato and Araki 1969) is probably a form of reflex epilepsy and may respond to treatment with carbamazepine. Familial paroxysmal dystonic choreoathetosis (Lance 1977) is different, in that attacks, lasting for up to four hours, may be precipitated by alcohol, emotion, or fatigue and are controlled by clonazepam, but not by phenytoin or its analogues.

Unilateral athetosis

Unilateral athetosis may also be congenital, being then usually associated with infantile hemiplegia. Often, the brain in such cases shows cerebral hemiatrophy, with an elective necrosis of the third cortical layer of the precentral gyrus, atrophy of the thalamus, and degeneration and gliosis or false porencephaly of the corpus striatum. Unilateral athetosis can also result from focal lesions involving the striatum at any age, due, for example, to acute encephalitis, encephalopathy, or infarction complicating the specific fevers in childhood, but senile chorea (see p. 348) or hemiballismus, which resemble it superficially, are also seen in late middle life and old age, due to focal atheromatous cerebral softening. A rare hereditary form of non-progressive athetotic hemiplegia has been described (Haar and Dyken 1977).

Symptoms and signs

Congenital athetosis is not usually noticed until the child is several months old, when abnormal postures or movements become evident. In the early months of life many such children are hypotonic ('floppy infants') and are thought to suffer from the flaccid or hypotonic form of cerebral palsy. Athetosis caused by an acute inflammatory or vascular lesion may develop rapidly within a few days of the lesion, or insidiously after an interval of several weeks, or even years.

Typical athetosis possesses the following features. One or both sides of the body may be involved. The muscles innervated by the cranial nerves are much more severely affected when the athetosis is bilateral than when unilateral. In bilateral athetosis the patient shows grimaces resembling caricatures of many normal facial expressions. Involuntary laughing and crying are common. The tongue shows writhing movements of protrusion and withdrawal, and the patient is often unable to maintain it protruded unless it is held between the teeth. Involuntary movements of the articulatory and pharyngeal muscles lead to dysarthria and dysphagia. The head may be rotated to one or other side, or extended. In unilateral athetosis the facial movements usually consist of little more than an exaggeration of normal expressions. In the upper limbs the peripheral segments are more involved in the involuntary movements than the proximal. The limb is usually adducted and internally rotated at the shoulder and semiflexed at the elbow. The characteristic posture of the hand is one of marked wrist flexion, with flexion at metacarpophalangeal and extension at the interphalangeal joints, and the thumb is usually adducted, and extended at its two distal joints. This posture is disturbed by slow, writhing movements of flexion and extension at the wrist and metacarpophalangeal joints, the fingers remaining extended at the interphalangeal joints, with varying degrees of adduction and abduction. Movements may also occur at the shoulder and elbow, leading sometimes to retraction and internal rotation at the shoulder and extension at the elbow. In severe unilateral cases the patient typically grasps the affected upper limb with the normal hand, to restrain the movement. He may even sit upon the affected hand or trap it behind his back in a chair for the same reason. Except in the mildest cases the movements interfere completely with voluntary use of the limb. The movements of the lower limb are usually less severe, and again are most marked distally. The foot is usually held in a position of talipes equinovarus, often with marked dorsiflexion of the great toe. Athetotic movements are always exaggerated by attempted voluntary movement and by nervousness and excitement. They diminish when the patient lies down and disappear during sleep. There is often associated hypotonia. In severe cases, especially of unilateral athetosis, muscular contractures usually develop and the peripheral parts of the limbs ultimately become fixed in their characteristic postures.

Double athetosis may be associated with spastic diplegia. Some patients show mild or moderate mental retardation but many with severe athetosis are normal intellectually.

Diagnosis

The involuntary movements are so distinctive that diagnosis is easy. Choreic movements are more rapid and jerky: those of dystonia slower and involve to a greater extent the long axis of the limbs and trunk. Athetosis, in fact, is midway between chorea and dystonia. The age and mode of onset distinguish the cause as either congenital abnormality, progressive degeneration, or acute focal lesion.

Prognosis and treatment

Medical treatment is disappointing. Benzhexol (*Artane*) and sedatives such as phenobarbitone, chlordiazepoxide (*Librium*), and diazepam (*Valium*) may slightly diminish the movements as may dopamine and serotonin antagonists such as tetrabenazine and thiopropazate, but the effect is usually short-lived and disappointing; improvement may follow re-educational exercises, as advocated by Phelps (1942), perseveringly carried out over a long period. Surgical measures tried in the past have included section of multiple dorsal roots, excision of a portion of the contralateral precentral gyrus (Bucy and Buchanan 1932; Bucy 1951), and anterolateral spinal tractotomy (Putnam 1933) but none has proved of lasting benefit. Cooper (1955) found that stereotaxic thalamotomy produced alleviation, but Paxton and Dow (1958) found it of no value and most authorities agree that these are the least rewarding cases for stereotaxic surgery.

References

Bucy, P. C. (1951). The surgical treatment of extrapyramidal diseases. *J. Neurol. Neurosurg. Psychiat.* **14**, 108.
—— and Buchanan, D. N. (1932). Athetosis. *Brain* **55**, 479.
Carpenter, M. B. (1950). Athetosis and the basal ganglia: Review of the literature and study of forty-two cases. *Arch. Neurol. Psychiat.*, *Chicago* **63**, 875.
Cooper, I. S. (1955). Relief of juvenile involuntary movement disorders by chemopallidectomy. *J. Am. med. Ass.* **164**, 1297.
Denny-Brown, D. (1946). *Diseases of the basal ganglia and subthalamic nuclei.* Oxford University Press, New York.
—— (1962). *The basal ganglia and their relation to disorders of movement.* Oxford University Press, Oxford.
Haar, F. and Dyken, P. (1977). Hereditary nonprogressive athetotic hemiplegia: a new syndrome. *Neurology*, *Minneapolis* **27**, 849.
Kato, M and Araki, S. (1969). Paroxysmal kinesigenic choreoathetosis. Report of a case relieved by carbamazepine. *Arch. Neurol.*, *Chicago* **20**, 508.
Lader, M. H. (1970). Drug-induced extrapyramidal syndromes. *J. R. Coll. Phycns.*, *London* **5**, 87.
Lance, J. W. (1977). Familial paroxysmal dystonic choreoathetosis and its differentiation from related syndromes. *Ann. Neurol.* **2**, 285.
Leibel, R. L., Shih, V. E., Goodman, S. I., Bauman, M. L., McCabe, E. R. B., Zwerdling, R. G., Bergman, I., and Costello, C. (1980). Glutaric acidemia: a metabolic disorder causing progressive choreoathetosis. *Neurology*, *Minneapolis* **30**, 1163.
Oppenheim, H. and Vogt, C. (1911). Nature et localisation de la paralysie pseudobulbaire congénitale et infantile. *J. Psychol. Neurol.*, *Leipzig* **18**, 293.
Paxton, H. D. and Dow, R. S. (1958). Two years' experience of chemopallidectomy. *J. Am. med. Ass.* **168**, 755.
Phelps, W. M. (1942). Evidences of improvement in cases of athetosis treated by re-education. *Res. Publ. Ass. nerv. ment. Dis.* **21**, 529.
Putnam, T. J. (1933). Treatment of athetosis and dystonia by section of extrapyramidal motor tracts. *Arch. Neurol. Psychiat.*, *Chicago* **29**, 504.
Singer, K. and Cheng, M. N. (1971). Thiopropazate hydrochloride in persistent dyskinesia. *Br. med. J.* **4**, 22.
Vogt, C. (1924–5). Sur l'état marbré du striatum. *Jb. Psychiat. Neurol.* **31**, 256.
—— and Vogt, O. (1919). Erster Versuch einer pathologisch-anatomischen Einteilungstriärer Motilitätsstörungen nebst Bemerkskungen über seine allgemeine wissenschaftliche Bedeutung. *J. Psychol. Neurol.*, *Leipzig* **24**, 1.

Chorea

Sydenham's chorea

Synonym. St. Vitus' dance.

Definition. An acute toxi-infective disorder of the nervous system, usually due to acute rheumatism, usually occurring in childhood and adolescence and giving involuntary movements as its most prominent manifestation.

Pathology

Cases of chorea which have come to autopsy have often shown diffuse changes in the brain. Macroscopically, oedema and congestion have been observed. Microscopically, changes have usually been most marked in the caudate nucleus, substantia nigra, and subthalamic nucleus, but cortical abnormalities have also been found. Vasodilatation is often conspicuous, but perivascular infiltration with lymphocytes and plasma cells is exceptional, though arteritis has been described. There is a diffuse loss of ganglion cells, involving not only the basal ganglia but also the cerebral cortex and cerebellum. Encephalitic changes have been described in acute rheumatism (Winkelman and Eckel 1932; Bruetsch and Bahr 1939). In about half of all cases, sera contain IgG antibodies that react with neuronal cytoplasmic antigens from the caudate and subthalamic nuclei (see Menkes 1980).

Aetiology

Most cases of chorea in childhood are due to acute rheumatism, as is evident from the frequency with which other rheumatic manifestations are present or subsequently develop. Other infections may rarely, however, be the cause, especially scarlet fever and diphtheria; and choreiform movements may be encountered as a symptom of encephalitis lethargica, as a rare complication of chickenpox, in systemic lupus erythematosus (Donaldson and Espiner 1971; Fermaglich, Streib, and Auth 1973), in patients taking oral contraceptives (Riddoch, Jefferson, and Bickerstaff 1971; Gamboa, Isaacs, and Harter 1971; Bickerstaff 1975), and in some individuals with chronic liver disease.

Heredity clearly plays a part in aetiology, since some families appear to be unusually susceptible to acute rheumatism, and there is a family history either of chorea or of acute rheumatism in 25 per cent of cases. However, no HLA antigen association has yet been identified. There seems to be a higher incidence of left-handedness among sufferers from chorea than among the general population.

The white race is more susceptible than the coloured races, and females suffer more than males in the proportion of about three to one. Chorea is rare before the age of 5 and after 20; four-fifths of all cases occur between the ages of 5 and 15.

Mental stress or emotional shock may play a part in precipitating the condition. In a few cases chorea occurs during pregnancy—chorea gravidarum. This usually occurs during a first pregnancy but may recur in subsequent pregnancies. It rarely occurs for the first time in a multipara or after the age of 25. Thyrotoxicosis is a rare association.

Symptoms and signs

Mode of onset

The onset is usually insidious, the first complaint often being that the child is clumsy and drops things. When the movements are noticed, he is described as restless, fidgety, or unable to keep still. Sometimes the onset is more abrupt and is then often ascribed to a fright.

Involuntary movements

Involuntary movements are the most prominent sign and are best described as quasi-purposive. Although they achieve no purpose, they often resemble fragments of purposive movements following one another in a disorderly fashion. In the face they are always bilateral. Frowning, raising the eyebrows, pursing the lips, smiling, and bizarre movements of the mouth and tongue occur. The protruded tongue may be held between the teeth to prevent its sudden withdrawal. The eyes may be rolled from one side to the other, the head turning in the same direction.

In mild cases speech is not affected; in severe cases there is considerable dysarthria, articulation is slurred, and words are sometimes jerked out explosively. Rarely, mastication and swallowing may be so much disturbed that the patient must be artificially fed.

In the upper limb, movements occur at all joints. At one moment the elbow is flexed with the fingers grasping the bedclothes; at the next the arm is flung out in full extension. Respiration is often jerky and irregular and is frequently impeded by movements involving the abdominal wall and movements of rotation or flexion of the spine. Movements of the lower limbs are usually less conspicuous and most evident at the periphery. Choreic movements are intensified by voluntary effort and by excitement. They disappear during sleep.

Associated movement

In chorea the involuntary muscular contractions normally associated with strong voluntary movement are exaggerated, and at the same time incoordinate. When the patient clenches his fist, vigorous associated movements may involve the face, trunk, and limbs. Despite this, the synergic extension of the wrist associated with strong flexion of the fingers is not normally performed. Contraction of the flexors may conflict with, and even overpower, that of the extensors, while the radial and ulnar extensors may not contract synchronously, so that the hand deviates from side to side.

This disorder of associated movement is an early sign which may antedate the involuntary movements, and can be elicited in suspected cases by asking the patient to clench his fists over the observer's fingers, while protruding the tongue.

Voluntary movement

In mild cases power is little impaired, though movements are abrupt. For example, if the patient be asked to stretch out the arms, he does so with a sudden movement as though he were flinging his hands away from him. In severe cases the involuntary movements cause considerable incoordination, and weakness may then be marked, as in so-called paralytic chorea, though total paralysis is never seen. Not uncommonly chorea is predominantly unilateral (hemichorea) in which case a diagnosis of hemiplegia may initially be entertained unless the hypotonia and involuntary movements are recognized.

Hypotonia and posture

Hypotonia is invariably present and is best demonstrated by passively extending the wrists and ankles, when abnormal hyperextension is obtainable. The so-called choreic posture of the hand, in which the thumb and fingers are hyperextended at the metacarpophalangeal joints and the wrist is flexed, is merely a manifestation of hypotonia, resulting from loss of tone in antagonistic muscles. The upper limbs are characteristically hyperpronated when outstretched and held above the head (the pronator sign).

Reflexes

The cutaneous reflexes in chorea are often exceptionally brisk; the plantar reflexes are flexor. When hypotonia is extreme, the tendon reflexes may be difficult to elicit, but they are usually obtainable and often show a typical repetition of the reflex movement, so that on tapping the quadriceps tendon with the leg dangling, it swings like a pendulum (the 'pendular' reflex).

Sensory changes do not occur, and there is no disturbance of the sphincters.

Mental state

Most choreic children exhibit some emotional lability. In severe cases there may be a persistent state of excitement with insomnia—so-called *maniacal chorea*.

The heart

As in most cases chorea is due to acute rheumatism, cardiac abnormalities are common. They are not, however, constant. When the heart is involved for the first time during the attack, the pulse rate is quickened, there is usually slight cardiac dilatation indicated by outward displacement of the apex beat, muffling of the apical first sound, and often a soft mitral systolic murmur suggesting myocarditis. When the heart has been affected in previous attacks of rheumatism, signs of valvular damage are more likely to be present. Pericarditis, arthritis, and rheumatic nodules are rarely associated with chorea. Pyrexia is usually absent, unless chorea is complicated by other manifestations of acute rheumatism.

Diagnosis

The diagnosis of chorea is usually easy, as the involuntary movements are distinctive. It is most likely to be confused with habit spasm, in which, however, the same movements are repeated again and again. In athetosis the movements are slower than in chorea and, in most cases, athetosis in childhood is congenital or is noticed before the age of 5, when chorea is very rare. Hysterical involuntary movements may simulate chorea but usually occur after the age of 15, and in females, and are an imitation of a case of true chorea. The imitation, however, is never exact. The movements are usually too jerky and sometimes rhythmical. There is neither exaggeration nor disorganization of associated movements, and the face usually escapes.

Paralytic chorea may simulate other forms of paralysis in childhood. It is distinguished from hemiplegia by the fact that the upper limb alone is paretic, and by the absence of signs of corticospinal-tract dysfunction. The absence of wasting and of EMG changes distinguishes it from poliomyelitis. A further diagnostic point is that even in the weak limb slight involuntary movements are present, and may also be observed elsewhere. Choreiform movements occurring in cerebral palsy are accompanied by other signs of brain damage; however, 'searching' movements superficially resembling those of chorea and sometimes misinterpreted as such, are often seen in 'clumsy children' with minimal cerebral dysfunction due to developmental apraxia (Gubbay 1975), when the underlying disorder is often difficult to recognize.

In maniacal chorea the mental state may overshadow the physical symptoms, but the history of involuntary movements or signs of rheumatic endocarditis may enable the correct diagnosis to be made.

Chorea having been diagnosed, the cause can usually be easily ascertained. Many patients show other evidence of rheumatism, but even if these are absent, this is the most likely cause. Confusion arose in the past from cases of encephalitis lethargica characterized by choreiform movements, but these have not been observed for many years. In such cases the characteristic lethargy was often absent, but the movements were often associated with a reversed sleep rhythm and ocular signs. In adult life, systemic lupus erythematosus, oral contraceptive medication, and chronic liver disease must all be excluded.

Huntington's chorea is distinguished by its onset in later life, usually after the age of 30, by its hereditary character, and its association with progressive dementia. When it does rarely occur in childhood, it usually presents with rigidity rather than chorea.

Prognosis

Death from chorea is rare and occurs in under 2 per cent of cases, usually due to cardiac involvement. It was once suggested that chorea gravidarum carries a less favourable prognosis (Matthews 1963) but this no longer seems to be the case (Lewis and Parsons 1966). Most patients recover in from two to three months, rarely in less than six weeks, and occasionally up to two years is needed (Menkes 1980). Recurrences occur in about one-third of all cases: a patient may have two, three, four, or even more attacks (Aron, Freeman and Carter 1965). The average interval between attacks is about one year; it is rarely more than two. The presence of other rheumatic manifestations, e.g. valvular lesions, does not influence recovery, but repeated attacks of chorea predispose to the development of rheumatic carditis and endocarditis. The illness usually leaves no serious sequels, though some mental lability may continue for a while, and minimal psychological and neurological residua occasionally persist (Bird, Palkes, and Prensky 1976); slight involuntary movements may be perpetuated as a habit.

Treatment

All patients suffering from chorea should be kept in bed for two or three weeks, and should then be allowed to get up only if the movements are considerably diminished in severity. Cardiac complications may necessitate longer bed rest, and the condition of the heart must be considered independently. Isolation is beneficial, and if possible the child should be nursed in a room alone. Excitement is to be avoided, but in all but the most severe cases some quiet occupation should be provided. If dysphagia is very severe, it is rarely necessary to tube-feed the patient. Salicylates and corticosteroid drugs are now known to have no influence upon the disease process. Traditional sedatives such as phenobarbitone, 30 mg three or four times daily, are sufficient in some cases but many patients are dramatically improved with chlorpromazine, 25–50 mg three or four times daily (Lewis and Parsons 1966), by haloperidol (Menkes 1980), or by diazepam.

During convalescence attention should be paid to re-education of limb movements. This is best promoted at first by occupational therapy with activities such as knitting, sewing, bead-threading, drawing, and painting. When the child is out of bed, and when his cardiac condition permits, remedial exercises may be added.

It was once customary to advise removal of infected tonsils but prophylactic penicillin is now preferred in an attempt to prevent recurrence. In chorea gravidarum there is no evidence that termination of pregnancy is beneficial.

References

Aron, A. M., Freeman, J. M., and Carter, S. (1965). The natural history of Sydenham's chorea. *Am. J. Med.* **38**, 83.

Bickerstaff, E. R. (1975). *Neurological complications of oral contraceptives*. Blackwell, Oxford.

Bird, M. T., Palkes, H., and Prensky, A. L. (1976). A follow-up study of Sydenham's chorea. *Neurology, Minneapolis* **26**, 601.

Brain, W. R. (1928). Posture of the hand in chorea and other states of muscular hypotonia. *Lancet* **i**, 439.

Bruetsch, W. L. and Bahr, M. A. (1939). Chronic rheumatic brain disease as a factor in the causation of mental illness. *J. Indiana med. Ass.* **32**, 4.

Donaldson, I. MacG. and Espiner, E. A. (1971). Disseminated lupus erythematosus presenting as chorea gravidarum. *Arch. Neurol., Chicago* **25**, 240.

Fermaglich, J., Streib, E., and Auth, T. (1973). Chorea associated with systemic lupus erythematosus: treatment with haloperidol. *Arch. Neurol., Chicago* **28**, 276.

Gamboa, E. G., Isaacs, G., and Harter, D. H. (1971). Chorea associated with oral contraceptive therapy. *Arch. Neurol., Chicago* **25**, 112.

Gubbay, S. S. (1975). *The clumsy child*. Saunders, London.

Lewis, B. V. and Parsons, M. (1966). Chorea gravidarum. *Lancet* **i**, 284.

Lhermitte, J. and Pagniez, P. (1930). Anatomie et physiologie pathologiques de la chorée de Sydenham. *Encéphale.* **25**, 24.

Matthews, W. B. (1963). *Practical neurology*. Blackwell, Oxford.

Menkes, J. H. (1980). *Textbook of child neurology*, 2nd edn. Lea and Febiger, Philadelphia.

Riddoch, D., Jefferson, M., and Bickerstaff, E. R. (1971). Chorea and the oral contraceptives. *Br. med. J.* **4**, 217.

Winkelman, N. W. and Eckel, J. L. (1932). The brain in acute rheumatic fever. *Arch. Neurol. Psychiat., Chicago* **28**, 844.

Huntington's chorea

Definition. A hereditary disorder characterized pathologically by degeneration of the ganglion cells of the forebrain and corpus striatum, and clinically by choreiform movements and progressive dementia, which usually begin during early middle life.

Pathology

The brain is small and of reduced weight, with marked atrophy affecting the gyri of the frontal lobes and the corpus striatum, especially the caudate. The ganglion cells in both the caudate nucleus and in the putamen are reduced in number and sometimes almost absent. Pallidal neurones also degenerate to a greater extent than is generally appreciated (Lange, Thörner, Hopf, and Schröder 1976). Foci of recent cell death in caudate and putamen are readily identified by immunohistochemical techniques (Averback 1980) and many of the biochemical and morphological changes in the striatum are qualitatively similar to those of normal ageing processes as seen in humans and rodents and in a rodent model of Huntington's chorea in which striatal neurones are destroyed by kainic acid (Finch 1980). Goebel, Heipertz, Scholz, Iqbal, and Tellez Nagel (1978) found increased lipofuscin and abnormal mitochondria ultrastructurally in cortical and striatal neurones and astrocytes. These degenerative changes are accompanied by an extensive proliferation of neuroglia. In four childhood cases Byers, Gilles, and Fung (1973) found loss of neurones and gliosis in both the globus pallidus and thalamus as well as substantial cerebellar atrophy. Rodda (1981) has also documented cerebellar atrophy with severe Purkinje-cell loss. Campbell, Corner, Norman, and Urich (1961), in a patient with the rigid form of the disease, found substantial loss of small nerve cells in the caudate nucleus and putamen with relative sparing of those in the globus pallidus and attributed rigidity to the putaminal lesion, chorea to that in the caudate nucleus. Bugiani, Tabaton, and Cammarata (1984) found relative sparing of large striatal neurones in the rigid variant. The ganglion cells of the frontal cortex are also shrunken in appearance, and the white matter of the cerebral hemispheres is reduced in amount.

Aetiology

Huntington's chorea is uncommon in Great Britain but less so in the United States of America. Though sporadic cases are rarely encountered, the disorder is almost invariably inherited as a Mendelian dominant trait. According to Davenport and Muncey (1917) its ancestral source in the United States can be traced to three brothers who migrated there in the seventeenth century. Of 1000 cases in some districts practically all could be traced to six individuals. Both sexes are affected and transmit the disease with equal frequency. The disease is one-third as common in blacks as in whites and is even less common in the Japanese (Kurtzke 1979). The age of onset of symptoms is usually between 30 and 45, but may be either later or earlier. Exceptionally members of affected sibships develop the disease in childhood and a unique infantile case has been reported (Haslam, Curry, and Johns 1983). In an extensive review of the disease in Queensland, Australia, however, Wallace, and Hall (1972) found evidence of considerable genetic heterogeneity and suggested that cases of adult and childhood onset may be due to different allelic genes. However, while cases beginning in childhood or adolescence usually display the rigid form of the disease, many such cases have been described in families in which affected individuals in earlier generations showed the typical onset with choreic movements in middle life and there is no essential difference in the pathological findings in the two varieties (Campbell *et al.* 1961; Oliver and Dewhurst 1969); families showing an onset with rigidity in adult life have been described (Bird and Paulson 1971). A suggestion that juvenile cases are more likely to inherit the gene from the father, late onset cases from the mother (Myers, Goldman, Bird, Sax, Merril, Schoenfeld, and Wolf 1983) has not been confirmed in Europe (Went, der Vlis, and Bruyn 1984). Of fundamental importance, however, has been the discovery by Gusella, Wexler, Conneally, Naylor, Anderson, Tanzi, Watkins, Ottina, Sakagushi, Young, Shoulson, Bonilla, and Martin (1983) that a cloned DNA sequence on chromosome 4 shows close linkage to the locus for Huntington's disease. This discovery seems likely to offer a reliable predictive test, a finding which raises important medical and ethical problems for sufferers and their families (Harper 1983, 1984).

Much work has been devoted to attempting to identify a specific biochemical abnormality. Suggestions that it may be due to a disorder of magnesium metabolism have not been confirmed (Fleming, Barker, and Stewart 1967). No significant abnormality in the lipid composition of white matter has been discovered (Hooghwinkel, Bruyn, and de Rooy 1968) and the erythrocyte glycolipids are normal (Wherrett and Brown 1969), but certain amino acids are reduced in the plasma and CSF of such patients (Perry, Hansen, Diamond, and Stedman 1969). Abnormalities of potassium-ATPase activity and of the fluidity of erythrocyte membranes have been reported (Butterfield, Oeswein, Prunty, Husle, and Markesbery 1978; Beverstock and Pearson 1981); low platelet monoamine oxidase activity (Mann and Chiu 1978), reduced uptake of dopamine by platelets (Butterworth, Gonce, and Barbeau 1977; McLean and Nihei 1980); abnormalities of lymphocyte capping (Noronha, Roos, Antel, and Arnason 1979) and in the growth of skin fibroblasts in culture (Barkley, Hardiwidjaja, and Menkes 1977) have all been described, as has a reduction in the activity of

angiotensin-converting enzyme in the corpus striatum (Arregui, Bennett, Bird, Yamamura, Iversen, and Snyder 1977). Impaired growth hormone (Keogh, Johnson, Nanda, and Sulaiman 1976) and prolactin (Hayden, Vinik, Paul, and Beighton 1977) release and other abnormalities of hypothalamic function (Lavin, Bone, and Sheridan 1981) are also found, but none of these changes has yet thrown light upon the fundamental biochemical abnormality. However, it is clear that there is imbalance between central dopamine and acetylcholine activity in such cases (Klawans and Rubovits 1972), and the enzymes glutamic acid decarboxylase, choline acetylase, and succinate dehydrogenase are all reduced in the corpus striatum of patients (McGeer, McGeer, and Fibiger 1973; Stahl and Swanson 1974). Enzymes of the pyruvate dehydrogenase complex have been found to be reduced in the caudate nucleus and putamen (Sorbi, Bird, and Blass 1983) while somatostatin appears to be increased (Aronin, Cooper, Lorenz, Bird, Sagar, Leeman, and Martin 1983), but there is no deficiency of cortical choline acetyltransferase nor is there an abnormality of the nucleus basalis such as occurs in Alzheimer's disease (Clark, Parhad, Folstein, Whitehouse, Hedreen, Price, and Chase 1983). There is a loss of GABA-containing neurones (Bird and Iverson 1974) so that increasing attention is being paid to the metabolism of gamma-aminobutyric acid (GABA) in this disease (Barbeau 1975). It is now known that GABA is greatly reduced in the nucleus accumbens, lateral pallidum, subthalamic nucleus, substantia nigra, and ventrolateral thalamic nucleus (Spokes, Garrett, Rossor, and Iversen 1980), but drugs which increase cerebral GABA concentrations (see below) have not been established as of proven benefit (*The Lancet* 1980). Positron emission tomography (PET scanning) demonstrates a clear decrease in glucose utilization in the caudate and putamen early in the course of the disease (Kuhl, Phelps, Markham, Metter, Riege, and Winter 1982).

Symptoms and signs

The first symptom is usually involuntary movements, which develop insidiously. They are most conspicuous in the face and upper limbs, and are usually more rapid and jerky than those of Sydenham's chorea. Impairment of ocular movement with reduced saccadic velocity and jerky following movements is common (Avanzini, Girotti, Caraceni, and Spreafico 1979). As the disorder progresses dysarthria and ataxia of the upper limbs and of the gait appear. Mental changes develop gradually, usually a few years after the involuntary movements. They consist of a progressive dementia. Most patients become inert, apathetic, and irritable. Delusions may occur, and outbursts of excitement are not uncommon. Suicide is exceptional.

However, the clinical picture does not always exhibit the classical features just described. Dementia may precede involuntary movements or the latter may never appear (Curran 1930). Alternatively, but rarely, the movements are not followed by dementia. Exceptionally parkinsonian rigidity (the 'rigid' form) takes the place of the involuntary movements (Campbell *et al.* 1961; Bird and Paulson 1971). An occasional onset in childhood has already been mentioned, and in such cases diffuse extrapyramidal rigidity, fits, and pseudobulbar palsy are often the presenting features.

Diagnosis

In typical cases with a family history the diagnosis is easy. In sporadic cases or in those where the family history is unknown, progressive dementia developing in middle life in association with involuntary movements may raise the possibility of general paresis, but this can easily be excluded by the absence of iridoplegia and by the negative serological reactions. Choreiform involuntary movements are rarely if ever seen in the other presenile dementias, in multi-infarct dementia, and in Creutzfeldt–Jakob disease, but when dementia is the presenting feature and when the family history is obscure, these other conditions may sometimes be considered before involuntary movements appear. The EEG in Huntington's chorea is often of low voltage (Scott, Heathfield, Toone, and Margerison 1972) but this is of little diagnostic value. In advanced cases the CT scan or pneumoencephalography may show a characteristic dilatation of the lateral ventricles with absence of the usual indentation due to the body of the caudate nucleus (Gath and Vinje 1968) but by the time this appearance is present the diagnosis is usually self-evident.

Prognosis

Save in rare cases, the disorder is progressive and terminates fatally, usually in from 10 to 15 years, though it may be much more acute; however, survival for 20 or 30 years is not uncommon.

Since it is a dominant trait, half the children of an affected person may be expected to develop and to be capable of transmitting the disease. Those who are unaffected will not transmit it, but, unfortunately, since symptoms usually do not develop until middle life, it is often impossible in the case of children of an affected parent to decide whether they will transmit the disorder until they have passed through their reproductive years. Much attention has therefore been devoted to a search for a reliable predictive test which will identify the presymptomatic carrier of the gene. The administration of levodopa, 800 mg and carbidopa 200 mg daily for 10 days, may evoke choreiform movements in some such cases (Klawans, Paulson, and Barbeau 1970) but this test is not totally reliable (Klawans, Goetz, and Perlik 1980); Esteban, Mateo, and Gimenez-Roldan (1981) prefer to measure the R2 response on the blink reflex after a single oral dose of levodopa and carbidopa. Other methods tried have included measurement of the radiosensitiviy of lymphoblastoid lines obtained from such patients (Moshell, Barrett, Tarone, and Robbins 1980; Arlett 1980), measurement of GABA in the CSF (Manyam, Hare, Katz, and Glaeser 1978), and PET scanning (Kuhl et al. 1982). Even if a totally reliable predictive test were available, which is clearly not yet the case, some have questioned the ethics of its application (Thomas 1982). However, there is evidence that even non-direct genetic counselling has already reduced family size in individuals at risk; nevertheless, the potential conflict between helping the family on the one hand and reducing the burden upon society imposed by an incurable disease on the other is very real (*The Lancet* 1982).

Treatment

Progressive dementia often ultimately necessitates institutional care. No form of treatment is known to arrest the progress of the dementia; choline is ineffective (Growdon, Cohen, and Wurtman 1977). Chlorpromazine or thiopropazate (*Dartalan*) may reduce slightly the involuntary movements. Lithium carbonate (Aminoff and Marshall 1974) and methysergide (Klawans, Rubovits, Ringel, and Weiner 1972) are among the many drugs which have been shown to be of no value. Tetrabenazine 25 mg three times daily is probably the most effective treatment (McLellan, Chalmers, and Johnson 1974), but its value is limited and its side-effects are often unacceptable. Isoniazid (Perry, Wright, Hansen, and Macleod 1979; Perry, Wright, Hansen, Thomas, Allan, Baird, and Diewold 1982) may increase brain GABA concentrations without producing clinical improvement, while muscimol, a GABA-mimetic drug (Shoulson, Goldblatt, Charlton, and Joynt 1978) and α-acetylenic GABA, an inhibitor of GABA-transaminase (Tell, Böhlen, Schechter, Koch-Weser, Agid, Bonnet, Coquillat, Chazot, and Fischer 1981) are also ineffective clinically. THIP, another putative GABA receptor agonist, also seems to be ineffective (Foster, Chase, Denaro, Hare, and Tamminga 1983), while lisuride 150 μg given by injection produces only transient alleviation of the involuntary movements (Frattola, Albizzati, Alemani, Bassi, Ferrarese, and Trabucchi 1983). Stereotaxic sur-

gery has been used but may accelerate dementia and is therefore contra-indicated.

A recent UK survey has suggested that neither neurologists nor general practitioners are giving adequate genetic counselling advice to patients and their families (Martindale and Yale 1983).

References

Aminoff, M. J. and Marshall, J. (1974). Treatment of Huntington's chorea with lithium carbonate: a double-blind trial. *Lancet* i, 107.

——, Trenchard, A., Turner, P., Wood, W. G., and Hills, M. (1974). Platelet uptake of dopamine and 5-hydroxy-tryptamine and plasma-catecholamine levels in patients with Huntington's chorea.*Lancet* ii, 1115.

Arlett, C. F. (1980). Presymptomatic diagnosis of Huntington's disease? *Lancet* i, 540.

Aronin, N., Cooper, P. E., Lorenz, L. J., Bird, E. D., Sagar, S. M., Leeman, S. E., and Martin, J. B. (1983). Somatostatin is increased in the basal ganglia in Huntington disease. *Ann. Neurol.* 13, 519.

Arregui, A., Bennett, J. P., Bird, E. D., Yamamura, H. I., Iversen, L. L., and Snyder, S. H. (1977). Huntington's chorea: selective depletion of activity of angiotensin converting enzyme in the corpus striatum. *Ann. Neurol.* 2, 294.

Avanzini, G., Girotti, F., Caraceni, T., and Spreafico, R. (1979). Oculomotor disorders in Huntington's chorea. *J. Neurol. Neurosurg. Psychiat.* 42, 581.

Averback, P. (1980). Immunohistochemical study of foci of recent cell death in Huntington's disease. *Can. J. neurol. Sci.* 7, 87.

Barbeau, A. (1975). Progress in understanding Huntington's chorea. *Can. J. neurol. Sci.* 2, 81.

——, Chase, T. N., and Paulson, G. W. (1972). *Huntington's Chorea, 1872–1972*, Advances in Neurology, Vol. 1. Raven Press, New York.

Barkley, D. S., Hardiwidjaja, S., and Menkes, J. H. (1977). Abnormalities in growth of skin fibroblasts of patients with Huntington's disease. *Ann. Neurol.* 1, 426.

Beverstock, G. C. and Pearson, P. L. (1981). Membrane fluidity measurements in peripheral cells from Huntington's disease patients. *J. Neurol. Neurosurg. Psychiat.* 44, 684.

Bird, E. D. and Iversen, L. L. (1974). Huntington's chorea—post-mortem measurement of glutamic acid decarboxylase, choline acetyltransferase and dopamine in basal ganglia. *Brain* 97, 457.

Bird, M. T. and Paulson, G. W. (1971). The rigid form of Huntington's chorea. *Neurology, Minneapolis* 21, 271.

Bugiani, O., Tabaton, M., and Cammarata, S. (1984). Huntington's disease: survival of large striatal neurons in the rigid variant. *Ann. Neurol.* 15, 154.

Butterfield, D. A., Oeswein, J. Q., Prunty, M. E., Husle, K. C., and Markesbery, W. R. (1978). Increased sodium plus potassium adenosine triphosphatase activity in erythrocyte membranes in Huntington's disease. *Ann. Neurol.* 4, 60.

Butterworth, R. F., Gonce, M., and Barbeau, A. (1977). Platelet dopamine uptake in Huntington's chorea and Gilles de la Tourette's syndrome: effect of haloperidol. *Can. J. neurol. Sci.* 4, 285.

Byers, R. K., Gilles, R. H., and Fung, C. (1973). Huntington's disease in children. Neuropathologic study of four cases. *Neurology, Minneapolis* 23, 561.

Campbell, A. M. G., Corner, B., Norman, R. M., and Urich, H. (1961). The rigid form of Huntington's disease. *J. Neurol. Neurosurg. Psychiat.* 24, 71.

Clark, A. W., Parhad, I. M., Folstein, S. E., Whitehouse, P. J., Hedreen, J. C., Price, D. L., and Chase, G. A. (1983). The nucleus basalis in Huntington's disease. *Neurology, Minneapolis* 33, 1262.

Curran, D. (1929–30). Huntington's chorea without choreiform movements. *J. Neurol. Psychopath.* 10, 305.

Davenport, C. B. and Muncey, E. B. (1916–17). Huntington's chorea in relation to heredity and eugenics. *Am. J. Insan.* 73, 195. (Also *Proc. Nat. Acad. Sci., Washington.* 1915 1, 283.)

Esteban, A., Mateo, D., and Gimenez-Roldan, S. (1981). Early detection of Huntington's disease. Blink reflex and levodopa load in presymptomatic and incipient subjects. *J. Neurol. Neurosurg. Psychiat.* 33, 43.

Finch, C. E. (1980). The relationships of aging changes in the basal ganglia to manifestations of Huntington's chorea. *Ann. Neurol.* 7, 406.

Fleming, L. W., Barker, M. G., and Stewart, W. K. (1967). Plasma and erythrocyte magnesium in Huntington's chorea. *J. Neurol. Neurosurg. Psychiat.* 30, 374.

Foster, N. L., Chase, T. N., Denaro, A., Hare, T. A., and Tamminga, C. A. (1983). THIP treatment of Huntington's disease. *Neurology, Minneapolis* **33**, 637

Frattola, L., Albizzati, M. G., Alemani, A., Bassi, S., Ferrarese, C., and Trabucchi, M. (1983). Acute treatment of Huntington's chorea with lisuride. *J. neurol. Sci.* **59**, 247.

Gath, I. and Vinje, B. (1968). Pneumoencephalographic findings in Huntington's chorea. *Neurology, Minneapolis* **18**, 991.

Goebel, H. H., Heipertz, R., Scholz, W., Iqbal, K., and Tellez-Nagel, I. (1978). Juvenile Huntington chorea: clinical, ultrastructural, and biochemical studies. *Neurology, Minneapolis* **28**, 23.

Growdon, J. H., Cohen, E. L., and Wurtman, R. J. (1977). Huntington's disease: clinical and chemical effects of choline administration. *Ann. Neurol.* **1**, 418.

Gusella, J. F., Wexler, N. S., Conneally, P. M., Naylor, S. L., Anderson, M. A., Tanzi, R. E., Watkins, P. C., Ottina, K., Wallace, M. R., Sakaguchi, A. Y., Young, A. B., Shoulson, I., Bonilla, E., and Martin, J. B. (1983). A polymorphic DNA marker genetically linked to Huntington's disease. *Nature* **306**, 234.

Harper, p. (1983). A genetic marker for Huntington's chorea. *Br. med. J.* **287**, 1567.

—— (1984). Localization of the gene for Huntington's chorea. *Trends Neuro. Sci.* **7**, 1.

Hayden, M. R., Vinik, A. I., Paul, M., and Beighton, P. (1977). Impaired prolactin release in Huntington's chorea: evidence for dopaminergic excess. *Lancet* **ii**, 423.

Hooghwinkel, G. J. M., Bruyn, G. W., and de Rooy, R. E. (1968). Biochemical studies in Huntington's chorea. VII. The lipid composition of the cerebral white matter and gray matter. *Neurology, Minneapolis* **18**, 408.

Keogh, H. J., Johnson, R. H., Nanda, R. N., and Sulaiman, W. R. (1976). Altered growth hormone release in Huntington's chorea. *J. Neurol. Neurosurg. Psychiat.* **39**, 244.

Klawans, H. L., Goetz, C. G., and Perlik, S. (1980). Presymptomatic and early detection in Huntington's disease. *Ann. Neurol.* **8**, 343.

——, Paulson, G. W., and Barbeau, A. (1970). Predictive test for Huntington's chorea. *Lancet* **ii**, 1185.

—— and Rubovits, R. (1972). Central cholinergic–anticholinergic antagonism in Huntington's chorea. *Neurology, Minneapolis* **22**, 107.

——, ——, Ringel, S. P., and Weiner, W. J. (1972). Observations on the use of methysergide in Huntington's chorea. *Neurology, Minneapolis* **22**, 929.

Kuhl, D. E., Phelps, M. E., Markham, C. H., Metter, E. J., Riege, W. H., and Winter, J. (1982). Cerebral metabolism and atrophy in Huntington's disease determined by ^{18}FDG and computed tomographic scan. *Ann. Neurol.* **12**, 425.

Kurtzke, J. F. (1979). Huntington's disease: mortality and morbidity data from outside the United States. In *Advances in neurology*, Vol. 23, (ed. T. N. Chase), p. 13. Raven Press, New York.

The Lancet (1980). Chemistry of Huntington's chorea. *Lancet* **i**, 1119.

—— (1982). Genetic counselling and the prevention of Huntington's chorea. *Lancet* **i**, 147.

Lange, H., Thörner, G., Hopf., A., and Schröder, K. F. (1976). Morphometric studies of the neuropathological changes in choreatic diseases. *J. neurol. Sci.* **28**, 401.

Lavin, P. J. M., Bone, I., and Sheridan, P. (1981). Studies of hypothalamic function in Huntington's chorea. *J. Neurol. Neurosurg. Psychiat.* **44**, 414.

Mann, J., and Chiu, E. (1978). Platelet monoamine oxidase activity in Huntington's chorea. *J. Neurol. Neurosurg. Psychiat.* **41**, 809.

Manyam, N. V. B., Hare, T. A., Katz, L., and Glaeser, B. S. (1978). Huntington's disease: cerebrospinal fluid GABA levels in at-risk individuals. *Arch. Neurol., Chicago* **35**, 728.

Martindale, B. and Yale, R. (1983). Huntington's chorea: neglected opportunities for preventive medicine. *Lancet* **i**, 634.

McGeer, P. L., McGeer, E. G., and Fibiger, H. C. (1973). Choline acetylase and glutamic acid decarboxylase in Huntington's chorea: a preliminary study. *Neurology, Minneapolis* **23**, 912.

McLean, D. R. and Nihei, T. (1980). Biochemical markers for Huntington's chorea. *Can. J. neurol. Sci.* **7**, 281.

McLellan, D. L., Chalmers, R. J., and Johnson, R. H. (1974). A double-blind trial of tetrabenazine, thiopropazate, and placebo in patients with chorea. *Lancet* **i**, 104.

McLeod, W. R. and Horne, D. J. de L. (1972). Huntington's chorea and tryptophan. *J. Neurol. Neurosurg. Psychiat.* **35**, 510.

Moshell, A. N., Barrett, S. F., Tarone, R. E., and Robbins, J. H. (1980). Radiosensitivity in Huntington's disease. Implications for pathogenesis and presymptomatic diagnosis. *Lancet* **i**, 9.

Myers, R. H., Goldman, D., Bird, E. D., Sax, D. S., Merril, C. R., Schoenfeld, M., and Wolf, P. A. (1983). Maternal transmission in Huntington's disease. *Lancet* **i**, 208.

Noronha, A. B. C., Roos, R. P., Antel, J. P., and Arnason, B. G. W. (1979). Huntington's disease: abnormality of lymphocyte capping. *Ann. Neurol.* **6**, 447.

Oliver, J. and Dewhurst, K. (1969). Childhood and adolescent forms of Huntington's disease. *J. Neurol. Neurosurg. Psychiat.* **32**, 455.

Perry, T. L., Hansen, S., Diamond, S., and Stedman, D. (1969). Plasma-aminoacid levels in Huntington's chorea. *Lancet* **i**, 806.

——, Wright, J. M., Hansen, S., and MacLeod, P. M. (1979). Isoniazid therapy of Huntington disease. *Neurology, Minneapolis* **29**, 370.

——, ——, ——, Thomas, S. M. B., Allan, B. M., Baird, P. A., and Diewold, P. A. (1982). A double-blind clinical trial of isoniazid in Huntington disease. *Neurology, Minneapolis* **32**, 354.

Rodda, R. A. (1981). Cerebellar atrophy in Huntington's disease. *J. neurol. Sci.* **50**, 147.

Scott, D. F., Heathfield, K. W. G., Toone, B., and Margerison, J. H. (1972). The EEG in Huntington's chorea: a clinical and neuropathological study. *J. Neurol. Neurosurg. Psychiat.* **35**, 97.

Shoulson, I., Goldblatt, D., Charlton, M., and Joynt, R. J. (1978). Huntington's disease: treatment with muscimol, a GABA-mimetic drug. *Ann. Neurol.* **4**, 279.

Sorbi, S., Bird, E. D., and Blass, J. P. (1983). Decreased pyruvate dehydrogenase complex activity in Huntington and Alzheimer brain. *Ann. Neurol.* **13** 72.

Spokes, E. G. S., Garrett, N. J., Rossor, M. N., and Iversen, L. L. (1980). Distribution of GABA in post-mortem brain tissue from control. psychotic and Huntington's chorea subjects. *J. neurol. Sci.* **48**, 303.

Stahl, W. L. and Swanson, P. D. (1974). Biochemical abnormalities in Huntington's chorea brains. *Neurology, Minneapolis* **24**, 813.

Tell, G., Böhlen, P., Schechter, P. J., Koch-Weser, J., Agid, Y., Bonnet, A. M., Coquillat, G., Chazot, G., and Fischer, C. (1981). Treatment of Huntington disease with γ-acetylenic GABA, an irreversible inhibitor of GABA-transaminase: increased CSF GABA and homocarnosine without clinical amelioration. *Neurology, Minneapolis* **31**, 207.

Thomas, S. (1982). Ethics of a predictive test for Huntington's chorea. *Br. med. J.* **284**, 1383.

Wallace, D. C. and Hall, A. C. (1974). Biochemical abnormalities in Huntington's chorea. *J. Neurol. Neurosurg. Psychiat.* **35**, 789.

Went, L. N., der Vlis, M. V., and Bruyn, G. W. (1984). Parental transmission in Huntington's disease. *Lancet* **i**, 1100.

Wherrett, J. R. and Brown, B. L. (1969). Erythrocyte glycolipids in Huntington's chorea. *Neurology, Minneapolis* **19**, 489.

Other forms of chorea

Choreiform movements, which are often unilateral, when they differ only in degree and severity from hemiballismus, may develop as a consequence of cerebral infarction in late life. When they are bilateral, they are often identified by the term *senile chorea*. The movements are troublesome but generally non-progressive and may be relieved to some extent by phenothiazines. Whether *dominantly inherited chorea without dementia* (Behan and Bone 1977) is a totally different disease from Huntington's chorea is still uncertain. Certainly different, however, is *familial degeneration of the basal ganglia with acanthocytosis* (Bird, Cederbaum, Valpey, and Stahl 1978), also called *chorea–acanthocytosis* (Limos, Ohnishi, Sakai, Fujii, Goto, and Kuroiwa 1982). This disease causes progressive chorea, oro-lingual–facial dyskinesia, and often polyneuropathy; it is usually fatal in the fourth or fifth decade and is of autosomal recessive inheritance. In another rare familial disorder of dominant inheritance, chorea is associated with myoclonic epilepsy, ataxia, major seizures, and dementia or mental retardation (Takahata, Ito, Yoshimura, Nishihori, and Suzuki 1978); in this condition, called *familial chorea with myoclonic epilepsy*, the principal nerve-cell loss is in the cerebellar dentate nuclei with gliosis in the pallidum.

Chorea as a manifestation of chronic liver disease, systemic lupus erythematosus and 'Moya-Moya disease' has already been mentioned, as has that which may complicate oral contraceptive medication (Nausieda, Koller, Weiner, and Klawans 1979). It can also appear transiently as a result of hypernatraemia (Sparacio, Anziska, and Schutta 1976) or during alcohol withdrawal (Fornazzari and Carlen 1982) and can be associated with polycythaemia and congenital heart disease (Edwards, Prosser, and Wells 1975). Congenital chorea in patients with hemiatrophy may be relieved by dantrolene sodium (Feit 1979).

Hemiballismus

Hemiballismus is a term applied to involuntary movements which affect the limbs unilaterally, though the face may rarely be involved. It differs from hemichorea only in degree, but the movements affect the proximal parts of the limbs to a greater extent, and hence lead to wide excursions, and they are practically continuous except during sleep. They are often so violent (Fig. 12.7) that the skin of the limbs may be excoriated. The lesion responsible is usually situated in the subthalamic nucleus (corpus Luysii) of the opposite side, but lesions have been observed elsewhere, especially in the corpus striatum and in the pathways connecting it to the subthalamic nucleus (see Whittier 1947; Meyers, Sweeney, and Schwidde 1950; Martin 1957).

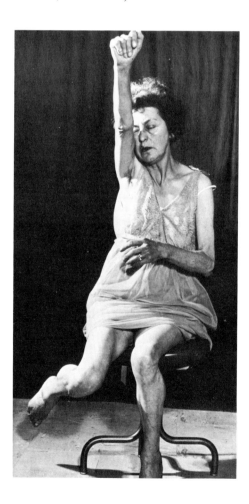

Fig. 12.7. Hemiballismus (photograph kindly supplied by Dr J.D. Spillane).

Spontaneous cessation of the movements is rare, and some patients have died from exhaustion. Phenothiazines such as tetrabenazine or perphenazine (Johnson and Fahn 1977) sometimes give partial relief, but when drugs are unsuccessful, stereotaxic thalamotomy, which is often justified, however elderly the patient, (Martin and McCaul 1959) may be dramatically successful.

Facial (tardive) dyskinesia

A parkinsoniam syndrome, choreiform movements, and/or segmental dystonia may develop in patients receiving long-term treatment with phenothiazine drugs for psychiatric conditions but usually improve when these drugs are withdrawn (*British Medical Journal* 1981). However, distressing facial dyskinetic movements with grimacing, chewing, and intermittent protrusion of the tongue are more disturbing complications of such treatment and unfortunately are often irreversible (Hunter, Earl, and Janz 1964; Evans 1965). Rarely, similar movements arise spontaneously in patients not taking drugs (Altrocchi 1972). Similar orofacial dyskinetic movements also develop in patients receiving levodopa for the treatment of parkinsonism, but unlike those due to phenothiazines they usually disappear when the dose of levodopa is reduced. Tetrabenazine, 25 mg four times daily (Godwin-Austen and Clark 1971; Asher and Aminoff 1981), thiopropazate (Singer and Cheng 1971) and sulpiride 300–1200 mg daily (Quinn and Marsden 1984) are among the remedies which have been found helpful in reducing these distressing movements.

Blepharospasm—oromandibular dystonia (Meige's syndrome)

This condition, also sometimes called Brueghel's syndrome (Marsden 1976; García-Albea, Franch, Múnoz, and Ricoy 1981) can, like the tardive dyskinesias described above, be a complication of long-term neuroleptic therapy (Weiner, Nausieda, and Glantz 1981) but more often develops without evident cause and is rarely familial (Nutt and Hammerstad 1981). It is characterized by blepharospasm and by repetitive sustained spasms or dystonic contractions of facial, mandibular, and lingual musculature, rarely spreading to the cervical, laryngeal, pharyngeal, and respiratory musculature. There is evidence in such cases of striatal dopaminergic preponderance (Tolosa and Lai 1979) with receptor hypersensitivity, and improvement may follow the use of haloperidol or deanol (Casey 1980), but lisuride seems likely to be even more effective (Micheli, Pardal, and Leiguarda 1982).

Palatal myoclonus

Palatal myoclonus is a condition in which rhythmical movements of the soft palate, occurring 60–180 times a minute, develop insidiously. They interfere with speech, swallowing, and respiration and usually persist during sleep. Rarely, after a few months, they resolve spontaneously (Jacobs, Newman, and Bozian 1981); more often they persist indefinitely. Often pathological examination reveals hypertrophy of the olivary nuclei (Koeppen, Barron, and Dentinger 1980); the condition appears to be a dysfunction of the olivocerebellar modulatory projection on to the rostral brainstem; the aetiology is unknown (Herrmann and Brown 1967). Ocular bobbing is a rare accompaniment (Yapa, Mayo, and Barron 1968). Usually no treatment is effective, but carbamazepine was helpful in one case (Sakai, Shiraishi, and Murakami 1981).

Gilles de la Tourette syndrome

This bizarre syndrome was first described in 1885 by Gilles de la Tourette who reported nine cases beginning in childhood with persistent multiple tics and coprolalia, a form of recurrent verbal utterance consisting of the expostulation of obscenities and swearwords. The disease is of unknown aetiology, has no known neuropathology and, to date, no consistent and precise abnormality of neurotransmitters has been identified (Friedhoff and Chase 1982). It is now thought that Dr Samuel Johnson suffered from the condition (*The Lancet* 1981). The vocal tics sometimes are associated with barks or grunts and some patients show echolalia and compulsive imitation of movements or gestures. The condition is often familial and has been noted especially in some Jewish families but certainly occurs in others (Eldridge, Sweet, Lake, Ziegler, and Shapiro 1977). While a psychiatric cause has been postulated, there can be little doubt that the condition is organic though it can be modified in its effects by psychogenic factors. The condition may resolve in females but tends to be more persistent in males. Haloperidol is the drug of choice, but clonazepam (Gonce and Barbeau 1977) and deanol (Finney, Christophersen, and Ziegler 1981) have proved to be of some benefit, and clonidine (Cohen, Young, Nathanson, and Shaywitz 1979) works in some patients resistant to haloperidol.

References

Altrocchi, P. H. (1972). Spontaneous oral-facial dyskinesia. *Arch. Neurol., Chicago* **26**, 506.

Asher, S. W. and Aminoff, M. J. (1981). Tetrabenazine and movement disorders. *Neurology, Minneapolis* **31**, 1051.

Behan, P. O. and Bone, I. (1977). Hereditary chorea without dementia. *J. Neurol. Neurosurg. Psychiat.* **40**, 687.

Bird, T. D., Cederbaum, S., Valpey, R. W., and Stahl, W. L. (1978). Familial degeneration of the basal ganglia with acanthocytosis: a clinical neuropathological, and neurochemical study. *Ann. Neurol.* **3**, 253.

British Medical Journal (1981). Tardive dyskinesia. *Br. med. J.* **282**, 1257.

Casey, D. E. (1980). Pharmacology of blepharospasm–oromandibular dystonia syndrome. *Neurology, Minneapolis* **30**, 690.

Cohen, D. J., Young, J. G., Nathanson, J. A., and Shaywitz, B. A. (1979). Clonidine in Tourette's syndrome. *Lancet* **ii**, 551.

Edwards, P. D., Prosser, R., and Wells, C. E. C. (1975). Chorea, polycythaemia, and cyanotic heart disease. *J. Neurol. Neurosurg. Psychiat.* **38**, 729.

Eldridge, R., Sweet, R., Lake, C. R., Ziegler, M., and Shapiro, A. K. (1977). Gilles de la Tourette's syndrome: clinical, genetic, psychologic, and biochemical aspects in 21 selected families. *Neurology, Minneapolis* **27**, 115.

Evans, J. H. (1965). Persistent oral dyskinesia in treatment with phenothiazine derivatives. *Lancet* **i**, 458.

Feit, H. (1979). A form of chorea that responds to dantrolene sodium. *Neurology, Minneapolis* **29**, 1631.

Finney, J. W., Christophersen, E. R., and Ziegler, D. K. (1981). Deanol and Tourette syndrome. *Lancet* **ii**, 989.

Fornazzari, L. and Carlen, P. (1982). Transient choreiform dyskinesias during alcohol withdrawal. *J. neurol. Sci.* **9**, 89.

Friedhoff, A. J. and Chase, T. N. (eds.) (1982). *Gilles de la Tourette syndrome*, Advances in Neurology, Vol. 35. Raven Press, New York.

García-Albea, E., Franch,O., Múnoz, D., and Ricoy, J. R. (1981). Brueghel's syndrome, report of a case with postmortem studies. *J. Neurol. Neurosurg. Psychiat.* **44**, 437.

Gilles de la Tourette, G. (1885). Étude sur une affection nerveuse caractérisée par l'incoordination motrice accompagnée d'écholalie et de coprolalie (jumping, latah, myriachit). *Arch. Neurol., Paris* **9**, 19, 158.

Godwin-Austen, R. B. and Clark, T. (1971). Persistent phenothiazine dyskinesia treated with tetrabenazine. *Br. med. J.* **4**, 25.

Gonce, M. and Barbeau, A. (1977). Seven cases of Gilles de la Tourette's syndrome: partial relief with clonazepam: a pilot study. *Can. J. neurol. Sci.* **4**, 279.

Herrmann, C., Jr. and Brown, J. W. (1967). Palatal myoclonus; a reappraisal. *J. neurol. Sci.* **5**, 473.

Hunter, R., Earl, C. J., and Janz, D. (1964). A syndrome of abnormal movements and dementia in leucotomized patients treated with phenothiazines. *J. Neurol. Psychiat.* **27**, 219.

Jacobs, L., Newman, R. P., and Bozian, D. (1981). Disappearing palatal myoclonus. *Neurology, Minneapolis* **31**, 748.

Johnson, W. G. and Fahn, S. (1977). Treatment of vascular hemiballism and hemichorea. *Neurology, Minneapolis* **27**, 634.

Koeppen, A. H., Barron, K. D., and Dentinger, M. P. (1980). Olivary hypertrophy: histochemical demonstration of hydrolytic enzymes. *Neurology, Minneapolis* **30**, 471.

The Lancet (1981). Tics and their treatment. *Lancet* **i**, 817.

Limos, L. C., Ohnishi, A., Sakai, T., Fujii, N., Goto, I., and Kuroiwa, Y. (1982). 'Myopathic' changes in chorea-acanthocytosis: clinical and histopathological studies. *J. neurol. Sci.* **55**, 49.

Marsden, C. D. (1976). Blepharospasm-oromandibular dystonia syndrome (Brueghel's syndrome). *J. Neurol. Neurosurg. Psychiat.* **39**, 1204.

Martin, J. P. (1927). Hemichorea resulting from a local lesion of the brain (the syndrome of the body of Luys). *Brain* **50**, 537.

—— (1957). Hemichorea (hemiballismus) without lesions in the corpus Luysii. *Brain* **80**, 1.

—— and McCaul, I. R. (1959). Acute hemiballismus treated by ventrolateral thalamotomy. *Brain* **82**, 104.

Meyers, R., Sweeney, D. B., and Schwidde, J. T. (1950). Hemiballismus. Aetiology and surgical treatment. *J. Neurol. Neurosurg. Psychiat.* **13**, 115.

Micheli, F., Pardal, M. M. F., and Leiguarda, R. C. (1982). Beneficial effects of lisuride in Meige disease. *Neurology, Minneapolis* **32**, 432.

Nausieda, P. A., Koller, W. C., Weiner, W. J., and Klawans, H. L. (1979). Chorea induced by oral contraceptives. *Neurology, Minneapolis* **29**, 1605.

Nutt, J. G. and Hammerstad, J. P. (1981). Blepharospasm and oromandibular dystonia (Meige's syndrome) in sisters. *Ann. Neurol.* **9**, 189.

Quinn, N. and Marsden, C. D. (1984). A double-blind trial of sulpiride in Huntington's disease and tardive dyskinesia. *J. Neurol. Neurosurg. Psychiat.* **47**, 844.

Sakai, T., Shiraishi, S., and Murakami,S. (1981). Palatal myoclonus responding to carbamazepine. *Ann. Neurol.* **9**, 199.

Singer, K. and Cheng, M. N. (1971).Thiopropazate hydrochloride in persistent dyskinesia. *Br. med. J.* **4**, 22.

Sparacio, R. R., Anziska, B., and Schutta, H. S. (1976). Hypernatremia and chorea: a report of two cases. *Neurology, Minneapolis* **26**, 46.

Takahata, N., Ito, K., Yoshimura, Y., Nishihori, K., and Suzuki, H. (1978). Familial chorea and myoclonus epilepsy. *Neurology, Minneapolis* **28**, 913.

Tolosa, E. S. and Lai, C. (1979). Meige disease: striatal dopaminergic preponderance. *Neurology, Minneapolis* **29**, 1126.

Weiner, W. J., Nausieda, P. A., and Glantz, R. H. (1981). Meige syndrome (blepharospasm–oromandibular dystonia) after long-term neuroleptic therapy. *Neurology, Minneapolis* **31**, 1555.

Whittier, J. R. (1947). Ballism and the subthalamic nucleus. *Arch. Neurol. Psychiat., Chicago* **58**, 672.

Yap, C. -B., Mayo, C., and Barron, K. (1968). 'Ocular bobbing' in palatal myoclonus. *Arch. Neurol., Chicago* **18**, 304.

13

Some congenital, developmental, and degenerative disorders

Cerebral palsy

The inclusive term 'cerebral palsy' was used by Ingram (1964) to identify a group of chronic non-progressive disorders of young children, present from birth, in which disease of the brain impairs motor function. The functional impairment may be the result of paresis, disorders of movement or incoordination, but motor disorders which are transient or are the result of maldevelopment or progressive disease of the brain or of abnormalities of the spinal cord are excluded.

The classification of conditions which fall into this group remains a matter of dispute but, modified from Ingram (1964) and Menkes (1980), the following is suggested as being reasonably satisfactory in the present state of knowledge:

Quadriplegia or tetraplegia
Diplegia (including hypotonic and rigid or spastic forms)
Hemiplegia and bilateral hemiplegia
Ataxia (cerebellar diplegia)
Dyskinesia (dystonic, choreoid, athetoid forms)
Mixed forms

To these groups may be added the disputed category of so-called 'minimal cerebral palsy' or 'minimal cerebral dysfunction' (Bax and MacKeith 1963). The dyskinetic forms of cerebral palsy have been considered in Chapter 12.

References

Bax, M. and MacKeith, R. (1963). Minimal cerebral dysfunction. *Little Club Clinics in Developmental Medicine*, No. 10. Heinemann, London.
Holt, K. S. (1965). *Assessment of cerebral palsy*. Lloyd-Luke, London.
Ingram, T. T. S. (1964). *Paediatric aspects of cerebral palsy*. Livingstone, Edinburgh.
Menkes, J. H. (1980). Textbook of child neurology, 2nd edn. Lea and Febiger, Philadelphia.

Congenital diplegia and quadriplegia

Synonyms. Congenital spastic paralysis; Little's disease.

Definition. The term 'congenital diplegia' is now used to include a group of cases characterized by bilateral and symmetrical disturbances of motility, which are present from birth and which subsequently remain stationary or show a tendency towards improvement. Though commonly the lesion involves chiefly the corticospinal tracts, causing weakness and spasticity, mental retardation, involuntary movements, and ataxia may be present in mixed cases in association with spastic weakness. Diplegia is the term traditionally used when all four limbs are affected but weakness and spasticity are more severe in the lower limbs, while quadriplegia or tetraplegia is the term employed when all four limbs are affected to an equal extent.

Aetiology and pathology

Cerebral palsy is found in between 1 and 2 per 1000 live births (Courville 1954; Department of Health 1970; Pharoah 1981). Of seven affected infants, one is likely to die, one will be grossly crippled physically, two severely mentally retarded, and one will be mildly affected with minor incapacity; the remaining two are likely to require special treatment (Menkes 1980).

There has been much dispute about the aetiology and pathogenesis of this condition. Plainly it is a disorder of multiple aetiology. Rarely it may be a consequence of traumatic intracranial haemorrhage resulting from precipitate, difficult, or instrumental delivery, whether due to tearing of dural venous sinuses or of cerebral veins and whether subarachnoid, subdural, or intracerebral (p. 235). Traumatic damage to the brainstem or upper cord is also uncommon (Towbin 1970). However, abnormal pregnancy, labour, or delivery (Ingram 1964) or prematurity and low birth weight (Polani 1958; Alberman, Benson and McDonald 1982) are clearly important factors leading to the birth of many diplegic infants. Prenatal or perinatal anoxia is plainly a major aetiological factor but complex neonatal metabolic abnormalities, especially hypoglycaemia, as well as disorders of cerebral perfusion resulting from brain swelling, increased vascular resistance, and hypotension all play a part in varying degree (Courville 1971; Menkes 1980). Kernicterus, usually due to Rh incompatibility and once a common cause of cerebral palsy, is now virtually a disease of the past (see below). Hyaline-membrane disease is associated with neonatal intracranial haemorrhage rather than directly with cerebral palsy (Leviton, Gilles and Strassfeld 1977), and chronic lung disease of prematurity is more often associated with progressive neurological deterioration and death (Ellison and Farino, 1980). Intracranial haemorrhage, neonatal seizures, and low birth weight are the risk factors most closely correlated with cerebral palsy (Nelson and Borman 1977; *British Medical Journal* 1978). There is a correlation between maternal epilepsy and various neurological abnormalities such as microcephaly, mental retardation, and febrile convulsions but not cerebral palsy (Nelson and Ellenberg 1982). There is no clear correlation with breech delivery (Faber-Nijholt, Huisjes, Touwen and Fidler 1983).

Severe anoxia alone may cause massive cystic degeneration of the central cerebral white matter, as Little (1862) originally showed, but this pathological change is rare in cerebral palsy. A more common finding, especially in premature infants, is periventricular encephalomalacia (Banker and Larroche 1962; DeReuck, Chattha and Richardson 1972), in which diminished arterial perfusion gives bilateral areas of necrosis and gliosis, sometimes but not invariably symmetrically distributed in the white and grey matter surrounding the lateral ventricles. In full-term infants multiple areas of cortical damage varying in distribution and severity and giving lobar or nodular cortical sclerosis (ulegyria), sometimes associated with cystic change (porencephaly) in the subjacent white matter are commoner. It is often difficult to distinguish between large intracerebral cysts (porencephaly) which may sometimes be developmental (Kramer 1956) and multilocular cystic encephalopathy (Crome 1958), often secondary to vascular damage. Severe neonatal polycystic encephalomalacia may, however, be a consequence of herpes simplex infection (Chutorian, Michener, Defendini, Hilal and Gamboa 1979). In the basal ganglia there may be spongiform degeneration (*status marmoratus*) or symmetrical demyelination with an appearance like the veining of marble (*état marbré* or *status dysmyelinatus*). The cortical changes are probably a result of infarction due to damage to small arteries or veins, but there is still dispute about the pathogenesis of the changes in the basal ganglia, although these, too, have been attributed to venous haemorrhage resulting from obstruction of the galenic venous system (Schwartz 1961). Lesions limited to the cerebellum with diffuse damage to the dentate nuclei and cerebellar cortex are seen in ataxic cerebral palsy but are much less common; clinical diagnosis from cerebellar agenesis, which, however, is often familial (Joubert, Eisenring, Robb, and Anderman 1969), may then be very difficult. Some indeed have questioned whether all such cases are due to maldevelopment, since many children have been found to have pathological changes in the cerebellum, without clinical manifestations and those with 'ataxic cerebral palsy' usually prove to have development anomalies (Menkes 1980). Perinatal damage to the brainstem due to compression of the vertebral arteries during delivery is even more rare (Yates 1959).

As will be seen, gross abnormalities of cerebral development, including anencephaly, schizencephaly, lissencephaly, macrogyria, micropolygyria, agenesis of the corpus callosum, and primary microcephaly may all produce some clinical features like those of cerebral palsy; infants with anencephaly do not survive, but the other disorders listed may all give mental retardation, seizures, and variable degrees of spastic paresis, sometimes compatible with long survival (see Menkes 1980). Many syndromes of mental retardation due to chromosomal anomalies (p. 471), specific metabolic defects (p. 452), and others of unknown cause may also be associated with variable neurological abnormalities.

Symptoms and signs

The symptoms depend upon the distribution of the degenerative changes in the brain. These may predominate in the prefrontal region, in the precentral gyri, or in subordinate centres concerned in motility and its co-ordination. Thus one function may be affected almost alone, producing types of congenital diplegia characterized by the predominance of: (1) mental retardation; (2) spastic weakness; (3) involuntary movements; and (4) ataxia. Mixed varieties, however, are common. Atonic cerebral palsy is a term applied to cases in which there is diffuse hypotonia in early infancy and childhood but often with brisk tendon reflexes and extensor plantar responses. In a few such patients spasticity develops later; many others develop ataxia or athetosis.

Frequently nothing abnormal is noticed about the child at birth and for some time afterwards, though diplegic infants are often difficult to feed. However, the increasing use of the Apgar scoring system in the assessment of the newborn (Drage and Berendes 1966; Nelson and Ellenberg 1981) and the examination of postural and other reflexes in young infants (Donovan, Coues and Paine 1962; Paine and Oppé 1966; Fenichel 1980) often assists in early identification, especially when primitive reflexes which normally disappear with maturation fail to do so (Menkes 1980). In some cases microcephaly and muscular rigidity are so marked that attention is drawn to them early. Sometimes the child is only thought to be abnormal on failing to reach a landmark of normal development at the expected time. Thus he may fail to take notice of his surroundings, to begin to raise his head when 3 months old, sit up at 6 months, and begin to walk and talk at the end of the first year of life. Diplegic children, too, are usually late in acquiring control of the sphincters.

Mental retardation (handicap)

Mental retardation can be the predominant symptom and may then occur without any gross disturbance of motility, except such clumsiness as results from inability to learn to control the limbs. In other cases retardation is associated with diplegia and may be severe, moderate, or mild. It is often severe in quadriplegic cases. Frequently the diplegic child seems more backward mentally than is actually the case, since his slowness in learning to walk, and his clumsiness in using his hands retard his mental development. Some children, though developing late, ultimately achieve high intelligence in spite of severe motor disabilities.

Weakness and spasticity

These symptoms, largely attributable to damage to corticospinal and extrapyramidal pathways, are usually remarkably symmetrical on the two sides. Rarely one side is more affected than the other. The lower limbs are usually more severely affected than the upper. The severity of the corticospinal defect varies greatly in different cases. When at its slightest, power and tone may be almost normal, the sole manifestations being exaggerated knee- and ankle-jerks, extensor plantar responses, and possibly slight contractures of the calf muscles, leading to moderate talipes equinovarus. Somewhat more severe changes cause a syndrome like that originally described by Little in 1862, in which weakness and spasticity are confined to the lower limbs and the muscles of the lower trunk. The lower limbs are rigid with plantar flexion of the ankle, extension at the knee, adduction and internal rotation at the hip, and with contractures in the spastic muscles. Voluntary power is often fairly strong, though hampered by the spasticity. The gait is characteristic, since the plantar flexion of the feet causes the child to walk on the toes; owing to adduction of the hips the knees may rub together, or may be actually crossed, the so-called 'scissors gait'. The tendon reflexes in the lower limbs are much exaggerated, the plantar reflexes extensor. The abdominal reflexes are often brisk despite the severe corticospinal lesion. Spinal deformities, such as lordosis and scoliosis, are common.

In the most severe cases (quadriplegia) the upper limbs and bulbar muscles as well as the lower limbs are severely involved and the posture may be decerebrate or decorticate, sometimes with preservation of tonic neck reflexes. In Ingram's (1964) series, no child with quadriplegia was found educable. In the upper limbs the rigidity is usually most marked in the flexor muscles; the involvement of bulbar muscles leads to spastic dysarthria and in severe cases to dysphagia. Dribbling of saliva is common.

Involuntary movements (extrapyramidal cerebral palsy)

Involuntary movements may be athetotic or choreiform, or may show features of both, being then described as choreo-athetoid. These movements are described on pages 322 and 342. In double athetosis, athetotic or choreiform movements are present on both sides of the body; in such cases there is no clinical evidence of damage to the corticospinal tracts and the plantar reflexes are flexor, but it is not uncommon to find athetotic or choreiform movements associated with spastic diplegia of the type described above.

Cerebellar diplegia

In this (ataxic) rare form of diplegia the symptoms are those of cerebellar deficiency, especially nystagmus, hypotonia, and ataxia (see Walsh 1963). In such cases hypotonia usually dominates the clinical picture at first; cerebellar diplegia is thus one cause of flaccid or atonic diplegia in early infancy although in some other cases with hypotonia and flaccidity the typical movements of chorea and/or athetosis appear in the second year of life.

Other symptoms

Optic atrophy, field defects, and cranial-nerve involvement are very rare but squint and nystagmus are common in diplegic children, and epilepsy occurs in about 27 per cent of cases (Ingram 1964) but in up to 50 per cent of those with quadriplegia (Menkes 1980). A moderate degree of skeletal infantilism is usually present, and puberty is often delayed.

Diagnosis

Usually diagnosis is easy, since the symptoms are clearly present from birth. The increased tone readily distinguishes spastic diplegia from benign congenital and progressive spinal muscular atrophy of infants, in both of which the muscles are flaccid. Difficulty may, however, be experienced in distinguishing these conditions from flaccid diplegia (due to ataxic or extrapyramidal diplegia) during the first 12 to 18 months of life. It is important to distinguish congenital diplegia from progressive cerebral disorders of early life, such as the lipidoses and the leucodystrophies, which also give bilateral spastic weakness. The distinction is based upon the fact that in such disorders the child is normal at birth and seems to develop normally in the early months, and symptoms, when they appear, become progressively worse, whereas in congenital diplegia the child is abnormal from the beginning and its condition remains stationary or slowly improves. This aspect of differential diagnosis has important genetic implications, as cerebral palsy is rarely familial while many leucodystrophies, etc. are inherited and may affect other sibs.

Prognosis

The prognosis of congenital diplegia depends upon its severity and especially upon the degree of mental handicap. In most severe quadriplegic cases the child may only survive for a year or two, often succumbing to pneumonia. Even when the disability is only moderate some affected individuals fail to survive beyond the early years of adult life. Although the condition sometimes remains stationary, there is often a very slow improvement in motor symptoms, both in those with spastic weakness and in those with voluntary movements, but this depends chiefly upon the mental state of the patient, and little improvement can be expected when severe mental handicap is present. In favourable cases it may be expected that a child will learn to walk, even though he may not do so until he is 5 or 6 years old.

Treatment

Treatment consists essentially in the education of movement, combined with the removal as far as possible of obstacles resulting from contractures and deformities. Much, therefore, depends upon the patience and care which are available for the education of the patient. Every effort must be made to help the child to learn to walk, and by means of simple games and occupations involving manipulative skill he must gradually be taught control over the movements of the upper limbs. Intensive physiotherapy is often of value but some specialized programmes of treatment in centres for the treatment of the cerebral palsied are based upon false concepts of neuromuscular function (Menkes 1980) and excessive physiotherapeutic effort must not be lavished on the hopeless case (Wilson 1969). In the United Kingdom, assessment and treatment centres established by the National Spastics Society play an invaluable role. Speech therapy often helps dysarthria. Treatment must be tailored to the needs of the individual case. Contractures may be dealt with by tenotomy, and in addition severe adductor spasm may be relieved by dividing the obturator nerve. Drugs such as diazepam, dantrolene and baclofen have some value in reducing spasticity and in occasional cases intrathecal phenol injections may relieve severe spasticity with flexor spasms. Levodopa has been thought to be beneficial in some cases of athetoid cerebral palsy (Rosenthal, McDowell and Cooper 1972) but its effects are marginal and other drugs such as tetrabenazine have been tried without benefit. Stereotaxic surgery is ineffective in athetosis but may be more helpful in cases with dystonia. Other surgical procedures designed to relieve spasticity and deformity have been utilized in selected cases (Samilson 1975). These operations, however, should be carried out only in children whose mental capacity and voluntary power will enable them to profit by them. Repeated electrical stimulation of the cerebellar cortex using platinum disc electrodes applied surgically to the exposed cortex with the aid of a portable receiver activated by an external transmitter has been claimed to reduce spasticity, athetosis, and dysarthria in many cases and to improve function and behaviour (Cooper, Riklan, Amin, Waltz and Cullinan 1976) but a recent controlled trial of such treatment failed to demonstrate benefit (Gahm, Russman,

Cerciello, Fiorentino and McGrath 1981). Epilepsy must be treated in the usual way.

References

Alberman, E., Benson, J. and McDonald, A. (1982). Cerebral palsy and severe educational subnormality in low-birthweight children: a comparison of births in 1951–53 and 1970–73. *Lancet* **i**, 606.

Baker, R. C. and Graves, G. O. (1931). Cerebellar agenesis. *Arch. Neurol. Psychiat., Chicago* **25**, 548.

Banker, B. Q. and Larroche, J. C. (1962). Periventricular leukomalacia of infancy: a form of neonatal anoxic encephalopathy. *Arch. Neurol., Chicago* **7**, 386.

British Medical Journal (1978). Preventing cerebral palsy. *Br. med. J.* **2**, 979.

Chutorian, A. M., Mitchener, R. C., Defendini, R., Hilal, S. K. and Gamboa, E. T. (1979). Neonatal polycystic encephalomalacia: four new cases and review of the literature. *J. Neurol. Neurosurg. Psychiat.* **42**, 154.

Collier, J. (1924). Pathogenesis of cerebral diplegia. *Brain* **47**, 1.

Cooper, I. S., Riklan, M., Amin, I., Waltz, J. M. and Cullinan, T. (1976). Chronic cerebellar stimulation in cerebral palsy. *Neurology, Minneapolis* **26**, 744.

Courville, C. B. (1954). *Cerebral palsy*. Courville, Los Angeles.

—— (1971). *Birth and brain damage*. Courville, Pasadena.

Crome, L. (1958). Multilocular cystic encephalopathy of infants. *J. Neurol. Neurosurg. Psychiat.* **21**, 146.

Department of Health (1970). *Cerebral palsy*. HMSO, London.

DeReuck, J., Chattha, A. G. and Richardson, E. P. (1972). Pathogenesis and evolution of periventricular leukomalacia in infancy. *Arch. Neurol., Chicago* **27**, 229.

Donovan, D. E., Coues, P. and Paine, R. S. (1962). The prognostic implications of neurologic abnormalities in the neonatal period. *Neurology, Minneapolis* **12**, 910.

Drage, J. S. and Berendes, H. (1966). Apgar scores and outcome of the newborn. *Pediat. Clin. N. Amer*, **13**, 636.

Ellison, P. H. and Farina, M. A. (1980). Progressive central nervous system deterioration: a complication of advanced chronic lung disease of prematurity. *Ann. Neurol.* **8**, 43.

Faber-Nijholt, R., Huisjes, H. J., Touwen, B. C. L. and Fidler, V. J. (1983). Neurological follow-up of 281 children born in breech presentation: a controlled study. *Br. med. J.* **286**, 9.

Fenichel, G. (1980). *Neonatal neurology*. Clinical Neurology and Neurosurgery Monographs, no. 2. Churchill-Livingstone, Edinburgh.

Gahm, N. H., Russman, B. S., Cerciello, R. L. Fiorentino, M. R. and McGrath, D. M. (1981). Chronic cerebellar stimulation for cerebral palsy: a double-blind study. *Neurology, Minneapolis* **31**, 87.

Holt, K. S. (1965). *Assessment of cerebral palsy*. Lloyd-Luke, London.

Ingram, T. T. S. (1964). *Paediatric aspects of cerebral palsy*. Livingstone, Edinburgh.

Joubert, M., Eisenring, J.–J., Robb, J. P. and Anderman, F. (1969). Familial agenesis of the cerebellar vermis: ataxia and retardation. *Neurology, Minneapolis* **19**, 813.

Kramer, W. (1956). Multilocular encephalomalacia. *J. Neurol. Neurosurg. Psychiat.* **19**, 209.

Leviton, A., Gilles, F. and Strassfeld, R. (1977). The influence of route of delivery and hyaline membranes on the risk of neonatal intracranial hemorrhages. *Ann. Neurol.* **2**, 451.

Little, W. J. (1862). On the influences of abnormal parturition, difficult labour, premature birth, and asphyxia neonatorum on the mental and physical condition of the child, especially in relation to deformities. *Trans. obstet. Soc., London* **3**, 293.

Menkes, J. H. (1980). *Textbook of child neurology*, 2nd edn. Lea and Febiger, Philadelphia.

Nelson, K. B. and Borman, S. H. (1977). Perinatal risk factors in children with serious motor and mental handicaps. *Ann. Neurol.* **2**, 371.

—— and Ellenberg, J. H. (1981). Apgar scores as predictors of chronic neurologic disability. *Pediatrics* **68**, 36.

—— and —— (1982). Maternal seizure disorder, outcome of pregnancy, and neurologic abnormalities in the children. *Neurology, Minneapolis* **32**, 1247.

Paine, R. S. and Oppé, T. E. (1966). Neurological examination of children. *Clin. Dev. Med.* **20/21**, 1.

Pharoah, P. O. D. (1981). Epidemiology of cerebral palsy: a review. *J. R. Soc. Med.* **74**, 516.

Polani, P. E. (1958). Prematurity and 'cerebral palsy'. *Br. med. J.* **2**, 1497.

Rosenthal, R. K., McDowell, F. H. and Cooper, W. (1972). Levodopa therapy in athetoid cerebral palsy. *Neurology, Minneapolis* **22**, 1.

Samilson, R. L. (1975). *Orthopaedic aspects of cerebral palsy*. Lippincott, London, Philadelphia.

Schwartz, P. (1961). *Birth injuries of the newborn*. Hafner, New York.

Towbin, A. (1970). Central nervous system damage in the human fetus and newborn infant. *Am. J. Dis. Child.* **119**, 529.

Walsh, E. G. (1963). Cerebellum, posture and cerebral palsy. *Little Club Clinics in Development Medicine*, No. 8. Heinemann, London.

Wilson, J. (1969). Chronic paediatric neurological disorders, *Br. med. J.* **4**, 152, 211.

Yates, P. O. (1959). Birth trauma to vertebral arteries. *Arch. Dis. Child.* **34**, 436.

Congenital and infantile hemiplegia

Definition. 'Congenital hemiplegia' is self-explanatory; 'infantile hemiplegia' is the term applied to hemiplegia which develops during the first few years of life Like hemiplegia in adult life, it is a symptom of many pathological states; the distinction between congenital and infantile varieties is largely artificial.

Aetiology

The cause of hemiplegia in childhood is often obscure, and there have been relatively few pathological studies of acute cases. The most convenient classification is one based upon the clinical features of hemiplegia, namely: (1) congenital hemiplegia; (2) hemiplegia complicating known infections; (3) hemiplegia of acute onset in the absence of any evident predisposing cause; (4) hemiplegia of slow onset.

1. Congenital hemiplegia is uncommon. There is a history of abnormal pregnancy or difficult labour in many cases, and the commonest cause is probably a vascular lesion occurring during birth. Norman, Urich and McMenemey (1957) discussed the aetiological factors, viz. a fall in systemic blood pressure, arterial compression owing to displacement of the cranial contents, and obstruction of the great cerebral vein. Ulegyria in the affected hemisphere is common (Benda 1952); almost as often the condition is due to a congenital malformation (Menkes 1980), such as true porencephaly or aplasia of one cerebral hemisphere. A cerebral vascular lesion or encephalitis occurring during fetal life are rare causes. Congenital double hemiplegia is distinguished from congenital quadriplegia by the more severe affection of the upper limbs.

2. Hemiplegia may complicate many acute infective disorders of childhood, but is commoner in some than in others. Whooping cough is a common association. Less frequently it occurs with measles, scarlet fever, diphtheria, chickenpox, smallpox, vaccinia, pneumonia, otitis media, septicaemia due to pyogenic organisms, typhoid fever, typhus, dysentery, or mumps. The relationship of the hemiplegia to the infection which it complicates is often obscure. Often the cerebral lesion is vascular. Thus meningeal and intracerebral haemorrhage have been described in whooping cough, and arterial thrombosis and embolism in diphtheria. Cerebral thrombosis, too, appears to be the commonest cause of hemiplegia in typhoid and typhus fevers and either cerebral venous thrombosis, cerebral abscess, or meningitis may cause hemiplegia in cases of otitis media. Acute haemorrhagic leucoencephalitis (p. 305) often, and acute post-infective encephalomyelitis (p. 300) less often, present with hemiplegia and may follow scarlet fever, smallpox, measles, or chickenpox. Sometimes there is a non-specific febrile illness of undetermined cause, heralded by recurrent fits or even epileptic status, with hemiplegia which becomes evident when consciousness is regained (Gordon 1976). Acute poliomyelitis, congenital syphilis, and tuberculous meningitis are rare causes.

3. Cases of hemiplegia occurring in early childhood without any obvious predisposing cause are slightly more frequent than those in the preceding group. Rarely it may be a manifestation of an encephalitis or toxic encephalopathy of unknown origin. In the majority, however, it is probably due to a vascular lesion, usually infarction, less often haemorrhage from an angioma or aneurysm, or subdural haematoma. Bickerstaff (1964) suggested that the condition is often due to internal carotid-artery thrombosis, perhaps as a result of carotid arteritis, resulting, for instance, from infected lymph nodes in the neck.

Infantile hemiplegia usually develops during the first three years of life and rarely after the age of 6.

4. Hemiplegia of slow onset is very rare in childhood. The causes include intracranial tumour, arising either in one cerebral hemisphere or in the pons, cerebral tuberculoma, and diffuse sclerosis.

Pathology

The pathological changes, as might be expected, are varied. Cases examined shortly after the onset often show focal vascular lesions, including meningeal and intracerebral haemorrhage or infarction. Ischaemic lesions within the fields of individual arteries or in the boundary zones between two arteries have been described. Sometimes the changes are those of 'acute haemorrhagic encephalitis', or post-infectious encephalomyelitis. In brains examined long after the onset of the hemiplegia, the changes commonly found are meningeal thickening, localized atrophic sclerosis, cysts, and pseudoporencephaly. The Sturge-Weber syndrome (p. 150) is a rare cause of infantile hemiplegia but the associated facial naevus and the characteristic intracranial calcification are distinctive.

Symptoms and signs

Congenital hemiplegia is usually detected at an early age, because the child does not move the affected arm and leg normally, or because these limbs feel rigid.

Infantile hemiplegia usually develops suddenly. When it occurs as a complication of an infective disease, hemiplegia does not usually develop until some days after the onset, usually during the second week and sometimes not until the patient is convalescent. Convulsions often occur at the onset. Consciousness is lost and the convulsive movements frequently predominate upon and may be confined to the side which subsequently becomes paralysed. Usually a series of attacks occurs during 24 hours and the patient remains comatose for a time, sometimes for several days after the convulsions stop. Headache, vomiting, delirium, and pyrexia frequently usher in the attacks. During the stage of coma the limbs on the affected side are flaccid and the plantar reflex is extensor. When the patient recovers consciousness, he is hemiplegic, and when the right side of the body is paralysed, usually aphasic also; sometimes there is intellectual impairment. In less severe cases hemiplegia may develop without convulsions and without loss of consciousness. The CSF may be normal or may show an increase in protein, red blood cells, or a leucocytosis, depending upon the nature of the cerebral lesion. In a patient with an intracranial angioma there may be a systolic bruit over the cranium or the carotid artery in the neck.

In favourable cases improvement occurs, and in a few weeks or months recovery may be complete. When the hemiplegia does not recover, flaccidity gives place to spasticity within a few weeks. The upper limb is severely affected as well as the lower and usually becomes spastic in an attitude of flexion, less often in extension. The signs of hemiplegia are described elsewhere (see p. 33). Disorders of sensation in the affected limbs are found on careful examination in about two-thirds of all patients (Tizard, Paine and Crothers 1954). Owing to the early onset, the development of the paralysed limbs is retarded and they remain smaller than those of the normal side; muscle fibres on the affected side are atrophic (Erbslöh, Reh, and Ziegler 1970). Contractures readily develop in both upper and lower limbs. When paralysis is incomplete, involuntary movements of an athetoid or choreic character may develop on the affected side and dystonic features develop in occasional cases many years after the onset. Homonymous hemianopia is present on the affected side in 17–27 per cent of cases (Menkes 1980). Facial weakness is common but involvement of cranial nerves is relatively rare. Epilepsy is much commoner than in cerebral diplegia, occurring in over 50 per cent of cases. The convulsions usually begin with tonic spasm or clonic movements of the paralysed side, but often later become generalized (Ford 1926) with loss of consciousness.

Diagnosis

Congenital hemiplegia is readily recognized: hemiplegia acquired in childhood must be distinguished from paralytic chorea, which is preceded by involuntary movements, and acute poliomyelitis which is rarely limited to one upper and lower limb and which is characterized by areflexia and muscular wasting without sensory loss. When the child is seen during an acute cerebral illness the subsequent development of hemiplegia cannot always be anticipated, but repeated convulsions, especially if these are predominantly unilateral, should suggest this possibility.

Hemiplegia of gradual onset is rare in childhood and is usually due to intracranial tumour. A CT scan and/or angiography may be needed in difficult cases.

Prognosis

Little improvement is likely to occur in severe congenital hemiplegia, but in mild cases careful education may enable the child to make some use of the paralysed limbs. It is exceptional for the lesion responsible for acquired infantile hemiplegia to prove fatal, but, if the child shows no signs of returning consciousness 48 hours after the onset of the convulsions, the outlook for recovery is poor. The more severe the symptoms of the acute stage, the more likely are mental handicap, aphasia, and hemiplegia to be persistent. Nevertheless, there are exceptions, and for several weeks after the acute stage there is no sure means of deciding to what extent recovery of function will occur. Some patients recover completely, but many remain intellectually impaired and hemiplegic, and of these more than half become epileptic. Less than a third become capable of an independent existence (Tizard 1953). The hope of considerable improvement should not be abandoned until at least a year has elapsed after the onset. Even after this interval some increase of power and co-ordination may occur in the paralysed limbs with treatment. Almost invariably the affected children eventually walk and lower limb function usually improves considerably but often little effective movement returns in the arm and hand.

Treatment

When the patient is unconscious the usual measures are needed (see p. 650). Otherwise treatment in the acute stage depends upon the cause. Cerebral oedema may require treatment with steroids, and hyperpyrexia with cooling. The after-treatment of hemiplegia, both of the congenital and of the acquired forms, includes active and passive movements to diminish the risks of contractures, and the correction of the latter by tenotomy when they develop. When any voluntary power remains, re-educational exercises should be instituted. Small doses of anticonvulsants should be given daily for several years in the hope of preventing epilepsy. Aphasia, when present, should be treated by speech therapy. In some cases with severe hemiplegia, intractable epilepsy, and behaviour disorder, the operation of hemispherectomy has been advocated and has resulted in marked reduction in the fits, improved behaviour and intellectual performance, and no significant increase in weakness of the affected limbs (Krynauw 1950; McKissock 1953; Wilson 1970). Unfortunately, follow-up studies of such cases have suggested that, save in cases of the Sturge–Weber syndrome (see p. 150), improvement after the operation may only be temporary and there is a high subsequent morbidity in over a third of cases, either due to persistent subdural haemorrhage, obstructive hydrocephalus, or haemosiderosis of the central nervous system due to chronic bleeding (Falconer and Wilson 1969). However, these long-term complications may be remediable so that the operation should still be considered in cases with intractable epilepsy, uncontrolled by adequate anticonvulsant therapy.

References

Benda, C. E. (1952). *Developmental disorders of mentation and cerebral palsies*. Gunne and Stratton, New York.

Bickerstaff, E. R. (1964). Aetiology of acute hemiplegia in childhood. *Br. med. J.* **2**, 82.

Erbslöh, F., Reh, H. E. and Ziegler, W. J. (1970). Kontrolaterale Hypotrophie de Skeletmuskulatur bei infantiler hemispastischer Cerebralparese. *Arch. Psychiat. Nervenkr.* **213**, 282.

Falconer, M. A. and Wilson, P. J. E. (1969). Complications related to delayed hemorrhage after hemispherectomy *J. Neurosurg.* **30**, 413.

Ford, F. R. (1926). Cerebral birth injuries and their results. *Medicine Baltimore* **5**, 122.

—— and Schaffer, A. J. (1927). The etiology of infantile acquired hemiplegia. *Arch. Neurol. Psychiat. Chicago* **18**, 323.

Gordon, N. (1976). *Pediatric neurology for the clinician*. Clinics in Developmental Medicine, nos. 59/60. Heinemann, London.

Krynauw, R. W. (1950). Infantile hemiplegia treated by removing one cerebral hemisphere *J. Neurol. Psychiat.* **12**, 243.

McKissock, W. (1953). Infantile hemiplegia. *Proc. R. Soc. Med.* **46**, 431.

Menkes, J. H. (1980). *Textbook of child neurology*, 2nd. edn. Lea and Febiger, Philadelphia.

Norman, R. M., Urich, H. and McMenemey, W. H. (1957). Vascular mechanisms of birth injury. *Brain* **80**, 49.

Tizard, J. P. M. (1953). The future of infantile hemiplegia. *Proc. Soc. Med.* **46**, 637.

——, Paine, R. S. and Crothers, B. (1954). Disturbances of sensation in children with hemiplegia. *J. Am. Med. Ass.* **155**, 628.

Wilson, P. J. E. (1970). Cerebral hemispherectomy for infantile hemiplegia: a report of 50 cases. *Brain* **93**, 147.

Minimal cerebral dysfunction

It has been suggested that in this condition, the cerebral abnormality, though not sufficient to cause easily identifiable syndromes of cerebral palsy, is severe enough to cause minor motor dysfunctions, epilepsy, learning difficulties, or abnormalities of behaviour (Bax and MacKeith 1963). The concept of minimal cerebral dysfunction was criticized as being 'an escape from making a diagnosis' (Ingram 1973; *The Lancet* 1973), and indeed many cases so diagnosed proved on careful scrutiny to be suffering from minor degrees of cerebral palsy in all its myriad forms. The hyperkinetic syndrome of infancy and early childhood (*British Medical Journal* 1975) has sometimes been considered erroneously under this heading. However, the term may still be usefully employed to identify those visuomotor disorders, abnormalities of cognition and execution, which may be found in minor degree in otherwise normal school children (Clements and Peters 1962; Brenner and Gillman 1966) and which may cause educational difficulties. Certainly there are some children who show no evidence of a lesion of the primary motor or sensory pathways but who have disorders of skilled movement (praxis), of the recognition and interpretation of sensory information (gnosis), or of speech and related faculties. Some such are the 'clumsy children' described by Gubbay, Ellis, Walton and Court (1965) who showed marked clumsiness of movement without paralysis, incoordination, or sensory loss. Improvement with increasing maturity was the rule but educational difficulties were striking initially in severely affected cases (p. 63) Many such patients also show semi-purposive involuntary movements, resembling those of chorea, and have also been identified by the term 'choreiform syndrome' (Kinsbourne 1980). It is still uncertain as to whether this syndrome of developmental apraxic or agnosic ataxia (Gubbay 1975), including the developmental Gerstmann syndrome (Benson and Geschwind 1970), is due to identifiable pathological changes in the brain, to a disorder of the physiological establishment of cerebral dominance, or sometimes to one cause or the other in different cases.

References

Bax, M. and MacKeith, R. (1963). Minimal cerebral dysfunction. *Little Club Clinics in Developmental Medicine*, No. 10. Heinemann, London.

Benson, D. F. and Geschwind, N. (1970). Developmental Gerstmann syndrome. *Neurology Minneapolis* **20**, 293.

Brenner, M. W. and Gillman, S. (1966). Visuomotor ability in schoolchildren—a survey. *Develop. Med. Child Neurol.* **8**, 686.

British Medical Journal (1975). Hyperactivity in children. *Br. med. J.* **4**, 123.

Clements, S. D. and Peters, J. E. (1962). Minimal brain dysfunctions in the school-age child. *Arch. Gen. Psychiat.* **6**, 185.

Gubbay, S. S. (1975). *The clumsy child.* Saunders, London.

——, Ellis, E., Walton, J. N. and Court, S. D. M. (1965). Clumsy children. *Brain* **88**, 295.

Ingram, T. T. S. (1973). Soft signs. *Develop. Med. Child Neurol.* **15**, 527.

Kinsbourne, M. (1980). Disorders of mental development. In *Textbook of child neurology* (ed. J. H. Menkes), 2nd. edn., p. 636. Lea and Febiger, Philadelphia.

The Lancet (1973). Minimal brain dysfunction. *Lancet* **2**, 487.

Kernicterus

This term has been applied to a disorder of infancy in which pathological examination of affected brains reveals canary-yellow staining of the meninges, choroid plexus, basal ganglia (especially the globus pallidus), the dentate nuclei, vermis, hippocampus, and medullary nuclei. In the affected areas there is widespread neuronal degeneration and secondary astrocytosis.

The condition is associated with an elevated blood level of indirect bilirubin to 20 mg per 100 ml or more in the neonatal period. Many reported cases were due to icterus gravis neonatorum (erythroblastosis fetalis or haemolytic disease of the newborn) due to Rh or other rarer forms of blood-group incompatibility in which, for instance, an Rh-positive infant with an Rh-positive father was affected by the passage of antibodies across the placenta from a previously sensitized but Rh-negative mother (Gerrard 1952). However, with at first exchange transfusion and, more recently, other methods of treatment and prevention, especially the use of anti-D immunoglobulin (see *British Medical Journal* 1981), kernicterus due to this cause has virtually disappeared. However, cases related to other factors, including prematurity, other forms of haemolytic anaemia, sepsis, acidosis, and the many causes of neonatal jaundice are still seen occasionally (Brown 1964; Menkes 1980). Experimental studies have shown, however, that a high bilirubin alone will not damage the developing brain (Vogel 1953) and it seems that only vulnerable nerve cells, perhaps abnormal as a result of various metabolic disturbances, such as anoxia, or exposure to drugs such a diazepam, vitamin K, or gentamicin, will be affected (Lathe 1955; Menkes 1980).

The affected infants are usually deeply jaundiced at birth, with bile in the stools and urine, hyperbilirubinaemia, and often haematological features of haemolytic anaemia. Many untreated cases were once fatal but few cases of neonatal haemolytic anaemia treated with early exchange transfusion developed kernicterus. Its development is usually heralded by coma, convulsions, and a decerebrate or decorticate posture with extensor spasms alternating with hypotonia. The survivors typically demonstrate nerve deafness, variable degrees of mental handicap, defects of vertical conjugate gaze, and neurological manifestations, resembling those

of bilateral choreoathetosis and/or dystonia (Evans and Polani 1950; Byers, Paine, and Crothers 1955; Schaffer and Avery 1977; Menkes 1980).

References

British Medical Journal (1981). Prevention of haemolytic disease of the newborn due to anti-D. *Br. med. J.* **282**, 676.

Brown, A. K. (1964). Management of neonatal hyperbilirubinemia. *Obstet. Gynec.* **7**, 985.

Byers, R. K., Paine, R. S. and Crothers, B. (1955). Extra-pyramidal cerebral palsy with hearing loss following erythroblastosis. *Pediatrics* **15**, 248.

Evans, P. R. and Polani, P. E. (1950). The neurological sequelae of Rh sensitisation. *Quart. J. Med.* **19**, 129.

Gerrard, J. (1952). Kernicterus. *Brain* **75**, 526.

Lathe, G. H. (1955). Exchange transfusion as a means of removing bilirubin in haemolytic disease of the newborn *Br. med. J.* **1**, 192.

Menkes, J. H. (1980). *Textbook of child neurology,* 2nd. edn, Lea and Febiger, Philadelphia.

Parsons, L. G. (1947). Haemolytic disease of the new-born. *Lancet* **i**, 534.

Schaffer, A. J. and Avery, M. E. (1977). *Disease of the newborn*, 4th edn. Saunders, Philadelphia.

Vogel, F. S. (1953). Studies on the pathogenesis of kernicterus. With special reference to the nature of kernicteric pigment and its deposition under natural and experimental conditions *J. exp. Med.* **98**, 509.

Zimmerman, H. M. and Yannet, H. (1935). Cerebral sequelae of icterus gravis neonatorum and their relation to kernikterus. *Am. J. Dis. Child.* **49**, 418.

Cerebral malformations

Infantile hydrocephalus has been considered in an earlier section of this book (pp. 137–142), while syringomyelia, spina bifida, and the conditions commonly associated with them will be described in Chapter 14 and developmental anomalies of the skull and skeleton will be dealt with in Chapter 21. It will, however, be convenient to mention here some of the commoner congenital malformations of the brain.

Anencephaly

This is the commonest major malformation of the CNS seen in the Western World, varying in incidence from 0.65 per 1000 live births in Japan to 3 per 1000 in the British Isles (Gabriel 1980). There has been a remarkable decline in its incidence in the Netherlands and Australia (Romijn and Treffers, 1983; Danks and Halliday 1983). It has been attributed to potato blight, hyperthermia, viral infection in the mother, anticonvulsant or phenothiazine medication, iodine deficiency, and softness of the water, but none of these theories has been proved scientifically. The cephalic neural folds fail to fuse into a neural tube with consequential degeneration of all forebrain germinal cells. The spinal cord, brainstem, and cerebellum are small, but the cord shows no descending tracts; above this level there are only a few glial and vascular tangles and remnants of midbrain. The eyes are normal but the optic nerves are absent and the calvarium is rudimentary. Fifty per cent of anencephalic fetuses are aborted spontaneously but if pregnancy goes to term the infants quickly succumb, showing only slow, sterotyped movements and frequent decerebrate posturing. Like spina bifida, anencephaly can be detected early in pregnancy by measuring alphafetoprotein (AFP) in the maternal serum or amniotic fluid (Brock and Sutcliffe 1972; Seller, Campbell, Coltart and Singer 1973; and see p. 419). After AFP estimation, the presence of anencephaly can be confirmed confidently by ultrasonic examination of the gravid uterus and indeed real-time scanning is generally regarded as mandatory prior to termination.

Holoprosencephaly

This defect, which varies in severity (Gabriel 1980) is one of failure of the primary cerebral vesicle (telencephalon) to divide and expand bilaterally. In its most severe form there is a single large cerebral ventricular cavity within an undivided prosencephalic vesicle and there is a single median eye (cyclopia). Less severe forms are associated with hypoplastic olfactory bulbs and tracts (arhinencephaly) and various midline facial malformations including hypertelorism and/or cleft lip and palate. The less severely affected infants show severe mental retardation, rigidity, seizures, and attacks of apnoea but few survive more than a few months.

Schizencephaly

The schizencephalies (Yakovelev and Wadsworth 1946a, b; Gabriel 1980) are a number of developmental defects in which there are bilateral congenital clefts in the cerebral mantle which extend from the cortical surface to the underlying ventricular cavities; the brain proximal to or below its clefts may be relatively normal, while that above is hypoplastic or rudimentary, so that the upper part of the cerebrum on both sides may be represented by a cyst covered with a paper-thin layer of nervous parenchyma. Differential diagnosis from *acquired porencephaly* (which is usually unilateral and due to focal infarction or other injury in fetal life or early infancy) may then arise, but that from *congenital porencephaly* (with absence of the corpus callosum and septum pellucidum and large ventricles) may be much more difficult. Transillumination of the infantile skull was often used in diagnosis but now the CT scan usually gives diagnostic findings. Affected individuals show spastic quadriparesis, seizures, and decerebration and rarely survive more than a few weeks.

Lissencephaly (agyria)

This very rare defect is one in which cortical sulci do not develop and the brain surface at birth remains smooth. The affected infants show decerebration, microcephaly, spastic tetraparesis, fits, and severe retardation. It may possibly be due to an autosomal recessive gene in some cases (Norman, Roberts, Sirois, and Tremblay 1976). Neuronal heterotopias in the white matter are common (Fenichel 1980).

Macrogyria (pachygyria)

In this rare disorder which is sometimes general, in which case severe mental retardation, spasticity, fits, and early death occur, or localized, when focal neurological signs may be seen, the gyri are excessively broad, coarse, and too few in number (Gabriel 1980).

Colpocephaly

In this uncommon condition a fetal configuration of the cerebral ventricles persists into postnatal life and the occipital horns are disproportionately large and dilated. The neurological manifestations are varied but tetraparesis, choreoathetosis, and optic atrophy are among the most frequent (Garg 1982).

Micropolygyria

In this condition there are too many tertiary and secondary gyri with neuronal heterotopias and abnormal lamination of cortical neurones. The clinical picture is either one of severe spasticity and mental retardation or of atonic cerebral palsy. There is also microcephaly (see below).

Microcephaly

This term, literally meaning small brain, is used to identify certain primary developmental anomalies (primary microcephaly) as well as secondary microcephaly which results from shrinkage of the brain (in neonatal hypoxia or encephalomalacia) or physical restriction of its development (as in craniostenosis, see p. 606). Primary microcephaly can be inherited as an autosomal recessive trait, in which case the brain at birth may weigh as little as 500 g, and may also show agyria, macrogyria, micropolygyria, corpus callosum agenesis, and neuronal heterotopias. Many such individuals demonstrate long survival, but with moderate mental retardation, fits and hyperkinetic behaviour, and variable spastic weakness of the limbs (Gabriel 1980). Microcephaly is also seen in some chromosomal disorders giving mental retardation and as a result of maternal irradiation or intrauterine infection with *toxoplasma*, cytomegalovirus, or rubella.

Rett's syndrome is a rare disorder causing developmental stagnation after apparent normal development for about 12 months followed by progressive dementia, autism, truncal ataxia, clumsiness of the hands, and acquired microcephaly: Subsequently prolonged arrest is common as is spastic paraparesis and epilepsy. The cause in unknown but as females are exclusively affected a dominant mutation on one X chromosome has been postulated (Hagberg, Aicardi, Dias and Ramos 1983).

Macrocephaly

This is a syndrome of diverse cause, defined as a head circumference more than two standard deviations greater than the mean for age, sex, race, and gestation (Gabriel 1980). It is most often due to hydrocephalus, however caused, in childhood, to Paget's disease or acromegaly in adults, but true *megalencephaly*, which implies an increase in the actual size of the brain as distinct from the skull, can be seen in various neuronal storage diseases and leukodystrophies, in tuberous sclerosis, and in the proliferative neurocutaneous syndromes as well as cerebral gigantism; these disorders are discussed in other parts of this volume. Primary megalencephaly, however, is a rare familial disorder, related to the phakomatoses such as tuberous sclerosis, and is often associated with abnormalities of cerebral cellular architecture and proliferation of glial cells and fibres. While many such patients are moderately retarded mentally and have epilepsy, the clinical picture is relatively non-specific. Some authors regard this condition as synonymous with cerebral gigantism (Fenichel, 1980). The CT scan is diagnostic.

Agenesis of the corpus callosum

This rare anomaly is often asymptomatic neurologically unless tests designed specifically to test the transfer of information from one cerebral hemisphere to the other can be employed. Even so, the deficit they show is less severe than that found after commisurotomy (Gott and Saul 1978). Various clinical syndromes, often resulting from associated developmental abnormalities such as hydrocephalus, microgyria, and corticospinal tract hypoplasia (Loeser and Alvord 1968 a, b; Parrish, Roessmann and Levinsohn 1979) have, however, been described, as has spontaneous recurrent hypothermia (Shapiro, Williams and Plum 1969). Ettlinger, Blakemore, Milner, and Wilson (1972) described behavioural studies which may be valuable in making the diagnosis, but if the anomaly is suspected, the CT scan is diagnostic. *Aicardi's syndrome* is a name which has been given to a group of cases, all female, in which severe mental retardation, flexor spasms, chorioretinal lacunae, vertebral and other developmental anomalies are associated with corpus callosum agenesis (de Jong, Delleman, Houben, Manschot, de Minjer, Mol, and Slooff 1976).

Cerebral white matter hypoplasia

This rare anomaly, in which the grey-matter structures of the brain are intact but there is gross hypoplasia of the white matter with consequential ventricular enlargement, was reported by Chattha and Richardson (1977) in 12 cases, three of them sisters. The affected individuals showed severe mental retardation, often spastic quadriparesis, and sometimes seizures.

References

Brock, D. J. H. and Sutcliffe, R. G. (1972). Alpha-fetoprotein in the antenatal diagnosis of anencephaly and spina bifida. *Lancet* ii, 197.
Chattha, A. S. and Richardson, E. P. (1977). Cerebral white-matter hypoplasia. *Arch. Neurol., Chicago* **34**, 137.

Danks, D. M. and Halliday, J. L. (1983). Incidence of neural tube defects in Victoria, Australia. *Lancet* **i**, 65.

deJong, J. G. Y., Delleman, J. W., Houben, M., Manschot, W. A., de Minjer, A., Mol, J. and Sloof, J. L. (1976). Agenesis of the corpus callosum, infantile spasms, ocular anomalies (Aicardi's syndrome). *Neurology, Minneapolis* **26**, 1152.

Ettlinger, G., Blakemore, C. B. Milner, A. D. and Wilson, J. (1972). Agenesis of the corpus callosum: behavioural investigation. *Brain* **95**, 327.

Fenichel, G. (1980). *Neonatal neurology*. Clinical Neurology and Neurosurgery Monographs, no. 2. Churchill Livingstone, Edinburgh.

Gabriel, R. S. (1980). Malformations of the central nervous system. In *Textbook of child neurology* (ed. J. H. Menkes) 2nd edn, p. 161. Lea and Febiger, Philadelphia

Garg, B. P. (1982). Colpocephaly: an error of morphogenesis. *Arch. Neurol., Chicago* **39**, 243.

Gott, P. S. and Saul, R. E. (1978). Agenesis of the corpus callosum: limits of functional compensation. *Neurology, Minneapolis* **28**, 1272.

Hagberg, B., Aicardi, J., Dias, K. and Ramos, R. (1983). A progressive syndrome of autism, dementia, ataxia and loss of purposeful hand use in girls: Rett's syndrome: report of 35 cases. *Ann. neurol.* **14**, 471.

Loeser, J. D. and Alvord, E. C. Jr. (1968 *a*). Agenesis of the corpus callosum. *Brain* **91** 553.

—— and —— (1968 *b*). Clinicopathological correlations in agenesis of the corpus callosum. *Neurology, Minneapolis* **18**, 745.

Norman, M. G., Roberts, M., Sirois, J. and Tremblay, L. J. M. (1976). Lissencephaly. *Can. J. neurol. Sci.* **2**, 39.

Parrish, M. L., Roessmann, U. and Levinsohn, M. W. (1979). Agenesis of the corpus callosum: a study of the frequency of associated malformations. *Ann. Neurol.* **6**, 439.

Romijn, J. A. and Treffers, P. E. (1983). Anencephaly in the Netherlands: a remarkable decline. *Lancet* **i**, 64.

Seller, M. J., Campbell, S., Coltart, T. M. and Singer, J. D. (1973). Early termination of anencephalic pregnancy after detection by raised alphafetoprotein levels. *Lancet* **ii**, 73.

Shapiro, W. R., Williams, G. H. and Plum, F. (1969). Spontaneous recurrent hypothermia accompanying agenesis of the corpus callosum. *Brain* **92**, 423.

Yakovlev, P. I. and Wadsworth, R. C. (1946*a*). Schizencephalies: a study of the congenital clefts in the cerebral mantle. I. Clefts with fused lips. *J. Neuropath. exp. Neurol.* **5**, 116.

—— and —— (1946*b*). Schizencephalies: a study of the congenital clefts in the cerebral mantle. II Clefts with hydrocephalus and lips separated. *J. Neuropath. exp. Neurol.* **5**, 169.

Tuberous sclerosis (Epiloia)

Synonyms. Bourneville's disease; Brushfield–Wyatt disease.

Definition. A rare congenital disorder characterized pathologically by sclerotic masses in the cerebral cortex, adenoma sebaceum, and tumours in various organs, and clinically by mental retardation and epilepsy.

Pathology

Macroscopically the brain may show microgyria or macrogyria, and absence of the corpus callosum has been described. The characteristic sclerotic patches to which the disease owes its name were first described by Bourneville and Brissaud in 1880. They are found in the cerebral cortex and are rare in the cerebellum. They are hard to the touch, and white in appearance, ranging from 0.5 to 2 cm in diameter. Microscopically they are composed of glial fibres, and also contain large cells, some of which are abnormal ganglion cells, while others are thought to be derived from spongioblasts. Tumour-like masses are also found in the cerebral ventricles and appear to be derived from ependyma. Occasionally a large glioblastoma or astrocytoma is found. Circular laminated bodies resembling corpora amylacea are found scattered throughout the cerebral cortex, cerebellum, choroid plexus, and the tumours themselves, and there is often cystic degeneration in the cerebral hemispheres and cerebellum, giving small cavities which

may be traversed by fine fibrils. The cerebral cortical ganglion cells are reduced in number and often atypical. The retinal tumours, phakomas, are composed of neuroglia. Adenoma sebaceum consists of hyperplasia of sebaceous glands embedded in a vascular matrix. Tumours in other situations include rhabdomyoma of the heart, teratoma, and adenosarcoma of the kidney, and growths have also been described in the thyroid, thymus, breast, and duodenum. Other occasional associated abnormalities include hydromyelia and spina bifida, and congenital cardiac malformations. The bones may show osteoporosis, cyst formation, and periosteal deposits which are visible radiologically (Holt and Dickerson 1952).

Aetiology

Beyond the fact that tuberous sclerosis is due to a congenital dysplasia arising in early embryonic life, little is known about its aetiology. In an analysis of 71 cases Bundey and Evans (1969) found evidence favouring simple autosomal dominant inheritance; sometimes the parent of an affected individual had adenoma sebaceum but no neurological abnormality, and involvement of more than one sib was relatively common. However, over 80 per cent of cases appeared to be due to new mutations. Marked discordance in a pair of monozygotic twins, one of whom was of normal intelligence, while the other was retarded, has been described (Gomez, Kuntz, and Westmoreland 1982) and was attributed to poor control of seizures in early life in the retarded twin. The condition is thought to be commoner in males than females and in the white races. It appears to be closely related to the syndrome of neurofibromatosis.

Symptoms and signs

The range of clinical manifestations has been reviewed by Nevin and Pearce (1968) and by Bundey and Evans (1969). In severe cases becoming manifest in early childhood, severe mental retardation and epilepsy are the rule and the fits often begin in the first year of life. Some young children present with 'infantile spasms' and with the EEG changes of so-called hypsarrhythmia (Pampiglione 1968; Pampiglione and Moynahan 1976). More often there are major convulsions, sometimes leading to status epilepticus, but minor and Jacksonian attacks may all occur. Focal neurological signs are uncommon except when a large intracranial neoplasm develops. In some mildly affected adults intelligence is normal but in others there is progressive dementia with psychotic episodes. Adenoma sebaceum, or epilepsy, or both may occur in patients of normal intelligence.

Adenoma sebaceum, which is not invariably present, manifests itself at about the fourth or fifth year of life as a pale pink, slightly raised rash, consisting of discrete spots, which fade on pressure, and appear first in the nasolabial folds, spreading over the face in a 'butterfly' pattern, sparing the upper lip (Fig. 13.1). A few scattered nodules may also appear on the forehead and neck, but rarely below the clavicles. After the second dentition the adenomas tend to coalesce and darken in colour to a deep red or brown hue. Exceptionally the cutaneous lesion does not appear until puberty or early adult life. Tumours in other situations occasionally grow large enough to cause symptoms. The retinal phakomas are flat, white, round or oval areas about half the size of the optic disc.

Diagnosis

Tuberous sclerosis can be distinguished from other causes of mental handicap associated with epilepsy only by the presence of adenoma sebaceum or retinal phakomas or of tumours elsewhere. The EEG is usually abnormal but the changes are variable and not diagnostic. Radiographs of the skull may show patchy calcification (Fig. 13.2) and pneumoencephalography is often diagnostic (Hudolin and Petrovčić 1957) showing protrusions ('candle-gut-

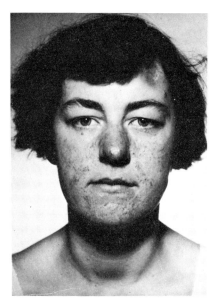

Fig. 13.1. Adenoma sebaceum in a patient with tuberous sclerosis. (Reproduced from Spillane (1975) by kind permission of the author.)

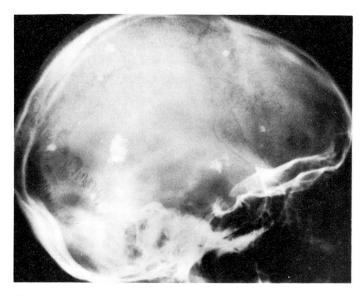

Fig. 13.2. Patchy intracranial calcification due to tuberous sclerosis in an adult.

tering') into the cerebral ventricles (Fig. 13.3). The CT scan can be equally informative.

Prognosis

Severely affected children often die between the ages of five and 15 years either from intercurrent disease or status epilepticus. Many mildly affected adults have a normal life span, but some die in middle life as a result of a tumour in the brain or in some other organ.

Treatment

Severe mental retardation may necessitate institutional treatment, and treatment appropriate for epilepsy should be given.

References

Bielschowsky, M. (1923–4). Zur Histopatholgie und Pathogenese der tuberösen Sklerose *J. Psychol. Neurol.* **30**, 167.

Brushfield, T. and Wyatt, W. (1926). Epiloia, parts I and II. *Br. J. Child Dis.* **23**, 178 and 254.

Bundey, S. and Evans, K. (1969). Tuberous sclerosis: a genetic entity *J. Neurol. Neurosurg. Psychiat.* **32**, 591.

Critchley, M. and Earl, C. J. C. (1932). Tuberose sclerosis and allied conditions. *Brain* **55**, 311.

Ferraro, A. and Doolittle, G. J. (1936). Tuberous sclerosis *Psychiat. Quart.* **10**, 365.

Gomez, M. R., Kuntz, N. L. and Westmoreland, B. F. (1982). Tuberous sclerosis, early onset of seizures, and mental subnormality: study of discordant monozygotic twins. *Neurology, Minneapolis* **32, 604.**

Holt, J. and Dickerson, W. (1952). Osseous lesions of tuberous sclerosis, *Radiology* **58**, 1.

Hudolin, V. and Petrovčić, F. (1957). A contribution to the diagnosis of tuberous sclerosis *J. Neurol. Neurosurg. Psychiat* **20**, 125.

Kessel, F. K. (1949). Some radiologic and neurosurgical aspects of tuberous sclerosis. *Acta psychiat. Kbh* **24**, 499.

Nevin, N. C. and Pearce, W. G. (1968). Diagnostic and genetical aspects of tuberous sclerosis *J. med. Genet* **5**, 273.

Pampiglione, G. (1968). Some inborn metabolic disorders affecting cerebral electrogenesis. In *Some advances in inborn errors of metabolism* (ed. K. S. Holt and V. P. Coffey,) Chapter 5. Livingstone, Edinburgh.

—— and Moynahan, E. J. (1976). Tuberous sclerosis syndrome: clinical and EEG studies in 100 children. *J. Neurol. Neurosurg. Psychiat.* **39**, 666.

Spillane, J. D. (1975). *An atlas of clinical neurology*, 2nd. edn. Oxford University Press, Oxford.

Neurofibromatosis

Synonyms. Neurofibroblastomatosis; von Recklinghausen's disease.

Definition. A disease of congenital origin, characterized by cutaneous pigmentation and tumour formation in various tissues. The commonest are cutaneous fibromas, mollusca fibrosa, and neurofibromas, but meningiomas and gliomas also occur. Combinations of these have been designated as separate syndromes. Thus Worster-Drought, Dickson, and McMenemey (1937) recognized the following:

1. Central type: (a) meningeal and perineurial—syndrome of Wishart (1822) which is rare. (b) Meningeal only—syndrome of Schultze (1880) which is the rarest. (c) Perineurial only—syndrome of Knoblauch (1843) which is the commonest.

2. Peripheral type. The peripheral neurofibromatosis of von Recklinghausen (1882) first described by Tilesius in 1793. The central and peripheral types may occur in combination. The condition is related to the other phakomatoses, including tuberous sclerosis.

Pathology

Neurofibromas are tumours usually situated upon peripheral nerves and composed of bundles of long spindle cells. There has been much controversy as to the nature of the cells of which they are composed. Russell and Rubinstein (1959) distinguished on histological grounds schwannomas, derived from cells of the neurilemma (sheath of Schwann), and neurofibromas, which they believed to be partly derived from fibroblasts as well as Schwann cells. Both may be found on peripheral and also upon cranial nerves, most often upon the vestibulocochlear nerve, but also upon others, especially the vagus, trigeminal, and hypoglossal, and they may occur upon spinal-nerve roots, usually the dorsal, or upon the cauda equina. Schwannomas particularly may be solitary. The cutaneous fibromas, or mollusca fibrosa, are formed from the connective-tissue elements of the cutaneous nerves. Nerve elements are absent, but there are characteristic whorls of spindle cells. The multiple cellular origin of most neurofibromas is demonstrated by the presence of glucose 6-phosphate dehydrogenase types A and B in many such tumours (Menkes 1980). No distinction is now generally made between Schwannoma and

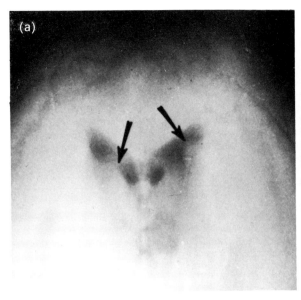 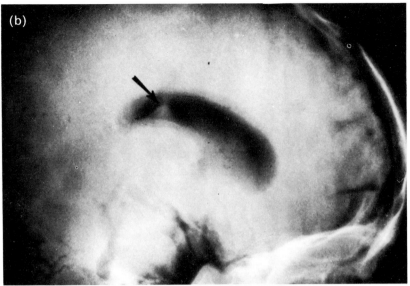

Fig. 13.3. Tuberous sclerosis: the pneumoencephalogram shows the characteristic lesions protruding into the cerebral ventricles. (a) Anteroposterior view; (b) lateral view.

neurofibroma (Kissel, Schmitt, and Andre 1975). It has been suggested that the serum of patients with this condition may contain increased nerve-growth-stimulating activity, but when a sensitive radioimmunoassay is used, this is only found in patients with central neurofibromatosis with bilateral acoustic neuromas (Siggers, Boyer, and Eldridge 1975). The bone changes associated with neurofibromatosis may consist either of hyperostosis or of rarefaction, with or without cyst formation. The cause of the 'scalloping' of vertebral bodies seen in some cases is unknown.

Neurofibromas may become sarcomatous. Abnormalities may also be present in the central as distinct from the peripheral nervous system. Patches of gliosis, neuronal heterotopias, and vascular malformations (Pearce 1967) and ependymal overgrowth may occur in the brain and spinal cord; syringomyelia, and even malignant tumours—glioma and ependymoma—may develop. Glioma of the optic chiasm is not uncommon and meningiomas are sometimes present. Pearce (1967), in a study of nine autopsied cases, found several intracranial gliomas which were clinically latent. Rodriguez and Berthrong (1966) reported a patient who had multiple intracranial meningiomas, an acoustic neuroma, multiple ependymomas, and syringomyelia. The condition has been described in association with Cockayne's syndrome (p. 464) (Felgenhauer and Ammann 1967) and with phaeochromocytoma. Neurofibromatosis is occasionally associated with other congenital abnormalities, such as spina bifida, cerebral meningocele, buphthalmos, syndactyly, and haemangiectatic naevi.

Aetiology

The disease appears to be due to a congenital abnormality of ectoderm and is inherited as an autosomal dominant trait. Some members of affected families show only cutaneous pigmentation, while others exhibit a more complete clinical picture. Bilateral acoustic neurofibromas sometimes occur in many members of a sibship in successive generations.

Symptoms and signs

Some of the signs of neurofibromatosis are present from birth, for example, cutaneous pigmentation. Others appear later, as a result of slow growth of the neurofibromas or of the reaction of other tissues to them. In some cases, however, the disorder is little, if at all progressive, and may be discovered accidentally. Except in those cases in which gross congenital abnormalities are present, the

patient does not usually seek medical advice until after the age of 20 years.

Cutaneous pigmentation

This is almost invariable. It consists of brownish spots, *café au lait* in colour, varying in size from a pin's head to areas the size of the palm. If five or more of these are present, even in the absence of cutaneous tumours, neurofibromatosis should be suspected. Unlike the *café au lait* spots of Albright's syndrome (polyostotic fibrous dysplasia) the patches of pigmentation in neurofibromatosis usually show a regular outline without deep indentations ('coast of California, rather than coast of Maine'). Occasionally a sheet of diffuse pigmentation is present on one or both sides of the trunk, corresponding to the cutaneous distribution of several spinal segments. Pigmentation is always most evident on the trunk and may be absent from the exposed parts.

Cutaneous fibromas

Cutaneous fibromas or mollusca fibrosa are soft, pinkish swellings, which may be sessile or pedunculated, and vary in size from a pin's head to an orange. They are often numerous and are found mainly on the trunk, but often there are some on the face (Fig. 13.4).

Neurofibromas

Neurofibromas are most easily found on superficial cutaneous nerves, especially those of the extremities and of the sides of the neck. They can be felt as moveable, bead-like nodules. They may be painful and are occasionally tender on pressure; sometimes they seem to grow within a nerve sheath, when pressure may produce pain along the nerve trunk and paraesthesiae in the appropriate dermatome.

Plexiform neuroma

'Plexiform neuroma' is the term applied to diffuse neurofibromatosis of nerve trunks, often associated with overgrowth of the skin and subcutaneous tissues. Large folds of skin may be formed, or there may be diffuse enlargement of the subcutaneous tissues of a limb, with or without underlying bony abnormality. The commonest sites are the temple, the upper lid, and the back of the neck. This hyperplasia has been called dermatolysis, pachydermatocele, and elephantiasis neuromatosa. Probably the famous 'Elephant

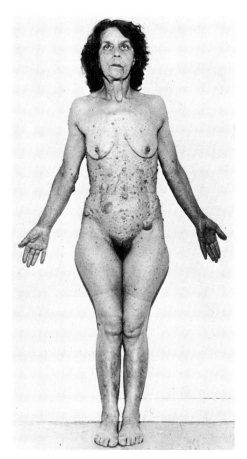

Fig. 13.4. Neurofibromatosis; note the multiple cutaneous tumours, especially on the trunk. (Reproduced from Spillane (1975) by kind permission of the author.)

Man' described by Treves was an example of this disorder. A similar hyperplasia may occur on one side of the tongue or gums.

Acoustic neuroma is described on pages 148 and 167.

Osseous manifestations

Kyphoscoliosis is often present and may be so severe as to cause spinal-cord compression. Even in the absence of intrathecal neurofibromas on nerve roots, characteristic concave 'scalloping' of the posterior borders of the vertebral bodies may be seen in radiographs of the spine. There may be marked hyperostosis of the bones of the face, with enlargement and rarefaction of the calvarium, often unilaterally. The long bones of the limbs may show subperiosteal hyperostosis, and their shafts may be curved.

Retinal manifestations

Phakomas, which are flat, white or grey, oval or circular masses, about half the size of the optic disc, may occur in the retina as in tuberous sclerosis (van der Hoeve 1923).

Visceral neurofibromas

Neurofibromas have been found on mucous membranes and in various viscera, including the adrenals. The vagus and sympathetic nerves may also be affected.

Mental retardation

About 10 per cent of patients are mentally retarded, often those with cerebral neuronal heterotopias.

Complications

Compression of the spinal cord may result from severe kyphoscoliosis or from a neurofibroma, or the scoliosis may lead to root pains. Neurofibromas within the skull may cause increased intracranial pressure, and focal compression of cranial nerves, especially the eighth (p. 167) or of the brain itself. Intracranial glioma or meningioma may be present. Sarcomatous change in a neurofibroma is manifested by a rapid increase in the size of the tumour, with compression and invasion of neighbouring structures. Epilepsy, acromegaly, adiposogenital dystrophy, infantilism of the Lorain type, phaeochromocytoma of the adrenal, and Addison's disease have all been encountered as complications (Saxena 1970). Optic atrophy may occur either as an associated finding or as a result of a glioma of an optic nerve or of the chiasm.

Diagnosis

The association of cutaneous pigmentation with neurofibromas and often with other associated abnormalities constitutes a unique clinical picture. Difficulties in diagnosis arise only when some of these clinical features are absent or inconspicuous. Thus a patient may present with symptoms of an intracranial tumour, spinal compression, scoliosis with root pains, hyperostosis, or localized elephantiasis. Careful examination of the skin for pigmentation, cutaneous and neural fibromas, will usually establish the correct diagnosis.

Prognosis

The disorder is not always progressive, but symptoms developing in a child or adolescent should lead to a guarded prognosis, as the disorder may later become fully developed. Pregnancy especially may cause exacerbation. Frequently the disease does not shorten life nor lead to marked discomfort. In severe cases death results from one of the complications described above, from intercurrent infection, or after a terminal phase of cachexia.

Treatment

Treatment is often palliative. Painful subcutaneous neurofibromas may be treated by excision. Suitable operative treatment may be required for associated intracranial or intraspinal tumours, or when a peripheral neurofibroma compresses a mixed nerve or becomes sarcomatous.

References

Bielschowsky, M. and Rose, M. (1927). Zur Kenntnis der zentralen Veränderungen bei Recklinghausenscher Krankheit. *J. Psychol. Neurol. Leipzig* **35**, 42.

Crome, L. (1962). Central neurofibromatosis. *Arch. Dis. Child.* **37**, 640.

Felgenhauer, W.–R.and Ammann, F. (1967). Syndrome de Cockayne fruste associé à la neurofibromatose de Recklinghausen. *J. Génét. hum.* **16**, 6.

Ford, F. R. (1966). *Diseases of the nervous system in infancy, childhood and adolescence*, 5th edn., p. 995. Thomas, Springfield, Illinois.

Kissel, P., Schmitt, J. and Andre, J. -M. (1975). Phacomatoses. *Encyclopédie Médico-Chirugicale* **1**, 79.

Lehman, E. P. (1926). Recklinghausen's neurofibromatosis and the skeleton. *Arch. Derm. Syph. Chicago* **14**, 178.

Menkes, J. J. (1980). *Textbook of child neurology*, 2nd edn. Lea and Febiger, Philadelphia.

Pearce, J. (1967). The central nervous system pathology in multiple neurofibromatosis. *Neurology Minneapolis* **17**, 691.

Penfield, W. and Young, A. W. (1930). The nature of von Recklinghausen's disease and the tumours associated with it. *Arch. Neurol. Psychiat., Chicago* **23**, 320.

Rodriguez, H. A. and Berthrong, M. (1966). Multiple intracranial tumours in von Recklinghausen's neurofibromatosis. *Arch. Neurol., Chicago* **14**, 467.

Russell, W. S. and Rubinstein, L. J. (1959). *Pathology of tumours of the nervous system*, pp. 236 et seq. Arnold, London.

Saxena, K. M. (1970). Endocrine manifestations of neurofibromatosis in children. *Am. J. Dis. Child.* **120**, 265.

Siggers D. C., Boyer, S. H. and Eldridge, R. (1975). Nerve-growth factor in disseminated neurofibromatosis. *New Engl. J. Med.* **292**, 1134.

Spillane, J. D. (1975). *An atlas of clinical neurology*, 2nd edn. Oxford University Press, Oxford.

van der Hoeve, J. (1923). Augengeschwülste bei der tuberösen Hirnsklerose (Bourneville) und verwandten Krankheiten. *Arch. Ophthal.* **111**, 1.

Weber, F. P. (1929–30). Periosteal neurofibromatosis, with a short consideration of the whole subject of neurofibromatosis. *Quart. J. Med.* **23**, 151.

Worster-Drought, C., Dickson, W. E. C. and McMenemey, W. H. (1937). Multiple meningeal and perineural tumours with analogous changes in the glia and ependyma. *Brain* **60**, 85.

Ataxia telangiectasia

This rare disorder, now classified with the phacomatoses, is of autosomal recessive inheritance and has been called the Louis–Bar syndrome. It is characterized by cerebellar ataxia with onset in infancy and with inability to walk by the age of 10 years. Telangiectasiae are seen in the bulbar conjunctivae and, later, on the skin. Most patients show a deficiency in serum gamma-globulin resulting in a diminished resistance to respiratory infections, one of which eventually proves fatal. Pathologically the Purkinje and granular cells of the cerebellum are selectively involved. Boder and Sedgwick (1963) reviewed 101 cases, Strich (1966) described the pathological findings in three cases, and McFarlin, Strober, and Waldmann (1972) reviewed its clinical features and immunology. The serum alphafetoprotein is raised to above 30 mg per ml in all cases, a finding suggesting widespread failure of tissue differentiation, especially in the liver, in such cases (Waldmann and McIntire 1972). Abnormalities of sensory and mixed evoked potentials have been demonstrated with other evidence of peripheral nerve involvement (Cruz Martínez, Barrio, Gutierrez, and López 1977). Recent work has shown that the condition is characterized by spontaneous chromosomal instability (confirmed by excessive radiosensitivity of cultured lymphocytes) and a proneness to develop cancer in addition to the severe immune deficiency and progressive neurological deterioration. There is also increasing evidence that these patients show a marked deficiency of DNA repair (Teplitz 1978; and see Bridges and Harnden 1982).

References

Boder, E. and Sedgwick, R. P. (1963). Ataxia telangiectasia: a review of 101 cases, *Little Club Clinics in Developmental Medicine* **8**, 110

Bridges, B. A. and Harnden, D. G. (1982). *Ataxia telangiectasia*. Wiley, Chichester and New York.

Cruz Martinez, A., Barrio, M., Gutierrez, A. M. and López, E. (1977). Abnormalities in sensory and mixed evoked potentials in ataxia-telangiectasia. *J. Neurol. Neurosurg. Psychiat.* **40**, 44.

McFarlin, D. E., Strober, W. and Waldmann, T. A. (1972). Ataxia-telangiectasia. *Medicine* **51**, 281.

Strich, S. J. (1966). Pathological findings in three cases of ataxia-telangiectasia. *J. Neurol. Neurosurg. Psychiat.* **29**, 487.

Teplitz, R. L. (1978). Ataxia telangiectasia. *Arch. Neurol., Chicago* **35**, 553.

Waldmann, T. A. and McIntire, K. R. (1972). Serum-alpha-fetoprotein levels in patients with ataxia telangiectasia. *Lancet* **ii**, 1112.

The hereditary ataxias

Definition. The term 'hereditary ataxia', though by no means completely descriptive, is a convenient one to apply to a group of closely related disorders, all genetically determined, and characterized pathologically by degeneration of some or all of the following parts of the nervous system—the optic nerves, the cerebellum, the olives, and the long ascending and descending tracts of the spinal cord. These localized degenerations occur in various combinations, with corresponding symptoms. Probably these disorders are closely related also to peroneal muscular atrophy and the other inherited neuropathies (see Chapter 18) with any of which they may, in occasional families, be combined. The age of onset

ranges from childhood to middle life, and the course is usually one of slow progression. Many different varieties have been described. Friedreich's ataxia is relatively common. Some forms have been described in only a single family. Each variety tends to breed true, but does not always do so, and more than one form may occur in the same family. In some families there is also a variable association with mental retardation, nerve deafness, and retinitis pigmentosa. By analogy with the storage disorders, including Refsum's disease and the disorders of amino-acid metabolism to be described in Chapter 15, it has been postulated that these conditions are each likely to be due to specific enzymatic defects; however, no such defect has yet been precisely identified and it is uncertain as to whether many different genes are involved or whether modification of the effects of only a small number of genes may account for the variable clinical manifestations and the frequency of transitional and hybrid cases. It would be impracticable to describe in detail all the forms of hereditary ataxia which have been described. The principal varieties were reviewed by Pratt (1967), Barbeau (1982), and Harding (1984). The following are the most important:

1. Hereditary spastic paraplegia.
2. Friedreich's ataxia.
3. The cerebellar degenerations, including the spastic ataxias.
4. Other miscellaneous heredoataxias.

Pathology

The pathology of the different varieties will be described in more detail in the appropriate sections. They present the following features in common.

There is degeneration of the ectodermal elements of the nervous system. The axons are usually affected more severely than the ganglion cells; in the later stages these also suffer, but it is difficult to say whether their degeneration is primary or secondary to axonal degeneration. The cerebellum and spinal cord are often smaller than normal and occasionally show congenital abnormalities. The brunt of the degenerative process usually falls either on the spinal cord or on the cerebellum but both may be involved. In the spinal forms some degenerative changes are usually found in all the long ascending and descending tracts, though predominant involvement of certain tracts determines the nature of the clinical picture. Thus the corticospinal tracts are most affected in hereditary spastic paraplegia; the corticospinal tracts, the posterior columns, the posterior spinocerebellar tracts, and the ganglion cells of the dorsal horns of grey matter in Friedreich's ataxia (Fig. 13.5); while the changes are most marked in the anterior columns in the various cerebellar ataxias. Degeneration is manifest in loss of both myelin and axons, with reactive gliosis. In many varieties there is also axonal degeneration in peripheral nerves (Hughes, Brownell and Hewer 1968).

Aetiology

The aetiology and pathogenesis of the hereditary ataxias is unknown. All appear to be genetically determined and most affect the sexes equally, but many cases are sporadic and even the individual disease entities vary considerably in their clinical presentation and course and in the mode of inheritance observed in different families (Bell 1939; Sjögren 1943; Pratt 1967; Barbeau *et al.* 1976, 1978, 1979, 1982). Hereditary spastic paraplegia is sometimes due to an autosomal recessive gene but is much more often dominant, while Friedreich's ataxia is usually recessive and less frequently dominant.

Many of the other cerebellar and/or spastic ataxias show recessive inheritance but, by contrast, the olivopontocerebellar degenerations are usually dominant, and so, too, may be some late-onset cerebellar ataxias (Harding 1981*a*). 'Pseudo-dominant' inheritance in Friedreich's ataxia may be due to homozygote–heterozygote mating (Harding and Zilkha 1981). In occasional families

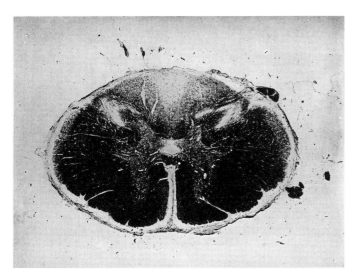

Fig. 13.5. Friedreich's ataxia. Spinal cord (myelin stain).

cerebellar degeneration may show X-linked recessive inheritance (Spira, McLeod, and Evans 1979) so that the position remains complicated. Linkage studies have suggested loose linkage between olivopontocerebellar atrophy and the HLA loci implying that both genes may be on the same chromosome (Nino, Noreen, Dubey, Resch, Namboodiri, Elston, and Yunis 1980), but in two other families van Rossum, Veenema, and Went (1981) were unable to find evidence that the ataxia locus was within measureable distance of the HLA locus on chromosome 6.

While, as indicated above, no specific biochemical abnormality has yet emerged in any of the hereditary ataxias, a defect of pyruvate metabolism associated with reduced serum and platelet lipoamide dehydrogenase (LAD) activity has been found in Friedreich's ataxia and other hereditary spastic ataxias (Kark and Rodriguez-Budelli 1979; Livingstone, Mastaglia, and Pennington 1980; Kark, Budelli, Becker, Weiner, and Forsythe 1981*a*) and it has been suggested that this may be useful in detecting heterozygous carriers of the gene and in preclinical diagnosis (Kark, Rodriguez-Budelli, Perlman, Gulley, and Torok 1980). Glutamate dehydrogenase deficiency has also been described in spinocerebellar degeneration (Plaitakis, Nicklas, and Desnick 1980). There is also some evidence of mitochondrial malic enzyme deficiency in such patients (Stumpf, Parks, Eguren, and Haas 1982) but the serum lipoproteins show normal fatty-acid profiles (Walker, Chamberlain, and Robinson 1980*a, b*). Reduced concentrations of aspartate in cerebellar cortex in some cerebellar degenerations (Perry, Kish, Hansen, and Currier 1981) probably reflect only loss of cerebellar neurones.

Clinical varieties

Hereditary spastic paraplegia

Families demonstrating both recessive and dominant inheritance have been described (Schwarz 1952; Schwarz, and Liu 1956) but in 22 families Harding (1981*b*) found that 19 showed dominant, three recessive inheritance. She identified two forms, one with an onset often in childhood (between 3 and 15 years and certainly before 35) (type I) and a second usually beginning after 35 (type II). However, the condition was genetically heterogeneous even within single families; Bone, Johnson, and Ferguson-Smith (1976) described the condition in only one of a pair of monozygous twins.

Pathology

The maximal degeneration is found in the corticospinal tracts of the spinal cord, especially from the upper thoracic region downwards. There are lesser degenerative changes in the posterior columns, especially the fasciculus gracilis, and in the large corticospinal cells of the precentral gyrus. While motor- and sensory-nerve conduction in peripheral nerves is normal, cortical and spinal somatosensory evoked potentials are markedly abnormal, confirming the posterior column dysfunction (Thomas, Jefferys, Smith, and Loulakakis 1981; Dimitrijevic, Lenman, Prevec, and Wheatly 1982).

Symptoms and signs

Symptoms of progressive destruction of the corticospinal tracts begin in the lower limbs. Attention is first attracted to the child on account of his stiff and clumsy gait. The lower limbs are weak and spastic, with exaggerated tendon reflexes and extensor plantar responses. The abdominal reflexes are diminished or lost, and pes cavus is usually present. Later the upper limbs are similarly affected, and finally, in some cases, the muscles innervated from the brainstem, with spastic dysarthria and dysphagia and loss of emotional control. The sphincters are usually slightly affected in the later stages. In spite of degeneration in the posterior columns, impairment of superficial or deep sensibility is usually slight. Intelligence is usually normal but mental retardation (Sutherland 1957), epilepsy (Bruyn and Mechelse 1962), cardiomyopathy with electrocardiographic abnormalities (Tyrer and Sutherland 1961), and optic atrophy with or without retinal pigmentation (Bickerstaff 1950; van Bogaert 1952) have been described.

Prognosis

The disease runs a slowly progressive course, weakness and contracture finally confining the patient to a wheelchair. However, despite the striking spasticity and clonus and grossly exaggerated lower limb reflexes, remarkably patients often manage to walk for 30 years or more after the onset. Death occurs after many years, usually from an intercurrent infection.

Friedreich's ataxia

This disorder is generally recessive and rarely dominant, but sporadic cases occur. The age of onset, interpreted as the age at which symptoms first bring the patient under observation, is usually between 5 and 15 years, though abnormalities such as pes cavus may be discovered in apparently normal members of affected families in early childhood. Exceptionally, symptoms first appear between the ages of 20 and 30 (Harding 1981*c*). There is no evidence of linkage between the causal gene and those responsible for any of the blood groups (Powell 1961) or with any HLA antigen (see Barbeau *et al.* 1976, 1978, 1979, 1982).

Pathology

The spinal cord is unusually small, but the cerebellum is usually normal. Histologically (Fig. 13.5), the degeneration is most marked in the posterior columns, especially in the fasciculus gracilis. It is most intense in the lower parts of the cord and diminishes towards the medulla. After the posterior columns, the lateral columns suffer most, especially the corticospinal tracts and the posterior spinocerebellar tracts, together with the cells of the dorsal nucleus, from which the latter are derived. The anterior spinocerebellar tracts usually escape. There is reactive gliosis. The dorsal-root fibres also degenerate, though their ganglion cells may be little affected. Sometimes there is some degeneration of anterior horn cells with resulting amyotrophy, often in distal-limb muscles.

The heart may show diffuse enlargement due to cardiomyopathy with diffuse fibrosis. Microscopically there is fatty degeneration of the myocardium with slight chronic inflammatory infiltration and fibrosis. Even when there is no involvement of lower motor neurones, large-diameter myelinated sensory fibres in the peripheral nerves usually show axonal degeneration with secondary demyelination (Hughes *et al.* 1968; Dyck and Lais 1972). Degeneration of vestibular and cochlear neurones occasionally occurs (Spoendlin 1974).

Symptoms and signs

As might be deduced from the pathological changes, the cardinal manifestations of Friedreich's ataxia are: ataxia, most marked in the lower limbs, with variable signs of spasticity; loss of deep reflexes; and, to a variable extent, impairment of sensibility, especially deep sensibility (vibration sense and position and joint sense). In addition, pes cavus and scoliosis are present, and nystagmus and dysarthria indicate a disturbance of cerebellar function at the level of the cranial nerves.

Signs appear first in the lower limbs, and it is the ataxic gait which usually first attracts attention. The patient walks on a broad base and tends to reel or stagger. In severe cases he is unable to walk without support on both sides. Standing is similarly affected, and he sways and may be unable to stand without support. The unsteadiness of stance is often intensified by eye closure. Ataxia of the lower limbs is usually less evident in movement of the limbs individually when the patient is lying in bed. In the later stages movements of the upper limbs also become ataxic, and intention tremor is occasionally seen. Slight involuntary movements, sometimes described as choreiform or myoclonic, are often present in the later stages. Irregular oscillations of the head are common. Nystagmus is present in 70 per cent of cases and is usually most marked on lateral gaze. Speech is invariably dysarthric in the later stages, the dysarthria being of cerebellar type. Speech is usually slow, monotonous, and slurred, and often scanning. It is frequently accompanied by vigorous grimaces and associated movements of the facial musculature. Corticospinal-tract degeneration leads to spastic weakness, most marked in the lower limbs, with loss of abdominal reflexes and extensor plantar responses. The tendon reflexes are lost owing to interruption of the reflex arcs on the afferent side but the jaw-jerk may be brisk (Salisachs 1979). The ankle-jerks are lost before the knee-jerks, and the latter may be exaggerated, owing to the corticospinal lesion, when the former are diminished. The limbs can be either hypotonic or slightly spastic, depending upon the relative severity of loss of afferent impulses, tending to diminish muscle tone, and of the corticospinal-tract lesion, tending to increase it. Sensory changes are variable. Shooting pains occasionally occur in the limbs. Postural sense and appreciation of passive movement and of vibration are usually impaired, especially in the lower limbs. In some cases all forms of sensibility are affected. The sphincters are usually unaffected, though incontinence of urine, and more rarely of faeces, rarely occurs in the late stages. Pes cavus and scoliosis are almost invariable, the former usually being associated with slight contracture of the Achilles tendon. Tyrer and Sutherland (1961) suggested that pes cavus is due to unbalanced action of the tibialis posterior muscle but the fact that it may be seen in otherwise unaffected sibs suggests that it and the scoliosis are more probably due to an associated abnormality of bony development.

Optic atrophy, retinal pigmentation, and deafness occasionally occur (van Bogaert and Martin 1974). Other rare ocular symptoms include ptosis, abnormalities of the pupillary reflexes, and ophthalmoplegia. Muscular atrophy is an uncommon complication but, when it occurs, resembles that of peroneal muscular atrophy. Harding (1981*b*) found such amyotrophy in up to 50 per cent of her cases. Associated congenital abnormalities include spina bifida occulta and infantilism.

Mentally, sufferers from Friedreich's ataxia are usually normal,

but schizophrenia has been described (Shepherd 1955) and mild dementia is occasionally seen in the later stages, leading to impaired intelligence and irritability. The CSF is normal. The EEG is frequently abnormal but the abnormality is nonspecific (Remillard, Andermann, Blitzer, and Andermann 1976). However, electroretinography and visual evoked potential recording (Carroll, Kriss, Baraitser, Barrett, and Halliday 1980; Kirkham and Coupland 1981) often demonstrate conduction abnormalities in the retina and in the visual pathways more posteriorly. Cortical somatosensory evoked responses following median-nerve stimulation also demonstrate impaired conduction in central sensory pathways in most cases (Jones, Baraitser, and Halliday 1980). Slight reduction in motor-conduction velocity in peripheral nerves, attributed to axonal degeneration in large-diameter myelinated fibres, has been described (Salisachs, Codina, and Pradas 1975) and abnormalities of sensory conduction and of evoked sensory potentials are more common (Dyck, Lambert, and Nichols 1974; Peyronnard, Lapointe, Bouchard, Lamontagne, Lemieux, and Barbeau 1976).

The cardiac changes may lead to heart failure, heart block, and electrocardiographic abnormalities (Evans and Wright 1942; Tyrer and Sutherland 1961); the echocardiogram may show evidence of cardiomyopathy and respiratory insufficiency is common (Cote, Bureau, Leger, Martin, Gattiker, Cimon, Larose, and Lemieux 1979). Diabetes mellitus may occur (Tyrer and Sutherland 1961) with an incidence varying from 8 per cent (Hewer and Robinson 1968) to 23 per cent (Hewer 1968) in different reports. Harding (1981*c*) found an incidence of 10 per cent.

Prognosis

Friedreich's disease is in most cases slowly but steadily progressive. Occasionally, however, it seems to arrest, and abortive cases are encountered, being discovered, for example, as non-progressive mild cases in apparently healthy members of affected families. Few patients, however, live more than 20 years after the onset; about three-quarters show evidence of cardiac dysfunction during life and over half die from heart failure, while diabetic ketosis and intercurrent infection are less common causes of death (Hewer 1968).

Treatment

Following the discovery of an abnormality of pyruvate oxidation in this condition, Barbeau (1978) suggested that there may be a deficiency of brain acetylcholine. In consequence, several trials of treatment have been conducted using the acetylcholine precursors choline (6–12 g daily) and lecithin (50–100 g daily). Lecithin failed to produce either clinical benefit or an increase in plasma free choline levels (Chamberlain, Robinson, Walker, Smith, Benton, Kennard, Swash, Kilkenny, and Bradbury 1980; Pentland, Martyn, Steer, and Christie 1981), but choline has produced limited clinical improvement in several trials (Barbeau 1978; Lawrence, Millac, Stout, and Ward 1980; Livingstone, Mastaglia, Pennington, and Skilbeck 1981), not only in Friedreich's ataxia but also in other forms of cerebellar degeneration. Oral physostigmine is also of minimal benefit (Kark, Budelli, and Wachsner 1981*b*). The place of these remedies in long-term treatment has yet to be defined, as has the role of lithium which, when given along with choline, increases blood levels of the latter.

The cerebellar degenerations including the spastic ataxias

Although the many forms of progressive cerebellar degeneration are very variable in clinical presentation and course, they show sufficient clinical and pathological similarity to justify their consideration together. The following are some of the more important varieties that have been described:

Sanger-Brown's (spinocerebellar) ataxia.
Marie's spastic ataxia.
Primary parenchymatous degeneration of the cerebellum (Holmes).
Olivopontocerebellar atrophy (Dejerine and Thomas).
Olivorubrocerebellar atrophy (Lhermitte and Lejonne).
Delayed cortical cerebellar atrophy (Rossi, Marie, Foix, and Alajouanine).

As their names imply, these forms of cerebellar degeneration differ in the precise localization of the degenerative process and its involvement of the brainstem. Their relationship was discussed by Critchley and Greenfield (1948) and Greenfield (1954).

Sanger-Brown's spinocerebellar ataxia

In 1892 Sanger-Brown described in 24 individuals, in five generations of the same family, a condition which usually began between 16 and 25 years with lower-limb ataxia and which later produced optic atrophy, ptosis, and diplopia (occasionally leading to complete external opthalmoplegia) with exaggerated tendon reflexes and ankle clonus but without nystagmus or pes cavus. Pathologically there was degeneration of the posterior columns and posterior spinocerebellar tracts with little change in the cerebellum and corticospinal tracts. Neff (1895) described a similar condition in another family, but beginning between the ages of 50 and 65 and sometimes producing dementia. While this condition is in retrospect somewhat reminiscent of the Kearns–Sayre syndrome (p. 579), there is no evidence that these patients showed retinal pigmentation which is virtually invariable in the latter disorder.

Marie's spastic ataxia

Marie, in 1893, under the title of 'hereditary cerebellar ataxia', described a group of patients suffering from cerebellar ataxia, progressive spasticity due to corticospinal-tract degeneration, and often optic atrophy. The onset was usually during adolescence. While some doubt has been cast upon whether this condition is a specific disease entity, spastic ataxia of this type with nystagmus, dysarthria, and optic atrophy certainly occurs in childhood or adolescence and runs a variable but progressive course (Hogan and Bauman 1977). Sometimes the syndrome is associated with paroxysmal dystonic choreoathetosis responsive to clonazepam (Mayeux and Fahn 1982).

Primary parenchymatous degeneration of the cerebellum

Holmes described four cases occurring in a single family, one studied pathologically. The cerebellum, pons, and medulla were abnormally small, especially the cerebellum, which histologically showed atrophy of all three cortical layers. There were also atrophy and gliosis of the olive and of olivocerebellar fibres in the medulla and inferior cerebellar peduncle. The midbrain, pons, and spinal cord were normal. The symptoms, which began in early middle life, between the ages of 33 and 40, were those of progressive cerebellar ataxia. Speech became explosive, and nystagmus and ataxia of the upper and lower limbs were present. Vision and the optic nerves were normal, the tendon reflexes were brisk, and there was no sensory disturbance.

Olivopontocerebellar atrophy

This was described by Dejerine and Thomas (1900). Some cases are sporadic but many families showing dominant inheritance have been reported.

The pathological changes consist of atrophy of olivary ganglion cells, and of the pontine grey matter, with degeneration of the middle cerebellar peduncles and to a lesser extent of the inferior peduncles. The cerebellum suffers mainly through atrophy of its afferent fibres. Purkinje and other ganglion cells of the cerebellar cortex are affected secondarily. It is the olive and the neocerebellum which undergo primary degeneration. The central nuclei of the cerebellum are relatively unaffected, but in *olivorubrocerebellar atrophy* these degenerate, as do the superior peduncles and the red nuclei. A detailed review of olivopontocerebellar degeneration and related disorders was given by Konigsmark and Weiner (1970). In a family with many affected members, Landis, Rosenberg, Landis, Schut, and Nyhan (1974) found in cerebellar biopsies from two patients severe degeneration of Purkinje cells, degeneration of cortical afferent fibres, and variable loss of granule cells. Tubular structures and crystalline inclusions were found on electron microscopy. Perry, Currier, Hansen, and MacLean (1977) found loss of cerebellar climbing fibres, reduced aspartate, and increased taurine in cerebellar cortex and dentate nuclei at autopsy.

The onset of symptoms usually occurs in late middle life up to the age of 60. Berciano (1982), reviewing 117 cases, found a significantly earlier age of onset in familial, as distinct from sporadic cases. The symptoms include dysarthria, ataxia and tremor of the limbs, ataxic gait, and sometimes muscular hypotonia. Nystagmus is usually absent. Voluntary power is well preserved and the reflexes may be normal; occasionally the ankle-jerks are lost. Parkinsonian features may develop, and dementia is common in the later stages. In some cases, spasticity, exaggerated reflexes, and extensor plantar responses rather than hypotonia occur and there is a static tremor superficially resembling that of Parkinson's disease. In some families there is also evidence of posterior-column dysfunction (Landis *et al.* 1974); Berciano (1982) stresses that ophthalmoplegia and involuntary movements are more severe in familial than sporadic cases and that dysphagia and incontinence are common in the later stages.

Dominant spino-pontine atrophy

This condition, described by Boller and Segarra (1969) and Taniguchi and Konigsmark (1971), gives severe progressive ataxia, nystagmus, dysarthria, hypotonia, hyperreflexia, and extensor plantar responses, beginning usually in adult life with preservation of the intellect and loss of vibration and tactile sensation occurring late. Affected individuals usually die between 30 and 57 years of age. Neuropathological examination shows marked degeneration of the nuclei of the basis pontis and of the cerebellar peduncles, spinocerebellar tracts, and posterior columns but the inferior olives are normal and the cerebellar cortex is preserved apart from minimal Purkinje-cell loss.

Delayed cortical cerebellar atrophy

Greenfield (1954) and Becker, Sabuncu, and Hopf (1971) considered that this condition is indistinguishable from the Holmes type of cerebellar degeneration (above). The condition is normally of late onset and dominant inheritance, presenting with truncal ataxia (Mauritz, Dichgans, and Hufschmidt 1979) and dysarthria followed by ataxia of the upper limbs. Pathologically there is atrophy of the vermis and cerebellar hemispheres with loss of Purkinje and granular cells and secondary degeneration of olivary nuclei (Hoffman, Stuart, Earle, and Brody 1971). The occurrence of tremor, brisk reflexes, posterior-column involvement, and extrapyramidal manifestations in some patients with a similar clinical presentation (Currier, Glover, Jackson, and Tipton 1972) makes differentiation from olivopontocerebellar atrophy (see above) difficult if not impossible. Indeed in a survey of adult-onset hereditary ataxia in Scotland, Koeppen, Hans, Shepherd, and Best (1977) found typical pathological findings of olivopontocerebellar degeneration at autopsy in two members of one family.

Cerebellar ataxia, corticospinal-tract and posterior-column involvement with ophthalmoplegia were the salient features of the so-called *Ferguson–Critchley type* of hereditary ataxia (Ferguson and Critchley 1929); in that family any single case would have been clinically indistinguishable from multiple sclerosis. Recently Harding (1981d, 1982) has concluded from a study of descendants of the family originally reported by Ferguson and Critchley (the Drew family of Walworth) that this condition should not be regarded as an independent disease entity. She concludes that the late-onset autosomal dominant cerebellar ataxias can be divided into four groups, namely: a pure cerebellar syndrome usually beginning at 60 years or later, corresponding to the Holmes type and to some of the cases described by Marie; cases of cerebellar ataxia with ophthalmoplegia, optic atrophy, dementia, extrapyramidal features, and amyotrophy (corresponding to some cases of the Sanger-Brown variety, some of olivopontocerebellar degeneration and some of spino-pontine atrophy); cases with pigmentary retinal degeneration with or without ophthalmoplegia, dementia, or extrapyramidal features (thus showing some resemblance to the Kearns–Sayre syndrome, apart from the age of onset); and cases with myoclonus and deafness (see below). Clearly in the absence of any indentifiable genetic markers and of any clear association with HLA haplotypes or other indices, classification remains arbitrary and uncertain.

Other miscellaneous heredoataxias

Many other variants of hereditary cerebellar ataxia have been described and the relationship of many of them to those described above is unclear.

The *Roussy–Lévy syndrome* (hereditary areflexia with distal amyotrophy and ataxia) shows certain affinities with Friedreich's ataxia on the one hand and with peroneal muscular atrophy on the other. Affected individuals have mild ataxia, pes cavus, distal amyotrophy in both the upper and lower limbs, and loss of the knee- and ankle-jerks, and the course is very slow with long periods of apparent arrest. The finding of multiple 'onion bulbs' in a nerve biopsy from one of the original cases described by Roussy and Lévy (1926) by Lapresle and Salisachs (1973) suggests that the condition is simply a variant of the hypertrophic variety of peroneal muscular atrophy.

A form of cerebellar ataxia of early onset with preserved tendon reflexes and without optic atrophy, cardiomyopathy, diabetes mellitus, or severe skeletal deformity, and with a much better prognosis than that of Friedreich's ataxia, has been described recently (Harding 1981e) and may prove to be a specific entity. An association of diabetes insipidus, diabetes mellitus, and optic atrophy (Page, Asmal, and Edwards 1976), of presumed recessive inheritance, but not accompanied by ataxia, has also been reported, as has hereditary optic atrophy, again without ataxia, associated with the A2 B8 haplotype (Stendahl-Brodin, Möller, and Link 1978). *Behr's syndrome* of heredofamilial optic atrophy beginning in early childhood and giving progressive visual failure, nystagmus, mild ataxia and spasticity, mental retardation, pes cavus, and urinary incontinence is thought on histological grounds to show some affinity with infantile neuroaxonal dystrophy (Horoupian, Zucker, Moshe, and Peterson 1979); it is usually recessive, rarely dominant.

An autosomal dominant form of hereditary ataxia identified first in Portuguese families in the Azores and in emigrants, but possibly existing in occasional families of non-Portuguese ancestry (Healton, Brust, Kerr, Resor, and Penn 1980) has been variously called *Joseph disease, Machado disease,* and *Azorean disease* (Sachdev, Forno, and Kane 1982). The clinical manifestations are somewhat variable but include various combinations of cerebellar ataxia, pyramidal and extrapyramidal signs, amyotrophy, dystonia, abnormal eye movements, and mild exophthalmos. Pathologically there is neuronal loss in the substantia nigra, cerebellar dentate nuclei, anterior horns, and Clarke's column, less often in the striatum. Abnormal protein patterns have been identified in

fibroblasts and in the brain (Rosenberg, Thomas, Baskin, Kirkpatrick, Bay, and Nyhan 1979; Rosenberg, Ivy, Kirkpatrick, Bay, Nyhan, and Baskin 1981).

Hereditary paroxysmal or periodic ataxia, sometimes beginning in childhood, sometimes in adult life, and usually of dominant inheritance, gives rise to episodes of severe ataxia, lasting for minutes or for a few hours and occurring every few days, weeks, or months. Vertical nystagmus may be seen during the attacks, less often between them. The cause is unknown although cerebellar dysfunction has been postulated and it is possible that sporadic cases may occur. The attacks may be completely abolished by acetazolamide, 250 mg twice daily (Griggs, Moxley, Lafrance, and McQuillen 1978; Donat and Auger 1979).

In *dyssynergia cerebellaris myoclonica* (the Ramsay–Hunt syndrome) progressive cerebellar ataxia with nystagmus and dysarthria is accompanied by repeated myoclonus and sometimes mental retardation, but the progressive dementia seen in progressive myoclonic epilepsy (p. 631) does not occur; no Lafora bodies are found in the brain at post-mortem examination, but there is severe degeneration of the dentate and red nuclei (Hunt 1921) and of the cerebral cortex and spinocerebellar tracts (Bird and Shaw 1978). Myoclonus may be precipitated by photic stimulation (Kreindler, Crighel, and Poilici 1959); a similar syndrome associated with nerve deafness has been described (May and White 1968).

Some cases also show a neuropathy with features of both Friedreich's ataxia and peroneal muscular atrophy, as well as myoclonic epilepsy (Smith, Espir, and Matthews 1978). Familial myoclonic epilepsy with dementia and choreoathetosis due to 'hereditary dentatorubral-pallidoluysian atrophy' is clearly closely related but may be pathologically distinct (Naito and Oyanagi 1982).

Other rare combinations include ataxia, nerve deafness, mental retardation, and signs of upper and lower motor-neurone lesions beginning in infancy (Berman, Haslam, Konigsmark, Capute, and Migeon 1973), familial agenesis of the vermis with episodic hypernoea, abnormal eye movements, and mental retardation (Joubert, Eisenring, and Robb 1969) and dominantly inherited cerebellar ataxia of late onset with defective optokinetic nystagmus and absent or abnormal oculovestibular reflexes but with preservation of cochlear function (Philcox, Sellars, Pamplett, and Beighton 1975). Similar abnormalities of eye movement and of vestibulo-ocular reflexes, with unstable fixation and dysmetria of voluntary saccades may, however, be found in many variants of hereditary ataxia, including Friedreich's ataxia (Baloh, Konrad, and Honrubia 1975).

In the rare autosomal recessive syndrome often called the *Marinesco–Sjögren syndrome* (Marinesco, Draganesco, and Vasiliu 1931; Sjögren 1950; Garland and Moorhouse 1953; Ron and Pearce 1971), somatic and mental retardation are accompanied by cerebellar ataxia, cataracts, and sometimes by epilepsy, microcephaly, and corticospinal-tract dysfunction.

The *Sjögren–Larsson syndrome*, which is also an autosomal recessive disorder (Sjögren and Larsson 1957), is characterized by congenital ichthyosis, mental retardation, spasticity, epilepsy, macular degeneration, abnormalities of the teeth, and hypertelorism (Guilleminault, Harpey, and Lafourcasde 1973). Amino-acid excretion may be abnormal (Ionasescu, Stegink, Mueller, and Weinstein 1973) and the condition may be due to an as yet unidentified disorder of lipid metabolism which may possibly be influenced favourably by giving a diet with medium-chain triglycerides.

Other rare disorders tentatively classified with the hereditary ataxias

Fahr's disease (familial calcification of the basal ganglia), a condition of autosomal dominant inheritance, has been described as beginning early in life with progressive dementia, convulsions, and rigidity. Calcification in the walls of the vessels of the lenticular and dentate nuclei may be seen on skull radiographs (Foley 1951).

Cerebellar ataxia and pigmentary macular degeneration occasionally occur (Strobos, de la Torre, and Martin 1957). However, the frequency with which basal-ganglia calcification is found incidentally in the CT scan (Brannan, Burger, and Chaudhary 1980) has cast doubt upon the significance of this finding. Certainly it is often seen in idiopathic hypoparathyroidism and related disorders and there may be a specific disorder, ferrocalcinosis, which can be identified as Fahr's disease. However, at least 24 conditions have been described in which this radiological abnormality has been seen and yet the majority of those who show it are asymptomatic (Harrington, MacPherson, McIntosh, Allam, and Bone 1981).

Other rare combinations of neurological features include neurofibromatosis, peroneal muscular atrophy, congenital deafness, partial albinism, and Axenfeld's defect of the iridocorneal angle occurring in several members of two generations of a family (Bradley, Richardson, and Frew 1974), optic atrophy, nerve deafness, and distal neurogenic atrophy (Iwashita, Inoue, Arati, and Kuroiwa 1970), and distal muscular atrophy, ataxia, retinitis pigmentosa, and diabetes mellitus of dominant inheritance without the biochemical features of Refsum's disease (Furukawa, Takagi, Nakao, Sugita, Tsukagoshi, and Tsubaki 1968).

Usher's syndrome is the name which has been given to the combination of congenital deafness and retinitis pigmentosa giving progressive blindness (Usher 1914; Vernon 1969); there is still dispute as to whether this condition is identical with or different from *Hallgren's syndrome*, in which the same two salient clinical features are sometimes associated with vestibulo-cerebellar ataxia and mental retardation in some members of affected families (Hallgren 1959; Merin, Abraham, and Auerbach 1974). Both are of autosomal recessive inheritance. Certainly, similar tapeto-retinal degeneration may be associated with many of the hereditary ataxias described above (François 1974).

Xeroderma pigmentosum is a rare autosomal recessive disease characterized by abnormal sensitivity to sunlight with pigmentary changes in the skin, telangiectases, keratoses, and eventually cutaneous carcinomata. Neurological complications include progressive dementia, chorea, nerve deafness, corticospinal-tract degeneration, peripheral neuropathy, and skeletal abnormalities (Waltimo, Iivanainen, and Hokkanen 1967; Thrush, Holti, Bradley, Campbell, and Walton 1974). *Köhlmeier–Degos disease* (*malignant atrophic papillosis*) is probably not familial but is a lethal cutaneosystemic vasculopathy of unknown aetiology which rarely affects the nervous system, giving dementia, progressive paresis, and sometimes subarachnoid haemorrhage (Petit, Saso, and Higman 1982).

Diagnosis

The diagnosis of the hereditary ataxias rests upon the development, often in early life, of progressive ataxia, often accompanied by symptoms of bilateral corticospinal-tract degeneration, sensory loss, pes cavus and scoliosis, and sometimes optic atrophy. When there is a clear family history it is usually easy to make a correct diagnosis. Sporadic cases, however, may give difficulty. Hereditary spastic paraplegia must be distinguished from congenital diplegia by the fact that the patient is normal at birth, and the disorder is progressive, whereas in diplegia the symptoms are congenital, and tend to improve. Friedreich's ataxia must be distinguished from multiple sclerosis. It frequently begins before the age of 15, when the onset of multiple sclerosis is rare. Both disorders are characterized by nystagmus, ataxia, and extensor plantar responses, but scoliosis, pes cavus, and loss of the knee- and ankle-jerks are peculiar to Friedreich's disease.

The progressive hereditary cerebellar degenerations of late middle life are to be distinguished from sporadic spinocerebellar degeneration arising as a complication of carcinoma in the lung or elsewhere; from tumours, by the absence of increased intracranial pressure; from tabes, by the usual preservation of the tendon reflexes, and the absence of sensory loss and of pupillary and serological abnormalities; and from subacute combined degeneration, by the absence of paraesthesiae, sensory loss, and a normal serum B_{12}. It should be remembered, too, that progressive multisystem degeneration, the Shy–Drager syndrome (p. 599) may present in middle or late life with cerebellar ataxia or extrapyramidal manifestations, and autonomic dysfunction may at first be difficult to detect.

From the bewildering variety of neurological symptoms and signs described above, it is apparent that until specific enzymatic or other biochemical defects underlying various manifestations of these syndromes are identified, classification will always be difficult. Many cases continue to occur which cannot readily be identified as belonging to any of the varieties listed. As knowledge extends, more and more of these disorders may eventually be identified as inborn errors of metabolism. For the present, however unsatisfactory it may be, ignorance of aetiology demands that they can only be classified by 'pattern recognition' of various complexes of symptoms and signs.

Treatment

Drug treatment of Friedreich's ataxia has been considered above (p. 364). Although many patients ultimately become bedridden, this should be postponed as long as possible and often a wheelchair and other appropriate aids are required. Physiotherapy and walking exercises may temporarily modify the ataxia and the help and advice of an occupational therapist may be invaluable. In Friedreich's ataxia the pes cavus may require surgical treatment or special shoes and a spinal support or Luque operation may be needed to control scoliosis. In the later stages respiratory and urinary infections will require appropriate measures.

References

Baloh, R. W., Konrad, H. R. and Honrubia, V. (1975). Vestibulo-ocular function in patients with cerebellar atrophy. *Neurology, Minneapolis* **25**, 160.

Barbeau, A. (1978). Emerging treatments: replacement therapy with choline or lecithin in neurological disease. *Can. J. neurol. Sci.* **5**, 157.

—— (1982). A tentative classification of recessively inherited ataxias. *Can. J. Neurol. Sci* **9**, 95.

—— et al. (1976). Quebec cooperative study of Friedreich's ataxia—phase one. *Can. J. neurol. Sci.* **3**, 269–397.

—— et al. (1978). Quebec cooperative study of Friedreich's ataxia—phase two, part one. *Can. J. neurol. Sci.* **5**, 53–165.

—— (1979). Quebec cooperative study of Friedreich's ataxia—phase two, part two. *Can. J. neurol. Sci.* **6**, 145–319.

—— et al. (1982). Quebec cooperative study of Friedreich's ataxia—phase three. *Can. J. neurol. Sci.* **9**, 91–263.

Becker, P. E., Sabuncu, N. and Hopf, H. C. (1971). Dominant erblicher Typ von 'cerebellarer Ataxia' *Z. Neurol.* **199**, 116.

Bell, J. (1939). Hereditary ataxia and spastic paraplegia. *Treasury of human inheritance*, Vol. iv, Pt. 3. University Press, Cambridge.

Berciano, J. (1982). Olivopontocerebellar atrophy: a review of 117 cases. *J. neurol. Sci.* **53**, 253.

Berman, W., Haslam, R. H. A., Konigsmark, B. W., Capute, A. J. and Migeon, C. J. (1973). A new familial syndrome with ataxia, hearing loss and mental retardation. *Arch. Neurol., Chicago* **29**, 258.

Bickerstaff, E. R. (1950). Hereditary spastic paraplegia. *J. Neurol. Neurosurg. Psychiat.* **13**, 134.

Bird, T. B. and Shaw, C. M. (1978). Progressive myoclonus and epilepsy with dentatorubral degeneration: a clinicopathological study of the Ramsay Hunt syndrome. *J. Neurol. Neurosurg. Psychiat.* **41**, 140.

Boller, F. and Segarra, J. M. (1969). Spino-pontine degeneration. *Eur. Neurol.* **42**, 356.

Bone, I., Johnson, R. H. and Ferguson-Smith, M. A. (1976). Occurrence of familial spastic paraplegia in only one of monozygous twins. *J. Neurol. Neurosurg. Psychiat.* **39**, 1129.

Bradley, W. G., Richardson, J. and Frew, I. J. C. (1974). The familial association of neurofibromatosis, peroneal muscular atrophy, congenital deafness, partial albinism, and Axenfeld's defect. *Brain* **97**, 521.

Brannan, T. S., Burger, A. A. and Chaudhary, M. Y. (1980). Bilateral basal ganglia calcifications visualised on CT scan. *J. Neurol. Neurosurg. Psychiat.* **43**, 403.

Bruyn, G. W. and Mechelse, K. (1962). The association of familial spastic paraplegia and epilepsy in one family. *Psychiat. Neurol. Neurochir.* **65**, 280.

Carroll, W. M., Kriss, A., Baraitser, M., Barrett, G. and Halliday, A. M. (1980). The incidence and nature of visual pathway involvement in Friedreich's ataxia. A clinical and visual evoked potential study of 22 patients. *Brain* **103**, 413.

Chamberlain, S., Robinson, N., Walker, J., Smith, C., Benton, S., Kennard, C., Swash, M., Kilkenny, B. and Bradbury, S. (1980). Effect of lecithin on disability and plasma free-choline levels in Friedreich's ataxia. *J. Neurol. Neurosurg. Psychiat.* **43**, 843.

Cote, M., Bureau, M., Leger, C., Martin, J., Gattiker, H., Cimon, M., Larose, A. and Lemieux, B. (1979). Evolution of cardio-pulmonary involvement in Friedreich's ataxia. *Can. J. Neurol. Sci.* **6**, 151.

Courville, C. B. and Friedman, A. P. (1940). Chronic progressive degeneration of the superior cerebellar cortex (parenchymatous cortical cerebellar atrophy). *Bull. Los Angeles neurol. Soc.* **5**, 171.

Critchley, M. and Greenfield, J. G. (1948). Olivo-pontocerebellar atrophy. *Brain* **71**, 343.

Currier, R. D., Glove, G., Jackson, J. F. and Tipton, A. C. (1972). Spinocerebellar ataxia: study of a large kindred. I. General information and genetics *Neurology, Minneapolis* **22**, 1040.

Dejerine, J. and Thomas, A. (1900). L'atrophie olivo-pontocérébelleuse. *N. Iconogr. Salpêt.* **13**, 330.

Dimitrijevic, M. R., Lenman, J. A. R., Prevec, T. and Wheatly, K. (1982). A study of posterior column function in familial spastic paraplegia. *J. Neurol. Neurosurg. Psychiat.* **45**, 46.

Donat, J. R. and Auger, R. (1979). Familial periodic ataxia. *Arch. Neurol., Chicago* **36**, 568.

Dyck, P. J. and Lais, A. C. (1972). Evidence for segmental demyelination secondary to axonal degeneration in Friedreich's ataxia. In *Clinical studies in myology* (International Congress Series No. 295), p. 253. Excerpta Medica, Amsterdam.

——, Lambert, E. H. and Nichols, P. C. (1974). Quantitative measurement of sensation related to compound action potential and number and sizes of myelinated and unmyelinated fibers of sural nerve in health, Friedreich's ataxia, hereditary sensory neuropathy, and tabes dorsalis. In *Handbook of electroencephalography and clinical neurophysiology*, Vol. 9, p. 83. North-Holland, Amsterdam.

Evans, W. and Wright, G. (1942). The electrocardiogram in Friedreich's disease. *Br. Heart J.* **4**, 91.

Ferguson, F. R. and Critchley, M. (1929). A clinical study of an heredofamilial disease resembling disseminated sclerosis. *Brain* **52**, 203.

Foley, J. (1951). Calcification of the corpus striatum and dentate nuclei occurring in a family. *J. Neurol. Neurosurg. Psychiat.* **14**, 253.

François, J. (1974). Tapetoretinal degeneration in spinocerebellar degenerations (heredoataxias). Proceedings of the Fourth International Congress of Neurogenetics and Neuro-ophthalmology. *Acta Genet. med., Roma* **23**, 3.

Friedreich, N. (1863). Ueber degenerative Atrophie de spinalen Hinterstrange. *Virchow's Arch. path. Anat.* **26**, 391.

—— (1876). Ueber Ataxie mit besonderer Berücksichtigung der hereditären Formen. *Virchow's Arch. path. Anat.* **68**, 145.

Furukawa, T., Takagi, A., Nakao, K., Sugita, H., Tsukagoshi, H. and Tsubaki, T. (1968). Hereditary muscular atrophy with ataxia, retinitis pigmentosa, and diabetes mellitus: a clinical report of a family. *Neurology, Minneapolis.* **18**, 942.

Garland, H. and Moorhouse, D. (1953). An extremely rare recessive hereditary syndrome including cerebellar ataxia, oligophrenia, cataract, and other features. *J. Neurol. Neurosurg. Psychiat.* **16**, 110.

Greenfield, J. G. (1954). *The spinocerebellar degenerations.* Blackwell, Oxford.

Griggs, R. C., Moxley, R. T., Lafrance, R. A. and McQuillen, J. (1978). Hereditary paroxysmal ataxia: response to acetazolamide. *Neurology Minneapolis.* **28**, 1259.

Guilleminault, C., Harpey, J. P. and Lafourcade, J. (1973). Sjögren–Larsson syndrome. Report of two cases in twins. *Neurology, Minneapolis.* **23**, 367.

Hallgren, B. (1959). Retinitis pigmentosa combined with congenital deafness; with vestibulo-cerebellar ataxia and mental abnormality in a proportion of cases. *Acta psychiat. scand.* **34**, Suppl. 138.

Harding, A. E. (1981a). Genetic aspects of autosomal dominant late onset cerebellar ataxia. *J. med. Genet.* **18**, 436.

—— (1981b). Hereditary 'pure' spastic paraplegia: a clinical and genetic study of 22 families. *J. Neurol. Neurosurg. Psychiat.* **44**, 871.

—— (1981c). Friedreich's ataxia: a clinical and genetic study of 90 families with an analysis of early diagnostic criteria and intrafamilial clustering of clinical features. *Brain* **104**, 589.

—— (1981d). 'Idiopathic' late onset cerebellar ataxia: a clinical and genetic study of 36 cases. *J. neurol. Sci.* **51**, 259.

—— (1981e). Early onset cerebellar ataxia with retained tendon reflexes: a clinical and genetic study of a disorder distinct from Friedreich's ataxia. *J. Neurol. Neurosurg. Psychiat.* **44**, 503.

—— (1982). The clinical features and classification of the late onset autosomal dominant cerebellar ataxias: a study of 11 families, including descendants of 'the Drew family of Walworth'. *Brain* **105**, 1.

—— and Zilkha, K. J. (1981). 'Pseudo-dominant' inheritance in Friedreich's ataxia. *J. med. Genet.* **18**, 285.

—— (1984). *The hereditary ataxias and related disorders.* Churchill–Livingstone, Edinburgh.

Harrington, M. G., Macpherson, P., McIntosh, W. B., Allam, B. F. and Bone, I. (1981). The significance of the incidental finding of basal ganglia calcification on computed tomography. *J. Neurol. Neurosurg. Psychiat.* **44**, 1168.

Healton, E. B., Brust, J. C. M., Kerr, D. L., Resor, S. and Penn, A. (1980). Presumably Azorean disease in a presumably non-Portuguese family. *Neurology, Minneapolis* **30**, 1084.

Hewer, R. L. (1968). Study of fatal cases of Friedreich's ataxia. *Br. med. J.* **3**, 649.

—— and Robinson, N. (1968). Diabetes mellitus in Friedreich's ataxia. *J. Neurol. Neurosurg. Psychiat.* **31**, 226.

Hoffmann, P. M., Stuart, W. H., Earle, K. M. and Brody, J. A. (1971). Hereditary late-onset cerebellar degeneration. *Neurology, Minneapolis* **21**, 771.

Hogan, G. R. and Bauman, M. L. (1977). Familial spastic ataxia: occurrence in childhood. *Neurology, Minneapolis* **27**, 520.

Holmes, G. (1907a). A form of familial degeneration of the cerebellum. *Brain* **30**, 466.

—— (1907b). An attempt to classify cerebellar disease, with a note on Marie's hereditary cerebellar ataxia. *Brain* **30**, 455.

Horoupian, D. S., Zucker, D. K., Moshe, S. and Paterson, H. de C. (1979). Behr syndrome: a clinicopathologic report. *Neurology, Minneapolis* **29**, 323.

Hughes, J. T., Brownell, B., and Hewer, R. L. (1968). The peripheral sensory pathway in Friedreich's ataxia: an examination by light and electron microscopy of the posterior nerve roots, posterior root ganglia, and peripheral sensory nerves in cases of Friedreich's ataxia. *Brain* **91**, 803.

Hunt, J. R. (1921). Dyssynergia cerebellaris myoclonica—primary atrophy of the dentate system: a contribution to the pathology and symptomatology of the cerebellum. *Brain* **44**, 490.

Ionasescu, V., Stegink, L., Mueller, S. and Weinstein, M. (1973). Amino acid abnormality in Sjögren–Larsson syndrome. *Arch. Neurol., Chicago* **28**, 197.

Iwashita, H., Inoue, N., Araki, S. and Kuroiwa, Y. (1970). Optic atrophy, nerve deafness and distal neurogenic amyotrophy. *Arch. Neurol., Chicago* **22**, 357.

Jones, S. J., Baraitser, M. and Halliday, A. M. (1980). Peripheral and central somatosensory nerve conduction defects in Friedreich's ataxia. *J. Neurol. Neurosurg. Psychiat.* **43**, 495.

Joubert, M., Eisenring, J. –J. and Robb, J. P. (1969). Familial agenesis of the cerebellar vermis. A syndrome of episodic hyperpnea, abnormal eye movements, ataxia and retardation. *Neurology, Minneapolis* **19**, 813.

Kark, R. A. P. and Rodriguez-Budelli, M. M. (1979). Clinical correlations of partial deficiency of lipoamide dehydrogenase. *Neurology, Minneapolis* **29**, 1006.

——, Budelli, M. M. R., Becker, D. M., Weiner, L. P. and Forsythe, A. B. (1981a). Lipoamide dehydrogenase: rapid heat inactivation in platelets of patients with recessively inherited ataxia. *Neurology, Minneapolis* **31**, 199.

——, —— and Wachsner, R. (1981b). Double-blind, triple-crossover trial of low doses of oral physostigmine in inherited ataxias. *Neurology, Minneapolis* **31**, 288.

——, Rodriguez-Budelli, M. M., Perlman, S., Gulley, W. F. and Torok, K. (1980). Preclinical diagnosis and carrier detection in ataxia associated with abnormalities of lipoamide dehydrogenase. *Neurology, Minneapolis* **30**, 502.

Kirkham, T. H. and Coupland, S. G. (1981). An electroretinal and visual evoked potential study in Friedreich's ataxia. *Can. J. Neurol. Sci.* **8**, 289.

Koeppen, A. H., Hans, M. B., Shepherd, D. I. and Best, P. V. (1977). Adult-onset hereditary ataxia in Scotland. *Arch. Neurol., Chicago* **34**, 611.

Konigsmark, G. and Weiner, L. (1970). The olivopontocerebellar atrophies: a review. *Medicine, Baltimore* **49**, 227.

Kreindler, A., Crighel, E. and Poilici, I. (1959). Clinical and electroencephalographic investigations in myoclonic cerebellar dyssynergia. *J. Neurol. Neurosurg. Psychiat.* **22**, 232.

Landis, D. M. D., Rosenburg, R. N., Landis, S. C., Schut, L. and Nyhan, W. L. (1974). Olivopontocerebellar degeneration. Clinical and ultrastructural abnormalities. *Arch. Neurol., Chicago* **31**, 295.

Lapresle, J. and Salisachs, P. (1973). Onion bulbs in a nerve biopsy specimen from an original case of Roussy–Lévy disease. *Arch. Neurol., Chicago* **29**, 346.

Lawrence, C. M., Millac, P., Stout, G. S. and Ward, J. W. (1980). The use of choline chloride in ataxic disorders. *J. Neurol. Neurosurg. Psychiat.* **43**, 452.

Livingstone, I. R., Mastaglia, F. L. and Pennington, R. J. T. (1980). An investigation of pyruvate metabolism in patients with cerebellar and spinocerebellar degeneration. *J. neurol. Sci.* **48**, 123.

——, ——, and Skilbeck, C. (1981). Choline chloride in the treatment of cerebellar and spinocerebellar ataxia. *J. neurol. Sci.* **50**, 161.

Marie, P., Foix, C. and Alajouanine, T. (1922). De l'atrophie cérébelleuse tardive à prédominance corticale. *Rev. neurol., Paris* **29**, 849, 1082.

Marinesco, G., Draganesco, S. and Vasiliu, D. (1931). Nouvelle maladie familiale, caractérisée par une cataracte congénitale et un arrêt du développement somatoneuropsychique. *Encéphale* **26**, 97.

—— and Tretiakoff, C. (1920). Étude histo-pathologique des centres nerveux dans trois cas de maladie de Friedreich. *Rev. neurol., Paris* **27**, 113.

Mathieu, P. and Bertrand, I. (1929). Études anatomo-cliniques sur les atrophies cérébelleuses. *Rev. neurol, Paris* **36**, 721.

Mauritz, K. H., Dichgans, J. and Hufschmidt, A. (1979). Quantitative analysis of stance in late cortical cerebellar atrophy of the anterior lobe and other forms of cerebellar ataxia. *Brain* **102**, 461.

May, D. L. and White, H. H. (1968). Familial myoclonus, cerebellar ataxia, and deafness: specific genetically-determined disease. *Arch. Neurol., Chicago* **19**, 331.

Mayeux, R. and Fahn, S. (1982). Paroxysmal dystonic choreoathetosis in a patient with familial ataxia. *Neurology, Minneapolis* **32**, 1184.

Merin, S., Abraham, F. A. and Auerbach, E. (1974). Usher's and Hallgren's syndrome. Proceedings of the Fourth International Congress of Neurogenetics and Neuroophthalmology. *Acta Genet. med., Roma* **23**, 49.

Naito, H. and Oyanagi, S. (1982). Familial myoclonus epilepsy and choreoathetosis: hereditary dentatorubral-pallidoluysian atrophy. *Neurology, Minneapolis.* **32**, 798.

Neff, I. H. (1895). A report of thirteen cases of ataxia in adults with hereditary history. *Am. J. Insan.* **51**, 365.

Nino, H. E., Noreen, H. J., Dubey, D. P., Resch, J. A., Namboodiri, K., Elston, R. C. and Yunis, E. J. (1980). A family with hereditary ataxia: HLA typing. *Neurology, Minneapolis* **30**, 12.

Page, M. McB., Asmal, A. C. and Edwards, C. R. W. (1976). Recessive inheritance of diabetes: the syndrome of diabetes insipidus, diabetes mellitus, optic atrophy and deafness. *Quart. J. Med.* **45**, 505.

Pentland, B., Martyn, C. N., Steer, C. R. and Christie, J. E. (1981). Lecithin treatment in Friedreich's ataxia. *Br. med. J.*, **282**, 1197.

Perry, T. L., Currier, R. D., Hansen, S. and MacLean, J. (1977). Aspartate–taurine imbalance in dominantly inherited olivopontocerebellar atrophy. *Neurology, Minneapolis* **27**, 257.

——, Kish, S. J., Hansen, S. and Currier, R. D. (1981). Neurotransmitter amino acids in dominantly inherited cerebellar disorders. *Neurology, Minneapolis* **31**, 237.

Petit, W. A., Soso, M. J. and Higman, H. (1982). Degos disease: neurologic complications and cerebral angiography. *Neurology, Minneapolis.* **32**, 1305.

Peyronnard, J. M., Lapointe, L., Bouchard, J. P., Lamontagne, A., Lemieux, B. and Barbeau, A. (1976). Nerve conduction studies and electromyography in Friedreich's ataxia. *Can. J. neurol. Sci.* **3**, 313.

Philcox, D. V., Sellars, S. L., Pamplett, R. and Beighton, P. (1975). Vestibular dysfunction in hereditary ataxia. *Brain* **98**, 309.

Plaitakis, A., Nicklas, W. J. and Desnick, R. J. (1980). Glutamate dehydrogenase deficiency in three patients with spinocerebellar syndrome. *Ann. Neurol* **7**, 297.

Powell, E. D. U. (1961). Blood-group studies in Friedreich's ataxia. *Br. med. J.* **1**, 868.

Pratt, R. T. C. (1967). *The genetics of neurological disorders.* Oxford Medical, London.

Remillard, G., Andermann, F., Blitzer, L. and Andermann, E. (1976). Electroencephalographic findings in Friedreich's ataxia. *Can. J. neurol. Sci.* **3**, 309.

Ron, M. A. and Pearce, J. (1971). Marinesco–Sjögren–Garland syndrome with unusual features. *J. neurol. Sci.* **13**, 175.

Rosenberg, R. N., Ivy, N., Kirkpatrick, J., Bay, C., Nyhan, W. L. and Baskin, F. (1981). Joseph disease and Huntington disease: protein patterns in fibroblasts and brain. *Neurology, Minneapolis* **31**, 1003.

——, Thomas, L., Baskin, F., Kirkpatrick, J., Bay, C. and Nyhan, W. L. (1979). Joseph disease: protein patterns in fibroblasts and brain. *Neurology, Minneapolis* **29**, 917.

Rossi, I. (1907). Atrophie parenchymateuse primitive du cervelet à localisation corticale. *N. Iconogr. Salpet.* **20**, 66.

Roussy, G. and Lévy, G. (1926). Sept cas d'une maladie familiale particulière. *Rev. neurol., Paris* **33**, 427.

Sachdev, H. S., Forno, L. S. and Kane, C. A. (1982). Joseph disease: a multisystem degenerative disorder of the nervous system. *Neurology, Minneapolis* **32**, 192.

Salisachs, P. (1979). Jaw reflex in Friedreich ataxia. *Neurology, Minneapolis* **29**, 1049.

——, Codina, M. and Paradas, J. (1975). Motor conduction velocity in patients with Friedreich's ataxia: report of 12 cases. *J. Neurol. Sci.* **24**, 331.

Schaffer, K. (1922). Zur pathologie und pathologischen Histologie de spastischen Heredodegeneration (hereditäre spastische Spinal paralysis). *Dtsch. Z. Nervenheilk.* **73**, 101.

Schwarz, G. A. (1952). Hereditary (familial) spastic paraplegia. *Arch. Neurol. Psychiat., Chicago* **68**, 655.

—— and Liu, C. -N. (1956). Hereditary (familial) spastic paraplegia: further clinical and pathologic observations. *Arch. Neurol. Psychiat., Chicago* **75**, 144.

Shepherd, M. (1955). Report of a family suffering from Friedreich's disease, peroneal muscular atrophy, and schizophrenia. *J. Neurol. Neurosurg. Psychiat.* **18**, 297.

Sjögren, T. (1943). Klinische und erbbiologische Unterschungen uber die Heredoataxien. *Acta psychiat., Kbh* Suppl. xxvii.

—— (1950). Hereditary congenital spinocerebellar ataxia accompanied by congenital cataract and oligophrenia. *Confin. neurol.*, **10**, 293.

—— and Larsson, T. (1957). Oligophrenia in combination with congenital ichthyosis and spastic disorders. A clinical and genetic study. *Acta psychiat. scand.* Suppl. 113, 1.

Smith, N. J., Espir, M. L. E. and Matthews, W. B. (1978). Familial myoclonic epilepsy with ataxia and neuropathy with additional features of Friedreich's ataxia and peroneal muscular atrophy. *Brain* **101**, 461.

Spira, P. J., McLeod, J. G. and Evans, W. A. (1979). A spinocerebellar degeneration with X-linked inheritance. *Brain* **102**, 27.

Spoendlin, H. (1974). Optic and cochleovestibular degenerations in the hereditary ataxias. II. Temporal bone pathology in two cases of Friedreich's ataxia with vestibulo-cochlear disorders. *Brain* **97**, 41.

Stendahl-Brodin, L., Möller, E. and Link, H. (1978). Hereditary optic atrophy with probable association with a specific HLA haplotype. *J. neurol. Sci.* **38**, 11.

Strobos, R. R. J., de la Torre, E. and Martin, J. F. (1957). Symmetrical calcification of the basal ganglia with familial ataxia and pigmentary macular degeneration. *Brain* **80**, 313.

Stumpf, D. A., Parks, J. K., Eguren, L. A. and Haas, R. (1982). Friedreich ataxia: III. Mitochondrial malic enzyme deficiency. *Neurology, Minneapolis* **32**, 221.

Sutherland, J. M. (1957). Familial spastic paraplegia: its relation to mental and cardiac abnormalities. *Lancet* **ii**, 169.

Taniguchi, R. and Konigsmark, B. W. (1971). Dominant spinopontine atrophy: report of a family through three generatons. *Brain* **94**, 349.

Thomas, P. K., Jefferys, J. G. R., Smith, I. S. and Loulakakis, D. (1981). Spinal somatosensory evoked potentials in hereditary spastic paraplegia. *J. Neurol. Neurosurg. Psychiat.* **44**, 243.

Thrush, D. C., Holti, G., Bradley, W. G., Campbell, M. J. and Walton, J. N. (1974). Neurological manifestations of xeroderma pigmentosum in two siblinga. *J. neurol. Sci.* **22**, 91.

Tyrer, J. H. and Sutherland, J. M. (1961). The primary spinocerebellar atrophies and their associated defects with a study of the foot deformity. *Brain* **84**, 289.

Usher, C. H. (1914). On the inheritance of retinitis pigmentosa, with notes of cases. *Royal London Ophth. Hosp. Rep.* **9**, 130.

van Bogaert, L. (1952). Études sur la paraplégie spasmodique familiale. V. Forme classique pure avec atrophie optique massive chez certains de ses membres. Considérations génétiques sur la paraplégie spasmodique familiale en général. *Acta neurol. belg.* **52**, 795.

—— and Martin, L. (1974). Optic and cochleovestibular degenerations in the hereditary ataxias I. Clinicopathological and genetic aspects. *Brain* **97**, 15.

van Rossum, J., Veenema, H. and Went, L. N. (1981). Linkage investigations in two families with hereditary ataxia. *J. Neurol. Neurosurg. Psychiat.* **44**, 516.

Vernon, M. (1969). Usher's syndrome—deafness and progressive blindness. *J. chron. Dis.* **22**, 133.

Walker, J. L., Chamberlain, S. and Robinson, N. (1980*a*). Lipids and lipoproteins in Friedreich's ataxia. *J. Neurol. Neurosurg. Psychiat.* **43**, 111.

——, —— and —— (1980*b*). Failure to detect abnormal fatty acid profiles in serum lipoproteins in Friedreich's ataxia. *Ann. Neurol.* **8**, 74.

Waltimo, O., Iivanainen, M. and Hokkanen, E. (1967). Xeroderma pigmentosum with neurological manifestations. *Acta neurol. scand.* **43**, Suppl. 31, 66.

Motor-neurone disease

Synonyms. Amyotrophic lateral sclerosis; progressive muscular atrophy; progressive bulbar palsy; motor-system disease.

Definition. A disease characterized pathologically by degenerative changes, most marked in the anterior horn cells of the spinal cord, the motor nuclei of the brainstem, and the corticospinal tracts, and clinically by progressive wasting of muscles, combined with symptoms of corticospinal-tract degeneration. The term 'progressive muscular atrophy' is associated especially with the names of Aran (1850) and Duchenne (1853). Charcot and Joffroy (1869) distinguished two varieties—progressive muscular atrophy of Aran and Duchenne, characterized only by lower motor-neurone lesions, and a form in which these were accompanied by signs of corticospinal-tract dysfunction, which he called 'amyotrophic lateral sclerosis'. These two varieties are now regarded as clinical variants of a single disease. When the lower motor-neurone lesions predominate, or, as more rarely happens, occur alone, the term 'progressive muscular atrophy' is still generally used and when muscles innervated from the medulla are first affected, it is called 'progressive bulbar palsy'. Many then use the term 'amyotrophic lateral sclerosis' for those cases in which signs of corticospinal-tract disease predominate at first and in which initially there is little or no evidence of lower motor-neurone involvement. In most cases, however, there is evidence of both upper and lower motor-neurone lesions though the latter are often more severe in the upper than in the lower limbs at first. Greenfield (1958) preferred the term amyotrophic lateral sclerosis to motor-neurone disease since pathological changes in the spinal cord are not confined to the motor neurones and many American authors use this term as an inclusive one, embracing all varieties of the disease. Motor-neurone disease, however, is a better inclusive term.

Pathology

The spinal cord
Naked-eye changes in the spinal cord are slight, but on section the grey matter of the anterior horns appears smaller than normal, and the ventral roots are wasted. Microscopically there is severe degeneration of anterior horn ganglion cells. This change is usually most marked in the cervical enlargement of the cord (Tsukagoshi, Yanagisawa, Oguchi, Nagushima, and Murakami 1979), but is always widespread. The ganglion cells exhibit chromatolysis, which is at first perinuclear and lipochrome is often present. The total number of ganglion cells is much reduced and the larger α-motor neurones are most severely affected. Relative preservation of a small group of sacral neurones (the X group of Onuf) may account for the preservation of sphincter control until

the late stages (Mannen, Iuata, Toyokura, and Nagashima 1977). Citrate synthase activity is reduced in the anterior horn cells (Hayashi and Tsubaki 1982), and so too is glycinergic receptor binding (Hayashi, Suga, Satake, and Tsubaki 1981). The degeneration is associated with a slight secondary gliosis, and rarely slight perivascular infiltration with round cells is observed. In the ventral roots large myelinated fibres of the α-motor neurones are selectively lost (Sobue, Matsuoka, Mukai, Takayanagi, and Sobue 1981) and glial-fibre bundles growing out from the spinal cord are often found (Ghatak and Nochlin 1982). Large axonal swellings containing many neurofilaments (spheroids) have been found in the anterior horns and in brainstem nuclei (Carpenter 1968). In the variety of amyotrophic lateral sclerosis which is common in the Mariana islands and in the Kii peninsula of Japan and which is often associated with the parkinsonism-dementia complex (p. 331), Alzheimer's neurofibrillary change is common in cortical neurones with granulovacuolar change in the cells of Ammon's horn of the hippocampus (Hirano, Kurland, and Sayre 1967), and neurofibrillary tangles have also been observed along with hyaline acidophilic bodies, superficially resembling Lewy bodies, in the anterior horn cells (*The Lancet* 1979). Similar changes have been reported in hereditary cases of motor-neurone disease occurring in racial groups other than the Chamorros and Japanese (Metcalf and Hirano 1971; Hughes and Jerome 1971; Takahashi, Nokamura, and Okada 1972) and even in occasional cases of the commoner sporadic form of the disease in adults (Schochet, Hardman, Ladewig, and Earle 1969; Meyers, Dorencamp, and Suzuki 1974; Queiroz, Nucci, and Filho 1977) as well as in juvenile cases (Nelson and Prensky 1972).

Myelin stains reveal degeneration of the spinal-cord white matter, most marked in, and often confined to, the anterolateral columns (Fig. 13.6). The corticospinal fibres suffer most, both the direct and the crossed tracts being affected. Corticospinal-tract degeneration is never equally severe at all levels. Often changes are severe in the lower thoracic and lumbosacral regions, while the upper thoracic region is but slightly affected, and severe changes are again found in the cervical enlargement, extending up to the medulla. The spinocerebellar tracts usually show degeneration, especially the anterior, and this varies in different segments. The rubrospinal, vestibulospinal, and tectospinal tracts also degenerate to a variable extent and, despite the well-known fact that sensory symptoms and signs are absent, slight degeneration is occasionally present in the posterior columns, especially in some familial cases (Engel, Kurland, and Klatzo 1959). The endogenous fibres of the spinal cord which lie close to the grey matter degenerate in the anterolateral but not in the posterior columns (Smith 1960).

The brainstem
The cells of the motor nuclei of the lower brainstem show degenerative changes similar to those in the anterior horn cells. These are most marked in the hypoglossal nucleus, the dorsal nucleus of the vagus, the nucleus ambiguus, and the trigeminal motor nucleus. The facial nucleus is usually less severely affected. There is usually marked corticospinal-tract degeneration. Bertrand and van Bogaert (1925) described a case in which this was severe in the medulla and negligible in the pons and cerebral peduncles. Degeneration has also been described in the inferior cerebellar peduncle, the medial longitudinal fasciculus, the medial and lateral lemnisci, and the reticular formation. The third-, fourth-, and sixth-nerve nuclei usually escape.

The cerebral hemispheres
Naked-eye changes are usually inconspicuous. Microscopic changes are most marked in the cerebral motor cortex. The typical lesion in subacute cases is degeneration of ganglion cells in the frontal and precentral regions. This is most marked in the third and fifth cortical layers, the latter of which contains the larger cor-

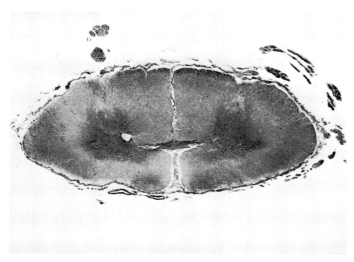

Fig. 13.6. Motor-neurone disease. Spinal cord.

ticospinal motor cells of Betz. Degeneration has also been found in cortical tangential fibres and some glial overgrowth is usually present in the affected regions. Degenerative changes are also found in the middle third of the corpus callosum and in corticospinal fibres in the posterior limb of the internal capsule (Brownell, Oppenheimer, and Hughes 1970).

Peripheral nerves and muscles

The peripheral nerves exhibit axonal degeneration, with secondary demyelination. Collateral sprouting of surviving motor axons occurs with reinnervation of groups of denervated muscle fibres which may subsequently become denervated again when the reinnervating neurone is involved in the disease process (Wohlfart 1957). Reinnervation commonly produces groups of muscle fibres of uniform histochemical type (Telerman-Toppet and Coërs 1978; Mastaglia and Walton 1982). Changes in the motor end-plates are non-specific (Bjornskov, Dekker, Norris, and Stuart 1975). In the affected muscles large (or sometimes small and scattered) groups of uniformly atrophic fibres typical of denervation atrophy are commonly seen; the larger the atrophic groups, the more rapid is likely to be the progress of the disease (Patten, Zito, and Harati 1979). In long-standing cases there may be so-called 'secondary myopathic change' (Drachman, Murphy, Nigam, and Hills 1967) with some random variation in fibre size, central nuclei, and degeneration or necrosis of individual fibres similar to that seen in myopathic disorders.

Aetiology

Motor-neurone disease is most often a disease of late middle life, usually beginning between the ages of 50 and 70, occasionally as early as the third decade or as late as the eighth. Cases occurring in early adult life may be difficult or impossible to distinguish clinically from chronic spinal muscular atrophy of the Kugelberg–Welander type (p. 384), unless signs of corticospinal-tract dysfunction are prominent. The sporadic disorder occurs world-wide and in all races (Edgar, Brody, and Detels 1973) and has an incidence of about 1.2–1.8 new cases in 100 000 of the population per year (Juergens, Kurland, Okazaki, and Mulder 1980; Buckley, Warlow, Smith, Hilton-Jones, Irvine, and Tew 1983) with a prevalence variably reported as between 2.5 and 7 per 100 000 (Kurland and Mulder 1954; Kurtzke 1969; Kahana, Alter, and Feldman 1976). It is generally more common in males than in females (Kurtzke 1982; Buckley *et al.* 1983), but not in Finland where geographical isolates of increased incidence have been reported (Jokelainen 1976); it may be less common in Mexicans (Olivares, San Esteban, and Alter 1972), but is relatively common in Filipinos (Matsumoto, Worth, Kurland, and Okazaki 1972) and in Niger-

ians, in whom it tends to run an unusually benign course (Osuntokun, Adueja, and Bademosi 1974). Clinically atypical varieties of the disease have been described in certain parts of India (the 'Madras type'—Valmikinathan, Mascreen, Meenakshisundaram, and Snehalatha 1973). Whether a form of sporadic spinal muscular atrophy restricted over many years to one upper limb and reported from Japan (Hashimoto, Asada, Ohta, and Kuroiwa 1976; Sobue, Saito, Iida, and Ando 1978) as well as from India (Gourie-Devi, Suresh and Shankar 1984) is a variant of motor-neurone disease or of the spinal muscular atrophies (p. 384) is still uncertain. The same doubts apply to those chronic, benign varieties of spinal muscular atrophy which sometimes remain asymmetrical or confined to the hands or both upper limbs for long periods (Harding, Bradbury, and Murray 1983). The sporadic variety is much the commonest, but many families showing dominant, recessive, or, rarely, X-linked recessive inheritance (Kennedy, Alter, and Sung 1968) have been described in many parts of the world (Pratt, Campbell and Liversedge 1967). In such familial cases many atypical variants have been reported including an onset in childhood or adolescence with chronic bulbar palsy (Fazio 1892; Londe 1893; Markand and Daly 1971) or benign proximal forms of the disease. A relatively benign X-linked variety involving bulbar and proximal limb muscles of late onset has also been reported (Barkhaus, Kennedy, Stern, and Harrington 1982). Horton, Eldridge, and Brody (1976) distinguished three different varieties, all of autosomal dominant transmission, one presenting as progressive muscular atrophy of comparatively rapid progression, another which is similar clinically but in which there is pathological involvement of the posterior columns, Clarke's column, and spinocerebellar pathways, and a third of very benign course, progressing slowly over 10, 20, or more years. Giménez-Roldán and Esteban (1977), however, found marked variability in clinical course within members of the same family, while Alberca, Castilla, and Gil-Peralta (1981) have described another relatively benign variant. Conjugal motor-neurone disease has also been reported in a single family (Chad, Mitsumoto, Adelman, Bradley, Munsat, and Zieper 1982).

Amyotrophic lateral sclerosis is endemic in the Chamorro people on the island of Guam and shows there a high familial incidence; it now seems unlikely that this condition, with which the so-called parkinsonism-dementia complex is often associated (Eldridge, Ryan, Rosario, and Brody 1969), is genetically determined (Kurland 1957, 1972; Hirano *et al.* 1967; Reed, Brody, and Holden 1975). The same syndromes occur in the Japanese Kii peninsula as noted above, but also in Filipino migrants to Guam (Garruto, Gajdusek, and Chen 1981) and in the Auyu and Jakai people of Western New Guinea (Gajdusek and Salazar 1982), often, in the latter location, in association with a subacute, recurrent, paralytic poliomyeloradiculitis. There is no convincing evidence of a viral aetiology and no definite environmental factor has yet been identified. Cycasin, present in cycad nuts, once thought to be responsible (Kurland 1972) is not the cause. Gajdusek (1982) points out that the condition occurs in populations which from birth have used drinking water containing insignificant quantities of calcium and magnesium, and in the areas concerned the content of these trace elements in the soil is also exceptionally low. However, the brains of such patients appear to contain excessive aluminium, calcium, and magnesium at autopsy. While these environmental factors are clearly important and while it is now apparent that neither a slow virus infection nor Mendelian inheritance can explain the condition, the part played by these trace elements is unexplained. Improved nutrition has resulted in a sharply decreased incidence (Garruto, Yanagihara, and Gajdusek 1985). This disorder plainly differs from sporadic motor-neurone disease as commonly observed in Europe and in America though it may be clinically indistinguishable. However, dementia has been reported in familial juvenile amyotrophic lateral sclerosis in Holland (Staal and Went 1968; Bots and Staal 1973) and, as mentioned above, pathological changes once thought to be confined to the Guam variety have been found in sporadic cases in other parts of the world, so that the nosological position remains uncertain. Indeed Alter and Schaumann (1976) described an American family with familial motor-neurone disease and parkinsonism which Hudson (1981) has equated with the amyotrophic variety of Creutzfeldt–Jakob disease; he also points out that dementia is commoner in familial and sporadic motor-neurone disease than is generally realized.

The condition was once regarded by some workers, especially in France, as a form of 'chronic poliomyelitis', but this hypothesis was not borne out by the histological appearances or by virological studies. Inflammatory infiltration is rare and scanty; exceptionally, however, the disease may develop in an individual who suffered many years earlier from acute anterior poliomyelitis and progressive atrophy often then begins in the limb or limbs most severely affected by the acute illness. Hallen, Brusis, and Pfisterer (1969) suggested that in such cases the process was indeed one of chronic poliomyelitis, but this view is not generally accepted. Wiechers and Hubbell (1981) suggest that this syndrome is due to disintegration with ageing in reinnervated motor units. The condition has also been reported to follow encephalitis lethargica (Milhorat 1946). Evidence to indicate that the causal virus is responsible for these sequelae is, however, lacking. It is, nevertheless, conceivable that injury to anterior horn cells caused by a virus may shorten the active life of some of these cells and the postulate that motor-neurone disease is due to a premature ageing process in such cells, perhaps precipitated by unknown environmental factors, has received some support (McComas, Upton, and Sica 1973). An abnormality of macrophage migration has been described (Urbánek and Jansa 1974) and a possible association with HLA–A3, especially in severe and rapidly progressive cases, has been reported (Antel, Arnason, Fuller, and Lehrich 1976), although others have found no association with any HLA antigen (Bartfeld, Pollack, Cunningham-Rundles, and Donnenfeld 1982) and abnormalities of humoral immunity in Guamian cases have been thought to be of no aetiological significance (Hoffman, Robbins, Oldstone, Gibbs, and Gajdusek 1981). However, a possible relationship with poliovirus has been revived by the finding of cell-mediated immunity to this virus in 21 of 33 patients, especially those with the HLA–A3 antigen (Kott, Livni, Zamir, and Kuritzky 1979).

If one seeks for risk factors and disease associations, exposure to lead or mercury and athletic participation were identified by Felmus, Patten, and Swanke (1976), while Kurtzke and Beebe (1980) and Kurtzke (1982) have found a significantly greater incidence of prior physical trauma or surgical operation in such patients; commonly the muscular weakness and wasting have begun in the limb or body part injured or operated upon. The significance of this relationship is obscure. Buckley *et al.* (1983), like Hawkes and Fox (1981), found an increased incidence in leather workers, but again the reason for this is unclear. Suggestions that the condition may be associated with a diffuse angiopathy (Störtebecker, Noordström, Pestény, Seeman, and Bjorkerud 1970; Urbánek and Jansa 1974), with disorders of lipid and carbohydrate metabolism (Ionasescu and Luca 1964; Gustafson and Störtebecker 1972), or with high concentrations of manganese and calcium in the central nervous system (Yase 1972) are either unsubstantiated as yet or have given no definite clues to the aetiology of the disease. Exocrine pancreatic dysfunction, found in certain cases, is probably an epiphenomenon. Campbell, Williams, and Barltrop (1970) suggested that the condition may be due to lead intoxication and certainly the neuronal effects of lead intoxication may mimic this disease (Boothby, de Jesus, and Rowland 1974). More recently, increased concentrations of lead have been found in the plasma (Conradi, Ronnevi, and Vesterberg 1978 *a*), skeletal muscle (Conradi, Ronnevi, and Vesterberg 1978 *b*), CSF (Conradi, Ronnevi, Nise, and Vesterberg 1980), and spinal cord (Kurlander and Patten 1979) of such patients, and there is also increased erythrocyte fragility (Ronnevi, Conradi, and Nise 1982)

and capillary fragility (Conradi, Kaijser, and Ronnevi 1978). Attempts to isolate a causal virus have been generally unsuccessful (Cremer, Oshiro, Norris, and Lennette 1973; Campbell and Liversedge 1981; *The Lancet* 1977; Weiner, Stohlman, and Davis 1980). However, Schu togavirus isolated from the CSF of a patient with an illness of seven years duration which resembled motor-neurone disease did produce anterior horn-cell degeneration in animals (Müller and Schaltenbrand 1979) and virus-like particles have been seen ultrastructurally in skeletal muscle from one such patient (Oshiro, Cremer, Norris, and Lennette 1976). It has been suggested that there is an association between this disorder and malignant disease (Brain, Croft, and Wilkinson 1965; Norris and Engel 1965; Vejjajiva, Foster and Miller 1967) and an identical clinical syndrome has been reported in association with macroglobulinaemia with improvement following treatment of the latter condition (Peters and Claltanoff 1968); but it now seems that the association with carcinoma is no more than could be accounted for by chance (Jokelainen 1976). The CSF homovallinic acid (HVA) is lower in such cases than in control subjects but levodopa is therapeutically ineffective (Mendell, Chase, and Engel 1971). The significance of CSF changes in such cases identified by isoelectric focusing and indicating a 'barrier-damage pattern' (Kjellin and Stibler 1976) has yet to be determined. It is well recognized that between a quarter and a third of all patients show an increase in the total protein content of the CSF (Guiloff, McGregor, Thompson, Blackwood, and Paul 1980). There is some evidence of disordered protein metabolism in neurones but not in myelin in such cases (Savolainen and Palo 1973) and of DNA-directed mRNA synthesis (Mann and Yates 1974), but whether these abnormalities indicate a fundamental aetiopathogenic mechanism is still uncertain.

The wobbler mouse mutant, upon which much research has been done, clearly differs from human motor-neurone disease (Murakami, Mastaglia, and Bradley 1980). Possibly hereditary canine spinal muscular atrophy of the Brittany spaniel (Cork, Griffin, Adams, and Price 1977), or the condition resembling motor-neurone disease which can be produced in animal models by inoculation of Theiler's virus (Duchen 1978) may prove more useful experimental models. While CSF from patients does not alter neurone-specific enolase in cultured motor neurones (Askanas, Marangos, and Engel 1981), sera show marked antineuronal cytotoxicity (Roisen, Bartfeld, Donnenfeld, and Baxter 1982). Festoff (1980) has postulated that in such cases there is continuous loss of nerve-muscle adherence resulting from collagen resorption at the neuromuscular junction, while Appel (1981) suggests that the disease is due to lack of a disorder-specific neurotrophic hormone, as yet unidentified. Indeed the aetiology remains as much an enigma as it was 30 years ago.

Symptoms and signs

Mode of onset
The disease is usually chronic, but may run a subacute course. The onset is generally insidious, but is rarely rapid. The nature of the earliest symptoms depends upon which region of the nervous system is first affected. Commonly the first abnormality is observed in the hands, where the patient becomes aware of weakness, stiffness, or clumsiness of movements of the fingers, or his attention may be drawn to the wasting, or he may perceive fascicular twitching. When the shoulder girdle and upper arm muscles are first affected, the first symptom is weakness of shoulder movements. When degeneration begins in the bulbar motor nuclei, the first symptom is usually dysarthria or dysphagia. Less often the disease begins with spastic paraplegia, or wasting of one or both lower limbs. Muscular cramp is often an early symptom.

Symptoms and signs of lower motor-neurone degeneration
Degeneration of neurones leads to weakness and wasting of the muscles which they innervate. Fasciculation is also conspicuous,

and occurs in those muscles supplied by ganglion cells undergoing active degeneration. It may be limited to a few groups of muscles, or be much more widespread, and its extent is an indication of the diffuseness of the degenerative process. Very rarely, widespread weakness and wasting occur in the absence of fasciculation. When this sign is not immediately evident it can often be evoked by sharply tapping the muscle. As a rule wasting begins in the hands, the muscles of the thenar eminences being first affected. Often one hand begins to waste some months or even a year before the other. In other cases the onset is symmetrical. Wasting tends to spread to the muscles innervated by the spinal-cord segment adjacent to that first affected. Hence, after the hands, the forearm muscles are involved, the flexors usually suffering before the extensors. Weakness and atrophy of hand muscles lead to clumsy finger movements, and some degree of claw-hand usually develops. This deformity is not as a rule severe, since the long flexors and extensors of the fingers, by which it is maintained, are soon themselves affected.

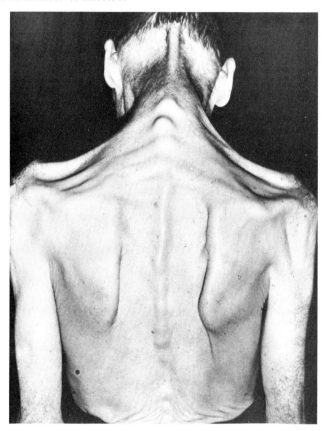

Fig. 13.7. Widespread wasting of shoulder girdle muscles in advanced motor-neurone disease.

Next in frequency the muscles of the shoulder girdle and upper arm are first involved, those innervated by the fifth cervical spinal segment, especially the deltoids, being earliest affected (Fig. 13.7). Those supplied by the sixth cervical segment, namely, triceps, latissimus dorsi, the sternal part of the pectoralis major and serratus anterior, are usually involved much later, as is the upper part of the trapezius. The muscles innervated by the medulla may be the first to suffer or may be affected simultaneously with, or shortly after, the upper limbs. The tongue then becomes shrunken and wrinkled with marked fasciculation (Fig. 13.8) The orbicularis oris also suffers early, but the orbicularis oculi and other facial muscles are affected later, and less severely. The palate is usually involved soon after the tongue, along with the extrinsic muscles of the pharynx and larynx. The intrinsic laryngeal muscles usually escape until late. The mandibu-

lar muscles usually suffer less severely than the tongue and orbicularis oris. Gradually pursing of the lips and whistling become impossible, and later saliva runs from the open lips. Protrusion of the tongue is at first weak and later lost. Speech suffers from paresis of the lips, tongue, and palate. The capacity to pronounce labials and dentals is impaired early, and later gutturals. Speech becomes slurred and finally unintelligible. Phonation, however, suffers late, if at all. Swallowing becomes increasingly difficult, and fluid may regurgitate through the nose. Patients usually find semi-solids easier to swallow than either solids or fluids. In progressive bulbar palsy, slurring of speech is often an early symptom and its cause may at first be difficult to identify, especially if there is no fasciculation in the tongue. Later, because of dysphagia, distressing episodes of choking may occur during meals. Ophthalmoplegia due to involvement of the third, fourth, and/or sixth nuclei is very rare but has been described (Harvey, Torack, and Rosenbaum 1979) and abnormalities of pursuit eye movements, less often of saccadic movements (Jacobs, Bozian, Heffner, and Barron 1981), and Bell's phenomenon on eyelid closure (Esteban, De Andrés, and Giménez-Roldán 1978) are also sometimes seen.

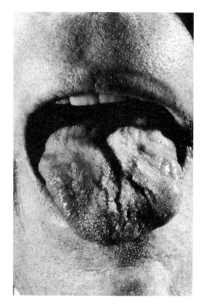

Fig. 13.8. Atrophy of the tongue in motor-neurone disease. (Reproduced from Spillane (1975) by kind permission of the author.)

Exceptionally the extensor muscles of the neck suffer early (Fig. 13.7), and when this occurs the head falls forwards. Early involvement of lower-limb muscles is rare. The anterior tibial group and peronei are usually first affected and unilateral or bilateral foot-drop results. This mode of onset, which simulates polyneuritis, especially when there is associated muscular pain, has sometimes been called the 'pseudopolyneuritic' form. Exceptionally, weakness begins in the proximal muscles of both the upper and lower limbs and, if fasciculation is at first inconspicuous, the condition resembles a proximal myopathy.

In whatever part of the body muscular wasting begins, in most cases it sooner or later becomes generalized, though progressive bulbar palsy may prove fatal before wasting becomes severe elsewhere. It is now well recognized that diaphragmatic paralysis with consequential respiratory insufficiency is an important complication (Parhad, Clark, Barron, and Staunton 1978) and indeed may develop acutely (Hill, Martin, and Hakim 1983). The onset may be insidious with severe unsuspected hypercapnia (Serisier, Mastaglia, and Gibson 1982) and rarely dyspnoea is the first symptom of the disease (Nightingale, Bates, Bateman, Hudgson, Ellis, and Gibson 1982).

Electrodiagnostic findings

Motor nerve conduction velocity is normal, if the limb temperature is controlled, up to a late stage, as surviving axons conduct at a normal rate but the amplitude of the compound muscle potential evoked by supramaximal stimulation of a motor nerve may be reduced. In the later stages, demyelination secondary to axonal degeneration may give modest slowing of conduction. Methods of estimating electrophysiologically the number of functioning motor units in the extensor digitorum brevis and thenar muscles reveal a rapid early decline in the number of such units in the early stages with early functional failure in surviving 'giant' units (Brown and Jaatoul 1974). Although there is some evidence of abnormal resistance of sensory nerves to ischaemia in such cases (Shahani, Davies-Jones, and Russell 1971), sensory nerve function when tested electrophysiologically is normal (Willison 1962).

Electromyography shows fibrillation potentials on mechanical stimulation by the exploring needle, spontaneous fibrillation and fasciculation potentials when the needle is stationary in the relaxed muscle, and a duration and amplitude of action-potentials greater than normal; even in cases of moderate weakness there may be a marked reduction in the number of spikes on maximal contraction and synchronization of the activity recorded by two separate electrodes within the same muscle (Buchthal and Pinelli 1953). 'Giant' motor units of long duration and greatly increased amplitude, presumed to result from the adoption of denervated muscle fibres by axonal sprouts from surviving neurones, are a common finding (Willison 1962; Barwick 1981). Fasciculaton potentials appear to originate in nerves proximal to the knee and elbow in most cases but are probably unrelated to collateral sprouting of neurones (Wettstein 1979). There is some evidence of impaired neuromuscular transmission as the disease progresses (Denys and Norris 1979) with a decremental response of the compound muscle action potential evoked by nerve stimulation, but this is probably an indication of degeneration of the lower motor neurone (Bernstein and Antel 1981). Single-fibre electromyography suggests that in the early stages certain motor unit pools in the spinal cord (Schwartz and Swash 1982), especially those supplying lower brachial myotomes (Swash 1980), are preferentially involved. Fibre density is not as high as in some other chronic neurogenic disorders (Swash and Schwartz 1982) and effective collateral reinnervation of denervated muscle fibres declines as the number of surviving motor units falls (Hansen and Ballantyne 1978).

Serum enzymes

It was once thought that neurogenic muscular atrophy in the spinal muscular atrophies, including motor-neurone disease, did not, unlike the myopathies, increase serum creatine kinase activity (Pearce, Pennington, and Walton 1964). However, it is now apparent that modest increases in the serum activity of this enzyme up to about 400 I.U./l (normal upper limit 75) are found in between 50 and 75 per cent of cases (Williams and Bruford 1970; Panitch and Franklin 1972; Welch and Goldberg 1972) and have been attributed to secondary myopathic change in the affected muscles (Achari and Anderson 1974). Acetylocholinesterase is also increased in plasma, but this is of no diagnostic value (Festoff and Fernandez 1981).

Symptoms and signs of upper motor-neurone degeneration

Save in those rare cases in which degeneration seems clinically confined to the lower motor neurones, there are manifestations of upper motor-neurone lesions which may be present from the beginning or may follow the muscular wasting. Since atrophy beginning in the lower limbs is relatively uncommon, the legs often present an uncomplicated picture of corticospinal-tract degeneration, with weakness and spasticity and extensor plantar responses. In the upper limbs the addition of an upper to a lower motor-neurone lesion causes a degree of weakness which is disproportionately great in comparison with the severity and the extent of the wasting, and the tendon reflexes are exaggerated in spite of the wasting. It is in the muscles innervated from the medulla that the effects of corticospinal-tract degeneration are of the greatest importance. Here we may encounter lower motor-neurone degeneration only—progressive bulbar palsy; upper motor-neurone degeneration only—'pseudobulbar palsy'; or a combination of the two, which is the most frequent. A lesion of both corticospinal tracts above the medulla, so-called 'pseudobulbar palsy', causes weakness and spasticity of the bulbar muscles and hence leads to dysarthria and dysphagia. The paretic or paralysed muscles are not wasted and hypotonic, as in progressive bulbar palsy, but spastic. The tongue may seem smaller than normal because of spasticity, but is not wrinkled and does not fasciculate. The jaw-jerk, palatal, and pharyngeal reflexes are exaggerated, and sneezing and coughing may be excited reflexly. Dysarthria is of the spastic or explosive type. Pseudobulbar palsy, when severe, also impairs voluntary control over emotional reactions, so that paroxysmal attacks of involuntary laughing and crying occur, often in the form of exaggeration or prolongation of a normal emotional response. Thus a patient laughs because he is amused, but having begun, is unable to stop. Alternatively, the emotional response may be quite inappropriate, such as uncontrollable laughter on hearing bad news, and does not correspond to, or express, the patient's emotional state. When pseudobulbar palsy and progressive bulbar palsy occur in the same individual, dysarthria and dysphagia are intensified, impairment of emotional control may be present, and an exaggerated jaw-jerk is obtained, in spite of manifest wasting of bulbar muscles.

The reflexes

The condition of the reflexes in a given case depends upon the relative preponderance of upper and lower motor-neurone degeneration. The palatal and pharyngeal reflexes tend to be lost in the later stages due to wasting of the muscles concerned. Owing to the corticospinal-tract degeneration, the abdominal reflexes, which are initially preserved much longer, for instance, than in multiple sclerosis, are eventually diminished or lost, and the plantar reflexes are extensor. The jaw-jerk and the tendon reflexes vary between exaggeration and abolition. Degeneration of the lower motor neurones causes impairment, and finally loss, of the relevant reflexes while corticospinal degeneration leads to exaggeration. Hence it is not uncommon to find exaggerated tendon-jerks in the upper limbs despite severe atrophy. Since in the lower limbs muscular wasting is usually late to develop, the knee- and ankle-jerks are generally exaggerated and the plantar responses extensor.

Other symptoms

In the early stages the sphincters are not as a rule affected, though slight precipitancy or difficulty of micturition is occasionally seen. Later retention or incontinence rarely occurs. Impotence often develops early. There is no sensory impairment. Horner's syndrome is a rare manifestation due to involvement of lateral horn cells in the dorsal cord.

The subcutaneous fat tends to disappear *pari passu* with the muscular wasting, and marked emaciation characterizes the later stages. Dementia with parkinsonian features is a common association in the Western Pacific form (see above) and probably occurs more often in sporadic cases than was previously appreciated (Hudson 1981).

Diagnosis

Motor-neurone disease must be distinguished from other conditions leading to muscular wasting and from other causes of bulbar palsy.

In syringomyelia muscular wasting in the upper limbs is often associated with spastic weakness of the lower limbs. Fasciculation, however, is rarely as striking as in motor-neurone disease, and the typical dissociated sensory loss, if not present at the outset, soon develops.

In syphilitic amyotrophy due to meningomyelitis the weakness and wasting is often accompanied by pain of radicular distribution. Signs of corticospinal-tract degeneration are often slight and sensory abnormalities are common; pupillary abnormalities may be present; the serological reactions are usually positive in either the blood or the CSF, in which other abnormalities characteristic of syphilis are usually found. Spinal pachymeningitis secondary to cysticercosis may rarely give a clinical picture indistinguishable from that of motor-neurone disease (Kahn 1972).

Spinal-cord tumour involving the cervical enlargement is likely to cause muscular wasting in one or both upper limbs, together with spastic paraplegia, but sensory loss is usual, and changes characterisitic of spinal block are often found in the CSF.

Cervical spondylosis may closely simulate motor-neurone disease when it causes muscular wasting and fasciculation in the upper limbs, and spastic weakness in the lower without sensory loss. The course, however, is usually much slower than that of motor-neurone disease, and the myelographic changes are characteristic. However, spondylosis and motor-neurone disease may co-exist.

Spinal radiculitis ('neuralgic amyotrophy') causes muscular wasting and weakness. The axillary nerve is most often affected. The onset is usually acute with severe pain in the neck and shoulder. The condition is not progressive, and any change is in the direction of improvement.

Cervical rib may give wasting of the small muscles of one or both hands. Muscular fasciculation, however, is usually absent, and pain along the ulnar border of the hand and forearm is often prominent, being frequently associated with relative anaesthesia and analgesia in this region, and sometimes with vascular changes. Moreover, cervical rib can be seen on X-ray, though it must be remembered that in the costoclavicular syndrome the same symptoms may be caused by pressure upon a normal first rib or fibrous band. However, digital pressure in the root of the neck often reproduces the patient's pain and paraesthesiae.

Lesions of peripheral nerves usually give little difficulty, since the distribution of the muscular wasting is restricted to the muscles supplied by the nerve and, in the case of the median and ulnar nerves, there are usually sensory abnormalities of equally distinctive distribution. A lesion of the deep branch of one ulnar nerve, giving wasting of small hand muscles without sensory loss, may cause difficulty, but nerve conduction velocity measurements (increased terminal latency) are usually diagnostic.

Polymyositis is usually too acute to cause problems, and can also be distinguished electromyographically and by muscle biopsy. Various myopathies of late onset, however, may be confused with progressive muscular atrophy. Their diagnosis is discussed on page 585.

The muscular dystrophies also are unlikely to give difficulty as they usually develop at a much earlier age. Dystrophia myotonica, however, is a disorder of adult life, but is readily distinguished by the peculiar distribution of the wasting, with its predilection for the sternomastoids, facial muscles, and the forearm and leg muscles, the presence of myotonia, the absence of fasciculation, and the association with cataract and other systemic abnormalities.

Peroneal muscular atrophy is distinguished by the typical distribution of the wasting, beginning in the periphery of the limbs, generally in the lower before the upper, and often with sensory impairment. This disease, moreover, is usually familial, and the first symptoms often appear in childhood. Scapuloperoneal muscular atrophy (p. 385) can also give difficulty but here again the pattern of weakness and wasting is distinctive.

It may sometimes be difficult or impossible to distinguish motor-neurone disease of unusually early onset from benign spinal muscular atrophy of adolescence or early adult life (*vide infra*) save by the age of onset and benign course of the latter disorder. Motor-neurone disease or spinal muscular atrophy localized to one upper limb, as described in Japan and India, is a rare but distinctive clinical picture (p. 371). Coarse and widespread fasciculation associated with muscular cramps and hyperhidrosis but without muscular wasting or hyperreflexia is a benign syndrome often confused with motor-neurone disease; in this condition, often called one variety of myokymia (Walton 1981), the electromyogram shows that many of the fasciculation potentials are like double or treble rather than single motor unit action potentials. A similar benign disorder with cramps and fasciculation may follow old poliomyelitis or myelitis (Fetell, Smallberg, Lewis, Lovelace, Hays, and Rowland 1982).

Pseudobulbar palsy may be due to bilateral vascular lesions involving the corticospinal tracts at any point above the medulla. When these are sudden in onset, the condition is unlikely to be confused with motor-neurone disease. When the onset is insidious, the distinction is based upon the absence of muscular wasting and the presence of hypertension and arterial disease. Myasthenia is distinguished by the characteristic fatigability, the response to edrophonium hydrochloride (*Tensilon*), and the absence of wasting and fasciculation. In syringobulbia the dissociated sensory loss over the face is a distinctive feature.

Prognosis

Motor-neurone disease is a progressive disease, but its rate of progress shows considerable variations. In a few cases the patient deteriorates rapidly, muscular weakness, wasting, and fasciculation early becoming widespread, and death may occur within a year. In cases of slower onset the prognosis is influenced by several factors. Those in which the degeneration is for a long time confined to the lower motor neurones do best. Early involvement of the bulbar muscles makes the outlook worse, especially when progressive bulbar palsy is combined with pseudobulbar palsy. Rosen (1978) found that 39.4 per cent of patients survive for five years, that young patients had a better prognosis than those over 50 years of age, and that the spinal form was associated with a threefold better five-year survival than the bulbar form. In general, patents with progressive bulbar palsy survive about 2–3 years, those with amyotrophic lateral sclerosis 3–5 years, and those with progressive muscular atrophy 3–10 years from the onset of symptoms, but there are many exceptions to this general guide. Temporary arrest may occur, but is uncommon.

Treatment

The cause of the disease being unknown, treatment is symptomatic. Every effort should be made, however, to exclude any form of chronic intoxication. Syphilis is excluded by the usual serological tests. The patient should avoid undue fatigue, but should be encouraged to continue in light employment as long as possible. Regular moderate exercise to maintain power in innervated muscles is probably beneficial provided the patient does not exhaust himself (*British Medical Journal* 1976a, b). Neostigmine, 15 mg orally, two, three, or four times daily with atropine, 0.6 mg, or propantheline, 15 mg twice daily, to overcome its side-effects, may have a temporary beneficial effect upon speech and swallowing in patients with bulbar weakness, and diazepam, 2–5 mg three times daily, or baclofen, may diminish spasticity. Antibiotics may be needed for respiratory and urinary infection. In the late stages tracheostomy may be necessary if dysphagia and choking attacks become severe and the usual attention is given to the bladder and skin. Temporary but substantial improvement in dysphagia due to pharyngeal paralysis may be achieved by the operation of cricopharyngeal sphincterotomy (Mills 1973; Loizou, Small, and Dalton 1980). Tube-feeding or gastrostomy are occasionally required to give appropriate nutriments. Some patients are helped by calipers and toe-springs if foot-drop is troublesome and later a wheel-chair may be necessary. In patients with respiratory insufficiency the use of portable respiratory-support devices

(Sivak, Gipson, and Hanson 1982) may prolong useful life and reduce disability in appropriate cases where mobility is reasonably preserved. Unfortunately no drug is known which has any influence upon the disease process. In the early stages, electrophysiological studies may indicate a diminished output of acetylcholine from affected axon terminals and this may explain transient improvement produced by giving neostigmine and its analogues. This suggested that guanidine hydrochloride, which increases acetylcholine output, might be of therapeutic benefit, but controlled trials have shown no clinical improvement (Norris, Calanchini, Fallat, Panchari, and Jewett 1974 a) and the drug sometimes causes a striking increase in weakness (Norris, Fallat, and Calanchini 1974 b). Lecithin given as an acetylcholine precursor is also ineffective (Kelemen, Hedlund, Murray-Douglas, and Munsat 1982). Antiviral agents are also of no benefit (Campbell and Liversedge 1981). Modified neurotoxin (Tyler 1979), as advocated by Sanders and Fellowes (1975), is also ineffective, as are transfer factor (Olarte, Gersten, Zabriskie, and Rowland 1979) and plasmapheresis (Schauf, Antel, Arnason, Davis, and Rooney 1980). Bovine brain gangliosides have also failed to produce benefit (Harrington, Hallett, and Tyler 1984). Transient improvement has, however, been reported after intravenous thyrotropin-releasing hormone (TRH) (see Rowland 1984). Useful advice on general management has been given by Newrick and Langton-Hewer (1984).

Opinions vary upon what the affected patient should be told. Certainly a responsible relative should be told the truth, while stressing the variability of the clinical course of the condition and emphasizing that some cases are more benign. It is my custom to tell the affected individual first that the condition is one which is well-recognized, if of unknown cause, and to explain something of research now in progress. In order not to destroy all hope, I prefer to say also that the condition progresses slowly up to a point but then usually becomes arrested, and may even subsequently improve spontaneously, while making it clear that no one can predict when and if arrest will occur. Comparatively few patients seem to be aware of the deception, even to the end.

References

Achari, A. N. and Anderson, M. S. (1974). Serum creatine phosphokinase in amyotrophic lateral sclerosis. *Neurology, Minneapolis* **24**, 834.

Alberca, R., Castilla, J. M. and Gil-Peralta, A. (1981). Hereditary amyotrophic lateral sclerosis. *J. neurol. Sci.* **50**, 201.

Alter, M. and Schaumann, B. (1976). A family with amyotrophic lateral sclerosis and Parkinsonism. *J. Neurol.* **212**, 281.

Antel, J. P., Arnason, B. G. W., Fuller, T. C. and Lehrich, J. R. (1976). Histocompatibility typing in amyotrophic lateral sclerosis. *Arch. Neurol., Chicago* **33**, 423.

Appel, S. H. (1981). A unifying hypothesis for the cause of amyotrophic lateral sclerosis, Parkinsonism, and Alzheimer disease. *Ann. Neurol.* **10**, 499.

Aran, F. A. (1850). Recherches sur une maladie non encore décrite du système musculaire. *Arch. gén. Méd.* **24**, 5.

Askanas, V., Marangos, P. J. and Engel, W. K. (1981). CSF from amyotrophic lateral sclerosis patients applied to motor neurons in culture fails to alter neuron-specific enolase. *Neurology, Minneapolis* **31**, 1196.

Barkhaus, P. E., Kennedy, W. R., Stern, L. Z. and Harrington, R. B. (1982). Hereditary proximal spinal and bulbar motor neuron disease of late onset: a report of six cases. *Arch. Neurol., Chicago* **39**, 112.

Bartfeld, H., Pollack, M. S., Cunningham-Rundles, S. and Donnenfeld, H. (1982). HLA frequencies in amyotrophic lateral sclerosis. *Arch. Neurol., Chicago* **39**, 270.

Barwick, D. D. (1981). Clinical electromyography. In *Disorders of voluntary muscle* (ed. J. N. Walton) 4th edn, p. 952. Churchill-Livingstone, Edinburgh.

Bernstein, L. P. and Antel, J. P. (1981). Motor neuron disease: decremental response to repetitive nerve stimulation. *Neurology, Minneapolis* **31**, 202.

Bertrand, I. and van Bogaert, L. (1925). Rapport sur la sclérose latérale amyotrophique. *Rev. Neurol., Paris* **32**, 779.

Bjornskov, E. K., Dekker, N. P., Norris, F. H. and Stuart, M. E. (1975). End-plate morphology in amyotrophic lateral sclerosis. *Arch. Neurol., Chicago* **32**, 711.

Boothby, J. A., de Jesus, P. V. and Rowland, L. P. (1974). Reversible forms of motor neuron disease: lead 'neuritis'. *Arch. Neurol., Chicago* **31**, 18.

Bots, G. T. A. M. and Staal, A. (1973). Amyotrophic lateral sclerosis–dementia complex, neuroaxonal dystrophy, and Hallervorden–Spatz disease, *Neurology, Minneapolis* **23**, 35.

Brain, Lord, Croft, P. B. and Wilkinson, M. (1965). Motor neurone disease as a manifestation of neoplasms (with a note on the course of classical motor neurone disease). *Brain* **88**, 479.

British Medical Journal (1976a). Management of motor neurone disease. *Br. med. J.* **1**, 1422.

—— (1976b). Symptomatic care in motor neurone disease. *Br. med. J.* **2**, 605.

Brown, W. F. and Jaatoul, N. (1974). Amyotrophic lateral sclerosis: electrophysiologic study (number of motor units and rate of decay of motor units). *Arch. Neurol., Chicago* **30**, 242.

Brownell, N., Oppenheimer, D. R. and Hughes, J. T. (1970). The central nervous system in motor neurone disease. *J. Neurol. Neurosurg. Psychiat.* **33**, 338.

Buchthal, F. and Pinelli, P. (1953). Action potentials in muscular atrophy of neurogenic origin. *Neurology, Minneapolis* **3**, 591.

Buckley, J., Warlow, C., Smith, P., Hilton-Jones, D., Irvine, S. and Tew, J. R. (1983). Motor neuron disease in England and Wales. *J. Neurol. Neurosurg. Psychiat.* **46**, 197.

Campbell, A. M. G., Williams, E. R. and Barltrop, D. (1970). Motor neurone disease and exposure to lead. *J. Neurol. Neurosurg. Psychiat.* **33**, 877.

Campbell, M. J. and Liversedge, L. A. (1981). The motor neurone diseases. In *Disorders of voluntary muscle* (ed. J. N. Walton) 4th edn, p. 725. Churchill-Livingstone, Edinburgh.

Carpenter, S. (1968). Proximal axonal enlargement in motor neuron disease. *Neurology, Minneapolis* **18**, 841.

Chad, D., Mitsumoto, H., Adelman, L. S., Bradley, W. G., Munsat, T. L. and Zieper, I. (1982). Conjugal motor neurone disease. *Neurology, Minneapolis* **32**, 306.

Charcot, J. M. and Joffroy, A. (1869). Deux cas d'atrophie musculaire progressive avec lésions de la substance grise et des faisceaux antéro-latéraux de la moelle épinière. *Arch. Physiol. norm. Path.* **2**, 354, 629, 744.

Conradi, S., Kaijser, L. and Ronnevi, L.-o. (1978). Capillary permeability in ALS, determined through transcapillary escape rate of ^{125}I-albumin. *Acta neurol. scand.* **57**, 257.

—— Ronnevi, L.-O., Nise, G. and Vesterberg, O. (1980). Abnormal distribution of lead in amyotrophic lateral sclerosis. *J. neurol. Sci.* **48**, 413.

——, ——, and Vesterberg, O. (1978a). Increased plasma levels of lead in patients with amyotrophic lateral sclerosis compared with control subjects as determined by flameless atomic absorption spectrophotometry. *J. Neurol. Neurosurg. Psychiat.* **41**, 389.

——, ——, and —— (1978b). Lead concentration in skeletal muscle in amyotrophic lateral sclerosis patients and control subjects. *J. Neurol. Neurosurg. Psychiat.* **41**, 1001.

Cork, L. C., Griffin, J. W., Adams, R. J. and Price, D. L. (1977). Hereditary spinal muscle atrophy in Brittany spaniels. *J. Neuropath. exp. Neurol.* **36**, 598.

Cremer, N. E., Oshiro, L. S., Norris, F. H. and Lennette, E. H. (1973). Cultures of tissues from patients with amyotrophic lateral sclerosis. *Arch. Neurol., Chicago* **29**, 331.

Denys, E. H. and Norris, F. H. (1979). Amyotrophic lateral sclerosis: impairment of neuromuscular transmission. *Arch. Neurol., Chicago* **36**, 202.

Drachman, D. B., Murphy, S. R., Nigam, M. P. and Hills, J. R. (1967). 'Myopathic' changes in chronically denervated muscle. *Arch. Neurol., Chicago* **16**, 14.

Duchen, L. W. (1978). Motor neuron diseases in man and animals, *Invest. Cell. Pathol.* **1**, 249.

Duchenne, G. B. (1853). Étude comparée des lésions anatomiques dans l'atrophie musculaire progressive et dans la paralysie générale. *Un. méd. Can.* **7**, 202.

Edgar, A. G., Brody, J. A. and Detels, R. (1973). Amyotrophic lateral sclerosis mortality among native-born and migrant residents of California and Washington. *Neurology, Minneapolis* **23**, 48.

Eldridge, R., Ryan, E., Rosario, J. and Brody, J. A. (1969). Amyotrophic lateral sclerosis and parkinsonism dementia in a migrant population from Guam. *Neurology, Minneapolis* **19**, 1029.

Engel, W. K., Kurland, L. T. and Klatzo, I. (1959). An inherited disease similar to amyotrophic lateral sclerosis with a pattern of posterior column involvement. An intermediate form? *Brain* **82**, 203.

Esteban, A., de Andres, C. and Giménez-Roldán, S. (1978). Abnormalities of Bell's phenomenon in amyotrophic lateral sclerosis. *J. Neurol. Neurosurg. Psychiat.* **41**, 690.

Fazio, M. (1892). Ereditarieta della parilisi bulbare progressiva. *Riforma. Med.* **8**, 327.

Felmus, M. T., Patten, B. M. and Swanke, L. (1976). Antecedent events in amyotrophic lateral sclerosis. *Neurology, Minneapolis* **26**, 167.

Festoff, B. W. (1980). Neuromuscular junction macromolecules in the pathogenesis of amyotrophic lateral sclerosis. *Med. Hypotheses* **6**, 121.

Festoff, B. W. and Fernandez, H. L. (1981). Plasma and red blood cell and acetylcholinesterase in amyotrophic lateral sclerosis. *Muscle & Nerve* **4**, 41.

Fetell, M. R., Smallberg, G., Lewis, L. D., Lovelace, R. E., Hays, A. P. and Rowland, L. P. (1982). A benign motor neuron disorder: delayed cramps and fasciculation after poliomyelitis or myelitis. *Ann. Neurol.* **11**, 423.

Gajdusek, D. C. (1982). Foci of motor neuron disease in high incidence in isolated populations of East Asia and the Western Pacific. In *Human motor neuron diseases* (ed. L. P. Rowland), p. 363. Raven Press, New York.

—— and Salazar, A. M. (1982). Amyotrophic lateral sclerosis and parkinsonian syndromes in high incidence among the Auyu and Jakai people of West New Guinea. *Neurology, Minneapolis* **32**, 107.

Garruto, R. M., Gajdusek, D. C. and Chen, K. -M. (1981). Amyotrophic lateral sclerosis and Parkinsonism–dementia among Filipino migrants to Guam. *Ann. Neurol.* **10**, 341.

——, Yanagihara, R. and Gajdusek, D. C. (1985). Disappearance of high-incidence ALS and parkinsonism-dementia on Guam. *Neurology, Cleveland* **35**, 193.

Ghatak, N. R. and Nochlin, D. (1982). Glial outgrowth along spinal nerve roots in amyotrophic lateral sclerosis. *Ann. Neurol.* **11**, 203.

Giménez-Roldan, S. and Esteban, A. (1977). Prognosis in hereditary amyotrophic lateral sclerosis. *Arch. Neurol., Chicago* **34**, 706.

Gourie-Devi, M., Suresh, T. G., and Shankar, S. K. (1984). Monomelic amyotrophy. *Arch. Neurol. Chicago* **41**, 388.

Greenfield, J. G. (1958). In *Neuropathology* (ed. J. G. Greenfield, W. Blackwood, W. H. McMenemey, A. Meyer and R. M. Normal), p. 545. Arnold, London.

Guiloff, R. J., McGregor, B., Thompson, E., Blackwood, W. and Paul, E. (1980). Motor neurone disease with elevated cerebrospinal fluid protein. *J. Neurol. Neurosurg. Psychiat.* **43**, 390.

Gustafson, A. and Störtebecker, P. (1972). Vascular and metabolic studies of amyotrophic lateral sclerosis. II. Lipid and carbohydrate metabolism. *Neurology, Minneapolis* **22**, 528.

Hallen, O., Brusis, T. and Pfisterer, H. (1969). Die Myatrophia spinalis postpoliomyelitica chronica. Ein Beitrag zum Problem der sog. Poliomyelitis anterior chronica. *Dtsch. Z. Nervenheilk.* **195**, 333.

Hansen, S. and Ballantyne, J. P. (1978). A quantitative electrophysiological study of motor neurone disease. *J. Neurol. Neurosurg. Psychiat.* **41**, 773.

Harding, A. E., Bradbury, P. G. and Murray, N. M. F. (1983). Chronic asymmetrical spinal muscular atrophy. *J. neurol. Sci.* **59**, 69.

Harrington, H., Hallett, M., and Tyler, H. R. (1984). Ganglioside therapy for amyotrophic lateral sclerosis. *Neurology, Cleveland* **34**, 1083.

Harvey, D. G., Torack, R. M. and Rosenbaum, H. E. (1979). Amyotrophic lateral sclerosis with ophthalmoplegia: a clinicopathologic study. *Arch. Neurol., Chicago* **36**, 615.

Hashimoto, O., Asada, M., Ohta, M. and Kuroiwa, Y. (1976). Clinical observations of juvenile nonprogressive muscular atrophy localized in hand and forearm. *J. Neurol.* **211**, 105.

Hawkes, C. H. and Fox, A. J. (1981). Motor neurone disease in leather workers. *Lancet* **i**, 507.

Hayashi, H. and Tsubaki, T. (1982). Enzymatic analysis of individual anterior horn cells in amyotrophic lateral sclerosis and Duchenne muscular dystrophy. *J. neurol. Sci.* **57**, 133.

——, Suga, M., Satake, M. and Tsubaki, T. (1981). Reduced glycine receptor in the spinal cord in amyotrophic lateral sclerosis. *Ann. Neurol.* **9**, 292.

Hill, R., Martin, J. and Hakim, A. (1983). Acute respiratory failure in motor neurone disease. *Arch. Neurol., Chicago* **40**, 30.

Hirano, A., Kurland, L. T. and Sayre, G. P. (1967). Familial amyotrophic lateral sclerosis. *Arch. Neurol., Chicago* **16**, 232.

Hoffman, P. M., Robbins, D. S., Oldstone, M. B. A., Gibbs, C. J. and Gajdusek, D. C. (1981). Humoral immunity in Guamanians with amyotrophic lateral sclerosis and Parkinsonism–dementia. *Ann. Neurol.* **10**, 193.

Horton, W. A., Eldridge, R. and Brody, J. A. (1976). Familial motor neuron disease: evidence for at least three different types. *Neurology, Minneapolis* **26**, 460.

Hudson, A. J. (1981). Amyotrophic lateral sclerosis and its association with dementia, Parkinsonism and other neurological disorders: a review. *Brain* **104**, 217.

Hughes, J. T. and Jerrome, D. (1971). Ultrastructure of anterior horn motor neurones in the Hirano–Kurland–Sayre type of combined neurological system degeneration. *J. neurol. Sci.* **13**, 389.

Ionasescu, V. and Luca, N. (1964). Studies on carbohydrate metabolism in amyotrophic lateral sclerosis and hereditary proximal spinal muscular atrophy. *Acta neurol. scand.* **40**, 47.

Jacobs, L., Bozian, D., Heffner, R. R. and Barron, S. A. (1981). An eye movement disorder in amyotrophic lateral sclerosis. *Neurology, Minneapolis* **31**, 1282.

Jokelainen, M. (1976). The epidemiology of amyotrophic lateral sclerosis in Finland. A study based on the death certificates of 421 patients. *J. neurol. Sci.* **29**, 55.

Juergens, S. M., Kurland, L. T., Okazaki, H. and Mulder, D. W. (1980). ALS in Rochester, Minnesota, 1925–1977. *Neurology, Minneapolis* **30**, 463.

Kahana, E., Alter, M. and Feldman, S. (1976). Amyotrophic lateral sclerosis: a population study. *J. Neurol.* **212**, 205.

Kahn, P. (1972). Cysticercosis of the central nervous system with amyotrophic lateral sclerosis: case report and review of the literature. *J. Neurol. Neurosurg. Psychiat.* **35**, 81.

Kelemen, J., Hedlund, W., Murray-Douglas, P. and Munsat, T. L. (1982). Lecithin is not effective in amyotrophic lateral sclerosis, *Neurology, Minneapolis* **32**, 315.

Kennedy, W. R., Alter, M. and Sung, J. H. (1968). Progressive proximal spinal and bulbar muscular atrophy of late onset. *Neurology, Minneapolis* **18**, 671.

Kjellin, K. G. and Stibler, H. (1976). Isoelectric focusing and electrophoresis of cerebrospinal fluid proteins in muscular dystrophies and spinal muscular atrophies. *J. neurol. Sci.* **27**, 45.

Kott, E., Livni, E., Zamir R. and Kuritzky, A. (1979). Cell-mediated immunity to polio and HLA antigens in amyotrophic lateral sclerosis. *Neurology, Minneapolis* **29**, 1040.

Kurland, L. T. (1957). Epidemiological investigations of amyotrophic lateral sclerosis. *Proc. Mayo Clin.* **32**, 449.

—— (1972). An appraisal of the neurotoxicity of cycad and the etiology of amyotrophic lateral sclerosis on Guam. *Fed. Proc.* **31**, 1540.

—— and Mulder, D. W. (1954). Epidemiologic investigations of amyotrophic lateral sclerosis. I. Preliminary report on geographic distribution, with special reference to the Mariana Islands, including clinical and pathologic observations. *Neurology, Minneapolis* **4**, 355.

Kurlander, H. M. and Patten, B. M. (1979). Metals in spinal cord tissue of patients dying of motor neuron disease. *Ann. Neurol.* **6**, 21.

Kurtzke, J. F. (1969). Comments on the epidemiology of amyotrophic lateral sclerosis (ALS). In *Motor neurone diseases* (ed. F. H. Norris and L. T. Kurland) p. 85. Grune & Stratton, New York.

—— (1982). Motor neuron(e) disease. *Br. med. J.* **284**, 141.

—— and Beebe, G. W. (1980). Epidemiology of amyotrophic lateral sclerosis: 1. A case-control comparison based on ALS deaths. *Neurology, Minneapolis* **30**, 453.

The Lancet (1977). Amyotrophic lateral sclerosis. *Lancet* **i**, 582.

—— (1979). Neuropathological normality in Guam. *Lancet* **ii**, 293.

Loizou, L. A., Small, M. and Dalton, G. A. (1980). Cricopharyngeal myotomy in motor neurone disease. *J. Neurol. Neurosurg. Psychiat.* **43**, 42.

Londe, P. (1983). Paralysie bulbaire progressive infantile et familiale. *Rev. Méd.* **13**, 1020.

Mann, D. M. A. and Yates, P. O. (1974). Motor neurone disease: the nature of the pathogenic mechanism. *J. Neurol. Neurosurg. Psychiat.* **37**, 1036.

Mannen, T., Iwata, M., Toyokura, Y. and Nagashima, K. (1977). Preservation of a certain motoneurone group of the sacral cord in amyotrophic lateral sclerosis. *J. Neurol. Neurosurg. Psychiat.* **40**, 464.

Markand, O. N. and Daly, D. D. (1971). Juvenile type of slowly progressive bulbar palsy: report of a case. *Neurology, Minnneapolis* **21**, 753.

Mastaglia, F. L. and Walton, J. N. (1982). (Eds.) *Skeletal muscle pathology*. Churchill-Livingstone, Edinburgh.

Matsumoto, N., Worth, R. M., Kurland, L. T. and Okazaki, H. (1972). Epidemiologic study of amyotrophic lateral sclerosis in Hawaii:

identification of high incidence among Filipino men. *Neurology, Minneapolis* **22**, 934.

McComas, A. J., Upton, A. R. M. and Sica, R. E. P. (1973). Motoneurone disease and ageing. *Lancet* **ii**, 1477.

Mendell, J. R., Chase, T. N. and Engel, W. K. (1971). Amyotrophic lateral sclerosis. A study of central monoamine metabolism and therapeutic trial of levodopa. *Arch. Neurol., Chicago* **25**, 320.

Metcalf, C. W. and Hirano, A. (1971). Amyotrophic lateral sclerosis. Clinicopathological studies of a family. *Arch. Neurol., Chicago* **24**, 518.

Meyers, K. R., Dorencamp, D. G. and Suzuki, K. (1974). Amyotrophic lateral sclerosis with diffuse neurofibrillary changes. *Arch. Neurol., Chicago* **30**, 84.

Milhorat, A. T. (1946). Studies in diseases of muscle. XV. Progressive spinal muscular atrophy as a late sequel of acute epidemic encephalitis: report of two cases. *Arch. Neurol. Psychiat., Chicago* **55**, 134.

Mills, C. P. (1973). Dysphagia in pharyngeal paralysis treated by cricopharyngeal sphincterotomy. *Lancet* **i**, 455.

Müller, W. K. and Schaltenbrand, G. (1979). Attempts to reproduce amyotrophic lateral sclerosis in laboratory animals by inoculation of Schu virus isolated from a patient with apparent amyotrophic lateral sclerosis. *J. Neurol.* **220**, 1.

Murakami, T., Mastaglia, F. L. and Bradley, W. G. (1980). Reduced protein synthesis in spinal anterior horn neurons in wobbler mouse mutant. *Exp. Neurol.* **67**, 423.

Nelson, J. S. and Prensky, A. L. (1972). Sporadic juvenile amyotrophic lateral sclerosis. A clinicopathological study of a case with neuronal cytoplasmic inclusions containing RNA. *Arch. Neurol., Chicago* **27**, 300.

Newrick, P.G. and Langton-Hewer, R. (1984). Motor neurone disease: can we do better? A study of 42 patients. *Br. med. J.* **289**, 539.

Nightingale, S., Bates, D., Bateman, D. E., Hudgson, P., Ellis, D. A. and Gibson, G. J. (1982). Enigmatic dyspnoea: an unusual presentation of motor-neurone disease. *Lancet* **i**, 933.

Norris, F. G., Calanchini, P. R., Fallat, R. J., Panchari, S. and Jewett, B. (1974*a*). The administration of guanidine in amyotrophic lateral sclerosis. *Neurology, Minneapolis* **24**, 721.

——, Fallat, R. J. and Calanchini, P. R. (1974*b*). Increased paralysis induced by guanidine in motor neuron disease. *Neurology, Minneapolis* **24**, 135.

—— and Engel, W. K. (1965). Carcinomatous amyotrophic lateral sclerosis. In *The remote effects of cancer on the nervous system* (ed. Lord Brain and F. H. Norris) p. 24. Grune & Stratton, New York.

Olarte, M. R., Gersten, J. C., Zabriskie, J. and Rowland, L. P. (1979). Transfer factor is ineffective in amyotrophic lateral sclerosis. *Ann. Neurol.* **5**, 385.

Olivares, L., San Esteban, E. and Alter, M. (1972). Mexican 'resistance' to amyotrophic lateral sclerosis. *Arch. Neurol., Chicago* **27**, 397.

Oshiro, L. S., Cremer, N. E., Norris, F. H. and Lennette, E. H. (1976). Virus-like particles in muscle from a patient with amyotrophic lateral sclerosis. *Neurology, Minneapolis* **26**, 57.

Osuntokun, B. O., Adeuja, A. O. G. and Bademosi, O. (1974). The prognosis of motor neuron disease in Nigerian Africans—a prospective study of 92 patients. *Brain* **97**, 385.

Panitch, H. S and Franklin, G. M. (1972). Elevation of serum creatine phosphokinase in amyotrophic lateral sclerosis. *Neurology, Minneapolis* **22**, 964.

Parhad, I. M., Clark, A. W., Barron, K. D. and Staunton, S. B. (1978). Diaphragmatic paralysis in motor neuron disease: report of two cases and a review of the literature. *Neurology, Minneapolis* **28**, 18.

Patten, B. M., Zito, G. and Harati, Y. (1979). Histologic findings in motor neuron disease: relation to clinically determined activity, duration, and severity of disease. *Arch. Neurol., Chicago* **36**, 560.

Pearce, J. M. S., Pennington, R. J. T. and Walton, J. N. (1964). Serum enzyme studies in muscle disease. Part II: Serum creatine kinase activity in muscular dystrophy and in other myopathic and neuropathic disorders. *J. Neurol. Neurosurg. Psychiat.* **27**, 96.

Peters, H. A. and Clatanoff, D. V. (1968). Spinal muscular atrophy secondary to macroglobulinemia. Reversal of symptoms with chlorambucil therapy. *Neurology, Minneapolis* **18**, 101.

Queiroz, L. de S., Nucci, A. and Filho, A. P. (1977). Motor neurone disease with neurofibrillary tangles in a Brazilian woman. *J. neurol. Sci.* **33**, 21.

Reed, D. M., Brody, J. A. and Holden, E. M. (1975). Predicting the duration of Guam amyotrophic lateral sclerosis. *Neurology, Minneapolis* **25**, 277.

Roisen, F. J., Bartfeld, H., Donnenfeld, H. and Baxter, J. (1982). Neuron specific in vitro cytotoxicity of sera from patients with amyotrophic lateral sclerosis. *Muscle & Nerve* **5**, 48.

Ronnevi, L. -O., Conradi, S. and Nise, G. (1982). Further studies on the erythrocyte uptake of lead in vitro in amyotrophic lateral sclerosis (ALS) patients and controls: abnormal erythrocyte fragility in ALS. *J. neurol. Sci.* **57**, 143.

Rosen, A. D. (1978). Amyotrophic lateral sclerosis. *Arch. Neurol., Chicago* **35**, 638.

Rowland, L. P. (1984). Motor neuron diseases and amyotrophic lateral sclerosis. *Trends Neurosci.* **7**, 110.

Sanders, M. and Fellowes, J. (1975). Use of detoxified snake neurotoxin as a partial treatment for amyotrophic lateral sclerosis. *Cancer Cytol.* **15**, 26.

Savolainen, H. and Palo, J. (1973). Amyotrophic lateral sclerosis: proteins of neuronal cell membranes, axons and myelin of the precentral gyrus and other cortical areas. *Brain* **96**, 537.

Schauf, C. L., Antel, J. P., Arnason, B. G. W., Davis, F. A. and Rooney, M. W. (1980). Neuroelectric blocking activity and plasmapheresis in amyotrophic lateral sclerosis. *Neurology, Minneapolis* **30**, 1011.

Schochet, S. S., Hardman, J. M., Ladewig, P. P. and Earle, K. M. (1969). Intraneuronal conglomerates in sporadic motor neuron disease. *Arch. Neurol., Chicago* **20**, 548.

Schwartz, M. S. and Swash, M. (1982). Pattern of involvement in the cervical segments in the early stage of motor neurone disease: a single fibre EMG study. *Acta neurol. scand.* **65**, 424.

Serisier, D. E., Mastaglia, F. L. and Gibson, G. J. (1982). Respiratory muscle function and ventilatory control: I in patients with motor neurone disease; II in patients with myotonic dystrophy. *Quart. J. Med.* **51**, 205.

Shahani, B., Davies-Jones, G. A. B. and Russell, W. R. (1971). Motor neurone disease. Further evidence for an abnormality of nerve metabolism. *J. Neurol. Neurosurg. Psychiat.* **34**, 185.

Sivak, E. D., Gipson, W. T. and Hanson, M. R. (1982). Long-term management of respiratory failure in amyotrophic lateral sclerosis. *Ann. Neurol.* **12**, 18.

Smith, M. A. (1960). Nerve fibre degeneration in the brain in amyotrophic lateral sclerosis. *J. Neurol. Neurosurg. Psychiat.* **23**, 269.

Sobue, G., Matsuoka, Y., Mukai, E., Takayanagi, T. and Sobue, I. (1981). Pathology of myelinated fibers in cervical and lumbar ventral spinal roots in amyotrophic lateral sclerosis. *J. neurol. Sci.* **50**, 413.

Sobue, I., Saito, N., Iida, . and Ando, K. (1978). Juvenile type of distal and segmental muscular atrophy of upper extremities. *Ann. Neurol.* **3**, 429.

Spillane, J. D. (1975). *An atlas of clinical neurology*, 2nd edn. Oxford University Press, Oxford.

Staal, A. and Went, L. N. (1968). Juvenile amyotrophic lateral sclerosis-dementia complex in a Dutch family. *Neurology, Minneapolis* **18**, 800.

Störtebecker, P., Nordström, G., Pestény, M. P. de, Seeman, T. and Bjorkerud, S. (1970). Vascular and metabolic studies of amyotrophic lateral sclerosis. I. Angiopathy in biopsy specimens of peripheral arteries. *Neurology, Minneapolis* **20**, 1157.

Swash, M. (1980). Vulnerability of lower brachial myotomes in motor neurone disease: a clinical and single fibre EMG study. *J. neurol. Sci.* **47**, 59.

—— and Schwartz, M. S. (1982). A longitudinal study of changes in motor units in motor neuron disease. *J. neurol. Sci.* **56**, 185.

Takahashi, K., Nakamura, Y. and Okada, E. (1972). Hereditary amyotrophic lateral sclerosis. Histochemical and electron microscopic study of hyaline inclusions in motor neurones. *Arch. Neurol., Chicago* **27**, 292.

Telerman-Toppet, N. and Coërs, C. (1978). Motor innervation and fiber type pattern in amyotrophic lateral sclerosis and in Charcot–Marie–Tooth disease, *Muscle & Nerve* **1**, 133.

Tsukagoshi, H., Yanagisawa, N., Oguchi, K., Nagashima, K. and Murakami, T. (1979). Morphometric quantification of the cervical limb motor cells in controls and in amyotrophic lateral sclerosis. *J. neurol. Sci.* **41**, 287.

Tyler, H. R. (1979). Double-blind study of modified neurotoxin in motor neuron disease. *Neurology, Minneapolis* **29**, 77.

Urbánek, K., Mascreen, M., Meenakshisundaram, E. and Snehalatha, C. (1973). Biochemical aspects of motor neurone disease—Madras pattern. *J. Neurol. Neurosurg. Psychiat.* **36**, 753.

Vejjajiva, A., Foster, J. B. and Miller, H. (1967). Motor neuron disease: a clinical study. *J. neurol. Sci.* **4**, 299.

Walton, J. N. (1981). Clinical examination of the neuromuscular system.

In *Disorders of voluntary muscle* (ed. J. N. Walton), 4th edn, p. 448. Churchill-Livingstone, Edinburgh.

Weiner, L. P., Stohlman, S. A. and Davis, R. L. (1980). Attempts to demonstrate virus in amyotrophic lateral sclerosis. *Neurology, Minneapolis* **30**, 1319.

Welch, K. M. A. and Goldberg, D. M. (1972). Serum creatine phosphokinase in motor neuron disease. *Neurology, Minneapolis* **22**, 697.

Wettstein, A. (1979). The origin of fasciculations in motoneuron disease. *Ann. Neurol.* **5**, 295.

Wiechers, D. O. and Hubbell, S. L. (1981). Late changes in the motor unit after acute poliomyelitis. *Muscle & Nerve* **4**, 524.

Williams, E. R. and Bruford, A. (1970). Creatine phosphokinase in motor neurone disease. *Clin. chim. Acta* **27**, 53.

Willison, R. G. (1962). Electrodiagnosis in motor neurone disease. *Proc. R. Soc. Med.* **55**, 1024.

Wohlfart, G. (1957). Collateral regeneration from residual motor nerve fibers in amyotrophic lateral sclerosis. *Neurology, Minneapolis* **7**, 124.

Yase, Y. (1972). The pathogenesis of amyotrophic lateral sclerosis. *Lancet* **ii**, 292.

Creutzfeldt–Jakob disease

In 1920 Creutzfeldt described a case of 'Peculiar focal disease of the central nervous system' and Jakob (1921, 1923) added further examples of what he called 'Spastic pseudosclerosis: encephalomyelopathy with disseminated neurogenic lesions'.

Since then there has been much confusion about the clinical and pathological features of Creutzfeldt–Jakob disease. For some years there was a tendency, particularly in the United Kingdom, to use this diagnostic label to identify groups of cases, sometimes involving more than one family member, in which clinical features of parkinsonism were accompanied by progressive dementia and evidence of corticospinal-tract dysfunction, sometimes with weakness, wasting, and fasciculation of muscles, similar to that seen in motor-neurone disease and due to progressive loss of anterior horn cells. These rare cases show clinical features resembling those of the parkinsonism-dementia complex, often associated with amyotrophic lateral sclerosis, which is endemic in the island of Guam (pp. 331 and 371). Some may represent variants of corticostriatonigral degeneration (p. 331) in which, however, dementia is usually absent, while others may represent variants of progressive multisystem degeneration (p. 599). Usually the course is relatively rapid with progressive dementia, dysarthria, spastic limb weakness, Parkinsonian rigidity, tremor, and muscular wasting. In most such cases the pathological changes differ from those now recognized as typical of Creutzfeldt–Jakob disease (see below) and correspond more closely to those of Alzheimer's disease on the one hand and of corticostriatonigral degeneration on the other. Diagnostic and nosological difficulty, however, was compounded by the use of the term corticostriatonigral degeneration (Silberman, Cravioto, and Feigin 1961) to identify a case with the classical pathological changes of Creutzfeldt–Jakob disease and by the fact that clinical features indistinguishable from those of motor-neuron disease of rapid progression have been noted in another case with similar pathological findings (Allen, Dermott, Connolly, and Hurwitz 1971). That the position with regard to familial cases remains difficult to define is increased by the following evidence: (1) familial striatal degeneration of childhood onset may cause rigidity, movement disorders, and dysphagia (Roessmann and Schwartz 1973); (2) striatonigral degeneration with primary putaminal degeneration and pigment deposition but without cortical changes appears to represent a supranigral parkinsonian syndrome responding poorly to dopamine precursors and agonists (Borit, Rubinstein, and Urich 1975); (3) autosomal dominant striatonigral degeneration has been reported beginning in the second to fourth decade with parkinsonian rigidity, spasticity, dysarthria, and eye movement disorders (Rosenberg, Nyhan, Bay, and Shore 1976); and (4) classical Creutzfeldt–Jakob disease

as described below may also be familial, demonstrating apparent dominant inheritance (May, Itabashi, and de Jong 1968; Haltia, Kovanen, van Crevel, Bots, and Stefanko 1979), but is nevertheless transmissible to primates (Cathala, Chatelain, Brown, Dumas, and Gajdusek 1980), suggesting vertical transmission of the disease either by genomic integration or transplacental passage. Case-to-case transmission of the disease, either by neurosurgery or possibly due to social contact is, of course, well-recognized (Will and Matthews 1982; Brown, Cathala, and Sadowsky 1983).

Foley and Denny-Brown (1955), however, described a case corresponding more closely to the clinical picture reported by Creutzfeldt and Jakob, and others were described by Brownell and Oppenheimer (1965) as examples of subacute presenile polioencephalopathy. The condition reported usually began in middle or late life with ataxia, dementia, abnormal movements (often myoclonus), and progressive deterioration leading to stupor with death within a few months. A similar picture was described by Jones and Nevin (1954) and Nevin, McMenemey, Behrman, and Jones (1960) under the title of subacute spongiform encephalopathy; they also noted visual failure and generalized convulsions in some cases as well as paroxysmal generalized sharp-wave complexes in the EEG associated with the myoclonus, with obliteration of normal background activity and widespread slow activity. Pathologically, Brownell and Oppenheimer (1965) found widespread cell loss and diffuse astrocytic hyperplasia in the cerebral cortex, striatum, and thalamus and granule-cell degeneration in the cerebellum, while Nevin *et al.* (1960) stressed the spongiform change with vacuolation and severe loss of nerve cells throughout the cerebral cortex. Subsequently it became clear that despite variations in the clinical and pathological picture, Creutzfeldt–Jakob disease and subacute spongiform encephalopathy are virtually identical (Goldhammer, Bubis, Sarovapinhas, and Broham 1972; Bunis, Goldhammer, and Brahamer 1972). Spongiform change is most striking in the more acute cases, which also show the typical EEG findings described by Jones and Nevin (1954) and by Burger, Rowan, and Goldensohn (1972); in such patients death has been known to occur within eight to 12 weeks from the onset (Brown and Cathala 1979). When the course extends to several months or even a year or more, diffuse neuronal loss and marked astrocytic hyperplasia is more common (Katzman, Kagan, and Zimmerman 1961). A case of 16 years' duration has been reported (Cutler, Brown, Narayan, Parisi, Janotta, and Baron 1984). No specific biochemical or ultrastructural abnormalities have been found in the brain (Korey, Katzman, and Orloff 1961; Robinson 1969; Allen *et al.* 1971) but transmission experiments have shown that the condition is due to a slow virus (p. 294) and that it can be transmitted to the chimpanzee (Beck, Daniel, Matthews, Stevens, Alpers, Asher, Gajdusek, and Gibbs 1969). Suggestions that a spiroplasma might be responsible have not been substantiated (Leach, Matthews, and Will 1983). Some authors have suggested that amantidine 100 mg twice daily may produce temporary improvement (Sanders and Dunn 1973) but others have found antiviral agents ineffective.

It may thus be concluded that Creutzfeldt–Jakob disease is due to an as yet unidentified slow virus infection which shows some affinities with kuru and that it may occur in cortical, corticostriatal, corticospinal, cortico-striato-spinal, and cortico-striato-cerebellar forms.

Familial cerebral amyloidosis

Familial amyloidosis of the nervous system usually causes peripheral neuropathy (p. 541), but sometimes involves the central nervous system and the vitreous of the eyes (Okayama, Goto, Ogata, Omae, Yoshida, and Inomata 1978). While amyloid angiopathy has also been reported to cause intracerebral haemorrhage in the elderly (Bruni, Bilbao, and Pritzker 1977), familial oculo-leptomeningeal amyloidosis (Goren, Steinberg, and Farboody 1980) can cause dementia, fits, strokes, coma, and visual loss with a lymphocytic pleocytosis and raised protein content in the CSF. In one reported family in which progressive cerebellar ataxia and dementia were the presenting features and in which autosomal dominant transmission was evident, there was some evidence of vascular amyloid deposition but the principal pathological changes were those of spongiform encephalopathy suggesting an association with Creutzfeldt–Jakob disease (Adam, Crow, Duchen, Scararilli, and Spokes 1982).

References

Adam, J., Crow, T. J., Duchen, L. W., Scaravilli, F. and Spokes, E. (1982). Familial cerebral amyloidosis and spongiform encephalopathy. *J. Neurol. Neurosurg. Psychiat.* **45**, 37.

Allen, I. V., Dermott, E., Connolly, J. H. and Hurwitz, L. J. (1971). A study of a patient with the amyotrophic form of Creutzfeld–Jakob disease. *Brain* **94**, 715.

Beck, E., Daniel, P. M., Matthews, W. B., Stevens, D. L., Alpers, M. P., Asher, D. M., Gajdusek, D. C. and Gibbs, C. J. (1969). Creutzfeld–Jakob disease. The neuropathology of a transmission experiment. *Brain* **92**, 699.

Borit, A., Rubinstein, L. J. and Urich, H. (1975). The striatonigral degenerations—putaminal pigments and nosology. *Brain* **98**, 101.

Brown, P. and Cathala, F. (1979). Creutzfeldt–Jakob disease in France: I. Retrospective study of the Paris area during the ten-year period 1968–1977. *Ann. Neurol.* **5**, 189.

——, —— and Sadowsky, D. (1983). Correlation between population density and the frequency of Creutzfeldt–Jakob disease in France. *J. neurol. Sci.* **60**, 169.

Brownell, B. and Oppenheimer, D. R. (1965). An ataxic form of subacute presenile polioencephalopathy (Creutzfeld–Jakob disease). *J. Neurol. Psychiat.* **28**, 350.

Bruni, J., Bilbao, J. M. and Pritzker, K. P. H. (1977). Vascular amyloid in the aging central nervous system: clinicopathological study and literature review. *Can. J. neurol. Sci.* **4**, 239.

Bubis, J. J., Goldhammer, Y. and Braham, J. (1972). Subacute spongiform encephalopathy. *J. Neurol. Neurosurg. Psychiat.* **35**, 881.

Burger, L. J., Rowan, A. J. and Goldensohn, E. S. (1972). Creutzfeld–Jakob disease. An electroencephalographic study. *Arch. Neurol., Chicago* **26**, 428.

Cathala, F., Chatelain, J., Brown, P., Dumas, M. and Gajdusek, D. C. (1980). Familial Creutzfeld–Jakob disease. Autosomal dominance in 14 members over 3 generations. *J. neurol. Sci.* **47**, 343.

Creutzfeldt, H. G. (1920). Über eine eigenartige herdförmige Erkrankung des Zentral-nervesystems. *Z. ges. Neurol. Psychiat.* **57**, 1.

Cutler, N. R., Brown, P. W., Narayan, T., Parisi, J. E., Janotta, F. and Baron, H. (1984). Creutzfeldt–Jakob disease: a case of 16 years' duration. *Ann. Neurol.* **15**, 107.

Foley, J. and Denny-Brown, D. (1955). Subacute progressive encephalopathy with bulbar myoclonus. *J. Neuropath.* **16**, 133.

Goldhammer, Y., Bubis, J. J., Sarovapinhas, I. and Braham, J. (1972). Subacute spongiform encephalopathy and its relation to Jakob–Creutzfeld disease: report on six cases. *J. Neurol. Neurosurg. Psychiat.* **35**, 1.

Goren, H., Steinberg, M. C. and Farboody, G. H. (1980). Familial oculoleptomeningeal amyloidosis. *Brain* **103**, 473.

Haltia, M., Kovanen, J., Van Crevel, H., Bots, G. T. A. M. and Stefanko, s. (1979). Familial Creutzfeldt–Jakob disease. *J. neurol. Sci.* **42**, 381.

Jakob, A. (1921). Über eigenartige Erkrankungen des Zentralnervensystems mit bemerkenswerten anatomischen Befunden. Spastische Pseudosklerose–Encephalomyelopathie mit disseminierten Degenerationsherden. *Z. ges. Neurol. Psychiat.* **64**, 146.

—— (1923). *Spastische Pseudosklerose; die extrapyramidalen Erkrangungen*, p. 215. Springer, Berlin.

Jones, D. P. and Nevin, S. (1954). Rapidly progressive cerebral degeneration (subacute vascular encephalopathy) with mental disorder, focal disturbances and myoclonic epilepsy. *J. Neurol. Neurosurg. Psychiat,* **7**, 148.

Katzman, R., Kagan, E. H. and Zimmerman, H. M. (1961). A case of Jakob–Creutzfeldt disease. 1. Clinicopathological analysis. *J. Neuropath. exp. Neurol.* **20**, 78.

Korey, S. R., Katzman, R. and Orloff, J. (1961). A case of Jakob–Creutz-

feldt disease. 2. Analysis of some constitutents of the brain of a patient with Jakob–Creutzfeldt disease. *J. Neuropath. exp. Neurol.* **20**, 95.

Leach, R. H., Matthews, W. B. and Will, R. (1983). Creutzfeldt–Jakob disease. Failure to detect spiroplasmas by cultivation and serological tests. *J. neurol. Sci.* **59**, 349.

May, W. W., Itabashi, H. H. and DeJong, R. N. (1968). Creutzfeldt–Jakob disease. II. Clinical, pathologic, and genetic study of a family. *Arch. Neurol., Chicago* **19**, 137.

Nevin, S., McMenemey, W. H., Behrman, S. and Jones, D. P. (1960). Subacute spongiform encephalopathy—a subacute form of encephalopathy attributable to vascular dysfunction (spongiform cerebral atrophy). *Brain* **83**, 519.

Okayama, M., Goto, I., Ogata, J., Omae, T., Yoshida, I. and Inomata, H. (1978). Primary amyloidosis with familial vitreous opacities: an unusual case and family. *Arch. intern. Med.* **138**, 105.

Robinson, N. (1969). Creutzfeldt–Jakob's disease: a histochemical study. *Brain* **92**, 581.

Roessmann, U. and Schwartz, J. F. (1973). Familial striatal degeneration. *Arch. Neurol., Chicago* **29**, 314.

Rosenberg, R. N., Nyhan, W. L., Bay, C. and Shore, P. (1976). Autosomal dominant striatonigral degeneration: a clinical, pathologic, and biochemical study of a new genetic disorder. *Neurology, Minneapolis* **26**, 703.

Sanders, W. L. and Dunn, T. L. (1973). Creutzfeldt–Jakob disease treated with amantidine. *J. Neurol. Neurosurg. Psychiat.* **35**, 581.

Silberman, J., Cravioto, H. and Feigin, I. (1961). Corticostriatal degeneration of the Creutzfeldt–Jakob type. *J. Neuropath. exp. Neurol.* **20**, 105.

Will, R. G. and Matthews, W. G. (1982). Evidence for case-to-case transmission of Creutzfeldt–Jakob disease. *J. Neurol. Neurosurg. Psychiat.* **45**, 235.

Peroneal muscular atrophy

Synonyms. Neural progressive muscular atrophy; Charcot–Marie–Tooth disease.

Definition. A hereditary form of progressive muscular atrophy first described in 1886 by Charcot and Marie and later in the same year by Tooth. Wasting usually begins in the small muscles of the feet and later in those of the hands, and is often restricted to the peripheral parts of the limbs. The condition is closely related to the Roussy–Lévy syndrome (p. 366) and to Dejerine–Sottas disease (p. 546).

Pathology and aetiology

Buzzard and Greenfield (1921) described 'interstitial neuritis' in branches of the peroneal nerve, and Alajouanine, Castaigne, Cambier, and Escourolle (1967) found proliferation of endoneurial connective tissue with secondary demyelination in lumbar roots. In some cases, there are also changes in the spinal cord, including degeneration of anterior horn cells and cells of the dorsal nuclei, together with posterior-column demyelination and rarely degeneration of the corticospinal tracts, a finding which emphasizes the relationship of the condition, at least in some families, to other disorders of the hereditary ataxia group.

New light was cast upon the classification of the variants of this disorder by the work of Dyck and Lambert (1968*a*, *b*), by Thomas, Calne, and Stewart (1974), by Behse and Buchthal (1977), by Bradley, Madrid, and Davis (1977), and by Madrid, Bradley, and Davis (1977). The commonest (and most benign) form of peroneal muscular atrophy, usually of dominant inheritance, is one in which there is a hypertrophic demyelinating neuropathy of the peripheral nerves, sometimes with palpable nerve enlargement but invariably with Schwann-cell proliferation and 'onion-bulb' formation in the affected nerves and gross slowing of motor and sensory nerve conduction velocity. Pathologically these changes are indistinguishable from those of the Roussy–Lévy syndrome. Ultrastructural studies of sural-nerve biopsies suggest an axolemmal abnormality (Waxman and Ouellette 1979). Dyck and Lambert (1968*a*) identified as a different disorder the severe Dejerine–

Sottas variety of hypertrophic neuropathy, usually of earlier onset and more rapid progression and due to an autosomal recessive trait, but Thomas *et al.* (1974), noting genetic heterogeneity and marked intrafamilial variation in clinical severity and course, doubted whether such a distinction is justified.

Much less common than the hypertrophic variety (Dyck and Lambert 1968*a*; Thomas *et al* 1974; Davis, Bradley, and Madrid 1978; Bradley 1981) is the dominant axonal variety, usually of later onset, involving the legs more than the arms, with normal rates of nerve condition and little sensory involvement. Dyck and Lambert (1968*a*) called the hypertrophic demyelinating variety 'hereditary sensory and motor neuropathy type 1' (HSMN I) and the axonal type HSMN II. Clearly, too, there is a third variety (dominant distal spinal muscular atrophy) with primary involvement of the anterior horn cells rather than of the motor axons of the peripheral nerves. This third variant (the neuronal type) accounts for those cases which have features of peroneal muscular atrophy without sensory loss and which show subsequent involvement of limb muscles more proximally than is usual in typical peroneal muscular atrophy. This third variant resembles but is distinct from scapuloperoneal muscular atrophy, a disorder which is usually neuropathic but rarely myopathic (Kaeser 1965) (see p. 385).

In the affected skeletal muscles the appearances are those of neurogenic atrophy (Mastaglia and Walton 1982) but 'secondary myopathic change' is often found (Haase and Shy 1960; Cazzato and Testa 1969). Nemaline rods are sometimes found (Danon, Sarpel, and Manaligod 1980).

The aetiology of the condition is unknown though Dyck, Ellefson, Lais, Smith, Taylor, and Van Dyke (1970) found an abnormality of ceramide hexoside metabolism in cases of severe hypertrophic neuropathy and abnormalities of pyruvate metabolism in cultured fibroblasts have been reported (Williams 1979) but no specific biochemical defect has yet been identified. An increased uptake of leucine into cytoplasmic protein (Monckton and Marusyk 1977) is probably non-specific. Sporadic cases of all varieties occur; dominant inheritance is commoner in all varieties (Davies *et al*, 1978) but autosomal recessive transmission is found in some families suffering from each form of the disease and rarely X-linked recessive inheritance has been described (Herringham 1889; Emery 1981). Homozygous expression of a dominant gene without increased clinical severity has also been reported (Killian and Kloepfer 1979). Members of affected families may show pes cavus and abnormalities of nerve conduction without other clinical symptoms or signs and probably represent a forme fruste of the disorder (Symonds and Shaw 1926; Dyck Lambert, and Mulder 1963; Dyck and Lambert 1968*a*).

Symptoms and signs

The first symptoms are muscular wasting and weakness, which usually begin in the peronei, extensor digitorum longus, or the small muscles of the foot, symmetrically on both sides. Usually the condition begins in adolescence or early adult life, occasionally in childhood (Vanasse and Dubowitz 1981). Paralysis of the peronei leads to talipes equinovarus, but when wasting begins in the intrinsic muscles of the feet, pes cavus results. However, there is some evidence from 'forme fruste' cases that the pes cavus may be an associated skeletal deformity. Difficulty in walking on the heels is a useful early sign. Often it is the deformity of the feet and the resulting laborious 'steppage' gait which bring the patient under observation. Wasting does not usually appear in the hands until some years after its onset in the feet. Occasionally, however, both upper and lower extremities are affected simultaneously; exceptionally the hands suffer first. The muscular atrophy, occasionally with fasciculation, tends to spread very slowly proximally, not involving the muscles longitudinally but transversely. It does not extend above the elbows nor above the junction of the middle and lower thirds of the thigh in the hypertrophic type but often spreads more proximally in the axonal type, and usually does so eventually in the neuronal type. This peculiar ascending distribution of the wasting leads to a striking appearance of the limbs. When the lower part of the calf is wasted, the 'fat bottle' calf is produced, and wasting of the lower third of the thigh leads to the so-called 'inverted champagne bottle' limb. Ultimately the feet become 'flail', neither dorsiflexion nor plantar flexion being possible. In the cases with a hypertrophic neuropathy which are the majority, motor and sensory nerve conduction are usually greatly slowed in the peroneal nerves and often in the median and ulnar nerves as well, especially if the hands are affected (Dyck *et al* 1963; Dyck and Lambert 1968*a* and *b*; Nielsen and Pilgaard 1972). In cases of the axonal and neuronal varieties, conduction is usually normal (Thomas and Calne 1974) but in surviving axons the amplitude of the compound motor and sensory evoked potentials (in the axonal type) and of the compound muscle action potential only, in the neuronal type, may be greatly reduced; sometimes it is difficult to be certain whether the primary process is demyelinating and hypertrophic or axonal (Salisachs 1974). Bradley *et al.* (1977) and Madrid *et al.* (1977) have suggested that an additional type intermediate between the hypertrophic and axonal varieties exists but this view has been disputed (Behse and Buchthal 1977). Contractures rarely occur, but are usually slight in proportion to the degree of wasting (Fig. 13.9)

Electromyography typically shows signs of denervation in muscles with large discrete motor-unit action potentials suggesting that the lesion responsible lies proximally in the motor neurones. Abnormalities of skin temperature control, of orthostatic control of blood pressure, of sweating in the lower extremities, and other features suggesting dysfunction of postganglionic sympathetic nerve fibres have been described (Jammes 1972).

The tendon reflexes are variable. They are usually diminished or lost in the wasted muscles in proportion to the degree of wasting, but may be lost before atrophy is marked. The plantar reflexes are also lost eventually.

Sensation may be unaffected, but there is generally loss of vibration sense at the ankles and occasionally some impairment of appreciation of light touch, pain, and temperature over the periphery of the limbs in the demyelinating and axonal, but not in the neuronal, varieties. Deep sensibility is less often affected. Charcot and Marie, in their original paper, described vasomotor changes in the extremities, and perforating ulcers may occur due to an associated hereditary sensory neuropathy (England and Denny-Brown 1952). Vertebral and other skeletal anomalies and other congenital malformations have been reported (Smith 1958); heart block occurred in several members of an affected family (Littler 1970). Sphincter control is unaffected. There is a clear association in some families with benign (essential) familial tremor (Salisachs 1976; Salisachs, Codina, Giménez-Raldán, and Zarranz 1979).

The cranial nerves are usually normal, but optic atrophy is occasionally seen (Serratrice, Tatossian, and Poinso 1964) and so, too, is inequality of the pupils, possibly due to involvement of ocular sympathetic fibres. Very occasionally the pupils are of the Argyll Robertson type (Alajouanine *et al* 1967). Trigeminal neuralgia and anaesthesia rarely occur and vestibular dysfunction has been described (Melgaard and Zilstorff 1979).

Diagnosis

The onset of muscular wasting in the legs, its symmetry and selectivity, and its peculiar ascent from the periphery are distinctive features which usually render the diagnosis easy. In the muscular dystrophies affected muscles waste longitudinally and selectively and the distribution of the wasting is characteristic and usually proximal in the various forms. In Welander's (1951) hereditary distal myopathy the age of onset is later than in peroneal atrophy, and there is no sensory loss, but distinction from distal spinal

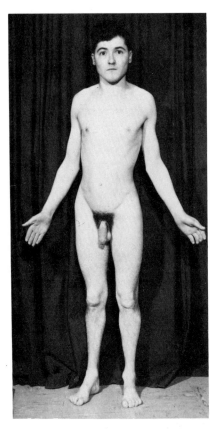

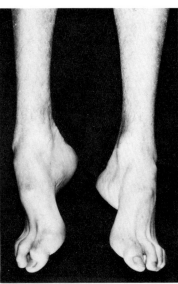

Fig. 13.9. A case of peroneal muscular atrophy; note the typical atrophy of the distal muscles of the lower limbs with bilateral pes cavus. There was also early wasting of the intrinsic muscles of both hands with complete loss of vibration sense below the knees. (Reproduced from Spillane (1975) by kind permission of the author.)

muscular atrophy (the neuronal variety) can be impossible without investigation. Dystrophia myotonica is distinguished by the presence of myotonia and by the distribution of the wasting, especially its selection of the sternomastoids and the long flexor and extensor muscles of the forearms rather than the small hand muscles. Progressive muscular atrophy usually begins in adult life, and the feet are rarely affected early; fasciculation is usually prominent, weakness and wasting less symmetrical, and the reflexes are often brisk. Friedreich's ataxia, like peroneal atrophy, is an hereditary dis-

order associated with pes cavus, but nystagmus, ataxia, and extensor plantar responses are peculiar to the former in which, moreover, muscular wasting is less common and overt. Diagnosis from other forms of polyneuropathy may sometimes be difficult; this is especially true of other demyelinating varieties with hypertrophy of peripheral nerves; in such cases, however, the clinical picture is less sterotyped and the course much more rapid, often with relapses and remissions. Whereas an increased CSF protein has been described in the more severe hypertrophic cases of peroneal muscular atrophy (Dyck and Lambert 1968a), this is rarely as great as in the varieties of steroid-responsive relapsing polyneuropathy which can cause similar peripheral-nerve hypertrophy. Other diseases which also give peripheral-nerve enlargement, including Refsum's disease, are identified by their other distinctive clinical features.

Prognosis

The disorder runs a very slow course and can arrest at any stage. Since the wasting always remains confined to the limbs, the disease does not shorten life and many patients have been reported alive 45 or 50 years after the onset. In the case reported by Alajouanine *et al.* (1967) the patient, whose condition was first diagnosed by Charcot, lived an active life for 60 years and eventually died at the age of 80. In spite of the deformities the degree of disability is often surprisingly slight. Generally, the prognosis is less good and ultimate disability more severe in the axonal and neuronal types and, as Thomas *et al.* (1974) and others have shown, there is sometimes remarkable heterogeneity of clinical presentation and course even within single families. Cases of early onset leading to severe disability with confinement to a wheelchair in late childhood or early adult life certainly occur but are relatively uncommon.

Treatment

No treatment will arrest the course of the disorder. Physiotherapy and various appliances often enable the patient to make the best use of his available resources (Harpin 1981). Appropriate boots or shoes and below-knee calipers with toe-springs or plastic moulded splints worn inside the shoes are often required.

References

Alajouanine, T., Castaigne, P., Cambier, J. and Escourolle, R. (1967). Maladie de Charcot–Marie. Étude anatomo-clinique. *Presse Méd.* **75**, 2745.

Behse, F. and Buchthal, F. (1977). Peroneal muscular atrophy (PMA) and related disorders. II. Histological findings in sural nerves. *Brain* **100**, 67.

Bradley, W. G. (1981). The neuropathies. In *Disorders of voluntary muscle* (ed. J. N. Walton) 4th edn, p. 753. Churchill-Livingstone, Edinburgh.

——, Madrid, R. and Davis, C. J. F. (1977). The peroneal muscular atrophy syndrome. Clinical, genetic, electrophysiological and nerve biopsy studies: Part 3. Clinical, electrophysiological and pathological correlations. *J. neurol. Sci.* **32**, 123.

Buzzard, E. F. and Greenfield, J. G. (1921). *Pathology of the nervous system.* Constable, London.

Cazzato, G. and Testa, G. (1969). Alterazioni miotessutali di tipo 'miopatico' in casi di atrofia muscolare progressiva nevritica di Charcot–Marie–Tooth. *Acta Neurol., Napoli* **24**, 171.

Charcot, J. M. and Marie, P. (1886). Sur une forme particulière d'atrophie musculaire progressive souvent familiale. *Rev. Médecine* **6**, 97.

Danon, M. R., Sarpel, G. and Manaligod, R. J. (1980). Nemaline rod myopathy and Charcot–Marie–Tooth disease: report of a case in a 10-year-old girl. *Arch. Neurol., Chicago* **37**, 123.

Davis, C. J. F., Bradley, W. G. and Madrid, R. (1978). The peroneal muscular atrophy syndrome. Clinical, genetic, electrophysiological and nerve biopsy studies: Part 1. Clinical, genetic and electrophysiological findings and classification. *J. Génét. hum.* **26**, 311.

Dyck, P. J., Ellefson, R. D., Lais, A. C., Smith, R. C., Taylor, W. F. and van Dyke, R. A. (1970). Histologic and lipid studies of sural nerves in inherited hypertrophic neuropathy: preliminary report of a lipid abnormality in nerve and liver in Dejerine–Sottas disease. *Proc. Mayo Clin.* **45**, 286.

—— and Lambert, E. H. (1968*a*). Lower motor and primary sensory neuron diseases with peroneal muscular atrophy. I. Neurologic, genetic, and electrophysiologic findings in hereditary polyneuropathies. *Arch. Neurol., Chicago* **18**, 603.

—— and —— (1968*b*). Lower motor and primary sensory neuron diseases with peroneal muscular atrophy. II. Neurologic, genetic, and electrophysiologic findings in various neuronal degenerations. *Arch. Neurol., Chicago* **18**, 619.

——, ——, and Mulder, D. W. (1963). Charcot–Marie–Tooth disease. Nerve conduction and clinical studies of a large sibship. *Neurology, Minneapolis* **13**, 1.

Emery, A. E. H. (1981). Genetic aspects of neuromuscular disease. In *Disorders of voluntary muscle* (ed. J. N. Walton) 4th edn, p. 785. Churchill-Livingstone, Edinburgh.

England, A. C. and Denny-Brown, D. (1952). Severe sensory changes, and trophic disorder, in peroneal muscular atrophy (Charcot–Marie–Tooth type). *Arch. Neurol., Chicago* **67**, 1.

Haase, G. R. and Shy, G. M. (1960). Pathological changes in muscle biopsies from patients with peroneal muscular atrophy. *Brain* **83**, 631.

Harpin, P. (1981). *With a little help*. Muscular Dystrophy Group of Great Britain, London.

Herringham, W. P. (1889). Muscular atrophy of the peroneal type affecting many members of a family. *Brain* **11**, 230.

Jammes, J. L. (1972). The autonomic nervous system in peroneal muscular atrophy. *Arch. Neurol., Chicago* **27**, 213.

Kaeser, H. E. (1965). Scapuloperoneal muscular atrophy. *Brain* **88**, 407.

Killian, J. M. and Kloepfer, H. W. (1979). Homozygous expression of a dominant gene for Charcot–Marie–Tooth neuropathy. *Ann. Neurol.* **5**, 515.

Littler, W. A. (1970). Heart block and peroneal muscular atrophy: a family study. *Quart. J. Med.* **39**. 431.

Madrid, R., Bradley, W. G. and Davis, C. J. F. (1977). The peroneal muscular atrophy syndrome. Clinical, genetic, electrophysiological and nerve biopsy studies: Part 2. Observations on pathological changes in sural nerve biopsies. *J. neurol. Sci.* **32**, 91.

Mastaglia, F. L. and Walton, J. N. (1982). *Skeletal muscle pathology*. Churchill-Livingstone, Edinburgh.

Melgaard, B. and Zilstorff, K. (1979). Central vestibular involvement in peroneal muscular atrophy: a preliminary report. *Ann. Neurol.* **5**, 118.

Monckton, G. and Marusyk, H. (1977). An autoradiographic study of muscular dystrophy, motor neuron disease and Charcot–Marie–Tooth disease. *Can. J. neurol. Sci.* **4**, 25.

Nielsen, V. K. and Pilgaard, S. (1972). On the pathogenesis of Charcot–Marie–Tooth disease: a study of the sensory and motor conduction velocity in the median nerve. *Acta orthop. scand.* **43**, 4.

Salisachs, P. (1974). Wide spectrum of motor conduction velocity in Charcot–Marie–Tooth disease: an anatomico-physiological interpretation. *J. neurol. Sci.* **23**, 25.

—— (1976). Charcot–Marie–Tooth disease associated with 'essential tremor': report of 7 cases and a review of the literature, *J. neurol. Sci.* **28**, 17.

——, Codina, A., Giménez-Roldán, S. and Zarranz, J. J. (1979). Charcot–Marie–Tooth disease associated with 'essential tremor' and normal and/or slightly diminished motor conduction velocity: report of 7 cases, *Eur. Neurol.* **18**, 49.

Serratrice, G., Tatossian, A. and Poinso, Y. (1964). Amyotrophie de Charcot–Marie associée à une atrophie optique bilatérale. *Presse Méd.* **72***a*, 2535.

Smith, C. K. (1958). Vertebral deformities and other anomalies in Charcot–Marie–Tooth disease. *Neurology, Minneapolis* **8**, 481.

Spillane, J. D. (1975). *An atlas of clinical neurology*, 2nd edn. Oxford University Press, Oxford.

Symonds, C. P. and Shaw, M. E. (1926). Familial claw-foot with absent tendon-jerks: a 'forme fruste' of the Charcot–Marie–Tooth disease. *Brain* **49**, 387.

Thomas, P. K. and Calne, D. B. (1974). Motor nerve conduction velocity in peroneal muscular atrophy: evidence for genetic heterogeneity. *J. Neurol. Neurosurg. Psychiat.* **37**, 68.

——, ——, and Stewart, G. (1974). Hereditary motor and sensory polyneuropathy (peroneal muscular atrophy). *Ann. hum. Genet.* **38**, 111.

Tooth, H. H. (1886). *The peroneal type of progressive muscular atrophy*. Cambridge University thesis, Cambridge.

Vanasse, M. and Dubowitz, V. (1981). Dominantly inherited peroneal muscular atrophy (hereditary motor and sensory neuropathy Type I) in infancy and childhood. *Muscle & Nerve* **4**, 26.

Waxman, S. G. and Ouellette, E. M. (1979). Ultrastructural and cytochemical observations in a case of dominantly inherited hypertrophic (Charcot–Marie–Tooth) neuropathy. *J. Neuropath. exp. Neurol.* **38**, 586.

Welander, L. (1951). Myopathia distalis tarda hereditaria. *Acta med. scand.* Suppl. 265.

Williams, L. L. (1979). Pyruvate oxidation in Charcot–Marie–Tooth disease. *Neurology, Minneapolis* **29**, 1492.

Infantile spinal muscular atrophy and related disorders

There was considerable discussion in the past as to the relationship between two muscular disorders of infancy, namely amyotonia congenita, or myatonia of Oppenheim (1900) on the one hand, and progressive spinal muscular atrophy of infancy on the other; the latter condition was first described by Werdnig (1890) and Hoffmann (1891). Spiller (1913), on clinical grounds, cast doubt upon the distinction between these conditions, and Greenfield and Stern (1927) pointed out that they were pathologically indistinguishable. But it is now clear that the diagnosis of amyotonia congenita was often wrongly made and that the progressive disorder which terminates fatally in infancy is always Werdnig–Hoffmann disease.

Confusion arose from the fact that infants showing severe hypotonia and weakness from the moment of birth were often diagnosed as examples of amyotonia congenita, while the diagnosis of Werdnig–Hoffmann disease was reserved for cases in which weakness and hypotonia developed during the first year of life. In fact, as Walton (1956) and Paine (1963) pointed out, the syndrome of diffuse muscular hypotonia and weakness developing early in infancy is one of multiple aetiology and the inclusive term 'amyotonia congenita', once utilized to identify the syndrome must be discarded as in every case an attempt must be made to identify the pathological basis of the disorder. Thus in many cases with severe weakness and hypotonia, even when present from birth, the condition is one of progressive spinal muscular atrophy; in others the hypotonia is symptomatic, being secondary to mental defect, flaccid cerebral diplegia, or to a variety of metabolic or nutritional disorders or to a number of congenital neuromuscular disorders including many varieties of congenital myopathy (see Chapter 19); there are, however, a few cases in which no cause for the hypotonia is discovered and in which slow improvement usually occurs—for the present these may be regarded as suffering from 'benign congenital hypotonia' (see below), but even this is almost certainly a disorder of multiple aetiology.

Acute progressive spinal muscular atrophy of infancy (Werdnig–Hoffman disease)

Pathology

There is atrophy and chromatolytic degeneration of the ganglion cells of the anterior horns of the spinal cord and, to a variable extent, of the cranial-nerve nuclei and of thalamic neurons (Thieffry, Arthuis, and Bargeton 1955) but the cortex is usually normal. Rarely there is vacuolation of affected neurones (Kohn 1971). The numbers of large motor neurones in the spinal cord are greatly reduced at autopsy, in contrast to a reduction in size but not in number in nemaline myopathy (Robertson, Kawamura, and Dyck 1978). Phrenic motor neurones are comparatively spared even in the late stages (Kuzuhara and Chou 1981). The ventral roots are small and largely demyelinated. The peripheral nerves show many small finely myelinated fibres, and the muscles show simple 'grouped' or neurogenic atrophy with large numbers of tiny fibres in groups with rounding and hypertrophy of surviving innervated fibres. The atrophic fibres are of both histochemical types and electron microscopy has shown only the changes of denervation though some atrophic fibres have a fetal appearance (Wechsler and Hager 1962; Shafiq, Milhorat, ad Gorycki 1967; Roy, Dubowitz, and Wolman 1971). The uptake of uridine by diseased chromatolytic neurones is normal and the nature of the defect in the diseased cells is unknown (Hogenhuis, Spaulding, and Engel 1967).

Aetiology

The fundamental cause is unknown, but the condition is due to an autosomal recessive gene and thus affects one in four offspring of either sex of two heterozygous carriers. The gene frequency in north-east England has been estimated to be 1 in 80 (Pearn 1973*a*). Unfortunately no method of detecting carriers is available and not infrequently two or three successive children of healthy parents may be affected. Although cases have been reported of apparent acute onset following acute infections, these are unlikely to play any part in aetiology. The finding of reduced concentrations of vitamin E in the plasma of affected infants (Shapira, Amit, and Rachmilewitz 1981) has raised the question as to whether deficiency of this vitamin plays any part in pathogenesis, but this substance was of no value in treatment when given by the same authors.

Symptoms and signs

Affected children are sometimes normal at birth and then may not show symptoms of the disorder until they are two or three months old. In other cases severe generalized weakness and hypotonia are present from birth, suggesting that the disease process began in fetal life. Reduced fetal movements in the third trimester of pregnancy are often noted by mothers of affected children (Pearn 1973*b*); when the condition begins in fetal life there may be variable distal contractures of the limbs at birth, so that the condition is one cause, but an uncommon one (*British Medical Journal* 1981) of the syndrome of arthrogryposis multiplex congenita (Smith, Bender, and Stover 1963; Gardner-Medwin and Tizard 1981). Muscular weakness usually begins in the muscles of the back, and the pelvic and shoulder girdles, whence it spreads to the proximal, and later to the distal, muscles of the limbs. The affected muscles waste rapidly: though the wasting may be obscured by subcutaneous fat, it may be shown by X-rays, ultrasound, or CT scanning. The affected children often adopt a typical posture with abduction and external rotation of the arms at the shoulder and similar abduction and external rotation at the hip joints. Muscular fasciculation is rarely seen in the limbs, but often in the tongue. The intercostal muscles usually become affected and the bulbar muscles may suffer also, but the diaphragm usually escapes until the later stages, so that indrawing of the lower ribs at the diaphragmatic attachment during inspiration is an invaluable diagnostic sign. The tendon reflexes are lost. Sensibility is unimpaired, and muscle biopsy shows the features of neurogenic atrophy as described above while electromyography reveals as a rule spontaneous fibrillation and discrete isolated motor-unit action potentials of normal or increased size on volition; motor nerve conduction velocity is normal (Buchthal and Zander Olsen 1970). The CSF is also normal.

Diagnosis

The condition must be distinguished from benign congenital hypotonia which is present at birth, is characterized by generalized muscular hypotonia with less wasting, preservation of the tendon reflexes, absence of complete paralysis, and of involvement of the intercostals, and in which there is a tendency to improvement; and from congenital myopathy, in which there may also be improvement. Muscle biopsy is generally distinctive in each case. Congenital diplegia and other causes of symptomatic hypotonia (see below) are usually easily recognized. Infantile polyneuropathy gives a similar picture rarely but is identifiable by a reduced conduction velocity in peripheral nerves and a rise in CSF protein.

Prognosis

The condition, as its name implies, is progressive, and usually terminates fatally in a few months, though temporary or even prolonged arrest has been described. It now seems likely that those in whom arrest occurs are more probably suffering from chronic spinal muscular atrophy and not true Werdnig–Hoffmann disease. In a review of 76 cases, Pearn and Wilson (1973) found that in one-third the disease was manifest at or before delivery; all cases showed delayed milestones by five months of age and 95 per cent were dead, usually as a result of respiratory infection, by the age of 18 months.

Treatment

No drug treatment of any value is known.

Chronic spinal muscular atrophy of childhood, adolescence, and early adult life

In 1956 Kugelberg and Welander described 12 patients occurring in six families, all of whom were suffering from a heredofamilial form of muscular atrophy simulating muscular dystrophy. They suggested that this condition, which appeared to be of autosomal recessive inheritance, might prove to be a new syndrome. Many subsequent reports have since appeared indicating that the condition may begin at any age from infancy, early childhood, or adolescence to early adult life. Proximal muscles of both the upper and lower limbs are usually affected first giving a clinical picture like that of muscular dystrophy, save for the presence of fasciculation in many cases; the electromyogram and muscle biopsy indicate denervation atrophy but the serum creatine kinase activity may be raised and secondary myopathic changes are common in muscle biopsy specimens (Mastaglia and Walton 1971) while 'myopathic' potentials may also be recorded in the electromyogram from some muscles (Gath, Sjaastad, and Looken 1969). The course of the condition is very variable from case to case but deterioration is usually slow and arrest frequently occurs. Apparent onset after a febrile illness, often reported (Gardner-Medwin, Hudgson, and Walton 1967), probably means simply that muscular weakness first became apparent after a period of bed rest.

There has been considerable controversy about the relationship of the Kugelberg–Welander syndrome (pseudomyopathic spinal muscular atrophy) to Werdnig–Hoffmann disease. Many authors, having noted the occurrence of severe and much milder cases in the same sibship, as well as apparent arrest, a subsequent benign course, and prolonged survival, even into adult life in some cases, concluded that the two conditions, each of autosomal recessive inheritance, were probably variants of the same disorder (Dubowitz 1964; Hausmanowa-Petrusewicz, Prot, and Sawicka 1966; Gardner-Medwin *et al.* 1967; Hausmanowa-Petrusewicz, Askanas, Badurska, Emeryk, Fidzianska, Garbalinska, Hetnarska, Jedrzejowska, Kamieniecka, Niebroj-Dobosz, Prot, and Sawicka 1968; Munsat, Woods, Fowler, and Pearson 1969). However, it is now evident that true Werdnig–Hoffmann disease, beginning at or before birth or, at the latest, before the sixth month of life, is an independent genetic entity (Pearn,

Carter, and Wilson 1973). Fried and Emery (1971) identified as a second variety, which they called spinal muscular atrophy type II, those cases previously regarded as examples of Werdnig–Hoffmann disease in which the onset was usually between 6 and 15 months of life, in which the disease process often arrested, and in which survival, though usually with severe disability, gross skeletal deformity, and multiple contractures, was possible into late childhood, adolescence, or even adult life. In their view this condition differed from spinal muscular atrophy type III (Kugelberg–Welander disease) in which the age of onset is usually later still, in which walking is usually possible, even if beginning late, and the course very much more benign. However, much recent work has failed to confirm this subdivision and there is now widespread agreement that, whereas acute Werdnig–Hoffmann disease is clinically and genetically distinct, all other cases of proximal spinal muscular atrophy, whether resulting in severe disability in infancy or early childhood or running a benign course in adolescence or adult life, are variants of a single disease process (Namba, Aberfeld, and Grob 1970; van Wijngaarden and Bethlem 1973; Bundey and Lovelace 1975; Emery, Hausmanowa-Petrusewicz, Davie, Holloway, Skinner, and Burkowska 1976a; Emery, Davie, Holloway, and Skinner 1976b; Pearn, Bundey, Carter, Wilson, Gardner-Medwin, and Walton 1978a; Hausmanowa-Petrusewicz, Zaremba, and Borkowska 1979; Pearn 1980). Some cases arising in adult life (Pearn, Hudgson, and Walton 1978b) may readily be confused clinically with the Becker type of muscular dystrophy, as muscle hypertrophy, especially in the calves (Bouwsma and van Wijngaarden 1980), is often seen. It is also clear that many patients previously diagnosed as cases of muscular dystrophy (usually of the limb-girdle and facioscapulohumeral varieties) are in fact suffering from chronic spinal muscular atrophy (Walton and Gardner-Medwin 1974; Tomlinson, Walton, and Irving 1974; Kazakov, Kovalenko, Skorometz, and Mikhailov 1977). It is also well recognized that a chronic form of the disease beginning in, and largely localized to, the distal muscles of both the upper and lower limbs (at least for some years) can be defined and can be equated with the neuronal form of peroneal muscular atrophy (see p. 380; Meadows, Marsden, and Harriman 1969; Mcleod and Prineas 1971; Pearn and Hudgson 1979; Harding and Thomas 1980). Rarely muscular wasting is limited to the hands (O'Sullivan and McLeod 1978) or remains markedly asymmetrical (Harding, Bradbury, and Murray 1983) and vocal-cord paralysis is another rare accompaniment (Young and Harper 1980).

Classification is not made easier by the fact that occasional families demonstrating autosomal dominant (Zellweger, Simpson, McCormick, and Ionaescu 1972; Pearn 1978) or X-linked recessive (Tsukagoshi, Shoji and Furukawa 1970) inheritance have been reported. A rare X-linked variety beginning in late adult life and giving dysarthria, dysphagia, and slowly progressive limb muscle weakness (combined spinal and bulbar atrophy) has also been reported (Ringel, Lava, Treihaft, Lubs, and Lubs 1978). In other similar families the onset is in adolescence giving severe disability in adult life (Dobkin and Verity 1976). X-linked infantile progressive bulbar palsy (Fazio–Londe disease) (Campbell and Liversedge 1981; Gardner-Medwin and Tizard 1981) is another rare variant. The relationship between this condition and neurogenic scapuloperoneal muscular atrophy (Ricker, Mertens, and Schimrigk 1968; Emery, Fenichel, and Engel 1968; Feigenbaum and Munsat 1970), which is occasionally X-linked (Thomas, Calne, and Elliott 1972), is still uncertain. Inconstant clinical manifestations reported in some cases and families include limb tremor, resembling essential tremor and obvious when the electrocardiogram is recorded (Russman and Fredericks 1979), called minipolymyoclonus by Spiro (1970), ocular or oculopharyngeal muscle involvement (Aberfeld and Namba 1969; Matsunaga, Inokuchi, Ohnishi, and Kuroiwa 1973), extensor plantar responses and other evidence of corticospinal-tract

dysfunction (Gardner-Medwin *et al.* 1967), pontocerebellar hypoplasia (Goutières, Aicardi, and Farkas 1977), cardiomyopathy (Mawatari and Katayama 1973; Tomlinson *et al.* 1974), hyperlipoproteinaemia (Quarfordt, De Vivo, Engel, Levy, and Fredrickson 1970; Dahl and Peters 1975), cystinuria and leucinuria (Radu, Tanase-Mogos, Rosu, Killyen, and Ionescu 1974), and chromosomal abnormalities (Ross, Simpson, and Styles 1974).

Clearly (see Gamstorp and Sarnat 1984), the prognosis of the condition is very variable and in a sporadic case arising in adult life diagnosis from motor-neurone disease can be difficult if not sometimes impossible, although in the more benign from of spinal muscular atrophy, weakness usually affects proximal muscles rather than distal in the beginning, the course is slow, and bulbar muscle weakness and signs of corticospinal-tract dysfunction are rare. The fact that arrest may occur even in severe cases of early onset underlines the necessity of employing measures (attention to posture, appropriate appliances such as spinal supports and splints, vigorous treatment of respiratory infection, etc.) to prevent skeletal deformity and contractures. Surgical correction of spinal deformity or contractures is sometimes justified. Physiotherapy (active exercise against resistance when possible), weight control, and moderate regular exercise play particular valuable roles in this disabling disease as muscle fibres which retain effective innervation may undergo hypertrophy; swimming under supervision may be especially helpful.

Scapuloperoneal muscular atrophy

This uncommon syndrome, previously mentioned on pages 375 and 381, shows some resemblance to chronic spinal muscular atrophy on the one hand and to facioscapulohumeral muscular dystrophy on the other. Usually of dominant inheritance, it is sometimes X-linked (Thomas *et al.* 1972) and sporadic cases are common. It usually begins in early adult life but an onset in childhood, adolescence (Mercelis, Demeester, and Martin, 1980), or middle life is sometimes seen. Muscular weakness and wasting in the legs is similar to that of peroneal muscular atrophy but in the upper limbs the involvement is proximal, usually with winging of the scapulae and variable affection of other shoulder girdle and upper-arm muscles. Early scapular winging and anterior tibial weakness give a picture like that of early facioscapulohumeral dystrophy but the face is spared and the condition is distinguished from the axonal and neuronal forms of peroneal muscular atrophy by the proximal involvement in the upper limbs and the sparing of the small hand muscles and from the hypertrophic form by the normal nerve conduction velocity. In most cases the condition appears to be due to a disorder of the anterior horn cells with neurogenic atrophy of muscle (Kaeser 1965), and there is no evidence of peripheral neuropathy. However, distal sensory loss (Davidenkow's syndrome) (Schwartz and Swash 1975) has been described, as has cardiopathy (Mawatari and Katayama 1973). In some cases and families, however, the same clinical syndrome has been shown to be due to a myopathy (Thomas, Schott, and Morgan-Hughes 1975). The course of the disorder is usually benign and many patients are greatly helped by appliances designed to correct bilateral foot-drop.

Benign congenital hypotonia

Symptoms and signs

This condition, a syndrome of multiple aetiology (Walton 1956, 1957; Paine 1963), is usually present at birth, though frequently it is not observed until the child is old enough to attempt to raise its head. The most striking feature is the extreme muscular hypotonia, which makes it possible for the limbs to be placed in bizarre attitudes. The muscles, though somewhat weak, are not paralysed, but the child may be unable to maintain any posture against the force of gravity. It is, therefore, at first unable to raise the head and, later, to sit or to stand, though able to move the legs if supported beneath the axillae. The tendon reflexes are usually present but may be depressed. The intercostal muscles and diaphragm usually escape. Electromyography may show no abnormality and muscle biopsy often shows no pathological change in muscle fibres though these may be smaller than normal or immature (Farkas-Bargeton, Aicardi, Arsenio-Nunes, and Wehrle 1978), while rarely they may all be of one histochemical type or else there may be marked disproportion in the number and size of fibres of the two principal histochemical types (so called 'fibre type disproportion') (Dubowitz and Brooke 1974).

Diagnosis

The diagnosis is not easy, as many conditions are characterized by muscular hypotonia in infancy (Brooke, Carroll, and Ringel 1979). Congenital laxity of the ligaments (as in families of contortionists) may result in excessive mobility at joints but the muscles are powerful. In Werdnig–Hoffmann disease the weakness and hypotonia are more severe, the tendon reflexes are lost, and there may be indrawing of the lower ribs during inspiration as a result of intercostal weakness. Mental defect and mild flaccid diplegia may be difficult to distinguish in the early stages as may other causes of symptomatic hypotonia (see the 'floppy infant syndrome', pp. 582–584). Serum enzyme studies, electromyography, and muscle biopsy are of particular value in excluding spinal muscular atrophy, muscular dystrophy, and other myopathies, while nerve conduction velocity measurement and lumbar puncture may be necessary to exclude infantile polyneuropathy. Even so the diagnosis will occasionally remain in doubt and may only be clarified by repeated observation and examination of the child over a period of months or years. Many of the benign congenital myopathies (Turner 1949; Gardner-Medwin and Tizard 1981) (see p. 583) may be indistinguishable from benign congenital hypotonia in the early stages. Indeed, as more such myopathies are being recognized by modern techniques of investigation, fewer cases of infantile hypotonia now remain unexplained than in the past.

Prognosis

The general tendency of the disorder is to improve, and, if the patient survives intercurrent infections, he may ultimately recover completely, though all physical milestones, including walking, are late; some patients have small, weak, and hypotonic muscles throughout life and are then tentatively classified as cases of 'benign congenital myopathy'.

Treatment

Treatment with graduated exercises must be directed to educating voluntary movement.

References

Aberfeld, D. C. and Namba, T. (1969). Progressive ophthalmoplegia in Kugelberg–Welander disease. *Arch. Neurol., Chicago* **20**, 253.

Batten, F. E. and Holmes, G. (1912–13). Progressive spinal muscular atrophy of infants (Werdnig–Hoffman type). *Brain* **35**, 38.

Bouwsma, G. and van Wijngaarden, G. K. (1980). Spinal muscular atrophy and hypertrophy of the calves. *J. neurol. Sci.* **44**, 275.

British Medical Journal (1981). Arthrogryposis multiplex congenita. *Br. med. J.* **283**, 2.

Brooke, M. H., Carroll, J. E. and Ringel, S. P. (1979). Congenital hypotonia revisited. *Muscle & Nerve* **2**, 84.

Buchthal, F. and Zander Olsen, P. (1970). Electromyography and muscle biopsy in infantile spinal muscular atrophy. *Brain* **93**, 15.

Bundey, S. and Lovelace, R. E. (1975). A clinical and genetic study of chronic proximal spinal muscular atrophy. *Brain* **98**, 455.

Campbell, M. J. and Liversedge, L. A. (1981). The motor neurone diseases. In *Disorders of voluntary muscle* (ed. J. N. Walton), 4th edn, p. 725. Churchill-Livingstone, Edinburgh.

Dahl, D. S. and Peters, H. A. (1975). Lipid disturbances associated with spinal muscular atrophy: clinical, electromyographic, histochemical, and lipid studies. *Arch. Neurol., Chicago* **32**, 195.

Dobkin, B. H. and Verity, M. A. (1976). Familial progressive bulbar and spinal muscular atrophy: juvenile onset and late morbidity with ragged-red fibers. *Neurology, Minneapolis* **26**, 754.

Dubowitz, V. (1964). Infantile muscular atrophy. A prospective study with particular reference to a slowly progressive variety, *Brain* **87**, 707.

—— and Brooke, M. H. (1974). *Muscle biopsy*, Major Problems in Neurology Series (ed. J. N. Walton). Saunders, London.

Emery, A. E. H., Davie, A. M., Holloway, S. and Skinner, R. (1976b). International collaborative study of the spinal muscular atrophies: Part 2. Analysis of genetic data. *J. neurol. Sci.* **30**, 375.

—— Hausmanowa-Petrusewicz, I., Davie, A. M., Holloway, S., Skinner, R. and Borkowska, J. (1976a). International collaborative study of the spinal muscular atrophies: Part 1. Analysis of clinical and laboratory data. *J. neurol. Sci.* **29**, 83.

Emery, E. S., Fenichel, G. M. and Eng, G. (1968). A spinal muscular atrophy with scapuloperoneal distribution. *Arch. Neurol., Chicago* **18**, 129.

Farkas-Bargeton, E., Aicardi, J., Arsenio-Nunes, M. L. and Wehrle, R. (1978). Delay in the maturation of muscle fibers in infants with congenital hypotonia. *J. neurol. sci.* **39**, 117.

Feigenbaum, J. A. and Munsat, T. L. (1970). A neuromuscular syndrome of scapuloperoneal distribution. *Bull. Los Angeles neurol. Soc.* **35**, 47.

Fried, K. and Emery, A. E. H. (1971). Spinal muscular atrophy type II. A separate genetic and clinical entity from type I (Werdnig–Hoffmann disease) and type III (Kugelberg–Welander disease). *Clin. Genet.* **2**, 203.

Gamstorp, I. and Sarnat, H. B. (1984). *Progressive spinal muscular atrophies*. Raven Press, New York.

Gardner-Medwin, D., Hudgson, P. and Walton, J. N. (1967). Benign spinal muscular atrophy arising in childhood and adolescence. *J. neurol. Sci.* **5**, 121.

—— and Tizard, J. P. M. (1981). Neuromuscular disorders in infancy and early childhood. In *Disorders of voluntary muscle* (ed. J. N. Walton), 4th edn, p. 625. Churchill-Livingstone, Edinburgh.

Gath, I., Sjaastad, O. and Loøken, A. C. (1969). Myopathic electromyographic changes correlated with histopathology in Wohlfart–Kugelberg–Welander disease. *Neurology, Minneapolis* **19**, 344.

Goutières, F., Aicardi, J. and Farkas, E. (1977). Anterior horn cell disease associated with pontocerebellar hypoplasia in infants. *J. Neurol. Neurosurg. Psychiat.* **40**, 370.

Greenfield, J. G. and Stern, R. O. (1927). The anatomical identity of the Werdnig–Hoffmann and Oppenheim forms of infantile spinal muscular atrophy. *Brain* **50**, 652.

Harding, A. E., Bradbury, P. G. and Murray, N. M. F. (1983). Chronic asymmetrical spinal muscular atrophy. *J. neurol. Sci.* **59**, 69.

—— and Thomas, P. K. (1980). Hereditary distal spinal muscular atrophy: a report on 34 cases and a review of the literature. *J. neurol. Sci.* **45**, 337.

Hausmanowa-Petrusewicz, I., Askanas, W., Badurska, B., Emeryk, B. Fidzianska, A., Garbalinska, W., Hetnarska, L., Jedrzejowska, H., Kamieniecka, Z., Niebroj-Dobosz, I., Prot, J. and Sawicka, E. (1968). Infantile and juvenile spinal muscular atrophy. *J. neurol. Sci.* **6**, 269.

——, Prot, J. and Sawicka, E. (1966). Le problème des formes infantiles et juvèniles de l'atrophie musculaire spinale. *Rev. Neurol.* **114**, 295.

——, Zaremba, J. and Borkowska, J. (1979). Chronic form of childhood spinal muscular atrophy: are the problems of its genetics really solved? *J. neurol. Sci.* **43**, 313.

Hoffmann, J. (1891). Weiterer Beitrag zur Lehre von der progressiven neurotischen Muskelatrophie. *Dtsch. Z. Nervenheilk.* **1**, 95.

—— (1893). Über chronische spinale Muskelatrophie im Kindesalter, *Dtsch. Z. Nervenheilk.* **3**, 427.

—— (1897). Weiterer Beitrag zur Lehre von der hereditären progressiven spinalen Muskelatrophie im Kindesalter. *Dtsch. Z. Nervenheilk.* **10**, 292.

Hogenhuis, L. A. H., Spaulding, S. W. and Engel, W. K. (1967). Neural RNA metabolism in infantile spinal muscular atrophy (Werdnig–Hoffmann disease) studied by radioautography. *J. Neuropath. exp. Neurol.* **26**, 335.

Kaeser, H. E. (1965). Scapuloperoneal muscular atrophy. *Brain* **88**, 407.

Kazokov, V. M., Kovalenko, T. M., Skorometz, A. A. and Mikhailov, E. P. (1977). Chronic spinal muscular atrophy simulating facioscapulo-humeral type and limb–girdle type of muscular dystrophy: report of two cases. *Eur. Neurol.* **16**, 90.

Kohn, R. (1971). Clinical and pathological findings in an unusual infantile motor neurone disease. *J. Neurol. Neurosurg. Psychiat.* **34**, 427.

Kugelberg, E. and Welander, L. (1956). Heredo-familial juvenile muscular atrophy simulating muscular dystrophy. *Arch. Neurol. Psychiat., Chicago* **15**, 500.

Kuzuhara, S. and Chou, S. M. (1981). Preservation of the phrenic motoneurons in Werdnig–Hoffmann disease. *Ann. Neurol.* **9**, 506.

Mastaglia, F. L. and Walton, J. N. (1971). Histological and histochemical changes in skeletal muscle from cases of chronic juvenile and early adult spinal muscular atrophy (the Kugelberg–Welander syndrome). *J. neurol. Sci.* **12**, 15.

Matsunaga, M., Inokuchi, T., Ohnishi, A. and Kuroiwa, Y. (1973). Oculopharyngeal involvement in familial neurogenic muscular atrophy. *J. Neurol. Neurosurg. Psychiat.* **36**, 104.

Mawatari, S. and Katayama, K. (1973). Scapuloperoneal muscular atrophy with cardiopathy: an X-linked recessive trait. *Arch. Neurol., Chicago* **28**, 55.

McLeod, J. G. and Prineas, J. W. (1971). Distal type of chronic spinal muscular atrophy: clinical, electrophysiological and pathological studies. *Brain* **94**, 703.

Meadows, J. C., Marsden, C. D. and Harriman, D. G. F. (1969). Chronic spinal muscular atrophy in adults. I. The Kugelberg–Welander syndrome. II. Other forms. *J. neurol. Sci.* **9**, 527, 551.

Mercelis, R., Demeester, J. and Martin, J. -J. (1980). Neurogenic scapuloperoneal syndrome in childhood. *J. Neurol. Neurosurg. Psychiat.* **43**, 888.

Munsat, T. L., Woods, R., Fowler, W. and Pearson, C. M. (1969). Neurogenic muscular atrophy of infancy with prolonged survival. The variable course of Werdnig–Hoffmann disease. *Brain* **92**, 9.

Namba, T., Aberfeld, D. C. and Grob, D. (1970). Chronic proximal spinal muscular atrophy. *J. neurol. Sci.* **11**, 401.

Oppenheim, H. (1900). Über allgemeine und localisierte Atonie der Muskulatur (Myatonie) im frühen Kindesalter. *Mschr. Psychiat. Neurol.* **8**, 232.

O'Sullivan, D. J. and McLeod, J. G. (1978). Distal chronic spinal muscular atrophy involving the hands. *J. Neurol. Neurosurg. Psychiat.* **41**, 653.

Paine, R. S. (1963). The future of the 'floppy infant'. A follow-up study of 133 patients. *Develop. med. Child Neurol.* **5**, 115.

Pearn, J. H. (1973*a*). The gene frequency of acute Werdnig–Hoffmann disease (SMA type I). A total population survey in North-East England. *J. med. Genet.* **10**, 260.

—— (1973*b*). Fetal movements and Werdnig–Hoffmann disease. *J. neurol. Sci.* **18**, 373.

—— (1978). Autosomal dominant spinal muscular atrophy: a clinical and genetic study. *J. neurol. Sci.* **38**, 263.

—— (1980). Classification of spinal muscular atrophies. *Lancet* **i**, 919.

——, Bundey, S., Carter, C. O., Wilson, J., Gardner-Medwin, D. and Walton, J. N. (1978*a*). A genetic study of subacute and chronic spinal muscular atrophy in childhood: a nosological analysis of 124 index patients. *J. neurol. Sci.* **37**, 227.

——, Carter, C. O. and Wilson, J. (1973). The genetic identity of acute infantile spinal muscular atrophy. *Brain* **96**, 463.

—— and Hudgson, P. (1979). Distal spinal muscular atrophy: a clinical and genetic study of 8 kindreds. *J. neurol. Sci.* **43**, 183.

——, ——, and Walton, J. N. (1978*b*). A clinical and genetic study of spinal muscular atrophy of adult onset: the autosomal recessive form as a discrete disease entity. *Brain* **101**, 591.

—— and Wilson, J. (1973). Werdnig–Hoffmann disease. Acute infantile spinal muscular atrophy. *Arch. Dis. Childh.* **48**, 425.

Quarfordt, S. G., DeVivo, D. C., Engel, W. K., Levy, R. I. and Fredrickson, D. S. (1970). Familial adult-onset proximal spinal muscular atrophy. Report of a family with type II hyperlipoproteinemia. *Arch. Neurol., Chicago* **22**, 541.

Radu, H., Tanase-Mogos, I., Rosu, A. M., Killyen, I. and Ionescu, V. (1974). A new polygenic disturbance: cystinuria, leucinuria and spinal muscular atrophy. *J. Neurol.* **207**, 73.

Ricker, K., Mertens, H.-G. and Schimrigk, K. (1968). The neurogenic scapulo-peroneal syndrome. *Eur. Neurol.* **1**, 257.

Ringel, S. P., Lava, N. S., Treihaft, M. M., Lubs, M. L. and Lubs, H. A. (1978). Late-onset X-linked recessive spinal and bulbar muscular atrophy. *Muscle & Nerve* **1**, 297.

Robertson, W. C., Kawamura, Y. and Dyck, P. J. (1978). Morphometric study of motoneurons in congenital nemaline myopathy and Werdnig–Hoffman disease. *Neurology, Minneapolis* **28**, 1057.

Ross, R. T., Simpson, C. A. and Styles, S. (1974). Wohlfart Kugelberg Welander syndrome. *Can. J. neurol. Sci.* **1**, 130.

Roy, S., Dubowitz, V. and Wolman, L. (1971). Ultrastructure of muscle in infantile spinal muscular atrophy. *J. neurol. Sci.* **12**, 219.

Russman, B. S. and Fredericks, E. J. (1979). Use of the ECG in the diagnosis of childhood spinal muscular atrophy. *Arch. Neurol., Chicago* **36**, 317.

Schwartz, M. S. and Swash, M. (1975). Scapuloperoneal atrophy with sensory involvement: Davidenkow's syndrome. *J. Neurol. Neurosurg. Psychiat.* **38**, 1063.

Shafiq, S. A., Milhorat, A. T. and Gorycki, M. A. (1967). Fine structure of human muscle in neurogenic atrophy. *Neurology, Minneapolis* **17**, 934.

Shapira, Y., Amit, R. and Rachmilewitz, E. (1981). Vitamin E deficiency in Werdnig–Hoffman disease. *Ann. Neurol.* **10**, 266.

Smith, E. M., Bender, L. F. and Stover, C. N. (1963). Lower motor neuron deficit in arthrogryposis: an EMG study. *Arch. Neurol., Chicago* **8**, 97.

Spiller, W. G. (1913). The relation of the myopathies. *Brain* **36**, 75.

Spiro, A. J. (1970). Minipolymyoclonus: a neglected sign in childhood spinal muscular atrophy. *Neurology, Minneapolis* **20**, 1124.

Thieffry, S., Arthuis, M. and Bargeton, E. (1955). Quarante cas de maladie de Werdnig–Hoffmann avec onze examens anatomiques. *Rev. Neurol.* **93**, 621.

Thomas, P. K., Calne, D. B. and Elliott, C. F. (1972). X-linked scapuloperoneal syndrome. *J. Neurol. Neurosurg. Psychiat.* **35**, 208.

—— Schott, G. D. and Morgan-Hughes, J. A. (1975). Adult onset scapuloperoneal myopathy. *J. Neurol. Neurosurg. Psychiat.* **38**, 1008.

Tomlinson, B. E., Walton, J. N. and Irving, D. (1974). Spinal cord limb motor neurones in muscular dystrophy. *J. neurol. Sci.* **22**, 305.

Tsukagoshi, H., Shoji, H. and Furakawa, T. (1970). Proximal neurogenic muscular atrophy in adolescence and adulthood with X-linked recessive inheritance. *Neurology, Minneapolis* **20**, 1188.

Turner, J. W. A. (1949). On amyotonia congenita. *Brain* **72**, 25.

van Wijngaarden, G. K. and Bethlem, J. (1973). Benign infantile spinal muscular atrophy—a prospective study. *Brain* **96**, 163.

Walton, J. N. (1956). Amyotonia congenita: a follow-up study. *Lancet* **i**, 1023.

—— (1957). The limp child. *J. Neurol. Psychiat.* **20**, 144.

—— and Gardner-Medwin, D. (1981). Progressive muscular dystrophy and the myotonic disorders. In *Disorders of voluntary muscle* (ed. J. N. Walton), 4th edn, p. 481. Churchill-Livingstone, Edinburgh.

Wechsler, W. and Hager, H. (1962). Elektronenmikroskopische Befunde an der Skeletmuskulatur bei progressiver spinaler Muskelatrophie. *Arch. Psychiat. Z. Neurol.* **203**, 111.

Werdnig, G. (1890). Über einen Fall von Dystrophia musculorum mit positiven Rückenmarksbefunde. *Wien med, Wschr.* **40**, 1796.

—— (1891). Zwei frühinfantile hereditäre Fälle von progressiver Muskelatrophie unter dem Bilde der Dystrophie, aber auf neurotischer Grundlage. *Arch. Psychiat.* **22**, 437.

Young, I. D. and Harper, P. S. (1980). Hereditary distal spinal muscular atrophy with vocal cord paralysis. *J. Neurol. Neurosurg. Psychiat.* **43**, 413.

Zellweger, H., Simpson, J., McCormick, W. F. and Ionasescu, V. (1972). Spinal muscular atrophy with autosomal dominant inheritance, *Neurology, Minneapolis* **22**, 957.

Facial hemiatrophy

Synonym. Parry–Romberg syndrome.

Definition. A disorder of uncertain aetiology, characterized by progressive wasting of some or all of the tissues of one side of the face and sometimes extending beyond these limits.

Pathology

Facial hemiatrophy, first described by Romberg in 1846, consists essentially of atrophy which usually involves all the tissues of the face—the skin, the subcutaneous fat and connective tissue, the muscles, cartilage, and bone. The muscular atrophy is due to disappearance, not of muscle but of fat and connective tissue. The tongue and soft palate are often affected. The cartilage of the nose is frequently atrophic: that of the ear, larynx, and tarsus is less often affected. The cerebral hemisphere on the affected side may be atrophic. Stief (1933) described vasodilatation in the ipsilateral hemisphere and round-cell infiltration of the cervical sympathetic on the affected side.

Aetiology

It is a disorder of early life, usually developing during the second decade, and is sometimes congenital. Several cases, however, have been observed with an onset in middle life or even old age. The cause of the condition is unknown. A relationship to morphoea (localized scleroderma) has been postulated but this could not explain the occasional involvement of other parts of the body on the affected side or the atrophy of the ipsilateral cerebral hemisphere. Various authors have attributed the condition to local trauma or infection, or to lesions of the ipsilateral trigeminal nerve or cervical sympathetic in which indefinite pathological changes have been found (Archambault and Fromm 1932) but pathological findings are very variable (Ford 1966) and pathogenesis remains obscure. In a recent report of three cases, Asher and Berg (1982) found changes in a CT scan suggestive of vascular malformation in the ipsilateral cerebral hemisphere in one, and an ill-defined abnormality in the opposite hemisphere in another; their third patient, who has been observed for 43 years, had had focal epilepsy since childhood and in middle life developed optic atrophy and dementia, other somatic asymmetries, amyotrophy, and areflexia but had a normal CT scan.

Symptoms and signs

Wasting may begin at any point of the face and may either remain limited to one region, sometimes corresponding to one division of the trigeminal nerve, or may spread, either slowly or quickly, to the whole face (Fig. 13.10), occasionally extending to the side of the neck and even, as in a case of Martin's, involving the breast on the same side. Cases of progressive hemiatrophy of the whole body are closely related. When the disorder is well developed the patient's appearance is striking, the affected half of the face being sunken and wrinkled with an appearance of old age, in marked contrast to the normal side. Very rarely both sides of the face are affected. The atrophy often involves the soft palate, tongue, and oral mucous membrane on the same side. There is no muscular weakness. Less hair on the face and scalp on the affected side is not uncommon. Pigmentary anomalies of the skin, such as vitiligo, frequently occur, and facial naevus has been described. Neuralgic facial pain, rarely true tic douloureux, is sometimes described. Sensory impairment is rare but cutaneous anaesthesia and analgesia have been reported. Sweating and lacrimal secretion may be either diminished or increased on the affected side. An ipsilateral Horner's syndrome is occasionally seen and Brain saw a case with a unilateral Argyll Robertson pupil. In other cases the pupil on the affected side has been larger than on the normal side.

Epileptic seizures, often Jacksonian but occasionally generalized, occur in some cases. Brain observed one such case in which left facial hemiatrophy was associated with right-sided epilepsy, hemiplegia, hemianaesthesia, hemianopia, and aphasia, and atrophy of the left cerebral hemisphere was demonstrated by encephalography. Migraine is common. Facial hemiatrophy is sometimes associated with syringomyelia, and morphoea has been noted elsewhere in the body.

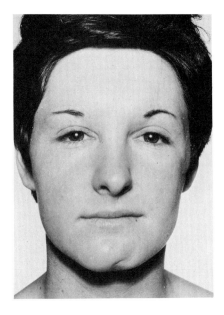

Fig. 13.10. Early left-sided facial hemiatrophy. (Kindly supplied by Dr J.D.Spillane.)

Diagnosis

The clinical picture is so striking that it can hardly be confused with anything else.

Prognosis

The wasting may become arrested before the whole face is involved, but there is no means of determining whether or not this will occur. In mild cases the disorder causes no disability apart from its cosmetic effect.

Treatment

No known treatment will arrest the progress of the disease. When trigeminal pain or epilepsy are present, carbamazepine should be tried but constant rather than paroxysmal pain is more likely to respond to standard analgesic remedies.

References

Archambault, L. and Fromm, N. K. (1932). Progressive facial hemiatrophy *Arch. Neurol. Psychiat. Chicago* **27**, 529.

Asher, S. W. and Berg, B. O. (1982). Progressive hemifacial atrophy. Report of three cases, including one observed over 43 years, and computed tomographic findings. *Arch. Neurol., Chicago* **39**, 44.

Ford, F. R. (1966). *Diseases of the nervous system in infancy, childhood and adolescence*, 5th edn, p. 310. Thomas, Springfield, Illinois.

Stief, A. (1933). Über einen Fall von Hemiatrophie des Gesichtes mit Sektionsbefund *Z. ges. Neurol. Psychiat.* **147**, 573.

Wartenberg, R. (1945). Progressive facial hemiatrophy. *Arch. Neurol. Psychiat., Chicago* **54**, 75.

Hemihypertrophy

In this rare condition there is hypertrophy of the tissues, including the long bones which are often longer than normal, on one half of the body. Associated anomalies may include congenital heart disease and chromosomal abnormalities (Henry, Louis, Hoeffel, and Pernot 1973). Focal neurological abnormalities on the affected side are uncommon but focal or generalized epileptic convulsions have been reported as well as congenital indifference to pain on the affected side (Fox and Huott 1974).

References

Fox, J. H. and Huott, A. D. (1974). Congenital hemihypertrophy with indifference to pain. *Arch. Neurol., Chicago* **30**, 490.

Henry, M., Louis, J. P., Hoeffel. J. C. and Pernot, C. (1973). Congenital hemihypertrophy with aortic, skeletal, and ocular abnormalities. *Br. med. J.* **1**, 87.

14

Disorders of the spinal cord and cauda equina

Anatomy of the spinal cord and cauda equina

The spinal cord lies within the vertebral canal, extending from the foramen magnum, where it joins the medulla oblongata, to the level of the first or second lumbar vertebra. It is oval in shape, being flattened from before backwards, and has two enlargements, in the cervical and lumbar regions, corresponding to the outflow of nerves to the limbs. At its lower end it terminates in the conus medullaris, from the end of which a delicate filament, the filum terminale, continues downwards to the posterior surface of the coccyx.

The surface of the cord shows several longitudinal grooves, the deep anterior median fissure and the shallower posterior median sulcus, while on the lateral aspect are two sulci, the anterolateral and the posterolateral. From each of the latter a series of root filaments emerge on each side. At intervals several filaments from the posterolateral sulcus unite to form a dorsal root, upon which is situated the dorsal-root ganglion; similarly those from the anterolateral sulcus unite to form a ventral root. One ventral and the corresponding dorsal root on each side join together just distal to the dorsal-root ganglion to form a spinal nerve. Thus there arise a series of spinal nerves, and the spinal cord is regarded as being organized into segments, one corresponding to each pair of spinal nerves. There are eight cervical, 12 dorsal or thoracic, five lumbar, five sacral segments, and one coccygeal. Since the spinal cord ends at the first or second lumbar vertebra, all the spinal nerves below the first lumbar descend to their respective foramina in a bundle of nerves known as the cauda equina.

The spinal cord, like the brain, is surrounded by three meninges. The pia mater, a fibrous membrane, forms the immediate covering of the cord, and from it fine septa penetrate into the cord substance. The arachnoid is a delicate, transparent membrane, which lies superficially to the pia mater, from which it is separated by the subarachnoid space; this contains CSF and is bridged by numerous trabeculae. The arachnoid extends as low as the second sacral vertebra. Outside the arachnoid lies the dura mater, which lines the vertebral canal, from which it is separated by the epidural space, containing fat and a thin-walled venous plexus. The dura extends a little lower than the arachnoid, to the second or third sacral vertebra. The spinal cord is suspended within its dural sheath by a series of ligamenta denticulata, which extend laterally from each side to terminate in tooth-like attachments to the inner aspect of the dura.

On transverse section the cord substance is seen to be divided into the central grey and peripheral white matter. The grey matter is composed of ganglion cells and nerve fibres, and the white matter of fibres and their myelin sheaths. The grey matter forms an H-shaped mass composed of an anterior and a posterior horn on each side, united by the grey commissure, in the middle of which lies the central canal. The anterior horns contain ganglion cells, whose axons enter the anterior roots and form the lower motor neurones. The cells which innervate the skeletal muscles (alpha motor neurones) measure between 30 and 70 μm in diameter (Truex and Carpenter 1969) and show certain histological characteristics which usually render their differentiation from the gamma motor neurones comparatively easy, as most of the latter are less than 30 μm in diameter (Tomlinson, Irving, and Rebeiz 1973). The large anterior horn cells (motor neurones) are arranged in definite groups (in transverse sections) and columns (in longitudinal sections) and Sharrard (1953, 1955) showed that specific groups and columns of cells in the cervical and lumbar enlargements consistently innervate various muscle groups and some individual muscles. The total number of limb motor neurones in the lumbosacral cord is remarkably consistent not only on the two sides of the cord but also in different individuals (Tomlinson *et al.* 1973).

The white matter, consisting of longitudinal bundles of nerve fibres, is regarded as being divided into three columns. The anterior column lies between the anterior fissure and the anterior horn of grey matter with its emerging roots. The lateral column lies lateral to the grey matter, between the ventral and dorsal roots, that is, between the anterolateral and posterolateral sulci. The posterior column lies between the posterior median septum and the posterior horn of grey matter and its dorsal root. The paths of the fibres entering the spinal cord by the posterior roots and the anatomical interrelationship of its fibre tracts were described earlier (see p. 19).

The blood supply of the spinal cord

Arteries. The spinal cord is richly supplied with blood. There are two posterior spinal arteries, each derived from the corresponding vertebral or posterior inferior cerebellar artery which pass downwards lateral to the medulla oblongata and throughout the whole length of the cord, where they lie either in front of, or behind, the dorsal-nerve roots. The single anterior spinal artery is formed by the union of a branch from each vertebral artery, and descends throughout the whole length of the cord in the anterior median fissure. The spinal arteries are reinforced by segmental arteries, which enter the intervertebral foramina and are derived from vertebral, intercostal, and lumbar arteries. The two most important of these are one in the lower cervical and one, the artery of Adamkiewicz, in the lower thoracic or upper lumbar region. The cord is also surrounded in each segment by a basocorona or arterial wreath, which unites the anterior and posterior spinal arteries and sends branches horizontally inwards to supply the white matter and most of the posterior horns of grey matter. The anterior horns are supplied by branches of the anterior spinal artery, distributed to the anterior horn on each side alternately.

The direction of blood flow in the anterior spinal artery may not be the same throughout. Bolton (1939) suggested that blood flows downwards in both the anterior and posterior spinal arteries as far as the lower cervical region; he also suggested that in the dorsal and lumbar regions flow was often upwards. Studies with spinal-cord angiography in animals and man (Di Chiro, Fried, and Doppman 1970; Di Chiro 1970; Fortuna, la Torre, and Occhipinti 1971; Di Chiro and Fried 1971; Treten 1976) have confirmed that flow is often in a rostral direction even in the lower cervical region but is variable from one individual to another and may be modified by vascular disease. Methods of measuring spinal-cord blood flow have been devised in animals (Griffiths 1973 *a*, *b*, *c*) and experimental work has shown that motor or sensory activity causes temporary vasodilatation and increased blood flow in the relevant portions of the cord and cauda equina (Blau and Rushworth 1958). Within the cord the anterior spinal artery supplies all but the posterior part of the posterior columns and posterior horns, which are supplied by the posterior spinal arteries. Descending branches from the spinal arteries also supply the cauda equina.

Syndromes of spinal-cord ischaemia and/or infarction (p. 423) may result from embolism or occlusion of the anterior spinal artery due to atheroma, aortic disease, or a drop in perfusion pressure (Herrick and Mills 1971; Silver and Buxton 1974) and may complicate aortography (*The Lancet* 1973). Posterior spinal-artery occlusion due to intrathecal phenol injection has also been described (Hughes 1970). The motor neurones and central grey matter are generally more vulnerable to ischaemia than white matter (Gilles and Nag 1971; Fried and Aparicio 1973).

Veins. The spinal veins derived from the spinal-cord substance terminate in a plexus in the pia mater, in which six longitudinal channels have been described. These pass upwards into the corresponding veins of the medulla oblongata and so drain into the intracranial venous sinuses. Segmental veins pass outwards along nerve roots to join the vertebral venous plexus, in which blood also flows upwards to the intracranial venous sinuses. The posterior half of the cord is drained by posterior medullary veins; the anterior medullary group has one lateral and two medial groups (Gillilan 1970) and the anatomical pattern helps to explain the clinical features of venous infarction of the cord (Hughes 1971, and see p. 423). Venous drainage through the intervertebral foramina is relatively unimportant, but thrombophlebitis may reach spinal veins by this route.

References

Blau, J. N. and Rushworth, G. (1958). Observations on the blood vessels of the spinal cord and their responses to motor activity. *Brain* **81**, 354.

Bolton, B. (1939). The blood supply of the spinal cord. *J. Neurol. Psychiat.* **2**, 137.

Corbin, J. L. (1961). *Anatomie, pathologie artérielle de la moelle.* Masson, Paris.

Di Chiro, G. (1970). Spinal cord angiography. *Proc. R. Soc. Med.* **63**, 184.

—— and Fried, L. C. (1971). Blood flow currents in spinal cord arteries. *Neurology Minneapolis* **21**, 1088.

——, Fried, L. C., and Doppman, J. L. (1970). Experimental spinal cord angiography. *Br. F. Radiol.* **43**, 19.

Fortuna, A., La Torre, E., and Occhipinti, E. (1971). The direction of blood flow in the cervical cord. *Eur. Neurol.* **5**, 335.

Fried, L. C. and Aparicio, O. (1973). Experimental ischemia of the spinal cord: histologic studies after anterior spinal artery occlusion. *Neurology, Minneapolis.* **23**, 289.

Gilles, F. H. and Nag, D. (1971). Vulnerability of human spinal cord in transient cardiac arrest. *Neurology, Minneapolis* **21**, 833.

Gillilan, L. A. (1970). Veins of the spinal cord: anatomic details; suggested clinical applications. *Neurology, Minneapolis* **20**, 860.

Griffiths, I. R. (1973 *a*). Spinal cord blood flow in dogs: 1. ;the 'normal' flow. *J. Neurol. Neurosurg. Psychiat.* **36**, 34.

——. (1973 *b*). Spinal cord blood flow in dogs: 2. The effect of the blood gases. *J. Neurol. Neurosurg. Psychiat.* **36**, 42.

——. (1973 *c*). Spinal cord blood flow in dogs: 3. The effect of blood pressure. *J. Neurol. Neurosurg. Psychiat.* **36**, 914.

Herrick, M. K. and Mills, P. E. (1971). Infarction of spinal cord. Two cases of selective gray matter involvement secondary to asymptomatic aortic disease. *Arch. Neurol, Chicago* **24**, 228.

Hughes, J. T. (1978). *Pathology of the spinal cord*, 2nd edn. Lloyd-Luke, London.

—— (1970). Thrombosis of the posterior spinal arteries: a complication of an intrathecal injection of phenol. *Neurology, Minneapolis* **20**, 659.

—— (1971). Venous infarction of the spinal cord. *Neurology, Minneapolis* **21**, 794.

The Lancet (1973). Spinal-cord damage after angiography. *Lancet.* **ii**, 1067.

Sharrard, W. J. W. (1953). Correlation between changes in the spinal cord and muscle paralysis in poliomyelitis—a preliminary report. *Proc. R. Soc. Med.* **46**, 346.

—— (1955). The histology of lesions in the lumbo-sacral spinal cord in convalescent and late poliomyelitis. *Proceedings of the Second International Congress of Neuropathology*, p. 437. Amsterdam.

Silver, J. R. and Buxton, P. H. (1974). Spinal stroke. *Brain* **97**, 539.

Tomlinson, B. E., Irving, D., and Rebeiz, J. J. (1973). Total numbers of limb motor neurones in the human lumbosacral cord and an analysis of the accuracy of various sampling procedures. *J. neurol. Sci.* **20**, 313.

Truex, R. C. and Carpenter, M. B. (1969). *Human neuroanatomy*, 6th edn. Williams and Wilkins, p. 247 Baltimore.

Treten, L. (1976). *A microangiographic and stereomicroscopic study of the spinal cord vascularity in man and rat.* University of Oslo, Oslo.

Paraplegia

Paraplegia means paralysis of the lower limbs. This may be caused by disorders of function at many different levels. It may be psychogenic—in hysteria. It may result from a cerebral lesion, when so placed as to damage corticospinal fibres from both leg areas of the motor cortex. Cerebral paraplegia may thus be caused by a meningioma arising in the falx (a parasagittal meningioma), by thrombosis of the superior sagittal sinus, by Little's disease (when it is more often called diplegia), and in rare instances by thrombosis of an unpaired anterior cerebral artery. In such cases the lower limbs are usually spastic in extension. Bilateral brainstem lesions usually cause tetraplegia rather than paraplegia. Paraplegia due to a spinal-cord lesion is very much commoner; it may be associated with increased tone in either extensor or flexor muscles of the legs, called paraplegia-in-extension or paraplegia-in-flexion. Paraplegia of lower rather than upper motor-neurone type may also be caused by a lesion of the anterior horn cells in the lumbosacral region as in poliomyelitis or, rarely, motor-neurone disease, by a lesion of the cauda equina, or of the peripheral nerves to the lower limbs, as in polyneuropathy, or of muscles, as in myopathy. We are concerned here mainly with paraplegia due to spinal-cord lesions.

After a partial cord lesion two mutually antagonistic reflex activities emerge, extensor hypertonia and the flexor withdrawal reflex (see p. 51). The former is recognized as physiologically equivalent to decerebrate rigidity, which depends upon intact connections between reticular formation nuclei and the spinal cord. The flexor withdrawal reflex, on the other hand, utilizes short spinal reflex arcs. After a lesion which involves corticospinal tracts only, both sets of reflexes are potentially active, but extensor hypertonia predominates as a persistent tonic activity, giving way only occasionally to the flexor withdrawal reflex when a noxious stimulus excites the latter. If, however, a spinal lesion involves sufficient of the cord to destroy not only corticospinal fibres but also the descending reticulospinal tracts upon which extensor hypertonia depends, the flexor reflex, freed from its antagonist, shows greatly increased activity and dominates the picture. Flexor spasms occur in the lower limbs, which in severe cases finally become fixed in an attitude of flexion. Paraplegia-in-flexion may be due to a slowly progressive lesion of the cord, in which case it follows paraplegia-in-extension after an intermediate phase. But after a traumatic lesion, causing immediate and complete severance of the cord, because the reticulospinal tract is interrupted from the beginning, as soon as the stage of spinal shock has passed, paraplegia-in-flexion will develop unless prevented.

Paraplegia-in-flexion

In paraplegia-in-flexion three main reflex activities are demonstrable: (1) the flexor withdrawal reflex; (2) excretory; and (3) sexual reflexes. We must also consider: (4) the 'mass reflex'; and (5) the tendon reflexes.

1. *The flexor withdrawal reflex* has already been described briefly (see p. 51). In paraplegia-in-flexion its activity is enhanced. Its receptive field is enlarged and it may be elicitable by a stimulus applied to any part of the lower limbs and abdominal wall, or even, with a high dorsal lesion, as high as the nipple. The motor response is vigorous, and strong flexion of the stimulated lower limb occurs at all joints, with upward movement of the great toe

and fanning of the other toes. The opposite lower limb may also flex. The activity of the flexor reflex is depressed by spinal shock and sometimes by cutaneous or urinary infection. It may then be obtainable only from the outer border of the sole with slight contraction of the hamstring muscles.

2. *Excretory reflexes.* When reflex activity of the divided spinal cord is well established, normally about three weeks after transection, reflex evacuation of the bladder and rectum, and reflex sweating occur. The volume of fluid required to evoke reflex contraction of the bladder varies in different cases, but is usually about 150–200 ml. Reflex emptying can be facilitated by deep breathing or by stimuli applied to the skin of the lower limbs. Reflex evacuation of the rectum occurs in response to a volume of from 100 to 180 ml. Sweating occurs reflexly in response to cutaneous stimuli from the areas of skin supplied by the fibres of the sympathetic nervous system which leave the cord below the level of the lesion.

3. *Sexual reflexes.* In paraplegia-in-flexion the cremasteric and bulbocavernosus reflexes are present, and reflex erection of the penis and seminal emission can be evoked by handling the organ. Spontaneous priapism may occur. These reflexes may be associated with contractions of the abdominal recti, the leg flexors, and the thigh adductors.

4. *The mass reflex.* Reflex facilitation probably accounts for the phenomenon named by Head and Riddoch (1917) the 'mass reflex', in which stimulation of the skin of the lower limbs or, when the lesion is high, of the lower abdominal wall, evokes reflex flexion of the lower limbs, evacuation of the bladder and rectum, and sweating.

5. *The tendon reflexes.* Tone in the extensor muscles is minimal in paraplegia-in-flexion, but the tendon reflexes can usually be elicited. Ankle clonus, however, is rarely elicitable.

Paraplegia-in-extension

In paraplegia-in-extension tone predominates in the hip adductors and in the extensors of the hips, knees, and ankles with resulting extension of the hip and knee and plantar-flexion at the ankles. The knee-and ankle-jerks are exaggerated, and patellar and ankle clonus are often present. Eliciting the knee-jerk may evoke sharp contraction of the adductors of the opposite hip, the crossed adductor-jerk. Reflex extension of the limb can often be obtained by applying a stimulus, such as a scratch from a pin, to the skin of the upper third of the thigh, and spontaneous extensor spasms may occur.

With this predominance of extensor tone the flexor withdrawal reflex is relatively inhibited. Its receptive field is small compared with that found in paraplegia-in-flexion. After it has been elicited, the limb rapidly regains its primary posture of extension. Flexor withdrawal of one limb is usually associated with increased extension of the other, the crossed extensor reflex. The excretory reflexes which accompany paraplegia-in-flexion are absent, and penile erection is followed by extension instead of flexion of the lower limbs.

Some recent developments

In occasional cases of paraplegia there is an apparent inconsistency between the degree of spasticity as assessed by flexion or extension of the limb on the one hand and the activity of the tendon reflexes on the other. Marsden, Merton, and Morton (1973) produced evidence to suggest that whereas the tendon jerks depend upon monosynaptic reflexes, the stretch reflex may be due to rapidly conducting long reflex pathways involving the cortex. Swash and Earl (1975) reported that in two patients with the Holmes–Adie syndrome and tabes dorsalis respectively, severe transverse-cord lesions caused a flaccid paraplegia with absent

tendon reflexes; both patients had flexor spasms but no spasticity. Measurement of the H-reflex is a useful method of assessing the excitability of spinal motor neurones in spinal shock and in spasticity and rigidity (Yap 1967; Diamantopoulos and Zander Olsen 1967). Experimental work in animals on conduction in demyelinated fibres (McDonald and Robertson 1972) and studies of demyelination, with subsequent Wallerian degeneration (in severe cases) or remyelination (when less severe) in experimental spinal-cord compression in the cat (Harrison and McDonald 1977; Griffiths and McCulloch 1983) have cast new light upon mechanisms of spinal-cord dysfunction and repair. Measurement of spinal evoked potentials following peripheral sensory stimulation (Cracco, Cracco, and Graziani 1975) has also proved useful in assessing the location and severity of spinal-cord lesions. In cases of traumatic paraplegia and quadriplegia, such potentials are present, even during spinal shock, below the lesion but, when the latter is complete, cortical evoked potentials are, of course, absent (Sedgwick, El-Negamy, and Frankel 1980); preservation of the latter is a useful means of distinguishing hysterical paraplegia. Above transverse-cord lesions in the mid-thoracic region, subtle abnormalities of cervical spinal evoked potentials may be found (Sedgwick *et al.* 1980). Sparing of the Onufrowicz nucleus in the second sacral anterior horn, as commonly found in cases of Werdnig–Hoffmann disease, has been interpreted as indicating that the cells of this nucleus innervate the external sphincter muscle of the urethra and anus (Iwata and Hirano 1978). The pathophysiology of paraplegia has recently been reviewed by Lance and McLeod (1981).

References

Cracco, J. B., Cracco, R. Q., and Graziani, L. J. (1975). The spinal evoked response in infants and children. *Neurology, Minneapolis*, **25**, 31.

Diamantopoulos, E. and Zander Olsen, P. (1967). Excitability of motor neurones in spinal shock in man. *J. Neurol. Neurosurg. Psychiat.* **30**, 427.

Griffiths, I. R. and McCulloch, M. C. (1983). Nerve fibres in spinal cord impact injuries: Part 1. Changes in the myelin sheath during the initial 5 weeks. *J. neurol. Sci.* **58**, 335.

Harrison, B. M. and McDonald, W. I. (1977). Remyelination after transient experimental compression of the spinal cord. *Ann. Neurol.* **1**, 542.

Head, H. and Riddoch, G. (1917). The automatic bladder, excessive sweating, and some other reflex conditions, in gross injuries of the spinal cord. *Brain* **40**, 188.

Iwata, M. and Hirano, A. (1978). Sparing of the Onufrowicz nucleus in sacral anterior horn lesions. *Ann. Neurol.* **4**, 245.

Lance, J. W. and McLeod, J. G. (1981). *A physiological approach to clinical neurology*, 3rd edn. Butterworths, London.

Marsden, C. D., Merton, P. A., and Morton, H. B. (1973). Is the human stretch reflex cortical rather than spinal? *Lancet* **i**, 759.

McDonald, W. I and Robertson, M. A. H. (1972). Changes in conduction during nerve fibre degeneration in the spinal cord. *Brain* **95**, 151.

Pedersen, E. (1 Ed.) (1962). Spasticity and neurological bladder disturbances. *Acta neurol. Kbh.* **38**, Suppl. 3.

Sedgwick, E. M., El-Negamy, E., and Frankel, H. (1980). Spinal-cord potentials in traumatic paraplegia and quadriplegia. *J. Neurol. Neurosurg. Psychiat.* **43**, 823.

Swash, M. and Earl, C. J. (1975). Flaccid paraplegia: a feature of spinal cord lesions in Holmes–Adie syndrome and tabes dorsalis. *J. Neurol. Neurosurg. Psychiat.* **38**, 317.

Walshe, F. M. R. (1914–15). The physiological significance of the reflex phenomena in spastic paralysis of the lower limbs. *Brain* **37**, 269.

—— (1919). On the genesis and physiological significance of spasticity and other disorders of motor innervation: with a consideration of the functional relationships of the pyramidal system. *Brain* **42**, 1.

—— (1923). On variations in the form of reflex movements, notably the Babinski plantar response, under different degrees of spasticity and under the influence of Magnus and de Kleijn's tonic neck reflex. *Brain* **46**, 281.

Yap, C.-B. (1967). Spinal segmental and long-loop reflexes and spinal motoneurone excitability in spasticity and rigidity. *Brain* **90**, 887.

The innervation of the bladder and rectum

Anatomy and physiology

The sympathetic fibres to the bladder arise chiefly from the first and second lumbar ganglia, with contributions from the third and fourth. These fibres unite to form the presacral nerve or superior hypogastric plexus, which lies in front of the aortic bifurcation. From this plexus come the two hypogastric nerves, each ending in the vesical plexuses on the lateral aspect of the bladder. The parasympathetic nerve supply from the second and third sacral nerves (the nervi erigentes) also joins the vesical plexuses. It is doubtful if there is a separately innervated internal sphincter. When the parasympathetic is stimulated, the longitudinal fibres of the detrusor pull the neck open and the circular fibres exert pressure on the bladder contents. The physiology of micturition is discussed by Yeates (1973), Johnson and Spalding (1974), Pearman and England (1976) and the pathophysiology of incontinence by Swash (1985).

In infancy, bladder evacuation occurs reflexly, the reflex arc running through the sacral cord segments. The development of control over bladder evacuation is associated with increasing ability to inhibit the evacuation reflex, control of the inhibitory impulses lies in the sympathetic system, which maintains closure of the sphincter and inhibits contraction of the detrusor muscles. At the same time it becomes possible voluntarily to overcome this inhibition and so to initiate the act of micturition, which is then completed reflexly. Thus there are three nervous mechanisms controlling bladder function—the sacral reflex arc for evacuation; the inhibitory influence of the sympathetic; and voluntary control overcoming the last-named and initiating micturition. In the 1950s it was in fact concluded by several workers that because so little effect upon bladder function was noted in man following sympathetic stimulation, the parasympathetic innervation of the detrusor was alone important. Now, however, it is recognized that there are indeed functional α- and β-adrenergic sympathetic fibres innervating the muscle of the bladder wall. β-receptors predominate in the bladder wall and stimulation of these allows the bladder to fill; α-receptors are more profuse in the neck of the organ and stimulation of these causes the internal sphincter to contract (Yeates 1974). Phenoxybenzamine, which blocks α-receptors, will open the bladder neck (Pearman and England 1976); it also has an effect in blocking muscarinic cholinergic receptors and so increases functional bladder capacity (Yeates 1982a).

Bladder sensation giving a feeling of fullness and a desire to micturate travels centrally in the spinothalamic tracts, as does that concerned with urethral pain (Nathan and Smith 1951), while urethral touch and pressure travel in the posterior columns. The descending motor pathway concerned with voluntary bladder evacuation lies in the lateral columns on an equatorial plane passing through the central canal (Nathan and Smith 1958). The voluntary initiation of micturition usually occurs in response to an awareness of bladder distension. The part of the postcentral gyrus lying at the vertex of the cerebral hemisphere is the cortical centre for bladder sensation, and the corresponding area of the precentral gyrus is probably the site of origin of motor impulses initiating the act of micturition. It is well recognized that parasagittal lesions which affect this region bilaterally can cause urinary retention. Andrew and Nathan (1964) showed that the area concerned lies in the superior frontal gyrus and that unilateral or, more often, bilateral lesions here may give urgency and frequency of micturition and incontinence or sometimes retention; the sensation giving rise to the desire to micturate is diminished or absent.

Investigation of bladder function

In order to diagnose the nature of a neurogenic disorder of bladder function and to treat it appropriately it is sometimes necessary to test bladder function quantitatively. *Cystometry* is a technique of measuring the rise of intravesical pressure induced by increasing volumes of fluid instilled into the bladder by catheter, recording with a manometer the intravesical pressure continuously or after the instillation of each 50 ml. The recording so obtained is called a *cystometrogram*; the principles of the method have been reviewed by Pearman and England (1976).

Disturbances of bladder function

Lesions involving the sacral reflex arc

Since the sacral reflex arc is concerned in evacuation of the bladder, its interruption usually causes retention of urine, owing to the unopposed action of the sympathetic. In tabes dorsalis the reflex is interrupted on its afferent side, because of degeneration of the afferent neurones. Lesions of the conus medullaris interrupt the central fibres of the reflex. Lesions of the cauda equina, if they destroy the second and third sacral nerves, interrupt both the afferent and the efferent paths of the reflex and hence usually cause retention of urine. Even after severe but incomplete lesions of the conus or cauda equina, however, 'reflex' evacuation of the bladder may occasionally develop. However, in cauda-equina lesions and in tabes the bladder is more usually atonic, that is, it accepts a very large volume of urine and slowly distends without contracting reflexly to raise the intravesical pressure.

Lesions of the spinal cord above the conus medullaris

Incomplete lesions of the spinal cord may affect principally either inhibitory fibres destined for the sympathetic outflow, or descending fibres concerned in the voluntary initiation of micturition. In the former case, the patient has difficulty in holding urine, and micturition is precipitate. This so-called urgency is a common symptom in the early stages of multiple sclerosis. Moderately severe but still incomplete lesions of the cord tend to impair voluntary control over micturition, so that urinary retention develops, owing to uninhibited action of the sympathetic. Retention is thus produced, for example, by spinal compression in its later stages, by transverse myelitis, and in the more advanced stages of multiple sclerosis.

After complete interruption of conduction in the spinal cord, either by transection or by severe transverse lesions above the conus, there is initially retention during the phase of spinal shock but subsequently enhancement of reflex activity develops in the distal portion, and reflex evacuation of the bladder then occurs through the agency of the sacral reflex arc. It may be facilitated by stimuli applied to the sacral cutaneous areas. But after some massive lesions of the sacral segments and/or cord the bladder remains atonic, presumably due to concurrent involvement of the cauda equina, perhaps as a result of ischaemia.

Cerebral lesions

The fibres concerned in the voluntary initiation of micturition may be interrupted above the spinal cord, and retention of urine may then develop, usually in association with severe bilateral corticospinal-tract lesions. Lesions involving the vertical region of the precentral cortex on both sides may also cause retention as Foerster first showed. Dysfunction of this part of the cerebral cortex or of pathways which descend from it probably account for retention of urine, or for urgency and incontinence (Andrew and Nathan 1964), which are not uncommon symptoms of intracranial tumour, anterior communicating artery aneurysm, or of diffuse cerebral lesions such as Alzheimer's disease, or other dementing processes.

Nocturnal enuresis in otherwise normal children probably arises in the first place as a result of delay in developing inhibition of reflex bladder evacuation. Later, for psychological reasons, the child acquires abnormal conditioned reflexes whereby bladder evacuation continues to occur during sleep (Kolvin, MacKeith, and Meadow 1973; Yeates 1982b). Rarely, however, enuresis in childhood is due to spinal-cord or cauda-equina lesions associated with spina bifida occulta.

Treatment of bladder disturbances

In the treatment of bladder dysfunction the underlying physiological principles must be borne in mind. When retention of urine occurs, adequate bladder drainage, usually with the aid of an indwelling catheter, becomes necessary, and steps must be taken to combat the risk of infection of the urinary tract and to treat it, when it develops, with appropriate urinary antiseptics or antibiotics. (See p. 395 for the care of the bladder in paraplegia.)

Since retention of urine is usually due to a relative preponderance of sympathetic influence, parasympathomimetic drugs may be very helpful. Injection of carbachol, B.P., 1 ml, may be given subcutaneously, or 1 mg of carbachol orally, but if, despite bladder contraction induced by this drug, by bethanechol 10–100 mg, or by distigmine (*Ubretid*), 0.5 mg by injection or 5 mg by mouth, there is no evacuation, catheterization will be required. Phenoxybenzamine 10–20 mg may relax the internal sphincter. In chronic cases division of the internal sphincter (bladder-neck resection) may help.

Interruption of the sympathetic supply to the bladder by resection of the presacral nerve has sometimes been carried out and good results have been claimed for this operation but its effect is rarely lasting. The same operation has been used to interrupt pain impulses from the bladder in painful conditions such as inoperable carcinoma.

In cases of frequency, urgency, or precipitancy due to predominant action of the parasympathetic, anticholinergic drugs may be helpful, and propantheline, 15 mg three or four times daily, is particularly useful. Emepromium 50 mg two or three times daily is an alternative. These drugs owe what little value they have in the treatment of nocturnal enuresis to their inhibitory effect upon the parasympathetic. Imipramine 50 mg at night (in the adult) or 25 mg (in children) is often more helpful in such cases, as are its derivatives, desimipramine and clomipramine. Drug treatment alone, however, is rarely successful in this condition and must be combined with the education of reflex inhibition produced by suggestion; hypnotism is sometimes helpful. Often too, the child needs help in solving his psychological problems at school or in the home. Deconditioning using a pad which, when moistened, causes ringing of a bell, has proved useful in some cases (see Kolvin *et al.* 1973).

In patients with incontinence after spinal-cord lesions every effort must be made to re-establish regular reflex bladder evacuation. Regular clamping and release of an indwelling catheter every 2–3 hours during the acute stage may help to initiate this process. The atonic bladder of cauda-equina lesions can usually be evacuated by suprapubic manual compression. Satisfactory incontinence apparatuses are available for the male but not, as yet, for the female patient.

The innervation of the rectum

The nerve supply of the rectum is identical with that of the bladder and micturition and defaecation are physiologically comparable except that in the rectum voluntary control is exerted over the external sphincter only and the rectum lacks voluntary inhibition.

After destruction of the sacral innervation of the rectum, automatic activity, dependent upon a parasympathetic plexus in its wall develops, the rectum contracting and the sphincter relaxing in response to a rise of tension within the viscus. This reflex activity is much more complete when the sacral innervation is intact, e.g. after complete transverse division of the spinal cord above the sacral enlargement. Owing to the relatively limited force of rectal contraction, however, it is at best not very efficient and there is a tendency for all disturbances of rectal innervation to cause constipation, though after complete transverse division of the spinal-cord, reflex defaecation sometimes occurs and may be facilitated by cutaneous stimuli applied to the sacral cutaneous areas. In most patients with spinal-cord or cauda-equina lesions, satisfactory control of the bowels is eventually achieved by means of twice-weekly enemas or suppositories or by manual evacuation of the faeces.

References

Andrew, J. and Nathan, P. W. (1964). Lesions of the anterior frontal lobes and disturbances of micturition and defaecation. *Brain* **87**, 233.

Denny-Brown, D. and Robertson, E. G. (1933). The state of the bladder and its sphincters in complete transverse lesions of the spinal cord and cauda equina. *Brain* **56**, 397.

—— and —— (1935). An investigation of the nervous control of defaecation. *Brain* **58**, 256.

Holmes, G. (1933). Observations on the paralysed bladder. *Brain* **56**, 383.

Johnson, R. H. and Spalding, J. M. K. (1974). *Disorders of the autonomic nervous system*. Blackwell, Oxford.

Kolvin, I., MacKeith, R. C., and Meadow, S. R. (1973). *Bladder control and enuresis*. Heinemann, London and Philadelphia.

Nathan, P. W. and Smith, M. C. (1951). Centripetal pathway from the bladder and urethra within the spinal cord. *J. Neurol. Neurosurg. Psychiat.* **14**, 262.

—— and —— (1958). The centrifugal pathway for micturition within the spinal cord. *J. Neurol. Neurosurg. Psychiat.* **21**, 177.

Pearman, J. W. and England, E. J. (1976). The urinary tract. In *Handbook of clinical neurology* (ed. P. J. Vinken and G. W. Bruyn) Vol. 26, p. 409. North-Holland, Amsterdam.

Pedersen, E. (Ed.) (1962). Spasticity and neurological bladder disturbances. *Acta neurol., Kbh.* **38**, Suppl. 3.

Swash, M. (1985). New concepts in incontinence. *Br. med. J.* **1**, 4.

Voris, H. C. and Landes, H. E. (1940). Cystometric studies in cases of neurologic disease. *Arch. Neurol. Psychiat. Chicago* **44**, 118.

Yeates, W. K. (1973). Bladder function in normal micturition. In *Bladder control and enuresis*. (ed. I. Kolvin, R. C. MacKeith, and S. R. Meadow) p. 28. Heinemann, London and Philadelphia.

—— (1974). Neurophysiology of the bladder. *Paraplegia* **12**, 73.

—— (1982 *a*). *Phenoxybenzamine in disorders of micturition*. Smith, Kline, and French, Welwyn Garden City.

—— (1982 *b*). Enuresis. In *Paediatric urology* (ed. D. I. Williams, and J. H. Johnston) 2nd edn. Butterworths, London.

The care of the paraplegic patient

The general management of a paraplegic patient requires much care and skill and is as important as is treatment of the cause of his disability, for his disorder renders him susceptible to complications which may prove fatal, and, even when less serious, may considerably retard recovery (see Vinken, Bruyn, and Braakmen 1976; Kao, Bunge, and Reier 1982).

Diet

The nutrition of the paraplegic patient is of the utmost importance: the daily caloric requirements are 3500, and the diet should include 125 g of protein, a high vitamin intake, and 3500–4000 ml of fluid. Milk should be given sparingly as its calcium content may increase the risk of urinary calculi. Anaemia may call for iron or even blood transfusion. When protein loss and wasting are severe, short courses of treatment with anabolic steroid drugs may be of value.

Care of the skin

In paraplegia the skin is very liable to injuries which are slow to heal and readily become infected. The factors which lead to bed-sores are—shock in the early stages after injury, vasomotor paralysis, repeated minor trauma, and above all, local ischaemia caused by pressure. Bed-sores are most likely to develop over the bony prominences, especially the heels, the tuber ischii, the sacrum, and the greater trochanter.

The paraplegic patient should be nursed if possible on a 'Ripple' bed or indeed on any type of bed which reduces or regularly transfers pressure. Care should be taken that the bed-clothes are warm and dry and free from rucks, and that a hot-water bottle or electric blanket is not placed in contact with the skin. The patient should be bathed daily, the skin being thoroughly cleansed with soap and water, and carefully dried. After this the back is well rubbed with spirit and dusted with a dusting powder. Areas of reddening of the skin or of loss of epidermis may heal quickly if protected by means of a waterproof spray of acrylic resin or by using a silicone barrier cream or plastic antiseptic spray. The posture of the patient should be changed every two hours both by day and night. If he develops an acute infection, the liability to bed-sores increases, and he should be moved every hour. The value of pads to protect pressure points is doubtful. The lower limbs should be kept extended and the calves should rest upon small pillows with the heels projecting beyond them. The weight of the bed-clothes is often taken from the lower limbs by means of a cradle. As far as possible, contact of the limbs with the bed-clothes should be reduced, and sedatives such as diazepam or nitrazepam may be given if necessary.

The treatment of pressure-sores

If an ulcer has already developed, all necrotic tissue should first be removed to allow free drainage, and swabs for bacterial culture should be taken regularly. At first the bed-sores may be cleaned with hydrogen peroxide or hypochlorite solutions which are still useful, and a dressing of penicillin (20 000 units in 10 ml of normal saline) or other appropriate antibiotic, once organisms have been identified, may be applied for a few days. After that saline dressings or sterile gauze impregnated with paraffin jelly and antibiotic should be used. The dressing should be well covered with adhesive plaster attached to skin some distance away from the pressure points and changed every day. Systemic antibiotic treatment is usually required. Occasionally skin-grafting is necessary (see Guttmann 1976).

Care of the bladder

When urinary retention occurs as a result of a lesion of the nervous system, cystitis almost invariably develops, and if untreated leads to ascending pyelonephritis. Retention of urine must therefore be treated by continuous catheter drainage of the bladder. Modern fine plastic catheters have reduced the incidence of infection. When urinary infection could not be otherwise controlled, suprapubic cystostomy was sometimes performed in the past but fortunately now it is rarely, if ever, needed. Manual control of catheter drainage can be obtained by a clip applied to the drainage tube, and operated by the patient, but continuous drainage into an appropriate bag, which may be strapped to the patient's thigh, is now usual. When the catheter has to be removed to be changed, it can be left out for several hours, during which time observations are made on the patient's ability to hold urine, which can be tested by abdominal straining or suprapubic manual pressure. In this way, and by estimations of residual urine, any evidence of recovery in the activity of the bladder can be assessed.

The greatest care must be taken that the catheter and all the vessels and apparatus employed are sterile, and the operator must be scrupulous in observing aseptic technique. If the urinary tract becomes infected, the organisms must be cultured and the appropriate chemotherapeutic or antibiotic agent is then used.

Cystoscopy and radiography of the urinary tract, including pyelography, may be necessary to exclude hydronephrosis and renal or vesical calculus; and estimation of renal function may also be needed.

The object to be aimed at is an automatic bladder voiding sterile urine. Neither the grossly atonic bladder nor an organ much contracted owing to infection will become automatic. Division of the internal sphincter (bladder-neck resection) is often carried out when the detrusor muscle is reflexly active but the sphincter does not relax (Thompson 1945). Various prostheses utilizing indwelling electrodes have been used in an attempt to stimulate a denervated bladder electrically or alternatively to cause contraction of the external sphincter in order to overcome incontinence, but none has yet entered into common use (see Boyarsky 1967). For further details of the care of the paralysed bladder see Johnson and Spalding (1974), Pearman and England (1976), Guttmann (1976), and Davidson and Lenman (1981).

Care of the rectum

The constipation which is often troublesome at first should be treated by giving an aperient and/or lubricant at night, two or three times a week, and by clearing the rectum the next day with a suppository, or more often an enema. In paraplegia the bowel empties itself very slowly after an enema and 'leaking' may occur for an hour or more, a point which is important to bear in mind in order to avoid the bed becoming wet and soiled. Often regular manual evacuation of faeces by the patient himself or by another family member (rubber gloves must be supplied to prevent paronychia and other skin sepsis on the hands) is useful.

Muscular spasms and spasticity

Involuntary spasms of the lower limbs are a troublesome and intractable symptom in many cases of paraplegia. Spasmodic extension may occur when extensor tone predominates. Spasmodic flexion, encountered in paraplegia-in-flexion, is much commoner. Flexor movements are excited reflexly by moving contact of the lower limbs with the bed-clothes, a slight movement being sufficient in many cases to excite a violent flexor spasm. As far as possible, contact of the limbs with the bed-clothes should therefore be reduced. The spasms may be diminished in frequency and severity by the use of relaxant drugs, of which the best are diazepam 5 mg three or four times a day, and baclofen 5 mg three times daily increasing by 5 mg steps every three or four days up to not more than 75 mg daily depending upon tolerance. Dantrolene, 25–50 mg twice daily, increasing up to not more than 800 mg daily, is helpful in some cases; mephenesin carbamate 1–3 g three to five times a day is generally less effective (Calne 1980).

In patients with no hope of recovery, flexor spasms have been treated by the intrathecal injection of alcohol or preferably of phenol in glycerin, or by anterior rhizotomy. In selected cases of partial paraplegia, injection of 1 ml of xylocaine, followed by 1–2 ml of 45 per cent alcohol into the motor points of selected muscles (e.g. hamstrings), after localization of the motor point or motor end-plate zone by electrical stimulation on the skin, is very helpful (Tardieu, Hariga, Tardieu, Gagnard, and Velin 1964). Anterior rhizotomy has the disadvantage of leading to muscular wasting and of increasing the risk of pressure-sores. In irrecoverable cases division of the obturator nerves and appropriate tenotomies may be helpful. Regular mechanical traction applied to the flexed limbs, combined with appropriate tenotomies were shown to be valuable by Platt, Russell, and Willison (1958). The use of intrathecal injections was described by Nathan (1959, 1965), by Kelly and Gautier-Smith (1959), and by Calne (1980).

Physiotherapy and compensatory training

There are few paraplegic patients who will not be able to get about in a wheelchair, and many more than was once thought possible can be taught to walk. Physiotherapy therefore aims at obtaining the maximum development of all those muscles in which voluntary power remains, and preventing flexor contractures of the lower limbs. Exercises are carried out at first with the help of slings as in the Guthrie-Smith apparatus, special attention being paid to the trunk muscles. Passive movements are carried out in the lower limbs once or twice daily. As soon as possible the patient is allowed to sit up in a wheel-chair, the need for frequent changes of posture still being borne in mind. In suitable cases walking is later attempted, and may be achieved even when no voluntary power remains in the lower limbs apart from hip flexion or 'rocking' movements of the pelvis. Appropriate walking instruments or full-length calipers will be necessary, locking at the knee and not coming high enough to exert pressure on the buttocks. A toe-raising spring can be incorporated. When trunk muscles are paralysed a spinal brace may be necessary. The patient must at first be supported by parallel bars; later he uses elbow-crutches. When the lower limbs are completely paralysed, the pelvis must be rotated and tilted by the abdominal muscles; first one leg, and then the other is swung forward in this way. It may be possible for a patient to learn to 'walk' on crutches by swinging his trunk using the pectoralis, latissimus dorsi, serratus anterior, and trapezius muscles if these are overdeveloped and if he has enough strength in his fingers to grasp the crutches, and can move them forward with his pectorals and deltoids. (For details see Guttmann 1973, 1976; Vinken *et al.* 1976.)

Other measures

In patients with complete transverse-cord lesions, temperature regulation is impaired due to inability to shiver below the level of the lesion as well as impairment of heat-loss mechanisms, so that hypothermia and hyperpyrexia are occasional complications which must be borne in mind (Johnson 1971). Blood-pressure control may also be defective with orthostatic hypotension when the lesion is in the cervical region, but substantial vascular adaptation eventually occurs in most chronic paraplegics (Johnson, Park, and Frankel 1971).

In cases of tetraplegia due to high cervical-cord lesions most deaths occur within the first three months; the prognosis has improved greatly with modern methods of care in patients surviving beyond that period. The use of electronic devices which enable the patient to control alarm systems and other electrical equipment with the aid of a mouthpiece, by eye movement, or by a simple manual switch ('POSSUM' or patient-operated selector mechanisms) has been a major advance in improving the level of independence and quality of life (Silver and Gibbon 1968).

Psychotherapy

Not the least important part of the physician's task is to help the patient to adjust himself to a new mode of life—a life not of inactivity but of different activities. At first he will need to be convinced that an active and useful life is still possible. Occupational therapy should be begun early: games such as archery and wheelchair football play an important part. In most cases the patient must be trained for a new occupation, and the co-operation of an employer sought. Family adjustments have also to be made. Coitus is not always impossible. An erection may be stimulated by handling the penis and, with the co-operation of an instructed wife, success may be achieved. Even when intercourse is impossible, in the case of a wife who is anxious to have a child, ejaculation may follow the intrathecal injection of small doses of neostigmine, following which artificial insemination may be possible (Guttmann 1973). Electroejaculation induced by stimulation with sinusoidal alternating current at 15 to 100 Hz via rigid intra-rectal electrodes is even more successful (Brindley 1981).

Injuries of the spinal cord

Aetiology

The spinal cord may be injured directly by penetrating wounds, for example, stabs or gun-shot wounds, when it may be penetrated by a missile or by fragments of bone. More often in civil life it suffers indirectly as a result of injuries of the vertebral column, either fractures, dislocations, or fracture-dislocations (see Vinken *et al.* 1976). The commonest sites of spinal injury in civil life are the lower cervical region and the thoracolumbar junction. The

upper cervical region suffers next in frequency (Jefferson 1928; Cloward 1980). The epidemiology of spinal-cord injury was fully reviewed by Kurtzke (1975). Though the spinal column may be injured as the result of a blow leading to fracture at the site of impact, more often it is injured by transmitted violence. Forcible extension of the neck may fracture the odontoid or contuse the cervical cord, but most spinal injuries are the result of forcible flexion. A blow on the head which does not cause a serious head injury may, by forcibly flexing the cervical spine, cause dislocation in the lower cervical region or acute central herniation of an intervertebral disc. Pre-existing cervical spondylosis with or without congenital narrowing of the cervical canal (Kessler 1975) greatly increases the risk of damage to the spinal cord by injuries which cause forcible neck extension. A blow on the forehead caused by diving into excessively shallow water, or a 'whiplash' injury such as may occur in a driver or passenger in a motor vehicle which is run into from behind when stationary, so that the head jerks forward and then backwards, are common causes of sudden hyperextension of the neck. Blows upon the shoulders, caused by heavy objects falling from a height, result in forcible flexion of the lower spine, which may yield at the thoracolumbar junction. This type of injury (as in a fall of stone in a mine) is produced chiefly by industrial accidents. Fracture-dislocation may also result from falls from a height on to the feet or buttocks. Lifting a heavy weight, falls, and strains may all cause prolapse of an intervertebral disc.

The spinal cord may be injured in the infant during birth as a result of violent traction. Such injuries may arise in three ways. Traction on the head may cause dislocation of the upper cervical spine, which is usually immediately fatal. Traction separating the head and shoulders, by exerting tension on the brachial plexus and cervical spinal roots, may injure the spinal cord while also producing a brachial plexus palsy. And in a breech presentation, violent traction may cause fracture-dislocation in the thoracic or lumbar regions.

Spontaneous fracture-dislocation of the spine may also occur when the vertebrae are diseased, as in tuberculous caries or in primary or secondary neoplasia of the vertebral column. The blast of a bomb or shell explosion may injure the spinal cord without damaging the spine.

A less common cause of spinal-cord injury is decompression sickness (Caisson disease or 'the bends'). Complete or partial paraplegia has been attributed in such cases to arterial infarction secondary to nitrogen-bubble emboli, but experimental studies in animals (Hallenbeck, Bore, and Elliott 1975; Hallenbeck 1976) indicate that venous infarction due to obstruction to cord venous drainage into the epidural vertebral venous system may be a more common mechanism.

Pathology

'*Concussion* of the spinal cord' is a term which has been employed when the cord is injured by transmitted violence without fracture or dislocation of the vertebral column. However, as in head injury (p. 226), it is now doubtful as to whether there is any genuine pathological distinction between concussion and *contusion*, defined as bruising of the cord without rupture of the pia mater, resulting from sudden displacement or compression. The contused cord is swollen and may show small haemorrhages. Microscopically, besides oedema and punctate haemorrhage there is swelling of axis cylinders and disintegration of their myelin sheaths. In severe cases both completely disappear and the cord may be markedly softened. Ascending and descending degeneration of the long tracts follows the focal lesion. The structural, vascular, physiological, and biochemical changes which follow experimental cord contusion were reviewed by Dohrmann (1972). In man acute contusion, especially in the cervical region, is often followed by progressive haemorrhagic necrosis or softening which is at a maximum in the centre of the cord; Nelson, Gertz, Rennels, Ducker, and Blaumanis (1977) postulate that this may result from vascular damage with the formation of mural thrombi in the affected vessels and with subsequent embolization of the central microvasculature of the cord. *Laceration* implies an injury of greater severity than contusion, with rupture of the pia mater and partial or complete transection of the cord. Barnett, Botterell, Jousse, and Wynn-Jones (1966) and Nurick, Russell, and Deck (1970) showed that a progressive myelopathy due to ascending cavitation of the cord above the level of the lesion may develop in some cases of traumatic paraplegia some years after the injury. The pathogenesis of this cystic degeneration or traumatic syringomyelia was reviewed by Barnett, Foster, and Hudgson (1973). When a wound penetrates the dura mater, meningitis is liable to occur as a complication of spinal injury. Rupture of the pia in such cases increases the risk of pyogenic myelitis. Injuries of the vertebral column may also damage spinal roots and nerves as they pass through the intervertebral foramina.

Symptoms and signs

The clinical manifestations of spinal injury depend upon the severity and situation of the lesion. Injury to the cord does not always follow damage to the vertebral column; thus, cervical dislocation without cord injury is not rare. An injury to the cord in the upper cervical region (above C4) is usually rapidly, if not immediately, fatal, as it paralyses both the diaphragm and the intercostal muscles but some such cases of traumatic tetraplegia now survive with assisted respiration (Silver and Gibbon 1968).

Complete interruption of the spinal cord leads immediately to flaccid paralysis with loss of all sensation and most reflex activity below the site of the lesion, with paralysis of the bladder and rectum. Muscular paralysis and sensory loss are irrecoverable, but, as the stage of spinal shock passes off after from one to four weeks, reflex activity develops in the divided portion of the cord and the patient develops paraplegia-in-flexion (see p. 391). For the motor symptoms of spinal-cord transection at different levels, see pages 406–7.

Lesions of the cord less severe than complete transection, such as contusion, may give an equally severe immediate disturbance of function, or symptoms may increase in severity for several days *pari passu* with the development of oedema or central softening in the cord. As oedema lessens or central softening reaches its fullest extent and as spinal shock passes off, there is often some improvement but the extent of the patient's ultimate motor or sensory disability is usually clear within about four weeks. If the injury is limited to one-half of the cord, a partial or complete Brown–Séquard syndrome may develop (see p. 45).

Injuries of the cauda equina. Fracture-dislocation of the spine below the first lumbar vertebra damages only the nerves of the cauda equina. In civil life unilateral injuries here are rare, though the severity and extent of the nerve damage may differ on the two sides. Paralysis of the bladder, rectum, and sexual functions follow immediately. The motor, sensory, and reflex disturbances are similar to those more gradually produced by slow compression of the cauda equina and are described on page 407.

Diagnosis

The diagnosis is usually obvious, the only question being the nature and extent of the cord injury. Myelography is rarely necessary in such cases but CT scanning may be helpful in indicating the extent of cord damage. Selective arteriography may help to exclude gross vascular change (Gargour, Wener, and Di Chiro 1972).

Prognosis

In high cervical-cord lesions the immediate risk is that of respiratory paralysis; assisted respiration, when needed, is invariably indicated as one cannot be certain at the outset as to how much recovery will subsequently take place. With modern methods of management, complications such as pneumonia, urinary and cutaneous infection, hypotension, and hypothermia, which were often fatal in the past, are no longer the hazards they once were. It is now possible for a patient with a completely divided cord to retain good general health indefinitely under careful supervision. When the cord has been incompletely divided, the prognosis is better, but, in the absence of infections of the bladder and skin, the limit of functional improvement can generally be predicted when the shock has passed off, certainly in two or three months after the injury. But even when it is clear that no further improvement in the limbs and trunk below the level of the lesion can be expected, remarkable degrees of functional improvement may yet be achieved through training and adaptation in an appropriate spinal injuries centre. After spinal contusion without actual division of the cord substantial recovery often follows over many months, though some residual disability is usual. The prognosis of cauda-equina injuries is often better than that of injuries of the cord itself, since the nerves of the cauda, if not divided, are capable of regeneration.

Treatment

Evidence derived from experiments upon animals suggests that dexamethasone 5 mg four times daily, if begun within an hour of injury, may reduce the extent of traumatic damage to the spinal cord; dimethyl sulphoxide is also of some value in animals (de la Torre, Johnson, Goode, and Mullan 1975). Recent work suggesting that endorphins are involved in the pathophysiology of spinal-cord injury has suggested that opiate antagonists such as naloxone might also be of benefit in spinal trauma in human subjects (Faden, Jacobs, Mougey, and Holday 1981).

The scope of surgery in the treatment of injuries of the spinal cord has been much discussed. Most surgeons now recommend immediate immobilization, combined, where appropriate, with traction in order to reduce a fracture-dislocation, and immediate transfer to a specialized spinal injuries unit. By contrast, Cloward (1980) is one of that minority of surgeons who recommends, especially in tetraplegia, immediate anterior decompression of injured cord and spinal fusion. However, in most cases the maximal injury has been produced at the time of the accident and the condition of the cord is both non-progressive and irreparable. Moreover, for several weeks after the injury, spinal shock may make it impossible to determine whether division of the cord is complete. When there is reason to believe that it has been completely divided, surgery cannot accomplish anything, and open operation may be contra-indicated by the presence of local sepsis or other complications. On the other hand, when there is radiographic evidence of gross bony deformity, massive disc protrusion, or the presence of a foreign body in the spinal canal, and clinical examination indicates that the cord has not been completely divided, and when in such cases recovery of function has begun but has become arrested, surgical intervention offers the hope of relieving compression which could be retarding recovery. In such cases an exploratory laminectomy may be indicated, and may also be needed to deal with severe persistent root pains, due to compression of dorsal roots or spinal nerves. The most important immediate single measure is immobilization on a flat bed, sometimes with continuous traction, but manipulation is rarely if ever indicated because of the risk of increasing damage to the cord. In cases of cauda-equina injury, the most that can be hoped for from operation is the relief of pressure which may be retarding regeneration of the nerves; suture of divided spinal nerves is rarely, if ever, possible. General management is described on page 394.

References

Barnett, H. J. M., Botterell, E. H., Jousse, A. T., and Wynn-Jones, M. (1966). Progressive myelopathy as a sequel to traumatic paraplegia. *Brain* **89**, 159.

—— Foster, J. B., and Hudgson, P. (1973). *Syringomyelia*. (Major Problems in Neurology Series ed. J. N. Walton). Saunders, London.

Bedford, P. D., Cosin, L. Z., and McCarthy, T. F. (1961). Bedsores. *Lancet* ii, 76.

Boyarsky, S. (1967). *The neurogenic bladder*. Williams and Wilkins, Baltimore.

Brindley, G. S. (1981). Electroejaculation: its technique, neurological implications and uses. *J. Neurol. Neurourg. Psychiat.* **44**, 9.

Byers, R. K. (1930). Late effects of obstetrical injuries at various levels of the nervous system. *New Engl. J. Med.* **203**, 507.

Calne, D. B. (1980). *Therapeutics in neurology*, 2nd edn. Blackwell, Oxford.

Cloward, R. B. (1980). Acute cervical spine injuries. *CIBA Clinical Symposia* **32**, 1.

Davidson, D. L. W. and Lenman, J. A. R. (1981). *Neurological therapeutics*. Pitman, London.

Deaver, G. G. and Brown, M. E. (1945). The challenge of crutches. *Arch. phys. Med.* **26**, 397, 515, 573, 747.

de la Torre, J. C., Johnson, C. M., Goode, D. J., and Mullan, S. (1975). Pharmacologic treatment and evaluation of permanent experimental spinal cord trauma. *Neurology, Minneapolis* **25**, 508.

Dohrmann, G. J. (1972). Experimental spinal cord trauma. *Arch. Neurol., Chicago* **27**, 468.

Elson, R. A. (1965). Anatomical aspects of pressure sores and their treatment. *Lancet* i, 884.

Faden, A. I., Jacobs, T. P., Mougey, E., and Holaday, J. W. (1981). Endorphins in experimental spinal injury: therapeutic effect of naloxone. *Ann. Neurol.* **10**, 326.

Ford, F. R. (1925). Breech delivery in its possible relations to injury of the spinal cord. *Arch. Neurol. Psychiat. Chicago* **14**, 742.

Gargour, G. W., Wener, L., and di Chiro, G. (1972). Selective arteriography of the spinal cord in post-traumatic paraplegia, *Neurology, Minneapolis* **22**, 131.

Guttmann, L. (1976). *Spinal cord injuries*, 2nd edn. Blackwell, Oxford.

Hallenbeck, J. M. (1976). Cinephotomicrography of dog spinal vessels during cord-damaging decompression sickness. *Neurology, Minneapolis* **26**, 190.

——, Bove, A. E., and Elliott, D. H. (1975). Mechanisms underlying spinal cord damage in decompression sickness. *Neurology, Minneapolis* **25**, 308.

Hamm, F. C. (1945). War wounds of the spinal cord. *J. Am. med. Ass.* **129**, 158.

Jefferson, G. (1927–8). Discussion on spinal injuries. *Proc. R. Soc. Med.* **21**, 625.

Joelson, J. J. (1945). War wounds of the spinal cord. *J. Am. med. Ass.* **129**, 157.

Johnson, R. H. (1971). Temperature regulation in paraplegia. *Paraplegia* **9**, 137.

——, Park, D., and Frankel, H. L. (1971). Orthostatic hypotension and the renin–angiotensin system in paraplegia. *Paraplegia* **9**, 146.

—— and Spalding, J. M. K. (1974). *Disorders of the autonomic nervous sytem*. Blackwell, Oxford.

Kao, C. C., Bunge, R., and Reier, P. J. (Eds.) (1982). *Spinal cord reconstruction*. Raven Press, New York.

Kelly, R. E. and Gautier Smith, P. C. (1959). Intrathecal phenol in the treatment of reflex spasms and spasticity. *Lancet* ii, 1102.

Kessler, J. T. (1975). Congenital narrowing of the cervical spinal canal. *J. Neurol. Neurosurg. Psychiat.* **38**, 1218.

Kurtzke, J. F. (1975). Epidemiology of spinal cord injury. *Exp. Neurol.* **48**, 163.

Lowman, E. W. (1947). Rehabilitation of the paraplegic patient. *Arch. Neurol. Psychiat., Chicago* **58**, 610.

Nathan, P. W. (1959). Intrathecal phenol to relieve spasticity in paraplegia. *Lancet* ii, 1099.

—— (1965). Chemical rhizotomy for relief of spasticity in ambulant patients. *Br. med. J.* **1**, 1096.

Nelson, E., Gertz, S. D., Rennels, M. L., Ducker, T. B., and Blaumanis, O. R. (1977). Spinal cord injury: the role of vasular damage in the pathogenesis of central hemorrhagic necrosis. *Arch. Neurol., Chicago* **34**, 332.

Nurick, S., Russell, J. A., and Deck, M. J. F. (1970). Cystic degeneration of the spinal cord following spinal cord injury. *Brain* **93**, 211.

Pearman, J. W. and England, E. J. (1976). The urinary tract. In *Handbook of clinical neurology* (ed. P. J. Vinken, G. W. Bruyn, and R. Braakman) Vol. 26, p. 409. North-Holland, Amsterdam.

Petkoff, B. P. (1945). War wounds of the spinal cord. *J. Am. med. Ass.* **129**, 154.

Platt, G., Russell, W. R., and Willison, R. G. (1958). Flexion spasms and contractures in spinal-cord disease. *Lancet* i, 757.

Silver, J. R. and Gibbon, N. O. K. (1968). Prognosis in tetraplegia. *Br. med. J.* **4**, 79.

Tardieu, G., Hariga, J., Tardieu, C., Gagnard, L., and Velin, J. (1964). Traitement de la spasticité par infiltration d'alcool dilué au point moteur ou par injection épidurale. *Rev. neurol.* **119**, 563.

Thompson, G. S. (1945). Restoration of function by transurethral operation. *Nav. med. Bull. Washington* **45**, 207.

Vinken, P. J., Bruyn, G. W., and Braakman, R. (Eds.) (1976). *Handbook of clinical neurology*, Vols 25 and 26. North-Holland, Amsterdam.

Haematomyelia and acute central cervical-cord injury

Definition. The term 'haematomyelia' implies bleeding within the spinal-cord substance. Haemorrhages occur in many pathological states. Petechial haemorrhages are found in acute inflammatory conditions, such as poliomyelitis, in toxic or hypersensitivity states, in blood diseases, especially those accompanied by purpura, and in asphyxia or other anoxic states. Haemorrhages also occur as a result of injury, in laceration of the cord following fracture-dislocation of the spine and penetration of the spinal canal by missiles. The term 'haematomyelia', however, is often reserved for a focal extravasation of blood developing within the spinal cord in the absence of any of these conditions.

Aetiology

Haematomyelia as just defined may develop without any obvious precipitating factor. Often, however, it follows an event which may have exposed the spinal cord to transmitted violence, though this often seems slight in proportion to the severity of the resulting symptoms. Blows on the spine and falls are sometimes held responsible. There is evidence that a congenital abnormality, such as an intramedullary telangiectasis or small angioma, may be one causal factor, and spontaneous haemorrhage into a syringomyelic cavity may occur. The condition has been described as the result of an intramedullary metastasis from a renal carcinoma (Kawakami and Mair 1973). Haematomyelia usually occurs in early adult life, and males are more often affected than females. It is now evident that, particularly in cases attributable to trauma, a syndrome similar to that produced by haematomyelia is more often due to central softening (haemorrhagic necrosis) within the spinal cord rather than simple haemorrhage, due to contusion of the cord such as may occur particularly in the cervical region in patients suffering from previously symptomless cervical spondylosis, often after acute flexion or hyperextension of the neck (Schneider, Thompson, and Bebin 1958; Cook 1959; Toglia 1976).

Pathology

The cervical enlargement is the commonest site of haemorrhage or central softening. Bleeding involves primarily the central grey matter and spreads upwards and downwards, assuming a round or oval form, according to its longitudinal extent. It may extend into the white matter, but usually this suffers from compression rather than from direct invasion by the haemorrhage. In the later stages the haemorrhage or softened area becomes brown and may finally be represented by a cystic cavity containing yellow fluid. Surrounding parts of the cord are invaded by activated microglial cells with subsequent gliosis. The distribution of central softening without haemorrhage is similar. There is destruction of ganglion cells of both the anterior and posterior horns of grey matter at the site of the lesion, and some degree of ascending and descending degeneration is usually found in long tracts of the white matter (Hughes 1978).

Symptoms and signs

The onset of symptoms in haematomyelia is usually rapid with sudden impairment of cord function, followed later by a progressive increase in symptoms. Sometimes the onset is more gradual, and the symptoms increase in severity over several days. In cases of central softening after acute flexion or hyperextension injuries to the neck, neurological disability is usually maximal immediately after the injury and progressive improvement occurs during the subsequent weeks or months (Symonds 1953). Since the cervical enlargement is the commonest site of haemorrhage, manifestations of a lesion in this situation will alone be described in detail. In some cases the patient complains at the onset of severe pain in the neck radiating down one or both upper limbs. Sometimes this pain (hyperpathia) is persistent (Hopkins and Rudge 1973). In other cases pain is absent, but there may be paraesthesiae, such as numbness and tingling. Muscular weakness develops rapidly. It is often marked in the upper limbs, one of which suffers more than the other. In the upper limbs it is due to destruction or compression of the anterior horn cells and hence may be associated later with muscular atrophy but immediately with diminution or loss of the tendon reflexes. It may be limited to the muscles innervated by the upper segments, cervical 5 and 6, or by the lower segments, cervical 8 and thoracic 1, of the cervical enlargement. Below the level of the lesion the motor symptoms are those of spastic paralysis which may be slight or severe in the lower limbs and may affect the two sides unequally. Sudden and severe tetraparesis after relatively minor flexion or extension of the neck, as in a so-called 'whiplash' injury, followed by rapid improvement, is not uncommon in the central cervical syndrome in cases of spondylosis with a narrow cervical canal.

The most prominent sensory changes are due to destruction of sensory fibres in the grey matter of the cord at the level of the lesion. When this extends into the posterior horns and destroys ganglion cells, all forms of sensibility will be impaired or lost over the whole or part of the upper limbs. When destruction is limited to the region of the anterior white commissure there is no loss of appreciation of light touch, posture, or passive movement, but analgesia and thermo-anaesthesia occur over several segmental cutaneous areas below the upper level of the haemorrhage, which interrupts the fibres subserving these forms of sensibility at their decussation. The picture is thus similar to that of syringomyelia and a 'cape-like' distribution of the dissociated anaesthesia is common. Often, too, there is also some impairment of appreciation of pain, heat, and cold, over the trunk or lower limbs on one or both sides, owing to compression of the spinothalamic tract. Postural sensibility may be impaired in the lower limbs, but not as a rule severely, owing to compression of the posterior columns. Some patients develop concomitant postural giddiness of vestibular origin (Toglia 1976).

The tendon reflexes effected by muscles which are the site of atrophic paralysis are diminished or lost. Those of the lower limbs are usually exaggerated. The abdominal reflexes are diminished or lost and the plantar reflexes are extensor when the corticospinal tracts are damaged. Sphincter disturbances are usual in the acute stage. Dorsal and lumbar haematomyelia are characterized by the rapid development of more or less complete paraplegia and sensory loss below the level of the lesion. Retention of urine is common.

The CSF may be normal or may show an increase in its protein content, with or without xanthochromia.

Diagnosis

Apart from traumatic lesions, there are few conditions in which a spinal-cord lesion develops so rapidly as in haematomyelia. The onset of transverse myelitis is usually less rapid, and it is often preceded by pains in the back. It is often associated with inflammatory changes in the CSF and when, as in a few cases, it is syphilitic, the serological reactions in the fluid and usually also in the blood are positive. Anterior poliomyelitis can be differentiated from haematomyelia by its febrile onset, by the wide but often asymmetrical distribution of the atrophic paralysis, by the absence of sensory loss and of corticospinal dysfunction, and by a pleocytosis in the CSF. Haemorrhage into a syringomyelic cavity constitutes a form of haematomyelia which it is important to recognize. However, this is a rare complication and haematomyelia is generally distinguishable from syringomyelia by virtue of its acute onset. The pre-existence of syringomyelia may be suggested by a history of painless injuries or trophic lesions of the fingers. Primary and secondary intramedullary tumours (see below) usually develop more insidiously. The very rare condition of intramedullary abscess of the spinal cord can give a clinical picture very similar to that of haematomyelia but there is usually fever and leucocytosis and evidence of a focus of pyogenic infection elsewhere. The acute central cervical-cord syndrome is usually recognized if the significance of the injury, however minor, is appreciated, especially if the radiographs of the cervical spine show spondylosis and a narrow canal.

Prognosis

The mortality is low, and most sufferers from haematomyelia survive. Death may rarely occur from upward extension of the haemorrhage giving paralysis of the diaphragm, through involvement of the spinal origin of the phrenic nerves, or from complications of paraplegia. In patients who survive, considerable improvement may be expected and is often particularly striking in traumatic cases with presumed central-cord softening in whom it may be concluded that much of the initial disability was due to a transient and reversible disturbance of function. Atrophic paralysis and sensory loss due to destruction of grey matter are permanent, but even these signs diminish in extent, as ganglion cells and fibres which have been compressed but not completely destroyed recover. Steady improvement may be expected in the power of the lower limbs and in many cases this returns to normal, even though exaggeration of tendon reflexes and extensor plantar responses may persist. When haemorrhage has occurred into a syringomyelitic cavity, much less improvement can be expected and the prognosis is that of syringomyelia.

Treatment

Complete rest is essential at first with immobilization of the cervical spine; a collar may be helpful later. When paraplegia is present this will require appropriate treatment. One or at the most two weeks after the onset, active rehabilitation can safely be started.

References

Benda, C. E. (1929). Zur Klinik der traumatischen Hämatomyelie. Zugleich ein Beitrag zur Differentialdiagnose zwischen Tumor Spinalis und Blutung *Nervenarzt.* **1**, 28.

Chevallier, P. and Desoile, H. (1930). L'hématomyélie des jeunes sujets (importance des lésions vasculaires herédo-syphilitiques). *Rev. Médecine* **47**, 486.

Cook, J. B. (1959). The relationship of spinal cord damage to cervical spinal injury. *Proc. R. Soc. Med.* **52**, 799.

Hopkins, A. and Rudge, P. (1973). Hyperpathia in the central cervical cord syndrome. *J. Neurol. Neurosurg. Psychiat.* **36**, 637.

Hughes, J. J. (1978). *Pathology of the spinal cord*, 2nd edn. Lloyd-Luke, London.

Kawakami, Y. and Mair, W. G. P. (1973). Haematomyelia due to secondary renal carcinoma. *Acta Neuropath., Berlin* **26**, 85.

Richardson, J. C. (1938). Spontaneous haematomyelia: a short review and a report of cases illustrating intramedullary angioma and syphilis of the spinal cord as possible causes. *Brain* **61**, 17.

Schneider, R. C., Thompson, J. M. and Bebin, J. (1958). The syndrome of acute central cervical spine cord injury. *J. Neurol. Neurosurg. Psychiat.* **21**, 216.

Symonds, C. P. (1953). The interrelation of trauma and cervical spondylosis in compression of the cervical cord. *Lancet* **i**, 451.

Toglia, J. U. (1976). Acute flexion–extension injury of the neck. Electronystagmographic study of 309 patients. *Neurology, Minneapolis* **26**, 808.

Compression of the spinal cord

Aetiology and pathology

Compression of the spinal cord may be due to:

Disease of the vertebral column. Among the conditions leading to spinal compression are secondary carcinoma and cervical spondylosis with protrusion of intervertebral discs (Fig. 14.1, p. 404). Less frequent causes include primary neoplasms arising from vertebrae, such as sarcoma, myeloma, osteoma, haemangioma, tuberculous and other forms of osteitis, such as staphylococcal osteitis, syphilitic osteitis, and osteitis deformans of Paget. Rarely, achondroplasia and severe kyphoscoliosis due to juvenile osteochondritis may have the same effect. The cord may occasionally be compressed by prolapse of an intervertebral disc elsewhere than the neck (e.g. in the dorsal region) or as a result of erosion of vertebrae from without by sarcoma, or by aneursym of the aorta. Compression due to trauma is described on page 396. High cervical-cord compression may result from bony or other anomalies of the craniovertebral junction (p. 607).

Other causes of compression. These include extradural abscess due either to metastatic infection or vertebral osteitis, arachnoiditis due to syphilis, tuberculosis, sarcoidosis or other granulomatous processes, infiltration of the meninges with reticulosis or leukaemic deposits, arachnoidal cysts, parasitic cysts, such as the hydatid and cysticercus, and extramedullary and intramedullary spinal tumours. Spinal subdural haematoma due to trauma or occurring after lumbar puncture in cases of thrombocytopenia is a rare cause (Edelson, Chernik, and Posner 1974). Spontaneous epidural haematoma, usually occurring in the dorsal region (Packer and Cummins 1978; Hernandez, Vinuela, and Feasby 1982) is also rare but is a surgical emergency; sometimes the bleeding is due to a vascular malformation and sometimes no cause is ever discovered. Cord compression is also a rare complication of thalassaemia, resulting from massive extension of bone marrow from vertebral bodies into the epidural space (*The Lancet* 1982).

Vertebral disease

1. *Separation of the odontoid process* of the axis, occurring either as a congenital abnormality or as the result of trauma or rheumatoid arthritis may, by permitting abnormal movement of the atlas on the axis, lead in time, sometimes after many years, to a delayed myelopathy resulting from compression of the spinal cord (Greenberg 1968; Stevens, Cartlidge, Appleby, Hall, and Shaw 1971). It is now recognized that whereas atlanto-axial dislocation is the commonest lesion in *rheumatoid cervical myelopathy*, some patients have subaxial subluxation alone, others subluxation in addition between other cervical vertebrae (Hughes 1977; Marks and Sharp 1981; McConkey 1982). The treatment now preferred is occipito-cervical fusion; operative decompression of the upper cervical cord in such cases is often complicated by haematomyelia (Dastur 1979).

2. *Intervertebral disc protrusion* is commonest in the cervical region. An acute central prolapse of a disc may give symptoms and signs of subacute cord compression and pain may not be prominent, whereas a lateral protusion will give pain in the arm due to root compression (brachial neuralgia). Chronic protrusions are the result of disc degeneration: they may be single or multiple, and are usually encountered during or after middle age. Such a slow, progressive degenerative process (*cervical spondylosis*) gives the condition of so-called spondylotic myelopathy. Its effect upon the spinal cord is complex: in addition to directly compressing it, the protruding discs may interfere with its blood supply; while, owing to tethering of the cord by the ligamenta denticulata and of the spinal roots by narrowing of the intervertebral foramina, ordinary neck movements may produce cumulative trauma. The result is a condition of patchy degeneration–cervical myelopathy (Wilkinson 1973).

3. *Neoplasms of the vertebral column.* Secondary carcinoma is the commonest vertebral neoplasm. It is rare before the age of 35. The primary growth is more often situated within the lung, breast, thyroid, or prostate, less frequently in the uterus, stomach, kidney, or elsewhere (Stark, Henson, and Evans 1982). Although the vertebral metastasis may be blood-borne, the spine is sometimes involved at the same segmental level as the primary growth, which in such cases may reach it via the perineural lymphatics. The carcinomatous deposits erode the spongy portions of the vertebral bodies, which finally collapse. The spinal cord may be compressed as a result of the spinal deformity or by an extradural extension of the growth. Usually the spinal roots are compressed earlier than the cord itself so that root and back pain may be present for some time before vertebral collapse gives acute cord compression.

Sarcoma can arise from a vertebra or invade the spinal column from neighbouring tissues. Cavernous haemangioma is a rare vertebral tumour but can cause spinal-cord or root compression and the radiological changes (accentuated vertical striation or a honeycomb pattern) are often, but not invariably, distinctive (McAllister 1975). Myeloma usually arises simultaneously in several vertebral bodies and often also in other bones, especially the ribs, but solitary myelomas of the spine giving cord compression are not uncommon (Clarke 1956). Osteomas are rare tumours which usually arise from the posterior part of a vertebral body and hence compress the cord anteriorly. So-called chondromas are usually intervertebral disc protrusions associated with spondylosis. Deposits of reticulosis and leukaemic metastases usually infiltrate the dura mater extensively on its outer surface but may occasionally invade the cord itself. In such cases pain and symptoms and signs of cord and root compression may occur without any abnormality on plain radiographs and a similar syndrome may result from extradural metastases of carcinoma, but myelography or CT scanning will usually demonstrate the extradural deposits with narrowing of the spinal canal (Gilbert, Kim, and Posner 1978).

4. *Tuberculous spinal osteitis* usually occurs in children and young adults but no age is exempt. It is now much less common in developed countries than it was 40 or 50 years ago as a result of pasteurization of milk, as most cases of skeletal tuberculosis were due to the bovine bacillus. However, it commonly results from the human bacillus in Asian, African, and South American countries and is still seen from time to time in Asian and West African immigrants to the United Kingdom, less often in the native-born. In northern Tanzania, Scrimgeour (1981) found that of 100 cases of non-traumatic paraplegia, 54 were due to tuberculosis, 13 to neoplasia, and six to schistosomiasis. The infective process generally begins in a vertebral body, and spreads to adjacent bodies leading to their collapse and an angular deformity of the spine. Typically the intervertebral discs are spared. It is rare for the deformity as such to be a major factor in compressing the cord, which is more often affected by either an extradural tuberculous abscess or tuberculous meningomyelitis (Freilich and Swash 1979). In addition to actual cord compression which may, however, be absent, interference with the vascular supply of subjacent segments, either by compression of radicular arteries or endarteritis, is an important factor in producing paraplegia. The dorsal cord is commonly affected.

5. *Syphilitic spinal osteitis* is now a very rare cause of spinal compression and produces effects similar to those of tuberculous caries. In Paget's *osteitis deformans*, softening and collapse of vertebrae occur without abscess formation. Slowly progressive

spastic weakness of the lower limbs due to spinal-cord compression may also occur in some *achondroplasic dwarfs* and in patients with severe *kyphoscoliosis* and resultant acute angulation of the vertebral column.

6. *Spinal extradural* or *epidural abscess* is due as a rule to staphylococcal infection, arising either through blood-borne invasion of the extradural space by the infecting organism or, more commonly, from vertebral osteomyelitis. In the early stages the symptoms are those of pain in the back and/or root pains with fever, leucocytosis, and spinal tenderness. If untreated, sensorimotor symptoms in the limbs and sphincter disturbance may herald irreversible paraplegia due to cord compression and interference with its blood supply. Surgical exploration and decompression of the spinal cord and treatment with the appropriate antibiotics must be carried out before this stage; the condition is a neurosurgical emergency. Spinal subdural abscess has also been described (Hirson 1965). Very rarely an intramedullary spinal abscess of metastatic origin develops and gives a clinical picture like that of intramedullary tumour of acute onset with pyrexia (see p. 421).

Spinal tumour

Spinal tumours are conveniently divided into extradural and intradural growths, the latter being further subdivided into those arising outside the spinal cord—extramedullary tumours, and within the cord—intramedullary tumours. Excluding secondary carcinoma of the vertebrae, Elsberg (1925) found that 10 per cent of spinal tumours were extradural, 67 per cent were extramedullary, and 14 per cent were intramedullary. More recent experience is variable (Alter 1975) but Oddsson (1947) found that of 144 spinal tumours, 18 per cent were extradural, 51 per cent extramedullary, 26 per cent intramedullary, and the remainder both extra- and intramedullary. Intramedullary tumours are commoner in childhood (Banna and Gryspeerdt 1971).

The origin and nature of extradural tumours have been described in earlier sections. The commonest extramedullary tumours are meningiomas and neurofibromas. Published figures of relative incidence vary but meningiomas seem to be slightly more common than neurofibromas (Alter 1975) while the two together are between two and three times as common as spinal gliomas. Neurofibromas usually arise from spinal roots, the posterior more frequently than the anterior. They may be single or multiple and may or may not be associated with generalized neurofibromatosis. Exceptionally, an extramedullary neurofibroma grows out through an intervertebral foramen, thus adopting a dumb-bell shape. The extraspinal portion may be palpable. Meningiomas may arise from arachnoid covering the roots or the cord. While neurofibromas develop at any level of the spinal canal and occur equally in the two sexes, meningiomas almost always lie in the dorsal region and much more often affect females than males. Sarcomatous changes in spinal meningiomas and primary extramedullary sarcomas are rare. Lipomas occasionally occur but usually in relation to occult spinal bifida and spinal dysraphism. Other developmental anomalies, not strictly tumours, but which may mimic growths in causing cord compression, include dorsal neurenteric cysts (Vinters and Gilbert 1981) and congenital extradural cysts (intraspinal meningoceles) (Parkinson, Chaudhuri, and Schwartz 1976). It has been suggested that intraspinal epidermoid cysts may follow several years after lumbar puncture due to implantation of fragments of epidermis into the spinal canal (see *The Lancet* 1977). Chordomas are rare malignant tumours arising from a remnant of the notochord. Spinal chordomas are almost invariably situated in the sacrococcygeal region (Gessaga 1973). Dermoid cysts and other forms of teratomatous growth may also develop within the spinal canal.

Kernohan, Woltman, and Adson (1931), who investigated the histology of intramedullary spinal tumours, claimed to have recognized varieties corresponding to most of the cerebral gliomas. Forty-two per cent of intramedullary tumours, according to these authors, are ependymomas, and the remainder includes spongioblastomas, astroblastomas, medulloblastomas, oligodendrogliomas, ganglioneuromas, very rare intramedullary metastases of carcinoma (Edelson, Deck, and Posner 1972), and haemangioblastomas (Browne, Adams, and Roberson 1976). Angiomatous malformations are not uncommon and may have a considerable longitudinal extent. They can cause spinal subarachnoid haemorrhage as well as cord compression (Aminoff and Logue 1974*a*; Logue 1979) and symptoms may first appear in pregnancy (Newman 1958); spinal subarachnoid bleeding is also occasionally seen in patients with neurofibromas, angioblastic meningiomas, and particularly with ependymomas of the filum terminale (Walton 1953). Leukaemic deposits may occur within the cord as well as in the extradural space, and gumma and tuberculoma are occasionally found. For some time it was thought that there was an unusually high incidence of cord tumours in patients with syringomyelia; it now seems more probable that ascending or descending cord cavitation arising as a complication of spinal tumour is a more likely explanation (Barnett, Foster, and Hudgson 1973). Systemic metastases from primary spinal neoplasms are rare but have been described in ependymoma of the filum terminale (Rubinstein and Logan 1970). By contrast, intra- and extramedullary spinal deposits resulting from intracranial gliomas, especially medulloblastomas, are not uncommon, particularly in children.

Both sexes are equally liable to spinal tumour, which may develop at any age, but in over 80 per cent of cases symptoms first appear between the ages of 20 and 60. There is no significant difference in incidence in different races (Alter 1975) but meningiomas and neurofibromas are relatively rare in childhood, as indeed are all spinal tumours in comparison to intracranial neoplasms (Ingraham and Matson 1954; Slooff 1964; Banna and Gryspeerdt 1971). The thoracic region of the cord is the commonest site of extradural and extramedullary tumours. Approximately two-thirds of extramedullary tumours are situated on the dorsal or dorsolateral aspects of the cord and approximately one-third on the ventral or ventrolateral aspects (Elsberg 1925; Alter 1975). In the cauda equina, ependymomas and neurofibromas are almost equally common, occurring more often in the male, while metastasis, reticulosis, meningioma, and lipoma in this situation are all rare (Fearnside and Adams 1978; *British Medical Journal* 1978 *a*).

Arachnoiditis

Pachymeningitis, involving both the dura and the arachnoid and resulting from meningovascular syphilis or from spread of infection from a staphylococcal or tuberculous arteritis of the vertebrae, was once common but is now very rare. Localized or diffuse arachnoiditis of variable aetiology is now seen more often, though it is still comparatively uncommon. Sometimes the arachnoidal adhesions enclose encysted collections of CSF. Meningococcal, pneumococcal, and viral meningitis have all been known to be followed by arachnoiditis but granulomatous processes such as syphilis, cryptococcosis (Davidson 1968), tuberculosis, and sarcoidosis are more often responsible, though the latter condition more commonly produces extra- or intramedullary mass lesions (Day and Sypert 1977). Trauma has also been implicated as a cause and there is evidence that lumbar intervertebral-disc prolapse is often responsible; in consequence, lumbo-sacral arachnoiditis causing a cauda-equina syndrome now appears substantially more common than cervical or dorsal involvement giving paraparesis (Shaw, Russell, and Grossart 1978; *British Medical Journal* 1978 *b*). In many cases, despite full investigation, aetiology remains obscure and the 'idiopathic' condition is rarely familial (Duke and Hashimoto 1974).

Tuberculous meningitis limited to the spinal cord is a cause of adhesive arachnoiditis in some tropical countries (Dastur and Wadia 1969), but tuberculous meningiomyelitis is also seen in Britain (Freilich and Swash 1979). Other occasional causes include epidural (Braham and Saia 1958) and spinal anaesthesia (Payne and Bergentz 1956), and rarely symptomatic arachnoiditis has been described as a sequel to myelography using oily contrast media (Shapiro 1975). Water-soluble media such as methylgluca-mine iocarmate may also be responsible (Jensen and Hein 1978), but the risk seems much less with metrizamide (*British Medical Journal* 1978 *b*). Blood in the theca and intrathecal injections of steroids or methotrexate have also been implicated (Esses and Morley 1983). Although arachnoiditis interferes with the function of both the cord and spinal roots, cord compression probably plays comparatively little part in its ill effects and interference with the blood supply of the cord seems more important.

Arachnoidal cysts

These cysts of presumed developmental origin, which differ from the neurenteric cysts mentioned above in not being associated with spina bifida, are an occasional cause of cord compression in children, adolescents, and young adults. Commonly they give episodes of radicular pain with signs of spinal-cord dysfunction which develop in a step-like manner. Most lie in the dorsal region posterior to the cord and communicate with the subarachnoid space by a narrow orifice which is only easily demonstrable by supine myelography (Nugent 1959; Raja and Hankinson 1970). They may be particularly common in cases of Marfan's syndrome (Newman and Tilley 1979).

Parasitic cysts

Hydatid cysts are not uncommon causes of spinal compression in some countries and are usually extradural. Cysticercus cysts also occasionally occur.

Effects of compression upon the cord

Spinal-cord compression, however caused, affects it in several ways. Direct pressure interferes with conduction in spinal roots and in the cord itself. Pressure upon the ascending longitudinal spinal veins leads to oedema of the cord below the site of compression. Taylor and Byrnes (1974) suggest that interference with venous drainage may explain symptoms and signs of low cervical-cord dysfunction arising in patients with high cervical-cord compression and this view has been supported by electromyographic studies (Stark, Kennard, and Swash 1981). Compression of the longitudinal and radicular spinal arteries also leads to ischaemia of the segments of the cord which they supply. These vascular disturbances cause local oedema and/or degeneration of ganglion cells and white matter. Areas of softening may develop—so-called compression 'myelitis'. In general, slow spinal compression affects the pyramidal (corticospinal) tracts first, the posterior columns next, and the spinothalamic tracts last but there are many exceptions to this rule. This may be due to the fact that the pyramidal tracts are supplied by terminal branches of the anterior spinal artery which are thus most susceptible to compression ischaemia. Alternatively it has been suggested that the pyramidal tract lies closest to the attachments of the ligamentum denticulatum which is subjected to traction when the cord is compressed. Finally, obstruction of the subarachnoid space causes loculation of the CSF below the point of compression and leads to characteristic changes in its composition.

Symptoms and signs

The clinical manifestations of compression of the spinal cord differ to some extent according to whether the lesion responsible is extradural, extramedullary, or intramedullary and according to its segmental level. However, it is so often difficult clinically to identify the site of cord compression before operation that the similarity of the symptoms produced by pressure in different situations becomes evident. It will be convenient, therefore, first to des-

cribed the general symptoms of spinal compression, and then to discuss how they may differ according to the site and segmental level of the lesion.

Mode of onset

The onset of symptoms is usually gradual, especially when they are due to a spinal tumour, but is often rapid in carcinoma of the vertebral column, in spinal extradural abscess, and in acute compression due to other causes. In Pott's disease it is usually gradual but paraplegia may develop acutely. About two-thirds of all sufferers from spinal tumour come to operation between the first and second years after the onset of symptoms. Sometimes the interval is considerably longer. The first symptoms are often sensory, the commonest being pain radiating in the distribution of one or more spinal roots. Root pains are usually severe in vertebral collapse from all causes, and sometimes in arachnoiditis. In the case of spinal tumours they are most often present when the tumour is extramedullary (particularly when it is a neurofibroma), and least in intramedullary tumours. Pain may be unilateral or bilateral, and is often described as burning or constricting and may be associated with soreness of the skin and tenderness of deeper structures. It is often intensified by movement of the spine, and by coughing and sneezing, and may be temporarily relieved by change in posture. Pain in the back may also occur, and is especially frequent in tumours of the cauda equina, and in malignant disease of the vertebral column. Compression of the spinothalamic tracts may cause pain of a peculiarly unpleasant character referred to the extremities. Thus pain in a lower limb can be a symptom of cervical-cord compression. Paraesthesiae may also be produced by compression of ascending sensory tracts, and take the form of numbness, coldness, or a sense of weight, swelling, or tightness in the limbs. Compression of the posterior columns often gives feelings as if the limb were enclosed in a tight bandage or stocking or as if constricted by a tight band or string.

Motor symptoms often develop later than sensory, though the reverse may occur. Weakness, stiffness, and clumsiness of one arm or dragging of one or both legs, especially when tired, are common. When the cervical cord is compressed, the order in which the limbs are affected is usually first one upper limb, then the lower limb on the same side, next the opposite lower limb, and finally the opposite upper limb, but cervical spondylotic myelopathy may present with paraparesis. When compression occurs below the cervical enlargement, motor symptoms are often confined to the lower limbs, one usually becoming weak before the other. Exceptionally, paraplegia develops rapidly. This is particularly common when an acute flexion or hyperextension injury of the neck afflicts an individual with previously asymptomatic cervical spondylosis. Sphincter disturbances are often late in appearing, even in the case of tumours of the conus medullaris and cauda equina.

The initial symptoms of a spinal angioma are variable and may not appear till middle age. They are rarely those of focal spinal compression, but more often indicate an insidiously progressive but rather patchy lesion in the thoracic or lumbar region. Most patients are middle-aged males, disturbances of micturition often appear early and symptoms may be modified by a change in posture (Aminoff and Logue 1974*a*). A systolic bruit may be heard over the spine. Unusual modes of onset are with subarachnoid haemorrhage or haematomyelia.

Schäfer (1975) gave a comprehensive review of the differential diagnosis of spinal compression syndromes.

Papilloedema

Papilloedema is an uncommon complication of spinal tumour (Raynor 1969; Alter 1975) and is attributed largely to the effects of the substantial rise in CSF protein which often accompanies these lesions. Communicating hydrocephalus or a syndrome resembling benign intracranial hyptertension is occasionally seen (Ridsdale and Moseley 1978).

Motor symptoms and signs
Compression of ventral roots or of the anterior horns of grey matter leads to a progressive lower motor-neurone lesion, with weakness, wasting, and sometimes fasciculation of the muscles innervated by the affected segments. These symptoms are most conspicuous when the cervical or lumbosacral regions are affected. Wasting of intercostal muscles is similarly produced by a lesion of the thoracic cord but may be very difficult to detect.

Compression of the corticospinal tracts causes spastic weakness of the trunk and limbs below the level of the lesion. One side of the body is often involved before the other, but later spastic paraplegia-in-extension develops and as interruption of conduction in the cord becomes complete this may give place to paraplegia-in-flexion.

Objective sensory changes
Compression of dorsal spinal roots at the level of the lesion may cause apparent hyperaesthesia and hyperalgesia (hyperpathia) or 'girdle pain' in the corresponding cutaneous areas. Anaesthesia and analgesia may follow. Compression of the long ascending sensory tracts also leads to objective sensory loss. Several forms of dissociated sensory loss are encountered. Compression of the spinothalamic tract causes impairment of appreciation of pain, heat, and cold on the opposite side of the body, but owing to lamination of the fibres of the tract there may also be a slow progressive ascent of the sensory 'level' and certain cutaneous areas may escape. Thus sensibility may be, for a time, unimpaired over the areas supplied by the sacral segments of the cord ('sacral sparing'). Less frequently the sacral segments are affected early, but an area of normal cutaneous sensibility intervenes between them and an area of sensory loss at a higher level. The final upper limit of the area of analgesia and thermo-anaesthesia often lies several segments below the level of the lesion. This discrepancy occurs when the uppermost sensory fibres compressed in the cord are those which have decussated several segments below. Only exceptionally is appreciation of pain, heat, and cold affected equally. Not uncommonly cold is still felt over an area which is anaesthetic to heat, and sometimes a cold object, though not recognized as cold, evokes an unpleasant painful sensation. Cutaneous anaesthesia to light touch is often absent until the late stages, probably on account of the bilateral paths of fibres subserving this form of sensibility. Loss of appreciation of posture, passive movement, and vibration is often impaired more upon one side then the other. Although these forms of sensation, which depend upon the integrity of the posterior columns, are likely to be affected early when the source of compression is posteriorly situated, they often also suffer when the cord is compressed from in front, probably due to pressure against the infolded ligamentum subflavum.

Tenderness of the spine on pressure or percussion may arise in two ways. When vertebrae are diseased, inflamed, or subjected to erosion by a tumour, their spinous processes are often tender. When the vertebrae are normal, however, compression of the spinal cord or dorsal roots may give tenderness of the spines of the vertebrae innervated by the segments affected. In this case the tender vertebra is not necessarily the one overlying the lesion, but is often situated at a lower level, since the segments of the spinal cord do not correspond with the vertebrae in relation to which they are situated (see below). When the cervical cord is compressed, flexing or extending the neck often causes pain, numbness, or tingling, radiating into the regions innervated by the affected part of the cord. This symptom (so-called 'electric shock-like' sensations or Lhermitte's sign) may occur with both extramedullary and intramedullary tumours, in cervical myelopathy due to spondylosis, and in multiple sclerosis.

The reflexes
Compression of the spinal cord at a given segmental level leads to diminution or loss of reflexes when the central portion of the reflex arc passes through the segment affected. When the corticospinal tract is simultaneously compressed, reflexes below the level of the lesion show the changes associated with corticospinal lesions, that is, the tendon reflexes are exaggerated, the cremasteric and abdominal reflexes are diminished or lost, and the plantar reflexes are extensor. The reflexes are often, therefore, of value in localizing a spinal lesion, especially when a reflex mediated by one spinal segment is diminished and one mediated by a slightly lower segment is exaggerated. For example, a lesion extending down to the fifth or even the sixth cervical segment but not involving the seventh is likely to give diminution or loss of the biceps– and radial-jerks, which depend upon the integrity of the former segments, while the triceps-jerk, of which the reflex arc passes through the seventh cervical segment, may be exaggerated. Thus a tap on the biceps tendon may fail to evoke a biceps jerk but instead gives contraction of triceps as the triceps jerk is exaggerated and can be obtained by stimulation over a wide field (inversion of the biceps jerk). Similarly, inversion of the radial jerk (finger flexion, occurring in the absence of a radial jerk, on tapping the tendon of the brachioradialis) is a useful clinical indication of a lesion at C5–6. The segmental levels of the various spinal reflexes are given on page 50.

The sphincters
The sphincters are not usually affected in the early stages of cord compression, but later precipitancy or hesitancy of micturition often develops, and later still urinary retention is common, or the bladder may empty automatically. Constipation is usual, but with severe paraplegia there may be incontinence of faeces. Sphincter changes often occur earlier in tumours involving the cauda equina and conus medullaris than when compression occurs at a higher level.

Autonomic symptoms
Autonomic symptoms are of limited value in the localization of a spinal lesion. When there is substantial interruption of descending spinal pathways, control by higher centres of autonomic function below the level of the lesion is impaired. In such cases excessive sweating is common over the parts of the body thus isolated from higher control and the regulation of body temperature and blood pressure may be impaired (p. 598). Since the sympathetic outflow from the spinal cord is limited to the region between the first thoracic and second lumbar segments, the upper level of cutaneous distribution of autonomic dysfunction does not as a rule correspond to the sensory 'level' caused by a lesion at a given spinal-cord segment see (p. 406). Oedema of the lower limbs often develops in cases of severe spinal compression, as in paraplegia due to other causes.

The spine
The spine may show angular deformity, local tenderness, or pain on movement when the vertebrae are diseased. In cervical spondylosis, however, both pain and restriction of movement are often slight. A spinal bruit may be heard when an angioma is present (Matthews 1959).

The cerebrospinal fluid
Examination of the CSF is of considerable diagnostic value when obstruction of the spinal subarachnoid space produces characteristic changes. However, in cases of suspected extradural abscess, lumbar puncture should not be performed at or near the site of spinal pain or tenderness in view of the risk of introducing organisms into the subarachnoid space. Furthermore, removal of CSF by lumbar puncture below a spinal block may render subsequent lumbar myelography impracticable, at least for several days,

because of shrinkage of the lumbar subarachnoid space. When there is strong clinical suspicion that the spinal cord is being compressed, therefore, it is wise to do a myelogram first (or even preferably a CT scan if available), examining a specimen of fluid removed at the time, without carrying out a preliminary diagnostic lumbar puncture.

The presence of a tumour of the cauda equina may lead to a failure to obtain CSF by lumbar puncture at the site of election below the fourth lumbar vertebra, if it completely fills the spinal canal at this point. Cisternal myelography may then be indicated.

Chemical changes. The principal chemical abnormality is a rise in the protein content of the fluid, usually to between 1.0 and 5.0 g/l but may be even higher if the block is complete. In addition the fluid is xanthochromic in about 40 per cent of cases, and may coagulate spontaneously. The fluid may contain an excess of mononuclear cells when the source of compression is inflammatory (e. g. spinal extradural abscess), and exceptionally in cases of tumour. The rise in CSF protein is most marked in cases of extramedullary spinal compression, and is often much less when the lesion is extradural or intramedullary. Cord compression in the cervical region without block often gives lesser rises than do lesions at lower levels. A rise of protein is also common in fluid removed *above* a tumour of the cauda equina.

Queckensteai's test and manometry. Before myelography was widely used, Queckenstedt's test was often utilized as a guide to the presence or absence of cord compression. However, the test gives so many false negative results in cases of cord compression without complete block that it has been largely discarded. Similarly, manometry, which may indicate subnormal pressure below an obstruction and the absence of normal variations in pressure corresponding to the pulse and respiration, is of limited diagnostic value. Nevertheless, Queckenstedt's test carried out in various head positions is still sometimes used to detect cervical-cord compression due to spondylosis; techniques of electromanometry were reviewed by Lakke (1975). But none of these techniques can supplant myelography and CT scanning in the diagnosis and localization of spinal lesions.

Exacerbation of symptoms following lumbar puncture. In cases of spinal subarachnoid block, especially due to a spinal tumour, withdrawal of CSF below the level of the block may lead to a shift in the position of the tumour and a temporary or even permanent intensification of the symptoms, especially root pains, weakness, and urinary retention. Thus hasty lumbar puncture is unwise when a spinal tumour is suspected. It is wiser to seek a neurosurgical opinion and to arrange myelography at a time when the neurosurgeon will be able to operate immediately, particularly if clinical deterioration follows the procedure.

Radiography
Radiography of the spine is obligatory in all cases of suspected spinal compression. When disease of the vertebral column is the cause, X-ray examination alone may enable the nature of the lesion to be identified (Burrows and Leeds 1981). It reveals the vertebral destruction due to tuberculous and other forms of osteitis, secondary carcinoma, primary vertebral neoplasm, and the changes resulting from trauma. However, a spinal extradural abscess due to acute vertebral osteitis may be present without visible radiological abnormalities in the early stages. Chronic disc protrusion is often associated with narrowing of the corresponding disc space (Fig. 14.1), and bony spurs from the bodies of adjacent vertebrae: its presence can be confirmed by myelography (Fig. 14.2). Many patients, particularly manual workers, have severe degenerative changes in the cervical spine without symptoms (Irvine, Foster, Newell, and Klukvin 1965; Wilkinson 1973) so that when radiological findings of spondylosis are present in a patient with signs of spinal-cord compression it cannot necessarily be assumed

that spondylosis is the cause and myelography is still necessary. A tumour within the vertebral canal may by erosion lead to its diffuse enlargement, in which case the pedicles may be eroded or the distance between them is increased, or it may extend outwards through an intervertebral foramen with local destruction of bone. Oblique views will then demonstrate enlargement of the foramen and a soft-tissue shadow of a 'dumb-bell' tumour may also be seen.

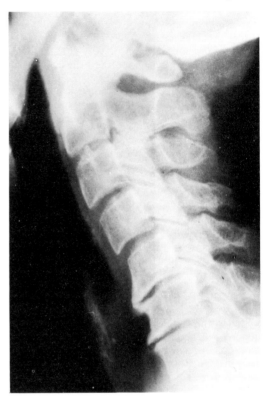

Fig. 14.1. A lateral radiograph of the cervical spine demonstrating anterior osteophytes and narrowing of disc spaces at C5−6 and C6−7.

Myelography
While some radiologists prefer to use air or oxygen injected intrathecally by lumbar puncture to demonstrate lesions causing spinal-cord compression, others still use an oily contrast medium made up of ethyl esters of isomeric iodophenidecyclic acids (*Myodil, Pantopaque*) of which 5–6 ml is usually injected by lumbar puncture with the patient in the sitting position. This preparation is often non-irritant and relatively few complications result from its use (Bull and McKissock 1962) although iodine sensitivity should be excluded before it is used. Occasionally low back pain, root pains in the legs, and even retention of urine may follow myelography but these complications are as a rule transient; untoward long-lasting sequelae (due to adhesive arachnoiditis—Davies 1956) are uncommon and in Great Britain no attempt is made to remove the injected oil (du Boulay 1975). In the United States, however, for medicolegal reasons, the lumbar puncture needle is generally left *in situ* and the oil is withdrawn when the examination has been completed. Water-soluble contrast media such as methylglucamine iothalamate (*Conray*) and methylglucamate iocarmate (*Dimer-X*) give excellent radiographs but produce acute reactions in an unacceptable proportion of patients (Shapiro 1975). However, the introduction of water-soluble metrizamide (*Amipaque*) has made it possible for the first time to demonstrate the entire spinal canal, as well as the intracranial subarachnoid space and the cerebral ventricles with contrast medium with relative safety, both in adults (Grainger and Lamb 1980) and in children (Swick, Sty and Haughton 1978; Pettersson and Harwood-

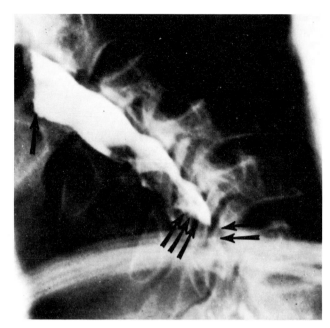

Fig. 14.2. A myelogram of a patient with cervical myelopathy due to spondylosis. There are a fluid level (the single arrow demonstrates hold-up due to a narrow canal), posterior osteophytes with a disc protrusion (double arrows) and corrugation of the ligamentum subflavum (triple arrows).

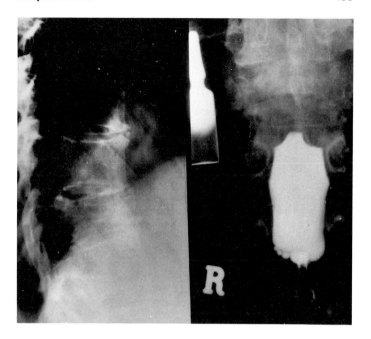

Fig. 14.3. A radiograph of the spine (on the left) showing collapse of a vertebral body due to a solitary myeloma with a complete block on myelography (on the right).

Nash 1982). Complications such as the arachnoiditis sometimes seen using oily contrast media are very rare with this agent, but headache is troublesome in some patients, epileptic seizures may follow the procedure, especially in susceptible individuals, and transient asterixis and encephalopathy have been reported (Bertoni, Schwartzman, van Horn and Partin 1981). Nevertheless, this preparation is now widely used and side-effects are few. Following injection the patient is examined on a tilting table under an X-ray screen and anteroposterior and lateral radiographs can be taken at appropriate spinal levels as the flow of contrast medium is observed. Usually the examination is carried out with the patient prone but supine myelography is also essential when a lesion at or near the foramen magnum or an arachnoid cyst lying posterior to the cord is suspected. If the contrast medium is arrested below a compressive lesion or when one in the cauda equina is suspected, it may be necessary to inject the medium by cisternal rather than lumbar puncture in order to outline its upper margins. In cases of suspected cervical myelopathy radiographs should be taken in several positions of the head. When a complete block is present, re-screening after 24 hours may show that some contrast medium has passed the obstruction. The appearances in the myelogram not only localize the compressive lesion but often also give an indication as to its nature (Figs. 14.3 and 14.4). In arachnoiditis there is usually a patchy hold-up of the medium, while in arteriovenous malformation of the cord, dilated vessels are often plainly outlined (Fig. 14.5).

CT Scanning

The introduction of the whole-body CT scanner (Haughton and Williams 1982; Pettersson and Harwood-Nash 1982) has transformed the radiological diagnosis of spinal lesions, both in adults and children. It can effectively demonstrate spinal soft tissues, detect metastases, prolapsed intervertebral discs, cord tumours, hypertrophy of the ligamentum subflavum, and also, as a rule, spinal stenosis, focal joint abnormalities, and many fractures. The expense of the equipment continues to restrict its wide availability, but as in the case of cranial CT scanning, its increasing use and availability will inevitably reduce the use of other techniques of radiological diagnosis, including myelography, in the future.

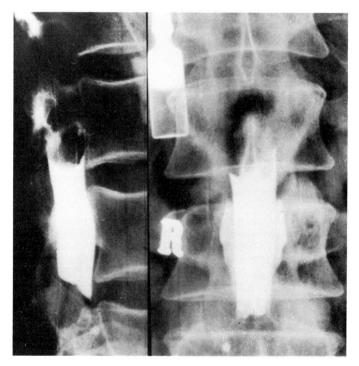

Fig. 14.4. Lateral and anteroposterior views of a myelogram demonstrating a rounded filling defect due to a neurofibroma of the cauda equina.

Electrophysiological studies

While, as mentioned above, the recording of spinal and cortical sensory evoked potentials is of considerable value in distinguishing organic from hysterical paraplegia, these methods are of less value in the investigation of suspected spinal-cord compression than they are, for example, in patients with suspected multiple sclerosis. Nevertheless, in cervical spondylosis causing radiculopathy and objective neurological•signs, these and related techniques can be helpful in identifying the site of root compression

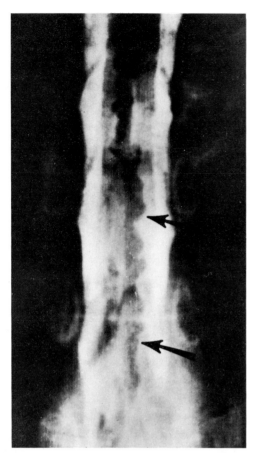

Fig. 14.5. A myelogram demonstrating an arteriovenous malformation of the dorsal cord; tortuous dilated veins are arrowed.

(Ganes 1980) and electromyography is also helpful in elucidating the cause of muscular wasting in such cases (Stark *et al.* 1981). Even when peripheral motor and sensory nerve conduction velocity is normal, recording the conduction velocity of the ulnar F-wave is also helpful in identifying root lesions, as in patients with epidural metastases (de Visser, Van der Sande and Kemp 1982).

Other methods of investigation

Spinal-cord angiography, as previously mentioned, is of particular value in the diagnosis of spinal vascular malformations but also has been used to help in demonstrating and identifying other spinal lesions (Di Chiro, Doppman, and Ommaya 1967; Doppman, Di Chiro, and Ommaya 1969; Vogelsang 1975; Djindjian, Merland, Djindjian, and Stoeter 1981). Digital subtraction angiography (Moseley 1982) may improve this image. Extradural venography and lumbar discography (a technique involving the direct injection of contrast medium into the intervertebral disc) are other methods used in some centres, especially to demonstrate herniated invertertebral discs, but are not yet a part of routine neuroradiological practice and certainly do not supplant myelography (Shapiro 1975). Isotope techniques (myeloscintography) are less valuable in identifying spinal lesions than gamma-encephalography, and indeed the increasing availability and use of whole-body CT scanning will undoubtedly reduce further the use of all of these techniques with the probable exception of myelography.

Symptoms and signs of spinal compression at different levels

The manifestations of spinal compression at a given level consist of: (1) those of a lower motor-neurone lesion, i.e. atrophic paralysis with diminution or loss of tendon reflexes in the muscles innervated by the affected segments; (2) those of an upper motor-neurone lesion, i.e. spastic paralysis with exaggeration of the tendon reflexes, diminution or loss of the abdominal and cremasteric reflexes and an extensor plantar reflex on one or both sides below the level of the compression; (3) those of dorsal-root irritation, such as girdle pain and hyperpathia, may be present, with a segmental distribution corresponding to the segments compressed; (4) various types of sensory loss as described above, with an upper level at or somewhat below the segmental level of the compression; (5) autonomic changes, e.g. excessive sweating below the level of the lesion. The following are the principal motor and reflex disturbances resulting from compression of the cord at different levels. The distribution of the sensory changes may be ascertained from the figures on page 43.

The upper cervical region. Spinal compression at this level or at the foramen magnum often, but not invariably, causes pain in the ;neck and occiput, intensified by movements of the cervical spine. Pain, paraesthesiae, and weakness in the upper limbs are early symptoms and loss of proprioceptive sensation in the hands may be particularly prominent. Wasting may occur in both upper limbs, even though the cervical enlargement is not compressed (Taylor and Byrnes 1974). Compression of the phrenic nerves or of their nuclei may impair the amplitude of diaphragmatic movements. A tumour in this region may extend upwards through the foramen magnum and cause symptoms by compressing the medulla and the lowest cranial nerves. Compression of the spinal tract and nucleus of the fifth nerve can give relative analgesia and thermo-anaesthesia over the face, and the ninth, tenth, and eleventh cranial nerves may also suffer. Signs of corticospinal-tract compression are present in both the upper and lower limbs with exaggeration of *all* deep tendon reflexes. Postural sense and appreciation of vibration are usually markedly impaired in one or both upper limbs and often in the legs as well. When a congenital anomaly (such as the Chiari type I malformation, basilar impression of the skull, or another craniovertebral developmental defect) or arachnoiditis is present in the region of the foramen magnum, this may lead to syringomyelia (p. 412). Much less often, the latter condition can develop as a result of a tumour (e.g. meningioma) in this region. Vertebrobasilar insufficiency has been described as a complication of rheumatoid atlantoaxial subluxation (Jones and Kaufmann 1976).

The fifth or sixth cervical segments. There is atrophy and weakness in the muscles innervated by these segments, namely, the rhomboids, deltoids, spinati, biceps and brachioradialis. There is spastic paralysis of the remaining muscles of the upper limbs and of the trunk and lower limbs. The biceps- and radial jerks are diminished or lost, but are often inverted, as already described (p. 403).

The eighth cervical and first thoracic segments. Weakness and atrophy involve the flexors of the wrist and fingers and the small hand muscles. A Horner's syndrome is rarely seen. The tendon reflexes of the upper limbs are preserved. There is spastic paralysis of the trunk and lower limbs. Compression of the cord at this level is virtually unknown in cervical spondylosis so that wasting of the small hand muscles rarely if ever occurs due to this cause, but can result from secondary venous stasis due to compression at a higher level (Taylor and Byrnes 1974; Start *et al.* 1981).

Mid-thoracic region. Atrophic paralysis is confined to the intercostals innervated by the segments involved. Movements of the diaphragm are normal. There is spastic paralysis of the muscles of the abdomen and lower limbs.

Ninth and tenth thoracic segments. The lower halves of the abdominal recti are paralysed; the upper halves are normal. Consequently the umbilicus is drawn upwards when the patient raises his head against resistance. The upper abdominal reflexes are preserved, while those of the lower segments are lost. There is spastic paralysis of the lower limbs.

Twelfth thoracic and first lumbar segments. The abdominal recti are normal, but the lower fibres of obliquus internus and transversus abdominis are paralysed. The abdominal reflexes are preserved, but the cremasteric reflexes are diminished or lost. There is spastic paralysis of the lower limbs.

Third and fourth lumbar segments. Flexion of the hip is preserved. There is weakness and wasting of quadriceps and of the hip adductors, with diminution or loss of the knee-jerks, and spastic paralysis of the remaining muscles of the lower limbs, with exaggeration of the ankle-jerks and extensor plantar responses.

First and second sacral segments. Flexion of the hip, adduction of the thigh, extension of the knee, and dorsiflexion of the foot are preserved. There is atrophic paralysis of the intrinsic muscles of the foot and those of the calf, with weakness of knee flexion and hip adduction and extension. The knee-jerks are preserved; the ankle-jerks and plantar reflexes are lost. The anal and bulbocavernosus reflexes are retained.

Third and fourth sacral segments. The large bowel and bladder are paralysed with retention of urine and faeces, due to the uninhibited action of the sympathetic. The external sphincters are paralysed and the anal and bulbocavernosus reflexes are lost. There is usually sensory loss in the perineum and buttocks in 'saddle' distribution. The motility and reflexes of the lower limbs are normal.

Compression of the cauda equina

Compression of the cauda equina is most often due to a neoplasm, (usually ependymoma or neurofibroma, rarely a chordoma), but the nerves may be compressed by an associated lipoma in cases of spina bifida occulta, by a constricting fibrous band (Léri 1926), or by chronic arachnoiditis. Perineurial cysts on posterior sacral roots (Tarlov 1948) are often asymptomatic but may cause sciatic pain; rarely if ever do they give other manifestations of cauda-equina compression. The cauda-equina syndrome which sometimes complicates ankylosing spondylitis (Matthews 1968), is of uncertain pathogenesis but may sometimes be due to arachnoiditis, more often to associated arachnoidal cysts (Hassan 1976). An important source of compression of a single root, or even of multiple roots, sometimes occurring acutely, is a displaced intervertebral disc (see p. 516). Rarely, spondylolisthesis may have the same effect, as may bony stenosis of the lumbar canal (Ehni 1975) which more often gives the syndrome of recurrent ischaemia or 'claudication' of the cauda equina on effort (see p. 423). The clinical picture is variable, depending upon the site and extent of the source of compression. It may be virtually impossible clinically to distinguish between a neoplasm arising in the cauda equina itself and one arising in the conus medullaris but extending into the cauda. A small tumour may for a long time compress only one or two roots on one side. A large and massive growth may involve the whole of the cauda. For anatomical reasons the lower roots are more likely to be compressed than the upper, since they suffer alone when a growth is situated in the lowest part of the spinal canal, but are also implicated, together with the upper roots, by tumours at a higher level.

In many cases of cauda-equina tumour, pain is the earliest symptom (Fearnside and Adams 1978). It is usually felt in the lumbar or sacral regions as a dull, aching pain which is liable to be exacerbated by jerky movements, coughing, and sneezing. Less often it is referred to one or both lower limbs in the distribution of the lower spinal nerves, or it may also be referred to the bladder, rectum, or testis.

Motor symptoms consist of weakness and wasting, in a distribution depending upon which nerves are affected. Most often there is paralysis of the muscles below the knee, though the tibialis anterior may escape, and of the hamstrings and glutei. In such cases the ankle-jerks are diminished or lost, and the plantar

reflexes may also be absent; but the knee-jerks are often preserved.

The distribution of the sensory loss also depends upon which spinal nerves are involved. Compression of the lower sacral dorsal roots or nerves gives a characteristic saddle-shaped area of anaesthesia and analgesia extending over the perineum, buttocks, and back of the thighs. Compression of the upper sacral and fifth lumbar nerves produces an area of sensory loss over the foot and over the posterior and outer aspect of the leg. When the lowest sacral segments are involved, though the external genitals are anaesthetic, and the patient may be unaware of the passage of a catheter, some bladder sensation usually remains, so that the patient is aware when it distends.

Disturbance of sphincter control is usual but may be unexpectedly late in developing. Compression of the third and fourth ventral and dorsal sacral roots interrupts the reflex arc upon which evacuation of the bladder and rectum depends. The result is retention of urine and faeces due to the unopposed contraction of the internal sphincters, even though the external sphincters are paralysed. Impotence occurs in the male. When the lowest sacral nerves are compressed, the anal and bulbocavernosus reflexes are lost.

Trophic changes may occur in the lower limbs, which are often cold and cyanosed, and tend to become oedematous. Slight injuries in the analgesic areas are apt to lead to sores which are slow to heal.

Diagnosis

The diagnosis of spinal compression involves four stages: (1) it must be distinguished from other lesions which may give rise to similar symptoms; (2) when its existence has been established, its segmental level must be determined; (3) an attempt should then be made to decide whether the compression is extradural, extramedullary, or intramedullary; and (4) its pathological nature must be considered.

Diagnosis from other disorders

When the earliest symptom is pain, spinal compression is liable to be confused with visceral disorders causing pain, such as pleurisy, angina pectoris, cholecystitis, gastric and duodenal ulcer, pancreatic carcinoma, and renal calculus. This error can only be avoided by a thorough examination of the nervous system, which will usually yield some indication of a lesion of the spinal cord, and also by the absence of physical signs of visceral disease. The girdle pain of pre–herpetic neuralgia (before the vesicles of herpes zoster appear) can also give rise to difficulty. Spinal compression must also be distinguished from intrinsic cord lesions, such as multiple sclerosis, syringomyelia, and motor-neurone disease, each of which may be simulated in certain respects by cervical myelopathy due to spondylosis. On clinical grounds this distinction can usually be made with considerable confidence, but the diagnosis can only be clinched by CT scanning and/or myelography and CSF analysis.

Localization of segmental level

In localizing the segmental level of spinal compression, segmental symptoms, especially atrophic paralysis and root pains and hyperpathia, are of the first importance. Next in value is the upper limit of the area of sensory loss, though this is not always easy to define. When it can be accurately determined, the segmental level of the upper limit of the analgesic area may be taken as indicating the lowest segment compressed but the sensory 'level' for pain sensation often suggests that the lesion is several segments lower than its actual site. Thus a level on the chest wall is commonly found in patients with cervical-cord lesions.

Clinical diagnosis between a tumour of the cauda equina and one of the conus medullaris is often difficult, and may be impossible. If, however, in spite of paralysis of the bladder and rectum, the anal and bulbocavernosus reflexes are preserved and if sensory loss is dissociated, with loss of pain, heat, and cold sensation, with preservation of light touch, it is likely that the lesion involves the conus rather than the cauda. An extensor plantar response on one or both sides indicates that the spinal cord is involved at least as high as the fifth lumbar segment.

Relationship of spinal segments to vertebrae. As the spinal cord terminates opposite the lower border of the first lumbar vertebra, spinal segments do not correspond numerically with the vertebral arches under which they lie. To ascertain which spinal segment is related to a given vertebra:

For the cervical vertebrae, add 1.
For thoracic 1–6, add 2.
For thoracic 7–9, add 3.
The tenth thoracic arch overlies lumbar 1 and 2 segments.
The eleventh thoracic arch overlies lumbar 3 and 4.
The twelfth thoracic arch overlies lumbar 5.
The first lumbar arch overlies the sacral and coccygeal segments.

It must also be noted that owing to the obliquity of the lower thoracic spinous processes a spinous process in this region is situated at the level of the body of the vertebra below. Despite these clinical guides it is, except in very exceptional or urgent circumstances, unwise to operate without confirmation of the level of the lesion by CT scanning or myelography.

The relationship of the source of compression to the cord

Angular deformity of the spine, and radiographic evidence of vertebral destruction may show clearly that vertebral disease is responsible. Without such evidence the clinical differentiation of extradural, extramedullary, and intramedullary sources of spinal compression is often difficult, and may be impossible. In extradural compression root pains often occur early, and symptoms of spinal compression are usually bilateral and symmetrical in their development. Motor symptoms usually appear first, to be followed later by sphincter disturbances, and sensory changes are frequently late. The distinction between extramedullary and intramedullary compression is sometimes impossible before operation but the myelographic findings and/or the CT scan usually differentiate between the two. The early onset of unilateral root pains and symptoms indicating that compression is mainly exerted upon one-half of the cord favour an extramedullary lesion. In such cases, moreover, blockage of the spinal subarachnoid space tends to occur early and the protein content of the spinal fluid is usually high. With intramedullary lesions, root pains are less frequent, motor symptoms are usually bilateral, and sphincter involvement occurs early. Dissociated sensory loss extending over several segments below the level of the lesion suggests an intramedullary growth. Subarachnoid blockage occurs later and the protein content of the fluid is usually lower in the case of intramedullary than in the case of extramedullary lesions.

Diagnosis of the cause

1. *Vertebral disease.* When spinal compression is due to vertebral collapse, there is usually considerable pain in, and rigidity of, the spine; angular deformity (a gibbus) is sometimes seen, and radiographic evidence of vertebral destruction is usually found. *Tuberculous caries* is to be suspected when these symptoms occur in a young patient who shows evidence of infection, such as pyrexia, sweating, and a raised sedimentation rate, with possibly in addition signs of a tuberculous focus elsewhere, but it may occur at any age and without general symptoms. Radiographically, vertebral-body destruction due to tuberculosis, unlike that resulting from malignant disease, commonly spares the intervertebral discs. *Secondary carcinoma* of the vertebral column is usually seen in middle-aged or elderly patients. The onset of the spinal symptoms is often rapid with considerable pain. There may be a history of an operation for carcinoma but, in the absence of this, careful clinical

and radiological examination often enable the primary growth to be found. The diagnosis of other forms of vertebral disease, for example, myelomatosis and Paget's disease can usually be established radiographically. When the former is suspected, the appropriate haematological tests should be carried out. *Cervical spondylosis* can also be demonstrated radiographically, but is so common after middle age that it is not always the cause of the patient's symptoms.

2. *Spinal tumour.* Spinal tumour is to be suspected whenever there is a gradual onset and subsequent slow progression of symptoms of spinal compression, in the absence of evident disease of the vertebral column. It is usually impossible to anticipate the nature of the spinal tumour, but cutaneous pigmentation and other manifestations of neurofibromatosis, which may be associated with an intrathecal neurofibroma, should be sought.

3. *Arachnoiditis.* It is often impossible to diagnose arachnoiditis clinically. The occurrence of multiple levels of segmental sensory disturbance, and a patchy or streaky arrest of contrast medium on myelography favour this condition.

Such rare causes of spinal compression as reticulosis, leukaemic deposits, extradural metastases, and parasitic cysts are often suspected only when clinical examination reveals evidence of the disease elsewhere.

Prognosis

General considerations

The prognosis of spinal compression depends upon: (1) the nature of the source of compression and the extent to which it can be relieved; (2) the severity and duration of the disturbance of function when the patient comes under observation; and (3) the level of the cord or cauda equina compressed. The influence of the nature of the compressing agent upon prognosis is considered below. The more severe the interruption of conduction in the cord, the less likely is recovery to be complete. Hence paraplegia-in-flexion, indicating a severe degree of cord damage, is of bad prognostic import, and little functional improvement can be expected in such cases. The longer the history, the less complete is recovery likely to be, though even when symptoms such as spastic weakness of the lower limbs have been present for two or more years, recovery may be remarkable if the cause can be removed. It cannot be stressed too strongly that rapidly-advancing spinal-cord compression demands immediate investigation and treatment so that appropriate measures can be taken before the circulation to the cord is irreversibly embarrassed. The outlook is best when the site of compression is in the middle or lower thoracic regions even though surgical operations in this region, particularly when carried out for the relief of anteriorly-situated lesions, such as the rare dorsal disc protrusions, are hazardous, first because the spinal canal is very narrow and secondly because the blood supply of the cord is at its most precarious at this point. When the upper cervical cord is compressed, the proximity of the spinal centres innervating the diaphragm adds to the risk both of the compression itself and of operations designed to relieve it. Compression of the lumbosacral region and cauda equina is especially liable to disturb the function of the bladder and bowel, and hence there is a high incidence of urinary infection in such cases. In all cases of spinal compression the presence of urinary infection and of bed-sores adds to the gravity of the prognosis.

Tuberculous spinal disease

The mortality rate of all forms of tuberculosis has been greatly reduced by modern chemotherapy. Spinal compression naturally increases the risks but about 70 per cent of patients with paraparesis recover completely if treated promptly. Others have some residual spastic weakness of the lower limbs. The prognosis both as to life and as to recovery of function is better in children than in adults. The sudden development of paraplegia rapidly becoming complete is usually due to 'concertina' collapse of a vertebral body or to thrombosis of vessels supplying the cord, and in each of these circumstances the outlook is poor. When severe long-standing paraplegia is present there is no hope of recovery.

Secondary carcinoma

In the past few patients survived more than 12 months after developing symptoms indicating the presence of metastatic carcinomatous deposits within the vertebral column, death occurring either as a direct result of the primary growth, or from cachexia due to widespread metastases. However, after prompt surgical decompression in appropriate cases followed by radiotherapy and/or chemotherapy, the prognosis is now much better and survival for five years or more is not uncommon in patients with reticulosis, myeloma, and prostatic or testicular tumours (Jameson 1974). High-dose corticosteroids given along with radiotherapy have markedly improved the outlook in patients with extradural metastases (Greenberg, Kim, and Posner 1980) and even in the rare cases of intramedullary metastasis some temporary improvement can be expected with such a regimen.

Spinal tumour

The prognosis of spinal tumour depends primarily upon the extent to which the growth can be removed. Accordingly, the outlook is much better with extramedullary tumours, many of which can be removed completely, than when the growth is intramedullary. Few intramedullary tumours can be successfully removed without considerable damage to the spinal cord although some ependymomas are encapsulated and can be 'shelled out' with subsequent improvement. The mortality rate of operations for spinal tumours is under 5 per cent in the best hands. Considerable functional improvement may be expected to follow the successful removal of a spinal tumour in all but the most advanced cases, even when symptoms of compression have been present for several years. Improvement, however, may be slow and may continue for up to two years after operation. Angiomas tend to be insidiously progressive in spite of all treatment but some show an unexpectedly benign and remittent course (Aminoff and Logue 1974) and many can now be removed in whole or in part (Shephard, Aminoff, and Kendall 1966; Logue 1974).

Acute intervertebral disc prolapse and cervical spondylosis

Acute central protrusion of a cervical intervertebral disc is usually best treated conservatively by immobilizing the neck in a plastic collar but if cord compression is severe, laminectomy and decompression may be needed; when carried out sufficiently early, the prognosis is good. Acute compression of the cauda equina, say by a central disc prolapse, demands immediate operation, especially if the sphincters are involved; here again the prognosis is good though some urinary difficulty may persist. Operative treatment is also indicated as a rule in cord compression due to prolapse of a dorsal intervertebral disc but the operation is risky, recovery is often incomplete, and irreversible paraplegia due to cord infarction is an all too frequent complication. In cervical myelopathy due to spondylosis the natural tendency of the disorder is to become arrested, but in some patients disability increases remorselessly, and most are left with a varying degree of residual disability.

Arachnoiditis and arachnoidal cysts

The response to operation in arachnoiditis is often disappointing and indeed operation is usually contra-indicated when the process is diffuse but the results of surgical removal of arachnoid cysts are usually excellent. Gourie-Devi and Satish (1979) suggest that the repeated intrathecal injection of 1500 I.U. of hyaluronidase may be beneficial in some cases.

Treatment

The treatment of compression of the spinal cord involves; (1) appropriate treatment of the compressive lesion; (2) when paraplegia is present, adequate care of the paralysed limbs, the skin, the urinary tract, and the bowels, along the lines laid down on page 394, for such treatment profoundly influences both survival and functional outcome.

Tuberculous spinal disease

A patient suffering from spinal tuberculosis requires appropriate chemotherapy and often orthopaedic treatment, such as immobilization in a plaster bed when the vertebral bodies are diseased.

Laminectomy is rarely desirable, since most patients rapidly improve on the treatment described. An exploratory operation, however, may be required when paraparesis fails to improve rapidly with treatment or suddenly increases in severity.

Cervical spondylosis

In some cases immobilization of the neck by means of a plaster or plastic collar has seemed to arrest the progress of cervical myelopathy but the value of this treatment is now recognized to be somewhat dubious in contrast to its confirmed beneficial effect in acute cervical intervertebral disc prolapse. Nevertheless, it is still widely used. In rapidly progressive cases, especially when the patient is relatively young, surgical decompression may be necessary. This is particularly likely to be indicated when myelography indicates that the cord is being compressed by significant disc protrusions at one or two levels and especially if there is infolding of the ligamentum subflavum and a narrow cervical canal (Bradley and Banna 1968). Surgery is often contra-indicated if three or more discs are involved. The choice between posterior decompression by laminectomy and anterior removal of the discs with spinal fusion (Cloward 1980) is a matter for decision depending upon clinical and myelographic findings in the individual case.

Lumbar spondylosis and spondylolisthesis

Operation in cases of lumbar spondylosis is indicated when chronic sciatic pain due to this cause has resisted conservative treatment or when the cauda equina is compressed by a large acute central disc protrusion. Laminectomy is of dubious value in cases of spondylolisthesis with compression of the cauda equina but spinal fusion may be beneficial, especially in the relief of pain.

Other spinal lesions

Surgical decompression is rarely feasible in cases of spinal-cord compression due to Paget's disease but is usually indicated in cases of vertebral haemangioma, and sometimes in kyphoscoliosis and achondroplasia.

Secondary carcinoma of vertebrae

When multiple vertebrae are involved, treatment can only be palliative as a rule, and morphine or its analogues should be given in doses adequate for pain relief. In many cases of acute compression at a single level, emergency laminectomy and decompression is indicated in order to relieve pressure and to obtain a surgical biopsy of the tumour as a preliminary to radiotherapy and chemotherapy. Decompression by an anterior approach now seems promising in many cases (Siegal, Siegal, Robin, Lubetzki-Korn, and Fuks 1982). The question as to whether the lesion should be irradiated depends upon the general condition of the patient and the situation and prognosis of the primary lesion, when known. Many patients have relief of pain as a result and in some cord compression is relieved; hence this treatment is usually indicated if the lesion is radiosensitive and unless the patient is in extremis as a result of the primary growth and/or multiple metastases elsewhere. Powerful analgesics and, in selected cases, surgical methods of pain relief (cordotomy, stereotaxic thalamotomy) may later be required.

Spinal tumour

Laminectomy should be performed, and when the tumour is extradural or extramedullary it should be removed as far as possible. Though many intramedullary tumours are inoperable, some, especially ependymomas, are extruded after incision of the cord and after removal of some of these lesions, cord damage is unexpectedly slight. The use of lasers or of ultrasonic scalpels (e. g. the *Cavitron*) has improved the results and lessened the complications of such procedures. When a spinal tumour cannot be removed for any reason, the operation of laminectomy may lead to a temporary improvement by diminishing the pressure upon the cord. X-ray irradiation may be of value as an accessory method of treatment following operation, especially for intramedullary tumours and sacral chordomas, which can rarely be removed. Angiomas show little if any response to radiotherapy; as already mentioned, removal is possible far more often than was thought likely in the past. Considerable benefit has been noted after excision of the superficial fistulous portion of the malformation, intradural ligation of feeding vessels, and excision of draining veins (Logue *et al.* 1974).

Meningitis, arachnoiditis, and extradural abscess

Chronic granulomatous meningitis, whatever its cause, may lead to softening of the spinal cord through interference with its vascular supply. In such cases little benefit can be expected to follow operation. At an earlier stage, however, when the symptoms are mainly due to constriction of the cord, improvement may follow laminectomy and removal of granulation tissue but in most cases (as in sarcoidosis) steroid drugs are the treatment of choice, with or without antibiotics if the lesion is infective; surgery is then better avoided. When arachnoiditis is found at operation, an attempt should be made to rupture or remove any cysts which may be present. Hyaluronidase (see above) may be of benefit. Tuberculous spinal meningitis requires the appropriate chemotherapy. Early decompression by laminectomy under antibiotic cover in cases of pyogenic spinal extradural abscess may be followed by complete recovery but if the patient is allowed to become paraplegic before operation is performed, it may be too late.

The rehabilitation of patients suffering from spinal compression who have undergone laminectomy, should include passive movements of the paretic limbs and exercises, in order to promote functional recovery (see p. 395).

References

Abrahamson, L., McConnell, A. A. and Wilson, G. R. (1934). Acute epidural spinal abscess. *Br. med. J.* **1**, 1114.

Adson, A. W. (1938). Intraspinal tumors; surgical consideration. Collective review. *Surg. Gynec. Obstet.* **67**, 225.

Alter, M. (1975). Statistical aspects of spinal cord tumors. In *Handbook of clinical neurology* (ed. P. J. Vinken and G. W.Bruyn) Vol. 19. North Holland, Amsterdam.

Aminoff, M. J. and Logue, V. (1974a). Clinical features of spinal vascular malformations. *Brain* **97**, 197.

—— and —— (1974b). The prognosis of patients with spinal vascular malformations. *Brain* **97**, 211.

Antoni, N. (1962). Spinal vascular malformations (angiomas) and myelomalacia. *Neurology, Minneapolis* **12**, 795.

Banna, M. and Gryspeerdt, G. L. (1971). Intraspinal tumours in children (excluding dysraphism). *Clin. Radiol.* **22**, 17.

Barnett, H. J. M., Foster, J. B. and Hudgson, P. (1973). *Syringomyelia.* (Major Problems in Neurology Series ed. J. N. Walton). Saunders, London.

Bertoni, J. M., Schwartzman, R. J., Van Horn, G. and Partin, J. (1981). Asterixis and encephalopathy following metrizamide myelography: investigations into possible mechanisms and review of the literature, *Ann. Neurol.* **9**, 366.

Blakeslee, G. A. (1928). Compression of the spinal cord in Hodgkin's disease. *Arch. Neurol. Psychiat., Chicago.* **20**, 130.

Bradley, W. G. and Banna, M. (1968). The cervical dural canal. A study of the 'tight dural canal' and of syringomyelia by prone and supine myelography. *Br. J. Radiol,* **41**, 608.

Braham, J. and Saia, A. (1958). Neurological complications of epidural anaesthesia. *Br. med. J.* **2**, 657.

Brain, W. R., Northfield, D. W. C. and Wilkinson, M. (1952). The neurological manifestations of cervical spondylosis. *Brain* **75**, 187.

Brice, J. and McKissock, W. (1965). Surgical treatment of malignant extradural spinal tumours. *Br. med. J.* **1**, 1341.

British Medical Journal (1978a). Cauda equina tumours. *Br. med. J.* **1**, 808.

—— (1978b). Chronic spinal arachnoiditis. *Br. med. J.* **2**, 518.

Browne, T. R., Adams, R. D. and Roberson, C. H. (1976). Hemangioblastoma of the spinal cord: review and report of five cases, *Arch. Neurol., Chicago.* **33**, 435.

Bucy, P. C. and Oberhill H. R. (1950). Intradural spinal granulomas, *J. Neurosurg,* **7**, 1.

Bull, J. W. D. and McKissock, W. (1962). *An atlas of positive contrast myelography.* Hoeber, New York.

Burrows, E. H. and Leeds, N. E. (1981). *Neuroradiology.* Churchill-Livingstone, Edinburgh.

Butler, R. W. (1934–5). Paraplegia in Pott's disease, with special reference to the pathology and aetiology. *Br. J. Surg.* **22**, 738.

Cairns, H. and Russell, D. S. (1931). Intracranial and spinal metastases in gliomas of the brain. *Brain* **54**, 377.

Campbell, A. M. G. and Phillips, D. G. (1960). Cervical disk lesions with neurological disorder. *Br. med. J.* **2**, 481.

Clarke, E. (1956). Spinal cord involvement in multiple myelomatosis. *Brain* **79**, 332.

Cloward, R. B. (1980). Acute cervical spine injuries. *CIBA Clinical Symposia* **32**, 1.

Dastur, D. K. (1979). Pathology and pathogenesis of chronic myelopathy in atlanto-axial dislocation, with operative or postoperative haematomyelia or other cord complications. *Clin. exp. Neurol.* **16**, 9.

—— and Wadia, N. H. (1969). Spinal meningitides with radiculo-myelopathy. Part 2—Pathology and pathogenesis. *J. neurol. Sci.* **8**, 261.

Davidson, S. (1968). Cryptococcal spinal arachnoiditis. *J. Neurol. Neurosurg. Psychiat.* **31**, 76.

Davies, F. C. (1956). Effect of unabsorbed radiographic contrast media on the central nervous system. *Lancet* **ii**, 747.

Day, A. L. and Sypert, G. W. (1977). Spinal cord sarcoidosis. *Ann. Neurol,* **1**, 79.

de Visser, B. W. O., Sande, J. J. Van Der and Kemp B. (1982). Ulnar F-wave conduction velocity in epidural metastatic root lesions. *Ann. Neurol.* **11**, 142.

Di Chiro, G., Doppman, J. and Ommaya, A. K. (1967). Selective arteriography of arteriovenous aneurysms of spinal cord. *Radiology* **88**, 1065.

Djindjian, R., Merland, J. J., Djindjian, M. and Stoeter, P. (1981). *Angiography of spinal column and spinal cord tumors.* Georg Thieme, Stuttgart.

Doppman, J. L., Di Chiro, G. and Ommaya, A. K. (1969). *Selective arteriography of the spinal cord.* Mosby, St. Louis.

Du Boulay, G. (1975). Myelography. In *Handbook of clinical neurology* (ed. P.J. Vinken, and G.W. Bruyn), Vol. 19, p. 179. North-Holland, Amsterdam.

Duke, R. J. and Hashimoto, S. A. (1974). Familial spinal arachnoiditis: a new entity. *Arch. Neurol., Chicago* **30**, 300.

Edelson, R. N., Chernik, N. L. and Posner, J. B. (1974). Spinal subdural hematomas complicating lumbar puncture: occurrence in thrombocytopenic patients. *Arch. Neurol., Chicago* **31**, 134.

Edelson, R. N., Deck, M. D. F. and Posner, J. B. (1972). Intramedullary spinal cord metastases. *Neurology, Minneapolis* **22**, 1222.

Ehni, G. (1975). Effects of certain degenerative diseases of the spine, especially spondylosis and disk protrusion, on the neural contents, particularly in the lumbar region. *Mayo Clin. Proc.* **50**, 327.

Elkington, J. St. C. (1936). Meningitis serosa circumscripta spinalis. *Brain.* **59**, 181.

Elsberg, C. A. (1925). *Tumors of the spinal cord.* Hoeber, New York.

Esses, S. I. and Morley, T. P. (1983). Spinal arachnoiditis. *Can. J. neurol. Sci.* **10**, 2.

Fearnside, M. R. and Adams, C. B. T. (1978). Tumours of the cauda equina. *J. Neurol. Neurosurg. Psychiat.* **41**, 24.

Freilich, D. and Swash, M. (1979). Diagnosis and management of tuberculous paraplegia with special reference to tuberculous radiculomyelitis. *J. Neurol. Neurosurg. Psychiat.* **42**, 12.

Ganes, T. (1980). Somatosensory conduction times and peripheral, cervical and cortical evoked potentials in patients with cervical spondylosis. *J. Neurol. Neurosurg. Psychiat.* **43**, 683.

Gessaga, E. C., Mair, W. G. P. and Grant, D. N. (1973). Ultrastructure of a sacrococcygeal chordoma. *Acta neuropath., Berlin* **25** 27.

Gilbert, R. W., Kim, J.-H. and Posner, J. B. (1978). Epidural spinal cord compression from metastatic tumor: diagnosis and treatment. *Ann. Neurol.* **3**, 40.

Gourie-Devi, M. and Satish, P. (1979). Enzyme therapy of spinal arachnoiditis—potential usefulness of hyaluronidase. *Curr. Sci.* **48**, 1017.

Grainger, R. G. and Lamb, J. T. (1980). *Myelographic techniques with metrizamide.* Nyegaard (UK), Birmingham.

Greenberg, A. D. (1968). Atlanto-axial dislocations. *Brain* **91**, 655.

Greenberg, H. S., Kim, J.-H. and Posner, J. B. (1980). Epidural spinal cord compression from metastatic tumor: results with a new treatment protocol. *Ann. Neurol.* **8**, 361.

Hassan, I. (1976). Cauda equina syndrome in ankylosing spondylitis: a report of six cases. *J. Neurol. Neurosurg. Psychiat.* **39**, 1172.

Hassin, G. B. (1928). Circumscribed suppurative nontuberculous peripachy-meningitis. *Arch. Neurol. Psychiat., Chicago* **20**, 110.

Haughton, V. and Williams, A. L. (1982). *Computed tomography of the spine.* Mosby, St. Louis.

Hernandez, D, Vinuela, F, and Feasby, T. E. (1982). Recurrent paraplegia with total recovery from spontaneous spinal epidural hematoma. *Ann. Neurol.* **11**, 623.

Hirson, C. (1965). Spinal subdural abscess. *Lancet* **ii**, 1215.

Hughes, J. T. (1977). Spinal cord involvement by C4–C5 vertebral subluxation in rheumatoid arthritis: a description of 2 cases examined at necropsy. *Ann. Neurol.* **1**, 575.

Ingraham, F. D, and Matson, D. D. (ed.) (1954). Intraspinal tumours in *Neurosurgery of infancy and childhood*, p. 345. Thomas, Springfield, Illinois.

Irvine, D. H., Foster, J. B., Newell, D. J. and Klukvin, B. N. (1965). Prevalence of cervical spondylosis in a general practice. *Lancet* **i**, 1089.

Jameson, R. M. (1974). Prolonged survival in paraplegia due to metastatic spinal tumours. *Lancet i*, 1209.

Jensen, T. S. and Hein, O. (1978). Intraspinal arachnoiditis and hydrocephalus after lumbar myelography using methylglucamine iocarmate. *J. Neurol. Neurosurg. Psychiat.* **41**, 108.

Jones, M. W. and Kaufmann, J. C. E. (1976). Vertebrobasilar artery insufficiency in rheumatoid atlantoaxial subluxation. *J. Neurol. Neurosurg. Psychiat.* **39**, 122.

Kernohan, J. W., Woltman, H. W. and Adson, A. W. (1931). Intramedullary tumors of the spinal cord. *Arch. Neurol. Psychiat., Chicago*, **25**, 679.

Lakke, J. P. W. F. (1975). Detection of obstruction of the spinal canal by CSF manometry. In *Handbook of clinical neurology*. (ed. P. J. Vinken and G. W. Bruyn) Vol. 19, p. 91. North-Holland, Amsterdam.

The Lancet (1977). Lumbar puncture and epidermoid tumours. *Lancet*. **i**, 635.

—— (1982). Spinal cord compression in thalassaemia. *Lancet i*, 664.

Leri, A. (1926) *Études sur les affections de la colonne vertébrale.* Paris.

Logue, V. (1979). Angiomas of the spinal cord: review of the pathogenesis, clinical features, and results of surgery, *J. Neurol. Neurosurg. Psychiat.* **42**, 1.

——, Aminoff, M. J. and Kendall, B. E. (1974). Results of surgical treatment for patients with a spinal angioma. *J. Neurol. Neurosurg. Psychiat.* **37**, 1074.

Marks, J. S. and Sharp, J. (1981). Rheumatoid cervical myelopathy. *Quart. J. Med.* **50**, 307.

Matthews, W. B. (1959). The spinal bruit. *Lancet* **ii**, 1117.

——, (1968). Neurological complications of ankylosing spondylitis. *J. neurol. Sci.*, **6**, 561.

McAllister, V. L., Kendall, B. E. and Bull, J. W. D. (1975). Symptomatic vertebral haemangiomas. *Brain* **98**, 71.

McConkey, B. (1982). Rheumatoid cervical myelopathy. *Br. med. J.*. **284**, 1731.

Moseley, I. (1982). Recent developments in imaging techniques. *Br. med J.* **284**, 1141.

Nassar, S. I. and Correll, J. W. (1968). Subarachnoid hemorrhage due to spinal cord tumours. *Neurology, Minneapolis* **18**, 87.

Newman, M. J. D. (1958). Spinal angioma with symptoms in pregnancy. *J. Neurol. Neurosurg. Psychiat.* **21**, 38.

Newman, P. K. and Tilley, P. J. B. (1979). Myelopathy in Marfan's syndrome. *J. Neurol. Neurosurg. Psychiat.* **42**, 176.

Nugent, G. R., Odom, G. L. and Woodhall, B. (1959). Spinal extradural cysts. *Neurology, Minneapolis* **9**, 397.

Oddsson, B. (1947). *Spinal meningioma.* Copenhagen.

Packer, N. P. and Cummins, B. H. (1978). Spontaneous epidural haemorrhage: a surgical emergency. *Lancet* **i**, 356.

Parkinson, D., Chaudhuri, A. and Shwartz, I. (1976). Congenital intraspinal extradural cysts (intraspinal meningocele). *Can. J. neurol. Sci*, **3**, 205.

Payne, J. P. and Bergentz, S. E. (1956). Paraplégia following spinal anaesthesia. *Lancet* **i**, 666.

Penning, L. (1961). Atlanto-axial instability and functional X-ray examination. *Medica-mundi* **7**, 113.

Pettersson, H. and Harwood-Nash, D. C. F. (1982). *CT and myelography of the spine and cord.* Springer-Verlag, Berlin.

Raja, I. A. and Hankinson, J. (1970). Congenital spinal arachnoid cysts. *J. Neurol. Neurosurg. Psychiat.* **33**, 105.

Raynor, R. B. (1969). Papilledema associated with tumors of the spinal cord. *Neurology, Minneapolis* **19**, 700.

Ridsdale, L. and Moseley, I. (1978). Thoracolumbar intraspinal tumours presenting features of raised intracranial pressure. *J. Neurol. Neurosurg. Psychiat.* **41**, 737.

Ross, J. C., Gibbon, N. O. K. and Damanski, M. (1964). Bladder dysfunction in non-traumatic paraplegia. *Lancet i*, 779.

Rubinstein, L. J. and Logan, W. J. (1970). Extraneural metastases in ependymoma of the cauda equina. *J. Neurol. Neurosurg. Psychiat.* **33**, 763.

Schäfer, E. –R. (1975). The spinal compression syndrome. In *Handbook of clinical neurology* (ed. P. J. Vinken and G. W. Bruyn) Vol. 19, p. 347, North-Holland, Amsterdam.

Scrimgeour, E. M. (1981). Non-traumatic paraplegia in northern Tanzania. *Br. med. J.* **283**, 975.

Seddon, H. J. (1934–5). Pott's paraplegia: prognosis and treatment. *Br. J. Surg.* **22**, 769.

Shapiro, R. (1975). *Myelography* 3rd edn. Yearbook Medical Publishers, Chicago.

Shaw, M. D. M., Russell, J. A. and Grossart, K. W. (1978). The changing pattern of spinal arachnoiditis. *J. Neurol. Neurosurg. Psychiat.* **41**, 97.

Shepherd, R. H. (1966). A reappraisal of spinal intradural angiomas with particular emphasis on treatment by excision. *Proc. R. Soc. Med.* (film) **59**, 796.

Siegal, T., Siegal, T., Robin, G., Lubetzki-Korn, I. and Fuks, Z. (1982). Anterior decompression of the spine for metastatic epidural cord compression: a promising avenue of therapy? *Ann Neurol.* **11**, 28.

Slooff, J. L., Kernohan, J. W. and MacCarty, C. S. (1964). *Primary intramedullary tumors of the spinal cord and filum terminale.* Saunders, Philadelphia and London.

Stark, R. J., Henson, R. A. and Evans, S. J. W. (1982). Spinal metastases. A retrospective survey from a general hospital. *Brain* **105**, 189.

——, Kennard, C. and Swash, M. (1981). Hand wasting in spondylotic high cord compression: an electromyographic study. *Ann Neurol.* **9**, 58.

Stevens, J. C., Cartlidge, N. E. F., Saunders, M., Appleby, A., Hall, M. and Shaw, D. A. (1971). Atlanto-axial subluxation and cervical myelopathy in rheumatoid arthritis. *Quart. J. Med.* **40**, 391.

Stookey, B. (1927). Adhesive spinal arachnoiditis simulating spinal cord tumor. *Arch. Neurol. Psychiat., Chicago*, **17**, 151.

Swick, H. M., Sty, J. R. and Haughton, V. M. (1978). Clinical evaluation of metrizamide for neuroradiology in children. *Ann. Neurol.* **3**, 409.

Symonds, C. P. and Meadows, S. P. (1937). Compression of the spinal cord in the neighbourhood of the foramen magnum. *Brain* **60**, 52.

Tarlov, I. M. (1948). Cysts (perineurial) of sacral roots. Another cause (nemovabre) of sciatic pain. *J. Am. med. Ass.* **138**, 740.

Taylor, A. R. and Byrnes, D. P. (1974). Foramen magnum and high cervical cord compression. *Brain* **97**, 473.

Vinters, H. V. and Gilbert, J. J. (1981). Neurenteric cysts of the spinal cord mimicking multiple sclerosis. *Can. J. neurol. Sci.* **8**, 159.

Vogelsang, H. (1975). Angiography. In *Handbook of clinical neurology* (ed. P. J. Vinken and G. W. Bruyn) Vol. 19, p. 229. North-Holland, Amsterdam.

Walton, J. N. (1953). Subarachnoid haemorrhage of unusual aetiology. *Neurology, Minneapolis.* **3**, 517.

Weil, A. (1931). Spinal cord changes in lymphogranulomatosis. *Arch. Neurol. Psychiat., Chicago* **26**, 1009.

Wilkinson, M. (1973). *Cervical spondylosis,* 2nd edn. Heinemann, London.

Woltman, H. W., Kernohan, J. W., Adson, A. W. and Craig, W. McK.

(1951). Intramedullary tumors of spinal cord and gliomas of intradural portion of filum terminale; fate of patients who have these tumors. *Arch. Neurol. Psychiat., Chicago* **65**, 378.

Syringomyelia

Definition. A chronic disorder characterized pathologically by the presence of long cavities, surrounded by gliosis, situated in the central part of the spinal cord and often extending up into the medulla (syringobulbia). The principal clinical features are cutaneous analgesia and thermoanaesthesia, often with preservation of light touch and postural sensibility, but with muscular wasting and trophic changes, especially in the upper limbs, and symptoms of corticospinal-tract dysfunction in the lower limbs. The term 'syringomyelia' was first used by Ollivier in 1824.

Pathology

The typical pathological changes are most frequently found in the lower cervical and upper thoracic regions of the cord. Extension to the medulla is common, and the process may reach the pons or even as high as the internal capsule. Thoracolumbar and lumbosacral syringomyelia is rare and is usually due to a true hydromyelia associated with developmental anomalies, although ascending cavitation following traumatic transverse lesions of the cord, or in association with cord tumours, is also seen.

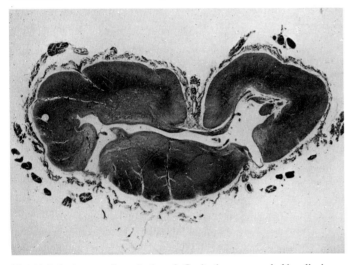

Fig. 14.6. Syringomyelia: spinal cord. Cavitation surrounded by gliosis.

The affected region of the cord is enlarged, mainly in the transverse plane (Fig. 14.6). In some cases the enlargement is sufficient to cause erosion of the bones of the spinal canal or at least widening of its anteroposterior diameter (Wells, Spillane, and Bligh 1959). Transverse section of the cord reveals a cavity surrounded by a zone of translucent gelatinous material which, microscopically, contains glial cells and fibres (Hughes 1978). The protein content of the fluid in the cavity is high. Barnett, Foster, and Hudgson (1973) distinguished between 'communicating' and noncommunicating syringomyelia; the pathogenesis of these two varieties will be discussed below. There is usually little difference, however, in the pathological characteristics of the cord cavities in the two varieties; the differences lie in the nature of the associated lesions.

The expanding cavity and surrounding gliosis, affecting the less resistant grey matter more severely than the dense white matter, at least in the first instance, invade the anterior horns of matter, thus causing atrophy of anterior horn cells, and degeneration of their axons in the ventral roots and peripheral nerves. Extension to the brainstem (syringobulbia) usually occurs first in the postero-lateral medulla near the spinal nucleus of the trigeminal nerve and the nucleus ambiguus, so that the earliest signs of brainstem dysfunction are usually due to the involvement of such nuclei. Compression of the long ascending and descending tracts of the cord or brainstem occurs rather later, giving secondary degeneration, most marked first in the corticospinal tracts, later in the spinothalamic tracts, and later still in the posterior columns. Haemorrhage into a syringomyelic cavity constitutes one uncommon form of haematomyelia.

Aetiology and pathogenesis

For many years it was thought that syringomyelia was due to a congenital abnormality perhaps causing abnormal closure of the central canal of the spinal cord in the embryo. Others took the view that the condition was a degenerative disorder of unknown cause. It is now evident that 'communicating syringomyelia' is the commoner variety (Barnett *et al*, 1973) and Gardner (Gardner and Angel 1958; Gardner 1965) was among the first to stress the relationship of the condition to congenital anomalies and other lesions in the neighbourhood of the foramen magnum, including the Chiari type I anomaly (congenital extension of the cerebellar tonsils below the foramen magnum), craniovertebral developmental abnormalities with or without occult hydrocephalus (Foster, Hudgson, and Pearce 1969), and basal arachnoiditis (Savoiardo 1976). Gardner suggested that abnormalities of this type, as well as the Dandy–Walker syndrome of closure of the foramina of Magendie and Luschka prevented, perhaps intermittently, the egress of CSF from the fourth ventricle into the subarachnoid space with the result that pressure waves of fluid were forced down into the central canal of the cord which thus became dilated (hydromyelia).

This view is now generally accepted, though opinions differ about the exact nature of the hydrodynamic mechanisms involved (Williams 1969, 1980*a*). The fact that a syringomyelic cavity is sometimes found to lie alongside an apparently normal spinal canal can be accounted for by the fact that, with dilatation of the canal, its ependymal lining quickly disappears and diverticula may form which dissect downwards (or sometimes upwards) alongside the canal in the central grey matter. In several large series of cases (Appleby, Foster, Hankinson, and Hudgson 1968; Barnett *et al.* 1973), the Chiari type I anomaly has been the commonest congenital anomaly to be found but basal arachnoiditis, developing either as a sequel to previous trauma, subarachnoid haemorrhage, or meningitis, or without evident cause, accounts for about a quarter of these cases. Arachnoiditis produced by cisternal injections of kaolin in dogs has been shown to produce experimental syringomyelia (Williams and Bentley 1980; Williams 1980*b*). It has also been suggested that perinatal trauma may either produce the cerebellar tonsillar ectopia (Williams 1977) or may induce syringomyelia in the presence of such a developmental anomaly (Newman, Terenty, and Foster 1981). However, it is also clear that primary cerebellar ectopia can be present without causing syringomyelia (Mohr, Strang, Sambrook, and Boddie 1977) but with other neurological signs such as hydrocephalus, paraparesis, or a cerebellar syndrome.

In 'non-communicating syringomyelia', by contrast (Barnett *et al.* 1973), the condition is more often due to or associated with spinal injury, with or without paraplegia (Shannon, Symon, Logue, Cull, Kang, and Kendall 1981), spinal arachnoiditis, or spinal tumour. In these cases the cavity may develop in the dorsal or lumbar cord first; indeed, except in cases of spina bifida (with which hydromyelia may be associated), the discovery of a lumbar syrinx in a patient without a history of injury should always raise the possiblity of a spinal glioma or ependymoma, though intramedullary metastases (Weitzner 1969) or extramedullary tumours are less common associations. In cases of traumatic paraplegia or arachnoiditis, the cavities usually ascend from the site of the lesion, but in upper cervical lesions downward cavitation is sometimes found. The cavitation has been attributed to a combination of factors including venous obstruction, exudation of protein, and ischaemia (Barnett *et al.* 1973), while oedema (Feigin, Ogota, and Budzilovich 1971) may be another factor. However, true communicating syringomyelia has been described as a complication of midbrain glioma (Williams and Timperley 1977).

Brewis, Poskanzer, Rolland, and Miller (1966) found the prevalence of syringomyelia to be 8.4 per 100 000 in an English city. The condition has been described in more than one member of a family (Bentley, Campbell, and Kaufmann 1975) and other congenital malformations, including spina bifida, have been found in families containing affected members. It is commoner in males than females and symptoms can appear at any age between 10 and 60 years but usually do so between 25 and 40.

Symptoms and signs

The symptoms of syringomyelia are readily interpreted as the outcome of the progressive lesion in the central region of the spinal cord.

Mode of onset

The onset is usually insidious but rarely develops rapidly over the course of a few weeks. Occasionally, indeed, the first symptoms may follow an episode of coughing, sneezing, or straining. Wasting and weakness of the small muscles of the hands are common early symptoms, but, alternatively, the patient may notice loss of feeling in the hands or the resulting injuries. Less often pain or trophic lesions first attract attention.

Sensory symptoms and signs

At the earliest stage there is an elongated cavity in the central grey matter extending longitudinally through several segments, usually in the lower cervical and upper thoracic cord segments. The lesion is often predominantly unilateral at first and therefore interrupts on one side the decussating sensory fibres derived from several consecutive dorsal roots. Since the fibres which decussate shortly after entering the cord are those which conduct impulses concerned in the appreciation of pain, heat, and cold, these forms of sensibility are impaired while other forms are preserved. This is the dissociated sensory loss described by Charcot, and usually appears first along the ulnar border of the hand, forearm, and arm, and on the upper part of the chest and back on one side in a 'half-cape' distribution with a horizontal lower border across the chest wall, ending sharply at the midline. Sometimes, however, sensation is impaired in a 'glove' area. When the lesion is centrally situated, or has extended from one side of the cord to the other, the area of dissociated sensory loss is bilateral. As it extends upwards and downwards in the cord, the area of sensory impairment extends to the radial sides of the upper limbs and neck, and downwards over the thorax, exhibiting at this stage a distribution *en cuirasse*. When the lesion reaches the upper cervical segments, it begins to involve the spinal tract and nucleus of the trigeminal nerve, which receives fibres conducting impulses concerned in the appreciation of pain, heat, and cold from the face. Progressive destruction of these fibres causes extension of the area of dissociated sensory loss in a concentric manner from behind forwards on the face, sensibility on the tip of the nose and upper lip sometimes being last affected. Exceptionally the disorder begins in the medulla, in which case sensory loss appears first on the face.

The progressive extension of the spinal lesion later causes compression of the lateral spinothalamic tracts on one or both sides, leading to loss of appreciation of pain, heat, and cold over the lower parts of the body. There is sometimes an area of normal sensibility over the abdomen intervening between the area of thoracic anaesthesia due to interruption of the decussating fibres and the area of sensory loss on one or both lower limbs due to compression of the spinothalamic tracts. When the spinothalamic tract is compressed at the level of the medulla, appreciation of pain, heat, and cold is impaired or lost over the whole of the opposite half of the body. The posterior columns are usually the last of the sensory pathways to suffer, but in the late stages appreciation of posture, passive movement, and vibration is likely to be impaired, especially in the lower limbs, and there may even be extensive anaesthesia to light touch.

Thermo-anaesthesia may be detected by the patient, since hot water no longer feels hot over the affected parts, and his analgesia exposes him to injuries, especially burns of the fingers, which he does not notice at the time, being painless. Spontaneous pains, though by no means invariable, are sometimes troublesome, and the patient may describe burning, aching, or shooting pains which rarely resemble the lightning pains of tabes; more often the pain is continuous and may then cause considerable distress. Such pains in one side of the face or in the upper limb may be the first symptom. When the lesion begins in the thoracolumbar or lumbosacral regions of the cord, the dissociated loss has an appropriate distribution. In non-communicating cases secondary to spinal-cord trauma or other lesions, an ascending sensory 'level' after months or years during which the neurological condition had been static will suggest the presence of an ascending syrinx.

Clinical manifestations of hydrocephalus develop in occasional cases.

Motor symptoms and signs

The earliest motor manifestations are usually muscular weakness and wasting, due to compression or destruction of anterior horn cells. Since the lesion usually begins in the cervicothoracic cord, muscular wasting usually first appears in the small hand muscles. It may be bilateral from the beginning, or one hand may suffer before the other. As the lesion extends, the wasting spreads to involve the forearms, and later the arms, shoulder girdles, and upper intercostals. It is often slight, and is never as severe as that seen in advanced motor-neurone disease. Fasciculation is uncommon. Contractures may develop, especially in hand and forearm muscles. Extension of the lesion to the posterolateral medulla often involves the nucleus ambiguus, causing paresis of the soft palate, pharynx, and vocal cord, occasionally giving laryngeal stridor (Alcala and Dodson 1975). The other motor functions of the cranial nerves are less often affected, though Brain observed paralysis of mandibular muscles, lateral rectus, facial muscles, and soft palate on one side as a result of haemorrhage into a syringomyelic cavity in the pons and medulla. The tongue is commonly involved and nystagmus is also common. It is variable in character, sometimes being phasic and present on lateral gaze, but may be dissociated in type, while vertical nystagmus on upward gaze is often seen (Thrush and Foster 1973); it has been ascribed to involvement of the cerebellar tonsils or of vestibular and cerebellar connections in the brainstem. Paralysis of the ocular sympathetic on one or both sides may be present, giving Horner's syndrome. The reaction to light is preserved.

Compression of the corticospinal tracts in the spinal cord causes weakness, with slight spasticity and extensor plantar responses in most cases in the later stages. The loss of power, however, is rarely severe. The tendon reflexes are exaggerated in the lower limbs, but are diminished or lost early in the upper limbs, particularly on the side of the dissociated anaesthesia, due to interruption of the reflex arc; only very rarely are they exaggerated in the arms, depending upon the predominance of the upper motor-neurone lesion. The sphincters are usually little affected. As with the sensory findings, ascending weakness of lower or upper motor-neurone type, or both, is an important feature of non-communicating syringomyelia, extending upwards from a spinal lesion.

Trophic symptoms and signs

Trophic symptoms are conspicuous. True hypertrophy involving all tissues may be present in one limb or one-half of the body or even the tongue. Loss of sweating or excessive sweating may occur, usually over the face and upper limbs. Excessive sweating may be spontaneous or may be excited reflexly when the patient takes hot or highly-seasoned food. Twenty per cent of patients exhibit osteoarthropathy—Charcot's joints. The shoulders, elbows, and cervical spine are most often affected, less often the joints of the hands, the temporomandibular joint, the sternoclavicular and acromioclavicular joints, and the joints of the lumbar spine or lower limbs. Atrophy and decalcification of bones around the joints with erosion of joint surfaces and subsequent bony destruction are the usual radiographic findings (Fig. 14.7). The joint changes are not usually associated with pain. The affected joint is often enlarged, and movement evokes loud crepitus but is generally painless. The long bones are often brittle. Trophic changes in the skin include cyanosis, hyperkeratosis, and thickening of the subcutaneous tissues, leading to a swelling of the fingers described as 'la main succulente'. The analgesia, as already described, renders the patient exceptionally liable to repeated minor injuries, and healing is often slow. Ulceration, whitlows, and necrosis of bone are not uncommon. Gangrene rarely occurs. The scars of former injuries are usually evident upon the palmar surface of the fingers (Fig. 14.8).

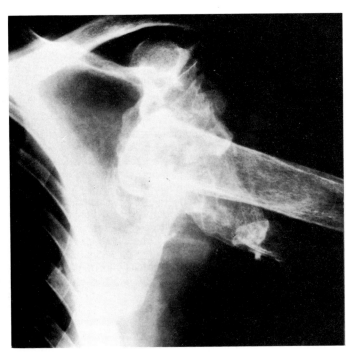

Fig. 14.7. A Charcot's shoulder joint in syringomyelia.

Syringobulbia
The medulla may be involved by upward extension from the cord, or may be the primary site of the disorder, when the onset of symptoms may be sudden or gradual. Trigeminal pain, vertigo, facial, palatal, or laryngeal palsy, or wasting of the tongue may each be the presenting symptom. The physical signs of syringobulbia have been described above.

Morvan's syndrome
Morvan (1883) described patients with painless whitlows on the fingers of both hands. Subsequently this title has been applied to cases in which there is progressive loss of pain sensation, ulceration, loss of soft tissue, and resorption of the phalanges with muscular atrophy, not only in the hands but sometimes also in the feet, with perforating ulcers. While it is clear that such changes in the hands do rarely occur in syringomyelia (Barnett *et al.* 1973), a similar syndrome may occur in leprosy; in most cases in which all four extremities are involved, the underlying pathology is one of hereditary sensory neuropathy or so-called acrodystrophic neuropathy (Spillane and Wells 1969; Bradley 1974).

Associated abnormalities
Many developmental and other abnormalities have been described in association with syringomyelia, occurring either in affected individuals or in members of their families. Bremer (1926) drew attention to the following: deformities of the sternum, kyphoscoliosis, a difference in the size of the breasts, increase in the ratio between arm and body length, acrocyanosis of the hands, curved fingers, enuresis, and anomalies of the hair and ears. Common abnormalities which may be added to Bremer's list include cervical rib, spina bifida, basilar impression of the skull, fusion of cervical vertebrae (the Klippel–Feil syndrome) with shortening of the neck, and other craniovertebral anomalies, hydrocephalus, and pes cavus (Barnett *et al.* 1973). Light brown pigmentation either in spots or diffuse sheets, often in a segmental distribution, is occasionally seen, especially on the shoulders.

The cerebrospinal fluid
The CSF usually shows no abnormality unless the cavity is large enough to cause a block when the protein content of the fluid is then raised.

Radiology
Straight radiographs of the cervical spine may show congenital anomalies (e.g. fusion of vertebral bodies) or may demonstrate that the anteroposterior diameter of the spinal canal is greater than normal. Prone myelography will usually confirm that the spinal cord itself is enlarged and is usually helpful in identifying the cause of non-communicating syringomyelia (such as a spinal tumour or arachnoiditis) but supine examination of the region of the foramen magnum using injected air or contrast medium is necessary to show the descent of the cerebellar tonsils (Chiari type I anomaly) with which many 'communicating' cases are associated (Fig. 14.9; Appleby *et al.* 1968; Barnett *et al.* 1973). When no such abnormality is demonstrated , air encephalography or even ventriculography with air or contrast medium is still very rarely needed to show closure of the exit foramina of the fourth ventricle or basal arachnoiditis. Much more often the appearances on CT scanning are diagnostic; however, metrizamide ventriculography carried out by injection of metrizamide into a ventriculoperitoneal shunt has demonstrated in such a case continuity of the syringomyelic cavity with the ventricular system (Foster, Wing, and Bray 1980).

Electromyography
Single-fibre EMG studies have shown a relatively constant pattern of involvement of cervical anterior horn cells in this condition (Schwartz, Stalberg, and Swash 1980).

Diagnosis
There is little difficulty in making a diagnosis of syringomyelia in advanced cases, since the association of wasting and trophic lesions of the hands with extensive dissociated sensory loss, and with signs of long tract dysfunction in the lower limbs, is distinctive. The diagnosis is more difficult in the early stages and must be made then if treatment is to be effective. Intramedullary tumour of the spinal cord (especially ependymoma) may closely simulate this condition. As a rule, however, it progresses more rapidly and blockage of the spinal subarachnoid space, with resulting CSF changes, soon occurs. The same is true of extramedullary spinal tumours, while pain is usually a more prominent symptom of these lesions than of syringomyelia. Haematomyelia, though it may produce similar signs, develops acutely; however, haemorrhage into a syringomyelic cavity constitutes one rare form of haematomyelia. Cervical spondylosis, though it may cause wasting of proximal

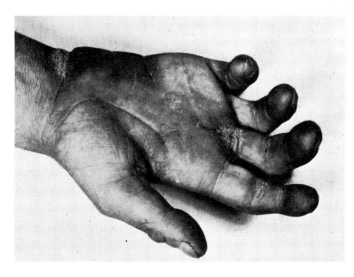

Fig. 14.8. Hand in syringomyelia, showing muscular wasting and fleshy fingers with scars of burns.

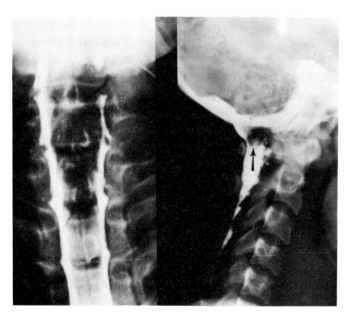

Fig. 14.9. The myelographic appearances of communicating syringomyelia in association with a Chiari type I anomaly. The anteroposterior view (on the left) shows marked widening of the upper cervical cord, while the lateral supine view demonstrates the ectopic cerebellar tonsils (arrow).

upper limb muscles and paraesthesiae in the hands as well as spastic weakness of the lower limbs, does not cause dissociated sensory loss in the arms and hands. Motor-neurone disease may simulate syringomyelia when it begins with wasting of small hand muscles, especially when corticospinal fibres to the lower limbs are simultaneously involved. Sensory loss, however, is absent, and muscular wasting develops more rapidly, while fasciculation is almost constantly present and usually widespread, whereas in syringomyelia it is less common. Cervical rib may cause symptoms which resemble those of early syringomyelia, and the distinction between the two is rendered difficult by the fact that they may coexist. Pain along the ulnar border of the hand and forearm is a common result of cervical rib, but rare in syringomyelia, and it is usual for the latter to become clinically overt when sensory loss is much more extensive than could be attributed to a cervical rib. Peroneal muscular atrophy is distinguished from syringomyelia by the fact that muscular wasting usually appears first in the lower

limbs. The trophic symptoms of Raynaud's disease may simulate syringomyelia, but dissociated sensory loss is absent in the former, while in the latter the attacks of blanching of the fingers seen in Raynaud's disease do not occur. Hereditary sensory neuropathy is distinguished by its early onset and by the distal loss of pain sensation in all four limbs.

Syringobulbia presents little diagnostic difficulty when it occurs as an upward extension of cervical syringomyelia. When it occurs alone, however, it must be distinguished from other medullary lesions. Thrombosis of the posterior inferior cerebellar artery, which may produce sensory loss similar to that found in syringobulbia, is distinguished by its acute onset. Tumours of the medulla may closely simulate syringobulbia, especially as symptoms of increased intracranial pressure may be slight or absent, but the onset is more rapid, and extension to the pons, leading to paralysis of the lateral rectus or conjugate ocular deviation and to facial paresis, is common in medullary tumours and rare in syringobulbia. Progressive bulbar palsy is distinguished by the lack of sensory loss. The diagnosis of basilar impression, which may closely simulate or be associated with syringomyelia, can be established only radiographically (see p. 607).

Prognosis

The course of syringomyelia, if untreated, is progressive, though progress is frequently slow, and prolonged arrest may occur, sometimes lasting for many years. A sudden intensification of symptoms may follow coughing, straining, or minor trauma (Barnett *et al.* 1973) or be produced by haemorrhage into a syringomyelic cavity, and exceptionally distension of the spinal cord may become so marked as to produce a complete transverse lesion leading to paraplegia. These events, however, are exceptional, and sufferers often live for many years, death occurring either from bulbar paralysis, leading to bronchopneumonia, or from some independent disease.

Treatment

In the past, apart from physiotherapeutic measures designed to reduce spasticity, delay contractures, and improve movement in weakened limbs, treatment of this condition was largely symptomatic. The protection of analgesic areas and early treatment of cutaneous lesions in order to promote healing were also regarded as essential and remain obligatory today. In some cases continuous pain has required powerful analgesics and rarely, if intractable, surgical methods (medullary tractotomy or stereotaxic thalamotomy), have been required for its relief. Some surgeons once recommended laminectomy for decompression of the swollen spinal cord with aspiration or incision and drainage of the cavity but the results were usually disappointing. However, in non-communicating cases secondary to spinal tumour or arachnoiditis, laminectomy with partial or complete removal of the causal tumour, decompression, the drainage of arachnoidal cysts or of the cavity itself, or the division of fibrous bands tethering the cord have all been helpful in some cases. When ascending cavitation follows a complete traumatic transverse lesion of the cord, the process may be arrested by total excision of a segment of the spinal cord at and just above the level of the injury (Barnett *et al.* 1973). For many years radiotherapy, introduced first in 1905, had a considerable vogue but is no longer used.

The discovery that in many communicating cases the condition is secondary to hydromyelia resulting from a developmental anomaly (Chiari malformation) in the region of the foramen magnum (Gardner 1965; Appleby *et al.* 1968) prompted many surgeons to recommend that the upper cervical cord and lower medulla should be decompressed at the foramen magnum and that if the exit foramina of the fourth ventricle were occluded they should be opened up and the upper end of the central canal should then be occluded with muscle or some other substance; aspiration of the central cavity may also be necessary (Hankinson 1970). If carried out sufficiently early in the course of the disease, the results of these procedures seem encouraging in that dissociated sensory loss may gradually disappear and reflex abnormalities may be reversed (Williams 1978; Logue and Edwards 1981; Pearce 1980); only rarely in very early cases is there complete recovery. Surgical treatment should thus be seriously considered in all such cases seen within a few years of the onset but is less likely to be helpful if the condition is long-established. When the condition is secondary to basal arachnoiditis or when a Chiari malformation is accompanied by arachnoiditis, the results of this operation are much less satisfactory. Some surgeons now recommend ventriculo-atrial drainage with a Spitz-Holter or other appropriate valve in such cases, but the results of this procedure are variable.

References

Alcala, H. and Dodson, W. E. (1975). Syringobulbia as a cause of laryngeal stridor in childhood. *Neurology, Minneapolis* **25**, 875.

Appleby, A., Foster, J. B., Hankinson, J. and Hudgson, P. (1968). The diagnosis and management of the Chiari anomalies in adult life. *Brain* **91**, 131.

Barnett, H. J. M., Foster, J. B., and Hudgson, P. (1973). *Syringomyelia*. Major Problems in Neurology series (ed. J. N. Walton). Saunders, London.

Bentley, S. J., Campbell, M. J. and Kaufmann, P. (1975). Familial syringomyelia. *J. Neurol. Neurosurg. Psychiat.* **38**, 346.

Bradley, W. G. (1974) *Disorders of peripheral nerves*. Blackwell, Oxford.

Bremer, F. W. (1926). Klinische Untersuchungen zur Ätiologie der Syringomyelie, der 'Status dysraphicus'. *Dtsch. Z. Nervenheilk.* **95**, 1.

Brewis, M., Poskanzer, D. C., Rolland, C. and Miller, H. G. (1966). Neurological disease in an English city. *Acta neurol. scand.* **42**, Suppl. 24.

Cruchet, R. and Delmas-Marsalet, P. (1939). Sur la maladie de Morvan. *Confin. neurol. Basel* **2**, 32.

Feigin, I., Ogata, J. and Budzilovich, G. (1971). Syringomyelia: the role of edema in its pathogenesis. *J. Neuropath. exp. Neurol.* **30**, 216.

Foster, J. B., Hudgson, P. and Pearce, G. W. (1969). The association of syringomyelia and congenital cervicomedullary anomalies: pathological evidence. *Brain* **92**, 25.

Foster, N. L., Wing, S. D. and Bray, P. F. (1980). Metrizamide ventriculography in syringomyelia. *Neurology, Minneapolis* **30**, 1323.

Gardner, W. J. (1965). Hydrodynamic mechanism of syringomyelia; its relationship to myelocele. *J. Neurol. Psychiat.* **28**, 247.

—— and Angel, J. (1958). The cause of syringomyelia and its surgical treatment. *Cleveland Clinic Quarterly* **25**, 4.

Hankinson, J. (1970). Syringomyelia and the surgeon. In *Modern trends in neurology* (ed. D. Williams), p. 127. Butterworths, London.

Hughes, J. T. (1978). *Pathology of the spinal cord*, 2nd edn. Lloyd-Luke, London.

Lassman, L. P., James, C. C. M., and Foster, J. B. (1968). Hydromyelia. *J. neurol. Sci.* **7**, 149l.

Logue, V. and Edwards, M. R. (1981). Syringomyelia and its surgical treatment—an analysis of 75 patients. *J. Neurol. Neurosurg. Psychiat.* **44**, 273.

Mohr, P. D., Strang, F. A., Sambrook, M. A. and Boddie, H. G. (1977). The clinical and surgical features in 40 patients with primary cerebellar ectopia (adult Chiari malformation). *Quart. J. Med.* **46**, 85.

Morvan, A. M. (1883). De la parésie analgésique à panaris des extrémitiés supérieures ou paréso-analgésie des extrémités supérieures. *Gazette Hebdomadaire Médecine et de Chirurgie* **35**, 580.

Newman, P. K., Terenty, T. R. and Foster, J. B. (1981). Some observations on the pathogenesis of syringomyelia. *J. Neurol. Neurosurg. Psychiat.* **44**, 964.

Pearce, J. M. S. (1981). Surgical management of syringomyelia. *Br. med. J.* **283**, 1204.

Savoiardo, M. (1976). Syringomyelia associated with postmeningitic spinal arachnoiditis. *Neurology, Minneapolis* **26**, 551.

Schwartz, M. S., Stalberg, E. and Swash, M. (1980). Pattern of segmental motor involvement in syringomyelia: a single fibre EMG study. *J. Neurol. Neurosurg. Psychiat.* **43**, 150.

Shannon, N., Symon, L., Logue, V., Cull, D., Kang, J and Kendall, B. E. (1981). Clinical features, investigation and treatment of post-traumatic syringomyelia. *J. Neurol. Neurosurg. Psychiat.* **44**, 35.

Spillane, J. D. and Wells, C. E. C. (1969). *Acrodystrophic neuropathy*. Oxford University Press, London.

Thrush, D. C. and Foster, J. B. (1973). An analysis of nystagmus in 100 consecutive patients with communicating syringomyelia. *J. neurol. Sci.* **20**, 381.

Weitzner, S. (1969). Coexistent intramedullary metastasis and syringomyelia of cervical spinal cord. *Neurology, Minneapolis* **19**, 674.

Wells, C. E. C., Spillane, J. D. and Bligh, A. S. (1959). The cervical spinal canal in syringomyelia. *Brain* **82**, 23.

Williams, B. (1969). Hypothesis: the distending force in the production of 'communicating syringomyelia'. *Lancet* **ii**, 189.

—— (1977). Difficult labour as a cause of communicating syringomyelia. *Lancet* **ii**, 51.

—— (1978). A critical appraisal of posterior fossa surgery for communicating syringomyelia. *Brain* **101**, 223.

—— (1980a). On the pathogenesis of syringomyelia: a review. *Proc. R. Soc. Med.* **73**, 798.

—— (1980b). Experimental communicating syringomyelia in dogs after cisternal kaolin injection. Part 2. Pressure studies. *J. neurol. Sci,* **48**, 109.

—— and Bentley, J. (1980). Experimental communicating syringomyelia in dogs after cisternal kaolin injection. Part 1. Morphology. *J. neurol. Sci.* **48**, 93.

—— and Timperley, W. R. (1977). Three cases of communicating syringomyelia secondary to midbrain gliomas. *J. Neurol. Neurosurg. Psychiat.* **40**, 80.

Myelodysplasia (spinal dysraphism)

Myelodysplasia was the term employed by Fuchs (1909) to describe a condition which he believed to be due to incomplete closure of the neural tube in the embryo. It is often familial and sometime hereditary, and may superficially simulate lumbar syringomyelia. However, it is often non-progressive. The symptoms usually indicate a disturbance of function of the lumbosacral region of the spinal cord, though other parts may be affected. Myelodysplasia is closely related to spina bifida, with which it is almost invariably associated.

Lumbosacral myelodysplasia may be responsible or associated with a variety of clinical manifestations. The following are the commonest: impairment of sphincter control, leading sometimes to enuresis; deformities of the feet such as pes cavus and syndactylism of the toes; wasting of muscles below the knees, often asymmetrical with impairment of one or both ankle-jerks; dissociated sensory loss like that of syringomyelia over one or both legs; and trophic changes in the feet, such as delayed healing of wounds, chronic ulceration, and gangrene. Symptoms usually appear in childhood but in less severe cases first become manifest in young or even middle-aged adults. Spina bifida may only be evident radiologically.

The commonest anatomical abnormality of the spinal cord is *diastematomyelia* (a bifid state of the lower cord). In many cases the spinal cords are contained within a single dural tube but in others each cord has its own dural sheath and the two are separated by a bony or fibrocartilaginous septum (Fig. 14.10) which may prevent the normal ascent of the cord as the vertebral column grows or else it may compress one or other spinal cord (James and Lassman 1964). Either this anomaly itself or other associated lesions within the spinal canal such as lipomas (Lassman and James 1967), which are commonly present in cases of 'spinal dysraphism' may demand surgical treatment which often gives considerable improvement. Other associated lesions found in some cases include intramedullary dermoids, adhesions in the cauda equina, and ectopic dorsal nerve roots (James and Lassman 1967), while a low conus medullaris, tethered by a fibrous band to the dura in the region of an occult spina bifida may give a similar clinical picture (James and Lassman 1972). Rarely a similar anatomical anomaly in the cervical region gives a clinical picture resembling that of syringomyelia. Myelography is invaluable in differential

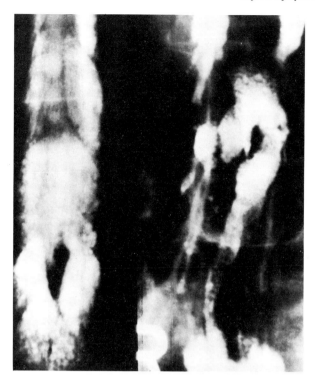

Fig. 14.10. A myelogram in a case of diastematomyelia; a prone antero-posterior view (on the left) shows diastematomyelia with a midline septum; the supine view (on the right) shows an intrathecal lipoma in the same case.

diagnosis but may have to be performed by the cisternal route under general anaesthesia in children (Gryspeerdt 1963). CT scanning and metrizamide myelography have greatly improved diagnostic accuracy (Haughton and Williams 1982; Pettersson and Harwood-Nash 1982). As there is a higher incidence of more overt neural-tube malformations such as spina bifida cystica and anencephaly in the families of such cases, mothers of children with spinal dysraphism should be offered prenatal screening during subsequent pregnancies (Carter, Evans, and Till 1976).

Myelodysplasia is distinguished from syringomyelia by the fact that it is occasionally familial and by its predominant effects upon the lower limbs. Other causes of muscular wasting and of trophic lesions of the feet must be excluded, especially peroneal muscular atrophy, hereditary sensory neuropathy, and ischaemia.

Although the spinal lesion is generally non-progressive, increasing pressure upon, or distortion of, the lower cord or cauda equina during growth produced by, say, a lipoma or fibrous band can give progressive muscular wasting, sensory loss, and trophic changes. Sometimes the condition first gives symptoms of a cauda-equina lesion, including urinary retention and impotence, in adult life.

There is no doubt, particularly when the lesion is in the lumbar region, that laminectomy with removal of lipomas or of bands which constrict or tether the spinal cord or its roots often gives considerable improvement.

References

Carter, C. O., Evans, K. A. and Till, K. (1976). Spinal dysraphism—genetic relation to neural tube malformations. *J. Med. Genet.* **13**, 343.
Fuchs, A. (1909). Über den klinischen Nachweis kongenitaler Defektbildungen in den unteren Rückenmarksabschnitten (Myelodysplasia). *Wien. med. Wschr.* **59**, 2142.
Gryspeerdt, L. (1963). Myelographic assessment of occult forms of spinal dysraphism. *Acta Radiol.* **1**, 702.
Haughton, V. M. and Williams, A. L. (1982). *Computed tomography of the spine.* Mosby, St Louis.

James, C. C. M. and Lassman, L. P. (1964). Diastematomyelia. *Arch. Dis. Childh.* **39**, 125.
—— and —— (1967). Results of treatment of progressive lesions in spina bifida occulta five to ten years after laminectomy. *Lancet* **ii**, 1277.
—— and —— (1972). *Spinal dysraphism (spina bifida occulta).* Butterworths, London.
Lassman, L. P. and James, C. C. M. (1967). Lumbosacral lipomas: critical survey of 26 cases submitted to laminectomy. *J. Neurol. Neurosurg. Psychiat.* **30**, 174.
Lichtenstein, B. W. (1940). Spinal dysraphism. Spina bifida and myelodysplasia. *Arch. Neurol. Psychiat., Chicago* **44**, 792.
Pettersson, H. and Harwood-Nash, D. C. F. (1982). *CT and myelography of the spine and cord.* Springer-Verlag, Berlin.
Riley, H. A. (1930). Syringomyelia or myelodysplasia. *J. nerv. ment. Dis.* **72**, 1.
Thévenard, A. (1942). L'arthropathie ulcéro-mutilante familiale. *Rev. neurol. Paris.* **74**, 193.

Caudal dysplasia (sacral agenesis)

This rare developmental anomaly, also called the caudal regression syndrome, is characterized by clinical and radiographic evidence of agenesis of the sacrococcygeal segments of the vertebral column and spinal cord; there is associated severe atrophy of the related spinal roots and nerves with grossly impaired innervation of the lower limb musculature (Price, Dooling, and Richardson 1970; Sarnat *et al.* 1976). Patients so affected have neurological abnormalities ranging in severity from mild impairment of bladder control to total motor and sensory paralysis below the level of the lesion. Other developmental anomalies (often of the cervical spine such as the Klippel–Feil deformity or multiple hemivertebrae) and of the abdominal viscera are often found in such cases.

References

Price, D. L., Dooling, E. C. and Richardson, E. P. (1970). Caudal dysplasia (caudal regression syndrome), *Arch. Neurol., Chicago* **23**, 212.
Sarnat, M. B., Case, M. E. and Graviss, R. (1976). Sacral agenesis; neurologic and neuropathologic features. *Neurology, Minneapolis* **26** 1124.

The Arnold–Chiari malformation

The common association between the Arnold–Chiari malformation and hyrocephalus and some of its clinical manifestations were considered on p. 138 and that between the Chiari type I anomaly and syringomyelia was described on p. 412. It may, however, be conveniently noted here that this malformation, and sometimes an encephalocele, may be produced in animals by excess vitamin A, arsenate, or clofibrate (Marin-Padilla 1980; Marin-Padilla and Marin-Padilla 1981). In human subjects, headache, ataxia, and dysphagia are sometimes the presenting symptoms, but so too in some cases are oscillopsia, diplopia, and blurred vision with vertical nystagmus (Spooner and Baloh 1981) or progressive upper-limb paralysis with sensory loss (Gol and Hellbusch 1978). In the former case suboccipital surgical decompression, in the latter re-routing of cervical nerve roots achieved by removal of part of the floor of the neural canal and/or facetectomy, may relieve the symptoms.

References

Gol, A. and Hellbusch, L. C. (1978). Surgical relief of progressive upper limb paralysis in Arnold–Chiari malformation. *J. Neurol. Neurosurg. Psychiat.* **41**, 433.
Marin-Padilla, M. (1980). Morphogenesis of experimental encephalocele (cranioschisis occulta). *J. neurol. Sci.* **46**, 83.
—— and Marin-Padilla, T. M. (1981). Morphogenesis of experimentally induced Arnold–Chiari malformation. *J. neurol. Sci,* **50**, 29.
Spooner, J. W. and Baloh, R. W. (1981). Arnold–Chiari malformation: improvement in eye movements after surgical treatment. *Brain* **104**, 51.

Congenital cervical spinal atrophy

Darwish, Sarnat, Archer, Brownell, and Kotagal (1981) described three children who at birth showed severe axial hypotonia, symmetrical flaccid paresis of the proximal and distal muscles of the upper limbs with poorly developed palmar flexion creases, and atrophy of small hand muscles. They postulate that this rare syndrome may have been due to a vascular insult involving the spinal cord during pregnancy as muscle biopsy revealed neurogenic atrophy of muscle and CT scanning showed greatly reduced density in several cervical cord segments.

Reference

Darwish, H., Sarnat, H., Archer, C., Brownell, K. and Kotagal, S. (1981). Congenital cervical spinal atrophy. *Muscle and Nerve* **4**, 106.

Spina bifida

Synonym. Rachischisis (an obsolete term)

Definition. Incomplete closure of the vertebral canal, which is usually associated with a similar anomaly of the spinal cord, or, when less severe, with other less striking intraspinal abnormalities.

Aetiology and pathology

In the early embryo the nervous system is represented by the neural groove, the lateral folds of which unite dorsally to form the neural tube. Arrest of this developmental process leads to defective closure of the neural tube, associated with a similar defect of closure of the bony vertebral canal—spina bifida. Several varieties of spina bifida are described, differing in respect of the nature and severity of the spinal defect. In the severe form a sac protrudes through the vertebral opening, yields an impulse on crying and coughing, and in the infant compression of the sac increases the tension of the fontanelle. The sac may contain meninges only—meningocele; in more severe cases it contains both meninges and the flattened, opened, or bifid spinal cord—myelocele or meningomyelocele. When the cutaneous covering is incomplete, there may be leakage of CSF. Very rarely the central canal of the cord is closed but dilated—syringomyelocele. Talwalker and Dastur (1970) distinguish six anatomical varieties of meningocele depending upon the association of such additional defects as fistulae, aberrant neural tissue, and tethering of the cord or roots, and three varieties of meningomyelocele which they prefer to call 'ectopic spinal cord'. In the least severe cases there is no protrusion, but a defect in the laminae may be palpable as a depression, which is sometimes covered by a dimple or a tuft of hair (spina bifida occulta). Often, however, there is no visible or palpable abnormality and the laminal defect is only then detected radiologically.

The commonest site of spina bifida is the lumbosacral region. Occasionally it is found in the thoracic region, very rarely in the cervical. In lumbosacral spina bifida the spinal cord often retains its fetal length and extends down to the sacrum. James and Lassman (1967, 1972) found in many cases of spina bifida occulta a variety of lesions including diastematomyelia, intramedullary dermoid, hydromyelia, cauda equina compression due to a fibrous band or to adhesions, ectopic dorsal nerve roots and subcutaneous lumbosacral lipoma communicating with a similar intraspinal lipoma. Spina bifida may be associated with other congenital abnormalities such as hydrocephalus due to atresia of the cerebral aqueduct or the Chiari type I (ectopia of the cerebellar tonsils) or type II (tonsillar ectopia with malformation of the medulla and cervical cord) anomalies (the latter is often called the Arnold–Chiari malformation—see above)(Spillane and Rogers 1959;

Emery and MacKenzie 1973). Other associated abnormalities in some cases include fusion of vertebral bodies or hemivertebrae, occipital meningocele, cervical hydromyelia or syringomyelia, hare lip, and cleft palate. Severe degrees of spina bifida may be incompatible with survival, the victim being stillborn or surviving birth only a short time. Paralysis of the lower limbs and of the sphincters is usually present in the latter type of case.

Renwick (1972) suggested that spina bifida and anencephaly might be related to the consumption of potatoes affected by 'blight', but this hypothesis was not supported by subsequent epidemiological studies which did, however, suggest a slightly increased incidence in females and a significant increase in incidence in Rochester, Minnesota in 1944 corresponding to a rubeola epidemic (Haynes, Gibson, and Kurland 1974). A possible relationship to hardness of water supplies is also unconfirmed to date (Lowe, Roberts, and Lloyd 1971). MacMahon and Yen (1971) noted a threefold increase in the incidence of these malformations in Boston, Massachusetts, in the years 1929–32, corresponding with the years of the great depression. It has been suggested that subclinical vitamin deficiency at conception and during early pregnancy is a possible cause and that periconceptual vitamin supplementation may prevent these malformations (Smithells, Sheppard, Schorah, Seller, Nevin, Harris, Read, and Fielding 1980); however, it is known that excess vitamin A may be a factor in producing anencephaly (*The Lancet* 1980). A recent proposal of the Medical Research Council(UK) to mount a controlled trial to investigate this problem aroused much ethical controversy (*The Lancet* 1982a) but the trial is proceeding. There is no evidence that a history of prior miscarriage is a significant factor (Laurence and Roberts 1977). Recently, some evidence has emerged to indicate that sodium valproate taken during pregnancy is significantly associated with neural-tube defects (Bjerkedal, Czeizel, Goujard, Kallen, Mastroiacova, Nevin, Oakley, and Robert 1982; Stanley and Chambers 1982; Jeavons 1982; *The Lancet* 1982b). Carter and Evans (1973) have estimated that the risk that a parent with spina bifida may transmit the condition to his or her offspring of either sex is about 3 per cent and it is also clear that there is an increased incidence of spina bifida in sibs of children with other malformations (Fraser, Czeizel, and Hanson 1982).

Symptoms and signs

Spina bifida occulta may give rise to no symptoms throughout life and may be an accidental discovery in the course of a routine examination. It is present in 17 per cent of all spines X-rayed (Curtius and Lorenz 1933). However, intradural lesions associated with it sometimes give rise to symptoms, of which the cause is not immediately evident. In such cases the history may reveal that symptoms were present at an early age, with later improvement, to be followed by a relapse in early adult life. However, in occasional cases, symptoms, say due to an intradural lipoma, may not appear until middle or late life. Such a relapse may be due to the effect of growth in causing tension upon the lower end of the cord and cauda equina, which are anchored at an abnormally low level, or to the compression of these structures by a lipoma, dermoid, or constricting band. The symptoms are those of a chronic lesion of the cauda equina, though one function is often more conspicuously affected than others.

Frequently is is noted that the patient was slow in learning to walk and walked clumsily at first. Muscular wasting and weakness may be present in the muscles below the knees, with impairment or loss of the ankle-jerks and contracture of the calf muscles, leading to pes cavus. James and Lassman (1967, 1972) drew particular attention to a milder syndrome of progressive muscular imbalance and neurological deficit resulting in deformity of one or both feet in childhood with, in some cases, trophic ulceration and incontinence, and pointed out that this syndrome resulting from minimal spinal dysraphism always demands investigation, as early treatment may prevent progressive deformity. Sensation may be impaired over the cutaneous areas innervated by the lowest sacral segments, with a typical saddle-shaped area of analgesia over the buttocks and posterior surface of the thighs. Pain is usually inconspicuous. Sphincter disturbances are often prominent. Enuresis may be present, either constantly or intermittently, from infancy. The patient may have been late in gaining control over the bladder as a child, and this may never have become complete. Often there is also precipitate micturition by day. Less often retention of urine develops with secondary hydro-ureter and hydronephrosis and impairment of renal function. The rectal sphincter is less often affected, though constipation or, less frequently, incontinence of faeces may occur. Impotence may be present in the male, either from the beginning of sexual life or after a period of normal potency. Trophic changes are conspicuous in some cases, and are rarely absent. In milder cases the feet are usually cold and cyanosed, and cutaneous injuries are slow to heal and tend to lead to ulceration, not only of the feet but also of the analgesic skin of the buttocks and thighs. Gangrene of the toes may occur and Charcot type arthropathy has been described in the feet. These more severe neurological and associated abnormalities, of all degrees of severity up to complete flaccid paraparesis with sphincter paralysis, are more often associated with overt spina bifida than with the occult form. Less common associated abnormalities include global atrophy or oedema of one lower limb, melanoleucoderma, and cutaneous naevi.

Cervical spina bifida occulta may be associated with hydromyelia or diastematomyelia causing symptoms resembling those of syringomyelia in the upper limbs, with wasting and trophic disturbances in the hands, and dissociated sensory loss.

The CSF usually shows no abnormality, though lumbar puncture may be difficult or impossible at the usual level. Radiography shows defective fusion of the laminae in the affected region, usually the first sacral and fifth lumbar. CT scanning may be diagnostic (Haughton and Williams 1982) but, if myelography is necessary it is best performed by the cisternal route in such cases and is often successful in demonstrating diastematomyelia, an unusually low position of the conus medullaris, a typical filling defect due to a lipoma, or even a fibrous band constricting the cauda equina (Gryspeerdt 1963).

Diagnosis

The diagnosis of spina bifida cystica with a protruding sac is easy. Spina bifida occulta, however, may be missed, if not borne in mind as a possible cause of the patient's symptoms. All cases of enuresis for which no cause can be found, especially when precipitate micturition occurs by day, should be carefully examined for the presence of minor neurological signs in the lower limbs, and radiographs of the lumbosacral spine should be taken. The more severe symptoms of spina bifida must be differentiated from those of a tumour of the cauda equina, while, when trophic lesions are prominent, it is necessary to exclude acrodystrophic neuropathy and peripheral vascular disease. The fact that in spina bifida symptoms have often been present since birth is an important diagnostic point, while the rarity of pain and the relatively nonprogressive nature of the condition will help to exclude tumour. The CSF protein content is much more often raised when a tumour is present than in dysraphism. And, of course, normal arterial pulses help to exclude arterial disease. X-ray examination of the spine, CT scanning (Pettersson and Harwood-Nash 1982), and myelography afford confirmatory evidence.

Antenatal diagnosis. An important development was the discovery that estimation of alpha-fetoprotein (AFP) in the amniotic fluid (Brock and Sutcliffe 1972; Allan, Ferguson-Smith, Donald, Sweet, and Gibson 1973; Seller Campbell, Coltart, and Singer 1973) or in the maternal serum (Brock, Bolton, and Scrimgeour 1974; Wald, Brock, and Bonnar 1974; UK Collaborative Study

1977, 1979) may successfully identify a fetus with a severe CNS malformation such as spina bifida cystica or anencephaly. It is now evident that AFP is an oncofetal antigen (*The Lancet* 1979); the mean serum AFP concentration in control pregnancies is about 54 mg/ml and a two- to 10-fold increase is seen at about 16 weeks in pregnancies in which the fetus has a major neural-tube defect. It is also clear that measurement of acetylcholinesterase (AChE) in amniotic fluid is an effective means of diagnosing open neural-tube defects (Smith, Wald, Cuckle, Stirrat, Bobrow, and Lagercrantz 1979; Hullin, Elder, Laurence, Roberts, and Newcombe 1981). Screening of pregnant women by means of serum alpha-fetoprotein estimation is therefore possible followed by ultrasonic examination and/or anmiocentesis with subsequent measurement of AFP and AChE in the fluid, leading in appropriate cases to therapeutic abortion. Ferguson-Smith, Rawlinson, May, Tait, Vince, Gibson, Robinson, and Ratcliffe (1978) showed that serum AFP screening was an effective means of identifying fetal neural-tube defects and in 11 585 pregnancies there were no terminations of normal pregnancies due to false–positive amniotic AFP results.

Prognosis

In the past, sufferers from the more severe degrees of spina bifida did not long survive. However, in recent years, early surgical treatment carried out in the first few days of life (see below) has resulted in there being many more survivors (Brocklehurst 1976). Laurence (1974) showed that without operation, in 100 patients with myelocele and meningocele, only 17 will survive into the teens with eight minimally handicapped and five dependent on wheelchairs. With aggressive early operative treatment 50 per cent will survive, 15 being minimally handicapped and 27 dependent on wheelchairs. There was a significantly higher incidence of mental handicap, usually due to hydrocephalus, in the survivors following operation.

In patients suffering complications of occult spina bifida the prognosis is generally very much better, especially now that ascending urinary infection and other renal complications can usually be treated effectively.

Treatment

Sharrard (1963) and others showed that the survival rate of sufferers from meningomyelocele may be greatly increased and subsequent disability greatly reduced by operative closure of the sac within the first 48 hours of life. Subsequent neurosurgical treatment may be required for associated hydrocephalus and various orthopaedic procedures may also be needed. Even if the lower limbs seem totally paralysed and anaesthetic, walking may eventually be possible with appropriate appliances if training is begun sufficiently early, usually towards the end of the second year of life. Incontinence of urine may be controlled in some cases by propantheline given in doses graded according to age (15 mg three times daily in the adult), while retention of urine may initially require catheterization followed later by bladder-neck resection. Urinary infection will require appropriate antibiotics and incontinence of faeces is usually controlled eventually by means of suppositories, regular enemas, or even, in some cases, manual evacuation as the child grows older. The selection of cases for early operation, depending upon the potential quality of life in the survivors and the prospect of independent existence, is still a fertile source of controversy and raises serious ethical problems. Lorber (1973, 1975) and Brocklehurst (1976) argued against a policy of operating upon all cases; in 37 newborn infants Lorber advised against operation in 25 because of the severity of the malformation and all died within nine months. Hunt, Lewin, Gleave, and Gairdner (1973) found the definition of predictive factors difficult but stressed the importance of defining the level of sensory impairment. Smith and Smith (1973) favoured operating early upon most infants with low lesions and a low sensory level, but postponing consideration of surgery for at least a month in more severe cases.

There is now good evidence that in cases of spina bifida occulta with neurological manifestations, operation carried out soon after symptoms first appear, to divide a constricting band, remove or decompress a lipoma or a dermoid cyst, may produce considerable improvement and prevent progressive deformity. This is particularly important in childhood so that growth of an affected limb will not be impaired, but operation may be equally successful if symptoms first develop in adult life.

References

Allan, L. D., Ferguson-Smith, M. A., Donald, I., Sweet, E. M. and Gibson, A. A. M. (1973). Amniotic-fluid alpha-fetoprotein in the antenatal diagnosis of spina bifida. *Lancet* ii, 522.

Bjerkedal, T., Czeizel, A., Goujard, J., Kallen, B., Mastroiacova, P., Nevin, N., Oakley, G. and Robert, E. (1982). Valproic acid and spina bifida. *Lancet* ii, 1096.

Brock, D. J. H., Bolton, A. E. and Scrimgeour, J. B. (1974). Prenatal diagnosis of spina bifida and anencephaly through maternal plasma-alpha-fetoprotein measurement. *Lancet* i, 767.

—— and Sutcliffe, R. G. (1972). Alpha-fetoprotein in the antenatal diagnosis of anencephaly and spina bifida. *Lancet* ii, 197.

Brocklehurst, G. (1976). *Spina bifida for the clinician.* Spastics International, No. 57. Heinemann, London.

Campbell, S., Pryse-Davies, J., Coltart, T. M., Seller, M. J. and Singer, J. D. (1975). Ultrasound in the diagnosis of spina bifida. *Lancet* i, 1065.

Carter, C. O. and Evans, K. (1973). Children of adult survivors with spina bifida cystica. *Lancet* ii, 924.

Curtius, F. and Lorenz, I. (1933).Über den Status dysraphicus, klinischer-bäiologische und rassenhygienische Untersuchungen an 35 Fällen von Status dysraphicus und 17 Fällen von Syringomyelie. *Z. ges. Neurol. Psychiat.* 149, 1.

Emery, J. L. and MacKenzie, N. (1973). Medullo-cervical dislocation deformity (Chiari II deformity) related to neurospinal dysraphism (meningomyelocele). *Brain* 96, 155.

Ferguson-Smith, M.A., Rawlinson, H. A., May, H. M., Tait, H. A., Vince, J. D., Gibson, A. A. M., Robinson, H. P. and Ratcliffe, J. G. (1978). Avoidance of anencephalic and spina bifida births by maternal serum-alphafetoprotein screening. *Lancet* i, 1330.

Fraser, F. C., Czeizel, A. and Hanson, C. (1982). Increased frequency of neural tube defects in sibs of children with other malformations. *Lancet* ii, 144.

Gryspeerdt, G. L. (1963). Myelographic assessment of occult forms of spinal dysraphism. *Acta radiol., Stockholm* 1, 702.

Hassin, G. B. (1925). Spina bifida occulta cervicalis. *Arch. Neurol. Psychiat., Chicago* 14, 813.

Haughton, V. M. and Williams, A. L. (1982). *Computed tomography of the spine.* Mosby, St. Louis.

Haynes, S. G., Gibson, J. B. and Kurland, L. T. (1974). Epidemiology of neural-tube defects and Down's syndrome in Rochester, Minnesota, 1935 – 1971. *Neurology, Minneapolis* 24, 691.

Hullin, D. A., Elder, G. H., Laurence, K. M., Roberts, A. and Newcombe, R. G. (1981). Amniotic fluid cholinesterase measurement as a rapid method for the exclusion of fetal neural-tube defects. *Lancet* ii, 325.

Hunt, G., Lewin, W., Gleave, I. and Gairdner, D. (1973). Predictive factors in open myelomeningocele with special reference to sensory levels. *Br. med. J.* 4, 197.

James, C. C. M. and Lassman, L. P. (1967). Results of treatment of progressive lesions in spina bifida occulta five to ten years after laminectomy. *Lancet* ii, 1277.

—— and —— (1972). *Spinal dysraphism (spina bifida occulta).* Butterworths, London.

Jeavons, P. M. (1982). Sodium valproate and neural tube defects. *Lancet* ii, 1282.

The Lancet (1979). Origin of maternal serum AFP. *Lancet* ii, 999.

—— (1980). Vitamins, neural-tube defects, and ethics committees. *Lancet* i, 1061.

—— (1982a). Vitamins to prevent neural tube defects. *Lancet* ii, 1255.

—— (1982b). Valproate and malformations. *Lancet* ii, 1313.

Lassman, L. P. and James,C. C. M. (1967). Lumbosacral lipomas: critical survey of 26 cases admitted to laminectomy. *J. Neurol. Psychiat.* 30, 174.

Laurence, K. M. (1974). Effect of early surgery for spina bifida cystica on survival and quality of life. *Lancet* i, 301.

—— and Roberts, C. J. (1977). Spina bifida and anencephaly: are miscarriages a possible cause? *Br. med. J.,* 2, 361.

Lorber, J. (1973). Early results of selective treatment of spina bifida cystica. *Br. med. J.* 3, 201.

—— (1975). Ethical problems in the management of myelomeningocele and hydrocephalus. *J. R. Coll. Phycns., London* 10, 47.

Lowe, C. R., Roberts, C. J. and Lloyd, S. (1971). Malformations of central nervous system and softness of local water supplies. *Br. med. J.* 2, 357.

MacMahon, B. and Yen, S. (1971). Unrecognized epidemic of anencephaly and spina bifida. *Lancet* i, 31.

Pettersson, H. and Harwood-Nash, D. C. F. (1982). *CT and myelography of the spine and cord.* Springer-Verlag, Berlin.

Renwick, J. H. (1972). Hypothesis: anencephaly and spina bifida are usually preventable by avoidance of a specific but unidentified substance present in certain potato tubers.*Br. J. prev. soc. Med.* 26, 67.

Roberts, J. B. M. (1962). Spina bifida and the urinary tract. *Ann. R. Coll. Surg., England* 31, 69.

Seller, M. J., Campbell, S., Coltart, T. M. and Singer, J. D. (1973). Early termination of anencephalic pregnancy after detection by raised alpha-fetoprotein levels. *Lancet* ii, 73.

Sharrard, W. J. W. (1963). Meningomyelocele: prognosis of immediate operative closure of the sac. *Proc. R. Soc. Med.* 56, 510.

Smith, A. D., Wald, N. J., Cuckle, H. S., Stirrat, G. M., Bobrow, M. and Lagercrantz, H. (1979). Amniotic-fluid acetylcholinesterase as a possible diagnostic test for neural-tube defects in early pregnancy. *Lancet* i, 685.

Smith, G. K. and Smith, E. D. (1973). Selection for treatment in spina bifida cystica. *Br. med. J.* 4, 189.

Smithells, R. W., Sheppard, S., Schorah, C. J., Seller, M. J., Nevin, N. C., Harris, R., Read, A. P. and Fielding, D. W. (1980). Possible prevention of neural-tube defects by periconceptional vitamin supplementation. *Lancet* i, 339.

Spillane, J. D. and Rogers, L. (1959). Lumbosacral spina bifida cystica with craniovertebral anomalies: report of two cases presenting with neurological disorder in adult life. *J. Neurol. Neurosurg. Psychiat.* 22, 144.

Stanley, O. H. and Chambers, T. L. (1982). Sodium valproate and neural tube defects. *Lancet* ii, 1282.

Talwalker, V. C. and Dastur, D. K. (19709). 'Meningoceles' and 'meningomyeloceles' (ectopic spinal cord). Clinicopathological basis of a new classification. *J. Neurol. Neurosurg. Psychiat.* 33, 251.

UK Collaborative Study (1977). Maternal serum-alpha-fetoprotein measurement in antenatal screening for anencephaly and spina bifida in early pregnancy. *Lancet* i, 1323.

—— (1979). Amniotic-fluid alpha-fetoprotein measurement in antenatal diagnosis of anencephaly and open spina bifida in early pregnancy. *Lancet* ii, 651.

Wald, N. J., Brock, D. J. H. and Bonnar, J. (1974). Prenatal diagnosis of spina bifida and anencephaly by maternal serum-alpha-fetoprotein measurement. *Lancet* i, 765.

Myelitis (myelopathy)

Definition. Inflammation of the spinal cord, usually involving both the grey and the white matter, in much of its transverse extent. When the process is limited longitudinally to a few segments, it is often described as transverse myelitis; when it spreads progressively upwards, as ascending myelitis. Since in this syndrome actual inflammation is not invariably present and demyelination, for example, may be the pathological substrate, some authors prefer to use the title myelopathy but myelitis is still generally favoured, provided this is not taken invariably to indicate an infective cause.

Aetiology

Myelitis may be a manifestation of meningovascular syphilis (see pp. 264–7). It may be due to involvement of the cord in acute or subacute viral encephalomyelitis or in acute encephalomyelitis, post-infective Devic's disease, and acute disseminated encephalo-myelitis complicating vaccination, smallpox, measles, chickenpox, or other specific fevers (p. 300). Thus it has been described as a complication of varicella (White 1962) and antirabies vaccination (Prussin and Katabi 1964), to name only two causes, and it may complicate infective mononucleosis (p. 258). In herpes zoster myelitis, the causal virus has been isolated from the spinal cord (Hogan and Krigman 1973). An episode indistinguishable from an attack of transverse myelitis may be one presentation of multiple sclerosis.

Myelitis may also be due to invasion of the cord by pyogenic organisms, which may reach it through a penetrating wound, by extension from osteomyelitis of an adjacent vertebra, by inward spread from pyogenic meningitis, or through the blood stream from a focus of infection in any part of the body, the latter being the route of infection in rare cases of intramedullary abscess or when myelitis rarely complicates typhoid fever or brucellosis. Tuberculous meningomyelitis also occurs, sometimes but by no means always as a result of tuberculosis of the spine. Schistosomal myelopathy due to *S. mansoni* (Cohen, Capildeo, Rose, and Pallis 1977) appears to be another rare cause of acute transverse myelitis due to an immune response to the parasite, and other granulomatous processes described elsewhere (e.g. connective tissue disease and sarcoidosis) sometimes cause the picture of acute or subacute myelitis.

Pathology

To the naked eye the spinal cord at the site of inflammation, usually the lower thoracic region, shows oedema and hyperaemia, and in severe cases actual softening – myelomalacia. Microscopically, the leptomeninges are congested and infiltrated with inflammatory cells. The cord substance exhibits congestion or thrombosis of vessels with perivascular inflammatory infiltration, and oedema. There is degeneration of ganglion cells, myelin sheaths, and axis cylinders. The cord is often diffusely infiltrated with inflammatory cells and with activated microglia. There is also gliosis in subacute cases. Ascending and descending degeneration can be traced in the long tracts. Abscess of the spinal cord is a very rare form of localized myelitis. The pus is encapsulated to a variable extent and, as it tends to spread longitudinally, the abscess usually has a spindle shape. When myelitis is due to pyogenic organisms, these may be demonstrable in films or on culture, and spirochaetes may be present in the syphilitic form, and, in the various granulomatous processes mentioned above, the specific histological changes, say, of sarcoidosis, may be found. Viral myelitis attacks primarily the grey matter, auto-immune post-infective myelitis the white, but often the pathological distinction between these two causes is not clear-cut, although the demonstration of viral particles by electron microscopy or fluorescent antibody techniques may help (Hughes 1978).

Symptoms and signs

The onset of symptoms is acute or subacute, often with pyrexia. There is usually considerable pain in the back at the level of the lesion. Flaccid paralysis, partial or complete, then develops more or less rapidly, being confined to part of the trunk and the lower limbs when the thoracic region of the cord is primarily involved. Sensory loss, which may be complete or incomplete, usually has an upper level corresponding to the segmental site of the lesion. There may be a zone of hyperpathia intervening between the area of sensory loss and that of normal sensibility above, and the spine may be tender in this region. There is impaired sphincter control often amounting to complete paralysis of the bladder and rectum. The tendon reflexes are usually at first diminished or lost due to spinal shock, and the abdominal reflexes are also lost below the level of the lesion. The plantar reflexes may be absent for a few days after the onset and later become extensor. In ascending mye-litis there is a more or less rapid upward progression of the paralysis and sensory loss (Landry's paralysis).

The CSF usually shows a considerable increase in protein content and cells, which are polymorphonuclear in the rare pyogenic cases, but usually exclusively or predominantly mononuclear in other forms. The VDRL and other serological reactions are negative, except in syphilitic cases. Gamma-globulin and specific immunoglobulins (especially IgG) are often raised, especially when an episode of 'transverse myelitis' is the first manifestation of multiple sclerosis.

Diagnosis

The rapid onset of the symptoms of a transverse or ascending lesion of the spinal cord usually renders the diagnosis easy, but CT scanning and/or myelography are usually obligatory in order to exclude acute cord compression. Myelitis is distinguished from acute post-infective polyneuritis (the Guillain–Barré syndrome) by the presence of extensor plantar reflexes, and of partial or complete sensory loss with a segmental upper level. Nevertheless, in the stage of spinal shock, when all reflexes, including the plantars, are absent, differentiation may not be easy; the CSF protein is raised, usually without a pleocytosis in the Guillain–Barré syndrome, in which the course is often less rapid, sensory loss less marked, and in which there is usually delayed conduction in peripheral nerves. Haematomyelia usually develops after injury; it usually involves the cervical enlargement and causes greater damage to the grey than to the white matter of the cord. Syphilitic myelitis is distinguished by positive serological reactions in the blood and CSF. When myelitis forms part of an attack of acute disseminated encephalomyelitis, cerebral symptoms may also be present, and in cases following vaccination and the specific fevers the causal condition is usually evident from the history. In disseminated myelitis with optic neuritis the diagnosis is clear when the latter precedes the former, but otherwise remains in doubt until optic neuritis develops. When myelitis rarely complicates poliomyelitis, the patient exhibits in addition the typical atrophic paralysis. In zoster myelitis the diagnosis is confirmed by the typical skin eruption. Though multiple sclerosis may be suspected as the cause of a transverse cord lesion, especially in a young adult, this diagnosis can only be established if there is a history of previous and characteristic lesions of the nervous system, or if signs of this—for example, pallor of the optic discs, nystagmus, or delayed visual evoked responses—are present. Serum and CSF antibody studies, viral culture, and/or immunofluorescent techniques may all assist in identifying a viral cause. The recording of visual, auditory, and of somatosensory evoked potentials has been found useful in distinguishing idiopathic cases from those in which the myelitis is due to multiple sclerosis (Ropper, Miett, and Chiappa 1982).

Prognosis

The prognosis depends upon the aetiology of the condition and its severity. Pyogenic myelitis is often fatal, but occasional cases of intramedullary abscess have been treated successfully with antibiotics and surgical drainage and mechanically-aided respiration has saved many patients who would previously have died of ascending myelitis. Any form of myelitis which is sufficiently severe to lead to a complete functional interruption of the cord must be considered grave, but nevertheless, if complications are prevented or treated effectively, recovery is possible. In myelitis forming part of acute disseminated encephalomyelitis the prognosis is often good, and if the patient survives the acute attack considerable functional recovery is the rule. In sporadic cases of myelitis the prognosis should be guarded in view of the possibility that the cord lesion may be the first symptom of multiple sclerosis. For the prognosis of syphilitic myelitis see page 267, and for that of acute disseminated myelitis with optic neuritis see page 306.

Treatment

General treatment is along the lines indicated for the treatment of paraplegia (see p. 394). Any specific cause must receive appropriate treatment. For the treatment of syphilitic myelitis see page 266 and for that of acute disseminated myelitis with optic neuritis see page 306.

In those cases in which no cause for the condition can be demonstrated (these are the majority) there is good evidence that treatment with ACTH, 80 units intramuscularly daily, when given in the acute phase and continued for several weeks or even months in diminishing dosage improves the outcome. Corticosteroid and immunosuppressive drugs are also used, but ACTH has been more generally favoured though no comparative controlled trials have been done.

References

Cohen, J., Capildeo, R., Rose, F. C. and Pallis, C. (1977). Schistosomal myelopathy. *Br. med. J.* **1,** 1258.

Davison, C. and Keschner,M. (1933). Myelitic and myelopathic lesions (a clinicopathologic study). 1. Myelitis. *Arch. Neurol. Psychiat., Chicago* **29,** 332.

Hogan, E.L. and Krigman, M. L. (1973). Herpes zoster myelitis. *Arch. Neurol., Chicago* **29,** 309.

Hughes, J. T. (1978). *Pathology of the spinal cord,* 2nd edn. Lloyd-Luke, London.

Prussin, G. and Katabi, G. (1964). Dorsolumbar myelitis following antirabies vaccination with duck embryo vaccine. *Ann. int. Med.* **60,** 114.

Ropper, A. H., Miett, T. and Chiappa, K. H. (1982). Absence of evoked potential abnormalities in acute transverse myelopathy.*Neurology, Minneapolis* **32,** 80.

Weller, R. O., Swash, M. and McLellan, C. L. (1983). *Clinical Neuropathology.* Springer-Verlag, Berlin.

White, W. H. (1962). Varicella myelopathy. *New Engl. J. Med.* **266, 2772.**

Radiation myelopathy

A syndrome of slowly progressive paraparesis, due to radiation injury to the spinal cord, may develop one to four years after a course of ionizing radiation given usually to the neck or mediastinum for the treatment of post-cricoid carcinoma or bronchial carcinoma with mediastinal spread. Weakness, spasticity, and sensory loss usually develop gradually, often with impairment of sphincter control (Palmer 1972) and the condition often becomes arrested. Lumbo-sacral radiculopathy may also occur (Ashenhurst, Quartey and Starreveld 1977). A transient myelopathy but without impairment of somatosensory evoked responses can occur during incidental cord exposure to radiotherapy but is usually followed by complete recovery (Lecky, Murray and Berry 1980). The CSF is usually normal and so, too, are myelography and CT scanning. However, occasionally cord swelling may result from radiation necrosis giving a myelographic appearance simulating an intramedullary tumour (Marty and Minckler 1973; Godwin-Austen, Howell and Worthington 1975). The dose of radiation given has almost always exceeded 4000 r (40 Gy) and is usually of the order of 6000–8000 r (60–80 Gy) (Pallis, Louis and Morgan 1961). Pathologically, vacuolation and degeneration of the neurones and white-matter degeneration are seen while the spinal arterioles and capillaries are usually greatly thickened and show narrowing of their lumina. Coagulative necrosis of the grey matter at the site of maximal exposure to radiation is sometimes seen (Burns, Jones and Robertson 1972) but vascular occlusion is usually prominent in addition (Palmer 1972). Similar pathological changes occur in the brain in late radiation encephalopathy (de Reuck and vander Eecken 1975). Experimental studies in animals (Mastaglia, McDonald, Watson and Yogendran 1976; Hopewell 1979) have shown that both vascular and glial damage may occur and the relative importance of these two pathological changes is

related to radiation dosage. The incidence of this complication can almost certainly be reduced by meticulous planning of radiation dosage (Sanyal, Pant, Subrahmaniyam, Agrawal and Mohanty 1979).

References

Ashenhurst, E. M., Quartey, G. R. C. and Starreveld, A. (1977). Lumbosacral radiculopathy induced by radiation.*Can. J. neurol. Sci.* **4,** 259.

Burns, R. J., Jones, A. N. and Robertson, J. S. (1972). Pathology of radiation myelopathy. *J. Neurol. Neurosurg. Psychiat.* **35,** 888.

De Reuck, J. and vander Eecken H. (1975). The anatomy of the late radiation encephalopathy. *Eur. Neurol.* **13,** 481.

Godwin-Austen, R. B.,Howell, D. A. and Worthington, B. (1975). Observations on radiation myelopathy. *Brain* **98,** 557.

Hopewell, J. W. (1979). Late radiation damage to the central nervous system: a radiobiological interpretation. *Neuropath. appl. Neurobiol.* **5,** 329.

Hughes, J. T. (1978). *Pathology of the spinal cord,.* 2nd edn. Lloyd-Luke, London.

Lecky, B. R. F., Murray, N. M. F. and Berry, R. J. (1980). Transient radiation myelopathy: spinal somatosensory evoked responses following incidental cord exposure during radiotherapy. *J. Neurol. Neurosurg. Psychiat.* **43,** 747.

Marty, R. and Minckler, D. S. (1973). Radiation myelitis simulating tumor, *Arch. Neurol., Chicago* g429, 352.

Mastaglia, F. L., McDonald, W. I., Watson, J. V. and Yogendran, K. (1976). Effects of X-radiation on the spinal cord: an experimental study of the morphological changes in central nerve fibres. *Brain* **84,** 460.

Palmer, J. J. (1972). Radiation myelopathy. *Brain* **95,** 109.

Sanyal, B., Pant, G. C.,Subrahmaniyam, K., Agrawal, M. S. and Mohanty, S. (1979). Radiation myelopathy. *J. Neurol. Neurosurg. Psychiat.* **42,** 413.

Subacute necrotic myelitis

This condition, first described by Foix and Alajouanine (1926) and subsequently by Greenfield and Turner (1939) and by Mair and Folkerts (1953) is commoner in men than in women and in older patients, particularly in those with chronic cor pulmonale. Clinically it is characterized by slowly progressive and ascending weakness of the lower extremities with variable sensory loss and sphincter disturbance; there are signs of combined upper and lower motor-neurone lesions and the clinical picture is that of a slowly progressive disorder of the cauda equina and lower cord continuing over several years. The protein content of the CSF is usually raised and myelography and/or CT scanning, which are necessary to exclude spinal tumour, are either negative or may demonstrate dilated blood vessels on the surface of the cord. Pathologically the cord is necrotic and there is widespread distension and often thrombosis of veins on the surface and within its substance. Some authors believe that the condition is due to a spinal thrombophlebitis (Blackwood 1963), others that there is venous angioma formation. No treatment is available though the condition is so rarely diagnosed in life that anticoagulants have not been given an adequate trial.

A disorder of similar clinical presentation, but different in its pathological characteristics and entitled 'subacute necrotic myelopathy', has been described as a complication of carcinoma (p. 487).

References

Blackwood, W. (1963). In *Greenfield's neuropathology,* 2nd edn (ed. W. Blackwood, W. H. McMenemey, A. Meyer, R. M. Norman and D. S. Russell). Chapter 15. Arnold, London.

Foix, C. and Alajouanine, T. (1926). La myélite nécrotique subaiguë. *Rev. neurol.* **2,** 1.

Greenfield, J. G. and Turner, J. W. A. (1939). Acute and subacute necrotic myelitis. *Brain* **62,** 227.

Mair, W. G. P. and Folkerts, J. F. (1953). Necrosis of the spinal cord due to thrombophlebitis (subacute necrotic myelitis). *Brain* **76,** 563.

'Landry's paralysis'

In 1859 Landry first described a condition of acute ascending paralysis and subsequently the name 'Landry's paralysis' was commonly given to cases with this clinical presentation. It is now well recognized that this is a syndrome and not a single disease entity and the use of this term as a definitive diagnosis is no longer justified. In very acute cases presenting with sensory disturbance in the limbs followed by the rapid development of flaccid areflexic paralysis and a fatal outcome, usually within a few days, the condition can usually be classified pathologically as one of *acute necrotic myelopathy* (Hughes 1978). *Transverse* or *ascending myelitis* as described above may also give a clinical picture of ascending paralysis of variable severity, while *post-infective polyneuritis* or *polyradiculopathy* (the Guillain–Barré syndrome) is yet another cause. The episodes of ascending paralysis which may follow acute exanthemata or inoculation, particularly with rabies vaccine, are plainly due to acute disseminated or ascending myelitis, while during epidemics, occasional cases of poliomyelitis may present in this way; so, too, may the acute polyneuropathy which complicates some cases of porphyria. A toxin produced by the bite of the Rocky Mountain wood tick has been known to produce similar symptoms which resolve when the tick is removed (Gibbes 1938) while Symonds (1949) described such a syndrome associated with a high serum potassium due to renal failure. Thus the prognosis and management of cases so-called 'Landry's paralysis' are dependent upon the elucidation of the cause of the syndrome in every case.

References

Gibbes, J. H. (1938). Tick paralysis in South Carolina. *J. Am. Med. Ass.* **111**, 1008.
Hughes, J. T. (1978). *Pathology of the spinal cord*, 2nd edn. Lloyd-Luke, London.
Landry, O. (1859). Note sur la paralysie ascendante aiguë. *Gaz. hebd. Méd.* **6**, 472.
Symonds, C. P. (1949). Reorientation in neurology. *Lancet* **i**, 677.

Some other spinal-cord lesions

Nutritional and metabolic disorders of the spinal cord including syndromes due to B$_{12}$ deficiency, tropical spastic paraplegia, and subacute myeloopticoneuropathy are described in Chapter 15, as are the effects of chemical and electrical injury. Myoclonus as a symptom of spinal-cord disease is considered on page 631.

Infarction and ischaemia of the spinal cord and cauda equina

The blood supply of the spinal cord and cauda equina

In the cervical and upper thoracic regions the major blood supply of the spinal cord is derived from the anterior spinal artery, formed by the union of the two anterior spinal branches which arise from the vertebral arteries within the cranial cavity. It runs in the anterior median fissure of the cord and receives small tributaries at different levels from the inferior thyroid arteries and from the costocervical trunk, each of which is derived from the corresponding subclavian artery. The anterior spinal artery supplies the anterior and lateral columns of the cord and the greater part of the spinal grey matter. The two small posterior spinal arteries also arise from the vertebrals intracranially and receive numerous small radicular tributaries entering the spinal cord along the posterior nerve roots; they supply the posterior columns of the cord. There are scanty circumferential vessels on the surface of the cord which form anastomoses between the anterior and posterior spinal vessels.

In the lower thoracic and lumbar regions the anterior and posterior spinal arteries receive large tributaries from the intercostal and lumbar branches of the aorta which contribute the major blood supply of the lower cord. One such vessel, the great anterior radicular artery of Adamkewicz (1882), which usually enters the spinal cord at about the T5–T8 segment but may do so at any level from T5 to L4, is of particular importance. The vessels in the lowest segments of the cord and the roots and nerves of the cauda equina receive tributaries from the iliolumbar and lateral sacral branches of the internal iliac arteries. Published work on the anatomy of the spinal-cord arterial tree and upon its variable and inconstant but profuse venous drainage has been reviewed by Garland, Greenberg and Harriman (1966), by Henson and Parsons (1967), Gillilan (1970), Di Chiro and Fried (1971), and by Hughes (1978). The contribution made by spinal-cord angiography to our understanding of spinal-cord blood supply and drainage is mentioned on page 390.

Infarction of the spinal cord and cauda equina

Occlusion of the *anterior spinal artery* in the cervical region was shown by Spiller (1909) to produce infarction of the anterior and lateral columns of the cord from the fourth cervical to the third thoracic segments. Clinically the onset is abrupt, often with pain in the neck and back and paraesthesiae in the upper limbs followed by flaccid paralysis of both arms with loss of pain and temperature sensation below a variable level in the cervical region but with preservation of light touch and position and joint sense. Initially there is usually also flaccid paralysis of the lower limbs (spinal shock) but, if the patient survives, spastic weakness of the lower limbs develops with increased reflexes and extensor plantar responses. There is usually retention of urine and of faeces in the early stages but automatic bladder and bowel control may eventually be achieved. In severe cases paralysis remains complete and the prognosis is grave, but when infarction is less extensive the lower limbs may show a variable degree of recovery.

Anterior spinal-artery occlusion ('spinal stroke') in the dorsal region is often a complication of dissecting aneurysm of the aorta, but may result from embolism as a result of disintegration of an atheromatous plaque in the aorta (Wolman and Bradshaw 1967) or from a drop in perfusion pressure (Silver and Buxton 1974), from transient cardiac arrest (Gilles and Nag 1971), or as a rare complication of spinal angiography (*The Lancet* 1973, 1974). Other rare causes include surgical correction of aortic coarctation (Darwish, Archer and Modin 1979), inadvertent injection of contrast into the thyrocervical trunk during cerebral angiography (Ramirez-Lassepas, McClelland, Snyder and Marsh 1977), fibrocartilagenous emboli from intervertebral-disc degeneration entering bone-marrow (Bots, Wattendorff, Buruma, Roos and Endtz 1981; Srigley, Lambert, Bilbao and Pritzker 1981), atrial myxoma (Hirose, Kosoegawa, Takado, Shimazaki and Murakami 1979), sickle-cell anaemia (Rothman and Nelson 1980), and non-compressive spinal Paget's disease giving a spinal-artery steal phenomenon reversible with calcitonin (Herzberg and Bayliss 1980). The central grey matter of the cord seems especially vulnerable to the effects of ischaemia (Herrick and Mills 1971). When dissecting aneurysm is the cause, and occasionally in other cases, there is severe pain in the back followed by total and permanent flaccid paralysis of the lower limbs, sphincter paralysis, and loss of pain and temperature sensation up to a sensory 'level' at about the umbilicus (corresponding to the T10 segment of the cord), but with preservation of some light touch sensation and of position and joint sense. Thrombosis of posterior spinal arteries complicating intrathecal phenol injection has been described (Hughes 1970) as has venous infarction of the cord (Hughes 1971), while infarction of the upper cervical cord, presumed to be due to spasm of spinal arteries, has been reported as a sequel of minor spinal trauma in childhood (Ahmann, Smith, Schwartz and Clark 1975).

While the clinical picture of anterior spinal-artery occlusion has been recognized for many years, there has been increasing attention of late to the fact that infarction of the cord may sometimes be much more restricted, possibly due to occlusion of one posterior spinal artery or of one or more feeding or radicular arteries (O'Moore 1978). In such cases weakness and sensory impairment may be restricted to one limb or may be asymmetrical in the two lower limbs and considerable or even complete recovery may take place after such a localized infarct. While rare by comparison with intermittent cerebral ischaemia, it also seems probable that transient episodes of weakness and of paraesthesiae in the lower extremities may well be due in many cases to *transient ischaemia of the spinal cord* or *cauda equina* (Wells 1966; Garland 1966; Henson and Parsons 1967). Furthermore, there is now pathological evidence to suggest that repeated episodes of ischaemia or focal infarction can cause slowly progressive spastic weakness of the lower limbs with variable sensory loss and signs of mixed upper and lower motor-neurone involvement. In such cases of *atherosclerotic myelopathy*, a step-wise clinical course with episodes of deterioration alternating with periods of apparent arrest may suggest the nature of the disease, as may associated clinical evidence of atherosclerosis, but inflammatory, demyelinating, and neoplastic disorders must be excluded by means of X-ray, CSF examination, serological tests to exclude syphilis, and CT scanning and/or myelography. Spinal-cord angiography (Di Chiro and Doppman 1969), while of value in diagnosing vascular malformations, may carry risks in suspected cord infarction or ischaemia, so that the diagnosis should usually be made in other ways. Rarely, collagen disease such as polyarteritis nodosa or systemic lupus erythematosus (Garcin 1955) may give episodes of spinal-cord infarction.

Spinal-cord embolism due to the causes listed above may give not only episodes of major infarction but also chronic ischaemic myelopathy as described above. Similar episodes may be seen in cases of subacute bacterial endocarditis; air and fat embolism of the cord appear to be very rare but decompression sickness (Caisson disease, p 442), occurring during decompression in divers and compressed-air workers, commonly gives transient episodes of spinal-cord dysfunction and occasionally incomplete or irreversible paraplegia (Haymaker 1957).

Treatment, other than the nursing care of patients with paraplegia, is of little value in spinal-cord infarction. Vasodilator drugs may reasonably be given, but seem to be of little value and in cases of intermittent ischaemia or progressive myelopathy there are theoretical reasons for suggesting that anticoagulant drugs may be worthy of a trial. Surgical treatment of an aortic dissecting aneurysm is of no value once cord infarction has occurred.

Intermittent claudication or ischaemia of the spinal cord or cauda equina

In 1906 Dejerine first suggested that transient weakness or numbness of one or both lower limbs occurring during exercise might be due to ischaemia of the spinal cord. It is now clear that in some patients the lower spinal cord or the nerves of the cauda equina may suffer a degree of compression which restricts their arterial blood supply but is not sufficient to give rise to any symptoms or abnormal physical signs at rest. However, when the patient begins to walk he often develops first aching pain in one or both calves similar to that of true intermittent claudication, but the peripheral pulses in the legs and feet are found to be normal. If he continues to walk, paraesthesiae in one or both feet may then supervene and often foot-drop follows (in ischaemia of the cauda equina) or spastic weakness of one or both legs (in ischaemia of the cord). In suspected cases the symptoms may be precipitated by appropriate exercise under supervision; when the cauda equina is principally affected, one or both ankle jerks may disappear, while if the lower

cord is being compressed, the plantar responses may become extensor.

The condition can usually be shown by radiography and myelography, which are obligatory investigations in such cases, to be due to either a central intervertebral disc protrusion (Blau and Logue 1961) or, in cases involving the cauda equina, a bony stenosis of the lumbar canal resulting from an overgrowth (of unknown aetiology) of the bony laminae (Verbiest 1954; Joffe, Appleby and Arjona 1966). Paget's disease and fluorosis are less common causes (Yates 1981). Diagnosis from claudication due to peripheral vascular disease depends upon the presence or absence of changes in the peripheral pulses, of bruits, and of neurological signs; pain in spinal or cauda-equina claudication is often made worse by standing (Hawkes and Roberts 1978). Generally the results of operative decompression are good with no mortality and few complications (Weir and de Leo 1981). In either event, laminectomy and decompression of the spinal canal usually produces complete relief of symptoms.

References

Ahmann, P. A.,Smith, S. A., Schwartz, J. F. and Clark, D. B. (1975). Spinal cord infarction due to minor trauma in children. *Neurology, Minneapolis* **25**, 301.

Blau, J. N. and Logue, V. (1961). Intermittent claudication of the cauda equina. *Lancet* **i**, 1081.

Bots, G. Th. A. M., Wattendorff, A. R., Buruma, O. J. S., Roos, R. A. C. and Endtz, L. J. (1981). Acute myelopathy caused by fibrocartilaginous emboli. *Neurology, Minneapolis* **31**, 1250.

Darwish, H., Archer, C. and Modin, J. (1979). The anterior spinal artery collateral in coarctation of the aorta: a clinical angiographic correlation. *Arch. Neurol., Chicago* **36**, 240.

Dejerine, J. (1906). Sur la claudication intermittente de la moelle épinière. *Rev. neurol.* **33**, 1.

Di Chiro, G. and Doppman, J. L. (1969). Differential angiographic features of hemangioblastomas and arteriovenous malformations of the spinal cord. *Radiology* **93**, 25.

—— and Fried, L. C. (1971). Blood flow currents in spinal cord arteries. *Neurology, Minneapolis* **21**, 1088.

Garcin, R. (1955). Aspects neurologiques du lupus érythémateux disséminé. *Rev. Neurol.* **92**, 511.

Garland, H., Greenberg, J. and Harriman, D. G. F. (1966). Infarction of the spinal cord. *Brain* **89**, 645.

Gilles, F. H. and Nag, D. (1971). Vulnerability of human spinal cord in transient cardiac arrest. *Neurology, Minneapolis* **21**, 833.

Gillilan, L. A. (1970). Veins of the spinal cord. Anatomic details: suggested clinical applications. *Neurology Minneapolis* **20**, 860.

Hawkes, C. H. and Roberts, G. M. (1978). Neurogenic and vascular claudication. *J. neurol. Sci.* **38**, 337.

Haymaker, W. (1957). Decompression sickness. In *Handbuch der Speziellen Pathologischen Anatomie und Histologie*, Vol.13 (ed. W. Scholz) p. 1600. Springer, Berlin.

Henson, R. A. and Parsons, M. (1967). Ischaemic lesions of the spinal cord: an illustrated review. *Quart. J. Med.* **36**, 205.

Herrick, M. K. and Milles, P. E. (1971). Infarction of spinal cord. Two cases of selective gray matter involvement secondary to asymptomatic aortic disease. *Arch. Neurol., Chicago* **24**, 228.

Herzberg, L. and Bayliss, E. (1980). Spinal-cord syndrome due to noncompressive Paget's disease of bone: a spinal-artery steal phenomenon reversible with calcitonin. *Lancet* **ii**, 13.

Hirose, G., Kosoegawa, H., Takado, M., Shimazaki, K. and Murakami, E. (1979). Spinal cord ischemia and left atrial myxoma. *Arch. Neurol., Chicago* **36**, 439.

Hughes, J. T. (1970). Thrombosis of the posterior spinal arteries. A complication of an intrathecal injection of phenol. *Neurology, Minneapolis* **20**, 659.

—— (1971). Venous infarction of the spinal cord, *Neurology, Minneapolis* **21**, 794.

—— (1978). *Pathology of the spinal cord*, 2nd edn. Lloyd-Luke, London.

Joffe, R., Appleby, A. and Arjona, V. (1966). 'Intermittent ischaemia' of the cauda equina due to stenosis of the lumbar canal. *J. Neurol. Neurosurg. Psychiat.* **29**, 315.

The Lancet (1974). Spinal stroke. *Lancet* **ii**, 1299.

O'Moore, B. (1978). Anterior spinal artery syndrome. *Acta neurol. scand.* **58,** 59.

Ramirez-Lassepas, M., McClelland, R. P., Snyder, B. D. and Marsh, D. G. (1977). Cervical myelopathy complicating cerebral angiography: report of a case and review of the literature. *Neurology, Minneapolis* **27,** 834.

Rothman, S. M. and Nelson, J. S. (1980). Spinal cord infarction in a patient with sickle cell anemia. *Neurology, Minneapolis* **30,** 1072.

Silver, J. R. and Buxton, P. H. (1974). Spinal stroke. *Brain* **97,** 539.

Spiller, W. G. (1909). Thrombosis of the cervical anterior median spinal artery: syphilitic acute anterior poliomyelitis. *J. nerv. ment. Dis.* **36,** 601.

Srigley, J. R., Lambert, C. D., Bilbao, J. M. and Pritzker, K. P. H. (1981). Spinal cord infarction secondary to intervertebral disc embolism. *Ann. Neurol.* **9,** 296.

Verbiest, H. (1954). A radicular syndrome from developmental narrowing of the lumbar vertebral canal. *J. Bone Jt. Surg.* **36b,** 230.

Weir, B. and de Leo, R. (1981). Lumbar stenosis: analysis of factors affecting outcome in 81 surgical cases. *Can. J. neurol. Sci.* **8,** 295.

Wells, C. E. C. (1966). Clinical aspects of spinovascular disease. *Proc. R. Soc. Med.* **59,** 790.

Wolman, L. and Bradshaw, P. (1967). Spinal cord embolism. *J. Neurol. Neurosurg. Psychiat.* **30,** 446.

Yates, D. A. H. (1981). Spinal stenosis. *J. R. Soc. Med.* **74,** 334.

15

Intoxications and metabolic disorders

Alcohol addiction

Aetiology

Alcohol addiction can be a symptom of many different mental disorders and every case requires careful psychological study. It is more common in males than in females, is comparatively rare before the age of 20, and most often occurs in middle life. A parental history of alcoholism is frequently present (*British Medical Journal* 1980). Alcoholism may be a symptom of loss of self-control associated with the early stages of dementia; it may occur in schizophrenia or in manic-depressive psychosis. Though alcoholism is less common in females than in males there appears to be a higher incidence of personality disorder in female alcoholics and its incidence in females and in young people is increasing. In some cases the periodicity of outbreaks of alcoholism is due to a periodically recurrent depression in an individual with cyclothymia. Alcohol addicts who are not frankly psychotic are often neurotic, and take alcohol as a means of escape from the difficulties of life. Business worries and domestic unhappiness are common secondary causes. The alcohol is often taken as spirits but beer or wine can also be addictive; and the alcoholic may also be a drug addict. Indeed there is some evidence that there are personality traits common to many of those who become addicted to any drug, of which alcohol is one.

The WHO definition of an alcoholic is: 'Alcoholics are those excessive drinkers whose dependence upon alcohol has attained such a degree that they show a noticeable mental disturbance or an interference with bodily and mental health, their interpersonal relations and their smooth economic and social functioning; or who show the prodromal signs of such development. They therefore need treatment' (DHSS 1973).

Incidence

It was estimated that in 1975 there were 4390 alcoholics per 100 000 in the USA and at least 1100 per 100 000 in Britain (Sim 1975). The Department of Health and Social Security (DHSS 1973) estimated that there were about 400 000 alcoholics in England and Wales. However, recent estimates are much higher, between 500 000 and 750 000 (*Office of Health Economics* 1981), and the annual economic cost of alcohol misuse has been estimated at about 650 million pounds sterling (Holtermann and Burchell 1981); truly the increase in alcohol-related disease has been termed an epidemic (*The Lancet* 1982). There are important and complex differences in the incidence observed in various racial and ethnic groups (Jellinek 1951; Williams and Glatt 1965) but almost every country appears to have its 'skid-row' where down-and-out intractable drinkers and those who consume methyl alcohol tend to congregate (Bourne, Alford, and Bowcock 1966; Edwards, Hawker, Williamson and Hensman 1966; Olin 1966).

Pathology

The prolonged consumption of alcohol produces degenerative changes in the central nervous system and in peripheral nerves. The brain is atrophied, and microscopically there is degeneration of cortical ganglion cells. Degeneration of the middle layers of the corpus callosum is said to be characteristic (Marchiafava 1933; Ironside, Bosanquet, and McMenemey 1961). In Wernicke's encephalopathy, which is usually associated with the Korsakow syndrome, there are proliferation of capillaries, gliosis, and often patchy small haemorrhages in the corpora mammillaria and midbrain (Victor and Adams 1953). In cases of polyneuropathy the peripheral nerves show degeneration of both myelin sheaths and of axis sylinders but it is clear that the axonal lesion is primary. There is evidence that the neuropathy, and the Wernicke–Korsakow syndrome, are not directly due to the alcohol, but to an associated deficiency of Vitamin B_1 (see p. 473). However, alcoholic pellagra also occurs with typical pathological changes (Ishii and Nishihara 1981). Victor and Adams (1961) concluded that whereas delirium tremens, alcoholic epilepsy, and alcoholic hallucinosis are due to habituation and alcohol withdrawal, and while the Wernicke–Korsakow syndrome, Korsakow's syndrome, polyneuropathy, retrobulbar neuropathy, and pellagra are due to nutritional deficiencies which are associated with alcoholism, the pathogenesis of alcoholic cerebellar degeneration, central pontine myelinolysis (see p. 319), of Marchiafava–Bignami disease and of alcoholic dementia is not yet fully understood and it is much more probable that these disorders are due or related to the direct toxic effect of long-continued ingestion of large quantities of alcohol. While there is no convincing evidence that alcohol damages the blood-brain barrier in animals (Phillips 1981), and a direct cytotoxic effect on cortical neurones is difficult to demonstrate (Phillips, Cragg, and Singh 1981), there is increasing evidence to show that progressive cerebral atrophy is related to excessive alcohol consumption (Harper and Krill 1985), especially in younger alcoholics, and can produce anything from minor cognitive and executive problems (*British Medical Journal* 1981; Paton, Potter, Lewis, Bissell, Ritson, Saunders, and Smerdon 1982) to moderate or severe global dementia (Lishman 1981). Even in alcoholics without clinically overt evidence of brain damage, CT scanning shows statistically significant cortical shrinkage and ventricular dilatation (Ron, Acker, Shaw and Lishman 1982). Brain damage can sometimes be correlated with the severity of liver damage (Lee, Møller, Hardt, Hanbek, and Jensen 1979; Acker, Aps, Majumdar, Shaw, and Thomson 1982) but also occurs in the absence of hepatic disease (Carlen, Wilkinson, Wortzman, Holgate, Cordingley, Lee, Huszar, Moddel, Singh, Kiraly, and Rankin 1981). While at autopsy in chronic alcoholics the changes of Wernicke's encephalopathy are still commonly found, cerebellar atrophy is even more common, being found in over a quarter, and there is a significant reduction in brain weight (Torvik, Lindboe, and Rogde 1982). There is also evidence that alcohol intoxication may precipitate cerebral infarction in young adults (Hillbom and Kaste 1978), and the relationship to head injury resulting from road traffic accidents or other forms of injury is very well known (*British Medical Journal* 1976). And while a fetal alcohol syndrome of low birth weight and other defects is well recognized in drinking mothers, severe maternal alcoholism can produce severe fetal malformations, ranging from spinal dysraphism, arhinencephaly, porencephaly, and corpus callosum agenesis to microdysplasias, congenital heart disease, and craniofacial dysmorphogenesis (Peiffer, Majewski, Fischbach, Bierich, Volk 1979). Cardiomyopathy and acute and chronic myopathic syndromes involving skeletal muscle have also been described in alcoholic patients (Ekbom, Hed, Kirstein, and Astrom 1964; Perkoff, Hardy, and Velez-Garcia 1966).

Chronic malnutrition is common in alcoholic subjects who substitute alcoholic beverages for food; breakfast is often discarded first and later other meals are regularly missed.

Symptoms and signs

Acute alcoholic intoxication

The action of alcohol upon the nervous system is paralytic, the highest functions being first affected. The earlier symptoms of intoxication, therefore are those of altered behaviour; the social value of alcohol in moderate doses rests upon its ability to release those inhibitions which cause shyness and to reduce in the individual who takes it, his critical capacity. In larger doses it produces irregularities of conduct, the nature of which depends upon the temperament of the individual, who may become excited, voluble, combative, depressed, or maudlin. There is impairment of memory, especially for recent events. The ability to carry out co-ordinated and complex motor acts is progressively impaired (Drew, Colquhoun, and Lond 1958) and since October 1967 in Great Britain it has been an offence in law to drive a motor vehicle when the blood alcohol exceeds 80 mg/100 ml. In Scandinavian countries the legal limit is very much lower. Eventually articulation becomes impaired; the conjunctivae are congested; the pupils are usually dilated, but may be contracted, and the pupillary reaction to light may be impaired; nystagmus is invariable and diplopia may occur. In still larger doses alcohol produces stupor, then coma, and finally death, through paralysis of vital centres.

The relationship between the alcoholic content of the blood and the state of the nervous system is variable. Much depends upon the body weight of the drinker, upon whether the simultaneous or previous ingestion of food delays absorption of the alcohol, and upon whether or not the individual is accustomed to taking alcoholic drinks. There are also significant racial differences in the rate of metabolism of alcohol, related to the concentration of the different isoenzymes of alcohol dehydrogenase in the liver. In general there are few if any signs of intoxication with a blood level of below 100 mg/100 ml, although between 50 and 100 mg/100 ml some lack of inhibition and impairment of motor skills, with a slowing of reaction time, are generally apparent. Intoxication is usually evident in conversation with or on examining an individual with a blood level of 150 mg/100 ml but he is usually still in reasonable control of his behaviour and faculties whereas at 200 mg/100 ml signs of drunkenness are usually apparent, and consciousness may be lost, except in habitual heavy drinkers or alcoholic subjects, at a level between 250 and 300 mg/100 ml. As a very rough guide, up to three single 'tots' of spirit or three half-pints of British beer will, in the average individual, give a blood level within an hour of between 50 and 75 mg/100 ml.

Methyl alcohol

The consumption of methyl alcohol in the form of methylated spirits, industrial alcohol, anti-freeze, and filtered metal polish is mainly seen in the poor countries where alcoholic drinks are expensive, or in exceptionally degenerate alcoholics. It may cause severe toxic confusional states, irreversible optic atrophy with bilateral central scotomata or even total blindness and sometimes rapid death. This poison has a selective myelinoclastic effect and retrolaminar demyelinating optic neuropathy is an early morphological correlate of visual loss (Sharpe, Hostovsky, Bilbao, and Rewcastle 1982). The mortality rate is related to the severe metabolic acidosis (lactate and formate) which develops 8–12 hours after ingestion (*The Lancet* 1983). A parkinsonian syndrome with bilateral infarction of the frontocentral white matter and putamen is a rare consequence of methanol poisoning (McLean, Jacobs, and Mielke 1980).

Pathological drunkenness

In some individuals, especially those who have suffered a severe head injury or other organic lesion of the brain, a comparatively small dose of alcohol may rapidly produce symptoms of acute intoxication; this may also occur in individuals taking barbiturate or benzodiazepine drugs regularly, in whom alcohol has an additive effect. It must also be remembered that personal injury is common in alcoholic subjects so that one must be careful not to attribute to intoxication the effects of closed head injuries occurring in such subjects. Uncharacteristic behaviour, out of keeping with a person's conduct when sober, and occurring during a drinking bout, is thought by some to be dependent upon latent personality or other constitutional traits or defects. Severe memory blackouts are also common, being periods of several hours during which a person was drinking, for which there is only patchy subsequent recollection or none at all (Cutting 1982).

Alcohol withdrawal

In those who are physically dependent upon alcohol but who are not yet alcoholics, and in some less severe chronic alcoholics, withdrawal of alcohol is followed within 12 hours by 'the shakes', often associated with nausea and sometimes with feelings of severe guilt, panic, apprehension, and transient visual or auditory illusions without clouding of consciousness. In more severe cases, delirium tremens occurs.

Delirium tremens

This is often seen after a prolonged debauch in the chronic alcoholic, but may be precipitated in such an individual by acute infection, surgical operation, or an accident. Sudden deprivation of alcohol is undoubtedly the most important factor.

The onset may be acute, but there is often prodromal nervousness, anorexia, and insomnia. The characteristic symptoms are tremor, and acute confusion, accompanied by hallucinations, which are principally visual. The tremor is coarse and generalized, and most evident in the face, tongue, and hands. The patient is completely disorientated, and experiences visual hallucinations, which often assume terrifying forms, especially of animals. Auditory hallucinations may also be present, and cutaneous sensations may be interpreted as insects crawling under the skin. The mood is usually one of terror, and the patient may attempt to escape from his surroundings, and attack with violence those around him. Convulsions may occur. In addition, symptoms of a severe toxaemia are generally present. Hyperpyrexia is not uncommon, and there may be albuminuria. The tongue is furred, the pulse rapid, and cardiac dilatation may occur. Delirium tremens runs an acute course, and in most cases recovery occurs in three or four days. In cases which end fatally, death may be due to heart failure in which dehydration plays an important part, or to intercurrent lobar pneumonia to which such individuals are peculiarly subject.

Acute alcoholic hallucinosis

This condition occurs in chronic alcoholics, either developing gradually or coming on suddenly after unusual excess. It is characterized by hallucinations which, unlike those in delirium tremens, are predominantly auditory and are often associated with delusions of persecution; signs of delirium are absent.

Dipsomania

This outmoded term was once used to identify alcoholic subjects who embarked upon recurrent drinking-bouts ('the lost weekend'). Such episodic heavy drinking may represent one step along the road to chronic alcoholism but in some individuals is a pattern which persists over many years, sometimes, but by no means invariably, in relation to the depressive phases of cyclothymic individuals.

Korsakow's psychosis

Korsakow's psychosis, though seen most frequently in chronic alcoholism with polyneuropathy, may be due to other causes (see p. 654). It is often associated with Wernicke's encephalopathy (see p. 475). Its most characteristic feature is a disturbance of attention and memory, leading to disorientation of the patient in space and time. His memory for recent events and his ability to retain new impressions are lost, and he fills the gap by confabulation, often bringing forward past events to fill gaps in his recent memory. For example, one who has been bedridden for weeks describes with a wealth of detail a walk which he took on the previous day. Many clinical varieties of Korsakow's psychosis have been described, chiefly in terms of variations of the emotional mood, which is usually euphoric.

Alcoholic cerebellar degeneration

Victor, Adams, and Mancall (1959) described 50 cases of this condition which is characterized by ataxia of stance and gait and of leg movements with little or no involvement of the arms (apart from action tremor which is seen in a few cases); nystagmus and dysarthria are usually absent. The condition seems to progress over a period of a few weeks or months and then to become arrested in most cases. Pathological observations reveal degeneration of all neurocellular elements of the cerebellar cortex, particularly of the Purkinje cells and also degeneration of the olivary nuclei. In the cerebellum changes are most striking in the anterior and superior aspects of the vermis and of the hemispheres (Torvik et al. 1982).

Marchiafava–Bignami disease

This rare condition, originally described in Italian drinkers of crude red wine, occurs occasionally in other alcoholic patients. It is characterized clinically by disorders of emotional control and cognitive function followed by variable delirium, fits, tremors, rigidity, and paralysis; most patients eventually become comatose and die within a few months. Symmetrical demyelination with subsequent cavitation and axonal destruction is found in the corpus callosum and often, in varying degree, in the central white matter of the cerebral hemispheres, the optic chiasm, and the middle cerebellar peduncles (Victor and Adams 1961).

Alcoholic dementia

Prolonged addiction to alcohol often leads to progressive mental deterioration. There is nothing distinctive about the resulting dementia, which is characterized, like other dementias, by impairment of memory and intellectual capacity, emotional instability, moral deterioration, and carelessness with regard to dress and person (Cutting 1982). Delusions may be present, a delusion of marital infidelity being particularly common. Alcoholic dementia may be associated with dysarthria, tremor, sluggish pupillary reactions, nystagmus, and myopathy. The full clinical picture of alcoholic polyneuropathy may be present, but even without this the tendon reflexes may be lost in the lower limbs.

Epilepsy

Epileptic attacks are not uncommon in chronic alcoholism, and are indistinguishable from the convulsions of idiopathic epilepsy. The convulsions of absinthe drinkers are due to the presence in the drink of the convulsant drug thujone. Fits may occur either at the height of a debauch, or much more often after withdrawal of alcohol ('rum fits') when they may be compared with the attacks which occur on the withdrawal of other drugs such as barbiturates.

Polyneuropathy

The symptoms of polyneuropathy which may complicate any form of chronic alcoholism are described on page 531 and pellagra is described on page 476.

Central pontine myelinolysis

This rare complication of alcoholism is considered on page 319.

Tobacco–alcohol amblyopia

This condition is considered on page 92. In Great Britain it is generally attributed to the effects of pipe tobacco, but American authors consider that heavy alcohol consumption is also a factor.

Alcoholic myopathy

In 1962 Hed, Lundmark, Fahlgren, and Orell described an acute muscular syndrome occurring in alcoholic patients after a debauch. Occasionally, muscle pain, tenderness, and oedema were curiously localized in these cases but in others many skeletal muscles were involved. In severely affected individuals widespread muscle fibre necrosis, myoglobinuria, renal damage, and hyperkalaemia were found. Perkoff et al. (1966) described a similar reversible acute muscular syndrome occurring in chronic alcoholic patients; painful cramps and muscular tenderness were usually found, the serum creatine kinase (CK) activity was often raised and in most cases the serum lactate failed to rise after ischaemic work suggesting that muscular glycogen utilization was impaired. A subacute painless myopathy resolving after the withdrawal of alcohol was also described by Ekbom et al. (1964). In a series of 44 cases, Oh (1972) found that 26 suffered from the acute syndrome while 18 had a subacute or chronic myopathy (also see Engel 1981). Konttinen, Härtel, and Louhija (1970) found increasing serum CK activity in 43 of 100 chronic alcoholic subjects.

Alcoholic cardiomyopathy

This condition, believed to be due to a direct toxic effect of alcohol upon cardiac mitochondria, and perhaps to interference with the metabolic degradation of noradrenaline, is characterized by cardiomegaly, increasing breathlessness, and often hepatomegaly. It is one of the commonest causes of congestive cardiac failure occurring under the age of 50 years in the absence of evidence of hypertension, ischaemia, or valvular disease (Lieber 1980).

Hepatic encephalopathy

This syndrome which may complicate cirrhosis of the liver is often seen in alcoholic patients and is described on page 451. Increases in serum ornithine carbamoyl transferase and glutamate dehydrogenase activity, indicating liver-cell and mitochondrial damage respectively, were found in many alcoholic patients by Konttinen et al. (1970), sometimes without other evidence of cirrhosis.

Other metabolic abnormalities

Severe hyponatraemia due to water intoxication giving rise to impaired consciousness, sometimes with epileptic attacks and/or signs of corticospinal-tract dysfunction, was reported in heavy beer drinkers by Demanet, Bonnyns, Bleiberg, and Stevens-Rocmans (1971). This may be a major factor in the pathogenesis of central pontine myelinolysis (p. 319). Merry and Marks (1972) drew attention to disorders of hypothalamic, pituitary, and adrenal function in alcoholic subjects in whom morning plasma cortisol levels were above normal but fell after the ingestion of moderate amounts of alcohol, in contrast to the findings in control subjects. Prolonged CSF acidosis persisting after alcohol withdrawal in chronic alcoholics has been described by Carlen, Kapur, Huszar, Lee, Moddel, Singh, and Wilkinson (1980) who speculate as to whether this may contribute to the progressive cerebral atrophy associated with alcoholic dementia.

Various haematological abnormalities, including disorders of haemopoiesis (Hillman 1975) and of platelet function (Cowan 1975) have also been described.

Diagnosis

The diagnosis of both acute and chronic alcoholic poisoning presents little difficulty if a reliable history is available. To determine whether an alcoholic who claims to have abstained from drinking is still imbibing, the most useful laboratory tests are to measure mean corpuscular volume (abnormal above 96 μm^3), the serum gamma glutamyl transpeptidase (abnormal above 55 u/l in the male, 35 u/l in the female), the blood alcohol (which may be raised even in the morning), and the serum uric acid (abnormal above 0.48 mmol/l). The early stages of acute intoxication must be distinguished from the effects of acute lesions of the nervous system, especially those following head injury, and a smell of alcohol in the breath is not proof that the symptoms are due to intoxication. The diagnosis of alcoholic coma is described on page 648. The clinical picture of delirium tremens is distinctive, though a similar picture follows withdrawal of barbiturates or amphetamines. Korsakow's psychosis may be associated with focal cerebral lesions as well as non-alcoholic forms of polyneuropathy, and these must be distinguished from alcoholism by the history and clinical features. Alcoholic dementia must be distinguished from general paresis and other dementias. A history of alcoholic excess does not necessarily mean that this is the cause of the dementia, as alcoholism may complicate other dementing diseases. In doubtful cases serological reactions in the blood and CSF, CT scanning, and other appropriate tests may be needed, but distinction between alcoholic and other forms of dementia may be impossible save on the basis of the history.

Alcoholic cerebellar degeneration must be distinguished from familial cerebellar ataxia and cerebellar degeneration secondary to carcinoma, while the Marchiafava–Bignami syndrome may simulate a tumour of the corpus callosum and central pontine myelinolysis can produce symptoms and signs similar to those which occur in brainstem tumour, demyelination due to other causes, or basilar artery thrombosis. Alcoholic myopathy must be distinguished from McArdle's syndrome of myophosphorylase deficiency and from other forms of endocrine and metabolic myopathy. In all of these conditions the history of excessive alcoholic intake is crucial and it must be remembered that some alcoholics are very adept at concealing the evidence of their heavy and often secret drinking so that even a spouse may be unaware of the true state of affairs at least for a time. Concealment of empty bottles and of evidence of excessive spending on drink are common.

Prognosis

The prognosis of alcohol addiction depends upon the underlying cause, and the stage at which treatment is begun. When the habit is the expression of a psychotic process or a serious personality defect, or when there is a strong hereditary tendency to alcoholism, the outlook is poor. A history of previous 'cures' and relapses also makes the outlook unsatisfactory. Voegtlin and his collaborators (1942) claimed that many patients treated by 'conditional reflex therapy' remained abstainers four years later. In a series of cases of delirium tremens reported by Tavel, Davidson, and Batterton (1961) the mortality rate was 11.8 per cent. The mortality rate in patients with Korsakow's psychosis is also high. In mild cases, however, with proper motivation, recovery may be complete. In more severe cases, and those of long standing, there is likely to be some permanent mental impairment.

The prognosis of chronic alcoholism and the results of treatment were reviewed by Victor and Adams (1974). Detailed reviews of the many medical consequences of alcoholism may also be found in Seixas, Williams, and Eggleston (1975) and Hore, Ritson, and Thomson (1982).

Alcoholic dementia runs a slow course in most cases, lasting for years. In the early stages withdrawal of alcohol leads to marked improvement, sometimes complete recovery, even with reversal of cerebral atrophy (Cutting 1982). In long-standing cases the brain has been permanently damaged, and recovery is incomplete. Exceptionally the course is much more rapid, and in a few weeks or months a rapidly progressive dementia terminates in coma and death, often preceded by terminal hyperpyrexia. Central pontine myelinolysis and Marchiafava–Bignami disease seem to be universally fatal within a few months. Alcoholic cerebellar degeneration usually becomes arrested after a period of deterioration and the various forms of myopathy slowly resolve when the alcohol is withdrawn.

Treatment

Alcohol addiction

The successful treatment of alcohol addiction requires thorough supervision, so that the amount of alcohol taken can be completely controlled. Often treatment can only be carried out successfully in an appropriate institution. Alcohol treatment centres for both out-patients and in-patients management have been established in many countries. Even so, many patients display remarkable cunning in obtaining access to supplies of alcohol and experience teaches that many alcoholics are accomplished and plausible liars. Complete and permanent abstinence from alcohol is the aim, but alcohol should never be suddenly withdrawn. Some psychiatrists prefer to use 'controlled drinking programmes' (Davies 1962) after control of the addiction, but are at present in the minority. The daily dose should be tapered, and in most cases the withdrawal can be accomplished within a week. Delirium tremens and other acute confusional states may follow the sudden withdrawal. Diazepam and other appropriate tranquillizers may be needed during the withdrawal period; drugs for the treatment of depression (amitriptyline, imipramine) are often necessary in addition. During the period of treatment a careful psychological assessment is needed to ascertain whether any underlying psychosis or neurosis is present, and in suitable cases the patient should receive psychotherapeutic treatment and/or appropriate drugs. The necessity for complete and permanent abstinence must be impressed upon the patient as the slightest lapse in this respect may be followed by relapse. Psychological help may be given by Alcoholics Anonymous (address in England, BM/AAL, London, W.C.1). It is a truism that chronic alcoholism is an incurable disease unless the patient really wishes to be cured when the association with others in a similar plight through A.A. may be invaluable. Various professional support groups (as for doctors and dentists) and other organizations are also helpful. Unfortunately some patients may forswear alcohol and then become addicted to other drugs

Voegtlin (1940) treated alcohol addiction by giving an injection of emetine and making the patient drink during the period of nausea, thus endeavouring to establish a conditional reflex of aversion, and aversion therapy has been used successfully by others. The drug disulfiram (*Antabuse*) acts by sensitizing the patient to even a small dose of alcohol (Hald and Jacobsen 1948; Martensen-Larsen 1948). The usual dose is 0.5 g daily; whenever a patient receiving this drug takes alcohol an unpleasant reaction with headache, intense flushing, and vomiting follows due to the release of acetaldehyde into the circulation. Unfortunately, some fatal reactions have been described and it is too easy for the patient to discontinue the drug on leaving hospital unless carefully supervised. This drug should only be given in the first instance in hospital; side-effects due to long-term administration include depression, confusion, impotence, peripheral neuropathy, and a metallic taste. Calcium carbimide (*Abstem*), 50 mg twice daily, is similar but less violent in its effects and also less toxic in long-term administration. Victor and Adams (1974), and Hore *et al.* (1982) have reviewed the literature of these and other modes of treatment.

Delirium tremens

The sufferer from delirium tremens should be treated as a patient with a severe toxaemia involving not only the nervous but also the cardiovascular system. Bed rest and careful nursing supervision are therefore indispensable. It is unnecessary to give alcohol, but a high fluid intake is important: Tavel *et al.* (1961) concluded that some severely ill patients may need up to 6 litres a day. Sedatives are also required: those most often used in the past were barbiturates but now chlordiazepoxide (*Librium*), 50 mg, or benzodiazepines are probably more effective (Sereny and Kalant 1965). Phenothiazine derivates are also valuable but may induce hypotension (Brown, Ryan, and McGrath 1959). Merry and Marks

(1972) recommended diazepam in doses up to 30 mg as required; this drug has less effect in suppressing cortisol activity than the barbiturates. Large doses of B and C vitamins should be given by injection, say in the form of *Parentrovite*. Smith (1949) recommended ACTH and this drug is still often given in a dosage of 20–40 units 8-hourly for at least 48 hours. Antibiotic cover to prevent pneumonia and other infections is also necessary for several days.

Acute alcoholic hallucinosis
Hallucinosis should be treated on the same lines as delirium tremens.

Other disorders
Korsakow's syndrome, Wernicke's encephalopathy, and alcoholic polyneuropathy should be treated by maintaining adequate nutrition and by giving large doses of thiamine and other vitamins. These measures are also appropriate in cases of alcoholic dementia but have little if any effect in conditions such as cerebellar degeneration or Marchiafava–Bignami disease.

References

Acker, W., Aps, E. J., Majumdar, S. K., Shaw, G. K. and Thomson, A. D. (1982). The relationship between brain and liver damage in chronic alcoholic patients. *J. Neurol. Neurosurg. Psychiat.* **45**, 984.

Bourne, P. G., Alford, J. A. and Bowcock, J. Z. (1966). Treatment of skid-row alcoholics. *Quart. J. Stud. Alcohol.* **27**, 242.

British Medical Journal (1976). Alcohol and the brain. *Br. med. J.* **1**, 1168.

—— (1980). Alcoholism: an inherited disease? *Br. med. J.* **281**, 1301.

—— (1981). Minor brain damage and alcoholism. *Bri. med. J.* **283**, 455.

Browne, I. W., Ryan, J. P. A. and McGrath, S. D. (1959). The management of the acute withdrawal phase in alcoholism. *Lancet* **i**, 959.

Carlen, P. L., Kapur, B., Huszar, L. A., Lee, M. A., Moddel, G., Singh, R. and Wilkinson, D. A. (1980). Prolonged cerebrospinal fluid acidosis in recently abstinent chronic alcoholics. *Neurology, Minneapolis* **30**, 956.

Silkinson, D. A., Wortzman, G., Holgate, R., Cordingley, J., Lee, M. A., Huszar, L., Moddel, G., Singh, R., Kiraly, L., Rankin, J. G. (1981). Cerebral atrophy and functional deficits in alcoholics without clinically apparent liver disease. *Neurology, Minneapolis* **31**, 377.

Carmichael, E. A. and Stern R. O. (1931). Korsakoff's syndrome: its histopathology. *Brain* **54**, 189.

Cowan, D. H. (1975). The platelet defect in alcoholism in *Medical Consequences of Alcoholism* (ed. F. A. Seixas, K. Williams and S. Eggleston. *Ann. NY Acad. Sci.* **252**, 328.

Cutting, J. (1982). Neuropsychiatric complications of alcoholism. *Br. J. Hosp. Med.* **28**, 335.

Davies, D. L. (1962). Normal drinking in recovered alcohol addicts. *Quart. J. stud. Alcohol.* **23**, 94.

Demanet, J. C., Bonnyns, M., Bleiberg, H. and Stevens-Rocmans, C. (1971). Coma due to water intoxication in beer drinkers. *Lancet* **ii**, 1115.

Department of Health and Social Security (DHSS) (1973). *Alcoholism*. Medical Memorandum, London.

Drew, G. C., Colquhoun, W. P. and Long, H. A. (1958). Effect of small doses of alcohol on a skill resembling driving. *Br. med. J.* **2**, 993.

Edwards, G., Hawker, A., Williamson, V. and Hensman, C. (1966). London's skid row. *Lancet* **i**, 249.

Ekbom, K., Hed, R., Kirstein, L. and Astrom, K. (1964). Muscular affections in chronic alcoholism. *Arch. Neurol., Chicago* **10**, 449.

Engel, A. G. (1981). Metabolic and endocrine myopathies. In *Disorders of voluntary muscle* (ed. J. N. Walton), 4th edn., p. 664. Churchill-Livingstone, Edinburgh.

Hald, J. and Jacobsen, E. (1948). A drug sensitizing the organism to ethyl alcohol. *Lancet* **ii**, 1001.

Harper, C. and Krill, J. (1985). Brain atrophy in chronic alcoholic patients. *J. Neurol. Neurosurg. Psychiat.* **48**, 211.

Hed, R., Lundmark, C., Fahlgren, H. and Orell, S. (1962). Acute muscular syndrome in chronic alcoholism. *New Engl. J. Med.* **274**, 1277.

Hillbom, M. and Kaste, M. (1978). Does ethanol intoxication promote brain infarction in young adults? *Lancet* **ii**, 1181.

Hillman, R. S. (1975). Alcohol and hematopoiesis. In *Medical Consequences of alcoholism* (ed. F. A. Seixas, K. Williams and S. Eggleston). *Ann. NY Acad. Sci.* **252**, 297.

Holtermann, S. and Burchell, A. (1981). *The costs of alcohol misuse* (Government Economic Service Working Paper No. 37). DHSS, London.

Hore, B. D., Ritson, E. B. and Thomson, A. D. (1982). *Alcohol and health: a handbook for medical students*. Medical Council on Alcoholism, London.

Ironside, R., Bosanquet, F. D. and McMenemey, W. H. (1961). Central demyelination of the corpus callosum (Marchiafava–Bignami disease). *Brain* **84**, 212.

Ishii, N. and Nishihara, Y. (1981). Pellagra among chronic alcoholics: clinical and pathological study of 20 necropsy cases. *J. Neurol. Neurosurg. Psychiat.* **44**, 209.

Jellinek, E. M. (1951). W. H. O. Expert Committee on Medical Health. Subcommittee on Alcoholism Report, *Wld. Hlth. Org., techn. Rep. Ser.* **42**, 20.

Konttinen, A., Härtel, G. and Louhija, A. (1970). Multiple serum enzyme analyses in chronic alcoholics. *Acta med. scand.* **188**, 257.

The Lancet (1982). Alcoholic disease. *Lancet* **i**, 1105.

—— (1983). Methanol poisoning. *Lancet* **i**, 910.

Lee, K., Møller, L., Hardt, F., Haubek, A. and Jensen, E. (1979). Alcohol-induced brain damage and liver damage in young males. *Lancet* **ii**, 759.

Leiber, C. S. (1980). Alcoholism—a medical approach. *Br. J. Alcohol & Alcoholism* **153**, 95.

Lishman, W. A. (1981). Cerebral disorder in alcoholism: syndromes of impairment. *Brain* **104**, 1.

Marchiafava, E. (1932–3). The degeneration of the brain in chronic alcoholism. *Proc. R. Soc. Med.* **26**, 1151.

Martensen-Larsen, O. (1948). Treatment of alcoholism with a sensitizing drug. *Lancet* **ii**, 1004.

McLean, D. R., Jacobs, H. and Mielke, B. W. (1980). Methanol poisoning: a clinical and pathological study. *Ann. Neurol.* **8**, 161.

Merry J. and Marks, V. (1972). The effect of alcohol, barbiturate and diazepam on hypothalamic/pituitary/adrenal function in chronic alcoholics. *Lancet* **ii**, 960.

Office of Health Economics (1981). *Alcohol: reducing the harm*. Office of Health Economics, London.

Oh, S. J. (1972). Alcoholic myopathy: initial review. *Alabama J. med. Sci.* **9**, 79.

Olin, J. W. (1966). 'Skid-row' syndrome: a medical profile of the chronic drunkenness offender. *Can. med. Ass. J.* **95**, 205.

Paton, A., Potter, J. F., Lewis, K. O., Bissell, D., Ritson, B., Saunders, J. B. and Smerdon, G. (1982). *ABC of Alcohol* (Articles published in the *British Medical Journal*). *British Medical Journal*, London.

Peiffer, J., Majewski, F., Fischbach, H., Bierich, J. R. and Volk, B. (1979). Alcohol embryo and fetopathy. *J. neurol. Sci.* **41**, 125.

Perkoff, G. T., Hardy, P., Velez-Garcia, E. (1966). Reversible acute muscular syndrome in chronic alcoholism. *New Engl. J. Med.* **274**, 1277.

Phillips, S. C. (1981). Does ethanol damage the blood-brain barrier? *J. neurol. Sci.* **50**, 81.

——, Cragg, B. G. and Singh, S. C. (1981). The short-term toxicity of ethanol to neurons in rat cerebral cortex tested by topical application in vivo and a note on a problem in estimating ethanol concentrations in tissue. *J. Neurol. Sci.* **49**, 353.

Ron, M. A., Acker, W., Shaw, G. K. and Lishman, W. A. (1982). Computerized tomography of the brain in chronic alcoholism: a survey and follow-up study. *Brain*, **105**, 497.

Seixas, F. A., Williams, K. and Eggleston, S. (Eds.) (1975). Medical consequences of alcoholism. *Ann. NY Acad. Sci.* **252**.

Sereny, G. and Kalant, H. (1965). Comparative clinical evaluation of chlordiazepoxide and promazine in treatment of alcohol-withdrawal syndrome, *Br. med. J.* **1**, 92.

Sharpe, J. A., Mostovsky, M., Bilbao, J. M. and Rewcastle, N. B. (1982). Methanol optic neuropathy: a histopathological study. *Neurology, Minneapolis* **32**, 1093.

Sim, M. (1975). *Guide to psychiatry*, 3rd edn. Churchill-Livingstone, Edinburgh.

Smith, J. J. (1949). The treatment of acute alcoholic states with A.C.T.H. (adrenocorticotrophic) and A.C.E. (adrenocortical) hormones. *Quart. J. Stud. Alcohol.* **11**, 190.

Tavel, M. E., Davidson, W. and Batterton, T. D. (1961). A critical analysis of mortality associated with delirium tremens. *Am. J. med. Sci.* **242**, 18.

Torvik, A., Lindboe, C. F. and Rogde, S. (1982). Brain lesions in alcoholics: a neuropathological study with clinical correlations. *J. neurol. Sci.* **56**, 233.

Victor, M. and Adams, R. D. (1953). The effect of alcohol on the nervous system. In *Metabolic and toxic diseases of the nervous system.* ARNMD Vol. 32, p. 526. Williams and Wilkins, Baltimore.

—— and —— (1961). On the etiology of the alcoholic neurologic diseases. *Am. J. clin. Nutr.* **9**, 379.

—— and —— (1974). Alcohol. *Harrison's Principles of Internal Medicine*, 7th edn (ed. M. M. Wintrobe *et al.*) Chapter 111. McGraw-Hill, New York.

——, —— and Mancall, E. L. (1959). A restricted form of cerebellar cortical degeneration occurring in alcoholic patients. *Arch. Neurol., Chicago* **1**, 579.

Voegtlin, W. L. (1940). The treatment of alcoholism by establishing a conditioned reflex. *Am. J. med. Sci.* **199**, 802.

——, Lemere, F., Broz, W. R. and O'Hollaren, P. (1942). Conditioned reflex therapy of alcoholic addiction: follow-up report of 1042 cases. *Am. J. med. Sci.* **203**, 525.

Williams, G. P. and Glatt, M. M. (1965). Unrecognized drinking. *Lancet* **ii**, 1294.

Drug addiction

General considerations

Drug addiction has been defined as the habitual use of a drug in order to modify the personality and diminish the strain of life. It is characterized by tolerance (increased doses are required to produce the desired effect), craving, and the development of severe symptoms on withdrawal. Drugs of addiction include opium and its derivatives, such as morphine and heroin and also pethidine (meperidine) and various other synthetic analgesic drugs; and cocaine. Within recent years addiction to barbiturates, amphetamine and its derivatives, and to lysergic acid diethylamide (LSD) and other hallucinogens has been recognized increasingly and, more rarely, addiction to anaesthetic and other volatile inhalants (e.g. glue sniffing) has been reported.

Drug habituation has been regarded as repeated use of a drug coupled with a desire to continue taking it but with little or no tendency to increase the dose. The dependence is psychological and not physical, hence there are no physical symptoms of deprivation. Bromides, nicotine, and marihuana (cannabis) are among the drugs traditionally regarded as leading to habituation. Millman (1982) suggests, however, that the phase of *psychological dependence* (habituation) is often followed by *compulsive drug abuse*, and then, in certain cases and with certain drugs, *physical dependence* or addiction.

Addiction to opiates and other synthetic analgesic drugs

Aetiology

The addict to morphine and to other analgesics may acquire his habit as a result of the legitimate administration of the drug for the relief of physical pain. As tolerance develops, increasing doses are required. After a time he becomes unable to relinquish the drug without developing the symptoms of abstinence described below. Moreover, to avoid this, he requires increasing doses. Morphine eventually gives the addict no pleasurable sensations. And De Quincey wrote: 'Opium had long ceased to found its empire upon spells of pleasure; it was solely by the tortures connected with the attempt to abjure it that it kept its hold.' Very few, however, who receive narcotics for the relief of pain become addicts. The drug, besides relieving pain, blunts the edge of reality: to the psychologically unstable, therefore, it affords a way of escape from life's difficulties. Having experienced the sedative effects of morphine, they continue to take it for the relief of mental pain or distress, and are thus fettered to their habit by a double bond, psychological and physiological.

Within recent years, addiction to many synthetic analgesic drugs has been reported and most of the remedies involved were listed by Victor and Adams (1974). They include diacetylmorphine (heroin), dihydromorphinone, codeine and its derivatives, dipipanone, pethidine (meperidine or *Demerol*), methadone, levorphan, *d*-propoxyphene, and phenazocine; these remedies resemble the opiates pharmacologically, but vary in their pattern of abuse and addictive properties. Pentazocine, another synthetic remedy, has a low addictive tendency, but occasional cases of physical dependency have been described (Wood, Moir, Campbell, Davidson, Gallon, Henney, and McAllion 1974).

Doctors and nurses once constituted the majority of addicts, as they have ready access to the drugs. Residence in a country where they are readily obtainable may also facilitate the acquisition of the habit. However, addiction to opiates, and especially to 'street' heroin sold by 'pushers', reached epidemic proportions in the United States, especially in young people, in the 1960s so that heroin addiction became a leading cause of death in urban males between 15 and 35 years of age. Most addicts were introduced to the habit by friends and most used intravenous injection ('mainlining'), often of impure preparations with obvious risks and complications. The number of drug addicts in the United States was officially said in 1955 to be 44 905 and Canada 3295 and in Great Britain about 470, but numbers have increased greatly within the last 20 years and Victor and Adams estimated in 1974 that there were over 400 000 addicts in New York city alone; the incidence in Great Britain and Europe was much less but nevertheless increased alarmingly.

There is some evidence to suggest that opiate addiction declined for a time as alcoholism increased in the young, but it is again increasing and remains an enormous social problem in many countries; in Britain there appears to have been an upsurge in the 1980s. There were 5116 registered opiate addicts in Britain in 1980 (Mitcheson 1983). Relatively few addicts are stable, leading useful lives on a fixed dose, even among those who become addicts accidentally during treatment of a painful disease. Many addicts to all drugs have defects of personality which makes treatment difficult; even if this is not the case initially, addiction often leads to disintegration of the personality and progressive degradation (Edwards and Busch 1981). Certainly, brain damage also occurs; to quote but one example, a severe spongiform leucoencephalopathy can result from the inhalation of impure heroin pyrolysate (Wolters, van Wijngaarden, Stam, Rengelink, Lousberg, Schipper, and Verbeeten 1982).

Symptoms of addiction

Most addicts show progressive mental deterioration, with loss of interest in the environment, of intellectual efficiency, and of self-respect. They become untrustworthy, and may commit almost any crime to obtain a supply of the drug, if faced with the prospect of deprivation. Physically the picture is one of chronic toxaemia, including specific symptoms attributable to the pharmacological action of the drug. The pupils are usually contracted, and react sluggishly to light. The alimentary tract suffers severely; the appetite is poor and constipation is always present. There is almost invariably weight loss and evidence of general neglect. There is severe fatigability, and muscular weakness, frequently with some ataxia. The pulse is often thin, and the extremities are cold. Slight albuminuria may be present. Carelessness leads to infection of the skin at the site of the injections; the resulting scars are usually evident, while in some cases abscesses or ulcers may be present when the patient comes under observation.

Symptoms of withdrawal (abstinence)

The addict suddenly deprived of his drug develops highly characteristic symptoms. As the time for his usual injection passes he becomes restless and apprehensive, and yawning and sneezing develop, followed by the symptoms like those of an acute coryza. He feels cold, and contraction of the smooth muscles of the skin produces the appearance of 'goose-flesh'. Later he complains of cramps in the abdomen, back, or lower limbs. His face is contracted in his distress; perspiration is excessive, and muscular spasms and twitching occur, most violently in the lower extremities. There is often a general tremor and the patient may be violent in his demand for the drug. Later, vomiting and diarrhoea occur, and lead to a stage of circulatory collapse, which can even terminate fatally.

Treatment

Not every drug addict requires withdrawal treatment. Some stabilized addicts leading useful lives on a fixed dose, especially when past middle age, may be best left untreated but nevertheless require regular supervision. In Great Britain, the right to every doctor to prescribe opiate for addicts has now been proscribed by law and all addicts must now obtain their drugs from licensed doctors, some working in psychiatric units or in specialized centres for the treatment of drug addiction, others working in private general or specialist practice.

Treatment can be conducted on an out-patient or in-patient basis, but for the severe addict of longstanding, treatment as an in-patient is preferable if an attempt is to be made, as is preferable, to withdraw the drug. This should not be done without substitution of another agent (unless the patient is addicted, for example, to methadone, which can be withdrawn gradually with few side-effects), since even gradual withdrawal of opiates can cause severe circulatory collapse and pulmonary oedema requiring assisted respiration (Clemmesen and Lassen 1963). The substitute drug of choice is in fact methadone (in all except methadone addicts who may require a benzodiazepine), given in a dose of 20–40 mg daily, where possible with subsequent reduction and gradual withdrawal over 10–14 days. Morphine antagonists such as naloxone may increase withdrawal symptoms and are contra-indicated. Clonidine may prove to be a useful adjuvant (Millman 1982).

Supportive psychotherapy and close social supervision after withdrawal are of crucial importance since there is a high incidence of relapse, partly due to the 'addictive personality', sometimes to the environment to which the individual returns. Some become addicted to other drugs, such as alcohol. Others are helped to overcome their craving for opiates only by means of long-term maintenance therapy with an appropriate dose of methadone. Medical and social management of all forms of addiction are matters for the expert.

Cocaine addiction

Coca leaves were once chewed in South America for their sedative effects and their power of abolishing fatigue. Cocaine as a drug of addiction may be injected subcutaneously, drunk as coca wine, smoked, or taken as snuff. It acts to some extent as a sexual stimulant, and is stated to produce a sense of internal peace. Addicts suffer from progressive mental deterioration, and, in severe cases, from confusional psychosis. Hallucinations, especially of insects crawling under the skin, are common, and fits may occur. Cocaine sniffing may lead to ulceration of the nasal septum. Addicts suddenly deprived of cocaine do not suffer, like morphine addicts, from severe deprivation symptoms. Treatment, therefore, is not required to counteract these, but is similar to the after-treatment of the morphine addict. Cocainism, however, is often more difficult to cure than morphine addiction.

References

Ball, J. C. and Chambers, C. K. (1970). *The epidemiology of opiate addiction in the United States*. Thomas, Springfield, Illinois.

Clemmesen, C. (1963). Treatment of narcotic intoxication. *Dan. med. Bull.* **10**, 97.

—— and Lassen, N. A. (1963). Treatment of circulatory shock in narcotic poisoning. *Dan. med. Bull.* **10**, 100.

Dole, V. P. and Byswander, M. E. (1968). Methadone maintenance and its implication for theories of narcotic addiction. *Res. Publ. Ass. nerv. ment. Dis.* **46**, 359.

Edwards, G. and Busch, C. (Eds.) (1981). *Drug problems in Britain: a review of ten years*. Academic Press, London.

Millman, R. B. (1982). Drug abuse, dependence and intoxication. In *Cecil textbook of medicine* (ed. J. B. Wyngaarden, and L. H. Smith, 16th edn, Chapter 446. Saunders, Philadelphia.

Mitcheson, M. (1983). Addiction. In *Oxford textbook of medicine* (ed. D. J. Weatherall, J. G. G. Ledingham and D. A. Warrell), p. 24.43. Oxford Medical, Oxford.

Vaillant, G. E. (1966). A 12-year follow-up of New York narcotic addicts. *Arch. gen. Psychiat.* **15**, 599.

Victor, M. and Adams, R. D. (1974). Opiates and other analgesic drugs. In *Harrison's principles of internal medicine*, 7th edn, Chapter 112, McGraw-Hill, New York.

Wolters, E. C., van Wijngaarden, G. K., Stam, F. C., Rengelink, H., Lousberg, R. J., Schipper, M. E. I. and Verbeeten, B. (1982). Leucoencephalopathy after inhaling "heroin" pyrolysate. *Lancet* **ii**, 1233.

Wood, A. J., Moir, D. C., Campbell, C., Davidson, J. F., Gallon, S. C., Henney, E. and McAllion, S. (1974). Medicines evaluation and monitoring group: central nervous system effects of pentazocine. *Br. med. J.* **1**, 305.

Sedatives and hypnotics

Barbiturates, chloral hydrate, the newer hypnotics and many allied drugs may be taken as drugs of habituation, either alone or with morphine, and addicts may become tolerant of enormous doses. All produce similar symptoms, both in cases of acute poisoning and in addicts, but some have additional individual peculiarities.

Habituation to synthetic hypnotics

When taken habitually (Glatt 1966) these drugs cause lethargy, dysarthria, nystagmus, muscular weakness, tremor, and incoordination. There is usually considerable emaciation. Chloral has a markedly toxic effect on the heart and on the skin, causing reddening of the face and a papular eruption. Treatment involves gradual withdrawal: sudden withdrawal may cause convulsions. The general management is similar to that of morphine addiction.

The introduction of many new sedative and tranquillizing remedies has been followed by reports of habituation to many of these including meprobamate, glutethimide, chlordiazepoxide, diazepam, and many more. When taken to excess, these drugs give symptoms like those of acute or chronic barbiturate intoxication (see below) and long-term habituation followed by withdrawal can result in withdrawal symptoms including hallucinations and delirium. The elderly are much more sensitive to the effects of the benzodiazepines than young subjects (Castleden, George, Marcer, and Hallett 1977) and the possibility has now been raised that long-continued and heavy use of these drugs may cause cerebral atrophy (Poser, Poser, Roscher, and Argyrakis 1983). Recent evidence (Ashton 1984; Tyrer 1984) clearly indicates that the problem of benzodiazepine (especially diazepam) dependence and the severity of withdrawal symptoms have both been underestimated.

The phenothiazines, by contrast, and related remedies such as reserpine and the butyrophenones (e.g. haloperidol) may cause cholestatic jaundice, agranulocytosis, epileptiform attacks, orthostatic hypotension, skin sensitivity reactions, and extrapyramidal manifestations including drug-induced parkinsonism and orofacial dyskinesia (see pp. 324 and 349 and Lader 1970).

Barbiturate poisoning

In Great Britain the increasing use of barbiturates and of other sedative drugs for suicidal attempts meant that in the 1950s and

1960s this group of drugs were more often used than coal-gas poisoning as a method of attempting suicide (Cumming 1961) and there were then more than 3000 hospital admissions annually due to this cause. Because of the frequency with which these drugs were used for suicidal attempts, extensive and successful efforts were made in Great Britain to reduce their use as many more satisfactory sedatives and hypnotics became available. However, even the benzodiazepines such as diazepam and nitrazepam are not without risk and are now often used, as are anti-depressive agents, in attempted (and successful) suicide.

In mild cases slurred speech, drowsiness, ataxia, and nystagmus are apparent but when the dose ingested is large patients are stuporose or comatose and there is eventually total areflexia with hypotension and oliguria. Small blisters filled with serum may appear on the limbs in severe cases. Hypothermia and cardiac arrest may occur (Fell, Gunning, Bardhan, and Triger 1968).

Management consists first in aspirating stomach contents, in identifying when possible the causative agent in these or in blood or urine (or by searching the patient's belongings or questioning the relatives or family doctor concerning drugs which were in the patient's possession). Maintenance of an adequate airway, often by intubation, of the blood pressure by the use of appropriate drugs (e.g. methedrine), of the fluid and electrolyte intake by intravenous therapy and the administration of appropriate antibiotics with intensive nursing care to prevent pulmonary collapse and bed-sores are all essential. The use of analeptic drugs such as bemegride and amiphenazole has been generally discarded in favour of elimination of the offending drug by dialysis with the artificial kidney in severe cases. Catheterization is usually necessary and assisted respiration may be required for several days. With such measures recovery from very severe poisoning is common (Kennedy, Lindsay, Briggs, Like, Young, and Campbell 1969; Millman 1982).

Chronic barbiturate intoxication is still relatively common (see Victor and Adams 1974). The clinical picture resembles that of alcoholism and chronic intoxication; as in alcoholism, delirium and withdrawal convulsions may follow withdrawal and treatment is similar to that of delirium tremens.

References

Ashton, H. (1984). Benzodiazepine withdrawal: an unfinished story. *Br. med. J.* **i**, 1135.

Castleden, C. M., George, C. F., Marcer, D. and Hallett, C. (1977). Increased sensitivity to nitrazepam in old age. *Br. med. J.* **1**, 10.

Cumming, G. (1961). *The medical management of acute poisoning*. Blackwell, London.

Essig, C. F. (1966). Non-narcotic addiction. *J. Am. med. Ass.* **196**, 714.

—— (1972). Chronic abuse of sedative-hypnotic drugs. In *Drug abuse* (ed. C. J. D. Zarafonetis) p. 205. Saunders, Philadelphia.

Fell, R. H., Gunning, A. J., Bardham, K. D. and Triger, D. R. (1968). Severe hypothermia as a result of barbiturate overdose complicated by cardiac arrest, *Lancet* **i**, 392.

Glatt, M. M. (1966). Controlled trials of non-barbiturate hypnotics and tranquillisers. *Psychiat. Neurol.* **152**, 28.

Kennedy, A. C., Lindsay, R. M., Briggs, J. D., Luke, R. G., Young, N. and Campbell D. (1969). Successful treatment of three cases of very severe barbiturate poisoning. *Lancet* **i**, 995.

Lader, M. H. (1970). Drug-induced extrapyramidal syndromes. *J. R. Coll. Phycns. London* **5**, 87.

Millman, R. B. (1982). Central nervous system depressants. In *Cecil textbook of medicine* (ed. J. B. Wyngaarden and L. H. Smith) 16th edn, Chapter 448. Saunders, Philadelphia.

Poser, W., Poser, S., Roscher, D. and Argyrakis, A. (1983). Do benzodiazepines cause cerebral atrophy? *Lancet* **i**, 715.

Tyrer, P.J. (1984). Benzodiazepines on trial. *Br. med. J.* **i**, 1101.

Victor M. and Adams, R. D. (1974). Barbiturates (Chapter 113). Depressants, stimulants and psychotegenic drugs (Chapter 114). In *Harrison's principles of internal medicine*, 7th edn. McGraw-Hill, New York.

Wright, J. T. (1955). The value of barbiturate estimations in the diagnosis and treatment of barbiturate intoxication. *Quart. J. Med.* **24**, 95.

Chronic bromide intoxication

Chronic bromide intoxication is now rare but occasionally results from the prolonged administration of bromide in proprietary headache preparations or in little-used sedatives such as carbromal.

Bromide tends to replace chlorides in the body, and more bromide will be absorbed by a person with a low chloride intake than by one who is taking more chloride. The blood bromide level is a rough index of intoxication, though individual susceptibility varies. The normal level of bromide in the blood is under 3 mg per 100 ml. According to Barbour, Pilkington, and Sargant (1936), levels of under 100 mg per 100 ml can be ignored; those between 100 and 200 mg per 100 ml are usually associated with symptoms of intoxication in the elderly or in those with impaired cardiac or renal function, and levels of over 200 mg per 100 ml produce symptoms in most cases. Bromide, like chloride, is excreted into the stomach and so may be reabsorbed.

In mild cases the symptoms are depression, fatigability, inability to concentrate, loss of memory, lack of appetite, and poor sleep. In more severe cases there is confusion with some disorientation. Terrifying hallucinations, especially occurring at night, are rather characteristic. Physical signs are variable: when severe they consist of slurred speech, tremor and ataxia of the upper limbs, a staggering gait, and diminution or loss of tendon reflexes. In more severe cases still the patient becomes stuporose. The rash often regarded as characteristic is frequently absent.

The bromide must be discontinued immediately and the patient given increases sodium chloride and fluid by mouth. In severe cases dialysis may be used. Restlessness is controlled if necessary by diazepam.

References

Barbour, R. F., Pilkington, F. and Sargant, W. (1936). Bromide intoxication *Br. med. J.* **2**, 957.

Minski, L. and Gillen, J. B. (1937). Blood bromide investigations in psychotic epileptics *Br. med. J.* **2**, 850.

Marihuana (hashish, Cannabis indica)

This drug (colloquially called 'grass') which has long been used by certain races in the Orient and in South America has recently been used extensively in Western countries, often being smoked in cigarettes ('joints'). Its use is still illegal in most developed countries; it is a drug of habituation and not of addiction and in itself it is usually thought to be a relatively minor nuisance rather than a serious social evil. It produces a transient sense of well-being and sometimes reversible hallucinations. One of its major dangers has been thought to be that for social reasons it may introduce its habitues to narcotics.

There has been considerable pressure in the United States and in Europe from certain groups who wish the social use of the drug to be legalized, partly on the grounds that its use is so widespread in many countries that existing laws are being continuously flouted, partly because it is believed by some that its very illegality encourages many young people to use it, and partly because there are many who believe it to be less of a social evil than alcohol. Clearly its occasional or intermittent use in low dosage does no lasting harm, but personality changes, loss of drive and purpose, academic failure, and various emotional symptoms have been reported in habitual users who may also show reversal of sleep rhythm and impairment of recent memory (Kolansky and Moore 1971). Campbell, Evans, Thomson and Williams (1971) suggested that heavy and prolonged smoking may lead to cerebral atrophy demonstrable by pneumoencephalography, but this important question remains unsolved even with CT scanning, although, on balance, it seems probable that like alcohol, severe abuse can cause dementia and definite atrophy (Edwards and Busch 1981). Cannabis smoke is also potentially carcinogenic.

Amphetamine addiction

Amphetamines and their derivatives are commonly taken by young people in order to obtain temporary uplift or mental alertness, or to reduce desire for sleep. Addiction has also occurred in young and middle-aged women who received these drugs in therapeutic doses for the treatment of depression or fatigue or obesity. Connell (1958) described acute psychotic states of paranoid and hallucinatory nature, while psychopathic and irresponsible behaviour is also common. Fits may occur as a result of intoxication or withdrawal. A common sign of addiction is continuous chewing, grinding of the teeth or licking of the lips, sometimes resulting in ulceration. A necrotizing vasculitis with frequent involvement of the nervous system leading to cerebral haemorrhage or infarction is an uncommon complication of amphetamine abuse and has also been described after ephedrine abuse (Wooten, Khangure, and Murphy 1983).

Other stimulants

Caffeine (a cup of tea or coffee contains 100–150 mg, and this drug is also a constituent of cola drinks) is a mild stimulant which, when taken to excess may cause insomnia, tachycardia, mild cardiac arrhythmias, and diuresis, but serious side-effects are rare. Cigarette smoking with consequent absorption of nicotine has a mild stimulant effect and may affect reaction time (Ashton, Savage, Telford, Thompson, and Watson 1972) and the 'contingent negative variation' in the EEG of human subjects (Ashton, Millman, Telford, and Thompson 1974) but there are no known long-term neurological ill-effects of smoking.

Monoamine oxidase inhibitors (e.g. phenelzine and tranylcypromine) have been widely used in the treatment of neurotic depression; in excess they have been known to cause insomnia, agitation, orthostatic hypotension, limb oedema, and even mania and convulsions. The principal danger of these remedies is that if they are taken along with tyramine-containing foods or beverages (cheese, 'Marmite', beer and red wine), severe hypertensive reactions may occur, sometimes causing intense headache, cardiac arrhythmias, cerebral vascular accidents, and even death. Similar cross-reactions may occur with phenothiazines and narcotic remedies.

Tricyclic antidepressive remedies, such as imipramine or amitryptiline and their derivatives, have proved invaluable in the treatment of depressive illness but may on occasion cause not only dryness of the mouth, constipation, blurring of vision, and other parasympathetomimetic effects, but sometimes orthostatic hypotension, agitation, restlessness and even ataxia, blood dyscrasia, and rarely, convulsions (especially in epileptics or individuals with a low convulsive threshold).

Hallucinogenic agents

The use of hallucinogenic drugs such as lysergic acid (LSD) and mescaline increased for a time and in some universities and other circles developed almost into a cult. The danger of these drugs is that the induced hallucinations are sometimes terrifying and rarely pleasurable and the view that they produce increased perception is a dangerous delusion. Irreversible psychosis may result and accidents have occurred during delusional episodes. Phencyclidine (PCP), a veterinary anaesthetic, has similar effects but is almost exclusively used for its hallucinatory effects in the USA (Mitcheson 1983). The abuse of these agents now seems to be on the decline and the users have become more sophisticated in avoiding the most severe adverse reactions. However, a recent disturbing development has been an 'epidemic' involving the use in Glasgow of hallucinogenic fungi (Young, Milroy, Hutchinson, and Kesson 1982).

Volatile inhalants

For some years it has been recognized that some doctors, particularly anaesthetists, may become addicted to some of the anaesthetic agents which they use in their clinical practice and which they inhale for their pleasurable effects. A myeloneuropathy has been reported to follow repeated and prolonged deliberate or accidental exposure to nitrous oxide in dentists (Layzer 1978). More recently in the USA, Britain, and in many other countries, children and adolescents have experimented with the inhalation of vapour given off by glues, especially those used in plastic modelling kits. When used in small amounts, the ill-effects of glue-sniffing are slight and transient, but sometimes confusional psychosis can occur and severe polyneuropathy sometimes results from the n-hexane which is a constituent of many glues (see p. 534). There is also evidence that toluene, present in many glues, can cause hallucinations, diplopia, convulsions, ataxia, and drowsiness leading to coma; while the encephalopathy is usually reversible, permanent brain damage may result (King, Day, Oliver, Lush, and Watson 1981).

References

Ashton, H., Millman, J. E., Telford, R. and Thompson, J. W. (1974). The effect of caffeine, nitrazepam and cigarette smoking on the contingent negative variation in man. *Electroenceph. clin. Neurophysiol.* **37**, 59.
——, Savage, R. D., Telford, R., Thompson, J. W. and Watson, D. W. (1972). The effect of cigarette smoking on the response to stress in a driving simulator. *Br. J. Pharmacol.* **45**, 546.
Campbell, A. M. G., Evans, M., Thomson, J. L. G. and Williams, M. J. (1971). Cerebral atrophy in young cannabis smokers. *Lancet*, **ii**, 1219.
Connell, P. H. (1958). *Amphetamine psychosis.* Maudsley Monographs, No. 5, London.
Edwards, G. and Busch, C. (eds.) (1981). *Drug problems in Britain: a review of ten years.* Academic Press, London.
King, M. D., Day, R. E., Oliver, J. S., Lush, M. and Watson, J. M. (1981). Solvent encephalopathy. *Br. med. J.* **283**, 486.
Kolansky, H. and Moore, W. T. (1971). Effects of marihuana on adolescents and young adults. *J. Am. med. Ass.* **216**, 486.
Layzer, R. B. (1978). Myeloneuropathy after prolonged exposure to nitrous oxide. *Lancet*, **ii**, 1227.
Mitcheson, M. (1983). Addiction. In *Oxford textbook of medicine* (ed. D. J. Weatherall, J. G. G. Ledingham, and D. A. Warrell) p. 24.43. Oxford Medical, Oxford.
Victor, M. and Adams, R. D. (1974). Depressants, stimulants and psychotogenic drugs. In *Harrison's principles of internal medicine*, 7th edn, Chapter 114. McGraw-Hill, New York.
Wooten, M. R., Khangure, M. S. and Murphy, M. J. (1983). Intracerebral hemorrhage and vasculitis related to ephedrine abuse. *Ann. Neurol.* **13**, 337.
Young, R. E., Milroy, R., Hutchison, S. and Kesson, C. M. (1982). The rising price of mushrooms. *Lancet* **i**, 213.

Anticonvulsant drugs

Anticonvulsants such as phenobarbitone, phenytoin, and primidone are occasionally used, especially by epileptic patients, for suicidal attempts. The symptoms and signs of acute poisoning and its management are similar to those described for barbiturate intoxication. During prolonged administration in the management of epilepsy the appearance of side-effects such as drowsiness, dysarthria, nystagmus, and ataxia may be due to variable absorption and utilization rates in different subjects or to changes in the excipient used in the preparation given (Tyrer, Eadie, Sutherland, and Hooper 1970) and can often be prevented by the estimation of blood levels (Kutt and Penry 1974; Eadie and Tyrer 1980). More troublesome side-effects include depression of folate metabolism with megaloblastic anaemia (Reynolds 1973), chronic lymphadenopathy, choreoathetosis and encephalopathy (McLellan and Swash 1974), and irreversible cerebellar degeneration (Dam 1970; Ghatak, Santoso, and McKinney 1976) which is fortunately rare. Phenytoin, carbamazepine, primidone, phenobarbitone, and sodium valproate may all cause asterixis, while phenytoin, but not the other remedies, can cause orofacial dyskinesia, limb chorea, and dystonia, possibly due to dopamine antagonism (Chadwick, Reynolds and Marsden 1976; Bodensteiner, Morris, and Golden 1981; Davies 1982), while valproate, which can impair oxidative phosphorylation (Haas, Stumpf, Parks, and Eguren 1981) can also cause a tremor like essential tremor (Karas, Wilder, Hammond, Bauman 1982) and hepatic dysfunction, with possible delayed brain maturation, in infant mice (Thurston, Hauhart, Schulz, Naccarato, Dodson, and Carroll 1981). Phenytoin may damage the cerebellum through its effect upon catecholamine metabolism (Snider and Snider 1977; McLain, Martin, and Allen 1980); it, too, can be hepatotoxic (Parker and Shearer 1979), it can depress thyroid function (Yoe, Bates, Howe, Ratcliffe, Schardt, Heath, and Evered 1978), and, like other anticonvulsants, sometimes causes osteomalacia (*British Medical Journal* 1976). Carbamazepine has been reported to precipitate an attack of non-hereditary acute porphyria (Laiwah, Rapeport, Thompson, MacPhee, Phillip, Moore, Brodie, and Goldberg 1983). The possibility that phenytoin may rarely be carcinogenic (*The Lancet* 1971) and that it and other anticonvulsants may have a teratogenic effect when taken during pregnancy (Annegers, Elveback, Hauser, an Kurland 1974) has also been raised. It now seems clear that long-continued use of phenytoin, for example, is associated with a slightly increased risk of developing lymphoma and that, taken during pregnancy, it increases the risk of congenital abnormalities in the fetus some two- to threefold (Eadie and Tyrer 1980; Laidlaw and Richens 1982). A fetal hydantoin syndrome with craniofacial and distal-limb dysmorphosis has also been described (Hansen and Smith 1975; *British Medical Journal* 1981).

References

Annegers, J. F., Elveback, L. R., Hauser, W. A. and Kurland, L. T. (1974). Do anticonvulsants have a teratogenic effect? *Arch. Neurol., Chicago* **31**, 364.

Bodensteiner, J. B., Morris, H. H. and Golden, G. S. (1981). Asterixis associated with sodium valproate. *Neurology, Minneapolis* **31**, 194.

British Medical Journal (1976). Anticonvulsant osteomalacia. *Br. med. J.* **2**, 1340.

—— (1981). Teratogenic risks of anti-epileptic drugs. *Br. med. J.* **283**, 515.

Chadwick, D., Reynolds, E. H. and Marsden, C. D. (1976). Anticonvulsant-induced dyskinesias: a comparison with dyskinesias induced by neuroleptics. *J. Neurol. Neurosurg. Psychiat.* **39**, 1210.

Dam. M. (1970). Number of Purkinje cells in patients with grand mal epilepsy treated with diphenylhydantoin. *Epilepsia*, **11**, 313.

Davies, D. M. (1982). *Textbook of adverse drug reactions*, 2nd edn. Oxford Medical, Oxford.

Eadie, M. J. and Tyrer, J. H. (1980). *Anticonvulsant therapy*, 2nd edn. Churchill-Livingstone, Edinburgh.

Ghatak, N. R., Santoso, R. A. and McKinney, W. M. (1976). Cerebellar degeneration following long-term phenytoin therapy. *Neurology, Minneapolis* **26**, 818.

Haas, R., Stumpf, D. A., Parks, J. K. and Eguren, L. (1981). Inhibitory effects of sodium valproate on oxidative phosphorylation. *Neurology, Minneapolis* **31**, 1473.

Hansen, J. W. and Smith, D. W. (1975). The fetal hydantoin syndrome. *J. Pediat.* **87**, 285.

Karas, B. J., Wilder, B. J., Hammond, E. J. and Bauman, A. W. (1982). Valproate tremors. *Neurology, Minneapolis* **32**, 428.

Kutt, H. and Penry, J. K. (1974). *A textbook of epilepsy*, 2nd edn. Churchill-Livingstone, Edinburgh.

Laiwah, A. A. C. Y., Rapeport, W. G., Thompson, G. G., MacPhee, G. J. A., Philip, M. F., Moore, M. R., Brodie, M. J., and Goldberg, A. (1983). Carbamazepine-induced non-hereditary acute porphyria. *Lancet* i, 790.

The Lancet (1971). Is phenytoin carcinogenic? *Lancet* ii, 1071.

Mclain, L. W., Martin, J. T. and Allen, J. H. (1980). Cerebellar degeneration due to chronic phenytoin therapy. *Ann. Neurol.* **7**, 18.

McLellan, D. L. and Swash, M. (1974). Choreo-athetosis and encephalopathy induced by phenytoin. *Br. med. J.* **2**, 204.

Parker, W. A. and Shearer, C. A. (1979). Phenytoin hepatotoxicity: a case report and review, *Neurology, Minneapolis* **29**, 175.

Reynolds, E. H. (1973). Anticonvulsants, folic acid, and epilepsy. *Lancet* i, 1376.

Snider, S. R. and Snider R. S. (1977). Phenytoin and cerebellar lesions. *Arch. Neurol. Chicago* **34**, 162.

Thurston, J. H., Hauhart, R. E. and Schulz, D. W., Naccarato, E. F., Dodson, W. E. and Carroll, J. E. (1981). Chronic valproate administration produces hepatic dysfunction and may delay brain maturation in infant mice. *Neurology, Minneapolis* **31**, 1063.

Tyrer, J. H., Eadie, M. J., Sutherland, J. M. and Hooper, W. D. (1970). Outbreak of anticonvulsant intoxication in an Australian city. *Br. med. J.* **4**, 271.

Yeo, P. O. B., Bates, D., Howe, J. G., ad Ratcliffe, W. A., Schardt, C. W., Heath, A. and Evered, D. C. (1978). Anticonvulsants and thyroid function. *Br. med. J.* **1**, 1581.

Lead poisoning

Aetiology

The nervous symptoms once entitled plumbism, are usually due to chronic poisoning with lead. Industrial lead poisoning was once common, but has been greatly reduced by legislative restrictions. Lead poisoning still occurs, however, especially among plumbers, battery-makers, and painters (Graham, Maxton, and Twort 1981; Le Quesne 1981, 1982). In such cases the principal route of absorption of the lead is probably the digestive tract, though some may enter the body though the lungs. Water passing through lead pipes was an occasional cause in the past, and beer and cider were sometimes similarly contaminated. The first glass of these beverages, which had stayed in a lead pipe all night, was particularly dangerous. Sucking lead paint or pica are still important causes of poisoning in children (Barltrop 1968). Cosmetics containing lead are an occasional source of poisoning, which may also follow the use of lead obtained from diachylon plaster as a home-made abortifacient. Lead tetra-ethyl is a highly poisonous substance which has caused encephalopathy in the United States (see Spencer and Schaumburg 1980). It is used in small quantities in some forms of petrol. Because of its potential environmental effect due to inhalation of vehicle exhaust fumes, many countries are now introducing legislation to reduce the lead content of motor fuel.

At least 90 per cent of ingested lead is not absorbed and adults excrete about 0.3 mg daily in the faeces, while the usual amount in infants is 0.3 mg daily with an upper limit of 0.18 mg (Barltrop and Killala 1967). That which is absorbed from the gut first enters the erythrocytes and is then stored in liver, kidney and bone; very little if any is laid down in brain or skeletal muscle; later that stored in liver and kidney is gradually transferred to bone (Barltrop 1968, 1969). In chronic lead poisoning 95 per cent of the lead is stored in the bones as insoluble phosphate and storage is facilitated by a diet rich in calcium. In acidosis stored lead is released into the blood stream, and its excretion in the faeces and urine is much increased. Mobilization and excretion of lead can be similarly effected by parathormone. Rapid mobilization of lead may precipitate an attack of encephalopathy.

It has long been known that in lead neuropathy the muscles paralysed are usually those most used in the patient's occupation (Hunter 1978). Fullerton (1966) showed that this heavy metal produces both axonal degeneration and demyelination in the peripheral nerves of guinea-pigs. Recent work suggests that there is a direct toxic effect upon Schwann cells (Dyck, O'Brien and Ohnishi 1977).

Pathology

Lead exerts a toxic action by combining with essential SH-groups of certain enzymes involved in porphyrin synthesis and carbohydrate metabolism; in particular it depresses delta-aminolaevulinic acid dehydratase activity. Enzymes concerned with haem synthesis are also suppressed, thus accounting for the high incidence of anaemia, and renal tubular function is also impaired. There is also evidence that mitochondrial energy is diverted to support the transport of lead by the mechanism involved in Ca^{++} transport, resulting in uncoupling of oxidative phosphorylation (Cammer 1980). In the central nervous system, early neuropathological studies suggested that the metal produced widespread degeneration of cerebral and spinal-cord neurones but this is now disputed and the oedema of lead encephalopathy is associated with relatively little deposition of lead in the brain when compared with other tissues (Kehoe 1961 a, b; Goldstein and Diamond 1974). In acute lead encephalopathy the brain is pale and oedematous and meningeal irritation may also occur (Smith, McLaurin, Nichols, and Asbury 1960). Possibly the oedema and vacuolation with reactive glial changes are due to microvascular lesions (Winder, Garten, and Lewis 1983). In guinea-pigs in which lead produced combined axonal degeneration and demyelination in peripheral nerves, epileptic seizures were also common and could be provoked by noise or movement (Fullerton 1966). Similar seizures, in the absence of any recognizable pathological changes in the brain other than oedema, were seen in the baboon (Hopkins 1970).

It is now evident that the encephalopathy and the neuropathy usually result from exposure to inorganic lead, while organic lead (such as tetraethyl lead present in petrol) produces a very different syndrome characterized by disturbed sleep, nightmares, agitation, and frank psychosis, usually followed by complete recovery after acute exposure (Le Quesne 1982). It should, however, be noted that tetraethyl lead in petrol is converted into inorganic lead by combustion, the latter being discharged in exhaust fumes. Neuronal loss in the hippocampus of rats has been produced experimentally by this agent (Seawright, Brown, Aldridge, Verschoyle, and Street 1980).

Much interest has also been aroused by the suggestion that high infantile lead levels in serum resulting from environmental exposure may cause mental retardation (Millar, Battistini, Cummings, Carswell, and Goldberg 1970; Beattie, Moore, Goldberg, Finlayson, Graham, Machie, Main, McLaren, Murdoch, and Stewart 1975). This question is still unsettled (*The Lancet* 1978), but though certain findings are contradictory, it appears that levels above 40 μg/100 ml may cause slight cognitive impairment and there possibly may be psychological and behavioural effects at lower levels (Rutter 1980).

Symptoms and signs

Acute encephalopathy

This is an acute cerebral disturbance which is rare in adults but is commonly seen in children aged 1 or 2, and is characterized by irritability, convulsions, delirium, and coma, often associated with papilloedema, and sometimes with neck stiffness. The CSF is often abnormal; its pressure is increased, and there is an excess of globulin and of cells, which in adults are usually lymphocytes, though in children polymorphs may be present. An increase in the sugar content of the fluid has also been described, and the presence of lead in it has been demonstrated. Between 20 and 30 per cent of children who suffer from this condition have recurring fits as a sequel (Coffin, Phillips, Stadles, and Spector 1966).

Chronic encephalopathy

Defects of memory and cognition and convulsions have been observed as chronic manifestations of lead poisoning. Primary optic atrophy occasionally occurs. Laryngeal palsy is a rare symptom described by Gowers and by Harris, who saw a case of bilateral abductor paralysis.

Lead neuropathy

This condition usually affects the extensor muscles of the wrist and fingers, as a rule bilaterally, though the right side may suffer alone, especially in right-handed individuals. Wrist- and finger-drop occur, and the loss of synergic extension of the wrist causes weakness of flexion of the fingers. The brachioradialis often escapes and so, as a rule, does abductor pollicis longus. If the upper-arm is involved the spinati, deltoid, biceps, brachialis, and brachioradialis muscles may be affected. This distribution of paralysis is seen in those using these muscles repeatedly, as, for example, in men making batteries. The lower limbs are occasionally affected, the muscles paralysed being those supplied by the common peroneal nerve, with the exception of the tibialis anterior, which often escapes. It is characteristic of lead neuropathy that it is predominantly motor, and sensory symptoms and signs are usually slight or absent. Rarely, the weakness and wasting is so widespread that it simulates progressive muscular atrophy but the evidence that lead intoxication plays a part in the pathogenesis of motor neurone disease is unconvincing (p. 372).

The paralysed muscles waste and show electrophysiological evidence of denervation with mild slowing of motor nerve conduction velocity, but fasciculation and sensory changes are absent.

Other symptoms and signs

Other symptoms and signs may be of diagnostic value. The blue line should be sought on the gums. There may be a history of colic and indeed lead colic is often a prominent symptom in adults. There is often a secondary anaemia, with stippling of the red cells—punctate basophilia. Cardiovascular hypertrophy with high blood pressure may be present, or symptoms of renal tubular dysfunction. Gout is now a rare complication. In chronic lead poisoning in children X-rays may show a 'lead line', a band of increased density, at the diaphysial end of the growing bones. The normal content of lead in the blood is 10–60 μg per litre. In lead encephalopathy there may be 100–800 μg in the blood, and 100–1000 μg or more per litre of urine.

Diagnosis

Acute lead encephalopathy must be distinguished from uraemia, in which there is always a high blood-urea content, and from hypertensive encephalopathy in which the blood pressure is usually higher. Meningitis may be simulated. Lead neuropathy is distinguished from a lesion of the radial nerve by the escape of the brachioradialis and by its gradual onset and by the involvement of muscles not supplied by the radial nerve. In various other forms of polyneuropathy, foot-drop is usually associated with wrist-drop; pain and/or paraesthesiae in the limbs are often prominent; and there is often sensory loss with a 'glove and stocking' distribution. Moreover, the blue line on the gums and other symptoms of lead poisoning are absent. In all doubtful cases the blood should be examined for evidence of anaemia and punctate basophilia and a raised lead level, and lead should be sought in the urine and faeces.

Patients with lead poisoning excrete increased quantities of coproporphyrin III and of delta-amino-laevulinic acid in the urine so that urinary screening tests should be performed when the diagnosis is suspected.

Prognosis

The outlook in acute encephalopathy is always serious, especially when convulsions occur, but with modern methods of treatment the prognosis has improved, and recovery, when it occurs, may be complete, but many patients are left mentally handicapped, blind, or epileptic (Krigman, Bouldin, and Mushak 1980). Little improvement is to be expected in chronic encephalopathy. In lead neuropathy the prognosis is good, provided the patient is removed from contact with lead. Recovery, however, is usually slow and may take one or two years.

Treatment

The patient with lead poisoning must be removed from contact with lead, and must not return to an occupation which exposes him to it. If he does so, whatever precautions are taken, relapse is almost inevitable. The first question to be settled is whether the patient requires active elimination of the lead or not. The treatment of lead poisoning has been revolutionized by the introduction of chelating agents. Disodium calcium ethylene-diamine-tetra-acetate (CaEDTA, *Versene*) forms with lead a chelate, which is a stable, water-soluble, and virtually non-ionized complex, and which is excreted by the kidneys. Its successful use was described by Browne (1955) and Sidbury (1955). The drug can be given both orally and intravenously. The oral dose used by Sidbury was 30 mg per kg of body weight given twice daily with liberal amounts of water. Two methods have been used for the intravenous route: slow infusion of 1 g on the first day and 2 g a day thereafter for a total of five days in divided doses, twice daily in 250 ml of 5 per cent glucose in water; or 400 mg was given once or twice a day in 5 or 10 ml of saline. For children the dose is 60–75 mg per kg of body weight, given similarly. Both seem equally satisfactory. There is usually marked improvement or even complete disappearance of symptoms even including those of lead encephalopathy, on about the third day of treatment, when blood and urine analyses show that most of the readily available lead has been excreted. An alternative method of treatment is BAL in doses of 2–4 mg per kg of body weight given every 4 hours for up to 10 days. Indeed many authorities suggest combined therapy with calcium versenate and BAL; in mild cases, penicillamine 1.0–1.5 g daily for three to five days may be sufficient (Poskanzer and Bennett 1974). Since lead is deposited in the bones, patients who have been exposed to lead for long periods cannot eliminate the metal rapidly. They may therefore relapse and require further courses of treatment. Wrist-drop and finger-drop will require appropriate splinting and physiotherapy. Dexamethasone, 5 mg or appropriate lower doses in children, given three or four times daily to reduce cerebral oedema, is helpful in the immediate treatment of encephalopathy and, if convulsions occur, anticonvulsants are required.

References

Barltrop, D. (1968). Lead poisoning in childhood. *Postgrad. med. J.* **44**, 537.

—— (1969) Environmental lead and its paediatric significance. *Postgrad. med. J.* **45**, 129.

—— and Killala, N. J. P. (1967). Faecal excretion of lead by children. *Lancet* **ii**, 1017.

Beattie, A. D., Moore, M. R., Goldberg, A., Finlayson, M. J. W., Graham, J. F., Mackie, E. M., Main, J. C., McLaren, D. A., Murdoch, R. M. and Stewart, G. T. (1975). Role of chronic low-level lead exposure in the aetiology of mental retardation. *Lancet* **i**, 589.

Browne R. C. (1955). Metallic poisons and the nervous system. *Lancet* **i**, 775.

Cammer, W. (1980). Toxic demyelination: biochemical studies and hypothetical mechanisms. In *Experimental and clinical neurotoxicology* (ed. P. S. Spencer and H. H. Schaumburg), Chapter 17. Williams and Wilkins, Baltimore.

Coffin, R., Phillips, J. L., Stadles, W. I. and Spector, S. (1966). Treatment of lead encephalopathy in children. *J. Pediat*, **69**, 198.

Dyck P. J., O'Brien, P. C. and Ohnishi, A. (1977). Lead neuropathy: II. Random distribution of segmental demyelination among "old internodes" of myelinated fibres. *J. Neuropath. exp. Neurol.* **36**, 570.

Fullerton, P. M. (1966). Chronic peripheral neuropathy produced by lead-poisoning in the guinea-pig. *J. Neuropath. exp. Neurol.* **25**, 214.

Goldstein, G. W. and Diamond, I. (1974). Metabolic basis of lead encephalopathy. In *Brain dysfunction in metabolic disorders* (ed. F. Plum), ARNMD, Vol. 53, Williams and Wilkins, New York.

Graham, J. A. G., Maxton, D. G. and Twort, C. H. C. (1981). Painter's palsy: a difficult case of lead poisoning. *Lancet* **ii**, 1159.

Hopkins, A. (1970). Experimental lead poisoning in the baboon. *Br. J. Indust. Med.* **27**, 130.

Hunter, D. (1978). *The diseases of occupations*, 6th edn. London University Press, London.

—— and Aub, J. C. (1926–7). Lead studies. XV. The effect of the parathyroid hormone and on the excretion of lead and of calcium in patients suffering from lead poisoning. *Quart. J. Med.* **20**, 123.

Kehoe, R. A. (1961a). The metabolism of lead in man in health and disease. 2. Metabolism under abnormal conditions. *J. R. Inst. publ. Hlth.* **24**, 101.

—— (1961b). Present hygienic problems relating to the absorption of lead. *J. R. Inst. publ. Hlth.* **24**, 177.

Krigman, M. R., Bouldin, T. W. and Mushak, P. (1980). Lead. In *Experimental and clinical neurotoxicology* (ed. P. S. Spencer and H. H. Schaumburg), Chapter 34. Williams and Wilkins, New York.

The Lancet (1978). Lead and mental handicap. *Lancet* **i**, 365.

Le Quesne, P. M. (1981). Commentary on contemporary neurotoxicity. Toxic substances and the nervous system: the role of clinical observation. *J. Neurol. Neurosurg. Psychiat.* **44**, 1.

—— (1982). Metal-induced diseases of the nervous system. *Br. J. Hosp. Med.* **28**, 534.

McKhann, C. F. (1932). Lead poisoning in children: the cerebral manifestations. *Arch. Neurol. Psychiat., Chicago* **27**, 294.

Millar, J. A., Battistini, V., Cumming, R. L. C., Carswell, F. and Goldberg, A. (1970). Lead and delta-aminolaevulinic acid dehydratase levels in mentally retarded children and in lead-poisoned suckling rats. *Lancet* **ii**, 695.

Morris, C. E., Heyman, A. and Pozefsky, T. (1964). Lead encephalopathy from whiskey. *Neurology, Minneapolis* **14**, 493.

Poskanzer, D. C. and Bennett, I. L., Jr. (1974). Heavy metals. In *Harrison's principles of internal medicine*, 7th edn, Chap. 110, McGraw-Hill, New York.

Rutter, M. (1980). Raised lead levels and impaired cognitive/behavioural functioning: a review of the evidence. *Develop. Med. Child Neurol.* **22**, suppl. 42.

Seawright, A. A., Brown, A. W., Aldridge, W. N., Verschoyle, R. D. and Street, B. W. (1980). In mechanisms of toxicity and hazard evaluation (ed. B. Holmstedt, R. Mercier and M. Roberfroid). Elsevier/North-Holland, Amsterdam.

Disbury J. B., Jr. (1955). Lead poisoning. *Am. J. Med.* **17**, 932.

Smith, J. F., McLaurin, R. L., Nichols, J. B. and Asbury, A. (1960). Studies in cerebral oedema and cerebral swelling. *Brain* **83**, 411.

Spencer, P. S. and Schaumburg, H. H. (Eds.) (1980). *Experimental and clinical neurotoxicology*. Williams and Wilkins, New York.

Sinder, C., Garten, L. L. and Lewis, P. D. (1983). The morphological effects of lead on the developing central nervous system. *Neuropath. appl. Biol.* **9**, 87.

Manganese poisoning

This is an industrial disease due to the inhalation of manganese dust and occurs particularly in manganese miners in Chile and in some parts of central Europe. The clinical features, which often appear within 6–9 months of exposure, are those of an extrapyramidal syndrome like parkinsonism with slurred, monotonous speech, slowness and clumsiness of movement, facial masking, and anteropulsion or retropulsion. Personality change in the form of irritability, emotional liability, and variable euphoria may be succeeded by intense fatigue, lethargy, and somnolence. Little improvement usually follows removal of the patient from exposure to the dust but chelating agents or BAL may be of some value and levodopa relieves the parkinsonian features (Politis, Schaumburg, and Spencer 1980).

Mercury poisoning

Acute mercurial poisoning may produce neurological symptoms and signs, but gastro-intestinal and renal damage usually dominate the clinical picture. Chronic mercurial poisoning in children may give 'pink disease' (p. 542) and one form in adults is Minamata disease (see below). Chronic exposure to this metal in industry and even in police officers exposed to mercurial finger-print powder (which is no longer used) may give rise to a syndrome of tremor, variable limb weakness and ataxia, and personality change often characterized by fatigability, insomnia, irritability, and erethism (childish over-emotionalism). In the central nervous system there is often selective damage to the granular-cell layer of the cerebellum. The condition may result either from organic or inorganic mercurial poisoning as in the inhalation of mercury vapour in thermometer workers (Vroom and Greer 1972), the excessive use of mercurous chloride laxatives (Davis, Wands, Weiss, Price, and Girling 1974), or through eating bread made from wheat treated with methyl mercury as in an epidemic in Iraq (Rustam and Hamdi 1974). Asymptomatic sensorimotor poly-neuropathy has also been reported in workers exposed to inorganic mercury vapour in chlor-alkali plants (Albers, Cavender, Levine, and Langolf 1982) and accidental ethyl mercury poisoning resulting from eating the meat of a pig which had eaten seeds treated with fungicides containing ethyl mercury chloride was fatal in two children who showed evidence at autopsy of severe damage to brain, spinal motor neurones, peripheral nerves, skeletal muscle, and the myocardium (Cinca, Dumitrescu, Onaca, Serbanescu, and Nestorescu 1980). Follow-up of poisoned Iraqui children showed improvement in ataxia and motor weakness in some, but many with visual loss remained permanently blind and only a few recovered partial sight (Amin-Zaki, Majeed, Clarkson, and Greenwood 1978); there was marked psychomotor retardation in children born to mothers exposed to methyl mercury (some of whom were themselves asymptomatic) in that epidemic (Marsh, Myers, Clarkson, Amin-Zaki, Tikriti, and Majeed 1980), confirming the view of Snyder and Seelinger (1976) that transplacental poisoning is especially serious in its effects. BAL or chelating agents should be given in such cases and penicillamine may also be effective.

Minamata disease

Between 1953 and 1956 a disorder characterized by symptoms and signs of peripheral neuropathy, cerebellar ataxia, visual and hearing loss, and inconstant pyramidal-tract involvement, and sometimes by the development of a progressive encephalopathy, was noted in villagers living near Minamata Bay in Kyushu Island, Japan. In fatal cases widespread neuronal damage was found in the granular layer of the cerebellum and in the cerebral cortex. The condition usually followed the ingestion of fish and circumstantial evidence suggested that it was due to the toxic action of a mercurial compound contained in the effluent which flowed into Minamata Bay from a fertilizer factory. A 20-year follow-up of 10 patients has shown that many had residual postural (action) tremor and CT scanning revealed bilateral, symmetrical, low-density areas in the visual cortex and diffuse cerebellar atrophy, involving especially the inferior vermis (Tokuomi, Uchino, Imamura, Yamanaga, Nakanishi, and Ideta 1982). A similar syndrome has been described in fish-eating Canadian Indians (Wheatley, Barbeau, Clarkson, and Lapham 1979).

References

Albers, J. W., Cavender, G. D., Levine, S. P. and Langolf G. D. (1982). Asymptomatic sensorimotor polyneuropathy in workers exposed to elemental mercury. *Neurology, Minneapolis* **32**, 1168.

Amin-Zaki, L., Majeed, M. A., Clarkson, T. W. and Greenwood, M. R. (1978). Methylmercury poisoning in Iraqi children: clinical observations over two years. *Br. med. J.* **1**, 597.

Cinca, I., Dumitrescu, I., Onaca, P., Serbanescu, A. and Nestorescu, B. (1980). Accidental ethyl mercury poisoning with nervous system, skeletal muscle, and myocardium injury. *J. Neurol. Neurosurg. Psychiat.* **43**, 143.

Davis, L. E., Wands, J. R., Weiss, S. A., Price, D. L. and Girling, E. F. (1974). Central nervous system intoxication from mercurous chloride laxatives. *Arch. Neurol., Chicago* **30**, 428.

Hunter, D. (1978). *The diseases of occupations*, 6th edn, London University Press, London.

Marsh, D. O., Myers, G. J., Clarkson, T. W., Amin-Zaki, L., Tikriti, S. and Majeed, M. A. (1980). Fatal methylmercury poisoning: clinical and toxicological data on 29 cases. *Ann. Neurol.* **7**, 348.

McAlpine, D. and Araki, S. (1958). Minamata disease. *Lancet* **ii**, 629.

Politis, M. J., Schaumburg, H. H. and Spencer, P. S. (1980). Neurotoxicity of selected chemicals. In *Experimental and Clinical neurotoxicology* (ed. P. S. Spencer and H. H. Schaumburg), Chapter 42. Williams and Wilkins, New York.

Poskanzer, D. C. and Bennett, I. L., Jr. (1974). Heavy metals. In *Harrison's principles of internal medicine*, 7th edn, Chapter 110. McGraw-Hill, New York.

Rustam, H. and Hamdi, T. (1974). Methyl mercury poisoning in Iraq—a neurological study. *Brain*, **97**, 499.

Snyder, R. D. and Seelinger D. F. (1976). Methylmercury poisoning: clinical follow-up and sensory nerve conduction studies. *J. Neurol. Neurosurg. Psychiat.* **39**, 701.

Tokuomi, H., Uchino, M., Imamura, S., Yamanaga, H., Nakanishi, R. and Ideta, T. (1982). Minamata disease (organic mercury poisoning): neuroradiologic and electrophysiologic studies. *Neurology, Minneapolis* **32**, 1369.

Vroom, F. Q. and Greer, M. (1972). Mercury vapour intoxication. *Brain* **95**, 305.

Wheatley, B., Barbeau, A., Clarkson, T. W. and Lapham. L. W. (1979). Methylmercury poisoning in Canadian Indians—the elusive diagnosis, *Can. J. neurol. Sci.* **6**, 417.

Other metals

Bismuth

An acute toxic encephalopathy, giving rise to confusion, ataxia, dysarthria, and myoclonic jerking, was first reported from France, in patients taking bismuth subnitrate orally for the treatment of gastrointestinal disorders, often for control of colostomy function (Supino-Viterbo, Sicard, Risvegliato, Rancurel, and Buge 1977; Martin Boyer 1978). The EEC showed monomorphic waves at 3–5 Hz in frontal and temporo-rolandic areas, unaffected by eye opening. Other cases have been reported from Australia (*The Lancet* 1980; Le Quesne 1982); the condition has virtually disappeared since the sale of bismuth has been controlled.

Organic tin

In France in 1954–55 (Alajouanine, Dérobert, and Thiéffry 1958) a drug (diethyl tin iodide) was used to treat boils but contained some triethyl tin as an impurity and the latter caused acute cerebral oedema, involving separation of the laminae of central nervous system myelin, with headaches, drowsiness, and papilloedema; some cases of paraplegia due to spinal-cord oedema also occurred. Epilepsy has also been reported after exposure to triethyl tin (Spencer and Schaumburg 1980; Le Quesne 1982).

Aluminium

Dialysis encephalopathy, characterized by epilepsy, often focal at the outset with variable localizing signs, goes on to cause progressive dementia eventually leading to a fatal termination (Burke, Alfrey, Huddlestone, Novenberg, and Lewin 1976). This disease was found to occur in patients undergoing renal dialysis only in certain units (Denver, Newcastle upon Tyne, Glasgow) where there was also a high incidence of renal bone disease, and was shown to be due to aluminium deposition in the brain due to a high concentration of this trace element in the public water supply

(McDermott, Smith, Ward, Parkinson, and Kerr 1978; Lederman and Henry 1978; Parkinson, Ward, Feest, Fawcett, and Kerr 1979; European Dialysis and Transplant Association 1980). Since aluminium was removed from the dialysis fluid this condition has virtually disappeared. Rejection encephalopathy following renal transplantation (Gross, Sweny, Pearson, Kennedy, Fernando, and Moorhead 1982) is a reversible disorder unrelated to aluminium intoxication.

Thallium

Thallium poisoning produces symptoms varying from mild polyneuropathy with alopecia to severe cranial and peripheral neuropathy, anuria, heart failure, and irreversible coma and death (Bank, Pleasure, Suzuki, Nigro, and Katz 1972; Kennedy and Cavanagh 1976; Davis, Standefer, Kornfeld, Abercrombie, and Butler 1981). In such cases there is primary axonal degeneration with secondary myelin loss; affected axons are swollen, containing distended mitochondria and vacuoles. Thallium is found in highest concentration in the brain in cerebral cortical and thalamic grey matter, but the neuropathological findings here are less distinctive.

Lithium

Lithium, used in the treatment of periodic depression, can give rise to severe intoxication, even in those receiving a stable dosage over long periods, unless blood levels are carefully monitored (Hansen and Amdisen 1978). Nephropathy with hypernatraemia may occur, but neurologically the principal manifestations are confusion, tremor, dysarthria, drowsiness, occasional fits, and rarely, acute generalized polyneuropathy (Brust, Hammer, Challenor, Healton, and Lesser 1979). Dialysis may be needed as emergency treatment.

References

Alajouanine, T., Dérobert, L. and Thieffry, S. (1958) Étude clinique d'ensemble de 210 cas d'intoxication par les sels organiques d'étain. *Rev. Neurol.* **98**, 85.

Bank, W. J., Pleasure, D. E., Suzuki, K., Nigro, M. and Katz R. (1972). Thallium poisoning. *Arch. Neurol., Chicago* **26**, 456.

Brust, J. C. M., Hammer, J. S., Challenor, Y., Healton, E. B. and Lesser, R. P. (1979). Acute generalized polyneuropathy accompanying lithium poisoning. *Ann. Neurol.* **6**, 360.

Burks, J. S., Alfrey, A. C., Huddlestone, J., Norenberg, M. D. and Lewin, E. (1976). A fatal encephalopathy in chronic haemodialysis patients. *Lancet* **i**, 764.

Davis, L. E., Standefer, J. C., Kornfeld, M., Abercrombie, D. M. and Butler, C. (1981). Acute thallium poisoning: toxicological and morphological studies of the nervous system. *Ann. Neurol.* **10**, 38.

European Dialysis and Transplant Association (1980). Dialysis dementia in Europe. *Lancet* **ii**, 190.

Gross, M. L. P., Sweny, P., Pearson, R. M., Kennedy, J., Fernando, O. N. and Moorhead, J. F. (1982). Rejection encephalopathy: an acute neurological syndrome complicating renal transplantation. *J. neurol. Sci.* **56**, 23.

Hansen, H. E. and Amdisen, A. (1978). Lithium intoxication (report of 23 cases and review of 100 cases from the literature). *Quart. J. Med.* **47**, 123.

Kennedy, P. and Cavanagh, J. B. (1976). Spinal changes in the neuropathy of thallium poisoning. *J. neurol. Sci.* **29**, 295.

The Lancet (1980). Idiosyncratic neurotoxicity: clioquinol and bismuth. *Lancet* **i**, 857.

Lederman, R. J. and Henry, C. E. (1978). Progressive dialysis encephalopathy, *Ann. Neurol.* **4**, 199.

Le Quesne, P. M. (1982). Metal-induced diseases of the nervous system. *Br. J. Hosp. Med.* **28**, 534.

Martin Boyer, G. (1978). Intoxications par les sels de bismuth administrés par voie orale. *Gastroenterol. Clin. Biol.* **2**, 349.

McDermott, J. R., Smith, A. I., Ward, M. K., Parkinson, I. S. and Kerr, D. N. S. (1978). Brain-aluminium concentration in dialysis encephalopathy. *Lancet* **i**, 901.

Parkinson, I. S., Ward, M. K., Feest, T. G., Fawcett, P. R. W. and Kerr, D. N. S. (1979). Fracturing dialysis osteodystrophy and dialysis encephalopathy: an epidemiological survey. *Lancet* **i**, 406.

Spencer, P. S. and Schaumburg, H. H., (Eds.) (1980). *Experimental and clinical neurotoxicology.* Williams & Wilkins, New York.

Supino-Viterbo V., Sicard, C., Risvegliato, M., Rancurel, G. and Buge, A. (1977). Toxic encephalopathy due to ingestion of bismuth salts: clinical and EEG studies of 45 patients. *J. Neurol. Neurosurg. Psychiat.* **40**, 748.

Poisoning with organophosphorus and organochlorine insecticides

Many organophosphorus insecticides in common use are powerful inhibitors of both cholinesterase and pseudocholinesterase and the compounds in this group most toxic to man are the so-called 'nerve gases'. The clinical features of mild poisoning include miosis and widespread muscular weakness and fasciculation. In more severe poisoning, respiratory distress, cardiac arrhythmia, widespread paralysis, and caridac arrest may occur (Namba, Greenfield, and Grob 1970; Namba, Nolte, Jackrel, and Grob 1971). The different preparations differ in their relative toxicity, but in many instances early treatment with pralidoxine 1 g intravenously followed by 0.5 g/hour by intravenous infusion with atropine sulphate 5 mg intravenously every 20–30 minutes is effective (Ladell 1958; Namba *et al.* 1971).

More recently the organochlorine insecticide, chlordecone, which can be absorbed through oral, respiratory, and dermal routes, has been shown to produce chronic intoxication in production workers giving rise to tremor, mental changes, opsoclonus, muscular weakness, ataxia, limb incoordination, and dysarthria (Taylor, Selhorst, Houff, and Martinez 1978). Neuropathological evidence suggests that this is a neurotoxic agent predominantly affecting Schwann cells and unmyelinated fibres in peripheral nerves (Martinez, Taylor, Dyck, Houff, and Isaacs 1978).

References

Ladell, W. S. S. (1958). Treatment of anticholinesterase poisoning. *Br. med. J.* **2**, 141.

Martinez, A. J., Taylor, J. R., Dyck, P. J., Houff, S. A. and Issacs, E. (1978). Chlordecone intoxication in man. II. Ultrastructure of peripheral nerves and skeletal muscle. *Neurology, Minneapolis* **28**, 631.

Namba, T., Greenfield, M. and Grob, D, (1970). Malathion poisoning. A fatal case with cardiac manifestations. *Arch. environm. Hlth., Chicago* **21**, 533.

——, Nolte, C. T., Jackrel, J. and Grob, D. (1971). Poisoning due to organophosphate insecticides. *Am. J. Med.* **50**, 475.

Taylor, J. R., Selhorst, J. B., Houff, S. A. and Martinez, A. J. (1978). Chlordecone intoxication in man. I. Clinical observations. *Neurology, Minneapolis* **28**, 626.

Subacute myelo-optico-neuropathy (SMON)

Since 1956 many cases of a neurological syndrome characterized by symptoms and signs of spinal-cord and peripheral-nerve involvement and optic atrophy, often with abdominal symptoms, have been reported, largely from Japan (Tsubaki, Tokokura, and Tsukagoshi 1965; Nakae, Yamamoto, and Igata 1971; Sobue, Mukoyama, Takayanagi, Nishigaki, Matsuoka, and Ando 1971) but also from Australia (Selby 1972), Singapore (Tay 1973), and the United Kingdom (Spillane 1971). A viral cause was initially postulated (Nakamura and Inoue 1971) but ample clinical, biochemical, and epidemiological evidence later became available (*The Lancet* 1971; Nakae, Yamamoto, Shingematsu, and Kono 1973) to indicate that the condition results from self-medication with clioquinol (*Entero-Vioform*) and/or related remedies, usually taken in large doses over a long period of time as a treatment for diarrhoea or other abdominal symptoms. A myeloncuropathy has been produced in dogs by the administration of this drug (Tateishi, Ikeda, Suito, Kuroda, and Otsuki 1972). Subsequently, especially outside Japan, it became apparent that acute reversible encephalopathy could follow ingestion of a large quantity of the drug over a short period. With long-term administration, optic atrophy was the commonest isolated manifestation with myelopathy and peripheral neuropathy being the next most common manifestations (Baumgartner, Gawel, Kaeser, Pallis, Rose, Schaumburg, Thomas, and Wadia 1979) and a fatal case with pathological findings has been reported from Spain in a woman who had taken clioquinol 200 mg daily for 27 years (Ricoy, Ortega and Cabello 1982). A striking fall in the incidence of these syndromes occurred when this drug and related remedies became available only on a doctor's prescription. However, optic atrophy is still an occasional complication in children treated with clioquinol for acrodermatitis enteropathica (Baumgartner et al. 1979).

References

Baumgartner, G., Gawel, M. J., Kaeser, H. E., Pallis, C. A., Rose, F. C., Schaumburg, H. H., Thomas, P. K. and Wadia, N. H., (1979). Neurotoxicity of halogenated hydroxyquinolines: clinical analysis of cases reported outside Japan. *J. Neurol. Neurosurg. Psychiat.* **42**, 1073.

The Lancet (1971). More on S.M.O.N. *Lancet* **ii**, 1244.

Nakae, K., Yamamoto, S. and Igata, A. (1971). Subacute myelo-optico-neuropathy (S.M.O.N.) in Japan. *Lancet* **ii**, 510.

——, ——, Shigematsu, I. and Kono, R. (1973). Relation between subacute myelo-optic neuropathy (S.M.O.N.) and clioquinol: nationwide survey. *Lancet* **i**, 171.

Nakamura, Y. and Inoue, Y. K. (1972). Pathogenicity of virus associated with subacute myelo-optico-neuropathy. *Lancet* **i**, 223.

Ricoy, J. R., Ortega, A. and Cabello, A. (1982). Subacute myelo-optic neuropathy (S.M.O.N.): first neuro-pathological report outside Japan. *J. neurol. Sci.* **53**, 241.

Selby, G. (1972). Subacute myelo-optic neuropathy in Australia. *Lancet* **ii**, 123.

Sobue, I., Mukoyama, M., Takayanagi, T., Nishigaki, S., Matsuoka, Y. and Ando, K. (1972). Myeloneuropathy with abdominal disorders in Japan. *Neurology, Minneapolis* **22**, 1034.

Spillane, J. D. (1971). S.M.O.N. *Lancet* **ii**, 1371.

Tateishi, J., Ikeda, H., Saito, A., Kuroda, S. and Otsuki, S. (1972). Myeloneuropathy in dogs induced by iodoxyquinoline. *Neurology, Minneapolis* **22**, 702.

Tay, C. H. (1973). S.M.O.N. in Singapore. *Lancet* **i**, 1519.

Tsubaki, T., Tokokura, Y. and Tsukagoshi, H. (1965). Subacute myelo-optico-neuropathy following abdominal symptoms. *Jap. J. Med.* **4**, 181.

Some other poisons with neurological effects

Certain other heavy metals including arsenic and gold, as well as many organic and inorganic chemicals, are known to produce polyneuropathy, sometimes associated with other neurological manifestations; they are considered in Chapter 17, while the effects of cyanide intoxication are described in Chapter 16 along with the nutritional disorders.

Podophyllum taken as an abortificient can cause disordered consciousness and polyneuropathy (Clark and Parsonage 1957) and hexachlorophene bathing of infants may cause a brain-stem vacuolar encephalopathy (Shuman, Leech, and Alvord 1975). An epidemic of poisoning in France giving rise to cutaneous ulceration and encephalopathy, fatal in 18 per cent of cases, resulted from contamination of a talc baby powder with 6.3 per cent hexachlorophene (Martin-Bouyer, Lebreton, Toga, Stolley, and Lockhart 1982; *The Lancet* 1982). Chloroquine has been noted sometimes to cause involuntary movements like orofacial dyskinesia or choreoathetosis (Umez-Eronini and Eronini 1977), solanine contaminating potatoes has produced confusion, paraesthesiae, abdominal and other anti-cholinesterase effects (McMillan and Thompson 1979), and cimetidine used in the treatment of peptic ulcer has been thought to cause confusion and muscular twitching

(Edmonds, Ashford, Brenner and Saunders 1979). Necrotizing encephalopathy has followed the intraventricular administration of methotrexate (Shapiro, Chernik and Posner 1973) and in Spain an epidemic of pneumonopathy, fever, headache, myalgia, and eosinophilia has followed the ingestion of denatured rape-seed oil; the toxic agent has not yet been identified (Toxic Epidemic Syndrome Study Group 1982). Skeletal fluorosis due to the excessive dietary ingestion of fluoride may produce spastic paraplegia due to spinal-cord compression (Singh, Jolly, and Bansal 1961). The many other drugs and chemicals which may have neurotoxic effects are reviewed by Spencer and Schaumburg (1980) and Davies (1982).

References

Clark, A. N. G. and Parsonage, M. J. (1957). A case of podophylum poisoning with involvement of the nervous system. *Br. med. J.* **2**, 1155.

Davies, D. M. (1982). *Textbook of adverse drug reactions*, 2nd edn. Oxford Medical, Oxford.

Edmonds, M. E., Ashford, R. F. U., Brenner, M. K. and Saunders, A. (1979). Cimetidine: does neurotoxicity occur? Report of three cases. *J. R. Soc. Med.* **72**, 172.

The Lancet (1982). Hexachlorophene today. *Lancet* **i**, 87.

Martin-Bouyer, G., Lebreton, R., Toga, M., Stolley, P. D. and Lockhart, J. (1982). Outbreak of accidental hexachlorophene poisoning in France. *Lancet* **i**, 91.

McMillan, M. and Thompson, J. C. (1979). An outbreak of suspected solanine poisoning in schoolboys: examination of criteria of solanine poisoning. *Quart. J. Med.* **48**, 227.

Shapiro, W. R., Chernik, N. L. and Posner, J. B. (1973). Necrotizing encephalopathy following intraventricular instillation of methotrexate. *Arch. Neurol., Chicago* **28**, 96.

Shuman, R. M., Leech, R. W. and Alvord, E. C. (1975). Neurotoxicity of hexachlorophene in humans. II. A clinicopathological study of 46 premature infants. *Arch. Neurol., Chicago* **32**, 320.

Singh, A., Jolly, S. S. and Bansal, B. C. (1961). Skeletal flourosis and its neurological complications. *Lancet* **i**, 197.

Spencer, P. S. and Schaumburg, H. H. (Eds.) (1980). *Experimental and clinical neurotoxicology*. Williams & Wilkins, New York.

Toxic Epidemic Syndrome Study Group (1982). Toxic epidemic syndrome, Spain, 1981. *Lancet*, **ii**, 697.

Umez-Eronini, E. M. and Eronini, E. A. (1977). Chloroquine-induced involuntary movements. *Br. med. J.* **1**, 945.

Oral contraceptives

Neurological side-effects of oral contraceptives include cerebral vascular accidents (Altshuler, McLaughlin, and Neubuerger 1968; and see p. 192) and choreiform movements which usually resolve when the drug is withdrawn (Lewis and Harrison 1969). An increased frequency and severity of attacks of migraine and epilepsy has also been described (Bickerstaff 1975).

References

Altshuler, J. H., McLaughlin, R. A. and Neubuerger, K. T. (1968). Neurological catastrophe related to oral contraceptives. *Arch. Neurol., Chicago* **19**, 264.

Bickerstaff, E. R. (1975). *Neurological complications of oral contraceptives*. Blackwell, Oxford.

Lewis, P. D. and Harrison, M. J. G. (1969). Involuntary movements in patients taking oral contraceptives. *Brit. med. J.* **4**, 404.

Cerebral anoxia and hypoxia

In clinical practice anoxia may result from deficient oxygenation of arterial blood due either to failure of adequate quantities of oxygen to reach the lungs (high altitudes, suffocation, drowning) or to diminished oxygenation resulting from pulmonary disease (emphysema); these causes are grouped together as examples of *anoxic anoxia.* Near-drowning accidents in children (Pearn, Nixon, and Wilkey 1976; Pearn 1977) (fresh-water immersion hypoxia) may rarely lead to spastic quadriplegia or even gross mental retardation, more often to permanent defects of visuo-motor skills. Transient hypoxaemia during sleep in patients with chronic bronchitis and emphysema may lead to pulmonary hypertension and secondary polycythaemia (Douglas, Calverley, Leggett, Brash, Flenley, and Brezinova 1979) and in such patients, perhaps paradoxically, venesection can result in improved cerebral blood flow with consequential improvement in mental function (Bornstein, Menon, York, Sproule, and Zak 1980).

Anaemic anoxia is that in which there is a deficiency in the circulating haemoglobin (as in severe anaemia, however caused) or else a chemical alteration in the haemoglobin which impairs its oxygen-carrying capacity (as in carbon-monoxide poisoning, described below).

Ischaemic anoxia may be focal, due to arterial disease, as in cerebral infarction (see pp. 192–4), or diffuse as in cardiac arrest, following open-heart surgery (Sotaniemi 1980*a*) or in fat embolism (in severe limb fractures) or diffuse arterial disease involving small arteries and arterioles.

In general, the clinical and pathological effects of these different varieties of anoxia upon the brain are similar. Indeed, the term anoxic-ischaemic brain injury is now commonly employed (*British Medical Journal* 1974: Dougherty, Rawlinson, Levy, and Plum 1981; Hill and Volpe 1981), implying that the casual factors are often multiple. In general, consciousness is lost after six seconds of total circulatory arrest and permanent brain damage occurs after five to eight minutes of total ischaemia or 15 minutes of substantial diffuse ischaemia or hypoxia. Brain damage may take the form of neocortical death (Brierley, Adams, Graham, and Simpson 1971) with prolonged coma or a persistent vegetative state (Bell and Hodgson 1974; Dougherty *et al.* 1981) or sometimes, alternatively, hypoxic-ischaemic leukoencephalopathy rather than cortical damage (Ginsberg, Hedley-Whyte, and Richardson 1976) or even cortical spongiform encephalopathy with periodic EEG discharges (Kuroiwa, Celesia, and Chung 1982). What determines the relative predominance and distribution of these differing pathological processes remains uncertain but synaptically released, neurotoxic amino acids seem to play a part (Meldrum 1985). In both adults (Snyder, Ramirez-Lassepas, and Lippert 1977; Sotaniemi 1980*b*) and children (Pampiglion, Chaloner, Harden, O'Brien 1978), the neurological sequelae may vary from mild cognitive and executive defects to prolonged and irreversible coma.

References

Bell, J. A. and Hodgson, H. J. F. (1974). Coma after cardiac arrest. *Brain* **97**, 361.

Bornstein, R., Menon, D., York, E., Sproule, B. and Zak, C. (1980). Effects of venesection on cerebral function in chronic lung disease. *Can. J. neurol. Sci.* **7**, 293.

Brierley, J. B., Adams, J. H., Graham, D. I. and Simpson, J. A. (1971). Neocortical death after cardiac arrest: a clinical neurophysiological and neuropathological report of two cases. *Lancet* **ii**, 560.

British Medical Journal (1974). Anoxic-ischaemic brain injury. *Br. med. J.* **3**, 73.

Dougherty, J. H. Jr., Rawlinson, D. G., Levy, D. E. and Plum, F. (1981). Hypoxic-ischemic brain injury and the vegetative state: clinical and neuropathologic correlation. *Neurology, Minneapolis* **31**, 991.

Douglas, N. J., Calverley, P. M. A., Leggatt, R. J. E., Brash, H. M., Flenley, D. C. and Brezinova, V. (1979). Transient hypoxaemia during sleep in chronic bronchitis and emphysema. *Lancet* **i**, 1.

Ginsberg, M. D., Hedley-Whyte, E. T. and Richardson, E. P. Jr. (1976). Hypoxic-ischemic leukoencephalopathy in man. *Arch. Neurol., Chicago* **33**, 5.

Hill, A. and Volpe, J. J. (1981). Seizures, hypoxic-ischemic brain injury and intraventricular hemorrhage in the newborn. *Ann. Neurol.* **10**, 109.

Kuroiwa, Y., Celesia, G. G. and Chung, H. D. (1982). Periodic EEG discharges and status spongiousus of the cerebral cortex in anoxic encephalopathy: a necropsy case report. *J. Neurol. Neurosurg. Psychiat.* **45**, 740.

Meldrum, B. (1985). Excitatory amino acids and anoxic-ischaemic brain damage. *Trends Neurosci.* **8**, 47.

Pampiglione, G., Chaloner, J., Harden, A. and O'Brien, J. (1978). Transitory ischemia/anoxia in young children and the prediction of quality of survival. *Ann. NY Acad. Sci.* **315**, 281.

Pearn, J. (1977). Neurological and psychometric studies in children surviving freshwater immersion accidents. *Lancet* **i**, 7.

——, Nixon, J. and Wilkey, I. (1976). Freshwater drowning and near-drowning accidents involving children: a five-year population study. *Med. J. Aust.* **2**, 942.

Snyder, B. D., Ramirez-Lassepas, M. and Lippert, D. M. (1977). Neurologic status and prognosis after cardiopulmonary arrest: 1. A retrospective study. *Neurology, Minneapolis* **27**, 807.

Sotaniemi, K. (1980*a*). Cerebral disorders in open-heart surgery patients: a neurological, electroencephalographic and neuropsychological follow-up study. *Acta Universitatis Ouluensis*, Series D, Medica No. 56, Neurologica No. 4.

—— (1980*b*). Brain damage and neurological outcome after open-heart surgery. *J. Neurol. Neurosurg. Psychiat.* **43**, 127.

Carbon monoxide poisoning

Carbon monoxide poisoning may result from the accidental or suicidal inhalation of coal-gas or of gas from a motor-car exhaust. Carbon monoxide may also be present in dangerous quantities in the air of coal-mines, especially after explosions or can result from the combustion of coal fires or braziers or gas or paraffin heaters in enclosed, inadequately ventilated rooms. By combining with haemoglobin to form carboxyhaemoglobin, carbon monoxide reduces the oxygen-carrying capacity of the blood, so leading to anoxaemia. Absorption of the gas is cumulative, so that a concentration of 0.1 per cent will saturate the blood up to 50 per cent. Effort increases absorption.

Pathology

In fatal cases the blood is cherry-red in colour and coagulates slowly. All the tissues are reddened. There is oedema of the lungs, and haemorrhages are found in the pleura and intestinal mucosa. Changes in the nervous system are of special importance and show a predilection for the cerebral cortex, the hippocampus, cerebellum, and corpus striatum. The changes are those of anoxia (see p. 11 and above).

However, there are some differences between the effects of hypoxic anoxia and those of carbon monoxide poisoning in relation to oxygen availability and utilization (Astrup and Pauli 1968), though the neurological effects are similar. There is a focal or laminar necrosis of the second and third cortical layers and often of the superficial white matter with striking degeneration of cerebellar Purkinje cells and of pyramidal neurones in Sommer's sector of Ammon's horn of the hippocampus. There may also be degeneration of the basal ganglia and patchy demyelination of central white matter. When the patient survives for several days there is often extensive ischaemic necrosis of the cerebral cortex and the lesions of the globus pallidus may progress to softening. CT scanning may show bilateral low-density areas in the pallidum in survivors for as long as three months after the initial exposure; when these are absent the outlook is good (Swada, Takahashi, Ohashi, Fusamoto, Maemura, Kobayashi, Yoshioka, and Sugimoto 1980). Chronic exposure to minimal concentrations of carbon monoxide in cigarette smoke is believed to contribute to atherogenesis (Wanstrup, Kieldscn, and Astrup 1969).

Symptoms and signs

McNally (1931) found that the severity of the symptoms was related to the degree of saturation of the blood. When this was less than 10 per cent there were no symptoms, at between 10 and 20 per cent the patient had slight headache and there was dilatation of cutaneous vessels, at between 30 and 50 per cent there was severe headache, weakness, giddiness, dimness of vision, nausea, vomiting, and collapse, at between 50 and 60 per cent the patient became comatose and convulsed. Tachycardia, tachypnoea, cyanosis, and, in some cases, glycosuria may be succeeded by rapidly deepening coma, and cardiac and respiratory arrest. Others may enter a persistent vegetative state, lasting for weeks, months, or rarely years (Plum and Posner 1980). However, if consciousness is regained within two or three days, recovery is often surprisingly complete, though in a minority of patients various cognitive and executive defects may persist.

Garland and Pearce (1967) drew particular attention to the striking variation in the clinical picture which may occur in such cases, including such features as major seizures, cortical blindness, dysphasia, apraxia, and various forms of agnosia with mental changes ranging from retardation to frank psychotic behaviour. Some patients seemed to recover after a few days only to relapse into coma in from one to three weeks, or into a state of akinetic stupor or confusion and visual agnosia with catatonic postures. Polyneuropathy is a rare complication (Snyder 1970) and may be associated with deafness (Goto, Miyoshi, and Ooya 1972). No convincing explanation has yet been advanced for this syndrome of post-anoxic encephalopathy but its incidence is reduced if activity is greatly limited in the early stages after poisoning (Plum, Posner, and Hain 1962). A mild parkinsonian syndrome may make its appearance within six weeks of recovery from the initial coma. Mild, or rarely severe, brain damage and/or malformation of the brain or limbs, or even stillbirth, can occur in the fetus as a result of maternal carbon monoxide intoxication (Ginsberg and Myers 1976).

Prognosis

In mild cases there is usually complete recovery, but in severe cases the patient may remain comatose for days or even weeks or months. Those who regain consciousness may exhibit symptoms of permanent damage to the nervous system, including dementia, deafness, blindness, aphasia, apraxia, choreo-athetoid movements, parkinsonian features, and polyneuropathy. Myoclonic jerking of the limbs precipitated by movement (post-anoxic action myoclonus—see p. 632) is also an occasional sequel. However, even a confusional state lasting for as long as two months does not necessarily mean that the patient will not recover completely (Garland and Pearce 1967).

Treatment

The patient should at once be moved from exposure to the gas, preferably to the open air. Oxygen should be given, if possible with 5 per cent of carbon dioxide, to increase the pulmonary ventilation, the object being as rapidly as possible to replace carboxyhaemoglobin by oxyhaemoglobin. If the patient is unconscious, artificial respiration may be needed. Smith, Ledingham, Sharp, Norman, and Bates (1962) recommended treatment with oxygen at two atmospheres pressure and exposure to hyperbaric oxygen in a pressure chamber, when available, is being used increasingly in severe cases; this is especially valuable when carbon monoxide poisoning is complicated by barbiturate poisoning or a cerebrovascular accident. Duncan and Gumpert (1983) reported that an intravenous infusion of dopamine in a dose of 17 μg/kg/min, given in order to increase the systemic blood pressure and, presumably, cerebral perfusion, resulted in the rapid restoration of vision in a patient who became virtually blind due to post-anoxic encephalopathy following accidental carbon monoxide poisoning.

References

Astrup, P. and Pauli, H. G. (1968). A comparison of prolonged exposure to carbon monoxide and hypoxia in man. *Scand. J. clin. Lab. Invest.* **22**, Suppl. 103.

Denny-Brown, D. (1960). Diseases of the basal ganglia. *Lancet* **ii**, 1105.

Duncan, J. S. and Gumpert, J. (1983). A case of blindness following carbon monoxide poisoning treated with dopamine. *J. Neurol. Neurosurg. Psychiat.* **46**, 459.

Garland, H. and Pearce, J. (1967). Neurological complications of carbon monoxide poisoning. *Quart. J. Med.* **36**, 445.

Ginsberg, M. D. and Myers, R. E. (1976). Fetal brain injury after maternal carbon monoxide intoxication: clinical and neuropathologic aspects. *Neurology, Minneapolis* **26**, 15.

Goto, I., Miyoshi, T. and Ooya, Y. (1972). Deafness and peripheral neuropathy following carbon monoxide intoxication—report of a case. *Folia Psychiat. Neurol. Jap.* **26**, 35.

McNally, W. D. (1931). Carbon monoxide poisoning. *Illinois med. J.* **59**, 383.

Medical Research Council (1958). Carbon monoxide poisoning. Use of carbon dioxide–oxygen mixture. *Br. med. J.* **2**, 1408.

Plum, F. and Posner, J. B. (1980). *Diagnosis of stupor and coma*, 3rd edn. Blackwell, Oxford.

——, —— and Hain, R. F. (1962). Post-anoxic encephalopathy. *Arch. intern. Med.* **110**, 18.

Swada, Y., Takahashi, M., Ohashi, N., Fusamoto, H., Maemura, K., Kobayashi, H., Yoshioka, T. and Sugimoto, T. (1980). Computerised tomography as an indication of long-term outcome after acute carbon monoxide poisoning. *Lancet* **i**, 783.

Smith, G., Ledingham, I. Mc.A., Sharp, G. P., Norman, J. N. and Bates, E. J. (1962). Treatment of coal-gas poisoning with oxygen at 2 atmospheres pressure. *Lancet* **i**, 816.

Snyder, R. D. (1970). Carbon monoxide intoxication with peripheral neuropathy. *Neurology, Minneapolis* **20**, 177.

Wanstrup, J., Kjeldsen, K. and Astrup, P. (1969). Acceleration of spontaneous intimal–subintimal changes in rabbit aorta by a prolonged moderate carbon monoxide exposure. *Acta path. microbiol. scand.* **75**, 353.

Caisson disease

Aetiology and pathology

Caisson disease, also known as compressed-air sickness, diver's paralysis, and 'the bends', first appeared when high-pressure caissons were introduced for submarine work. It also occurs in tunnel workers and others who work in compressed air. Divers once worked in caissons which were open at the bottom and in which the air was maintained at high pressure, usually 30 to 35 lb/in², to balance the pressure of the water, which increased in proportion to the depth. As a result of the increased air pressure in such circumstances the tissues of those working in it absorb the gases of the air. If such individuals are suddenly transferred to normal atmospheric pressure these gases, especially the nitrogen, are liberated in the tissues as small bubbles, in a manner comparable to the liberation of bubbles of carbon dioxide in a bottle of soda water when the cork is removed. The nitrogen is especially soluble in lipid, and is thus liberated in large amounts in the nervous system. For this reason also obese individuals are more liable to develop caisson disease than those of spare build. The liberation of bubbles of gas not only damages tissue directly but also interferes with its blood supply through blockage of small vessels.

Symptoms and signs

The first symptom is usually pain in the limbs, trunk, and epigastrium, sometimes associated with vomiting. The pain often begins in the knees and hips and aseptic necrosis of one or both femoral heads is an important sequel. Headache and vertigo may occur and in severe cases the patient rapidly becomes comatose. Scintillating scotomata and paraesthesiae in the extremities are important premonitory symptoms (Behnke 1974). Hemiplegia or paraplegia with sensory loss may occur. Indeed it is commonly assumed that spinal-cord damage with paraparesis is the commonest neurological complication, but Peters, Levin, and Kelly (1977) found severe neuropsychological deficits on psychometric testing in seven out of 10 divers who had suffered episodes of decompression sickness and concluded that this condition causes multiple and diffuse lesions in the nervous system.

Prognosis

In severe cases the condition is fatal. In less severe cases recovery usually occurs, sometimes in a few hours, but disability may persist for days, weeks, or months. In some cases, symptoms and signs of paraparesis may persist indefinitely (p. 424).

Treatment

Prophylaxis consists in the slow decompression of workers exposed to high pressures. When symptoms have developed, immediate recompression is necessary, the patient being placed in an air lock for this purpose, and restoration to normal pressure must be extremely slow. Otherwise treatment is symptomatic.

Mountain sickness

Fatigue, dyspnoea, clubbing of the fingers, cyanosis, and somnolence with polycythaemia and a haematocrit often exceeding 70 per cent are the usual manifestations of this disorder (Monge's disease) and are readily relieved by a return to lower altitudes. Pulmonary oedema is a less common manifestation.

References

Behnke, A. R. (1974). Disorders due to alterations in barometric pressure. In *Harrison's principles of internal medicine*, 7th edn, Chapter 117. McGraw-Hill, New York.

Hallenbeck, J. M., Bove, A. A. and Elliott, D. H. (1975). Mechanisms underlying spinal cord damage in decompression sickness. *Neurology, Minneapolis* 25, 308.

Hultgren, H. N. and Grover, R. F. (1968). Circulatory adaptation to high altitude. *Ann. rev. Med.* 19, 119.

Paton, W. D. M. and Walder, D. N. (1954). *Compressed air illness*. MRC Special Report Series, No. 281. HMSO, London.

Peters, B. H., Levin, H. S. and Kelly P. J. (1977). Neurologic and psychologic manifestations of decompression illness in divers. *Neurology, Minneapolis* 27, 125.

Electric shock

Pathology

The pathological changes in the nervous system produced by electric shock are characteristic. They consist of chromatolysis of ganglion cells, multifocal vacuolation, often due to dilatation of perivascular spaces, vascular lesions ranging from focal petechial haemorrhages to actual disruption of large vessels, changes in the peripheral nerves such as fragmentation of axons and neurilemma, and a peculiar spiral-like appearance of muscle fibres. These changes may be associated with electrical burns of the skin and resemble those of hyperpyrexia or heat stroke (Farrell and Starr 1968).

Aetiology and pathogenesis

There has been much discussion as to how electric shock injures the nervous system. The heating effect of the current may in itself cause severe damage, as in legal electrocution or lightning stroke. Bodily tissues vary considerably in their resistance to the flow of electricity whether due to electrocution or lightning. Bone and skin are relatively resistant, whereas blood, muscle, and nervous tissue are good conductors (Wallace and Petersdorf 1974). The point of contact with earth is important, as is the pathway of current through the body; thus contact with the leg or foot is likely to be less harmful than if the shock enters via the head or hand and is then conducted to one or both feet; the duration of contact is also

important. Cardiac arrhythmia and arrest and tetanic muscular contraction followed sometimes by muscle necrosis and consequent myoglobinuria are important complications.

Changes in the central nervous system most often occur when the current has been applied directly to the skull. The extreme variability of the circumstances in which electric shock may occur must explain the unpredictability of the results of exposure. Eleven thousand volts may cause only slight injury (Critchley 1934). On the other hand 40 volts has been known to prove fatal. Death from electric shock, however, is now relatively rare. The increasing safety-consciousness of designers of electrical fittings and appliances has greatly reduced electrical injuries in children. However, the use of portable electrical heaters in bathrooms is still a serious danger and the immersion of such a heater in bath-water has been used for both suicide and homicide. And there have been some notable lightning strikes, occasionally fatal, afflicting golfers, for example, during thunderstorms.

Symptoms and signs

A severe electric shock usually causes immediate loss of consciousness. If the patient remains conscious there is often severe pain associated with bizarre sensory disturbances, especially visual hallucinations. A typical immediate sequel is a transitory flaccid paraplegia with objective sensory disturbance, both disappearing after about 12 hours. Critchley classified the neurological sequelae of electric shock as: (1) cerebral; (2) spinal; (4) mixed cerebrospinal affection; (4) peripheral-nerve lesions, isolated or multiple; and (5) psychological disorders, hysteria being particularly common. Symptoms of an isolated cerebral lesion are rare, but basilar artery occlusion has been reported (Farrell and Starr 1968) and spinal atrophic paralyses leading to a clinical picture resembling motor-neurone disease is not uncommon. Both immediate spastic tetraplegia (So and Lee 1973) and delayed myelopathy (Holbrook, Beech, and Silver 1970), giving wasting of muscles in the upper limbs and paraparesis have been described. Brachial neuropathy may follow a shock to the upper limbs and Critchley described a lasting polyneuropathic syndrome following lightning stroke. Both paraparesis and radicular- or peripheral-nerve lesions are sometimes delayed, first appearing days, rarely months, after the initial insult (Farrell and Starr 1968).

Prognosis

Generalizations about prognosis are virtually impossible as the clinical picture is so varied.

Treatment

The first essential is to turn off the current if the patient is still in contact and then to give immediate artificial respiration and, if necessary, external cardiac massage, since it may be possible to revive a victim even after cardiac arrest. It is difficult to know how long artificial respiration should be carried on in the absence of any response, but if the heart is still beating resuscitation has sometimes been effective after several hours.

References

Critchley, M. (1934). Neurological effects of lightning and of electricity. *Lancet* i, 68.

Farrell, D. F. and Starr, A. (1968). Delayed neurological sequelae of electrical injuries. *Neurology, Minneapolis* 18, 601.

Holbrook, L. A., Beach, F. X. M. and Silver, J. R. (1970). Delayed myelopathy: a rare complication of severe electrical burns. *Br. med. J.* 4, 659.

Morrison, L. R., Weeks, A. and Cobb, S. (1930). Histopathology of different types of electric shock on mammalian brains. *J. Industr. Hyg.* 12, 324.

Pritchard, E. A. B. (1934). Changes in the central nervous system due to electrocution. *Lancet* i, 1163.

So, S. C. and Lee, M. L. K. (1973). Spastic quadriplegia due to electric shock. *Br. med. J.* 2, 590.

Wallace, J. F. and Petersdore, R. G. (1974). Electrical injuries. In *Harrison's principles of internal medicine*, 7th edn. Chapter 120. McGraw-Hill, New York.

Heat stroke

Heat stroke is characterized by partial or complete loss of consciousness, hyperpyrexia, convulsions, and delirium following excessive exposure to sun or heat. It has been reported in athletes, such as racing cyclists, undertaking prolonged exertion in hot conditions and may be precipitated by the use of amphetamines or by psychotropic drugs such as prophenazine and amitriptyline (Lefkowitz, Ford, Rich, Biller, and McHenry 1983). The body temperature usually exceeds 41.1 °C; there is lack of sweating and circulatory collapse (Climatic Physiology Committee 1958). Occasional cases have been described with permanent neurological sequelae after recovery, including cerebellar ataxia, dysarthria, mild dementia, and polyneuropathy (Mehta and Baker 1970). Acute rhabdomyolysis, myoglobinuria, and renal failure has also been reported (Lefkowitz et al 1983). The condition is a medical emergency, requiring rapid cooling either with ice or with cold tap water while the skin is fanned in evaporative conditions. Chlorpromazine is also helpful with diazepam given intravenously (if possible) for the treatment or prevention of convulsions (*The Lancet* 1982).

References

Climatic Physiology Committee (1958). A classification of heat illness. *Br. med. J.* **1**, 1533.
The Lancet (1982). Management of heatstroke. *Lancet* **ii**, 910.
Lefkowitz, D., Ford, C. S., Rich, C., Biller, J. and McHenry, L. C. (1983). Cerebellar syndrome following neuroleptic induced heat stroke. *J. Neurol. Neurosurg. Psychiat.* **46**, 183.
Mehta, A. C. and Baker, R. N. (1970). Persistent neurological deficits in heat stroke. *Neurology, Minneapolis* **20**, 336.

Accidental hypothermia

Accidental hypothermia as a cause of coma is described on p. 647. It is sometimes seen as a complication of myxoedema (p. 470) or may follow the use of phenothiazines, especially in elderly subjects living in poorly heated rooms in winter conditions. Both physiological and behavioural changes contribute to the vulnerability of old people in such conditions (Collins, Exton-Smith, and Doré 1981). However, in younger subjects, alcoholic abuse and Wernicke's encephalopathy are prominent causes of accidental hypothermia; the heart rate, blood pressure, and respiratory rate all decline as the temperature falls in such subjects, as do awareness, pupillary reflexes, tendon reflexes, and muscle tone; nevertheless, verbal responsiveness and retention of reflexes may be seen with body temperatures as low as 20–27 °C (Fischbeck and Simon 1981) and there is no correlation between the degree of hypothermia on the one hand and eye movement abnormalities or extensor plantar responses on the other.

References

Collins, K. J., Exton-Smith, A. N., and Doré, C. (1981). Urban hypothermia: preferred temperature and thermal perception in old age. *Br. med. J.* **282**, 175.
Fischbeck, K. H. and Simon, R. P. (1981). Neurological manifestations of accidental hypothermia. *Ann. Neurol.* **10**, 384.

Snake bite

Snake-venom neurotoxins comprise a heterogeneous group of proteins, their neurotoxic fractions being closely associated with,

but distinct from, the cholinesterase, ribonuclease, and deoxyribonuclease fractions of the venom (Porges 1953; Pearn 1971). The bites of many venomous snakes may be followed by widespread muscular weakness and above all by respiratory paralysis, though sea-snake bites may be followed by widespread necrosis of skeletal muscle and hepatic and renal damage (Marsden and Reid 1961). The neurotoxic and myotoxic effects of various snake venoms have been reviewed in detail by Harris (1982 *a b*) and by Harris and Maltin (1982). Treatment is based upon the use of assisted respiration and intravenous injections of polyvalent antivenene (Pearn 1971).

References

Harris, J. B. (1982*a*). Toxic constituents of animal venoms and poisons. 1. Incidence of poisoning, clinical and experimental studies, and reptile venoms. *Adv. Drug React. Accid. Pois. Rev.* **1**, 65.
—— (1982*b*). Toxic constituents of animal venoms and poisons. 2. Spiders, scorpions, marine animals, non-venomous animals, reactions to antivenoms. *Adv. Drug React Accid Pois. Rev.* **1**, 143.
—— and Maltin, C.A. (1982). Myotoxic activity of the crude venom and the principal neurotoxin, taipoxin, of the Australian taipan, *Oxyuranus scutellatus*. *Br. J. Pharmacol.* **76**, 61.
Marsden, A. T. H. and Reid, H. A. (1961). Pathology of sea-snake poisoning. *Br. med. J.* **1**, 1290.
Pearn, J. H. (1971). Survival after snake-bite with prolonged neurotoxic envenomation. *Med. J. Aust.* **2**, 259.
Porges, N. (1953). Snake venoms, their biochemistry and mode of action. *Science* **117**, 47.

Tetanus

Definition. Tetanus is an intoxication of the nervous system with the exotoxin of the tetanus bacillus. It is characterized by the progressive development of muscular rigidity with paroxysmal exacerbations.

Aetiology

Tetanus is due to infection with the *Clostridium tetani*, a gram-positive, anaerobic organism which bears spores. The spore is oval or rounded, and develops at one end of the bacillus, which then presents the appearance of a drumstick. The *Cl. tetani* is actively motile, its movement being due to flagella.

The *Cl. tetani* is widely distributed in the soil; it is also found in the faeces of many animals, especially horses, and of a very few normal human beings. The disease arises in man through contamination of wounds with the spores of the organism, especially as a result of accidents in which road dust or soil is introduced into the wound. Other, less common, sources of tetanus infection have included vaccination, infection of wounds by contaminated dressings or catgut, and the injection of infected drugs, especially in narcotic addicts. Tetanus neonatorum, due to infection of the stump of the umbilical cord in new-born infants, and puerperal tetanus are common in some tropical countries.

The mere introduction of tetanus spores into a wound is not sufficient to cause the disease. Often it seems necessary that other organisms should also be present and a foreign body, such as a splinter, is commonly present. The *Cl. tetani* do not spread beyond the wound, but produce an exotoxin, which reaches the nervous system by ascending the axis cylinders of the peripheral nerves. The dorsal-root ganglia act as a filter which prevents the toxin from entering the cord by the dorsal roots so that its portal of entry is confined to the ventral roots. There is, however, some evidence to suggest that the toxin may also spread by the blood stream; Zacks and Sheff (1966) found that it could be isolated from brain, spinal cord, skeletal muscle, and spleen after being injected into mice. Zacks, Hall, and Sheff also found vesicles and dense intra-mitochondrial inclusions in the skeletal muscle of such animals. In human subjects there is also widespread myopathic change in affected skeletal muscles with a concomitant rise in serum creatine kinase activity; electron microscopy reveals post-synaptic damage at the motor end-plates (Eyrich, Agostini, Schulz, Müller, Noetzel, Reichenmiller, and Wiemers 1967). In experimental tetanus, chromatolysis of anterior horn cells with hyperaemia and spinal-cord haemorrhages are seen, but spinal synaptic endings are morphologically normal (Tarlov, Ling, and Yamada 1973). Having reached the brain stem and spinal cord, the toxin produces its characteristic effects by blocking inhibitory neurones and thus disturbing the normal regulation of the reflex arc. Afferent stimuli not only produce an exaggerated effect, but reciprocal innervation is also abolished and both prime movers and antagonists contract, thus causing spasms.

When a small amount of toxin is slowly absorbed, it reaches the anterior horn cells by the route described. In such cases the first symptom is local spasm of the muscles in the neighbourhood of the wound. When a slightly larger amount of toxin is produced, it enters the circulation and reaches the nervous system diffusely by ascending all the motor nerves. The larger the volume of toxin, the more remains unabsorbed by the anterior horn cells and is thus available to attack distant synapses and ultimately the vital centres. There is then no local tetanus; trismus is usually the first symptom and the spasm subsequently spreads rapidly, to involve the arms, trunk, and legs.

Pathology

Tetanus is essentially a disorder of function of the nervous system and no constant structural changes are found, though hyperaemia is common in the spinal cord and brain, especially in the anterior horns of grey matter and there may be rupture of muscle fibres with haemorrhages and consequent myopathic change (Eyrich *et al.* 1967) in those muscles which have been subjected to violent spasms.

Symptoms

Incubation period

The incubation period varies, but in acute generalized cases is usually seven or eight days. In patients who have had prophylactic inoculations of toxoid it may extend to several weeks. Exceptionally it is as short as one or two days or, conversely, it may seem, on occasion, to be as long as two or three weeks, when the clinical syndrome may be milder than in the average case, or the spasms may even be localized in one or more limbs (local tetanus). Such a prolonged incubation period is commonest in those previously immunized.

Descending form

A prodromal phase of restlessness and irritability is common. The first motor symptom is usually trismus, which is rapidly followed, or may be preceded, by stiffness of the neck. Within a few hours, however, the spasm extends to other muscles and dysphagia is often an early complaint. Spasm of facial muscles may lead either to pursing of the lips or to retraction of the angles of the mouth—the risus sardonicus. The eyes may be partly closed through contraction of the orbicularis oculi, or the eyebrows may be elevated by spasm of the frontalis. Examination reveals rigidity of the musculature of the limbs and trunk. There may be slight opisthotonos. The muscles of the abdominal wall are rigid, and the lower limbs, which are usually affected more than the upper, are fixed in extension. As the disease progresses, this persisting general rigidity undergoes paroxysmal exacerbations attended by severe cramp-like pains. Opisthotonic spasm usually occurs in these attacks, but in some cases the spine is bent in other directions, for example, forwards or laterally. Spasm of the larynx and respiratory muscles leads to dyspnoea and/or stridor, and profuse sweating occurs. These convulsive paroxysms may be excited by external stimuli,

for example, by attempting to feed the patient. Between paroxysms the general muscular rigidity persists. The tendon reflexes are exaggerated, but, with some exceptions described below, there are usually no other signs of organic lesions of the nervous system. Consciousness is retained to the end.

Death may occur in a convulsive attack from asphyxia, or, when severe spasms recur frequently, from sudden cardiac arrest. The illness may be apyrexial, but some fever is not uncommon, and hyperpyrexia is an important and serious complication in severe cases, the temperature even continuing to rise after death. Other risks include a negative nitrogen balance leading to uraemia, hypotension, and gastric dilatation, all most liable to occur between the 7th and 14th days, and motor paresis. Laryngeal spasm, apnoea, and pneumonia are also risks. In favourable cases the severity and frequency of the spasms gradually diminish, but the general rigidity frequently persists for several weeks, trismus often being the last sign to disappear.

Ascending or local form

In this form the first symptom is local spasm of the muscles near the wound, whence persistent or intermittent spasm spreads to neighbouring muscles and in severe cases to the other limbs, head, and trunk. After recovery from this form of the disease the original local spasm may persist for days or weeks. In one reported case due to injury by a porcupine quill, severe rigidity was present in one upper limb only (though trismus was also present in the early stages) for over five months, and in the first few months any attempt to use the limb produced severe spasms localized to it— 'recruitment spasm' (Struppler, Struppler, and Adams 1963).

Cephalic tetanus

Cephalic tetanus is a rare variety of the ascending form and follows wounds of the head, face, and neck. Muscular paralysis is frequently present, usually involving the facial muscles on one side (Vakil, Singhal, Pandya, and Irani 1973) and may be associated with facial spasm on the opposite side. Trismus and pharyngeal spasm usually develop. When the wound involves the orbit, ptosis, external ophthalmoplegia, and iridoplegia may occur on one or both sides. Cephalic tetanus can remain localized or become generalized. It is rarely fatal, but, when recovery occurs, facial paralysis and spasm may persist for weeks. The lower motor-neur-one paralysis has been attributed to a high concentration of toxin in brainstem motor nuclei (Dastur, Shahani, Dastour, Kohiyar, Bharucha, Mondkar, Kashyap, and Nair 1977).

Tetanus neonatorum

When the tetanus spores infect the umbilical cord, the neonate frequently shows intense pharyngeal spasm, with difficulty in feeding and subsequent spasms and opisthotonos. The mortality rate in new-born infants is very high; permanent tetraplegia due to anterior horn-cell damage is a rare sequel (Gadoth, Dagan, Sandbank, Levy, and Moses 1981).

Splanchnic tetanus

This term has been given to a variety which follows abdominal wounds and in which the bulbar and respiratory muscles are affected early and severely.

Autonomic manifestations

Common autonomic manifestations include tachycardia, irregularities of cardiac rhythm, peripheral vasoconstriction, profuse sweating, hyperpyrexia, and increased urinary catecholamine excretion, presumed to be due to involvement of the sympathetic nervous system (Kerr, Corbett, Prys-Roberts, Smith, and Spalding 1968), while episodes of profound arterial hypotension, responsive to carbon dioxide inhalation, have also been recorded (Corbett, Spalding, and Harris 1973).

Modified tetanus

The symptoms of tetanus may be considerably modified by previous immunization or by a prophylactic inoculation of antitoxin in a non-immunized individual. The incubation period in such cases is usually longer than normal. There is a tendency for the spasms to remain localized, and often, if generalized tetanus ensues, spasms are absent, and if they occur are likely to be slight.

Diagnosis

Other conditions causing trismus may be confused with tetanus. Trismus is sometimes produced by painful lesions in the region of the jaw such as dental abscess, or may follow mandibular block with local anaesthetics. The presence of the causative lesion and the localized character of the spasm enable these cases to be distinguished from tetanus. Trismus may also occur in encephalitis, and in the past, post-vaccinal encephalitis in which trismus was a prominent symptom was sometimes at first regarded as tetanus. Signs of dysfunction of the brain and spinal cord are always present in such cases and distinguish them from tetanus. The convulsions of strychnine poisoning superficially resemble those of tetanus, but develop more rapidly. Moreover, the fact that they follow reflex excitation is apparent from the beginning, whereas this is a late feature in tetanus. Strychnine poisoning also differs from tetanus in that muscular relaxation is complete between the paroxysms, and the upper limbs are more severely affected. A history of poisoning can usually be obtained. Rabies may also be confused with tetanus, but in this condition trismus is absent and dysphagia is the most conspicuous symptom. Further, muscular relaxation occurs between the paroxysms and there is almost always a history of a bite by a rabid animal. Tetany is distinguished from tetanus by the fact that the muscular spasm always begins in the periphery of the limbs and by the typical carpopedal spasm. Trismus occurs only in the most severe attacks. Hysteria may cause either trismus or generalized rigidity associated with opisthotonos. Hysterical trismus, however, is not always associated with rigidity elsewhere, while hysterical opisthotonos usually forms part of a hysterical convulsion which develops suddenly without pre-existing rigidity, is attended by apparent impairment of consciousness, and is often accompanied by other signs of hysteria. Nevertheless, hysterical trismus with associated spasms is sufficiently common, often after minor injury, to give diagnostic difficulty in some cases; electromyography may be useful in such cases. In describing a syndrome of 'pseudo-tetanus', Stoddart (1979) pointed out that not only hysteria, with or without hyperventilation and tetany, but also drug-induced muscular spasms in the head and neck, usually due to the administration of phenothiazines, may closely simulate tetanus, so that careful enquiry about drug-taking is essential.

Prognosis

The prognosis of tetanus unmodified by immunization or prophylactic inoculation of antitoxin is always grave, though the outlook was somewhat improved when treatment with antitoxin was introduced. In a series of cases from the London Hospital quoted by Fildes (1929), the mortality before antitoxin was used was 81.7 per cent and afterwards it was 71.8 per cent. In general, the shorter the incubation period the worse is the prognosis, and few patients with an incubation period of less than six days used to recover in the past. The interval between the first symptom and the first generalized reflex spasms is clearly important but so, too, is the severity of the condition when treatment is begun, and five grades of increasing severity and increasingly poor prognosis (Grades I–V) were defined by Patel and Joag (1959). Nevertheless, the new methods of treatment recently introduced offer the hope of saving life even when the incubation period is short and the illness severe; the overall mortality rate is now 30 per cent or less. There may be some persistent motor weakness for many months after recovery. Illis and Taylor (1971), in a follow-up study, found that many patients suffered from irritability, sleep disorders, fits, myoclonus, decreased libido, or postural hypotension, and many showed EEG abnormalities.

Treatment

The patient should be nursed in isolation, if possible in an intensive care unit, and should be kept as quiet as possible. The value of antitoxin is limited by the fact that the nervous system is largely impenetrable by immune bodies even though antitoxin can neutralize circulating toxin. Many authorities still advise that a massive dose (10 000 units) should be given intravenously but an increasing number doubt whether antitoxin is of any value. However, many still recommend surgical toilet of the wound, if identified, in an attempt to remove the tetanus bacilli and spores. In early cases, prior to the development of severe generalized spasms, there is some evidence that 250 IU of human tetanus immune globulin (TIG), given intrathecally, may greatly improve the outcome, while intramuscular TIG seems to be of less value (Gupta, Kapoor, Goyal, Batra, and Jain 1980). However, 500 units of the latter, given either intramuscularly or intravenously, is commonly recommended as being much safer and more effective than antitoxin (Adams 1983).

The modern treatment of severe tetanus is based upon the elimination of muscle spasm by tubocurarine chloride in doses of 15 mg repeated as necessary up to a daily total of 150–650 mg, while artificial respiration is carried out with intermittent positive-pressure equipment through a tracheostomy tube, and naso-oesophageal feeding is employed.

Chlorpromazine may be helpful in the control of spasms when given in a dosage of 100–150 mg four- or six-hourly intramuscularly or, in neonates, 25 mg four-or six-hourly but diazepam given intravenously is now preferred to chlorpromazine by most authors. Antibiotics are given to prevent pulmonary infection. The continuous supervision of an anaesthetist is required. Nutrition and fluid and electrolyte balance must be watched, and many nursing difficulties need to be overcome (Shackleton 1954; Forbes and Auld, Wright, Berman, and Laurence 1955; Smith 1958; Adams *et al.* 1959; Adams 1983).

References

Abel, J. J. and others. Researches on tetanus. *Bull. Johns Hopk. Hosp. 1935*, **56**, 84; III, 1935, **56**, 317; IV, 1935, **57**, 343; V, 1936, **59**, 307; VI, 1938, **62**, 91; VII, 1938, **62**, 522; VIII, 1938, **62**, 610.

Adams, E. B. (1983). Tetanus. In *Oxford textbook of medicine* (ed. D. J. Weatherall, J. G., Ledingham, and D. A., Warrell) Chapter 5, p. 228. Oxford University Press, Oxford.

——, Wright, R., Berman, E. and Laurence, D. R. (1959). Treatment of tetanus with chlorpromazine and barbiturates. *Lancet* **i**, 755.

Corbett, J. L., Spalding, J. M. K. and Harris, P. J. (1973). Hypotension in tetanus. *Br. med. J.* **3**, 423.

Dastur, F. D., Shahani, M. T., Dastour, D. H., Kohiyar, F. N., Bharucha, E. P., Mondkar, V. P., Kashyap, G. H. and Nair, K.G. (1977). Cephalic tetanus: demonstration of a dual lesion. *J. Neurol. Neurosurg. Psychiat.* **40**, 782.

Eyrich, K., Agostini, B., Schulz, A., Müller, E., Noetzel, H., Reichenmiller, H. E. and Wiemers, K. (1967). Clinical and morphological studies of skeletal muscle changes in tetanus. *Germ. med. Mth.* **12**, 469.

Fildes, P. (1929). Bacillus tetani. In *A system of bacteriology*, Vol 3, p. 298. London.

Forbes, G. R. and Auld, M. (1955). Management of tetanus. *Am. J. Med.* **18**, 947.

Gadoth, N., Dagan, R., Sandbank, U., Levy, D. and Moses, S. W. (1981). Permanent tetraplegia as a consequence of tetanus neonatorum: evidence for widespread lower motor neuron damage. *J. neurol. Sci.* **51**, 273.

Gupta, P. S., Kapoor, R., Goyal, S., Batra, V. K. and Jain, B. K. (1980). Intrathecal human tetanus immunoglobulin in early tetanus. *Lancet* **ii**, 439.

Illis, L. S. and Taylor, F. M. (1971). Neurological and electro-encephalographic sequelae of tetanus. *Lancet* **i**, 826.

Kerr, J. H., Corbett, J. L., Prys-Roberts, C., Smith, A. C. and Spalding, J. M. K. (1968). Involvement of the sympathetic nervous system in tetanus. *Lancet* **ii**, 236.

Patel, J. C. and Joag, G. G. (1959). Grading of tetanus to evaluate prognosis. *Indian J. Med. Sci.* **13**, 834.

Shackleton, P. (1954). The treatment of tetanus. *Lancet* **ii**, 155.

Sherrington, C. S. (1917). Observations with antitetanus serum in the monkey. *Lancet* **ii**, 964.

Smith, A. C. (1958). The treatment of severe tetanus by paralysing drugs and intermittent pressure respiration. *Proc. R. Soc. Med.* **51**, 1006.

Stoddart, J. C. (1979). Pseudo-tetanus. *Anaesthesia* **34**, 877.

Struppler, A., Struppler, E. and Adams, R. D. (1963). Local tetanus in man. *Arch. Neurol., Chicago* **8**, 162.

Tarlov, I. M., Ling, H. and Yamada, H. (1973). Neuronal pathology in experimental local tetanus. *Neurology, Minneapolis* **23**, 580.

Vakil, B. J., Singhal, B. S., Pandya, S. S. and Irani, P. F. (1973). Cephalic tetanus. *Neurology, Minneapolis* **23**, 1091.

Zacks, S. I., Hall, J. A. S. and Sheff, M. F. (1966). Studies in tetanus. IV. Intramitochondrial dense granules in skeletal muscles from human cases of tetanus intoxication. *Am. J. Path.* **48**, 811.

—— and Sheff, M. F. (1966). Studies on tetanus. V. *In vivo* localization of purified tetanus neurotoxin in mice with fluorescein-labelled tetanus antitoxin. *J. Neuropath. exp. Neurol.* **25**, 422.

Botulism

Definition. A form of food poisoning due to intoxication with the exotoxin of the *Clostridium botulinum* derived from infected foodstuffs, especially those preserved in tins, and characterized by extreme weakness and fatigability of both striated and unstriated muscle.

Aetiology

The *Cl. botulinum* is a large, gram-positive, anaerobic, spore-bearing organism, which is an inhabitant of the soil in certain regions and may contaminate food. It finds a most congenial environment in tinned food, especially vegetables and fruit, and both bought and home-preserved foodstuffs may be contaminated with it. The commonest type is so-called Type E, and Type E spores have been shown to be plentiful in North American soil and littoral waters (Meyers 1956). It produces a powerful exotoxin, to which its toxic effects are due. Tinned food infected with the bacillus can often be detected as tainted. Production of gas in the tin may abolish the normal vacuum, and the food often has a peculiar rancid odour and taste. This, however, may be disguised by sauces and dressings. There are many examples of severe and fatal poisoning occurring in a person who simply tasted food to see if it was tainted. Cooking at boiling temperature for a few minutes destroys the toxin, but boiling at high altitudes may be less effective (Cherington 1974). There have been outbreaks of botulism in many countries, especially in Germany, where it was first attributed to eating infected sausages—hence the name, derived from 'botulus', a sausage—and in the United States. An outbreak leading to a number of deaths occurred at Loch Maree in Scotland in 1922 and in a more recent outbreak in Birmingham, England (Ball, Hopkinson, Farrell, Hutchison, Paul, Watson, Page, Parker, Edwards, Snow, Scott, Leone-Ganado, Hastings, Ghosh, and Gilbert 1979) it followed the ingestion of contaminated tinned Alaskan salmon. Botulism has frequently been observed in domestic animals which have eaten the remains of tainted food, and fowls which have been thus intoxicated may die before symptoms appear in human beings who have eaten the same food. Contamination of fish by Type E may occur before they are caught and Whittaker (1964) reported eight simultaneous cases due to eating white chubb fish from the Great Lakes area, fish which was contaminated with Type E spores. Infant botulism, first fully characterized in California in the 1970s, even though a case reported in 1931 was recognized in retrospect, has been shown to occur in infants usually between one and six months of age, and to be due to colonization of the gut by spores which subsequently multiply and produce botulinum toxin (Midura and Arnon 1976; Arnon 1980). The condition in infants may be one cause of the sudden infant death syndrome (Arnon, Midura, Damus, Wood, and Chin 1978), but breast feeding may be partially protective (Arnon, Damus, Thompson, Midura, and Chin 1982). While the spores may be derived from dust, soil, or from eating honey, host factors, as yet unidentified, may be important. The condition has been described in infants in England (Turner, Brett, Gilbert, Ghosh, and Liebeschuetz 1978) and Australia (Shield, Wilkinson, and Ritchie 1978), but is still largely confined to California (Johnson, Clay, and Arnon 1979).

Botulinus toxin acts presynaptically, by abolishing the release of acetylcholine at cholinergic nerve endings (Burgen, Dickens, and Zatman 1949; Zacks 1964).

Pathology

The changes in the nervous system consist of severe congestion of both the brain and meninges, leading to oedema and perivascular haemorrhages.

Symptoms and signs

In man, symptoms usually develop between 18 and 36 hours after eating the tainted food, less often as early as 12 hours or as late as 48 hours or longer afterwards. In up to one-third of all cases an acute gastrointestinal disturbance, characterized by nausea, vomiting, and diarrhoea, occurs, but in most cases this is absent, constipation, probably due to paresis of the smooth muscle of the intestines, occurring early and persisting throughout the illness.

The earliest symptoms of muscular weakness may be visual. Dimness of vision results from paresis of accommodation; the pupils sometimes become dilated, and lose their reaction to light, and ptosis usually develops early. Paresis of external ocular muscles leads to diplopia, and nystagmus may be present. In some cases complete ocular immobility occurs. Vertigo is not uncommon. Owing to weakness of the muscles concerned, swallowing and talking become difficult; attempts to swallow lead to choking and regurgitation of food through the nose; and there may be complete aphonia. Weakness of jaw muscles renders mastication difficult or impossible, the muscles of the trunk and limbs also become extremely weak, and respiratory insufficiency or paralysis may follow. The muscular disturbance often resembles extreme fatigability, rather than actual paralysis, as the patient may be able to carry out a movement moderately well on one occasion but is then unable to repeat it. The tendon reflexes are preserved and the plantar reflexes flexor. There is usually no sensory disturbance. In most cases consciousness remains unimpaired up to the end, though occasionally there is terminal coma, and terminal convulsions have been described.

Other than in cases of sudden infant death, the prognosis of infant botulism is often surprisingly good. The condition presents as a rule with poor sucking, difficulty in swallowing, a weak cry, and weak head movements, but with variable weakness of the limbs and trunk and of respiratory muscles with little if any oculomotor involvement. Gradual recovery over a few weeks is usual (Johnson *et al.* 1979).

The CSF is usually normal. The temperature remains normal, unless a complicating infection, such as bronchopneumonia, develops. Death occurs either from respiratory paralysis or broncho-pneumonia.

Diagnosis

The most useful diagnostic features are: (1) a previously healthy patient; (2) absence of fever; (3) abdominal symptoms; (4) weakness, malaise, and fatigability; (5) cranial-nerve signs; and (6) a likely food source.

In cases in which an acute gastro-intestinal disturbance occurs, the diagnosis from other forms of acute gastro-enteritis cannot usually be made before muscular weakness appears, unless domestic animals have already shown signs of poisoning. The dilated pupils may suggest atropine poisoning, but the unclouded mental condition enables this to be excluded. Clinically and neurophysiologically, the condition may show resemblances to the Eaton–Lambert myasthenic syndrome which, however, is less acute in its onset and usually causes areflexia. In infancy, infantile myasthenia may be simulated but there is little if any response to edrophonium. When the diagnosis is doubtful it may be confirmed by the demonstration of the *Cl. botulinum* or of its toxin in the faeces or in the remains of food which has been consumed.

Supramaximal stimulation of a peripheral nerve with recording of the evoked muscle action potential may give a decremental response at low rates of stimulation but an increase in amplitude during stimulation at 50 Hz, as in the Eaton–Lambert syndrome (p. 571) (Cherington 1974). Single-fibre electromyography helps to confirm the known disorder of acetylcholine release (Schiller and Stålberg 1978).

Prognosis

The mortality varies in different outbreaks; in the past it often ranged between 16 and 65 per cent but the outlook is much better with modern treatment and many milder cases, especially the infantile variety, are now recognized. Death usually occurs between the fourth and eighth day. Convalescence is very slow but in those who survive eventual recovery is usually complete.

Treatment

Prophylaxis consists in the careful scrutiny of all tinned foods, and the rejection, without tasting, of any which seem tainted. The cooking of tinned products for 10 minutes before use abolishes all risk of botulism. Antitoxin appears to possess greater prophylactic than curative value and can seldom be used before the onset of muscular symptoms. Fifty thousand units of a polyvalent serum should nevertheless be given. Antibiotics should also be given orally and parenterally, penicillin being the drug of choice, in order to destroy surviving organisms in the gastrointestinal tract which may still be producing exotoxin. Complete rest is needed to protect the muscles from undue fatigue, and sedatives may be necessary. Nasal feeding and artificial respiration may be required.

Sustained improvement usually results from guanidine hydrochloride given in a dosage of 250 mg every four hours for several days (Cherington 1974). However, 4-aminopyridine, given by single or repeated intravenous injections in a dose of 0.35–0.5 mg/kg body weight, may be even more effective (Ball *et al.* 1979).

References

Arnon, S. S. (1980). Infant botulism. *Ann. Rev. Med.* **31,** 541.
—— Damus, K., Thompson, B., Midura, T. F. and Chin, J. (1982). Protective role of human milk against sudden death from infant botulism. *J. Pediat.* **100,** 568.
——, Midura, T. F., Damus, K., Wood, R. M. and Chin, J. (1978). Intestinal infection and toxin production by clostridium botulinum as one cause of sudden infant death syndrome. *Lancet* **i,** 1973.
Ball, A. P., Hopkinson, R. B., Farrell, I. D., Hutchinson, J. G. P., Paul, R., Watson, R. D. S., Page, A. J. F., Parker, R. G. F., Edwards, C. W., Snow, M., Scott, D. K., Leone-Ganado, A., Hastings, A., Ghosh, A. C. and Gilbert, R. J. (1979). Human botulism caused by clostridium botulinum type E: the Birmingham outbreak. *Quart. J. Med.* **48,** 473.
Burgen, A. S. V., Dickens, F. and Zatman, L. J. (1949). Action of botulinum toxin on the neuro-muscular junction. *J. Physiol. (Lond.)* **109,** 10.
Cherington, M. (1974). Botulism: ten-year experience. *Arch. Neurol., Chicago* **30,** 432.
Johnson, R. O., Clay, S.A. and Arnon, S. S. (1979). Diagnosis and management of infant botulism. *Am. J. Dis. Child* **133,** 586.
Meyers, K. F. (1956). The status of botulism as a world health problem. *Bull. Wld. Hlth Org.* **15,** 28.
Midura, T. F. and Arnon, S. S. (1976). Infant botulism: identification of clostridium botulinum and its toxins in faeces. *Lancet* **ii,** 934.
Monro, T. K. and Knox, W. W. N. (1923). Remarks on botulism as seen in Scotland in 1922. *Br. med. J.* **1,** 279.
Petty, C. J. (1965). Botulism: the disease and the toxin. *Am. J. med. Sci.* **249,** 345.
Schiller, H. H. and Stålberg, E. (1978). Human botulism studied with single-fiber electromyography. *Arch. Neurol., Chicago* **35,** 346.
Shield, L. K., Wilkinson, R. G. and Ritchie, M. (1978). Infant botulism in Australia. *Med. J. Aust.* **1,** 157.
Turner, H. D., Brett, E. M., Gilbert, R. J., Ghosh, A. C. and Liebeschuetz, H. J. (1978). Infant botulism in England. *Lancet* **i,** 1277.
Whittaker, R. L., Gilbertson, R. B. and Garrett, A. S. (1964). Botulism, Type E. Report of 8 simultaneous cases. *Ann. intern. Med.* **61,** 448.
Zacks, S. I. (1964). *The motor end-plate.* Saunders, Philadelphia.

Saxitoxin poisoning

Saxitoxin, a powerful neurotoxic agent, may produce symptoms in human subjects eating mussels or other shellfish which have been contaminated by dinoflagellates of the genus *Gonyaulax* which only occur in the sea at certain times of the year and in certain weather conditions (the 'red tide'). Epidemics have been reported from the Pacific coast of the USA and from many places in Europe. An outbreak in Northumberland affecting 78 individuals was described by McCollum, Pearson, Ingham, Wood, and Dewar (1968); while the condition has been known to be fatal, all patients in this series recovered. Symptoms, which usually developed within 30 minutes to 12 hours after eating mussels, included paraesthesiae in the limbs and in circumoral distribution, muscular weakness, ataxia, headache, vomiting, and choking sensations. Recovery was usually complete within 24–72 hours.

Somewhat similar symptoms can result from poisoning with tetrodotoxin (the toxin of the puffer fish) and from a variety of other venoms and toxins produced by, for example, scorpions and sea anemones (Narahashi 1980).

References

McCollum, J. P. K., Pearson, R. C. M., Ingham, H. R., Wood, P. C. and Dewar, H. A. (1968). An epidemic of mussel poisoning in North-East England. *Lancet* **ii,** 767.
Narahashi, T. (1980). Nerve membrane as a target for environmental toxicants. In *Experimental and clinical neurotoxicology* (ed. P. S. Spencer and H. H. Schaumburg) Chapter 16. Williams and Wilkins, New York.

Ergotism

'Ergotism' is a term applied to poisoning with the toxins produced by the fungus *Claviceps purpurea* of rye. Two forms occur, one characterized by gangrene—the gangrenous form—the other by muscular spasms and generalized convulsions—the convulsive form, which is now very rare.

Poisoning with ergot was usually due in the past to the consumption of bread made from contaminated flour. The gangrenous form was occasionally caused by the administration of ergot as an abortifacient. Very rarely it may follow the excessive use of ergotamine tartrate in the treatment of migraine (Hudgson and Hart 1964; Dige-Peterson, Lassen, Noer, Tønnesen, and Olesen 1977) or of the closely-related drug dimethysergide (*Deseril*) given as a prophylactic in this condition, though retroperitoneal fibrosis is a more important complication of treatment with the latter remedy. Many patients who take abnormally large amounts of these drugs may develop pains in the limbs and paraesthesiae, blanching of digits, and coldness in the extremities but fully-developed ergotism is now rare. It was always rare in Britain, but commoner on the continent of Europe, where it was especially prevalent during the Middle Ages. Epidemics occurred in France, Germany, Sweden, Norway, Finland, Russia, and elsewhere, and in Russia it is apparently still endemic. The gangrenous and convulsive forms differed in geographical distribution, the former occurring to the west, and the latter to the east, of the Rhine, though mixed epidemics were sometimes observed where these regions met. It seems that the gangrenous form was due to poisoning with ergotoxin or ergotamine, but the convulsive form appeared to depend upon the coexistence of two factors, namely consumption of an unknown constituent of ergot, not the alkaloid, and a lack of vitamin A in the diet (Mellanby 1931; Barger 1931).

Convulsive ergotism was associated with degeneration of the spinal cord, especially the dorsal columns, and also of peripheral nerves. Thickening of the media and hyaline degeneration of the intima of the arteries, sometimes with thrombosis, are the changes found in the gangrenous form.

The onset of gangrenous ergotism may be insidious or rapid. Gangrene is often preceded by severe burning pains, hence the name St. Anthony's fire. Gangrene might involve only the fingers or toes or whole limbs. Convulsive ergotism began with muscular fasciculation, followed by clonic and tonic muscular spasms, leading to abnormal postures and finally, in severe cases, generalized convulsions. Anaesthesia of the limbs, hemiplegia, and paraplegia sometimes occurred.

References

Barger, G. (1931). *Ergot and ergotism.* Gurney and Jackson, London.

Dige-Petersen, H., Lassesn, N., Noer, I., Tønnesen, K. H. and Olesen, J. (1977). Subclinical ergotism. *Lancet* ii, 65.

Hudgson, P. and Hart, J. A. L. (1964). Acute ergotism: report of a case and a review of the literature. *Med. J. Aust.* 2, 589.

Mellanby, E. (1931). The experimental production and prevention of degeneration in the spinal cord. *Brain,* 54, 247.

Von Storch, T. J. C. (1938). Complications following the use of ergotamine tartrate. Their relation to the treatment of migraine headache. *J. Am. med. Ass.* 111, 293.

The neurological manifestations of acute porphyria

The porphyrias are disorders of the metabolism of porphyrins and porphyrin precursors (Dean 1969). They may be symptomless, may cause cutaneous lesions, or may be responsible for an acute illness (acute porphyria) which gives psychological, neurological, and abdominal symptoms. Dean divided this group of conditions first into the three varieties of hepatic porphyria, namely porphyria variegata (protocoproporphyria, the South African type), acute intermittent porphyria (pyrroloporphyria, the Swedish type), and coproporphyria (Goldberg, Rimington, and Lochhead 1967; Brodie, Moore, and Goldberg 1977). In addition there are other rare varieties of non-hepatic porphyria including the erythropoietic type (congenital porphyria) in which there are anaemia, splenomegaly, and pink staining of the teeth and of bones without neurological manifestations, and symptomatic porphyria which presents largely with cutaneous manifestations precipitated often by alcoholism but not by barbiturates, or else by eating bread made from wheat grain treated with hexachlorophene (Peters, Gocmen, Cripps, Bryan, and Dogramaci 1982).

Macalpine, Hunter, and Rimington (1968) suggested that King George III of England suffered from a psychotic illness due to porphyria and gave reasons for suggesting that the disorder was present in many members of the Royal Houses of Stuart, Hanover, and Prussia.

Aetiology and pathology

The South African and Swedish types of porphyria and coproporphyria are all inherited as autosomal dominant traits. The Swedish type is commonest in Europe (Waldenstrom 1957) and is seen most often in females between 16 and 50 years. Acute attacks are often precipitated by drugs, especially barbiturates, light sensitivity does not occur, and there is a high excretion of porphobilinogen G and of delta-amino-laevulinic acid during the acute attacks and for a long time afterwards. It has been suggested that delta-amino-laevulinic acid may act by inhibiting GABA binding to its receptors (Müller and Snyder 1977). In the South African type (Dean and Barnes 1958) the age and sex incidence is similar; acute attacks are always precipitated by drugs and are often fatal, light sensitivity (porphyria variegata) is found in many affected individuals, particularly males, and there is a high excretion of porphobilinogen in the acute attack but this returns to normal as the patient recovers. Faecal protoporphyrin excretion is normal in acute intermittent porphyria but is raised in the South African variety. Coproporphyria is less common than the other two types; there is excessive excretion of coproporphyrin in the stools, acute attacks of neurological dysfunction may be precipitated by barbiturates but there are no skin changes, and both urinary coproporphyrin and uroporphyrin are increased in the attacks. In acute attacks, especially in the Swedish type, there is a greatly increased activity of delta-amino-laevulinic acid synthetase, the rate-limiting enzyme of haem biosynthesis, in liver biopsy specimens, along with excessive urinary exretion of certain porphyrogenic steroids (Goldberg, Moore, Beattice, Hall, McCallum, and Grant 1969; Sweeney, Pathak, and Asbury 1970; *The Lancet* 1972). Badawy (1978) suggested that measurement of haem utilization by rat-liver tryptophan pyrrolase may be helpful in predicting which drugs may precipitate attacks. Apart from barbiturates, this test identified chlordiazepoxide, chloroquine, phenytoin, phenylbutazone, tolbutamide, and several other drugs as potential precipitants, while cortisone, morphine, paracetamol, pethidine, propranolol, salicylate, and imipramine, among others, did not have this effect. A complete list of unsafe drugs is given by Goldberg, Moore, McColl, and Brodie (1983). In many cases uroporphyrinogen-I synthetase activity is reduced in the red blood cells and coproporphyrimogen oxidase is greatly reduced in fibroblasts in coproporphyria but not in the other types (Elder, Evans, Thomas, Cox, Brodie, Moore, Goldberg, and Nicholson 1976).

The pathological changes in the nervous system were studied by Hierons (1957) who found evidence of demyelination in peripheral nerves and abnormalities of the anterior horn cells. Vesicular dissolution of peripheral-nerve myelin similar to that seen in diphtheritic neuropathy has been described subsequently (Anzil and Dozic 1978). The mental disturbances observed in acute attacks seem to be of metabolic origin and no specific pathological changes have been found in the brain. Dagg, Goldberg, Lochhead, and Smith (1965) drew attention to the similarity of lead poisoning to acute porphyria. In both conditions there is a considerable increase in the excretion of delta-amino-laevulinic acid. They suggested that the abdominal, cardiovascular, and neurological manifestations might be explained on a neurogenic basis with focal demyelination of peripheral and autonomic nerves. However, Cavanagh and Mellick (1065) studied four fatal cases and concluded that the peripheral-nerve lesion was predominantly axonal. Mustajoki and Seppäläinen (1975) found slowing of sensory and to a lesser extent of motor nerve conduction in 20 patients with the Swedish and 5 with the South African variety of porphyria between attacks. The current view is that the neuropathy of this condition is primarily axonal but that there is usually secondary demyelination (Weller and Cervós-Navarro 1977;

Asbury and Johnson 1978; Thorner, Bilbao, Sima, and Briggs 1981).

Symptoms and signs

The syndrome of acute intermittent porphyria may present with the acute clinical picture, or with cutaneous lesions alone, or with a combination of the two. The biochemical abnormality may also be symptomless, particularly in the sibs of affected patients.

The onset is usually in adolescence or early adult life, and the acute manifestations are frequently precipitated by the administration of barbiturates, sulphonamides, chloroquine, and many other drugs (Garcin 1964 and see above), or by over-indulgence in alcohol.

Early symptoms of nervous involvement include restlessness, emotional instability and mood disorder, sometimes leading a confusional state. Epileptic attacks are common, and are sometimes the presenting feature. In severe cases there may be stupor or coma, or status epilepticus.

The other characteristic clinical picture is a polyneuropathy, usually predominantly motor, with muscular weakness, initially chiefly proximal in the limbs, but becoming generalized and sometimes involving respiratory and bulbar muscles. Though subjective sensory symptoms are common, objective sensory loss is rare.

General symptoms often usher in the attacks, especially acute abdominal pain with nausea and vomiting. Hypertension may occur, and there may be impairment of renal function. In the South African type the skin may show scars, erosions, or bullae, and bronze pigmentation and hirsutism are common.

During the acute attack, the urine contains large amounts of delta-amino-laevulinic acid and porphobilinogen. In the Swedish type, there is very little increase in urinary and faecal porphyrin excretion except in the acute attack, while in the South African type urinary and faecal porphyrins show a much greater increase, again particularly during an attack. The urine is not invariably abnormal in colour, even during the attack, but often the patient will have noted it to be dark, with the typical 'port-wine' colour which darkens on standing.

Diagnosis

Porphyria should be considered as a possible cause of otherwise unexplained confusional states, coma, epilepsy, or polyneuropathy occurring in early adult life, especially if the symptoms have been precipitated by any of the drugs known to be apt to precipitate it. On suspicion of the diagnosis, estimation of urinary porphyrin excretion is indicated. The Watson–Schwartz test is a useful screening test for the Swedish variety between attacks (Dean 1969). Measurement of erythrocyte uroporphinogen-I-synthase is invaluable in the diagnosis of acute intermittent porphyria of all types and that of coproporphyrinogen-oxidase for the diagnosis of coproporphyria (*The Lancet* 1978).

Prognosis

Acute porphyria is always a serious disease but the mortality rate fell after intermittent positive pressure respiration was introduced (Dean 1969). In Berman's (1961) series of 81 cases, there were 22 deaths, only 12 of which were attributed solely to the porphyria. In 10 the cause of death was cardio-respiratory failure, and in 2 cardiac arrest—a mortality rate of 15.6 per cent. All these patients had severe paralysis. However, even in gravely ill patients, complete recovery may still occur.

Treatment

Prophylaxis obviously includes the avoidance of the drugs known to precipitate attacks in the case of known sufferers, and the investigation of sibs for evidence of asymptomatic porphyria. Treatment is primarily symptomatic, and the usual treatment of bulbar and respiratory paralysis may be needed. Otherwise, chlorpromazine seems to be of particular value for relief of pain and other symptoms. It may be given in a dose of 25–50 mg three or four times a day, and a single dose of 100 mg is reported to have been followed by a complete remission (Welby, Street, and Watson 1956). Of greater benefit is a high-carbohydrate diet, and intravenous infusions of laevulose (400 g daily) reduce delta-aminolaevulinic acid synthetase activity and may produce marked clinical improvement (*The Lancet* 1978). Intravenous infusions of haematin may be even more successful in terminating acute attacks (Pierach and Watson 1978), the usual dose being 4 mg/kg body weight infused slowly over 30 minutes, repeated daily for several days (Goldberg *et al.* 1983).

References

Anzil, A. P. and Dozic, S. (1978). Peripheral nerve changes in porphyric neuropathy. *Acta Neuropath.* **42**, 12.

Asbury, A. K. and Johnson, P. C. (1978). *Pathology of peripheral nerve.* Saunders, Philadelphia.

Badawy, A. A.-B. Treatment of acute hepatic porphyria. *Lancet* i, 1361.

Berman, S. (1961). Neurologic disorders in porphyria. A brief clinical survey of 81 cases. *Reports at the VII International Congress in Neurology*, Rome, p. 33.

Brodie, M. J., Moore, M. R. and Goldberg, A. (1977). Enzyme abnormalities in the porphyrias. *Lancet,* **ii**, 699.

Cavanagh, J. B. and Mellick, R. S. (1965). On the nature of the peripheral nerve lesions associated with acute intermittent porphyria. *J. Neurol. Psychiat.* **28**, 320.

Dagg, J. H., Goldberg, A., Lochhead, A. and Smith, J. A. (1965). The relationship of lead poisoning to acute intermittent porphyria. *Quart. J. Med.* **34**, 163.

Dean, G. (1969). The porphyrias. *Br. med. Bull.* **25**, 48.

—— and Barnes, H. D. (1955). The inheritance of porphyria acuta, cutanea tarda, and symptomless porphyrinuria. *Br. med. J.* **2**, 89.

—— and —— (1958). Porphyria. A South African screening experiment. *Br. med. J.* **1**, 298.

Bobriner, K. and Rhoads, C. P. (1940). The porphyrins in health and disease. *Physiol. Rev.* **20**, 416.

Eales, L. (1960). Cutaneous porphyria. *S. Afr. J. Lab. clin. Med.* **6**, 63.

Elder, G. H., Evans, J. O., Thomas, N., Cox, R., Brodie, M. J., Moore, M.R., Goldberg, A. and Nicholson, D. C. (1976). The primary enzyme defect in hereditary coproporphyria. *Lancet* **ii**, 1217.

Garcin, R. (1964). Porphyries aiguës. Introduction générale. *Soc. Med. Hôp., Paris* **115**, 1089.

Goldberg, A. (1959). Acute intermittent porphyria. *Quart. J. Med.* **28**, 183.

—— Moore, M. J., Beattie, A. D., Hall, P. E., McCallum, J. and Grant, J. K. (1969). Excessive urinary excretion of certain porphyrinogenic steroids in human acute intermittent porphyria. *Lancet* i, 115.

——, ——, McColl, K. E. L. and Brodie, M. J. (1983). Porphyrin metabolism and the porphyrias. In *Oxford textbook of medicine* (ed. D. J. Weatherall, J. G. G. Ledingham and D. A. Warrell) Chapter 9.81. Oxford University Press, Oxford.

——, Rimington, C. and Lochhead, A. C. (1967). Hereditary coproporphyria. *Lancet,* i, 632.

Haeger, B. (1958). Urinary δ-aminolaevulinic acid and porphobilinogen in different types of porphyria. *Lancet,* **ii**, 606.

Hierons, R. (1957). Changes in the nervous system in acute porphyria. *Brain* **80**, 176.

The Lancet (1972). Enzymes in the hepatic porphyrias. *Lancet* **ii**, 121.

—— (1978). Treatment of acute hepatic porphyria. *Lancet* i, 1024.

MacAlpine, I., Hunter, R. and Rimington, C. (1968). Porphyria in the Royal Houses of Stuart, Hanover and Prussia. *Br. med. J.* **1**, 7.

Müller, W. E. and Snyder, S. H. (1977). δ-Aminolaevulinic acid: influences on synaptic GABA receptor binding may explain CNS symptoms of porphyria. *Ann. Neurol.* **2**, 340.

Mustajoki, P. and Seppäläinen, A. M. (1975). Neuropathy in latent hereditary hepatic porphyria. *Br. med. J.,* **2**, 310.

Peters, H. A., Gocmen, A., Cripps, D. J., Bryan, G. T. and Dogramaci, I. (1982). Epidemiology of hexachlorobenzene-induced porphyria in Turkey: clinical and laboratory follow-up after 25 years. *Arch. Neurol., Chicago* **39**, 744.

Pierach, C. A. and Watson, C. J. (1978). Treatment of acute hepatic porphyria. *Lancet* i, 1361.

Sweeney, V. P., Pathak, M. A. and Asbury, A. K. (1970). Acute intermittent porphyria. Increased ALA-synthetase activity during an acute attack. *Brain* **93**, 369.

Thorner, P. S., Bilbao, J. M., Sima, A. A. F. and Briggs, S. (1981). Porphyric neuropathy: an ultrastructural and quantitative case study. *Can. J. neurol. Sci.* **8**, 281.

Waldenstrom, J. (1957). The porphyrias as inborn errors of metabolism. *Am. J. Med.* **22**, 758.

Welby, J. C., Street, J. P. and Watson, C. J. (1956). Chlorpromazine in the treatment of porphyria. *J. Am. med. Ass.* **162**, 174.

Weller, R. and Cervos-Navarro, J. (1977). *Pathology of peripheral nerves.* Butterworths, London.

The neurological manifestations of hepatic failure

Neurological symptoms may appear as the result of hepatic failure from any cause, e.g. acute virus hepatitis, eclampsia, portal cirrhosis, Wilson's disease, haemochromatosis, acute chemical poisoning, or the terminal stages of biliary cirrhosis. They may arise spontaneously or be precipitated in patients with chronic liver disease by gastrointestinal haemorrhage, acute alcoholic intoxication, the administration of morphine, barbiturates or benzodiazepines, paracentesis, diuretics, or surgery. They may also follow the operation of portacaval anastomosis (Sherlock 1981). The hepatic damage of Reye's syndrome in childhood, which may possibly be the consequence of salicylate intoxication (Partin, Parton, Schubert, and Hammond 1982; *The Lancet* 1982*a*; Starko and Mullick 1983; and see p. 254), contributes to the neurological manifestations of that disorder, but probably does not account for the striking cytotoxic cerebral oedema.

The causes of the disturbances of central nervous function are complex, and were discussed by Summerskill, Davidson, Sherlock and Steiner (1956), Victor (1974) and Sherlock (1981). One essential factor is that as a result of abnormal anastomoses between the portal and systemic arterial systems, either arising naturally or produced by surgery, nitrogenous material intended for the liver enters the systemic circulation. Similar symptoms may be observed after liver transplantation (Parkes, Murray-Lyon, and Williams 1970*a*). Measurement of the blood ammonia gives a rough index of the severity of the condition which is now called porto-systemic encephalopathy. Duffy, Vergara, and Plum (1974) showed that alpha-ketoglutaramate, a metabolite of glutamine not previously demonstrated in mammalian tissue, is increased four-to tenfold in patients with hepatic encephalopathy. Experimental portocaval anastomosis results in increased permeability of the cerebral blood-brain barrier (Laursen and Westergaard 1977) and Schafer and Jones (1982) suggest that GABA derived from the gut crosses this barrier and induces increased numbers of GABA and benzodiazine receptors in the brain. There is also evidence that hyperammonaemia and increased circulating aromatic amino acids together induce cerebral depletion of dopamine and nor-adrenaline and also cause an accumulation of false neurotransmitters (octopamine and phenylethanolamine) (*The Lancet* 1982*b*, 1983).

One of the most constant pathological changes in the brain is the presence in the cortex and in the basal ganglia of Alzheimer type 2 astrocytes which show no cytoplasm with ordinary staining methods (Adams and Foley 1953). These cells are also present in Wilson's disease. Cavanagh and Kyu (1969) suggested that the astrocytic abnormality may be due to a defect in function of the mitotic spindle and there is also evidence of microtubular dysfunction (*The Lancet* 1971; Cavanagh 1974) but Laursen and Westerguard (1977) postulate that the astrocytic change results from an accumulation of intracellular material due to increased permeability of the blood-brain barrier.

Neurological symptoms in chronic hepatic disease may be inter-mittent, and sometimes predominantly psychiatric, for long periods. In other cases, and in acute hepatic failure, they develop rapidly and progressively. Psychiatric symptoms consist of personality changes, abnormalities of mood and behaviour, and drowsiness deepening into stupor and coma. Speech is likely to be slurred, and there may be dysphasia. A 'flapping' tremor (so-called asterixis) is rather characteristic when the arms are outstretched, but may occur in other toxic states also and even in midbrain infarction (Bril, Sharpe, and Ashby 1979). Neurological signs suggestive of focal cerebral damage or dysfunction are occasionally seen (Pearce 1963). Extrapyramidal rigidity and tremor may be present with or without signs of corticospinal lesions or cerebellar deficiency. Muscle twitching may occur. Myelopathy with spasticity and increased limb reflexes but with flexor plantar responses was described by Rawson and Liversedge (1966) but Plant, Rebeiz, and Richardson (1968), on the basis of neuropathological studies, suggested that this syndrome is more properly due to a restricted form of encephalopathy with descending degeneration of the corticospinal tracts. An increased terminal latency or diminution in the size of the sensory evoked response in electrophysiological studies of peripheral-nerve function (Seneviratne and Peiris 1970) indicates the presence of a subclinical peripheral neuropathy in many cases. A syndrome of chronic choreo-athetosis has also been observed (Toghill, Johnston, and Smith 1967).

In severe cases triphasic delta waves are often present in the EEG. In milder cases there is slowing of the dominant frequency. The EEG can be used as a sensitive indicator of the response to treatment as well as for diagnosis (Laidlaw and Read 1961; Parkes, Sharpstone, and Williams 1970*b*). The CSF is usually normal. Measurement of the blood ammonia is still most widely used for biochemical monitoring but the blood mercaptan is also a helpful index of the response to treatment (McClain, Zieve, Doizaki, Gilberstadt, and Onstad 1980).

The clinical and biochemical signs of the causal hepatic disorder will be present. Jaundice may be slight or absent in chronic hepatic failure due to cirrhosis.

Treatment consists first in reducing the absorption of nitrogenous substances from the bowel. Hence a protein intake of less than 20 g daily is recommended and neomycin, 1–2.5 g daily (Dawson, McLaren, and Sherlock 1957), has been given in an attempt to reduce absorption. *Lactobacillus acidophilus* has been used for the same purpose (Macbeth, Kass, and McDermott 1965) while surgical exclusion of the colon has also been successful (Walker, Emlyn-Williams, Craigie, Rosenoer, Agnew, and Sherlock 1965). However, a high-carbohydrate diet, including lactulose, is also helpful, and few now recommend neomycin (Zieve 1981), but it has been suggested that vegetable protein is less harmful than that derived from animal sources (Greenberger, Carley, Schenker, Bettinger, Stamnes, and Beyer 1977). In acute hepatic coma, extracorporeal perfusion of a baboon liver was shown to relieve the symptoms (Abouna, Fisher, Still, and Humel 1972). Levodopa 5 g given by gastric tube in 100 ml water (Parkes *et al.* 1970*b*) has been shown to produce striking temporary improvement in the level of consciousness and in the EEG in hepatic coma and bromocriptine has a similar effect (Morgan, Jakobovits, James, and Sherlock 1980), while the cognitive deficits of chronic hepatic encephalopathy are also improved by treatment with this drug in standard dosage (Elithorn, Lunzer, and Weinman 1975). It has recently been suggested that oral zinc supplementation (zinc acetate 600 mg daily) may also be helpful but this remains to be substantiated (Reding, Duchateau, and Bataille 1984).

References

Abouna, G. M., Fisher, L. McA., Still, W. J., and Hume, D. M. (1972). Acute hepatic coma successfully treated by extracorporeal baboon liver perfusions. *Br. med. J.* **1**, 23.

Adams, R. D. and Foley, J. M. (1953). The neurological disorder associated with liver disease in *Metabolic disorders of the nervous system.* ARNMD, **32**, 198. Baltimore, Maryland.

Bril, V., Sharpe, J. A. and Ashby, P. (1979). Midbrain asterixis. *Ann. Neurol.* **6**, 362.

Cavanagh, J. B. (1974). Liver bypass and the glia. In *Brain dysfunction in metabolic disorders* (ed. F. Plum) Vol. 53. ARNMD. New York.

—— and Kyu, M. H. (1969). Colchicine-like effect on astrocytes after portocaval shunt in rats. *Lancet* **ii**, 620.

Dawson, A. M., McLaren, J. and Sherlock, S. (1957). Neomycin in the treatment of hepatic coma. *Lancet* **ii**, 1263.

Duffy, T. E., Vergara, F. and Plum, F. (1974). δ-Ketoglutaramate in hepatic encephalopathy. In *Brain dysfunction in metabolic disorders*, (ed. F. Plum). ARNMD, New York.

Elithorn, A., Lunzer, M. and Weinman, J. (1975). Cognitive deficits associated with chronic hepatic encephalopathy and their response to levodopa. *J. Neurol. Neurosurg. Psychiat.* **38**, 794.

Greenberger, N. J., Carley, J., Schenker, S., Bettinger, I., Stamnes, C. and Beyer, P. (1977). Effect of vegetable and animal protein diets in chronic hepatic encephalopathy. *Am. J. Dig. Dis.* **22**, 845.

Laidlaw, J. and Read, A.E. (1961). The EEG diagnosis of manifest and latent delirium. *J. Neurol. Psychiat.* **24**, 58.

The Lancet (1971). The astrocyte in liver disease. *Lancet* **ii**, 1189.

—— (1982*a*). Reye's syndrome—epidemiological considerations. *Lancet* **i**, 941.

—— (1982*b*). False neurotransmitters and hepatic failure. *Lancet* **i**, 86.

—— (1983). Diet and hepatic encephalopathy. *Lancet* **i**, 625.

Laursen, H. and Westergaard, E. (1977). Enhanced permeability to horseradish peroxidase across cerebral vessels in the rat after portocaval anastomosis. *Neuropath. appl. Neurobiol.* **3**, 29.

Liversedge, L. A. and Rawson, M. D. (1966). Myelopathy in hepatic disease and portacaval anastomosis. *Lancet* **i**, 277.

Macbeth, W. A. A. G., Kass, E. H., and McDermott, W. V. (1965). Treatment of hepatic encephalopathy by alteration of intestinal flora with *Lactobacillus acidophilus*. *Lancet* **i**, 399.

McClain, C. J., Zieve, L., Doizaki, W. M., Gilberstadt, S., and Onstad, G. R. (1980). Blood methanethiol in alcoholic liver disease with and without hepatic encephalopathy. *Gut* **21**, 318.

Morgan, M. Y., Jakobovits, A. W., James, I. M., and Sherlock, S. (1980). Successful use of bromocriptine in the treatment of chronic hepatic encephalopathy. *Gastroenterology* **78**, 663.

Pant, S. S., Rebeiz, J. J., and Richardson, E. P. (1968). Spastic paraparesis following portacaval shunts. *Neurology, Minneapolis* **18**, 134.

Parkes, J. D., Murray-Lyon, I. M., and Williams, R. (1970(*a*)). Neuropsychiatric and electroencephalographic changes after transplantation of the liver. *Quart. J. Med.* **39**, 515.

——, Sharpstone, P., and Williams, R. (1970(*b*)). Levodopa in hepatic coma. *Lancet* **ii**, 1341.

Partin, J. S., Partin, J. C., Schubert, W.K., and Hammond, J. G. (1982). Serum salicylate concentrations in Reye's disease: a study of 130 biopsy-proven cases. *Lancet* **i**, 191.

Pearce, J. M. S. (1963). Focal neurological syndromes in hepatic failure. *Postgrad, med. J.* **39**, 653.

Read, A. E., Laidlaw, J., and Sherlock, S. (1961). Neuropsychiatric complications of portacaval anastomosis. *Lancet* **i**, 961.

Reding, P., Duchateau, J., and Bataille, C. (1984). Oral zinc supplementation improves hepatic encephalopathy. *Lancet* **ii**, 493.

Schafer, D. F. and Jones, E. A. (1982). Hepatic encephalopathy and the ν-aminobutyric-acid neurotransmitter system. *Lancet* **i**, 18.

Seneviratne, K. N. and Peiris, O. A. (1970). Peripheral nerve function in chronic liver disease. *J. Neurol. Neurosurg. Psychiat.* **33**, 609.

Sherlock, S. (1981). *Diseases of the liver and biliary system*, 6th edn. Blackwell, Oxford.

Starko, K. M. and Mullick, F. G. (1983). Hepatic and cerebral pathology findings in children with fatal salicylate intoxication: further evidence for a causal relation between salicylate and Reye's syndrome. *Lancet* **i**, 326.

Summerskill, W. H. J., Davidson, E. A., Sherlock, S., and Steiner, R. E. (1956). The neurospsychiatric syndrome associated with hepatic cirrhosis and an extensive portal collateral circulation. *Quart. J. Med.* **25**, 245.

Toghill, P. J., Johnston, A. W., and Smith, J. F. (1967). Choreoathetosis in portosystemic encephalopathy. *J. Neurol. Psychiat.* **30**, 358.

Victor, M. (1974). Neurologic changes in liver disease. In *Brain dysfunction in metabolic disorders* (ed. F. Plum) Vol. 53. ARNMD, New York.

Walker, J. G., Emlyn-Williams, A., Craigie, A., Rosenoer, W. M., Agnew, J., and Sherlock, S. (1965). Treatment of chronic portal-

systemic encephalopathy by surgical exclusion of the colon. *Lancet* **ii**, 861.

Zieve, L. (1981). The mechanisms of hepatic coma. *Hepatology* **1**, 360.

Inborn errors of metabolism including the neuronal storage disorders

There are a great many disorders of the nervous system of which some, until very recently, were classified as being degenerative, since their cause was unknown, which are now recognized to be due to specific inborn errors of metabolism and which are usually, if not invariably, genetically determined. In many of these, abnormal material is stored in the neurones, glial cells, myelin, or supporting tissues of the central and/or peripheral nervous system and in some a specific enzymatic defect has been identified. Developments in this field are occurring so rapidly that virtually any classification becomes outdated as soon as it is formulated. Useful reviews have been provided by Menkes (1980) and by Rosenberg and Pettegrew (1984). Many, but by no means all of these conditions are classified among the biochemical causes of mental retardation. The following is a simple working classification according to present knowledge.

A. Urea-cycle disorders;
B. Amino-acid disorders;
C. Disorders of lipid metabolism;
D. Disorders of serum lipoproteins;
E. Disorders of purine metabolism;
F. Disorders of carbohydrate metabolism;
G. Disorders of mucopolysaccharide metabolism;
H. Miscellaneous disorders of unknown aetiology.

Urea-cycle disorders

As Hutchison and Diamond (1981) have pointed out, urea-cycle defects are prominent among the metabolic disorders that cause symptomatic hyperammonaemia in neonates and young infants. There are five enzymes which convert ammonia to urea for excretion in the urine and each may be defective, so that the diseases which have been described have been respectively entitled argininaemia, arginosuccinicaciduria, ornithine transcarbamoylase deficiency, citrullinaemia, and hyperornithinaemia. Although these syndromes have different clinical courses, all usually produce moderate-to-severe mental retardation with intermittent ataxia and hyperammonaemia, commonly with recurrent episodes of lethargy and vomiting, and often epileptic seizures (Freeman, Nicholson, Schimke, Rowland, and Carter 1970; Farriaux, Cartigny, Dhondt, Kint, Louis, Delattre, and Fontaine 1974). Protein meals may lead in severe cases to uncontrolled seizures and decerebrate rigidity; children who survive the first few weeks of life usually develop spongy degeneration of the cerebral white matter with increasing paralysis and spasticity. In argininaemia there is some evidence that restriction of dietary arginine may improve the prognosis and various dietary regimes have been introduced in the other varieties, though little practical benefit has yet been observed. Ornithine carbamoyl transferase deficiency is probably the commonest defect and is usually rapidly fatal in male infants; as the disease is X-linked, it is much milder when it occurs in female carriers of the gene and should be considered as a possible cause of recurrent acute encephalopathy, sometimes reminiscent of Reye's disease, in young infants (Kendall, Kingsley, Leonard, Lingam, and Oberholzer 1983).

References

Adams, R. D., and Lyon, G. (1982). *Neurology of hereditary metabolic diseases of children*. Hemisphere Publishing, Washington.

Farriaux, J. -P., Cartigny, B., Dhondt, J.-L., Kint, J., Louis, J., Delattre, P., and Fontaine, G. (1974). A propos d'une observation d'arginino-succinylurie néo-natale. *Acta paediat. belg.* **28**, 193.

Freeman, J. M., Nicholson, J. F., Schimke, R. T., Rowland, L. P., and Carter, S. (1970). Congenital hyperammonemia: association with hyperglycinemia and decreased levels of carbamyl phosphate synthetase. *Arch. Neurol., Chicago* **23**, 430.

Hutchison, H. T. and Diamond, I. (1981). Metabolic disorders. In *Current Neurology* (ed. S. H. Appel), Vol. 3. Chapter 8, John Wiley, New York.

Kendall, B. E., Kingsley, D. P. E., Leonard, J. V., Lingam, S., and Oberholzer, V. G., (1983). Neurological features and computed tomography of the brain in children with ornithine carbamoyl transferase deficiency. *J. Neurol. Neurosurg. Psychiat.*, **46**, 28.

Menkes, J. H. (1980). *Textbook of child neurology*, 2nd edn. Lea and Febiger, Philadephia.

Rosenberg, R.N. and Pettegrew, J. W. (1984). Genetic neurologic diseases, Chapter 2 in *The clinical neurosciences* (ed. R. N. Rosenberg). Churchill-Livingstone, New York.

Amino-acid disorders

Crome and Stern in 1972 tabulated over 100 metabolic disorders, over 30 involving amino-acid metabolism, which may be associated with mental retardation and since then many others have been described. Many of these can only be recognized by means of highly specialized chromatographic techniques applied to the examination of infants' urine (Kalodny and Cable 1982). Ideally, were it not for the many difficulties, such screening tests should be carried out in all new-born infants. In addition, prenatal diagnosis through amniocentesis, allowing selective abortion, is now utilized increasingly in the case of those inborn errors of metabolism or chromosomal abnormalities which can be identified in amniotic cells in culture (Harris 1975). Only some of the commoner and more important conditions will be considered here.

The organic acidaemias

In this group of disorders, the toxic metabolites which accumulate are water-soluble organic acids. In virtually all of them, attacks of acute encephalopathy, resembling those of the Reye syndrome, and usually associated with hyperammonaemia, occur intermittently, often apparently related to sudden increases in these metabolites secondary to dietary intake or increased catabolism (Hutchison and Diamond 1981). Among the commonest are the three ketotic hyperglycinaemias, namely propionic acidaemia, methylmalonic acidaemia, and β-ketothiolase deficiency. These give rise to recurrent episodes of encephalopathy with lethargy, vomiting, and ketoacidosis, usually beginning in the neonatal period. The clinical manifestations are occasionally mild but more often lead to severe brain damage or death in infancy. Non-ketotic hyperglycinaemia, by contrast (Agamanolis, Potter, Kerrick, and Sternberger 1982), which is also called "glycine encephalopathy," produces elevated levels of glycine in urine, serum, CSF, and brain, without ketosis, thrombocytopenia, or neutropenia; although mild cases occur, the condition is often rapidly fatal in infancy. Children who survive show severe mental retardation, lethargy, hypotonia, and scizures with a hypsarrhythmic EEG (Markand, Garg, and Brandt 1982). In milder cases a spinal-cord syndrome with combined upper and lower motor-neurone signs has been described (Bank and Morrow 1972).

Isovaleric acidaemia is an inborn error of leucine metabolism, usually leading to coma within the first week of life. During acute crises of ketoacidosis, the urine and perspiration of affected children smell like sweaty feet; dietary leucine restriction may produce clinical improvement (Hutchison and Diamond 1981). Two other syndromes in which mental retardation is associated with aminoaciduria have been called "the oast-house syndrome" and maple-syrup urine disease. Oast-house disease (Hooft, Timmer-

mans, Snoeck, Antener, Oyaert, and van den Hende 1964) causes convulsions, hypotonia, oedema, and diarrhoea as well as mental retardation and is due to methionine malabsorption. In maple-syrup urine disease, convulsions, vomiting, opisthotonos, and severe retardation occur due to leucinosis (Westall 1964); a variant with valine intoxication has been reported (Hutchison and Diamond 1981). Cases which respond to treatment with thiamine have been described (Scriver, Mackenzie, Clow, and Delvin 1971). Other less common disorders include hydroxymethylglutamyl-coenzyme A lyase deficiency, characterized by acidosis, severe hypoglycaemic episodes, and disordered leucine metabolism (Leonard, Seakins, and Griffin 1979) and glutaric acidaemia which may give dystonia, encephalopathy, and acidosis.

Phenylketonuria

Phenylketonuria, also known as phenylpyruvic oligophrenia, is an autosomal recessive metabolic disorder first described by Folling in 1934. It is characterized by a defect in the hydroxylation of phenylalanine to tyrosine, which leads to the urinary excretion of phenylpyruvic acid. The deficiency is one of liver phenylalanine hydroxylase, which is absent in severe cases and reduced in milder or variant cases which may only become apparent in adult life with mild subnormality. Unless the condition is detected and treated during the first few weeks of life, mental retardation is severe. It has been estimated (Brimblecombe, Blainey, Stoneman, and Wood 1961) that there are about 40 new cases in the United Kingdom every year. The importance of recognizing mild cases is that they may transmit the disease in its more severe form to their children. Even heterozygous parents of severe cases may respond abnormally to a phenylalanine load (Ford and Berman 1977).

The child usually appears normal at birth, but subsequently fails to develop and may suffer from convulsions. Most such children have blonde hair and a fair complexion, and skin changes have been described, often due to diminished skin pigmentation. Mental retardation is usually severe; it is associated with a non-specific clumsiness of gait and movement, and often with stereotyped repetitive movements. The EEG shows "a marked generalized abnormality with poverty of rhythmic activity, excess of large irregular slow waves, and large discharges with variable focal distribution" (Pampiglione 1961).

The presence of phenylpyruvic acid in the urine is demonstrated by adding to the acidified urine a few drops of fresh 5 per cent ferric chloride solution, which produces a deep bluish-green colour. A simple and more reliable paper-strip test is now available (Brimblecome *et al.* 1961). A level of phenylalanine in the serum exceeding 20 mg/100 ml is usually associated with moderate or severe mental retardation, while a figure below that level may be compatible with normal intellectual development, but there are marginal cases in which management presents a difficult problem (*British Medical Journal* 1971).

Treatment consists in putting the child as early as possible on a diet containing a restricted amount of phenylalanine. This was discussed in detail by Brimblecombe *et al.* (1961). Of all 10 cases they reported in which treatment was begun by the age of six weeks, and in which the dietary control of phenylalanine was satisfactory, there was no example of mental deficiency. They also pointed out the dangers of excessive phenylalanine restriction. Fisch, Torres, Gravem, Greenwood, and Anderson (1969), reviewing 12 years of experience, confirmed that affected children treated at an early age had significantly higher developmental and intelligence quotients than those treated later. Berry, O'Grady, Perlmutter, and Bofinger (1979) found that discontinuing the diet reduced achievement.

Hartnup disease

Baron, Dent, Harris, Hart, and Jepson (1956) first described this hereditary metabolic disorder. Milne, Crawford, Girao, and

Loughridge (1960) collected from the literature 11 patients who were members of seven unrelated familites. The disease is inherited as an autosomal recessive trait. It is characterized by renal amino-aciduria and an excessive excretion of indican and indolic acids. The condition is a disorder of cellular transport of monocarboxylic neutral amino acids in the kidney and intestine. At autopsy cerebral atrophy with neuronal cell loss in the cerebral cortex and Purkinje-cell loss in the cerebellum is found (Tahmoush, Alpers, Feigin, Armbrustmacher, and Prensky 1976).

A curious feature of the disorder is the episodic character of the symptoms. The main clinical features are a photosensitive rash typical of pellagra, mental deterioration, and attacks of cerebellar ataxia. The disease occurs in childhood and tends to improve with increasing age, and in some patients the clinical manifestations have been very mild. The rash may respond to nicotinamide therapy and the attacks of ataxia recover spontaneously. It is suggested that the cerebellar ataxia may be due to intoxication by retained indolic acids, in which case alkalinization of the urine by sodium bicarbonate will increase the excretion of indolic acids and provide an easy method of therapy.

Fanconi syndrome

In patients with the Fanconi syndrome of multiple renal tubular defects and aminoaciduria presenting in adult life, the commonest clinical manifestation is hypophosphataemic osteomalacia (Milkman's syndrome) which may respond to treatment with dietary phosphate supplements (Smith, Lindenbaum, and Walton 1976). In such cases severe muscular weakness (osteomalacic myopathy) is common but neurogenic muscular atrophy has been reported (Mallette and Patten 1977).

Other syndromes associated with amino-acid disorders

A number of other syndromes, mostly rare, have been found to be associated with disorders of the metabolism of amino acids. The term *oculo-cerebral dystrophy* (Lowe's syndrome or cerebro-oculorenal syndrome) is characterized by eye changes, such as cataract, enophthalmos and corneal opacities, mental retardation, and amino-aciduria. Other disorders include carnosinaemia with fits and mental retardation due to carnosinase deficiency (Terplan and Cares 1972); homocystinuria with mental retardation, epilepsy, ectopia lentis, and a Marfanoid appearance (Carson and Raine 1971); and many more. Amino-aciduria is also characteristic of Wilson's disease. Abnormalities of myelin development in the amino-acidurias were reviewed by Prensky, Carr, and Moser (1968), and the neuropathological changes in several of these diseases by Martin, van Bogaert, and Guazzi (1968). The disorders now recognized with their clinical and biochemical manifestations are reviewed comprehensively by Crome and Stern (1972) and Menkes (1980).

References

Agamonolis, D. P., Potter, J. L., Kerrick, M. K., and Sternberger, N. H. (1982). The neuropathology of glycine encephalopathy: a report of five cases with immunohistochemical and ultrastructural observations. *Neurology, Minneapolis* **32**, 975.

Bank, W. J., and Morrow, G. (1972). A familial spinal cord disorder with hyperglycinemia. *Arch. Neurol., Chicago* **27**, 136.

Baron, D. N., Dent, C. E., Harris, H., Hart, E. W., and Jepson, J. B. (1956). Hereditary pellagra-like skin rash with temporary cerebellar ataxia, constant renal amino-aciduria, and other bizarre biochemical features. *Lancet* **ii**, 421.

Berry, H. K., O'Grady, D. J., Perlmutter, L. J., and Bofinger, M. K. (1979). Intellectual development and academic achievement in children treated early for phenylketonuria. *Develop. Med. Child Neurol.* **21**, 311.

Brimblecombe, F. S. W., Blainey, J. D., Stoneman, M. E. R., and Wood,

B. S. B. (1961). Dietary and biochemical control of phenylketonuria. *Br. med. J.* **2**, 793.

British Medical Journal (1971). Problems of phenylketonuria. *Br. med. J.* **4**, 695.

Carson, N. A. J. and Raine, D. N. (1971). *Inherited disorders of sulphur metabolism*. Williams & Wilkins, Edinburgh.

Crome, L. C. and Stern, J. (1972). *Pathology of mental retardation*, 2nd edn. Churchill-Livingstone, London.

Farriaux, J. -P., Cartigny, B., Dhondt, J. -L., Kint, J., Louis, J., Delattre, P., and Fontaine, G. (1974). A propos d'une observation d'arginino-succinylurie néo-natale. *Acta paediat. belg.*, **28**, 193.

Fisch, R. O., Torres, F., Gravem, H. J., Greenwood, C. S., and Anderson, J. A. (1969). Twelve years of clinical experience with phenylketonuria. A statistical evaluation of symptoms, growth, mental development, electroencephalographic records, serum phenylalanine levels, and results of dietary management. *Neurology, Minneapolis* **19**, 659.

Fölling, A. (1934). Über Ausscheidung von Phenylbrenztraubensäure in den Harn als Stoffwechselanomalie in Verbindung mit Imbezillaïat. *Z. physiol. Chem.* **227**, 169.

Ford, R. C. and Berman, J. L. (1977). Phenylalanine metabolism and intellectual functioning among carriers of phenylketonuria and hyper-phenylalaninaemia. *Lancet* **i**, 767.

Freeman, J. M., Nicholson, J. F., Schimke, R. T., Rowland, L. P., and Carter, S. (1970). Congenital hyperammonemia: association with hyperglycinemia and decreased levels of carbamyl phosphate synthetase. *Arch. Neurol., Chicago* **23**, 430.

Harris, H. (1975). *Prenatal diagnosis and selective abortion*. Harvard University Press, Cambridge, Massachusetts.

Hooft, C., Timmermans, J., Snoeck, J., Antener, I., Oyaert, W., and van den Hende, C. (1964). Methionine malabsorption in a mentally defective child. *Lancet*, **ii**, 20.

Hutchison, H. T. and Diamond, I. (1981). Metabolic disorders. In *Current neurology* (ed. S. H. Appel) Vol. 3, Chapter 8. John Wiley, New York.

Kolodny, E. H. and Cable, W. J. L., (1982). Inborn errors of metabolism. *Ann. Neurol.* **11**, 221.

Leonard, J. V., Seakins, J. W. T., and Griffin, N. K. (1979). Beta-hydroxy-beta-methylglutaric-aciduria presenting as Reye's syndrome. *Lancet* **i**, 680.

Mallette, L. E. and Patten, B. M. (1977). Neurogenic muscle atrophy and osteomalacia in adult Fanconi syndrome. *Ann. Neurol.* **1**, 131.

Markand, O. N., Garg. B. P., and Brandt. I. K. (1982). Nonketotic hyperglycinemia: electroencephalographic and evoked potential abnormalities. *Neurology, Minneapolis* **32**, 151.

Martin, J. J., van Bogaert, L., and Guazzi, G. C. (1968). Déterminations cérebrales des amino-aciduries. *Confin. neurol.* **30**, 97.

Menkes, J. H. (1980). *Textbook of child neurology*, 2nd edn. Lea and Febiger, Philadelphia.

Milne, M. D., Crawford, M. A., Girao, C. B., and Loughridge, L. W. (1960). The metabolic disorder in Hartnup disease. *Quart. J. Med.*, **29**, 407.

Pampiglione, G. (1961). EEG in inborn errors of metabolism. *Reports at the VII International Congress of Neurology*, Rome, P. 15.

Prensky, A. L., Carr, S., and Moser, H. W. (1968). Development of myelin in inherited disorders of amino acid metabolism. *Arch. Neurol., Chicago* **19**, 552.

Raine, D. N. (1972). Management of inherited metabolic disease. *Br. med. J.* **2**, 329.

Scriver, C. R., Mackenzie, S., Clow, C. L., and Delvin, E. (1971). Rhiamine-responsive maple-syrup-urine disease. *Lancet* **i**, 310.

Smith, R., Lindenbaum, R. H., and Walton, R. J. (1976). Hypophosphataemic osteomalacia and Fanconi syndrome of adult onset with dominant inheritance. *Quart. J. Med.* **45** 387.

Tahmoush, A. J., Alpers, D. H., Feigin, R. D., Armbrustmacher, V., and Prensky, A. L. (1976). Hartnup disease: clinical, pathological, and biochemical observations. *Arch. Neurol., Chicago* **33**, **797**.

Terplan, K. L. and Cares, H. L. (1972). Histopathology of the nervous system in carnosine enzyme deficiency with mental retardation. *Neurology, Minneapolis* **22**, 644.

Westall, R. G. (1964). Dietary treatment of a child with maple syrup urine disease (branched-chain ketoaciduria). In *Neurometabolic disorders in childhood* (ed. K. S. Holt and J. Milner), p. 94. Livingstone, Edinburgh.

The lipidoses (lipid storage diseases)

Many inherited diseases which cause the deposition of abnormal lipid in the central and/or peripheral nervous system and sometimes in other tissues or organs are now recognized. We have recently moved away from a clinical classification of these disorders, towards one based upon the nature of the material which is stored in abnormal amount and/or upon the nature of the enzymatic defect which is responsible. Unfortunately the phenotypical presentation of many different metabolic defects may be very similar, while, on the other hand, apparently identical biochemical defects occasionally produce very different clinical manifestations so that no single classification is uniformly satisfactory. Thus, while Menkes (1980) continues to classify these diseases as disorders of lipid storage, Adams and Lyon (1982) suggest that they should be called the *lysosomal storage diseases* as in most of them a particular lysosomal enzyme is defective or lacking, so that a particular cellular metabolite cannot be degraded and the cell in consequence becomes packed with this substance. However, since the lysosomal storage disorders also include some glycogen storage diseases and the mucopolysaccharidoses, which are diseases of carbohydrate metabolism, the term lipid storage disease is retained here, while appreciating that some of the diseases provisionally classified in this group (Table 15.1) may yet prove not to be truly lipidoses. In fact, as Table 15.1 shows, at least 10 sphingolipid storage diseases are at present recognized. An even more complex tabulation, including additional sub-varieties, is given by Kolodny and Cable (1982). The basic unit of the material stored in cells is a ceramide, a long-chain amino alcohol, sphingosine, linked to a fatty acid of 16–26 carbon atoms. The individual sphingolipids are of four types, *viz.*: sphingomyelin, neutral glycosphingolipids, sulphoglycosphingolipids, and gangliosides (Adams and Lyon 1982). While the gangliosidoses are generally characterized by progressive cerebral degeneration and often by visual loss, in the metachromatic and globoid-cell leucodystrophies there is severe destruction of myelin in the central and peripheral nervous system with relatively little storage in restricted neuronal groups. The lesions of Fabry's disease are largely non-neuronal, while those of Farber's disease involve neurones but also joints and connective tissue.

Infantile amaurotic family idiocy (Tay–Sachs and Sandhoff disease)

Synonyms. Cerebromacular degeneration; Tay–Sachs disease, and Sandhoff's disease.

Definition. Two diseases of early life, often occurring in several members of the same family, characterized pathologically by widespread deposit of gangliosides in the ganglion cells of the brain and retina, and clinically by progressive dementia, blindness, and paralysis.

Pathology

The pathological changes in Tay–Sachs disease (Tay 1881; Sachs 1887) and in Sandhoff's disease (Sandhoff, Andreae, and Jatzkewitz 1968) are identical although in the former ganglioside GM_2 alone accumulates in neurones and in the latter there is also accumulation of globoside. The neurones of the cerebral cortex, the Purkinje cells of the cerebellum, the retinal ganglion cells, and, to a lesser extent, the neurones of the brainstem and spinal cord become ballooned due to the accumulation of lipid, usually with peripheral displacement of the nucleus. Macroscopically the brain is often atrophic with ventricular dilatation and secondary demyelination, sometimes with cavitation of white matter, but paradoxically in the late stages megalencephaly has been des-

Table 15.1. *Classification of the commoner lipid storage and related diseases (modified from White (1973) and Menkes (1980))*

Disease	Lipid accumulated	Enzyme defect
Infantile amaurotic idiocy		
Tay–Sachs disease	Ganglioside GM_2	Hexosaminidase A
Sandhoff's disease	Ganglioside GM_2 plus globoside	Hexosaminidase A and B
Late infantile amaurotic idiocy (Batten–Bielschowsky group)		
Generalized GM_1 gangliosidosis	GM_1 ganglioside	β-galactosidase
Juvenile GM_2 gangliosidosis	GM_2 ganglioside	Hexosaminidase A (partial)
Late infantile form with curvilinear bodies	Ceroid and lipofuscin	Unknown
Juvenile amaurotic idiocy (Spielmeyer–Vogt)	Often ceroid and lipofuscin (in occasional cases GM_2 ganglioside)	Usually unknown (in occasional cases hexosaminidase A—partial)
Neuronal ceroid–lipofuscinosis	Ceroid and lipofuscin	Unknown
Late onset lipidosis (Kufs)	Lipofuscin	Unknown
Niemann–Pick disease, type A	Sphingomyelin	Sphingomyelinase
Gaucher's disease, infantile	Glucocerebroside	Glucocerebrosidase
Gaucher's disease, juvenile	Lactosylceramide, GM_3 ganglioside, and glucocerebroside	Lactosylceramide β–galactosidase
Krabbe's disease	Galactocerebroside	β–galactosidase
Metachromatic leucodystrophy (sulphatide lipidosis)	Sulphatide	Arylsulphatase A
Xanthomatoses		
Hand–Schuller–Christian disease	Cholesterol	Unknown
Farber's disease	Ceramide and gangliosides	Ceramidase
Wolman's disease	Triglyceride and esterified cholesterol	Unknown
Sialidosis, type 1	Sialylated oligosaccharides	α–neuraminidase
Sialidosis, type 2	Sialylated oligosaccharides	α–neuraminidase and β–galactosidase
Fabry's disease	Trihexosyl ceramide	α–galactosidase
Refsum's disease	Phytanic acid	Phytanic acid α–hydroxylase
Pelizaeus–Merzbacher disease	Unknown	Unknown
Alexander's disease	Unknown	Unknown
Canavan–van Bogaert–Bertrand disease	Unknown	Unknown

cribed (Crome and Stern 1972). Electron microscopic examination of affected nerves, dendrites, and some glial cells shows "membranous cytoplasmic bodies" (Terry and Weiss 1963), sometimes called "zebra bodies" because of the typical concentric laminations which they show due to the accumulation of gangliosides in the presence of phospholipids and cholesterol.

Aetiology

Tay–Sachs disease is largely confined to infants of Ashkenazic Jewish ancestry, but Sandhoff's disease occurs in non-Jewish children. Both disorders are of autosomal recessive inheritance; the former is due to hexosaminidase A deficiency, while in the latter hexosaminidase B is also deficient (Suzuki, Jacob, Suzuki, Kutty, and Suzuki 1971). While total deficiency of hexosaminidase A gives Tay–Sachs disease and concomitant deficiency of the B enzyme Sandhoff's disease, partial hexosaminidase A deficiency can cause an adult and much more benign form of Tay–Sachs disease (Kolodny and Cable 1982). Indeed, partial hexosaminidase deficiencies have been found in patients with clinical pictures resembling those of hereditary ataxia, motor-neurone disease, and spinal or peroneal muscular atrophy (Johnson 1981). And in four families with chronic GM$_2$ gangliosidosis and hexosaminidase A deficiency, the clinical picture was strongly suggestive of Friedreich's ataxia (Willner, Grabowski, Gordon, Bender, and Desnick 1981). In another family, two adults with partial enzyme deficiency who presented with proximal muscular weakness in the lower limbs and stammering each had children with severe Tay–Sachs disease (Navon, Argov, Brand, and Sandbank 1981)

Symptoms and signs

The child is usually normal at birth but between three and six months of age listlessness and apathy develop with failure to reach normal developmental milestones. Convulsions subsequently develop in many cases, often with myoclonic jerking in response to "startle". Progressive flaccid paralysis of all four limbs usually develops but in the later stages may be replaced by spasticity and opisthotonos. There is a cherry-red spot at the macula and in early infancy this is almost pathognomonic; atrophy of the optic disc and retina progress rapidly and eventually there is total blindness, but the pupil reactions are often preserved until relatively late. Progressive enlargement of the head occasionally occurs as a late manifestation; the disease is unresponsive to any form of treatment and invariably terminates fatally in the second or third year of life.

Diagnosis

This is generally easy as no other disease causes such a progressive cerebral degeneration in early infancy in the absence of hepatosplenomegaly and with a cherry-red spot at the macula. However, the 'cherry-red spot—myoclonus syndrome' due to sialidosis, type 1 (Thomas, Abrams, Swallow, and Stewart 1979) must also be considered as an alternative, but the latter patients are of normal intelligence, often show cataracts, and generally present later in childhood or even adult life. A similar cherry-red spot may also be seen in some cases of Niemann–Pick and Gaucher's diseases but in these cases it usually appears later and is accompanied by enlargement of the liver and spleen; it is also occasionally found in generalized GM$_1$ gangliosidosis (see below) in which there are also systemic manifestations. Schilder's disease may also cause progressive blindness, dementia, and paralysis in infancy but is of later onset, of variable clinical course, and does not as a rule cause optic atrophy or myoclonus. The EEG in Tay–Sachs disease often shows irregular, generalized spike and wave discharges (Cobb, Martin, and Pampiglione 1952) while in Schilder's disease and other leucodystrophies the changes are non-specific.

An assay of hexosaminidase in the serum will confirm the diagnosis and may also be used to detect heterozygous carriers (Okada and O'Brien 1969). Antenatal diagnosis is possible by measuring the hexosaminidase activity of amniotic cells obtained by amniocentesis (O'Brien, Okada, Chen, and Fillerup 1970).

References

Adams, R. D. and Lyon, G. (1982). *Neurology of hereditary metabolic diseases of children*. Hemisphere Publishing, Washington.

Cobb, W., Martin, F., and Pampiglione, G. (1952). Cerebral lipidosis: an electroencephalographic study. *Brain* **75**, 343.

Crome, L. and Stern, J. (1972). *Pathology of mental retardation*, 2nd edn. Livingstone, Edinburgh.

Greenfield, J. G. and Holmes, G. (1925). The histology of juvenile amaurotic idiocy. *Brain* **48**, 183.

Johnson, W. G. (1981). The clinical spectrum of hexosaminidase deficiency diseases. *Neurology, Minneapolis* **31**, 1453.

Kolodny, E. H. and Cable, W. J. L. (1982). Inborn errors of metabolism. *Ann. Neurol.* **11**, 221.

Menkes, J. H. (1980). *Textbook of child neurology*, 2nd edn. Lea and Febiger, Philadelphia.

Navon, R., Argov, Z., Brand, N., and Sandbank, U. (1981). Adult GM$_2$ gangliosidosis in association with Tay-Sachs disease: a new phenotype, *Neurology, Minneapolis* **31**, 1397.

O'Brien, J. S., Okada, S., Chen, A., and Fillerup, D. L. (1970). Tay-Sachs disease: detection of heterozygotes and homozygotes by serum hexosaminidase assay. *New Engl. J. Med.* **283**, 15.

Okada, S. and O'Brien, J. S. (1969). Tay–Sachs disease: generalized absence of a beta-D-N-acctylhexosaminidase component. *Science* **165**, 698.

Sachs, B. (1887). On arrested cerebral development, with special reference to its cortical pathology. *J. nerv. ment. Dis.* **15**, 541.

Sandhoff, K., Andreae, V., and Jatzkewitz, H. (1968). Deficient hexosaminidase activity in an exceptional case of Tay–Sachs disease with additional storage of kidney globoside in visceral organs. *Life Sci.* **7**, 283.

Suzuki, Y., Jacob, J. C., Suzuki, K., Kutty, K. M., and Suzuki, K. (1971). GM$_2$-gangliosidosis with total hexosaminidase deficiency. *Neurology, Minneapolis* **21**, 313.

Tay, W. (1881). Symmetrical changes in the region of the yellow spot in each eye of an infant. *Trans. ophthal. Soc. UK* **1**, 55.

Terry, R. D. and Weiss, M. (1963). Studies in Tay–Sachs disease: ultrastructure of cerebrum. *J. Neuropath. exp. Neurol.* **22**, 18.

Thomas, P. K., Abrams, J. D., Swallow, d., and Stewart, G. (1979). Sialidosis type 1: cherry red spot-myoclonus syndrome with sialidase deficiency and altered electrophoretic mobilities of some enzymes known to be glycoproteins. *J. Neurol. Neurosurg. Psychiat.* **42**, 873.

White, H. H. (1973). Diseases due to inborn metabolic defects. In *A textbook of neurology* (ed. H. H. Merritt) p. 652. Lea and Febiger, Philadelphia.

Willner, J. P., Grabowski, G. A., Gordon, R. E., Bender, A. N., and Desnick, R. J. (1981). Chronic GM$_2$ gangliosidosis masquerading as atypical Friedreich ataxia: clinical, morphologic, and biochemical studies of nine cases. *Neurology, Minneapolis* **31**, 787.

Late-infantile, juvenile, and late-onset amaurotic idiocy

This group of disorders, previously entitled the cerebromacular or cerebroretinal degenerations, and originally described by Vogt (1905), Spielmeyer (1906), Jansky (1909), Bielschowsky (1914), Batten (1914), and Kufs (1925), among others, is now known to embrace many different disorders, all characterized by a progressive course, all familial and due as a rule to autosomal recessive inheritance, but resulting from a variety of different metabolic abnormalities, some identified comparatively recently and some as yet unknown. As Menkes (1980) points out, some have been identified as independent disease entities solely by ultrastructural studies. Zeman and Dyken (1969) suggested that age of onset alone is an unsafe guide to classification but Adams and Lyon (1982) suggest that it may still be useful to consider early-infantile, late-infantile, childhood (juvenile), and adult forms independently.

Generalized GM$_1$ gangliosidosis

This condition, also called familial neurovisceral lipidosis, occurs in two main forms. Type I (Norman, Urich, Tingey, and Goodbody 1959), also known as pseudoHurler's disease, resembles Hurler's disease clinically in that the affected infants are hypotonic at birth, show severe developmental delay, and usually have large frontal bosses, depressed nasal bones, macroglossia, low-set ears, and generalized skeletal deformities. Hepatosplenomegaly is usually found at about six months of age and a cherry-red spot is present in about 50 per cent of cases. In type II, progressive mental deterioration, often with convulsions, begins at about 8 to 16 months of age and a cherry-red spot is usually present but bony abnormalities are absent and there is no enlargement of the liver or spleen. It is now apparent, too, that chronic GM$_1$ gangliosidosis can present in childhood with relatively benign but progressive dystonia, with only mild intellectual deterioration, and without myoclonus, fits, or cherry-red spots (Goldman, Katz, Rapin, Purpura, and Suzuki 1981; Kobayashi and Suzuki 1981). A similar case has been described in an adult (Longstreth, Daven, Farrell, Bolen, and Bird 1982).

In both varieties the neurones are distended with lipid as in Tay–Sachs disease and membranous cytoplasmic bodies as well as abnormal lysosomal accumulations are usually found ultrastructurally (Suzuki, Suzuki, and Chen 1968; Derry, Fawcett, Andermann, and Wolfe 1968). As in Hurler's disease, β-galactosidase is absent in leukocytes and fibroblasts but unlike the latter condition there is no abnormality of mucopolysaccharides.

Other late-infantile, juvenile, and adult forms
The principal problem in attempting to classify this group of disorders upon any rational basis is that, if one excludes the cases of chronic GM$_1$ and GM$_2$ gangliosidosis described above (Suzuki and Suzuki 1970; Menkes, O'Brien, Okada, Grippo, Andrews, and Cancilla 1971; Adams and Lyon 1982; Kolodny and Cable 1982), the nature of the accumulated lipid in the remaining cases and of the causal enzymatic defect is still unknown. Some, at least, of these conditions clearly belong to the group of neuronal ceroid-lipofuscinoses (see below) but classification remains fluid as long as biochemical uncertainty persists.

In the late-infantile cases (Batten–Bielschowsky) there is no racial predominance, a cherry-red spot at the macula is not usually found, and the affected children are usually normal until two to four years of age. The condition usually begins with myoclonic jerking, sometimes with generalized convulsions, and there is progressive ataxia, paralysis, and retinal degeneration with optic atrophy. Parkinsonian features occasionally appear; in most cases there is eventual spastic paralysis, but progression is slow with death usually occurring in late childhood.

By contrast, the juvenile cases (Spielmeyer–Vogt) usually present with progressive impairment of vision and intellect between six and 14 years of age with retinal pigmentation and optic atrophy and slowly developing spastic paralysis without fits or ataxia. A presentation with progressive dystonia (juvenile dystonic lipidosis) has been described (Elfenbein 1968); this may have been GM$_1$ gangliosidosis (see above).

The adult variety (Kufs' disease) which is rare (Kornfeld 1972) does not usually cause blindness but generally presents with progressive spastic weakness and with epilepsy and/or dementia.

In many disorders within this group, vacuolated lymphocytes or cells sometimes resembling the "sea-blue histiocytes" of Niemann–Pick disease may be found in the peripheral blood. The CSF protein may be slightly raised. In contrast to the usual finding in Tay–Sachs disease, the electroretinogram (ERG) is grossly abnormal or absent and the occipital visual evoked response (VER) is greatly increased in amplitude (Harden, Pampiglione, and Picton-Robinson 1973). The EEG may show the irregular spike and wave discharge previously thought typical of "cerebral lipidosis" (Cobb, Martin, and Pampiglione 1952) with an abnormal response to photic stimulation and is indeed more abnormal in these cases as a rule than in Tay–Sachs disease (Pampiglione and Harden 1973). Visual and sensory evoked potential recording is often helpful in diagnosing GM$_1$ gangliosidosis (Harden, Martinovic, and Pampiglione 1982).

Pathological examination of brain material obtained from such cases shows neuronal swelling less marked than in the gangliosidoses and the material stored is PAS-positive but is not dissolved by the usual lipid solvents. In some cases Zeman and Donahue (1963) found curvilinear cytoplasmic bodies showing a granular or multiloculated appearance on electron microscopy (Andrews, Sorenson, Cancilla, Price, and Menkes 1971). Subsequent histochemical studies (Zeman and Dyken 1969) found that much of the

abnormal material was ceroid and lipofuscin and now many such cases are classified under the inclusive title of neuronal ceroid-lipofuscinosis (Pellissier, Hassoun, Gambarelli, Tripier, Roger, and Toga 1974). Indeed Zeman (1969) suggested that if one excludes the gangliosidoses, all of the conditions in this group represent varying manifestations of this primary pathological change, but this view is not universally accepted. Indeed Carpenter, Karpati, Andermann, Jacob, and Andermann (1977) prefer to call some of the accumulated material granular osmiophilic deposits rather than lipofuscin (see Menkes 1980). However, others have shown that the characteristic cytoplasmic bodies and/or "fingerprint profiles" may be found in skeletal muscle, peripheral nerve, and skin examined ultrastructurally (Carpenter, Karpati, and Andermann 1972; Lyon 1975) and in the appendix (Rapola and Haltia 1973). Certainly this type of pathological change has been discovered frequently in cases of late-infantile amaurotic idiocy (Santavuori, Haltia, Rapola, and Raitta 1973; Haltia, Rapola, Santavuori, and Kaŕanen 1973). Kufs' disease is often now classified as adult ceroid-lipofuscinosis (Vercruyssen, Martin, Ceuterick, Jacobs, and Swerts 1982). Sea-blue histiocytes may be found in bone marrow along with finger-print curvilinear profiles in ultrastructural preparations of cultured fibroblasts, bone-marrow cells, or vacuolated lymphocytes (Miley, Gilbert, France, O'Brien, and Chun 1978; Baumann and Markesbery 1978). Similar neuronal cytoplasmic bodies have been found in the brains of patients with Morquio's syndrome, one of the mucopolysaccharidoses (Gilles and Deuel 1971).

References

Adams, R. D. and Lyon, G. (1982). *Neurology of hereditary metabolic diseases of children*. Hemisphere Publishing, Washington.

Andrews, J. M., Sorenson, V., Cancilla, P. A., Price, H. M., and Menkes, J. H. (1971). Late infantile neurovisceral storage disease with curvilinear bodies. *Neurology, Minneapolis* **21**, 207.

Batten, F. E. (1914). Family cerebral degeneration with macular change (so-called juvenile form of family amaurotic idiocy). *Quart. J. Med.* **7**, 444.

Baumann, R. J. and Markesbery, W. R. (1978). Juvenile amaurotic idiocy (neuronal ceroid lipufuscinosis) and lymphocyte fingerprint profiles. *Ann. Neurol.* **4**, 531.

Bielschowsky, M. (1914). Uber spatinfantile familiare amaurotische Idiotie mit Kleinhirnsymptomen. *Deutsch. Z. Nervenheilk.* **50**, 7.

Carpenter, S., Karpati, G., and Andermann, F. (1972). Specific involvement of muscle, nerve, and skin in late infantile and juvenile amaurotic idiocy. *Neurology, Minneapolis* **22**, 170.

——, ——, ——, Jacob, J. C., and Andermann, E. (1977). The ultrastructural characteristics of the abnormal cytosomes in Batten–Kufs' disease. *Brain* **100**, 137.

Cobb, W., Martin, F., and Pampiglione, G. (1952). Cerebral lipidosis: an electro-encephalographic study *Brain* **75**, 343.

Derry, D. M., Fawcett, J. S., Andermann, F., and Wolfe, L. S. (1968). Late infantile systemic lipidosis. Major monosialogangliosidosis: delineation of two types. *Neurology, Minneapolis* **18**, 340.

Elfenbein, I. B. (1968). Dystonic juvenile idiocy without amaurosis, a new syndrome: light and electron microscopic observations of cerebrum. *Johns Hopk. Med. J.* **123**, 205.

Gilles, F. H. and Deuel, R. K. (1971). Neuronal cytoplasmic globules in the brain in Morquio's syndrome. *Arch. Neurol., Chicago* **25**, 393.

Goldman, J. E., Katz, D., Rapin, I., Purpura, D. P., and Suzuki, K. (1981). Chronic GM$_1$ gangliosidosis presenting as dystonia: I. Clinical and pathological features. *Ann. Neurol.* **9**, 465.

Haltia, M., Rapola, J., Santavuori, P., Keränen, A. (1973). Infantile type of so-called neuronal ceroid-lipofuscinosis. Part 2. Morphological and biochemical studies. *J. neurol. Sci.* **18**, 269.

Harden, A., Martinovic, Z., and Pampiglione, G. (1982). Neurophysiological studies in GM$_1$ gangliosidosis. *Ital. J. neurol. Sci.* **3**, 201.

——, Pampiglione, G., and Picton-Robinson, N. (1973). Electroretinogram and visual evoked response in a form of 'neuronal lipidosis' with diagnostic EEG features. *J. Neurol. Neurosurg. Psychiat.* **36**, 61.

Jansky, J. (1909). Uber einen noch nicht bescriebenen Fall der familiaren amaurotischen idiotie mit Hypoplasie des Kleinhirns. *Z. Erforsch. Behandl. Jugendlich. Schwachsinns* **3**, 86.

Kobayashi, T. and Suzuki, K. (1981). Chronic GM$_1$ gangliosidosis presenting as dystonia: II. Biochemical studies. *Ann. Neurol.* **9**, 476.

Kolodny, E. H. and Cable, W. J. L. (1982). Inborn errors of metabolism. *Ann. Neurol.* **11**, 221.

Kornfell, M. (1972). Generalized lipofuscinosis (generalized Kufs' disease). *J. Neuropath. exp. Neurol.* **31**, 668.

Kufs, M. (1925). Uber eine Spatform der amaurotischen Idiotie und ihre heredofamiliaren Grundlagen *Z. Ges. Neurol. Psychiat.* **95**, 169.

Longstreth, W. T. Jr., Daven, J. R., Farrell, D. F., Bolen, J. W., and Bird, T. D. (1982). Adult dystonic lipidosis: clinical, histologic, and biochemical findings of a neurovisceral storage disease. *Neurology, Minneapolis* **32**, 1295.

Lyons, B. B. (1975). Peripheral nerve involvement in Batten–Spielmeyer–Vogt's disease. *J. Neurol. Neurosurg. Psychiat.* **38**, 175.

Menkes, J. H. (1980). *Textbook of child neurology*, 2nd edn. Lea and Febiger, Philadelphia.

——, O'Brien, J. S., Okada, S., Grippo, J., Andrews, J. M., and Cancilla, P. A. (1971). Juvenile GM$_2$ gangliosidosis, *Arch. Neurol., Chicago* **25**, 14.

Miley, C. E., Gilbert, E. F., France T. D., O'Brien, J. F., and Chun, R. W. M. (1978). Clinical and extraneural histological diagnosis of neuronal ceroid-lipofuscinosis. *Neurology, Minneapolis* **28**, 1008.

Norman, R. M., Urich, H., Tingey, A. H., and Goodbody, R. A. (1959). Tay–Sachs disease with visceral involvement and its relationship to Niemann–Pick disease. *J. Path. Bact.* **78**, 409.

Pampiglione, G. and Harden, A. (1973). Neurophysiological identification of a late infantile form of 'neuronal lipidosis'. *J. Neurol. Neurosurg. Psychiat.* **36**, 68.

Pellissier, J. F., Hassoun, J., Gambarelli, D., Tripier, M. F., Roger, J., and Toga, M. (1974). Céroide-lipofuscinose neuronale. Etude ultrastructurale de deux biopsies cérébrales. *Acta Neuropath., Berlin* **28**, 353.

Rapola, J. and Haltia, M. (1973). Cytoplasmic inclusions in the vermiform appendix and skeletal muscle in two types of so-called neuronal ceroid-lipofuscinosis. *Brain.* **96**, 833.

Santavuori, P., Haltia, M., Rapola, J., and Raitta, C. (1973). Infantile type of so-called neuronal ceroid-lipofuscinosis. Part 1. A clinical study of 15 patients. *J. neurol. Sci.* **18**, 257.

Spielmeyer, W. (1906). Ueber eine besondere Form von familiaere amaurotischen Idiotie. *Neurol. Zbl.* **25**, 51.

Suzuki, K., Suzuki, K., and Chen, G. C. (1968). Morphological, histochemical and biochemical studies on a case of systemic late infantile lipidosis (generalized gangliosidosis). *J. Neuropath. exp. Neurol.* **27**, 15.

Suzuki, Y. and Suzuki K. (1970). Partial deficiency of hexosaminidase component A in juvenile GM$_2$-gangliosidosis. *Neurology, Minneapolis* **20**, 848.

Vercruyssen, A., Martin, J. J., Ceuterick, C., Jacobs, K., and Swerts, L. (1982). Adult ceroid-lipofuscinosis: diagnostic values of biopsies and of neurophysiological manifestations. *J. Neurol. Neurosurg. Psychiat.* **45**, 1056.

Vogt, H. (1905). Ueber familiaere amaurotische Idiotie und verwandte Krankheitsbilder. *Mschr. Psychiat. Neurol* **18**, 161, 310.

Zeman, W. (1969). What is amaurotic idiocy? *Lipids* **4**, 76.

—— and Donahue, S. (1963). Fine structure of the lipid bodies in juvenile amaurotic idiocy *Acta Neuropath.* **3**, 144.

—— and Dyken, P. (1969). Neuronal ceroid-lipofuscinosis (Batten's disease): relationship to amaurotic family idiocy? *Pediatrics* **44**, 570.

Niemann–Pick disease

Described by Niemann in 1914, this disorder, characterized by storage of sphingomyelin in the cells of the reticuloendothelial system and sometimes in the brain, is now known to occur in four distinct forms, all of autosomal recessive inheritance, which have been called types A to D (see Menkes 1980 and Kolodny and Cable 1982). The classical form of the disease (type A) which is the commonest, usually affects Jewish children. Many show a cherry-red spot in the retina, and they develop hepatosplenomegaly and intellectual deterioration, usually in the first years of life, accompanied often by jaundice, anaemia, abdominal enlargement and poor physical development. Myoclonus or generalized seizures are common and progressive spastic paralysis usually develops with death before the age of five years (Frederickson and Sloan 1972). In some cases, supranuclear ophthalmoplegia occurs (Neville, Lake, Stephens, and Sanders 1973). In type B, the viscera are involved but the nervous system is spared, while in type C neurological symptoms do not usually appear until two to four years of age and the clinical course is slower; in type D symptoms of nervous-system involvement do not appear until even later in childhood and the course is slower still.

Pathologically the brain and retina show ballooned ganglion cells with a characteristic vacuolated foamy appearance which contain large amounts of sphingomyelin (Croker 1961; Lynn and Terry 1964). Diagnosis can be made by bone-marrow examination, which often reveals 'sea-blue histiocytes' (Neville *et al.* 1973), by rectal biopsy, or by the assay of sphingomyelinase in leucocytes, in skin or bone-marrow cultures (Kampine, Brady, and Kaufer 1967; Sloan, Uhlendorf, and Kaufer 1969), and prenatally in amniotic-cell cultures in types A and B, but not in types C and D.

References

Crocker, A. C. (1961). The cerebral defect in Tay–Sachs disease and Niemann–Pick disease. *J. Neurochem.* **7**, 69.

Frederickson, D. S. and Sloan, H. R. (1972). Sphingomyelin lipidoses: Niemann–Pick disease. In *The metabolic basis of inherited disease*, 3rd edn (ed. J. B. Stanbury, J. B. Wyngaarden, and D. S. Fredrickson), p. 783. McGraw-Hill, New York.

Kampine, J., Brady, R., and Kanfer, J. (1967). Diagnosis of Gaucher's disease and Niemann–Pick disease with small samples of venous blood. *Science* **155**, 86.

Kolodny, E. H. and Cable, W. J. L. (1982). Inborn errors of metabolism. *Ann. Neurol.* **11**, 221.

Lynn, R. and Terry, R. D. (1964). Lipid histochemistry and electron microscopy in adult Niemann–Pick disease. *Am. J. Med.* **37**, 987.

Menkes, J. H. (1980). *Textbook of child neurology* 2nd edn. Lea and Febiger Philadelphia.

Neville, B. G. R., Lake, B. D., Stephens, R., and Sanders, M. D. (1973). A neurovisceral storage disease with vertical supranuclear ophthalmoplegia and its relationship to Niemann–Pick disease—a report of nine patients. *Brain* **96**, 97.

Niemann, A. (1914). Ein unbekanntes Krankheitsbild. *Jahrb. Kinderheilk.* **79**. 1.

Sloan, H. R., Uhlendore, B. W., and Kanfer, J. N. (1969). Deficiency of sphingomyelin-cleaving enzyme activity in tissue cultures derived from patients with Niemann–Pick disease. *Biochem. Biophys. Res. Commun.* **34**, 582.

Gaucher's disease

This rare disease, first described by Gaucher in 1882, is usually due to an autosomal recessive gene but occasional families show dominant inheritance (Pratt 1967). It is due to the storage of cerebroside in the cells of the reticuloendothelial system and sometimes in the brain, resulting from a deficiency of glucocerebrosidase, but so-called juvenile Gaucher's disease is now regarded by some as GM$_3$ gangliosidosis (Menkes 1980). Adams and Lyon (1982), however, regard the latter view as unproven and simply classify the varieties of later onset as Gaucher's disease types II and III, while indicating that these forms are less precisely defined clinically and pathologically and that typical Gaucher cells may, for instance, be found in some cases of Niemann–Pick disease. In the commonest chronic form there is marked progressive enlargement of the liver and spleen but the nervous system is not involved. In the less common infantile cases (Barlow 1957; Bogaert 1957) there is severe involvement of the brain with progressive apathy, sometimes strabismus, and pseudobulbar palsy with progressive spastic paralysis of the limbs and decerebrate rigidity. Convulsions sometimes occur and the disease is usually fatal before the end of the first year. Radiography of long bones may show areas of rarefaction, particularly in the lower ends of the femora.

Pathologically the characteristic feature in the cells of the spleen, bone marrow, or brain is the presence of large spherical or oval Gaucher cells which show a lacy, striated appearance of the cytoplasm. In the infantile cases the defective enzyme is probably glucosyl ceramide β-glucosidase (Brady, Kanfer, Bradley, Shapiro 1966). The diagnosis may also be made by estimating this enzyme in cultures of leucocytes or skin fibroblasts.

Splenectomy is sometimes performed simply because of the massive splenic enlargement and the risk of rupture in chronic cases but has no influence upon the course of the disease. Improvement in a single case was thought to have followed treatment with lysosome-entrapped glucocerebroside β-glucosidase (Belchetz, Crawley, Braidman, and Gregoriadis 1977).

References

Adams, R. D. and Lyon, G. (1982). *Neurology of hereditary metabolic disease of children*. Hemisphere Publishing, Washington.

Barlow, C. (1957). Neuropathological findings in a case of Gaucher's disease. *J. Neuropath. exp. Neurol.* **16**, 239.

Belchetz, P. E., Crawley, J. C. W., Braidman, I. P., and Gregoriadis, G. (1977). Treatment of Gaucher's disease. *Lancet* ii, 116.

Brady, R. O., Kanfer, J. N., Bradley, R. M., and Shapiro, D. (1966). Demonstration of a deficiency of glucocerebroside-cleaving enzyme in Gaucher's disease. *J. clin. Invest.* **45**, 1112.

Gaucher, P. (1882). *De l'epithelioma primitif de la rate*. Thèse, Paris.

Menkes, J. H. (1980). *Textbook of child neurology*, 2nd edn. Lea and Febiger, Philadelphia.

Pratt, R. T. C. (1967). *The genetics of neurological disorders*. Oxford University Press, London.

van Bogaert, L. (1957). *Cerebral lipidoses*. Thomas, Springfield, Illinois.

Other rare lipid storage diseases

Sialidosis type 1 (or the cherry-red spot–myoclonus syndrome) is the name which has been given to a disorder of adult onset and autosomal recessive inheritance characterized by cherry-red spots and non-pigmentary retinal degeneration, progressive ataxia, intention myoclonus, and visual failure but with normal intelligence (O'Brien 1977, 1978; Rapin, Goldfischer, Katzman, Engel and O'Brien 1978; Thomas, Abrams, Swallow, and Stewart 1979; Swallow, Evans, Stewart, Thomas, and Abrams 1979; Miyatake, Atsumi, Obayashi, Mizuno, Ando, Ariga, Matsui-Nakamura, and Yamada 1979; Federico, Cecio, Apponi Battini, Michalski, Strecker, and Guazzi 1980). Peripheral neuropathy is an occasional manifestation (Steinman, Tharp, Dorfman, Forno, Sogg, Kelts, and O'Brien 1980). These patients have high levels of sialylated oligosaccharides in their urine and a deficiency of sialidase (α-neuraminidase) in their cultured fibroblasts. In sialidosis type 2 (Matsuo, Egawa, Okada, Suetsugu, Yamamoto, and Watanabe 1983), intelligence is again normal, cherry-red spots and myoclonus occur, but unlike type 1 the affected patients show cerebellar ataxia, coarse facies, and vertebral deformities; lymphocytes and bone-barrow cells are vacuolated. β-galactosidase as well as α-neuraminidase is reduced in leucocytes and fibroblasts. Whether "Salla disease", a lysosomal storage disease identified in Finland by Aula, Autio, Raivio, Rapola, Thoden, Koskela, and Yamashina (1979), giving rise to severe mental retardation, coarse facial features, clumsiness, and loss of speech, without a specific identifiable enzyme defect, is an independent disease entity is not yet certain. It appears to be a disorder of sialic-acid metabolism but differs from sialidosis types 1 and 2 (Renlund, Aula, Raivio, Autio, Sainio, Rapola, and Koskela 1983). Another syndrome not yet characterized fully is one giving failure to thrive, retinitis pigmentosa, sensorineural deafness, mental retardation, distal spinal muscular atrophy, hepatosplenomegaly, and adrenocortical deficiency with *reduced arachidonic acid* in the tissues (Dyck, Yao, Knickerbocker, Holman, Gomez, Hayles, and Lambert 1981). It must also be noted that in many *mitochondrial disorders*, which often present primarily as myopathies (see Chapter 19), brain mitochondria may also be abnormal. One such is carnitine acetyltransferase deficiency which may produce a fatal ataxic encephalopathy in early childhood (DiDonato, Rimoldi, Moise, Bertagnoglio, and Uziel 1979). Some such disorders therefore affect both lipid and carbohydrate metabolism.

References

Aula, P., Autio, S., Raivio, K. O., Rapola, J., Thoden, C.-J., Koskela, S.-L., and Yamashina, I. (1979). "Salla disease": a new lysosomal storage disorder. *Arch. Neurol., Chicago* **36**, 88.

DiDonato, S., Rimoldi, M., Moise, A., Bertagnoglio, B., and Uziel, G. (1979). Fatal ataxic encephalopathy and carnitine acetyltransferase deficiency: a functional defect of pyruvate oxidation? *Neurology, Minneapolis* **29**, 1578.

Dyck, P. J., Yao, J. K., Knickerbocker, . E., Holman, R. T., Gomez, M. R., Hayles, A. B., and Lambert, E. H. (1981). Multisystem neuronal degeneration, hepatosplenomegaly and adrenocortical deficiency associated with reduced tissue arachidonic acid. *Neurology, Minneapolis* **31**, 925.

Federico, A., Cecio, A., Apponi Battini, G., Michalski, J. C., Strecker, G., and Guazzi, G. C. (1980). Macular cherry-red spot and myoclonus syndrome: juvenile form of sialidosis, *J. neurol. Sci.*, **48**, 157.

Matsuo, T., Egawa, I., Okada, S., Suetsugu, M., Yamamoto, K., and Watanabe, M. (1983). Sialidosis type 2 in Japan: clinical study in two siblings' cases and review of literature. *J. neurol. Sci.*, **45**, 55.

Miyatake, T., Atsumi, T., Obayashi, T., Mizuno, Y., Ando, S., Ariga, T., Matsui-Nakamura, K., and Yamada, T. (1979). Adult type neuronal storage disease with neuraminidase deficiency. *Ann. Neurol.* **6**, 232.

O'Brien, J. S. (1977). Neuraminidase deficiency in the cherry-red spot myoclonus syndrome. *Biochem. biophys. Res. Commun.* **79**, 1136.

—— (1978). The cherry-red spot myoclonus syndrome: a newly recognised inherited lysosomal storage disease due to acid neuraminidase deficiency *Clin. Genet.* **14**, 55.

Rapin, I., Goldfischer, S., Katzman, R., Engel, J., and O'Brien, J. S. (1978). The cherry-red spot–myoclonus syndrome. *Ann. Neurol.* **3**, 234.

Renlund, M., Aula, P., Raivio, K. O., Autio, S., Sainio, K., Rapola, J., and Koskela, S. -L. (1983). Salla disease: a new lysosomal storage disorder with disturbed sialic acid metabolism. *Neurology, Minneapolis* **33**, 57.

Steinman, L., Tharp, B. R., Dorfman, L. J., Forno, L. S., Sogg, R. L., Kelts, K. A., and O'Brien, J. S. (1980). Peripheral neuropathy in the cherry-red spot–myoclonus syndrome (sialidosis type I). *Ann. Neurol.* **7**, 450.

Swallow, D. M., Evans, L., Stewart, G., Thomas, P. K., and Abrams, J. D. (1979). Sialidosis type 1: cherry red spot–myoclonus syndrome with sialidase deficiency and altered electrophoretic mobility of some enzymes known to be glycoproteins. II. Enzyme studies. *Ann. hum. Genet.* **43**, 27.

Thomas, P. K., Abrams, J. D., Swallow, D., and Stewart, G. (1979). Sialidosis type I: cherry red spot–myoclonus syndrome with sialidase deficiency and altered electrophoretic mobilities of some enzymes known to be glycoproteins. *J. Neurol. Neurosurg. Psychiat.* **42**, 873.

Krabbe's disease

This condition, also called globoid-cell leucodystrophy or galactosylceramide lipidosis (Adams and Lyon 1982), was first delineated by Krabbe in 1916. Galactocerebroside accumulates in the brain and peripheral nerves and sulphatide is reduced, probably due to a deficiency of galactocerebroside β-galactosidase (Austin, Suzuki, Armstrong, Brady, Bachhawat, Schlenker, and Stumpf 1970). It usually begins at four to six months of age with convulsions, restlessness, and irritability followed by progressive rigidity and ultimately bulbar paralysis. Tonic spasms induced by noise or other forms of sensory stimulation are common. Optic atrophy is sometimes seen. Because of the neuropathy the tendon reflexes are usually depressed. The disease is uninfluenced by treatment and is invariably fatal within a few months or years, though rare cases with survival into adult life have been described. The CSF protein is invariably raised and motor and sensory conduction in the peripheral nerves is delayed (Bischoff and Ulrich 1969; Dunn, Lake, Dolman, and Wilson 1969). A similar disorder has been reported in dogs (Roszel, Steinberg, and McGrath 1972).

The characteristic pathological change is one of widespread demyelination of the white matter of the cerebrum, cerebellum, and spinal cord; the brain shows minimal sparing of the subcortical arcuate fibres. Thus the pathological changes are those of a demyelinating disease (see Chapter 11) and not of a neuronal storage disorder. In the demyelinated areas epithelioid cells and large multinuclear, PAS-positive, globoid cells, 20–50 μm in diameter, are seen and may also be found in peripheral nerves (Hogan, Gutmann, and Chou 1969). Ultrastructurally these cells show cytoplasmic inclusions which are tubular in longitudinal section but irregularly crystalloid in transverse section (Suzuki and Grover 1970; Liu 1970; Andrews, Cancilla, Grippo, and Menkes 1971).

References

Adams, R. D. and Lyon, G. (1982), *Neurology of hereditary metabolic diseases of children*, Hemisphere Publishing, Washington.

Andrews, J. M., Cancilla, P. A., Grippo, J., and Menkes, J. H. (1971). Globoid cell leukodystrophy (Krabbe's disease): morphological and biochemical studies. *Neurology, Minneapolis* **21**, 337.

Austin, J., Suzuki, K., Armstrong, D., Brady, R., Bachhawat, B.K., Schlenker, J., and Stumpf, D. (1970). Studies in globoid (Krabbe) leukodystrophy (GLD). V. Controlled enzymic studies in ten human cases. *Arch. Neurol., Chicago* **23**, 502.

Bischoff, A. and Ulrich, J. (1969). Peripheral neuropathy in globoid cell leukodystrophy (Krabbe's disease). Ultrastructural and histochemical findings. *Brain* **92**, 861.

Dunn, H. G., Lake, B. D., Dolman, C. L., and Wilson, J. (1969). The neuropathy of Krabbe's infantile cerebral sclerosis (globoid cell leukodystrophy). *Brain* **92**, 329.

Hogan, G. R., Gutmann, L., and Chou, S. M. (1969). The peripheral neuropathy of Krabbe's (globoid) leukodystrophy. *Neurology, Minneapolis* **19**, 1094.

Krabbe, K. (1916). A new familial, infantile form of diffuse brain sclerosis. *Brain* **39**, 74.

Liu, H. M. (1970). Ultrastructure of globoid leukodystrophy (Krabbe's disease) with reference to the origin of globoid cells. *J. Neuropath. exp. Neurol.* **29**, 441.

Roszel, J. F., Steinberg, S. A., and McGrath, J. T. (1972). Periodic acid-Schiff-positive cells in cerebrospinal fluid of dogs with globoid cell leukodystrophy, *Neurology, Minneapolis* **22**, 738.

Suzuki K. and Grover, W. D. (1970). Krabbe's leukodystrophy (globoid cell leukodystrophy): an ultrastructural study. *Arch. Neurol., Chicago* **22**, 385.

Metachromatic leucodystrophy (sulphatide lipidosis)

This disorder was first described by Greenfield in 1933 and in 1950 Brain and Greenfield identified it as a form of diffuse cerebral sclerosis which they called "late infantile metachromatic leucoencephalopathy with primary degeneration of the interfascicular oligodendroglia." In 1960 Austin showed that it was due to the accumulation of sulphatide (cerebroside sulphate) in neurones but more particularly in myelin and glial cells in the cerebral white matter and peripheral nerves; hence the condition is now classified with the lipidoses. Subsequently he demonstrated a primary deficiency of arylsulphatase A (Austin, Armstrong, and Shearer 1965).

The commonest variety of this autosomal recessive condition is the late infantile, which usually develops in the second or third year of life with progressive difficulty in walking, clumsiness in the upper limbs, occasional strabismus, and later progressive spastic (or flaccid) paralysis, dementia, and bulbar paralysis. Death is usual within six months to four years. Convulsions are uncommon, occurring late if at all, but optic atrophy is not infrequent. The ten-

don reflexes are often lost due to the neuropathy, motor and sensory nerve conduction velocity is usually slowed (Fullerton 1964), and the CSF protein is usually increased.

The juvenile form of the condition (Austin 1965; Menkes 1966) begins between five and seven years of age and progresses slowly. An adult variety is also relatively common (Austin, Armstrong, Fouch, Mitchell, Stumpf, Shearer, and Briner 1968; Betts, Smith, and Kelly 1968; Hirose and Bass 1972) and usually gives a progressive facile euphoric dementia, occasionally with psychotic features, and ultimately with slowly developing signs of corticospinal tract dysfunction and variable evidence of subclinical polyneuropathy. The CT scan is especially useful in diagnosis in late-infantile cases (Buonanno, Ball, Laster, Moody, and McLean 1978).

Pathologically there is diffuse demyelination of the white matter of the brain, spinal cord, and peripheral nerves with loss of oligodendroglia and with the accumulation of metachromatic granules due to the accumulation of sulphatide in neurones and glial cells but more particularly in the demyelinated areas. These granules stain brown rather than blue with stains such as cresyl violet or thionine. Similar metachromatic granules may be found in the renal tubules and may thus be isolated from centrifuged specimens of urine, or found in saliva. At autopsy they are also present in gall bladder, pancreas, and liver. Ultrastructurally they are seen as compact "myelin bodies" in brain or as torpedo-like structures in peripheral nerve (Liu 1968). There are minor ultrastructural differences between infantile, late-infantile, and adult cases (Thomas, King, Kocen, and Brett 1977). Diagnosis was made in the past by examining the urine, by brain, peripheral-nerve, or rectal biopsy (Julius, Buehler, Aylsworth, Petery, Rennert, and Greer 1971), or by measurement or urinary arylsulphatase A (Austin, Armstrong, Shearer, and McAfee 1966; Stumpf and Austin 1971) but the simplest and most reliable test is to estimate the enzyme in leucocytes obtained from venous blood (Percy and Brady 1968). The enzyme deficiency was once thought to be the same in infantile, juvenile, and adult cases, but isoelectric focusing has shown that the enzyme has 6–8 bands of activity and variations in the deficiency are seen in relation to age of onset (Farrell, MacMartin, and Clark 1979). This test is also scessful in identifying heterozygous carriers (Bass, Witmer, and Freifuss 1970) but treatment of the condition with purified arylsulphatase does not produce clinical benefit (Greene, Hug, and Schubert 1969). A rare variant has been described in which the clinical picture is typical of the adult form and urinary sulphatide excretion is raised but *in vitro* activity of arylsulphatase A and B and cerebroside sulphatase activity are normal; nevertheless, there appears to be an unidentified defect of sulphatide hydrolysis *in vivo* (Hahn, Gordon, Feleki, Hinton, and Gilbert 1982). A link with the mucopolysaccharidoses is evident from the finding of arylsulphatase B deficiency in a case of the Maroteaux–Lamy syndrome (Pilz, von Figura, and Goebel 1979, and see p. 467).

References

Austin, J. (1960). Metachromatic form of diffuse sclerosis: III. Significance of sulfatide and other lipid abnormalities in white matter and kidney. *Neurology, Minneapolis* **10**, 470.

—— Armstrong, D., Fouch S., Mitchell, C., Stumpf, D., Shearer, I., and Briner, O. (1968). Metachromatic leukodystrophy (MLD). VIII. MLD in adults: diagnosis and pathogenesis. *Arch. Neurol., Chicago* **18**, 225.

——, ——, and Shearer, L. (1965). Metachromatic form of diffuse cerebral sclerosis. V. The nature and significance of low sulfatase activity: a controlled study of brain, liver and kidney in four patients with metachromatic leukodystrophy (MLD) *Arch. Neurol., Chicago* **13**, 593.

——, ——, ——, and McAfee, D. (1966). Metachromatic form of diffuse cerebral sclerosis. VI. A rapid test for the sulfatase A deficiency in metachromatic leukodystrophy (MLD) urine. *Arch. Neurol., Chicago* **14**, 259.

Bass, N. H., Witmer, E. J., and Dreifuss, F. E. (1970). A pedigree study of metachromatic leukodystrophy. Biochemical identification of the carrier state. *Neurology, Minneapolis* **20**, 52.

Betts, T. A., Smith, W. T., and Kelly, . E. (1968). Adult metachromatic leukodystrophy (sulphatide lipidosis) simulating acute schizophrenia: report of a case. *Neurology, Minneapolis* **18**, 1140.

Brain, W. R. and Greenfield, J. G. (1950). Late infantile metachromatic leucoencephalopathy with primary degeneration of the interfascicular oligodendroglia. *Brain* **73**, 291.

Buonanno, F. S., Ball, M. R., Laster, D. W., Moody, D. M., and McLean, W. T. (1978). Computed tomography in late-infantile metachromatic leukodystrophy. *Ann. Neurol.* **4**, 43.

Farrell, D. F., MacMartin, M. P., and Clark, A. F. (1979). Multiple molecular forms of arylsulfatase A in different forms of metachromatic leukodystrophy (MLD). *Neurology, Minneapolis* **29**, 16.

Fullerton, P. M. (1964). Peripheral nerve conduction in metachromatic leucoencephalopathy (sulphatide lipidosis). *J. Neurol. Psychiat.* **27**, 100.

Greene, H. L., Hug, G., and Schubert, W. K. (1969). Metachromatic leukodystrophy. Treatment with arylsulfatase-A. *Arch. Neurol., Chicago* **20**, 147.

Greenfield, J. G. (1933). A form of progressive cerebral sclerosis in infants associated with primary degeneration of the interfascicular glia. *J. Neurol. Psychopath.* **13**, 289.

Hahn, A. F., Gordon, B. A., Feleki, V., Hinton, G. G., and Gilbert, J. J. (1982). A variant form of metachromatic leukodystrophy without arylsulfatase deficiency. *Ann. Neurol.* **12**, 33.

Hirose, G. and Bass, N. H. (1972). Metachromatic leukodystrophy in the adult. A biochemical study. *Neurology, Minneapolis* **22**, 312.

Julius, R., Buehler, B., Aylsworth, A., Petery, L. S., Rennert, O., and Greer, M. (1971). Diagnostic techniques in metachromatic leukodystrophy. *Neurology, Minneapolis* **21**, 15.

Liu, H. M. (1968). Ultrastructure of central nervous system lesions in metachromatic leukodystrophy with special reference to morphogenesis. *J. Neuropath. exp. Neurol.* **27**, 624.

Menkes, J. H. (1966). Chemical studies of two cerebral biopsies in juvenile metachromatic leukodystrophy: the molecular composition of cerebrosides and sulfatides. *J. Pediat.* **69**, 422.

Percy, A. K., and Brady, R. O. (1968). Metachromatic leukodystrophy: diagnosis with samples of venous blood. *Science* **161**, 594.

Pilz, H., von Figura, K., and Goebel, H. H. (1979). Deficiency of arylsulfatase B in 2 brothers aged 40 and 38 years (Maroteaux–Lamy syndrome, type B). *Ann. Neurol.* **6**, 315.

Stumpf, D. and Austin, J. (1971). Metachromatic leukodystrophy (MLD). IX. Qualitative and quantitative differences in urinary arylsulfatase A in different forms of MLD. *Arch. Neurol., Chicago* **24**, 117.

Thomas, P. K., King, R. H. M., Kocen, R. S., and Brett, E. M. (1977). Comparative ultrastructural observations on peripheral nerve abnormalities in the late infantile, juvenile and late onset forms of metachromatic leukodystrophy. *Acta neuropath., Berlin* **39**, 237.

Xanthomatoses

Hand–Schüller–Christian disease. In this rare disease described by Hand (1893), Schüller (1915), and Christian (1919) there is a massive accumulation of cholesterol in cells of the reticuloendothelial system and in the skull bones. The cholesterol-containing cells show a typical foamy appearance histologically; the liver and spleen are often enlarged and the lymph nodes, lungs, and pleura may be involved. X-rays of the skull and pelvis commonly show extensive areas of rarefaction in membranous bones.

The usual neurological manifestations are diabetes insipidus due to invasion of the pituitary and tuber cinereum by xanthomatous deposits and exophthalmos due to involvement of the orbital tissues. However, plaques of demyelination with foam cells in the brain were described by Davison (1933) and Feigin (1956), and Elian, Barnstein, Matz, Askenasy, and Sandbank (1969) reported an adult male in whom a large dural xanthoma produced signs of an intracranial space-occupying lesion. Diabetes insipidus usually responds to treatment with pitressin but retardation of growth and mental development are common and the disease is ultimately fatal.

Farber's disease. This rare disorder, also called lipogranulomatosis (Farber, Cohen, and Uzman 1957) causes irritability and hoarseness of the cry within the first few weeks of life. Subcutaneous nodules and erythematous swellings develop, usually in relationship to joints, mental and motor retardation are both severe, and the condition is usually fatal before the age of two years. Ceramides and gangliosides accumulate in neurones and glial cells in the central nervous system and in mesenchymal cells in the subcutaneous tissue due to a deficiency of ceramidase (Sugita, Dulaney, and Moser 1972).

Wolman's disease. In 1956 Abramov, Schorr, and Wolman described this rare syndrome which resembles clinically Niemann–Pick disease type A and is also characterized by failure to gain weight, malabsorption, and adrenal insufficiency. There is massive hepatosplenomegaly and adrenal calcification (Wolman, Sterk, Gatt, and Frenkel 1961; Guazzi, Martin, Philippart, Roels, van der Eecken, Vrints, Delbeke, and Hooft 1968). Mental retardation is usual but other neurological manifestations are usually absent. Sudanophilic lipid (triglyceride and free and esterified cholesterol) is stored in the leptomeninges and in liver, spleen, intestine, adrenals, and lymph nodes. Acanthocytosis of red blood cells is common. A defect of acid lipase is responsible.

Cerebrotendinous xanthomatosis. This rare disease (van Bogaert, Scherer, and Epstein 1937; Menkes, Schimschock, and Swanson 1968), due to cholestanol (dihydrocholesterol) deposition in the nervous system, gives rise to cataracts, cerebellar ataxia, and dementia, associated with xanthomas of tendons and in the lungs. It is very slowly progressive and can be diagnosed by estimation of cholestanol in the serum and red cells. The CT scan may show a diffuse reduction in white matter density in the cerebrum and cerebellum. Treatment with the missing bile acid (chenodeoxycholic acid) has given encouraging results (Berginer, Berginer, Salen, Shefer, and Zimmerman 1981).

References

Abramov, A., Schorr, S., and Wolman, M. (1956). Generalized xanthomatosis with calcified adrenals. *Am. J. Dis. Child.* **91**, 282.

Berginer, V. M., Berginer, J., Salen, G., Shefer, S., and Zimmerman, R. D. (1981). Computed tomography in cerebrotendinous xanthomatosis. *Neurology, Minneapolis* **31**, 1463.

Christian, H. A. (1919). Defects in membranous bones, exophthalmos, and diabetes insipidus. *Contr. Med. Biol. Res.* **1**, 390, New York.

Davison, C. (1933). Xanthomatosis and the central nervous system. *Arch. Neurol. Psychiat., Chicago* **30**, 75.

Elian, M., Bornstein, B., Matz, S., Askenasy, H. M., and Sandbank, U. (1969). Neurological manifestations of general xanthomatosis. Hand–Schüller–Christian disease. *Arch. Neurol., Chicago* **21**, 115.

Farber, S., Cohen, J., and Uzman, L. L. (1957). Lipogranulomatosis: a new lipoglycoprotein "storage" disease. *J. Mount Sinai Hosp. N.Y.* **24**, 816.

Feigin, I. (1956). Xanthomatosis of nervous system. *J. Neuropath. Exp. Neurol.* **15**, 400.

Guazzi, G. C., Martin, J. J., Philippart, M., Roels, H., van der Eecken, H., Vrints, L., Delbeke, M. J., and Hooft, C. (1968). Wolman's disease. *Eur. Neurol.* **1**, 334.

Menkes, J. H., Schimschock, J. R., and Swanson, P. D. (1968) Cerebrotendinous xanthomatosis: the storage of cholesterol within the nervous system. *Arch. Neurol., Chicago* **19**, 47.

Schüller, A. (1915). Uber eigenartige Schädeldefekte im Jugendalter. *Fortschr. Röntgenstr.* **23**, 12.

Sugita, M., Dulaney, J. T., and Moser, H. W. (1972). Ceramidase deficiency in Farber's disease (lipogranulomatosis) *Science* **178**, 1100.

van Bogaert, L., Scherer, H. J., and Epstein, E. (1937). *Une forme cerebrale de la cholesterinose generalisée.* Masson, Paris.

Wolman, M., Sterk, V. V., Gatt, S., and Frenkel, M. (1961). Primary familial xanthomatosis with involvement and calcification of the adrenals. *Pediatrics* **28**, 742.

Fabry's disease

This rare disorder (angiokeratoma corporis diffusum) is inherited as an X-linked recessive trait and rarely produces symptoms in heterozygous females (Wise, Wallace, and Jellinek, 1962; Bird and Langunoff 1978). It is due to the deposition of ceramide tri- and di-hexosides in vacuolated foamy cells in smooth, cardiac, and striated muscle, in bone marrow, in reticuloendothelial cells, and in renal glomeruli, resulting from a deficiency of α-galactosidase. In the central nervous system the lipid storage is usually confined to blood-vessel walls, sometimes resulting in thrombosis, but autonomic neurones are sometimes directly involved (Christensen-Kou and Reske-Nielsen 1971). Intradermal nerve fibres show swollen axons, dense lipid inclusions, and degeneration of unmyelinated fibres (Cable, McCluer, Kolodny, and Ullman 1982).

In childhood the presenting feature is usually a punctate rash on the face, buttocks, and genitalia, and fever, abdominal and joint pain as well as weight loss are common. Painful paraesthesiae in the extremities are also common as well as excruciating episodes of abdominal, chest, and muscle pain which may be relieved by diphenylhydantoin (Lockman, Hunninghake, Krivit, and Desnick 1973); the pain is probably due to involvement of both dorsal-root ganglion cells (Kahn 1973) and peripheral nerves (Kocen and Thomas 1970). Corneal opacities may be found on slit-lamp examination. Hypertension and episodes of cerebral infarction or haemorrhage are not uncommon when the condition presents first in adult life. The disease is progressive and is uninfluenced by treatment including intravenous infusion of purified α-galactosidase (Mapes, Anderson, and Sweeley 1970). Death is usually due to renal failure.

The diagnosis can be made by renal biopsy or by the demonstration of specific crystalline inclusions on electron microscopy of skin fibroblasts grown in tissue culture (McLean and Stewart 1974). Motor and sensory conduction in peripheral nerves is often slowed (Sheth and Swick 1980) and this method, as well as the examination of urinary sediment for glycolipids (Cable *et al.* 1982) may be helpful in identifying female heterozygous carriers; α-galactosidase activity in carriers overlaps the norml range.

References

Bird, T. D. and Langunoff, D. (1978). Neurological manifestations of Fabry disease in female carriers. *Ann. Neurol.* **4**, 537.

Cable, W. J. L., McCluer, R. H., Kolodny, E. H., and Ullman, M. D. (1982). Fabry disease: detection of heterozygotes by examination of glycolipids in urinary sediment. *Neurology, Minneapolis* **32**, 1139.

Christensen-Lou, H. O. and Reske-Nielsen, E. (1971). The central nervous system in Fabry's disease. A clinical, pathological and biochemical investigation. *Arch. Neurol., Chicago* **25**, 351.

Kahn, P. (1973). Anderson–Fabry disease: a histopathological study of three cases with observations on the mechanism of production of pain. *J. Neurol. Neurosurg. Psychiat.* **36**, 1053.

Kocen, R. S. and Thomas P. K. (1970). Peripheral nerve involvement in Fabry's disease. *Arch. Neurol., Chicago* **22**, 81.

Lockman, L. A., Hunninghake, D. B., Krivit, W., and Desnick, R. J. (1973). Relief of pain of Fabry's disease by diphenylhydantoin. *Neurology, Minneapolis* **23**, 871.

Mapes, C. A., Anderson, R. L., and Sweeley, C. C. (1970). Enzyme replacement in Fabry's disease: an inborn error of metabolism. *Science* **169**, 987.

McLean, J., and Stewart, G. (1974). Fabry's disease; specific inclusions found on electron microscopy of fibroblast cultures. *J. med. Genet.* **11**, 133.

Sheth, K. J. and Swick, H. M. (1980). Peripheral nerve conduction in Fabry disease. *Ann. Neurol.* **7**, 319.

Wise, D., Wallace, H. J., and Jellinek, E. H. (1962). Angiokeratoma corporis diffusum. *Quart. J. Med.* **31**, 177.

Refsum's disease (heredopathia atactica polyneuritiformis)

This progressive degenerative disorder of the nervous system was described in 1946 by Refsum in two families; the affected individuals showed retinal pigmentation, nerve deafness, ataxia, muscular atrophy, and other evidence of peripheral neuropathy. Cammermeyer in 1956 showed that lipid was deposited in neurones and in macrophages in areas of central and peripheral demyelination, and in 1965 Richterich, van Mechelen, and Rossi showed that the lipid which accumulated was 3,7,11,15–tetramethyl hexadecanoic acid (phytanic acid) due to a block in the alpha-oxidation of phytanic to pristanic acid. The enzyme, phytanic acid α-hydroxylase is absent; this is normally responsible for β-hydroxylation and decarboxylation. In such patients, however, a daily intake of less than 10 mg phytanic acid can be handled by ω-oxidation (Billimoria, Clemens, Gibberd, and Whitelaw 1982). The condition is due to an autosomal recessive gene; it usually begins between the ages of four and seven years with symptoms and signs of a polyneuropathy followed by visual deterioration and ataxia. The eyes show optic atrophy and retinal pigmention without the vascular changes of true retinitis pigmentosa. Less constant features are fixed pupils, nerve deafness, ichthyosis, cataracts, bony abnormalities, and a cardiomyopathy wih prolongation of the QT segment and QRS complex in the electrocardiogram. The peripheral nerves often become hypertrophied and show 'onion-bulb' formation.

The CSF protein is usually raised to between 1.0 and 6.0 g/l and the serum phytanic acid (normal 2.0 mg/l) is raised to 0.1—0.5 g/l. Motor and sensory nerve conduction in peripheral nerves is markedly slowed. Nerve biopsy is sometimes used to confirm the diagnosis.

The condition runs an indolent course with slow deterioration over many years. A diet devoid of phytol (a derivative of chlorophyll which is a phytanic acid precursor) has been shown to produce striking improvement (Eldjarn, Try, Stokke, Munthe-Kaas, Refsum, Steinberg, Auigun, and Mize 1966; Steinberg, Mize, Herndon, Fales, Engel, and Vroom 1970; Lundberg, Lilja, Lundberg, and Try 1972; Eldjarn, Stokke, and Try 1976; Refsum 1979). Butter and animal fat restriction is particularly important (Refsum 1981). Plasmapheresis is helpful in removing phytanic acid from the circulation in some cases (Billimoria *et al.* 1982).

References

Billimoria, J. D., Clemens, M. E., Gibberd, F., and Whitelaw, M. N. (1982). Metabolism of phytanic acid and Refsum's disease. *Lancet* i, 194.

Cammermeyer, J. (1956). Neuropathological changes in hereditary neuropathies; manifestations of the syndrome heredopathia atactica polyneuritiformis in the presence of interstitial hypertrophic polyneuropathy. *J. Neuropath. exp. Neurol* **15**, 340.

Eldjarn, L., Stokke, O., and Try, K. (1976). Biochemical aspects of Refsum's disease and principles for the dietary treatment. In *Handbook of clinical neurology* (ed. P. J. Vinken and G. W. Bruyn) Vol. 27, Chapter 23. North-Holland, Amsterdam.

—— Try, K., Stokke, O., Munthe-Kaas, A. W., Refsum, S., Steinberg, D., Auigun, J., and Mize, C. (1966). Dietary effects on serum phytanic-acid levels and on clinical manifestations in heredopathia atactica polyneuritiformis. *Lancet* i, 691.

Lundberg, A., Lilja, L. G., Lundberg, P. O., and Try, K. (1972). Heredopathia atactica polyneuritiformis (Refsum's disease): experience of dietary treatment and plasmapheresis. *Eur. Neurol.* **8**, 309.

Refsum, S. (1946). Heredopathia atactica polyneuritiformis. *Acta psychiat. Kbh.* Suppl. 38.

—— (1979). Heredopathia atactica polyneuritiformis—phytanic acid storage disease. Therapeutic and pathogenetic aspects. In *Peroneal atrophies and related disorders* (ed. G. Serratrice and H. Roux) p. 277. Masson, Paris.

—— (1981). Heredopathia atactica polyneuritiformis. Phytanic-acid storage disease, Refsum's disease: a biochemically well-defined disease with a specific dietary treatment. *Arch. Neurol., Chicago* **38**, 605.

Richterich, R., Van Mechelen, D., and Rossi, E. (1965). Refsum's disease. An inborn error of lipid metabolism with storage of 3,7,11,15–tetramethyl hexadecanoic acid. *Am. J. Med.* **39**, 230.

Steinberg, D., Mize, C. E., Herndon, J. H., Fales, H. M., Engel, W. K., and Vroom, F. Q. (1970). Phytanic acid in patients with Refsum's syndrome and response to dietary treatment. *Arch. intern. Med.* **125**, 75.

Pelizaeus–Merzbacher disease

This rare demyelinating disorder first described by Pelizaeus (1885) and Merzbacher (1910) usually presents before three months of age as an X-linked recessive disorder with jerky head movements, disorganized eye movements, and irregular nystagmus followed by the gradual development of cerebellar ataxia, involuntary movements, and ultimately spasticity in all four limbs (Tyler 1958). The CSF is normal and the diagnosis is rarely made during life. There is a less common form of the disease of later onset and dominant inheritance (Camp and Lowenberg, De Meyer, and Falls 1941; Zeman 1964), and an atypical family with late onset and probable autosomal recessive inheritance has been described (Fahmy, Carter, Paulson, and Nance 1969). Pathologically there is patchy demyelination of cerebral white matter, often in perivascular distribution, with accumulation of sphingomyelin but not of cholesterol esters. Seitelberger (1970) postulated a disorder of glycerophosphatide metabolism but the pathogenesis and biochemical basis of the condition are both unknown. The EEG is abnormal with disordered REM sleep activity (Niakan, Belluomini, Lemmi, Summitt, and Ch'ien 1979) and visual, auditory, and somatosensory evoked potential recordings also assist diagnosis (Wilkus and Farrell 1976; Adams and Lyon 1982).

References

Adams, R. D. and Lyon, G. (1982). *Neurology of hereditary metabolic diseases of children*. Hemisphere Publishing, Washington.

Camp, C. D. and Lowenberg, K. (1941). An American family with Pelizaeus-Merzbacher disease. *Arch. Neurol. Psychiat., Chicago* **45**, 261.

Fahmy, A., Carter, T., Paulson, G., and Nance, W. E. (1969). A 'new' form of hereditary cerebral sclerosis. *Arch. Neurol., Chicago* **20**, 468.

Merzbacher, L. (1910). Eine eigenartige familiär-hereditäre Erkrankungsform. *Z. Ges. Neurol. Psychiat.* **3**, 1.

Niakan, E., Belluomini, J., Lemmi, H., Summitt, R. L., and Ch'ien, L. (1979). Disturbances of rapid-eye-movement sleep in 3 brothers with Pelizaeus–Merzbacher disease. *Ann. Neurol.* 6, 253.

Pelizaeus, F. (1885). Ueber eine eigentümliche Form spastischer Lähmung mit Cerebralerscheinungen auf hereditärer Grundlage. *Arch. Psychiat. Nervenkr.* **16**, 698.

Seitelberger, F. (1970). Pelizaeus–Merzbacher's disease. In *Handbook of clinical neurology* (ed. P. J. Vinken and G. Bruyn) Vol. 10, p. 151. North Holland, Amsterdam.

Tyler, H. R. (1958). Pelizaeus–Merzbacher disease. *Arch. Neurol. Psychiat., Chicago* **80**, 162.

Wilkus, R. J. and Farrell, D. F. (1976). Electrophysiologic observations in the classical form of Pelizaeus–Merzbacher disease. *Neurology, Minneapolis* **26, 1042.**

Zeman, W., DeMyer, W., and Falls, H. F. (1964). Pelizaeus–Merzbacher's disease: a study in nosology. *J. Neuropath. exp. Neurol.* **23**, 334.

Alexander's disease

In 1949, Alexander reported a degenerative neurological disorder in an infant characterized by mental retardation and progressive megalencephaly. Pathologically the condition is characterized by eosinophilic hyaline bodies (Rosenthal fibres) deposited in subpial and perivascular bands distributed randomly throughout the cerebral white matter (Schochet, Lampert, and Earle 1968; Russo, Aron, and Anderson 1976). On electron microscopy these bodies consist of granular osmophilic masses resulting from the conglutination of altered glial filaments. An onset in adult life has been described (Seil, Schochet, and Earle 1968) though the condition usually begins in infancy or early childhood. It has also been called hyaline panneuropathy or dysmyelinogenic leucodystrophy. It may be genetically determined; though spasticity and seizures are common, there is no consistent clinical picture but death is usual in the second or third year (Adams and Lyon 1982).

References

Adams, R. D. and Lyon, G. (1982). *Neurology of hereditary metabolic diseases of children*. Hemisphere Publishing, Washington.

Alexander, W. S. (1949). Progressive fibrinoid degeneration of fibrillary astrocytes associated with mental retardation in a hydrocephalic infant. *Brain* **72**, 373.

Russo, L. S. Jr., Aron, A., and Anderson, P. J. (1976). Alexander's disease: a report and reappraisal. *Neurology, Minneapolis* **26**, 607.

Schochet, S. S., Lampert, P. W., and Earle, K. M. (1968). Alexander's disease: a case report with electron microscopic observations. *Neurology, Minneapolis* **18**, 543.

Seil, F. J., Schochet, S. S., and Earle, K. M. (1968). Alexander's disease in an adult: report of a case. *Arch. Neurol., Chicago* **19**, 494.

Canavan's diffuse sclerosis (van Bogaert–Bertrand)

Canavan in 1931 described a rare degenerative disorder of early infancy, probably of autosomal recessive inheritance, characterized by progressive mental deterioration, megalencephaly, and optic atrophy. van Bogaert and Bertrand (1949) noted the occurrence of the disorder in Jewish families and pointed out that many patients became totally blind and also showed bilateral spastic weakness. Pathologically the condition is characterized by spongy degeneration of the brain with vacuolation in the deeper layers of the cerebral cortex and subjacent white matter; there is also total myelin loss in the white matter of the cerebral and cerebellar hemispheres with relative preservation of neurones and axons and ballooning of astrocytes (Kamoshita, Reed, and Aguilar 1967; Kamoshita, Rapin, Suzuki, and Suzuki 1968). Most affected children die before the age of two years. The pathogenesis is unknown although lysosomal enzyme activity is increased in skin fibroblasts cultured from such cases (Milunsky, Kanfer, Spielvogel, and Shahood 1972). The CSF is usually normal. Menkes (1980) suggests that mitochondrial dysfunction may lead to chronic cerebral oedema which is a feature of such cases; the condition should probably be classified as a dysmyelinating disorder but its pathogenesis is still unknown.

References

Canavan, M. M. (1931). Schilder's encephalitis periaxalis diffusa. *Acta Neurol. Psychiat., Chicago* **25**, 299.

Kamoshita, S., Rapin, I., Suzuki, K., and Suzuki, K. (1968). Spongy degeneration of the brain: a chemical study of two cases including isolation and characterization of myelin. *Neurology, Minneapolis* **18**, 975.

——, Reed, G. B., and Aguilar, M. J. (1967). Axonal dystrophy in a case of Canavan's spongy degeneration. *Neurology, Minneapolis* **17**, 895.

Menkes, J. H. (1980). *Textbook of child neurology*, 2nd edn. Lea and Febiger, Philadelphia.

Milunsky, A., Kanfer, J. N., Spielvogel, C., and Shahood, J. M. (1972). Elevated lysosomal enzyme activities in Canavan's disease. *Pediat. Res.* **6**, 425.

van Bogaert, L. and Bertrand, L. (1949). Sur une idiotie familiale avec dégénérescence spongieuse du nevraxe. *Acta neurol. belg.* **49**, 572.

Cockayne's syndrome

This rare disorder (Cockayne 1936, 1946; Rowlatt 1969) of recessive inheritance but unknown aetiology gives mental and physical retardation beginning usually after the first year of life. Clinically it causes microcephaly, dwarfism, a so-called 'bird facies', retinal pigmentation, deafness, large hands and feet, and a thick skull vault and small pituitary fossa as well as mental retardation. Pathologically there is extensive hypomyelination, demyelination, and atrophy of cerebral, cerebellar, brain-stem, and spinal-cord white matter with calcification of the cortex and basal ganglia. Peripheral neuropathy is an occasional manifestation (Moosa and Dubowitz 1970). Rarely the onset is later and one patient aged 25 years had a successful pregnancy (Kennedy, Rowe, and Kepes 1980).

References

Cockayne, E. A. (1936). Dwarfism with retinal atrophy and deafness. *Arch. Dis. Child.* **11**, 1.
——, (1946). Dwarfism with retinal atrophy and deafness. *Arch. Dis. Child.* **21**, 52.
Kennedy, R. M., Rowe, V. D., and Kepes, J. J. (1980). Cockayne syndrome: an atypical case. *Neurology, Minneapolis* **30**, 1268.
Moosa, A. and Dubowitz, V. (1970). Peripheral neuropathy in Cockayne's syndrome. *Arch. Dis. Child.* **45**, 674.
Rowlatt, U. (1969). Cockayne's syndrome: report of a case with necropsy findings. *Acta Neuropath., Berlin* **14**, 52.

Chediak–Hegashi syndrome

Chediak (1952) described this syndrome characterized by partial albinism, hepatosplenomegaly, lymphadenopathy, mental retardation, and cerebellar degeneration with nystagmus. Peripheral neuropathy is often present (Donohue and Bain 1957; Sheramata, Kott, and Cyr 1971; Adams and Lyon 1982); the polymorphonuclear leucocytes show peroxidase-positive granules and cytoplasmic inclusions are found in neurones as well as perivascular cellular infiltration in pons, cerebellum, and peripheral nerves.

References

Adams, R. D. and Lyon, G. (1982). *Neurology of hereditary metabolic diseases of children.* Hemisphere Publishing, Washington.
Chediak, M. (1952. Nouvelle anomalie leucocytaire de caractère constitutionnel et familial. *Rev. Hemat.* **7**, 362.
Donohue, W. L. and Bain, H. W. (1957). Chediak–Higashi syndrome. *Pediatrics* **20**, 416.
Sheramata, W., Kott, S., and Cyr, D. P. (1971). The Chediak–Higashi–Steinbrinck syndrome. *Arch. Neurol., Chicago* **25**, 289.

Disorders of serum lipoproteins

A-beta-lipoproteinaemia (the Bassen–Kornzweig syndrome)

This autosomal recessive condition, first described by Bassen and Kornzweig in 1950, presents in childhood, usually between the ages of two and 16 years, with atypical retinitis pigmentosa, progressive cerebellar ataxia, mental retardation, peripheral neuropathy, and steatorrhoea. The red blood cells show a typical 'thorny' malformation (acanthocytosis) and the serum levels of cholesterol, carotenoids, vitamin A, and phospholipids are invariably depressed, with absence of the β-lipoprotein moiety. Acanthocytosis is not, however, absolutely specific for this syndrome, having been reported in patients with normal serum lipoproteins, including some with anaemia and cirrhosis (Menkes 1980) and others with various neurological manifestations including Hallervorden–Spatz disease, and adults with mental retardation, extrapyramidal manifestations, and areflexia (Critchley, Clark, and

Wickler 1968). Indeed a specific recessive disorder called *choreaacanthocytosis*, sometimes associated with spinal muscular atrophy, has been defined (Ohnishi, Sato, Nagara, Sakai, Iwashita, Kuroiwa, Nakamura, and Shida 1981; Yamamoto, Hirose, Shimazaki, Takado, Koseogawa, and Saeki 1982). Pathologically there is demyelination of the spinocerebellar tracts and posterior columns and neuronal loss in the cerebral cortex and anterior horns of the spinal cord (Sobrevilla, Goodman, and Kane 1964). The steatorrhoea may improve on a low-fat diet but the neurological disorder was in the past progressive and ultimately fatal. However, there is now evidence that early treatment with vitamin E may prevent or delay the development of neurological manifestations, while in patients with established disease this remedy can arrest or reverse the manifestations of neuropathy (Muller, Lloyd, and Wolff 1983).

Hypo-alpha-lipoproteinaemia (Tangier disease)

This rare autosomal recessive disorder usually gives rise to peripheral neuropathy and retinitis pigmentosa (Engel, Dorman, Levy, and Frederickson 1967). The neuropathy may be progressive or recurrent with loss of both myelin sheaths and axons (Bradley 1981). There is almost total absence of high-density plasma lipoproteins; the liver, spleen, lymph nodes, and tonsils are usually enlarged and demonstrate storage of cholesterol esters.

References

Bassen, F. A. and Kornzweig, A. L. (1950). Malformation of erythrocytes in a case of atypical retinitis pigmentosa. *Blood* **5**, 381.
Bradley, W. G. (1981). The neuropathies. In *Disorders of Voluntary Muscle* (ed. J. N. Walton) 4th edn, p. 753. Churchill-Livingstone, Edinburgh.
Critchley, E. M. R., Clark, D. B., and Wikler, A. (1968). Acanthocytosis and neurological disorder without beta-lipoproteinemia. *Arch. Neurol., Chicago* **18**, 134.
Engel, W. K., Dorman, D. D., Levy, R. I., and Frederickson, D. S. (1967). Neuropathy in Tangier disease. *Arch. Neurol., Chicago* **17**, 1.
Menkes, J. H. (1980). *Textbook of child neurology*, 2nd edn. Lea and Febiger, Philadelphia.
Muller, D. P. R., Lloyd, J. K., and Wolff, O. H. (1983). Vitamin E and neurological function. *Lancet* **i**, 225.
Ohnishi, A., Sato, Y., Nagara, H., Sakai, T., Iwashita, H., Kuroiwa, Y., Nakamura, T., and Shida, K. (1981). Neurogenic muscular atrophy and low density of large myelinated fibres of sural nerve in chorea-acanthocytosis. *J. Neurol. Neurosurg. Psychiat.* **44**, 645.
Sobrevilla, L. A., Goodman, M. L., and Kane, C. A. (1964). Demyelinating central nervous system disease, muscular atrophy, and acanthocytosis (Bassen-Kornzweig syndrome). *Am. J. Med.* **37**, 821.
Yamamoto, T., Hirose, G., Shimazaki, K., Takado, S., Koseogawa, H., and Saeki, M. (1982). Movement disorders of familial neuroacanthocytosis syndrome. *Arch. Neurol., Chicago* **39**, 298.

Disorders of purine metabolism

Hyperuricaemia (the Lesch–Nyhan syndrome)

Catel and Schmidt (1959) first described severe choreoathetosis and spasticity in childhood with hyperuricaemia, and in 1964 Lesch and Nyhan defined the usual neurological characteristics of this rare X-linked disorder which is thus confined to males. The affected boys usually show mild-to-moderate mental retardation and choreoathetosis or dystonia which usually begins in the second year of life; this may be followed by the development of spasticity in all four limbs, but this is not invariable (Watts, Spellacy, Gibbs, Allsop, McKevan, and Slavin 1982). A typical but unexplained feature is self-mutilation with biting of the tongue, lips, and fingers leading to progressive destruction unless the fingers, in particular, are protected. Renal calculi and haematuria ultimately develop and most patients die from renal failure.

The serum uric acid is usually raised and the urinary uric acid: creatine ratio is greater than two (Berman, Balis, and Dancis 1968). The condition is due to a deficiency of hypoxanthine-guanine phosphoribosyl transferase (Seegmiller, Rosenbloom, and Kelley 1967), a defect which can be identified in fibroblasts in culture. Identification of this enzymatic abnormality can be used for the identification of heterozygous female carriers (Migeon, der Kaloustian, and Nyhan 1968; McKeran, Andrews, Howell, Gibbs, Chinn, and Watts 1975) and for antenatal diagnosis in amniotic-cell cultures. Allopurinol may reduce the serum uric acid and may delay the development of renal failure but has little or no effect upon the neurological manifestations which have not been explained neuropathologically (Sass, Itabashi, and Dexter 1965; Berman, Balis, and Dancis 1969; Menkes 1980). The CT scan is normal (Watts *et al.* 1982). While treatment with 5-hydroxytryptophan was thought in one trial to improve the choreoathetosis (Frith, Johnstone, Joseph, Powell, and Watts 1976), more recent observations suggest that neither this drug nor phenothiazines, pimozide or carbidopa are of significant benefit (Watts *et al.* 1982).

References

Berman, P. H., Balis, M. E., and Dancis, J. (1968). Diagnostic test for congenital hyperuricemia with central nervous system dysfunction. *J. Lab. clin. Med.* **71**, 247.

——, ——, and —— (1969). Congenital hyperuricemia. *Arch. Neurol., Chicago* **20**, 44.

Catel, W. and Schmidt, J. (1959). Über familiäre gichtische Diathese in Verbindung mit zerebalen und renalen Symptomen bei einen Kleinkind. *Deutsche Med. Wschr.* **84**, 2145.

Frith, C. D., Johnstone, E. C., Joseph, M. H., Powell, R. J., and Watts, R. W. E. (1976). Double-blind clinical trial of 5-hydroxytryptophan in a case of Lesch-Nyhan syndrome. *J. Neurol. Neurosurg. Psychiat.* **39**, 656.

Lesch, M. and Nyhan, W. L. (1964). A familial disorder of uric acid metabolism and central nervous sytem function. *Am. J. Med.* **36**, 561.

McKeran, R. O., Andrews, T. M., Howell, A., Gibbs, D. A., Chinn, S., and Watts, R. W. E. (1975). The diagnosis of the carrier state for the Lesch-Nyhan syndrome. *Quart. J. Med.* **44**, 189.

Menkes, J. H. (1980). *Textbook of child neurology*, 2nd edn. Lea and Febiger, Philadelphia.

Migeon, B. R., der Kaloustian, V. M., and Nyhan, W. L. (1968). X-linked hypoxanthine-guanine phosphoribosyl transferase deficiency: heterozygote has two clonal populations. *Science* **160**, 425.

Sass, J. K., Itabashi, H. H., and Dexter, R. A. (1965). Juvenile gout with brain involvement. *Arch. Neurol., Chicago* **13**, 639.

Seegmiller, J. E., Rosenbloom, F. M., and Kelley, W. N. (1967). Enzyme defect associated with a sex-linked human neurological disorder and excessive purine synthesis. *Science* **155**, 1682.

Watts, R. W. E., Spellacy, E., Gibbs, D. A., Allsop, J., McKeran, R. O., and Slavin, G. E. (1982). Clinical, post-mortem, biochemical and therapeutic observations on the Lesch–Nyhan syndrome with particular reference to the neurological manifestations. *Quart. J. Med.* **51**, 43.

Disorders of carbohydrate metabolism

Glycogen storage disease

Of all the many disorders of glycogen storage which have been described, only one, namely Pompe's glycogenosis (Cori type II—Cori, 1952–3), a disorder of autosomal recessive inheritance due to amylo-1, 4-glucosidase (acid maltase) deficiency, affects the central nervous system directly, although seizures due to hypoglycaemia often occur in the other varieties and focal neurological signs of undetermined cause are rarely seen in type I glycogenosis (von Gierke's disease) (Menkes 1980). In addition, marked glycogen accumulation in the brain may occur in the *cerebro-hepato-renal syndrome*, a disorder of autosomal recessive inheritance but unknown pathogenesis, which is characterized by cranio-facial dysmorphia, generalized hypotonia, renal cysts, and hepatic and skeletal abnormalities (Agamanolis and Patre 1979). Usually the condition presents shortly after birth with generalized muscular weakness, hypotonia, and cardiomegaly. At autopsy there is evidence of diffuse glycogen storage in the neurones of the cerebral cortex and spinal cord (Crome, Cummings, and Duckett 1963) but the muscular and cardiac involvement predominate and the condition is usually fatal within the first few months of life. Lysosomal and free cytoplasmic glycogen may be found in a biopsy of sural nerve (Goebel, Lenard, Kohlschütter, and Pilz 1977). An identical enzymatic defect may cause an acquired myopathy first developing in late childhood, adolescence, or even adult life (see p. 576).

Glycoprotein storage (polyglucosan body disease)

It has long been known that the Lafora bodies found in the brain of patients with progressive myoclonic epilepsy (p. 632) contain glycoprotein, and it is now evident that this material, found also in corpora amylacea, is largely made up of glucose polymers or polyglucosans. Robitaille, Carpenter, Karpati, and Di Mauro (1980) have shown that these polyglucosan bodies are found in the central nervous system in classical myoclonic epilepsy (Lafora body disease) but also in the ageing brain, in type II glycogenosis, in rare cases of bilateral athetosis or amyotrophic lateral sclerosis. They described four patients in whom there was evidence of progressive upper and lower motor-neurone dysfunction, sensory loss in the legs, a 'neurogenic bladder', and dementia (in two) and in whom the polyglucosan bodies were found in neuronal and astrocytic processes throughout the nervous system.

References

Agamanolis, D. P. and Patre, S. (1979). Glycogen accumulation in the central nervous system in the cerebro-hepato-renal syndrome. *J. neurol. Sci.* **41**, 325.

Cori, G. T. (1952–3). Glycogen structure and enzyme deficiencies in glycogen storage disease. *Harvey Lect.* **48**, 145.

Crome, L., Cumings, J. N., and Duckett, S. (1963). Neuropathological and neurochemical aspects of generalized glycogen storage disease. *J. Neurol. Neurosurg. Psychiat.* **26**, 422.

Goebel, H. H., Lenard, H. G., Kohlschütter, A., and Pilz, H. (1977). The ultrastructure of the sural nerve in Pompe's disease. *Ann. Neurol.* **2**, 111.

Menkes, J. H. (1980). *Textbook of child neurology*, 2nd edn. Lea and Febiger, Philadelphia.

Robitaille, Y., Carpenter, S., Karpati, G., and DiMauro, S. (1980). A distinct form of adult polyglucosan body disease with massive involvement of central and peripheral neuronal processes and astrocytes. *Brain* **103**, 315.

Galactosaemia

Mental retardation can be associated with an abnormal metabolism of lactose, due to a defect of the enzyme galactose-1-phosphate uridyl transferase, inherited as an autosomal recessive factor. The mental defect occurs with varying degrees of severity, and in severe cases enlargement of the liver is associated with jaundice, and the child later develops cataracts. A reducing substance will be found in the urine, and the diagnosis is established by incubating red blood cells obtained from the umbilical cord with galactose. In affected babies an accumulation of galactose-1-phosphate can be demonstrated. In such cases a lactose-free diet appears to give good results (Menkes 1980).

Fructosuria

Two metabolic disorders are associated with fructosuria. The first is essential fructosuria, which is symptomless, and was once confused with diabetes mellitus because of the positive result of testing the urine with Benedict's solution. The other syndrome is known as fructose intolerance, a hereditary disorder in which the absorption of fructose leads to an abnormally high blood fructose associated with hypoglycaemia. There is a deficiency of fructose-1-phosphate aldolase in liver, kidney, and small intestinal mucosa. This condition may be, but is not always, associated with mental retardation, and spastic paraparesis has been described (Rennert and Greer 1970). Dormandy and Porter (1961) reported a case of familial fructose and galactose intolerance. Treatment simply consists of a fructose-free diet (Menkes 1980).

Hypoglycaemia

There are many causes of hypoglycaemia in childhood, and as a result of repeated or prolonged hypoglycaemic attacks severe cerebral damage may occur, with mental deterioration (Moncrieff 1960). The pathological changes in such cases are similar to those of anoxia (see p. 440) with widespread neuronal damage (Anderson, Milner, and Strich 1967) but the Purkinje cells of the cerebellum are peculiarly sensitive to hypoglycaemia so that surviving children are often ataxic. Ingram, Stark and Blackburn (1967) reviewed 26 children who suffered from hypoglycaemic coma between the ages of 10 weeks and 11 years. Twelve were diabetic, one had islet-cell adenomatosis, and in 13 the cause of the hypoglycaemia was unknown. Nine of the 23 children seen at follow-up were mentally retarded, four were epileptic, and 10 showed signs of ataxia or ataxic diplegia. In addition to the idiopathic type, and hypoglycaemia in diabetes and islet-cell adenomatosis, episodes of hypoglycaemia can occur with a raised blood fructose, and the same may happen in galactosaemia. As mentioned above, episodic hypoglycinaemia is a common feature of several of the urea-cycle disorders and amino-acidurias (Adams and Lyon 1982) and it may occur in systemic carnitine deficiency (see below).

References

Adams, R. D. and Lyon, G. (1982), *Neurology of hereditary metabolic diseases of children*. Hemisphere Publications, Washington.

Anderson, J. M., Milner, R. D. G., and Strich, S. J. (1967). Effects of neonatal hypoglycaemia on the nervous system: a pathological study. *J. Neurol. Neurosurg. Psychiat.* **30**, 295.

Dormandy, T. L. and Porter, R. J. (1961). Familial fructose and galactose intolerance *Lancet.* **i,** 1189.

Ingram, T. T. S., Stark, G. D., and Blackburn, I. (1967). Ataxia and other neurological disorders as sequels of severe hypoglycaemia in childhood. *Brain* **90,** 851.

Menkes, J. H. (1980). *Textbook of child neurology*, 2nd edn. Lea and Febiger, Philadelphia.

Moncrieff, A. (1960). Biochemistry of mental defect. *Lancet* **ii**, 273.

Rennert, O. M. and Greer, M. (1970). Hereditary fructosemia. *Neurology, Minneapolis* **20**, 421.

Subacute necrotizing encephalomyelopathy (Leigh's disease)

This rare condition, first described by Leigh in 1951, is inherited by an autosomal recessive mechanism and its clinical and pathological features strongly suggest that it is due to an inherited enzyme defect, but no specific abnormality has yet been identified. At first the diagnosis was usually made only at post-mortem but subsequently many cases were diagnosed during life and were found to show raised blood pyruvate levels and a metabolic acidosis. Hommes, Polman, and Reerink (1968) found in such cases a marked reduction in serum pyruvate carboxylase, the enzyme which converts pyruvate to oxalacetate but in other cases the activity of this enzyme has been normal. Recently, Sorbi and Blass (1982) have found abnormal activation of pyruvate dehydrogenase in fibroblasts derived from such cases. Pathologically the brains of affected individuals show widespread cellular necrosis with capillary proliferation in the optic nerves and chiasm, basal ganglia, and brain-stem. The appearances are similar to those of Wernicke's encephalopathy, but the distribution of the lesions is somewhat different, the corpora mammillaria usually being spared (Richter 1968). The CT scan may demonstrate symmetrical focal lesions in medial thalamus and midbrain (Schwartz, Hutchison, and Berg 1981). Biochemically there is often pyruvic and lactic acidaemia and in the affected brains there is an accumulation of thiamine pyrophosphate and a deficiency of thiamine triphosphate (TTP) (Murphy and Craig 1975). An inhibitor which inhibits adenosine triphosphate (ATP)-thiamine diphosphate (TDP) phosphoryltransferase, thus blocking the synthesis of TTP, has been identified in blood, urine, and CSF (Plaitakis, Whersell, Cooper, and Yahr 1980). Crome (1970) reported a typical case in which the kidneys showed nephrosis and changes in the glomeruli and renal tubules as well as the accumulation of adventitious lipid material in the intima of many arteries and arterioles. Clinically the affected children show failure to thrive, poverty of movement, hypotonia and spasticity, loss of tendon reflexes, nystagmus, and optic atrophy; convulsions sometimes occur and the condition is usually fatal in six to 12 months. Occasional cases have been reported in adolescence (Hardman, Allen, Baughman, and Waterman 1968) and adult life. In adult cases the clinical manifestations are remarkably variable, sometimes being minimal (Plaitakis *et al.* 1980) and in other cases more severe with optic atrophy, ataxia, spastic paresis, myoclonus, major fits, emotional lability, and mild dementia (Kalimo, Lundberg, and Olsson 1979). In some cases there has been thought to be temporary arrest of the disease process following treatment with lipoic acid (0.7 mg/kg body weight) (Worsley, Brookfield, Elwood, Noble, and Taylor 1965). However, there is no convincing evidence that any treatment is of long-term value, though the control of acidosis, if acute and severe, may require appropriate measures.

References

Crome, L. (1964). Neuropathological changes in diseases caused by inborn errors of metabolism. In *Neurometabolic disorders in childhood* (ed. K. S. Holt and J. Milner) Chapter 4. Livingstone, Edinburgh.

——, (1970). Subacute necrotizing encephalomyelopathy associated with renal and arterial lesions, *Brain* **93**, 709.

Greenhouse, A. H. and Schneck, S. A. (1968). Subacute necrotizing encephalomyelopathy. A reappraisal of the thiamine deficiency hypothesis. *Neurology, Minneapolis* **18**, 1.

Hardman, J. M. Allen, L. W., Baughman, F. A., and Waterman, D. F. (1968). Subacute necrotizing encephalopathy in late adolescence. *Arch. Neurol., Chicago* **18**, 478.

Hommes, F. A., Polman, H. A., and Reerink, J. D. (1968). Leigh's encephalomyelopathy: an inborn error of gluconeogenesis. *Arch. Dis. Child.*, **43**, 423.

Kalimo, H., Lundberg, P. O., and Olsson, Y. (1979). Familial subacute necrotizing encephalomyelopathy of the adult form (adult Leigh syndrome). *Ann. Neurol.* **6**, 200.

Leigh, D. (1951). Subacute necrotizing encephalomyelopathy in an infant. *J. Neurol. Neurosurg. Psychiat.* **14**, 216.

Murphy, J. V. and Craig, L. (1975). Leigh's disease: significance of the biochemical changes in brain. *J. Neurol. Neurosurg. Psychiat.* **38**, 1100.

Plaitakis, A., Whersell, W. O., Cooper, J. R., and Yahr, M. D. (1980). Chronic Leigh disease: a genetic and biochemical study. *Ann Neurol.* **7**, 304.

Richter, R. R. (1968). Infantile subacute necrotizing encephalopathy (Leigh's disease). Its relationship to Wernicke's encephalopathy. *Neurology, Minneapolis* **18**, 1125.

Schwartz, W. J., Hutchison, H. T., and Berg, B. O. (1981). Computerized tomography in subacute necrotizing encephalomyelopathy (Leigh disease). *Ann. Neurol.* **10**, 268.

Sorbi, S. and Blass, J. P. (1982). Abnormal activation of pyruvate dehydrogenase in Leigh disease fibroblasts. *Neurology, Minneapolis* **32**, 555.

Worsley, H. E., Brookfield, R. W., Elwood, J. S., Noble, R. L., and Taylor, W. H. (1965). Lactic acidosis with necrotizing encephalopathy in two sibs. *Arch. Dis. Childh.* **40**, 492.

Other disorders of carbohydrate metabolism

Intermittent cerebellar ataxia and choreoathetosis provoked by fever and/or excitement with an absence of neurological abnormality between attacks has now been reported as a consequence of pyruvate decarboxylase deficiency (Blass, Kark, and Engel 1971). Aspartylglucosaminuria, a rare condition causing structural abnormalities, hyperactivity, skin changes, recurrent infection, infantile diarrhoea (in some cases), and moderate or severe retardation may be especially common in Finland (Palo and Mattsson 1970; Arstila, Palo, Haltia, Riekkinen, and Autio 1972). A progressive poliodystrophy with hypomyelination resembling Alpers' disease and giving psychomotor retardation, hypotonia, seizures, and respiratory insufficiency has been shown to be due to pyruvate dehydrogenase deficiency restricted to the brain (Prick, Gabreëls, Renier, Trijbels, Jaspar, Lamers, and Kok 1981).

References

Arstila, A. U., Palo, J., Haltia, M., Riekkinen, P., and Autio, S. (1972). Aspartylglucosaminuria I: fine structural studies on liver, kidney and brain. *Acta neuropath., Berlin* **20**, 207.

Blass, J. P., Kark, R. A. P., and Engel, W. K. (1971). Clinical studies of a patient with pyruvate decarboxylase deficiency. *Arch. Neurol., Chicago* **25**, 449.

Crome, L. C. and Stern, J. (1972). *Pathology of mental retardation*, 2nd edn. Churchill Livingstone, London.

Palo, J. and Mattsson, K. (1970). Eleven new cases of aspartylglucosaminuria. *J. ment. Defic. Res.* **14**, 168.

Prick, M., Gabreëls, F., Renier, W., Trijbels, F., Jaspar, H., Lamers, K., and Kok, J. (1981). Pyruvate dehydrogenase deficiency restricted to brain. *Neurology, Minneapolis* **31**, 398.

Disorders of mucopolysaccharide metabolism

Gargoylism (Hurler's disease)

This syndrome, which is characterized by mental and physical retardation, hepatosplenomegaly, clouding of the cornea, a characteristic facial appearance, and multiple skeletal deformities, is now known to embrace at least six and more probably seven (Menkes 1980) different disorders, each characterized by varying degrees of storage of chondroitin (dermatan) sulphate and heparan sulphate in various tissues and organs of the body including the central nervous system (McKusick 1969; Dorfman 1972). All save the so-called Hunter syndrome (Hunter 1917), which is inherited as an X-linked recessive trait, are of autosomal recessive inheritance.

Patients with the typical Hurler syndrome often seem normal at birth but towards the end of the first year show evidence of mental retardation, corneal clouding, widely spaced eyes, flattening of the nasal bridge, thickening of the lips, and an open mouth. The skin is often coarse, an umbilical hernia is common with a protuberant abdomen, the hands are large with short and stubby fingers, and there is often hepatosplenomegaly. Radiological changes are particularly common in the humerus with cortical thickening and medullary enlargement but many long bones may be abnormal. (Caffey 1952). Progressive spasticity and dementia, sometimes with deafness and optic atrophy, develop and death usually results from bronchopneumonia in childhood. Skin fibroblasts contain excess mucopolysaccharides and typical inclusions are seen ultrastructurally (Lyon, Hors-Cayla, Jonsson, and Maroteaux 1973) while urinary mucopolysaccharide excretion is increased (Renuart 1966). The lymphocytes often contain metachromatically staining cytoplasmic inclusions (Reilly granules) (Belcher 1972).

The Hunter type usually spares the cornea and runs a milder course, the Sanfilippo variety affects the nervous system severely but often gives mild somatic manifestations, the Morquio variety (Gilles and Deuel 1971), in which keratosulphate is stored in abnormal amounts, causes severe skeletal abnormalities and often less severe nervous-system involvement, and the Scheie and Maroteaux–Lamy variants usually spare the nervous system and the intellect (see Menkes 1980). Antenatal diagnosis through amniotic-cell culture is now possible. No drug treatment is of any value but bone-marrow transplantation may reverse the abnormal clinical features and give biochemical improvement (Hobbs,

Hugh-Jones, Barrett, Byrom, Chambers, Henry, James, Lucas, Rogers, Benson, Tansley, Patrick, Mossman, and Young 1981).

As already noted (p. 456), GM_1 gangliosidosis (pseudo-Hurler's disease) gives similar clinical features (mental retardation, hepatosplenomegaly, abnormal facies, and bony abnormalities) but the urinary mucopolysaccharide excretion is normal.

References

Belcher, R. W. (1972). Ultrastructure and cytochemistry of lymphocytes in the genetic mucopolysaccharidoses. *Arch. Path.* **93**, 1.

Caffey, J. (1952). Gargoylism: prenatal and postnatal bone lesions and their early postnatal evolution. *Am. J. Roentgen.* **67**, 715.

Dorfman, A. (1972). The molecular basis of the mucopolysaccharidoses: current status of knowledge. *Triangle* **11**, .43.

Gilles, F. H. and Deuel, R. K. (1971). Neuronal cytoplasmic globules in the brain in Morquio's syndrome. *Arch. Neurol., Chicago* **25**, 393.

Hobbs, J. R., Hugh-Jones, K., Barrett, A. J., Byrom, N., Chambers, D., Henry, K., James, D. C. O., Lucas, C. F., Rogers, T. R., Benson, P. F., Tansley, L. R., Patrick, A. C., Mossman, J., and Young, E. P. (1981). Reversal of clinical features of Hurler's disease and biochemical improvement after treatment by bone-marrow transplantation. *Lancet* **ii**, 709.

Hunter, C. (1917). A rare disease in two brothers. *Proc. R. Soc. Med.* **10**, 104.

Lyon, G., Hors-Cayla, M. C., Jonsson, V., and Maroteaux, P. (1973). Aspects ultrastructuraux et signification biochimique des granulations metachromatiques et autres inclusions dans les fibroblastes en culture provenant de lipidoses et de mucopolysaccharidoses. *J. neurol. Sci.* **19**, 235.

McKusick, V. A. (1969). The nosology of the mucopolysaccharidoses. *Am. J. Med.* **47**, 730.

Menkes, J. H. (1980). *Textbook of child neurology*, 2nd edn. Lea and Febiger, Philadelphia.

Renuart, A. W. (1966). Screening for inborn errors of metabolism associated with mental deficiency or neurologic disorders or both. *New Engl. J. Med.* **274**, 384.

Miscellaneous disorders of varied or unknown aetiology

Menkes' kinky-hair disease (trichopoliodystrophy)

In 1962 Menkes, Alter, and Steigleder described an X-linked recessive disorder characterized by early and severe retardation of growth, peculiar white and 'kinky' hair, frequent epileptic seizures, and focal cerebral and cerebellar degneration involving particularly the grey matter. The condition is usually fatal in early childhood; French, Sherard, Lubell, Brotz, and Moore (1972) and Ghatak, Hirano, Poon, and French (1972) suggested that it should be entitled 'trichopoliodystrophy' and identified pathological changes in skeletal muscle as well as in the central nervous system. Danks, Campbell, Stevens, Mayne, and Cartwright (1972) suggested that the condition is due to diminished copper absorption as they found low serum copper and caeruloplasmin levels in such cases. It is now postulated that neonatal copper deficiency causes the pathological changes which take the form of nerve-cell loss and gliosis in cerebral and cerebellar cortex and thalamic relay nuclei (Williams, Marshall, Lott, and Caviness 1978; Iwata, Hirano, and French 1979 a, b). Serum, hepatic, and brain copper levels are all low, there is reduced cytochrome oxidase A1 and A3 in liver, brain, and white blood cells and an increased affinity for copper by metallothioneines in fibroblasts from affected patients (Grover, Henkin, Schwartz, Brodsky, Hobdell, and Stolk 1982); the incorporation of ^{64}Cu into cultured amniotic cells can be used for antenatal diagnosis (Horn 1976). Dopamine β-hydroxylase activity is also reduced in the blood and CSF. The EEG is usually grossly abnormal with appearances resembling those of hypsarrhythmia, and visual evoked potentials are reduced or absent (Friedman, Harden, Koivikko, and Pampiglione 1978). Copper injections appear to have no influence on the course of the disease.

A similar X-linked syndrome with diminished copper absorption from the gut, giving mental retardation, seizures, and low serum copper and caeruloplasmin with normal hair and relatively non-progressive hypotonia and choreoathetosis has been described (Haas, Robinson, Evans, Lascelles, and Dubowitz 1981).

Alpers' disease (progressive cerebral poliodystrophy)

This condition, described by Alpers in 1931, is still poorly defined, being thought by some to be a heredodegenerative disorder but attributed by others to anoxia (Norman 1958) or an inflammatory process (Dreifuss and Netsky 1964). However, evidence has emerged to indicate that it is an inherited process of autosomal recessive inheritance and unknown aetiology; it has been described in three sibs (Sandbank and Lerman 1972). It may begin in early infancy or in the first few years of life and leads to progressive dementia, seizures, spasticity, and opisthotonos. It can be diagnosed in life only by brain biopsy which shows almost total neuronal loss in the grey matter of the cerebral cortex with astrogliosis and microgliosis; large disorganized mitochondria may be found (Sandbank and Lerman 1972). There is increasing evidence to suggest that the condition may be a diffuse mitochondrial disease leading to disturbed pyruvate oxidation in muscle, liver, and brain with abnormal nicotinamide adenine dinucleotide oxidation (Prick, Gabreëls, Renier, Trijbels, Sengers, and Slooff 1981).

Cerebral gigantism

In 1964 Sotos, Dodge, Muirhead, Crawford, and Talbot described five mentally retarded patients with large faces, large dolicocephalic skulls, widely spaced eyes, high arched palates, and large hands and feet. They showed excessive growth up to about the fifth year of life and subsequently their height, weight, and bone age were two to four years in advance of normal (Gardner-Medwin 1969). Precocious puberty has been described in some cases subsequently reported but the syndrome has no known aetiology, and no specific endocrinological or neuropathological features have been identified.

Urbach–Wiethe's disease (lipoid proteinosis)

This rare disorder, probably of autosomal recessive inheritance, is characterized by hoarseness of the voice, cutaneous and mucosal lesions, intracranial calcification, alopecia, ocular and dental abnormalities, photosensitivity, and short stature. In two sibs reported by Newton, Rosenberg, Lampery, and O'Brien (1971) rage attacks, epilepsy, and severe loss of recent memory were prominent. The chemical composition of the abnormal material stored in the brain is unknown. The disease may present in childhood, but the course is usually prolonged well into adult life.

Infantile neuroaxonal dystrophy

This rare disorder, which seems to be due to an autosomal recessive gene, was first described by Seitelberger in 1952. Pathologically it is characterized by the accumulation of large axonal swellings in the grey matter of the brain and spinal cord and by degeneration of the globus pallidus, cerebellum, and long spinal tracts. Optic atrophy and partial denervation of skeletal muscles may also occur. Ultrastructural studies of sections of frontal cortex have shown that the axonal spheroids contain a sponge-like network of tubular structures and that presynaptic terminals are particularly involved (Hedley-Whyte, Gilles, and Uzman 1968; Herman, Huttenlocher, and Bensch 1969; Coster, Roels, and Vander Eecken 1971). Similar changes are found in muscle biopsy sections involving extra- and intrafusal axons and motor end-plates (Martin and Martin 1972). Sural-nerve biopsy usually shows ballooned axons with accumulations of membranous profiles, vesicles, and a homogenous centre with masses of 90Å filaments in endothelial, endoneurial, perineurial, and Schwann cells, resembling the findings seen in giant axonal neuropathy (Shimono, Ohta, Asada, and Kruoiwa 1976; Begeer, Houthoff, Van Weerden, de Groot, Blaauw, and Peloultre 1979).

The condition usually begins between the ages of one and three years with arrest of development and motor weakness progressing to paralysis due to a combination of pyramidal-tract and lower motor-neurone dysfunction; there may be loss of pain sensation in the legs. Convulsions are rare but progressive optic atrophy leads to blindness and most patients die before the end of the first decade. A juvenile form beginning in the second decade with clinical features of progressive myoclonic epilepsy has been described (Dorfman, Pedley, Tharp, and Scheithauer 1978).

The EEG usually shows diffuse fast activity, the EMG confirms the presence of denervation (Aicardi and Castelein 1979), and the serum and CSF lactate dehydrogenase activity may be raised. Certain features of the condition resemble those of experimental tocopherol deficiency in animals but no specific biochemical abnormality has yet been detected and no effective treatment has yet been introduced. Some authorities believe that the condition is identical with, or closely related to, Hallervorden–Spatz disease (see p. 339) but most are confident that it is an independent entity (Indravasu and Dexter 1968; Martin and Martin 1972; Adams and Lyon 1982).

References

Adams, R. D. and Lyon, G. (1982). *Neurology of hereditary metabolic diseases of children*. Hemisphere Publishing, Washington.

Aicardi, J. and Castelein, P. (1979). Infantile neuroaxonal dystrophy. *Brain* **102**, 727.

Alpers, B. J. (1931). Diffuse progressive degeneration of the gray matter of the cerebrum. *Arch. Neurol. Psychiat., Chicago* **25**, 469.

Begeer, J. H., Houthoff, H. J., Van Weerden, T.W., de Groot, C.J., Blaauw, E. H., and le Coultre, R. (1979). Infantile neuroaxonal dystrophy and giant axonal neuropathy: are they related? *Ann. Neurol.* **6**, 540.

Coster, W. de, Roels, H., and Vander Eecken, H. (1971). Electron microscopical study of neuroaxonal dystrophy. *Eur. Neurol.* **5**, 65.

Cowen, D. and Olmstead, E. V. (1963). Infantile neuroaxonal dystrophy. *J. Neuropath. exp. Neurol.* **22**, 175.

Danks, D. M., Campbell, P. E., Stevens, B. J., Mayne, V., and Cartwright, E. (1972). Menkes' kinky hair syndrome: defect in copper absorption. *Pediatrics* **50**, 188.

Dorfman, L. J., Pedley, T. A., Tharp, B. R., and Scheithauer, B. W. (1978). Juvenile neuroaxonal dystrophy: clinical, electrophysiological, and neuropathological features. *Ann. Neurol.* **3**, 419.

Dreifuss, F. E. and Netsky, M. G. (1964). Progressive poliodystrophy. *Am. J. Dis. Child.* **107**, 649.

French, J. H., Sherard, E. S., Lubell, H., Brotz, M., and Moore, C.L. (1972). Trichopoliodystrophy. I. Report of a case and biochemical studies. *Arch. Neurol., Chicago* **26**, 229.

Friedman, E., Harden, A., Koivikko, M., and Pampiglione, G. (1978). Menkes' disease: neurophysiological aspects. *J. Neurol. Neurosurg. Psychiat.* **41**, 505.

Gardner-Medwin, D. (1969). Cerebral gigantism? *Develop. Med. Child Neurol.* **11**, 796.

Ghatak, N. R., Hirano, A., Poon, T. P., and French, J. H. (1972). Trichopoliodystrophy. II. Pathological changes in skeletal muscle and nervous system. *Arch. Neurol., Chicago* **26**, 60.

Grover, W. D., Henkin, R. I., Schwartz, M., Brodsky, N., Hobell, E., and Stolk, J.M. (1982). A defect in catecholamine metabolism in kinky-hair disease. *Ann. Neurol.* **12**, 263.

Haas, R. H., Robinson, A., Evans, K., Lascelles, P.T., and Dubowitz, V. (1981). An X-linked disease of the nervous system with disordered copper metabolism and features differing from Menkes disease. *Neurology, Minneapolis* **31**, 852.

Hedley-Whyte, E. T., Gilles, F. H., and Uzman, B. G. (1968). Infantile neuroaxonal dystrophy: a disease characterized by altered terminal axons and synaptic endings. *Neurology, Minneapolis* **18**, 891.

Herman, M. M., Huttenlocher, P. R., and Bensch, K. G. (1969). Electron microscopic observations in infantile neuroaxonal dystrophy: report of a cortical biopsy and review of the recent literature. *Arch. Neurol., Chicago* **20**, 19.

Horn, N. (1976). Copper incorporation studies on cultured cells for pre-natal diagnosis of Menkes' disease. *Lancet* i, 1156.

Huttenlocher, P. R. and Gilles, F. H. (1967). Infantile neuroaxonal dystrophy. Clinical, pathological and histochemical findings in a family with 3 affected siblings. *Neurology, Minneapolis* 17, 1174.

Indravasu, S. and Dexter, R. A. (1968). Infantile neuroaxonal dystrophy and its relationship to Hallervorden–Spatz disease. *Neurology, Minneapolis* 18, 693.

Iwata, M., Hirano, A., and French, J. H. (1979 a). Thalamic degeneration in X-chromosome-linked copper malabsorption. *Ann. Neurol.* 5, 359.

——, ——, and —— (1979 b). Degeneration of the cerebellar system in X-chromosome-linked copper malabsorption. *Ann. Neurol.* 5. 542.

Martin, J. J. and Martin, L. (1972). Infantile neuroaxonal dystrophy. Ultrastructural study of the peripheral nerves and of the motor end plates. *Eur. Neurol.* 8, 239.

Menkes, J. H., Alter, M., and Steigleder, G. K. (1962). A sex-linked recessive disorder with growth retardation, peculiar hair, and focal cerebral and cerebellar degeneration. *Pediatrics* 29, 674.

Newton, F. H., Rosenberg, R. N., Lampery, P. W., and O'Brien, J.S. (1971). Neurologic involvement in Urbach-Wiethe's disease (lipoid proteinosis). *Neurology, Minneapolis* 21, 1205.

Norman, R. M. (1958). Alpers' disease. In *Neuropathology* (ed. J. Greenfied, W. Blackwood, W. H. McMenemey, A. Meyer, and R. M. Norman), p. 378. Arnold, London.

Prick, M. J. J., Gabreëls, F. J. M., Renier, W. O., Trijbels, J. M. F., Sengers, R. C. A., and Slooff, J. L. (1981). Progressive infantile poliodystrophy. Association with disturbed pyruvate oxidation in muscle and liver. *Arch. Neurol.*, Chicago 38, 767.

Sandbank, U. and Lerman, P. (1972). Progressive cerebral poliodystrophy–Alpers' disease. *J. Neurol. Neurosurg. Psychiat.* 35, 749.

Seitelberger, F. (1952). Eine unbekannte Form von infantiler lipoidopercher Krankheit des Gehirns. Proceedings of the *First International Congress of Neuropathology*, Vol. 3, p. 323. Turin.

Shimono, M., Ohta, M., Asada, M., and Kuroiwa, Y. (1976). Infantile neuroaxonal dystrophy: ultrastructural study of peripheral nerve. *Acta neuropath.*, Berlin 36 71.

Sotos, J. F., Dodge, P. R., Muirhead, D., Crawford, J.D., and Talbot, N.B. (1964). Cerebral gigantism in childhood. *New Engl. J. Med.* 271, 109.

Williams, R. S., Marshall, P. C., Lott, I. T., and Caviness, V. S. (1978). The cellular pathology of Menkes steely hair syndrome. *Neurology, Minneapolis* 28, 575.

Some other metabolic disorders

Serious infantile protein–calorie malnutrition, as in kwashiorkor, has a profound effect upon brain development and may be associated with deficits in intelligence and delayed physical growth (Elliott and Knight 1972; *The Lancet* 1972). There are clearly periods in early brain development when it is particularly vulnerable (*British Medical Journal* 1978; Dastur, Manghani, Osuntokun, Sourander, and Kondo 1982). Endemic cretinism due to maternal iodine deficiency is another important cause (Pharoah, Buttfield, and Hetzel 1971) and fetal iodine deficiency may impair subsequent motor development and performance (Connolly, Pharoah, and Hetzel 1979). Hypercalcaemia of infancy due to hyperreactivity to vitamin D or overdosage with this vitamin (Seelig 1969) may also cause mental retardation.

Systemic carnitine deficiency

While carnitine deficiency restricted to skeletal muscle is well known to produce lipid storage myopathy, and carnitine palmityl transferase deficiency can produce a syndrome of muscle pain and myoglobinuria (see Chapter 19), systemic carnitine deficiency is well recognized to cause not only muscle weakness but also episodes of acute encephalopathy with vomiting, confusion, stupor, seizures, and then coma, often with nonketotic hypoglycaemia precipitated by fasting and often leading to a fatal outcome (Slonim, Borum, Mrak, Najjar, Richardson, and Diamond 1983). Another fatal disease causing intermittent ataxia, oculomotor pal-

sies, hypotonia, confusion, stupor, and hepatic dysfunction has been shown to be due to carnitine acetyltransferase deficiency (DiDonata, Rimoldi, Moise, Bertagnoglio, and Uziel 1979).

Neurological complications of gastrointestinal disease

The many neurological and neuromuscular disorders which may complicate gastrointestinal disease were reviewed by Pallis and Lewis (1974); many, such as the Korsakow–Wernicke syndrome following partial gastrectomy and some other malabsorption syndromes, are due to vitamin deficiency (Chapter 16) but others are unexplained. Thus in coeliac disease (nontropical sprue) in childhood, but more often in adult life, neurological complications may occur in up to 10 per cent of cases and include peripheral neuropathy, myelopathy, encephalopathy, cerebellar ataxia, progressive multifocal leukoencephalopathy, basilar impression, tetany, and seizures (Finelli, McEntee, Ambler, and Kestenbaum, 1980; Kinney, Burger, Hurwitz, Hijmans, and Grant 1982). Degeneration of the posterior columns of the spinal cord has also been reported in cystic fibrosis (Geller, Gilles, and Shwachman 1977). Whipple's disease, too, which usually presents with gastrointestinal symptoms, can sometimes produce lesions which are confined to the nervous system, producing seizures, intermittent fever, and progressive dementia leading to coma and death (Romanul, Radvany, and Rosales 1977; Pollock, Lewis, and Kendall 1981); peripheral neuropathy may also occur and the cerebral lesions are usually identifiable on the CT scan (Halperin, Landis, and Kleinman 1982).

References

British Medical Journal (1978). Nutrition and the brain. *Br. Med. J.* 1, 1569.

Connolly, K. J., Pharoah, P. O. D., and Hetzel, B. S. (1979). Fetal iodine deficiency and motor performance during childhood. *Lancet* ii, 1149.

Dastur, D. K., Manghani, D. K., Osuntokun, B. O., Sourander, P., and Kondo, K. (1982). Neuromuscular and related changes in malnutrition: a review. *J. neurol. Sci.* 55, 207.

DiDonato, S., Rimoldi, M., Moise, A., Bertagnoglio, B., and Uziel, G. (1979). Fatal ataxic encephalopathy and carnitine acetyltransferase deficiency: a functional defect of pyruvate oxidation? *Neurology, Minneapolis* 29, 1578.

Elliott, K. and Knight, J. (1972). *Lipids, malnutrition and the developing brain.* Elsevier, New York.

Finelli, P. F., McEntee, W. J., Ambler, M., and Kestenbaum, D. (1980). Adult celiac disease presenting as cerebellar syndrome. *Neurology, Minneapolis* 30, 245.

Geller, A., Gilles, F., and Shwachman, H. (1977). Degeneration of fasciculus gracilis in cystic fibrosis. *Neurology, Minneapolis* 27, 185.

Halperin, J. J., Landis, D. M. D., and Kelinman, G. M. (1982). Whipple disease of the nervous system. *Neurology, Minneapolis* 32, 612.

Kinney, H. C., Burger, P. C., Hurwitz, B. J., Hijmans, J. C., and Grant, J. P. (1982). Degeneration of the central nervous system associated with celiac disease. *J. neurol. Sci.* 53, 9.

The Lancet (1972). Nutrition and the developing brain. *Lancet* ii, 1349.

Pallis, C. and Lewis, P. D. (1974). *Neurology of gastrointestinal disease.* Saunders, London.

Pharoah, P. O. D., Buttfield, I. H., and Hetzel, B. (1971). Neurological damage to the fetus resulting from severe iodine deficiency during pregnancy. *Lancet* i, 308.

Pollock, S., Lewis, P. D., and Kendall, B. (1981). Whipple's disease confined to the nervous system. *J. Neurol. Neurosurg. Psychiat.* 44, 1104.

Romanul, F. C. A., Radvany, J., and Rosales, R. K. (1977). Whipple's disease confined to the brain: a case studied clinically and pathologically. *J. Neurol. Neurosurg. Psychiat.* 40, 901.

Seelig, M. S. (1969). Vitamin D and cardiovascular, renal, and brain damage in infancy and childhood. *Ann. NY Acad. Sci.* 147 537.

Slonim, A. E., Borum, P. R., Mrak, R. E., Najjar, J., Richardson, D., and Diamond, M. P. (1983). Nonketotic hypoglycemia: an early indicator of systemic carnitine deficiency. *Neurology, Minneapolis* 33, 29.

Some endocrine causes of mental retardation and of other neurological symptoms

A *diencephalic syndrome* of infancy has been described giving severe emaciation and growth retardation but intellect is usually normal and in most cases hypothalamic gliomas or gliomas of the optic nerve are eventually demonstrated (Pelc and Flament-Durand 1973).

In *diabetes insipidus* due to lesions of the neurohypophysis or of its afferent neurosecretory cells originating in the supraoptic and paraventricular nuclei of the hypothalamus, thirst and polyuria result from a diminished output of antidiuretic hormone (ADH); the condition may be hereditary or idiopathic and usually responds to treatment with vasopressin (Green, Buchan, Alvord, and Swanson 1967); the intellect is well preserved. However, in *nephrogenic diabetes insipidus* the renal tubules cannot respond to ADH, the affected infants excrete large quantities of very dilute urine with a specific gravity usually below 1.006, and the polyuria leads to severe hypertonic dehydration which, if untreated, is rapidly fatal. Massive and frequent administration of fluid is necessary to correct the dehydration and associated hypernatraemia; even so, the survivors are often mentally retarded (Ruess and Rosenthal 1963). The condition, being inherited as an X-linked recessive trait, usually affects only males; it is resistant to vasopressin treatment because of a defect in the specific adenyl cyclase of the renal tubules (Thorn 1970).

Other causes of *hypernatraemia* in infancy, including excessive sodium intake resulting from the use of certain dried milks in early life, may cause convulsions, disordered consciousness, and, if severe, permanent brain damage (Morris-Jones, Houston, and Evans 1967). In adults, hypernatraemia, hypodipsia, and hypovolaemia have been described as an effect of hypothalamic or suprasellar tumours (Vejjajiva, Sitprija, and Shuangshoti 1969; Lascelles and Lewis 1972). By contrast, *hyperosmolal coma* with *hyponatraemia* and associated hyperglycaemia, often causing cerebral oedema with a raised CSF pressure, is a well-recognised complication of diabetic ketosis (Espinas and Poser 1969; Clements, Blumenthal, Morrison and Winegrad 1971; *The Lancet* 1972) but has also been described as a consequence of severe burns, during peritoneal dialysis, and in steroid therapy; it sometimes causes focal epileptic seizures (Meccario, Messis, and Vastola 1965; Boyer 1967; Boyer, Gill, and Epstein 1967). By contrast, *hyponatraemia* and *hypo-osmolality* in patients with head injury or brain disease are often ascribed to inappropriate secretion of ADH, but Bouzarth and Shenkin (1982) argue that the ADH secretion is often appropriate and occurs as a response to the excessive administration of intravenous fluids. It should also be noted that central pontine myelinolysis (p. 319), commonly associated with hyponatraemia (Tomlinson, Pierides, and Bradley 1976; Burcar, Norenberg, and Karnell 1977; Wright, Laureno, and Victor 1979) is now thought in many cases to result from over-rapid correction of hyponatraemia following the excessive administration of intravenous saline (Norenberg, Leslie, and Robertson 1982; Laureno 1983). A probable case, with recovery, has been described in a patient with Addison's disease (Kandt, Heldrich, and Moser 1983). Confusion and mild delirium and even coma with hyponatraemia and hypoglycaemia may also occur in Addison's disease, especially during crises (Plum and Posner 1980), while psychotic symptoms are common in Cushing's disease (Spillane 1951) but coma is rare.

Hypopituitarism (p. 150) is usually associated with symptoms and signs of adrenal and/or thyroid insufficiency and with gonadal dysfunction (Fraser 1970), and the form which may occur in childhood after traumatic infarction of the interior lobe of the pituitary (Daniel, Prichard, and Treip 1959) may cause prolonged coma after minor head injury. When it is secondary to tumours in the pituitary region, the symptoms of the tumour itself often dominate the clinical picture and the same is true of *acromegaly* in which, however, the endocrine abnormality *per se* is sometimes associated with minor mental changes (Kanis, Gillingham, Harris, Horn, Hunter, Redpath, and Strong 1979) and with neuromuscular dysfunction (p. 575). As stated above, cretinism in infancy is an important cause of mental retardation; in adult life *myxoedema* may be associated with profound mental symptoms ("myxoedematous madness"), with hypothermic coma (Macdonald 1958; Plum and Posner 1980), or with cerebellar ataxia (Bernard, Campbell, and McDonald 1971). Both cretinism and myxoedema may also give symptoms of muscular dysfunction (p. 575). *Thyrotoxicosis* is usually associated with anxiety, tremor, and hyperactivity but is a rare cause of stupor and coma in hyperacute cases, while by contrast, apathetic thyrotoxicosis with depression and apathy in elderly subjects has been described (Thomas, Mazzaferri, and Skillman 1970).

Finally, it should be mentioned that in *idiopathic hypoparathyroidism* (Simpson 1952), mental retardation, epilepsy, and incipient tetany are common, and epilepsy and papilloedema have also been reported in true hypoparathyroidism after thyroid surgery (Willison and Whitty 1957. Mental defect with epilepsy and intracranial calcification is also common in *pseudohypoparathyroidism* but mental defect alone is more often seen in pseudo-pseudohypoparathyroidism (Dickson, Morita, Cowsert, Graves, and Meyer 1970). Spinal-cord compression due to ectopic calcification has been reported in pseudohypoparathyroidism (Cullen and Pearce 1964). The neuromuscular disorders commonly observed in disorders of calcium metabolism are described on page 576.

References

Barnard, R. O., Campbell, M.J., and McDonald, W.I. (1971). Pathological findings in a case of hypothyroidism with ataxia. *J. Neurol. Neurosurg. Psychiat.* **34**, 755.

Berman, P. H., Balis, M. E., and Dancis, J. (1969). Congenital hyperuricemia: an inborn error of purine metabolism associated with psychomotor retardation, athetosis and self-mutilation. *Arch. Neurol., Chicago* **20**, 44.

Bouzarth, W. F. and Shenkin, H. A. (1982). Is 'cerebral hyponatraemia' iatrogenic? *Lancet* **i**, 1061.

Boyer, J., Gill, G. N., and Epstein, F.H. (1967). Hyperglycemia and hyperosmolarity complicating peritoneal dialysis. *Ann. intern. Med.* **67**, 568.

Boyer, M. H. (1967). Hyperosmolar anacidotic coma in association with glucocorticoid therapy. *J. Am. med. Ass.* **202**, 1007.

Burcar, P. J., Norenberg, M. D., and Yarnell, P. R. (1977). Hyponatremia and central pontine myelinolysis. *Neurology, Minneapolis* **27**, 223.

Clements, R. S., Blumenthal, S. A., Morrison, A. D., and Winegrad, A. I. (1971). Increased cerebrospinal-fluid pressure during treatment of diabetic ketosis. *Lancet* **ii**, 671.

Cullen, D. R. and Pearce, J. M. S. (1964). Spinal cord compression in pseudohypoparathyroidism. *J. Neurol. Neurosurg. Psychiat.* **27** 459.

Daniel, P. M., Prichard, M. M. L., and Treip, C. S. (1959). Traumatic infarction of the anterior lobe of the pituitary gland. *Lancet* **ii**, 927.

Dickson, L. G., Morita, Y., Cowsert, E. J., Graves, J., and Meyer, J. S. (1960). Neurological, electroencephalographic and heredo-familial aspects of pseudohypoparathyroidism and pseudo-pseudohypoparathyroidism. *J. Neurol. Neurosurg. Psychiat.* **23**, 33.

Espinas, O.E. and Posner, C. M. (1969). Blood hyperosmolality and neurologic deficit. *Arch. Neurol., Chicago* **20**, 182.

Fraser, R. (1970). Human pituitary disease. *Br. med. J.* **4**, 449.

Green, J. R., Buchan, G. C., Alvord, E. C., and Swanson, A. G. (1967). Hereditary and idiopathic types of diabetes insipidus. *Brain.* **90**, 707.

Kandt, R.S., Heldrich, F. J., and Moser, H. W. (1983). Recovery from probable pontine myelinolysis associated with Addison's disease. *Arch. Neurol., Chicago* **40**, 118.

Kanis, J. A., Gillingham, F. J., Harris, P., Horn, D. B., Hunter, W.M., Redpath, A. T., and Strong, J. A. (1974). Clinical and laboratory study of acromegaly: assessment before and one year after treatment. *Quart. J. Med.* **43** 409.

The Lancet (1972). Hyperosmolal coma. *Lancet* **ii**, 1071.

Lascelles, P. T. and Lewis, P. D. (1972). Hypodipsia and hypernatraemia associated with hypothalamic and suprasellar lesions. *Brain* **95** 249.

Laureno, R. (1983). Central pontine myelinolysis following rapid correction of hyponatremia. *Ann. Neurol.* **13**, 232.

Maccario, M., Messis, C. P., and Vastola, E. F. (1965). Focal seizures as a manifestation of hyperglycemia, without ketoacidosis. *Neurology, Minneapolis* **15**, 195.

Macdonald, D. W. (1958). Hypothermic myxoedema coma. *Br. med. J.*, **2**, 1144.

Morris-Jones, P. H., Houston, I. B., and Evans, R. C. (1967). Prognosis of the neurological complications of acute hypernatraemia. *Lancet* **ii**, 1385.

Norenberg, M. D., Leslie, K. O. and Robertson, A. S. (1982). Association between rise in serum sodium and central pontine myelinolysis. *Ann. Neurol.* **11**, 128.

Pelc, S. and Flament-Durand, J. (1973). Histological evidence of optic chiasma glioma in the 'diencephalic syndrome', *Arch. Neurol., Chicago* **28**, 139.

Plum, F. and Posner, J.B. (1980). *The diagnosis of stupor and coma*, 3rd edn. Davis, Philadelphia.

Ruess, A. L. and Rosenthal, I. M. (1963). Intelligence in nephrogenic diabetes insipidus. *Am. J. dis. Child.* **105**, 358.

Simpson, J. A. (1952). The neurological manifestations of idiopathic hypoparathyroidism. *Brain* **75**, 76.

Spillane, J. D. (1951). Nervous and mental disorders in Cushing's syndrome. *Brain* **74**, 72.

Thomas, F. B., Mazzaferri, E. L., and Skillman, T. G. (1970). Apathetic thyrotoxicosis. *Ann. intern. Med.* **72** 679.

Thorn, N. A. (1970). Antidiuretic hormone synthesis, release and action under normal and pathological circumstances. *Advances in Metabolic Disorders*. **4**, 39.

Tomlinson, B. E., Pierides, A. M., and Bradley, W. G. (1976). Central pontine myelinolysis: two cases with associated electrolyte disturbance. *Quart. J. Med.* **45**, 373.

Vejjajiva, A., Sitprija, V., and Shuangshoti, S. (1969). Chronic sustained hypernatraemia and hypovolaemia in hypothalamic tumour. *Neurology, Minneapolis* **19**, 161.

Willison, R. G. and Whitty, C. W. M. (1957). Parathyroid deficiency presenting as epilepsy. *Br. med. J.* **1**, 802.

Wright, D. G., Laureno, R., and Victor, M. (1979). Pontine and extrapontine myelinolysis. *Brain* **102**, 361.

Some non-metabolic causes of mental retardation

Microbial causes of mental retardation, including cytomegalovirus infection, rubella, and toxoplasmosis (Stern, Elek, Booth, and Fleck 1969), are considered on pages 258 and 293.

Chromosomal anomalies

Crome and Stern (1972) listed 22 chromosomal anomalies which may be associated with mental retardation and more have been described subsequently (Menkes 1980). A detailed review of these disorders would be out of place in a textbook of neurology. Among the commoner syndromes are the 'Cri du chat' syndrome due to partial deletion of the short arm of chromosome S, characterized by low birth weight, microcephaly, cat-like cry, severe retardation, and hypertelorism; Klinefelter's syndrome with hypogenitalism, dwarfism, and a eunuchoid appearance and an XXY or XXXY chromosome constitution; Turner's syndrome or ovarian dysgenesis, with retarded growth, webbed neck, amenorrhoea, deafness in many cases, and an XO chromosomal pattern; and Down's syndrome (mongolism). Severe neuropathological abnormalities have also been reported in the Trisomy E (17–18) syndrome (Michaelson and Gilles 1972).

Down's syndrome (mongolism)
This is the commonest syndrome associated with mental retardation, occurring in about 1 in 650 live births. It is usually due to trisomy of chromosome 21, occasionally to translocation or mosaicism. Accurate diagnosis of the nature of the chromosomal anomaly is important in order to be able to advise the parents upon the risk of involvement of further children. There is clear association with increasing maternal age, and screening by amniocentesis should ideally be offered to all pregnant women over the age of 40 years, and if possible, over 35 (Fairweather 1982). A decrease in gamma-glutamyl transpeptidase activity in the amniotic fluid occurs in some cases but is by no means diagnostic, though it may be very helpful in diagnosis of the fetal trisomy 18 syndrome (Jalanko and Aula 1982).

The principal clinical features are mental and physical retardation (often relatively mild but varying in severity) and a typical mongoloid appearance of the face with abnormalities of the skull, skeleton, hands, and feet and of the palmar creases. Congenital heart lesions and other visceral abnormalities are often present. The patients are usually simple and affectionate, may sometimes be capable of benefiting from limited education, and may also be able to undertake relatively menial tasks. Those patients who survive beyond the age of 40 years usually show clinical and neuropathological evidence of Alzheimer's disease (Ohara 1972; Ellis, McCulloch, and Corley 1974).

References

Crome, L. C. and Stern, J. (1972). *Pathology of mental retardation*, 2nd edn. Churchill-Livingstone, London.

Ellis, W. G., McCulloch, J. R., and Corley, C. L. (1974). Presenile dementia in Down's syndrome. *Neurology, Minneapolis* **24**, 101.

Fairweather, D. V. I. (1982). Screening in pregnancy for congenital abnormality. *Br. J. Hosp. Med.* **28**, 602.

Jalanko, H. and Aula, P. (1982). Decrease in gamma-glutamyl transpeptidase activity in early amniotic fluid in fetal trisomy 18 syndrome. *Br. med. J.* **284**, 1593.

Menkes, J. H. (1980). *Textbook of child neurology*, 2nd edn. Lea and Febiger, Philadelphia.

Michaelson, P. S., and Gilles, F. H. (1972). Central nervous system abnormalities in Trisomy E (17–18) syndrome. *J. neurol. Sci.* **15**, 193.

Ohara, P. T. (1972). Electron microscopical study of the brain in Down's syndrome. *Brain* **95**, 681.

Stern, H., Elek, S. D., Booth, J. C., and Fleck, D. G. (1969). Microbial causes of mental retardation: the role of prenatal infections with cytomegalovirus, rubella virus, and toxoplasma. *Lancet*, **ii**, 443.

Mental retardation syndromes of undetermined cause

Many other syndromes of mental retardation accompanied by morphological changes in the nervous system and skeleton have been described in which no specific chromosomal or biochemical anomaly has yet been discovered. Crome and Stern (1972) listed over 50 syndromes which had identified including the de Lange syndrome (retardation, dwarfism, and characteristic facial and cranial appearances), Donohue's syndrome or leprechaunism, the Treacher Collins syndrome (craniofacial deformity, malar hypoplasia, microgenitalia, deafness), Cockayne's syndrome with impaired DNA repair, (p. 464), Menkes kinky hair disease (p. 467), the Prader–Willi syndrome (hypotonia, hypometria, hypogonadism, and mental retardation), the Riley–Day syndrome of dysautonomia (p. 599), and Sotos' syndrome of cerebral gigantism (p. 468).

Despite the enormous number of syndromes associated with mental retardation which are now recognized, it is still the case that the commonest cause remains that of so-called 'non-specific retardation' (Benton 1969; Menkes 1980) which may sometimes be familial (Dekaban and Klein 1968), a fact which constitutes a major public health problem and a challenge to future research. In many such cases there is evidence of some degree of microcephaly which may be due to manifold causes, including exposure to radiation or treatment of the mother with methyldopa for hypertension during pregnancy, among others (*The Lancet* 1979). The fact that non-specific retardation is commoner in males than females has led to the discovery that an X-linked recessive gene with a secondary constriction or fragile site on the X-chromosome (Sutherland 1977; *The Lancet* 1981) appears to be a common cause of the condition, being almost as common as Down's syndrome (Herbst and Millar 1980).

References

Benton, A. L. (1969). Neuropsychological aspects of mental retardation. *J. spec. Educ.* **4**, 3.

Crome, L. C. and Stern, J. (1972). *Pathology of mental retardation*, 2nd edn. Churchill-Livingstone, London.

Dekaban, A.S. and Klein, D. (1968). Familial mental retardation. *Acta genet., Basel* **18**, 206.

Herbst, D. S. and Miller, J. R. (1980). Non-specific X-linked mental retardation. II. The frequency in British Columbia. *Am. J. Med. Genet.* **7**, 461.

The Lancet (1979). Unclassified mental retardation. *Lancet* **i**, 250.

—— (1981). X-linked mental retardation. *Lancet* **i**, 1–86.

Menkes, J. H. (1980). *Textbook of child neurology*, 2nd edn. Lea and Febiger, Philadelphia.

Sutherland, G. R. (1977). Fragile sites on human chromosomes: demonstration of their dependence on the type of tissue culture medium. *Science* **197**, 265.

Carbon dioxide intoxication

In patients with chronic respiratory disease, especially chronic bronchitis and emphysema, it is now evident that neurological manifestations may result from the fact that the respiratory centre appears to become insensitive to carbon dioxide which is retained in the circulation as bicarbonate as a result of chronic alveolar hypoventilation. Chronic alveolar hypoventilation is also being recognized increasingly as a complication of various neuromuscular disorders including myasthenia gravis, muscular dystrophy, motor-neurone disease, and dystrophia myotonica (Buchsbaum, Martin, Turino, and Rowland 1968; Walton 1981); often in such cases severe diaphragmatic weakness can be demonstrated. In some such cases a chronic syndrome characterized by headache, lethargy, drowsiness, and fluctuating confusion persists for many weeks or months. In other cases, however, an acute syndrome characterized by severe headache and vomiting, convulsions, papilloedema, and rapid impairment of consciousness has been described, due to increasing cerebral oedema, and may be precipitated by the administration of oxygen. In many such patients it is necessary to give steroid drugs and diuretics to reduce brain swelling but intermittent positive-pressure respiration, monitored by measurements of the blood $p(O_2)$ and $p(CO_2)$ is the most effective treatment, in order to remove the accumulated CO_2 and, in time, to restore the sensitivity of the respiratory centre. In cases of neuromuscular disease with chronic respiratory insufficiency and CO_2 retention it may be difficult to decide whether or not assisted respiration is justified on ethical grounds. In muscular dystrophy of the Duchenne type this treatment is rarely justified in order briefly to prolong life in the presence of severe disability, but in other patients, suffering for instance from limb-girdle dystrophy, spinal muscular atrophy, or motor-neurone disease, severe respiratory insufficiency may develop at a time when the patient is still mobile. Intermittent external pulmonary insufflation with a respirator of the Bird type may be very effective in some such cases and may prolong useful life for many years.

Sleep apnoea syndromes, variants of the above, have been increasingly recognized in recent years (*The Lancet* 1979; Stradling 1982). The commonest cause is the obstructive type in which there is cessation of air flow because of passive collapse of the pharyngeal walls despite vigorous abdominal and thoracic inspiratory movements. Most such patients are obese and demonstrate loud snoring and daytime somnolence (the Pickwickian syndrome of hypersomnia with periodic apnoea) (Guilleminault, Cummiskey, and Dement 1980). In other cases there is central apnoea with transitory cessation of respiratory motor activity and nocturnal alveolar hypoventilation, usually due to one of the conditions mentioned above, though the syndrome may also occur in patients with chronic bronchitis and emphysema or with Ondine's curse (Dooling and Richardson 1977) as well as the Shy–Drager syndrome (Chokroverty, Sharp, and Barron 1978). This syndrome may be an occasional cause of sudden infant death (Armstrong, Sachis, Bryan, and Becker 1982; *The Lancet* 1984) and may certainly account for sudden unexpected death in adults. Removal of any lesion (e.g. enlarged tonsils) which obstructs the respiratory pathway may be beneficial in obstructive cases.

References

Armstrong, D., Sachis, P., Bryan, C., and Becker, L. (1982). Pathological features of persistent infantile sleep apnea with reference to the pathology of sudden infant death syndrome. *Ann. Neurol.* **12**, 169.

Buchsbaum, H. W., Martin, W. A., Turino, G. M., and Rowland, L. P. (1968). Chronic alveolar hypoventilation due to muscular dystrophy. *Neurology, Minneapolis* **18**, 319.

Chokroverty, S., Sharp, J. T., and Barron, K. D. (1978). Periodic respiration in erect posture in Shy–Drager syndrome. *J. Neurol. Neurosurg. Psychiat.* **41**, 980.

Dooling, E. C. and Richardson, E. P. (1977). Ophthalmoplegia and Ondine's curse. *Arch. Ophthalmol.* **95**, 1790.

Fishman, A. P., Turino, G. M., and Bergofolly, E. H. (1957). The syndrome of alveolar hypoventilation. *Am. J. Med.* **23**, 333.

Guilleminault, C., Cummiskey, J., and Dement, W. C. (1980). Sleep apnea syndrome: recent advances. *Adv. intern. Med.* **26**, 347.

The Lancet (1979). Sleep apnoea syndrome. *Lancet* **i**, 25.

—— (1984) Ventilatory dysfunction and sudden infant death syndrome. *Lancet* **ii**, 558.

Manfredi, F., Fieker, H. O., Spoto, A. P., and Saltzman, H. A. (1960). Severe carbon dioxide intoxication. *J. Am. med. Ass.* **173**, 999.

Plum, F. and Posner, J. B. (1980). *The diagnosis of stupor and coma*, 3rd edn. Davis, Philadelphia.

Stradling, J. R. (1982). Obstructive sleep apnoea syndrome. *Br. med. J.* **285**, 528.

Walton, J. N. (1981). Clinical examination of the neuromuscular system. In *Disorders of voluntary muscle* (ed. J. N. Walton), 4th edn. Chapter 13, Churchill-Livingstone, Edinburgh.

16

Deficiency disorders

The isolation of the vitamins and the study of their physiological properties and of the effects of their lack upon animals in experimental conditions led to the hope that vitamin deficiency in man would be recognizable in a similarly clear-cut manner; but greater clinical experience of nutritional disorders during the Second World War resulted in a more critical attitude to a problem which is now seen to be more complex than was first thought. The patient suffering from nutritional deficiency has usually been partially starved for a long time. His disorder is often chronic; different vitamins are likely to have been lacking in varying proportions in different circumstances; other dietary elements may well also have been inadequate; acute and chronic gastrointestinal and other infections are complicating factors acting both through the toxins they produce and also by interfering with food absorption. We are thus presented with variable and often overlapping clinical pictures which cannot often be correlated with specific deficiencies. It seems best, therefore, first to review the physiology of those vitamins whose lack is believed to cause nervous disorders and then to describe the chief syndromes which appear to be caused by nutritional deficiency.

Vitamins A and D
Vitamin A deficiency causes night blindness, xerophthalmia, and keratomalacia and usually occurs in association with protein–calorie malnutrition in young children in tropical countries, a condition which can also be associated with impaired cerebral development and/or myopathy and polyneuropathy (Dastur, Manghani, Osuntokun, Sourander, and Kondo 1982). Secondary deficiency can occur in malabsorption syndromes and liver disease (see McLaren 1983). Vitamin D deficiency, whether due to lack of exposure to sunlight, to malnutrition or malabsorption, or to the many disorders which secondarily affect calcium metabolism (see Kanis 1983), gives rise to rickets in young children or osteomalacia in adults and can cause a severe but reversible proximal myopathy at any age (p. 576).

Excessive intake of these vitamins may also be harmful. Hypervitaminosis A due to excessive consumption of polar bear or seal liver (in Arctic explorers) or to excess consumption of cod liver oil or vitamin tablets, has been known to cause headache, drowsiness, vomiting, generalized weakness, and dryness of the skin. A possible relationship between vitamin A and hydrocephalus is mentioned on p. 137. Excess vitamin D can cause hypercalcaemia (p. 489).

The B group of vitamins
Experimental work has led to the isolation of a number of factors in the vitamin B complex, five of which need especially to be considered in relation to nervous disease: these are vitamins B_1 (thiamine or aneurine), nicotinic acid (niacin), B_2 (riboflavine), B_6 (pyridoxine), and B_{12}. The B group of vitamins are present in greatest amount in brewers' yeast, in the germ and aleurone layer of ripe wheat, and also in egg yolk and mammalian liver, and in smaller amounts (except for B_{12}, present in greater quantities) in milk, green vegetables, potatoes, and meat.

Vitamin B_1 (thiamine)
This vitamin plays an important part in the glycolytic and pentose phosphate pathways of glucose metabolism. It forms a compound with pyrophosphoric acid which acts as co-enzyme A to the enzyme which breaks down pyruvic acid, an intermediate product in the breakdown of glucose. A deficiency of thiamine, by interfering with the breakdown of pyruvic acid, leads to an accumulation of pyruvic acid in the blood. A rise in serum pyruvate may therefore be helpful diagnostically, but measurement of erythrocyte transketolase activity before and after the addition of thiamine pyrophosphate (TPP) is more sensitive. There is a close biochemical relationship between the effects of thiamine deficiency and the changes occuring in Leigh's subacute necrotizing encephalopathy (see p. 466), in which there is defective activation of pyruvate dehydrogenase in both affected children and adults (DeVivo, Haymond, Obert, Nelson, and Pagliara 1979; Kalimo, Lundberg, and Olsen 1979; Plaitakis, Whetsell, Cooper, and Yahr 1980; Sorbi and Blass 1982) and in which thiamine pyrophosphate accumulates in affected areas of the brain (Pincus, Solitaire, and Cooper 1976). Acute experimental deficiency in pigeons causes opisthotonos, chronic deficiency 'locomotor ataxia', weakness of the legs, cardiac failure, peripheral neuropathy, and brain haemorrhages. Experimental thiamine deficiency in rats caused 'ragged-red' muscle fibres with abnormal mitochondria and lipid droplets as well as demyelination in peripheral nerves (Kark, Brown, Edgerton, Reynolds, and Gibson 1975).

The minimum requirement of thiamine in the day's food is not more than 1.5–3 mg. Thiamine deficiency may be detected by a subnormal blood level (less than 3 μg per 100 ml), diminished urinary excretion after a test dose, or by the biochemical methods mentioned above.

Nicotinic acid
Nicotinic acid or niacin acts as a co-enzyme in intracellular oxidation processes. The daily requirements of an adult are probably about 20 mg. The essential amino acid tryptophan is a niacin precursor and hence phaeochromocytoma of the adrenal can cause pellagra by converting tryptophan into 5-hydroxytryptamine, while in Hartnup disease (p. 453) pellagra results from failure of tryptophan absorption. Deficiency of nicotinic acid produces in dogs a condition known as 'black-tongue', which is very similar to human pellagra. There is diminished excretion of N-methylnicotinamide and its pyridones in the urine.

Riboflavine
Riboflavine also acts as a co-enzyme in carbohydrate breakdown. It is the precursor of two flavoprotein co-enzymes, namely flavin mononucleotide and flavine adenine dinucleotide, and thus plays a part in many important metabolic processes (Rivlin 1970; Van Itallie and Follis 1974). The daily minimal requirement in man is probably 2–3 mg. Riboflavine deficiency causes angular stomatitis, glossitis, injection of the limbus of the cornea, and in some cases abnormal corneal vascularization.

Pyridoxine
Vitamin B_6 is a combination of three naturally occurring pyridines, namely pyridoxine, pyridoxal, and pyridoxinine. The first is found mainly in plant foods, the latter two in animal products; in the average diet, pyridoxine is the main source of vitamin activity. Pyridoxine aids the conversion of tryptophan to N-methyl nicotinamide. In infants reared on a pyridoxine-deficient diet, convulsions and anaemia were noted. In adults living on a diet deficient in this vitamin or in those receiving desoxypyridoxine, or more often, isoniazid, hydrallazine, or penicillamine (these substances are pyridoxine antagonists), symmetrical polyneuropathy, optic

atrophy and/or microcyic anaemia may develop and each can be corrected by administration of this vitamin. Pyridoxine also antagonizes the action of levodopa. Pyridoxine deficiency can best be detected by measuring it in the serum (a figure of less than 25 ng/ml indicates deficiency) or by finding an excretion of xanthurenic acid of more than 50 mg/day in the urine after a 2 g load of tryptophan.

Vitamin E

While vitamin E deficiency in animals is known to cause myopathy, until recently there was little evidence to implicate vitamin E in the pathogenesis of human disease. However, as Muller, Lloyd, and Wolff (1983) point out, early therapy with vitamin E in abetalipoproteinaemia delays or may even prevent neurological complications, and in established cases it may arrest or reverse the neuropathy. Secondly, in disorders of fat absorption with severe vitamin E deficiency, neurological manifestations may be improved by vitamin E. Finally, neuropathological abnormalities have been described in vitamin E deficiency states (such as cystic fibrosis) in man which resemble those of experimental vitamin E deficiency in animals. Spinocerebellar degeneration giving dysarthria, ataxia, severe proprioceptive loss, and diminished tendon reflexes has been described as a complication of chronic fat malabsorption and has been shown to be due to vitamin E deficiency (Harding, Muller, Thomas, and Willison 1982).

References

Beaupre, E. M. and Grouney, P. M. (1963). Pyridoxine-responsive anaemia with neuropathy. *Ann. intern. Med.* **59**, 724.

Dastur, D. K., Manghani, D. K., Osuntokun, B. O., Sourander, P. and Kondo, K. (1982). Neuromuscular and related changes in malnutrition: a review. *J. neurol. Sci.* **55**, 207.

DiVivo, D. C., Haymond, M. W., Obert, K. A., Nelson, J. S. and Pagliara, A. S. (1979). Defective activation of the pyruvate dehydrogenase complex in subacute necrotizing encephalomyelopathy (Leigh disease). *Ann. Neurol.* **6**, 483.

Harding, A. E., Muller, D. P. R., Thomas, P. K. and Willison, H. J. (1982). Spinocerebellar degeneration secondary to chronic intestinal malabsorption: a vitamin E deficiency syndrome. *Ann. Neurol.* **12**, 419.

Kalimo, H., Lundberg, P. O. and Olsson, Y. (1979). Familial subacute necrotizing encephalomyelopathy of the adult form (adult Leigh syndrome). *Ann. Neurol.* **6**, 200.

Kanis, J. A. (1983). Disorders of calcium metabolism. In *Oxford textbook of medicine* (ed. D. J. Weatherall, J. G. G. Ledingham and D. A. Warrell), p. 10.4. Oxford University Press, Oxford.

Kark, R. A. P., Brown, W. J., Edgerton, V. R., Reynolds, S. F. and Gibson, G. (1975). Experimental thiamine deficiency. Neuropathic and mitochondrial changes induced in rat muscle. *Arch. Neurol., Chicago* **32**, 818.

McLaren, D. S. (1983). Vitamins and trace elements. In *Oxford textbook of medicine* (ed. D. J. Weatherall, J. G. G. Ledingham, and D. A. Warrell) p 8.21. Oxford University Press, Oxford.

Muller, D. P. R., Lloyd, J. K. and Wolff, P. H. (1983). Vitamin E and neurological function. *Lancet* i, 225.

Pincus, J. H., Solitare, G. B. and Cooper, J. R. (1976). Thiamine triphosphate levels and histopathology. *Arch. Neurol., Chicago* **33**, 759.

Plaitakis, A., Whetsell, W. O., Cooper, J. R. and Yahr, M. D. (1980). Chronic Leigh disease: a genetic and biochemical study. *Ann. Neurol.* **7**, 304.

Rivlin, R. S. (1970). Riboflavin metabolism. *New Engl. J. Med.* **283**, 463.

Sorbi, S. and Blass, J. P. (1982). Abnormal activation of pyruvate dehydrogenase in Leigh disease fibroblasts. *Neurology, Minneapolis* **32**, 555.

Stannus, H. S. (1944). Some problems in riboflavin and allied deficiencies. *Br. med. J.* **2**, 103, 140.

Swank, R. L. (1940). Avian thiamine deficiency. A correlation of pathology and clinical behaviour. *J. exp. Med.* **71**, 683.

—— and Prados, M. (1942). Avian thiamine deficiency, *Arch. Neurol. Psychiat., Chicago* **47**, 97.

Van Itallie, T. B. and Follis, R. H. (1974). Thiamine deficiency, ariboflavinosis and vitamin B₆ deficiency. In *Harrison's principles of internal medicine*, 7th edn. Chapter 78. McGraw-Hill, New York.

Vilter, R. W., Mueller, J. E., Glazer, H. S., Jarrold, A. J., Thompson, C.

and Hawkins, V. R. (1963). The effect of vitamin B₆ deficiency produced by desoxypyridoxine in human beings. *J. Lab. clin. Med.* **42**, 335.

Beriberi

Aetiology

The discovery that beriberi was due to dietary deficiency of vitamin B₁, or thiamine, which was contained in the germinal layer discarded from polished rice, was of major importance in preventing and treating the disease. There are, however, problems in the aetiology of beriberi which still remain unsolved. Thiamine is not just an antineuritic vitamin in the sense that its absence from the diet necessarily causes neuritis, for this does not occur in animals unless they are also given carbohydrates, and in man a fall in the ratio of thiamine to carbohydrate and protein in the diet is also a causal factor, beriberi occurring when the ratio of mg of thiamine per 1000 non-fat calories falls below 0.3. Since thiamine is necessary for normal carbohydrate metabolism, these observations suggest that the nervous system and heart suffer in beriberi either from an inability to metabolize carbohydrates normally or because the pentose phosphate pathway is needed not only for carbohydrate metabolism but also for lipid synthesis. Other causal factors are chronic diarrhoea which interferes with the absorption of thiamine, liver disease which probably impairs its storage, and physical exertion which increases the need of the tissues for it.

Any or all of these factors may combine with dietary deficiency to cause beriberi among prisoners of war or under-nourished people. There is no doubt that it can also occur in patients whose diet is not deficient in thiamine but who suffer from gastrointestinal disorders which impair its absorption, such as pyloric stenosis, gastro-enterostomy, ulcerative colitis, dysentery, and steatorrhoea. Chronic alcoholism may cause beriberi by leading to both a defective intake and impaired absorption of thiamine, while the high calorie value of the alcohol increases the need for thiamine and hence the relative deficiency. Pregnancy also increases the demand for the vitamin. Vitamin B deficiency is also seen, even in highly-developed countries, in elderly people living alone on inadequate diets and may even result from the anorexia which sometimes accompanies chronic endogenous depression or anorexia nervosa (Kanis, Brown, Fitzpatrick, Hibbert, Horn, Nairn, Shirling, Strong and Alton 1974).

Pathology

The changes in the peripheral nervous system are those of axonal neuropathy with secondary demyelination (Prineas 1970; Takahashi and Nakamura 1976; Ohnishi, Tsuji, Igisu, Murai, Goto, Kuroiwa, Tsujihata and Takamori 1980) (see p. 524), involving both the somatic and autonomic nerves. This is the so-called 'dry' form. There may be chromatolysis in the ganglion cells of the anterior horns and dorsal root ganglia of the spinal cord, and of the motor nuclei of the cranial nerves. The changes in the muscles are those of denervation. In the 'wet' form of beriberi there is also myocardial degeneration, with enlargement of the right side of the heart, chronic venous congestion of the liver and spleen, effusions in the pleural cavities and pericardium, ascites, and oedema of the skin and subcutaneous tissues. Patients dying in the acute stage show congestion and haemorrhagic injection of the pyloric antrum and duodenum.

Symptoms and signs

The onset in some cases is very rapid, especially in infants, but fulminating beriberi is occasionally seen in the adult (Baron and Oliver 1958). In others it is more gradual, and mild cases occur. In the most acute cases symptoms of polyneuropathy develop within 24 or 48 hours. These consist of paraesthesiae and tenderness of the limbs, sensory loss, and progressive atrophic paralysis, with loss of reflexes. The paralysis may spread rapidly to involve all the muscles of both the upper and lower limbs and finally the laryngeal muscles, intercostals, and diaphragm. Manifestations of cardiac involvement include dyspnoea and palpitations, tachycardia, cardiac dilatation, and signs of heart failure. Oedema may be slight or extreme. Gastrointestinal dysfunction can cause either constipation or diarrhoea.

In chronic cases the clinical picture is that of a polyneuropathy with or without cardiac failure.

Diagnosis

The diagnosis of polyneuropathy is discussed on page 524. In wet beriberi the combination of polyneuropathy and cardiac failure is unique. The dry form must be distinguished from neuropathy due to other causes. Tenderness of the calves and excessive sensitivity of the skin on the soles of the feet are often more striking in B_1-deficiency neuropathy than in any other. Beriberi should be suspected when the diet has been deficient for any reason or there is evidence of malabsorption. The pyruvic acid in the blood is often raised in beriberi above the normal content of 0.4–1.0 mg per dl, and a pyruvate tolerance test may be helpful (Joiner, McArdle and Thompson 1950) but measurement of urinary thiamine (less than 65 μg per g creatinine is considered abnormal) and of erythrocyte transketolase activity is more reliable. Since many heavy metals produce polyneuropathy by acting as competitive inhibitors of co-enzyme A or by combining with SH groups which are necessary in this reaction, the possibility of occult heavy metal poisoning should be borne in mind.

Prognosis

In untreated fulminating cases death may occur within a few days from heart failure. Patients who survive the acute stage without treatment are left with evidence of a chronic polyneuropathy with or without heart failure. Most patients who receive early and thorough treatment during the acute stage make a complete recovery, and remain well as long as they continue to take an adequate diet and/or are able to absorb thiamine. Treatment may produce some improvement even in the chronic stage, but these patients may not recover completely.

Treatment

The heart failure must be treated by bed rest. The diet should consist of frequent small feeds with a minimum of carbohydrates and fluid. Thiamine, 50 mg should be injected intramuscularly at once. There is usually an immediate response, but diuretics and digoxin may also be needed. Oral treatment with 50 mg thiamine three times daily should be continued for some days, the dose later being reduced to a maintenance level of 5–10 mg daily. The usual physiotherapeutic treatment of polyneuropathy should be carried out, and a diet rich in thiamine and other B vitamins should be given. Indeed, it is wise to give nicotinic acid, riboflavine, and pyridoxine as well and to be sure that there is no evidence of associated vitamin B_{12} deficiency. Chronic alcoholics should be treated for alcohol addiction. Patients in whom deficiency is secondary to gastrointestinal disease or to endogenous depression will need appropriate treatment.

References

Baron, J. H. and Oliver, L. C. (1958). Fulminating beriberi. *Lancet* i, 354.
Goodhart, R. S. and Sinclair, H. M. (1940). Deficiency of vitamin B_1 in man as determined by the blood cocarboxylase. *J. biol. Chem.* **132**, 11.
Joiner, C. L., McArdle, B. and Thompson, R. H. S. (1950). Blood pyruvate estimations in the diagnosis and treatment of polyneuritis. *Brain* **73**, 431.
Kanis, J. A., Brown, P., Fitzpatrick, K., Hibbert, D. J., Horn, D. B., Nairn, I. M., Shirling, D., Strong, J. A. and Walton, H. J. (1974). Anorexia nervosa: a clinical, psychiatric and laboratory study. *Quart. J. Med.* **43**, 321.
Ohnishi, A., Tsuji, S., Igisu, H., Murai, Y., Goto, I., Kuroiwa, Y., Tsujihata, M. and Takamori, M. (1980). Beriberi neuropathy: morphometric study of sural nerve. *J. neurol. Sci.* **45**, 17.
Prineas, J. (1970). Peripheral nerve changes in thiamine-deficient rats. *Arch. Neurol., Chicago* **23**, 541.
Spillane, J. D. (1973). *Tropical neurology.* Oxford Medical, London.
Takahashi, K. and Nakamura, H. (1976). Axonal degeneration in beriberi neuropathy. *Arch. Neurol., Chicago* **33**, 836.
Victor, M. and Adams, R. D. (1961). On the etiology of the alcoholic neurological diseases. *Am. J. clin. Nutr.* **9**, 379.
Walshe, F. M. R. (1918–19). On the 'deficiency theory' of the origin of beri-beri in the light of clinical and experimental observations on the disease with an account of a series of 40 cases. *Quart. J. Med.* **12**, 320.
Williams, R. R. (1961). *Toward the conquest of beriberi.* Harvard University Press, Cambridge, Massachusetts.

Wernicke's encephalopathy

Synonym. Polio-encephalitis haemorrhagica superior (an obsolete term).

Definition. An acute or subacute disorder affecting chiefly the midbrain and hypothalamus, caused by thiamine deficiency and characterized pathologically by congestion, capillary proliferation, and petechial haemorrhages, and clinically by disorders of memory and consciousness, ophthalmoplegia, and ataxia.

Aetiology

Experimental work has shown that a condition identical with Wernicke's encephalopathy can be produced in animals fed a diet deficient in thiamine. In man the fasting level of pyruvate in the blood has been found to be invariably elevated, and to return to normal after the administration of thiamine parallel with clinical improvement.

The deficiency may be due to various causes. An inadequate diet was the cause of Wernicke's encephalopathy in prisoners of war, and in civil life the causes are the same as those which produce beriberi, namely, inadequate diet, chronic alcoholism (Victor and Adams 1961), gastrointestinal disorders, especially carcinoma of the stomach, persistent vomiting of pregnancy, and anorexia nervosa (Handler and Perkin 1982). The condition has also been recorded after gastrectomy, as a complication of the vomiting due to digitalis poisoning (Richmond 1959), and of chronic haemodialysis (Lopez and Collins 1968). The condition is more common than is generally realized; in one series of 51 cases, only seven were diagnosed during life (Harper 1979; *British Medical Journal* 1979).

Pathology

In confirmation of Wernicke's original description of the pathology, the essential lesion consists of foci of marked congestion with many small petechial haemorrhages affecting particularly the hypothalamus and the grey matter of the upper brainstem. The corpora mammillaria are constantly involved (Harper 1979), and often there is also a zone of congestion with petechiae in the grey matter immediately surrounding the third ventricle, i.e. throughout the hypothalamus and medial part of the thalamus on each side. Foci are also seen often in the posterior colliculi of the midbrain, and less frequently in the grey matter of the floor of the fourth ventricle and other regions. They have also been described in the optic nerves. Histologically the essential lesion seems to be one of dilatation and proliferation of capillaries with small perivascular haemorrhages. Pathological changes are similar in vitamin-deficient alcoholic patients with the Korsakow syndrome but without the clinical features of Wernicke's disease (Mair, Warrington and Weiskrantz 1979). Damage to nerve cells is usually surprisingly slight. Some chronic and atypical cases have been reported with less widespread pathological changes (Grunnet 1969).

Symptoms and signs

The onset is usually insidious. Vomiting and nystagmus are early symptoms. The patient may experience a sense of unreality; he has difficulty in concentrating and sleeps badly. This condition passes into a confusional state which ends in stupor and coma (Wallis, Willoughby and Baker 1978). Hypothermia presumed to be due to posterior hypothalamic involvement has been reported (Philip and Smith 1973). In less severe and acute cases the mental changes are usually those of Korsakow's syndrome with defects of recent memory and confabulation. The ophthalmoplegia usually begins with weakness of the lateral recti and horizontal and/or vertical nystagmus with variable defects of conjugate gaze are common (Cogan and Victor 1954). There is usually some limb ataxia. Retinal haemorrhages may be present. Often Wernicke's encephalopathy is accompanied by polyneuropathy, but not invariably.

Diagnosis

The diagnosis is suggested by the occurrence of cerebral symptoms in a patient in whom one of the predisposing causes already mentioned is present, and may be confirmed by other chemical and biochemical evidence of thiamine deficiency. Wernicke's encephalopathy is most often confused with acute encephalitis in which, however, fever is present, with a pleocytosis in the CSF. Associated features of the Korsakow syndrome and polyneuropathy will clinch the diagnosis.

Prognosis

Wernicke's encephalopathy if untreated is often fatal. In prisoner-of-war camps the condition when diagnosed early and treated with the inadequate supplies of thiamine usually available had a mortality rate of 50 per cent. Intensive early treatment, however, usually leads to rapid and complete recovery, but in some cases the Korsakow syndrome may persist for months or occasionally for years after recovery from the acute stage. The latter does not respond to thiamine as completely and promptly as Wernicke's encephalopathy and recovery from it may be incomplete (see p. 654).

Treatment

The treatment is that of beriberi (see p. 475). As other deficiencies besides that of thiamine may be present it is advisable to give other B group vitamins in addition.

References

British Medical Journal (1979). Wernicke's encephalopathy. *Br. med. J.* **2**, 291.

Campbell, A. C. P. and Biggart, J. H. (1939). Wernicke's encephalopathy (polioencephalitis haemorrhagica superior): its alcoholic and non-alcoholic incidence. *J. Path. Bact.* **48**, 245.

—— and Russell, W. R. (1941). Wernicke's encephalopathy: the clinical features and their probable relationship to vitamin B deficiency. *Quart. J. Med.* **10**, 41.

Cogan, D. G. and Victor, M. (1954). Ocular signs of Wernicke's disease. *Arch. Ophthal.* **51**, 204.

Grunnet, M. L. (1969). Changing incidence, distribution and histopathology of Wernicke's polioencephalopathy. *Neurology, Minneapolis* **19**, 1135.

Handler, C. E. and Perkin, G. D. (1982). Anorexia nervosa and Wernicke's encephalopathy: an underdiagnosed association. *Lancet* **ii**, 771.

Harper, C. (1979). Wernicke's encephalopathy: a more common disease than realised. *J. Neurol. Neurosurg. Psychiat.* **42**, 226.

Lopez, R. I. and Collins, G. H. (1968). Wernicke's encephalopathy, *Arch. Neurol., Chicago* **18**, 248.

Mair, W. G. P., Warrington, E. K. and Weiskrantz, L. (1979). Memory disorder in Korsakoff's psychosis: a neuropathological and neuropsychological investigation of two cases. *Brain* **102**, 749.

Philip, G. and Smith, J. F. (1973). Hypothermia and Wernicke's encephalopathy. *Lancet* **ii**, 122.

Prados, M. and Swank, R. L. (1942). Vascular and interstitial cell changes in thiamine-deficient animals. *Arch. Neurol. Psychiat., Chicago* **47**, 626.

Richmond, J. (1959). Wernicke's encephalopathy associated with digitalis poisoning. *Lancet* **i**, 344.

Victor, M. and Adams, R. D. (1961). On the etiology of the alcoholic neurological diseases. *Am. J. clin. Nutr.* **9**, 379.

Wallis, W. E., Willoughby, E. and Baker, P. (1978). Coma in the Wernicke-Korsakoff syndrome. *Lancet* **ii**, 400.

Pellagra

Definition. A disease caused chiefly by deficiency of nicotinic acid (niacin), though lack of other essential food factors may contribute. It is characterized by cutaneous lesions, mental changes, glossitis, diarrhoea, and degeneration of the brain, spinal cord, and peripheral nerves.

Aetiology

Pellagra was once endemic in the poorer strata of the population in some South European countries, in Africa, and especially in the southern states of the USA. It is rare in Great Britain, where it is seen most often in elderly individuals living alone and in alcoholics. It can occur at any age and affects both sexes with equal frequency. It was once commonly, but not exclusively, found among white maize-eaters. The amino acid, tryptophan, is a nicotinic-acid precursor and dietary deficiency of tryptophan or nicotinic acid or both may produce the syndrome. The administration of nicotinic acid produces immediate improvement in affected patients, and will prevent the development of pellagra if added to a diet which otherwise produces it. As with other deficiency diseases, defective intestinal absorption of nicotinic acid is sometimes the cause of 'secondary' pellagra which may occur even though there is ample nicotinic acid in the diet. 'Secondary' pellagra may thus occur after dysentery or long-continued diarrhoea, after operation or cancer involving the stomach or small intestine, and in alcohol addicts. The combination of alcoholism and a deficient diet is an important cause of pellagra in some countries. In India, a high-leucine content in sorghum (jowar) contributes to the occurrence of pellagra but can be prevented by adding isoleucine to the diet (Krishnaswamy and Gopalan 1971). Pellagra-like skin lesions may be seen in Hartnup disease (p. 453). Rarely, similar skin lesions also appear in patients treated with isoniazid, a pyridoxine inhibitor, while in patients with the carcinoid syndrome (malignant argentaffinoma), the circulating serotonin may cause tryptophan deficiency and a pellagra-like syndrome. The disease of dogs, canine black tongue, like human pellagra, can be prevented and cured by nicotinic acid. Maize has been thought to contain an antivitamin to nicotinic acid.

Pathology

The meninges are thickened and the brain may be oedematous or atrophic. Chromatolysis and pigmentation are found in ganglion cells throughout the central nervous system and in autonomic ganglia. The spinal cord shows demyelination in many long tracts. This is most marked in the posterior columns in the upper thoracic and cervical regions, but the corticospinal and spinocerebellar tracts also suffer. Changes in peripheral nerves are less conspicuous, and consist mainly of patchy demyelination. Pigmentation and hyaline degeneration have been described in cerebral arterioles and capillaries.

The principal extraneural lesions are atrophy of the stomach and intestine and ulceration of the large bowel.

Symptoms and signs

In endemic areas the disease may run a protracted course over many years. The first attack and subsequent exacerbations tend to occur in the spring. The early attacks are characterized by gastro-intestinal disturbances, especially diarrhoea, associated with development of the cutaneous lesions. The latter begin with erythema in the parts of the body exposed to light, while later the deeper layers of the skin are involved, leading to desquamation, thickening, and finally atrophy. Exceptionally cutaneous lesions are absent. The tongue shows glossitis, with loss of epithelium, and similar changes occur in the pharynx. Gastric achylia is the rule and porphyrinuria is sometimes present. Nervous changes develop later. Many abnormal mental states occur, depending in part on the psychological constitution of the patient. Mania and melancholia are seen, the latter sometimes leading to suicide. Often the terminal state is dementia. Visual impairment and diplopia may occur. Dysarthria and dysphagia may develop in the later stages, together with tremor and ataxia, especially in the lower limbs. The tendon jerks may be increased at first, but are later lost. The plantar reflexes may be extensor, but spastic paraparesis is relatively rare. Sensory symptoms consist of pain in the limbs with tender muscles and superficial anaesthesia and analgesia, often with loss of appreciation of passive movements of the toes. Nicotinic-acid deficiency has also been regarded as the cause of an encephalopathy leading to stupor or coma. As mentioned above, decreased excretion of N-methylnicotinamide in the urine may assist in diagnosis (see McLaren 1983).

Diagnosis

The clinical picture is unique, and can hardly be confused with anything else, but in the absence of the cutaneous lesions the nervous condition may resemble subacute combined degeneration.

Prognosis

The prognosis in the past was poor, many patients ending their days in mental hospitals. Early treatment, however, is curative in most cases.

Treatment

Treatment is primarily dietetic. However, in acutely ill patients, water and electrolyte disturbances may demand intravenous fluid. Nicotinamide should be given rather than nicotinic acid to avoid vasomotor side-effects of the latter. In the early stages 100 mg may be given if need be intravenously or intramuscularly; later 200 mg two or three times a day by mouth is sufficient. Frequent small meals should be given at first followed by a high-calorie diet; as many vitamin deficiencies are multiple, other B group vitamins should usually be given as well.

References

Ellinger, P., Benesch, R. and Hardwick, S. W. (1945). Nicotinamide methochloride elimination tests on normal and nicotinamide-deficient persons. *Lancet* **ii**, 197.
Greenfield, J. G. and Holmes, J. M. (1939). A case of pellagra. The pathological changes in the spinal cord. *Br. med. J.* **1**, 815.
Jolliffe, N., Bowman, K. M., Rosenblum, L. A. and Fein, H. D. (1940). Nicotinic acid and deficiency encephalopathy. *J. Am. med. Ass.* **114**, 307.
Krishnaswamy, K. and Gopalan, C. (1971). Effect of isoleucine on skin and electroencephalogram in pellagra. *Lancet* **ii**, 1167.
Langworth, O. R. (1931). Lesions of the central nervous system characteristic of pellagra. *Brain* **54**, 291.
McLaren, D. S. (1983). Vitamins and trace elements. In *Oxford textbook of medicine* (ed. D. J. Weatherall, J. G. G. Ledingham and D. A. Warrell), p. 8.21. Oxford University Press, Oxford.
Moser, H., Victor, M. and Adams, R. D. (1974). Metabolic and nutritional diseases of the nervous system. In *Harrison's principles of internal medicine*, 7th edn., Chapter 332. McGraw-Hill, New York.
Spillane, J. D. (1947). *Nutritional disorders of the nervous system.* Livingstone, Edinburgh.
—— (1973). *Tropical neurology.* Oxford Medical, London.
Sydenstricker, V. P. (1958). The history of pellagra, its recognition as a disorder of nutrition and its conquest. *Am. J. clin. Nutr.* **6**, 409.
—— and Cleckley, H. M. (1941). Effects of nicotinic acid in stupor, lethargy and various other psychiatric disorders. *Am. J. Psychiat.* **98**, 83.

Nutritional neuropathies of obscure origin

For many years doctors practising in the tropics (Spillane 1973) have been familiar with syndromes which occurred either alone or in association with beriberi, pellagra, or ariboflavinosis. Fresh attention was directed to these during the Spanish Civil War and the Second World War. They appear to be due to malnutrition though some may be due to toxic substances in food; various views are held about their causation. Treatment with riboflavine, thiamine, and nicotinic acid has not afforded conclusive evidence that any of these alone is the deficient factor and it seems probable that there are often multiple deficiencies as well as some imbalance between various constituents of the diet.

Painful feet. There are burning sensations in the soles, especially severe at night and accompanied by hyperalgesia and sweating, and later by a changeable and patchy hyperaesthesia. Hyperkeratosis and itching of scrotal skin is a common accompaniment. This syndrome has been attributed to deficiency of nicotinic acid, but deficiency of pantothenic acid also seems likely to be a most important factor.

Nutritional neuropathy in former prisoners of war. Gibberd and Simmons (1980) studied 4684 former Far-East prisoners of war and found evidence of optic atrophy and peripheral neuropathy in 679 of them. In 89 cases, however, signs of spinal-cord dysfunction or Parkinson's disease, with an incidence far higher than in the general population, developed many years after the end of the Second World War. Gill and Bell (1982), in a similar group, noted optic atrophy, peripheral neuropathy (of the 'burning feet' type), and sensorineural deafness, persisting for up to 36 years after the original period of malnutrition (Le Quesne 1983).

Tropical ataxic neuropathy. This begins with dysaesthesiae in the feet, gradually followed by unsteadiness of gait. Sensory loss is prominent. Appreciation of vibration is lost first in the lower limbs, then awareness of passive movement, first in the toes, then more proximally. Cutaneous sensory loss appears and spreads up to the knees or even the waist. The knee- and ankle-jerks are usually exaggerated but the plantar reflexes are flexor. The condition has been reported from West Africa (Money 1961; Monekosso 1964), from Tanganyika (Haddock, Ebrahim, and Kapur 1962), and from Senegal (Collomb, Quere, Cros, and Giordono 1967). In many cases the clinical picture is purely one of sensory ataxia, often of sudden onset, but amblyopia and optic atrophy and pyramidal tract involvement have been found in some cases. Collomb et al. (1967) pointed out that in Senegal polyneuropathy occurred in 63 per cent of cases, spastic paraparesis in 21 per cent, and a combination of spasticity and ataxia in 16 per cent. Optic and auditory nerve involvement were present in 32 per cent; most sufferers had severe protein–calorie malnutrition and evidence of nicotinic acid and riboflavine deficiency.

Osuntokun (1968) reported 84 cases from Western Nigeria and found plasma and urinary thiocyanate levels to be raised in such patients. He concluded that the condition was due to chronic exposure to dietary cyanide, obtained from culinary derivatives of cassava, the tuber of manioc. Pathological changes included extensive demyelination in peripheral nerves; similar ultrastructural changes were found in the peripheral nerves of rats treated with cyanide (Williams and Osuntokun 1969). However, treatment with riboflavine and hydroxocobalamin had no effect upon the course of the illness (Osuntokun, Langman, Wilson, and Alidetoyinbo 1970). It is still uncertain as to whether this Nigerian ataxic neuropathy is the same condition as that which presents with very similar clinical manifestations in Senegal and other tropical countries (Spillane 1969, 1973).

Cranial nerve disorders. The commonest of these is acute or subacute retrobulbar neuropathy. Nerve-deafness, laryngeal palsy, anosmia, and trigeminal anaesthesia may also occur, with or without spinal ataxia. Monekosso and Ashby (1963) found an association of nutritional amblyopia and spinal ataxia in occasional cases.

In the West Indian amblyopia described by McKenzie and Phillips (1968), optic-disc pallor is accompanied by central or paracentral scotomata and the authors considered that cyanide intoxication was a causal factor. Plainly the condition shows close affinities to tropical ataxic neuropathy as described above, in which optic atrophy, nerve deafness, and sensory spinal ataxia are the commonest three manifestations (Osuntokun, Monekosso, and Wilson 1969).

Strachan's syndrome

This unexplained disorder, rarely reported in alcoholics in Jamaica and in the United States, or occurring as a complication of chronic liver disease or non-tropical sprue, is almost certainly of nutritional origin though no single deficiency factor has been identified (Moser, Victor, and Adams 1974). Progressive optic atrophy and peripheral paraesthesiae are the predominant symptoms with progressive ataxia and loss of both superficial and deep sensation associated with degeneration of sensory neurones and posterior root ganglia and ascending demyelination of the posterior columns of the cord. Motor involvement is uncommon, vertigo and deafness occur occasionally, and in some cases glossitis, corneal ulceration, and genital dermatitis are seen (the so-called orogenital syndrome). This rare syndrome, too, shows several similarities clinically to tropical ataxic neuropathy.

Spastic paraplegia. This was the rarest of these disorders among prisoners of war. Spillane (1947) pointed out its resemblances to lathyrism. Cruickshank, Montgomery, and Spillane (1961) reported cases of paraplegia of gradual or sudden onset in Jamaica associated with loss of posterior-column sensibility, retrobulbar neuritis, nerve-deafness, and occasionally distal wasting of limb muscles. Montgomery, Cruickshank, Robertson, and McMenemy (1964) analysed the clinical findings in 206 cases and the pathological findings in 10. There were 25 cases with ataxia, optic atrophy, and nerve-deafness resembling the other tropical neuropathies described above, and almost certainly due to malnutrition. In 181 cases, however, the picture was one of spastic paraparesis; most patients showed positive blood tests for syphilis, but these were negative in the CSF. Pathologically the affected spinal cords often showed evidence of chronic meningomyelitis. They considered that toxic food substances (bush tea) or nutritional deficiencies might in some way modify the clinical and pathological picture of neurosyphilis and so produce this syndrome. Mani and Montgomery (1969) described 35 cases from Southern India which resembled those observed in Jamaica. They found no evidence of cynaide intoxication in their cases and nothing to indicate that syphilis was responsible. They raised the possibility that the condition could be due to a slow virus infection.

Amblyopia (Behrman 1962) and spastic paraplegia (Jefferson 1963) have been reported in West Indian immigrants to the United Kingdom but in these cases, too, the aetiology remains unexplained (Spillane 1973). Spastic paraparesis certainly occurs in some cases of Nigerian tropical neuropathy but there the pathological changes in the spinal cord seem different from those found in the West Indies. On the other hand the amblyopic, auditory, and sensory ataxic syndromes observed in many tropical countries show many similarities. Much further work will be required to determine how many different syndromes exist and to identify the causal factors in each of them.

Treatment

The treatment of these tropical neuropathies must include the provision of a full balanced diet with vitamin supplements, particularly of the B group. If given before irreversible pathological changes have occurred there is sometimes, but not always, an encouraging response; in cases of West Indian or South Indian spastic paraplegia the usual treatment for syphilis should also be given but improvement, if any, is usually slight.

Lathyrism

The consumption of lathyrus peas, which are often eaten in India, may produce a slowly-progressive spastic paraplegia, especially when the peas are contaminated with seeds of the weed akta (*vicia sativa*) which contain certain alkaloids and a cyanogenetic glycoside. The toxic principle was identified as B-(N)oxalyl aminoalanine. The seed can be detoxified by steeping it in hot water or by parboiling it before cooking, which removes the substance (Wadia 1973).

References

Behrman, S. (1962). African race-influenced bilateral amblyopia among West Indian immigrants in the United Kingdom. *Br. J. Opthal.* **46**, 554.
Brain, W. R. (1947). Malnutrition of the nervous system. *Br. med. J.* **2**, 763.
Collomb, H., Quere, M. A., Cros, J., and Giordano, G. (1967). Les neuropathies dites nutritionnelles au Sénégal. *J. neurol. Sci.* **5**, 159.
Cruickshank, E. K., Montgomery, R. D., and Spillane, J. D. (1961). Obscure neurologic disorders in Jamaica. *Wld Neurol.* **2**, 99.
Denny-Brown, D. (1947). Neurological conditions resulting from prolonged and severe dietary restriction. *Medicine, Baltimore.* **26**, 41.
Gibberd, F. B. and Simmonds, J. P. (1980). Neurological disease in ex-Far-East prisoners of war. *Lancet* **ii**, 135.
Gill, G. V. and Bell, D. R. (1982). Persisting nutritional neuropathy amongst former war prisoners. *J. Neurol. Neurosurg. Psychiat.* **45**, 861.
Haddock, D. R. W., Ebrahim, G. J. and Kapur, B. B. (1962). Ataxic neurological syndrome found in Tanganyika. *Br. med. J.* **2**, 1442.
Jefferson, J. M. (1963). Jamaican neuromyelopathy. *Midl. med. Rev.* **3**, 37.
Le Quesne, P. M. (1983). Persisting nutritional neuropathy in former war prisoners. *Br. med. J.* **286**, 917.
Mani, K., Mani, A. and Montgomery, R. D. (1969). A spastic paraplegic syndrome in South India. *J. neurol. Sci.* **9**, 179.
McKenzie, A. D. and Phillips, C. I. (1968). West Indian amblyopia. *Brain* **91**, 249.
Monekosso, G. L. (1964). Clinical survey of a Yoruba village. *W. Afr. med. J.* **13**, 47.
—— and Ashby, P. H. (1963). The natural history of an amblyopia syndrome in Western Nigeria. *W. Afr. med. J.* **12**, 226.
Money, G. L. (1961). Etiology of funicular myelopathies in Tropical Africa. *Wld Neurol.* **2**, 526.
Montgomery, R. D., Cruickshank, E. K., Robertson, W. B. and McMenemey, W. H. (1964). Clinical and pathological observatons on Jamaican neuropathies—a report on 206 cases. *Brain* **87**, 425.
Moser, H., Victor, M. and Adams R. D. (1974). Metabolic and nutritional diseases of the nervous system. In *Harrison's principles of internal medicine*, 7th edn, Chapter 332. McGraw-Hill, New York.
Osuntokun, B. O. (1968). An ataxic neuropathy in Nigeria. A clinical, biochemical and electrophysiological study. *Brain* **91**, 215.
——, Langman, M. J. S., Wilson, J. and Aladetoyinbo, A. (1970).Controlled trial of hydroxocobalamin and riboflavine in Nigerian ataxic neuropathy. *J. Neurol. Neurosurg. Psychiat.* **33**, 663.
——, Monekosso, G. L. and Wilson, J. (1969). Relationship of a degenerative tropical neuropathy to diet: report of a field survey. *Br. med. J.* **1**, 547.
Spillane, J. D. (1947). *Nutritional disorders of the nervous system.* Livingstone, Edinburgh.
Spillane, J. D. (1973). *Tropical neurology.* Oxford Medical, London.
Spillane, J. D. and Scott, G. I. (1945). Obscure neuropathy in the Middle East. *Lancet* **ii**, 262.

Wadia, N. H. (1973). An introduction to neurology in India. In *Tropical neurology* (ed. J. D. Spillane), Chapter 1. Oxford Medical, London.

Williams, A. O. and Osuntokun, B. O. (1969). Peripheral neuropathy in tropical (nutritional) ataxia in Nigeria. *Arch. Neurol., Chicago* **21**, 475.

Vitamin B₁₂ neuropathy (subacute combined degeneration of the spinal cord and brain)

Synonyms. Posterolateral sclerosis; combined system disease.

Definition. A deficiency disease, usually associated with pernicious anaemia, and characterized pathologically by degeneration of the white matter of the spinal cord, most evident in the posterior and lateral columns, and of the peripheral nerves and brain, and clinically by paraesthesiae, impairment of position and joint sense, sensory ataxia, and paraparesis. Subacute combined degeneration was described by Leichtenstern in 1884, and the spinal-cord changes were associated with anaemia by Lichtheim in 1887. The first complete clinical and pathological account was given by Russell, Batten, and Collier (1900). Minot and Murphy discovered the therapeutic value of liver in 1926 and this led to the recognition of extrinsic and intrinsic factors by Castle and his collaborators. Lester Smith in England and Rickes, Brink, Koniuszy, Wood, and Folkers in America isolated the essential factor, cyanocobalamin, vitamin B₁₂, from the liver in 1948. Richmond and Davidson (1958) suggested that vitamin B₁₂ neuropathy is a better name than subacute combined degeneration.

Pathology

Macroscopic changes in the nervous system are slight. Slight cerebral atrophy may be seen, and on section of the cord demyelination is evident from the greyish appearance of the white matter. The principal pathological change is one of focal demyelination in localized areas widely scattered throughout the white matter, giving a 'spongy' appearance; often this is associated with an accumulation of lipid-filled macrophages and gemistocytic astrocytes. The lesions, which closely resemble those seen in experimental vitamin B₁₂ deficiency in animals, are most striking in the heavily myelinated fibres of the posterior columns but also involve the lateral columns, and axonal degeneration follows (Kunze and Leitenmaier 1976; Agamanolis, Chester, Victor, Kark, Hines, and Harris 1976; Davies-Jones, Preston, and Timperley 1980). Secondary degeneration of long tracts, especially involving the posterior columns and corticospinal tracts, follows. In the most severely affected regions both the myelin sheaths and the axis cylinders disappear, leaving vacuolated spaces separated by a fine glial meshwork (Fig. 16.1). Similar focal areas of degeneration may be found in the white matter of the brain, with degenerative changes especially in the cerebral association fibres (Adams and Kubik 1944). Peripheral-nerve lesions are also invariable with loss of the larger myelinated fibres in distal sensory nerves and evidence of axonal degeneration in teased single fibres (McLeod, Walsh, and Little 1969; Bradley 1974; Weller and Cervós-Navarro 1977; Asbury and Johnson 1978) although in experimental vitamin B₁₂ deficiency in monkeys, segmental demyelination predominates (Torres, Smith, and Oxnard 1971).

Usually the pathological changes of pernicious anaemia are found in fatal cases, now fortunately rare. These include glossitis, anaemia, hyperplasia of bone marrow in long bones, slight or moderate enlargement of the spleen, and excess iron in the reticulo-endothelial system. Magnus and Ungley (1938) found a profound atrophy of all coats of the stomach wall, localized to the body and sparing the pyloroduodenal region. The sera of about 60 per cent of patients with pernicious anaemia contain gastric parietal-cell antibodies which can interfere with the ability of intrinsic factor to promote normal physiological handling of vitamin B₁₂.

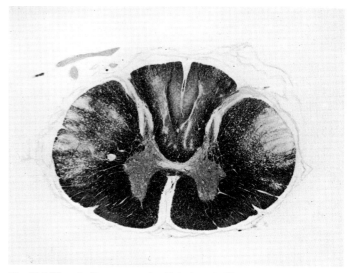

Fig. 16.1 Vitamin B₁₂ neuropathy. Spinal cord; C3.

Aetiology

Vitamin B₁₂ neuropathy is a disease of middle life, the average age of onset being about 50. It may, however, begin in the 20s or as late as 70. Both sexes are equally affected. Its familial ocurrence is uncommon, but well authenticated, and families have been described in which multiple cases of vitamin B₁₂ neuropathy and pernicious anaemia have occurred, sometimes in more than one generation.

In most cases vitamin B₁₂ neuropathy is associated with megaloblastic anaemia, but the relationship is a complicated one. At first it was thought that the spinal-cord degeneration was secondary to the anaemia, but the anaemia may be slight or even, exceptionally, absent, when the spinal degeneration is severe, while only 10–15 per cent of patients with Addisonian anaemia suffer from vitamin B₁₂ neuropathy (Waters and Mollin 1961; Reynolds 1976). And psychiatric syndromes of confusion, depression, and dementia have been observed as a result of avitaminosis B₁₂ with normal findings in the peripheral blood and marrow (Strachan and Henderson 1965). There is also evidence to suggest that tobacco amblyopia may be due to traces of cyanide in tobacco smoke which interfere with the utilization of vitamin B₁₂ and that the condition may be corrected by the administration of hydroxocobalamin but not by cyanocobalamin (Chisholm, Bronte-Stewart, and Foulds 1967).

The importance of gastric achylia lies not in the absence of gastric acidity but in the lack of an intrinsic factor, secreted by the normal stomach, which facilitates the absorption of an extrinsic factor, contained in the food. This is cyanocobalamin, a cobalt-containing complex isolated in a red crystalline form from the liver by Smith (1948) and Rickes *et al.* (1948) and called by the latter vitamin B₁₂. The only function of intrinsic factor is to render possible the absorption of extrinsic factor; this occurs in the terminal ileum; it is neccssary for normal haemopoiesis and the maintenance of the nutrition of the nervous system. The fact that absence of intrinsic factor is often associated with circulating serum antibodies against the gastric parietal cells which normally produce it is one of the several facts which suggest that pernicious anaemia is an auto-immune disease (Kunze and Leitenmaier 1976). There is also considerable evidence that methyl group transfer, necessary in the metabolism of myelin, requires the presence of both vitamin B₁₂ and methyltetrahydrofolic acid via the methionine synthetase reaction which is dependent upon B₁₂; methionine may possibly have a protective effect (Reynolds 1981). While failure to secrete intrinsic factor is thc usual fault, impaired absorption may also cause vitamin B_{12} neuropathy; so, too, may inadequate intake, as in vegans, a sect of strict vegetarians, who refuse to eat any animal products (Smith 1962).

Although vitamin B_{12} neuropathy is usually associated with pernicious anaemia, the blood count may be normal. Vitamin B_{12} neuropathy may also follow partial or total gastrectomy (Williams, Hall, Thompson, and Cooke 1969), intestinal disease, such as idiopathic steatorrhoea, regional ileitis, tropical sprue (Iyer, Taori, Kapadia, Mathan, and Baker 1973), and resections, diverticulosis and fistulae of the small intestine (Pallis and Lewis 1974). In such cases a megaloblastic anaemia may be due to either folic acid or vitamin B_{12} deficiency, and folic acid given for the anaemia may aggravate the neurological symptoms of B_{12} deficiency. Another rare cause of B_{12} neuropathy is inherited (autosomal recessive) congenital malabsorption of vitamin B_{12}. Malabsorption due to biologically inert intrinsic factor, to pancreatic disease, or to the effects of drugs (Kunze and Leitenmaier 1976) has also been described but no cases of neurological dysfunction due to these rare causes have been reported (Pallis and Lewis 1974).

Symptoms and signs

Neurological manifestations
The clinical picture is usually due to combined features of posterior-column, corticospinal-tract, and peripheral-nerve degeneration, but involvement of the optic nerves and brain is not uncommon.

The onset of symptoms is usually gradual, but is sometimes rapid. Indeed coma, myelopathy, and neuropathy of rapid onset with rapid improvement in many, but not all, symptoms following cyanocobalamin administration has been reported in a 23-year-old woman (Kosik, Mullins, Bradley, Tempelis, and Cretella 1980). The first symptoms are generally paraesthesiae, with tingling sensations, first felt in the tips of the toes, and later in the fingers. Less often both upper and lower extremities are involved simultaneously, or both hands may be first affected. Other paraesthesiae often described include sensations of numbness, coldness, and tightness, while sharp stabbing pains occasionally occur and many patients describe sensations as if the extremities were swollen or encased in tight bandages or constricting bands. The paraesthesiae, which usually begin in the feet and legs, tend to spread slowly up the trunk, and a sense of constriction around the chest or abdomen is common. Motor weakness and ataxia develop at a variable interval afterwards. The patient may first notice that he easily tires when walking, or that he walks unsteadily and tends to stumble.

Objective sensory changes are almost always present, involving first the forms of sensibility mediated by the posterior columns. Postural sensibility and appreciation of passive movement and of vibration are impaired first in the lower, and later in the upper limbs. Cutaneous sensibility to light touch, pin-prick, heat, and cold is impaired at first in the periphery, leading to the characteristic 'glove and stocking' distribution of superficial sensory loss. The calves may be tender on pressure. The proximal border of the anaesthetic areas may then ascend gradually.

In some cases weakness and spasticity, in others sensory ataxia, predominate in the lower limbs, but both weakness and sensory ataxia are usually present in all four limbs, and are most severe in the lower with a positive Romberg's sign. Moderate muscular wasting in the later stages due to the peripheral neuropathy, especially in the peripheral muscles, may develop.

The reflexes vary considerably. In about 50 per cent of cases the ankle-jerks are absent when the patient is first seen; the knee-jerks are lost rather less frequently; in other cases both are exaggerated. The plantar reflexes are flexor at first in about half the cases, but later become extensor in all but a few. When the degeneration is confined to the posterior columns, ataxia is the predominant symptom throughout and signs of corticospinal defect are lacking. Conversely, spastic paraplegia may alone be present while in yet other cases signs of peripheral neuropathy predominate.

Sphincter disturbances first give difficult or precipitate micturition, and later retention of urine or incontinence. Impotence sometimes occurs early.

Bilateral primary optic atrophy with some visual impairment is observed in about 5 per cent of cases and may even be the presenting feature with central scotomata (Freeman and Heaton 1961) (see p. 92); nystagmus is common. The pupils may be small, but react normally. Otherwise the cranial nerves are usually normal, though dysarthria occurs rarely.

Mental changes are common and their importance has been stressed by Holmes (1956), Fraser (1960), Strachan and Henderson (1965), Pallis and Lewis (1974), and Davies-Jones et al. (1980). They may be present without anaemia or signs of spinal-cord disease. There may be a mild dementia, with impaired memory and intellectual capacity, or a confusional psychosis with disorientation and paranoid tendencies, or Korsakow's syndrome; or the mental disorder may be predominantly affective, manifesting itself in irritability or severe depression. The CSF is normal. In pernicious anaemia, with or without symptoms and signs of involvement of the brain and spinal cord, the EEG may show diffuse slow activity and returns to normal after appropriate treatment (Samson, Swisher, Christian, and Engel 1952; Walton, Kiloh, Osselton, and Farrall 1954; Kunze and Leitenmaier 1976).

Associated manifestations
Gastric achlorhydria is constantly present in Addisonian anaemia, but free acid may be present in the gastric juice when the neuropathy is due to nutritional deficiency or malabsorption. There is usually macrocytic anaemia with a high mean cell volume, megalocytes or even megaloblasts in the circulating blood, poikilocytosis, anisocytosis, polychromatophilia, and leucopenia, with a relative lymphocytosis. Even when the peripheral blood count is normal, the bone marrow may be abnormal on sternal puncture. Glossitis is common, but may be slight or absent when the anaemia is not severe. Other symptoms may be present if anaemia is severe and include dyspnoea, the characteristic lemon tint of the skin, cardiac dilatation, haemic murmurs, and oedema, most marked in the lower limbs. The spleen is palpable in only a few cases. Gastrointestinal symptoms are common, especially anorexia, flatulence, and diarrhoea, particularly when the neuropathy is secondary to intestinal disease.

Diagnosis

The neurological picture must be distinguished from tabes, multiple sclerosis, spinal-cord compression, polyneuropathy, and Strachan's syndrome (p. 478). Reflex iridoplegia is usually present in tabes and the plantar responses are flexor (except in taboparesis), while in most cases the VDRL and other seriological reactions are positive in either the blood or the CSF if not in both.

In multiple sclerosis there is often evidence of multiple lesions with pallor of the optic discs and nystagmus. The ankle-jerks are usually exaggerated and very rarely diminished. Difficulty in diagnosis is most likely to arise in those cases characterized by progressive spastic paraplegia as is common in middle-aged patients. This disease, however, usually runs a much more chronic course than subacute combined degeneration, while anaemia is absent and the serum B_{12} normal.

Spinal compression may lead to an ataxic paraplegia of gradual onset. Careful examination, however, often indicates a well-defined upper level of the motor disability and sensory loss, a finding which is rare in B_{12} deficiency, while characteristic changes are usually found in the CSF and on myelography. Cervical spondylotic myelopathy may closely resemble the spinal lesions of vitamin B_{12} neuropathy, while cervical spondylosis and the neuropathy may coexist, in which case careful investigation of both will be required to assess their relative importance. When peripheral neuropathy due to vitamin B_{12} deficiency is associated with symptoms and signs of spinal-cord disease, distinction from other forms of peripheral neuropathy is not difficult, but when peripheral neuropathy is the sole or the predominant manifestation, this distinction may be wholly dependent upon estimation of the serum B_{12} and upon other diagnostic tests. Rarely there may be a coexistent deficiency of vitamin B_1 (Hornabrook and Marks 1960; Cox-Klazinga and Endtz 1980). Usually in B_{12} deficiency sensory manifestations are more severe than motor; the electrophysiological findings are predominantly those of an axonal neuropathy with evidence of partial denervation of distal limb muscles (Kosik et al. 1980). Visual evoked potentials may also show significant conduction delay (Troncoso, Mancall, and Schatz 1979).

When vitamin B_{12} neuropathy is suspected on neurological grounds and indeed, in any case in which this possibility exists, a blood count should be made and serum B_{12} should be estimated. The normal range is from 100 to 960 pg per ml. In vitamin B_{12} neuropathy the serum vitamin B_{12} is usually below 80 pg per ml. It should be noted that chlorpromazine and some other drugs may interfere with estimation of the serum B_{12}, giving falsely low levels (Herbert, Gottlieb, and Altschule 1965). Another useful test is the investigation of vitamin B_{12} absorption using radioactive B_{12} (Berlyne, Liversedge, and Emery 1957). In pernicious anaemia the absorption is almost nil, but if intrinsic factor is given as well it becomes normal. When doubt remains as to whether a low serum B_{12} is due to Addisonian pernicious anaemia or to some other cause, the Schilling test (measurement of the urinary output of radioactive vitamin B_{12} after oral administration) is diagnostic; a rise in gastric parietal-cell antibodies in the serum gives useful confirmatory evidence (Wintrobe and Lee 1974).

Prognosis

The average survival of patients with pernicious anaemia before the introduction of liver treatment was about two years. Now it is possible with cyanocobalamin or hydroxocobalamin to restore the blood to normal and maintain the patient in good health indefinitely. Such patients need never develop vitamin B_{12} neuropathy. When this has already developed, it can always be arrested, but the degree of recovery depends upon the stage which the disease has reached. The peripheral nerves can regenerate; this is not possible in the spinal cord, but some remyelination is possible. Striking improvement may therefore be expected in the symptoms of polyneuropathy with disappearance of paraesthesiae and pains in the limbs, sensory loss of the 'glove and stocking' distribution, and muscular wasting if present, and with return of the tendon reflexes and improvement in co-ordination. Extensor plantar reflexes and spastic weakness and gross loss of postural sensibility, however, usually improve much less and, if severe, may persist unchanged. Even when the disease has been arrested by treatment, intercurrent infection may lead to an exacerbation.

Treatment

Vitamin B_{12} must be given intramuscularly; oral treatment requires very large doses and the results are inconstant. Ungley (1949) thought that a larger dose should be given to treat B_{12} neuropathy than in anaemia without nervous manifestations but this view is no longer held (Davies-Jones et al. 1980).

Treatment should be begun with 1000 μg of vitamin B_{12} given every 2 or 3 days for 5 doses to restore the tissue stores. After this 100 μg should be given weekly for 6 months, after which 100 μg a month is usually sufficient but may need to be increased if infection or renal insufficiency develops. Vitamin B_{12} must be given for the rest of the patient's life. Folic acid is not only ineffective in treating vitamin B_{12} neuropathy but may be deleterious as the administration of a folate load can produce a secondary B_{12} deficiency with exacerbation of neurological symptoms.

The diet should be ample and well supplied with vitamins. If

there is any suspicion of B_1 deficiency, thiamine should also be given. Physiotherapy is of some value in severe cases.

References

Adams, R. D. and Kubik, C. S. (1944). Subacute combined degeneration of the brain. New Engl. J. Med. **231** 1.

Agamanolis, D. P., Chester, E. M., Victor, M., Kark, J. A., Hines, J. D. and Harris, J. W. (1976). Neuropathology of experimental vitamin B_{12} deficiency in monkeys. Neurology, Minneapolis **26**, 905.

Asbury, A. K. and Johnson, P. C. (1978). Pathology of peripheral nerve. Saunders, Philadelphia.

Berk, L., Denny-Brown, D., Findland, M. and Castle, W. B. (1948). Effectiveness of vitamin B_{12} in combined system disease. New Engl. J. Med. **239**, 328.

Berlyne, G. M., Liversedge, L. A. and Emery, E. W. (1957). Radioactive vitamin B_{12} in the diagnosis of neurological disorders. Lancet i, 294.

Bradley, W. G. (1974). Disorders of peripheral nerves. Blackwell, Oxford.

Chisholm, I. A., Bronte-Stewart, J. and Foulds, W. S. (1967). Hydroxocobalamin versus cyanocobalamin in the treatment of tobacco amblyopia. Lancet ii, 450.

Cox-Klazinga, M. and Endtz, L. J. (1980). Peripheral nerve involvement in pernicious anaemia. J. neurol. Sci. **45**, 367.

Davies-Jones, G. A. B., Preston, F. E. and Timperley, W. R. (1980). Neurological complications in clinical haematology. Blackwell, Oxford.

Fraser, T. N. (1960). Cerebral manifestations of Addisonian pernicious anaemia. Lancet. ii, 458.

Freeman, A. G. and Heaton, J. M. (1961). The aetiology of retrobulbar neuritis in Addisonian pernicious anaemia. Lancet i, 908.

Gildea, E. F., Kattwinkel, E. E. and Castle, W. B. (1930). Experimental combined system disease. New Engl. J. Med. **202**, 523.

Greenfield, J. G. and Carmichael, E. A. (1935). The peripheral nerves in cases of subacute combined degeneration of the cord. Brain **58**, 483.

Herbert, V., Gottlieb, C. W. and Altschule, M. D. (1965). Apparent low serum-vitamin-B_{12} levels associated with chlorpromazine. Lancet ii, 1652.

Holmes, J. M. (1956). Cerebral manifestations of vitamin B_{12} deficiency. Br. med. J. **2**, 1394.

Hornabrook, R. W. and Marks, V. (1960). The effect of vitamin B_1 therapy on blood-pyruvate levels in subacute combined degeneration of the cord. Lancet ii, 893.

Iyer, G. V., Taori, G. M., Kapadia, C. R., Mathan, V. I. and Baker, S. J. (1973). Neurologic manifestations in tropical sprue. Neurology, Minneapolis **23**, 959.

Kosik, K. S., Mullins, T. F., Bradley, W. G., Tempelis, L. D. and Cretella, A. J. (1980). Coma and axonal degeneration in vitamin B_{12} deficiency. Arch. Neurol., Chicago **37**, 590.

Kunze, K. and Leitenmaier, K. (1976). Vitamin B_{12} deficiency and subacute spinal disease. In Handbook of clinical neurology, Vol. 28, (ed. P. J. Vinken and G. W. Bruyn), Chapter 6. North-Holland, Amsterdam.

Magnus, H. A. and Ungley, C. C. (1938). The gastric lesion in pernicious anaemia. Lancet i, 420.

McLeod, J. G., Walsh, J. C. and Little, J. M. (1969). Sural nerve biopsy. Med. J. Austral. **2**, 1092.

Mollin, D. L. (1959). Radioactive B_{12} in the study of blood diseases. Br. med. Bull. **15**, 8.

Mooney, F. S. and Heathcote, J. G. (1963). Oral treatment of subacute combined degeneration of spinal cord. Br. med. J. **1**, 1585.

Pallis, C. A. and Lewis, P. D. (1974). The neurology of gastrointestinal disease. Saunders, London.

Reynolds, E. H. (1976). The neurology of vitamin B_{12} deficiency: metabolic mechanisms. Lancet ii, 832.

—— (1981). Pathogenesis of subacute combined degeneration. Lancet ii, 1109.

Richmond, J. and Davidson, S. (1958). Subacute combined degeneration of the spinal cord in non-Addisonian anaemia. Quart. J. Med. **27**, 517.

Rickes, E. L., Brink, N. G., Koniuszy, F. R., Wood, T. R. and Folkers, K. (1948). Crystalline vitamin B_{12}. Science **107**, 396.

Russell, J. S. R., Batten, F. E. and Collier, J. (1900). Subacute combined degeneration of the spinal cord. Brain **23**, 39.

Samson, D. C., Swisher, S. N., Christian, R. M. and Engel, G. L. (1952). Cerebral metabolic disturbance and delirium in pernicious anaemia. Arch. int. Med. **90**, 4.

Smith, A. D. M. (1962). Veganism: a clinical survey with observations on vitamin B_{12} metabolism. Br. med. J. **1**, 1655.

Smith, E. L. (1948). Purification of anti-pernicious anaemia factors from liver. *Nature, London* **161**, 638.

Strachan, R. W. and Henderson, J. G. (1965). Psychiatric syndromes due to avitaminosis B$_{12}$ with normal blood and marrow. *Quart. J. Med.* **34**, 303.

Strauss, M. B. and Castle, W. B. (1932). The extrinsic (deficiency) factor in pernicious and related anaemias. *Lancet* **ii**, 111.

Torres, I., Smith, W. T. and Oxnard, C. E. (1971). Peripheral neuropathy associated with vitamin B$_{12}$ deficiency in captive monkeys. *J. Path.* **105**, 125.

Troncoso, J., Mancall, E. L. and Schatz, N. J. (1979). Visual evoked responses in pernicious anaemia. *Arch. Neurol., Chicago* **36**, 168.

Ungley, C. C. (1949). Subacute combined degeneration of the cord. *Brain* **72**, 382.

Walton, J. N., Kiloh, L. G., Osselton, J. W. and Farrall, J. (1954). The electroencephalogram in pernicious anaemia and subacute combined degeneration of the cord. *Electroenceph. clin. Neurophysiol.* **6**, 45.

Walter, A. H. and Mollin, D. L. (1961). Studies on the folic acid activity of human serum. *J. clin. Path.* **14**, 335.

Weller, R. O. and Cervós-Navarro, J. (1977). *Pathology of peripheral nerves.* Butterworth, London.

Williams, J. A., Hall, G. S., Thompson, A. G. and Cooke, W. T. (1969). Neurological disease after partial gastrectomy. *Br. med. J.* **3**, 210.

Wintrobe, M. M. and Lee, G. R. (1974). Pernicious anaemia and other megaloblastic anaemias. In *Harrison's principles of internal medicine*, 7th edn, Chapter 305. McGraw-Hill, New York.

Folate deficiency

Folate deficiency produced by malabsorption (as in steatorrhoea and intestinal 'blind-loop' syndromes) or by the use of anticonvulsant drugs, causes haematological abnormalities identical with those of pernicious anaemia, but until comparatively recently was not thought to cause neurological manifestations. However, it has been shown that some patients with polyneuropathy and myelopathy (Grant, Hoffbrand, and Wells 1965; Reynolds, Rothfeld, and Pincus 1973) and others with mental illness, including dementia (Carney 1967) are folate-deficient with serum values of less than 2 μg/ml. In some such cases improvement was noted after the administration of folic acid, 5 mg three times daily. In epileptic patients who develop folate deficiency and megaloblastic anaemia due to anticonvulsant therapy, the administration of folic acid may lower blood anticonvulsant levels (Baylis, Crowley, Preece, Sylvester, and Marks 1971) with consequential aggravation of the epilepsy (Reynolds 1976). While the exact role of folate in the aetiology of neurological disorders remains uncertain, it is reasonable to estimate the serum folate in cases of unexplained polyneuropathy, myelopathy, and dementia. Pallis and Lewis (1974) found much of the evidence relating neurological symptomatology on the one hand to folate deficiency on the other unconvincing. Nevertheless, reports of a possible association continue to appear. Botez (1976) suggested that the 'restless legs' syndrome may sometimes be due to folate deficiency, and the evidence of an association with an organic brain syndrome seems reasonably conclusive (Reynolds 1976; *The Lancet* 1976; Davies-Jones, Preston and Timperley 1980).

References

Baylis, E. M., Crowley, J. M., Preece, J. M., Silvester, P. E. and Marks, V. (1971). Influence of folic acid on blood–phenytoin levels. *Lancet* **i**, 62.

Botez, M. I. (1976). Folate deficiency and neurological disorders in adults. *Medical Hypotheses* **2**, 135.

Carney, M. W. P. (1967). Serum folate values in 423 psychiatric patients. *Br. med. J.* **2**, 512.

Davies-Jones, G. A. B., Preston, F. E. and Timperley, W. R. (1980). *Neurological Complications in clinical haematology.* Blackwell, Oxford.

Grant, H. C., Hoffbrand, A. V. and Wells, D. G. (1965). Folate deficiency and neurological disease. *Lancet* **ii**, 763.

Herbert, V. (1964). Studies of folate deficiency in man. *Proc. R. Soc. Med.* **57**, 377.

The Lancet (1976). Folic acid and the nervous system. *Lancet* **ii**, 836.

Pallis, C. A. and Lewis, P. D. (1974). *The neurology of gastrointestinal disease.* Saunders, London.

Reynolds, E. H. (1976). Neurological aspects of folate and vitamin B$_{12}$ metabolism. *Clinics in Haematology* **5**, 661.

——, Rothfeld, P. and Pincus, J. H. (1973). Neurological disease associated with folate deficiency. *Br. med. J.* **2**, 398.

Neurological complications of other haematological disorders

The neurological complications which may occur in a variety of blood diseases are mentioned in many sections of this book. Thus the complications of leukaemia, myeloma, and reticulosis are described in Chapter 17. The neurological manifestations of infectious mononucleosis are described on page 258 and were reviewed by Silverstein, Steinberg and Nathanson (1972). Polycythaemia vera, which may present with symptoms suggesting cerebral haemorrhage, cerebrovascular insufficiency, or even intracranial neoplasm (Kremer, Lambert, and Lawton 1972) is mentioned on page 189. It may also be complicated by polyneuropathy (Yiannikas, McLeod, and Walsh 1983). Intracerebral, subdural, or subarachnoid haemorrhage may also complicate the bleeding diseases including haemophilia and the various forms of thrombocytopenic purpura (p. 214), while symptoms and signs of cerebral dysfunction are common in thrombotic microangiopathy (p. 221). These and the neurological effects of other microangiopathies, including vascular involvement in the collagen diseases, in scurvy and vitamin K deficiency, as a consequence of anticoagulant therapy and as a rare complication of hereditary haemorrhagic telangiectasia, as well as the anoxic consequences of profound anaemia have been reviewed by Lumsden (1970) and Davies-Jones, Preston, and Timperley (1980). Relatively little attention has been paid in the literature to the fact that in sickle-cell anaemia, in thalassaemia (Cooley's anaemia), and in other inherited haemoglobinopathies accompanied by haemolytic anaemia of varying severity, neurological manifestations are not uncommon and may even be the presenting clinical features. Complications of *sickle-cell disease* include mental changes, disordered consciousness, convulsions, meningism, or frank meningitis (often pneumococcal), while cranial-nerve palsies, cerebrovascular accidents, and paraparesis have all been described (Adeloye and Odeku 1970). The commonest vaso-occlusive disorders occurring in this disease are hemiplegia, coma, convulsions, and optic atrophy (or visual loss due to ischaemic retinitis proliferans) but paraplegia due to cord infarction may occur, while radiculopathy and mononeuropathy due to ischaemia are less common (Davies-Jones *et al.* 1980). An organic mental syndrome occurring in childhood and responding to exchange transfusion has also been described (Haruda, Friedman, Ganti, Hoffman, and Chutorian 1981). In *thalassaemia*, strokes and/or convulsions occasionally occur as well as recurrent attacks of focal cerebral ischaemia, and proximal myopathy is relatively common (Logothetis, Constantoulakis, Economidou, Stefanis, Hakes, Augoustaki, Sofroniadou, Loewenson, and Bilek 1972). Cerebral arterial or venous infarction is also an occasional complication of paroxysmal nocturnal haemoglobinuria, especially after episodes of increased haemolysis (Johnson, Kaplan, and Brailock 1970). Kernicterus resulting from Rh incompatibility has been described on p. 356; this complication has been greatly reduced by the use of prophylactic anti-D immunoglobulin (*British Medical Journal* 1981). *Acanthocytosis* of the red cells is a well-known accompaniment of α-beta-lipoproteinaemia (the Bassen–Kornzweig syndrome) (p. 464) but has also been described in patients with involuntary movements, evidence of proximal myopathy, areflexia, and bladder dysfunction in whom the serum lipoproteins were normal (Aminoff 1972).

References

Adeloye, A. and Odeku, E. L. (1970). The nervous system in sickle cell disease. *Afr. J. med. Sci.* **1**, 33.

Aminoff, M. J. (1972). Acanthocytosis and neurological disease. *Brain* **95**, 749.

British Medical Journal (1981). Prevention of haemolytic diseases of the newborn due to anti-D. *Br. med. J.* **282**, 676.

Davies-Jones, G. A. B., Preston, F. E., and Timperley, W. R. (1980). *Neurological complications in clinical haematology.* Blackwell, Oxford.

Haruda, F., Friedman, J. H., Ganti, S. R., Hoffman, N., and Chutorian, A. M. (1981). Rapid resolution of organic mental syndrome in sickle cell anaemia in response to exchange transfusion. *Neurology, Minneapolis* **31**, 1015.

Johnson, R. V., Kaplan, S. R., and Blailock, Z. R. (1970). Cerebral venous thrombosis in paroxysmal nocturnal haemoglobinuria. *Neurology, Minneapolis* **20**, 681.

Kremer, M., Lambert, C. D., and Lawton, N. (1972). Progressive neurological deficits in primary polycythaemia. *Br. med. J.* **3**, 216.

Logothetis, J., Constantoulakis, M., Economidou, J., Stefanis, C., Hakas, P., Augoustaki, O., Sofroniadou, K., Loewenson, R., and Bilek, M. (1972). Thalassemia major (homozygous beta-thalassemia). *Neurology, Minneapolis* **22**, 294.

Lumsden, C. E. (1970). Pathogenetic mechanisms in the leucoencephalopathies in anoxic–ischaemic processes, in disorders of the blood and in intoxications. In *Handbook of clinical neurology* (ed. P. J. Vinken and G. W. Bruyn.) Vol. 9, Chapter 20. North-Holland, Amsterdam.

Silverstein, A., Steinberg, G., and Nathanson, M. (1972). Nervous system involvement in infectious mononucleosis. *Arch. Neurol., Chicago* **26**, 353.

Yiannikas, C., McLeod, J. G., and Walsh, J. C. (1983). Peripheral neuropathy associated with polycythemia vera. *Neurology, Minneapolis* **33**, 139.

17

The neurological manifestations of neoplasms arising outside the nervous system

A neoplasm elsewhere in the body may affect the nervous system in several different ways. The most familiar is by the spread of metastases to the nervous system itself, or to the structures by which it is contained. Many non-metastatic neurological complications of systemic cancer are, however, recognized. The effects of cancer upon the nervous system have been comprehensively reviewed by Henson and Urich (1982).

Cerebral metastatic neoplasms

The commonest sites of a primary carcinoma, likely to give cerebral metastases, are the bronchus, breast, kidney, stomach, prostate, and thyroid. Often it is the symptoms of a cerebral metastasis which first bring the patient under medical observation. This is particularly common in the case of lung carcinoma when, indeed, the primary growth may be so small as not to be evident on plain X-rays of the lung. At the other extreme there may be a latent interval of many years between the removal of the primary growth and the development of a cerebral metastasis, as in the case of breast cancer.

The clinical features, diagnosis, and management of secondary carcinoma of the brain and cord are described elsewhere (pp. 151 and 409). Two diagnostic points are of importance: it may be possible to demonstrate the presence of neoplastic cells in the CSF, especially when there is dural infiltration at the base of the brain as commonly occurs in breast cancer (Horton, Means, Cunningham, and Olson 1973) or in carcinomatosis of the meninges (Olson, Chernik, and Posner 1974); and CT scanning may demonstrate multiple metastases when only one may be causing clinical symptoms (Strang and Ajmone-Marsan 1961). It is also worth recalling first that neoplastic angioendotheliosis (in which small arterioles and capillaries are clogged with malignant cells thus causing multifocal infarction of brain, spinal cord, or peripheral nerve) is a rare manifestation of systemic cancer (Dolman, Sweeney, and Magil 1979); and secondly that the finding of malignant cells in the CSF containing melanin may indicate that intracranial metastases of malignant melanoma are present, or alternatively that there may be a primary melanoma of the brain, cord, or leptomeninges (Hayward 1976).

The likelihood that a cerebral metastasis is solitary is of obvious importance in relation to treatment. Russell and Rubinstein (1959), in a series of 117 cases of cerebral metastasis from bronchial carcinoma, found a solitary secondary in the brain in 30 per cent, but in all but two of these cases secondary growths were found elsewhere in the body, though in six the extracranial deposits were restricted to the hilar glands.

Direct invasion of the nervous system by tumour

The commoner tumours which arise outside the nervous system, but within the skull or spinal canal, are considered in the sections dealing with intracranial and spinal tumours. Tumours arising from other neighbouring structures which directly invade the nervous system are comparatively rare. They include chordomas, osteomas, chondromas and sarcomas of bone, glomus jugulare tumours, malignant tumours arising in the orbit, nasal sinuses, and nasopharynx. Myeloma is considered below.

Carcinomatous meningitis

Sometimes metastatic carcinoma of the nervous system presents with the clinical features of subacute meningitis through spread of metastases to the basal leptomeninges. The identification of tumour cells in the CSF is a valuable aid to diagnosis (see p. 69 and Olson *et al.* 1974).

Cranial metastases

The main clinical importance of metastatic growths in the cranial bones is that such tumours readily spread to the dura and may then lead to a subdural haematoma. Deposits in the bones of the base of the skull often cause intractable headache and cranial-nerve palsies, especially of the fifth and sixth nerves (Henson and Urich 1982).

Spinal metastases

Metastatic carcinoma of the spine is discussed elsewhere (see p. 409).

Direct invasion of plexuses, peripheral nerves, and skeletal muscle

Nerve plexuses or peripheral nerves are sometimes invaded either by a primary tumour or by metastatic growths in neighbouring lymph nodes. Brachial plexus, phrenic, or recurrent laryngeal-nerve involvement is particularly likely to occur in the case of tumours of the apex of the lung (Pancoast's tumour) but also in carcinoma of the thyroid and breast. Infiltration of the lumbosacral plexus by pelvic cancer, often of uterus or rectum, giving lower limb pain, weakness, and sensory loss, is well recognized. Involvement of peripheral nerves by haematogenous metastases is rare except in lymphoma, although it does occasionally occur, as do isolated metastases in skeletal muscle or even diffuse microscopic infiltration of muscle (Henson and Urich 1982). An isolated mental nerve neuropathy ('the numb chin syndrome') is a rare manifestation of systemic cancer (Massey, Moore, and Schold 1981).

Myeloma (plasmacytoma)

Myelomas may arise within the bones of the skull, orbit, or spine (Clarke 1954), and may then invade the nervous system secondarily (see p. 152). Headache, nausea and vomiting, and general malaise are common symptoms in multiple myelomatosis and are sometimes misconstrued as being due to intracranial disease. Compression of the spinal cord, cauda equina, and spinal roots are common and symptomatic herpes zoster, hypercalcaemic encephalopathy, and the carpal tunnel syndrome have all been described (Currie and Henson 1971).

Polyneuropathy is a common complication of multiple myeloma (Victor, Banker, and Adams 1958) and may also be seen in patients with solitary myeloma (Read and Warlow 1978); it is not the result of compression of nervous structures by tumour tissue. The lower limbs may be affected alone, or with the upper as well. Thickened carpal ligaments may lead to a carpal tunnel syndrome. While systemic amyloidosis may rarely complicate multiple myeloma and it has been suggested by some workers that amyloid or 'pseudo-amyloid' is often laid down in the peripheral nerves in myelomatosis, it is now evident that the peripheral neuropathy in such cases is clinically heterogeneous, and that it is sometimes predominantly axonal, sometimes predominantly demyelinating in type; amyloid deposition in nerves is only rarely responsible. Chemotherapy does not usually improve the neuropathy but irradiation of solitary myelomas often does so (Read and Warlow 1978; Kelly, Kyle, Miles, O'Brien, and Dyck 1981). Radiation is also helpful in osteosclerotic myeloma complicated by polyneuropathy (Kelly, Kyle, Miles, and Dyck 1983).

Neurological complications of the reticuloses

Macroglobulinaemia (Waldenström's syndrome)
Some 25 per cent of patients with macroglobulinaemia suffer from neurological complications, many of which appear to be due to increased serum viscosity and macroglobulin levels. The subject was reviewed by Solomon (1965). The principal abnormalities are retinopathy, with papilloedema and haemorrhages in some cases, various manifestations of encephalopathy, including strokes, with headache, auditory symptoms, such as tinnitus, deafness, and vertigo, and postural hypotension. When there is also evidence of associated subacute meningitis of lymphocytic type, the condition is sometimes called the Berg–Neel syndrome (see Henson and Urich 1982). A progressive cerebellar ataxia in a patient with macroglobulinaemia but without hyperviscosity improved when the myeloproliferative disorder was treated with chlorambucil (Spencer and Moench 1980). Peripheral neuropathy, usually with both demyelination and axonal degeneration, occurs in about 8 per cent of cases; there may be deposition of macroglobulin and of monoclonal globulin (M component) within the myelin sheaths of the nerve fibres (Julien, Vital, Vallat, Lagueny, Deminiere, and Darriet 1978). Peripheral neuropathy is also seen in some benign monoclonal gammopathies (Kahn, Riches, and Kahn 1980). A relationship between cryoglobulinaemia, malignant disease, and neuropathy is much more questionable (Henson and Urich 1982). Symptoms due to increased blood viscosity may be relieved by plasmapheresis but it is now more usual to treat the condition with cyclophosphamide or other cytotoxic agents which may produce some improvement (Bouroncle, Dalta, and Frajola 1964).

Progressive multifocal leuco-encephalopathy
Progressive multifocal leuco-encephalopathy was originally described by Aström, Mancall, and Richardson (1958) and by Cavanagh, Greenbaum, Marshall, and Rubinstein (1959). The subject has been reviewed by Richardson (1965) and by Henson and Urich (1982).

It is characterized by foci of demyelination in the white matter of the cerebral hemispheres, sometimes also involving the brainstem and cerebellum and, sparsely, the spinal cord. These areas range in size from some just visible to the naked eye to large confluent areas. Usually the myelin sheaths disappear with preservation of the axis cylinders. Inflammatory infiltration is often absent but there is usually a characteristic change in the astrocytes, which are enlarged with bizarre nuclei, often showing mitoses, and in all cases, the nuclei of the oligodendrocytes are paler than normal and contain inclusion bodies (Martin and Banker 1969). The CT scan usually shows multiple low-attenuation areas (Carroll, Lane, and Norman 1977; Lane, Carroll, and Pedley 1978).

Progressive multifocal leuco-encephalopathy is a rare disorder, usually occurring as a terminal event in patients suffering from the reticuloses and the leukaemias (Davies, Hughes, and Oppenheimer 1973). It has also been reported in sarcoidosis, tuberculosis, and in a few cases of carcinomatosis and other disorders but rarely arises spontaneously in apparently healthy individuals (Fermaglich, Hardman, and Earle 1970). It was suggested initially that it was due to invasion of the nervous system by a virus in patients with defective immune responses, and this view was confirmed by the observations of Zu Rhein and Chou (1965), Silverman and Rubinstein (1965), and Howatson, Nagai, and Zu Rhein (1965),

who, with the electron microscope, identified in the oligodendrocytes particles of polyoma virus. The virus may be identified in paraffin-embedded tissues (Morecki and Porro 1970); it was isolated and identified in culture as being a member of the polyoma SV_{40} subgroup of papova viruses (Padgett, Walker, Zu Rhein, and Eckroade 1971), now generally called the JC type (Weiner, Narayan, Penney, Herndon, Feringa, Tourtellotte, and Johnson 1973). The demyelination is attributed to destruction of the oligodendrocytes by the virus and the changes in the nuclei of the astrocytes to viral invasion.

The disorder usually terminates fatally in three to six months from the onset, but remission and survival for five years have both been reported (Hedley-Whyte, Smith, Tyler, and Peterson 1966; Price, Nielsen, Horten, Rubino, Padgett, and Walker 1983). It is characterized by symptoms of massive destruction of the white matter of the cerebral hemispheres and/or cerebellum, i.e. hemiplegia, quadriplegia, aphasia, visual-field defects or blindness, dysarthria, and ataxia. Convulsions are uncommon. The patient dies in coma. The CSF is usually normal. Sometimes other opportunistic infections (cryptococcosis, listeriosis) which may occur in immunocompromised patients complicate the clinical picture. While treatment with cytarabine was though to be helpful in one case (Marriott, O'Brien, Mackenzie, and Janota 1975), another patient failed to improve when treated with this drug and transfer factor (van Horn, Bastian, and Moake 1978).

Subacute 'poliomyelitis'
Walton, Tomlinson, and Pearce (1968) reported a patient with Hodgkin's disease who developed subacute muscular weakness and wasting and in whom pathological examination revealed inflammatory changes like those of poliomyelitis in the anterior horns of the spinal cord; no virus was identified. Probably this motor neuronopathy represented a variant of subacute myelopathy (see below).

Leukaemia
Neurological complications of acute leukaemia in childhood have been reported with increasing frequency and have been attributed to the longer survival achieved with modern treatment; they are seen most often in lymphoblastic leukaemia but also in the other varieties (West, Graham-Pole, Hardisty, and Pike 1972). Unilateral or bilateral facial palsy is a well-recognized manifestation. However, other symptoms may include those of subacute meningitis, multiple cranial-nerve palsies, or even cerebellar or uncal herniation (Sinniah, Loui, Ortega, Siegel, and Landing 1982); the frequency of the latter syndrome stresses that lumbar puncture for the identification of leukaemic cells in the CSF must be used with caution and only as a rule if the absence of papilloedema and the findings in the CT scan suggest that it is likely to be safe. Central pontine myelinolysis and diffuse cerebral atrophy are important late complications (Crosley, Rorke, Evans, and Nigro 1978), as is atypical measles encephalopathy (Pullan, Noble, Scott, Wisniewski, and Gardner 1976). Cerebral involvement has been attributed to the entry of leukaemic cells into the brain at the sites of intracranal petechial haemorrhage. Currie and Henson (1971) pointed out that focal symptoms and signs indicative of intracranial as well as less-common intraspinal lesions may occur in acute leukaemia in adults as well as in children and in patients with chronic lymphatic and myeloid leukaemia. Leukaemic cells can often be identified in the CSF. Intrathecal methotrexate (8 mg/m^2 of body surface weekly for five weeks) or cytosine arabinoside (30 mg/m^2) (*The Lancet* 1972) and/or craniospinal irradiation with 24 Gy (*British Medical Journal* 1973) have been employed in treatment but a necrotizing encephalopathy has been reported as a consequence of intraventricular methotrexate (Shapiro, Chernik, and Posner 1973). In children with acute lymphoblastic leukaemia, the outlook is worse when the central nervous system is involved early and relapse rates are lower when effective prophy-

Table 17.1. *Type of 'neuromyopathy' in cases of cancer**

	Cerebellar degeneration	Motorneurone type	Sensory neuropathy	Mixed peripheral neuropathy	Myasthenic	Neuromuscular	Other	Total
Unselected series	3 (2.9%)	3 (2.9%)	—	15 (14.6%)	2 (1.9%)	72 (70%)	8 (7.7%)	103
Selected group	6 (13.6%)	3 (6.8%)	6 (13.6%)	14 (31.8%)	—	10 (22.8%)	5 (11.4%)	44
All patients	9 (6.1%)	6 (4.1%)	6 (4.1%)	29 (19.7%)	2 (1.4%)	82 (55.8%)	13 (8.8%)	147

From Croft and Wilkinson (1965)

lactic treatment is given to the nervous system before neurological symptoms arise (Nesbit, D'Angio, Sather, Robison, Ortega, Donaldson, and Hammond 1981). The combination of intrathecal methotrexate with 24 Gy craniospinal irradiation is probably more effective for such prophylaxis than either alone (Green, Freeman, Suther, Sallan, Nesbit, Cassady, Sinks, Hammond, and Frei 1980). Unfortunately, however, there is growing evidence to suggest that the 'somnolence syndrome' with increasing slow-wave activity in the EEG, may be a long-term consequence of irradiation (Chi'en, Aur, Stagner, Cavallo, Wood, Goff, Pitner, Hustu, Seifert, and Simone 1980), while a progressive leucoencephalopathy may also follow irradiation and the use of folic acid antagonists such as pyrimethamine and methotrexate (DeVivo, Malas, Nelson, and Land 1977; Henson and Urich 1982). Bone-marrow transplantation seems unlikely to avoid these complications once the nervous system is involved.

The lymphomas

It has long been recognized that intracerebral deposits of Hodgkin's lymphoma, follicular lymphoma, reticulum-cell sarcoma, and lymphosarcoma may produce the symptoms and signs of an intracranial space-occupying lesion (John and Nabarro 1955; Whisnant, Siekert, and Sayre 1956; Sokal and Glaser 1956; Hutchinson, Leonard, Mawdsley, and Yates 1958; Sohn, Valensi, and Miller 1967), while spinal-cord, cauda equina or root compression, symptomatic herpes zoster, and peripheral-nerve or plexus lesions are even more common than intracranial lesions (Currie and Henson 1971). Lymphomatous meningitis is commoner in non-Hodgkin's lymphoma than are intracerebral deposits, and multiple cranial-nerve palsies are a common clinical presentation (Venables, Proctor, Bates, Cartlidge, and Shaw 1980; Teoh, Barnard, and Gautier-Smith 1980). Intracerebral Burkitt's lymphoma has also been described (Magrath, Mugerwa, Bailey, Olweny, and Kiryabwire 1974). Multifocal leukoencephalopathy has been described above. Polyneuropathy similar to that which may complicate carcinoma (see below) (Walsh 1971) or motor neuropathy (Schold, Cho, Somasundaram, and Posner 1979) and polymyositis (Rose and Walton 1966) are also well-documented complications, as is hypercalcaemic stupor (Schott 1975).

Paraneoplastic neurological syndromes

Many neurological syndromes are recognized to occur in association with neoplasms of the viscera, but unrelated to the presence of metastases. Denny-Brown (1948) under the heading 'Primary sensory neuropathy with muscular changes associated with carcinoma' described two cases of bronchial carcinoma in patients whose predominant neurological symptoms were gross loss of sen-

sibility and an associated ataxia. Lennox and Prichard (1950) reported five cases of peripheral neuritis among 299 cases of carcinoma of the bronchus. Brain, Daniel, and Greenfield (1951) reported four cases of subacute cortical cerebellar degeneration associated with carcinoma of the bronchus in two and of the ovary in one.

Brain and Adams (1965) provided a comprehensive classification of these disorders in terms of the anatomical level involved. However, Henson and Urich (1982) point out that the Brain–Adams classification, still widely used, was mainly topographical and further research has led to the grouping of these conditions according to the pattern of pathological changes, association with specific types of tumour, and, where known, pathogenetic mechanisms. In their view it is now possible to isolate four, or possibly five, major groups of disorders, largely of unknown aetiology, which are, respectively:

1. Encephalomyelitis, encephalitis (of various types) and myelitis;
2. Subacute cerebellar cortical degeneration;
3. Peripheral neuropathy;
4. Myopathy.
5. Complications which are difficult to classify (some of which are debatable), including subacute necrotic myelitis and various neurometabolic disorders.

The incidence of non-metastatic complications of carcinoma

Croft and Wilkinson (1965) published a survey of the incidence of carcinomatous neuromyopathy in a series of patients with carcinoma in various sites. It should be noted that in many such earlier reports, the term 'carcinomatous neuromyopathy' was used in an inclusive manner, embracing not only the neuromuscular complications but also those involving the central nervous system. This inclusive use of the term has now been dropped and neuromyopathy is used only for the syndrome of combined peripheral neuropathy and myopathy. Croft and Wilkinson showed that in a consecutive series of 1476 cases of cancer in various sites, there was an over-all incidence of 'neuromyopathy' of 6.6 per cent, the highest figures being 16.4 per cent for carcinoma of the ovary, 14.2 per cent for carcinoma of the lung, and 9 per cent for carcinoma of the stomach, compared with 4.4 per cent for carcinoma of the breast. Table 17.1 shows the incidence of the various neurological syndromes encountered in the unselected series of 1476 patients with cancer and in 44 cases specifically referred to them as suffering from neuromyopathy (the selected group).

Croft and Wilkinson used the term 'neuromuscular' here to cover a large group of cases of muscular wasting in which it was impossible to be sure on clinical grounds whether the condition was primarily myopathic or neuropathic, or both combined. Thus their figures showed that lung carcinoma is responsible for over 50 per cent of all cases of non-metastatic neurological disease associated with carcinoma and that evidence of such a complication is found in 14.2 per cent of all patients with breast carcinoma. Neuromuscular dysfunction accounted for approximately 50 per cent of all such cases irrespective of the site of the primary growth. Campbell and Paty (1974) also found a high incidence of asymptomatic neuromuscular disease in patients with lung cancer. More than half the patients they studied showed electromyographic evidence of neuromyopathy (i.e. a combination of 'myopathic' motor units with spontaneous and other activity suggesting nerve fibre loss but with normal nerve conduction: an axonal neuropathy was postulated).

Pathology

Neuropathology

Progressive multifocal leuco-encephalopathy has already been described (p. 485). Apart from this, when the central nervous system is involved as a remote effect of carcinoma and in the absence of metastases, the pathological picture may be described as a polio-encephalomyelopathy, that is, it is characterized by neuronal destruction and inflammatory infiltration, both diffuse and perivascular, the neuronal degeneration and inflammatory infiltration varying independently of one another. These changes are always to some extent diffuse, but when the damage falls predominantly upon one particular part of the nervous system, this determines the clinical picture; this relative selectivity in many cases accounts for the recognizable clinical syndromes. In the brain the inflammatory changes may affect predominantly the limbic lobe, the brainstem, or the cerebellum, when loss of Purkinje cells is always a striking feature, but in some cases no evidence of inflammation can be found (Henson and Urich 1982). Vick, Schulman, and Dau (1969), in reporting a case of carcinomatous cerebellar degeneration with associated evidence of diffuse encephalomyelitis and radiculitis of sensory neurones, suggested that the degeneration of Purkinje cells might well be of toxic or metabolic origin and that the diffuse inflammatory changes were possibly due to an unidentified virus. In the spinal cord the anterior horn cells may be destroyed at varying levels, and there may be ascending and descending degeneration of long tracts. In some cases many cells of the posterior root ganglia are destroyed, with consequential Wallerian degeneration in the posterior columns and peripheral nerves (sensory neuropathy). Sagittal sinus thrombosis, probably due to 'hypercoagulability' of the blood, is an occasional complication (Sigsbee, Deck, and Posner 1979), and diffuse vasculitis leading to mononeuritis multiplex has been reported (Johnson, Rolak, Hamilton, and Laguna 1979).

The peripheral nerves are more often diffusely involved, leading to a peripheral sensorimotor neuropathy, studied by Croft, Urich, and Wilkinson (1967), Trojaborg, Frantzen, and Andersen (1969), Campbell and Paty (1974), and Henson and Urich (1982). Croft et al. (1967) found both axonal loss and demyelination in affected nerves, sometimes with sparse lymphocytic infiltration, but it is now generally agreed that the primary lesion is axonal and that any demyelination is secondary.

Many attempts have been made, so far without success, in an effort to show that these neurological complications of neoplasia are immunological or infective in origin (Henson and Urich 1982). Paty, Campbell, and Hughes (1974) found some evidence of cellular sensitivity to peripheral-nerve antigens in patients with neuromyopathy but concluded that this probably resulted from a secondary reaction to previously sequestrated neural antigens. Nevertheless, a carcinomatous myopathy in a patient who showed a marked leukaemoid reaction with medullary plasmocytosis and progressive hypergammaglobulinaemia has been described (Bruyn and Joshua 1971) and various other abnormalities of the immune system and of the serum globulins are occasionally seen but are the exception rather than the rule. There appears to be some association between the appearance of neuromyopathy on the one hand and weight loss on the other (Hawley, Cohen, Saini, and Armbrustmacher 1980).

The pathology of the muscles

The pathological changes in the muscles are often slight in proportion to the degre of muscular weakness. Shy and Silverstein (1965) reported changes suggestive of a myopathy, i.e. loss of cross-striations, floccular, cloudy and granular changes, and internally placed nuclei with an increase of endomysial connective tissue. Many cases showed basophilic fibres with large vesicular nuclei, and prominent nucleoli characteristic of regeneration of muscle. Inflammatory changes were inconstant and rarely marked. Polymyositis and dermatomyositis developing after middle life are often associated with occult or overt malignant disease (Rose and Walton 1966; Astrom and Adams 1981; Currie 1981), but it now seems evident that the acute necrotizing myopathy without phagocytosis or inflammatory change which is sometimes found in patients with carcinoma (Brownell and Hughes 1975) and the even commoner non-specific cachexia (Henson and Urich 1982) are both different from polymyositis in the accepted sense of the term and their pathogenesis remains obscure.

Cerebrospinal fluid

Both in patients with involvement of the central nervous system and in those with polyneuropathy the CSF is often normal, but a moderate rise in protein and of gamma-globulin is sometimes seen, though a pleocytosis is uncommon.

Clinical features

Encephalitic form

When the brain is chiefly involved, symptoms will depend upon the region chiefly affected. The onset of symptoms is often insidious and may cover a wide range of psychiatric disorders, such as dementia, deterioration of memory, or disorder of mood, such as depression, anxiety, or agitation. When the brainstem is chiefly affected ('brainstem encephalitis'), the symptoms will depend upon the distribution of the lesions, ranging from ophthalmoplegia to bulbar palsy, often with nystagmus, ataxia, sometimes involuntary movements, and evidence of bilateral pyramidal-tract damage. Rarely a cerebellar encephalitis (different from cerebellar cortical degeneration) is seen (Henson and Urich 1982), in which case ataxia can develop acutely. Limbic encephalitis, largely limited to the hippocampus and amygdala (Henson, Hoffman, and Urich 1965; Corsellis, Goldberg and Norton 1968) may be an incidental finding at post-mortem; in some cases, however, it presents with a profound impairment of recent memory reminiscent of the Korsakow syndrome, while in others it is more severe with epileptic seizures, hallucinations, and dementia. Severe central hypoventilation has been described in a case in which neuronal intracytoplasmic inclusions were demonstrated in the cerebral cortex but no virus could be isolated (Kaplan and Itabashi 1974).

Myelopathy (myelitis)

The symptoms may resemble those of motor-neurone disease. The patient may present with symptoms of bulbar palsy, weakness of one or both upper limbs or of the lower limbs, or of generalized weakness and lassitude. Wasting and fasciculation are found in the affected muscles. The tendon reflexes may be exaggerated or diminished and the plantar reflexes may be flexor or extensor. Brain, Croft, and Wilkinson (1965) thought that 'carcinomatous motor-neurone disease' often ran a more benign course than the classical disorder. In fact all of the available evidence now indicates that there is no association between classical motor-neurone disease (amyotrophic lateral sclerosis) and malignancy (Henson and Urich 1982). But the myelitis or myelopathy which commonly occurs in association with cancer seems selectively to affect the anterior horn cells, giving a predominantly motor neuronopathy (Schold *et al.* 1979). While the pathological changes are those of inflammation, the condition is quite distinct from subacute necrotizing myelopathy (see below).

Subacute cerebellar degeneration
This syndrome has been reviewed by Brain and Wilkinson (1965), Vick *et al.* (1969) and Henson and Urich (1982). The onset is usually subacute with progressive loss of cerebellar function, leading to ataxia in both upper and lower limbs and dysarthria. Nystagmus, however, is absent in half the cases. Vertigo, dysarthria, and diplopia may all occur, and ataxia can ultimately be so severe that the patient is unable to sit unsupported; myoclonus occasionally occurs. The tendon reflexes may be diminished or lost, and the plantar reflexes extensor.

Sensory neuropathy
This is the clinical condition associated with degeneration of the posterior-root ganglion cells which Henson and Urich (1982) have called posterior-root ganglionitis. The patient develops, usually subacutely, sensory impairment, which tends to involve all forms of sensation in both upper and lower limbs, and is often accompanied by distressing paraesthesiae (Harwich, Cho, Parro, and Posner 1977). There is sensory ataxia, and the tendon reflexes are likely to be diminished or lost. Muscular wasting and weakness may also be present.

Peripheral sensorimotor neuropathy (polyneuropathy)
Croft *et al.* (1967) divided their patients into three groups. These were: (1) a mild and often terminal peripheral neuropathy occurring in the course of known malignant disease; (2) subacute or acute severe peripheral neuropathy, often occurring before any evidence of malignant disease is present; and (3) patients similar to those in the second group but in whom the neuropathy follows a remitting, or sometimes relapsing, course.

The symptoms and signs are typical of a polyneuropathy with distal weakness and wasting and sensory loss, symmetrical in the upper and lower limbs with diminution or loss of tendon reflexes.

Sometimes the clinical and investigative features point in such cases to an isolated polyneuropathy, but much more often there is also electromyographic evidence of myopathy (Campbell and Paty 1974). While slowing of motor nerve conduction velocity suggesting demyelination of peripheral nerves has been reported (Croft *et al.* 1967), in most cases motor and sensory conduction is normal or only slightly reduced (Trojaborg *et al.* 1969; Campbell and Paty 1974).

Myopathy and neuromyopathy
The carcinomatous neuromyopathies are by far the commonest of the remote effects of malignant disease. Symptoms of muscular weakness may, and often do, antedate the symptoms of malignancy, sometimes by several years. The predominant complaints of all patients are difficulty in standing and walking, in rising from a sitting position, and in climbing stairs, sometimes with pain in the legs and peripheral paraesthesiae. While both the muscles and the peripheral nerves are affected in many cases (hence the neuromyopathy), the manifestations of myopathy (muscular weakness and wasting) usually predominate. The muscles most frequently involved are the proximal ones. Involvement of the bulbar muscles occurs rarely. The tendon reflexes in the affected muscles are diminished or lost and very occasionally fasciculation is seen. The symptoms of a neuromyopathy may be accompanied by those of one of the central nervous-system syndromes described above.

The electromyographic findings indicate a myopathy. There is a short mean action-potential duration and a marked increase in the number of short polyphasic potentials. Many patients may show electrical evidence of neuropathic involvement as well.

The myasthenic syndrome
One of the rarer manifestations of malignancy is the myasthenic (Eaton–Lambert) syndrome, usually associated with bronchogenic carcinoma (see Lambert and Rooke 1965 and page 571). However, it has also been reported in patients with rectal, renal, gastric, and cutaneous cancer, in leukaemia, reticulum-cell sarcoma, and malignant thymoma (Lauritzen, Smith, Fischer-Hansen, Sparup, and Olesen 1980), and in patients with auto-immune disorders such as hypo- and hyperthyroidism, Sjögren disease, and sarcoidosis. In some cases no associated disease is found (Brown and Johns 1974); it is now thought to be due to an auto-immune mechanism (see p. 572). The initial symptom is weakness and easy fatigability of the legs, less frequently the arms; some patients may have blurring of vision or ptosis. The tendon reflexes are almost invariably absent. There is an appreciable delay in developing a strong and maximal voluntary contraction of affected muscles, but with prolonged exertion weakness subsequently develops more rapidly than in normal persons. The fatigability may not respond at all to edrophonium or neostigmine or does so to a lesser extent than in myasthenia gravis; it is, however, corrected by guanidine in a dose of 30–45 mg/kg body weight per day in four divided doses. The response of such patients to various muscle relaxant drugs is different from that of patients with myasthenia gravis (Croft 1958; Simpson 1981).

There are characteristic electrical reactions. The action potential and the twitch evoked in a muscle by a single supramaximal stimulus are greatly reduced in amplitude even though the strength of voluntary contraction may be normal or nearly so. Repetitive supramaximal stimulation of a peripheral nerve at slow rates gives a further decrease in amplitude but stimulation at fast rates leads to a progressive increase in the amplitude of the evoked potential (paradoxical potentiation). Electromyography often shows evidence of a myopathy but the true diagnosis can easily be missed if studies of neuromuscular transmission are not performed.

Subacute necrotizing myelopathy
This rare disorder is characterized clinically by a subacute onset of the symptoms of an ascending lesion of the spinal cord, partial or complete, and usually terminating fatally in days or weeks. The patient develops paraplegia with some impairment of sensibility and loss of sphincter control. The CSF may be normal but more frequently there is a rise of protein with an excess of cells, either mononuclear or polymorphs. Pathologically there is a massive and symmetrical necrosis which may extend to the whole spinal cord or involve principally the thoracic region. The blood vessels show adventitial thickening and fibrosis, or sometimes even necrosis.

Mancall and Rosales (1964) found nine cases in the literature and added two more of their own. In 10 out of 11 cases the myelopathy was associated with a carcinoma. In the 11th case there was a sarcoma, and the condition may be associated with reticulum-cell sarcoma or lymphoma (Henson and Urich 1982).

Neurometabolic disorders associated with neoplasms

Tumours of many different kinds may produce metabolic disorders leading to neurological symptoms which may bring the patient under observation. The most important of such symptoms are mental disturbances and muscular weakness. The principal syndromes of this kind were reviewed by Brain and Norris (1965), by Brain and Adams (1965) and more recently by Henson and Urich (1982).

Hypercalcaemia

The production of hypercalcaemia by a tumour of the parathyroid gland has long been recognized. However, there are several other ways in which tumours arising elsewhere may produce hypercalcaemia. Tumours arising in some organ other than the parathyroid gland may produce a parathormone-like substance which leads to hypercalcaemia, while genuine primary hyperparathyroidism has been reported in patients with carcinoma and leukaemia (Wang, Steier, Aunt, and Tobin 1978). There is also some evidence that prostaglandin release from tumour cells may play a part (Henson and Urich 1982). Sarcoidosis may also produce hypercalcaemia in a manner not fully understood. When a tumour metastasizes widely to bones the resulting bone destruction may liberate calcium into the blood stream faster than it can be excreted, and so cause a hypercalcaemia. Myelomatosis may also produce this effect. Hypercalcaemia, however produced, may lead to symptoms of a non-specific encephalopathy, such as drowsiness, confusion or stupor, or to muscular weakness (Lemann and Donatelli 1964; Dent and Watson 1964; Currie and Henson 1971; Schott 1975).

Adrenal hypercorticism

Various tumours, including bronchial adenoma, bronchogenic carcinoma, thymoma, or pancreatic carcinoma, may secrete ACTH (Williams, Oluhy, and Thorn 1974) and so lead to adrenal hypercorticism. There is, indeed, evidence that virtually all oat-cell carcinomas of bronchus and bronchial carcinoids secrete ACTH-like materials (*British Medical Journal* 1977). This may not in the early stages lead to the typical symptoms of Cushing's syndrome, but may give hypokalaemic alkalosis, the symptoms of Cushing's syndrome developing only later. Clinically this syndrome may present with symptoms of a confusional psychosis or dementia, or those of a myopathy (O'Riodan, Blanshard, Moxham, and Nabarro 1966; Friedman, Marshall-Jones, and Ross 1966).

Hypoglycaemia

Some tumours other than those arising in the pancreas may produce hypoglycaemia. Kahn (1980) found that mesenchymal tumours were responsible for this complication in 45 per cent of cases, hepatomas in 23 per cent, and adrenocortical carcinoma in 10 per cent. It is thought that in some cases the tumour elaborates a material with insulin-like activity which nevertheless differs in structure from insulin, while in other cases it is possible that rapid consumption of glucose by the tumour may play a part. The presenting symptoms are likely to be those familiar as a result of hypoglycaemia, namely, an encephalopathy characterized by stupor, coma, and convulsions.

Hyponatraemia

Hyponatraemia is most likely to occur in association with a bronchogenic carcinoma or adenoma which secretes a substance like vasopressin with the effects of antidiuretic hormone (inappropriate ADH secretion). The result is hyponatraemia, hypotonicity of extracellular fluid, and a hypertonic urine with sodium loss. The patient usually presents with water intoxication and encephalopathy characterized by coma, convulsions, and a raised CSF pressure. Treatment depends upon fluid restriction (see Welt 1974 and Henson and Urich 1982).

Other neurological complications of malignancy

Apart from the many metastatic and non-metastatic complications of malignant disease reviewed above, patients with cancer may develop various nutritional deficiencies causing either the neurological manifestations of specific vitamin lack (such as the Wernicke–Korsakow syndrome, beriberi, pellagra, and the like) or those associated with chronic malnutrition. Because of impaired immune responses they are also at risk from many opportunistic infections such as, for example, cryptococcosis and many other fungal infections, protozoal infections such as toxoplasmosis, and/or unusual and severe manifestations of viral infection with herpes (zoster or simplex), measles, cytomegalovirus, and many more (see Henson and Urich 1982).

References

Adams, R. D., Denny-Brown, D., and Pearson, C. M. (1953). *Diseases of muscle.* Hoeber, London.

Aström, K.-E. and Adams, R. D. (1981). Pathological reactions of the skeletal muscle fibre in man. In *Disorders of voluntary muscle* (ed. J. N. Walton) 4th edn, Chapter 5. Churchill-Livingstone, Edinburgh.

——, Mancall, E. L., and Richardson, E. P. (1958). Progressive multifocal leuko-encephalopathy. *Brain* **81**, 93.

Bouroncle, B. A., Dalta, P., and Frajola, W. J. (1964). Waldenström's macroglobulinaemia: report of three patients treated with cyclophosphamide. *J. Am. med. Ass.* **189**, 729.

Brain, W. R. and Adams, R. D. (1965). A guide to the classification and investigation of neurological disorders associated with neoplasms. In *The remote effects of cancer on the nervous system* (ed. W. R. Brain and F. Norris), Chapter 21 Grune and Stratton, New York.

——, Croft, P. B., and Wilkinson, M. (1965). Motor neurone disease as a manifestation of neoplasm (with a note on the course of classical motor neurone disease). *Brain* **88**, 479.

——, Daniel, P. M., and Greenfield, J. G. (1951). Subacute cerebellar degeneration and its relation to carcinoma. *J. Neurol. Neurosurg. Psychiat.* **14**, 59.

—— and Henson, R. A (1958). Neurological syndromes associated with carcinoma. *Lancet* **ii**, 971.

—— and Norris, F. (1965). *The remote effects of cancer on the nervous system.* Grune and Stratton, New York.

—— and Wilkinson, M. (1965). Subacute cerebellar degeneration associated with neoplasms. *Brain* **88**, 465.

British Medical Journal (1973). Irradiation of C.N.S. in leukaemia. *Br. med. J.* **2**, 377.

—— (1977). ACTH-secreting lung tumours. *Br. med. J.* **1**, 1047.

Brown, J. C. and Johns, R. J. (1974). Diagnostic difficulties encountered in the myasthenic syndrome sometimes associated with carcinoma. *J. Neurol. Neurosurg. Psychiat.* **37**, 1214.

Brownell, B. and Hughes, J. T. (1975). Degeneration of muscle in association with carcinoma of the bronchus. *J. Neurol. Neurosurg. Psychiat.* **38**, 363.

Bruyn, C. W. and Joshua, D. (1971). Myopathy with leukemoid reaction secondary to alveolar–bronchiolar cell carcinoma. *Neurology, Minneapolis* **21**, 1114.

Campbell, M. J. and Paty, D. W. (1974). Carcinomatous neuromyopathy: 1. Electrophysiological studies. *J. Neurol. Neurosurg. Psychiat.* **37**, 131.

Carroll, N. A., Lane, B., and Norman, D. (1977). Diagnosis of progressive multifocal leukoencephalopathy by computed tomography. *Radiology* **122**, 137.

Cavanagh, J. B., Greenbaum, D., Marshall, A. H. E., and Rubinstein, L. J. (1959). Cerebral demyelination associated with disorders of the reticuloendothelial system. *Lancet* **ii**, 524.

Ch'ien, L. T., Aur, R. J. A., Stagner, S., Cavallo, K., Wood, A., Goff, J. V. (1980). Long-term neurological implications of somnolence syndrome in children with acute lymphocytic leukemia. *Ann. Neurol.* **8**, 273.

Clarke, E. (1954). Cranial and intracranial myelomas. *Brain* **71**, 61.

Corsellis, J. A. N., Goldberg, G. J., and Norton, A. R. (1968). 'Limbic encephalitis' and its association with carcinoma. *Brain* **91**, 481.

Croft, P. B. (1958). Abnormal responses to muscle relaxants in carcinomatous neuropathy. *Br. med. J.* **1**, 181.

——, Urich, H., and Wilkinson, M. (1967). Peripheral neuropathy of sensorimotor type associated with malignant disease. *Brain* **90**, 31.

—— and Wilkinson, M. (1965). The incidence of carcinomatous neuromyopathy with special reference to carcinoma of the lung and the breast. In *The remote effects of cancer on the nervous system* (ed. W. R. Brain and F. Norris, Chapter 6. Grune and Stratton, New York.

—— and —— (1969). The course and prognosis in some types of carcinomatous neuromyopathy. *Brain* **92**, 1.

Crosley, C. J., Rorke, L. B., Evans, A., and Nigro, M. (1978). Central nervous system lesions in childhood leukemia. *Neurology, Minneapolis* **28**, 678.

Currie, S. (1981). Inflammatory myopathies—Part I: Polymyositis and related disorders. In *Disorders of voluntary muscle* (ed. J. N. Walton) 4th edn, Chapter 15. Churchill-Livingstone, Edinburgh.

—— and Henson, R. A. (1971). Neurological syndromes in the reticuloses. *Brain* **94**, 307.

Davies, J. A., Hughes, J. T., and Oppenheimer, D. R. (1973). Richardson's disease (progressive multifocal leukoencephalopathy). *Quart. J. Med.* **42**, 481.

Denny-Brown, D. (1948). Primary sensory neuropathy with muscular changes associated with carcinoma. *J. Neurol. Neurosurg. Psychiat.* **11**, 73.

Dent, C. E. and Watson, L. C. A. (1964). Hyperparathyroidism and cancer. *Br. med. J.* **2**, 218.

DeVivo, D. C., Malas, D., Nelson, J. S., and Land, V. J. (1977). Leukoencephalopathy in childhood leukemia. *Neurology, Minneapolis* **27**, 609.

Dolman, C. L., Sweeney, V. P., and Magil, A. (1979). Neoplastic angioendotheliosis: the case of the missed primary? *Arch. Neurol., Chicago* **36**, 5.

Fermaglich, J., Hardman, J. M., and Earle, K. M. (1970). Spontaneous progressive multifocal leukoencephalopathy. *Neurology, Minneapolis* **20**, 479.

Friedman, M., Marshall-Jones, P., and Ross, E. J. (1966). Cushing's syndrome: adrenocortical hyperactivity secondary to neoplasms arising outside the pituitary–adrenal system. *Quart. J. Med.* **35**, 193.

Gotham, J. E., Wein, H., and Meyer, J. S. (1963). Clinical studies of neuropathy due to macroglobulinaemia (Waldenström's syndrome). *Can. med. Ass. J.* **89**, 806.

Green, D. M., Freeman, A. I., Sather, H. N., Sallan, S. E., Nesbit, M. E., Cassady, J. R., Sinks, L. F., Hammond, D., and Frei, E. (1980). Comparison of three methods of central-nervous-system prophylaxis in childhood acute lymphoblastic leukaemia. *Lancet* i, 1398.

Hawley, R. H., Cohen, M. H., Saint, N., and Armbrustmacher, V. W. (1980). The carcinomatous neuromyopathy of oat cell lung cancer. *Ann. Neurol.* **7**, 65.

Hayward, R. D. (1976). Malignant melanoma and the central nervous system. *J. Neurol. Neurosurg. Psychiat.* **39**, 526.

Hedley-Whye, E. T., Smith, B. P., Tyler, H. R., and Peterson, W. P. (1966). Multifocal leukoencephalopathy with remission and five year survival. *J. Neuropath. exp. Neurol.* **25**, 107.

Henson, R. A., Hoffman, H. L., and Urich, H. (1965). Encephalomyelitis with carcinoma. *Brain* **88**, 449.

——, Russell, D. S., and Wilkinson, M. (1954). Carcinomatous neuropathy and myopathy. *Brain* **77**, 82.

—— and Urich, H. (1982). *Cancer and the nervous system. The neurological manifestations of systemic malignant disease.* Blackwell, Oxford.

Horton, J., Means, E. D., Cunningham, T. J., and Olson, K. B. (1973). The numb chin in breast cancer. *J. Neurol. Neurosurg. Psychiat.* **35**, 211.

Horwich, M. S., Cho, L., Porro, R. S., and Posner, J. B. (1977). Subacute sensory neuropathy: a remote effect of carcinoma. *Ann. Neurol.* **2**, 7.

Howatson, A. F., Nagai, M., and Zu Rhein, G. (1965). Polyoma-like virions in human demyelinating brain disease. *Can. med. Ass. J.* **93**, 379.

Hutchinson, E. C., Leonard, B. J., Mawdsley, C., and Yates, P. O. (1958). Neurological complications of the reticuloses. *Brain* **81**, 75.

John H. T. and Nabarro, J. D. N. (1955). Intracranial manifestations of malignant lymphoma. *Br. J. Cancer* **9**, 386.

Johnson, P. C., Rolak, L. A., Hamilton, R. H., and Laguna, J. F. (1979). Paraneoplastic vasculitis of nerve: a remote effect of cancer. *Ann. Neurol.* **5**, 437.

Julien, J., Vital, C., Vallat, J.-M., Lagueny, A., Deminiere, C., and Darriet, D. (1978). Polyneuropathy in Waldenström's macroglobulinemia: deposition of M component on myelin sheaths. *Arch. Neurol., Chicago*, **35**, 423.

Kahn, C. R. (1980). The riddle of tumour hypoglycaemia revisited. *Clinics in Endocrinology and Metabolism. Endocrinology and Cancer* **9**, 335.

Kahn, S. N., Riches, P. G., and Kohn, J. (1980). Paraproteinaemia in neurological disease: incidence, associations and classification of monoclonal immunoglobulins. *J. clin. Path.* **33**, 617.

Kaplan, A. M. and Itabashi, H. H (1974). Encephalitis associated with carcinoma. *J. Neurol. Neurosurg. Psychiat.* **37**, 1166.

Kelly, J. J., Kyle, R. A., Miles, J. M., and Dyck, P. J. (1983). Osteosclerotic myeloma and peripheral neuropathy. *Neurology, Minneapolis* **33**, 202.

——, ——, ——, O'Brien, P. C., and Dyck, P. J. (1981). The spectrum of peripheral neuropathy in myeloma. *Neurology, Minneapolis* **31**, 24.

Lambert, E. H. and Rooke, E. D. (1965). Myasthenic state and lung cancer. In *The remote effects of cancer on the nervous system* (ed. W. R. Brain and F. Norris) Chapter 8. Grune and Stratton, New York.

The Lancet (1972). Treating the nervous system in acute leukaemia. *Lancet* i, 297.

Lane, B., Carroll, B. A., and Pedley, T. A. (1978). Computerized cranial tomography in cerebral diseases of white matter. *Neurology, Minneapolis* **28**, 534.

Lauritzen, M., Smith, T., Fisher-Hansen, B., Sparup, J., and Olesen, J. (1980). Eaton–Lambert syndrome and malignant thymoma. *Neurology, Minneapolis* **30**, 634.

Lemann, J. and Donatelli, A. A. (1964). Calcium intoxication due to primary hyperparathyroidism: a medical and surgical emergency. *Ann. intern. Med.* **60**, 447.

Lennox, B and Prichard, S. (1950). The association of bronchial carcinoma and peripheral neuritis. *Quart. J. Med.* **19**, 97.

Lloyd, O. C. and Urich, H. (1959). Acute disseminated demyelination of the brain associated with lymphosarcoma. *Lancet* ii, 529.

Magrath, I. T., Mugerwa, J., Bailey, I., Olweny, C., and Kiryabwire, Y. (1974). Intracerebral Burkitt's lymphoma: pathology, clinical features and treatment. *Quart. J. Med.* **43**, 489.

Mancall, E. L. and Rosales, R. K. (1964). Necrotizing myelopathy associated with visceral carcinoma. *Brain* **87**, 639.

Marriott, P. J., O'Brien, M. D., Mackenzie, I. C. K., and Janota, I. (1975). Progressive multifocal leucoencephalopathy. *J. Neurol. Neurosurg. Psychiat.* **38**, 205.

Martin, J. B. and Banker, B. Q. (1969). Subacute multifocal leukoencephalopathy with widespread intranuclear inclusions. *Arch. Neurol., Chicago* **21**, 590.

Massey, E. W., Moore, J., and Schold, S. C. (1981). Mental neuropathy from systemic cancer. *Neurology, Minneapolis* **31**, 1277.

Morecki, R. and Porro, R. S. (1970). Progressive multifocal leukoencephalopathy: identification of virions in paraffin-embedded tissues. *Arch. Neurol., Chicago* **22**, 253.

Nesbit, M. E., D'Angio, G. J., Sather, H. N., Robison, L. L., Ortega, J., Donaldson, M., and Hammond, G. D. (1981). Effect of isolated central nervous system leukaemia on bone marrow remission and survival in childhood acute lymphoblastic leukaemia: a report for Children's Cancer Study Group. *Lancet* i, 1386.

Olson, M. E., Chernik, N. L., and Posner, J. B. (1974). Infiltration of the leptomeninges by systemic cancer. *Arch. Neurol, Chicago* **30**, 122.

O'Riordan, J. L., Blanshard, G. P., Moxham, A., and Nabarro, S. (1966). Corticotrophin-secreting carcinomas. *Quart. J. Med.* **35**, 137.

Padgett, B. L., Walker, D. L., Zu Rhein, G. M., and Eckroade, R. J. (1971). Cultivation of papova-like virus from human brain with progressive multifocal leucoencephalopathy. *Lancet* i, 1257.

Paty, D. W., Campbell, M. J., and Hughes, D. (1974). Carcinomatous neuromyopathy: immunological studies. *J. Neurol. Neurosurg. Psychiat.* **37**, 142.

Price, R. W., Neilsen, S., Horten, B., Rubino, M., Padgett, B., and Walker, D. (1983). Progressive multifocal leukoencephalopathy: a burnt-out case. *Ann. Neurol.* **13**, 485.

Pillan, C. R., Noble, T. C., Scott, D. J., Wisniewski, K., and Gardner, P. S. (1976). Atypical measles infections in leukaemic children on immunosuppressive treatment. *Br. med. J.* **1**, 1562.

Read, D. and Warlow, C. (1978). Peripheral neuropathy and solitary plasmacytoma. *J. Neurol. Neurosurg. Psychiat.* **41**, 177.

Richardson, E. P. (1965). Progressive multifocal leukoencephalopathy. In *The remote effects of cancer on the nervous system* (ed. W. R. Brain and F. Norris) Chapter 2. Grune and Stratton, New York.

Rose, A. L. and Walton, J. N. (1966). Polymyositis: a survey of 89 cases with particular reference to treatment and prognosis. *Brain* **89**, 747.

Russell, D. S. and Rubinstein, L. J. (1959). *Pathology of tumours of the nervous system*, p. 213. Arnold, London.

Schold, S. C., Cho, E.-S., Somasundaram, M., and Posner, J. B. (1979). Subacute motor neuronopathy: a remote effect of lymphoma. *Ann. Neurol.* **5**, 271.

Schott, G. D. (1975). Hypercalcaemic stupor as a presentation of lymphosarcoma. *J. Neurol. Neurosurg. Psychiat.* **38**, 382.

Shapiro, W. R., Chernik, N. L., and Posner, J. B. (1973). Necrotizing encephalopathy following intraventricular instillation of methotrexate. *Arch. Neurol., Chicago* **28**, 96.

Shy, G. M. and Silverstein, I. (1965). A study of the effects upon the motor unit by remote malignancy. *Brain* **88**, 515.

Sigsbee, B., Deck, M. D. F., and Posner, J. B. (1979). Nonmetastatic superior sagittal sinus thrombosis complicating systemic cancer. *Neurology, Minneapolis* **29**, 139.

Silverman, L. and Rubinstein, L. J. (1965). Electron microscopic observations on a case of progressive multifocal leukoencephalopathy. *Acta neuropath., Berlin* **5**, 215.

Simpson, J. A. (1981). Myasthenia gravis and myasthenic syndromes. In *Disorders of voluntary muscle* (ed. J. N. Walton) 4th edn, Chapter 16. Churchill-Livingstone, Edinburgh.

Sinniah, D., Looi, L. M., Ortega, J. A., Siegel, S. E. and Landing B. (1982). Cerebellar coning and uncal herniation in childhood acute leukaemia. *Lancet* **ii**, 702.

Solomon, A. (1965). Neurological manifestations of macroglobulinemia. In *The remote effects of cancer on the nervous system* (ed. W. R. Brain and F. Norris), Chapter 12. Grune and Stratton, New York.

Spencer, S. S. and Moench, J. C. (1980). Progressive and treatable cerebellar ataxia in macroglobulinemia. *Neurology, Minneapolis* **30**, 536.

Strang, R. and Ajmone-Marsan, C. (1961). Brain metastases. *Arch. Neurol., Chicago* **4**, 8.

Swash, M., Perrin, J., and Schwartz, M. S. (1979). Significance of immunoglobulin deposition in peripheral nerve in neuropathies associated with paraproteinaemia. *J. Neurol. Neurosurg. Psychiat.* **42**, 179.

Teoh, R., Barnard, R. O., and Gautier-Smith, P. C. (1980). Polyneuritis cranialis as a presentation of malignant lymphoma. *J. neurol. Sci.* **48**, 399.

Trojaborg, W., Frantzen, E., and Andersen, I. (1969). Peripheral neuropathy and myopathy associated with carcinoma of the lung. *Brain* **92**, 71.

van Horn, G., Bastian, F. O., and Moake, J. L. (1978). Progressive multifocal leukoencephalopathy: failure of transfer factor and cytarabine. *Neurology, Minneapolis* **28**, 794.

Venables, G. S., Proctor, S. J., Bates, D., Cartlidge, N. E. F., and Shaw, D. A. (1980). Intracranial disease in non-Hodgkin's lymphoma. *Quart. J. Med.* **49**, 111.

Vick, N., Schulman, S., and Dau, P. (1969). Carcinomatous cerebellar degeneration, encephalomyelitis and sensory neuropathy (radiculitis). *Neurology, Minneapolis* **19**, 425.

Victor, M., Banker, B. Q., and Adams, R. D. (1958). The neuropathy of multiple myeloma. *J. Neurol. Neurosurg. Psychiat.* **21**, 73.

Walsh, J. C. (1971). Neuropathy associated with lymphoma. *J. Neurol. Neurosurg. Psychiat.* **34**, 42.

Walton, J. N., Tomlinson, B. E., and Pearce, G. W. (1968). Subacute 'poliomyelitis' and Hodgkin's disease. *J. neurol. Sci.* **6**, 435.

Wang, J. C., Steier, W., Aunt, M. K., and Tobin, M. S. (1978). Primary hyperparathyroidism and chronic lymphocytic leukemia. *Cancer* **42**, 1964.

Weiner, L. P., Narayan, O., Penney, J. B., Herndon, R. M., Feringa, E. R., Tourtellotte, W. W., and Johnson, R. T. (1973). Papovavirus of JC type in progressive multifocal leukoencephalopathy. *Arch. Neurol., Chicago* **29**, 1.

Welt, L. G. (1974). Disorders of fluids and electrolytes. In *Harrison's principles of internal medicine*, 7th edn, Chapter 264. McGraw-Hill, New York.

West, R. J., Graham-pole, J., Hardisty, R. M., and Pike, M. C. (1972). Factors in pathogenesis of central-nervous-system leukaemia. *Br. med. J.* **3**, 311.

Whisnant, J. P., Siekert, R. G., and Sayre, G. P. (1956). Neurologic manifestations of the lymphomas. *Medical Clinics of North America* **40**, 1151.

Williams, G. H., Oluhy, A. G., and Thorn, G. W. (1974). Diseases of the adrenal cortex. In *Harrison's principles of internal medicine*, 7th edn, Chapter 86. McGraw-Hill, New York.

Zu Rhein, G. and Chou, S. M. (1965). Particles resembling papova viruses in human cerebral demyelinating disease. *Science* **148**, 1477.

18

Disorders of peripheral nerves

Tumours of nerves

The connective tissue of a peripheral nerve may be the site of a tumour, either benign—a fibroma, or malignant—a sarcoma. Such growths do not differ from similar tumours elsewhere. Tumours peculiar to peripheral nerves are those arising from the nerve elements and those arising from the nerve sheaths. Classification is still a matter of some dispute (Kramer 1970; Dyck, Thomas, and Lambert 1975; Weller and Cervós-Navarro 1977; Asbury and Johnson 1978) but it is generally agreed that there are three principal groups which are first, non-neoplastic tumour-like growths or pseudotumours (e.g. traumatic or compression 'neuromas') secondly tumours of the nerve sheath (the benign neurinoma or Schwannoma and the neurofibroma, as well as the malignant sarcoma), and thirdly rare tumours arising from neural elements themselves (the neuroblastomas, ganglioneuroblastomas, and ganglioneurofibromas). Other rare tumours include the paraganglioma or chromaffinoma (which usually grow from the carotid body, glomus jugulare, the adrenal or retroperitoneal tissues), the rare granular-cell tumour (usually solitary, but rarely multifocal and occasionally malignant) which can arise from the perineurium and may be derived from Schwann cells, and metastases which can very rarely be found within nerve trunks. The neurinoma, Schwannoma, or neurilemmoma arises from nerve sheaths either on peripheral or cranial nerves or nerve roots and may be single or miltuple. Neurofibromas on peripheral nerves may be single but are much more often seen in von Recklinghausen's neurofibromatosis (p. 359). Peripheral nerves may, of course, be compressed or invaded by primary or secondary tumours arising in other tissues.

Traumatic and allied lesions of peripheral nerves

The work of Seddon and his collaborators did much to elucidate the nature of the different types of nerve injury. Seddon (1944) described three well-defined varieties. *Neurotmesis* is complete anatomical division. *Axonotmesis* is a 'lesion in continuity' in which the supporting structure of the nerve is preserved in whole or in part but there is nevertheless such extensive division of axons that true Wallerian degeneration occurs peripherally. *Neurapraxia* is the term applies to a 'transient block', a less severe lesion producing paralysis which is often incomplete, is unaccompanied by peripheral degeneration, and recovers rapidly and completely. The subject was reviewed in the light of experience gained in the Second World War in *Medical Research Council Special Report Series,* No. 282 (1954) and subsequently by Sunderland (1978) and Seddon (1975).

Ischaemic lesions. Ischaemic lesions may involve motor and sensory nerves and also the muscles. They may occur as a result of arterial injury or occlusion, as in tourniquet paralysis; or closed limb fractures, giving arterial injury which may cause, for example, Volkmann's ischaemic paralysis. The anterior tibial syndrome is a form of ischaemic paralysis of the muscles in which the anterior tibial muscles, after being subjected to unaccustomed effort, swell within their tight fascial compartment and may undergo partial or complete infarction. Richards (1951) reviewed the effects of ischaemia upon peripheral nerves, pointing out as

Seddon (1975) has done, that arterial occlusion involves muscle, peripheral nerve, and even bone, to an equal extent; he also stressed the importance of chronic ischaemic neuropathy due to more gradual ischaemia resulting from progressive arterial disease. Nerve ischaemia and infarction due to narrowing or occlusion of vasa nervorum also account, for example, for isolated cranial-nerve lesions (usually of one third or sixth nerve) in diabetes, and for mononeuritis multiplex or more diffuse polyneuropathy in various auto-immune vasculitides such as polyarteritis nodosa. Ischaemia of the lumbosacral plexus has also been described following intragluteal injections with inadvertent intra-arterial injection of a vasotoxic drug into a gluteal artery (Stöhr, Dichgans, and Dorstelmann 1980). Ischaemic monomelic neuropathy (Wilbourn, Furlan, Hulley, and Ruschhaupt 1983) is also an important complication of peripheral vascular disease and/or of vascular surgery on limb arteries. Fullerton (1963) and others have also shown that local ischaemia due to pressure is one factor giving rise to symptoms and signs when peripheral nerves or roots are compressed. So-called 'tourniquet paralysis' is due to a combination of ischaemia and pressure (Bolton and McFarlane 1978; Yamada, Muroga, and Kimura 1981).

Pressure neuropathy Repeated or prolonged pressure upon a nerve leads to ischaemia, but also to mechanical deformation of the myelin sheath with local oedema (Rudge, Ochoa, and Gilliatt 1974; Neary and Eames 1975). The initial disturbance of function is neurapraxial but this may be followed by axonotmesis, and, if the pressure is not relieved, perineurial fibrosis develops and prevents recovery. This is the lesion underlying the neuropathy caused by herniated intervertebral disc, narrowed intervertebral foramen, cervical rib, median-nerve compression in the carpal tunnel, ulnar-nerve compression at the elbow, meralgia paraesthetica, and other so-called entrapment neuropathies.

Neurotmesis

Neurotmesis occurs as a result of open wounds, direct blunt injuries, severe traction upon a nerve, and some forms of local chemical poisoning, e.g. by misplaced injections (Gentili, Hudson, and Hunter 1980). Retrograde degeneration occurs in the central stump for 2 or 3 cm and the peripheral stump undergoes Wallerian degeneration. The axons of the central end soon sprout, and form a neuroma composed of nerve fibres and scar tissue on the central stump (Spencer 1974; Sunderland 1978).

Symptoms and signs of complete division

Complete division of a mixed peripheral nerve causes motor, sensory, vasomotor, sudomotor, and trophic manifestations corresponding in anatomical distribution to the region in which these functions are mediated by the divided nerve.

Motor symptoms
Interruption of the motor fibres of a nerve leads to paralysis of lower motor-neurone type in the muscles which it innervates. The denervated muscles exhibit flaccid paralysis, and rapidly waste. The reflexes in which they participate are diminished or lost. Investigation of the motor functions of a nerve involves testing the patient's power to contract muscles both as prime movers and also as synergists (MRC 1976). The observer must be on his guard to

detect trick movements, for it is often possible for a movement which is normally effected by a paralysed muscle to be carried out by another muscle when the paralysed limb is first placed in an appropriate position. Electromyography is particularly valuable in identifying the paralysed muscles, while if the divided nerve is one in which conduction can be measured electrically, soon after the injury conduction in the segment distal to the lesion becomes greatly slowed and is later lost.

Sensation

Methods of testing sensation are described elsewhere (p. 76). Division of a sensory nerve causes complete loss of cutaneous sensibility only over the area exclusively supplied by the nerve, the *autonomous zone*. This is surrounded by an *intermediate zone*, which is the area of the nerve's territory overlapped by the supply of adjacent nerves. The autonomous and intermediate zones together constitute the *maximal zone* which is the full extent of the nerve's distribution. The cutaneous area over which appreciation of light touch is lost is usually larger than that characterized by loss of appreciation of pin-prick. The latter area is often ill-defined and merges gradually into the intermediate zone in which the appreciation of pin-prick is present, though impaired. In some cases, even after complete division of a nerve, the completely analgesic area is surrounded by a zone in which, although a stronger stimulus than normal is necessary to evoke pain, the painful sensation is more than usually disagreeable ('hyperpathia'). The term 'deep sensibility' is used to embrace the appreciation and localization of pressure, of the pain induced by deep pressure, and the recognition of posture and passive movements at the joints. When deep sensibility is impaired as a result of nerve division, this is confined to an area which is less extensive than that anaesthetic to light touch.

Vasomotor, sudomotor, and trophic functions

Vasomotor and trophic disturbances which follow destruction of a motor or a mixed nerve are probably due, at least in part, to the interruption of efferent sympathetic fibres concerned in vasoconstriction. These changes are most marked after injuries of the median, ulnar, and sciatic nerves. After complete division the analgesic area of skin becomes dry and inelastic, and ceases to sweat. The surface becomes scaly owing to retarded desquamation; the affected area is blue and colder than normal, especially in cold weather; and the limb becomes oedematous when dependent. The analgesic area is liable to suffer injury, and when damaged heals slowly, so that ulcers may develop. The growth of the nails and hair is retarded (Simpson 1970). Adhesions between tendons and their sheaths, and fibrous changes in the muscles and joints are to be regarded as complications rather than as direct results of the nerve injury, since they can usually be prevented by repeated passive movements of the joints; however, pericapsulitis of the shoulder joint, or 'frozen shoulder', is in some cases very difficult to prevent (Jayson 1981).

Axonotmesis

This type of lesion is best illustrated by the experimental crushing of a peripheral nerve with forceps, after which all or most of the axons are broken but the supporting sheath of the nerve largely survives (Seddon 1975). It may be the result of open wounds or direct blunt injuries, such as fractures and dislocations, traction or compression, as well as local action by physical and chemical agents. Peripheral to the injury degeneration is complete, but in acute cases regeneration always occurs, and functional recovery is more rapid and more complete than after complete division and

suture. At first, however, the effects are the same as those of neurotmesis.

Neurapraxia

In neurapraxia, although the functions of the nerve are temporarily impaired and sometimes seem completely lost, recovery occurs so quickly that it could not possibly have resulted from regeneration. Lesions of this type may be produced by any of the causes of axonotmesis, provided the axons are not actually severed. Pressure is the commonest cause, but ischaemia is another important cause as in tourniquet paralysis (Bolton and McFarlane 1978; Yamada *et al.* 1981). In neurapraxia according to Seddon: (*a*) the loss of function is predominantly motor; (*b*) there is little wasting, and the electrical reactions of the muscles persist unchanged; (*c*) subjective sensory disturbances—numbness, tingling and burning—are common; (*d*) objective sensory disturbances are generally partial, and often minimal as far as touch, pain, heat, and cold are concerned; (*e*) loss of postural sensibility and vibration sense are common; (*f*) loss of sweating is unusual; and nerve conduction distal to the lesion is preserved. The lesion is usually therefore dissociated, the motor and proprioceptive fibres suffering most, probably because the largest fibres are the most vulnerable, but in occasional cases all motor and sensory function is temporarily lost. Recovery is fairly rapid, usually beginning after a few days or weeks, and becoming complete within six or eight weeks, though, occasionally, complete restoration of function may be delayed until the sixth month. Recovery progresses irregularly and follows no anatomical order, but is always complete.

Diagnosis of the nature of a nerve lesion

The appropriate treatment of a peripheral-nerve lesion depends upon an accurate diagnosis of its nature and severity. The symptoms of neurotmesis and axonotmesis are for a long time indistinguishable. It is possible to wait until sufficient time has elapsed for regeneration to occur and, if it does not, to conclude that the nerve has been completely divided, but if suture is delayed more than five or six months the prospects of recovery are poor. Moreover, the whole transverse extent of a nerve may not be equally severely injured and combinations of neurotmesis, axonotmesis, and neurapraxia occur. It is always necessary to take account of the nature of the injury since experience will often suggest the type of nerve damage to be expected. It is often possible to recognize neurapraxia by the features described above. Electromyography and studies of nerve conduction, to be described below, are of considerable value. However, as Bradley (1974) pointed out, these tests are of little value in distinguishing between neurotmesis and axonotmesis and when the lesion is proximal or when it is probable, from the nature of the injury, that actual division of the nerve has taken place, exploration within the succeeding two or three months is probably indicated. Particular difficulties may arise in distinguishing between traction injuries of the brachial plexus (in which, after axonotmesis, regeneration and some degree of functional recovery may be anticipated) on the one hand, and avulsion of roots from the spinal cord on the other. The recording of peripheral and spinal somatosensory evoked potentials can be helpful (Jones 1979; Synek and Cowan 1982). Myelography (demonstrating abnormal filling of 'root sleeves') may also be useful in making this distinction, as may loss of the axon 'flare' response and of sensory nerve action potentials evoked from the anaesthetic area; if both are lost, the lesion probably lies proximal to the posterior root ganglia so that avulsion is likely and recovery impossible.

Special methods in the diagnosis of nerve lesions

In many cases clinical examination and electromyography will suffice to diagnose peripheral lesions and to follow their progress towards recovery, but methods of measuring both motor and sensory conduction velocity have greatly increased diagnostic precision. Other methods are occasionally helpful. Gilliatt and Wilson (1954) and Fullerton (1963) drew attention to the increase in sensory symptoms produced by temporary ischaemia obtained by applying a pneumatic tourniquet to the limb. *Sweating* responses after exposure to heat may be used to demarcate a denervated area (Gutmann 1940) (see p. 598). This may be particularly useful in distinguishing between lesions of spinal roots, plexuses, and peripheral nerves, e.g. between cervical rib and ulnar neuropathy, and in demonstrating a peripheral-nerve lesion coexisting with a lesion of the spinal cord, e.g. a common peroneal nerve lesion in a patient anaesthetic from a spinal injury. However, Seddon (1975) found this method of little value in clinical practice. *Procaine nerve-block* (Highet 1942b) may be applied either to an injured nerve or to neighbouring nerves when the diagnosis is complicated by anomalous muscle movements or when it is uncertain to which nerve a sensory area belongs; however, this technique is now rarely, if ever, necessary.

Electrophysiological techniques

The older electrical methods (e.g. Erb's 'reaction of degeneration') and even the charting of strength duration curves (Brown and Wynn-Parry 1974) once widely used to detect evidence of partial or complete denervation of skeletal muscle, have now been largely supplanted by more sophisticated diagnostic methods, including electromyography and measurement of motor and sensory nerve conduction velocity. Methods of studying neuromuscular transmission, of particular importance in the diagnosis of myasthenia gravis and the myasthenic-myopathic syndrome, are described on pages 586–7.

Electromyography (EMG)

This technique normally involves recording the electrical activity of muscle at rest, during minimal voluntary contraction, and during full contraction. Surface electrodes may be used in order to identify which muscle or muscle groups are participating in voluntary movement, but for diagnostic work it is necessary to insert a concentric needle electrode into the muscle, to amplify the activity and to display it on a cathode ray oscilloscope, while simultaneously rendering the potentials audible in a loudspeaker (see Licht 1971; Mayo Clinic 1981; Barwick 1981; Lenman and Ritchie 1983). Additional sophistications of diagnostic techniques have been used by some workers utilizing methods such as integration of the EMG (Lenman 1959, 1981), automatic frequency analysis (Walton 1952; Fex and Krakau 1957; Rose and Willison 1967; Dowling, Fitch, and Willison 1968), single-fibre electromyography (Ekstedt 1964), and intracellular recording (Brooks and Hongdalarom 1968; McComas and Johns 1981).

Normal muscle. When a normal muscle is tested at rest there is no evidence of electrical activity. On slight voluntary contraction motor-unit potentials of 300–2000 μV in amplitude, and 4–8 ms in duration, are recorded. These are usually monophasic, biphasic, or triphasic in shape, but up to five per cent of potentials recorded from normal muscle may be polyphasic. On vigorous voluntary contraction of the muscle an interference pattern develops. Since the patient recruits as many motor units as possible, and they fire asynchronously, each one interferes with the ones which precede and follow it (Fig. 18.1).

One method of quantitative electromyography depends upon the measurement of mean action potential duration and ampli-

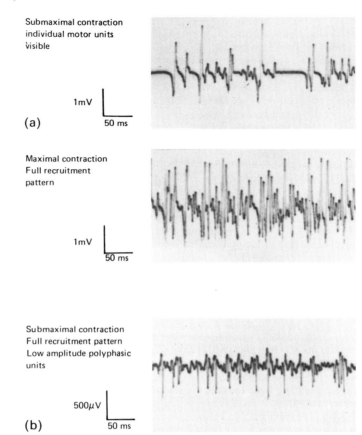

Submaximal contraction
individual motor units
visible

1mV

(a)   50 ms

Maximal contraction
Full recruitment
pattern

1mV

50 ms

Submaximal contraction
Full recruitment pattern
Low amplitude polyphasic
units

500μV

(b)   50 ms

Fig. 18.1. (a) The normal electromyogram. *Upper*: Submaximal contraction. Note that the individual motor units here vary between 1.5 and 3 mV in amplitude and are of approximately 5–7ms duration. *Lower*: During maximal contraction there is a full 'interference pattern'; the spikes of greater amplitude represent action potentials derived from motor units lying relatively close to the recording electrode, while those of lower amplitude are derived from motor units lying some distance away.

(b) The electromyogram in myopathy. The constituent motor units are greatly reduced in amplitude and duration and many are polyphasic.

tude, based upon the accurate measurement of at least 20 single action potentials recorded during voluntary contraction (Kugelberg 1949; Buchthal, Pinelli, and Rosenfalck 1954; Lenman 1981); the amplitude and duration of such potentials increases with age.

Additional information can now be obtained by techniques which have been introduced to estimate the numbers and sizes of motor units in certain limb muscles and especially in the extensor digitorum brevis muscle of the foot (McComas, Fawcett, Campbell and Sica 1971; Campbell, McComas, and Petito 1973; Ballantyne and Hansen 1974; McComas 1977). Information relating to the integrity of the reflex arc, motor-neurone excitability, and the activity of the muscle spindles can be obtained by recording the H and F reflexes or by studying the tonic contraction evoked by vibration applied to the muscle (Magladery, Porter, Park and Teasdall 1951; Lance, de Gail, and Nielson 1966; Marsden, Meadows, and Hodgson 1969; Lenman 1981; Lance and McLeod 1981).

Completely denervated muscle After complete transection of a nerve, and when sufficient time—about two weeks—has elapsed to allow the distal segment to degenerate, fibrillation potentials can be recorded from the resting muscle. A fibrillation potential, resulting from the spontaneous contraction of a single muscle fibre, is usually 50–100 μV in amplitude, 1–2 ms in duration, and monophasic or biphasic in shape. On attempted voluntary contraction no motor unit action potentials are produced. A total absence of such potentials on attempted volition is found whether

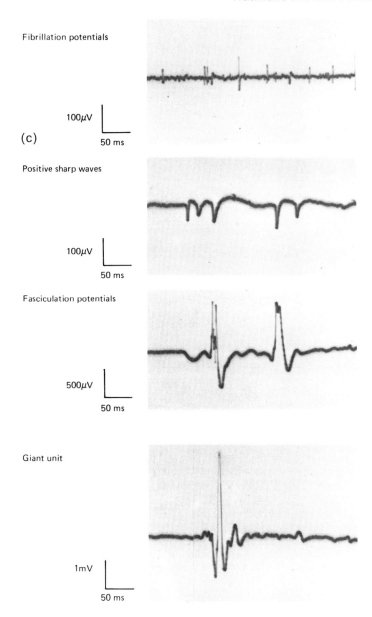

Fibrillation potentials

100μV

50 ms

(c)

Positive sharp waves

100μV

50 ms

Fasciculation potentials

500μV

50 ms

Giant unit

1mV

50 ms

Fig. 18.1. (c) The electromyogram in denervation. From top to bottom:
(i) Spontaneous fibrillation; this is recorded from relaxed resting muscle; the individual potentials measure no more than about 100 μV in amplitude and are about 1 ms duration.
(ii) Positive sharp waves (saw tooth potentials) also recorded from relaxed resting muscle; this phenomenon is occasionally seen in denervated muscle.
(iii) Fasciculation potentials firing spontaneously, also recorded from relaxed resting muscle in a patient with motor-neurone disease; these potentials are morphologically indistinguishable from motor unit action potentials.
(iv) A giant motor unit action potential of approximately 5 mV in amplitude occurring during volitional activity in a patient with motor-neurone disease.
(Fig.18.1 (a), (b), and (c) kindly provided by Dr R. Weiser.)

the lesion is neurapraxial or due to neurotmesis or axonotmesis; however, in neurapraxia, unlike the other two types of lesion, fibrillation does not occur. Hence if no fibrillation potentials appear two or three weeks after apparent total denervation of a muscle, the lesion is probably neurapraxial. On the other hand, when fibrillation potentials are recorded this does not necessarily mean that all motor axons have been divided; it simply indicates

that this is true of some. Another type of spontaneous activity sometimes recorded from resting denervated muscle is that of so-called positive sharp waves or 'saw-tooth' potentials.

Partially denervated muscle. The EMG recorded from partially denervated muscle shows what might be expected from a combination of degeneration of some lower motor neurones with preservation of others. If the needle tip lies near muscle fibres denervated due to axonal division, fibrillation potentials will be observed. On slight voluntary contraction intact motor units will fire, and the size, shape, and duration of their motor unit potentials will be normal, but vigorous muscular contraction will not bring into action a sufficient number of additional units to produce a full interference pattern (Fig. 18.1). Thus the latter is reduced.

While the above description applies to acute partial denervation due, for instance, to an incomplete lesion of a motor root or peripheral nerve, there are certain essential differences between this pattern of activity and that more often observed in diseases giving rise to chronic progressive denervation, such as, for instance, motor-neurone disease or spinal muscular atrophy. If the denervating process is active, fibrillation and positive sharp waves are often found but such activity may be absent or difficult to find if the process is very chronic or has become arrested. However, in such cases, *fasciculation potentials* may be recorded, occurring spontaneously and repetitively when the muscle is at rest; these potentials are morphologically indistinguishable from motor unit action potentials. They usually indicate the presence of a lesion situated proximally in the motor neurone (e.g. in the anterior horn cell) and axon reflexes may play a part in their pathogenesis (Stalberg and Trontelj 1970). Fasciculation may also be a benign phenomenon (Trojaborg and Buchthal 1965) and can be exceptionally profuse in one form of myokymia.

It is also evident that in chronic denervating processes, surviving axons often produce collateral sprouts which then 'adopt' and reinnervate denervated muscle fibres so that some surviving motor units become much larger than normal in both amplitude and duration (so-called 'giant motor units', which are particularly common in motor-neurone disease).

Myopathic muscle. In myopathy the disorder of function is not based on the pattern of innervation. Fasciculation does not occur and often there is no spontaneous fibrillation either but in some cases of myopathy (and especially in polymyositis) the disease process may affect intramuscular nerve endings or alternatively focal necrosis of part of a muscle fibre may separate the remainder of the fibre from its motor end-plate so that fibrillation potentials are then seen. On slight voluntary contraction there may be some normal muscle fibres which respond, but these will be few. Consequently the population of muscle fibres within individual motor units is randomly reduced so that the duration and amplitude of the motor unit potentials is diminished and many are broken-up or polyphasic. On maximal contraction more motor units may fire, but as these contain diseased muscle fibres there is a low-voltage and complex interference pattern made up of many short-duration and polyphasic potentials (Fig. 18.1).

Myotonia is associated with characteristic chains of oscillations of high frequency which are evoked by movement of the exploring needle within the muscle and which produce a typical recurring 'dive-bomber' sound in the loud-speaker. Myotonic discharges wax and wane, beginning slowly, building up to a crescendo, and then fading gradually. They must be distinguished from other bizarre high-frequency discharges (sometimes called 'pseudomyotonic') which begin and end abruptly and give a sound which is more constant; the pathophysiology of these discharges is poorly understood and they often appear as spontaneous activity in disorders as diverse as motor-neurone disease, polyneuropathy, muscular dystrophy, and many metabolic myopathies, so that, unlike true myotonic discharges, they lack diagnostic specificity.

Single-fibre electromyography. The technique of single-fibre electromyography, introduced comparatively recently, involves the use of a needle multi-electrode which has many tiny openings in its 'shell', so that the different exposed parts of the core each function as electrodes recording from the surface of the individual muscle fibres with which they come into contact. If one supposes that the axon derived from one anterior horn cell divides within the muscle so that each terminal branch innervates a single muscle fibre, this type of electrode can be used to record contraction of the individual fibres. If for some reason the nerve impulse in one nerve twig arrives after that in another branch has reached the adjacent muscle fibre, then there will be an interval between the potentials derived from each of the muscle fibres; this interval is known as jitter. And if, during repeated muscular contraction, whether voluntary or electrically induced, one such potential disappears, this is known as blocking and may indicate either a failure of conduction in the nerve branch concerned, or more probably a failure of neuromuscular transmission at its motor end-plate, as in myasthenia gravis. The measurement of these phenomena has proved to be of considerable diagnostic value (Walton 1982).

Measurement of nerve conduction velocity

Techniques of measuring motor and sensory nerve conduction velocity have been greatly refined in recent years and have added considerable precision to the diagnosis of peripheral-nerve lesions, nerve entrapment syndromes, and diseases of peripheral nerve, especially polyneuropathy (see Kaeser 1970; Bradley 1974; Fawcett and Barwick 1981; Kimura 1983). Motor conduction in the fastest-conducting fibres is usually measured by applying a supramaximal stimulus to a motor nerve at two or more different points along its course through bipolar electrodes applied to the skin over the trunk of the nerve and then recording the evoked muscle action potential from an appropriate muscle supplied by the nerve (Fig. 18.2(a)). The latency from the stimulus to the initial rise of the muscle action potential is measured in milliseconds for each stimulus, as is the distance between the pairs of stimulating electrodes so that the conduction velocity in m/s in various segments of the trunk of the nerve may readily be calculated. In the case of the median nerve (Fig. 18.2(a)) the interval between the stimulus applied at the wrist and the initial rise of the muscle action potential in the abductor pollicis brevis of opponens pollicis is known as the terminal latency. Temperature has a profound effect upon nerve conduction so that the skin temperature of the limb must be carefully maintained at 20–25 °C. Sensory conduction can be measured similarly by applying stimuli to ring electrodes upon a finger (Fig. 18.2(b)) and then recording the sensory-nerve action potential through cutaneous electrodes applied over the trunk of the nerve (orthodromic conduction) or by stimulating the nerve trunk and recording from the digital ring electrodes (antidromic conduction). The sensory-nerve action potential is small so that averaging techniques (Gilliatt, Melville, Velate, and Willison 1965; Buchthal and Rosenfalck 1966) or the use of needle recording electrodes inserted close to the nerve are sometimes required. Well-established methods are now available for studying conduction in the median, ulnar, radial, and digital nerves in the upper limb (Trojaborg 1970; Casey and Le Quesne 1972; Bradley 1974; Fawcett and Barwick 1981) and in the common peroneal, posterior tibial, and sural nerves in the lower (Gilliatt, Goodman, and Willison 1961; Behse and Buchthal 1971; Kimura 1983). Conduction velocity is normally lower in children than in adults (Wagner and Buchthal 1972). In the median nerve, maximum motor conduction velocity is normally 49–68 m/s, sensory conduction 60–70 m/s, and the terminal motor latency 2.0–4.5 ms. Conduction velocity in the ulnar nerve is similar, while in the common peroneal nerve maximum motor conduction is 45–55 m/s, sensory conduction 45–70 m/s, and terminal motor latency 3.4–6.8 ms.

As previously mentioned, conduction distal to a neurapraxial

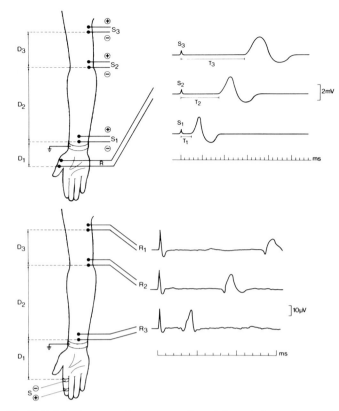

Fig. 18.2. (a) Diagrammatic representation of the technique of measuring maximum motor conduction velocity in the median nerve.

(b) Diagrammatic representation of the technique for measuring maximum sensory conduction velocity in the median nerve by orthodromic stimulation. (For fuller details see text. Fig.18.2 (a) and (b) are reproduced from Bradley (1974) by kind permission of the author and publisher.)

lesion of a peripheral nerve may remain normal at a time when its function is severely impaired. When a nerve is compressed, as in entrapment neuropathies, the speed of motor and sensory conduction across the site of the lesion may be either lost or greatly reduced, while, for instance, in median-nerve compression in the carpal tunnel, terminal latency is greatly increased. Techniques are now available for measuring conduction over short segments of nerve in presumed entrapment neuropathies (Brown and Yates 1982). In demyelinating neuropathies, conduction is markedly delayed along affected nerve trunks, while in axonal neuropathies conduction velocity in surviving axons may be normal, but as the number of axons responding to stimulation is reduced, the evoked muscle or sensory action potentials are greatly reduced in amplitude or dispersed, while in 'dying-back' axonal neuropathies, terminal motor and sensory latency may be prolonged.

Changes in the EMG, in tactile sensibility, and in nerve conduction after suture or compression of peripheral nerves in human subjects have been studied longitudinally by Buchthal and Kühl (1979); they found, as did Borenstein and Desmedt (1980), that enlargement of reinnervated motor units and marked dispersion of motor unit action potentials persisted long after suture; the sensory potential recovered five times, and tactile sensibility 10 times, as quickly after correction of a compressive lesion as after suture. In compressive lesions which were relieved, maximum motor and sensory conduction velocity recovered to 80–90 per cent of normal within one year, but in adults after nerve suture it had only reached 65–75 per cent of normal after 40 months. Recovery of conduction in autogenous sural-nerve grafts is similar (Talis, Staniforth, and Fisher 1978).

The measurement of spinal *somatosensory evoked potentials* is useful in determining whether lesions of the brachial plexus lie proximal or distal to the dorsal root ganglia (Jones 1979), and Tamada *et al.* (1981) have shown that because of selective involvement of different groups of nerve fibres, depending upon the thickness of their myelin sheaths, selective abnormalities of early peaks with relative preservation of late peaks may be seen in the cerebral somatosensory evoked potential in some peripheral-nerve lesions.

Symptoms and signs of recovery

Recovery of function after complete division of a nerve occurs by means of an outgrowth of nerve fibres from the central end, and can therefore take place only when the divided ends lie in apposition or have been brought together by suture. The time required for recovery depends principally upon the distance which the regenerating fibres have to travel from the site of injury to their destinations and also upon the integrity of the distal sheaths of Schwann cells into which the regenerating axons must grow. Mechanisms of regeneration in myelinated nerves were studed by Thomas (1966, 1970) and by Orgel, Aguayo, and Williams (1972) and in unmyelinated nerves by Dyck and Hopkins (1972), Aguayo, Peyronnard, and Bray (1973), and Thomas and King (1974). After complete division and suture many axons are misdirected so that recovery is often incomplete. The average rate of motor nerve regeneration in man is 1.5 mm per day. There has been much theoretical discussion about the interpretation of sensory changes which characterize returning function, but there is considerable agreement as to the facts. The first indication that nerve fibres have passed into the distal part of the nerve may be a peculiar sensitivity of the nerve trunk below the site of the union. Mechanical stimulation readily evokes a tingling sensation, which is referred into the cutaneous territory of the nerve (Tinel's sign). Before other objective signs of recovery appear, the patient may say that the part feels more life-like or is less numb. The first objective sign of returning function is a diminution in the area of impaired deep sensibility. Painful sensibility returns next, but for a long time has characteristics which distinguish it from normal pain. During this stage of recovery, a stronger stimulus than normal may be required to evoke pain, but the response is of a peculiarly unpleasant quality, and is diffuse and badly localized ('hyperpathia' or the stage of 'protopathic sensation' according to Head). Somewhat later the affected area becomes especially sensitive to extremes of heat and cold. The appreciation of light touch, and its accurate localization and tactile discrimination—Head's 'epicritic sensation'—do not recover until many months after the return of pain sensation, and may never recovery completely. When recovery of appreciation of light touch occurs the uncomfortable and irradiating painful sensibility disappears. However, when a peripheral-nerve lesion gives rise to chronic pain, resection and subsequent grafting of that nerve may not relieve it (see causalgia, and Noordenbos and Wall 1981).

With the return of pain sensation, vasomotor changes become less conspicuous and the skin heals more readily. There is often considerable sensory recovery before there is any return of motor power. In testing voluntary power the limb should always be placed in such a position that the movement to be carried out is not opposed by the force of gravity. Further, when a muscle can act both as a prime mover and as a synergist it should be tested in both capacities, as return of power may be demonstrated in one before the other.

The above description of recovery applies only to a nerve which has been completely divided and sutured. After axonotmesis recovery is slightly more rapid and much more often complete; after neurapraxia, as stated above, it is more rapid still, and always complete.

The following scheme was recommended by the Medical Research Council to assess recovery, both motor (voluntary power) and sensory:

I. Motor recovery

Stage 0. No contraction.
Stage 1. Return of perceptible contraction in the proximal muscles.
Stage 2. Return of perceptible contraction in both proximal and distal muscles.
Stage 3. Return of function in both proximal and distal muscles of such an extent that all *important* muscles are of sufficient power to act against resistance.
Stage 4. Return of function as in stage 3 with the addition that *all* synergic and isolated movements are possible.
Stage 5. Complete recovery.

II. Sensory recovery

Stage 0. Absence of sensibility in the autonomous zone.
Stage 1. Recovery of deep cutaneous pain sensibility within the autonomous zone.
Stage 2. Return of some degree of superficial cutaneous pain and touch sensibility within the autonomous zone.
Stage 3. Return of superficial cutaneous pain and touch sensibility throughout the autonomous zone with disappearance of any over-response.
Stage 4. Return of sensibility as in stage 3 with the addition that there is recovery of 2-point discrimination within the autonomous zone.

Donoso, Ballantyne, and Hansen (1979) suggest that if there is no voluntary EMG activity in a muscle supplied by a sutured nerve within seven months (12 months for grafts), or measurable motor conduction distal to the suture by 10 months (14 months for grafts), or of clinically detectable muscle movement by 10 months, re-exploration is indicated.

Treatment

Non-operative treatment

Treatment is directed to avoiding swelling of the paralysed part, to maintaining the nutrition of the paralysed muscles, preventing contractures in their antagonists, and keeping the joints mobile, so that when regeneration of nerve fibres occurs the limb may be in the best possible condition to profit by the return of nervous function. Even if operation on the nerve is required, the treatment of the limb is the same before and after the operation. In the past, firm splinting was commonly employed in order to keep a paralysed muscle in a relaxed position and to preclude movement which was thought to promote contracture of antagonists. Seddon (1975) reviewed the objective evidence in detail and concluded that except in cases of Erb's paralysis, when the arm should be splinted at the shoulder in a position of abduction and external rotation, splinting generally has little to commend it, as immobilized muscles tend to atrophy and become fibrotic more quickly. Hence while over-stretching of paralysed muscles must be avoided, regular passive movement is generally indicated and only those light spring-loaded devices which allow movement against slight resistance in the initially paralysed muscles once they begin to show evidence of voluntary contraction are indicated. There is also some dispute about the value of regular electrical stimulation, but Seddon (1975) concluded that repetitive square-wave stimulation of paralysed muscles at a frequency of about 40 stimuli per minute is of some value. As soon as voluntary power begins to return, the patient is encouraged to assist recovery by active exercises, in which at first the movement is assisted by the physiotherapist. Later re-education in skilled movements is an important part of the treatment, and the patient must be prevented from relying upon 'trick movements'. Sensory rehabilitation, especially in the hand after lesions of the median and/or ulnar nerves, may be even more crucial functionally than return of full motor power (*The Lancet* 1981), and formal sensory retraining exercises help patients to realise their full sensory potential (Wynn-Parry and Salter 1975).

Operative treatment

The techniques of peripheral-nerve surgery do not fall within the scope of this book, but it is desirable to consider the indications for surgical treatment, which were considerably clarified by experience during the Second World War. On the whole, recovery is more complete after secondary than after primary suture. In all open wounds, therefore, when there is a risk of infection, primary suture should never be performed. If the nerve is seen, its condition should be noted, and if it has been divided, steps taken to prevent retraction of the stumps. Secondary suture can then be performed two or three months later. There is good evidence to show that direct and detailed reconstruction of the intraneural architecture with matching and suture of individual nerve fasciculi under the operating microscope (so-called funicular repair) is preferred by many surgeons, but there is still dispute as to whether this method, or traditional epineurial repair, gives better results (*British Medical Journal* 1979a). An exception to this rule was made by some surgeons in the case of small penetrating war wounds and clean glass cuts which almost invariably heal well after suture, but Seddon (1975) recommended secondary suture for these injuries also. When the patient presents with a healed wound and the past treatment of the nerve injury is unknown, the nerve should be explored, unless the clinical condition and electrophysiological tests suggest that the lesion is neurapraxial. After closed injuries with fractures medical treatment should be carried out for long enough to permit regenerating nerve fibres to reach the most proximal muscle supplied by the nerve, calculating the rate of regeneration at 1 mm a day and allowing a slight margin. If there is then no recovery of function in that muscle, the nerve should be explored. Ballantyne and Campbell (1973), who carried out serial electrophysiological studies after segmental repair of selected human peripheral nerves, found that maximum improvement of sensory function was observed at 15 months after suture but improvement in conduction in motor fibres sometimes continued for up to 47 months. Cragg and Thomas (1964) studied experimentally the conduction velocity in regenerated peripheral-nerve fibres.

In severe traction injuries of the brachial plexus, when there is evidence (p. 500) of distraction of roots or spinal nerves, surgical treatment is valueless. For many years nerve grafting has been used to bridge large defects in peripheral nerves. Autografts may be successful but their use is limited by the size of the nerve and the length of the graft required. Allografts were often unsuccessful in the past because of rejection of the grafted nerve segment, but Gye, McLeod, Hargrave, Pollard, Loewenthal, and Booth (1972), among others, showed that the use of allografts combined with immunosuppression with drugs such as azathioprine may be much more successful after severe injury or even in diseases such as leprosy (McLeod, Hargrave, Gye, Pollard, Walsh, Little, and Booth 1975).

Causalgia

Symptoms

Causalgia is a distressing symptom, usually associated with incomplete lesions of a peripheral nerve. Though it may follow a lesion of any nerve, it is most often seen when the inner cord of the brachial plexus or the median or the sciatic nerve is damaged. It consists of intense and persistent burning pain, subject to paroxysmal exacerbations; this may be excited not only by actual contact with the limb but also by any event which excites an emotional reaction in the patient. The pain usually begins a week or two after the injury. The appearance of the affected limb is characteristic. In median-nerve causalgia the hand is pink and sweating; the skin is tight and glossy; the nails are curved, grow rapidly, and are tender; the finger pads are wasted, so that the nail-beds protrude; the joints are stiff and swollen, and the bones rarefied and brittle. Tenderness may be evoked either by superficial or by deep stimulation or both, in a few cases only by the latter. Superficial tenderness usually extends over the whole cutaneous area innervated by the nerve, and thus is more extensive than the area of anaesthesia produced by nerve section, which corresponds to the area exclusively supplied by the nerve. The affected nerve may be tender throughout the whole length of the limb, even as high as the brachial plexus. There may be little or no associated muscular paralysis. Owing to the extreme tenderness of the affected part the patient makes every effort to protect the limb from all forms of external stimulation. Similar symptoms may be referred to the stump following amputation.

Many attempts have been made in the past to explain causalgia; the most plausible explanation has been elaborated on the basis of the 'gate theory' of sensation of Melzack and Wall (1965) (p. 46). If large-diameter sensory fibres are selectively damaged by injury, the 'gate' mechanism is then biased in favour of small-fibre influences (*The Lancet* 1972) so that all somatic input from the affected area of skin produces hyperpathia. It has also been suggested that there may be false synapses (ephapses) between afferent fibres subserving pain in sympathetic nerves with somatic sensory afferents, but this is much less certain and the exact role played by the autonomic system has not yet been established.

Treatment

The most effective treatment appears to be sympathetic block with local anaesthetic, followed by sympathectomy if the pain is relieved. Surgical excision of the affected segment of nerve followed by resuturing and/or procaine block of somatic afferents and even cordotomy have been shown as a rule to be ineffective. Noordenbos and Wall (1981) reported seven patients who suffered chronic pain after partial peripheral-nerve lesions (with causalgia representing the most extreme variety) in whom neurolysis, local anaesthesia, sympathetic block, guanethidine, percutaneous electrical stimulation, and powerful analgesics had all failed to give relief; all underwent resection of the affected nerve segment followed by grafting, and in all pain of similar intensity, character, and distribution recurred. They suggest that peripheral-nerve damage may produce pathophysiological changes in the central nervous system which are not reversed by treatment directed at the site of the original injury. Nevertheless, there are some cases in which repetitive percutaneous electrical stimulation of large sensory fibres does give relief (Meyer and Fields 1972), as does sympathectomy, but no single form of treatment is invariably successful.

Symptoms superficially resembling those of causalgia sometimes develop in amputation stumps in which painful neuromata on the distal ends of severed nerves develop. In such cases, the severe spontaneous pain may be reproduced by pressure upon the neuroma. Excision of the neuroma or repeated injection of local anaesthetic or phenol may give relief but repeated percussion of the neuroma in the amputation stump with an appropriate instrument may also be effective in some cases.

Algodystrophy (the shoulder–hand syndrome)

Algodystrophy or 'reflex dystrophy of the upper extremity' is the name commonly used in France to identify a syndrome thought by some to be related to causalgia, which is more often known in Anglo-American terminology as the 'shoulder–hand syndrome'. Algodystrophy is probably the more appropriate term since rarely a similar syndrome may involve the foot. The condition is characterized by intense, ill-defined pain and hyperpathia in the affected extremity, often with swelling, smooth shiny skin, increased sweating, vasomotor changes, and, in chronic cases, atrophy and osteoporosis of the bones (Sudeck's atrophy) (*British Medical Journal* 1978). Pericapsulitis of the shoulder joint (a 'frozen shoulder') is almost always present; in a series of 23 patients with frozen shoulder, three developed the associated changes in the hand (Bruckner and Nye 1981). While many cases follow trauma to the affected limb, the condition can also follow hemiplegia, myocardial infarction, herpes zoster, or treatment with barbiturates. The cause is unknown; sympathectomy may be effective in relieving the condition, as may guanethidine infusions; local corticosteroid injections into the shoulder joint capsule can also be helpful.

Symptoms, signs and treatment of individual nerve lesions

Entrapment neuropathies (and other lesions of individual peripheral nerves)

While isolated lesions of individual peripheral nerves can result from ischaemia or inflammation ('mononeuritis multiplex'), from trauma, or from infiltration or compression by malignant processes, to quote but a few examples, most such lesions seen in clinical practice are due to compression or entrapment by other anatomical structures. The entrapment neuropathies have been comprehensively reviewed by Nakano (1978) and by Dawson, Hallett, and Millender (1983). Congenital ring constrictions of the trunk and limbs are a rare cause (Marlow, Jarratt, and Hosking 1981).

The phrenic nerve

The phrenic nerve is derived from the anterior primary divisions of the third, fourth, and fifth cervical spinal nerves, the main contribution coming from the fourth. It is the motor nerve to the diaphragm. Irritation of this nerve causes a dry, unproductive, 'barking' cough: rarely it may cause hiccup. Paralysis causes loss of movement of the diaphragm on the affected side. The effects are most evident when the lesion is bilateral. The diaphragm fails to descend on inspiration and may actually be drawn upwards. There is increased eversion of the costal margins with indrawing of the upper abdominal wall on inspiration. Diaphragmatic paralysis alone causes no symptoms as long as the patient is at rest, but dyspnoea may occur on exertion. Bilateral paralysis in patients with spinal muscular atrophy or limb-girdle muscular dystrophy, in whom the intercostal muscles are also involved, may sometimes give severe alveolar hypventilation with hypercapnia, requiring assisted respiration. Diminished expansion of the bases of the lungs renders the patient liable to develop a basal bronchopneumonia.

Diaphragmatic paralysis is most often produced by lesions involving the anterior horn cells of the spinal cord in the third, fourth, and fifth cervical segments, for example, direct trauma, poliomyelitis, transverse myelitis, and tumours of the spinal cord. The phrenic nerve was once intentionally divided for the treatment of tuberculosis; it may be injured during operations on the neck, or compressed by aneurysm of the aorta, by intrathoracic neoplasms, or by enlarged mediastinal glands. It may be involved in polyneuropathy due to alcohol, diphtheria, lead, or other toxins

or in post-infective polyneuropathy (the Guillain–Barré syndrome). In such cases conduction velocity in the nerve, which can be measured electrically (Davis 1967), is usually reduced.

The nerves of the upper limb

The brachial plexus

The brachial plexus (Fig. 18.3) is formed from the anterior primary divisions of the fifth, sixth, seventh, and eighth cervical and the first thoracic spinal nerves. It sometimes receives a contribution from the second thoracic nerve. Variations in the composition of the plexus are not uncommon. In the so-called 'prefixed' type there is a contribution from the fourth cervical nerve; the fifth cervical branch is large and there may be no branch from the second thoracic. In the 'post-fixed' type there may be no branch from the fourth cervical, and that from the fifth is comparatively small, whereas the second thoracic branch is quite distinct. The spinal segmental representation of muscles may be slightly higher or slightly lower than normal, according to whether the plexus is prefixed or post-fixed.

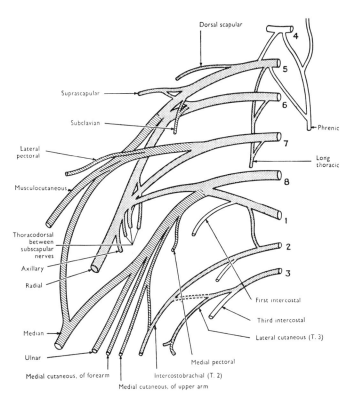

Fig. 18.3. Right brachial plexus. The anterior trunks are shaded, the posterior stippled.

The contributions to the plexus from the anterior primary divisions soon divide into anterior and posterior trunks, and from these its three cords are formed. The lateral cord is formed by a union of anterior trunks of the fifth, sixth, and seventh nerves. From it arise the lateral anterior thoracic (pectoral) and musculocutaneous nerves and the lateral head of the median nerve. The medial or inner cord is formed by a combination of the anterior trunk of the eighth cervical with the contribution of the first thoracic nerve to the plexus. It gives origin to the medial head of the median nerve, the ulnar nerve, the medial cutaneous nerves of the arm and forearm, and the medial anterior thoracic (pectoral) nerve. The posterior cord is formed by the union of the posterior trunks from the fifth, sixth, seventh, and eighth cervical and sometimes the first thoracic nerves. It gives rise to the axillary and radial nerves, the two subscapular nerves, and the nerve to teres major.

Certain muscles are innervated by nerves which leave the plexus proximal to the formation of the three cords. The most important are: the dorsal scapular nerve, from the fifth cervical, which supplies the levator scapulae and the rhomboid muscles; the long or posterior thoracic nerve, from the fifth, sixth, and seventh cervical nerves, which supplies the serratus anterior; and the suprascapular nerve, from the fifth and sixth cervical nerves, which supplies the supraspinatus and the infraspinatus. For details of methods of examination of individual muscles and their innervation by roots and peripheral nerves, see Medical Research Council (1976).

Lesions of the brachial plexus

If we consider with the brachial plexus the spinal nerves from which it is derived, we find that it is liable to damage at many points and from many causes. One or more spinal nerves may be involved by a lesion of the cervical spine, including congenital abnormality such as fusion of vertebrae—the Klippel–Feil syndrome—fracture-dislocation, herniated intervertebral disc, spondylosis occurring alone or with any of the latter, and, rarely, tuberculous or syphilitic caries or malignant deposits. The plexus itself may be damaged by stabs or gun-shot wounds, by fracture of the clavicle, and by dislocation of the upper end of the humerus. Its component parts may be torn by forcible separation of the head and shoulder or by abduction of the arm, or compressed by abnormalities in the thoracic outlet (the space between the clavicle and first rib). The plexus is occasionally invaded by neoplastic deposits in cervical lymph nodes or by apical pulmonary neoplasm, and it can be compressed by a neurofibroma. The character of the motor and sensory disturbances resulting from such lesions depends upon their situation and the part(s) of the plexus involved.

Total plexus paralysis

This is rare. When the lesion is close to the vertebral column, all the muscles supplied by the plexus are paralysed and the cervical sympathetic may also be involved. When the plexus is involved at the level of the cords, the spinati, rhomboids, serratus anterior, pectorals, and cervical sympathetic may escape. Appreciation of light touch, pain, and temperature is lost over the forearm and hand and over the outer surface of the arm in its lower two-thirds. Postural sensibility and appreciation of passive movement are lost in the fingers. All upper-limb tendon reflexes are absent.

Upper plexus paralysis (Erb–Duchenne type)

This is due to a lesion of the branch from the fifth cervical nerve to the brachial plexus. Occasionally the sixth cervical contribution is involved but this is exceptional. Upper plexus paralysis is usually the result of indirect violence, the nerve being torn by undue separation of the head and shoulder. It was once a common form of birth injury resulting from traction on the head when there was difficulty in delivering one shoulder. It may occur in adults as a result of a fall on the shoulder forcing the head to one side as on falling violently from a motor cycle, and occasionally follows general anaesthesia in patients in whom, during the operation, the arm has been held abducted and externally rotated. The muscles paralysed as a result of interruption of the fifth cervical nerve are the biceps, deltoid, brachialis, brachioradialis, supraspinatus, infraspinatus, and the rhomboids. When the sixth cervical is also involved there may be weakness, but not usually complete paralysis, of serratus anterior, latissimus dorsi, triceps, pectoralis major, and extensor carpi radialis.

The position of the limb is characteristic. It hangs at the side internally rotated at the shoulder, with the elbow extended and the forearm pronated. There is wasting of the paralysed muscles. Paralysis of the deltoid renders abduction at the shoulder impossible. The elbow cannot be flexed because of paralysis of the flexors. External rotation at the shoulder is lost owing to paralysis of the spinati. Movements of the wrist and fingers are unaffected. The biceps and supinator jerks are lost. There is usually no sensory loss, but occasionally a small area of anaesthesia and analgesia is found overlying the deltoid.

The results of operative treatment are disappointing and surgical intervention is inadvisable, except in those rare instances in which the upper plexus has been injured by a stab or gun-shot wound. It is contra-indicated if the lesion is shown to be proximal to the dorsal-root ganglia (Bonney 1954; Seddon 1975). The 'flare' response which follows local scratching of the skin is an axon reflex which is lost in lesions occurring distal to the ganglia. Thus if the 'flare' response is present, and particularly if myelography demonstrates a traumatic meningocele (Seddon 1975) or a pattern of root-sleeve filling which indicates that the fifth root or spinal nerve has been torn from its origin from the spinal cord, the prognosis is very poor. The arm should be put up in an adjustable abduction splint with a movable joint at the elbow, and the usual after-treatment of peripheral nerve lesions should be carried out. When the lesion is distal to the ganglia, however, the prognosis is generally better as actual division or tearing of the nerve is then less common, especially when the cause of the paralysis is birth injury. Complete recovery occurs in at least 50 per cent of cases. In infants recovery is often rapid and may be complete in from three to six months. In adults it may take as long as two years. Seddon (1975) gave detailed advice about splints, prostheses, and operations involving muscle transplantation which may be of value in such cases. Holler and Hopf (1968) drew attention to aberrant reinnervation after partial recovery due to regeneration which may give rise to synkinetic movements of shoulder girdle muscles and one-half of the diaphragm.

Lower plexus paralysis (Dejerine–Klumpke type)

The contribution of the first thoracic nerve to the brachial plexus may be torn as a result of traction on the arm when in an abducted position. Lower plexus paralysis sometimes results from birth injury, or may be produced by a fall during which the patient endeavours to save himself by clutching something with the hand. The first thoracic nerve is usually affected alone, but the eighth cervical may also be involved. The resulting paralysis and wasting involves all the small hand muscles, a claw-hand resulting from the unopposed action of the long flexors and extensors of the fingers. When the eighth cervical nerve is also involved there may be wasting and weakness of the ulnar flexors of the wrist and fingers. Cutaneous anaesthesia and analgesia are present in a narrow zone along the ulnar border of the hand and for a variable distance up the forearm. There is often an associated paralysis of the cervical sympathetic.

Lesions of the cords of the plexus

The effects of lesions of the cords of the plexus can readily be deduced from the anatomical information given above.

The lateral cord. The lateral cord is occasionally injured in dislocations of the humerus. Its interruption causes paralysis of the biceps, coracobrachialis, and of all the muscles supplied by the median nerve, except those of the thenar eminence. Sensation is affected to a variable extent on the radial aspect of the forearm.

The posterior cord. This is rarely damaged, but when it is there is paralysis of the muscles supplied by the axillary and radial nerves, and loss of sensibility over the areas of their cutaneous supply.

Middle plexus paralysis. This is also rare and is equivalent to interruption of the posterior cord with, in addition, paralysis of the latissimus dorsi as a result of involvement of the thoracodorsal nerve.

The inner medial cord. Injury to the inner cord of the plexus is most often produced by subcoracoid dislocation of the humerus. It causes paralysis of the muscles supplied by the ulnar nerve, and of those intrinsic muscles of the hand supplied by the median. Sensory loss occurs along the ulnar border of the hand and forearm. Treatment is that appropriate to the individual nerves involved.

Recently it has been reported that coronary-artery bypass surgery may be complicated by peripheral-nerve lesions, of which the commonest is a brachial plexopathy, usually involving the lower trunk or fibres of the inner cord, and thought possibly to be related to needle trauma during jugular-vein cannulation (Lederman, Breuer, Hanson, Fulan, Loop, Cosgrove, Estafanous, and Greenstreet 1982). Other mononeuropathies seen in such cases have included lesions of the saphenous, common peroneal, ulnar, phrenic, and recurrent laryngeal nerves, as well as Horner's syndrome. Most deficits were transient and lasting disability was rare.

Diagnosis of the site of the lesion
It is important in relation to both prognosis and treatment to decide the precise site of the lesion. Axon responses to histamine and reflex vasodilatation to cold help to decide this, being absent when the lesion is distal to the dorsal-root ganglion and present when it is proximal (Bonney 1954; Seddon 1975). Myelography and somatosensory evoked potential recording may also be needed (see above).

Costoclavicular syndromes including cervical rib

Aetiology and pathology

The adoption by man of an upright posture and the release of his upper limb as an organ of prehension has imposed certain stresses upon the nervous and vascular supply of the limb, and rendered the bony structure of the upper thoracic outlet liable to congenital abnormalities which may interfere with nerves and blood vessels. There may be a rudimentary rib derived from the seventh cervical vertebra—cervical rib, which is sometimes associated with a pre-fixed brachial plexus. The first true rib may be congenitally abnormal. The brachial plexus may alternatively be post-fixed, and the contribution from the first thoracic nerve is then unusually large, often with an addition from the second thoracic segment.

The production of symptoms by these factors is complex (Lascelles, Mohr, Neary, and Bloor 1977). The eighth cervical and first thoracic contributions to the plexus may rest upon, and be compressed by, a cervical rib, an enlarged seventh cervical transverse process, a fibrous band uniting this process to the first rib or by the edge of the scalenus anterior or medius muscles. Or it may be compressed by an abnormal or even a normal first rib. The subclavian artery in such cases often arises at a higher level than normal, and may be similarly compressed, or, on abducting the arm, by the clavicle, as it lies between the clavicle and the first rib.

While the scalenus anterior and medius muscles may play a part in the production of symptoms there seems to be no justification for identifying a specific 'scalenus anterior syndrome'. The mutual relations of the various structures of the upper thoracic outlet are constantly being altered by the respiratory movements and by movements of the upper limb, which contribute a cumulative traumatic factor, which may in time lead to the production of fibrous tissue—an additional element in compression. The third part of the subclavian artery may become the site of aneurysmal dilatation (Naylor 1958), in which thrombosis may be a source of embolism in the upper limb (Rob and Standeven 1958) or even in the vertebral artery giving brainstem ischaemia, or the artery itself may become thrombosed. Finally, loss of tone in the shoulder girdle, traction due to carrying heavy weights, or drooping of the shoulder-girdle after thoracoplasty, may precipitate symptoms in middle life even though the bony abnormalities are congenital, or may cause symptoms even when the bony structures are normal. These factors probably explain why in right-handed persons symptoms usually occur on the right side, though cervical ribs are generally bilateral, and why women are more prone than men to develop symptoms in middle life.

Symptoms may be either neurological or vascular, or both, the latter being due to intermittent or persistent vascular occlusion. The occasional coexistence of Horner's syndrome is difficult to explain except as a result of traction upon the cervicothoracic ganglion. Cervical ribs are fairly common, and are often present without causing symptoms: in fact it has been estimated that symptoms occur in only 5 to 10 per cent of cases. They may also be associated with other developmental abnormalities, notably syringomyelia.

Symptoms rarely arise in childhood, but occur with increasing frequency between the third and fifth decades of life.

Symptoms and signs

With structural abnormalities. The onset is usually gradual, and the symptoms of which the patient complains may be mainly sensory, motor, or vascular, or a combination of these. The commonest sensory symptom is pain, referred to the ulnar border of the hand and distal half of the forearm and often associated with numbness, tingling, or other paraesthesiae. Typically the pain is relieved by raising the hand above the head, which diminishes the pressure upon the nerve. Sensory examination often reveals either hyperalgesia or relative analgesia in a narrow zone corresponding to the cutaneous distribution of the eighth cervical or first thoracic segment along the ulnar border of the hand and lower forearm or occasionally on the medial aspect of the upper arm. Exceptionally, pain in the neck at the site of the rib is the only symptom. Motor manifestations consist of weakness and wasting, the distribution of which depends in part upon the position of the plexus. It is usually confined to the small muscles of the hand (Gilliatt, le Quesne, Logue, and Sumner 1970), and may begin either in those supplied by the median or in those supplied by the ulnar nerve. Less frequently the muscles of the ulnar side of the forearm are affected, often most when the plexus is post-fixed. Horner's syndrome may be present.

Vascular symptoms are due to compression of the subclavian artery. Attacks of blanching or cyanosis of the fingers occur, and sometimes even gangrene. The radial pulses are frequently unequal, being of smaller volume upon the affected side, and can sometimes be obliterated when the shoulder is retracted. The course of the subclavian arteries is frequently abnormal when cervical ribs are present, and the artery can be felt passing obliquely across the posterior triangle of the neck to a point behind the middle of the clavicle. Thrombosis or stenosis of the artery may occur, and there is often a systolic bruit or palpable thrill over the vessel. Symonds reported a case in which the thrombus extended from the subclavian artery on the right side into the right common carotid, and caused embolism of the right internal carotid; vertebral artery embolism is commoner (Gunning, Pickering, Robb-Smith, and Ross Russell 1964). There may also be an aneurysm distal to the point of pressure with embolism of digital arteries.

The cervical rib may be visible or palpable as a bony swelling in the neck, pressure over which may cause pain or tingling referred to the ulnar border of the hand and forearm, or obliteration of the radial pulse. Cervical ribs can be demonstrated radiographically, but the symptoms may be due to a fibrous band, which will not be seen in radiograms, or to a normal first rib. The whole cervical and upper thoracic spine should be included in the X-rays.

Without overt structural abnormalities. Though the symptoms may be as severe as in the former group they tend to be less so, to be sensory rather than motor, and subjective rather than objective. Pain and paraesthesiae are referred along the ulnar border of the forearm and hand. Nocturnal acroparaesthesiae (pain and tingling in the hands, occurring especially at night, and often in middle-aged women) (Heathfield 1957; Dick and Zadik 1958) were once attributed to this 'costoclavicular outlet syndrome' but are now known in practically all cases to be due to compression of the median nerve in the carpal tunnel.

Diagnosis

The effects of a cervical rib are distinguished from those of motor-neurone disease by the presence of pain and analgesia. In syringomyelia, wasting of the small hand muscles is associated with analgesia and thermo-anaesthesia, but the sensory loss is usually much more extensive than that associated with a cervical rib, and signs of corticospinal-tract degeneration are likely to be present; however, the two conditions may coexist. The radiographic demonstration of a rib must not, therefore, be taken as proof that it is the cause of the patient's symptoms. Tumour of the lung apex will usually be visible radiographically. Lesions of the median or ulnar nerves may be confused with cervical rib, but the diagnosis is established by the characteristic distribution of the motor and sensory symptoms of lesions of these nerves. Clinically, the single most useful diagnostic sign is that of reproducing the patient's pain and paraesthesiae on the affected side by rolling the cords of the brachial plexus under the examiner's fingers in the supraclavicular fossa. Measurement of nerve conduction velocity is invaluable in distinguishing the condition from peripheral-nerve lesions; thus conduction in the median nerve excludes a carpal tunnel syndrome and, in the ulnar nerve, entrapment at the elbow (Gilliatt, Willison, Dietz, and Williams 1978). Often in compression of the inner cord of the plexus due to cervical rib or a constricting fibrous band, the sensory evoked potential normally produced by stimulating the little finger on the affected side is lost (Gilliatt *et al.* 1970). Recording of somatosensory evoked potentials may also be helpful (Yiannikas and Walsh 1983). For other causes of wasting in the hands see page 507.

Treatment

Only surgical treatment affords permanent relief from a structural abnormality, and to obtain the best results it should be undertaken early. The precise operation required depends upon the nature of the abnormality present (Lascelles *et al.* 1977) but the characteristic clinical syndrome described above, even in the absence of any radiological abnormality, demands exploration of the root of the neck. It may be necessary simply to divide a constricting fibrous band or to remove a cervical rib or a large seventh cervical transverse process, or a portion of the first rib, depending upon the lesion. It may alternatively be sufficient to divide the scalenus anterior or medius muscle, thus allowing the first rib to drop. Following operation there is rapid relief of sensory symptoms, and considerable improvement in muscular power may be expected. If there is severe muscular atrophy before operation, it is unlikely that full recovery will occur; hence the importance of operating early.

The long thoracic nerve

The long thoracic nerve is derived by three roots from the fifth, sixth and seventh cervical nerves. The upper two roots pass through the scalenus medius muscle. The nerve, which supplies serratus anterior, is injured alone most frequently as a result of pressure upon the shoulder, either from a sudden blow or from the prolonged pressure of carrying weights on the shoulder. Occasionally it is involved in shoulder-girdle neuritis ('neuralgic amyotrophy') (see p. 521), and it is rarely involved in inflammation secondary to apical pleurisy. Isolated lesions of this nerve are comparatively rare but 'winging' of the scapula, presumably due to this cause, occasionally follows pneumonia or other infective illnesses or rarely arises spontaneously for no obvious cause.

The serratus anterior fixes the scapula to the chest wall when forward pressure is exerted with the upper limb. It brings the scapula forward when the upper limb is thrust forward, as in a fencing lunge, and it assists in elevating the limb above the head by rotating the scapula and arm when the latter is held abducted at the shoulder joint by contraction of deltoid. Paralysis of the serratus anterior causes no deformity of the scapula when the limb is at rest. If, however, the patient is asked to push the limb forward against resistance, the inner border of the scapula becomes winged, especially in its lower two-thirds (Fig. 18.4). He cannot

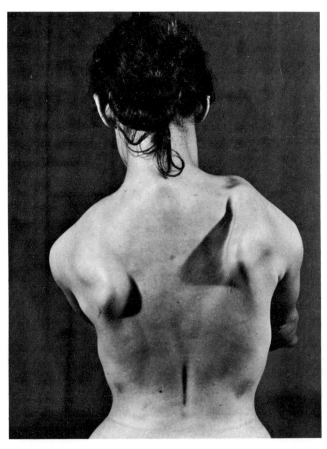

Fig. 18.4. Winging of the scapula due to paralysis of the left serratus anterior.

raise the limb above the head in front of him and on abducting the arm the scapula rides up on the posterior chest wall on the affected side and can be seen to do so when facing the patient. Electrical stimulation of the nerve at Erb's point with recording of the evoked action potential in serratus anterior can be used to measure latency (normally 3.9 ± 0.6 ms) and this technique is useful in assessing lesions of the nerve (Kaplan 1980). Relatively few isolated lesions of this nerve recover.

Compression of the *dorsal scapular nerve* by scalenus medius is a rare cause of winging of the scapula on wide abduction of the arm (Nakano 1978).

The suprascapular nerve

This nerve supplies the infraspinatus and supraspinatus. Because of its relatively short course following its origin from the brachial plexus, isolated traumatic lesions of this nerve are rare (Sunderland 1978) though it is occasionally damaged as a sequel of scapular fracture (Seddon 1975). Kopell and Thompson (1963) suggested that the nerve may suffer entrapment as it passes through the suprascapular foramen and that this is an often unrecognized source of shoulder pain following upper extremity injury. In most cases there is a 'frozen shoulder' due to pericapsulitis of the joint and motor paralysis and weakness are relatively slight. However, compression of the nerve by a hypertrophied inferior transverse scapular ligament is now well documented (Aiello, Serra, Traina, and Tugnoli 1982) and can cause paresis of the infraspinatus or supraspinatus, or both (Nakano 1978).

The axillary (circumflex) nerve

The axillary nerve arises from the posterior cord of the brachial plexus. It innervates the teres minor and deltoid muscles, and supplies cutaneous sensibility to an oval area, the long axis of which extends from the acromion process to half-way down the outer aspect of the arm (Fig. 1.33; p. 43). Injury to the axillary nerve, therefore, causes wasting and weakness of the deltoid with paralysis of abduction of the arm and anaesthesia and analgesia corresponding to its cutaneous supply, though in clinical practice the actual area of sensory loss is often no more than a small area near the insertion of the deltoid. The axillary nerve may be involved by injuries in the region of the neck of the humerus and is the nerve most often involved in shoulder girdle neuritis ('neuralgic amyotrophy'), in which case there is usually severe and persistent pain in the shoulder region for several hours or even for one or two days before the paralysis is noted. The usual treatment for peripheral-nerve lesions (p. 497) is given.

The radial or musculospiral nerve

The radial nerve constitutes the termination of the posterior cord of the brachial plexus and is derived from the fifth, sixth, seventh, and eighth cervical spinal nerves. It innervates the following muscles in the order given: triceps, anconeus, brachioradialis, extensor carpi radialis longus, and, through the posterior interosseous nerve, extensor carpi radialis brevis, supinator, extensor digitorum, extensor digiti minimi, extensor carpi ulnaris, the three extensors of the thumb, and extensor indicis. It carries sensation from the lower half of the radial aspect of the arm, and the middle of the posterior aspect of the forearm also from a variable area on the dorsum of the hand extending from the wrist distally as far as the interphalangeal joint of the thumb and the metacarpophalangeal joints of the index and middle fingers, and bounded laterally by the radial border of the thumb, and medially by the axis of the middle metacarpal (Fig. 1.33; p. 43).

Complete interruption of the radial nerve in or above the axilla causes paralysis and wasting of all the muscles it supplies. Paralysis of triceps gives inability to extend the elbow. Paralysis of brachioradialis is detected through failure of this muscle to contract when the patient flexes the elbow with the forearm midway between pronation and supination, the muscle then acting as a flexor of the elbow and not as a supinator. Paralysis of the supinator causes loss of supination. Paralysis of the extensors of the wrist and fingers gives wrist-drop and finger-drop. Not only is the patient unable to extend the wrist as a primary movement, but synergic extension of the wrist fails to occur in association with flexion of the fingers, thus secondarily impairing the power of flexion. In investigating

thumb extension special attention must be paid to extension at the carpometacarpal and metacarpophalangeal joints, since extension at the terminal joint may be carried out by some of the intrinsic hand muscles. The long extensors of the fingers produce extension only at the metacarpophalangeal joints, extension at the other joints being brought about by the interossei and lumbricals. In a case of radial paralysis, when the patient attempts to extend the fingers, the latter muscles contract synergically and give flexion at the metacarpophalangeal and extension at the interphalangeal joints. Following a pressure palsy of the radial nerve, sensory loss is variable and may be absent but if present is found usually on the dorsum of the hand between the thumb and index finger. Radial-nerve conduction studies may be helpful in determining the site of the lesion (p. 496); antidromic latency measurement may be especially helpful (Critchlow, Seybold, and Jablecki 1980).

When the nerve is injured in the lower third of the arm, as is most common, the triceps usually escapes paralysis, and the branch to brachioradialis, and less often that to extensor carpi radialis longus, may also escape, the distribution of the paralysis coinciding with that following a lesion of the *posterior interosseous nerve*. The radial nerve is often injured where it winds round the humerus as a result of fractures of that bone. It may also be compressed in the axilla through the use of a crutch, or when the arm of an anaesthetized patient is allowed to hang over the edge of the operating table, or during sleep, especially when the patient is intoxicated. In such cases pressure may be due to the arm hanging over the back of a chair ('Saturday-night paralysis'). As Kopell and Thompson (1963) pointed out, the deep branch of the radial nerve can be compressed by the fibrous edge of the extensor carpi radialis brevis, or as it passes through a slit in the supinator muscle, giving signs comparable to those of radial-nerve palsy without sensory loss, the picture being effectively that of a posterior interosseous nerve lesion. This may follow trauma and is commonly associated with a 'tennis elbow' syndrome. However, there have been many reports of 'idiopathic' posterior interosseous-nerve lesions occurring without trauma and resulting from entrapment in the supinator or compression by a fibrous band (Hustead, Mulder, and MacCarty 1958; Goldman, Honet, Sobel, and Goldstein 1969; Spinner 1972).

In such cases a light splint must be used to maintain extension of the wrist, but although extension at the metacarpophalangeal joints may be ensured, these joints should not be rigidly fixed. A system of spring extension should, therefore, be used for the fingers (a 'spring-loaded' splint); this maintains extension, while allowing flexion against slight resistance.

The prognosis of lesions of the radial nerve is often good as most are due to simple pressure and are thus neurapraxial. Even after complete division and suture, signs of returning muscular function are usually evident in from four to eight months, according to the level of the lesion. When the posterior interosseous nerve is involved and electrical tests indicate a complete lesion the nerve should be explored and if possible decompressed.

The musculocutaneous nerve

The musculocutaneous nerve is a branch of the lateral cord of the brachial plexus, its fibres being derived from the fifth and sixth cervical spinal nerves. It supplies the biceps and part of the brachialis, the principal flexors of the elbow, and its sensory distribution is to the radial border of the forearm as low as the carpometacarpal joint of the thumb (Fig. 1.33; p. 43).

Division of the musculocutaneous nerve, therefore, causes weakness of flexion of the elbow-joint, though some flexion can still be carried out by the brachioradialis and that part of the brachialis which is innervated by the radial nerve. Sensation is impaired over the cutaneous distribution of the nerve. The musculocutaneous nerve is rarely injured alone, but may be damaged by dislocation of the head of the humerus or by penetrating wounds. Very rarely it may, like the radial nerve, be affected by simple pressure of the coracobrachialis muscle (Nakano 1978) and transient paralysis of the biceps has been known to occur in a man falling asleep with his wife's head lying across his upper arm.

The forearm should be supported in a sling and the usual treatment of a peripheral-nerve lesion is given.

The median nerve

The fibres of the median nerve are derived from the sixth, seventh, and eighth cervical and first thoracic spinal segments. It is formed by the union of two heads from the inner and outer cords of the brachial plexus. In the forearm it supplies the following muscles, with branches given off in the order named: pronator teres, flexor carpi radialis, palmaris longus, flexor digitorum superficialis, flexor pollicis longus, flexor digitorum profundus, pronator quadratus. In the hand it usually supplies the two radial lumbricals, opponens pollicis, abductor pollicis brevis, and the outer head of the flexor pollicis brevis. Sometimes it supplies the first dorsal interosseous. Seddon (1975) described the commoner anomalies in the nerve supply of the muscles of the hand.

Traumatic lesions. After a complete lesion of the median nerve above its highest muscular branch there is, therefore, paralysis of pronation of the forearm. Occasionally this is due to compression of one or both heads which form the nerve as a result of sclerosis in the wall of the axillary artery to which they are closely related in the axilla. More often the nerve can be trapped or compressed as it passes through the pronator teres muscle at the elbow (the pronator syndrome—Spinner 1972) or kinked against the fibrous edge of the flexor digitorum superficialis (Kopell and Thompson 1963). Less often it is entrapped by a ligament of Struthers (a fibrous band from a supratrochlear spur or supracondylar process at the distal, anteromedial part of the humerus) (see Nakano 1978). The radial flexor of the wrist is paralysed, so that when the wrist is flexed against resistance, the hand deviates to the ulnar side. There is inability to flex the terminal phalanx of the thumb and the phalanges of the index finger. There is weakness of flexion of the phalanges of the remaining fingers, especially the middle finger, but not complete paralysis, since the ulnar half of the flexor digitorum profundus is supplied by the ulnar nerve. Flexion at the metacarpophalangeal joints is carried out by the interossei and lumbricals, of which only the two outer lumbricals are innervated by the median. Paralysis of the muscles of the thenar eminence supplied by the median nerve leads to weakness of thumb abduction, a movement which must be tested in a plane at right angles to the palm, and opposition of the thumb is lost. There is wasting of the paralysed muscles, especially conspicuous in the lateral half of the thenar eminence, rendering the first metacarpal unduly prominent (Fig. 18.5). A lesion of the median nerve or of the anterior interosseous nerve in the middle of the forearm may paralyse the superficial flexors of the thumb and index finger, while allowing those of the other three fingers, the branches to which leave the nerve at a higher level, to escape. When the nerve is injured at the wrist, paralysis is confined to the hand. When investigating muscular power after a median-nerve lesion it must be remembered that the abductor pollicis longus may be used in a trick movement as a radial flexor of the wrist, and that opposition of the thumb may be simulated by the combined action of the abductors and the flexor pollicis longus.

Sensory loss following a median-nerve lesion is somewhat variable, especially in regard to the appreciation of pin-prick (see Fig. 1.33; p. 43). Loss of this modality may be confined to the skin over the terminal phalanges of the index and middle fingers, the affected area being somewhat more extensive on their palmar than on their dorsal aspect. However, pain and temperature loss

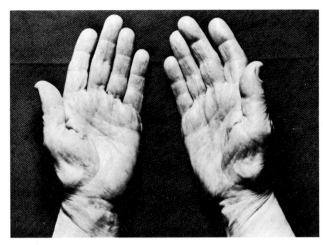

Fig. 18.5. Partial thenar atrophy due to compression of both median nerves in the carpal tunnel.

often covers a somewhat larger area, including the palmar aspect of the terminal phalanx of the thumb. Loss of appreciation of light touch is more constant in its outline, which runs along the radial border of the thumb to the base of the thenar eminence, thence across the palm to the cleft between the middle and ring fingers, including about half of the palmar aspect of the ring finger on the radial side. On the dorsum it includes the radial aspect of the terminal two-thirds of the ring finger and the dorsal aspect of the middle and index fingers as far proximally as the middle of the proximal phalanges. From the radial side of the index finger the border passes along the fold of the first interosseous space and up the inner border of the thumb as far as the ulnar edge of the nail. Deep sensibility is usually lost in the terminal phalanges of the index and middle fingers. The median nerve is the commonest site of causalgia, which only occurs, however, when the lesion is incomplete. Nerve conduction velocity measurement (p. 496) is invaluable in localizing accurately the site of the lesion (Buchthal, Rosenfalck, and Trojaborg 1974).

The median nerve may be injured at any point of its course by stab or gunshot wounds. It is occasionally damaged in dislocation of the shoulder. The commonest acute traumatic lesion in civil life is a cut at the wrist, usually the result of the hand having been put through a window pane. In such cases the ulnar nerve may also be damaged. Painful lesions of the median nerve and/or of the medial and lateral cutaneous nerves of the forearm are an occasional complication of venepuncture in the antecubital fossa (Berry and Wallis 1977).

The anterior interosseous nerve
Isolated lesions of this nerve, developing apparently spontaneously, are not uncommon (Kiloh and Nevin 1952) and usually give rise simply to paralysis of flexion of the terminal phalanges of the thumb and index finger (Smith and Herbst 1974). The diagnosis can readily be confirmed electrophysiologically (O'Brien and Upton 1972) and the latency of conduction from the elbow to pronator quadratus is usually prolonged (Nakano, Lundergan, and Okihiro 1977). While the paresis may recover spontaneously (Gardner-Thorpe 1974), if there is no recovery in a few months, exploration may be indicated, as a fibrous band constricting the nerve or compression by a tendon or aberrant muscle belly may be found (Spinner 1972).

Treatment

To prevent stretching of the paralysed muscles the thumb may be held in a position of palmar abduction and opposition by a splint consisting of a leather or plastic cuff at the wrist to which are attached two light springs which run to a moulded cylinder fitted over the matacarpophalangeal joint and made from a cast of the thumb (Highet 1942a; Seddon 1975). The usual treatment for the paralysed muscles is carried out. Causalgia requires special treatment (see p. 498). Signs of returning sensibility usually precede motor recovery. After suture of the nerve the latter occurs in from three months to a year, depending upon the situation of the lesion and the distance of individual muscles below it. Voluntary power usually reappears first in pronator teres and in flexor carpi radialis. Sensory recovery is often incomplete, especially in respect of appreciation of light touch upon the index finger, but the proportion of useful motor and sensory recoveries is high—88 and 79 per cent respectively (Seddon 1949).

The carpal tunnel syndrome

Compression of the median nerve in the carpal tunnel (Brain, Wright, and Wilkinson 1947) occurs spontaneously, chiefly in middle-aged women, and in pregnancy (Wilkinson 1960). It may also occur after fractures and arthritis involving the wrist-joint, in acromegaly, myxoedema (Murray and Simpson 1958), the nephrotic syndrome and amyloidosis, and in pyogenic infections of the hand. It results either from lesions which reduce the size of the carpal tunnel, from tenosynovitis with swelling of flexor tendon sheaths due to over-use. or from soft tissue swelling due to fluid retention (as in pregnancy or myxodema). It has been described, possibly due to ischaemia resulting from a 'steal' phenomenon, after the surgical establishment of a Cimino–Brescia fistula in patients undergoing repeated haemodialysis (Harding and Le Fanu 1977). There is also a relationship between cervical spondylosis, pericapsulitis of the shoulder joint (frozen shoulder), tennis elbow, and the carpal tunnel syndrome (Murray-Leslie and Wright 1976). It is rarely familial, due to an abnormally small size of the carpal tunnel (Danta 1975), so-called primary carpal stenosis (Dekel and Coates 1979). A similar syndrome has been noted to develop spontaneously in guinea pigs (Fullerton and Gilliatt 1967). Pain and tingling are felt in the cutaneous distribution of the nerve to the digits, often awakening the patient at night, and constituting the commonest form of acroparaesthesiae. Cutaneous sensory loss over the digits makes it difficult to handle small objects, and is sometimes accompanied by wasting and weakness of abductor brevis and opponens pollicis, with hollowing of the outer thenar eminence (Fig. 18.5). Often, however, pain and paraesthesiae may be the only symptoms for many months and years and are accentuated by using the hand or by warmth. The only abnormal physical signs may be some blunting of sensation in the thumb and fingers supplied by the median nerve and/or tingling in the appropriate distribution produced by a sharp tap over the carpal ligament. The application of a tourniquet to the upper arm above arterial blood pressure may quickly produce ischaemic paraesthesiae in the affected fingers (Gilliatt and Wilson 1954; Fullerton 1963). The demonstration of increased terminal latency on stimulation of the median nerve at the wrist and recording the muscle action potential from abductor pollicis brevis is a valuable diagnostic sign (Simpson 1956; Fullerton 1963; Preswick 1963; McLeod 1966). Studies of antidromic sensory conduction from the fingers supplied by the median nerve when compared with sensory conduction in the ulnar nerve may be even more useful (Keble 1968; Buchthal and Rosenfalck 1971; Loong and Seah 1971) and the ratio of the amplitudes of the sensory-nerve action potentials recorded from the ulnar and median nerves after stimulating the little and middle fingers is especially helpful; however, occasional patients with carpal tunnel syndrome have been found to have a subclinical ulnar neuropathy (Sedal, McLeod, and Walsh 1973). Spontaneous rhythmic motor unit potentials are occasionally found in the thenar muscles (Spaans, 1982). Rarely a normal proximal median-nerve latency is found with prolonged distal latency because of an anastomosis between the median and ulnar

nerves in the forearm (the Martin–Gruber anastomosis) (Iyer and Fenichel 1976).

The carpal tunnel syndrome in pregnancy may be expected to recover after labour (Wilkinson 1960). Diuretics, immobilization, and local injections of hydrocortisone (Foster 1960) may produce temporary improvement, but in most long-standing cases only surgical division of the transverse carpal ligament is likely to be effective.

The ulnar nerve

The ulnar nerve is derived from the eighth cervical and first thoracic spinal nerves. It gives off no branches above the elbow, where it lies behind the medial condyle of the humerus. It supplies branches to the flexor carpi ulnaris and the inner half of flexor digitorum profundus. In the hand it usually supplies the palmaris brevis, the muscles of the hypothenar eminence, the two medial lumbricals, the palmar and dorsal interossei, the transverse and oblique heads of the adductor pollicis, and the medial head of the flexor pollicis brevis. The first dorsal interosseous muscle is sometimes supplied by the median. Seddon (1954a) described some common anomalies in the nerve supply of the muscles of the hand.

Interruption of the nerve at or above the elbow causes paralysis of these muscles. As a result of paralysis of flexor carpis ulnaris the hand deviates to the radial side on flexion of the wrist against resistance. Weakness of this muscle can also be demonstrated when the patient closes his hand and the examiner adducts it, placing his finger on the tendon of the flexor carpi ulnaris; this tendon can normally be felt to tighten when the fingers are extended, but in ulnar palsy it does not do so. Paralysis of the ulnar half of the flexor digitorum profundus abolishes flexion of the little finger at the interphalangeal joints, and weakens flexion of the ring finger at these joints. Paralysis of the muscles of the hypothenar eminence abolishes abduction of the little finger, and impairs flexion of this finger at the metacarpophalangeal joint. Paralysis of the interossei abolishes abduction and adduction of the fingers. In examining these movements the hand should be kept with the palm pressed against a flat surface, as the long extensors and flexors of the fingers act to some extent as abductors and adductors. Further, when the interossei are paralysed the fingers cannot be held with the metacarpophalangeal joints flexed and the interphalangeal joints extended. Paralysis of the transverse and oblique heads of the adductor pollicis weakens adduction of the thumb, most evident when the patient attempts to press the thumb firmly against the index finger. Lumbrical weakness specifically impairs extension of terminal phalanges.

Wasting of the paralysed muscles is evident on the ulnar side of the front of the forearm, in the hypothenar eminence, the interosseous spaces, and the ulnar half of the thenar eminence (Fig. 18.6). Paralysis of the small muscles of the hand causes 'claw-hand', this posture being produced by the unopposed action of their antagonists. Since the interossei cause flexion of the fingers at the metacarpophalangeal joints and extension at the interphalangeal joints, when these muscles are paralysed the opposite posture is maintained by the long flexors and extensors, namely, hyperextension at the metacarpophalangeal joints and flexion at the interphalangeal joints. This is usually most marked in the ring and little fingers, as the two radial lumbricals, which are supplied by the median nerve, partially compensate for loss of action of the interossei on the index and middle fingers.

After a lesion of the ulnar nerve at or above the elbow, loss of deep sensibility is usually limited to the little finger. The area of analgesia to pin-prick is variable, but usually covers the little finger, the ulnar border of the palm, and often the ulnar half of the ring finger. The area of anaesthesia to light touch usually includes the little finger and the ulnar half of the ring finger, along with the ulnar border of the hand, both on its dorsal and palmar aspects as

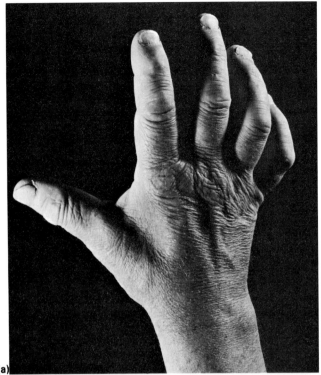

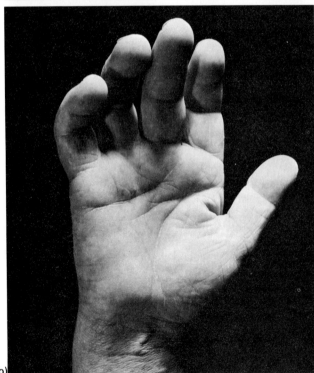

Fig.18.6. The hand in right ulnar-nerve paralysis.

far as the wrist, the area being bounded on the radial side by a line continuous with the axis of the ring finger (Fig. 1.33; p. 43).

When the ulnar nerve is divided at the wrist, the flexor carpi ulnaris and the ulnar half of the flexor digitorum profundus escape and paralysis is confined to the small muscles of the hand supplied by the nerve. When the lesion is below the point of origin of the dorsal branch, the area of sensory loss is less than that described above. On the palmar aspect of the hand the area is the same as when the nerve is divided above the wrist, but on the dorsal aspect

appreciation of light touch is lost over the terminal two phalanges of the little finger, and the ulnar half of these phalanges of the ring finger, while loss of appreciation of pin-prick is usually confined to the terminal phalanx of the little finger. In such cases all the muscles supplied by the ulnar nerve in the hand are likely to be affected. When the deep palmar branch alone is involved there is no sensory loss and the hypothenar muscles escape.

Ulnar nerve lesions

Lesions of the ulnar nerve above the elbow are rare, but it may be involved in a penetrating wound. At the elbow it may suffer as a result of fractures and dislocations involving the lower end of the humerus, and the elbow-joint. The injury to the nerve may then be immediate. Occasionally, however, it is involved years after an injury leading to cubitus valgus ('tardy ulnar palsy'—Gilliatt 1975). Similarly the nerve may be damaged by osteophytic outgrowths from arthritis of the elbow-joint, by a ganglion, or by a Charcot elbow. However, the commonest site of chronic irritation or compression of the nerve in this situation is as it passes between the humeral and ulnar heads of the flexor carpi ulnaris (the cubital tunnel syndrome) (Kopell and Thompson 1963; Spinner 1972; Eisen and Danon 1974; Miller 1979; *British Medical Journal* 1979*b*; Dawson *et al.* 1983).

In individuals who have a shallow groove for the nerve behind the inner condyle of the humerus or an unusual degree of physiological cubitus valgus, the nerve may be unduly mobile, tending to slip forwards over the inner condyle when the elbow is flexed. Occupations involving repeated elbow flexion occasionally cause symptoms through the long-continued minor trauma involved. In such cases of chronic injury of the nerve at the elbow-joint the lesion is a localized pressure neuropathy associated with fibrous thickening of the nerve at the site of trauma, where a spindle-shaped swelling can often be felt. The earliest symptoms are pain and paraesthesiae referred to the cutaneous distribution of the nerve, often first apparent only when the patient awakens in the morning after sleeping with the elbow flexed. In long-standing cases there are usually weakness and wasting of muscles innervated by the nerve as well. Pressure on the nerve behind the elbow, or where it enters the cubital tunel, may then reproduce the patient's paraesthesiae. Ulnar paralysis occasionally results from pressure on the nerve at the elbow during sleep or from repeated pressure of the elbow on a table or desk during work or study. At the wrist the ulnar nerve may be injured by cuts, and the median nerve may be simultaneously involved. The entire palmar branch of the nerve, including its superficial sensory component, is occasionally compressed or injured on the anterior aspect of the wrist. A pressure neuropathy of the deep palmar branch of the ulnar nerve sometimes occurs in individuals whose occupation involves prolonged or recurrent pressure upon the outer part of the palm and an isolated lesion of this branch has been described in a diabetic subject (Finelli 1975). Rarely, too, benign tumours may compress the deep branch in childhood (Cavanagh and Pincott 1977). In such cases the muscles of the hypothenar eminence usually escape damage and there is no sensory loss. Both at the wrist and in the palm the cause of compression may be a ganglion.

Motor and sensory nerve conduction studies may be valuable in localizing the lesion, estimating its severity, and assessing recovery (Ebeling, Gilliatt, and Thomas 1960; Gilliatt and Thomas 1960; Payan 1970; Odusote and Eisen 1979). When the lesion is at the elbow, motor conduction is markedly slowed in the segment of the nerve around the elbow, while in lesions of the deep palmar branch of the nerve, conduction in the forearm is normal but terminal latency is increased. Conduction block may persist for several months after a simple pressure palsy (Harrison 1976).

Treatment

The treatment of lesions of the ulnar nerve is similar to that of other peripheral-nerve lesions. Highet's 'knuckle-duster' splint was designed to maintain the hand in a posture of flexion at the metacarpophalangeal and extension at the interphalangeal joints (Highet 1942*a*). It was modified in order to restore the metacarpal arch (Bowden 1954*b*), and even better spring-loaded splints which do not prevent voluntary contraction in recovering muscles are now available (Seddon 1975). When the nerve is the site of pressure neuropathy as a result of abnormalities of the elbow-joint or wrist, an appropriate decompression operation is required (Miller and Hammel 1980). When the nerve suffers from chronic irritation, it must be transposed to lie in front of the inner condyle of the humerus. In such cases operation rapidly relieves sensory symptoms, but recovery of voluntary power is necessarily slower. In a series of 23 cases, good functional recovery took place in 74 per cent but muscle wasting was least likely to improve (Harrison and Nurick 1970). In lesions of the deep palmar branch, exploration is usually indicated, as it may be possible to remove a ganglion or even a small benign tumour which is compressing the nerve. After suture of the nerve, sensibility usually begins to recover before voluntary power. Motor recovery, which occurs to a useful extent in about 80 per cent of cases (Seddon 1949), usually begins in the flexor carpi ulnaris and flexor digitorum profundus, and is most complete in these muscles and in the abductor digit minimi. It may take two years after suture at the elbow.

Digital-nerve neuropathy

As Kopell and Thompson (1963) pointed out, one or more digital nerves in the hand may be compressed in the intermetacarpal tunnel. This gives burning pain and sensory impairment on the contiguous halves of two adjacent digits. Repeated digital nerve blocks with local anaesthetic agents may relieve the discomfort but not the sensory impairment.

Diagnosis of wasting of the muscles of the hand

Lesions of the median and ulnar nerves must be distinguished from other causes of wasting of small hand muscles. These muscles are innervated by the anterior horn cells of the first thoracic segment of the spinal cord, with an occasional minimal contribution from the eighth cervical. The causes of wasting, therefore, include lesions of the lower motor neurones at any point between this spinal segment and the muscles, together with certain other conditions in which primary muscular degeneration or reflex muscular wasting occurs.

Lesions of acute onset involving the anterior horns

The commonest causes are acute poliomyelitis and related viral infections. These are usually easily distinguished by the acute onset, the non-progressive character of the wasting, the presence of muscular weakness and wasting of patchy and asymmetrical distribution elsewhere in the body, and the absence of sensory loss. *Herpes zoster* is a rare cause but here the pain, rash, and sensory loss are distinctive. Acute post-infective polyradiculopathy (the Guillain–Barré syndrome) usually affects proximal limb muscles more severely than distal, at least at first, and like other forms of polyneuropathy (see below) it usually affects all four limbs. *Vascular lesions of the spinal cord* are a rare cause. Thrombosis of a branch of the anterior spinal artery can destroy anterior horn cells, but in such cases the corticospinal and spinothalamic tracts are usually damaged simultaneously. *Haematomyelia* or cord contusion following acute hyperextension injuries of the neck may also damage anterior horn cells in the cervical enlargement. Wasting is not usually confined to muscles innervated by the first thoracic segment and is generally associated with extensive sensory loss over the upper limbs and with involvement of long ascending and descending tracts of the cord.

Lesions of slow onset involving the anterior horns

The commonest chronic lesion is *motor-neurone disease*, which often begins with wasting of the small muscles in one or both hands. This condition is distinguished by its progressive course, the presence of fasciculation and, sooner or later, wasting of other muscle groups, the frequent coexistence of corticospinal-tract degeneration, and the absence of sensory loss. Genetically determined *spinal muscular atrophy* of the distal type can begin in the small muscles of the hands, and often in the feet as well; rarely, this condition remains restricted to one extremity for many years. In *syringomyelia* wasting of the hand muscles is often an early symptom. The diagnosis depends upon the characteristic associated analgesia and thermo-anaesthesia, trophic lesions, and the frequent involvement of the corticospinal tracts. In *tumour of the spinal cord* the signs of a progressive focal lesion at the cervical enlargement are usually accompanied by pain and evidence of involvement of long ascending and descending tracts.

Lesions of the ventral roots

The ventral roots are occasionally involved in localized *syphilitic meningomyelitis*, or in *arachnoiditis* in which the cord substance usually also suffers. The ventral root lesion can be distinguished from a lesion of the anterior horn cells only when the dorsal roots are also involved, giving root pain and impairment of sensation over the affected segmental cutaneous areas.

Lesions of the spinal nerve

The spinal nerve results from a fusion of the ventral and dorsal roots, and a lesion of the first thoracic nerve, therefore, causes root-pain and often sensory loss along the ulnar border of the hand and forearm, in addition to muscular wasting of the small muscles of the hand. The spinal nerve may be compressed by spinal lesions, though this is rare in the case of the first thoracic nerve which is rarely affected by intervertebral disc disease or spondylosis, in which conditions, contrary to widespread misconceptions, wasting of small hand muscles is exceptional; it can, however, result occasionally when vascular changes in the first thoracic segment follow cord compression at a higher level. It can also be compressed as a result of vertebral body collapse or extradural deposits of carcinoma or reticulosis. A traumatic lesion of the first thoracic spinal nerve is reponsible for the *Dejerine–Klumpke type of birth palsy*. Lesions involving the first dorsal segment of the spinal cord, its ventral roots and spinal nerve, usually cause paralysis of the cervical sympathetic, as its pre-ganglionic fibres leave the cord at this level.

Lesions of the medial cord of the brachial plexus

Lesions of the medial cord of the plexus, for example the pressure of a *cervical rib*, cause wasting of some or all the muscles supplied by the ulnar nerve, including those in the forearm as well as the small hand muscles supplied by the median. Often weakness and wasting are confined to the hand. The distribution of pain and sensory loss involves the eighth cervical and first thoracic segmental areas, that is, roughly, the supply of the ulnar nerve, together with part of the ulnar border of the forearm and arm.

Lesions of the median and ulnar nerves

All lesions situated between the anterior horn cells of the first thoracic segment and the medial cord of the brachial plexus, inclusive, cause wasting of the small hand muscles. Distally to the medial cord of the plexus the innervation of these muscles is divided between the ulnar and median nerves. Lesions of these nerves, as already described, are distinguished by the characteristic distribution of muscular wasting and sensory loss. Apart from localized lesions of these nerves, wasting in the hand may occur in various forms of *polyneuropathy* in which sensory loss of peripheral distribution and tenderness of the muscles are usually present, and the same symptoms and signs are usually found in the lower limbs. In *peroneal muscular atrophy* wasting of the hands usually follows that of the legs and feet but not invariably. The onset of the wasting in early life, its gradual ascent of the limbs stopping short at the elbows and knees, and the associated peripheral sensory impairment (in some cases) are distinguishing features.

Muscular dystrophy

Wasting of the small hand muscles is found in some forms of *muscular dystrophy*, especially the so-called *distal* type of *myopathy*, and much less often in *dystrophia myotonica* in which forearm muscles are wasted but not so much those of the hands. The diagnosis depends upon the age of onset, the symmetrical character, distribution, and progressive course of the wasting, the absence of fasciculation, sensory loss, and signs of involvement of the central nervous system, the familial nature of the disorder and the electrophysiological findings.

Trophic disorders

Muscular wasting secondary to disuse in *arthritis* of the joints of the hand must not be overlooked. It is easily recognized on account of pain, swelling, and bony changes in the joints. In the so-called *shoulder–hand syndrome* or *algodystrophy*, pericapsulitis of the shoulder-joint is often associated initially with painful swelling of the hand but subsequently there may be atrophy of the small hand muscles and even of the bones (Sudeck's atrophy). *Ischaemia* due to arteriosclerosis or thromboangiitis is a rare cause of muscular wasting, more often in the lower than in the upper limb. *Ischaemic contracture* caused by fractures in the region of the elbow or other major arterial lesions leads to paralysis, wasting, and contracture of the muscles of the forearm and hand, with or without sensory loss.

Electrodiagnosis

Electromyography, measurement of motor and sensory nerve conduction velocity and of distal latency (pp. 494–7) have greatly improved diagnostic precision in lesions causing wasting of the small hand muscles and studies of multisegmental efferent and afferent conduction velocity are particularly valuable (Jušić and Milić 1972).

The nerves of the lower limb

The lumbosacral plexus

The lumbar plexus is formed by contributions from the twelfth thoracic and the first, second, third, and fourth lumbar spinal nerves; the sacral plexus, from the fourth and fifth lumbar and the first, second, and third sacral nerves. The principal nerves derived from the lumbar plexus are the femoral and the obturator, and from the sacral plexus the sciatic and the superior and inferior gluteal nerves. The lumbosacral plexus may be compressed by pelvic metastases or one of its spinal nerves by a prolapsed intervertebral disc. It may be injured by the pressure of the fetal head or obstetric forceps during delivery (Donaldson 1977) and it is occasionally affected by pelvic deposits of endometriosis; either the obturator or the sciatic nerves may thus be damaged on one or both sides. The lumbosacral cord is most frequently affected, leading to unilateral or bilateral paralysis of the anterior tibial and peroneal muscles. (See also under the sciatic nerve, p. 509) Acute idiopathic lumbosacral neuropathy comparable to the much commoner brachial plexus syndrome ('neuralgic amyotrophy') (p.521) has also been described (Evans, Stevens, and Dyck 1981).

The lateral cutaneous nerve of the thigh

The lateral cutaneous nerve of the thigh is derived from the dorsal divisions of the second and third lumbar nerves. Passing through the psoas major muscle it enters the thigh beneath the lateral end of the inguinal ligament, and, piercing the fascia lata of the thigh about 4 inches distal to the anterior superior iliac spine, divides into an anterior and a posterior branch which carry sensation from the lateral aspect of the thigh and the lateral part of its anterior aspect from the buttock almost down to the knee (Fig. 1.33; p. 43). Either where the nerve emerges from the pelvis or where it passes through or beneath the inguinal ligament or through the fascia lata it may be constricted by fibrous tissue with the production of pain, numbness, and paraesthesiae referred to the cutaneous distribution of the nerve, especially of its anterior branch. Much less often there is also pain radiating along the groin, due to a connection with the ilioinguinal nerve (Teng 1972). Evidence of subclinical entrapment at the inguinal ligament is a common autopsy finding (Jefferson and Eames 1979). When symptoms occur the syndrome is known as 'meralgia paraesthetica'; it usually afflicts middle-aged men but also occurs in women, particularly when overweight. It may follow application of a plaster jacket or corset and occasionally develops secondarily to tilting of the pelvis in patients suffering from lumbar intervertebral disc prolapse. The pain and numbness are often brought on by walking or standing for long periods. The site of the pain, which is usually associated with relative anaesthesia and analgesia of the skin of the outer aspect of the thigh, is distinctive. The disorder is usually benign, has little more than a nuisance value, and may remit spontaneously. When pain is more troublesome repeated infiltration of local anaesthetic around the lateral half of the inguinal ligament may relieve symptoms, but if this is unsuccessful, operative decompression or division of the nerve may be indicated (Stevens 1957; Teng 1972).

The obturator nerve

The obturator nerve is derived from the second, third, and fourth lumbar nerves by branches which lie anteriorly to those forming the femoral nerve. The union of these roots occurs in the psoas muscle and the nerve emerges from the pelvis by the obturator foramen. It gives a branch to the hip-joint and supplies adductor longus and gracilis, adductor brevis usually, and sometimes pectineus, obturator externus, and adductor magnus. Its cutaneous supply is variable and is distributed to the skin of the distal two-thirds of the medial aspect of the thigh (Fig. 1.33; p. 43). It also supplies a branch to the knee joint.

Injury to the obturator nerve causes paralysis of the thigh adductors except for the flexor fibres of the adductor magnus, which are innervated by the sciatic. Sensory loss is usually absent. The nerve is most often injured in the course of a difficult labour, or occasionally as a result of hip dislocation. The usual treatment of lower motor-neurone paralysis is applied to the paralysed muscles.

The nerve may occasionally be compressed in the obturator canal by an obturator hernia or as a result of osteitis pubis following genito-urinary surgery and an isolated obturator neuropathy is an occasional complication of hip replacement (Melamed and Satya-Murti 1983). Pain down the medial aspect of the thigh is the most prominent symptom and sometimes demands intrapelvic section of the nerve at the expense of permanent adductor paralysis (Kopell and Thompson 1963).

The ilioinguinal nerve

This nerve, derived from the first and second lumbar roots, innervates a narrow band of skin across the upper thigh, inguinal region, iliac crest, and the base of the scrotum (or labia). It contains motor fibres to the lower portions of the transversalis and internal oblique muscles. It is rarely affected by direct injury or by a misplaced herniorrhaphy incision and is an occasional untoward complication of other forms of lower abdominal surgery (Stulz and Pfeiffer 1982); it may suffer entrapment near to the anterior superior iliac spine, especially in patients with abnormalities of the hip joint, and dysfunction of this nerve is thought sometimes to play a part in the pathogenesis of direct inguinal hernia. Pain in the groin, sometimes causing the patient to adopt a flexed posture, is the usual manifestation and injection of local anaesthetic around the nerve or division of it usually affords relief (Kopell and Thompson 1963).

The genitofemoral nerve

This nerve may be entrapped by intra-abdominal adhesions (especially after appendicectomy) or may be damaged by injury to the groin (Nakano 1978). There is pain in the internal inguinal ring, relieved by hip flexion, and there may be sensory impairment in the skin of the femoral triangle. Surgical decompression is occasionally needed.

The saphenous nerve

This terminal sensory branch of the femoral nerve (see below) is sometimes compressed as it leaves Hunter's canal, deep to the sartorius muscle, and this causes pain down the medial aspect of the knee and leg, often aggravated by climbing stairs (Nakano 1978). Knee extension and thigh adduction may increase the pain, as may digital pressure over the saphenous opening in the subsartorial fascia (about 5–6 cm above the medial femoral condyle). Surgery is rarely necessary and the condition is often self-limiting.

The femoral nerve

The femoral nerve is derived from the lumbar plexus, arising from the dorsal parts of the second, third, and fourth lumbar nerves, posterior to the obturator nerve. The nerve is formed in the psoas major muscle, and after passing through the pelvis enters the thigh beneath the inguinal ligament, lateral to the femoral sheath and femoral vessels. In the abdomen it sends a branch to the iliacus and in the femoral triangle divides into terminal branches which supply the pectineus, sartorius, and quadriceps. It gives articular branches to the hip- and knee-joints. Its intermediate and medial cutaneous branches supply the anterior and medial aspects of the thigh in its lower two-thirds, and by the saphenous nerve it supplies sensibility to the inner aspect of the leg and foot as far distally as midway between the medial malleolus and the base of the great toe (Fig. 1.33; p. 43).

After a lesion of the femoral nerve there may be slight weakness of hip flexion due to paralysis of iliacus, but the principal motor disturbance is weakness of knee extension owing to paralysis of quadriceps, which is wasted. In consequence the leg gives way in walking and climbing stairs is difficult. The knee-jerk is lost, and sensibility is lost over the cutaneous area innervated by the nerve. Causalgia may occur in the distribution of the saphenous nerve after partial lesions.

The femoral nerve may be damaged by psoas abscess or by pelvic neoplasia, or be injured in fractures of the pelvis or of the femur, or by hip dislocation. Lesions of this nerve are rarely seen as a result of gun-shot wounds of the thigh, as the proximity of the femoral artery renders most such injuries rapidly fatal. The commonest lesion is a neuropathy which is sometimes secondary to diabetes ('diabetic amyotrophy'), to lumbar spondylosis or stenosis, or may be of unknown aetiology. Bilateral neurogenic quadriceps amyotrophy is often a *forme fruste* of spinal muscular atrophy

(Furukawa, Akagami, and Maruyama 1977). In a series of 23 unilateral cases, Thage (1965) found that seven were due to diabetes, two were traumatic, one was due to neurinoma, five to lumbar disc lesions, and eight were idiopathic. Measurement of femoral nerve conduction velocity and terminal latency are invaluable in diagnosis (Thage 1974).

The sciatic nerve

The sciatic nerve is derived from the sacral plexus, which is formed by a fusion of the ventral primary divisions of the fourth and fifth lumbar and of the first, second, and third sacral spinal nerves. The nerve is composed of two divisions which are destined to form the tibial (medial popliteal) and common peroneal (lateral popliteal) nerves. These two divisions, though bound together by connective tissue, are separable up to the sacral plexus from which they are separately derived, the tibial coming from the ventral divisions of the fourth and fifth lumbar and first, second, and third sacral nerves, while the common peroneal comes from the dorsal divisions of the fourth and fifth lumbar and first and second sacral nerves. The sciatic nerve, in addition to these principal components, contains nerves to the hamstrings and a nerve to the short head of the biceps muscle. It leaves the pelvis by passing through the great sciatic notch below the piriformis muscle into the buttock and then descends in the back of the thigh, lying midway between the great trochanter of the femur and the ischial tuberosity. It terminates at a variable point between the sciatic notch and the proximal part of the popliteal fossa by dividing into the common peroneal and tibial nerves.

In addition to supplying motor nerves to semitendinosus, semimembranosus, the long and short heads of the biceps, and part of adductor magnus, the sciatic is the motor nerve to all muscles below the knee. The superficial peroneal branch of the common peroneal nerve supplies the peronei longus and brevis; the deep peroneal nerve supplies tibialis anterior, extensor digitorum longus, extensor hallucis longus, peroneus tertius, and extensor digitorum brevis. The tibial nerve supplies gastrocnemius, popliteus, plantaris, and soleus as well as tibialis posterior, flexor digitorum longus, and flexor hallucis longus. The medial and lateral plantar nerves supply the small muscles of the feet.

After complete interruption of the sciatic nerve there is paralysis of flexion of the knee, which is carried out by the hamstrings, and of all the muscles below the knee. Foot-drop occurs as a result of paralysis of the anterior tibial group of muscles and the peronei. The patient can stand and walk, but drags the toes of the affected foot and is unable to stand on his toes or heel on the paralysed side.

The sensory distribution of the sciatic nerve lies entirely below the knee (Fig. 1.33; p. 43). After complete division of the nerve, light touch is the form of sensation which is lost most extensively. Anaesthesia to cotton wool extends over the whole of the foot, with the exception of a zone about 4 cm wide along its inner aspect, extending about 5 cm distal to the internal malleolus; this is supplied by the saphenous nerve. On the leg the area of anaesthesia to light touch includes the outer aspect, roughly from the midline in front to the midline behind up to about 5 cm below the upper end of the fibula. Analgesia to pin-prick is less extensive than anaesthesia to light touch. Appreciation of pressure and of vibration is lost over the whole of the foot, except for the proximal two-thirds of its inner aspect, and position and joint sense are lost in the toes.

The knee-jerk is unaffected, but the ankle-jerk is lost and so too is the plantar reflex. Vasomotor and trophic changes are usually conspicuous after complete division. The leg is often oedematous, especially when dependent. The skin is dry, and sweating is lost over the foot, except in the saphenous area along its inner border. Perforating ulcers may develop on the sole.

The sciatic nerve may be damaged as a result of fractures of the pelvis or femur, and gunshot wounds of the buttock and thigh. In civil life a common cause of a sciatic-nerve lesion is a misplaced injection given too far medially in the buttock, and there is evidence that rarely the nerve may undergo entrapment or compression by the pyriformis muscle as it transverses the sciatic notch. It may be compressed within the pelvis by neoplasms, or by the fetal head during delivery. Sciatic-nerve dysfunction appearing during exercise and recovering after rest ('claudication' of the sciatic nerve) can be due to ischaemia of the nerve due to insufficiency of its arterial supply and this may be correctable by arterial surgery (Lamerton, Bannister, Withrington, Seifert, and Eastcott 1983). The nerve or one or both of its two major divisions can also be compressed by a popliteal (Baker's) cyst in rheumatoid arthritis or other conditions affecting the knee joint which cause such a synovial cystic swelling (Nakano 1978). The common peroneal division is much more susceptible to injury than the tibial. Complete division of the nerve is rare. Differential diagnosis is discussed in the section on sciatica.

The common peroneal (lateral popliteal) nerve

After division of the common peroneal nerve there is paralysis with wasting of the peronei and of the anterior tibial group of muscles. The power of dorsiflexion of the foot and toes and of eversion of the foot is lost, and foot-drop results. Inversion is lost when the foot is dorsiflexed, but weak inversion is possible in association with plantar-flexion. When the nerve is divided above the point of origin of its lateral cutaneous branch, sensation is impaired over the dorsum of the foot, including the first phalanges of the toes, and over the antero-lateral aspect of the leg in its lower half or two-thirds, the area of anaesthesia to light touch being somewhat more extensive than the area of analgesia (Fig. 1.33; p. 43). When the lesion lies below the origin of the lateral cutaneous branch, sensation is impaired only over the dorsum of the foot, and the anaesthetic area is usually bounded by a line passing upwards from the space between the fourth and fifth toes parallel with the outer border of the foot. Deep sensibility is unimpaired.

The common peroneal nerve may be injured by penetrating wounds in the neighbourhood of the knee-joint, or by fractures involving the upper end of the fibula. It is sometimes entrapped, compressed, or irritated by fibrous, constricting bands as it winds round the neck of the fibula and may suffer from compression by a tight bandage applied to the knee, or by pressure during sleep. In some occupations, as in slaters working on roofs, the nerve may be compressed if the individual habitually works with one leg flexed and lying under the other with its outer aspect against the roof surface. In such cases of entrapment or compression neuropathy, the muscles which the nerve innervates do not always suffer equally. The peronei are usually more severely affected than the anterior tibial group, and the area of sensory loss is often less than that found after complete division.

A common peroneal-nerve palsy, of which the most striking symptom is foot-drop, may result from the causes mentioned and often recovers in two or three months but sometimes surgical exploration of the nerve at the fibular neck is required (Sidey 1969). Sometimes no cause is identified (Berry and Richardson 1976). The diagnosis can be confirmed by measurements of nerve conduction velocity in the nerve. Slowing of sensory conduction across the segment of the nerve which passes around the neck of the fibula localized the lesion accurately in 64 per cent of a series of 47 patients (Singh, Behse, and Buchthal 1974).

It is important to note that the amplitude of the compound muscle action potential recorded by surface electrodes over the extensor digitorum brevis muscle during supramaximal stimulation of the nerve may be larger on stimulation at the knee than at the ankle. This may result from the fact that an anomalous branch of the superficial peroneal nerve (the accessory deep peroneal nerve), which passes alongside the peroneus brevis muscle and behind the lateral malleolus, may supply the lateral part of the extensor digitorum brevis (Lambert 1969; Gutmann 1970; Infante and Kennedy 1970). Palpable atrophy of the extensor digitorum brevis is a useful sign of lower-limb neuropathy and especially of a common peroneal-nerve lesion (Kirkpatrick 1982). It is also seen particularly in the rare 'anterior' tarsal tunnel syndrome in which the anterior tibial nerve suffers entrapment on entering the foot; there may also be sensory loss on the dorsum of the foot, especially between the first and second toes.

The tibial (medial popliteal) nerve

After division of the tibial nerve the calf muscles and those of the sole are paralysed and wasted and the foot assumes a position of talipes calcaneovalgus. The ankle-jerk is lost, and the plantar reflex may also be inelicitable. There is usually no loss of deep sensibility. There is anaesthesia to light touch over the skin of the sole, including the plantar aspect of the toes and the dorsal aspect of their terminal phalanges. The area of analgesia is less extensive and spares the toes (Fig. 1.33; p. 43).

Posterior tibial nerve

Rarely the posterior tibial nerve may be compressed behind and below the medial malleolus giving rise to burning pain in the sole of the foot and toes and sensory loss over almost the entire sole of the foot (the 'posterior' tarsal tunnel syndrome). If the condition is due to an abnormal posture of the foot, the use of an appropriate support may be helpful, but if it results from venous engorgement (in patients with varicose veins) or tenosynovitis, surgical decompression is occasionally required unless the causative factors can be relieved by other measures (Kopell and Thompson 1963). The condition has been described in hypothyroidism (Schwartz, Mackworth-Young, and McKeran 1983), and in hyperlipidaemia, with relief after plasmapheresis (Ruderman, Palmer, Olarte, Lovelace, Haas, and Rowland 1983). Measurement of terminal latency and of sensory conduction velocity in the medial and lateral plantar nerves are both of value in diagnosis, but sensory studies are more sensitive (Oh, Sarala, Kuba, and Elmore 1979).

Plantar and interdigital nerves

Plantar nerves may occasionally be compressed as they enter the medial aspect of the sole of the foot giving a picture of sensory loss slightly less extensive than that of posterior tibial-nerve compression (Kopell and Thompson 1963; Nakano 1978). Neuropathies of plantar interdigital nerves causing pain and analgesia in the adjacent halves of two contiguous toes have also been described and are rarely associated with neuroma formation.

Treatment

After lesions of the sciatic nerve and of the common peroneal nerve it is important to prevent contracture of the Achilles tendon. The patient should, therefore, wear a night-splint, and during the day the foot-drop should be overcome by wearing a shoe with a toe-raising spring or a light moulded plastic splint worn inside the shoe. The usual treatment of peripheral-nerve lesions should be carried out, including passive and active movement. Recovery is always slow after complete division of the nerve and suture (Seddon 1975). When the sciatic-nerve trunk has been divided, return of voluntary power cannot be expected for from a year to 18 months, and may take much longer. It may be necessary to carry out treatment for three years. In division of the common peroneal nerve some return of power may be expected to be demonstrable in from nine months to a year, but it is likely to be at least two years before maximum recovery is attained. Useful motor recovery occurs in about 50 per cent of cases after suture. In the case of the tibial nerve motor recovery is better than sensory. In the rare cases of posterior tibial or plantar-nerve compression, surgical decompression is indicated in intractable cases and in some cases of interdigital neuropathy, excision of a neuroma or division of the affected nerves may be necessary to relieve persistent pain.

References

Aguayo, A. J., Peyronnard, J. M., and Bray, G. M. (1973). A quantitative ultrastructural study of regeneration from isolated proximal stumps of transected unmyelinated nerves. *J. Neuropath. exp. Neurol.* **32**, 256.

Aiello, I., Serra, G., Traina, G. C.,, and Tugnolu, V. (1982). Entrapment of the suprascapular nerve at the spinoglenoid notch. *Ann. Neurol.* **12**, 314.

Asbury, A. K. and Johnson, P. C. (1978). *Pathology of peripheral nerve.* Saunders, Philadelphia.

Ballantyne, J. P. and Campbell, M. J. (1973). Electrophysiological study after surgical repair of sectioned human peripheral nerves, *J. Neurol. Neurosurg. Psychiat.* **36**, 797.

—— and Hansen, S. (1974). Computer method for the analysis of evoked motor unit potentials. I. Control subjects and patients with myasthenia gravis. *J. Neurol. Neurosurg. Psychiat.* **37**, 1187.

Barnes, R. (1954). Peripheral nerve injuries. *Spec. Rep. Ser. med. Res. Coun., London 282, 156.*

Barwick, D. D. (1981). Clinical electromyography, in *Disorders of Voluntary Muscle* (ed. J. N. Walton), 4th edn. Chapter 28, Churchill-Livingstone, Edinburgh.

Behse, F. and Buchthal, F. (1971). Normal sensory conduction in the nerves of the leg in man. *J. Neurol. Neurosurg. Psychiat.* **34**, 404.

Berry, H. and Richardson, P. M. (1976). Common peroneal nerve palsy: a clinical and electrophysiological review. *J. Neurol. Neurosurg. Psychiat.* **39**, 1162.

Berry, P. R. and Wallis, W. E. (1977). Venepuncture nerve injuries. *Lancet* **i**, 1236.

Bolton, C. F. and McFarlane, R. M. (1978). Human pneumatic tourniquet paralysis. *Neurology, Minneapolis* **28**, 787.

Bonney, G. (1954). The value of axon responses in determining the site of lesion in traction injuries of the brachial plexus. *Brain* **77**, 588.

Borenstein, S. and Desmedt, J. E. (1980). Range of variations in motor unit potentials during reinnervation after traumatic nerve lesions in humans. *Ann. Neurol.* **8**, 460.

Bowden, R. E. M. (1954*a*). Peripheral nerve injuries. *Spec. Rep. Ser. med. Res. Coun. London 282, 263.*

—— (1954*b*). Peripheral nerve injuries. *Spec. Rep. Ser. med. Res. Coun. London 282, 298.*

Bradley, W. G. (1974). *Disorders of peripheral nerves.* Blackwell, Oxford.

Brain, W. R., Wright, A. D., and Wilkinson, M. (1947). Spontaneous compression of both median nerves in the carpal tunnel, *Lancet* **i**, 277.

British Medical Journal (1978). Algodystrophy. *Br. med. J.* **1**, 461.

—— (1979*a*). Regeneration of peripheral nerves after injury. *Br. med. J.* **2**, 624.

—— (1979*b*). Cubital tunnel syndrome. *Brit. med. J.* **2**, 460.

Brooks, J. E. and Hongdalarom, T. (1968). Intracellular electromyography. Resting and action potentials in normal human muscle. *Arch. Neurol., Chicago.* **18**, 291.

Brown, J. C. and Wynn-Parry, C. B. (1981). Neuromuscular stimulation and transmission. In *Disorders of voluntary muscle* (ed. J. N. Walton) 4th edn, Chapter 26. Churchill-Livingstone, Edinburgh.

Brown, W. F. and Yates, S. K. (1982). Percutaneous localization of conduction abnormalities in human entrapment neuropathies. *Can. J. neurol. Sci.* **9**, 391.

Bruckner, F. E. and Nye, C. J. S. (1981). A prospective study of adhesive capsulitis of the shoulder ('frozen shoulder') in a high risk population. *Quart. J. Med.* **50**, 191.

Buchthal, F. and Kühl, V. (1979). Nerve conduction, tactile sensibility, and the electromyogram after suture or compression of peripheral nerve: a longitudinal study in man. *J. Neurol. Neurosurg. Psychiat.* **42**, 436.

——, Pinelli, P. and Rosenfalck, P. (1954). Action potential parameters in normal human muscle and their physiological determinants. *Acta physiol. scand.* **32**, 219.

—— and Rosenfalck, A. (1966). Evoked action potentials and conduction velocity in human sensory nerves. *Brain Research* **3**, special issue.

—— and —— (1971). Sensory conduction from digit to palm and from palm to wrist in the carpal tunnel syndrome. *J. Neurol. Neurosurg. Psychiat.* **34**, 243.

——, ——, and Trojaborg, W. (1974). Electrophysiological findings in entrapment of the median nerve at wrist and elbow. *J. Neurol. Neurosurg. Psychiat.* **37**, 340.

Campbell, M. J., McComas, A. J. and Petito, F. (1973). Physiological changes in ageing muscles. *J. Neurol. Neurosurg. Psychiat.* **36**, 174.

Casey, E. B. and Le Quesne, P. M. (1972). Digital nerve action potentials in healthy subjects, and in carpal tunnel and diabetic patients. *J. Neurol. Neurosurg. Psychiat.* **35**, 612.

Cavanagh, N. P. C. and Pincott, J. R. (1977). Ulnar nerve tumours of the hand in childhood. *J. Neurol. Neurosurg. Psychiat.* **40**, 795.

Cragg, B. G. and Thomas, P. K. (1964). The conduction velocity of regenerated peripheral nerve fibres, *J. Physiol.* **171**, 164.

Critchlow, J. F., Sybold, M. E., and Jablecki, C. J. (1980). The superficial radial nerve: techniques for evaluation. *J. Neurol. Neurosurg. Psychiat.* **43**, 929.

Danta, G. (1975). Familial carpal tunnel syndrome with onset in childhood. *J. Neurol. Neurosurg. Psychait.* **38**, 350.

Davis, J. N. (1967). Phrenic nerve conduction in man. *J. Neurol. Neurosurg. Psychiat.* **30**, 420.

Dawson, D. M., Hallett, M., and Millender, L. H. (1983). *Entrapment neuropathies.* Little Brown, Boston.

Dekel, S. and Coates, R. (1979). Primary carpal stenosis as a cause of "idiopathic" carpal-tunnel syndrome. *Lancet* **ii**, 1024.

Dick, T. B. S. and Zadik, F. R. (1958). Acroparaesthesiae and the carpal tunnel. *Br. med. J.* **2**, 288.

Donaldson, J. (1977). *The neurology of pregnancy.* Saunders, Philadelphia.

Donoso, R. S., Ballantyne, J. P., and Hansen, S. (1979). Regeneration of sutured human peripheral nerves: an electrophysiological study. *J. Neurol. Neurosurg. Phsychiat.* **42**, 97.

Dowling, M. H., Fitch, P., and Willison, R. G. (1968). A special purpose digital computer (Biomac 500) used in the analysis of the human electromyogram. *Electroenceph. clin. Neurohysiol.* **25**, 570.

Downie, A. W. and Scott, T. R. (1967). An improved technique for radial nerve conduction studies. *J. Neurol. Neurosurg. Psychiat.* **30**, 332.

Dyck, P. J. and Hopkins, A. P. (1972). Electron microscopic observations on degeneration and regeneration of unmyelinated fibres. *Brain* **95**, 223.

—— Thomas, P. K. and Lambert, E. H. (1975). *Peripheral Neuropathy.* Saunders, Philadelphia.

Ebeling, P., Gilliatt, R. W., and Thomas, P. K. (1960). A clinical and electrical study of ulnar nerve lesions in the hand. *J. Neurol. Neurosurg. Psychiat.* **23**, 1.

Eisen, A. and Danon, J. (1974). The mild cubital tunnel syndrome. *Neurology, Minneapolis* **24**, 608.

Ekstedt, J. (1964). Human single muscle fiber action potentials. *Acta physiol. scand.* **61**, Suppl. 226.

Evans, B. A. Stevens, J. C., and Dyck, P. J. (1981). Lumbosacral plexus neuropathy. *Neurology, Minneapolis* **31**, 1327.

Fawcett, P. R. W. and Barwick, D. D. (1981). Studies in nerve conduction. In *Disorders of voluntary muscle* (ed. J. N. Walton) 4th edn, Chapter 27. Churchill-Livingstone, Edinburgh.

Fex J. and Krakau, C. E. T. (1957). Some experiences with Walton's frequency analysis of the electromyogram. *J. Neurol. Neurosurg. Psychiat.* **20**, 178.

Finelli, P. F. (1975). Mononeuropathy of the deep palmar branch of the ulnar nerve. *Arch. Neurol., Chicago* **37**, 564.

Foerster, O. (1929). In Lewandowsky's *Handbuch der Neurologie*, Ergänzungsband, 2. Teil 1. Abschnitt. Spezielle Anatomie und Physiologie der peripheren Nerven Berlin.

—— (1929). In Lewandowsky's *Handbuch der Neurologie*, Ergänzungsband, 2. Teil 2. Abschnitt. Die Symptomatologie der Schussverletzungen der peripheren Nerven, Berlin.

—— (1929). In Lewandowsky's *Handbuch der Neurologie*, Ergänzungsband, 2. Teil 3. Abschnitt. Die Therapie der Schussverletzungen der peripheren Nerven. Berlin.

Foster, J. B. (1960). Hydrocortisone and the carpal-tunnel syndrome. *Lancet* i, 454.

Fullerton, P. M. (1963). The effect of ischaemia on nerve conduction in the carpal tunnel syndrome. *J. Neurol. Neurosurg. Psychait.* **26**, 385.

—— and Gilliatt, R. W. (1967). Median and ulnar neuropathy in the guinea-pig. *J. Neurol. Neurosurg. Psychiat.* **30**, 393.

Furukawa, T., Akagami, N., and Maruyama, S. (1977). Chronic neurogenic quadriceps amyotrophy. *Ann. Neurol.* **2**, 528.

Gardner-Thorpe, C. (1974). Anterior interosseous nerve palsy: spontaneous recovery in two patients. *J. Neurol. Neurosurg. Psychiat.* **37**, 1146.

Gentili, F., Hudson, A. R., and Hunter, D. (1980). Clinical and experimental aspects of injection injuries of peripheral nerves. *Can. J. neurol. Sci.* **7**, 143.

Gilliatt, R. W. (1975). Peripheral nerve compression and entrapment. *Eleventh Symposium on Advanced Medicine.* Pitman, London.

——, Goodman, H. V., and Willison, R. G. (1961). The recording of lateral popliteal nerve action potentials in man. *J. Neurol. Neurosurg. Psychiat.* **24**, 305.

——, Le Quesne, P. M., Logue, V., and Sumner, A. J. (1970). Wasting of the hand associated with a cervical rib or band. *J. Neurol. Neurosurg. Psychiat.* **33**, 615.

——, Melville, I. D., Velate, A. S., and Willison, R. G. (1965). A study of normal nerve action potentials using an averaging technique (barrier grid storage tube), *J. Neurol. Neurosurg. Psychiat.* **28**, 191.

—— and Sears, T. A. (1958). Sensory nerve action potentials in patients with peripheral nerve lesions. *J. Neurol. Neurosurg. Psychiat.* **21**, 109.

—— and Thomas P. K. (1960). Changes in nerve conduction with ulnar lesions at the elbow. *J. Neurol. Neurosurg. Psychiat.* **23**, 312.

——, Willison, R. G., Dietx, V., and Williams, I. R. (1978). Peripheral nerve conduction in patients with a cervical rib and band. *Ann. Neurol.* **4**, 124.

—— and Wilson, T. G. (1954). Ischaemic sensory loss in patients with peripheral nerve lesions. *J. Neurol. Neurosurg. Psychiat.* **17**, 104.

Goldman, S., Honet, J. C., Sobel, R., and Goldstein, A. S. (1969). Posterior interosseous nerve palsy in the absence of trauma. *Arch. Neurol., Chicago* **21**, 435.

Gunning, A. J., Pickering, G. W., Robb-Smith, A. H. T., and Ross Russell, R. (1964). Mural thrombosis of the subclavian artery and subsequent embolism in cervical rib. *Quart. J. Med.* **33**, 133.

Gutmann, L. (1940). Topographic studies of disturbances of sweat secretion after complete lesions of peripheral nerves. *J. Neurol. Psychiat.* **3**, 197.

—— (1970). Atypical deep peroneal neuropathy. *J. Neurol. Neurosurg. Psychiat.* **33**, 453.

Gye, R. S., McLeod, J. G., Hargrave, J. C., Pollard, J. D., Loewenthal, J., and Booth, G. C. (1972). Use of immunosuppressive agents in human nerve grafting. *Lancet* i, 647.

Harding, A. E. and Le Fanu, J. (1977). Carpal tunnel syndrome related to antebrachial Cimino-Brescia fistula. *J. Neurol. Neurosurg. Psychiat.* **40**, 511.

Harrison, M. J. G. (1976). Pressure palsy of the ulnar nerve with prolonged conduction block. *J. Neurol. Neurosurg. Psychiat.* **39**, 96.

—— and Nurick, S. (1970) Results of anterior transposition of the ulnar nerve for ulnar neuritis. *Br. med. J.* **1**, 27.

Heathfield, K. W. G. (1957). Acroparaesthesiae and the carpal-tunnel syndrome. *Lancet* ii, 663.

Highet, W. B. (1942a). Splintage of peripheral nerve injuries. *Lancet* i, 555.

—— (1942b). Procaine nerve block in the investigation of peripheral nerve injuries. *J. Neurol. Psychiat.* **5**, 101.

Holler, M. and Hopf, H. C. (1968). Posttraumatische Synkinesien zwischen Zwerchfell und Muskeln des Plexus brachialis. *Dtsch. Z. Nervenheilk.* **193**, 141.

Hustead, A. P., Mulder, D. W., and MacCarthy, C. S. (1958). Non traumatic, progressive paralysis of the deep radial (posterior interosseous) nerve. *Arch. Neurol. Psychiat., Chicago* **79**, 269.

Infante, E. and Kennedy, W. R. (1970). Anomalous branch of the peroneal nerve detected by electromyography. *Arch. Neurol., Chicago* **22**, 162.

Iyer, V. and Fenichel, G. M. (1976). Normal median nerve proximal latency in carpal tunnel syndrome: a clue to coexisting Martin–Gruber anastomosis. *J. Neurol. Neurosurg. Psychiat.* **39**, 449.

Jayson, M. I. V. (1981). Frozen shoulder: adhesive capsulitis. *Br. med. J.* **283**, 1005.

Jefferson, D. and Eames, R. A. (1979). Subclinical entrapment of the lateral femoral cutaneous nerve: an autopsy study. *Muscle & Nerve* **2**, 145.

Jones, S. J. (1979). Investigation of brachial plexus traction lesions by peripheral and spinal somatosensory evoked potentials, *J. Neurol. Neurosurg. Psychiat.* **42**, 107.

Jušić, A. and Milić, S. (1972). Nerve potentials and afferent conduction velocities in the differential diagnosis of amyotrophy of the hand. *J. Neurol. Neurosurg. Psychiat.* **35**, 861.

Kaeser, H. E. (1970). Nerve conduction velocity measurements. In *Handbook of Clinical Neurology* (ed. P. J. Vinken and G. W. Bruyn) Vol. 7, Chapter 5. North-Holland, Amsterdam.

Kaplan, P. E. (1980). Electrodiagnostic confirmation of long thoracic nerve palsy. *J. Neurol. Neurosurg. Psychiat.* **43**, 50.

Kemble, F. (1968). Electrodiagnosis of the carpal tunnel syndrome. *J. Neurol. Neurosurg. Psychiat.* **31**, 23.

Kiloh, L. G. and Nevin, S. (1952). Isolated neuritis of the anterior interosseous nerve. *Br. med. J.* **850**.

Kimura, J. (1983). *Electrodiagnosis in diseases of nerve and muscle.* Davis, Philadelphia.

Kirkpatrick, C. T. (1982). Extensor digitorum brevis—a predictor of neuropathy in the leg? *Br. med. J.* **284**, 238.

Kopell, H. P. and Thompson, W. A. L. (1963). *Peripheral entrapment neuropathies.* Williams and Wilkins, Baltimore.

Kramer, W. (1970). Tumours of nerves. In *Handbook of clinical neurology* (ed. P. J. Vinken and G. W. Bruyn) Volume 8, Chapter 23. North-Holland, Amsterdam.

Kugelberg, E. (1947). Electromyograms in muscular disorders. *J. Neurol. Neurosurg. Psychiat.* **10**, 122.

—— (1949). Electromyography in muscular dystrophies. *J. Neurol. Neurosurg. Psychiat.* **12**, 129.

Lambert, E. H. (1969). The accessory deep peroneal nerve: a common variation in innervation of extensor digitorum brevis. *Neurology, Minneapolis.* **19**, 1169.

Lamerton, A. J., Bannister, R., Withrington, R., Seifert, M. H., and Eastcott, H. H. G. (1983). "Claudication" of the sciatic nerve. *Br. med. J.* **286**, 1785.

Lance, J. W., De Gail, P., and Nielson, P. D. (1966). Tonic and phasic spinal cord mechanisms in man. *J. Neurol. Neurosurg. Psychiat.* **29**, 535.

—— and McLeod, J. G. (1981). *A physiological approach to clinical neurology*, 3rd edn. Butterworths, London.

The Lancet (1972). Causalgia. *Lancet* i, 1170.

—— (1981). Sensory rehabilitation of the hand. *Lancet* i, 135.

Lascelles, R. G., Mohr, P. D., Neary, D., and Bloor, K. (1977). The thoracic outlet syndrome, *Brain* **100**, 601.

Lederman, R. J., Breuer, A. C. Hanson, M. R., Furlan, A. J., Loope, F. D., Cosgrove, D. M., Estafanous, F. G., and Greenstreet, R. L. (1982). Peripheral nervous system complications of coronary artery bypass graft surgery. *Ann. Neurol.* **12**, 297.

Lenman, J. A. R. (1959). A clinical and experimental study of the effects of exercise on motor weakness in neurological disease. *J. Neurol. Neurosurg. Psychiat.* **22**, 182.

—— (1981). Integration and analysis of the electromyogram and related techniques. In *Disorders of voluntary muscle* (ed. J. N. Walton) Chapter 29. Churchill-Livingstone, Edinburgh.

—— and Ritchie, A. E. (1983) *Clinical electromyography.* 3rd edn. Blackwell, Oxford.

Licht, S. (Ed.) (1971). *Electrodiagnosis and electromyography.* 3rd edn. Licht, New Haven.

Loong, S. C. and Seah, C. S. (1971). Compression of median and ulnar sensory nerve action potentials in the diagnosis of the carpal tunnel syndrome. *J. Neurol. Neurosurg. Psychiat.* **34**, 750.

Magladery, J. W., Porter, W. E. Park, A. M., and Teasdall, R. D. (1951). Electrophysiological studies of nerve and reflex activity in normal man. *Bull. Johns Hopk. Hosp.* **88**, 499.

Marlow, N., Jarratt, J., and Hosking, G. (1981). Congenital ring constrictions with entrapment neuropathies. *J. Neurol. Neurosurg. Psychiat.* **44**, 247.

Marsden, C. D., Meadows, J. C., and Hodgson, H. J. F. (1969). Observations on the reflex response to muscle vibrations in man and its voluntary control. *Brain* **92**, 829.

Mayo Clinic (1981). *Clinical examinations in neurology.* 5th edn. Saunders, Philadelphia.

McComas, A. J. (1977). *Neuromuscular function and disorders.* Butterworths London.

——, Fawcett, P. R. W., Campbell, M. J., and Sica, R. E. P. (1971). Electrophysiological estimation of the number of motor units within a human muscle. *J. Neurol. Neurosurg. Psychiat.* **34**, 121.

—— and Johns, R. J. (1981). Potential changes in the normal and diseased muscle cell. In *Disorders of voluntary muscle* (ed. J. N. Walton) 4th edn, Chapter 30. Churchill-Livingstone, Edinburgh.

McLeod, J. G. (1966). Digital nerve conduction in the carpal tunnel syndrome after mechanical stimulation of the finger. *J. Neurol. Neurosurg. Psychiat.* **29**, 12.

——, Hargrave, J. C., Gye, R. S., Pollard, J. D., Walsh, J. C., Little, J. M., and Booth, G. C. (1975). Nerve grafting in leprosy. *Brain* **98**, 203.

Medical Research Council (1976). *Aids to the examination of the peripheral nervous system*, 3rd ed. H.M.S.O., London.

Melamed, N. B. and Satya-Murti, S. (1983). Obturator neuropathy after total hip replacement. *Ann. Neurol.* **13**, 578.

Melzack, R. and Wall, P. D. (1965). Pain mechanisms: a new theory. *Science* **150**, 971.

Meyer, G. A. and Fields, H. L. (1972). Causalgia treated by selective large fibre stimulation of peripheral nerve. *Brain* **95**, 163.

Miller, R. G. (1979). The cubital tunnel syndrome: diagnosis and precise localization. *Ann. Neurol.* **6**, 56.

—— and Hummel, E. E. (1980). The cubital tunnel syndrome: treatment with simple decompression. *Ann. Neurol.* **7**, 567.

Murray, I. P. C. and Simpson, J. A. (1958). Acroparaesthesiae in myxoedema. *Lancet* **i**, 1360.

Murray-Leslie, C. F. and Wright, V. (1976). Carpal tunnel syndrome, humeral epicondylitis, and the cervical spine: a study of clinical and dimensional relations. *Brit. med. J.* **1**, 1439.

Nakano, K. K. (1978). The entrapment neuropathies. *Muscle & Nerve* **1**, 264.

——, Lundergan, C., and Okihiro, M. M. (1977). Anterior interosseous nerve syndromes: diagnostic methods and alternative treatments. *Arch. Neurol., Chicago* **34**, 477.

Naylor, A. (1958). Two cases of subclavian aneurysm associated with cervical rib. *Br. med. J.* **2**, 142.

Neary, D. and Eames, R. A. (1975). The pathology of ulnar nerve compression in man. *Neuropath. appl. Neurol.* **1**, 69.

Noordenbos, W. and Wall, P. D. (1981). Implications of the failure of nerve resection and graft to cure chronic pain produced by nerve lesions. *J. Neurol. Neurosurg. Psychiat.* **44**, 1068.

O'Brien, M. D. and Upton, A. R. M. (1972). Anterior interosseous nerve syndrome. *J. Neurol. Neurosurg. Psychiat.* **35**, 531.

Odusote, K. and Eisen, A. (1979). An electrophysiological quantitation of the cubital tunnel syndrome. *Can. J. neurol. Sci.* **6**, 403.

Oh, S. J. Sarala, P. K., Kuba, T., and Elmore, R. S. (1979). Tarsal tunnel syndrome: electrophysiological study. *Ann. Neurol.* **5**, 327.

Orgel, M., Aguayo, A. J., and Williams, H. B. (1972). Sensory nerve regeneration: an experimental study of skin grafts in the rabbit. *J. Anat.* **111**, 121.

Payan, J. (1970). Anterior transposition of the ulnar nerve: an electrophysiological study. *J. Neurol. Neurosurg. Psychiat.* **33**, 157.

Preswick, G. (1963). The effect of stimulus intensity on motor latency in the carpal tunnel syndrome. *J. Neurol. Neurosurg. Psychiat.* **26**, 398.

Rasmussen, T. B. and Freedman, H. (1946). Treatment of causalgia: analysis of 10 cases. *J. Neurosurg.* **3**, 165.

Richards, R. L. (1951). Ischaemic lesions of peripheral nerves: a review. *J. Neurol. Neurosurg. Psychiat.* **14**, 76.

—— (1954). Peripheral nerve injuries. *Spec. Rep. Ser. med. Res. Coun. London* **282**, 186.

Rob, C. G. and Standeven, A. (1958). Arterial occlusion complicating thoracic outlet compression syndrome. *Br. med. J.* **2**, 709.

Rose, A. L. and Willison, R. G. (1967). Quantitative electro-myography using automatic analysis: studies in healthy subjects and patients with primary muscle disease. *J. Neurol. Neurosurg. Psychiat.* **30**, 403.

Ruderman, M. I., Palmer, R. H., Olarte, M. R., Lovelace, R. E., Haas, R., and Rowland, L. P. (1983). Tarsal tunnel syndrome caused by hyperlipidemia: reversal after plasmapheresis. *Arch. Neurol., Chicago* **40**, 124.

Rudge, P., Ochoa, J., and Gilliatt, R. W. (1974). Acute peripheral nerve compression in the baboon. *J. neurol. Sci.* **23**, 403.

Schwartz, M. S., Mackwroth-Young, C. G., and NcKeran, R. O. (1983). The tarsal tunnel syndrome in hypothyroidism. *J. Neurol. Neurosurg. Psychiat.* **46**, 440.

Sedal, L., McLeod, J. G., and Walsh, J. C. (1973). Ulnar nerve lesions associated with the carpal tunnel syndrome. *J. Neurol. Neurosurg. Psychiat.* **36**, 118.

Seddon, H. J. (1944). Three types of nerve injury. *Brain* **66**, 237.

—— (1949). The practical value of peripheral nerve repair. *Proc. R. Soc. Med.* **42**, 427.

—— (1954a). Peripheral nerve injuries. *Spec. Rep. Ser. med. Res. Coun. London* **282**, 1.

—— (1954b). Peripheral nerve injuries. *Spec. Rep. Ser. med. Res. Coun. London* **282**, 389.

—— (1975). *Surgical disorders of peripheral nerves*, 2nd edn. Churchill-Livingstone, Edinburgh.

——, Medawar, P. B., and Smith, H. (1943). Rate of regeneration of peripheral nerves in man. *J. Physiol., London* **102**, 191.

Sidey, J. D. (1969). Weak ankles. A study of common peroneal entrapment neuropathy. *Br. med. J.* **3**, 623.

Simpson, J. A. (1956). Electrical signs in the diagnosis of carpal tunnel and related syndromes. *J. Neurol. Neurosurg. Psychiat.* **19**, 275.

—— (1970). Nerve injuries. General aspects. In *Handbook of clinical neurology* (ed. P. J. Vinken and G. W. Bruyn) Vol. 7, Chapter 7. North-Holland, Amsterdam.

Singh, N., Behse, F., and Buchthal, F. (1974). Electrophysiological study of peroneal palsy. *J. Neurol. Neurosurg. Psychiat.* **37**, 1202.

Smith, B. H. and Herbst, B. A. (1974). Anterior interosseous nerve palsy. *Arch. Neurol. Chicago* **30**, 330.

Spaans, F. (1982). Spontaneous rhythmic motor unit potentials in the carpal tunnel syndrome. *J. Neurol. Neurosurg. Psychait.* **45**, 19.

Spencer, P. S. (1974). The traumatic neuroma and proximal stump. *Bull. Hosp. Jt. Dis.* **35**, 85.

Spinner, M. (1972). *Injuries to the major branches of peripheral nerves of the forearm.* Saunders, Philadelphia.

Stalberg, E. and Trontelj, J. V. (1970). Demonstration of axon reflexes in human motor nerve fibres. *J. Neurol. Neurosurg. Psychiat.* **33**, 571.

Stevens, H. (1957). Meralgia paraesthetica. *Arch. Neurol. Psychiat., Chicago* **77**, 557.

Stöhr, M., Dichgans, J., and Dorstelmann, D. (1980). Ischaemic neuropathy of the lumbrosacral plexus following intragluteal injection. *J. Neurol. Neurosurg. Psychiat.* **43**, 489.

Stulz, P. and Pfeiffer, K. M. (1982). Peripheral nerve injuries resulting from common surgical procedures in the lower portion of the abdomen. *Arch. Surg.* **117**, 324.

Sunderland, S. (1978). *Nerves and Nerve Injuries*, 2nd edn. Churchill-Livingstone, Edinburgh.

Synek, V. M. and Cowan, J. C. (1982). Somatosensory evoked potentials in patients with supraclavicular brachial plexus injuries. *Neurology Minneapolis* **32**, 1347.

Tallis, R., Staniforth, P., and Fisher, T. R. (1978). Neurophysiological studies of autogenous sural nerve grafts. *J. Neurol. Neurosurg. Psychiat.* **41**, 677.

Telford, E. D. and Mottershead, S. (1947). The 'costoclavicular syndrome'. *Br. med. J.* **1**, 325.

Teng, P. (1972). Meralgia paraesthetica. *Bull. Los Angeles Neurol. Soc.* **37**, 75.

Thage, O. (1965). The 'quadriceps syndrome'. *Acta neurol. scand. 41*, Suppl. **13**, 245.

—— (1974). *Quadriceps weakness and wasting. A neurological, electrophysiological and histological study.* Munksgaard, Copenhagen.

Thomas, P. K. (1966). The cellular response to nerve injury. 1. The cellular outgrowth from the distal stump of transected nerve. *J. Anat.* **100**, 287.

—— (1970). The cellular response to nerve injury. 3. The effect of repeated crush injuries. *J. Anat.* **106**, 463.

—— and King, R. H. M. (1974). The degeneration of unmyelinated axons following nerve section: an ultrastructural study. *J. Neurocytol.* **3**, 497.

Trojaborg, W. (1970). Rate of recovery in motor and sensory fibres of the radial nerve: clinical and electrophysiological aspects. *J. Neurol. Neurosurg. Psychiat.* **33**, 625.

—— and Buchthal, F. (1965). Malignant and benign fasciculations. *Acta neurol. scand. 41*, Suppl. **13**, 251.

Wagner, A. L. and Buchthal, F. (1972). Motor and sensory conduction in infancy and childhood: reappraisal. *Develop. Med. Child Neurol.* **14**, 189.

Walshe, F. M. R. (1942). The anatomy and physiology of cutaneous sensibility: a critical review. *Brain* **65**, 48.

——, Jackson, H., and Wyburn-Mason, R. (1944). On some pressure effects associated with cervical and with rudimentary and 'normal' first ribs, and the factors entering into their causation. *Brain* **67**, 141.

Walton, J. N. (1952). The electroyogram in myopathy: analysis with the audio-frequency spectrometer. *J. Neurol. Neurosurg. Psychiat.* **15**, 219.

—— (1982). *Essentials of neurology*, 5th edn. Pitman, London.

Weller, R. O. and Cervós-Navarro, J. (1977). *Pathology of peripheral nerves*. Butterworth, London.

Wilbourn, A. J., Furlan, A. J., Hulley, W., and Ruschhaupt, W. (1983). Ischaemic monomelic neuropathy. *Neurology, Minneapolis* **33**, 447.

Wilkinson, M. (1960). The carpal-tunnel syndrome in pregnancy. *Lancet*, **i**, 453.

Wynn Parry, C. B. and Salter, M. (1975). Sensory re-education after median nerve lesions. *Hand* 250.

Yamada, T., Muroga, T., and Kimura, J. (1981). Tourniquet-induced ischemia and somatosensory evoked potentials. *Neurology, Minneapolis* **31**, 1524.

Yiannikas, C. and Walsh, J. C. (1983). Somatosensory evoked responses in the diagnosis of thoracic outlet syndrome. *J. Neurol. Neurosurg. Psychiat.* **46**, 234.

Zachary, R. B. (1945). Thenar palsy due to compression of the median nerve in the carpal tunnel. *Surg. Gynec. Obstet.*, **81**, 213.

—— (1954). Peripheral nerve injuries. *Spec. Rep. Ser. med. Res. Coun., London* **282**, 354.

Spinal radiculitis and radiculopathy

In the cervical region the ventral and dorsal spinal roots of each segment lie close together within the intervertebral foramen. The dorsal-root ganglion lies just peripherally in the gutter of the transverse process. Beyond that the two roots fuse to form the spinal nerve. In the lumbar region the ganglia lie in the foramina. Each pair of roots has an investment of dura mater and the leptomeninges.

Lesions of dorsal roots are commoner than those of ventral roots. Either or both may be involved in inflammatory lesions of spinal meninges such as arachnoiditis. The dorsal roots degenerate, and are inflamed in herpes zoster and occasionally in various forms of encephalomyelitis. Spinal roots and nerves may also be involved in granulomatous processes involving the meninges such as sarcoidosis, in Behçet's syndrome and in leukaemia and reticulosis. In post-infective polyradiculopathy (the Guillain–Barré syndrome) these structures are often affected more severely than the more distal portions of the peripheral nerves. They may be compressed by extramedullary spinal tumour, or irritated by abnormal constituents of the CSF, such as blood after subarachnoid haemorrhage, or substances introduced for diagnostic or therapeutic purposes. A radiculitis limited to the cauda equina has been described and is an uncommon complication of ankylosing spondylitis (Matthews 1968).

Diseases of the vertebral column may damage either spinal roots or spinal nerves. A growth which invades the spinal theca or a herniated intervertebral disc may compress spinal roots, but when there is vertebral collapse, due to primary or secondary neoplasm, tuberculous or other infection, Paget's disease, or traumatic fracture-dislocation, it is usually the roots and spinal nerves which are compressed together in or near the intervertebral foramina. They are also occasionally compressed in severe scoliosis or spondylosis, and may be the site of presumed allergic neuropathy in serum sickness or 'neuralgic amyotrophy' (p. 521).

An irritative lesion of a single dorsal root causes pain of a lancinating or burning character, often precipitated or intensified by coughing or sneezing and sometimes by movements of the spine, and often associated with hyperaesthesia and hyperalgesia over the full segmental distribution of the root. According to Foerster, no detectable sensory loss is produced by surgical division of a single dorsal root, owing to the overlapping of adjacent root areas. When more than one adjacent root is interrupted, the area of sensory loss is that area exclusively supplied by the combined roots involved, and the area of analgesia is larger than that of anaesthe-

sia to light touch. A lesion of a ventral root causes atrophic paralysis of any muscle exclusively supplied by that root, and a partial lower motor-neurone lesion of any muscle to whose innervation it contributes. Fasciculation may occur in affected muscles. A lesion of a spinal nerve produces the same manifestations as a lesion of the corresponding ventral and dorsal root combined. Details of the muscles innervated by different spinal roots and the dermatomes which they supply are given on pages 32 and 43 and by the Medical Research Council (1976).

The diagnosis of radiculopathy depends first upon recognizing the segmental character of the sensory and motor symptoms. The nature of the lesion can be ascertained only by taking into account the whole clinical picture; the presence of associated symptoms of a lesion of the spinal cord and vertebral column, and the results of spinal X-rays, especially of the intervertebral foramina, and often examination of the CSF and myelography or CT scanning. Broadly speaking, an acute onset of root symptoms alone suggests an inflammatory lesion or acute disc protrusion, an insidious onset of root symptoms with or without symptoms of a lesion of the spinal cord at the same level suggests compression, and the coexistence of pain in the back, limitation of movements of the spine, and local spinal tenderness or deformity at the same level points to disease of the spine as the cause.

Sensory neuropathy due to degeneration of the dorsal-root ganglia

This is an unusual but striking syndrome characterized clinically by the subacute onset of a severe sensory ataxia with gross sensory loss, particularly of posterior column sensibility, but often of all forms, with loss of reflexes. The causes are various including carcinoma (see p. 488), syphilis, diabetes, and unknown factors. Pathologically there is a selective loss of dorsal-root ganglion cells and their fibres in dorsal roots, posterior columns of the spinal cord, and peripheral nerves (McAlpine and Page 1951; Bosanquet and Henson 1957). An acute sensory neuronopathy of this type giving rise to numbness, pain, and sensory impairment over the face and entire body and showing no significant improvement over a five-year period has been described following the treatment of an acute non-specific febrile illness with antibiotics (Sterman, Schaumburg, and Asbury 1980); sensory conduction was slowed or absent and the CSF protein was raised.

Hereditary sensory neuropathy is a disorder often included in the hereditary ataxia group (p. 362) in which there is progressive peripheral impairment of all forms of sensibility but especially of pain and temperature, beginning early in life due to degeneration of dorsal-root ganglia; it is inherited as an autosomal recessive trait. It may be associated with increased synthesis of immunoglobulin A (Whitaker, Falchuk, Engel, Blaese, and Strober 1974). Insensitivity to pain may be so extensive in the trunk and extremities that a diagnosis of congenital insensitivity to pain may be made erroneously; painless perforating ulcers of the feet commonly result, with painless fracture or resorption of bones in the feet and even in the phalanges (Morvan's syndrome).

Spinal radiculopathy due to intervertebral-disc disease

Disorders of the spinal column and especially lesions of the intervertebral discs are by far the commonest cause of painful root compression. Such lesions are found chiefly in the cervical and lumbar regions of the spine, though they occur occasionally in the thoracic region (Logue 1952; Carson, Gumpert, and Jefferson 1971). The principal cause is undoubtedly a tendency of the intervertebral discs to degenerate with increasing age which no doubt explains the common occurrence of degeneration of both cervical and lumbar invertebral discs in the same patient. Other factors, especially trauma, also play a part.

The intervertebral disc consists of a semi-fluid central portion, the nucleus pulposus, which is surrounded by the annulus fibrosus, a strong fibro-cartilaginous and elastic structure binding the bodies of the vertebrae together. When force is exerted upon the disc it is distributed laterally in all directions, and, if the force is too strong for the resistance of the annulus fibrosus, the nucleus pulposus will herniate through it. Such protrusions may occur either in the midline or posterolaterally into the spinal canal (Fig. 14.2; p. 405), or more laterally into the intervertebral foramen (Fig. 18.7). These

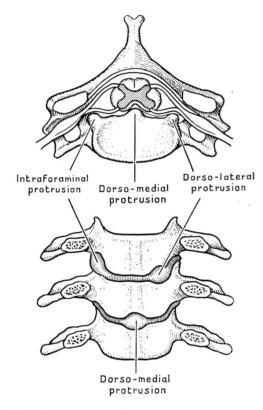

Fig. 18.7. Sites of intervertebral-disc protrusion.

are called nuclear herniations. There is, however, another type of disc protrusion, the annular protrusion, which is produced in a different way. A degenerated intervertebral disc tends to collapse, in which case the annulus bulges in all directions. The protruded material becomes vascularized and its fibrous elements increase. Nuclear herniation is originally soft, but in time undergoes a similar transformation into fibrocartilage, so that the end result of both a nuclear and an annular protrusion may be a hard calcified boss. For anatomical reasons the effects of cervical and lumbar protrusions are somewhat different and must be considered separately.

Cervical-disc lesions and brachial radiculopathy

Cervical intervertebral discs are bounded on their lateral margins by an articulation known as the apophyseal joint which lies on the anteromedial side of the intervertebral foramen, the posterior boundary of which is formed by the articulation between the pedicles of the two adjacent vertebrae. The cervical spinal roots may therefore be compressed, either by posterolateral protrusions of

the intervertebral disc into the spinal canal or within the intervertebral foramen, either by an acute disc protrusion or by osteophytes which narrow the foramen; these largely arise from apophyseal joints. Such pressure, as Frykholm (1951) showed, leads to fibrosis of the root sheaths.

The pathological changes of the chronic syndrome of cervical spondylosis may involve one pair of intervertebral joints or more than one and are often related to single or multiple annular protrusions with eventual bony boss formation, though this process may occur in patients who have suffered previous acute protrusions; when the joint lesions are multiple the joints affected may be adjacent to one another or they may not. Since age, manual labour, and recurrent minor trauma are the chief factors causing degeneration of the intervertebral discs, most patients are middle-aged or older, but acute cervical-disc protrusion may occur at an earlier age.

Acute protrusions
Acute protrusions can occur spontaneously or be the result of trauma. A patient suffering from an acute protrusion may give a history of recurrent attacks of pain in the neck often diagnosed as 'fibrositis'. Suddenly a pain which is severe and lasting occurs. The neck may feel as though it is fixed, and both active and passive movements intensify the pain, which may be very severe. Antero-posterior movements of the head (which occur mainly at the atlanto-occipital joints) and rotation (which occurs largely at the atlanto-axial joint) are restricted only by protective muscle spasm. It is lateral movements which are particularly painful, especially towards the side of the lesion (Spurling's sign). The pain is also referred within the distribution of the spinal nerve which is compressed. On examination the neck is usually held rigidly, and sometimes, slightly flexed towards the side of the lesion. The muscles innervated by the affected spinal nerve may be somewhat weak and hypotonic, but severe muscular weakness and wasting are unusual. The tendon reflexes mediated by the affected segment are diminished, and sometimes lost. It may be possible to find some hyperpathia within the corresponding dermatome, or some diminution of cutaneous sensibility. Plain X-rays usually show little abnormality, though there may be slight narrowing of the affected intervertebral disc. Myelography may show an indentation of the column of contrast medium or obliteration of the corresponding root sheath. Discography (p. 406) is now often used in the diagnosis of lumbar-disc protrusions but its potential risks still outweigh its advantages in the diagnosis of cervical lesions.

The treatment of spontaneous acute cervical-disc protrusion may, in certain cases, involve cervical traction, but much more often immobilization is sufficient. In the acute phase a soft 'Gamgee' tissue collar or one made of newspaper may be helpful and powerful analgesics are usually required. After this phase has passed, immobilization may be continued by means of a plastic collar for a few days or weeks. If these methods fail surgical exploration may be required (Yoss, Corbin, MacCarty, and Love 1957) but this is rarely necessary in acute cervical-disc lesions most of which respond quickly to conservative treatment. Acute central protrusions causing spinal-cord compression (p. 400) also respond rapidly, as a rule, to immobilization, but laminectomy is occasionally needed if symptoms and signs of cord dysfunction are severe and do not quickly improve.

It is important also to recognize that the prognosis of acute cervical-disc protrusions may be unpredictable after industrial injury where financial compensation is involved. In such cases pain in the neck and arm, if not responding rapidly to treatment, may breed tension and anxiety which in turn increase pain which may be very persistent, especially if the position is complicated by the motive of possible financial gain. In such cases 'hysterical' weakness and sensory loss may develop in the affected limb and it is difficult to distinguish with confidence between a genuine hysterical overlay (subconscious motivation) and malingering (conscious motivation). 'Collar-dependence' is also common with resultant stiffness of cervical muscles. While tranquillizing and muscle-relaxant drugs such as diazepam are often helpful in such cases, rehabilitation and persuasion to discard the collar are often very diffcult, at least until the compensation claim is settled; the longer settlement is delayed, the worse the prognosis.

Cervical spondylosis

The duration and the history of symptoms of cervical spondylosis are very variable and radicular symptoms may be acute, subacute, or insidious in their onset. To avoid confusion, the term spondylosis should be reserved for the syndrome resulting from subacute or chronic central and lateral protrusion of cervical intervertebral discs and should not be used in cases of acute protrusion as described above. In fact, radicular symptoms are often absent in cases of cervical-cord compression (myelopathy) (Phillips 1975); this syndrome is described on page 400. Involvement of one spinal nerve leads to symptoms resembling those of a spontaneous acute protrusion of a single intervertebral disc into the intervertebral foramen, as described above. Pain, however, is not always limited to one dermatome, but may extend down the upper limb to involve several digits, in which case a clinical picture which used to be called 'brachial neuritis or neuralgia' is produced. An insidious onset is characterized by dysaesthesiae with burning and tingling sensations, sometimes accompanied by pain, radiating down the upper limb into one or more digits and tending sometimes to be particularly troublesome at night. Motor symptoms and signs are usually slight or absent and only exceptionally is there a complaint of weakness, but, rarely, localized wasting with fasciculation may be severe enough to simulate motor-neurone disease.

On examining the patient there is commonly some diminution of the appreciation of light touch and pin-prick within the distribution of the dermatomes corresponding to the affected spinal nerves. There may also be localized areas of spinal tenderness in the corresponding muscles. Appreciation of posture and passive movement is usually unimpaired. There may be slight muscular wasting of muscles innervated by the affected spinal nerves, but weakness is usually slight. Pseudomyotonia in the affected hand has been reported (Satoyoshi, Doi, and Kinoshita 1972). The tendon reflexes innervated from the affected segments are often diminished or lost and, if there is evidence of associated myelopathy, 'inversion' of the biceps or radial reflexes may be observed (p. 403). Active and passive movements of the neck may be somewhat restricted, but are usually relatively painless. There may be some local tenderness on pressure.

Plain X-rays usually show narrowing of intervertebral discs with posterior osteophytes, and, in the oblique views, the intervertebral foramina are encroached upon by osteophytes from the apophyseal joints.

It is uncommon to find evidence of spondylotic radiculopathy without some evidence of associated myelopathy, while, by contrast, myelopathy often occurs without evidence of root involvement. Nevertheless, myelography, while demonstrating a central bulge of one or more intervertebral discs, a narrow spinal canal (*The Lancet* 1972), or posterior indentation due to infolding of the ligamentum subflavum (Taylor 1953), may also demonstrate associated lateral protrusions of the affected discs. The effect of cervical movement upon spinal cord and root compression was reviewed by Adams and Logue (1971*a, b*).

Treatment

In some cases a simple radiculopathy responds to immobilization in a plaster or plastic collar which is usually required for two or three months. Both traction and manipulation have their advocates, but the latter carries a risk of cord damage. Surgical decom-

pression of the intervertebral foramina is rarely required. Laminectomy and posterior decompression continues to be useful in cases with associated myelopathy (Bishara 1971; Adams and Logue 1971*c*) but there is increasing evidence that in selected cases of myelopathy without substantial root or spinal-nerve involvement the anterior operation of removal of the affected disc or discs, followed by spinal fusion (the Cloward operation) gives superior results (Phillips 1973). Various forms of physiotherapy are useful adjuvants to treatment. In the acute stage analgesic drugs and bed rest with the arm supported on a pillow may be needed, but care must be taken that immobilization does not lead to a 'frozen shoulder'.

Lumbar disc lesions and sciatica

The term sciatica is applied to a benign syndrome characterized especially by pain beginning in the lumbar region and spreading down the back of one lower limb to the ankle and sometimes the foot; it is usually intensified by coughing or sneezing; there is usually little weakness or sensory loss but sometimes diminution or loss of the ankle-jerk. In most cases spontaneous recovery occurs rather slowly with some liability to recurrence. Sciatica thus defined is usually due to herniation of one or more of the lumbar intervertebral discs. It seems best, therefore, to discuss sciatica under this heading and to consider other causes of sciatic pain in relation to diagnosis.

Aetiology

Lumbar-disc protrusion often follows trauma, a history of which is obtainable in about half of all cases. The commonest type of stress is that produced by lifting a heavy object with the lumbar spine flexed or by a fall in a similar posture. Since 75 per cent of patients are in or beyond the fourth decade it seems that degenerative changes which begin in early adult life predispose towards herniation but the syndrome is not uncommon in adolescents and even in children. The changes in the lumbar spine associated with pregnancy may also precipitate it. Thickening of the ligamentum subflavum is often noted in addition.

The age-incidence shows a peak with 35 per cent of cases in the fourth decade, and between 75 and 80 per cent of patients are males. Most lumbar herniations occur between the fourth and fifth lumbar or fifth lumbar and first sacral bodies, with a relative frequency of two to three. A disc protrusion compresses the spinal nerve which is running to the foramen one segment below, the fourth lumbar disc the fifth lumbar nerve, and the fifth lumbar disc the first sacral nerve. Sometimes there are protrusions from two or more discs. The compressed nerve becomes swollen and tense. Occasionally an acute central lumbar-disc protrusion results in the sequestration into the spinal extradural space of a large portion of the disc; this can act as a major space-occupying lesion in the lumbar canal, compressing multiple spinal nerves in the cauda equina.

Symptoms and signs

In most cases the onset is subacute, and sciatica is often preceded by backache, which may have occurred intermittently for years (see *The Lancet* 1981). The pain may immediately follow an injury such as a strain or a fall, or there may be a latent interval of days or even weeks. After two or three days of pain in the lumbar spine the pain radiates down the back of one leg from the buttock to the ankle and sometimes into the foot. It is often possible to distinguish three elements: (1) pain in the back, aching in character and intensified by spinal movement; (2) pain deep in the buttock and thigh, also aching or gnawing in character and influenced by the posture of the limb; and (3) pain radiating to the leg and foot, momentarily increased by coughing and sneezing. When the first sacral root is compressed, pain radiates to the outer border of the foot. When the pressure is upon the fifth lumbar root, it spreads from the outer aspect of the leg to the dorsum or inner border of the foot. In general the pain is intensified by stooping, sitting, lifting, and walking. The patient is usually most comfortable lying in bed on the sound side with the affected leg slightly flexed at the hip and knee. The pain interferes with sleep and when very severe slight relief may be obtained only by getting up and walking about. There is often a feeling of numbness, heaviness, or deadness in the leg, especially along the top or outer side of the foot.

There may be muscular weakness and slight wasting, not only of muscles supplied by the sciatic nerve, but sometimes also of other lower-limb muscles. Compression of the first sacral root causes weakness of the small muscles of the foot and those of the calf, while the ankle-jerk is diminished or lost. Very rarely an S1 radiculopathy causes, paradoxically, calf hypertrophy (Mielke, Ricker, Emser, and Boxler 1982). Compression of the fifth lumbar root causes weakness of the tibialis anterior and peronei—occasionally complete foot-drop—and the ankle-jerk is preserved. If the fourth lumbar root is involved, the knee-jerk may be diminished. The plantar reflex is flexor. Weakness of extension of the hallux on the affected side is a valuable sign of a fifth lumbar-root lesion and examination of the 'great-toe reflex', evoked by a sharp tap with a tendon hammer upon a finger which is so placed upon the dorsum of the proximal phalanx of the toe that it stretches slightly the extensor hallucis longus, is also useful in diagnosis (Taylor and Wienir 1969). There is tenderness on pressure in the buttock and thigh, straight-leg-raising is limited by pain, and stretching the sciatic nerve by extending the knee with the hip flexed causes severe pain—Lasègue's sign. Sensory loss is often slight, but commonly there is some blunting of light touch and pin-prick over the outer half of the foot and three outer toes and the lower part of the outer aspect of the leg when the first sacral root is involved. The fourth and fifth lumbar cutaneous areas are shown in Fig 1.33, p. 43. Scoliosis is often associated with sciatica, the lumbar spine being laterally flexed, usually towards the affected side, less frequently towards the opposite side. Some rigidity of the lumbar spine is usually present, and there may be a tender spot at the level of the fifth lumbar transverse process. In the case of large central-disc protrusions in the lumbar region, pain is sometimes bilateral though often more severe on one side, muscular weakness is more widespread, several tendon reflexes may be lost (e.g. one knee-jerk and both ankle-jerks), sensory loss is more extensive, indicating involvement of multiple roots, and sphincter control may be impaired. Such a cauda equina syndrome (Shephard 1959) should be regarded as a neurosurgical emergency. An excess of protein, up to 0.7–0.8 g/l is present in the CSF in about 80 per cent of cases, but the cell count is normal.

X-ray examination should be carried out in all cases of sciatica, since many causes of sciatic pain are associated with bony changes visible in radiographs. Straight X-rays are not always of value in the diagnosis of herniated disc. The L5–S1 disc space is normally often narrower than that of the other lumbar discs, so that little stress can be laid upon minor degrees of narrowing at this level. Narrowing of the L4–5 space is more likely to be significant especially if associated with sclerosis of adjacent vertebral bodies. Spondylolisthesis at L4–5, but more often at L5–S1, may give not only low back pain but also symptoms and signs of root compression resembling those of intervertebral-disc prolapse and is usually readily demonstrable by X-ray. Myelography may demonstrate a filling defect, but is only indicated as a rule if pain is unusually persistent despite adequate rest or immobilization or if there are physical signs of such a degree and extent that surgical treatment is contemplated; a herniated disc may be present in spite of a negative myelogram. There is considerable evidence, however, that small 'buttonhole' posterior protrusions of the nucleus can produce severe back pain without distortion of the dural sac (Hilton, Ball, and Benn 1980) and in suspected cases discography (p. 406) may be the only effective method of demonstrating such a lesion

or fissuring of the annulus (Park, McCall, O'Brien, and Webb 1979). Protrusion of the lumbar posterior longitudinal ligament, which is often apparent on myelography, may give symptoms simulating those of disc prolapse (Beatty, Sugar, and Fox 1968), as may cysts on sacral nerve roots (Tarlov 1938; Plewes and Jacobson 1970) and lumbar canal stenosis (see pp. 407 and 424); the latter is often associated with symptoms of cauda equina dysfunction which develop during exertion and are relieved by rest; it, too, is readily demonstrated by this technique. Increasing attention has also been paid of late to the fact that sciatic or femoral neuropathy, due to root and spinal-nerve compression, is a common consequence of root canal stenosis, often associated with osteoarthrosis and hypertrophy of facet joints, and this can mimic exactly lumbar-disc prolapse (Choudhury and Taylor 1977; Critchley 1982). In such cases, electromyography and measurement of motor and sensory conduction velocity, with recording of H and F responses, can be valuable in identifying evidence of radicular lesions (Fisher, Shivde, Teixera, and Grainer 1978) and spinal CT scanning is sometimes more helpful than myelography (Critchley 1982).

Diagnosis

Sciatica due to a lumbar-disc protrusion must be distinguished from: (1) compression of nerve roots by a tumour within the spinal canal; (2) root compression resulting from spondylolisthesis, sacral cysts, other developmental anomalies, or lumbar canal stenosis; (3) inflammatory or granulomatous processes involving the cauda equina; (4) inflammatory, degenerative, and neoplastic lesions of the spine and pelvis involving the roots; and (5) neoplasms of the pelvic viscera. The principal points of distinction are that in prolapsed disc the onset of symptoms is fairly rapid, the buttock and posterior aspect of the thigh over the course of the sciatic nerve are usually tender on pressure, muscular wasting and sensory loss are usually slight, and the course of the disorder during the first few weeks or months is stationary or often one of improvement. In the other lesions mentioned the onset is usually more gradual, the nerve is not tender on pressure, and muscular wasting and sensory loss are usually more pronounced. Further, these symptoms are progressive.

In such cases the abdomen and pelvis must be thoroughly examined for sources of compression, and the lumbar spine and pelvis should be X-rayed. Attention must also be paid to the patient's general condition, and inquiry made for symptoms suggestive of pelvic neoplasm or recent loss of weight. Rectal examination should never be omitted; and in women vaginal examination may also be advisable. A complete examination of the nervous system is required to exclude spinal tumours or arachnoiditis as a cause of sciatic pain and, if these are suspected, CT scanning and/or myelography are usually indicated.

Herniated disc must be distinguished from arthritis of the hip-joint with which pain resembling sciatica may be associated. In herniated disc, movements of the hip-joint are painless, provided the sciatic nerve is not stretched. The lower limb can be rotated and abducted without pain, whereas these movements are painful and often limited in arthritis of the hip, in which disuse atrophy of muscles may be seen but there are no reflex changes or sensory loss. X-rays will confirm the diagnosis.

Congenital abnormalities of the lumbosacral junction, such as spondyloslisthesis or sacralization of the fifth lumbar vertebra, may cause low back pain but only occasionally true sciatica, unless the fifth lumbar root is compressed. These conditions will be apparent on X-ray. Other causes of low back pain which must be considered in differential diagnosis include contusion due to local injury to the back or one buttock, sometimes associated with transient sciatic pain, osteoarthrosis of apophyseal or neurocentral joints without significant disc protrusion, sacro-iliac strain, and ankylosing spondylitis which will usually be apparent radiologically (see Keim and Kirkcaldy-Willis 1980). Local lumbar pain is not uncommon in some women during menstruation and/or pregnancy and in patients in the paramenopausal age group similar symptoms but without, as a rule, radiation to the legs, may be the result of muscular tension associated with anxiety and/or depression and may respond to treatment with appropriate remedies. As in the case of industrial injuries to the cervical region (see p. 396) symptoms of low back strain with or without intervertebral-disc protrusion may be aggravated and perpetuated and the clinical picture clouded by the compensation issue.

Peripheral arterial disease involving the femoral artery and/or its branches are occasional causes of pain in the leg in middle age and later life: intermittent claudication is not always present. The diagnosis is readily established by absence or diminution of the femoral, dorsalis pedis, or posterior tibial pulses. The syndrome of intermittent ischaemia of the cauda equina with pain, paraesthesiae, or weakness of the leg occurring only on exertion and relieved by rest can usually be distinguished from sciatica, due to a single lateral-disc protrusion, by myelography (see p. 404).

Abnormalities of motor and/or sensory nerve conduction and EMG evidence of denervation of muscles innervated by the affected root is also of considerable value in some cases.

Prognosis

In mild cases the stage of severe pain lasts only two or three weeks and the patient recovers in a month or two, but may from time to time experience aching along the course of the nerve and stooping may still excite some pain in the affected leg. In more severe cases there may be slight improvement after several weeks, but the condition then becomes stationary and the patient continues to suffer from considerable pain which fluctuates in severity for a number of months or even years. Recovery, however, ultimately occurs in most cases, except for the residual symptoms just mentioned. In a study of 73 unselected cases treated with bed rest alone, Pearce and Moll (1967) found that 70 per cent recovered satisfactorily but the remaining 30 per cent required other measures. Recovery of symptoms may occur even though the disc protrusion persists. For this reason, perhaps, relapses are common. In some cases they occur at frequent intervals, so that the patient is hardly ever free from pain over a period of several years. In other cases the second attack may be delayed until 10 or more years after the first. Operation gives good results in 90 per cent of cases operated upon, but even after operation a relapse may occur. Reported recurrence rates in larger series vary between two and 10 per cent; there is no evidence that the weight of disc removed is related to the outcome (Shannon and Paul 1979).

Treatment

Many patients with lumbar intervertebral-disc protrusion recover completely if treated conservatively. Operation should therefore be reserved for those with large central protrusions involving multiple roots (in whom it is obligatory, especially if the sphincters are involved), for those with intractable pain unresponsive to conservative measures, and for those with marked motor weakness (e.g. foot-drop) present from the outset. It is probably indicated also in those whose symptoms remain severe and become chronic, those who relapse, and in any with gross and persistent symptoms of root compression, sufficiently severe to cause disability. Probably not more than 10 per cent require operation, but the percentage will be higher among manual workers, in whom inability to do the necessary physical work may itself constitute an indication for surgery.

Conservative treatment consists of rest in bed and analgesics, to which may be added various measures designed to immobilize the lower part of the spine and the affected lower limb. Green (1975) recommended intramuscular dexamethasone, beginning with 64 mg on the first day, 32 mg on the second, 24 mg on the third,

and so on, over a seven-day period, and reported dramatic relief of pain, presumed to be due to relief of oedema in or around the root being compressed, but these findings have not been confirmed. When rest in bed for two or three weeks has been tried and failed, immediate relief is sometimes given by the application of a plaster jacket which fixes the lumbar spine in slight extension. The patient, who is allowed to walk about, should wear this for three months. Alternatively many patients are relieved by the application of continuous lumbar traction for two or three weeks followed by the provision of a light lumbar support or corset which is worn for three months or longer. Manipulation also has its advocates and is remarkably successful in some patients with intractable pain but the outcome is difficult to predict in advance (Doran and Newell 1975). An 'overlay' of depression and anxiety commonly occurs in patients with lumbar-disc disease and as a result of tension in the lumbar muscles accentuates and perpetuates pain. Antidepressive remedies and tranquillizing drugs such as amitriptyline and diazepam are particularly valuable in some patients. About 70 per cent of patients respond satisfactorily to conservative treatment (Pearce and Moll 1967) but in those who continue to have pain, provided there is no evidence of a severe 'functional overlay', surgical treatment is probably indicated.

Sacral epidural injection
In some cases considerable benefit follows stretching the nerve roots by giving an epidural injection at the sacral hiatus. This can readily be palpated at the lower end of the sacrum, where it is covered by the dorsal sacrococcygeal ligament. The foramen is bounded above by the concave lower border of the sacrum in the midline and at the sides by the two lateral tubercles. The patient either lies on one side or assumes the knee-elbow position. The site of the injection is cleaned with antiseptic and anaesthetized with procaine, and a fine lumbar puncture needle is passed through the ligament upwards and slightly forwards. Twenty ml of 1 per cent lignocaine or bupivicaine (150 mg in 4 hours) are first injected, and this may be followed by an injection of normal saline, of which 80 ml or more can sometimes be injected, the solution being at body temperature. Coomes (1961) used 50 ml of 0.5 per cent procaine and found the effects of such an injection to be superior to those of bed rest alone. Epidural injection yields relief of pain in about 50 per cent of cases. Sometimes the result is dramatic, the patient being completely and permanently relieved. A second injection may be given after an interval of two or three days if necessary.

Lumbar extradural injection
Another form of treatment sometimes used is that of giving an extradural injection of a corticosteroid preparation; the technique of lumbar injection was described by Barry and Kendall (1962). In a controlled trial Dilke, Burry, and Grahame (1973) found that the effects of 80 mg of methylprednisolone injected in 10 ml of normal saline gave excellent relief of pain and other symptoms.

Chemonucleolysis
Chymopapain, a proteolytic enzyme derived from papaya latex, can break down mucopolysaccharide-protein complexes which form an important part of the structure of intervertebral discs. Smith and Brown (1967) carried out discography by injecting contrast medium through a lateral approach directly into the nucleus pulposus of the affected disc or discs and followed this with an injection of 2 mg of chymopapain in 0.5 ml of distilled water. The injection caused severe pain in the back for 12–24 hours but sciatic pain was usually relieved in 24 hours. Potential risks of the method include sensitivity reactions and disc space infection but others have shown that the technique is effective in relieving symptoms rapidly (Nordby and Lucas 1973; Graham 1974). No controlled trial has yet been reported (*British Medical Journal* 1974) and Maroon, Holst, and Osgood (1976) reported severe anaphylactic

reactions in two patients; the results in others were not demonstrably superior to those of other conservative measures.

Physiotherapy

Local heat, diathermy, massage, and other traditional forms of treatment commonly used in cases of sciatica and various forms of low back pain have a useful palliative effect in some cases. Once the phase of acute pain has passed, graduated exercises are of considerable value in improving the mobility of the affected portion of the spine, in relieving muscular spasm or secondary scoliosis, and in improving power in weakened muscles.

Radiculitis of the cauda equina

Rarely the cauda equina is the site of a radiculopathy of obscure origin, of subacute or insidious onset. The symptoms and signs are those of a cauda equina lesion (see p. 407), and the inflammatory nature of the process may be suggested by a pleocytosis, usually mononuclear, in the CSF with some rise in protein. Such a syndrome has been described in ankylosing spondylitis (Matthews 1968) but in most instances, repeated investigation or the eventual pathological findings in such cases have shown that the condition is due either to tumour (e.g. ependymoma of the filum terminale), to mechanical compression of roots, or to ischaemia of roots resulting from atherosclerosis or stenosis of the lumbar canal. Other neurological disorders occasionally associated with ankylosing spondylitis include multiple sclerosis, focal epilepsy, and peripheral-nerve lesions, but a cauda equina syndrome is probably the commonest (Thomas, Kendall, and Whitfield 1974).

References

Adams, C. B. T. and Logue, V. (1971*a*). Studies in cervical spondylotic myelopathy. I. Movement of the cervical roots, dura and cord, and their relation to the course taken by the extrathecal roots. *Brain* **94**, 557.

—— and —— (1971*b*). Studies in cervical spondylotic myelopathy. II. Observations on the movement and contour of the cervical spine in relation to the neural complications of cervical spondylosis. *Brain* **94**, 569.

—— and —— (1971*c*). Studies in cervical spondylotic myelopathy. III. Some functional effects of operations for cervical spondylotic myelopathy. *Brain* **94**, 587.

Barry, P. J. C. and Kendall, P. H. (1962). Corticosteroid infiltration of the extradural space. *Ann. phys. Med.* **6**, 267.

Beatty, R. S., Sugar, O., and Fox, T. A. (1968). Protrusion of the posterior longitudinal ligament simulating herniated lumbar intervertebral disc. *J. Neurol. Neurosurg. Psychiat.* **31**, 61.

Bishara, S. N. (1971). The posterior operation in treatment of cervical spondylosis with myelopathy: a long-term follow-up study. *J. Neurol. Neurosurg. Psychiat.* **34**, 393.

Bosanquet, F. D. and Henson, R. A. (1957). Sensory neuropathy in diabetes mellitus. *Folia psychiat. neerl.* **60**, 107.

Bradford, F. K. and Spurling, R. G. (1941). *The intervertebral disk*. Thomas, Springfield, Illinois.

British Medical Journal (1974). Dissolving discs. *Br. med. J.* **2**, 625.

Carson, J., Gumpert, J., and Jefferson, A. (1971). Diagnosis and treatment of thoracic intervertebral disc protrusions. *J. Neurol. Neurosurg. Psychiat.* **34**, 68.

Choudhury, A. R. and Taylor, J. C. (1977). Occult lumbar spinal stenosis. *J. Neurol. Neurosurg. Psychiat.* **40**, 506.

Coomes, E. N. (1961). A comparison between epidural anaesthesia and bed rest in sciatica. *Br. med. J.* **1**, 20.

Critchley, E. M. R. (1982). Lumbar spinal stenosis. *Br. med. J.* **284**, 1588.

Dandy, W. E. (1944). Newer aspects of ruptured intervertebral disks. *Ann. Surg.* **119**, 481.

Dilke, T. F. W., Burry, H. C., and Grahame, R. (1973). Extradural corticosteroid injection in management of lumbar nerve root compression. *Br. med. J.* **2**, 635.

Doran, D. M. L. and Newell, D. J. (1975). Manipulation in the treatment of low back pain: a multi-centre study. *Br. med. J.* **2**, 161.

Fisher, M. S., Shivde, A.J., Teixera, C., and Grainer, L. S. (1978). Clini-

cal and electrophysiological appraisal of the significance of radicular injury in back pain. *J. Neurol. Neurosurg. Psychiat.* **41**, 303.

Frykholm, R. (1951). Cervical nerve root compression resulting from disc degeneration and root-sleeve fibrosis. *Acta chir. scand.* Supp. 160.

Graham, C. E. (1974). Backache, and sciatica. A report of 90 patients treated by intradiscal injection of chymopapain (discase). *Med. J. Aust.* **1**, 5.

Green, L. N. (1975). Dexamethasone in the management of symptoms due to herniated lumbar disc. *J. Neurol. Neurosurg. Psychiat.* **38**, 1211.

Hilton, R. C., Ball, J., and Benn, R. T. (1980). Annular tears in the dorso-lumbar spine. *Ann. Rheumat. Dis.* **39**, 533.

Keim, H. A. and Kirkaldy-Willis, W. H. (1980). Low back pain. *CIBA Clinical Symposia* **32** (6).

The Lancet (1972). Signs and symptoms in cervical spondylosis. *Lancet* **ii**, 70.

—— (1981). Progress in back pain? *Lancet* **i**, 977.

Logue, V. (1952). Thoracic intervertebral disc prolapse with spinal cord compression. *J. Neurol. Neurosurg. Psychiat.* **15**, 227.

Love, J. G. and Schorn, V. G. (1965). Thoracic disk protrusions. *J. Am. med. Ass.* **191**, 627.

Maroon, J. C., Holst, R. A., and Osgood, C. P. (1976). Chymopapain in the treatment of ruptured lumbar discs. *J. Neurol. Neurosurg. Psychiat.* **39**, 508.

Matthews, W. B. (1968). The neurological complications of ankylosing spondylitis. *J. neurol. Sci.* **6**, 561.

McAlpine, D. and Page, F. (1951). Sensory neuropathy due to posterior root ganglion degeneration. *Arch. Mddx. Hosp.* **1**, 250.

Medical Research Council (1976). *Aids to the examination of the peripheral nervous system*, 3rd edn. HMSO, London.

Mielke, U., Ricker, K., Emser, W., and Boxler, K. (1982). Unilateral calf enlargement following S_1 radiculopathy. *Muscle & Nerve* **5**, 434.

Nordby, E. J. and Lucas, G. L. (1973). A comparative analysis of lumbar disk disease treated by laminectomy or chemonucleolysis. *Clinical Orthopaedics and Related Research* **90**, 119.

O'Connell, J. E. A. (1944). Maternal obstetrical paralysis. *Surg. Gynec. Obstet.* **29**, 374.

—— (1950). The indications for and results of the excision of lumbar intervertebral disk protrusions, a review of 500 cases. *Ann. R. Coll. Surg. Engl.* **6**, 403.

Park, W. M., McCall, I. W., O'Brien, J. P., and Webb, J. K. (1979). Fissuring of the posterior annulus fibrosus in the lumbar spine. *Br. J. Radiol.* **52**, 382.

Pearce, J. and Moll, J. M. H. (1967). Conservative treatment and natural history of acute lumbar disc lesions. *J. Neurol. Neurosurg. Psychiat.* **30**, 13.

Phillips, D. G. (1973). Surgical treatment of myelopathy with cervical spondylosis. *J. Neurol. Neurosurg. Psychiat.* **36**, 879.

—— (1975). Upper limb involvement in cervical spondylosis. *J. Neurol. Neurosurg. Psychiat.* **38**, 386.

Plewes, J. L. and Jacobsen, I. (1970). Sciatica caused by sacral-nerve-root cysts. *Lancet* **ii**, 799.

Satoyoshi, E., Doi, Y., and Kinoshita, M. (1972). Pseudomyotonia in cervical root lesions with myelopathy. *Arch. Neurol., Chicago* **27**, 307.

Shannon, N. and Paul, E. A. (1979). L4/5 and L5/S1 disc protrusions: analysis of 323 cases operated on over 12 years. *J. Neurol. Neurosurg. Psychiat.* **42**, 804.

Shephard, R. H. (1959). Diagnosis and prognosis of cauda equina syndrome produced by protrusion of lumbar disk. *Br. med. J.* **2**, 1434.

Shinners, B. M. and Hamby, W. B. (1949). Protruded lumbar intervertebral discs. *J. Neurosurg.* **6**, 450.

Smith, L. and Brown, J. E. (1967). Treatment of lumbar intervertebral disc lesions by direct injection of chymopapain. *J. Bone Jt Surg.* **49B** 502.

Spurling, R. G. and Grantham, E. G. (1940). Neurologic picture of herniations of the nucleus pulposus in the lower part of the lumbar region. *Arch. Surg., Chicago,* **40**, 375.

Sterman, A. B., Schaumburg, H. H., and Asbury, A. K. (1980). The acute sensory neuronopathy syndrome: a distinct clinical entity. *Ann. Neurol.* **7**, 354.

Tarlov, I. M. (1938). Perineurial cysts of the spinal nerve roots. *Arch. Neurol. Psychiat., Chicago* **40**, 1067.

Taylor, A. R.. (1953). Mechanism and treatment of spinal-cord disorders associated with cervical spondylosis. *Lancet* **i**, 717.

Taylor, T. K. F. and Wienir, M. (1969). Great-toe reflexes in the diagnosis of lumbar disc disorder. *Br. med. J.* **2**, 487.

Thomas, D. J. Kendall, M. J., and Whitfield, A. G. W. (1974). Nervous system involvement in ankylosing spondylitis. *Br. med. J.* **1**, 148.

Whitaker, J. N., Falchuck, Z. M., Engel, W. K., Blaese, R. M., and Strober, W. (1974). Hereditary sensory neuropathy: association with increased synthesis of immunoglobulin A. *Arch. Neurol., Chicago* **30**, 359.

Wilkinson, M. (1960). The morbid anatomy of cervical spondylosis and myelopathy. *Brain* **83**, 589.

Yoss, R. E., Corbin, K. B., MacCarty, C. S., and Love, J. G. (1957). Significance of symptoms and signs in localization of involved root in cervical disk protrusion. *Neurology, Minneapolis* **7**, 673.

Other forms of mononeuropathy

'Interstital neuritis' was a diagnosis often made in the past to explain a lesion of a single peripheral or spinal nerve for which no obvious cause could be demonstrated, but it is now evident that no such inflammatory process exists as a specific pathological entity. In most cases so diagnosed it is now apparent that the condition resulted either from mechanical compression of the nerve in question or of its component roots, or from ischaemia, due either to peripheral vascular disease (Richards 1951; Gairns, Garven, and Smith 1960), diabetes, or to a diffuse inflammatory disorder of arteries such as polyarteritis nodosa (Lovshin and Kernohan 1948) in which an arteritis of the vasa nervorum may occur resulting in a 'mononeuritis multiplex'. It is also evident that *ischaemic monomelic neuropathy*, usually taking the form of multiple axonal mononeuropathies developing acutely and simultaneously in several peripheral nerves in the distal part of a limb, can be thromboembolic or can follow vascular surgery. It is produced by the shunting of blood away from, or the acute non-compressive occlusion of, a major proximal limb artery (Wilbourn, Furlan, Hulley, and Ruschhaupt 1983). It is also well recognized that some individuals have a peculiar liability to develop peripheral-nerve lesions (of the lateral popliteal, ulnar, or median nerves and less frequently of other mixed nerves) as a result of transient and minimal trauma; these patients may develop recurrent palsies of the affected nerve or nerves and this liability often appears to be inherited (Earl, Fullerton, Wakefield, and Schutta 1964). The pathogenesis of this form of '*hereditary neuropathy with liability to pressure palsy*', in which there is evidence of some loss of myelinated fibres and extensive segmental demyelination with marked slowing of conduction in many peripheral nerves at a time when symptoms may be absent (Davies 1954; Behse, Buchthal, Carlsen, and Knappeis 1972), is unknown. Sometimes the brachial plexus, rather than a peripheral nerve, may be involved, as in a case in which the neuropathy followed removal of one first rib (Bosch, Chui, Martin, and Cancilla 1980). In many such cases nerve biopsy demonstrates multifocal thickening of the myelin sheath (Debruyne, Dehaene, and Martin 1980) which Madrid and Bradley (1975) called tomaculous ('sausage-like') neuropathy and which suggests a morphological abnormality of myelination rendering peripheral nerves unduly sensitive to pressure or traction (Bosch *et al* 1980). Manifestations of multiple peripheral-nerve entrapment are also seen occasionally in rare inherited metabolic disorders including amyloidosis and mucopolysaccharidosis (Karpati, Carpenter, Eisen, Wolfe, and Feindel 1974).

References

Behse, F., Buchthal, F., Carlsen, F., and Knappeis, G. G. (1972). Hereditary neuropathy with liability to pressure palsies: electrophysiological and histopathological aspects. *Brain* **95**, 777.

Bosch, E. P., Chui, H. C., Martin, M. A., and Cancilla, P. A. (1980). Brachial plexus involvement in familial pressure-sensitive neuropathy: electrophysiological and morphological findings. *Ann. Neurol.* **8**, 620.

Davies, D. M. (1954). Recurrent peripheral-nerve palsies in a family. *Lancet* **ii**, 266.

Debruyne, J., Dehaene, I., and Martin, J. J. (1980). Hereditary pressure-sensitive neuropathy. *J. neurol. Sci.* **47**, 385.

Earl, C. J., Fullerton, P. M., Wakefield, G. S., and Schutta, H. S. (1964). Hereditary neuropathy with liability to pressure palsies. *Quart. J. Med.* **33**, 481.

Gairns, F. W., Garven, H. S. D., and Smith, G. (1960). The digital nerves and the nerve endings in progressive obliterative vascular disease. *Scot. med. J.* **5**, 382.

Karpati, G., Carpenter, S., Eisen, A. A., Wolfe, L. S., and Feindel, W. (1974). Multiple peripheral nerve entrapments. *Arch. Neurol., Chicago* **31**, 418.

Lovshin, L. L. and Kernohan, J. W. (1948). Peripheral neuritis in periarteritis nodosa. *Arch. intern. Med.* **82**, 321.

Madrid, R. and Bradley, W. G. (1975). The pathology of neuropathies with focal thickening of the myelin sheath (tomaculous neuropathy). *J. neurol. Sci.* **25**, 415.

Richards, R. L. (1951). Ischaemic lesions of peripheral nerves: a review. *J. Neurol. Psychiat.* **14** 76.

Wilbourn, A. J., Furlan, A. J., Hulley, W., and Ruschhaupt, W. (1983). Ischemic monomelic neuropathy. *Neurology, Minneapolis* **33**, 447.

Neuropathy of the face, neck, and scalp

Pain is commonly experienced in the distribution of one or more of the cutaneous nerves of the face, neck, and scalp and has been attributed to neuropathy, but the nature of the pathological process in some such cases is speculative. Sometimes there may well be mechanical compression of the affected nerve, but in other cases emotional and muscular tension is clearly a factor. The term 'neuritis' once used in some cases is now outmoded. Occasionally the territory of all the divisions of one trigeminal nerve is involved. More often symptoms are limited to the distribution of one branch, usually the supra-orbital or auriculotemporal, less often the infra-orbital. The cutaneous distribution of the great occipital nerve is also a common site of pain.

Symptoms and signs

The onset may be acute, and the pain may come on after a cold, tonsillitis, or an attack of influenza. Pain following the distribution of the affected nerve may occur in paroxysms lasting for several hours, most frequently towards the close of the day, when the patient is fatigued. An attack of pain may also be precipitated by exposure to cold. When the pain is severe it interferes with sleep. It is of a dull, aching character, intensified by exacerbations in which it seems to shoot along the course of the nerve. There is often hyperpathia in the area of skin supplied by the nerve, and when this includes the scalp it is noticed on combing and brushing the hair. The nerve trunk may be tender on pressure.

Diagnosis

There are many causes of paroxysmal pain in the face and scalp, and care must be taken to exclude other conditions before falling back on a diagnosis of unexplained neuropathy.

Infection of the nasal air sinuses is a common cause, frontal sinusitis being associated with supra-orbital pain, and infection of the maxillary antrum with pain in approximately the distribution of the infra-orbital nerve. In ethmoiditis the pain is chiefly at the root of the nose, and in infection of the sphenoidal sinus is usually referred to the forehead or occiput. In acute cases there is usually a history of catarrh or a cold in the head with or without a purulent nasal discharge. There may be visible oedema over the frontal sinus or antrum. X-rays will usually reveal the site of infection. The tympanic membranes should always be examined to exclude latent otitis media.

The teeth are a common cause of facial pain. Search should be made for dental disease, and the possibility that there is an unerupted tooth (especially a wisdom tooth) must always be considered. This may be present, as may also a buried root, in an apparently edentulous patient, and can be detected only by X-ray examination. Pain of dental origin is often accentuated by chewing or by the ingestion of hot or cold foods. Pain on chewing, and radiating into the temple or down over the mandible is also a feature of some cases of temporomandibular arthrosis due to dental malocclusion (Costen's syndrome). The pharynx should also be examined for the presence of a growth, which may occasionally cause pain referred to the ear and neck.

The eye is occasionally a source of referred neuralgic pain, the commonest ocular cause being glaucoma, which is easily missed unless considered. Pain may also be referred to the face in disease of the heart and lungs as in the case of lower-jaw pain developing on exertion in angina pectoris.

Intractable neuralgia may follow herpes zoster involving the first division of the trigeminal nerve. The history of the eruption and the residual scars render the diagnosis easy. Trigeminal neuralgia, by contrast, is distinguished by the brevity of the attacks of pain and the characteristic precipitating factors. Trigeminal neuropathy, usually giving numbness, but occasionally pain, is a rare manifestation of connective-tissue disease, such as systemic lupus (Ashworth and Tait 1971).

In migraine the headache occurs in attacks or paroxysms which are often associated with vomiting and preceded by the characteristic aura. There is usually a long history. Periodic migrainous neuralgia ('cluster headache') gives attacks of severe pain in and around the eye, lasting for up to two hours and occurring daily or twice daily in bouts lasting for several weeks or months.

Temporal or cranial arteritis occurs in the elderly and often causes pain and tenderness in the scalp, particularly in the temporal and occipital regions; the temporal arteries are usually tortuous and tender and the erythrocyte sedimentation rate is raised.

Tabes is an occasional cause of paroxysmal pain in the face or scalp, but is readily recognized by its other clinical features.

The various intracranial causes of pain in the face and head must also be borne in mind, especially lesions of the trigeminal fibres in the brainstem such as syringobulbia, and thrombosis of the posterior inferior cerebellar artery, in both of which pain is usually associated with analgesia and thermo-anaesthesia.

Occipital pain may be due to lesions of the cervical region of the spinal cord or of the vertebral column at this level, especially cervical spondylosis. Traumatic neuropathy of the second cervical nerve can also give occipital neuralgia and sensory impairment and can follow forcible approximation of the arches of the atlas and axis with excessive rotation (Behrman 1983). The 'neck–tongue syndrome', in which sudden rotatory movements of the head cause unilateral sub-occipital pain and ipsilateral numbness of the tongue (Lance and Anthony 1980) is probably due to subluxation of one lateral atlanto-axial joint (Bogduk 1981). Pain and stiffness in the neck and occipital muscles ('stiff neck') is often a banal, self-limiting disorder of undetermined cause, but has been noted occasionally to occur in epidemic forms ('epidemic cervical myalgia'—Davies 1960); a viral aetiology has been postulated but remains unproven.

Psychogenic pain is distinguished by its lack of relation to a specific nerve, its failure, often, to respond to analgesic drugs, and by the patient's exaggerated emotional reaction to the pain. However, chronic tension of the muscles attached to the scalp, occurring in association with anxiety and/or depression, may give rise to pain of exactly the type described, and this is not infrequently unilateral. This is particularly true of the so-called 'atypical facial pain' which usually occurs in the upper jaw in young or middle-aged women and which is often attributed erroneously to 'neuritis' but which in most cases is of purely psychogenic origin. Other aspects of the differential diagnosis of facial pain are considered on page 111.

Prognosis

In most cases the prognosis in patients with acute episodes of pain in the face and scalp is good and there is a rapid spontaneous recovery or response to treatment. Occasionally, however, especially in neurotic patients, the pain proves intractable.

Treatment

The first essential is to exclude the organic causes of facial pain referred to above by means of appropriate investigations. Simple analgesic drugs are often effective but the fact that many cases respond even more satisfactorily to a combination of antidepressive and tranquillizing remedies is sufficient to indicate that in many such cases there is no organic cause for the pain.

If pain persists despite the measures outlined and no organic lesion compressing the nerve can be identified, it is occasionally necessary to inject the affected nerve trunk with local anaesthetic, the supra-orbital nerve being injected at the supra-orbital notch, the infra-orbital at its foramen, by the methods described in the section on trigeminal neuralgia. The great occipital nerve can be similarly injected, and when occipital pain is due to cervical myalgia relief may sometimes be obtained from similar injection of any tender spots in the muscles. Posterior cervical and/or occipital pain in spondylosis will sometimes require temporary immobilization in a cervical collar.

Shoulder-girdle neuritis (neuralgic amyotrophy)

Localized neuritis of one or more nerves innervating the shoulder-girdle muscles was well recognized before the Second World War and also during the war, especially in the Near East (Spillane 1943; Parsonage and Turner 1948). The patients were often in hospital after an operation or acute infection such as pneumonia. Pain is usually the initial symptom; it may be intense for several days and is followed by muscular wasting and weakness. The muscles most often affected are the serratus anterior, spinati, deltoid, and trapezius in that order. When the deltoid is involved there may be sensory loss over the distribution of the axillary (circumflex) nerve. More recent experience has shown that in more than a third of cases there is no history of antecedent illness, infection, or trauma, that other muscles including biceps and forearm muscles are less commonly involved, that clinical and/or electrophysiological evidence (slowing of nerve conduction with electromyographic evidence of denervation) gives evidence of bilateral brachial plexus involvement in about one-quarter of all cases, and that very rarely there is a mild lymphocytic pleocytosis or rise in protein in the CSF (Weikers and Mattson 1969; Tsairis, Dyck, and Mulder 1972). The condition occasionally occurs in pregnancy, is rarely bilateral clinically (Lane and Dewar 1978) and has been described in more than one member of a family (Geiger, Mancall, Penn, and Tucker 1974). Very rarely an identical syndrome may be painless (Schott 1983); signs of root compression or irritation are generally absent but exceptionally a flexion-adduction sign (radicular pain evoked by abduction and lateral rotation of the arm with the elbow extended) can be elicited (Waxman 1979). Rarely a comparable syndrome involves the lumbosacral plexus (Evans, Stevens, and Dyck 1981). Despite the severity of the initial pain and/or paralysis, recovery of muscle power is usually excellent, beginning within one or two months, but complete functional recovery may take up to three years or longer (Tsairis et al. 1972); only occasionally is paralysis permanent, especially in deltoid or serratus anterior. The cause is unknown but an identical syndrome may follow 7–10 days after the injection of foreign serum ('serum neuropathy') and the condition is presumed to be an auto-immune brachial-plexus neuropathy. Treatment is symptomatic; in the first few days pain of an intense burning character in the shoulder and arm may be so severe that powerful analgesics are required. When the acute phase is over, active exercises should be encouraged as soon as possible.

Intercostal neuropathy

Intercostal neuropathy is a rare disorder which is diagnosed more often than it occurs. It is characterized by paroxysmal pain throughout the distribution of an intercostal nerve, frequently associated with cutaneous tenderness in the area it supplies, especially at the point of emergence of its lateral cutaneous branch. Before diagnosing this condition care must be taken to exclude the many other disorders which may be associated with similar pain which can be due to inflammation or compression of spinal dorsal roots, especially by syphilis or arachnoiditis, or by a neoplasm of the spinal cord. It may precede or follow an attack of herpes zoster. The spinal nerve may be compressed as a result of localized collapse of the vertebral column, most often due to tuberculous caries, secondary carcinoma, or trauma. Spondylosis is often associated with root pains, which may also be produced by scoliosis. Pleurisy, both tuberculous and neoplastic, is sometimes mistakenly diagnosed as intercostal neuralgia, and the thorax is a common site of referred pain in visceral disease, especially diseases of the upper abdominal viscera including cholecystitis and carcinoma of the body or tail of the pancreas. Pain in the distribution of an intercostal nerve is also seen in some patients after thoracotomy and may be intractable. Another important, if uncommon, cause of this syndrome is the so-called 'rib-tip' syndrome due to increased mobility of the anterior ends of the lower ribs (*British Medical Journal* 1976).

Treatment

Intercostal neuropathy should be treated with analgesics. Local anaesthetic injections may give temporary relief and if all else fails the nerve may be injected with alcohol or phenol, care being taken that the needle does not penetrate the pleura. In occasional cases, surgical division of two or three intercostal nerves close to the spine may be needed but even after this operation pain may recur after a few months. Even posterior rhizotomy at the appropriate levels does not always afford permanent relief.

References

Ashworth, B. and Tait, G. B. W. (1971). Trigeminal neuropathy in connective tissue disease. *Neurology, Minneapolis* **21**, 609.

Behrman, S. (1983). Traumatic neuropathy of second cervical spinal nerves. *Br. med. J.* **286** 1312.

Bogduk, N. (1981). An anatomical basis for the neck-tongue syndrome. *J. Neurol. Neurosurg. Psychiat.* **44**, 202.

Bradley, W. G. (1974). *Disorders of peripheral nerves.* Blackwell, Oxford.

British Medical Journal (1976). Rib pain. *Br. med. J.* **1**, 358.

Davies, D. M. (1960). Epidemic cervical myalgia. *Lancet* **i**, 1275.

Evans, B. A., Stevens, J. C., and Dyck, P. J. (1981). Lumbosacral plexus neuropathy. *Neurology, Minneapolis* **31**, 1327.

Geiger, L. R., Mancall, E. L., Penn, A. S., and Tucker, S. H. (1974). Familial neuralgic amyotrophy—report of three families with review of the literature. *Brain* **97**, 87.

Lance, J. W. and Anthony, M. (1980). Neck–tongue syndrome on sudden turning of the head. *J. Neurol. Neurosurg. Psychiat.* **43**, 97.

Lane, R. J. M. and Dewar, J. A. (1978). Bilateral aneuralgic amyotrophy. *Br. med. J.* **1**, 895.

Parsonage, M. J. and Turner, J. W. A. (1948). Neuralgic amyotrophy. The shoulder-girdle syndrome. *Lancet* **i**, 973.

Schott, G. D. (1983). A chronic and painless form of idiopathic brachial plexus neuropathy. *J. Neurol. Neurosurg. Psychiat.* **46**, 555.

Spillane, J. D. (1943). Localized neuritis of the shoulder girdle. *Lancet* **ii**, 532.

Sunderland, S. (1978). *Nerves and nerve injuries,* 2nd edn. Churchill-Livingstone, Edinburgh.

Taylor, R. A. (1960). Heredofamilial mononeuritis multiplex with brachial predilection. *Brain* **83**, 113.

Thage, O. (1974). *Quadriceps weakness and wasting. A neurological, electrophysiological and histological study.* Munksgaard, Copenhagen.

Tsairis, P., Dyck, P. J., and Mulder, D. W. (1972). Natural history of brachial plexus neuropathy. *Arch. Neurol., Chicago* **27**, 109.

Waxman, S. G. (1979). The flexion-adduction sign in neuralgic amyotrophy, *Neurology, Minneapolis* **29**, 1301.

Weikers, N. J. and Mattson, R. H. (1969). Acute paralytic brachial neuritis. *Neurology, Minneapolis* **19**, 1153.

Polyneuritis (polyneuropathy)

Synonyms. Multiple symmetrical peripheral neuritis; multiple neuritis.

Definition. Polyneuritis is a clinical syndrome, of which the essential feature is simultaneous impairment of function of many peripheral nerves, often resulting in symmetrical flaccid muscular weakness, and usually also sensory abnormalities, affecting as a rule the distal more than the proximal segments of the limbs, and sometimes also involving the cranial nerves. Polyneuritis thus defined has very many causes, which may operate in many different ways and may involve different parts of the peripheral nerves. Among the causes are numerous endogenous and exogenous toxins, acute inflammatory processes which directly attack the nerves, ischaemia, and many metabolic disorders including vitamin deficiency.

History. Peripheral neuritis was recorded by Lettsom in 1789 and an epidemic in Paris was described by Robert Graves in 1828. Todd first conceived that the terminal branches of the peripheral nerves might undergo degeneration, and this was demonstrated pathologically by Dumenil in 1864. Joffroy in 1879 contributed to the classification of polyneuritis and Grainger Stewart gave it the name multiple symmetrical peripheral neuritis in 1881. Korsakow described the mental changes sometimes associated with alcoholic polyneuritis in 1889.

As Simpson (1962) pointed out, except in the case of leprosy and the auto-immune neuropathies, true inflammation in peripheral nerves is relatively uncommon and most such disorders are more correctly termed 'neuropathy'. Pathological studies have shown that many polyneuropathies are mainly demyelinating (the myelin sheath and/or Schwann cell are attacked by the disease) but some are due to axonal degeneration, often with secondary demyelination. In demyelinating neuropathies nerve conduction is usually markedly delayed, while in axonal degenerations there may be no conduction at all, or, if denervation is partial, the surviving axons conduct at a normal rate but the amplitude of evoked muscle or sensory potentials is reduced since fewer axons respond.

While many forms of polyneuropathy affect both sensory and motor fibres, some appear to involve motor fibres selectively and others sensory fibres, while it is also evident that sometimes heavily myelinated, rapidly conducting fibres are predominantly involved, while in other cases finely myelinated or even unmyelinated fibres are attacked. Some processes which involve the axon primarily seem to involve its entire length, others begin distally ('dying-back' neuropathies). The factors which determine such selective involvement of Schwann cells, myelin, axons, and different classes of fibres are still poorly understood (Bradley 1974; Dyck, Thomas, and Lambert 1983).

Aetiology

The following classification includes the most important causes (see also the classification by Research Group in Neuromuscular Diseases 1968 and as revised by Walton 1981):

1. Toxic substances

(*a*) *Metals*: Antimony, arsenic, bismuth, copper, lead, mercury (pink disease, Minimata disease), phosphorus, thallium.

(b) *Drugs, organic chemicals, and other toxic substances*: Acrylamide, amiodarone, aniline, BHMH, buckthorn (coyotillo fruit), 'bush tea', calcium carbimide, carbamazepine, carbon monoxide, carbon disulphide, carbon tetrachloride, chloral, chloretone, chloroquine, clioquinol, cyanogenetic glycosides, cytotoxic agents including vincristine sulphate, dapsone, DDT, dinitrobenzol, disulfiram, emetine, ethionamide, ethylene oxide, glutethimide, hydrallazine, hexachlorophane, immune sera, indomethacin, isoniazid, methaqualone, metronidazole, misonidazole, n-hexane, nitrofurantoin, parathion, pentachlorphenol, perhexiline, phenytoin, stilbamidine, streptomycin, sulphanilamide, and its compounds, sulphonal, tetrachlorethane, thalidomide, trichlorethylene, triorthocresylphosphate (ginger paralysis and apiol paralysis) (see Argov and Mastaglia 1979).

2. Deficiency, metabolic, and haematological disorders

Beriberi, chronic alcoholism, chronic obstructive pulmonary disease, famine oedema, folic acid deficiency, liver disease and chronic disease of (including coeliac disease), or operations upon, the gastrointestinal tract, pellagra, pregnancy, protein–calorie malnutrition, tropical neuropathy, vitamin B_{12} neuropathy.

Acromegaly, diabetes, hyperinsulinism, myxoedema, porphyria, uraemia.

Neuropathy in A-alpha and beta-lipoproteinaemia, in dysglobulinaemia, monoclonal gammopathy, and various paraproteinaemias.

Neuropathy in polycythaemia vera, leukaemia, multiple myeloma, and haemorrhagic disorders (see also 7, 8, and 9).

3. Infective conditions

(a) *Local infection of nerves*: Brucellosis, leprosy, leptospirosis, and infective mononucleosis, very rarely syphilis.
(b) *Polyneuritis complicating acute or chronic infections*: Dysentery, focal infection, gonorrhoea, influenza, malaria, measles, meningitis, mumps, paratyphoid, puerperal sepsis, scarlet fever, septicaemia, smallpox, syphilis, tuberculosis, typhoid, typhus.
(c) *Infections with organisms whose exotoxins have an affinity for the peripheral nerves*: Diphtheria, dysentery, tetanus.

4. Post-infective (?allergic) polyneuropathy

(a) Acute post-infective polyradiculoneuropathy (the Guillain–Barré syndrome).
(b) Some cases of subacute and chronic polyneuropathy.
(c) ?Recurrent polyneuropathy.

5. Trauma

Physical injury and nerve entrapment, electric shock, cold, and radiation injury.

6. Ischaemic neuropathies

Neuropathies due to ischaemia or infarction of peripheral nerves as in peripheral vascular disease (other than in the auto-immune arteritides—see 7).

7. Connective-tissue and allied disorders

Giant-cell arteritis, polyarteritis nodosa, rheumatoid polyneuritis, sarcoidosis, systemic lupus erythematosus, systemic sclerosis, other vascular neuropathies including peripheral vascular disease.

8. Genetically determined polyneuropathy

Peroneal muscular atrophy, the Roussy–Levy syndrome, progressive hypertrophic polyneuritis of Dejerine and Sottas, Refsum's disease, hereditary neuropathy with liability to pressure palsies, neuropathy in metachromatic leucodystrophy, in the Krabbe form of diffuse sclerosis and in other leukodystrophies and storage disorders, in primary amyloidosis, in porphyria, in Fabry's disease, in A-alpha and beta-lipoproteinaemia and various other obscure varieties of hereditary neuropathy including neuropathic arthrogryposis multiplex congenita, so-called "globular" neuropathy, giant axonal neuropathy, neuropathy with optic atrophy, nerve deafness and/or paraproteinaemia (see Bradley 1974; Walton 1981; Dyck *et al.* 1983, pp. 380–3 and 548).

9. Polyneuropathy of obscure origin

Recurrent polyneuritis. Chronic progressive polyneuritis.
Carcinomatous neuropathy and the other paraneoplastic neuropathies.
Congenital hypomyelination neuropathy.
Neuropathies of undetermined cause.

General considerations

In some cases a toxin is introduced into the body from without. In others it is formed within the body as a result of bacterial action or of various metabolic disturbances, or the source may be impossible to define. Many drugs and toxins appear to have a specific affinity for the peripheral nerves; some damage the axons while others combine with and affect the function of the phospholipids of the myelin sheaths. Many such toxins ascend the peripheral nerves, thus causing first a local neuropathy involving the nerves in the region in which the toxin originates, as in palatal paralysis in diphtheria, and later generalized polyneuropathy, in which the toxin is disseminated in the blood stream and so reaches peripheral nerves throughout the body.

The role of avitaminosis and of other deficiencies in the causation of polyneuritis is more complex than was once thought and is discussed on page 473. In the infective disorders listed above, there is little direct clinical or experimental evidence, except in leprosy, to show that axons, Schwann cells, or myelin sheaths are directly damaged by the infecting organisms; in many such disorders the injury to peripheral nerves is presumed to be either toxic or due to a hypersensitivity reaction, either cell-mediated or humoral in type. Certainly, both cytotoxic factors in serum and immunoglobulin abnormalities (Rosenberg, Aung, Tindall, Molenich, Baskin, Capra, and Toben 1975) on the one hand and evidence of cell-mediated immunity to neural antigens on the other (Abramsky, Webb, Teitelbaum, and Arnon 1975) have been found in many forms of polyneuropathy (see p. 527). In neuropathy secondary to the various connective-tissue disorders, ischaemia resulting from arteritis of the vasa nervorum certainly plays an important role. In the group of genetically determined polyneuropathies the primary enzymatic defect responsible for the storage of identifiable material in peripheral nerves and in other organs has been identified in some disorders such as Refsum's disease and several of the leukodystrophies (see pp. 460 and 462). However, in many other conditions the nature of the underlying abnormality is still unknown despite recent advances in knowledge of the biochemical composition of normal and abnormal nerves (Bradley 1974; Dyck *et al.* 1983) and despite experimental studies in animals of the axoplasmic flow of radioactive protein in the normal state and in various forms of toxic neuropathy (Bradley and Williams 1973). Some recent evidence about the part played by viruses and other organisms and by disordered immunity in the Guillain–Barré syndrome and in various subacute and chronic demyelinating neuropathies will be reviewed below. In the axonal neuropathies, Spencer, Sabri, Schaumburg, and Moore (1979) suggest that many neurotoxic compounds deplete energy supplies in the axon by inhibiting nerve-fibre enzymes required for the maintenance of energy synthesis.

Pathology

There have been important recent advances in knowledge concerning the pathology of peripheral neuropathy (polyneuritis) of various types. These have come partly from post-mortem studies but have been based more particularly on experimental studies in animals and upon nerve biopsy studies in patients (Thomas 1970; Stevens, Lofgren, and Dyck 1973; Weller and Cervós-Navarro 1977; Asbury and Johnson 1978; Dyck *et al*, 1983), utilizing techniques for the examination of single teased nerve fibres stained with osmic acid. Measurement of internodal length (the distance between nodes of Ranvier) in such teased fibres is an important part of the examination. Methods involving osmic acid staining of transverse sections of nerves in which fibres can be counted and their diameters measured have also made valuable contributions (Figs. 18.8–18.12) as has electron microscopy. The sural nerve is

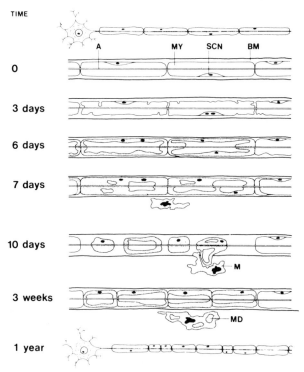

Fig. 18.8. Diagrammatic representation of the successive changes occurring during segmental demyelination and remyelination as in diphtheritic neuropathy. The axon (A) remains intact throughout but the myelin (MY) breaks down. There is activation of Schwann cells with division of their nuclei (SCN). Regeneration occurs within the basement membrane (BM). Both activated Schwann cells and macrophages (M) take part in the digestion of myelin debris (MD). Some internodes (sections of myelin between nodes of Ranvier) remain intact, others are damaged, and after remyelination abnormally short internodes are formed so that the nerve, after recovery, shows marked variation in internodal length. (Diagram reproduced from Bradley (1974) by kind permission of the author and publishers.)

the one most conveniently biopsied but has the occasional disadvantage that, being wholly sensory, it is not invariably diseased in neuropathies which are predominantly motor in type. The information derived from these studies must be carefully assessed in relation to known changes in fibre number and diameter and in internodal length observed in various peripheral nerves in subjects of varying age (Swallow 1966; Lascelles and Thomas 1966; O'Sullivan and Swallow 1968; Ochoa and Mair 1969 *a*, *b*). The ultrastructural abnormalities seen in both Wallerian degeneration (Thomas 1964; Ballin and Thomas 1969) and segmental demyelination (Weller and Nester 1972) must also be carefully assessed with special techniques required to avoid artefact and in the knowledge of variations which may be observed in normal appearances. The importance of examining unmyelinated as well as myelinated fibres has also been stressed (Peyronnard, Aguayo, and Bray 1973; Behse, Buchthal, Carlsen, and Knappeis 1975) and attention must also be paid to changes in Schwann cells (in myeli-

nated fibres) and Remak cells (in unmyelinated fibres). Such studies have demonstrated that in many forms of neuropathy (in diphtheria, the Guillain–Barré syndrome, carcinomatous neuropathy, familial hypertrophic neuropathy, and metachromatic leucodystrophy, for example) the disease process affects predominantly the Schwann cells and results in segmental demyelination of peripheral nerves, with a progressive shrinkage of the myelin away from the nodes of Ranvier and the eventual denuding of axons which frequently remain intact. In this phase, conduction in the affected nerves is markedly slowed. Occasionally in demyelination, sausage-shaped myelin swellings (so-called 'tomaculous neuropathy') are found, but the specificity of this change is in doubt (Madrid and Bradley 1975). Recovery is accompanied by remyelination but the newly-formed myelin is often thinner than normal and the internodal distances are shorter; however, nerve conduction velocity may recover eventually to normal. Repeated demyelination and remyelination may lead to Schwann-cell proliferation, 'onion-bulb' formation (Fig. 18.12, p. 525), and ultimately to palpable hypertrophy of nerves (Thomas and Lascelles 1967). In other forms of neuropathy (Gilliatt 1966), including, for example, those due to alcoholism, porphyria, triorthocresylphosphate, isoniazid, vincristine, and thalidomide, the process appears to be one of axonal degeneration which either involves the axon diffusely or may begin distally and then spread proximally ('dying-back neuropathies'); segmental demyelination is slight or absent at first so that nerve conduction velocity is reduced comparatively little. In the neuropathies due to lead and acrylamide (Fullerton 1966; Fullerton and Barnes 1966) both the axons and their myelin sheaths may be affected simultaneously. In diabetes, too, segmental demyelination may come first but is quickly followed by axonal degeneration. In some axonal neuropathies ultrastructural studies have identified specific changes in the fine structure of the axons and neurofilaments, as, for example, in giant axonal neuropathy, while in some demyelinating varieties, lysosomes and other inclusions accumulate in Schwann cells. Such changes will be mentioned below in relation to the individual disease entities. Recent studies have plainly indicated that the distinction between demyelinating and axonal neuropathies is often less precise than was once thought to be the case, especially when the process is advanced, as axonal degeneration is often followed quickly by secondary demyelination and vice versa (Bradley 1974; Weller and Cervés-Navarro 1977; Asbury and Johnson 1978; Dyck *et al.* 1983). Nevertheless, in early cases the distinction remains valid and is often of some diagnostic value.

Symptoms, signs, and prognosis

The symptoms, signs and prognosis and further details of the pathology of the commoner and more important forms of polyneuropathy are described under their respective headings.

Diagnosis

As a rule the diagnosis of polyneuropathy is easy, owing to the characteristic symmetrical and peripheral distribution of the muscular weakness and wasting, pain, tenderness, and sensory impairment. The position is not so straight-forward when the symptoms and signs are predominantly motor or sensory, or asymmetrical, or predominant in the lower limbs, or in those occasional cases in which proximal muscular weakness is more striking at first, when a variety of other neurological disorders may be mimicked. Electrical measurements of motor and sensory nerve conduction are invaluable in establishing the perpheral nerves as the site of the lesion and in indicating whether it is predominantly demyelinating or axonal. Occasional and uncommon manifestations which may give rise to diagnostic difficulty include impulse-induced repetitive discharges in motor nerves ('neurotonia', with delayed muscular relaxation after voluntary contraction resembling myotonia) which is thought to be due to slow waning of heightened excitability of a motor nerve after passage of an impulse (Warmolts and

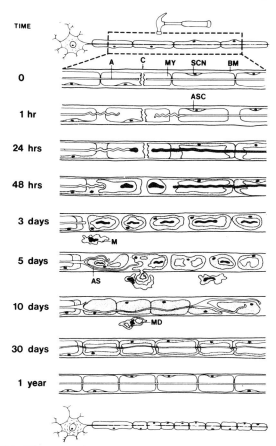

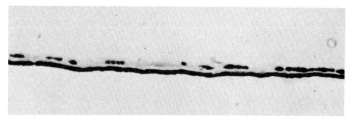

Fig. 18.11. A pair of teased myelinated nerve fibres stained with osmic acid. The upper fibre is fragmented into myelin ovoids as a result of axonal degeneration; the lower fibre is intact. (Reproduced from Bradley (1974) by kind permission of the author and publishers.)

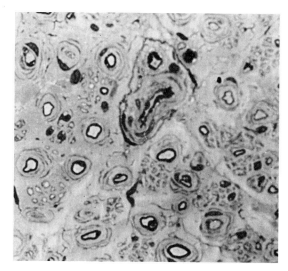

Fig. 18.9. Diagrammatic representation of changes occurring in a peripheral nerve distal to a traumatic lesion causing axonotmesis. At the level of the lesion (C) (e.g. a crush) there is disruption of the axon with fragmentation both of the axon and of the myelin sheath. The Schwann cells are activated and broken down myelin is digested by both Schwann cells and macrophages. The axon sprouts from the fifth day onwards and the Schwann cells begin to form new myelin sheaths from the tenth day. After regeneration, distal to the crush, all internodes are abnormally short. (Reproduced from Bradley (1974) by kind permission of the author and publishers.)

Fig. 18.12. Transverse section of a 1 μm araldite section of peripheral nerve stained with toluidine blue showing multiple 'onion-bulbs'; sural-nerve biopsy from a case of hypertrophic neuropathy. (Kindly supplied by Dr R. Madrid.)

Fig. 18.10. A single teased nerve fibre, stained with osmic acid, from a case of hypertrophic neuropathy. Consecutive lengths of the single fibre are mounted below one another. Arrowheads mark the position of the nodes of Ranvier. None of the internodes is of normal length (about 1.00 mm in a fibre of 10 μm diameter) and there is extensive demyelination and remyelination with marked variation in internodal length. (Reproduced from Bradley (1974) by kind permission of the author and publishers.)

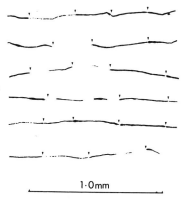

1·0mm

(1978) have shown that, in general, motor and sensory nerve conduction velocity measurement is of greater diagnostic value than sural-nerve biopsy in most cases, even though the latter sometimes yields specific diagnostic information. Thus sural-nerve biopsy must be used for diagnostic purposes only when the nature of the neuropathy remains in doubt and when all other available techniques of investigation have been employed. Careful clinical evaluation, especially of sensory abnormalities, and examination of other family members often improves the diagnostic "yield" (Dyck, Oviatt, and Lambert 1981).

The clinical association of pain, ataxia, and loss of tendon reflexes in the lower limbs may simulate tabes. The pain of polyneuropathy, however, when present, is of a persistent, burning character and differs from the lightning pains of tabes; it is usually associated with tenderness of the deep tissues on pressure, whereas in tabes these are insensitive. Although the pupillary reaction to light may be sluggish in polyneuropathy, especially in the alcoholic and diabetic forms, a true Argyll Robertson pupil is rarely, if ever found (except in peroneal muscular atrophy), and the VDRL reaction is negative, except in patients who happen to suffer both from syphilis and from polyneuropathy. As stated elsewhere, some of the symptoms of subacute combined degeneration in B_{12} deficiency are due to an associated neuropathy. The true cause of these symptoms, however, is usually easily established by the presence of extensor plantar responses, impairment of appreciation of vibration over the trunk as well as the limbs, and the presence of anaemia, glossitis, and a low concentration of vitamin B_{12} in the serum. When weakness predominates in proximal limb muscles as in some cases of the Guillain–Barré syndrome, diagnosis from polymyositis or motor-neurone disease may not be easy

Mendell 1980) and continuous muscle-fibre activity with myokymia ('neuromyotonia') (Vasilescu and Florescu 1982), sometimes associated with lysosomal abnormalities in cultured Schwann cells (Askanas, Engel, Berginer, Odenwald, and Galdi 1981). The syndrome of 'painful legs and moving toes' is also associated with similar clinical phenomena and with a neuropathy involving the posterior-nerve roots (Nathan 1978). However, Schoener, Gonce, and Delwaide (1984) found evidence of lumbar-root dysfunction in some such cases but of more proximal sensorimotor dysfunction in others. Buchthal and Behse (1978) and Behse and Buchthal clinically but is usually helped greatly by electromyography, nerve conduction velocity measurement, and examination of the CSF. When a diagnosis of polyneuropathy has been made, the diagnosis of the cause is based upon distinctive features of the history and symptoms peculiar to the different varieties, and upon investigative findings which are described under their respective headings.

Treatment

The first step in treatment is to prevent further exposure to the causal drug or toxin, if this can be identified, and its elimination from the body, or the correction of abnormal metabolic states or vitamin deficiency. The necessary steps are described in the sections dealing with the various forms of neuropathy. In certain acute forms (e.g. the Guillain–Barré syndrome) assisted respiration and intensive care may be needed if the respiratory muscles are involved. Some varieties (as in connective-tissues disease) are steroid-responsive and a course of treatment with prednisone or ACTH may reasonably be given in any case of subacute, predominantly demyelinating polyneuropathy for which no cause can be found, especially if the protein content of the CSF is raised. This treatment is now thought to be ineffective in the acute Guillain–Barré syndrome.

Rest in bed is essential only when the severity of the muscular weakness is such that the patient cannot walk or in those forms of polyneuropathy (such as beriberi) in which the heart is also involved. In most cases, continuing activity is important.

Local treatment consists of the prevention of muscular contractures, maintenance of the nutrition of the muscles, and promotion of recovery in voluntary power. Wrist-drop and foot-drop must be prevented by the use of appropriate splints. As long as muscular tenderness is severe, splints may not be tolerated and the feet must then be supported by a board placed beneath the soles, the weight of the bed-clothes being taken by a cradle. Later, moulded metal or plastic splints may be used to support the feet at a right angle. When contractures have already developed they must be overcome by appropriate physical means. Daily active and passive movements should be instituted as soon as the patient is able to bear them. Analgesic drugs will be required when the pain is severe. A useful review of the principles of treatment was given by Bradley (1975).

References

Abramsky, O., Webb, C., Teitelbaum, D., and Arnon, R. (1975). Cell-mediated immunity to neural antigens in idiopathic polyneuritis and myeloradiculitis. *Neurology, Minneapolis* **25**, 1154.

Argov, Z. and Mastaglia, F. L. (1979). Drug-induced peripheral neuropathies. *Br. med. J.* **1**, 663.

Asbury, A. K. and Johnson, P. C. (1978). *Pathology of peripheral nerve.* Saunders, Philadelphia.

Askanas, V., Engel, W. K., Berginer, V. M., Odenwald, W. F., and Galdi, A. (1981). Lysosomal abnormalities in cultured Schwann cells from a patient with peripheral neuropathy and continuous muscle fiber activity. *Ann. Neurol.* **10**, 238.

Ballin, R. H. M. and Thomas, P. K. (1969). Changes at the nodes of Ranvier during Wallerian degeneration: an electron microscopic study. *Acta neuropath. (Berlin)* **14**, 237.

——, ——, Carlsen, F., and Knappeis, G. G. (1975). Unmyelinated fibres and Schwann cells of sural nerve in neuropathy. *Brain* **98**, 493.

Bradley, W. G. (1974). *Disorders of peripheral nerves.* Blackwell, Oxford.

—— (1975). The treatment of polyneuropathy. *The Practitioner* **215**, 452.

—— and Williams, M. H. (1973). Axoplasmic flow in axonal neuropathies 1. Axoplasmic flow in cats with toxic neuropathies. *Brain* **96**, 235.

Buchthal, F. and Behse, F. (1978). Polyneuropathy. In *Contemporary clinical neurophysiology*, (EEG Suppl. No. 34) (ed. W. A. Cobb and H. Van Duijn) p. 373. Elsevier, Amsterdam.

Dyck, P. J., Oviatt, K. F., and Lambert, E. H. (1981). Intensive evaluation of referred unclassified neuropathies yields improved diagnosis. *Ann. Neurol.* **10**, 222.

——, Thomas, P. K., and Lambert, E. H. (1983). *Peripheral neuropathy*, 2nd edn. Saunders, Philadelphia.

Fullerton, P. M. (1966). Chronic peripheral neuropathy produced by lead poisoning in guinea-pigs. *J. Neuropath, exp. Neurol.* **25**, 214.

—— and Barnes, J. M. (1966). Peripheral neuropathy in rats produced by acrylamide. *Br. J. indust. Med.* **23**, 210.

Gilliatt, R. W. (1966). Nerve conduction in human experimental neuropathies. *Proc. Roy. Soc. Med.* **59**, 989.

Lascelles, R. G. and Thomas, P. K. (1966). Changes due to age in internodal length in the sural nerve in man. *J. Neurol. Neurosurg. Psychiat.* **29**, 40.

Madrid, R. and Bradley, W. G. (1975). The pathology of neuropathies with focal thickening of the myelin sheath (tomaculous neuropathy). *J. neurol. Sci.* **25**, 415.

Nathan, P. W. (1978). Painful legs and moving toes: evidence on the site of the lesion. *J. neurol. Neurosurg. Psychiat.* **41**, 934.

Ochoa, J. and Mair, W. G. P. (1969a). The normal sural nerve in man. I. Ultrastructure and numbers of fibres and cells. *Acta neuropath. (Berlin)* **13**, 197.

—— and —— (1969b). The normal sural nerve in man. II. Changes in the axons and Schwann cells due to ageing. *Acta Neuropath. (Berlin)* **13**, 217.

O'Sullivan, D.J. and Swallow, M. (1968). The fibre size and content of the radial and sural nerves. *J. Neurol. Neurosurg. Psychiat.* **31**, 464.

Peyronnard, J.-M., Aguayo, A. J., and Bray, G. M. (1973). Schwann cell internuclear distances in normal and regenerating unmyelinated nerve fibres. *Arch. Neurol, Chicago* **29**, 56.

Research Group on Neuromuscular Diseases (1968). Classification of the neuromuscular disorders. *J. neurol. Sci.* **6**, 165.

Rosenberg, R. N., Aung, M. H., Tindall, R. S. A., Molenich, S., Baskin, F., Capra, J. D., and Toben, H. R. (1975). Idiopathic polyneuropathy associated with cytotoxic anti-neuroblastoma serum. *Neurology, Minneapolis* **25**, 1101.

Schoenen, J, Gonce, M, and Delwaide P. J. (1984). Painful legs and moving toes: a syndrome with different physiopathologic mechanisms. *Neurology, Minneapolis* **34**, 1108.

Simpson, J. A. (1962). The neuropathies. In *Modern trends in neurology*, 3rd series (ed. D. Williams) p. 245. Butterworths, London.

—— (1964). Biology and disease of peripheral nerves. *Br. med. J.* **2**, 709.

Spencer, P. S., Sabri, M. I., Schaumburg, H. H., and Moore, C. L. (1979). Does a defect of energy metabolism in the nerve fiber underlie axonal degeneration in polyneuropathies? *Ann. Neurol.* **5**, 501.

Stevens, J. C., Lofgren, E. P., and Dyck, P. J. (1973). Histometric evaluation of branches of peroneal nerve: technique for combined biopsy of muscle nerve and cutaneous nerve. *Brain Res.* 52, 37.

Swallow, M. (1966). Fibre size and content of the anterior tibial nerve of the foot. *J. Neurol. Neurosurg. Psychiat.* **29**, 205.

Thage, O., Trojaborg, W. and Buchthal, F. (1963). Electromyographic findings in polyneuropathy. *Neurology, Minneapolis* **13**, 273.

Thomas, P. K. (1964). Changes in the endoneurial sheaths of peripheral myelinated nerve fibres during Wallerian degeneration. *J. Anat. (London)* **98**, 175.

—— (1970). The quantitation of nerve biopsy findings. *J. neurol. Sci.* **11**, 285.

—— and Lascelles, R. G. (1967). Hypertrophic neuropathy. *Quart. J. Med.* **36**, 223.

Vasilescu, C. and Florescu, A. (1982). Peripheral neuropathy with a syndrome of continuous motor unit activity. *J. Neurol.* **226**, 275.

Walton, J. N. (1981). Appendix to 'Clinical examination of the neuromuscular system.' In *Disorders of voluntary muscle* (ed. J. N. Walton) 4th edn, Chapter 13. Churchill-Livingstone, Edinburgh.

Warmolts, J. R. and Mendell, J. R. (1980). Neurotonia: impulse-induced repetitive discharges in motor nerves in peripheral neuropathy. *Ann. Neurol.* **7**, 245.

Weller, R. O. and Cervos-Navarro, J. (1977). *Pathology of peripheral nerves.* Butterworths, London.

—— and Nester, B. (1972). Early changes at the node of Ranvier in segmental demyelination: histochemical and electron microscopic observations. *Acta neuropath., Berlin* **95**, 665.

The Guillain–Barré syndrome (acute post-infective polyradiculoneuropathy)

Synonyms. Acute infectious polyneuritis; febrile polyneuritis; acute post-infective polyneuritis.

Definition. An acute and diffuse post-infective disorder of the nervous system involving the spinal roots and peripheral nerves, and occasionally the cranial nerves.

Aetiology

Acute post-infective polyneuritis or polyradiculoneuropathy is now one of the commonest forms of polyneuropathy in Great Britain. Many cases were observed among troops during the 1914–18 war (Guillain, Barré, and Strohl 1916; Holmes 1917; Bradford, Bashford, and Wilson 1918). The condition may occur in either sex and at any age but is uncommon in early childhood (Rossi, Mumenthaler, Lütschg, and Ludin 1976), and often has a peak incidence between 20 and 50 years of age (Marshall 1963) but a bimodal age distribution has been noted in some reported series of cases (McFarland and Heller 1966; Eisen and Humphreys 1974) with one group occurring between 15 and 30 years, another between 40 and 65. Kaplan, Schonberger, Hurwitz, and Katona (1983) reviewed 2575 US cases and found the peak incidence to be between 50 and 74 years of age with a lesser peak between 15 and 35. There is no obvious seasonal clustering of cases (Soffer, Feldman, and Alter 1978). In Olmsted County, Minnesota, the mean annual incidence was 1.6 per 100 000 of the population (Lesser, Hauser, Kurland, and Mulder 1973). Although this syndrome is clearly defined it is by no means certain that all cases are of uniform aetiology. In the past it was known as acute infective polyneuritis but no infecting organism has been isolated consistently from such cases though there is a significantly increased incidence of antecedent specific and non-specific infective illnesses (Kaplan *et al.* 1983); however, it may arise apparently spontaneously. Associations with infectious mononucleosis (Raftery, Schumacher, Grain, and Quinn 1954) or subclinical Epstein–Barr virus infection (Grose and Feorina 1972), measles (Lidin-Janson and Strannegard 1972), cytomegalovirus infection (Leonard and Tobin 1971; Dowling, Menonna, and Cook 1977), mycoplasma infection (Goldschmidt, Menonna, Fortunato, Dowling, and Cook 1980) water pollution (Sliman 1978), herpesvirus infection (Dowling and Cook 1981), and immune complex nephritis (Behan, Lowenstein, Stilmant, and Sax 1973) have been described and the condition has been reported to follow surgical operations (Arnason and Asbury 1968). Following a nationwide immunization campaign in the United States in 1976, more than 40 million adults were vaccinated with swine influenza virus vaccine (A/New Jersey/76) and more than 500 cases of the Guillain–Barré syndrome occurred among vaccinated individuals with 25 deaths (Langmuir 1979; Keenlyside, Schonberger, Bregman, and Bolyai 1980), the incidence being 7.5 times as great in the vaccinated as in those who were not. Subsequently, however, Kaplan *et al.* (1983) produced figures to cast doubt upon the significance of the association (see also *The Lancet* 1984). An uncommon association with Hodgkin's disease has also been reported suggesting that rarely transient immunosuppression may be a factor (Lisak, Mitchell, Zweiman, Orrechio, and Asbury 1977). The current view is that it is an inflammatory disorder due to disordered immunity, perhaps as a result of a variety of unidentified allergens, but the possibility still exists that some cases could be due to the direct invasion of peripheral nerves by one or more viruses. There is a possible association with the HLA-A1, B8, DRW3, and DW3 haplotypes (Adams, Festenstein, Gibson, Hughes, Jaraquemada, Papasteriadis, Sachs, and Thomas 1979) and Waksman and Adams (1955) produced a similar condition in animals by injecting an emulsion of peripheral nerve to which they had been sensitized, while Asbury and Arnason (1968), Pollard, King, and Thomas (1975) and King, Pollard, and Thomas (1975), among others, studied monophasic and relapsing or recurrent experimental allergic neuritis. Lymphocyte sensitization to human sciatic nerve extract and to muscle has been described (Caspary, Currie, Walton, and Field 1971) and immunocytes have been identified in the circulating blood (Whitaker, Hirano, Cook, and Dowling 1970; Cook, Dowling, and Whitaker 1970), but sera obtained from such patients may produce demyelination of cultures of peripheral nervous tissue *in vitro* (Cook, Dowling, Murray, and Whitaker 1971; Hiraro, Cook, Whitaker, Dowling, and Murray 1971) so that it seems probable that humoral as well as cellular immune processes play a part in pathogenesis. There is also evidence of serum-mediated Schwann cell cytotoxicity in such cases (Lisak, Kuchmy, Armati-Gulson, Brown, and Sumner 1984). Complement-fixing antibodies against peripheral nerve may also be detected in the serum (Latov, Gross, Kastelman, Flanogan, Lamme, Alkaitis, Olarte, Sherman, Chess, and Penn 1981); the *in vivo* demyelinating effect of serum from such patients (Saida, Saida, Lisak, Brown, Silberberg, and Asbury 1981; Low, Schmelzer, Dyck, and Kelly 1982) shows some correlation with disease activity; there is evidence that P_0 glycoprotein, P_1 and P_2 basic proteins, and myelin-associated glycoprotein may all be involved in antibody formation (Schober, Itoyama, Sternberger, Trapp, Richardson, Asbury, Quarles, and Webster 1981), and the evidence supporting the major importance of auto-antibodies and of immune complexes in pathogenesis continues to increase (Cook and Dowling 1981). A similar disorder has been observed in dogs following the bite of a racoon, so-called 'coonhound paralysis' (Cummings and Haas 1967) and this can be produced experimentally (Holmes, Schultz, Cummings, and de Lahanta 1979).

Pathology

Naked-eye abnormalities are slight and consist of variable congestion of the meninges; in fatal cases there may be petechial haemorrhages in the substance of the spinal cord. Microsopically the cord may show chromatolysis of ganglion cells, both of the anterior horns and of the dorsal roots, with slight perivascular infiltration with small, round cells. The spinal roots and peripheral nerves show marked demyelination, with proliferation of Schwann cells, and in some cases swelling and fragmentation of the axons (Dyck, Thomas, and Lambert 1983). There is a marked focal, perivascular lymphocytic inflammatory exudate (Asbury, Arnason, and Adams 1969) and a net-like or vesicular pattern of myelin disruption with relative sparing of axons and phagocytosis of myelin by macrophages (Wisniewski, Terry, Whitaker, Cook, and Dowling 1969). Inflammatory cells and macrophages appear to strip off lamellae of myelin (Asbury and Johnson 1978). In long-standing cases denervation atrophy is found in the muscles. Perivascular inflammatory infiltration has been observed in the brain, and infiltration with round cells may be present in the liver, kidneys, and lungs; the kidneys sometimes show evidence of immune complex nephritis (Behan *et al.* 1973).

Symptoms and signs

There is often an initial febrile illness in which no nervous symptoms appear, followed by a period of latency, lasting from a few days to several weeks, after which paralysis develops. More often the patient is first seen in the paralytic stage, prodomal symptoms being slight or absent. There is much evidence to indicate that some cases of subacute or chronic polyneuropathy are aetiologically similar (p. 530).

More often symptoms of increasing muscular weakness come on suddenly. Less often, weakness develops more slowly over a few days instead of increasing rapidly over a single day. The paralysis may affect all four limbs simultaneously or may begin in the lower limbs and spread to the upper. In contrast with other forms of polyneuropathy, all the muscles of a limb are usually affected, those of the proximal segments suffering as much as, or even more severely than, those of the distal segments. Occasionally weakness is even limited to proximal limb muscles and may be asymmetrical. In severe cases the muscles of the neck and trunk are also involved, and there is often paralysis of the facial muscles on both sides, though this is occasionally unilateral (Kimura 1971). Facial myokymia with pathological changes in the facial nerve has been reported (Zandycke, Martin, Vande Gaer, and Van den Heyning 1982). Dysphagia may occur as a result of pharyngeal paralysis, but the palate usually escapes; respiratory muscle involvement requiring assisted respiration is an important complication in severe cases (Hewer Hilton, Crampton Smith, and Spalding 1968). External ophthalmoplegia is occasionally seen, especially in the so-called Miller–Fisher variant (see below). Rarely ophthalmoplegia antedotes diffuse neuropathy (see p. 531). In occasional cases the affection is confined to the cranial nerves (cranial polyneuritis or *polyneuritis cranialis*) and 'locked-in coma' has been described (Carroll and Mastaglia 1979). The paralysed muscles are flaccid, but severe wasting is exceptional. Superficial and deep reflexes are usually diminished or lost, but are rarely retained in spite of weakness of voluntary movement in the muscles concerned. The sensory symptoms characteristic of polyneuropathy are usually but not invariably present, and in the early stages the patient may complain of pain, numbness, and tingling in the limbs. All forms of sensibility may be impaired over the peripheral segments of the limbs and the muscles may be tender but when even typical paraesthesiae are described, sensory abnormalities on examination are often conspicuous by their absence. Bilateral optic neuritis leading to visual impairment is rare but papilloedema is seen occasionally and is usually attributed to the greatly increased protein content of the CSF with impaired absorption (Reid and Draper 1980): bilateral deafness is even rarer. The sphincters are rarely involved and never to a severe extent, though there may at times be retention of urine necessitating catheterization. Cerebral symptoms are usually absent and consciousness is usually unclouded throughout, but a confusional state or even coma may rarely develop.

General symptoms of toxaemia may be present, including tachycardia and slight cardiac dilatation (Clarke, Bayliss, and Cooper 1954), or albuminuria and an erythematous rash. Autonomic manifestations include arterial hypertension (Davidson and Jellinek 1977), postural hypotension, localized anhidrosis, and impaired baroreflex sensitivity (Tuck and McLead 1981); hyponatraemia in such cases may be due to an abnormally low 'resetting' of osmoreceptor responses (Penney, Murphy, and Walters 1979). The blood may show a moderate polymorphonuclear leucocytosis. The characteristic change in the CSF is a great excess of protein (occasionally up to 10 g/l) with either a normal cell count, or at most only a moderate excess of mononuclear cells. This is the 'dissociation albumino-cytologique' stressed by Guillain *et al.* (1916). The fluid is rarely yellow or brown and may clot spontaneously. The high protein with increased oligoclonal IgG may persist for many weeks even after recovery. Nevertheless the same clinical picture may coexist with a spinal fluid that is virtually normal, particularly in the early stages.

Diagnosis

Acute post-infective polyneuritis is readily distinguished from other forms of polyneuropathy by the acute onset, the rapid development of the paralysis, and the severe involvement of the proximal limb muscles. It is distinguished from poliomyelitis by the symmetrical character of the paralysis, the presence of sensory loss, by the CSF changes, and by the slightness or absence of muscular wasting in the later stages. Diagnostic criteria of many kinds, some excessively flexible, others excessively restrictive, have been suggested, but those laid down by an *ad hoc* NINCDS committee in 1978 and later revised by Asbury (1981) are now generally accepted. He believes that the Miller Fisher syndrome (see below) can properly be regarded as being embraced by this syndrome, that sensory loss and areflexia with typical CSF and electrophysiological findings, thus excluding sensory neuronopathy, also represents an acceptable variant, as do many cases of polyneuritis cranialis. However, pure pandysautonomia is probably a distinct

and different entity; the most difficult problem is to decide where the diagnostic features of the subacute Guillain–Barrè syndrome end and those of chronic inflammatory demyelinating neuropathy (see below) begin.

Other conditions which may occasionally cause diagnostic difficulty are tick paralysis (p. 256) and Bannwarth's syndrome (multiple mononeuritis with cutaneous erythema, radiculitis, pain, and facial-nerve involvement) (Wulff, Hansen, Strange, and Trojaborg 1983) which is, however, distinguished by the finding of CSF pleocytosis as well as a rise in protein. The term Landry's paralysis, once applied to cases of acute ascending paralysis, is now outmoded. Acute myelitis, especially the ascending form, may also cause widespread flaccid paralysis, but in this condition the plantar reflexes are usually extensor, sensory loss is more extensive and involves the whole body below the level of the lesion, and sphincter disturbances are invariably present. Measurement of motor and sensory condition velocity (Buchthal and Rosenfalck 1971; Eisen and Humphreys 1974; Burke, Skuse, and Lethlean 1974) is an invaluable aid to diagnosis, demonstrating slowing of conduction in the great majority of cases soon after the onset, and abnormalities of the F-wave (Kimura and Butzer 1975) may help to confirm that the central segments of the peripheral nerves are predominantly involved. The recording of somatosensory evoked potentials (McLeod 1981) helps to confirm the involvement of roots and proximal segments of peripheral nerves, while the changes in terminal latency, areas, amplitudes, and durations of individual motor unit potentials, suggest that there is significant axonal damage as well as demyelination in the acute phase in many cases (Martinez-Figueroa, Hansen, and Ballantyne 1977).

Prognosis

The mortality rate of the disease was high in the past in some epidemics, death usually resulting from respiratory paralysis, with or without terminal bronchopneumonia. Slight and temporary remissions sometimes occurred, but were often followed by severe relapses. In sporadic cases, however, the ultimate outlook is usually good, though improvement is often slow and the paralysis, having reached its peak, may remain stationary for some weeks. Sometimes recovery is incomplete. Even in the most favourable cases the patient is not likely to be convalescent in less than three to six months and in occasional cases the condition may smoulder on for one or two years but may nevertheless recover completely. Pleasure, Lovelace and Duvoisin (1968) found that more than half of a series of 49 patients followed on average for 11 years showed some persistent evidence of peripheral-nerve damage and 16 per cent had a significant residual disability. Oppenheimer and Spalding (1973) suggested that if recovery had not occurred within two years it was unlikely to be complete, but Osuntokun and Agbebi (1973) reported that 27 of a series of 34 Nigerian patients recovered completely, two died, and five improved. Plainly some confusion has arisen in the past because of the varying diagnostic criteria used in different series of cases. If one restricts the definition of the Guillain–Barrè syndrome to acute cases with the peak of disability being reached as a rule in two to three weeks and not more than four after the clinical onset (Asbury 1981), there is plainly a significant mortality of 5–10 per cent even with modern intensive care and assisted respiration when appropriate, but most of those who survive the first six to eight weeks recover, usually completely, after many months, though up to 20 per cent have some persistent weakness and/or sensory impairment.

Treatment

Among others, Graveson (1957) and Jackson, Miller, and Schapira (1957) suggested that the condition could be effectively controlled by cortisone or corticotrophin (ACTH). While many neurologists have continued to use these drugs in all cases, others are equally adamant that such treatment does not modify the natural history of the illness (Goodall, Kosmidis, and Geddes 1974). The use of immunosuppressive agents has not been strikingly successful either (Drachman, Paterson, Berlin, and Roguska 1970) but others have found azathioprine helpful (Yuill, Swinburn, and Liversedge 1970). In fact while it is now apparent that chronic and relapsing cases of auto-immune polyneuropathy (see below) which have often been classed erroneously in the past as variants of the Guillain–Barré syndrome, are sometimes dramatically controlled by steroids, recent well-designed controlled trials in the acute syndrome have failed to show any benefit from steroids (Hughes, Newsom Davis, Perkin, and Pearce 1978). The same appears to be true of plasmapheresis (Asbury, Fisher, McKhann, Mobley, and Server 1980; Osterman, Fagius, Säfwenberg, Danersund, Wallin, and Nordesjö 1982; Kennard, Newland, and Ridley 1983). Much depends upon good nursing and physiotherapy. Bulbar and respiratory paralysis should be treated with intermittent positive-pressure respiration as in poliomyelitis (p. 284).

Complications including respiratory infections will demand appropriate antibiotics. Hypernatraemia with water retension which occurs in occasional cases may demand diuretics (Posner, Ertel, Kossmann, and Scheinberg 1967). The principles of management are well outlined by Hughes *et al.* (1981).

References

Adams, D., Festenstein, H., Gibson, J. D., Hughes, R. A. C., Jaraquemada, J., Papasteriadis, C., Sachs, J., and Thomas, P. K. (1979). HLA antigens in chronic relapsing idiopathic inflammatory polyneuropathy. *J. Neurol. Neurosurg. Psychiat.* **42**, 184.

Arnason, B. G. and Asbury, A. K. (1968). Idiopathic polyneuritis after surgery. *Arch. Neurol., Chicago* **18**, 500.

Asbury, A. K. (1981). Diagnostic consderations in Guillain–Barré syndrome. *Ann. Neurol*, **9** (suppl), 1.

—— and Arnason, B. G. (1968). Experimental allergic neuritis: a radioautographic study. *J. Neuropath. exp. Neurol.* **27**, 581.

——, —— and Adams, R. D. (1969). The inflammatory lesion in idiopathic polyneuritis. *Medicine, Baltimore* **48**, 173.

——, Fisher, R., McKhann, G. M., Mobley, W., and Server, A. (1980). Guillain–Barré syndrome: is there a role for plasmapheresis? *Neurology, Minneapolis* **30**, 1112.

—— and Johnson, P. C. (1978). *Pathology of peripheral nerve.* Saunders, Philadelphia.

Behan, P. O., Lowestein, L. M., Stilmant, M., and Sax, D. S. (1973). Landry–Guillain–Barré-Strohl syndrome and immune-complex nephritis. *Lancet* **i**, 850.

Bradford, J. B., Bashford, E. F., and Wilson, J. A. (1918–19). Acute infective polyneuritis. *Quart. J. Med.* **12**, 88.

Buchthal, F. and Rosenfalck, A. (1971). Sensory potentials in polyneuropathy. *Brain* **94**, 241.

Burke, D., Skuse, N. F., and Lethlean, A. K. (1974). Sensory conduction of the sural nerve in polyneuropathy. *J. Neurol. Neurosurg. Psychiat.* **37**, 647.

Carroll, W. M. and Mastaglia, F. L. (1979). 'Locked-in coma' in postinfective polyneuropathy. *Arch. Neurol., Chicago* **36**, 46.

Caspary, E. A., Currie, S., Walton, J. N., and Field, E. J. (1971). Lymphocyte sensitization to nervous tissue and muscle in patients with the Guillain–Barré syndrome. *J. Neurol. Neurosurg. Psychiat.* **34**, 179.

Clarke, E. S., Bayliss, R. I. S., and Cooper, R. (1954). Cardiovascular manifestations of the Guillain–Barré syndrome. *Br. med. J.* **2**, 1504.

Cook, S. D. and Dowling, P. C. (1981). The role of autoantibody and immune complexes in the pathogenesis of Guillain–Barré syndrome. *Ann. Neurol.* **9** (suppl.), 70.

——, ——, Murray, M. R., and Whitaker, J. N. (1971). Circulating demyelinating factors in acute idiopathic polyneuropathy. *Arch. Neurol., Chicago* **24**, 136.

——, ——, and Whitaker, J. N. (1970). The Guillain–Barré syndrome: relationship of circulating immunocytes to disease activity. *Arch. Neurol., Chicago* **22**, 470.

Cummings, J. F. and Haas, D. C. (1967). Coonhound paralysis. An acute idiopathic polyradiculoneuritis in dogs resembling the Landry–Guillain–Barré syndrome. *J. neurol. Sci.* **4**, 51.

Davidson, D. L. W. and Jellinek, E. H. (1977). Hypertension and papilloedema in the Guillain–Barré syndrome. *J. Neurol. Neurosurg. Psychiat.* **40**, 144.

Dowling, P. C. and Cook, S.D. (1981). Role of infection in Guillain–Barré syndrome: laboratory confirmation of herpesviruses in 41 cases. *Ann. Neurol.* **9** (supp.), 44.

——, Menonna, J., and Cook, S. D. (1977). Cytomegalovirus complement fixation antibody in Guillain–Barré syndrome. *Neurology, Minneapolis* **27**, 1153.

Drachman, D. A., Paterson, P. Y., Berlin, B. S., and Roguska, J. (1970). Immunosuppression and the Guillain–Barré syndrome. *Arch. Neurol., Chicago* **23**, 385.

Dyck, P. J., Thomas, P. K., and Lambert, E. H. (1983). *Peripheral neuropathy*, 2nd edn. Saunders, Philadelphia.

Eisen, A. and Humphreys, P. (1974). The Guillain–Barré syndrome: a clinical and electrodiagnostic study of 25 cases. *Arch. Neurol., Chicago* **30**, 438.

Goldschmidt, B., Menonna, J., Fortunato, J., Dowling, P. C., and Cook, S. D. (1980). Mycoplasma antibody in Guillain–Barré syndrome and other neurological disorders. *Ann. Neurol.* **7**, 108.

Goodall, J. A. D., Kosmidis, J. C., and Geddes, A. M. (1974). Effect of corticosteroids on course of Guillain–Barré syndrome. *Lancet* **i**, 524.

Graveson, G. S. (1957). Acute polyneuritis treated with cortisone. *Lancet* **i**, 340.

Grose, C. and Feorino, P. M. (1972). Epstein–Barr virus and Guillain–Barré syndrome. *Lancet* **ii**, 1285.

Guillain, G., Barré, J. A., and Strohl, A. (1916). Sur un syndrome de radiculo-névrite avec hyperalbuminose du liquide céphalorachidien sans réaction cellulaire. Remarques sur les caractères cliniques et graphiques des réflexes tendineux. *Bull Soc. méd. Hôp. Paris* **40**, 1462.

Haymaker, W. and Kernohan, J. W. (1949). The Landry–Guillain–Barré syndrome. *Medicine, Baltimore* **28**, 59.

Hewer, R. L., Hilton, P. J., Crampton Smith, A., and Spalding, J. M. K. (1968). Acute polyneuritis requiring artificial respiration. *Quart. J. Med.* **37**, 479.

Hirano, A., Cook, S. D., Whitaker, J. N., Dowling, P. C., and Murray, M. R. (1971). Fine structural aspects of demyelination *in vitro*. The effects of Guillain–Barré serum. *J. Neuropath. exp. Neurol.* **30**, 249.

Holmes, D. F., Schultz, R. D., Cummings, J. F., and deLahunta, A. (1979). Experimental coonhound paralysis: animal model of Guillain–Barré syndrome. *Neurology, Minneapolis* **29**, 1186.

Holmes, G. (1917). Acute febrile polyneuritis. *Br. med. J.* **2**, 37.

Hughes, R. A. C., Kadlubowski, M., and Hufschmidt A. (1981). Treatment of acute inflammatory polyneuropathy. *Ann. Neurol.* **9**, (suppl.), 125.

——, Newsom Davis, J. M., Perkins, J. D., and Pearce, J. M. (1978). Controlled trial of prednisone in polyneuropathy. *Lancet* **ii**, 750.

Jackson, R. H., Miller, H., and Schapira, K. (1957). Polyradiculitis (Landry–Guillain–Barré syndrome). Treatment with cortisone and corticotrophin. *Br. med. J.* **1**, 480.

Janeway, R. and Kelly D. (1966). Papilledema and hydrocephalus associated with recurrent polyneuritis. *Arch. Neurol., Chicago* **15**, 507.

Kaplan, J. E., Schonberger, L. B., Hurwitz, E. S., and Katona P. (1983). Guillain–Barré syndrome in the United States, 1978–1981: additional observations from the national surveillance system. *Neurology, Minneapolis* **33**, 633.

Keenlyside, R. A., Schonberger, L. B., Bergman, D. J., and Bolyai, J. Z. S. (1980). Fatal Guillain–Barré syndrome after the national influenza immunization program. *Neurology, Minneapolis* **30**, 929.

Kennard, C., Newland, A. C., and Ridley A. (1982). Treatment of the Guillain–Barré syndrome by plasma exchange. *J. Neurol. Neurosurg. Psychiat.* **45**, 847.

Kimura, J. (1971). An evaluation of the facial and trigeminal nerves in polyneuropathy: electrodiagnostic study in Charcot–Marie–Tooth disease, Guillain–Barré syndrome and diabetic neuropathy. *Neurology, Minneapolis* **21**, 745.

—— and Butzer, J. F. (1975). F-wave conduction velocity in Guillain–Barré syndrome. *Arch. Neurol. Chicago* **32**, 524.

King, R. H. M., Pollard, J. D., and Thomas, P. K. (1975). Aberrant remyelination in chronic relapsing experimental allergic neuritis. *Neuropath. Appl. Neurobiol.* **1**, 367.

The Lancet, (1984). Influenza and the Guillain–Barré syndrome. *Lancet* **ii**, 850.

Langmuir, A. D. (1979). Guillain–Barré syndrome: the swine influenza virus vaccine incident in the United States of America, 1976–77: preliminary communication. *J. R. Soc. Med.* **72**, 660.

Latov, N., Gross, R. B., Kastelman, J., Flanagan, T., Lamme, S., Alkaitis, D. A., Olarte, M. R., Sherman, W. H., Chess, L., and Penn, A. S. (1981). Complement-fixing antiperipheral nerve myelin antibodies in patients with inflammatory polyneuritis and with polyneuropathy and paraproteinemia. *Neurology, Minneapolis* **31**, 1530.

Leonard, J. C. and Tobin, J. O'H. (1971). Polyneuritis associated with cytomegalovirus infections. *Quart. J. Med.* **40, 435.**

Lesser, R. P., Hauser, W. A., Kurland, L. T., and Mulder, D. W. (1973). Epidemiologic features of the Guillain–Barré syndrome: experience in Olmsted County, Minnesota, 1935 through 1968. *Neurology, Minneapolis* **23**, 1269.

Lidin-Janson, G. and Strannegard, O. (1972). Two cases of Guillain–Barré syndrome and encephalitis after measles. *Br. med. J.* **2**, 572.

Lisak, R. P., Mitchell, M., Zweiman, B., Orrechio, E., and Asbury, A. K. (1977). Guillain–Barré syndrome and Hodgkin's disease: three cases with immunological studies. *Ann. Neurol.* **1**, 72.

——, Kuchmy, D., Armati-Gulson, P. J., Brown, M. J., and Sumner, A. J. (1984). Serum-mediated Schwann cell cytotoxicity in the Guillain–Barré syndrome. *Neurology, Minneapolis* **34**, 1240.

Low, P. A. and Schmelzer, J., Dyck, P. J., and Kelly, J. J. (1982). Endoneurial effects of sera from patients with acute inflammatory polyradiculoneuropathy: electrophysiologic studies on normal and demyelinated rat nerves. *Neurology, Minneapolis* **32**, 720.

Marshall, J. (1963). The Landry–Guillain–Barré syndrome. *Brain* **86**, 55.

Martinez-Figueroa, A., Hansen, S., and Ballantyne, J. P. (1977). A quantitative electrophysiological study of acute idiopathic polyneuritis. *J. Neurol. Neurosurg. Psychiat.* **40**, 156.

McFarland, H. R. and Heller, G. L. (1966). Guillain–Barré disease complex: a statement of diagnostic criteria and analysis of 100 cases. *Arch. Neurol. Chicago* **14**, 196.

McLeod, J. G. (1981). Electrophysiological studies in the Guillain–Barré syndrome. *Ann. Neurol.* **9**, (suppl.), 20.

NINCDS Ad Hoc Committee (1978). Criteria for diagnosis of Guillain–Barré syndrome. *Ann. Neurol.* **3**, 565.

Oppenheimer, D. R. and Spalding, J. M. K. (1973). Late residua of acute idiopathic polyneuritis. *J. Neurol. Neurosurg. Psychiat.* **36**, 978.

Osterman, P. O., Fagius, J., Säwenberg, J., Danersund, A., Wallin, G., and Nordesjo, L.-O. (1982). Treatment of the Guillain–Barré syndrome by plasmapheresis. *Arch. Neurol., Chicago* **39**, 148.

Osuntokun, B. O. and Agbebi, K. (1973). Prognosis of Guillain–Barré syndrome in the African: the Nigerian experience. *J. Neurol. Neurosurg. Psychiat.* **36**, 478.

Penney, M. D., Murphy, D., and Walters, G. (1979). Resetting of osmoreceptor response as cause of hyponatraemia in acute idiopathic polyneuritis. *Br. med. J.* **2**, 1474.

Pleasure, D. E., Lovelace, R. E., and Duvoisin, R. C. (1968). The prognosis of acute polyradiculoneuritis. *Neurology, Minneapolis* **18**, 1143.

Pollard, J. D., King, R. H. M., and Thomas, P. K. (1975). Recurrent experimental allergic neuritis: an electron microscope study. *J. neurol. Sci.* **24**, 365.

Posner, J., Ertel, N. H., Kossmann, R. J., and Scheinberg, L. C. (1967). Hyponatremia in acute polyneuropathy. *Arch. Neurol., Chicago* **17**, 530.

Raftery, M., Schumacher, E. E., Grain, G. O., and Quinn, E. L. (1954). Infectious mononucleosis and Guillain–Barré syndrome. *Arch. intern. Med.* **93**, 246.

Reid, A. C. and Draper, I. T. (1980). Pathogenesis of papilloedema and raised intracranial pressure in Guillain–Barré syndrome. *Br. med. J.* **281**, 1393.

Rossi, L. N., Mumenthaler, M., Lütschig, J., and Ludin, H. P. (1976). Guillain–Barré syndrome in children with special reference to the natural history of 38 personal cases. *Neuropädiatrie* **7**, 42.

Saida, T., Saida, K., Lisak, R. P., Brown, M. J., Silberberg, D. H., and Asbury, A. K. (1982) In vivo demyelinating activity of sera from patients with Guillain–Barré syndrome. *Ann. Neurol.* **11**, 69.

Schober, R., Itoyama, Y., Sternberger, N. H., Trapp, B. D., Richardson, E. P., Asbury, A. K., Quarles, R. H., and Webster, H. de F. (1981). Immunocytochemical study of P_0 glycoprotein, P_1 and P_2 basic proteins, and myelin-associated glycoprotein (MAG) in lesions of idiopathic polyneuritis. *Neuropath. Appl. Neurobiol.* **7**, 421.

Sliman, N. A. (1978). Outbreak of Guillain–Barré syndrome associated with water pollution. *Br. med. J.* **1**, 751.

Soffer, D., Feldman, S., and Alter, M. (1978). Epidemiology of Guillain–Barré syndrome. *Neurology, Minneapolis* **28**, 686.

Tuck, R. R. and McLeod, J. G. (1981). Autonomic dysfunction in Guillain–Barré syndrome. *J. Neurol. Neurosurg. Psychiat.* **44**, 983.

Waksman, B. H. and Adams, R. W. (1955). Allergic neuritis, an experimental disease of rabbits induced by the injection of peripheral nerve tissue and adjuvants. *J. exp. Med.* **102**, 213.

Whitaker, J. N., Hirano, A., Cook, S. D., and Dowling, P. C. (197). The ultrastructure of circulating immunocytes in Guillain–Barré syndrome. *Neurology, Minneapolis* **20**, 765.

Wisniewski, H., Terry, R. D., Whitaker, J. N., Cook, S. D., and Dowling, P. C. (1969). Landry–Guillain–Barré syndrome: a primary demyelinating disease. *Arch. Neurol., Chicago* **21**, 269.

Wulff, C. H., Hansen, K., Strange, P., and Trojaborg, W. (1983). Multiple mononeuritis and radiculitis with erythema, pain, elevated CSF protein and pleocytosis (Bannwarth's syndrome). *J. Neurol. Neurosurg. Psychiat.* **46**, 485.

Yuill, G. M., Swinburn, W. R., and Liversedge, L. A. (1970). Treatment of polyneuropathy with azathioprine. *Lancet* **ii**, 854.

Zandycke, M. Van, Martin, J.-J., Vande Gaer, L., and Van Den Heyning, P. (1982). Facial myokymia in the Guillain–Barré syndrome: a clinicopathologic study. *Neurology, Minneapolis* **32**, 744.

The Miller Fisher syndrome

In 1956 Miller Fisher described a syndrome of opthalmoplegia, ataxia, and areflexia which he believed was an unusual variant of 'acute idiopathic polyneuritis'. Many cases have been reported since in adults (see Asbury 1981; Ropper 1983) and children (Becker, Watters, and Humphreys 1981) and it is generally agreed that the finding of a high CSF protein content, of slowed conduction velocity in peripheral nerves, and of variable limb muscle weakness in acute cases allow the condition to be accepted as a variant of the Guillain–Barré syndrome. However, in some cases there are also impaired consciousness, supranuclear eye movement disorders (Meinenberg and Ryffel 1983), and other evidence of involvement of the brainstem parenchyma which justify separate identification of this syndrome (Becker *et al.* 1981).

References

Asbury, A. K. (1981). Diagnostic considerations in Guillain–Barré syndrome. *Ann. Neurol.* **9**, (Suppl.), 1.

Becker, W. J., Watters, G. V., and Humphreys, P. (1981). Fisher syndrome in childhood. *Neurology, Minneapolis* **31**, 555.

Fisher, M. (1956). An unusual variant of acute idiopathic polyneuritis (syndrome of ophthalmoplegia, ataxia and areflexia). *New Engl. J. Med.* **255**, 57.

Meinenberg, O. and Ryffel E. (1983). Supranuclear eye movement disorders in Fisher's syndrome of ophthalmoplegia, ataxia, and areflexia: report of a case and literature review. *Arch. Neurol., Chicago* **40**, 402.

Ropper, A. H. (1983). The CNS in Guillain–Barré syndrome. *Arch. Neurol., Chicago* **40**, 397.

Recurrent and relapsing polyneuropathy

Since Nattrass (1921) reported a case of recurrent hypertrophic neuritis in which the patient suffered recurrent acute episodes of polyneuropathy with apparent complete recovery in between, there has been considerable controversy about the relationship of this syndrome and of subacute and chronic steroid-responsive demyelinating neuropathies with eventual peripheral-nerve hypertrophy on the one hand to the Guillain–Barré syndrome on the other (Swash 1979). Austin (1958) reviewed the literature in detail and reported a patient who suffered 20 recurrent episodes of polyneuropathy over a five-year period, each apparently responding to steroid treatment. Certainly any recurrent demyelinating neuropathy, whatever its cause, may lead to peripheral-nerve enlargement resulting from Schwann-cell proliferation giving rise to 'onion-bulb' formation (Webster, Schröder, Asbury, and Adams 1967; Zacks, Lipshutz, and Elliott 1968; Dyck, Lais, Ohta, Bastron, Okazaki, and Groover 1975). Recurrent polyneuropathy or mononeuropathy may sometimes be a dominantly inherited disorder (Roos and Thygesen 1972) but this familial disorder does not usually result in peripheral-nerve hypertrophy or an increase in the CSF protein content and is probably related to the so-called familial recurrent palsies of peripheral nerves (p. 520). Recurrent episodes of brachial plexus neuropathy (neuralgic amyotrophy) have also been noted sometimes to be familial (Taylor 1960; Gieger, Mancall, Penn, and Tucker 1974; Bradley, Madrid, Thrush, and Campbell 1975). Rarely, ophthalmoplegia may antedate the signs of diffuse neuropathy (Donaghy and Earl 1985).

Clearly there exists a group of patients who present with either acute recurrent episodes of polyneuropathy or a subacute or chronic progressive syndrome (Dyck *et al.* 1975), in whom peripheral-nerve conduction is slowed, the CSF protein is raised, and nerve biopsy demonstrates segmental demyelination and often eventually a hypertrophic process, and in whom there is an unequivocal response to steroid therapy so that some become steroid-dependent; a similar syndrome has been reported in a patient who showed evidence at autopsy of neurolymphomatosis (Borit and Altrocchi 1971). Thomas, Lascelles, Hallpike, and Hewer (1969) believed that this condition is a subacute or chronic variant of the Guillain–Barré syndrome. Dyck *et al.* (1975) found that about 60 per cent of such patients improved and were able to work, 25 per cent became confined to a wheelchair, and 10 per cent died of their disease. There is increasing evidence that this condition, in which myokymia, muscle hypertrophy, and delayed relaxation due to irritability of intramuscular nerve terminals is occasionally seen (Valenstein, Watson, and Parker 1978) can be greatly benefited not only by steroid treatment but also by immunosuppressive remedies such as azathioprine and by repeated plasmapheresis (Oh 1978; Dalakas and Engel 1981; Gross and Thomas 1981; Toyka, Augspach, Wietholter, Besinger, Haveveld, Liebert, Heininger, Schwendemann, Reiners, and Grabensee 1982; Pollard, 1983). Engel, Cuneo, and Levy (1978) found that polyinosinic-polycytidylic acid poly-L-lysine stabilized with carboxymethyl cellulose (poly-I.C.L.C.), which induces interferon in primates, was dramatically successful in treating a single resistant case, but the value of this substance has not yet been fully evaluated.

References

Austin, J. H. (1958). Recurrent polyneuropathies and their corticosteroid treatment. *Brain* **81**, 157.

Borit, A. and Altrocchi, P. H. (1971). Recurrent polyneuropathy and neurolymphomatosis. *Arch. Neurol., Chicago* **24**, 40.

Bradley, W. G., Madrid, R., Thrush, D. C., and Campbell, M. J. (1975). Recurrent brachial plexus neuropathy. *Brain* **98**, 381.

Dalakas, M. C. and Engel, W. K. (1981). Chronic relapsing (dysimmune) polyneuropathy: pathogenesis and treatment. *Ann. Neurol.* **9** (suppl.), 134.

Donaghy, M. and Earl, C. J. (1985). Ocular palsy preceding chronic relapsing polyneuropathy by several weeks. *Ann. Neurol.* **17**, 49.

Dyck, P. J. (1969). Experimental hypertrophic neuropathy: pathogenesis of onion-bulb formations produced by repeated tourniquet applications. *Arch. Neurol. Chicago* **21**, 73.

——, Lais, A. C., Ohta, M., Bastron, J. A., Okazaki, H., and, Groover, R. V. (1975). Chronic inflammatory polyradiculopathy. *Mayo Clin. Proc.* **50**, 621.

Engel, W. K., Cuneo, R. A., and Levy, H. B. (1978). Polyinosinic-polycytidilic acid treatment of neuropathy. *Lancet* **i**, 503.

Geiger, L. R., Mancell, E. L., Penn, A. S., and Tucker, S. H. (1974). Familial neuralgic amyotrophy—report of three families with review of the literature. *Brain* **97**, 87.

Gross, M. L. P. and Thomas, P. K. (1981). The treatment of chronic relapsing and chronic progressive idiopathic inflammatory polyneuropathy by plasma exchange. *J. neurol. Sci.* **52**, 69.

Nattrass, F. J. (1921). Recurrent hypertrophic neuritis. *J. Neurol. Psychopathol.* **2**, 159.

Oh, S. J. (1978). Subacute demyelinating polyneuropathy responding to corticosteroid treatment. *Arch. Neurol., Chicago* **35**, 509.

Pollard, J. D., McLeod, J. G., Gatenby, P., and Kronenberg, H. (1983). Prediction of response to plasma exchange in chronic relapsing polyneuropathy: a clinico-pathological correlation. *J. neurol. Sci.* **58**, 269.

Roos, D. and Thygesen, P. (1972). Familial recurrent polyneuropathy. *Brain* **95**, 235.

Swash, M. (1979). Clinical aspects of Guillain–Barré syndrome: a review. *J. R. Soc. Med.* **72**, 670.

Taylor, R. A. (1960). Heredofamilial mononeuritis multiplex with brachial predilection. *Brain* **83**, 113.

Thomas, P. K., Lascelles, R. G., Hallpike, J. F., and Hewer, R. L. (1969). Recurrent and chronic relapsing Guillain–Barré polyneuritis. *Brain* **92**, 589.

Toyka, K. V., Augspach, R., Weitholter, H., Besinger, U. A., Haveveld, F., Liebert, U. G., Heininger, K., Schwendemann, G., Reiners, K., and Grabensee, B. (1982). Plasma exchange in chronic inflammatory polyneuropathy: evidence suggestive of a pathogenic humoral factor. *Muscle & Nerve* **5**, 479.

Valenstein, E., Watson, R. T., and Parker, L. (1978). Myokymia, muscle hypertrophy and percussion "myotonia" in chronic recurrent polyneuropathy. *Neurology, Minneapolis* **28**, 1130.

Webster, H. De F., Schröder, J. M., Asbury, A. K., and Adams, R. D. (1967). The role of Schwann cells in the formation of 'onion bulbs' found in chronic neuropathies. *J. Neuropath. exp. Neurol.* **26**, 276.

Zacks, S. I., Lipshutz, H., and Elliott, F. (1968). Histochemical and electron microscopic observations on 'onion bulb' formation in a case of hypertrophic neuritis of 25 years duration with onset in childhood. *Acta Neuropath., Berlin* **11**, 157.

Alcoholic polyneuropathy

Aetiology

The cause of alcoholic polyneuropathy is still not fully understood. It has been thought to be a form of beriberi, the deficiency of thiamine being due to a combination of defective diet, impaired absorption owing to gastrointestinal irritation, and increased need caused by the high calorie value of the alcohol. It has been said that if the thiamine deficiency is corrected the patient may improve while still drinking. The fact that thiamine does not invariably produce improvement (Brown 1941) does not exclude nutritional deficiency as the cause as chronic polyneuropathy in beriberi also responds poorly. Novak and Victor (1974), in a comprehensive neuropathological study, give cogent reasons for concluding first that thiamine deficiency is the primary causal factor and that the pathological changes in affected nerves are identical with those of beriberi. However, Behse, and Buchthal (1977) reported findings which suggested that in addition to the deficiency of thiamine, there is a direct toxic action of alcohol on peripheral nerve and this question is still not settled (Asbury and Johnson 1978; Spencer and Schaumburg 1980). The sex and age incidence are those of alcoholic addiction, most patients being middle-aged, and males being affected more often than females.

Pathology

The changes in the nervous system are those of a predominantly axonal polyneuropathy of the 'dying-back' type (Prineas 1970), involving the somatic peripheral nerves and sometimes the vagus and sympathetic nerves (Novak and Victor 1974; Duncan, Johnson, Lambie, and Whiteside 1980). However, the greater splanchnic nerve is usually spared (Low, Walsh, Huang, and McLeod 1975) so that postural hypotension is rare and blood-pressure control is usually normal. Although there is some slowing of conduction in peripheral nerves (Mawdsley and Mayer 1965) this is rarely severe and there is relatively little segmental demyelination (Gilliatt 1966; Behse and Buchthal 1977). Electrophysiological evidence confirms that the neuronal lesion is predominantly distal (Casey and Le Quesne 1972) and there is good evidence that slowing of nerve conduction and reduced amplitudes of sensory nerve action potentials are a consequence of axonal loss, as surviving axons conduct at normal rates (Ballantyne, Hansen, Weir,

Whitehead, and Mullin 1980). The affected neurones show axonal degeneration especially at the periphery, and chromatolysis is found in ganglion cells of the anterior horns and spinal dorsal-root ganglia and ganglia of the motor nuclei of the cranial nerves. The changes in the muscles are those of denervation, sometimes with an associated alcoholic myopathy (p. 578).

Symptoms and signs

Sensory disturbances are usually prominent in the clinical picture. In the early stages the patient complains of numbness, tingling, and paraesthesiae in the hands and feet, and especially pain in the extremities. The pain may be severe and described as burning or 'like tearing flesh off the bones'. Cramp-like pains occur in the calves and are especially severe at night. Following the early sensory disturbances the limbs become weak, the lower limbs usually being more severely affected than the upper.

As is the rule in polyneuropathy, both motor and sensory symptoms affect predominantly the periphery of the limbs symmetrically. In severe cases both wrist-drop and foot-drop are present, the latter causing a 'steppage' gait, and there is some wasting of peripheral limb muscles. If the patient can move his limbs, sensory ataxia can usually be demonstrated, and in one form of the disorder—the so-called pseudotabetic variety—ataxia of gait is conspicuous and is due to loss of postural sensibility. There is a blunting of all forms of sensibility in the periphery, cutaneous anaesthesia and analgesia usually extending up to the elbows and knees. Postural sensibility and appreciation of passive movements are impaired in the fingers and toes. Often pressure upon the muscles, especially those of the calves, is painful, and scratching the sole may also be very painful, but yet pain perception may be delayed. Exceptionally pain and tenderness are slight or absent.

The tendon reflexes are diminished or lost, the ankle-jerks disappear before the knee-jerks. The plantar reflexes may also be lost, but if present are flexor. The skin of the extremities is often oedematous and sweating. Muscular contractures rarely develop in severe cases. The sphincters are usually unaffected.

Abnormalities in the cranial nerves are inconstant. The pupils tend to be contracted and may react sluggishly to light. Nystagmus is common. The cranial nerves may be affected, the vagus being most often involved, with resulting tachycardia and impaired baroreceptor responses, and the facial next in frequency. Korsakow's psychosis, Wernicke's encephalopathy (see p. 475), or alcoholic dementia may complicate the picture. The CSF may be normal, or its protein content may be moderately increased. Other symptoms and signs of alcoholism (hepatic cirrhosis, gastritis) are often present. Myocardial failure due to alcoholic cardiomyopathy may also occur, and pulmonary tuberculosis is a not uncommon complication. The neurological and electromyographic findings are sometimes complicated by the presence of an associated alcoholic myopathy (p. 578). Patients are often obese and florid but are occasionally wasted due to malnutrition.

Diagnosis

The diagnosis of polyneuropathy has been described on page 524.

Prognosis

The prognosis of alcoholic polyneuropathy depends upon how early treatment is begun, and how far it is possible to remove or prevent the causal factors. With early treatment the prognosis is good, and in mild cases the symptoms disappear in a few weeks. In more severe cases recovery takes several months, and in chronic cases recovery may be incomplete, especially with respect to return of power in the peripheral muscles. In some cases, despite early treatment and the withdrawal of alcohol. the disorder runs a rapidly progressive course with increasing mental confusion, terminating either by death in coma or heart failure or from intercurrent pneumonia.

Treatment

Vitamin B$_1$ (thiamine) should certainly be given and may usefully be combined with other vitamins in an intramuscular injection of *Parentrovite* or of some similar multi-vitamin preparation. Subsequently a vitamin-rich diet is necessary but should for some time be supplemented by giving thiamine, 50 mg daily. The treatment of alcohol addiction must be combined with that of the polyneuropathy (see p. 526).

References

Asbury, A. K. and Johnson, P. C. (1978). *Pathology of peripheral nerve*. Saunders, Philadelphia.

Ballantyne, J. P., Hansen, S., Weir, A., Whitehead, J. R. G., and Mullin, P. J. (1980). Quantitative electrophysiological study of alcoholic neuropathy. *J. Neurol. Neurosurg. Psychiat.* **43**, 427.

Behse, F. and Buchthal, F. (1977). Alcoholic neuropathy: clinical electrophysiological, and biopsy findings. *Ann. Neurol.* **2**, 95.

Brown, M. R. (1941). Alcoholic polyneuritis. *J. Am. med. Ass.* **116**, 1615.

Casey, E. B. and Le Quesne, P. M. (1972). Electrophysiological evidence for a distal lesion in alcoholic neuropathy. *J. Neurol. Neurosurg. Psychiat.* **35**, 624.

Duncan, G., Johnson, R. H., Lambie, D. G., and Whiteside, E. A. (1980). Evidence of vagal neuropathy in chronic alcoholics. *Lancet* **ii**, 1053.

Gilliatt, R. (1966). Nerve conduction in human and experimental neuropathies. *Proc. R. Soc. Med.* **59**, 989.

Low, P. A., Walsh, J. C., Huang, C. Y., and McLeod, J. G. (1975). The sympathetic nervous system in alcoholic neuropathy—a clinical and pathological study. *Brain* **98**, 357.

Mawdsley, C. and Mayer, R. F. (1965). Nerve conduction in alcoholic polyneuropathy. *Brain* **88**, 335.

Novak, D. J. and Victor, M. (1974). The vagus and sympathetic nerves in alcoholic polyneuropathy. *Arch. Neurol., Chicago* **30**, 273.

Prineas, J. (1970). Peripheral nerve changes in thiamine-deficient rats. *Arch. Neurol., Chicago* **23**, 541.

Spencer, R. S. and Schaumburg, H. (1980). *Experimental and clinical neurotoxicology*. Williams & Wilkins, New York.

Victor, M. and Adams, R. D. (1953). The effect of alcohol on the nervous system. *Res. Publ. Ass. nerv. ment. Dis.* **32**, 526.

Isoniazid neuropathy

A sensorimotor neuropathy may occur in patients receiving isoniazid, usually in doses of 300 mg daily or more, for the treatment of tuberculosis, and may rarely be accompanied by the mental symptoms and skin changes of pellagra. It is due to a conditioned pyridoxine deficiency and can often be prevented by the administration of pyridoxine, 25–50 mg daily. It has been shown that the neuropathy occurs in individuals who detoxicate isoniazid slowly and that the ability to detoxicate the drug slowly or rapidly is genetically determined. Sural-nerve biopsy in such cases has confirmed that the neuropathy is predominantly axonal in type, involving myelinated and unmyelinated fibres (Ochoa 1970).

References

Carlson, H. B., Anthony, E. M., Russell, W. F., and Middlebrook G. (1956). Prophylaxis of isoniazid neuropathy with pyridoxine. *New Engl. J. Med.* **255**, 118.

Clarke, C. A., Price Evans, D. A., Harris, R., McConnell, R. B., and Woodrow, J. C. (1968). Genetics in medicine. A review. Part II. Pharmacogenetics. *Quart. J. Med.* **37**, 183.

McConnell, R. B. and Cheetham, H. D. (1952). Acute pellagra during isoniazed therapy. *Lancet* **ii**, 959.

Ochoa, J. (1970). Isoniazid neuropathy in man: quantitative electron microscope study. *Brain* **93**, 831.

Arsenical polyneuropathy (and that due to some other heavy metals)

Aetiology

Polyneuropathy may follow either acute or chronic arsenic poisoning, more usually the latter. The arsenic may have been administered with intent to murder or in an attempt at suicide. In murder attempts white arsenic or sodium arsenite, which is contained in certain rat-poisons and weed-killers, have usually been employed. Arsenic was also obtained from old-fashioned fly-papers for this purpose. Accidental arsenical poisoning may occur in occupations involving handling arsenic (such as arsenical sprays used in agriculture—Heyman, Pfeiffer, Willett, and Taylor 1956), though this is rare, or as a result of ingesting contaminated food or drink, as in the Manchester epidemic in 1900, when poisoning was produced by the consumption of beer brewed with glucose containing arsenic. Exposure to arsenic trioxide in a copper-smelting factory has accounted for some cases (Feldman, Niles, Kelly-Hayes, Sax, Dixon, Thompson, and Laudau 1979). Poisoning has also been produced by inhalation of arsenic from wallpaper dyes, as a result of licking golf balls when arsenical weedkiller has been used on the course, and from the ingestion of bootleg alcohol. Medicinal arsenical poisoning is now rare but was once frequent when Fowler's solution was often given over long periods in the treatment of chorea, multiple sclerosis, and pernicious anaemia. Polyneuropathy was, however, rare after treatment with arsenobenzene derivatives, once extensively used in treating syphilis.

The observation that arsenical poisoning causes an accumulation of pyruvate in the blood suggested that arsenic, like other heavy metals, acts by reacting with a thiol group which is an essential component of co-enzyme A; this provides a link between arsenical polyneuropathy and polyneuropathy due to thiamine deficiency (Peters, Stocken, and Thompson 1945).

A sensorimotor polyneuropathy virtually identical with that due to arsenic may be produced on occasion by other heavy metals including gold, mercury, zinc, bismuth, antimony, and thallium and the mechanism is similar. In a recent report of three cases due to gold given for the treatment of rheumatoid arthritis, myokymia as well as signs of progressive polyneuropathy were prominent and there was spontaneous improvement when gold treatment was discontinued (Katrak, Pollock, O'Brien, Nukada, Allpress, Calder, Palmer McCormack, and Laurent 1980). Thallium used commercially as a rat poison and as an insecticide or as a depilatory, has been responsible for a number of cases (p. 439).

Pathology

This neuropathy is axonal as in thiamine deficiency.

Symptoms and signs

The symptoms resemble those of the alcoholic variety. As in the latter paraesthesiae are conspicuous, and pain is usually severe. Muscular weakness is usually more marked in the lower than in the upper limbs. Korsakow's psychosis or a confusional state may be present. In clinical diagnosis the presence of abnormalities outside the nervous system is important. In chronic arsenical poisoning gastro-intestinal symptoms may be absent, but excessive salivation is not uncommon, and there is often a secondary anaemia. Cutaneous changes are common. These may consist of erythema or even of exfoliative dermatitis. In long-standing cases there is often pigmentation which is absent from the exposed parts and consists of a fine mottling of the skin, with patches of light chocolate colour, the intervening areas being white. Hyperkeratosis of the palms and soles is often found, the thickened skin having a smooth, somewhat waxy appearance. Herpes zoster is a common complication. The blood pyruvate is raised and even when the resting level is normal, a pyruvate tolerance curve demonstrates that the serum pyruvate rises well above the normal upper limit of 13 mg/l after a loading dose of glucose, but this finding lacks specificity.

Diagnosis

The diagnosis of arsenical from other forms of polyneuropathy (p. 524) depends upon the presence of other abnormalities just described, especially those in the skin, and upon the demonstration by appropriate toxicological tests of arsenic in the hair, nails, urine, or faeces. The normal upper limit of arsenic in the hair is 0.1 mg/100 g hair (Heyman et al. 1956).

Prognosis

The prognosis is good, provided that the general symptoms of arsenical poisoning are not too far advanced when the patient begins treatment. Recovery of voluntary power, however, is slow and may take one or two years.

Treatment

Dimercaprol was the first drug shown to be of value (Heyman et al. 1956) and is still widely used; calcium versenate, another chelating agent, is also effective in promoting the excretion of arsenic as is penicillamine (Simpson 1962). In addition the general treatment of polyneuropathy is required (see p. 526).

References

Feldman, R. G., Niles, C. A., Kelly-Hayes, M., Sax, D. S., Dixon, W. J., Thompson, D. J., and Landau, E. (1979). Peripheral neuropathy in arsenic smelter workers. *Neurology, Minneapolis* **29**, 939.

Heyman, A. Pfeiffer, J. B., Willett, R. W., and Taylor, H. M. (1956). Peripheral neuropathy caused by arsenical intoxication. *New Engl. J. Med.* **254**, 401.

Katrak, S. M., Pollock, M., O'Brien, C. P., Nukada, H., Allpress, S., Calder, C., Palmer, D. G., Grennan, D. M., McCormack, P. L., and Laurent, M. R. (1980). Clinical and morphological features of gold neuropathy. *Brain* **103**, 671.

Peters, R. A., Stocken, L. A., and Thompson, R. H. S. (1945). British Anti-Lewisite (BAL). *Nature, Lond.* **156**, 616.

Simpson, J. A. (1962). The neuropathies. In *Modern Trends in neurology*, 3rd series (ed. D. Williams) p. 245. Butterworths, London.

Organic chlorine compounds used as insecticides

Campbell (1952) reported five cases of polyneuropathy and three of retrobulbar neuritis following the use of an insecticide containing ortho-and para-dichloro-benzene, DDT, and pentachlorophenol. He suggested that the last might be the toxic factor. (For neurological complication of organophosphorus insecticides see page 439). Fullerton (1969) pointed out that, whereas peripheral neuropathy is the predominant complication of industrial poisoning with lead, acrylamide, organophosphates, and thallium, substances such as tetrachlorethane, pentachlorophenol, and DDT produce polyneuropathy only after gross overdosage. A recent example was the report of delayed polyneuropathy after the massive ingestion in a suicidal attempt of parathion, a cholinesterase inhibitor which is not normally neurotoxic in man (de Jager, Van Weerden, Houthoff, and de Monchy 1981). Hexachlorophene, widely used as a skin antiseptic, may produce vacuolar degeneration in the central nervous system in infants (p. 440) but also causes axonal degeneration and demyelination in peripheral nerves in animals (de Jesus and Pleasure 1973; Pleasure, Towfight, Silberberg, and Parris 1974; Maxwell and le Quesne 1979) but no convincing cases of human polyneuropathy due to this substance have yet been described.

References

Campbell, A. M. G. (1952). Neurological complications associated with insecticides and fungicides. *Br. med. J.* **2**, 415.

De Jager, A. E. J., Van Weerden, T. W., Houthoff, H. J., and De Monchy, J. G. R. (1981). Polyneuropathy after massive exposure to parathion. *Neurology, Minneapolis* **31**, 603.

Fullerton, P. M. (1969). Toxic chemicals and peripheral neuropathy: clinical and epidemiological features. *Proc. R. Soc. Med.* **62**, 201.

Maxwell, I. C. and Le Quesne, P. M. (1979). Conduction velocity in hexochlorophane neuropathy: correlation between electrophysiological and histological findings. *J. neurol. Sci.* **43**, 95.

Pleasure, D. E., Towfight, J., Silberberg, D., and Parris, J. (1974). The pathogenesis of hexachlorophene neuropathy: in vivo and in vitro studies. *Neurology, Minneapolis* **24**, 1068.

Lead neuropathy

Lead poisoning was considered in detail on page 435. Lead may produce a predominantly motor type of polyneuropathy, often affecting mainly those muscles in common use in the individual's occupation (e.g. wrist-drop in battery-makers). Subclinical neuropathy, identifiable by nerve conduction studies, is not uncommon in lead workers (Catton, Harrison, Fullerton, and Kazantzis 1970; Feldman, Hayes, Younes, and Aldrich 1977). In experimental studies in the guinea-pig, Fullerton (1966) found that lead produced a combination of segmental demyelination and axonal degeneration but Lampert and Schochet (1968) found that demyelination and Schwann-cell proliferation predominated.

References

Catton, M. J., Harrison, M. J. G., Fullerton, P. M., and Kazantzis, G. (1970). Subclinical neuropathy in lead workers *Br. med. J.* **2**, 80.

Feldman, R. G., Hayes, M. K., Younes, R., and Aldrich, F. D. (1977). Lead neuropathy in adults and children. *Arch. Neurol., Chicago* **34**, 481.

Fullerton, P. M. (1966). Chronic peripheral neuropathy produced by lead poisoning in guinea-pigs. *J. Neuropath. exp. Neurol.* **25**, 214.

Lampert, P. W. and Schochet, S. S. (1968). Demyelination and remyelination in lead neuropathy. *J. Neuropath. exp. Neurol.* **27**, 527.

Organic solvents

Trichloroethylene when used as an anaethetic agent rarely if ever produces neurological complications, but its industrial use has been shown sometimes to cause polyneuropathy and other complications including confusion and even dementia (Mitchell and Parsons-Smith 1969). Chronic exposure to ethylene oxide gas in workers manufacturing ethylene oxide sterilizers can also cause polyneuropathy, while acute intoxication more often gives skin lesions, dyspnoea, cyanosis, pulmonary oedema, headache, nausea, vomiting, and drowsiness (Kuzuhara, Kanazawa, Nakanishi, and Egashira 1983). *Carbon tetrachloride*, too, like carbon monoxide poisoning, has occasionally caused polyneuropathy but the symptoms of poisoning by these agents are dominated by evidence of involvement of other organs (e.g. the liver or brain) (Fullerton 1969a). Industrial exposure to *methyl-n-butyl ketone*, a solvent widely used in printing synthetic fabrics, has also caused an axonal dying-back type of neuropathy in animals (Spencer and Schaumburg 1975; Spencer, Schaumburg, Raleigh, and Terhaar 1975) and a moderately severe sensorimotor polyneuropathy in human subjects in a large industrial outbreak (Allen, Mendell, Billnaier, Fontaine, and O'Neill 1975). Sensorimotor neuropathy, visual dysfunction and emotional lability has followed exposure to a foaming catalyst, *2-t-butylazo-2-hydroxy-5-methylhexane* (BHMH) (Spencer, Beaubernard, Bischoff-Fenton, and Kurt 1985).

n-Hexane, principally employed as a cement solvent, has caused polyneuropathy in Japan and in the United States (Herskowitz, Ishii, and Schaumburg 1971) and is also responsible for a predominantly motor type of polyneuropathy, though with minor sensory manifestations, which has been reported to follow the habitual inhalation of vapour produced from certain glues widely used in plastic modelling (glue-sniffer's neuropathy) (Goto, Matsumura, Inoue, Murai, Shida, Santa, and Kuroiwa 1974; also see p. 434). Experimentally this substance also damages the brain as well as peripheral nerves (Schaumburg and Spencer 1976).

Acrylamide, a chemical widely used in the polymer industry, was reported to cause sensorimotor polyneuropathy in factory workers by Garland and Patterson (1967). It has also done so in those drinking contaminated well water (Igisu, Goto, Kawamura, Kato, Izumi, and Kuroiwa 1975). Often the neurological manifestations are preceded by evidence of contact dermatitis on the hands followed by coldness, blueness and excessive sweating of the extremities (Spencer and Schaumburg 1974a, b). Severe ataxia is common and has been thought to indicate associated cerebellar damage (Fullerton 1969b). Electrophysiological and pathological studies in man and animals (Fullerton and Barnes 1966; Bradley and Asbury 1970; Hopkins and Gilliatt 1971) suggest that this is predominantly a 'dying-back' axonal neuropathy. However, Jennekens, Veldman, Schotman, and Gispen (1979) found evidence of multifocal axonal degeneration and Davenport, Farrell, and Sumi (1976) found that acrylamide and methyl-n-butyl ketone together produced a giant axonal neuropathy with neurofilamentous axonal masses in sural-nerve biopsies.

In all these disorders recovery usually occurs gradually after removal from exposure to the causal agent.

References

Allen, N., Mendell, J. R., Billmaier, D. J., Fontaine, R. E., and O'Neill J. (1975). Toxic polyneuropathy due to methyl-n-butyl ketone. *Arch. Neurol., Chicago* **32**, 209.

Bradley, W. G. and Asbury, A. K. (1970). Radioautographic studies of Schwann cell behaviour: 1 Acrylamide neuropathy in the mouse. *J. Neuropath, exp. Neurol.* **29**, 500.

Davenport, J. G., Farrell, D. F., and Sumi, S. M. (1976). 'Giant axonal neuropathy' caused by industrial chemicals: neurofilamentous axonal masses in man. *Neurology, Minneapolis* 26, 919.

Fullerton, P. M. (1969a). Toxic chemicals and peripheral neuropathy: clinical and epidemiological features. *Proc. R. Soc. Med.* **62**, 201.

—— (1969b). Electrophysiological and histological observations on peripheral nerves in acrylamide poisoning in man. *J. Neurol. Neurosurg. Psychiat.* **32**, 186.

—— and Barnes, J. M. (1966). Peripheral neuropathy in rats produced by acrylamide. *Br. J. indust. Med.* **23**, 210.

Garland, T. O. and Patterson M. W. H. (1967). Six cases of acrylamide poisoning. *Br. med. J.* **4**, 134.

Goto, I. Matsumura, M., Inoue, N., Murai, Y., Shida, K., Santa, T., and Kuroiwa, Y. (1974). Toxic polyneuropathy due to glue sniffing. *J. Neurol. Neurosurg. Psychiat.* **37**, 848.

Herskowitz, A., Ishii, N., and Schaumburg, H. (1971). n-Hexane neuropathy. *New Engl. J. Med.* **285**, 82.

Hopkins, A. P. and Gilliatt, R. W. (1971). Motor and sensory nerve conduction velocity in the baboon: normal values and changes during acrylamide neuropathy. *J. Neurol. Neurosurg. Psychiat.* **34**, 415.

Igishu, H., Goto, I., Kawamura, Y., Kato, M., Izumi, K., and Kuroiwa, Y. (1975). Acrylamide encephaloneuropathy due to well water pollution. *J. Neurol. Neurosurg. Psychiat.* **38**, 581.

Jennekens, F. G. I., Veldman, H., Schotman, P., and Gispen, W. H. (1979). Sequence of motor nerve terminal involvement in acrylamide neuropathy. *Acta Neuropath., Berlin* **46**, 57.

Kuzuhara, S., Kanazawa, I., Nakanishi, T., and Egashira, T. (1983). Ethylene oxide polyneuropathy. *Neurology, Minneapolis* **33**, 377.

Mitchell, A. B. S. and Parsons-Smith B. G. (1969). Trichloroethylene neuropathy. *Br. med. J.* **1**, 422.

Schaumburg, H. H. and Spencer, P. S. (1976). Degeneration in central and peripheral nervous systems produced by pure n-hexane: an experimental study. *Brain* **99**, 183.

Spencer, P. S. and Schaumburg, H. H. (1974a). A review of acrylamide neurotoxicity. Part I. Properties, uses and human exposure. *Can. J. neurol. Sci.* **1**, 143.

——, and —— (1974b). A review of acrylamide neurotoxicity. Part II.

Experimental animal neurotoxicity and pathologic mechanisms. *Can. J. neurol. Sci.* **1**, 152.

——, and —— (1975). Experimental neuropathy produced by 2, 5-hexa-nedione—a major metabolite of the neurotoxic industrial solvent methyl n-butyl ketone. *J. Neurol. Neurosurg. Psychiat.* **38**, 771.

——, ——, Raleigh, R. L., and Terhaar, C. J. (1975). Nervous system degeneration produced by the industrial solvent methyl n-butyl ketone. *Arch. Neurol., Chicago* **32**, 219.

——, Beaubernard, C. M., Bischoff-Fenton, M. C., and Kurt, T. L. (1985). Clinical and experimental toxicity of BHMH. *Ann. Neurol.* **17**, 28.

Thalidomide neuropathy

Thalidomide, used some years ago as a hypnotic in Britain and in Europe, was withdrawn from the market when it was found to produce phocomelia in the fetus if taken by the mother in early pregnancy. After regular ingestion of the drug for several months many patients developed a predominantly sensory neuropathy giving unpleasant burning dysaesthesiae in the hands and feet accompanied by peripheral impairment of pain sensation, often restricted to the digits (Fullerton and Kremer 1961). While in milder cases slow recovery often followed withdrawal of the drug, in severe cases painful paraesthesiae and sensory loss often persisted for many years. The neuropathy was found to be due to selective involvement of large diameter fibres in peripheral nerves and was predominantly axonal in type. In a follow-up study, Fullerton and O'Sullivan (1968) found that 50 per cent of patients (usually those most severely affected initially) remained unchanged for many years, but the others improved or recovered.

Later it was suspected that *methaqualone* (a constituent of *Mandrax*) also caused peripheral neuropathy (*British Medical Journal* 1973) but this drug was also withdrawn from the market because of other toxic effects.

References

British Medical Journal (1973). Does methaqualone cause neuropathy? *Br. med. J.* **3**, 307.

Fullerton, P. M. and Kremer, M. (1961). Neuropathy after intake of thalidomide (Distaval) *Br. med. J.* **2**, 855.

—— and O'Sullivan, D. J. (1968). Thalidomide neuropathy: a clinical, electrophysiological and histological follow-up study. *J. Neurol. Neurosurg. Psychiat.* **31**. 543.

Polyneuropathy due to triorthocresylphosphate

During the spring of 1930 thousands of cases of polyneuropathy, some fatal, occurred in the United States, owing to the consumption of fluid extract of ginger used in the manufacture of bootleg alcohol which was adulterated with triorthocresylphosphate. The condition became known as 'ginger paralysis'. More recent outbreaks of polyneuropathy in South Africa, Germany, Morocco, and the Merseyside area have been traced to cresyl esters in cooking oil (Hotston 1946; Spencer and Schaumburg 1980). The same toxic substance was responsible for causing polyneuropathy in women who took apiol as an abortifacient. Triorthocresylphosphate irreversibly inhibits pseudocholinesterase, but not all inhibitors of pseudocholinesterase produce degeneration of peripheral nerves. There may also be inhibition of true cholinesterase (Hern 1967). The so-called Spanish toxic oil syndrome (p. 440) is not due to triorthocresylphosphate.

Both in man and in experimental animals triorthocresylphosphate produces chromatolysis of the anterior horn cells of the spinal cord and of the ganglion cells of brainstem motor nuclei, degeneration of the fasciculus gracilis and the corticospinal tracts in the spinal cord, and destruction of both myelin and axons in the peripheral nerves. Cavanagh (1953, 1964) showed that changes occur initially in those nerve fibres which are longest and of the greatest diameter, both in the peripheral and central nervous system and hence that the primary pathological process is one of 'dying-back' of the axon. Symptoms of polyneuropathy develop from 10 to 20 days after the consumption of adulterated food or drink, and consist of bilateral wrist-drop and foot-drop, with wasting of distal limb muscles. Pain in the limbs is common, but sensory loss is inconstant. In many cases the paralysis proves permanent. Acute retrobulbar neuritis has been described in apiol poisoning. For treatment see page 526.

References

Aring, C. D. (1942). The systemic nervous affinity of triorthocresylphosphate (Jamaica ginger palsy). *Brain* **65**, 34.

Cavanagh, J. B. (1954). The toxic effects of tri-ortho-cresyl phosphate on the nervous system. *J. Neurol. Neurosurg. Psychiat.* **17**, 163.

—— (1953). Organo-phosphorus neurotoxicity: a model 'dying-back' process comparable to certain human neurological disorders *Guy's Hosp. Rep.* **112**, 303.

—— (1964). Peripheral nerve changes in ortho-cresyl phosphate poisoning in the cat. *J. Path. Bact.* **87**, 365.

Hern, J. E. C. (1967). Inhibition of true cholinesterase in TOCP poisoning with potentiation by 'Tween 80' *Nature, Lond.* **215**, 963.

Hotston, R. D. (1946). Outbreak of polyneuritis due to orthotricresyl phosphate poisoning *Lancet* **i**, 207.

Smith, M. I., Elvolve, E., and Frazier, W. H. (1930). Pharmacological action of certain phenol esters, with special reference to the etiology of so-called ginger paralysis. *Publ. Hlth. Rep. Washington* **45**, 2509.

Spencer, P. S. and Schaumburg, H. H. (1980). *Experimental and clinical neurotoxicology.* Williams and Wilkins, New York.

Weber, M. L. 1936–7). Follow-up study of thirty five cases of paralysis caused by adulterated Jamaica ginger extract. *Med. Bull. Veterans' Adm. Washington* **13**, 228.

Nitrofurantoin neuropathy

Nitrofurantoin (*Furadantin*) is a drug now widely used in the treatment of urinary infection. Cases have been reported in which a symmetrical sensorimotor peripheral neuropathy developed during treatment with this drug and was shown to occur only in those with severe impairment of renal function (Ellis 1962; Loughridge 1962). It is now clear that this drug should be used with great caution if the blood urea (or non-protein nitrogen) is above normal or if there are other indications of renal dysfunction. Even in normal persons the drug may cause reduction in motor and/or sensory nerve conduction velocity (Toole, Gergen, Hayes, and Felts 1968) but clinical polyneuropathy is uncommon when the drug is given for short periods, if renal function is unimpaired.

References

Ellis, F. G. (1962). Acute polyneuritis after nitrofurantoin therapy. *Lancet* **ii**, 1136.

Loughridge, L. W. (1962). Peripheral neuropathy due to nitrofurantoin. *Lancet* **ii**, 1133.

Toole, J. F., Gergen, J. A., Hayes, D. M., and Felts, J. H. (1968). Neural effects of nitrofurantoin. *Arch. Neurol., Chicago* **18**, 680.

Uraemic polyneuropathy

Since the original report of Asbury, Victor, and Adams (1962) it has become abundantly clear that a mixed sensorimotor polyneuropathy may occur frequently in patients who are uraemic as a result of chronic renal failure. 'Restless legs' (Ekbom 1944) is an occasional manifestation (Banerji and Hurwitz 1970; Thomas, Hollinrake, Lascelles, O'Sullivan, Baillod, Moorhead, and Mackenzie 1971) and may presage the development of neuropathy in patients under chronic haemodialysis (Thomas 1978). The neuropathy may be especially prominent in patients on dialysis who develope type B hepatitis (Davison, Williams, Mawdsley, and Robson 1972). In many cases improvement follows treatment of the renal disease, as by intermittent dialysis (Stanley, Brown, and

Pryor 1977), but this is not invariable (Nielsen 1974*a*). Improvement or even recovery may, however, follow renal transplantation (Nielsen 1974*b*; Ibrahim, Barnes, Crosland, Dawson-Edwards, Honigsberger, Nerman, and Robinson 1974; Bolton 1976). The finding of slowing of motor and sensory nerve conduction velocity in such cases (Nielsen 1973) and nerve-biopsy studies led to an initial conclusion that the neuropathy is demyelinating, but Dyck, Johnson, Lambert, and O'Brien (1971) suggested that in such cases the prominent demyelination is secondary to primary axonal degeneration. Hansen and Ballantyne (1978) found electrophysiological evidence of a 'dying-back' type of axonal neuropathy. Recently, however, Said, Boudier, Selva, Zingraff, and Drueke (1983) have found that three different forms of neuropathy, namely acute axonal neuropathy, progressive axonal neuropathy with secondary segmental demyelination, and predominantly demyelinative neuropathy, may each occur in uraemic patients. The factors determining which form develops in an individual case are unclear. Polyneuropathy has also been described as a complication of primary hyperoxaluria (Moorhead, Cooper, and Timperley 1975).

References

Asbury, A. K., Victor, M., and Adams, R. D. (1962). Uremic polyneuropathy. *Trans. Am. neurol. Ass.* **87**, 100.

Banerji, N. K. and Hurwitz, L. J. (1970). Restless legs syndrome, with particular reference to its occurrence after gastric surgery. *Br. med. J.* **4**, 774.

Bolton, C. F. (1976). Electrophysiologic changes in uremic neuropathy after successful renal transplantation. *Neurology Minneapolis* **26**, 152.

Davison, A. M., Williams, I. R., Mawdsley, C., and Robson, J. S. (1972). Neuropathy associated with hepatitis in patients maintained on haemodialysis. *Brit. med. J.* **1**, 409.

Dyck, P. J., Johnson, W. J., Lambert, E. H., and O'Brien, P. C. (1971). Segmental demyelination secondary to axonal degeneration in uremic neuropathy. *Mayo Clin. Proc.* **46**, 400.

Ekbom, K. (1944). Asthenia crurum paraesthetica (irritable legs). *Acta med. scand.* **118**, 197.

Hansen, S. and Ballantyne, J. P. (1978). A quantitative electro-physiological study of uraemic neuropathy. *J. Neurol. Neurosurg. Psychiat.* **41**, 128.

Ibrahim, M. M., Barnes, A. D., Crosland, J. M., Dawson-Edwards, P., Honigsberger, L., Nerman, C. E., and Robinson, B. H. B. (1974). Effect of renal transplantation on uraemic neuropathy. *Lancet* **ii**, 739.

Moorhead, P. J., Cooper, D. J., and Timperley, W. R. (1975). Progressive peripheral neuropathy in patients with primary hyperoxaluria. *Br. med. J.* **2**, 312.

Nielsen, V. K. (1973). The peripheral nerve function in chronic renal failure. V. Sensory and motor conduction velocity. *Acta med. scand.* **194**, 445.

—— (1974*a*). The peripheral nerve function in chronic renal failure. VII. Longitudinal course during terminal renal failure and regular haemodialysis. *Acta med. scand.* **195**, 155.

—— (1974*b*). The peripheral nerve function in chronic renal failure. IX. Recovery after renal transplantation. Electrophysiological aspects (sensory and motor nerve conduction). *Acta med. scand.* **195**, 171.

Said, G., Boudier, L., Selva, J., Zingraff, J., and Drueke, T. (1983). Different patterns of uraemic polyneuropathy: clinicopathologic study. *Neurology, Minneapolis* **33**, 567.

Stanley, E., Brown, J. C., and Pryor, J. S. (1977). Altered peripheral nerve function resulting from haemodialysis. *J. Neurol. Neurosurg. Psychiat.* **40**, 39.

Thomas, P. K. (1978). Screening for peripheral neuropathy in patients treated by chronic hemodialysis. *Muscle & Nerve* **1**, 396.

—— Hollinrake, K., Lascelles, R. G., O'Sullivan, D. J., Baillod, R. A., Moorhead, J. F., and Mackenzie, J. C. (1971). The polyneuropathy of chronic renal failure. *Brain* **94**, 761.

Chloroquine neuromyopathy

A motor polyneuropathy, unaccompanied by symptoms or signs of sensory dysfunction, may develop in patients receiving treatment with chloroquine, usually in doses of 500 mg daily or more for one year or longer. Histological studies indicate that the muscle fibres are also affected as they commonly show striking vacuolation which appears to be due to the accumulation of glycogen. The nerve lesion seems to affect mainly the terminal axons and recovery is usually rapid after withdrawal of the drug (Gérard, Stoupel, Collier, and Flament-Durand 1973).

References

Gérard, J. M., Stroupel, N., Collier, A., and Flament-Durand, J. (1973). Morphologic study of a neuromyopathy caused by prolonged chloroquine treatment. *Eur. Neurol.* **9**, 363.

Whisnant, J. P., Espinosa, R. E., Kierland, R. R., and Lambert, E. H. (1963). Chloroquine neuromyopathy. *Mayo Clin. Proc.* **38**, 501.

Vincristine neuromyopathy

Vincristine sulphate, widely used for the treatment of leukaemia, of lymphoma, of medulloblastoma in childhood and of intracranial gliomas in adult life, has been found to produce in many cases a sensorimotor polyneuropathy (Sandler, Tobin, and Henderson 1969; McLeod and Penny 1969). Pathological and electrophysiological studies suggest that the damage is primarily axonal and of the 'dying-back' type (Casey, Jelliffe, Le Quesne, and Millett 1973) but secondary demyelination with consequent slowing of nerve conduction also occurs (Gottschalk, Dyck, and Kiely 1968; Bradley 1970) and focal necrosis of muscle fibres is sometimes found (Bradley, Lassman, Pearce, and Walton 1970). The incidence of neuropathy seems to be higher in patients treated for lymphoma than in those with leukaemia or non-lymphoid cancer (Watkins and Griffin 1978). Now that vincristine has been largely supplanted by more effective agents, the incidence of this condition is declining. Intrathecal vincristine may produce extensive neuronal damage in the central nervous system (Schochet, Lampert, and Earle 1968).

References

Bradley, W. G. (1970). The neuromyopathy of vincristine in the guinea pig: an electrophysiological and pathological study *J. neurol. Sci.* **10**, 133.

—— Lassman, L. P., Pearce, G. W., and Walton, J. N. (1970). The neuromyopathy of vincristine in man. *J. neurol. Sci.* **10**, 107.

Casey, E. B., Jelliffe, A. M., Le Quesne, P. M., and Millett, Y. L. (1973). Vincristine neuropathy—clinical and electrophysiological observations. *Brain* **96**, 69.

Gottschalk, P. G., Dyck, P. J., and Kiely, J. M. (1968). Vinca alkaloid neuropathy: nerve biopsy studies in rats and in man. *Neurology, Minneapolis* **18**, 875.

McLeod, J. G. and Penny, R. (1969). Vincristine neuropathy: an electrophysiological and histological study. *J. Neurol. Neurosurg. Psychiat.* **32**, 297.

Sandler, S. G., Tobin, W., and Henderson, E. S. (1969). Vincristine-induced neuropathy: a clinical study of fifty leukemic patients. *Neurology, Minneapolis* **19**, 367.

Schochet, S. S., Lampert, P. W., and Earle, K. M. (1968). Neuronal changes induced by intrathecal vincristine sulfate. *J. Neuropath. exp. Neurol.* **27**, 645.

Watkins, S. M. and Griffin, J. P. (1978). High incidence of vincristine-induced neuropathy in lymphomas. *Br. med. J.* **1**, 610.

Misonidazole neuropathy

The radiosensitizing drug misonidazole, widely used as an adjuvant to radiotherapy, has been found to produce a polyneuropathy largely affecting the lower limbs, and improving after withdrawal of the drug, in patients under treatment for pharyngeal, laryngeal, and bronchial carcinoma (Melgaard, Hansen, Kamieniecka, Paulson, Pedersen, Tang, and Trojaborg 1982). The neurotoxic properties of this drug limit its therapeutic use.

Reference

Melgaard, B., Hansen, H. S., Kamieniecka, Z., Paulson, O. B., Pedersen, A. G., Tang, X., and Trojaborg, W. (1982). Misonidazole neuropathy: a clinical, electrophysiological, and histological study. *Ann. Neurol.* **12**, 10.

Ethambutol neuropathy

It is well known that ethambutol, one of the most effective antituberculous drugs, can occasionally cause optic neuritis (Carr and Henkind 1962), but it may also cause sensorimotor polyneuropathy (Sobue, Ando, Mukoyama, and Matsuoka 1973). Experimentally, in rats, it produces an axonal neuropathy which is more severe in proximal rather than distal segments of peripheral nerves (Matsuoka, Takayanagi, and Sobue 1981).

References

Carr, R. E., and Henkind, P. (1962). Ocular manifestations of ethambutol—toxic amblyopia after administration of an experimental antituberculous drug. *Arch. Ophthal.* **67**, 566.
Matsuoka, Y., Takayanagi, T., and Sobue, I. (1981). Experimental ethambutol neuropathy in rats: morphometric and teased-fiber studies. *J. neurol. Sci.* **51**, 89.
Sobue, I., Ando, K., Mukoyama, M., and Matsuoka, Y. (1973). Antituberculous drug neuropathy—comparison of ethambutol neuropathy with SMON. *Adv. neurol. Sci.* **17**, 106.

Perhexilene and amiodarone neuropathy

Perhexilene maleate, a drug introduced for the long-term treatment of angina pectoris, which dilates the coronary arteries and slows the heart rate through a direct action on the sinoatrial node, may cause severe weight loss, hypo-glycaemia, hepatic dysfunction, and polyneuropathy after long-term treatment (Bousser, Bouche, Brochard, and Herreman 1976; Fardeau, Tomé, and Simon 1979). While the neuropathy is sometimes mild, it can be severe but usually recovers within a few months after withdrawal of the drug. While there may be severe axonal loss, demyelination seems to be the primary process (unusual in drug-induced neuropathies) (Said 1978) and electrophysiological evidence of slowed conduction velocity may predict the development of this complication in patients receiving the drug (Wigesekera, Critchley, Fahim, Lynch, and Wright 1980). In addition to segmental demyelination, electron microscopy may show polymorphic cytoplasmic inclusions (Fardeau *et al.* 1979). A similar neuropathy, sometimes with cerebellar ataxia may follow the use of the anti-arrhythmic remedy amiodarone (Mizon, Rosa, Betermiez, and Sevestre 1985).

References

Bousser, M. G., Bouche, P., Brochard, C., and Herreman, G. (1976). Neuropathies périphériques au maléate de perhexiline, a propos de 7 observations. *Coeur de Médecine interne* **15**, 181.
Fardeau, M., Tomé, F. M. S., and Simon, P. (1979). Muscle and nerve changes induced by perhexiline maleate in man and mice. *Muscle & Nerve* **2**, 24.
Mizon, J. P., Rosa, A., Betermiez, P., and Sevestre, H. (1985). Neuropathie et syndrome cérébelleux a l'amiodarone. *Rev. Neurol.* **141**, 2, 146.
Said, G. (1978). Perhexiline neuropathy: a clinicopathological study. *Ann. Neurol.* **3**, 259.
Wijesekera, J. C., Critchley, E. M. R., Fahim, Y., Lynch, P. G., and Wright, J. S. (1980). Peripheral neuropathy due to perhexiline maleate. *J. neurol. Sci.* **46**, 303.

Disulfiram neuropathy

Sensorimotor polyneuropathy, improving slowly and often recovering completely after withdrawal of the drug, is an occasional complication of prolonged disulfiram (*Antabuse*) medication (Hayman and Wilkins 1956; Bradley and Hewer 1966). Clinical, electrophysiological, and pathological evidence suggests that the drug has a direct dose-related effect upon axons (Mokri, Ohnishi, and Dyck 1981), causing a neurofilamentous distal axonopathy due to enzymatic conversion to carbon disulphide which produces such changes experimentally in animals (Ansbacher, Bosch, and Cancilla 1982). Nukada and Pollock (1981) also found evidence of extensive segmental demyelination and postulated a direct toxic effect on Schwann cells in addition. Optic neuritis occasionally occurs (Dent 1950; Gardner-Thorpe and Benjamin 1971).

References

Ansbacher, L. E., Bosch, E. P., and Cancilla, P. A. (1982). Disulfiram neuropathy: a neurofilamentous distal axonopathy. *Neurology, Minneapolis* **32**, 424.
Bradley, W. G., and Hewer, R. L. (1966). Peripheral neuropathy due to disulfiram. *Br. med. J.* **2**, 449.
Dent, J. Y. (1950). Discussion following paper of A. S. Paterson. *Br. J. Addict.* **47**.
Gardner-Thorpe, C., and Benjamin, S. (1971). Peripheral neuropathy after disulfiram administration. *J. Neurol. Neurosurg. Psychiat.* **34**, 253.
Hayman, M., and Wilkins, P. A. (1956). Polyneuropathy as a complication of disulfiram therapy of alcoholism. *Quart. J. Stud. Alcohol* **17**, 601.
Mokri, B., Ohnishi, A., and Dyck, P. J. (1981). Disulfiram neuropathy. *Neurology, Minneapolis* **31**, 730.
Nukada, H. and Pollock, M. (1981). Disulfiram neuropathy: a morphometric study of sural nerve. *J. neurol. Sci.* **51**, 51.
Paterson, A. S. (1950). Modern techniques for the treatment of acute and prolonged alcoholism. *Br. J. Addict.* **47**, 3.

Diphenylhydantoin (anticonvulsant) neuropathy

Lovelace and Horwitz (1968) described developing polyneuropathy in 26 patients after long-term administration of diphenylhydantoin for the treatment of epilepsy, and Eisen, Woods, and Sherwin (1974) confirmed that in such epileptic patients, even in the absence of symptoms, there may be some slowing of motor and sensory nerve conduction velocity especially if the plasma level of the drug exceeds 20 μg/l. Fortunately this complication is uncommon and rarely clinically severe. Martinez-Figueroa, Johnson, Lambie, and Shakir (1980) gave reasons for suggesting that folate deficiency may be involved and found that treatment with folate reversed abnormalities of distal latency in motor and sensory nerves. Shorvon and Reynolds (1982) found that this complication was uncommon in patients treated with phenytoin, rare in those given barbiturates for anticonvulsant purposes, and that it did not occur in their patients treated with carbamazepine.

References

Eisen, A., Woods, J. F., and Sherwin, A. L. (1974). Peripheral nerve function in long-term therapy with diphenylhydantoin. *Neurology, Minneapolis* **24**, 411.
Lovelace, R. E., and Horwitz, S. J. (1968). Peripheral neuropathy in long-term diphenylhydantoin therapy. *Arch. Neurol., Chicago* **18**, 69.
Martinez-Figueroa, A., Johnson, R. H., Lambie, D. G., and Shakir, R. A. (1980). The role of folate deficiency in the development of peripheral neuropathy caused by anti-convulsants. *J. neurol. Sci.* **48**, 315.
Shorvon, S. D., and Reynolds, E. H. (1982). Anticonvulsant peripheral neuropathy: a clinical and electrophysiological study of patients on single drug treatment with phenytoin, carbamazepine or barbiturates. *J. Neurol. Neurosurg. Psychiat.* **45**, 620.

Sodium cyanate neuropathy

When sickle cell anaemia is treated with sodium cyanate, polyneuropathy with evidence of axonal degeneration and demyelination may develop (Ohnishi, Peterson, and Dyck 1975). This condition may be related in certain respects to tropical ataxic neuropathy due to the ingestion of cyanogenetic glycosides (see Osuntokun, Matthews, Hussein, Wise, and Linnell 1974, and p. 477).

References

Ohnishi, A., Peterson, C. M., and Dyck, P. J. (1975). Axonal degeneration in sodium cyanate-induced neuropathy. *Arch. Neurol. Chicago* **32**, 530.

Osuntokun, B. O., Matthews, D. M., Hussein, H. A.-A., Wise, I. J., and Linnell, J. C. (1974). Plasma and hepatic cobalamins in tropical ataxic neuropathy. *Clin. Sci. Molec. Med.* **46**, 563.

Serum neuropathy

Neuropathy is a rare sequel of serotherapy, most often seen after the administration of antiserum in the treatment of tetanus and diphtheria. Nervous symptoms usually appear two or three days after the onset of serum sickness. The commonest lesion is radiculopathy, the fifth cervical spinal nerve being most often affected on one or both sides, with pain in the corresponding segmental distribution and paralysis of the relevant muscles, especially the deltoid. This syndrome is almost identical with that of 'shoulder-girdle neuritis' (neuralgic amyotrophy) (see p. 521). Less often the whole brachial plexus is involved, or a more diffuse polyneuropathy occurs. Cerebral symptoms of encephalopathy are rare. Optic neuritis has been described. Complete recovery usually occurs in from one to 18 months, though occasionally some muscular weakness persists. Treatment appropriate to the situation of the lesion is indicated.

References

Allen, I. M. (1931). The neurological complcations of serum therapy, with report of a case. *Lancet* **ii**, 1128.

Baron, J. H. (1958). A. T. S. cervical polyradiculitis treated by cortisone. *Br. med. J.* **2**, 678.

Polyneuropathy in pregnancy

It is better to speak of polyneuropathy in rather than of pregnancy since any form of neuropathy can occur in pregnant patients (Donaldson 1977). Persistent vomiting, unsuitable diet, and increased requirements due to the needs of the fetus may all contribute to nutritional deficiency in pregnancy. Where beriberi is endemic, pregnancy appears to predispose to it. Bilateral retrobulbar neuritis resembling that due to vitamin deficiency was observed by Ballantyne (1941) in hyperemesis gravidarum. Ungley (1933) decribed recurrent neuritis in pregnancy and the puerperium in three members of the same family.

When there is reason to suspect nutritional deficiency, food and vitamin supplements should be given.

References

Ballantyne, A. J. (1941). Ocular complcations in hyperemesis gravidarum. *J. Obstet. Gynec.* **48**, 206.

Donaldson, J. (1977). *The neurology of pregnancy*. Saunders, Philadelphia.

Strauss, M. B. and McDonald, W. J. (1933). Polyneuritis of pregnancy. *J. Am. med. Ass.* **100**, 1320.

Ungley, C. C. (1933). Recurrent polyneuritis. *J. Neurol. Psychiat.* **14**, 15.

—— (1938). On some deficiences of nutrition and their relation to disease. *Lancet* **i**, 925.

Buckthorn neuropathy

Ingestion of the fruit of the Tullidora or Coyotillo plant, a poisonous shrub of the buckthorn family which grows in central or northern Mexico and the south-western United States, may cause an ascending paralysis leading to death in the acute stage. More often, however, buckthorn polyneuropathy (Calderon-Gonzales and Rizzi-Hernandez 1967) regresses slowly with eventual complete recovery. The neurotoxic compounds T496 and T544 have been isolated from the endocarp of the fruit; experimentally in animals they produce intramyelin vacuoles and segmental demyelination in peripheral nerve, presumed to bc duc to an effect upon Schwann-cell metabolism (Mitchell, Weller, Evans, Arai, and Davies 1978).

References

Calderon-Gonzales, R. and Rizzi-Hernandez, H. (1967). Buckthorn polyneuropathy. *New Engl. J. Med.* **277**, 69.

Mitchell, J., Weller, R. O., Evans, H., Arai, I., and Davies, G. D. (1978). Buckthorn neuropathy: effects of intraneural injection of *Karwinskia humboldtiana* toxins. *Neuropath. appl. Neurobiol.* **4**, 85.

Diabetic polyneuropathy

Aetiology

The aetiology of diabetic neuropathy is still controversial and was reviewed by Watkins (1983) and Dyck, Thomas, and Lambert (1983). The incidence of this complication has varied enormously in different series. Goodman, Baumoel, Frankel, Marcus, and Wassermann (1953) noted pain and paraesthesiae in 40 per cent of cases but found weakness and objective sensory loss in under 10 per cent. In other series the incidence has been substantially greater, and electrophysiological evidence of subclinical neuropathy can be detected in many diabetic subjects (Waxman 1980). The condition is uncommon in childhood and its incidence rises steadily with increasing age. It is found in early-onset insulin-sensitive diabetes, in maturity-onset cases, and also in diabetes secondary to pancreatitis (Osuntokun 1970) or haemochromatosis; a hereditary predisposition has been postulated (Chopra and Fannin 1971).

There has been much dispute about the relative roles of metabolic factors on the one hand and of atherosclerosis of the vasa nervorum on the other; while the latter may play a part, especially in the pathogenesis of mononeuropathies, there is now general agreement that the polyneuropathy is of metabolic origin in most cases. It cannot be correlated simply with hyperglycaemia, though neuropathy occurs in alloxan- or streptozotocin-induced diabetes in animals (Sharma and Thomas 1974, 1975). Disorders of pantothenic acid (Bosanquet and Henson 1957) and pyruvate (Butterfield and Thompson 1957) metabolism have been found but do not correlate with the severity of the neuropathy. Abnormalities of lipid composition (Eliasson 1966; Brown, Iwamori, Kishimoto, Rapoport, Moser, and Asbury 1979), of myelin protein (Palo, Savolainen, and Haltia 1972), or of the ionic permeability of nodal gap substance (Seneviratne and Weerasuriya 1974) have been found in diabetic peripheral nerves, and there is also evidence of disordered sorbitol metabolism (Thomas and Ward 1975). In streptozotocin-diabetic rats there is an impairment of retrograde axonal flux of glycoproteins (Jefferys and Thomas 1981). Overhydration of Schwann cells, alterations in calcium binding on plasma membranes resulting from interconversions between different inositol lipids, and increased endoneurial water in diabetic nerves, which are commonly resistant to ischaemia, have all been postulated as possible contributory mechanisms (Thomas 1978), but no single causative biochemical abnormality has yet been identified.

Pathology

Motor and sensory nerve conduction studies and single-fibre electromyography (Downie and Newell 1961; Gilliatt and Willison 1962; Chopra and Hurwitz 1969a; Lamontagne and Buchthal 1970; Thiele and Stalberg 1975), and autopsy as well as sural-nerve biopsy studies (Thomas and Lascelles 1965; Chopra and Fannin 1971) indicate that the neuropathy is demyelinating with Schwann-cell abnormalities, reduction in the density of myelinated fibres of all sizes (Chopra and Hurwitz 1969b), and sometimes 'onion-bulb' hypertrophy (Ballin and Thomas 1968). Segmental demyelination and remyelination may be found in lumbar spinal roots as well as in peripheral nerves (Ohnishi, Harada, Tateishi, Ogata, and Kawanami 1983). Despite the predominance of demyelination there is substantial electrophysiological evidence of axonal dysfunction and concomitant collateral reinnervation (Hansen and Ballantyne 1977). In diabetic autonomic neuropathy, reflex latencies and conduction velocities in post-ganglionic sympathetic fibres are normal as long as the fibres conduct (Fagius and Wallin 1980) but even when autonomic manifestations dominate the clinical picture, slowed motor and sensory conduction in somatic nerves is commonly found (Ewing, Burt, Williams, Campbell, and Clarke 1976a). When isolated peripheral-nerve lesions occur, however (mononeuropathy), especially in cranial nerves, pathological evidence has indicated that ischaemia with localized infarction of nerve trunks is the cause (Raff, Sangalang, and Asbury 1968). Nevertheless, measurement of conduction velocity and of F-wave latencies suggest that diabetic (proximal) amyotrophy, once thought to be due to ischaemia of one or both femoral nerves, is more probably due to a proximal metabolic neuropathy (Chokroverty 1982).

Symptoms and signs

The main varieties of diabetic neuropathy which have been described include generalized sensorimotor polyneuropathy (the commonest, and often predominantly sensory), proximal amyotrophy, autonomic neuropathy, and mononeuropathy (of peripheral or cranial nerves). Much less common is diabetic truncal neuropathy, often giving a band- or girdle-like area of sensory loss on the anterior trunk around the chest wall in the distribution of thoracic intercostal nerves; this is usually seen in patients with severe associated distal neuropathy in the limbs as well as autonomic neuropathy (Sabin, Geschwind, and Waxman 1978). Possibly similar in its pathogenesis but different in its clinical manifestations is diabetic thoracic radiculopathy (Kikta, Breuer, and Wilbourn 1982), giving severe chest or abdominal pain with associated dysaesthesia and sensory loss, again corresponding to intercostal nerve distribution, but often unilateral and associated with EMG evidence of denervation. Another syndrome recently described is that of acute painful neuropathy developing in males after severe weight loss, causing continuous burning lower-limb pain and dysaesthesiae with little sensory loss, preserved reflexes, no motor weakness but with impotence and depression, recovering in a few months with good control of the diabetes and weight gain (Archer, Watkins, Thomas, Sharma, and Payan 1983).

Loss of tendon reflexes and of vibration sense in the lower limbs is very common in diabetes in the absence of other clinical signs of neuropathy and in such cases nerve conduction is usually slowed. Severe polyneuropathy is exceptional but when it occurs sensory symptoms usually predominate over motor, and the lower limbs are more affected than the upper. Severe oedema of the legs occasionally occurs. Pure sensory neuropathy may been seen (p. 514). Pain in the calves may be considerable, and loss of postural sensibility is often marked in the lower limbs, leading to severe ataxia. Charcot's arthropathy is rarely seen. 'Diabetic amyotrophy' (Garland 1957; Casey and Harrison 1972), characterized by pain, tenderness, and weakness of muscles, usually limited to the anterior aspect of one or both thighs, is often due to a unilateral or bilateral femoral nerve neuropathy but is not due to mononeuritis multiplex as there is generally evidence of a subclinical generalized neuropathy (Williams and Mayer 1976) and the condition seems to be metabolic rather than vascular (Chokroverty, Reyes, Rubino, and Tonaki 1977). Isolated lesions of other peripheral nerves, particularly the lateral popliteal, also occur. Ocular palsies occurring in diabetes are almost invariably mononeuropathies due to infarction of the nerve trunks (usually) or midbrain (rarely) (see p. 107). They usually resolve in three to six months. In elderly diabetics the pupils are often contracted and may react sluggishly to light ('diabetic pseudotabes'). Primary optic atrophy may occur.

The importance and remarkable prevalence of diabetic autonomic neuropathy due to degeneration of sympathetic fibres has become increasingly evident in recent years (Ewing, Campbell, and Clarke 1980; Ewing and Clarke 1982). Absent circulatory reflexes, and particularly an abnormal response to the Valsalva manoeuvre (Sharpey-Schafer and Taylor 1960) are common as is postural hypotension (Low, Walsh, Huang, and McLeod 1975). Chronic diarrhoea, often nocturnal, steatorrhoea and impotence are also common and so too are disorders of sweating including facial sweating after food (Watkins 1973). Sudden cardiorespiratory arrest is well documented (Page and Watkins 1978) and in general when autonomic neuropathy is well-established the prognosis is poor (see below). Other complications of diabetes may be present, including peripheral vascular disease due to atheroma, which may lead to gangrene of the extremities or perforating ulcer.

Diagnosis

The diagnosis of polyneuropathy is described on page 524. The diabetic origin of the condition is usually confirmed by the discovery of glycosuria and hyperglycaemia but other forms of neuropathy occasionally occur in diabetic subjects. The manifestations of metabolic neuropathy must be distinguished from those of vascular occlusion with resultant ischaemic neuropathy as generally indicated above.

Prognosis

The prognosis of many forms of diabetic neuropathy is good, provided that the patient responds satisfactorily to treatment for diabetes, and that associated arterial or renal disease is not severe. As mentioned above, vascular mononeuropathies usually recover spontaneously, while acute, subacute, and chronic forms of polyneuropathy, as well as amyotrophy, usually improve with adequate control of the diabetes. However, autonomic neuropathy carries a poor prognosis; of a series of diabetics with such a neuropathy and abnormal tests of autonomic function reviewed by Ewing, Campbell, and Clarke (1976b, 1980) 44 per cent died within two years and six months, 56 per cent within five years.

Treatment

The usual treatment of diabetes must be carried out and it is clear that the adequacy of control can be closely correlated with arrest of, or actual improvement in, the symptoms and signs of polyneuropathy (*The Lancet* 1972). In addition, myo-inositol, 500 mg twice daily, has been found to increase the amplitude of evoked action potentials in peripheral nerves in diabetic sensorimotor neuropathy (Salway, Whitehead, Finnegan, Karunanayaka, Barnett, and Payne 1978), and aldose reductase inhibitor treatment may also be of some value (Fagius and Jameson 1981). Ephedrine, 30 mg four times daily, is effective in the relief of diabetic neuropathic oedema (Edmonds, Archer, and Watkins 1983). Whether the increasing use of the artificial pancreas (Service, Daube, O'Brien, and Dyck 1981) will improve the prognosis is still uncertain.

Measures appropriate to the usual management of poly-neuropathy may be needed (p. 526).

References

Archer, A. G., Watkins, P. J., Thomas, P. K., Sharma, A. K., and Payan, J. (1983). The natural history of acute painful neuropathy in diabetes mellitus. *J. Neurol. Neurosurg. Psychiat.* **46**, 491.

Ballin, R. H. M and Thomas, P. K. (1968). Hypertrophic changes in diabetic neuropathy. *Acta Neuropath., Berlin* **11**, 93.

Bosanquet, F. D., and Henson, R. A. (1957). Sensory neuropathy in diabetes mellitus. *Psychiat. Neurol. Neurochirurg.* **60**, 107.

Brown, M. J., Iwamori, M., Kishimoto, Y., Rapoport, B., Moser, H. W., and Asbury, A. K. (1979). Nerve lipid abnormalities in human diabetic neuropathy: a correlative study. *Ann. Neurol.* **5**, 245.

Butterfield, W. J. H. and Thompson, R. H. S. (1957). The effect of dimercaprol (BAL) on blood sugar and pyruvate levels in diabetes mellitus. *Clin. Sci.* **16**, 679.

Casey, E. B. and Harrison, M. J. G. (1972). Diabetic amyotrophy: a follow-up study. *Br. med. J.* **1**, 656.

Chokroverty, S. (1982). Proximal nerve dysfunction in diabetic proximal amyotrophy: electrophysiology and electron microscopy. *Arch. Neurol., Chicago* **39**, 403.

—— Reyes, M. G., Rubino, F. A., and Tonaki, H. (1977). The syndrome of diabetic amyotrophy. *Ann. Neurol.* **2**, 181.

Chopra, J. S. and Fannin, T. (1971). Pathology of diabetic neuropathy. *J. Path.* **104**, 175.

—— and Hurwitz, L. J. (1969a). A comparative study of peripheral nerve conduction in diabetes and non-diabetic chronic occlusive peripheral vascular disease. *Brain* **92**, 83.

—— and —— (1969b). Sural nerve myelinated fibre density and size in diabetics. *J. Neurol. Neurosurg. Psychiat.* **32**, 149.

Downie, A. W. and Newell, D. J. (1961). Sensory nerve conduction in patients with diabetes mellitus and controls. *Neurology, Minneapolis* **11**, 876.

Dyck, P. J., Thomas, P. K., and Lambert, E. H. (1983). *Peripheral neuropathy*, 2nd edn. Saunders, Philadelphia.

Edmonds, M. E., Archer, A. G., and Watkins, P. J. (1983). Ephedrine: a new treatment for diabetic neuropathic oedema. *Lancet* **i**, 548.

Eliasson, S. G. (1966). Lipid synthesis in peripheral nerve from alloxan diabetic rats. *Lipids* **1**, 237.

Ewing, D. J., Burt, A. A., Williams, I. R., Campbell, I. W., and Clarke, B. F. (1976a). Peripheral motor nerve function in diabetic autonomic neuropathy. *J. Neurol. Neurosurg. Psychiat.* **39**, 453.

——, Campbell, I. W., and Clarke, B. F. (1976b). Mortality in diabetic autonomic neuropathy. *Lancet* **i**, 601.

——, ——, and —— (1980). The natural history of diabetic autonomic neuropathy. *Quart. J. Med.* **49**, 95.

—— and Clarke, B. F. (1982). Diagnosis and management of diabetic autonomic neuropathy. *Br. med. J.* **285**, 916.

Fagius, J. and Jameson, S. (1981). Effects of aldose reductase inhibitor treatment in diabetic polyneuropathy—a clinical and neurophysiological study. *J. Neurol. Neurosurg. Psychiat.* **44**, 991.

—— and Wallin, B. G. (1980). Sympathetic reflex latencies and conduction velocities in patients with polyneuropathy. *J. neurol. Sci.* **47**, 449.

Garland, H. (1957). Diabetic amyotrophy. In *Modern trends in neurology*, 2nd series (ed. D. Williams) p. 229. Butterworths, London.

Gilliatt, R. W. and Willison, R. G. (1962). Peripheral nerve conduction in diabetic neuropathy. *J. Neurol. Neurosurg. Psychiat.* **25**, 11.

Goodman, J. I., Baumoel, S., Frankel, L., Marcus, L. J., and Wassermann, S. (1953). *The diabetic neuropathies.* Thomas, Springfield, Illinois.

Hansen, S. and Ballantyne, J. P. (1977). Axonal dysfunction in the neuropathy of diabetes mellitus; a quantitative electrophysiological study. *J. Neurol. Neurosurg. Psychiat.* **40**, 555.

Jefferys, J. G. R. and Thomas, P. K. (1981). Diabetic neuropathy update. *Trends in Neurosci.* **4**, 1.

Jordan, W. R. (1936). Neuritic manifestations in diabetes mellitus. *Arch. intern. Med.* **57**, 307.

Kikta, D. G., Breuer, A. C., and Wilbourn, A. J. (1982). Thoracic root pain in diabetes: the spectrum of clinical and electromyographic findings. *Ann. Neurol.* **11**, 80.

Lamontagne, A. and Buchthal, F. (1970). Electrophysiological studies in diabetic neuropathy. *J. Neurol. Neurosurg. Psychiat.* **33**, 442.

The Lancet (1972). Diabetic neuropathy: a preventable complication. *Lancet* **ii**, 583.

—— (1983). Diabetic neuropathy—where are we now? *Lancet* **i**, 1366.

Low, P. A., Walsh, J. C., Huang, C. Y., and McLeod, J. G. (1975). The sympathetic nervous system in diabetic neuropathy—a clinical and pathological study. *Brain* **98**, 341.

Ohnishi, A., Harada, M., Tateishi, J., Ogata, J., and Kawanami, S. (1983). Segmental demyelination and remyelination in lumbar spinal roots of patients dying with diabetes mellitus. *Ann. Neurol.* **13**, 541.

Osuntokun, B. O. (1970). The neurology of non-alcoholic pancreatic diabetes mellitus in Nigerians. *J. neurol. Sci.* **11**, 17.

Page, M. McB., and Watkins, P. J. (1978). Cardiorespiratory arrest and diabetic autonomic neuropathy. *Lancet* **i**, 14.

Palo, J., Savolainen, H., and Haltia, M. (1972). Proteins of peripheral nerve myelin in diabetic neuropathy. *J. neurol. Sci.* **16**, 193.

Raff, M. C., Sangalang, V., and Asbury, A. K. (1968). Ischaemic mononeuropathy multiplex associated with diabetes mellitus. *Arch. Neurol., Chicago* **18**, 487.

Rundles, R. W. (1945). Diabetic neuropathy. *Medicine, Baltimore* **24**, 111.

Sabin, T. D., Geschwind, N., and Waxman, S. G. (1978). Patterns of clinical deficits in peripheral nerve disease. In *Physiology and pathobiology of axons* (ed. S. G. Waxman), p. 431. Raven Press, New York.

Salway, J. G., Whitehead, L., Finnegan, J. A., Karunanayaka, A., Barnett, D., and Payne, . B. (1978). Effect of myo-inositol on peripheral-nerve function in diabetes. *Lancet* **ii**, 1282.

Seneviratne, K. N. and Weerasuriya, A. (1974). Nodal gap substance in diabetic nerve. *J. Neurol. Neurosurg. Psychiat.* **37**, 502.

Service, F. J., Daube, J. R., O'Brien, P. C., and Dyck, P. J. (1981). Effect of artifical pancreas treatment on peripheral nerve function in diabetes. *Neurology, Minneapolis* **31**, 1375.

Sharma, A. K. and Thomas, P. K. (1974). Peripheral nerve structure and function in experimental diabetes. *J. neurol. Sci.* **23**, 1.

—— and —— (1975). Peripheral nerve regeneration in experimental diabetes. *J. neurol. Sci.* **24**, 417.

Sharpey-Schafer, E. P. and Taylor, P. J. (1960). Absent circulatory reflexes in diabetic neuritis. *Lancet*, **i**, 559.

Thiele, B. and Stalberg, E. (1975). Single fibre EMG findings in polyneuropathies of different aetiology. *J. Neurol. Neurosurg. Psychiat.* **38**, 881.

Thomas, P. K. (1978). Human and experimental diabetic neuropathy. In *Peripheral neuropathies* (ed. N. Canal and G. Pozza). p. 239. Elsevier/North-Holland, Amsterdam.

—— and Lascelles, R. G. (1965). Schwann-cell abnormalities in diabetic neuropathy. *Lancet* **i**, 1355.

—— and Ward, J. D. (1975). Diabetic neuropathy. In *Complications of diabetes* (ed. H. Keen and J. Jarrett) p. 151. London.

Watkins, P. J. (1973). Facial sweating after food: a new sign of diabetic autonomic neuropathy. *Br. med. J.* **i**, 583.

—— (1983). ABC of diabetes. *Br. med. J.*, suppl.

Waxman, S. G. (1980). Pathophysiology of nerve conduction: relation to diabetic neuropathy. *Ann. intern. Med.* **92**, 297.

Williams, I. R. and Mayer, R. R. (1976). Subacute proximal diabetic neuropathy. *Neurology, Minneapolis* **26**, 108.

Woltman, H. W. and Wilder, R. M. (1929). Diabetes mellitus. Pathologic changes in the spinal cord and peripheral nerves. *Arch. intern. Med.* **44**, 576.

Hypoglycaemic neuropathy

In patients with an insulin-secreting pancreatic islet-cell adenoma, motor weakness may occur and can occasionally be accompanied by peripheral paraesthesiae. It has been suggested that this syndrome is due to a peripheral neuropathy (Lambert, Mulder, and Bastron 1960) and this now seems well-established, the neuropathy being distal, symmetrical, and predominantly motor (Jaspan, Wellman, Bernstein, and Rubenstein 1982; *The Lancet* 1982), even though Danta (1969) found 22 reported cases in which there were some sensory symptoms and signs. However, Tom and Richardson (1951) suggested that hyperinsulinism more often damages the anterior horn cells of the spinal cord rather than the peripheral nerves and Harrison (1976) found evidence suggesting damage to anterior horn cells or motor roots in a patient who developed distal muscular wasting after prolonged hypoglycaemic coma.

References

Danta, G. (1969). Hypoglycemic peripheral neuropathy. *Arch. Neurol., Chicago* 21, 121.

Harrison, M. J. G. (1976). Muscle wasting after prolonged hypoglycaemic coma; case report with electrophysiological data. *J. Neurol. Neurosurg. Psychiat.* 39, 465.

Jaspan, J. B., Wellman, R. L., Bernstein, L., and Rubenstein, A. H. (1982). Hypoglycemic peripheral neuropathy in association with insulinoma: implication of glucopenia rather than hyperinsulinism. *Medicine* 61, 33.

Lambert, E. H., Mulder, D. W., and Bastron, D. W. (1960). Regeneration of peripheral nerves with hyperinsulinism neuropathy. Report of a case. *Neurology, Minneapolis* 11, 125.

The Lancet (1982). Hypoglycaemic peripheral neuropathy. *Lancet* i, 1447.

Tom, M. I. and Richardson, J. C. (1951). Hypoglycaemia from islet-cell tumour of pancreas with amyotrophy and cerebrospinal nerve cell changes; a case report. *J. Neuropath.* 10, 57.

Neuropathy in myxoedema and pituitary disorders

Bilateral compression of the median nerves in the carpal tunnels is a common complication of myxoedema (Murray and Simpson 1958) but Nickel, Frame, Bebin, Tourtelotte, Parker, and Hughes (1961) described a symmetrical, predominantly sensory, neuropathy involving all four limbs which in such cases responded to treatment with L-thyroxine. Subsequently, Fincham and Cape (1968) and Dyck and Lambert (1970) reported that a diffuse demyelinating sensorimotor neuropathy may indeed complicate hypothyroidism, and Shirabe, Tawara, Terao, and Araki (1975) postulated a disorder of Schwann-cell metabolism. However, recent evidence from electrophysiological studies and sural-nerve biopsy in two cases favours a predominantly axonal lesion (Pollard, McLeod, Honnibal, and Verheijden 1982), while Mohr and Reid (1977) reported extensor plantar responses in such a case, so that the exact pathogenesis remains uncertain.

The carpal-tunnel syndrome is also well known to complicate acromegaly but in this disorder, too, polyneuropathy has been described (Low, McLeod, Turtle, Donnelly, and Wright 1974), as is also the case in thyrotropic hormone deficiency (Grabow and Chou 1968) and pituitary gigantism (Lewis 1972).

References

Dyck, P. J., and Lambert, E. H. (1970). Polyneuropathy associated with hypothyroidism. *J. Neuropath, exp. Neurol.* 29, 631.

Fincham, R. W. and Cape, C. A. (1968). Neuropathy in myxedema: a study of sensory nerve conduction in the upper extremities. *Arch. Neurol., Chicago* 19, 464.

Grabow, J. D. and Chou, S. M. (1968). Thyrotropin hormone deficiency with a peripheral neuropathy. *Arch. Neurol., Chicago* 19, 284.

Lewis, P. D., (1972). Neuromuscular involvement in pituitary gigantism. *Br. med. J.* 2, 499.

Low, P. A., McLeod, J. G., Turtle, J. R., Donnelly, P., and Wright, R. G. (1974). Peripheral neuropathy in acromegaly. *Brain* 97, 139.

Mohr, P. D. and Reid, H. (1977). Myeloneuropathy associated with hypothyroidism. *Br. med. J.* 1, 1005.

Murray, I. P. C. and Simpson, J. A. (1958). Acroparaesthesiae in myxoedema. *Lancet* i, 1360.

Nickel, S. N., Frame, B., Bebin, J., Tourtelotte, W. W., Parker, J. A., and Hughes, B. R. (1961). Myxoedema neuropathy and myopathy. A clinical and pathological study. *Neurology, Minneapolis* 11, 125.

Pollard, J. D., McLeod, J. G., Honnibal, T. G. A., and Verheijden, M. A. (1982). Hypothyroid polyneuropathy: clinical, electrophysiological and nerve biopsy findings in two cases. *J. neurol. Sci.* 53, 461.

Shirable, T., Tawara, S., Terao, A., and Araki, S. (1975). Myxoedematous polyneuropathy: a light and electron microscopic study of the peripheral nerve and muscle. *J. Neurol. Neurosurg. Psychiat.* 38, 241.

Liver disease, xanthomatosis, and polyneuropathy

Hepatic encephalopathy (p. 451) has been recognized for many years but the recognition of polyneuropathy as a complication of hepatic cirrhosis, active chronic hepatitis, and haemochromatosis (not secondary, in the latter condition, to diabetes) is comparatively recent (*British Medical Journal* 1972). Knill-Jones, Goodwill, Dayan, and Williams (1972) found evidence of an indolent, predominantly demyelinating polyneuropathy in 13 out of a series of 70 unselected patients with chronic liver disease, and Thomas and Walker (1965) described polyneuropathy resulting from xanthomatous deposits in peripheral nerves in primary biliary cirrhosis. Clinical and electrophysiological evidence of peripheral neuropathy as well as the well-recognized central nervous system manifestations of dementia, ataxia, and other long-tract signs, is also commonly found in the rare hereditary disorder, cerebrotendinous xanthomatosis (Kuritzky, Berginer, and Korczyn 1979).

References

British Medical Journal (1972). Peripheral neuropathy and chronic liver diseases. *Br. med. J.* 2, 607.

Knill-Jones, R. P., Goodwill, C. J., Dayan, A. D., and Williams, R. (1972). Peripheral neuropathy in chronic liver disease: clinical, electrodiagnostic, and nerve biopsy findings. *J. Neurol. Neurosurg. Psychiat.* 35, 22.

Kuritzky, A., Berginer, V. M., and Korczyn, A. D., (1979). Peripheral neuropathy in cerebrotendinous xanthomatosis. *Neurology, Minneapolis*, 29, 880.

Thomas, P. K., and Walker, J. G. (1965). Xanthomatous neuropathy in primary biliary cirrhosis. *Brain* 88, 1079.

Amyloid neuropathy

Amyloidosis was in the past divided into primary and secondary forms. Secondary amyloidosis was thought to be associated with chronic suppuration, other chronic infective conditions, and occasionally with malignant disease, particularly plasmacytoma. Primary amyloidosis occurred in the absence of any of these predisposing causes and was usually familial. So far as the amyloidosis itself is concerned it is doubtful whether the two forms are genuinely different, but in secondary amylodiosis the conspicuous features have usually been those of diffuse visceral involvement by amyloid, while primary amyloidosis is likely to present more selectively, and not uncommonly with symptoms resulting from involvement of peripheral nerves. There is also evidence that a 'primary' but non-hereditary form of anyloidosis may cause a predominantly sensory, painful, and hyperaesthetic distal neuropathy in middle-aged or elderly patients with orthostatic hypotension, diarrhoea or constipation, cardiac dysfunction, and impotence (in the male) in the absence of diabetes; usually the condition is secondary to a plasma-cell-originating dysproteinaemia (Trotter, Engel, and Ignaczak 1977). Kelly, Kyle, O'Brien, and Dyck (1979) have also pointed out that primary systemic amyloidosis which is not inherited can give a combined somatic, painful, axonal sensorimotor, and autonomic neuropathy, usually in older men, and in such cases, too, there may be plasma-cell dyscrasias and marked changes in serum and urinary proteins. While such a neuropathy is usually progressive, it is often overshadowed by the renal, cardiac, haematological, and gastrointestinal manifestations and most patients die from one or other of the latter effects of the amyloidosis.

Three main varieties of inherited amyloid neuropathy, all of dominant inheritance (Andrade, Canijo, Klein, and Kaelin 1969; Andrade, Araki, Block, Cohen, Jackson, Kuroiwa, McKusick, Nissim, Sohar, and Van Allen 1970), have been described. The commonest in many parts of the world is the so-called Portuguese type (Andrade 1952) which presents as a rule with a diffuse polyneuropathy and has also been reported in Japan (Araki, Mawatari, Ohta, Nakajima, and Kuroiwa 1968). The so-called Indiana type (Rukavina, Block, Jackson, Falls, Carey, and Curtis 1956; Mahloudji, Teasdall, Adamkiewicz, Hartman, Lambird, and McKusick 1969) usually presents with evidence of a bilateral carpal-tunnel syndrome due to deposition of amyloid beneath the carpal ligament, a syndrome also described in amyloidosis secondary to myelomatosis (Dayan, Urich, and Gardner-Thorpe 1971). In the Iowa type (van Allen, Frohlich, and Davis 1969) the affected family members showed evidence of progressive sensorimotor neuropathy, nephropathy, and peptic ulcer. The descriptions given below apply to the manifestations of the polyneuropathy as seen in the Portuguese and Iowa varieties; these closely resemble the findings often observed in sporadic, non-familial, primary amyloidosis as described above.

The first symptoms are usually sensory, and consist of painful dysaesthesiae in the distal parts of the upper or lower limbs. The physical signs are those of a polyneuropathy with distal sensory loss, muscular wasting and weakness, and diminution or loss of tendon reflexes. Hyperpathia is sometimes prominent and pain is more severely impaired than other forms of sensation (Dyck and Lambert 1969). Nevertheless painless ulcers may occur. The peripheral nerves are characteristically thickened, and firmer than normal. Histological and electron-microscopic studies have shown that deposits of amyloid are usually interfascicular but also occur in the endoneurium and perineurium and there is severe loss of unmyelinated axons and of smaller-diameter myelinated fibres (Coimbra and Andrade 1971a, b; Thomas and King 1974).

There is often an increase of protein, less often a pleocytosis in the CSF. Other manifestations of amyloidosis, notably macroglossia, myocardial involvement, and impaired renal function may be present. Involvement of autonomic nerves often causes gastrointestinal symptoms, orthostatic hypotension, and impotence (Munsat and Poussaint 1962).

In the blood, serum electrophoresis shows that hypogammaglobulinaemia is common, polyclonal and monoclonal spikes are much less frequent, and lambda light chains of IgG and IgD are more common than kappa. Amyloid fibril protein from familial amyloid neuropathy shows certain differences from that obtained from primary systemic or secondary amyloidosis (Shoji and Okano 1981). The Congo-red test may or may not be positive. Biopsy is the best method of confirming the diagnosis and may be carried out on the skin, gum, rectum, liver, kidney, or, most suitably in neurological cases, on a palpably thickened cutaneous nerve running from an area of abnormal sensation.

The diagnosis must be made from other forms of peripheral neuropathy, especially those associated with thickening of the peripheral nerves, e.g. leprosy, and the various forms of hypertrophic neuropathy.

Death usually occurs in from one to five years from cardiac failure. Treatment is symptomatic.

References

Andrade, C. (1952). A peculiar form of peripheral neuropathy. *Brain* **75**, 408.

Araki, S., Block, W. D., Cohen, A. S., Jackson, C. E., Kuroiwa, Y., McKusick, V. A., Nissim, J., Sohar, E., and Van Allen, M. W. (1970). Hereditary amyloidosis. *Arthritis and Rheumatism* **13**, 902.

Canijo, M., Klein, D., and Kaelin, A. (1969). The genetic aspect of the familial amyloidotic polyneuropathy. *Humangenetik* **7**, 163.

Araki, S., Mawatari, S., Ohta, M., Nakajima, A., and Kuroiwa, Y. (1968). Polyneuritic amyloidosis in a Japanese family. *Arch. Neurol., Chicago* **18**, 593.

Coimbra, A. and Andrade, C. (1971a). Familial amyloid polyneuropathy: an electron microscope study of the peripheral nerve in five cases. I. Interstitial changes. *Brain* **94**, 199.

—— , and —— (1971b). Familial amyloid polyneuropathy: an electron

microscope study of the peripheral nerve in five cases. II. Nerve fibre changes. *Brain* **94**, 207.

Dayan, A. D., Urich, H., and Gardner-Thorpe, C. (1971). Peripheral neuropathy and myeloma. *J. neurol. Sci.* **14**, 21.

Dyck, P. J. and Lambert, E. H. (1969). Dissociated sensation in amyloidosis: compound action potential, quantitative histologic and teased-fiber, and electron microscopic studies of sural nerve biopsies. *Arch. Neurol., Chicago* **20**, 490.

Kelly, J. J., Kyle, R. A., O'Brien, P. C., and Dyck, P. J. (1979). The natural history of peripheral neuropathy in primary systemic amyloidosis. *Ann. Neurol.* **6**, 1.

Mahloudji, M., Teasdall, R. D., Adamkiewicz, J. J., Hartman, W. H., Lambird, P. A., and McKusick, V. A. (1969). The genetic amyloidoses: with particular reference to hereditary neuropathic amyloidosis, type II (Indiana or Rukavina type). *Medicine, Baltimore* **48**, 1.

Munsat, T. L. and Poussaint, A. F. (1962). Clinical manifestations and diagnosis of amyloid polyneuropathy. *Neurology, Minneapolis* **12**, 413.

Rukavina, J. G., Block, W. D., Jackson, C. E., Falls, H. F., Carey, J. H., and Curtin, A. C. (1956). Primary systemic amyloidosis: a review and an experimental, genetic and clinical study of 29 cases with particular emphasis on the familial form. *Medicine, Baltimore* **35**, 239.

Shoji, S. and Okano, A. (1981). Amyloid fibril protein in familial amyloid polyneuropathy. *Neurology, Minneapolis* **31**, 186.

Thomas, P. K. and King, R. H. M. (1974). Peripheral nerve changes in amyloid neuropathy. *Brain* **97**, 395.

Trotter, J. L., Engel, W. K., and Ignaczak, T. F. (1977). Amyloidosis with plasma cell dyscrasia: an overlooked cause of adult onset sensorimotor neuropathy. *Arch. Neurol., Chicago* **34**, 209.

Van Allen, M. W., Frohlich, J. A., and Davis, J. R. (1969). Inherited predisposition to generalized amyloidosis. *Neurology, Minneapolis* **19**, 10.

Pink disease

Synonyms. Erythroedema polyneuritis; acrodynia.

Definition. A disease affecting young children, now virtually unknown, characterized by irritability, photophobia, and red discoloration with slight swelling of the hands and feet, and of polyneuropathy.

Pathology

Paterson and Greenfield (1924) and Wyllie and Stern (1931) found degeneration of peripheral nerves and chromatolysis of anterior horn cells in the spinal cord. Histologically the cutaneous lesions consisted of hyperkeratosis, hypertrophy of sweat glands, and lymphocytic infiltration of the corium, with oedema.

Aetiology

The victims of the disease were young children between the ages of 4 months and 7 years, the onset usually being between the ages of 6 and 18 months. The disease was once widely prevalent, especially in Australia, Britain, and North America and most cases occurred between the autumn and early spring. Warkany and Hubbard (1948) first suggested that mercury given in teething powders or ointments was the causal agent (see mercury poisoning, pp. 438 and 543) and since these powders and calomel were withdrawn from the market, the disease has disappeared.

Symptoms and signs

The earliest symptoms were often those of mild nasal discharge and congestion or diarrhoea. Shortly afterwards the child became miserable and irritable, with insomnia and loss of appetite. The hands and feet became bluish-red, slightly swollen and cold, and there was often an erythematous rash over the face, trunk, and extremities. There was always excessive sweating, with cutaneous desquamation on the hands and feet. In severe cases there were also oral ulceration and falling-out of teeth, nails, and hair.

There was no paralysis, but the muscles were hypotonic, and in chronic cases the tendon reflexes were lost and peripheral analgesia was sometimes demonstrable. The pulse was rapid and the blood pressure often slightly raised. The urine often contained excess protein and detectable amounts of mercury but the CSF was normal.

Diagnosis

This combination of symptoms occurring in early childhood was unique.

Prognosis

The mortality was low, approximately 5 per cent, death being due to cardiac failure, or more often to intercurrent infection, such as bronchopneumonia. The disease ran a chronic course, usually from three months to a year.

Treatment

Treatment was mainly symptomatic. Bower (1954) found ganglion-blocking drugs worthy of a trial when autonomic symptoms predominated. Feeding was often difficult because of anorexia and irritability and sedatives were generally required. Slow improvement followed withdrawal of drugs containing mercury and chelating agents were rarely required.

References

Bower, B. D., (1954). Pink disease: the autonomic disorder and its treatment with ganglion-blocking agents. *Quart. J. Med.* N. S. **23**, 215.
Paterson, D. and Greenfield, J. G. (1923–4). Erythroedema polyneuritis. *Quart. J. Med.* **17**, 6.
Warkany, J. and Hubbard, D. M. (1948). Mercury in the urine of children with acrodynia. *Lancet* **i**, 829.
Wyllie, W. G. and Stern, R. O. (1931). Pink disease: its morbid anatomy, with a note on treatment. *Arch. Dis. Childh.* **6**, 137.

Mercury poisoning

The symptoms of methyl mercury poisoning in adults (p. 438) are usually dominated by manifestations of central nervous system damage but sensory symptoms in the extremities are common in such cases. However, electrophysiological studies have shown no evidence of peripheral-nerve damage and the sensory symptoms are therefore believed to be of central origin (Le Quesne, Damluji, and Rustam 1974) though abnormalities of neuromuscular transmission have been found in some cases (Von Burg and Rustam 1974). On recording somatosensory evoked potentials, most cases show absence of the N20 component, the potential of the somatic sensory area (Tokuomi, Uchino, Imamura, Yamanaga, Nakanishi, and Ideta 1982). Unlike organic (methyl mercury) poisoning, however, exposure to inorganic mercury vapour (as in chlor-alkali plant workers) can cause an axonal sensorimotor polyneuropathy, the severity of which is related to the magnitude and duration of exposure (Albers, Cavender, Levine, and Langolf 1982).

References

Albers, J. W., Cavender, G. D., Levine, S. P., and Langolf, G. D. (1982). Asymptomatic sensorimotor polyneuropathy in workers exposed to elemental mercury. *Neurology, Minneapolis* **32**, 1168.
Le Quesne, P. M., Damluji, S. F., and Rustam, H. (1974). Electrophysiological studies of peripheral nerves in patients with organic mercury poisoning. *J. Neurol. Neurosurg. Psychiat.* **37**, 333.
Tokuomi, H., Uchino, M., Imamura, S., Yamanaga, H., Nakanishi, R., and Ideta, T. (1982). Minamata disease (organic mercury poisoning): neuroradiologic and electrophysiologic studies. *Neurology, Minneapolis* **32**, 1369.
Von Burg, R. and Rustam, H. (1974). Electrophysiological investigations of methyl-mercury intoxication in humans. Evaluation of peripheral nerve by conduction velocity and electromyography. *Electroenceph. clin. Neurophysiol.* **37**, 381.

Diphtheritic neuropathy

Aetiology

Polyneuropathy is the commonest and most important nervous complication of diphtheria, the exotoxin of *Corynebacterium diphtheriae* having an affinity for peripheral nerves. Diphtheria is now rare but in the past polyneuropathy was commonest in childhood and rare in adult life. It was shown in 1929 that the paralysis bore a definite relationship to the severity of the local infection, which is usually faucial but may be extrafaucial. Antitoxin reduced greatly the incidence of paralysis, which was almost unknown in patients who received it on the first day of the illness, and became progressively more frequent the longer such treatment was delayed

Palatal paralysis is due to the ascent of toxin from the faucial site of infection to the medulla. Local ascent of nerves by the toxin accounts for localized paralysis following a cutaneous infection, the muscles paralysed being those supplied by the spinal segment from which the infected region is innervated (Walshe 1918–19). Localized neuropathy in one or more extremities was often seen after diphtheritic infection of wounds in the Middle East in the Second World War. Paralysis of accommodation and generalized polyneuropathy are due to the dissemination of the toxin by the blood stream to the ciliary muscles and peripheral nerves.

Pathology

The primary lesion in the peripheral nerves is segmental demyelination (Fisher and Adams 1956; Morgan-Hughes 1965, 1968) accompanied by typical slowing of motor nerve conduction, which may persist for some time after clinical recovery. Secondary axonal degeneration can be produced in experimental animals (Bradley and Jennekens 1971) and the demyelinated nerves are excessively sensitive to pressure (Hopkins and Morgan-Hughes 1969). The neuropathic effects of the toxin are dose-dependent; the toxin becomes unavailable for inactivation by antitoxin within one hour and small-diameter nerve fibres are more severely affected (Cavanagh and Jacobs 1964). Hemiplegia, a rare complication of diphtheria, is usually due to either embolism or thrombosis of a cerebral artery, or to acute post-infective encephalitis.

Symptoms and signs

Paralysis of the palate, usually the earliest nervous symptom, may appear within a few days of the onset. Usually, however, it develops in the second or third week. It is generally bilateral but may be unilateral. The voice becomes nasal and there is regurgitation of fluids through the nose on swallowing. The palatal reflex is usually lost.

Paralysis of accommodation often develops as a rule during the third or fourth week giving dimness of vision for near objects. It is usually bilateral, rarely unilateral, and may pass unnoticed in myopic subjects who do not need to accommodate for near vision. The pupillary reactions to light and on convergence are unimpaired. Paresis of external ocular muscles is not very rare, the lateral rectus being most often affected.

The symptoms of generalized polyneuropathy, not always preceded by paralysis of the palate and of accommodation, do not develop until between the fifth and seventh week. At this stage paralysis of the pharyngeal constrictors, of the laryngeal intrinsic muscles, with laryngeal anaesthesia, and diaphragmatic paralysis are the most serious complications, because of the dysphagia and dyspnoea which they cause. The vocal-cord adductors are more often paralysed than the abductors. Paralysis of neck muscles may occur.

The lower limbs are usually more severely affected than the

upper, and distal muscles suffer more than proximal. Sensory loss is common, cutaneous anaesthesia and analgesia of the 'glove and stocking' distribution being associated with tenderness of muscles on pressure. Postural sensibility is often grossly impaired, giving marked ataxia, the so-called 'pseudotabetic form' of diphtheritic paralysis.

The tendon reflexes are lost early and may be absent for months or even years. Loss of the tendon reflexes may occur without other signs and, with or without palatal palsy, may constitute the only nervous manifestations of diphtheria. The plantar reflexes may be unobtainable but are usually flexor, though Rolleston noted extensor plantar responses, an indication that the corticospinal tracts are rarely involved. The sphincters are usually unaffected, but impotence has been described. The 'cardiac paralysis' of the early stages is probably due to toxic cardiomyopathy, but tachycardia may also result from vagal paralysis. The CSF may be normal or its protein content may be increased.

Diphtheritic hemiplegia is fortunately rare. Its effects are similar to those of other acquired forms of infantile hemiplegia (see p. 354). Meningism was once common in the acute stage with cervical rigidity or opisthotonos and rigidity of the limbs, so-called 'spasmodic diphtheria'. The CSF in such cases of presumed encephalopathy is usually normal in composition. Permanent bulbar palsy is a rare sequel.

Diagnosis

For the diagnosis of polyneuropathy see page 524. The diphtheritic form is usually easily recognized on account of the age of the patient and the occurrence of such characteristic features as palatal paralysis and paralysis of accommodation. The diphtheria bacillus should always be sought at the site of infection, but may be absent.

Prognosis

The prognosis of the paralysis is usually good if the child survives. Paralysis of the palate and of accommodation disappears in from three to six weeks, and recovery from limb paralysis is usually complete, though it may take several months. Paralysis of the pharynx, larynx, and diaphragm, though equally recoverable, is more serious owing to the risk of bronchopneumonia. Permanent paralysis is fortunately very rare. Hemiplegia is a serious complication, as it may not only be fatal, but in patients who survive, recovery is usually incomplete, and epilepsy and dementia may follow.

Treatment

The routine treatment of diphtheria includes injection of adequate doses of antitoxin as early as possible. If this has been given, administration of further doses when paralysis develops is of doubtful value. Paralysis of the limbs should be treated as indicated for the treatment of polyneuritis (see p. 526). Paralysis of the pharynx and larynx necessitates special care in feeding. Food should be soft and semi-fluid, and if, in spite of this, coughing or choking occurs, it will be necessary to employ tube feeding and/or tracheostomy. Bulbar and respiratory paralysis should be treated as in poliomyelitis (see p. 284).

References

Bradley, W. G. and Jennekens, F. G. I. (1971). Axonal degeneration in diphtheritic neuropathy *J. neurol. Sci.* **13**, 415.

Cavanagh, J. B. and Jacobs, J. M. (1964). Some quantitative aspects of diphtheritic neuropathy. *Br. J. exp. Path.* **45**, 309.

Fisher, C. M. and Adams, R. D. (1956). Diphtheritic polyneuritis: a pathological study. *J. Neuropath. exp. Neurol.* **15**, 243.

Hopkins, A. P. and Morgan-Hughes, J. A. (1969). The effect of local pressure in diphtheritic neuropathy. *J. Neurol. Neurosurg. Psychiat.* **32**, 614.

Maher, R. M. (1948). Significance of palatal movements in diphtheria. *Lancet* **i**, 57.

Morgan-Hughes, J. A. (1965). Changes in motor nerve conduction velocity in diphtheritic polyneuritis. *Rev. Pat. nerv. ment.* **86**, 253.

——— (1968). Experimental diphtheritic neuropathy: a pathological and electrophysiological study. *J. neurol. Sci.* **7**, 157.

Rolleston, J. D. (1913). Diphtheritic hemiplegia. *Clin. J.* **42**, 12.

Rolleston, J. D. (1929). *Acute diseases*, 2nd edn. London.

Walshe, F. M. R. (1917–18). On the pathogenesis of diphtheritic paralysis, Part I. *Quart. F. Med.* **11**, 191.

——— (1918–19). On the pathogenesis of diphtheritic paralysis, Part II. *Quart. J. Med.* **12**, 14.

Polyneuropathy in collagen and other auto-immune disorders

Polyneuropathy occuring in association with sarcoidosis, systemic lupus erythematosus, scleroderma, and rheumatoid arthritis raises problems of pathogenesis which are not yet completely solved (Hart and Golding 1960; Kibler and Rose 1960; Steinberg 1960; Asbury and Johnson 1978). In polyarteritis nodosa it is due to vascular lesions of the peripheral nerves, a mononeuritis multiplex, and the same appears to be the case in systemic lupus (Bailey, Sayre, and Clark 1956). Indeed it seems probable that involvement of the vasa nervorum is the pathological process common to all of the disorders in this group. Dyck, Conn, and Okazaki (1972) described a neuropathy secondary to necrotizing angiitis in a patient with rheumatoid arthritis and found no essential difference between the lesions observed in this case and those seen in polyarteritis nodosa. Mononeuropathy may also occur in the necrotizing angiitis, virtually identical with polyarteritis nodosa, which may result from drug sensitivity or from the abuse of drugs such as amphetamine (Stafford, Bogdanoff, Green, and Spector 1975). Polyneuropathy secondary to sarcoidosis may be associated with sarcoid myopathy (Garcin and Lapresle 1967) but in many cases symmetrical sensorimotor polyneuropathy occurs apparently alone, there is evidence both of axonal damage and demyelination, and sural-nerve biopsy shows multiple noncaseous sarcoid granulomas in the epineurial and perineurial spaces with panangiitis; the condition is often steroid-responsive (Oh 1980; Nemni, Galassi, Cohen, Hays, Gould, Singh, Bressman, and Gamboa 1981). An inflammatory sensory perineuritis of unknown aetiology, principally involving cutaneous nerves, has also been described (Asbury, Picard, and Baringer 1972). In systemic lupus, systemic sclerosis, and polyarteritis nodosa, as in sarcoid, the neuropathy may show some improvement with steroids. In rheumatoid arthritis, Pallis and Scott (1965) identified five different types of peripheral neuropathy. Isolated lesions of major peripheral nerves in either the upper or lower limbs, digital neuropathy in the upper limbs, and distal sensory neuropathy in the lower limbs are in their view relatively benign and often recover. However, the syndrome of distal sensorimotor polyneuropathy involving all four limbs carries a uniformly poor prognosis. It seems to arise more commonly in patients who have been treated with steroid drugs given for their rheumatoid disease and most affected individuals die of a diffuse vasculitis. Conn, McDuffie, and Dyck (1972) pointed out that in such cases treated with steroids there was pathological evidence of proliferative endarteritis suggesting a healing process secondary to acute arteritis. In milder cases of rheumatoid neuropathy there is evidence of segmental demyelination of peripheral nerves with less evidence of vascular damage (Weller, Bruckner, and Chamberlain 1970; Haslock, Wright, and Harriman 1970; Beckett and Dinn 1972).

Whereas in many cases of polyneuropathy due to the causes listed above the nature of the primary disease is self-evident, in any subacute or chronic sensorimotor polyneuropathy with marked slowing of motor and/or sensory nerve conduction, particularly when the erythrocyte sedimentation rate is raised, the possibility of an underlying collagen or connective-tissue disease should be considered. Much recent evidence has also emerged to indicate that in some cases of subacute or chronic, demyelinating, non-familial, sensorimotor neuropathy there may be associated abnormalities of serum proteins, especially the immunoglobulins, but without any evidence of malignant disease or myelomatosis. Such cases have been reported with monoclonal gammopathy (Dalakas and Engel 1981), cryoglobulinaemia (Chad, Pariser, Bradley, Adelman, and Pinn 1982), IgM plasma-cell dyscrasia (Nemni, Galassi, Latov, Sherman, Olarte, and Hays 1983), and benign IgG paraproteinaemia (Read, Vanhegan, and Matthews 1978; Smith, Kahn, Lacey, King, Eames, Whybrew, and Thomas 1983; Leibowitz, Gregson, Kennedy, and Kahn 1983). However, cryoglobulinaemic polyneuropathy may also be seen in multiple myeloma (Vallat, Desproges-Gotterton, Leboutet, Loubet, Gualde, and Treves 1980) and a motor neuropathy resembling motor-neurone disease has been reported in association with macroglobulinaemia and IgM plasma-cell dyscrasia (Rowland, Defendini, Sherman, Hirano, Olarte, Latov, Lovelace, Inoue, and Osserman 1982).

References

Asbury, A. K. and Johnson, P. C. (1978). *Pathology of peripheral nerve.* Saunders, Philadelphia.
——, Picard, E. H., and Baringer, J. R. (1972). Sensory perineuritis. *Arch. Neurol. (Chicago)* **26**, 302.
Bailey, A. A., Sayre, G. P., and Clark, E. C. (1956). Neuritis associated with systemic lupus erythematosus. *Arch Neurol. Psychiat., Chicago* **75**, 251.
Beckett, V. L. and Dinn, J. J. (1972). Segmental demyelination in rheumatoid arthritis. *Quart. J. Med.* **41**, 71.
Chad, D., Pariser, K., Bradley, W. G., Adelman, L. S., and Pinn, V. W. (1982). The pathogenesis of cryoglobulinemic neuropathy. *Neurology, Minneapolis* **32**, 725.
Conn, D. L., McDuffie, F. C., and Dyck, P. J. (1972). Immuno-pathologic study of sural nerves in rheumatoid arthritis. *Arthritis and Rheumatism* **15**, 135.
Dalakas, M. C. and Engel, W. K. (1981). Polyneuropathy with monoclonal gammopathy: studies of 11 patients. *Ann. Neurol.* **10**, 45.
Dyck, P. J., Conn, D. L., and Okazaki, H. (1972). Necrotizing angiopathic neuropathy: three-dimensional morphology of fiber degeneration related to sites of occluded vessels. *Mayo Clin. Proc.* **47**, 461.
Garcin, R. and Lapresle, J. (1967). Syndrome multinévritique avec lesions de sarcoidose a la biopsie musculaire. *Neurological problems*, p. 299. Masson, Paris.
Hart, F. D. and Golding, J. R. (1960). Rheumatoid neuropathy. *Br. med. J.* **1**, 1594.
Haslock, D. I., Wright, V., and Harriman, D. G. F. (1970). Neuromuscular disorders in rheumatoid arthritis. *Quart. J. Med.* **39**, 335.
Kibler, R. F. and Rose, F. C. (1960). Peripheral neuropathy in collagen diseases. *Br. med. J.* **1**, 1781.
Leibowitz, S., Gregson, N. A., Kennedy, M., and Kahn, S. N. (1983). IgM paraproteins with immunological specificity for a Schwann cell component and peripheral nerve myelin in patients with polyneuropathy. *J. neurol. Sci.* **59**, 153.
Nemni, R., Galassi, G., Cohen, M., Hays, A. P., Gould, R., Singh, N., Bressman, S., and Gamboa, E. T. (1981). Symmetric sarcoid polyneuropathy: analysis of a sural nerve biopsy. *Neurology, Minneapolis* **31**, 1217.
——, ——, Latov, N., Sherman, W. H., Olarte, M. R., and Hays, A. P. (1983). Polyneuropathy in nonmalignant IgM plasma cell dyscrasia: a morphological study. *Ann. Neurol.* **14**, 43.
Oh, S. J. (1980). Sarcoid polyneuropathy: a histologically proved case. *Ann Neurol.* **7**, 178.
Pallis, C. A. and Scott, J. T. (1965). Peripheral neuropathy in rheumatoid arthritis. *Br. med. J.* **1**, 1141.
Read, D. J., Vanhegan, R. I., and Matthews, W. B. (1978). Peripheral neuropathy and benign IgG paraproteinaemia. *J. Neurol. Neurosurg. Psychiat.* **41**, 215.
Rowland, L. P., Defendini, R., Sherman, W., Hirano, A., Olarte, M. R., Latov, M., Lovelace, R. E., Inoue, K., and Osserman, E. F. (1982).

Macroglobulinemia with peripheral neuropathy simulating motor neuron disease. *Ann Neurol.* **11**, 532.
Smith, I. S., Kahn, S. N., Lacey, B. W., King, R. H. M., Eames, R. A., Whybrew, D. J., and Thomas, P. K. (1983). Chronic demyelinating neuropathy associated with benign IgM paraproteinaemia. *Brain* **106**, 169.
Stafford, C. R., Bogdanoff, N. M. Green, L., and Spector, H. B. (1975). Mononeuropathy multiplex as a complication of amphetamine angiitis. *Neurology, Minneapolis* **25**, 570.
Steinberg, V. L. (1960). Neuropathy in rheumatoid diseases. *Br. med. J.* **1**, 1600.
Vallat, J. M., Desproges-Gotterton, R., Leboutet, M. J., Loubet, A., Gualde, N., and Treves, R. (1980). Cryoglobulinemic neuropathy: a pathological study. *Ann Neurol.* **8**, 179.
Weller, R. O., Bruckner, F. E., and Chamberlain, M. A. (1970). Rheumatoid neuropathy: a histological and electrophysiological study. *J. Neurol. Neurosurg. Psychiat.* **33**, 592.

Leprous neuritis

Aetiology

Leprosy is due to infection with the *Mycobacterium leprae* of Hansen, an acid-fast bacillus, staining like the tubercle bacillus by Ziehl–Neelsen's method. The disease is certainly contagious but prolonged contact with one or more affected patients may be needed for infection to occur. In parts of the United States there may be a potential animal source of infection in the armadillo (see Dastur 1978). The organism has a predilection for the mucous membranes, skin, and peripheral nerves.

Pathology

The characteristic lesion is a granuloma, the leprous nodule, composed of large connective-tissue cells, the lepra-cells, containing lepra bacilli and surrounded by epithelioid and plasma cells and fibroblasts. Two main varieties of pathological change may be found in peripheral nerves. In tuberculoid neuritis, which can occur without skin lesions (Jopling and Morgan-Hughes 1965), the powerful immune responses of the host represented by focal masses of epithelioid cells in the lesions keep the bacilli in abeyance, but the entire nerve parenchyma undergoes damage at sites of predilection so that there is extensive Wallerian degeneration distal to these lesions (Dastur and Kabholkar 1974). In lepromatous neuritis, on the other hand, the immune response is suppressed, bacilli are present in large numbers, especially in Schwann cells, there are usually extensive associated skin lesions, and there is more diffuse damage to both peripheral-nerve myelin and axons (Dastur 1967). There is marked activation of phagolysosomes (Dastur and Porwal 1979). The dorsal-root ganglia, the trigeminal ganglia, the sympathetic ganglia, and the anterior horns of the spinal cord may be invaded, and within the cord fibres derived from the dorsal-root ganglia degenerate. There is often an associated lepromatous myositis (Sebille and Gray 1979).

Symptoms and signs

The onset of symptoms is gradual. Prodromal toxaemic symptoms may occur and are followed by limb pains referred to the distribution of the peripheral nerves and often by a sense of numbness of the extremities. Symptoms tend to be symmetrical, anaesthesia of the 'glove and stocking' distribution developing, together with atrophic paralysis of peripheral-limb muscles. Pure neural tuberculoid leprosy without skin lesions is uncommon. In advanced lepromatous leprosy there may be bizarre patterns of sensory impairment in the skin of the upper limbs, with comparative sparing of sensation in the palms and antecubital fossae but dense sensory loss on the dorsum of the hands and forearms; this seems to be due to the fact that fine cutaneous nerve endings are most extensively damaged in cooler skin areas (Sabin 1969). Facial anaesthesia nd paralysis due to involvement of the fifth and seventh cranial nerves are common (Antia, Divekar, and Dastur 1966; Dastur, Antia, and Divekar 1966). Trophic changes are conspicuous in the limbs. Bullae, ulceration, and necrosis of the phalanges occur, and the digits may ultimately be destroyed. Thickening of the peripheral nerves is usually, but not invariably, palpable, conduction velocity is slowed, and the EMG indicates denervation (Sebille and Gray 1979).

Diagnosis

Leprous neuritis must be distinguished from other forms of neuropathy, especially from the chronic demyelinating and progressive hypertrophic forms, in which palpable thickening of peripheral nerves may also occur, from syringomyelia, and from Raynaud's disease. Bacteriological examination and cutaneous-nerve biopsy may be necessary.

Prognosis

Modern chemotherapy with sulphone drugs has much improved the prognosis. Recovery is usually complete in a few years in cases treated early, but there may be evidence of residual nerve damage.

Treatment

For the treatment of leprosy the reader is referred to textbooks of tropical medicine. Shepard (1974) gives a useful revew and confirms, as does Dastur (1978), that diamino-diphenyl-sulphone (DDS), given in a dose of up to 100 mg daily for five years or more, remains the standard treatment. Pressure-sensitive devices which are of value in management are discussed by Brand and Ebner (1969) and nerve grafting is helpful in selected cases (McLeod, Hargrave, Gye, Pollard, Walsh, Little, and Booth 1975).

References

Antia, N. H., Divekar, S. C., and Dastur, D. K. (1966). The facial nerve in leprosy. 1. Clinical and operative aspects. *Int. J. Leprosy* **34**, 103.

Brand, P. W. and Ebner, J. D. (1969). Pressure sensitive devices for denervated hands and feet. *J. Bone Jt Surg.* **51A**, 109.

Cochrane, R. G. (1954). In *Modern trends in dermatology* (ed. R. M. B. MacKenna) p. 153, Butterworths, London.

Dastur, D. K. (1967). The peripheral neuropathology of leprosy. In *Symposium on leprosy* (ed. N. H. Antia, and D. K. Dastur). Bombay University Press, Bombay.

—— (1978). Leprosy (an infectious and immunological disorder of the nervous system). In *Handbook of clinical neurology*, Vol. 33 (ed. P. J. Vinken and G. W. Bruyn) Chapter 19. North-Holland, Amsterdam.

——, Antia, N. H., and Divekar, S. C. (1966). The facial nerve in leprosy. 2. Pathology, pathogenesis, electromyography and clinical correlations. *Int. J. Leprosy* **34**, 118.

—— and Dabholkar, A. S. (1974). Histochemistry of leprous nerves and skin lesions *J. Path.* **113**, 69.

—— and Porwal, G. L. (1979). Lepromatous leprosy. as a model of Schwann cell pathology and lysosomal activity. In *Clinical and experimental neurology*, Proceedings of the Australian Association of Neurologists, Vol. 16 (ed. J. M. Tyrer and M. J. Eadie) p. 277. ADIS Health Science Press, Sydney.

Jopling, W. H. and Morgan-Hughes, J. A. (1965). Pure neural tuberculoid leprosy. *Br. med. J.* **2**, 799.

Khanolkar, V. R. (1951). Studies in the histology of early lesions of leprosy. *Indian Council of Med. Res. Spec. Rep. Series*, 19.

McLeod, J. G., Hargrave, J. C., Gye, R. S., Pollard, J. D., Walsh, J. C., Little, J. M., and Booth, G. C. (1975). Nerve grafting in leprosy. *Brain* **98**, 203.

Sabin, T. D. (1969). Temperature-linked sensory loss: a unique pattern in leprosy. *Arch. Neurol., Chicago* **20**, 257.

Sebille, A. and Gray, F. (1979). Electromyographic recording and muscle biopsy in lepromatous leprosy. *J. neurol. Sci.* **40**, 3.

Shepard, C. C. (1974). Leprosy, in *Harrison's principles of internal medicine*, 7th edn, Chap. 157, McGraw-Hill, New York.

Progressive hypertrophic polyneuropathy

Definition and classification. As originally described, this was a rare syndrome, often familial, characterized by enlargement of the peripheral nerves, associated with symptoms of slowly progressive polyneuropathy, and often with other abnormalities. It was first described in 1889 by Gombault and Mallet, but is usually associated with the names of Dejerine and Sottas, who reported two cases in 1893. However, hypertrophy of peripheral nerves is simply a result of chronic recurrent demyelination and remyelination with Schwann-cell proliferation. It may occur in relapsing steroid-responsive polyneuropathy (p. 530), in diabetes (p. 538), in multiple sclerosis (Schoene, Carpenter, Behan, and Geschwind 1977), in leprosy, and in many disorders in which abnormal metabolites are laid down within the nerves, as previously noted. Thus it is a typical feature of Refsum's disease (see Campbell and Williams 1967, Try 1969, and p. 462).

However, the term progressive hypertrophic polyneuropathy has usually been used to identify an inherited disorder of unknown aetiology (Thomas, Lascelles, and Stewart 1975). It is now evident that peroneal muscular atrophy (p. 383) is a syndrome and not a single disease and that the distinction once made between the latter condition and Dejerine–Sottas disease is imprecise. Indeed, following Dyck and Lambert (1968*a*, *b*), Harding and Thomas (1980*a*, *b*, *c*) and many others now suggest that the hereditary motor and sensory neuropathies can be divided into three separate groups, namely HMSN types I, II, and III. Types I and II correspond to the clinical syndrome of peroneal muscular atrophy and represent the hypertrophic demyelinating and axonal varieties of this condition respectively; a third, purely motor, form of peroneal atrophy, the neuronal type, equates with distal spinal muscular atrophy. However, the complexity of the situation is underlined by the fact that a severe neuronal motor and sensory neuropathy beginning in early childhood, thought to be different from HMSN types I-III, has been described (Ouvrier, McLeod, Morgan, Wide, and Conchin 1981). Inheritance in both types I and II is usually autosomal dominant (Mongia, Ghanem, Preston, Lewis, and Atack 1978), much less often autosomal recessive (Harding and Thomas 1980*b*), very rarely X-linked. The onset in type I is usually in the first decade, the tendon reflexes are usually absent, foot deformity is common, as is distal sensory loss, and there is often palpable hypertrophy of peripheral nerves with a motor conduction velocity of less than 38 m/s. In type II the condition is usually milder, foot deformity and sensory loss are less overt, the onset is usually in the second decade, the tendon reflexes are better preserved, and motor conduction velocity is often normal, or at least greater than 38 m/s, even though sensory conduction is always abnormal.

Dyck and Lambert (1968 *a*, *b*) proposed that the term Dejerine–Sottas disease (HMSN III) should be reserved for patients with an onset in infancy of severe, progressive, and disabling hypertrophic sensorimotor neuropathy. Dyck, Lambert, Sanders, and O'Brien (1971) noted that the condition in such families was usually of autosomal recessive inheritance, that the changes in the peripheral nerves showed hypomyelination as well as recurrent demyelination, and that the CSF protein content was usually raised. Sometimes infantile neuropathies of this type give a clinical picture closely resembling that of Werdnig–Hoffmann's disease; a rise in CSF protein is an invaluable diagnostic finding (Kasman, Bernstein, and Schulman 1976).

There seems to be some evidence that congenital hypomyelination neuropathy (Kennedy, Sung, and Berry 1977; Guzzetta, Ferrière, and Lyon 1982) may be a variant of this condition.

Clearly, therefore, progressive, genetically-determined, hypertrophic polyneuropathy is most often due to HMSN type I, less often to HMSN type III, but can occasionally result from other inherited disorders such as Refsum's disease.

Pathology

There is a marked increase in the diameter of the peripheral nerves, though some are affected more than others. The sciatic nerve in a case reported by Harris and Newcomb (1929) measured 4 cm in diameter. The cranial nerves may be involved, and similar changes have been described in sympathetic nerves, the cauda equina, and in spinal roots. This 'onion-bulb' hypertrophy, largely due to Schwann-cell proliferation, was studied with the electron microscope by Weller (1967), Thomas and Lascelles (1967), Weller and das Gupta (1968), and Weller and Herzog (1970), among others. The interfibrillar connective tissue also hypertrophies, though to a lesser extent. There is extensive segmental demyelination with secondary damage to axons (Dyck and Gomez 1968; Dyck, Lais, and Offord 1974) and abnormalities of the lipid constitution of the peripheral nerves, once though to be specific, were described in such cases (Dyck, Ellefson, Lais, Smith, Taylor, and Van Dyke 1970; Koeppen, Messmore, and Stehbens 1971). However, recent work (Yao and Dyck 1981) has failed to confirm that there is a specific systemic glycosphingolipid abnormality. Involvement of a single peripheral nerve (hypertrophic mononeuropathy) is rarely seen (Hawkes, Jefferson, Jones, and Smith 1974). Within the spinal cord degeneration of the posterior columns is usually present, and is secondary to changes in the nerves. It is most marked in the lumbosacral region and in the cervical cord is more severe in the fasciculus gracilis. Compression of the spinal cord giving rise to 'long-tract signs' is occasionally seen in severe hypertrophic neuropathy and seems to be a mechanical effect produced by hypertrophied spinal roots (Symonds and Blackwood 1962). The muscles show denervation atrophy. The pathological changes in Refsum's syndrome are similar, and a cardiomyopathy was described in that disease by Cammermeyer (1956) and Gordon and Hudson (1959).

Symptoms and signs

Sensory symptoms are often prominent and some patients complain of shooting pains in the limbs, with a sense of numbness in the hands and feet. Difficulty in walking is usually the earliest complaint. Muscular weakness and wasting develop symmetrically in the peripheral limb muscles. Pseudomyotonia with muscle hypertrophy is a rare manifestation (Korczyn, Kuritzky, and Sandbank 1978). Either the hands or the feet may be first affected, or both may suffer simultaneously. The wasting rarely extends above the knees or the elbows. Coarse fasciculation may be present in affected muscles. Claw-hand and claw-foot can result from the muscular atrophy, but pes cavus may be present as a congenital abnormality.

Cutaneous sensory loss of 'glove and stocking' distribution is often found, and postural sensibility is also impaired.

Argyll Robertson pupils have been described in a few cases. Nystagmus is not uncommon and cataracts have been described (Gold and Hoganhuis 1968). The deep reflexes are diminished or lost in affected muscles; the plantar reflexes may be absent, exceptionally they are extensor but this is probably due to mechanical compression of the spinal cord (Symonds and Blackwood 1962). Kyphoscoliosis is sometimes present, and arthropathic changes occasionally develop in limb joints. Palpable thickening of peripheral nerves is a valuable diagnostic sign but is not invariably present. It is usually identified most easily in the ulnar, common peroneal, or greater auricular nerves or in cutaneous nerves crossing the sternomastoid when the head is turned to one side. The CSF protein may be raised.

Diagnosis

There is often little difficulty in making a correct diagnosis in a patient with manifestations of a slowly progressive polyneuropathy in whom the peripheral nerves are thickened. In neurofibromatosis, which may cause focal thickening of nerves, it is rare to find palpable thickening of multiple nerves. Leprosy and sarcoidosis are unlikely to cause confusion. The inherited disorder must, however, be distinguished from other forms of demyelinating polyneuropathy (e.g. diabetic and amyloid neuropathy, Refsum's disease, and recurrent or subacute post-infective polyneuropathy) in which enlargement of nerves may occur. Electrophysiological studies are often helpful (Lewis and Sumner 1982) in that chronic or recurrent acquired demyelinating neuropathy usually gives multifocal slowing of nerve conduction velocity, whereas in HMSN types I and III there is uniform slowing of conduction along the whole length of the nerve.

Prognosis

The course of the disease is extremely slow and usually steadily progressive, though temporary arrest may occur. When the onset is in childhood patients usually survive to adult life, becoming increasingly crippled, and finally confined to a wheelchair. Death results from intercurrent disease.

Treatment

No treatment is known to influence the course of the disease, but management along the lines indicated for polyneuropathy will help to maintain the power of the limbs as long as possible.

References

Cammermeyer, J. (1956). Neuropathological changes in hereditary neuropathies: manifestations of the syndrome heredopathia atactica polyneuritiformis in the presence of interstitial hypertrophic polyneuritis. *J. Neuropath. exp. Neurol.* **15**, 340.

Campbell, A. M. G. and Williams, E. R. (1967). Natural history of Refsum's syndrome in a Gloucestershire family. *Br. med. J.* **3**, 777.

Croft, P. B., and Wadia, N. H. (1957). Familial hypertrophic polyneuritis. *Neurology, Minneapolis* **7**, 356.

Dejerine, J. and Sottas, J. (1893). Sur la névrite interstitielle hypertrophique et progressive de l'enfance. *C. R. Soc. Biol., Paris* **50**, 63.

Dyck, P. J., Ellefson, R. D., Lais, A. C., Smith, R. C., Taylor, W. F., and Van Dyke, R. A. (1970). Histologic and lipid studies of sural nerves in inherited hypertrophic neuropathy: preliminary report of a lipid abnormality in nerve and liver in Dejerine-Sottas disease. *Mayo Clin. Proc.* **45**, 286.

——, and Gomez, M. R. (1968). Segmental demyelinization in Dejerine–Sottas disease: light, phase-contrast, and electron microscopic studies. *Mayo Clin. Proc.* **43**, 280.

——, Lais, A. C., and Offord, K. P. (1974). The nature of myelinated nerve fiber degeneration in dominantly inherited hypertrophic neuropathy. *Mayo Clin. Proc.* **49**, 34.

——, and Lambert, E. H. (1968*a*). Lower motor and primary sensory neuron diseases with peroneal muscular atrophy. I. Neurologic, genetic and electrophysiologic findings in hereditary polyneuropathy. *Arch. Neurol., Chicago* **18**, 603.

——, and ——, (1968*b*). Lower motor and primary sensory neuron diseases with peroneal muscular atrophy. II. Neurologic, genetic and electrophysiologic findings in various neuronal degenerations. *Arch. Neurol., Chicago* **18**, 619.

——, ——, Sanders, K., and O'Brien, P. C. (1971). Severe hypomyelination and marked abnormality of conduction in Dejerine–Sottas hypertrophic neuropathy: myelin thickness and compound action potential of sural nerve in vitro. *Mayo Clin. Proc.* **46**, 432.

Gold, G. N. and Hogenhuis, L. A. H. (1968). Hypertrophic interstitial neuropathy and cataracts. *Neurology, Minneapolis* **18**, 526.

Gordon, N. and Hudson, R. E. B. (1959). Refsum's syndrome—heredopathia atactica polyneuritiformis. *Brain* **82**, 41.

Guzzetta, F., Ferrière, G., and Lyon, G. (1982). Congenital hypomyelination polyneuropathy: pathological findings compared with polyneuropathies starting later in life. *Brain* **105**, 395.

Harding, A. E. and Thomas, P. K. (1980*a*). The clinical features of hereditary motor and sensory neuropathy types I and II. *Brain* **103**, 259.

——, and ——, (1980*b*). Autosomal recessive forms of hereditary motor and sensory neuropathy. *J. Neurol. Neurosurg. Psychiat.* **43**, 669.

——, and ——, (1980*c*). Genetic aspects of hereditary motor and sensory neuropathy (types I and II). *J. Med. Genet.* **17**,, 329.

Harris, W. and Newcomb, W. D. (1929). A case of relapsing interstitial hypertrophic polyneuritis. *Brain* **52**, 108.

Hawkes, C. H., Jefferson, J. M., Jones, E. L., and Smith, W. T. (1974). Hypertrophic mononeuropathy. *J. Neurol. Neurosurg. Psychiat.* **37**, 76.

Kasman, M., Bernstein, L., and Schulman, S. (1976). Chronic polyradiculoneuropathy of infancy: a report of three cases with familial incidence. *Neurology, Minneapolis* **26**, 565.

Kennedy, W. R., Sung, J. H., and Berry, J. F. (1977). A case of congenital hypomyelination neuropathy. *Arch. Neurol., Chicago* **34**, 337.

Koeppen, A. H., Messmore, H., and Stehbens, W. E. (1971). Interstitial hypertrophic neuropathy: biochemical study of the peripheral nervous system. *Arch. Neurol., Chicago* **24**, 340.

Korczyn, A. D., Kuritzky, A., and Sandbank, U. (1978). Muscle hypertrophy with neuropathy. *J. neurol. Sci.* **36**, 399.

Kriel, R. L., Cliffer, K. D., Berry J., Sung, J. H., and Bland, C. S. (1974). Investigation of a family with hypertrophic neuropathy resembling Roussy-Levy syndrome. *Neurology, Minneapolis* **24**, 801.

Lewis, R. A., and Sumner, A. J. (1982). The electrodiagnostic distinctions between chronic familial and acquired demyelinative neuropathies. *Neurology, Minneapolis* **32**, 592.

Mongia, S. K., Ghanem, Q., Preston, D., Lewis, A. J., and Atack, E. A. (1978). Dominantly inherited hypertrophic neuropathy. *Can. J. neurol. Sci.* **5**, 239.

Ouvrier, R. A., McLeod, J. G., Morgan, G. J., Wise, G. A., and Conchin, T. E. (1981). Hereditary motor and sensory neuropathy of neuronal type with onset in early childhood. *J. neurol. Sci.* **51**, 181.

Refsum, S. (1946). Heredopathia atactica polyneuritiformis. *Acta psychiat. scand.*, Suppl. 38.

Schoene, W. C., Carpenter, S., Behan, P. O., and Geschwind, N. (1977). "Onion bulb" formations in the central and peripheral nervous system in association with multiple sclerosis and hypertrophic polyneuropathy. *Brain* **100**, 755.

Symonds, C. P. and Blackwood, W. (1962). Spinal cord compression in hypertrophic neuritis. *Brain* **85, 251.**

Thomas, P. K., and Lascelles, R. G. (1967). Hypertrophic neuritis. *Quart. J. Med.* **36**, 223.

——, ——, and Stewart, G. (1975). Hypertrophic neuropathy. In *Handbook of clinical neurology*, Vol. 21 (ed. P. J. Vinken and G. W. Bruyn), Chapter 8. North-Holland, Amsterdam.

Try, K. (1969). Heredopathia atactica polyneuritiformis (Refsum's disease): the diagnostic value of phytanic acid determination in serum lipids. *Eur. Neurol.* **2**, 1.

Weller, R. O. (1967). An electron microscopic study of hypertrophic neuropathy of Dejerine and Sottas. *J. Neurol. Neurosurg. Psychiat.* **30**, 111.

——, and Das Gupta, T. K. (1968). Experimental hypertrophic neuropathy: an electron microscope study. *J. Neurol. Neurosurg. Psychiat.* **31**, 34.

——, and Herzog, I. (1970). Schwann cell lysosomes in hypertrophic neuropathy and in normal human nerves. *Brain* **93**, 347.

Yao, J. K. and Dyck, P. J. (1981). Lipid abnormalities in hereditary neuropathy. Part 4. Endoneurial and liver lipids of HMSN-III (Dejerine–Sottas disease). *J. neurol. Sci.* **52**, 179.

Other inherited polyneuropathies

Many inherited disorders of the nervous system described elsewhere in this volume may also involve the peripheral nerves, giving manifestations of polyneuropathy. This is the case in several leukodystrophies, especially metachromatic leukodystrophy (p. 460) and Krabbe's disease (p. 459). Other rare degenerative diseases such as neuroaxonal dystrophy (Duncan, Strub, McGarry, and Duncan 1970 and p. 468) and Cockayne's syndrome (Moosa and Dubowitz 1970 and p. 464) may also cause polyneuropathy. Loss of small sensory neurones is found in Fabry's disease (Ohnishi and Dyck 1974 and p. 462) and sensory neuropathy has been reported in acrodermatitis chronica atrophicans (Hopf 1975). Disorders of lipid metabolism, some clearly identifiable, such as Tangier disease or alpha-lipoprotein deficiency (Engel, Dorman, Levy, and Fredrickson 1967; Kocen, King, Thomas, and Haas 1973; and p. 464) and some unidentified (Fessel 1971) also give clinical manifestations of peripheral-nerve disease. In the rare condition of *giant axonal neuropathy* (Car-penter, Karpati, Andermann, and Gold 1974; Igisu, Ohta, Tabira, Hosokawa, Goto, and Kuroiwa 1975), the affected children show tight, curly, and pale scalp hair and progressive weakness and sensory loss in the lower extremities with difficulty in walking; sural-nerve biopsy in such cases shows giant axons containing a massive increase in neurofilaments; the cause is unknown. That the condition is due to a disorder of cytoplasmic neurofilaments seems clear (Koch, Schultz, Williams, and Lampert 1977); visual function may be impaired and so, too, is oculomotor function in some cases (Kirkham, Guitton, and Coupland 1980). A similar inherited disorder has been reported in dogs (Duncan, Griffiths, Carmichael, and Henderson 1981); while the protein composition of the neurofilaments appears to be normal (Ionasescu, Searby, Rubenstein, Sandra, Cancilla, and Robillard 1983), there is evidence that the condition may be due to an inborn error of the organization of intermediate filaments (Pena 1982).

In the hereditary ataxias, peripheral-nerve involvement is constant in peroneal muscular atrophy and other related disorders (pp. 380-3), and hereditary sensory neuropathy (Ohta, Ellefson, Lambert, and Dyck 1973; Murray 1973 and see p. 514), which may be associated with increased synthesis of immunoglobulin A (Whitaker, Falchuck, Engel, Blaese, and Strober 1974) is also well defined. Rarely the hereditary syndrome is associated with spastic paraplegia (Cavanagh, Eames, Galvin, Brett, and Kelly 1979); and, while non-hereditary sensory neuropathy is well-recognized as a non-metastatic complication of carcinoma (p. 488), the latter condition is also known to occur in patients without malignant disease (Kaufman, Hopkins, and Hurwitz 1981). A variant of the hereditary syndrome causing corneal ulceration, painless fractures, and mutilation of the extremities has been described in Navajo children (Appenzeller, Kornfeld, and Snyder 1976). While congenital insensitivity to pain is a disorder of multiple pathogenesis, being observed in dysautonomia (p. 599) and in some cases being probably due to central nervous system dysfunction (Thrush 1973), evidence of sensory peripheral neuropathy with abnormal Schwann cells has been reported (Appenzeller and Kornfeld 1972) and a specific metabolic defect involving neuromelanin has been postulated (Lau, Raw, Schmidt, and Piva 1977).

Finally, in certain well-recognised metabolic disorders including porphyria (Ridley, Hierons, and Cavanagh 1968; Ridley 1969 and see p. 449), polyneuropathy is a well-recognized complication.

References

Appenzeller, O. and Kornfeld, M. (1972). Indifference to pain; a chronic peripheral neuropathy with mosaic Schwann cells. *Arch. Neurol., Chicago* **27**, 322.

——, ——, and Snyder, R. (1976). Acromutilating, paralyzing neuropathy with corneal ulceration in Navajo children. *Arch. Neurol., Chicago* **33**, 733.

Carpenter, S., Karpati, G., Andermann, F., and Gold, R. (1974). Giant axonal neuropathy. *Arch. Neurol., Chicago* **31**, 312.

Cavanagh, N. P. C., Eames, R. A., Galvin, R. J., Brett, E. M., and Kelly, R. E. (1979). Hereditary sensory neuropathy with spastic paraplegia. *Brain* **102**, 79.

Duncan, C., Strub, R., McGarry, P., and Duncan, D. (1970). Peripheral nerve biopsy as an aid to diagnosis in infantile neuroaxonal dystrophy. *Neurology, Minneapolis* **20**, 1024.

Duncan, I. D., Griffiths, I. R., Carmichael, S., and Henderson, S. (1981). Inherited canine giant axonal neuropathy. *Muscle & Nerve* **4**, 223.

Engel, W. K., Dorman, J. D., Levy, R. I., and Fredrickson, D. S. (1967). Neuropathy in Tangier disease. Alpha-lipoprotein deficiency manifesting as familial recurrent neuropathy with interstitial lipid storage. *Arch. Neurol., Chicago*, **17**, 1.

Fessel, W. J. (1971). Fat disorders and peripheral neuropathy. *Brain* **94**, 531.

Hopf, H. C. (1975). Peripheral neuropathy in acrodermatitis chronica atrophicans (Herxheimer). *J. Neurol. Neurosurg. Psychiat.* **38**, 452.

Igisu, H., Ohta, M., Tabira, T., Hosokawa, S., Goto, I., and Kuroiwa, Y.

(1975). Giant axonal neuropathy: a clinical entity affecting the central as well as the peripheral nervous system. *Neurology, Minneapolis* 25, 717.

Ionasescu, V., Searby, C., Rubenstein, P., Sandra, A., Cancilla, P., and Robillard, J. (1983). Giant axonal neuropathy: normal protein composition of neurofilaments. *J. Neurol. Neurosurg. Psychiat.* 46, 551.

Kaufman, M. D., Hopkins, L. C., and Hurwitz, B. J. (1981). Progressive sensory neuropathy in patients without carcinoma: a disorder with distinctive clinical and electrophysiological findings. *Ann. Neurol.* 9, 237.

Kirkham, T. H., Guitton, D., and Coupland, S. G. (1980). Giant axonal neuropathy: visual and oculomotor deficits. *Can. J. neurol. Sci.* 7, 177.

Kocen, R. S., King, R. H. M., Thomas, P. K., and Haas, L. F. (1973). Nerve biopsy findings in two cases of Tangier disease. *Acta neuropath., Berlin* 26, 317.

Koch, T., Schultz, P., Williams, R., and Lampert, P. (1977). Giant axonal neuropathy: a childhood disorder of microfilaments. *Ann. Neurol.* 1, 438.

Lau, T., Raw, I., Schmidt, B. J., and Piva, S. (1977). Pain insensitivity a metabolic disease. *Lancet* i, 598.

Moosa, A., and Dubowitz, V. (1970). Peripheral neuropathy in Cockayne's syndrome. *Arch. Dis. Childh.* 45, 598.

Murray, T. J. (1973). Congenital sensory neuropathy. *Brain* 96, 387.

Ohnishi, A., and Dyck, P. J. (1974). Loss of small peripheral sensory neurons in Fabry disease. *Arch. Neurol., Chicago.* 31, 120.

Ohta, M., Ellefson, R. D., Lambert, E. H., and Dyck, P. J. (1973). Hereditary sensory neuropathy, type II. *Arch. Neurol., Chicago* 29, 23.

Pena, S. D. J. (1982). Giant axonal neuropathy; an inborn error of organization of intermediate filaments. *Muscle & Nerve* 5, 166.

Ridley, A. (1969). The neuropathy of acute intermittent porphyria. *Quart. J. Med.* 38, 307.

——, Hierons, R., and Cavanagh, J. B. (1968). Tachycardia and the neuropathy of porphyria. *Lancet* ii, 798.

Thrush, D. C. (1973). Congenital insensitivity to pain—a clinical, genetic and neurophysiological study of four children from the same family. *Brain* 96, 369.

Whitaker, J. N., Falchuck, Z. M., Engel, W. K., Blaese, R. M., and Strober, W. (1974). Hereditary sensory neuropathy: association with increased synthesis of immunoglobulin A. *Arch. Neurol., Chicago* 30, 359.

Other uncommon causes of polyneuropathy

Panautonomic neuropathy not due to diabetes (Low, Dyck, Lambert, Brimijoin, Trautmann, Malagelada, Fealey, and Barrett 1983) will be further considered in Chapter 20. Among other uncommon causes of polyneuropathy are chronic obstructive pulmonary disease in cigarette smokers (Faden, Mendoza, and Flynn 1981) and cold injury as in trench or immersion foot (Peyronnard, Pedneault, and Aguayo 1977). Radiation injury may also involve not only the spinal cord (radiation myelopathy) but the brachial or lumbosacral plexuses (Horowitz and Stewart 1983).

References

Faden, A., Mendoza, E., and Flynn, F. (1981). Subclinical neuropathy associated with chronic obstructive pulmonary disease: possible pathophysiologic role of smoking. *Arch. Neurol., Chicago* 38, 639.

Horowitz, S. L., and Stewart, J. D. (1983). Lower motor neuron syndrome following radiotherapy. *Can. J. neurol. Sci.* 10, 56.

Low, P. A., Dyck, P. J., Lambert, E. H., Brimijoin, W. S., Trautmann, J. C., Malagelada, J. R., Fealey, R. D., and Barrett, D. M. (1983). Acute panautonomic neuropathy. *Ann. Neurol.* 13, 412.

Peyronnard, J. M., Pedneault, M., and Aguayo, A. G. (1977). Neuropathies due to cold: quantitative studies of structural changes in human and animal nerves. In *Neurology* (Proceedings of the 11th World Congress of Neurology p. 144). Excerpta Medica, Amsterdam.

Chronic progressive polyneuropathy

The term 'chronic progressive polyneuritis' or 'slow chronic polyneuritis' (Harris 1935) was once applied to rare cases of polyneuritis which could not be attributed to any of the common toxic causes and which ran a slowly progressive course. In all such cases, if the many causes of polyneuropathy as described above can reasonably be excluded, it is important to bear in mind the possibility, especially if the neuropathy is shown by electrophysiological studies to be predominantly of the axonal type, that it may be a manifestation of underlying malignant disease (p. 488) or of a reticulosis or blood disease (p. 485). However, whereas the neuropathy of multiple myeloma (Victor, Banker, and Adams 1958; Walsh 1971), which may recover after effective treatment of the primary disorder (Davis and Drachman 1972), is, like other paraneoplastic neuropathies, predominantly axonal, that which may be the presenting symptom of Waldenström's macroglobulinaemia (Propp, Means, Deibel, Sherer, and Barron 1975) is predominantly demyelinating. Another possible cause of axonal neuropathy to be considered in obscure cases is occult intestinal malabsorption, as in gluten sensitivity (Pallis and Lewis 1974). Even if these and other obscure causes of polyneuropathy are considered, there remain some cases in which the cause of the neuropathy cannot be explained, especially in late life (Fisher 1982).

When the polyneuropathy, by contrast, is predominantly demyelinating, with marked slowing of motor and sensory nerve conduction and especially if the protein content of the CSF is raised, or if there is peripheral nerve enlargement, the possibility must always be considered that the condition is related to recurrent or relapsing polyneuropathy (p. 530). The possibility of a response to treatment with steroid drugs must then be entertained and a therapeutic trial with prednisone given in full dosage at least for several weeks or even, in diminishing dosage, for several months, monitoring progress by serial measurement of nerve conduction velocity, is usually justified. Measurement of serum immunoglobulin and complement (Whitaker, Sciabbarrasi, Engel, Warmolts, and Strober 1973) may be of limited value in identifying cases in which immune mechanisms are disordered.

References

Davis, L. E. and Drachman, D. B. (1972). Myeloma neuropathy: successful treatment of two patients and review of cases. *Arch. Neurol., Chicago* 27, 507.

Fisher, C. M. (1982). Late-life chronic peripheral neuropathy of obscure nature. *Arch. Neurol., Chicago* 39, 234.

Harris, W. (1935). Chronic progressive (endotoxic) polyneuritis. *Brain* 58, 368.

Pallis, C. A. and Lewis, P. D. (1974). *The neurology of gastrointestinal disease.* Saunders, London.

Propp, R. P., Means, E., Deibel, R., Sherer, G., and Barron, K. (1975). Waldenström's macroglobulinemia and neuropathy. *Neurology, Minneapolis* 25, 980.

Victor, M., Banker, B. Q., and Adams, R. D. (1958). The neuropathy of multiple myeloma. *J. Neurol. Neurosurg. Psychiat.* 21, 73.

Walsh, J. C. (1971). The neuropathy of multiple myeloma: an electrophysiological and histological study. *Arch. Neurol., Chicago* 25, 404.

Whitaker, J. N., Sciabbarrasi, J., Engel, W. K., Warmolts, J. R., and Strober, W. (1973). Serum immunoglobulin and complement (C3) levels. *Neurology, Minneapolis* 23, 1164.

Polyneuritis cranialis

The term 'polyneuritis cranialis' has been used in two senses.

1. Some cranial nerves may be involved in polyneuropathy as well as the nerves of the limbs. The cranial nerves are often affected in acute post-infective polyneuropathy, but there is probably no form of neuropathy in which cranial nerves invariably escape. When they are affected this is usually symmetrical. The facial nerve is most often involved, leading to facial paralysis, usually bilateral, and next in frequency the bulbar nerves, leading to dysphagia, and the trigeminal. The oculomotor nerves are less frequently affected (Fisher 1956) and the optic nerves usually escape, though bilateral optic neuritis rarely occurs. Exceptionally the

cranial nerves may be affected alone or there may be only slight involvement of the nerves of the limbs, indicated by paraesthesiae or diminution in the tendon reflexes. Donaghy and Earl (1985) reported three cases in which extraocular muscle palsies developed several weeks before chronic relapsing polyneuropathy affected the limbs.

2. The term 'polyneuritis cranialis' has also been applied to an inflammatory lesion of multiple cranial nerves within the skull. This can follow osteomyelitis of the bones of the skull base or basal pachymeningitis secondary to nasal sinusitis or chronic otitis media. The lesion may involve the anterior group, the third, fourth, fifth, and sixth nerves on one or both sides, or the posterior group, the seventh to twelfth usually on one side only, but in some cases almost all the nerves are affected. This condition must be distinguished from involvement of multiple cranial nerves in carcinomatosis of the meninges. It must also be distinguished from the syndrome of multiple cranial nerve involvement, often beginning unilaterally, which may be seen in patients with nasopharyngeal carcinoma, in sarcoidosis or in other granulomatous meningitides including syphilis and torulosis. Unilateral or bilateral facial-nerve palsy has been described as a complication of acute leukaemia, while recurrent (often familial) unilateral or bilateral facial palsy, often associated with a congenitally fissured tongue, is often referred to as Melkersson's syndrome (Stevens 1965).

References

Donaghy, M. J. and Earl, C. J. (1985). Ocular palsy preceding chronic relapsing polyneuropathy by several weeks. *Ann. Neurol.* **17**, 49.

Fisher, M. (1956). An unusual variant of acute idiopathic polyneuritis (syndrome of ophthalmoplegia, ataxia and areflexia). *New Engl. J. Med.* **255**, 57.

Forster, F. M., Brown, M., and Merritt, H. H. (1941). Polyneuritis with facial diplegia. *New Engl. J. Med.* **225**, 51.

Stevens, H. (1965). Melkersson's syndrome. *Neurology, Minneapolis* **15**, 263.

Viets, H. R. (1927). Acute polyneuritis with facial diplegia. *Arch. Neurol. Psychiat., Chicago* **17**, 794.

19

Disorders of muscle

The anatomy and physiology of muscle

A voluntary muscle is composed of muscle fibres, each of which is a multinucleate cell, consisting of myofibrils, sarcoplasm, and a number of discrete intracellular organelles including mitochondria, ribosomes, and the sarcotubular system. Each fibre is enclosed within a sarcolemmal sheath, deep to which the muscle nuclei are situated and each has a motor end-plate in which the nerve fibre terminates. The sarcolemma has three layers, an innermost plasma membrane, a middle layer of basement membrane, and an outer layer of collagen. The amorphous basement membrane, about 50 nm thick, acts as the microskeleton for the muscle fibre and is more specialized at the end-plate region where it contains acetylcholinesterase (see below). The 10-nm thick plasma membrane is a more specialized lipoprotein bilayer which is differentially permeable to various ions, thus exercising control over the relative ionic composition of the intracellular and extracellular fluids and hence over the resting membrane potential of the muscle fibre. Under normal conditions muscle fibres never contract singly, but the functional unit of muscle activity is known as the motor unit, being that group of muscle fibres supplied by a single anterior horn cell and its motor nerve axon. Discharge of such a single anterior horn cell results in the simultaneous contraction of all the muscle fibres which it innervates.

For many years it was thought (see Lewis and Ridge 1981; Landon 1982) that the constituent fibres of motor units in mammalian skeletal muscle were gathered into groups or fasciculi, but the work of Edström and Kugelberg (1968) and others showed that the fibres of a single unit are usually widely scattered throughout a muscle when examined in transverse section. Only after denervation and subsequent reinnervation by regenerating neurones are fibres innervated by a single anterior horn cell or by one of its axonal branches gathered into groups (Kugelberg, Edström, and Abbruzzese 1970). Contraction of the muscle fibres which make up a motor unit produces action potentials which can be recorded in the electromyogram (EMG). The morphology of this electrical activity in the EMG depends on physical factors such as the dimensions of the electrode used, as well as on the muscle chosen for examination. For example, in the biceps brachii of a healthy young adult, the electrical activity of a single motor unit usually appears as a di- or triphasic wave with a duration of 5-10 ms and an amplitude of less than 250 μV; however, the variation in form, amplitude, and duration is considerable (see p. 494; Barwick 1981; Lenman 1981; Kimura 1983). Probably these so-called motor unit action potentials are often produced not by the electrical activity of the entire motor unit, but simply by the summated electrical activity of a number of its component fibres regarded as constituting a subunit.

An important advance in our knowledge of the physiology of muscular contraction was the discovery of humoral transmission of the nerve impulse at the myoneural junction. It was Dale (1934) who first showed that acetylcholine (ACh) is the transmitter. It is now evident that the synaptic vesicles in the motor nerve terminal are actually packets of ACh. Single packets of ACh are continually being released spontaneously and give rise to small depolarizations (miniature end-plate potentials) which can be recorded electrically with a micro-electrode in the region of the end-plate. Once released, the ACh diffuses through the synaptic clefts of the end-plate to combine with the specialized ACh receptors on the post-junctional plasma membrane. Each ACh receptor is made up of a number of glycosylated polypeptide chains organized into five subunits and spans the lipid bilayer of the plasma membrane. The arrival of a nerve impulse at the end-plate results in the synchronous release of many packets of ACh which produce a localized depolarization of the muscle fibre membrane in the end-plate region; this is the end-plate potential. When this potential reaches a certain critical size it triggers off an excitatory wave, the action potential, which then travels away from the end-plate along the plasma membrane of the fibre (see Lewis and Ridge 1981; Zaimis and Wray 1981). At rest the inside of the membrane is some 80 mV negative with respect to the outside (the resting potential), but during the action potential the polarization of the membrane momentarily reverses, so that for about 1 ms the inside of the fibre becomes positive. This reversal of electrical polarity is caused by increased sodium permeability of the membrane. The wave of excitation spreads inwards into the substance of the muscle fibre along the transverse system of tubules, the 'T' system (see Huxley 1964) and the consequent mobilization of calcium ions in the sarcoplasmic reticulum initiates contraction of the myofibrils.

Ultrastructural studies of skeletal muscle (see Landon 1982) have demonstrated that the unit of structure of the individual myofibril is the sarcomere, extending from one Z-line (situated in the midst of the 'I'-band) to the next. Attached to each Z-line are many thin filaments of the protein actin. There is also a second type of filament which is thicker and is composed of myosin; these filaments correspond to the dark (birefringent) A-bands of the myofibrils. Each filament of myosin is surrounded by a hexagonal array of actin filaments; in addition, molecular cross-bridges reach out from the myosin to the actin filaments. During contraction, the cross-bridges repeatedly disengage and re-engage at successive sites on the actin filaments. The propulsion imparted to the actin filaments causes them to slide over the myosin filaments so as to interdigitate more fully with the latter; in this way the whole myofibril, and consequently its parent fibre, shortens. The biochemical changes which accompany muscle contraction are very complex (for reviews see Peachey, 1968 and Gergely 1981) but it is plain that among the many biochemical reactions which occur, creatine phosphate is broken down in the presence of calcium to creatine and phosphate, and adenosine triphosphate (ATP) is broken down to adenosine diphosphate (ADP). The release of high-energy phosphate bonds provides much of the energy required for muscular contraction.

It is also important to note that skeletal muscle fibres are not homogeneous and contain at least two main types of muscle fibre which are morphologically and histochemically distinct. One fibre type, called Type I, tends to be somewhat smaller than the second type; it contains myofibrils which are generally somewhat slender and a high concentration of mitochondria. Histochemical stains demonstrate that this type of fibre contains a high concentration of enzymes such as succinic dehydrogenase which are concerned with aerobic metabolism. In the larger Type II fibre, whose myofibrils are generally more coarse and more widely dispersed, there are fewer mitochondria and histochemical studies indicate that these fibres contain a higher concentration of glycogen and of enzymes such as phosphorylase and myofibrillar adenosine triphosphatase which are concerned with anaerobic metabolism. In man, all skeletal muscles contain an admixture of Type I and Type II fibres, so that in transverse sections stained histochemically, a characteristic checkerboard pattern is observed (see Dubowitz 1968, 1981; Landon 1982). Physiological experiments also indicate that these fibres are functionally different. Thus in many animals there are certain muscles such as soleus which are made up predominantly of Type I fibres (so-called red muscle). These muscles are concerned largely with the maintenance of posture and, upon stimulation, are found to contract and relax relatively slowly. By contrast, other muscles concerned more directly with motor activity, such as the flexor digitorum longus, are made up predominantly of Type II fibres (white muscle) and are more rapidly contracting (fast 'twitch' muscles). Subdivision of Type II fibres into Types IIa and IIb is also possible on the basis of their intensity of staining with myofibrillar ATPase reaction at different acid pHs and their oxidative enzyme content (Table 19.1), the Type IIa fibres showing inhibition of ATPase activity at pH 4.6 and a relatively higher content of oxidative enzymes than the Type IIb fibres in which the ATPase activity is only inhibited at pH 4.3. Both subtypes are physiologically fast-twitch fibres, but because of their greater oxidative metabolic activity, those of Type IIa are more fatigue-resistant than those of Type IIb. The two major types are also distinguishable through the properties of their myosin light chains and through the tropomyosin and troponin which they contain, the respective protein in the two fibre types being immunochemically distinct. It is also evident (see Dubowitz 1968, 1981) that in some manner, apparently related to firing rate, the motor nerve controls not only the physiological behaviour, but also the histochemical structure, of the muscle fibres in that transposition of motor nerve from a fast muscle to a slow muscle, and vice versa, may completely alter the physiological and histochemical characteristics of the muscle fibres. Thus in effect it is the neurones which control the behaviour of the muscle fibres which make up their motor units so that one can speak of Type I and Type II neurones. Thus when a group of denervated muscle fibres are reinnervated by a sprouting neurone they become of uniform histochemical type (so-called 'type-grouping'—see Karpati and Engel 1968 and Dubowitz and Brooke 1974).

Table 19.1. *Histochemical and physiological characteristics of the three major muscle fibre types**

	Fibre type		
	I	IIa	IIb
Enzyme reactions			
NADH–tetrazolium reductase and SDH	+++	++	+
Myofibrillar ATPase			
pH 9.4	+	+++	+++
pH 4.6	+++	−	+++
pH 4.3	+++	−	−
Phosphorylase	+	+++	+++
Physiological properties			
Twitch speed	Slow	Fast	Fast
Fatigue resistance	+++	++	+
Nomenclature			
Peter *et al.* (1972)	Slow-twitch oxidative	Fast-twitch oxidative-glycolytic	Fast-twitch glycolytic
Burke *et al.* (1971)	S (slow contracting)	FR (fast contracting fatigue resistant)	FF (fast contracting fast fatigue)

* From Walton and Mastaglia (1980a).

Finally, before commenting upon individual diseases of muscle, it is important to mention briefly some drugs which act upon the neuromuscular junction. ACh, when released at the neuromuscular junction, is broken down by acetylcholinesterase which is normally present in the subneural basement membrane and can be demonstrated histochemically. The drug curare acts on the postjunctional membrane, where it reduces or prevents the depolarizing effect of the transmitter excited by the nerve impulse (Hunt and Kuffler 1950; Riker 1953). Drugs such as physostigmine and neostigmine destroy cholinesterase and allow ACh liberated at the myoneural junction to accumulate. Guanidine hydrochloride acts by increasing the output of ACh at the nerve endings. Initially the accumulation of ACh produces muscular contraction as a result of depolarization of the muscle fibre membrane, but if it accumulates in excess, the depolarization persists and may result in blockage of the muscle action potential (depolarization block). Whereas drugs such as tubocurarine and gallamine compete with ACh for the end-plate chemical receptors and are thus known as competitive inhibitors, drugs such as decamethonium and suxamethonium produce muscle paralysis first as a result of depolarization block but subsequently also produce competitive block so that they are said to have a 'dual' action (see Zaimis and Wray 1981).

References

Barwick, D. D. (1981). Clinical electromyography. In *Disorders of voluntary muscle* (ed. J. N. Walton) 4th edn, Ch. 28. Churchill-Livingstone, Edinburgh.

Burke, R. E., Levine, D. H., Zajac, F. C., Tsairis, P., and Engel, W. K. (1971). Mammalian motor units: physiological correlation in three types of rat gastrocenemius. *Science* **174**, 709.

Dale, H. (1934). Chemical transmission of the effects of nerve impulses. *Br. med. J.* **2**, 835.

Dubowitz, V. (1968). *Developing and diseased muscle*, Heinemann, London.

——. (1981). Histochemical aspects of muscle disease. In *Disorders of voluntary muscle* (ed. J. N. Walton) 4th edn, Ch. 8. Churchill-Livingstone, Edinburgh.

—— and Brooke, M. H. (1974). *Muscle biopsy*. Saunders, London.

Edström, L. and Kugelberg, E. (1968). Histochemical composition, distribution of fibres and fatiguability of single motor units. *J. Neurol. Neurosurg. Psychiat.* **31**, 424.

Gergely, J. (1981). Biochemical aspects of muscular structure and function. In *Disorders of voluntary muscle* (ed. J. N. Walton) 4th edn, Ch. 4. Churchill-Livingstone, Edinburgh.

Hunt, C. C. and Kuffler, S. W. (1950). Pharmacology of the neuromuscular junction. *Pharmacol. Rev.* **2**, 96.

Huxley, A. F. (1964). Muscle. *Ann. Rev. Physiol.* **26**, 131.

Karpati, G. and Engel, W. K. (1968). 'Type grouping' in skeletal muscles after experimental reinnervation. *Neurology, Minneapolis* **18**, 447.

Kimura, J. (1983). *Electrodiagnosis in diseases of nerve and muscle*. Davis, Philadelphia.

Kugelberg, E., Edström, L. and Abbruzzese, M. (1970). Mapping of motor units in experimentally reinnervated rat muscle. Interpretation of histochemical and atrophic fibre patterns in neurogenic lesions. *J. Neurol. Neurosurg. Psychiat.* **33**, 319.

Landon, D. N. (1982). Skeletal muscle—normal morphology, development and innervation. In *Skeletal muscle pathology* (ed. F. L. Mastaglia and J. N. Walton) Ch. 1. Churchill-Livingstone, Edinburgh.

Lenman, J. A. R. (1981). Integration and analysis of the electromyogram and related techniques. In *Disorders of voluntary muscle* (ed. J. N. Walton) 4th edn, Ch. 29. Churchill-Livingstone, Edinburgh.

Lewis, D. M. and Ridge, R. M. A. P. (1981). The anatomy and physiology of the motor unit. In *Disorders of voluntary muscle* (ed. J. N. Walton), 4th edn, Ch. 1. Churchill-Livingstone, Edinburgh.

Peachey, L. D. (1968). Muscle. *Ann. Rev. Physiol.* **30**, 401.

Peter, J. B., Barnard, R. J., Edgerton, V. R., Gillespie, C. A. and Stempel, K. E. (1972). Metabolic profiles of three fibre types of skeletal muscle in guinea pigs and rabbits. *Biochemistry* **11**, 2627.

Riker, W. F. (1953). Excitatory and anticurare properties of acetylcholine and related quaternary ammonium compounds at the neuromuscular junction. *Pharmacol. Rev.* **5**, 1.

Walton, J. N. (1983). Diseases of voluntary muscle. In *Oxford textbook of medicine* (ed. D. J. Weatherall, J. G. G. Ledingham, and D. A. Warrell) section 22. Oxford University Press, Oxford.

—— and Mastaglia, F. L. (1980 *a*). The molecular basis of muscle diseases. In *The molecular basis of neuropathology* (ed. R. H. S. Thompson and A. N. Davison) Ch. 17. Arnold, London.

—— and —— (Eds.) (1980 *b*). The muscular dystrophies. *Br. med. Bull.* **36** (2).

Zaimis, E. and Wray, D. (1981). General physiology and pharmacology of neuromuscular transmission. In *Disorders of voluntary muscle* (ed. J. N. Walton) 4th edn, Ch. 3. Churchill-Livingston, Edinburgh.

General comments on disorders of muscle

The past 30 years have seen increasing world-wide interest in diseases of muscle. A comprehensive classification of the neuromuscular disorders was produced by the Research Group on Neuromuscular Diseases of the World Federation of Neurology (1968) and was modified by Walton (1981). It includes, however, many disorders which affect muscle through disease of the spinal cord, anterior horn cells, and peripheral nerves which have been dealt with in other parts of this volume (see Chapters 13, 14, and 18). This chapter will therefore be concerned with those disorders which primarily affect voluntary muscle and the myoneural junction. The term 'myopathy' may reasonably be used (Walton 1966) to define any disease or syndrome in which the patient's symptoms and/or physical signs can be attributed to pathological, biochemical, or electrophysiological changes which are occurring in the muscle fibres or in the interstitial tissues of the voluntary musculature and in which there is no evidence that the symptoms related to the muscular system are in any way secondary to disordered function of the central or peripheral nervous system. Within this group, therefore, are to be included many degenerative disorders which appear to be genetically determined, as well as others of a primary biochemical character and yet others in which the disease process appears to be inflammatory or due to disordered immunity. The construction of this chapter will be different from many others in this book in that the clinical and genetic aspects of the conditions to be considered are first described in turn, and the chapter concludes with commentaries upon differential diagnosis by means of clinical and investigative methods.

References

Research Group on Neuromuscular Diseases (1968). Classification of the neuromuscular disorders *J. neurol. Sci* **6**, 165.

Walton, J. N. (1966). Diseases of muscle. *Abstr. Wld Med.* **40**, 1,81.

—— (1981). The clinical examination of the voluntary muscles. In *Disorders of voluntary muscle* (ed. J. N. Walton) 4th edn, Ch. 13. Churchill-Livingstone, Edinburgh.

Progressive muscular dystrophy

Muscular dystrophy has been defined as genetically-determined primary degenerative myopathy (Walton 1966), but this definition can no longer be accepted as wholly satisfactory as there are several other myopathies, to be mentioned in this chapter, which are genetically determined but are not normally regarded as being muscular dystrophies in the accepted sense of the term. However, this definition is nevertheless reasonable, with exclusions, as muscular dystrophy appears to be due to some factor or factors present in the individual's genetic constitution from birth; pathological and other evidence indicates that the disease is primarily one of the muscle cell and the process is still classified as degenerative as there is no evidence available to indicate its cause, though there is much evidence to suggest that an abnormality of the plasma membrane of the muscle fibre is an important factor (see Walton and Mastaglia 1980). Innumerable hypotheses have been advanced to explain the pathogenesis of the muscular dystrophies including a failure of the muscle cell to regenerate following injury, the absence of an unidentified enzyme within the muscle cell, a primary abnormality of collagen leading to excessive fibrosis within muscle, and many more, but none of these has been supported by

clinical and experimental study. The 'vascular hypothesis' postulating functional ischaemia of muscle (Mendell, Engel, and Derrer 1971) has been disproved (Paulson, Engel, and Gomez 1974; Jerusalem, Engel, and Gomez 1974; Musch, Papapetropoulos, McQueen, Hudgson, and Weightman 1975), while the 'neurogenic hypothesis', suggesting a trophic defect of the motor neurone as being an important factor (McComas, Sica, and Campbell 1971), appears to have been due in part to certain deficiencies in the technique used to count motor unit numbers (Ballantyne and Hansen 1974) and in part to the fact that some of the patients examined may have been suffering from spinal muscular atrophy closely resembling muscular dystrophy clinically.

The most convincing evidence now available suggests that in Duchenne dystrophy, in particular, there is a defect in the plasma membrane of the muscle fibre which allows the uncontrolled entry of calcium. This in turn causes areas of hypercontraction of myofibrils (Cullen and Fulthorpe 1975; Mokri and Engel 1975) and activation of calcium-activated neutral proteases leading to muscle-fibre necrosis (Rowland 1976; Ebashi and Sugita 1978). The present position has been reviewed by Pennington (1981) and Cullen and Mastaglia (1982). It is also important to note that current work on the mapping of the X-chromosome (Williamson 1983: *The Lancet* 1983; Bakker *et al.* 1985) makes it likely that the gene responsible for Duchenne muscular dystrophy will soon be isolated and characterized.

Classification

Classification of the muscular dystrophies is by no means academic as it is the only safe guide to prognosis and genetic counselling. The traditional clinico-anatomic classification of this group of diseases into the pseudohypertrophic, pelvic girdle atrophic, facio-scapulohumeral, juvenile scapulohumeral, distal, ocular, late-life, and congenital forms proved unsatisfactory both clinically and genetically, since if, for instance, one classifies all cases showing pseudohypertrophy into one group, this is then shown to be heterogeneous with several different forms of inheritance and little clinical uniformity. Important contributions were made by Tyler and Wintrobe (1950), Stevenson (1953), Becker (1953, 1957), Walton and Nattrass (1954), Morton and Chung (1959), Dubowitz (1960), and Emery and Walton (1967). A useful clinico-genetic classification based upon current knowledge is given below, modified from Walton and Gardner-Medwin (1981).

The 'pure' muscular dystrophies:
(*a*) X-linked muscular dystrophy
    Severe (Duchenne)
    Benign (Becker)
    Benign with early contractures (Emery–Dreifuss)
    Scapuloperoneal (rare)
(*b*) Autosomal recessive muscular dystrophy
    Limb-girdle (usually scapulohumeral, rarely pelvifemoral)
    Childhood type, resembling Duchenne
    Congenital muscular dystrophy
(*c*) Autosomal dominant muscular dystrophy
    Facioscapulohumeral
    Scapuloperoneal
    Late-onset proximal
    Distal
    Ocular
    Oculopharyngeal

Although this classification would seem to be the most satisfactory that can be devised based upon present knowledge, there are still cases which are difficult to fit into any of the groups described. Many more detailed family studies will be required, using rigid clinical, genetic, and investigative criteria, or, alternatively, precise techniques of gene identification, before a final and definitive classification can be achieved. Though the nature of the pathological process causing muscular weakness and wasting in these cases is broadly similar in character, if different in tempo and in various other characteristics, in the various types, there are other features such as differences in the pattern of muscular involvement and in the degree to which enzymes such as creatine kinase leak into the serum in the different varieties, which strongly suggest that they will in the end prove to be different diseases.

It will now be convenient to consider the general clinical features of the muscular dystrophies, before describing the distinctive clinical characteristics of the various sub-varieties.

Clinical features of the muscular dystrophies

These depend upon which muscles are first involved by the disease process and upon the rate of progress of the disease. Weakness in the muscles around the pelvic girdle characteristically gives slowness in walking, inability to run, frequent falling, and difficulty in climbing stairs or in rising from the floor. Eventually the patients develop an accentuated lumbar lordosis and a characteristic waddling gait. Climbing up the legs on rising from the floor (Gowers' sign) is a characteristic feature of the conditions (Fig. 19.1) but is by no means specific for muscular dystrophy, as it occurs in any condition in which pelvic girdle muscles are weak and may thus be seen in various forms of spinal muscular atrophy, congenital myopathy, and polymyositis. Weakness in the shoulder girdles gives

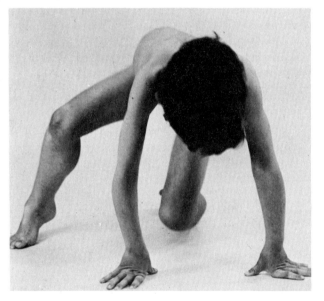

Fig. 19.1. A boy suffering from the Duchenne type muscular dystrophy rising from the floor.

an unusually sloping appearance of the shoulders with a tendency for the scapulae to rise prominently when the patient attempts to abduct the arms. Many patients utilize trick movements by placing one hand beneath the other elbow in an attempt to lift the hand to the face or head. Facial weakness in its characteristic form, as seen in the facioscapulohumeral variety, causes inability to whistle and to pout the lips or to close the eyes, while distal weakness (as seen in the distal variety) gives weakness of grip and fine finger movements and foot-drop. Contractures are common in all forms of muscular dystrophy in the late stages, but are seen particularly in the severe Duchenne type. They may result from weakness of a group of muscles whose antagonists remain comparatively powerful (this explains the partial foot-drop with turning in of the feet and toes which is seen in advancing cases of the Duchenne type and which typically causes the children to walk on their toes; it results from progressive weakness of the anterior tibial group at a time when the calf muscles remain powerful). Contractures may also be due to the posture adopted by a patient once confined to a

wheelchair; then the biceps brachii, and hamstrings show a particular tendency to shorten. A most important clinical characteristic of all forms of muscular dystrophy is that muscles are picked out by the disease in a curiously selective manner; this is also a most difficult feature to explain on any theory of pathogenesis. Though there are certain differences in the patterns of muscular involvement seen in the various sub-varieties, it is common in the upper limbs, for instance, to find that the serrati and pectoral muscles are weakened and atrophic, as are biceps and brachioradialis, while deltoid and triceps remain relatively powerful. In the lower limbs quadriceps and anterior tibials are particularly weakened and the calf muscles are spared, but in some cases of limb-girdle muscular dystrophy the hamstrings and quadriceps are affected equally. Such a selective pattern of muscular involvement is strongly suggestive of muscular dystrophy, but a similar affection of individual muscles with sparing of others is also seen in the more benign varieties of spinal muscular atrophy (p. 383) though in some cases of the latter condition the pattern is somewhat different (e.g. the deltoid is often involved).

The severe X-linked (Duchenne) type

Although it is clear that this condition is due to an X-linked recessive gene, about one-third of the affected boys appear to be isolated cases and in these individuals the disease is presumed to have resulted from genetic mutation occurring perhaps in the cells of one segment of the ovary in either the patient's mother or maternal grandmother (Gardner-Medwin 1970). The evidence indicating X-linked recessive inheritance comes first from the inspection of pedigrees, secondly from the fact that several women have been known to have affected children by more than one male, and thirdly from the fact that three cases of the disease have now been reported in patients of female morphology suffering from Turner's syndrome (ovarian agenesis) with an XO chromosome constitution (Walton 1956a; Ferrier, Bamatter, and Klein 1965; Jalbert, Mouriquand, Beaudoing, and Jalliard 1966; Emery and Walton 1967). The condition is found in about one in 3500 liveborn males but can also be manifest very rarely in females in whom there is a translocation between the short arm of the X chromosome and a part of chromosome 21 or another autosome (Gomez, Engel, Dewald, and Peterson 1977); such translocations have proved very helpful in mapping the X chromosome and the position of the Duchenne gene has now been identified within narrow limits (Williamson 1983; Roses, Pericak-Vance, Yamaoka, Stubblefield, Stajich, Vance, Roses and Carter 1983; *The Lancet* 1983).

The condition usually first becomes clinically apparent towards the end of the third year of life with difficulty in walking, frequent falling, and difficulty in climbing stairs, but some boys are hypotonic in infancy and do not walk until after 18 months of age. The pelvic-girdle muscles are thus first affected, but involvement of the shoulder girdles soon follows. Enlargement of the calf muscles and sometimes of quadriceps, deltoids, and other muscles as well, occurs in about 90 per cent of cases at some stage but later disappears as the disease advances.

This enlargement was once referred to as pseudohypertrophy in view of the fact that muscle biopsy demonstrated, in some such muscles, marked infiltration with fat, but there is now good histological evidence that more often early enlargement is due to true muscular hypertrophy with enlargement of individual muscle fibres. Most patients show slow progressive deterioration and become unable to walk by the time they are 10 years old. False or apparent clinical improvement may occur between the ages of 5 and 8 years, when the rate of deterioration due to the disease is apparently outstripped by the processes of normal physical development. Once the child is confined to a wheelchair, progressive deformity with muscular contractures and skeletal distortion and atrophy occur, and death usually results from inanition, respiratory infection, or cardiac failure towards the end of the second decade. Some children waste progressively, but others become markedly obese and there is no convincing explanation for this discrepancy. Macroglossia is not infrequent and occasionally certain incisor teeth are absent. The intelligence quotient in these cases is 10 per cent or more lower than in a group of control children of comparable age and sex (Dubowitz 1965; Murphy, Thompson, Corey, and Conen 1965). Marked skeletal atrophy and deformity occur and the shafts of long bones may become pencil-thin and fracture on minimal trauma (Walton and Warrick 1954). Cardiac involvement is invariable, but may not be detectable in the early stages. Persistent tachycardia is common and there is a characteristic electrocardiogram which shows tall R waves in the right precordial leads and deep Q waves in the limb leads and left precordial leads (Skyring and McKusick 1961; Emery 1972).

While no effective treatment for this tragic progressive disorder has yet been discovered, and methods of management will be discussed later, an important advance was the discovery that the female carriers of the gene can usually be detected by means of serum creatine (CK) kinase estimation, perhaps with assistance from the radioimmunoassay of serum myoglobin (Nicholson 1981), quantitative EMG, and muscle biopsy (Walton and Gardner-Medwin 1981). Many other refined techniques of detection have been tested including the measurement of protein synthesis by muscle polyribosomes *in vitro* (Ionasescu, Zellweger, and Conway 1971), the estimation of serum pyruvate kinase activity (Alberts and Samaha 1974), and studies of phosphorylation in erythrocte membranes (Roses, Roses, Miller, Hull, and Appel 1976), but serum CK estimation, employing Bayesian methods to determine the probability that the young woman is or is not a carrier (Emery and Morton 1968; Emery 1981) is still the most reliable and is best carried out in adolescent girls (Nicholson, Gardner-Medwin, Pennington, and Walton 1979). This fact is of particular importance to the sisters of dystrophic boys, who have approximately a 50-50 chance of being carriers. A carrier female, who may rarely show clinical evidence of minor degrees of muscle weakness (a manifesting carrier), is likely to pass the disease on to half of her sons, and half her daughters will themselves be carriers; it is not, therefore, surprising that most young women identified as carriers decide not to have children. Selective abortion of male fetuses identified by amniocentesis (Emery, Watt, and Clack 1972) is widely practised. Unfortunately methods of antenatal diagnosis of affected males (as by fetal blood sampling by fetoscopy, followed by serum CK estimation) have not yet proved sufficiently reliable for one to abort only affected males, but once the Duchenne gene is isolated this will be feasible (Bakker *et al.* 1985). If most carriers are detected by identifying the gene marker, and if most do not reproduce or produce male infants, then undoubtedly the incidence of the disease will fall in the future, though cases will continue to arise as a result of mutation.The principles of carrier detection and the recent literature on this topic have been reviewed by Emery (1981) and by Walton and Gardner-Medwin (1981).

Another important development has been the introduction of simple techniques for serum CK estimation using a single drop of blood on a filter paper, allowing the introduction of neonatal screening programmes. Many now favour the performance of such a test on all new-born males in order to identify preclinical cases of the disease, if only to prevent the birth of a second affected male before the disease has been diagnosed in the first-born.

The benign X-linked (Becker) type of muscular dystrophy
The existence of a distinct benign X-linked recessive form of muscular dystrophy was first suggested by Becker and Kiener (1955) and subsequent reports made it clear that the benign cases are distinct and not simply part of a spectrum of severity related to the Duchenne type. This disorder differs from the severe Duchenne variety in that the onset of the disease is usually between the fifth and twenty-fifth year; the disorder may be transmitted by affected males through carrier daughters to their grandsons, there is gradually progressive weakness and wasting of the pelvic and later of the

pectoral muscles, and most patients become unable to walk 25 years or more after the onset. Cardiac involvement is common in these families (Markland, North, D'Agostino, and Daly 1969), contractures and skeletal deformity occur late, if at all, and some such patients, though severely disabled, survive to a normal age. Crossing-over with deutan colour blindness and the Xg blood group has been described (Emery, Smith, and Sanger 1969) and the locus for this form of X-linked dystrophy is probably different from that of the Duchenne gene. The detection of female carriers of this gene is sometimes possible (Emery, Clack, and Taylor 1967) but is less reliable than in the Duchenne type (Walton and Gardner-Medwin 1981). The X-linked condition described by Dreifuss and Hogan (1961) and by Emery and Dreifuss (1966) may well be a variant of the Becker type; the onset was early (at about four to five years), the course benign, contractures developed early, and myocardial involvement was invariable.

X-linked scapuloperoneal muscular dystrophy
While scapuloperoneal muscular atrophy (p. 385) is usually neurogenic rather than myopathic, and more often dominant than X-linked, families in which the condition is due to a primary myopathy and in which the inheritance was plainly X-linked have been reported by Rotthauwe, Martier, and Beyer (1972) and Thomas, Calne, and Elliott (1972). The question as to whether such cases could possibly have been examples of spinal muscular atrophy with secondary myopathic change remains as yet unanswered (Walton and Gardner-Medwin 1981).

Limb-girdle muscular dystrophy
This form of the disease occurs equally in the two sexes and usually begins in the second or third decade of life, but occasionally first appears in middle life. Though genetic evidence plainly indicates that in most families the condition is inherited by an autosomal recessive mechanism and that its incidence is therefore considerably increased by consanguinity, many cases are sporadic and it has been suggested that some may be due to manifestation in the heterozygote (Morton and Chung 1959; Chung and Morton 1959). In most of the cases, muscle weakness begins in the shoulder-girdle muscles (Fig. 19.2) and may then remain limited to these for many years before eventually spreading to involve the pelvic girdle. In a much smaller number, by contrast, the pelvic-girdle muscles are first involved and the weakness usually spreads to the shoulders in about 10 years. Enlargement of calf muscles is not uncommon. The severity of the disease varies a good deal from case to case and from family to family. Often muscular weakness and wasting are asymmetrical initially, and sometimes the disease process appears temporarily to arrest, but in most patients the degree of disability is severe within 20 years of the onset. There is some evidence to suggest that in the patients in whom weakness begins in the upper limbs (the scapulohumeral form) the disease runs a more benign course than in those in whom the pelvic-girdle muscles are first involved. There may be considerable difficulty in distinguishing sporadic cases beginning in the pelvic girdle on purely clinical grounds from cases of benign spinal muscular atrophy, from Becker dystrophy, and from various forms of metabolic myopathy; the EMG and muscle biopsy are of particular value in making the distinction. Indeed a review of patients previously diagnosed as cases of limb-girdle muscular dystrophy in Newcastle upon Tyne, using quantitative EMG, estimation of the numbers of functioning motor units and histochemical studies applied to muscle biopsy sections, showed that half were in fact suffering from chronic spinal muscular atrophy of the Kugelberg–Welander type (Mastaglia and Walton 1971; Walton 1973) and in one case coming to autopsy (Tomlinson, Walton, and Irving 1974) the number of limb motor neurones in the spinal cord was greatly reduced, confirming the neuronal origin of the disorder. A neurogenic cause is much commoner in patients presenting with pelvic girdle rather than scapulohumeral weakness and in those with so-called 'myopathy restricted to the quadriceps muscles'.

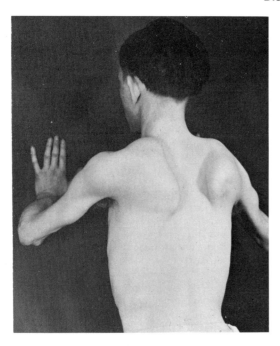

Fig. 19.2. A patient suffering from limb-girdle muscular dystrophy, demonstrating bilateral winging of the scapulae.

Indeed it is now usual to talk of the 'limb-girdle syndrome', though undoubtedly cases of true limb-girdle muscular dystrophy (especially of scapulohumeral distribution) do occur. Contractures and skeletal deformity occur late in the course of this disease by comparison with the Duchenne type, but progress much more rapidly when the patient is unable to walk. Most sufferers are severly disabled in middle life and many die before the normal age.

Childhood muscular dystrophy with autosomal recessive inheritance

This is one of the most difficult categories of muscular dystrophy to characterize. Proof of autosomal recessive inheritance is rarely possible and the arguments for the very existence of this condition have largely depended upon the occasional occurrence of muscular dystrophy in young girls and in a few families in which parental consanguinity made autosomal recessive inheritance likely. Even though some reported cases (Kloepfer and Talley 1958; Jackson and Carey 1961; Johnston 1964) seemed reasonably convincing, few if any of those reported were investigated in sufficient depth to exclude spinal muscular atrophy of the Kugelberg–Welander type (Penn, Lisak, and Rowland 1970; Mastaglia and Walton 1971) which often mimics muscular dystrophy closely, especially if there is extensive secondary myopathic change in the affected muscles superimposed upon evidence of the primary devervating process. However, increasing evidence has emerged of late to indicate that an autosomal recessive form of true muscular dystrophy of early onset does occur and follows a more benign course than that demonstrated by males with typical Duchenne dystrophy. While it certainly occurs rarely in Britain and in the USA, this condition seems to be particularly common in North Africa and in the Middle East (Ben Hamida, Fardeau, and Attia 1983). The onset may be in the second year or as late as the fourteenth, but is most often in the second half of the first decade. Progression is comparatively slow and patients usually become unable to walk in their early twenties, but sometimes as early as 15 years or as late as 40 years. The pattern of weakness may be very similar to that observed in the typical severe X-linked Duchenne type (Walton and Gardner-Medwin 1981) and so too are the histological changes seen in muscle-biopsy samples, though less severe.

Congenital muscular dystrophy

It was Batten who in 1909 suggested that the syndrome of amyotonia congenita, as first described by Oppenheim (1900), might be due to a simple congenital atrophic myopathy. However, he was probably describing the condition which has been variously entitled benign congenital myopathy (Turner 1940, 1949; Turner and Lees 1962) or benign congenital hypotonia with incomplete recovery (Walton 1956 b), a syndrome which differs from the muscular dystrophies in its relatively non-progressive course and in the absence of specific histological abnormalities in the muscle fibres (see p. 582). However, Banker, Victor, and Adams (1957), Pearson and Fowler (1963), Gubbay, Walton, and Pearce (1966), Zellweger, Afifi, McCormick, and Mergner (1967), and Denner, Rapole, and Somer (1975) described cases with congenital hypotonia and severe, but relatively non-progressive, muscular weakness in which the muscle histology was typical of muscular dystrophy. In several children there were widespread contractures suggesting arthrogryposis multiplex congenita. The exact nosological status of these non-progressive muscle disorders remains uncertain, but in a few cases congenital muscular dystrophy is rapidly progressive and terminates fatally within the first year of life (Wharton 1965). Patients with congenital dystrophy intermediate in severity between the static and rapidly progressive groups make it unlikely that subdivision on the grounds of severity alone is justifiable.

The essential features of this disorder are severe hypotonia present from birth with the subsequent development of more or less progressive muscular wasting and weakness, often followed by apparent arrest. Facial and neck muscle weakness is common (Donner et al. 1975). A form of congenital dystrophy reported from Japan is associated with malformation of the central nervous system and severe mental retardation (Kamoshita, Konishi, Segawa, and Fukuyama 1976). The diagnosis from spinal muscular atrophy of infancy can only be made with confidence by means of electromyography, serum enzyme studies, and muscle biopsy. Sibs are commonly affected, and autosomal recessive inheritance seems likely in many families.

Facioscapulohumeral muscular dystrophy

This form, which is inherited by an autosomal dominant mechanism (Tyler and Wintrobe 1950; Stevenson 1953), occurs equally in the two sexes and can begin at any age from childhood until adult life, though it is usually recognized first in adolescence. Autosomal recessive inheritance has been suggested in certain families, but if this does occur it is very uncommon. Facial involvement is apparent at an early stage and is generally accompanied by weakness of shoulder-girdle muscles; this is often remarkably selective with bilateral winging of the scapulae and involvement of the pectoral muscles but with sparing of others. Biceps and brachioradiales are often selectively involved and there is difficulty in raising the arms above the head. Muscular hypertrophy is uncommon but occasionally is seen in the calves and deltoids. In the lower limbs most such patients show selective involvement of the anterior tibial muscles with bilateral foot-drop and some few, showing unusually rapid progress, demonstrate a particularly severe accentuation of the lumbar lordosis at a comparatively early stage of the disease. Scapuloperoneal muscular dystrophy is very similar but without facial weakness; however, most cases of scapuloperoneal muscular atrophy have been shown to be due to a neuropathic, as distinct from a myopathic, process (p. 385). In most patients with facioscapulohumeral dystrophy the condition is benign, runs a prolonged course with periods of apparent arrest, and muscular contractures and skeletal deformity are late in developing. There are some patients in whom the disease process is apparently abortive and after certain muscles are selectively involved, the spread of weakness seems to cease spontaneously. Indeed, substantial variation in the severity of the condition in affected members in a single family is common. Most patients show a very characteristic pouting appearance of the lips with a typical transverse smile; most affected individuals survive and remain active until a normal age. Cardiac involvement is rare and the range of intelligence is normal.

As in limb-girdle muscular dystrophy, recent studies have shown that this condition is probably a syndrome of multiple aetiology rather than a single disease entity. Thus facioscapulo-humeral muscular atrophy has been described (Fenichel, Emery, and Hunt 1967) and a study in Newcastle (Walton 1973) showed evidence of denervation in many patients. Inflammatory changes in muscle biopsy sections, resembling those of polymyositis, have also been reported in many cases (Munsat, Piper, Cancilla, and Mednick 1972) but there is no clinical response to prednisone and this clinical syndrome may also be produced by a mitochondrial myopathy (Hudgson, Bradley, and Jenkinson 1972). In infancy, the so-called Möbius syndrome may be mimicked (Hanson and Rowland 1971).

Distal muscular dystrophy

This form of the disease is rare in Britain and in the United States, but Welander (1951, 1957) reported her experience of over 250 cases in Sweden. In her series the condition was inherited as an autosomal dominant trait, began usually between the ages of 40 and 60 years and affected both sexes, though it seemed to be commoner in men than in women. Weakness began in the small muscles of the hands and in the anterior tibial muscles and calves, but eventually spread proximally, in contradistinction to the weakness observed in peroneal muscular atrophy (Charcot–Marie–Tooth disease) with which this disorder is most often confused. The condition in Sweden is comparatively benign and slowly progressive, but sporadic cases seen in other countries of the world tend to show a rather more rapid course and more severe disability (see Sumner, Crawford, and Harriman 1971 and Walton and Gardner-Medwin 1981). The difficulty of differential diagnosis from distal spinal muscular atrophy should not be underestimated.

Ocular myopathy

This disorder usually begins with progressive bilateral ptosis (Hutchinson 1879; Fuchs 1890; Kiloh and Nevin 1951). It used to be referred to in the literature as progressive nuclear ophthalmoplegia, but it has been shown that it is often due to a true myopathy of the external ocular muscles. However, Drachman, Wetzel, Wasserman, and Naito (1969) suggested that in some such cases the primary process is indeed one of denervation, and Roseberg, Schotland, Lovelace, and Rowland (1968), in reporting 28 cases, of which nine showed evidence of concomitant disease in the central nervous system (including ataxia, paraplegia, retinitis pigmentosa, and peripheral neuropathy), suggest that the condition is better called progressive ophthalmoplegia and that it is probably a syndrome of multiple pathogenesis. Certainly it is commonly associated with mitochondrial abnormalities not only in ocular muscles (Zintz and Villiger 1967) but also in the skeletal musculature (Olson, Engel, Walsh, and Einaugler 1972) in which the Type I muscle fibres may be of the so-called 'ragged-red' type, with excessive lipid droplets. Similar mitochondrial abnormalities may be found in cases of oculopharyngeal muscular dystrophy (see below) and have also been found in the cerebellum in cases of the Kearns-Sayre syndrome (Schneck, Adachi, Briet, Wolintz, and Volk 1973) in which ophthalmoplegia, retinitis pigmentosa, and cerebellar ataxia occur. Often such cases have been called 'ophthalmoplegia plus'. The complexity of the situation has been underlined by autopsy studies which have shown normal brainstem nuclei in some cases of presumed ocular myopathy (Cogan, Kuwabara, and Richardson 1962; Ross 1963), loss of neurones from the oculomotor nuclei in a case associated with spinal muscular atrophy (Aberfeld and Namba 1969), and mitochondrial abnormalities in many others. There is clear evidence of dominant inheritance in mny families but other cases are sporadic. Excessive curare sensitivity has also been reported in some cases of ocular 'myopathy' (Ross 1963; Mathew, Jacob, and Chandy 1970). Diplopia is uncommon and in most cases bilateral external ophthalmoplegia develops slowly and progressively over a period of many years. Usually there is also some weakness of the upper facial muscles and often the neck and shoulder-girdle muscles are affected to some extent. The facial weakness is particularly severe in the orbicularis oculi, but is not as intense as that seen in facio-scapulohumeral muscular dystrophy.

Oculopharyngeal muscular dystrophy

Victor, Hayes, and Adams (1962) separated a group of cases of ocular myopathy with dysphagia to which they gave the name oculopharyngeal myopathy. Bray, Kaarsoo, and Ross (1965) supported this subdivision and defined the other distinguishing clinical features, of which the most valuable is the age of onset (mean 23 years for the ocular cases and 40 for the oculopharyngeal). Many of the reported cases were of French-Canadian stock (see Barbeau 1966) and occasional cases, often sporadic, have occurred elsewhere. The inheritance in familial cases is usually dominant, but families with recessive inheritance have been described (Fried, Arlozorov, and Spira 1975). The disorder bears some slight resemblances to dystrophia myotonica, not only in some of its clinical and genetic features, but in the probable involvement of smooth muscle (Lewis 1966) and reports of abnormalities of immunoglobulins (Russe, Busey, and Barbeau 1969) in some families. Sometimes the histological appearances in the affected muscles are those of muscular dystrophy (Rebeiz, Caulfield, and Adams 1969), sometimes those of a mitochondrial myopathy (Julien, Vital, Vallat, Vallat, and le Blanc 1974).

Myotonic disorders

Myotonia, which occurs not only in man but also in certain goats (Brown and Harvey 1919), is the continued active contraction of a muscle persisting after the cessation of voluntary effort or electrical stimulation; an electrical after-discharge in the EMG accompanies the phenomenon. Clinically, it is best demonstrated as a slowness in relaxation of the grip or by a persistent dimpling after a sharp blow on a muscle belly (e.g. in the thenar eminence or tongue). It appears to be due to an abnormality of the muscle fibre itself as it persists after section or blocking of the motor nerve and after curarization (Denny-Brown and Nevin 1941). The phenomenon appears to be associated with reduced chloride conductance and permeability of the plasma membrane of the muscle fibres (Lipicky and Bryant 1966; Adrian and Marshall 1976). Three hereditary syndromes, all with autosomal dominant inheritance, have been described, namely myotonia congenita, dystrophia myotonica, and paramyotonia congenita. Only in one of these, namely dystrophia myotonica, are dystrophic changes observed within some of the affected muscles. Transitional cases may be seen suggesting a close relationship between the three disorders, but the difference in course and prognosis of typical cases of dystrophia myotonica on the one hand and of myotonia congenita on the other, and the fact that in most families the conditions breed true, confirms that they are different diseases (Caughey and Myriantho-poulos 1963). Further nosological problems arise over the close relationship between paramyotonia and the periodic paralyses. It seems clear that all of these disorders are more closely related to each other than they are to the pure muscular dystrophies.

In a rare and little-understood syndrome, sometimes called neuromyotonia, a clinically similar but probably distinct phenomenon is associated with myokymia (benign coarse fasciculation), cramps, hyperhidrosis, and sometimes muscle wasting (Gamstorp and Wohlfart 1959; Greenhouse, Bicknell, Pesch, and Seelinger 1967). The cases of continuous muscle fibre activity described by

Isaacs (1967) and Mertens and Zschocke (1965) seem to be similar. Although the failure of relaxation in these cases is similar to myotonia, no dimple is induced by percussion and electromyography shows that the after-discharge is different in form. Phenytoin is often beneficial in such cases (Gardner-Medwin and Walton 1969; Wallis, Van Poznaik, and Plum 1970).

Myotonia may also be produced experimentally by the administration of diazocholesterol and dichlorophenoxyacetic acid (Kuhn and Stein 1966; Somers and Winer 1966; Schröder and Kuhn 1968; Wallis *et al.* 1970). Symptomatic myotonia, both clinical and electrical, has been observed rarely in polyneuropathy and polymyositis (see Walton and Gardner-Medwin 1981). It must be distinguished from electrical pseudomyotonia (bizarre high-frequency discharges) commonly seen in the EMG in many metabolic myopathies and in various denervating diseases (Buchthal and Rosenfalck 1962) and from clinical pseudomyotonia (slow contraction as well as relaxation) seen in hypothyroidism (Wilson and Walton 1959; Norris and Panner 1966).

Myotonia congenita

Myotonia congenita (Thomsen 1876; Nissen 1923; Thomasen 1948) is usually present from birth. Myotonia is usually generalized, giving painless stiffness which is accentuated by rest and cold and gradually relieved by exercise. In infancy it can cause feeding difficulty and a typical 'strangled' cry. Rarely this autosomal dominant form first gives symptoms later in childhood. The EMG invariably shows typical myotonic discharges even in infancy. It is particularly easy to demonstrate myotonia by asking the patient to grip firmly and then to relax, when difficulty in opening the hand will be experienced. The phenomenon can also be demonstrated by percussion of affected muscles and is often well seen in the thenar eminence and tongue; percussion in either situation results in the formation of a dimple in the muscle which only slowly disappears. Diffuse hypertrophy of muscles usually persists throughout life in these cases, though the myotonia tends to improve. There has been evidence of an associated psychosis in some individuals and families (Johnson 1967). Rarely myotonia may increase during exertion (myotonia paradoxa) when it must be distinguished from the cramping stiffness of McArdle's disease. Hypertrophia musculorum vera (Friedreich 1863; Spiller 1913) may well be a variant of this condition.

Recessively inherited myotonia congenita (Becker 1966; Harper and Johnston 1972) now seems to be commoner than dominantly inherited Thomsen's disease and may account for most cases in which symptoms and signs are not present at birth but develop in late infancy or childhood. In these cases myotonia may be more severe than in classical Thomsen's disease.

Dystrophia myotonica

Dystrophia myotonica (myotonia atrophica) was described by Steinert (1909) and Batten and Gibb (1909) and has been reviewed by Thomasen (1948), Caughey and Myrianthopoulos (1963), and Harper (1979). It is a diffuse systemic disorder with an incidence of about 13.5 per 100 000 live births, in which myotonia and distal musular atrophy are accompanied by cataracts, frontal baldness in the male (Fig. 19.3), gonadal atrophy, cardiomyopathy, impaired pulmonary ventilation, mild endocrine anomalies, bone changes, mental defect or dementia, hypersomnia and abnormalities of the serum immunoglobulins. The affected families show progressive social decline in successive generations, diminished fertility, and an increased infantile mortality rate. The presenting symptom of the condition is usually weakness in the hands, difficulty in walking and frequent falling and myotonia is only rarely obtrusive. Poor vision, loss of weight, impotence or loss of libido, ptosis and increased sweating are common. The condition is usually observed to begin between the ages of 20 and 50 but typical clinical features of the disorder may be recognized in offspring of affected individuals in the second decade. The condition may also present in early infancy with severe muscular weakness and hypotonia and developmental delay, both physical and mental; these children may erroneously be regarded as examples of benign congenital hypotonia unless the existence of myotonic dystrophy in other members of the family is recognized (Dodge, Gamstorp, Byers, and Russell 1965; Pruzanski, 1966). The fact that infantile hypotonia due to myotonic dystrophy occurs almost exclusively with an affected female rather than male parent argues in favour of an as yet unidentified maternal environmental factor (Harper and Dyken 1972; Dyken and Harper 1973; Harper 1979).

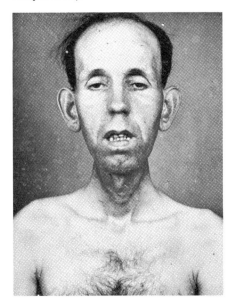

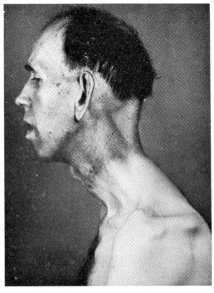

Fig. 19.3. Dystrophia myotonica. Note the frontal alopecia, myopathic facies, and wasting of the sternomastoids.

The facial appearance is characteristic (Fig. 19.3); ptosis is usual and involvement of other external ocular muscles may be seen. Wasting of the masseters, temporal muscles, and sternomastoids is almost invariable and in the extremities there is distal weakness and wasting involving mainly forearm muscles, the anterior tibial groups and the calves and peronei. Slit-lamp examination reveals cataracts in about 90 per cent of cases. Cardiac involvement is very common (Kennel, Titus, and Merideth 1974) and the pulmonary vital capacity and maximum expiratory pressure are often impaired (Kilburn, Eagan, Sieker, and Heyman 1959; Kaufman 1965); as a result, many patients tolerate barbiturate anaesthesia poorly and hypersomnia may occur (Gillam, Heaf, Kaufman, and Lucas 1964; Coccagna, Mantovani, Parchi, Mironi, and Lugaresi 1975). Disordered oesophageal contraction can often be demonstrated by contrast radiography or manometry (Gleeson, Swann, Hughes, and Lee 1967). The smooth muscle of the colon may be affected, giving severe constipation, especially in congenital cases (Lenard, Goebel, and Weigel 1977). The testes are usually small and histologically the changes in these organs resemble those of Klinefelter's syndrome though the nuclear sex is male. Irregular menstruation and infertility and prolonged parturition are common in affected females (Shore 1975). Pituitary function is usually normal but there may be a selective failure of adrenal androgenic function and occasionally thyroid activity and glucose utilization are impaired (Marshall 1959; Caughey and Myrianthopoulos 1963). Hyperostosis of the skull vault, localized or diffuse, and a small sella turcica are frequent radiological findings (Jequier 1950; Walton and Warrick 1954). Both mental defect and progressive dementia occur. Rosman and Kakulas (1966) described neuronal heterotopias in the brain at autopsy in four cases and investigation in life may reveal a high incidence of abnormality in the EEG (Barwick, Osselton, and Walton 1965; Lundervold, Refsum, and Jacobsen 1969) or progressive cerebral ventricular englargement (Refsum, Lounum, Sjaastad, and Engeset 1967). Excessive catabolism of immunoglobulin-G has been demonstrated by Wochner, Drews, Strober, and Waldmann (1966) and Jensen, Jensen, and Jarnum (1971). Abnormalities of insulin secretion have also been described in such cases (Walsh, Turtle, Miller, and McLeod 1970) and in recent years, abnormalities in the sensitivity of blood platelets to adrenaline (Bousser, Conrad, Lecrubier, and Samama 1975) and of the erythrocyte membrane (Roses and Appel 1973; Buterfield, Chesnut, Roses, and Appel 1974; Appel and Roses 1977). Myotonic discharges in the EMG may apparently be restricted to very few muscles in many patients (Streib and Sun 1983). A generalized disorder of cell membranes has been postulated (see Walton and Gardner-Medwin 1981; Aström and Adams 1982).

In genetic counselling the early recognition of affected individuals, if possible before they have a family, is of considerable importance. Slit-lamp examination and electromyography, in addition to a careful clinical examination are the most useful methods (Bundey, Carter, and Soothill 1970; Polgar, Bradley, Upton, Anderson, Howet, Petita, Roberts, and Scopa 1972; Harper 1973). The demonstration of linkage between the gene responsible for myotonic dystrophy, ABH secretor, and the Lutheran blood group (Harper, Bias, Hutchinson, and McKusick 1971; Harper, Rivas, Bias, Hutchinson, Dyken, and McKusick 1972), which all lie on chromosome 19 (see Roses et al. 1983), has allowed antenatal diagnosis by amniocentesis in some families, but unfortunately linkage is not close enough for this method to be universally applicable as yet (Harper 1979).

Most patients show progressive deterioration and become severely disabled and unable to walk within 15 to 20 years of the onset. Death from respiratory infection or cardiac failure usually occurs well before the normal age.

Paramyotonia congenita

This condition, first described by Eulenburg (1886), is characterized by myotonia which is apparent only on exposure to cold, and in addition the patients experience attacks of generalized muscular weakness similar to those of familial periodic paralysis. The condition is closely related to hyperkalaemic periodic paralysis or adynamia episodica hereditaria (Gamstorp 1956). Resnick and Engel (1967) have, however, described patients with myotonia who suffered attacks of periodic paralysis of the hypokalaemic variety. Thus although the nosological status of paramyotonia congenita remains confused (Pratt 1967) it remains a useful diagnostic category for patients in whom myotonia and episodic weakness are induced by cold, so long as it is recognized that the particular precipitants and any associated electrolyte changes in each family must be worked out if useful advice and treatment are to be given (Thrush, Morris, and Salmon 1972). It is best reserved for patients in whom the myotonia is severe, sometimes paradoxical (increased by muscular contraction) and clearly worsened by cold. Cases at the other end of the spectrum with very mild myotonia but with severe episodes of muscular weakness are probably best called myotonic periodic paralysis (van't Hoff 1962; Riggs, Griggs, and Moxley 1977).

Chondrodystrophic myotonia (the Schwartz–Jampel syndrome)

This rare syndrome, presumed to be of autosomal recessive inheritance, is characterized by generalized myotonia, dwarfism, skeletal abnormalities with hip contractures or dislocations, and a peculiar facial appearance with tense puckering of the mouth, blepharospasm, and narrow palpebral fissures (Schwartz and Jampel 1962; Aberfeld, Hinterbuchner, and Schneider 1965; Aberfeld, Namba, Vye, and Grob 1970). Some patients show continuous muscle-fibre activity in the EMG (Cao, Cianchetti, Calisti, De Virgiliis, Ferreli, and Tangheroni 1978). Intelligence is usually normal; the myotonia may be relieved by procaine amide (Huttenlocher, Landwirth, Hanson, Gallacher, and Bensch 1969).

Treatment

Muscular dystrophy

Regrettably there is no evidence that any form of drug treatment has any influence upon the course of muscular dystrophy. Many remedies have been tried in the past and have been found wanting and none is to be recommended for routine administration, though complications such as respiratory infection may demand appropriate antibiotics. Dubowitz and Heckmatt (1980) have reviewed drug trials carried out in the past and methods of assessment of the clinical response. Despite recent advances in knowledge of pathogenesis, there is no convincing evidence that calcium antagonists have any influence on the disease process or that protease inhibitors are yet likely to be safe or effective in human subjects (Walton 1983). There is good evidence to suggest that physical exercise is of value in delaying the march of the weakness (Vignos and Watkins 1966) and the onset of contractures and it is advisable to institute a regular programme of exercise, which may be started under the supervision of a skilled physiotherapist and subsequently continued at home by the patients, who, like their parents and other relatives, should be given appropriate instructions. Passive stretching of those tendons, such as the tendons of Achilles, which show a tendency to shorten, should also be carried out regularly, particularly in Duchenne type cases (Vignos, Spencer, and Archibald 1963). In certain selected cases the wearing of light spinal supports is helpful in delaying skeletal deformity and occasionally calipers and night-splints are successful in helping affected individuals to walk for longer periods than they would otherwise be able to do. There is evidence that surgical division of the Achilles tendons in selected cases, a procedure which has long been regarded as being contra-indicated, and certain other surgical procedures may be beneficial in selected cases, provided these are followed by immediate mobilization of the patient in walking plasters or calipers (Siegel, Miller, and Ray 1968; Siegel 1972). Immobilization of patients with muscular dystrophy is in general to be avoided as far as ever possible as this frequently causes deterioration. Walton and Gardner-Medwin (1981) point out that the use of radical surgical measures is controversial. Certainly patients with Duchenne dystrophy may be helped to walk for two or three years longer than without surgery, but many at this stage take to a wheelchair with relief and the time comes when adjustment to a wheelchair life may be preferred to aggressive physiotherapeutic measures. Many types of appliance are of great value in improving the quality of life at all ages and the advice of a skilled occupational therapist may be invaluable (Harpin 1981). Physical methods of treatment have been reviewed by Vignos (1983). Not least in importance is the psychological management of these patients which may demand considerable reserves of patience and understanding on the part of parents, doctors, nurses, and social workers. Optimism and encouragement, however unjustifiable in the face of continuing deterioration, are greatly needed.

Myotonia

In dystrophia myotonica, no treatment is known which will influence the progressive muscular wasting and weakness which eventually develops. In paramyotonia, treatment of the attacks of periodic paralysis is similar to that required in patients with familial periodic paralysis and depends upon whether the paralysis is shown to be hypo- or hyperkalaemic in type. Myotonia itself may, however, be substantially relieved by means of appropriate drugs. These are particularly valuable in patients with myotonia congenita, but are also helpful in some with myotonic dystrophy in whom the myotonia is severe. Of drugs used in the past, including quinine, prednisone, and procainamide, the latter is one of the most successful in a dosage of 250-500 mg three or four times daily, depending upon tolerance (Leyburn and Walton 1959). Later it was shown (Munsat 1967) that, if anything, phenytoin sodium (*Epanutin* or *Dilantin*) is sometimes even more successful in a dosage of 100 mg three times daily.

References

Aberfeld, D. C., Hinterbuchner, L. P., and Schneider, M. (1965). Myotonia, dwarfism, diffuse bone disease and unusual ocular and facial abnormalities (a new syndrome). *Brain* 88, 313.
—— and Namba, T. (1969). Progressive ophthalmoplegia in Kugelberg-Welander disease: report of a case, *Arch. Neurol., Chicago* 20, 253.
——, ——, Vye, M. V., and Grob, D. (1970). Chondrodystrophic myotonia: report of two cases. *Arch. Neurol., Chicago* 22, 455.
Adrian, R. H. and Marshall, M. W. (1976). Action potentals reconstructed in normal and myotonic muscle fibres. *J. Physiol.* 258, 125.
Alberts, M. C. and Samaha, F. J. (1974). Serum pyruvate kinase in muscle disease and carrier states. *Neurology, Minneapolis* 24, 462.
Appel, S. H. and Roses, A. D. (1977). Membranes and myotonia. In *Pathogenesis of human muscular dystrophies* (ed. L. P. Rowland), p. 747. Excerpta Medica, Amsterdam.
Aström, K. E. and Adams, R. D. (1982). Myotonic disorders. In *Skeletal muscle pathology* (ed. F. L. Mastaglia and J. N. Walton) Ch. 7. Churchill-Livingstone, Edinburgh.
Bakker, E. and 15 others (1985). Prenatal diagnosis and carrier detection of Duchenne muscular dystrophy with closely linked RFLPs. *Lancet* i, 655.
Ballantyne, J. P. and Hansen, S. (1974). Myopathies: the neurogenic hypothesis. *Lancet* ii, 588.
Banker, B. O., Victor, M., and Adams, R. D. (1975). Arthrogryposis multiplex due to congenital muscular dystrophy. *Brain* 80, 319.
Barbeau, A. (1966). The syndrome of hereditary late onset ptosis and dysphagia in French Canada. In *Progressive muskeldystrophie, myotonie, myasthenie* (ed. E. Kuhn) p. 102. Springer, New York.
Barwick, D. D., Osselton, J. W., and Walton, J. N. (1965). Electroencephalographic studies in hereditary myopathy. *J. Neurol. Neurosurg. Psychiat.* 28, 109.

Batten, F. E. (1909). The myopathies or muscular dystrophies; critical review. *Quart. J. Med.* 3, 313.
—— and Gibb, H. P. (1909). Myotonia atrophica. *Brain* 32, 187.
Becker, P. E. (1953). *Dystrophia musculorum progressiva*. Thieme, Stuttgart.
—— (1957). Neue Ergebnisse der Genetik der Muskeldystrophien. *Acta Genet. med. Roma* 7, 303.
—— (1966). Zur Genetik der Myotonien. In *Progressive muskeldystrophie, myotonie, myasthenie* (ed. E. Kuhn), p. 247. Springer, New York.
—— and Kiener, F. (1955). Eine neue x-chromosomale Muskeldystrophie. *Arch. Psychiat. Nervenkr.* 193 427.
Ben Hamida, M., Fardeau, M., and Attia, N. (1983). Severe childhood muscular dystrophy affecting both sexes and frequent in Tunisia. *Muscle & Nerve* 6, 469.
Bousser, M. G., Conrad, J., Lecrubier, C., and Samama, M. (1975). Increased sensitivity of platelets to adrenaline in human myotonic dystrophy. *Lancet* ii, 307.
Bray, G. M., Kaarsoo, M., and Ross, R. T. (1965). Ocular myopathy with dysphagia. *Neurology, Minneapolis* 15, 678.
Brown, G. L. and Harvey, A. M. (1939). Congenital myotonia in the goat. *Brain* 62, 341.
Buchthal, F. and Rosenfalck, P. (1962). Electrophysiological aspects of myopathy with particular reference to progressive muscular dystrophy. In *Muscular dystrophy in man and animals* (ed. G. H. Bourne and N. Golarz) Ch. 7. Karger, Basle.
Bundey, S., Carter, C. O. and Soothill, J. F. (1970). Early recognition of heterozygotes for the gene for dystrophia myotonica. *J. Neurol. Neurosurg. Psychiat.* 33, 279.
Butterfield, D. A., Chesnut, D. B., Roses, A. D., and Appel, S. H. (1974). Electron spin resonance studies of erythrocytes from patients with myotonic muscular dystrophy. *Proc. Nat. Acad. Sci.* 71, 909.
Cao, A., Cinchetti, C., Calisti, L., de Virgiliis, S., Ferreli, A., and Tangheroni, W. (1978) Schwartz–Jampel syndrome: clinical, electrophysiological and histopathological study of a severe variant. *J. neurol. sci.* 35, 175.
Caughey, J. E. and Myrianthopoulos, N. C. (1963. *Dystrophia myotonica and related disorders*. Thomas, Springfield, Illinois.
Chung, C. S. and Morton, N. E. (1959). Discrimination of genetic entities in muscular dystrophy. *Am. J. hum. Genet.* 11, 339.
Coccagna, G., Mantovani, M., Parchi, C., Mironi, F., and Lugaresi, E. (1975). Alveolar hypoventilation and hypersomnia in myotonic dystrophy. *J. Neurol. Neurosurg. Psychiat.* 38, 977.
Cogan, D. G., Kuwabara, T., and Richardson, E. P. (1962). Pathology of abiotrophic ophthalmoplegia externa. *Bull. Johns Hopk. Hosp.* 111, 42.
Cullen, M. J. and Fulthorpe, J. J. (1975). Stages in fibre breakdown in Duchenne muscular dystrophy. An electron microscopic study. *J. neurol. Sci.* 24, 179.
—— and Mastaglia, F. L. (1982). Pathological reactions of skeletal muscle. In *Skeletal muscle pathology* (ed. F. L. Mastaglia and J. N. Walton) Ch. 2. Churchill-Livingstone, Edinburgh.
Denny-Brown, D. and Nevin, S. (1941). The phenomenon of myotonia. *Brain* 64, 1.
Dodge, P. R., Gamstorp, I., Byers, R. K., and Russell, P. (1965). Myotonic dystrophy in infancy and childhood. *Pediatrics* 35, 3.
Donner, M., Rapola, J., and Somer, H. (1975). Congenital muscular dystrophy: a clinicopathological and follow-up study of 15 patients. *Neuropädiatrie* 6, 239.
Drachman, D. A., Wetzel, N., Wasserman, M., and Naito, H. (1969). Experimental denervation of ocular muscles. *Arch. Neurol., Chicago* 21, 170.
Dreifuss, F. E. and Hogan, G. R. (1961). Survival in x-chromosomal muscular dystrophy. *Neurology, Minneapolis* 11, 734.
Dubowitz, V. (1960). Progressive muscular dystrophy of the Duchenne type in females and its mode of inheritance. *Brain* 83, 432.
—— (1965). Intellectual impairment in muscular dystrophy. *Arch. Dis. Childh.* 40, 296.
—— and Heckmatt, J. (1980). Management of muscular dystrophy. *Br. med. Bull.* 36, 139.
Dyken, P. R. and Harper, P. S. (1973). Congenital dystrophia myotonica. *Neurology, Minneapolis* 23, 465.
Ebashi, S. and Sugati, H. (1978). The role of calcium in physiological and pathological processes of skeletal muscle. In *Abstracts of the IVth International Congress on Neuromuscular Diseases*, Montreal. Excerpta Medica, 1CS 455.
Emery, A. E. H. (1972). Abnormalities of the electrocardiogram in hereditary myopathies. *J. med. Genet.* 9, 8.

—— (1981). Genetic aspects of neuromuscular disease. In *Disorders of voluntary muscle* (ed J. N. Walton) 4th edn. Ch. 22. Churchill-Livingstone, Edinburgh.

—— Clack, E. R., and Taylor, J. L. (1967). Detection of carriers of benign X-linked muscular dystrophy. *Br. med. J.* **4**, 522.

—— and Dreifuss, F. E. (1966). Unusual type of benign X-linked muscular dystrophy. *J. Neurol. Neurosurg. Psychiat.* **29**, 338.

—— and Morton, R. (1968). Genetic counselling in lethal X-linked disorders. *Acta genet., Basel* **18**, 534.

—— Smith, C. A. B., and Sanger, R. (1969). The linkage relations of the loci for benign (Becker type) X-borne muscular dystrophy, colour blindness and the Xg blood group. *Ann. hum. Genet., London* **32**, 261.

—— and Walton, J. N. (1967). The genetics of muscular dystrophy. In *Progress in medical genetics* (ed. A. G. Steinberg and A. G. Bearn), Vol V, p. 116. Grune & Stratton, New York.

—— Watt, M. S., and Clack, E. R. (1972). The effect of genetic counselling in Duchenne muscular dystrophy. *Clin. Genet.* **3**, 147.

Eulenberg, A. (1886). Ueber eine familiäre, durch sechs Generationen verfolgbare Form congenitaler Paramyotonie. *Neurol. Zbl.* **5**, 265.

Fenichel, G. M., Emcry, E. S. and Hunt, P. (1967). Neurogenic atrophy simulating facioscapulohumeral muscular dystrophy: a dominant form. *Arch. Neurol., Chicago* **17**, 257.

Ferrier, P., Bamatter, F., and Klein, D. (1965). Muscular dystrophy (Duchenne) in a girl with Turner's syndrome. *J. med. Genet.* **2**, 38.

Fried, K., Arlozorov, A., and Spira, R. (1975). Autosomal recessive oculopharyngeal muscular dystrophy. *J. med. Genet.* **12**, 416.

Friedreich, N. (1863). Ueber congenitale halbseitige Kopfhypertrophie. *Virchows Arch. path. Anat.* **38**, 474.

Fuchs, E. (1890). Ueber isolierte doppelseitige Ptosia. *Arch. Ophthal., Chicago* **36**, 234.

Gamstorp, I. (1956). Adynamia episodica hereditaria. *Arch. paediat., Uppsala* Suppl. 108.

—— and Wohlfart, G. (1959). A syndrome characterised by myokymia, myotonia, muscular wasting and increased perspiration. *Acta psychiat. scand.* **34**, 181.

Gardner-Medwin, D. (1970). Mutation rate in Duchenne type of muscular dystrophy. *J. med. Genet.* **7**, 334.

—— and Walton, J. N. (1969). Myokymia with impaired muscular relaxation. *Lancet* **i**, 127.

Gillam, P. M. S., Heaf, P. J. D., Kaufman, L., and Lucas, B.G.B. (1964). Respiration in dystrophia myotonica. *Thorax* **19**, 112.

Gleeson, J. A., Swann, J. C., Hughes, D. T. D., and Lee, F. I. (1967). Dystrophia myotonica—a radiological survey. *Br. J. Radiol.* **40**, 96.

Gomez, M. R., Engel, A. G., Dewald, G., and Peterson, H. A. (1977). Failure of inactivation of Duchenne dystrophy X-chromosome in one of female identical twins. *Neurology, Minneapolis* **27**, 537.

Greenhouse, A. H., Bicknell, J. M., Pesch, R. N., and Seelinger, D. F. (1967). Myotonia, myokymia, hyperhidrosis and wasting of muscle. *Neurology, Minneapolis* **17**, 263.

Gubbay, S. S., Walton, J. N., and Pearce, G. W. (1966). Clinical and pathological study of a case of congenital muscular dystrophy. *J. Neurol. Neurosurg. Psychiat.* **29**, 500.

Hanson, P. A. and Rowland, L. P. (1971). Möbius syndrome and facioscapulohumeral muscular dystrophy. *Arch. Neurol., Chicago* **24**, 31.

Harper, P. S. (1973). Pre-symptomatic detection and genetic counselling in myotonic dystrophy. *Clin. Genet.* **4**, 1.

—— (1979). *Myotonic dystrophy*. Saunders, London.

—— Bias, W. B., Hutchinson, J. R., and McKusick, V. A. (1971). ABH secretor status of the fetus: a genetic marker identifiable by amniocentesis. *J. med. Genet.* **8**, 438.

—— and Dyken, P. R. (1972). Early-onset dystrophia myotonica: evidence supporting a maternal environmental factor. *Lancet* **ii**, 53.

—— and Johnston, D. M. (1972). Recessively inherited myotonia congenita. *J. med. Genet.* **9**, 213.

—— Rivas, M. L., Bias, W. B., Hutchinson, J. R., Dyken, P. R., and McKusick, V. A. (1972). Genetic linkage confirmed between the locus for myotonic dystrophy and the ABH-secretor and Lutheran blood group loci. *Am. J. hum. Genet.* **24**, 310.

Harpin, P. (1981). *With a little help*. Muscular Dystrophy Group of Great Britain, London.

Hudgson, P., Bradley, W. G., and Jenkinson, M. (1972). Familial 'mitochondrial' myopathy: a myopathy associated with disordered oxidative metabolism in muscle fibres. Part I—Clinical, electrophysiological and pathological findings. *J. neurol. Sci.* **16**, 343.

Hutchinson, J. (1879). An ophthalmoplegia externa or symmetrical immobility (partial) of the eye with ptosis. *Trans. med.-chir. Soc., Edinburgh* **62**, 307.

Huttenlocher, P. R., Landwirth, J., Hanson, V., Gallacher, B.B., and Bensch, K. (1969). Osteochondro-muscular dystrophy: a disorder manifested by multiple skeletal deformities, myotonia and dystrophic changes in muscle. *Pediatrics* **44**, 945.

Ionasescu, V., Zellweger, H., and Conway, T. W. (1971). A new approach for carrier detection in Duchenne muscular dystrophy. *Neurology, Minneapolis* **21**, 703.

Isaacs, H. (1967). Continuous muscle fibre activity in an Indian male with additional evidence of terminal motor fibre abnormality. *J.Neurol. Neurosurg. Psychiat.* **30**, 126.

Jackson, C. E. and Carey, J. H. (1961). Progressive muscular dystrophy: autosomal recessive type. *Pediatrics* **28**, 77.

Jalbert, P., Mouriquand, C., Beaudoing, A., and Jalliard, M. (1966). Myopathie progressive de type Duchenne et mosaique XO/XX/XXX: considerations sur la genèse de la fibre musculaire striée. *Ann. Génét.* **9**, 104.

Jensen, H., Jensen, K. B., and Jarnum, S. (1971). Turnover of IgG and IgM in myotonic dystrophy. *Neurology, Minneapolis* **21**, 68.

Jequier, M. (1950). Dystrophie myotonique et hyperostose cranienne. *Schweiz. med. Wschr.* **80**, 593.

Jerusalem, F., Engel, A. G., and Gomez, M. R. (1974). Duchenne dystrophy—I. Morphometric study of the muscle microvasculature. *Brain* **97**, 115.

Johnson, J. (1967). Myotonia congenita (Thomsen's disease) and hereditary psychosis. *Br. J. Psychiat.* **113**, 1025.

Johnston, H. A. (1964). Severe muscular dystrophy in girls. *J. med. Genet.* **1**, 79.

Julien, J., Vital, C., Vallat, J. M., Vallat, M., and le Blanc, M. (1974). Oculopharyngeal muscular dystrophy: a case with abnormal mitochondria and 'fingerprint' inclusions. *J. neurol. Sci.* **21**, 165.

Kamoshita, S., Konishi, Y., Segawa, M., and Fukuyama, Y. (1976). Congenital muscular dystrophy as a disease of the central nervous system. *Arch. Neurol., Chicago* **33**, 513.

Kaufman, L. (1965). Respiratory function in muscular dystrophy. In *Research in muscular dystrophy*, 3rd series p. 79. Pitman, London.

Kennel, A. J., Titus, J. L., and Merideth, J. (1974). Pathologic findings in the atrioventricular conduction system in myotonic dystrophy. *Mayo Clin. Proc.* **49**, 838.

Kilburn, K. H., Eagan, J. T., Sieker, H. O., and Heyman, A. (1959). Cardiopulmonary insufficiency in myotonic and progressive muscular dystrophy. *New Engl. J. Med.* **261**, 1089.

Kiloh, L. G. and Nevin, S. (1951). Progressive dystrophy of external ocular muscles (ocular myopathy). *Brain* **74**, 115.

Kloepfer, H. W. and Talley, C. (1958). Autosomal recessive inheritance of Duchenne type muscular dystrophy. *Ann. hum. Genet.* **22**, 138.

Kuhn, E. and Stein, W. (1966). Modellmyotonie nach 2,4-dichlorphenoxyacetat (2,4-D). *Klin. Wschr.* **44**, 700.

The Lancet (1983). DNA probes for the Duchenne carrier. *Lancet* **ii**, 497.

Lenard, H.-G., Goebel, H. H., and Weigel, W. (1977). Smooth muscle involvement in congenital myotonic dystrophy *Neuropädiatrie* **8**, 42.

Lewis, I. (1966). Late-onset muscular dystrophy: oculopharyngo-oesophageal variety. *Can. med. Ass. J.* **95**, 146.

Leyburn, P. and Walton, J. N. (1959). The treatment of myotonia: a controlled trial. *Brain* **82**, 81.

Lipicky, R. J. and Bryant, S. H. (1966). Sodium, potassium and chloride fluxes in intercostal muscle from normal goats with hereditary myotonia. *J. Gen. Physiol.* **50**, 89.

Lundervold, A., Refsum, S., and Jacobsen, W. (1969). The EEG in dystrophia myotonica. *Eur. Neurol.* **2**, 279.

Markand, O. N., North, R. R., D'Agostina, A. N., and Daly, D. D. (1969). Benign sex-linked muscular dystrophy. *Neurology, Minneapolis,* **19**, 617.

Marshall, J. (1959). Observations on endocrine function in dystrophia myotonica. *Brain* **82**, 221.

Mastaglia, F.L. and Walton, J. N. (1971). Histological and histochemical changes in skeletal muscle from cases of chronic juvenile and early adult spinal muscular atrophy (the Kugelberg–Welander syndrome). *J. neurol. Sci.* **12**, 15.

Mathew, N. T., Jacob, J. C., and Chandy, J. (1970). Familial ocular myopathy with curare sensitivity. *Arch. Neurol., Chicago.* **22**, 68.

McComas, A. J., Sica, R. E. P., and Campbell, M. J. (1971). 'Sick' motoneurones: a unifying concept of muscle disease. *Lancet* **i**, 321.

Mendell, J. R., Engel, W. K., and Derrier, E. C. (1971). Duchenne muscular dystrophy: functional ischemia reproduces its characteristic lesions. *Science* **172**, 1143.

Mertens, H. G. and Zschocke, S. (1965). Neuromyotonie. *Klin. Wschr.* **43**, 917.

Mokri, B. and Engel, A. G. (1975). Duchenne dystrophy: electron microscopic findings pointing to a basic or early abnormality in the plasma membrane of the muscle fibre. *Neurology, Minneapolis* **25**, 1111.

Morton, N. E., and Chung, C. S. (1959). Formal genetics of muscular dystrophy, *Amer. J. hum. Genet.* **11**, 360.

Munsat, T. L. (1967). Therapy of myotonia: a double-blind evaluation of diphenyl-hydantoin, procainamide and placebo. *Neurology, Minneapolis*, **17**, 359.

—— Piper, D., Cancilla, P., and Mednick, J. (1972. Inflammatory myopathy with facioscapulohumeral distribution. *Neurology, Minneapolis*, **22**, 335.

Murphy, E. G., Thompson, M. W., Corey, P. N. J., and Conen, P. E. (1965). Varying manifestations of Duchenne muscular dystrophy in a family with affected females. In *Muscle* (ed. W. M. Paul, E. E. Daniel, C. M. Kay, and G. Monckton). Pergamon, New York.

Musch, B. C., Papapetropoulos, T. A., McQueen, D. A., Hudgson, P., and Weightman, D. (1975). A comparison of the structure of small blood vessels in normal, denervated and dystrophic human muscle. *J. neurol. Sci.*, **26**, 221.

Nicholson, G. A., Gardner-Medwin, D., Pennington, R. J. T., and Walton, J. N. (1979). Carrier detection in Duchenne muscular dystrophy: assessment of the effect of age on detection rate with serum-creatine-kinase activity. *Lancet* **i**, 692.

Nicholson, L. (1981). Serum myoglobin in muscular dystrophy and carrier detection. *J. neurol. Sci.* **51**, 411.

Nissen, K. (1923). Beiträge zur Kenntnis der Thomsen'schen Krankheit (myotonia congenita) mit besonderer Berücksichtigung des hereditären Momentes und seiner Beziehungen zu den Mendelschen Vererbungsregiln. *Z. klin. Med.* **496**, 58.

Norris, F. H. and Panner, B.J. (1966). Hypothyroid myopathy: clinical, electromyographical and ultrastructural observations. *Arch. Neurol., Chicago* **14**, 574.

Olson, W., Engel, W. K., Walsh, G. O., and Einaugler, R. (1972). Oculocraniosomatic neuromuscular disease with 'ragged-red' fibers: histochemical and ultrastructural changes in limb muscles of a group of patients with idiopathic progressive external ophthalmoplegia. *Arch. Neurol., Chicago* **26**, 193.

Oppenheim, H. (1900). Ueber allgemeine und localisierte Atonie der Musculatur (myatonie) in frühen Kindesalter. *Mschr. Psychiat. Neurol.* **8**, 232.

Paulson, O. B., Engel, A. G., and Gomez, M. R. (1974). Muscle blood flow in Duchenne type muscular dystrophy, limb-girdle dystrophy, polymyositis, and in normal controls. *J. Neurol. Neurosurg. Psychiat.* **37**, 685.

Pearson, C. M. and Fowler, W. G. (1963). Hereditary non-progressive muscular dystrophy inducing arthrogryposis syndrome. *Brain* **86**, 75.

Penn, A. S., Lisak, R.P., and Rowland, L. P. (1970). Muscular dystrophy in young girls. *Neurology, Minneapolis* **20**, 147.

Pennington, R. J. T. (1981). Biochemical aspects of muscle disease. In *Disorders of voluntary muscle* (ed. J. N. Walton) 4th edn, Ch. 12. Churchill-Livingstone, Edinburgh.

Polgar, J. G., Bradley, W. G., Upton, A. R. M., Anderson, J., Howat, J. M. L., Petito, F., Roberts, D. F., and Scopa, J. (1972). The early detection of dystrophia myotonica. *Brain* **95**, 761.

Pratt, R. T. C. (1967). *The genetics of neurological disorders*. Oxford Medical, London.

Pruzanksi, W. (1966). Variants of myotonic dystrophy in pre-adolescent life (the syndrome of myotonic dysembryoplasia). *Brain* **89**, 563.

Rebeiz, J. J., Caulfield, J. B., and Adams, R. D. (1969). Oculopharyngeal dystrophy—a presenescent myopathy: a clinicopathologic study. In *Progress in neuro-ophthalmology*, Excerpta Medica International Congress Series No. 176. Excerpta Medica, Amsterdam.

Refsum, S., Lounum, A., Sjaastad, O., and Engeset, A. (1967). Dystrophia myotonica: repeated pneumoencephalographic studies in ten patients. *Neurology, Minneapolis* **17**, 345.

Resnick, J. S. and Engel, W.K. (1967). Myotonic lid lag in hypokalaemic periodic paralysis. *J. Neurol. Neurosurg. Psychiat* **30**, 47.

Riggs, J. E., Griggs, R. C., and Moxley, R. T. (1977). Acetazolamide induced weakness in paramyotonia congenita. *Ann. intern. Med.* **86**, 169.

Rosenberg, R. N., Schotland, D.L., Lovelace, R. E., and Rowland, L. P. (1968). Progressive ophthalmoplegia. *Arch. Neurol., Chicago* **19**, 362.

Roses, A. D. and Appel, S.H. (1973). Protein kinase activity in erythrocyte ghosts of patients with myotonic muscular dystrophy. *Proc. Nat. Acad. Sci.* **70**, 1855.

——, Pericak-Vance, M. A., Yamaoka, L. H., Stubblefield, E., Stajich, J., Vance, J. M., Roses, M. J., and Carter, D.B. (1983). Recombinant DNA strategies in genetic neurological disease. *Muscle & Nerve* **6**, 339.

——, Roses, M. J., Miller, S. E., Hull, K. L., and Appel, S. H. (1976). Carrier detection in Duchenne muscular dystrophy. *New Engl. J.Med.* **294**. 193.

Rosman, N. P. and Kakulas, B. A. (1966). Mental deficiency associated with muscular dystrophy. A neuropathological study. *Brain* **89**, 769.

Ross, R. T. (1963). Ocular myopathy sensitive to curare. *Brain* **86**, 67.

Rotthauwe, H. -W., Mortier, W., and Beyer, H. (1972). Neuer Typ einer recessiv X-chromosomal vererbten Muskeldystrophie: Scapulo-humerodistale Muskeldystrophie mit frühzeitigen Kontrakturen und Herzrythmusstörungen. *Humangenetik* **16**, 181.

Rowland, L. P. (1976). Pathogenesis of muscular dystrophies. *Arch. Neurol., Chicago* **33**, 315.

Russe, H., Busey, H., and Barbeau, A. (1969). Immunoglobulin changes in oculopharyngeal muscular dystrophy. *Proc. 3nd Internat. Congr. Neurogenetics*. Montreal. Excerpta Medica, ICS 175.

Schneck, L., Adachi, M., Briet, P., Wolintz, A., and Volk, B. W. (1973). Ophthalmoplegia plus with morphological and chemical studies of cerebellar and muscle tissue. *J. neurol. Sci.* **19**, 37.

Schröder, J. M. and Kuhn, E. (1968). Zur Ultrastruktur der Muskelfaser bei der experimentellen 'Myotonie' mit 20, 25-Diazacholesterin. *Virchows Arch. Abt. A Path. Anat.* **344**, 181.

Schwartz, O. and Jampel, R. S. (1962). Congenital blepharophimosis associated with a unique generalized myopathy. *Arch. Ophthalmol.* **68**, 52.

Shore, R.N. (1975). Myotonic dystrophy: hazards of pregnancy and infancy. *Develop. Med. Child Neurol.* **17**, 356.

Siegel, I. (1972). Equinocavovarus in muscular dystrophy: its treatment by percutaneous tarsal medullostomy and soft tissue release. *Arch. Surg.* **104**, 644.

——, Miller, J. E., and Ray, R. D. (1968). Subcutaneous lower limb tenotomy in the treatment of pseudohypertrophic muscular dystrophy. *J. Surg.* **50-A**, 1437.

Skyring, A. and McKusick, V. A. (1961). Clinical, genetic and electrocardiographic studies in childhood muscular dystrophy. *Am. J. med. Sci.* **242**, 534.

Somers, J. E. and Winer, N. (1966). Reversible myopathy and myotonia following administration of a hypocholesterolemic agent. *Neurology, Minneapolis* **16**, 761.

Steinert, H.(1909). Myopatholigische Beiträge: I. Ueber das klinische und anatomische Bild des Muskelschwunds der Myotoniker. *Dtsch Z. Nervenheilk.* **37**, 58.

Stevenson, A. C. (1953). Muscular dystrophy in Northern Ireland. *Ann. Eugen., London* **18**, 50.

Streib, E. W. and Sun, S. F. (1983). Distribution of electrical myotonia in myotonic muscular dystrophy. *Ann. Neurol.* **14**, 80.

Sumner, D., Crawfurd, M. D'A., and Harriman, D.G.F. (1971). Distal muscle dystrophy in an English family. *Brain* **94**, 51.

Thomas, P. K., Calne, D. B., and Elliott, C. F. (1972). X-linked scapuloperoneal syndrome. *J. Neurol. Neurosurg. Psychiat.* **35**, 208.

Thomasen, E. (1948). *Thomsen's disease, paramyotonia, dystrophia myotonica*. Universitetsforlaget, Aahus.

Thomsen, J. (1876). Tonische Krämpfe inwillkürlich beweglichen Muskeln in Folge von ererbter psychischer Disposition (ataxia muscularis?). *Arch. Psychiat. Nervenkr.* **6**, 706.

Thrush, D. C., Morris, C.J., and Salmon, M. V. (1972). Paramyotonia congenita—a clinical, histochemical and pathological study. *Brain* **95**, 536.

Tomlinson, B. E., Walton, J. N., and Irving, D. (1974). Spinal cord limb motor neurones in muscular dystrophy. *J. neurol. Sci.* **22**, 305.

Turner, J. W. A. (1940). The relationship between amyotonia congenita and congenital myopathy. *Brain* **63**, 163.

—— (1949). On amyotonia congenita. *Brain* **74**, 25.

—— and Lees, F. (1962). Congenital myopathy—a fifty year follow-up. *Brain* **85**, 733.

Tyler, F. H. and Wintrobe, M. M. (1950). Studies in disorders of muscle. I. The problem of progressive muscular dystrophy. *Ann. intern. Med.* **32**, 72.

van't Hoff, W. (1962). Familial myotonic periodic paralysis. *Quart. J. Med.* **31**, 385.

Victor, M., Hayes, R., and Adams, R. D. (1962). Oculopharyngeal muscular dystrophy. A familial disease of late life characterised by dysphagia and progressive ptosis of the eyelids. *New Engl. J. Med.* **267**, 1267.

Vignos, P. J. (1983). Physical models of rehabilitation in neuromuscular disease. *Muscle & Nerve* **6**, 323.

——, Spencer, G. E., and Archibald, K. C. (1963). Management of progressive muscular dystrophy of childhood. *J. Am. med. Ass.* **184**, 89.

—— and Watkins, M. P. (1966). The effect of exercise in muscular dystrophy. *J. Am. med. Ass.* **197**, 843.

Wallis, W. E., Van Poznak, A., and Plum, F. (1970). Generalized muscular stiffness, fasciculations, and myokymia of peripheral nerve origin. *Arch. Neurol.*, *Chicago* **22**, 430.

Walsh, J. C., Turtle, J. R., Miller, S., and McLeod, J. G. (1970). Abnormalities of insulin secretion in dystrophia myotonica. *Brain* **93**, 731.

Walton, J. N. (1956 *a*). The inheritance of muscular dystrophy: further observations. *Ann. hum. Genet.* **21**, 40.

—— (1956*b*). Amyotonia congenita: a follow-up study. *Lancet* **i**, 1023.

—— (1966). Diseases of muscle. *Abstr. Wld Med.* **40**, 1, 81.

—— (1973). Some changing concepts in neuromuscular disease. In *Clinical studies in myology*, Proceedings of the Second International Congress on Muscle Diseases, Part 2, ed. B. A. Kakulas, p. 429. Excerpta Medica, Amsterdam.

—— (1983). Changing concepts of neuromuscular disease. *Hosp. Update* **9**, 949.

—— and Gardner-Medwin, D. (1981). Progressive muscular dystrophy and the myotonic disorders. In *Disorders of voluntary muscle* (ed. J. N. Walton) 4th edn, Ch. 14. Churchill-Livingstone, Edinburgh.

—— and Mastaglia, F. L. (Eds.) (1980). The muscular dystrophies. *Br. med. Bull.* **36**, (2).

—— and Nattrass, F. J. (1954). On the classification, natural history and treatment of the myopathies. *Brain* **77**, 169.

—— and Warrick, C. K. (1954). Osseous changes in myopathy. *Br. J. Radiol.* **27**, 1.

Welander, L. (1951). Myopathia distalis tarda hereditaria. *Acta med. scand.* Suppl. 264, 1.

—— (1957). Homozygous appearance of distal myopathy. *Acta genet. med.*, *Roma* **7**, 321.

Wharton, B.A. (1965). An unusual variety of muscular dystrophy. *Lancet* **i**, 603.

Williamson, R. (1983). Cloned gene probes and the study of human inherited disease. *Hosp. Update* **9**, 25.

Wilson, J. and Walton, J. N. (1959). The muscular manifestations of hypothyroidism. *J. Neurol. Psychiat.* **22**, 320.

Wochner, R. D., Drews, G., Strober, W., and Waldmann, T. A. (1966). Accelerated breakdown of immunoglobulin G (IgG) in myotonic dystrophy: a hereditary error of immunoglobulin catabolism. *J. clin. Invest.* **45**, 321.

Zellweger, H., Afifi, A., McCormick, W. F., and Mergner, W. (1967). Severe congenital muscular dystrophy. *Am. J. Dis. Child* **114**, 591.

Zintz, Von R. and Villiger, W. (1967). Elektronenmikroskopische Befunde bei 3 Fällen von chronisch progressiver okulärer Muskeldystrophie. *Ophthalmologica Basel* **153**, 439.

Inflammatory disorders of muscle

Specific infections

Voluntary muscle may be involved as a secondary effect of suppuration arising in skin, bone, or connective tissue and widespread necrosis frequently occurs following trauma as a result of infection with the anaerobic organism of gas gangrene. Some viral infections may give rise to an acute myositis; this is particularly common in infection with certain viruses of the Coxsackie type. Thus in epidemic pleurodynia, often called Bornholm disease, due to Coxsackie virus B5, pain in the muscles of the trunk and diaphragmatic involvement, giving pain on deep breathing and coughing, occur but the disorder is self-limiting and usually recovers within a few days. However, acute and fulminant polymyositis with rhabdomyolysis and myoglobinuria has been reported due to infection with Coxsackie B6 and Echo 9 viruses (Fakuyama, Ando, and

Yokota 1977; Josselson, Pula, and Sadler 1980) while it has also been suggested that these and many other individual viruses may sometimes precipitate auto-immune polymyositis (Walton 1983). Acute myositis has also been described in influenza (Middleton, Alexander, and Szymanski 1970). In addition the influenza virus, both influenza A and B and especially the A2 Hong Kong virus, have been reported to cause an acute or subacute necrotizing inflammatory myopathy, usually in children but also in adults (Mejlszenkier, Safran, Healy, Embree, and Quellette 1973; Dietzman, Schaller, Ray, and Reed 1976; Congy, Hauw, Wang, and Moulias 1980) and the virus has been isolated from skeletal muscle (Gamboa, Eastwood, Hays, Maxwell, and Penn 1979).

Acute suppurative myositis is rare in developed countries, except after crush injuries or complicating pressure sores, but in the tropics staphylococcal pyomyositis (*tropical myositis*) is relatively common, usually affecting men (Chiedozi 1979). Single or multiple abscesses occur in muscle, usually in glutei and/or quadriceps, and recovery is usually complete after systemic antibiotic therapy and surgical drainage (*British Medical Journal* 1979). Muscle is only rarely involved in parasitic infestations, but muscular pain and weakness may occur in toxoplasmosis (Chandler, Mair, and Mair 1968), in South American trypanosomiasis, and in trichinosis, which usually develops after the ingestion of infested pork. Fleeting muscle pain and tenderness may be accompanied by peri-orbital oedema and *Trichinella spiralis* may be detected on muscle biopsy (Adams 1975). Rarely, severe generalized muscular pain and weakness can give a picture simulating acute polymyositis (Gross and Ochoa 1979). Cysticercosis, too, can cause acute myalgia, fever, and eosinophilia but has also been reported to produce a diffuse hypertrophic myopathy (Sawnhey, Chopra, Banerji, and Wahi 1976; Pallis and Lewis 1981) while other rare parasitic infections of skeletal muscle include echinococcosis, sarcosporidiosis, and actinomycosis (Mastaglia and Walton 1982; Walton 1983).

Muscular involvement in collagen or connective-tissue diseases and sarcoidosis

In cases of rheumatoid arthritis and other connective-tissue diseases, examination of muscle biopsy sections often demonstrates foci of inflammatory cells, but this focal nodular myositis is rarely accompanied by muscular wasting and weakness save for that resulting secondarily from joint disease. In sarcoidosis, however, muscular involvement may be so widespread that some patients with this affliction present with subacute weakness and wasting of proximal muscles and typical sarcoid granulomas may be found on muscle biopsy (see Currie 1981). Sometimes this occurs in patients with established sarcoidosis (Silverstein and Sitzbach 1969; Jerusalem and Imback 1970; Douglas, McLeod, and Matthews 1973), but sometimes the myopathy is the presenting feature. However, it is now clear that a diffuse granulomatous myopathy, often with histological changes in the muscle indistinguishable from those of sarcoidosis, may occur without any other clinical or investigative evidence of the latter condition (Gardner-Thorpe 1972; Hewlett and Brownell 1975) and that this granulomatous disorder is a form of polymyositis unrelated to sarcoidosis. Eosinophilic myositis, usually presenting as a localized tender swelling in one calf or thigh, sometimes followed by a difuse proximal myopathy, is one component of the rare hypereosinophilic syndrome, also characterized by eosinophilia, anaemia, hypergammaglobulinaemia, cardiac and pulmonary involvement, skin changes, peripheral neuropathy, and encephalopathy (Layzer, Shearn, and Satya-Murti 1977; Stark 1979). It may be accompanied by eosinophilic fasciitis (Thornell and Bjelle 1981). These cases, like other forms of polymyositis, are usually steroid-responsive.

In polyarteritis nodosa, severe localized muscle pain, subcutaneous oedema, and tenderness may occur as a result of muscle infarction. Focal nodular myositis may also occur in systemic lupus erythematosus, but in some cases muscular involvement is more severe and diffuse and this syndrome becomes one of polymyositis, although histological investigation sometimes reveals a vacuolar myopathy (Pearson and Yamazaki 1958). The diffuse muscular involvement often seen with progressive systemic sclerosis is also clearly due to an associated polymyositis (see below) and indeed some children and adolescents with polymyositis show acrosclerosis, dysphagia, and a Raynaud's syndrome. Localized muscular abnormalities indistinguishable from those of polymyositis may also be noted in the muscles underlying areas of linear morphoea or scleroderma (Stern, Payne, Alvarez, and Hannapel 1975).

Polymyositis

The classification and nosological status of polymyositis remains controversial. This name is usually given to identify a group of cases in which muscular wasting and weakness occur and are sometimes, but not invariably, associated with muscle pain and tenderness and/or skin changes or with evidence of some form of connective-tissue or collagen disease. Muscle biopsy generally demonstrates areas of muscle fibre necrosis accompanied by interstitial, perifascicular, or perivascular cellular infiltrates or both, though these are not invariable. The term is commonly used to include cases with florid skin change, which are more properly called dermatomyositis; it is usually taken to indicate the so-called idiopathic syndrome and excludes disorders such as polymyalgia rheumatica (see below) and also acute myositis resulting from infections with micro-organisms, parasites, fungi, and viruses. The relationship of the myopathies seen in sarcoidosis, Sjogren's disease, and bronchogenic carcinoma to polymyositis is still somewhat obscure (Currie 1981; Mastaglia and Walton 1982), though with the exception of the specific myasthenic-myopathic syndrome (see below) sometimes observed in patients with lung cancer and cases with clear evidence of peripheral neuropathy as well as myopathy, it seems that many patients with so-called carcinomatous myopathy in reality are suffering from polymyositis (Rose and Walton 1966). Shy (1962) suggested that all such polymyopathies should be identified according to their aetiology and pathological characteristics. However, Mastaglia and Walton (1982) conclude that the term 'polymyositis' should be retained as in many cases the aetiology of the condition remains obscure despite full investigation. Furthermore, a response to steroids occurs in many patients in whom muscle biopsy findings are non-specific. There is evidence that in occasional cases, there is involvement of distal branches of peripheral nerves as well as muscle fibres, and these cases may be regarded as examples of neuromyositis (McEntee and Mancall 1965), though this term is now little used. Polymyositis and polyneuritis are both, of course, well-recognized manifestations of systemic lupus erythematosus and may occur together.

Aetiology

The work of Dawkins (1965), Kakulas (1966), and Currie (1971), which showed that polymyositis may be produced in animals by injecting muscle homogenates with Freund's adjuvant, suggested that this syndrome in man may well be the result of a cell-mediated auto-immune process. One can thus suggest that polymyositis in which there is no clinical evidence to suggest that any tissue other than muscle is involved may be an organ-specific auto-immune disease, while in cases showing involvement of skin or joints it may be regarded as being a feature of non-organ-specific auto-immune disease (Mastaglia and Walton 1982). The clear-cut relationship between polymyositis and dermatomyositis on the

one hand, and malignant disease on the other, also suggests that the condition is sometimes the result of a conditioned auto-immune response in patients suffering from cancer. The close relationship of the condition to other disorders of the connective-tissue group is underlined by the occurrence of certain cases which successively present manifestations of polymyositis, systemic lupus erythematosus, and/or scleroderma or systemic sclerosis.

There is increasing evidence to support the auto-immune hypothesis. Thus Currie, Saunders, Knowles, and Brown (1971) found an increased incidence of lymphocyte transformation in response to muscle antigen in cells obtained from cases of polymyositis and demonstrated that these cells were cytotoxic to muscle cells in tissue culture; confirmatory evidence was later reported by Mastaglia and Currie (1971), Esiri, MacLennan, and Hazleman (1973), and Haas and Arnason (1974), though Lisak and Zweiman (1975) reported contrary findings. Whitaker and Engel (1972) found vascular deposits of immunoglobulin and complement in muscle biopsies obtained from such patients and Dawkins and Zilko (1975) found evidence of subtle immunodeficiency in patients with both polymyositis and myasthenia gravis. That disordered humoral immunity may play a part was confirmed by Behan and Behan (1977) who found positive serum anticomplementary activity, but the major part played by killer T lymphocytes in causing muscle-fibre destruction has been confirmed by the studies of Rowe, Isenberg, McDougall, and Beverley (1981), Cambridge and Stern (1981), and Isenberg and Cambridge (1982).

There have also been several reports of the detection by electron microscopy of picornavirus (Chou and Gutmann 1970), myxovirus (Chou 1968; Sato, Walker, Peters, Reese, and Chou 1971), and Coxsackie virus-like (Mastaglia and Walton 1971) particles in muscle biopsies from such patients (Mastaglia and Hudgson 1981) but virus isolation is rarely successful (Mastaglia and Walton 1982). Thus it seems likely that polymyositis is due to a lymphocyte-mediated auto-immune process and that viral infection may be one factor which is capable of initiating it.

Classification

The clinical classification proposed by Walton and Adams (1958), as modified by Rose and Walton (1966), has been found useful for clinical assessment.

Group I:
    Polymyositis
        Acute, with myoglobinuria
            in childhood
        Subacute or chronic–in early adult life
            in middle and late life

Group II: Polymyositis with dominant muscular weakness but with some evidence of an associated collagen disease or dermatomyositis with severe muscular disability and with minimal or transient skin changes.

Group III: Polymyositis complicating severe collagen disease, e.g. rheumatoid arthritis, or dermatomyositis with florid skin changes and minor muscle weakness.

Group IV: Polymyositis and/or dermatomyositis complicating malignant disease.

In the classification of the World Federation of Neurology (see Walton 1981; Mastaglia and Walton 1982) the organ-specific auto-immune cases (Group I) are classified as type α, Groups II and III (non-organ-specific) are classified together as type β, and Group IV becomes type γ.

Incidence

Polymyositis is world-wide, occurs in many races and appears to be commoner in women. It is more common in adult life than muscular dystrophy, but is less common than the latter in childhood. About 15 per cent of cases occur under the age of 15, another 15 per cent between the ages of 16 and 30, about 25 per cent between 31 and 45, and 30 per cent between the ages of 46 and 60. The condition usually occurs spontaneously, but may follow a variety of febrile illnesses and has been known to develop after the administration of various drugs, including sulphonamides and penicillamine (Schraeder, Peters, and Dahl 1972; Mastaglia and Argov 1981) or following exposure to sunlight. It is rarely familial (Lewkonia and Buxton 1973), but if there is any genetic susceptibility this is slight and no convincing association with any HLA haplotype has been discovered (Walker, Mastaglia, and Roberts 1982).

Clinical manifestations

Detailed analyses of the clinical manifestations of polymyositis have been given by many authors (Eaton 1954; Garcin, Lapresle, Gruner, and Scherrer 1955; Pearson and Rose 1960; Barwick and Walton 1963; Currie 1981; Walton 1983). Muscle pain and tenderness occur in approximately 50 per cent of cases, as does dysphagia. In about a third of all cases the condition presents simply as a subacute proximal myopathy with no other manifestations; rarely there is a hyperacute onset with widespread muscle destruction and myoglobinuria. Cutaneous manifestations are seen in about two-thirds of all patients and may take the form of widespread erythema with desquamation seen particularly on the face and on the other exposed areas of the trunk, but occasionally involving almost the whole body. A particularly characteristic heliotrope erythema around the eyes, together with periorbital oedema, is seen in some patients, as is congestion of the nail beds. Sometimes the skin changes are slight and may take the form of no more than a faint butterfly-type rash on the face, while in others, particularly in childhood, there may be ulceration over bony prominences with subcutaneous calcification; the latter is occasionally very extensive (calcinosis universalis). Raynaud's syndrome is a common association and many younger patients develop thickening and loss of elasticity of the skin over the fingers, face, and anterior chest wall resembling those of generalized scleroderma or acrosclerosis.

About a quarter of all patients have some joint pain and stiffness. Proximal limb muscles are almost invariably involved and it is characteristic that the neck muscles are weak in many cases so that patients may have difficulty in holding up the head. Specific involvement of distal limb muscles, without proximal weakness, is uncommon (except in inclusion body myositis—see below), but weakness may be generalized in about a third of all cases, and in under a third contractures eventually develop. Facial weakness and involvement of external ocular muscles occur rarely (Rothstein, Carlson, and Sumi 1981; Bates, Stevens, and Hudgson 1973; Susac, Garcia-Mallin, and Glaser 1973). Occasionally myasthenic fatigability is striking and is partially responsive to edrophonium or neostigmine, but treatment with these and related drugs produces only slight and temporary improvement. The deep tendon reflexes may be depressed in the affected muscles but are often surprisingly brisk despite the severity of the muscular weakness. In a few patients with so-called localized nodular myositis, the condition presents with severe localized muscle pain, swelling, or tenderness, often in one muscle group of a single limb (e.g. quadriceps or calf) or even of the head and neck (e.g. masseter), only evolving much later into a more diffuse muscular affliction (Cumming, Weiser, Teoh, Hudgson, and Walton 1977).

Pulmonary involvement with chronic respiratory insufficiency has been described (Camp, Lane, and Mowat 1972) and myocardial damage with pericarditis also occurs rarely (Walton and Adams 1958), but these and other forms of visceral affection are usually, but not invariably, indicative of associated systemic sclerosis or systemic lupus.

Prognosis

Even without treatment the course of the illness is variable. Sometimes it runs a fluctuating course with spontaneous exacerbations and remissions; progressive deterioration with a fatal termination within a few weeks or months of the onset is seen particularly in acute dermatomyositis, but in some patients spontaneous arrest occurs. However, before the introduction of steroid drugs, the over-all mortality of the disease was about 50 per cent. Slow insidious progression is also seen, particularly in middle age, but spontaneous recovery may occur in childhood (Nattrass 1954; Rose 1974).

In a review of 89 cases observed and studied in north-east England, Rose and Walton (1966) found that 16 per cent of their patients had associated malignant disease. Seventy-five patients in their series had received adequate steroid therapy and in the great majority the treatment produced subjective and objective clinical improvement accompanied by a progressive reduction in serum creatine kinase activity (see p. 587). Withdrawal of treatment during the first two years after the onset sometimes resulted in relapse. Most patients required treatment for at least three to five years and no deaths occurred under the age of 30. Most children and young adults recovered completely, but after the age of 30 a number of patients went on to develop evidence of diffuse connective-tissue disease unresponsive to treatment, while after the age of 50 malignant disease which was present in many cases adversely affected the prognosis. An even more extensive follow-up study reported by De Vere and Bradley (1975) amply confirmed the benefits of steroid treatment. They also showed that about 50 per cent of men over the age of 45 years with dermatomyositis were ultimately found to have malignant disease.

Treatment

The condition is best treated with 60 mg of prednisone daily, given for two or three weeks, thereafter reducing the dose to 40 mg daily when clinical improvement appears and subsequently regulating the maintenance dose according to the level of serum creatine kinase activity and the clinical response. Occasionally even higher doses of prednisone (up to 120 mg daily) may be required for short periods. Once there is an adequate clinical response, alternate-day treatment has considerable advantages. Maintenance therapy may have to be continued for many years before the drug can be withdrawn. There is now increasing evidence that immunosuppressive remedies such as cyclophosphamide or azathioprine, 2–2.5 mg/kg body weight daily, have an adjuvant effect when combined with prednisone, and it is now usual to combine prednisone and immunosuppressive treatment from the onset (Currie and Walton 1971; Haas 1973; De Vere and Bradley 1975; Currie 1981). While some workers prefer methotrexate or chlorambucil, prednisone and azathioprine (the former continued in maintenance doses for several years, the latter for 12–18 months, with the usual precautions being taken to identify potentially harmful bone-marrow suppression) is the commonest combination. Thymectomy has not found general favour (Behan and Currie 1978) and plasmapheresis is of doubtful benefit. In steroid-resistant cases, whole-body irradiation has been found to be dramatically successful (Engel, Lichter, and Galdi 1981) and cyclosporin is under test. Respiratory and urinary infection should be treated with appropriate antibiotics and in occasional severe cases intermittent positive-pressure respiration is necessary. Following the acute stage, active and passive movements carried out under the supervision of a skilled physiotherapist are valuable.

Inclusion body myositis

This condition is a relatively benign and chronic form of myopathy, not associated with connective-tissue disease or malignancy, which occurs particularly in elderly men but occasionally afflicts younger patients (Carpenter and Karpati 1981). Slowly progressive painless weakness involves distal muscles more severely than proximal, there is often associated dysphagia, and the condition is usually progressive, giving severe handicap in about two years. Typically bluish granular inclusions are found along the edge of slit-like vacuoles within muscle fibres stained by haematoxylin and eosin, but in addition there are masses of filaments or filamentous microtubules, 15–18 nm in diameter, within the nuclei and cytoplasm of the fibres, while interstitial inflammatory-cell infiltrates are also seen (Chou 1968; Carpenter, Karpati, Heller, and Eisen 1978). Treatment with steroids and immunosuppressive agents is usually ineffective. Eisen, Berry, and Gibson (1983) suggest that this curious condition is sometimes neurogenic.

Polymyalgia rheumatica

Polymyalgia rheumatica (Bagratuni 1953; Gordon 1960; Todd 1961; Hart 1969) occurs almost always in elderly patients whose principal complaint is one of widespread muscular pain, often with local tenderness, minor constitutional upset, and sometimes general malaise. Muscle weakness is not usually present, though pain may be so severe that movement is restricted and many patients are wrongly diagnosed as suffering from polymyositis. Difficulty in getting out of a bath or out of a low chair without help is characteristic. Muscle biopsy usually reveals normal muscle. Some patients develop rheumatoid arthritis but Paulley and Hughes (1960) and others have suggested that there is a close relationship between this condition and cranial arteritis, which develops in some others. Indeed, there is increasing evidence that a diffuse giant-cell arteritis is present in many cases (Brooke and Kaplan 1972) and subclinical hepatic dysfunction, improving with treatment, has been described (Long and James 1974). In all patients the ESR is substantially raised, but the EMG, serum enzyme studies, and muscle biopsy are usually negative. The response to steroid therapy is usually immediate and dramatic (Bird, Esselinck, Dixon, Mowat, and Wood 1979).

References

Adams, R. D. (1975). *Diseases of muscle*, 3rd edn. Hoeber, New York.

Bagratuni, L. (1953). Polymyalgia rheumatica. *Ann. Rheum. Dis.* **12**, 98.

Barwick, D. D. and Walton, J. N. (1963). Polymyositis. *Am. J. Med.* **35**, 646.

Bates, D., Stevens, J. C. and Hudgson, P. (1973). 'Polymyositis' with involvement of facial and distal musculature: one form of the facio-scapulohumeral syndrome? *J. neurol. Sci.* **19**, 105.

Behan, P. O. and Currie, S. (1978). *Neuroimmunology*. Saunders, Eastbourne.

Behan, W. M. H. and Behan, P. O. (1977). Complement abnormalities in polymyositis. *J. neurol. Sci.* **34**, 241.

Bird, H. A., Esselinck, W., Dixon, A. St. J., Mowat, A. G. and Wood, P. H. N. (1979). An evaluation of criteria for polymyalgia rheumatica. *Ann. rheum. Dis.* **38**, 434.

British Medical Journal (1979). Pyomyositis. *Br. med. J.* **1**, 1047.

Brooke, M. H. and Kaplan, H. (1972). Muscle pathology in rheumatoid arthritis, polymyalgia rheumatica, and polymyositis. A histochemical study. *Arch. Path.* **94**, 101.

Cambridge, G. and Stern, C. M. (1981). The uptake of tritium-labelled carnitine by monolayer cultures of human fetal muscle and its potential as a label in cytotoxicity studies. *Clin. exp. Immunol.* **43**, 211.

Camp, A. V., Lang, D. J. and Mowat, A. G. (1972). Dermatomyositis with parenchymal lung involvement. *Br. med. J.* **1**, 155.

Carpenter, S. and Karpati, G. (1981). The major inflammatory myopathies of unknown cause. In *Pathology annual* (ed. S. C. Sommers and P. R. Rosen) p. 205. Appleton-Century-Crofts, New York.

——, ——, Heller, I. and Eisen, A. (1978). Inclusion body myositis: distinct variety of idiopathic inflammatory myopathy. *Neurology, Minneapolis* **28**, 8.

Chandar, K., Mair, H. J. and Mair, N. S. (1968). Case of toxoplasma polymyositis. *Br. med. J.* **1**, 158.

Chiedozi, L. (1979). Pyomyositis. Review of 205 cases in 112 patients. *Am. J. Surg.* **137**, 255.

Chou, S. M. (1968). Myxovirus-like structures and accompanying nuclear changes in chronic polymyositis. *Arch. Path.* **86**, 649.

—— and Gutmann, L. (1970). Picornavirus-like crystals in subacute polymyositis. *Neurology, Minneapolis* **20**, 205.

Congy, F., Hauw, J. J., Wang, A. and Moulias, R. (1980). Influenzal acute myositis in the elderly. *Neurology, Minneapolis* **30**, 877.

Cumming, W. J. K., Weiser, R., Teoh, R., Hudgson, P. and Walton, J. N. (1977). Localised nodular myositis: a clinical and pathological variant of polymyositis. *Quart. J. Med.* **184**, 531.

Currie, S. (1971). Experimental myositis: the in-vivo and in-vitro activity of lymph-node cells. *J. Path.* **105**, 169.

—— (1981). Inflammatory myopathies: polymyositis and related disorders. In *Disorders of voluntary muscle* (ed. J. N. Walton), 4th edn, Ch 1. Churchill-Livingstone, Edinburgh.

——, Saunders, M., Knowles, M. and Brown, A. E. (1971). Immunological aspects of polymyositis: the in-vitro activity of lymphocytes on incubation with muscle antigen and with muscle cultures. *Quart. J. Med.* **40**, 63.

—— and Walton, J. N. (1971). Immunosuppressive therapy in polymyositis. *J. Neurol. Neurosurg. Psychiat.* **34**, 447.

Dawkins, R. L. (1965). Experimental myositis associated with hypersensitivity to muscle. *J. Path. Bact.* **90**, 619.

——, Garlepp, M. and McDonald, B. (1982). Immunopathology of muscle. In *Skeletal muscle pathology* (ed. F. L. Mastaglia and J. N. Walton) Ch. 15. Churchill-Livingstone, Edinburgh.

—— and Zilko, P. J. (1975). Polymyositis and myasthenia gravis: immunodeficiency disorders involving skeletal muscle. *Lancet* i, 200.

DeVere, R. and Bradley, W. G. (1975). Polymyositis: its presentation, morbidity and mortality. *Brain* **98**, 637.

Dietzman, D. E., Schaller, J. G., Ray, C. G. and Reed, M. E. (1976). Acute myositis associated with influenza B infection. *Arch. Dis. Child.* **51**, 135.

Douglas, A. C., McLeod, J. G. and Matthews, J. D. (1973). Symptomatic sarcoidosis of skeletal muscle. *J. Neurol. Neurosurg. Psychiat.* **36**, 1034.

Eaton, L. M. (1954). The perspective of neurology in regard to polymyositis: study of 41 cases. *Neurology, Minneapolis* **4**, 245.

Eisen, A., Berry, K. and Gibson, G. (1983). Inclusion body myositis (IBM): myopathy or neuropathy? *Neurology, Minneapolis* **33**, 1109.

Engel, W. K., Lichter, A. S. and Galdi, A. P. (1981). Polymyositis: remarkable response to total body irradiation. *Lancet* i, 658.

Esiri, M. M., MacLennan, I. C. M. and Hazleman, B. L. (1973). Lymphocyte sensitivity to skeletal muscle in patients with polymyositis and other disorders. *Clin. exp. Immunol.* **14**, 25.

Fukuyama, Y., Ando, T. and Yokota, J. (1977). Acute fulminant myoglobinuric polymyositis with picornavirus-like crystals. *J. Neurol. Neurosurg. Psychiat.* **40**, 775.

Gamboa, E. T., Eastwood, A. B., Hays, A. P., Maxwell, J. and Penn, A. S. (1979). Isolation of influenza virus from muscle in myoglobinuric polymyositis. *Neurology, Minneapolis* **29**, 1323.

Garcin, R., Lapresle, J., Gruner, J. and Scherrer, J. (1955). Les polymyosites. *Rev. Neurol.* **92**, 465.

Gardner-Thorpe, C. (1972). Muscle weakness due to sarcoid myopathy. *Neurology, Minneapolis* **22**, 917.

Gordon, I. (1960). Polymyalgia rheumatica. *Quart. J. Med.* **116**, 473.

Gross, B. and Ochoa, J. (1979). Trichinosis: clinical report and histochemistry of muscle. *Muscle & Nerve* **2**, 394.

Haas, D. C. (1973). Treatment of polymyositis with immunosuppressive drugs. *Neurology, Minneapolis* **23**, 55.

—— and Arnason, B. G. W. (1974). Cell-mediated immunity in polymyositis. *Arch. Neurol., Chicago* **31**, 192.

Hart, F. D. (1969). Polymyalgia rheumatica. *Br. med. J.* **2**, 99.

Hewlett, R. H. and Brownell, B. (1975). Granulomatous myopathy: its relationship to sarcoidosis and polymyositis. *J. Neurol. Neurosurg. Psychiat.* **38**, 1090.

Isenberg, D. and Cambridge, G. (1982). Polymyositis. *Hosp. Update* **8**, 639.

Jerusalem, F. and Imbach, P. (1970). Granulomatöse myositis und muskelsarkoidose. *Dtsch. med. Wschr.* **43**, 2184.

Josselson, J., Pula, T. and Sadler, J. H. (1980). Acute rhabdomyolysis associated with an Echo virus-9 infection. *Arch. intern. Med.* **140**, 1671.

Kakulas, B. A. (1966). Destruction of differentiated muscle cultures by sensitized cells. *J. Path. Bact.* **91**, 495.

Layzer, R. B., Shearn, M. A. and Satya-Murti, S. (1977). Eosinophilic polymyositis. *Ann. Neurol.* **1**, 65.

Lewkonia, R. M. and Buxton, P. H. (1973). Myositis in father and daughter. *J. Neurol. Neurosurg. Psychiat.* **36**, 820.

Lisak, R. P. and Zweiman, B. (1975). Mitogen and muscle extract induced in vitro proliferative responses in myasthenia gravis, dermatomyositis and polymyositis. *J. Neurol. Neurosurg. Psychiat.* **38**, 521.

Long, R. and James, O. (1974). Polymyalgia rheumatica and liver disease. *Lancet* i, 77.

Mastaglia, F. L. and Argov, Z. (1981). Drug-induced neuromuscular disorders in man. In *Disorders of voluntary muscle* (ed. J. N. Walton), 4th edn, Ch. 25. Churchill-Livingstone, Edinburgh.

—— and Currie, S. (1971). Immunological and ultrastructural observations on the role of lymphoid cells in the pathogenesis of polymyositis. *Acta Neuropath., Berlin* **18**, 1.

—— and Hudgson, P. (1981). Ultrastructural studies of diseased muscle. In *Disorders of voluntary muscle* (ed. J. N. Walton) 4th edn, Ch. 9. Churchill-Livingstone, Edinburgh.

—— and Walton, J. N. (1971). Coxsackie virus-like particles in skeletal muscle from a case of polymyositis. *J. neurol. Sci.* **11**, 593.

—— and —— (1982). Inflammatory myopathies. In *Skeletal muscle pathology* (ed. F. L. Mastaglia and J. N. Walton) Ch. 11. Churchill-Livingstone, Edinburgh.

McEntee, W. J. and Mancall, E. L. (1965). Neuromyositis: a reappraisal. *Neurology, Minneapolis* **15**, 69.

Mejlszenkier, J. D., Safran, A. P., Healy, J. J., Embree, L. and Quellette, E. M. (1973). The myositis of influenza. *Arch. Neurol., Chicago* **29**, 441.

Middleton, P. J., Alexander, R. M. and Szymanski, M. T. (1970). Severe myositis during recovery from influenza. *Lancet* ii, 533.

Nattrass, F. J. (1954). Recovery from muscular dystrophy. *Brain* **77**, 549.

Pallis, C. and Lewis, P. D. (1981). Inflammatory myopathies: polymyositis and related disorders. In *Disorders of voluntary muscle* (ed. J. N. Walton) 4th edn, Ch. 15 Part II. Churchill-Livingstone, Edinburgh.

Paulley, J. W. and Hughes, J. P. (1960). Giant-cell arteritis, or arteritis of the aged. *Br. med. J.* **2**, 1562.

Pearson, C. M. and Rose, A. S. (1960). Myositis, the inflammatory disorders of muscle. *Res. publ. Ass. nerv. ment. Dis.* **38**, 422.

—— and Yamazaki, J. N. (1958). Vacuolar myopathy in systemic lupus erythematosis. *Am. J. clin. Path.* **29**, 455.

Rose, A. L. (1974). Childhood polymyositis. A follow-up study with special reference to treatment with corticosteroids. *Am. J. Dis. Child.* **127**, 518.

—— and Walton, J. N. (1966). Polymyositis: a survey of 89 cases with particular reference to treatment and prognosis. *Brain*, **89**, 747.

Rothstein, T. L., Carlson, C. B. and Sumi, S. M. (1971). Polymyositis with facioscapulohumeral distribution. *Arch. Neurol., Chicago* **25**, 313.

Rowe, D., Isenberg, D. A., McDougall, J. and Beverley, P. C. L. (1981). Characterization of polymyositis infiltrates using monoclonal antibodies to human leucocyte antigens. *Clin. exp. Immunol.* **45**, 290.

Sato, T., Walker, D. L., Peters, H. A., Reese, H. H. and Chou, S. M. (1971). Chronic polymyositis and myxovirus-like inclusions. *Arch. Neurol., Chicago* **24**, 409.

Sawhney, B. B., Chopra, J. S., Banerji, A. K. and Wahi, P. L. (1976). Pseudohypertrophic myopathy in cysticercosis. *Neurology, Minneapolis* **26**, 270.

Schraeder, P. L., Peters, H. A. and Dahl, D. S. (1972). Polymyositis and penicillamine. *Arch. Neurol., Chicago* **27**, 456.

Shy, G. M. (1962). The late onset myopathy. *Wld. Neurol.* **3**, 149.

Silverstein, A. and Sitzbach, L. E. (1969). Muscle involvement in sarcoidosis. *Arch. Neurol., Chicago* **21**, 235.

Stark, R. J. (1979). Eosinophilic polymyositis. *Arch. Neurol., Chicago* **36**, 721.

Stern, G. M., Rose, A. L. and Jacobs, K. (1967). Circulating antibodies in polymyositis. *J. neurol. Sci.* **5**, 181.

Stern, L. Z., Payne, C. M., Alvarez, J. T. and Hannapel, L. K. (1975). Myopathy associated with linear scleroderma. *Neurology, Minneapolis* **25**, 114.

Susac, J. O., Garcia-Mullin, R. and Glaser, J. S. (1973). Ophthalmoplegia in dermatomyositis. *Neurology, Minneapolis* **23**, 305.

Thornell, L. E. and Bjelle, A. (1981). Eosinophilic fasciitis: an ultrastructural and immunohistochemical study of the intermediate filament protein skeletin in regenerating muscle fibres. *Neuropath. appl. Neurobiol.* **7**, 435.

Todd, J. W. (1961). Polymyalgia rheumatica. *Lancet* ii, 1111.

Walker, G. L., Mastaglia, F. L. and Roberts, D. F. (1982). Search for genetic influence in idiopathic inflammatory myopathy. *Acta Neurol. scand.* **66**, 432.

Walton, J. N. (1981). Clinical examination of the neuromuscular system. In *Disorders of voluntary muscle* (ed. J. N. Walton), 4th edn, Ch. 13. Churchill-Livingstone, Edinburgh.

—— (1983). The inflammatory myopathies. *J. R. Soc. Med.* **76**, 1.

—— and Adams, R. D. (1958). *Polymyositis*. Livingstone, Edinburgh.

Whitaker, J. N. and Engel, W. K. (1972). Vascular deposits of immunoglobulin and complement in idiopathic inflammatory myopathy. *New Engl. J. Med.* **286**, 333.

Myasthenia gravis

Definition. A chronic disease with a tendency to remit and to relapse, characterized by abnormal muscular fatigability which may for a long time be confined to, or be predominant in, an isolated group of muscles and is later associated in many cases with permanent weakness of some muscles. The fatigability is due to an auto-immune process in which circulating antibodies against the acetylcholine receptor (AChR) cause a disorder of conduction at the myoneural junction; this can be temporarily relieved by neostigmine and similar drugs or by steroids and immunosuppressive agents, and in some cases permanently by removal of the thymus gland. Early descriptions were given by Wilks (1877) and Erb (1879), while the present name was coined by Jolly (1895). Walker (1934) was the first to describe the beneficial effect of physostigmine, and the first successful thymectomy was performed by Blalock in 1936.

Classification

As Simpson (1981) points out, the symptom of myasthenia is not peculiar to one disease. Similar fatigability can be observed in muscles affected by polymyositis, systemic lupus, dermatomyositis, and one type of carcinomatous myopathy (see below). However, a therapeutic response to anticholinesterase drugs, and now the identification of circulating antibodies against AChR, are necessary for the definition of true myasthenia gravis; and although some response may be found in the symptomatic myasthenias, it is rarely dramatic and often fails within a few weeks. Myasthenia gravis is therefore a clearly recognizable disease in which the response to appropriate drugs is dramatic and sustained and it is one which has an individual natural history and pathology.

There is increasing evidence that congenital, as distinct from neonatal (see below) myasthenia gravis and the familial form, is a different disease (see Lisak and Barchi 1982; Dawkins, Garlepp, and McDonald 1982; Chou 1982). Thus in one congenital variety Engel, Lambert, and Gomez (1977) described a marked decrease in nerve terminal size, increased synaptic vesicle density, degenerative postsynaptic changes, and absent acetylcholinesterase and four distinct forms of congenital myasthenia are now recognized (Engel 1984). Antibodies to AChR are not found in such congenital and familial cases (Vincent and Newsom Davis 1979) which seem somewhat heterogeneous (Vincent, Cull-Candy, Newsom Davis, Trautmann, Molenaar, and Polak 1981). The clinical classification or grading of cases of true myasthenia in most common use is that of Osserman (1958):

I Ocular myasthenia.

IIA Mild generalized myasthenia with slow progression; no crises; drug-responsive.

IIB Moderate generalized myasthenia; severe skeletal and bulbar involvement, but no crises; drug response is less satisfactory.

III Acute fulminating myasthenia; rapid progression of severe symptoms with respiratory crises and poor drug response; high incidence of thymoma; high mortality.

IV Late severe myasthenia; same as III, but takes two years to progress from Classes I or II; crises; high mortality.

Incidence and natural history

Myasthenia occurs in all races and affects both sexes, but is seen in women twice as often as in men (Osserman 1958). Its prevalence in Finland is about 50 cases per million of the population (Hokkanen 1969) but world-wide its incidence is about 0.4/100 000 (Kurtzke 1978). Only occasionally is it seen in more than one member of the same family but it has been reported in twins (Namba, Shapiro, Brunner, and Grob 1971*a*), and there is a form showing an onset in early childhood which may be of autosomal recessive inheritance (Bundey 1972). Jacob, Clack, and Emery (1968) found no familial incidence in a series of 70 cases, but others (Namba, Brunner, Brown, Muguruma, and Grob 1971*b*) have found a substantially increased familial incidence and noted that familial cases generally showed a much earlier age of onset. Although the relationship between myasthenia gravis and various HLA antigens remains somewhat unclear, there is little doubt that in Caucasians there is a significant association with A1, B8, and DRW3 in patients with thymic hyperplasia (Simpson 1981; Lisak and Barchi 1982; Dawkins *et al.* 1982). There is some evidence that patients with thymoma and high AChR antibody titres have no clear-cut HLA association, that females under 40 without thymoma have a high incidence of HLA-A1, B8, and/or DRW3, and that patients over 40 without thymoma with low antibody titres are more often male with A3, B7, or DRW2 (Compston, Vincent, Newsom Davis, and Batchelor 1980). An association with A2 in patients with thymoma (Feltkamp, Van den Berg-Loonen, Nijenhuis, Engelfriet, Van Rossum, Van Loghem, and Oosterhuis 1974; Fritze, Herrmann, Naeim, Smith, and Walford 1974) has not been confirmed, but in Japanese patients, though not in Caucasians, thymoma and/or elevated titres of anti-AChR antibody have been found associated with $GM^{1.2.21}$ (Nakao, Matsumoto, Miyazaki, Nishitani, Ota, Fujita, and Tsuji 1980). The mean age of onset is about 26 years in women and 30 years in men, but the condition may sometimes arise for the first time in childhood and occasionally as late as 80 years. It often arises without apparent cause, but occasionally follows emotional upset, physical stress, febrile illness, or pregnancy. Most remissions occur within the first five years and most deaths also occur within this period. After the disease has been in progress for 10 years, death from myasthenia itself is rare and in some instances the disease is apparently burnt out by then (Simpson 1981).

There is a close relationship between myasthenia gravis and thyrotoxicosis and the two diseases occur in combination in the same individual far more often than can be accounted for by chance (Schlezinger and Corin 1968; Namba and Grob 1971). The condition which has been called acute thyrotoxic bulbar palsy is almost certainly due in most cases to myasthenia affecting bulbar muscles in a thyrotoxic individual. There is also a less clear-cut relationship with systemic lupus, biliary cirrhosis, rheumatoid arthritis, and multiple sclerosis in some cases (Lisak and Barchi 1982).

Neonatal myasthenia is seen in about one in seven of the children born to myasthenic mothers, but in those who survive it usually recovers in between a week and three months after birth and does not recur (Wise and McQuillen 1970; Namba, Brown, and Grob 1970). Myasthenia has also been reported in dogs (Fraser, Palmer, Senior, Parkes, and Yealland 1970), and a myasthenic syndrome in man has been noted during the administration of various drugs including phenytoin (Brumlik and Jacobs 1974), antibiotics, especially streptomycin (Hokkanen and Toivakka 1969), kanamycin and colistimethate (McQuillen, Cantor, and O'Rourke 1968; Decker and Fincham 1971), and penicillamine (Bucknall, Dixon, Glick, Woodland, and Zutshi 1975). The many drugs which may induce myasthenia have been reviewed by Mastaglia and Argov (1981) who also point out that penicillamine-induced myasthenia in particular may be associated with a rise in circulating anti-AChR antibodies and does not resolve when the drug is withdrawn. There are data which suggest a genetic susceptibility to penicillamine-induced myasthenia (Garlepp, Dawkins, and Christiansen 1983).

Symptoms and signs

The muscles most often affected are the external ocular, bulbar, neck, and shoulder-girdle muscles in this descending order, but not uncommonly those of respiration and the proximal muscles of the lower extremities are also involved. The onset is usually gradual; ptosis of one or both upper lids is often the first symptom and is soon associated with diplopia due to paralysis of one or more of the external ocular muscles. These symptoms typically appear in the evening when the patient is tired and disappear after a night's rest. When bulbar muscles are first involved, difficulty in swallowing and/or in chewing is described, often most evident during a meal, and speech may become indistinct when the patient is tired.

On examination unilateral or bilateral ptosis is often found and is intensified by asking the patient to gaze upwards. Weakness of the external ocular muscles is usually asymmetrical and may progress to complete external ophthalmoplegia in one or both eyes. Occasionally conjugate ocular movements seem to be affected, but more often there is no functional relationship between the muscles involved in the two eyes and weakness of a single muscle (e.g. lateral rectus) is not uncommon. Paresis of accommodation has been described and the pupillary reflexes are usually normal but may be sluggish or exhibit fatigability.

The facial muscles are almost always affected (Fig. 19.4). Weakness of the orbicularis oculi is relatively constant; in the lower face the retractors of the angles of the mouth tend to suffer more than the elevators, so that a characteristic 'myasthenic snarl' is seen on smiling. Weakness of jaw muscles leads to difficulty in chewing, and weakness of the muscles of the soft palate, pharynx, tongue and larynx to difficulty in swallowing and in articulation. The characteristic fatigability of speech may be demonstrated by asking the patient to count up to 50, when speech becomes progressively less distinct; palatal weakness gives a nasal character to the voice and occasional regurgitation of fluid through the nose on swallowing. Typically, weakness of the neck muscles may cause the head to fall forward, a sign seen most often in myasthenia gravis but also in some cases of polymyositis. In severe cases the weakness of the upper limbs is such that the hands cannot be lifted to the mouth and it is characteristic that muscle power may initially be reasonably satisfactory, but after testing a particular movement on several occasions, the strength rapidly declines. Breathlessness is always a sinister symptom, as respiratory weakness may develop rapidly and may even cause sudden death. Sudden respiratory failure is often called a myasthenic crisis (Szobor 1970).

Muscular wasting is not usually found in the the early stages, but in long-standing cases permanent weakness and wasting, irreversible by drugs, are common in the external ocular muscles and in certain limb muscles, particularly triceps brachii. The term 'myasthenic myopathy' is sometimes used to identify this irreversible muscular weakness, but as the term is also utilized to describe rare cases of myopathy of undetermined cause in which weakness is improved, if only partially or transiently, by neostigmine, its meaning is imprecise (Rowland, Lisak, Schotland, de Jesus, and Berg 1973). While in most cases muscular weakness eventually becomes widespread throughout the muscles of the head and neck, trunk and limbs, Grob (1953) and Ferguson, Hutchinson, and Liversedge (1955), showed that in some the disease remains limited clinically to the external ocular muscles and never spreads to those of the bulb or limbs.

It is a notable feature of myasthenia gravis that the tendon reflexes almost always remain brisk, even when weakness is severe.

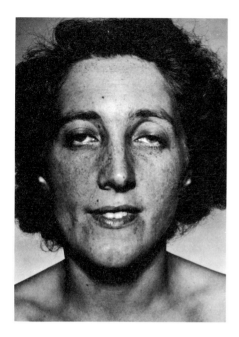

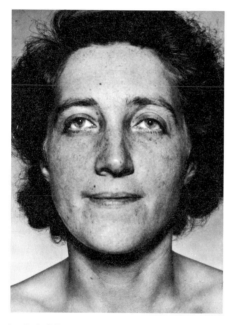

Fig. 19.4. Myasthenia gravis. *Left*, bilateral ptosis and weakness of facial muscles; *right*, the change in facial expression after an injection of neostigmine. (Reproduced from Spillane (1975) by kind permission of the author and publishers.)

Diagnosis

The diagnosis of myasthenia depends first upon the characteristic clinical picture, secondly upon electrical tests of neuromuscular transmission, thirdly upon the clinical response to an intravenous injection of edrophonium hydrochloride, and fourthly upon the measurement in the blood of circulating antibodies to AChR.

The demonstration of fatigability by means of repetitive supramaximal stimulation of a nerve such as the ulnar with simultaneous recording of the evoked muscle potential from the hypothenar muscles (Figs. 19.5 and 19.6) has often proved useful in the past (Johns, Grob, and Harvey 1955; Slomić, Rosenfalck, and Buchthal 1968; Desmedt and Borenstein 1970; Brown and Wynn Parry 1981) but is only useful if the muscles being tested are affected by the disease. This technique has been largely sup-

planted by the measurement in single-fibre electromyography of jitter and blocking, both of which are increased in myasthenia (Stalberg, Trontemj, and Schwartz 1976; Barwick 1981). Ocular tonometry (Campbell, Simpson, Crombie, and Walton 1970; Wray and Pavan-Langston 1971) or nystagmography (Spector, Daroff, and Birkett 1975) carried out before and after the injection of edrophonium are also of some value in the diagnosis of ocular myasthenia.

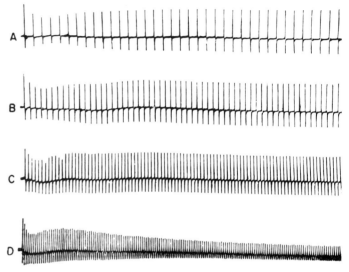

Fig. 19.5. Neuromuscular transmission in myasthenia gravis. The muscle action potentials recorded from the hypothenar muscles during supramaximal stimulation of the ulnar nerve at different frequencies. (A) Stimulus frequency, 5 Hz; (B) 10 Hz; (C) 25 Hz; (D) 50 Hz. The response to initial stimulus measures 6.2 mV. (Illustration kindly provided by Dr R. J. Johns; reproduced from Johns, Grob, and Harvey (1956). by kind permission of the author and publishers.)

However, the simplest clinical diagnostic test is still assessment of the clinical response to an injection of edrophonium hydrochloride (*Tensilon*). This quick-acting drug, which is given initially in a dosage of 2 mg, followed immediately by a further 8 mg intravenously if there is no severe reaction, has supplanted neostigmine for diagnostic purposes (Osserman and Kaplan 1953). Provocative tests designed to increase myasthenia, utilizing drugs such as curare and quinine, are dangerous and largely outmoded. However, methods involving regional perfusion with curare of certain muscle groups are safer and have been helpful in some doubtful cases (Brown and Charlton 1975; Brown, Charlton, and White 1975; Horowitz, Genkins, Kornfeld, and Papatestas 1975). Churchill-Davidson and Richardson (1952) showed that myasthenic patients are abnormally resistant to depolarizing neuromuscular blocking drugs such as decamethonium and that tolerance is particularly marked in clinically unaffected muscles. However, depolarization block, if it occurs at all, is brief and soon changes to a longer competitive (curare-like) type of block. This dual response in the child or adult is characteristic of myasthenia gravis, though the response obtained in normal neonates is similar (Churchill-Davidson and Wise 1963). This provocative test, too, is not now needed for diagnosis.

Much the most sensitive diagnostic test is now the measurement of anti-AChR antibody in the circulating blood using human AChR (Lindstrom 1977; Lisak and Barchi 1982; Dawkins *et al.* 1982) in a radioimmunoassay technique. Antibodies are found in practically all patients with adult-onset generalized active myasthenia gravis and in neonatal myasthenia, much less often in ocular cases, and practically never in congenital or familial cases of early onset. The titres are often exceptionally high in patients with thymoma. The lack of any close correlation between the titres and disease severity (Newsom Davis, Pinching, Vincent, and Wilson 1978) may be due to the fact that the receptor contains five subunits and possibly more sensitive assays for individual subunits may have to be developed to detect antibodies in some cases.

An important point in clinical management is to remember the frequency with which myasthenia gravis may be associated with benign thymic hyperplasia or malignant thymoma (Goldman, Herrmann, Keesey, Mulder, and Brown 1975) so that tomography of the anterior mediastinum is essential in all cases. Radiographs of the chest should also be done to exclude bronchial carcinoma, but the myasthenic syndrome which may complicate malignant disease (see below) shows clinical and electrophysiological features which are in many respects different from those of myasthenia gravis. Tests designed to exclude associated thyrotoxicosis or other auto-immune disorders (Hausmanowa-Petrusewicz, Chorzelski, and Strugalska 1969), including rheumatoid arthritis (Aarli, Milde, and Thunold 1975) may also be indicated.

Aetiology

Simpson (1960) first drew attention to the interrelationship between myasthenia gravis and other auto-immune diseases, including thyroid disorders, diabetes, rheumatoid arthritis, systemic lupus, and sarcoidosis. He suggested that the thymus might produce an antibody against muscle end-plate protein. Strauss, Seegal, Hsu, Burkholder, Nastuk, and Osserman (1960) demonstrated a muscle-binding globulin in myasthenic serum and Marshall and White (1961) showed that direct injection of bacterial antigen into the guinea-pig thymus produced a histological reaction similar to that of myasthenia. Goldstein and Hofmann (1968) claimed to have produced a syndrome resembling myasthenia in animals by injecting thymus extract and producing an auto-immune thymitis, but Vetters, Simpson, and Folkarde (1969) failed to confirm these findings. Desmedt (1957, 1966) suggested that the lesion was presynaptic and Dahlbäck, Elmquist, Johns, Radner, and Thesleff (1961) showed in isolated intercostal muscles removed from myasthenic and control patients, that there seemed to be a disturbance of transmitter formation or release. Subsequently many workers found circulating antibodies to muscle (Namba and Grob 1966; Namba, Himei, and Grob 1967; Oosterhuis, Bethlem, and Feltkamp 1968) and to neuronal extracts (Kornguth, Hanson, and Chun 1970; Martin, Herr, Wanamaker, and Kornguth 1974), lymphocyte transformation in response to muscle antigens (Kott, Genkins, and Rule 1973), and to acetylcholine receptor (Abramsky, Aharonov, Teitelbaum, and Fuchs 1975) in patients with myasthenia. Probably the most important developments were first the demonstration by Fambrough, Drachman, and Satyamurti (1973) of reduced receptors for α-bungarotoxin in myasthenic muscle, and secondly the production by Patrick and Lindstrom (1973) of experimental myasthenia in animals immunized with AChR, followed by the demonstration of circulating antibodies to AChR in such animals and in the very great majority of human subjects with myasthenia (Tarrab-Hazdai, Aharonov, Silman, and Fuchs 1975; Aharonov, Abramsky, Tarrab-Hazdai, and Fuchs 1975; Newsom-Davis 1979; Roses, Olanow, McAdams, and Lane 1981). Antibodies were also demonstrated by immunofluorescent techniques in myasthenic end-plates and it was shown that a defect of neuromuscular transmission could be produced in mice injected with serum from human myasthenic subjects. New developments in the immunology and immunopathology of myasthenia and in the histochemical and ultrastructural study of the end-plate region (Bjornskov, Norris, and Mower-Kuby 1982) now emerge almost daily, but there is evidence first that AChR antibody is present in all four IgG subclasses and sometimes in IgM and that sensitized T cells of thymic origin play an important part in the process in addition (see Lisak and Barchi 1982). The morphological abnormalities in terminal nerve endings in myasthenic muscle (Coërs

and Desmedt 1959; Bickerstaff and Woolf 1960), abnormalities of the fine structure, immunopathology, and geometry of the motor end-plates (Simpson 1971; Santa, Engel, and Lambert 1972a; Engel, Tsijihata, Lindstrom, and Lennon 1976; Lindstrom 1978) and occasional evidence of neurogenic muscular atrophy (Brownell 1972; Oosterhuis and Bethlem 1973) are the result of the auto-immune process. Thus it appears that both cellular immunity, mediated by T lymphocytes of thymic origin, and humoral factors contribute to pathogenesis. Suggestions that a putative thymic hormone or toxin (thymosin) (Wilson, Obrist, and Wilson 1953; Bach, Dardenne, Papiernik, Barois, Levasseur, and le Brigand 1972), other than anti-AChR antibody, actively plays a part in pathogenesis now seem unlikely.

Treatment

The standard treatment for myasthenia gravis for many years was neostigmine or the closely related drug pyridostigmine (*Mestinon*). The usual dosage of neostigmine was to begin with a 15-mg tablet three or four times a day, and usually it was necessary to give in addition atropine, 0.6 mg twice daily, to overcome the muscarinic side-effects. Later evidence indicated that the long-acting *Mestinon*, which was initially used by many workers in combination with neostigmine which acts more quickly, is probably preferable as the standard medication and the initial dosage is 60 mg three or four times daily, again often with atropine or propantheline unless muscarinic side-effects are absent. The dosage is then steadily increased until maximum benefit is obtained. Some patients find that it is best to take the tablets every two hours, while some require them three-hourly. Other drugs which were subsequently tried included ambenonium hydrochloride (*Mytelase*) of which the usual dosage is 10–25 mg three or four times daily and aldosterone inhibitors but these remedies seem to have no advantage over the more traditional medication and adjuvants commonly employed in the past including potassium chloride and ephedrine (see Simpson 1981; Lisak and Barchi 1982) have been largely abandoned. Occasional cases of myasthenia with failure to respond to cholinergic drugs have been described (Black, Brait, de Jesus, Horner, and Rowland 1973) and long-term treatment has even been thought to be a possible factor in causing irreversible myopathy (Fenichel, Kibler, Olsen, and Dettbarn 1972) and changes in the motor end-plates (Engel, Lambert, and Santa 1973). Many patients. especially those with mild myasthenia or symptoms restricted to only a limited number of muscles, continue to do well on anticholinesterase drugs alone, but within recent years there has been a substantial swing towards treatment with steroids and immunosuppressive remedies, with recurrent plasmapheresis, designed to remove circulating antibodies, being increasingly used in an emergency.

Initially corticotrophin (ACTH) was given in a 10-day course of treatment which often produced initial deterioration followed by prolonged improvement (Namba, Brunner, Shapiro, and Grob 1971c) and some preferred maintenance therapy (Cape and Utterback 1972). Subsequently it became clear that prednisone given daily, or more often on alternate days, often in an initial dosage of 50–60 mg daily or 100–120 mg on alternate days, followed by gradual reduction to an appropriate long-term maintenance dose, is equally, if not more, effective (Warmolts and Engel 1972; Pinelli, Tonali, and Scoppetta 1974) and this treatment is now used in most cases (Johns 1977; Drachman 1978; Patten 1978; Simpson 1981; Lisak and Barchi 1982). Indeed in ocular cases, prednisone is generally regarded as the drug of choice; in many other patients, anticholinesterase drugs are still required as well, though often in diminished dosage. Some workers prefer immunosuppressive agents such as azathioprine or cyclophosphamide, either with or instead of prednisone. Often the clinical response to either or both is dramatic or at least very satisfactory, but paradoxically some patients, even those with high concentrations of circulating AChR antibodies, show little or no response. Thoracic duct drainage, once recommended (Bergström, Franksson, Matell, Nilsson, Persson, Ven Reis, and Stensman 1975), has now been largely abandoned, but plasmapheresis (one or two courses given over 10–14 days) has been found to be remarkably beneficial in some cases (Dau, Lindstrom, Cassel, and Clark 1979) and has been recommended for routine treatment, as long-term benefit has been claimed. Others, however, believe that the effect is only temporary (Newsom Davis *et al.* 1978) and the majority view is that this form of treatment should be reserved for use in cases resisting other forms of treatment or in an emergency or when preparing a patient for thymectomy (Lisak and Barchi 1982; Engel 1984).

Differential diagnosis between myasthenic and cholinergic crises, in patients receiving anticholinesterase medication, in which rapidly increasing muscular weakness occurs and in which serious respiratory weakness may threaten life, can be difficult. The most useful single test is to give an intravenous injection of edrophonium. If this increases muscle power, then it is likely that the weakness is myasthenic and requires more treatment, while if it reduces power, the weakness is probably cholinergic and treatment must be reduced. Any hint of impending respiratory insufficiency may be an indication for withdrawal of all drugs and for assisted respiration with positive pressure apparatus and tracheotomy, possibly with plasmapheresis. Unfortunately some patients show a differential sensitivity of different muscles to various anticholinesterase drugs. It is not unknown to find that a dose of pyridostigmine which improves power in the limb muscles may be sufficient to cause cholinergic paralysis of the diaphragm.

The place of thymectomy has been controversial, but now seems much clearer. Simpson (1958, 1974) reviewed the problem in detail and pointed out that thymectomy benefits both sexes but that the extent of improvement is greatest in women, who would otherwise have a worse prognosis than men. Benefit following the operation may occur at any time, but he found the results to be best in young women with a short history suffering from severe myasthenia. They are also good in juvenile myasthenia (Hansson, Johansson, Stalberg, and Westerholm 1972). Perlo, Arnason, Poskanzer, Castleman, Schwab, Osserman, Papatestis, Alpert, and Kark (1971) found remission or improvement after operation in 76 per cent of a series of 267 patients and Buckingham, Howard, Bernatz, Payne, Harrison, O'Brien, and Weiland (1976) reported results which were similar. While the operation is not generally justified in purely ocular cases, it is now regarded as obligatory in all patients with radiological evidence of thymic enlargement (who may prove to have a thymoma) and it is now generally agreed that unless age, intercurrent illness, or other factors contra-indicate the procedure, it carries such a low operative mortality in experienced hands and gives such good results if removal is complete, that virtually all patients should be offered the procedure under the cover of steroids and (if necessary) anticholinesterase medication. Recent evidence suggests that men do just as well as women postoperatively (Lisak and Barchi 1982). The prognosis is worse if a thymoma is present; radiotherapy, once widely recommended to the thymus before operation, is now rarely given but may be required postoperatively. Even after thymectomy, two out of three patients with a thymoma die within five years, but the survivors may benefit to the same extent as those without a tumour. As some thymomas are malignant, death is sometimes due to metastases, but even a non-neoplastic thymus may regrow after operation (Joseph and Johns 1973).

The myasthenic-myopathic syndrome (the Eaton–Lambert syndrome)

This syndrome is often associated with oat-cell carcinoma of the bronchus, but has also been described occasionally in patients with

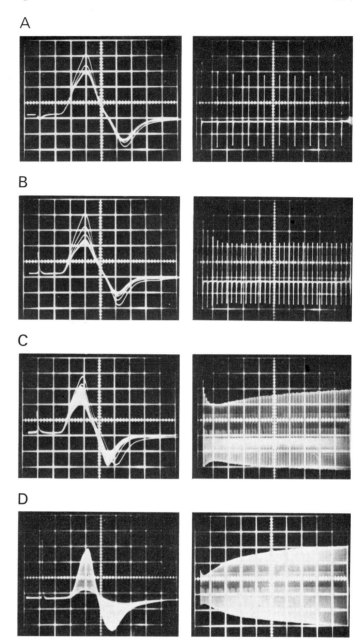

Fig. 19.6 Neuromuscular transmission in the Eaton-Lambert syndrome. Recording of motor unit action potentials from one hypothenar eminence during supramaximal stimulation of the ulnar nerve. (A) Stimulus frequency, 1 Hz; (B) 3 Hz; (C) 10 Hz; (D) 30 Hz. At each frequency the left panel represents superimposed responses, with each horizontal division representing 2 ms; on the right are sequential responses, each horizontal division representing 1 s. On the vertical scale each division in A, B and C represents 1 mV, in D 5 mV. (Illustration kindly provided by Dr J. C. Brown.)

carcinoma in other sites and rarely presents with the clinical picture of a subacute proximal myopathy in young patients without malignant disease (Brown and Johns 1974 and see p. 488). The clinical picture is usually one of subacute muscular weakness and wasting affecting the proximal parts of the limbs and trunk with some fatigability, not usually as striking as in myasthenia gravis; only occasionally are the external ocular and bulbar muscles involved (Rooke, Eaton, Lambert, and Hodgson 1960; Oh 1974). The weakness is thus myasthenic in the sense that the patient complains of increased enfeeblement after exertion, but in many such cases muscle power actually increases after brief exercise, a reversed myasthenic effect. In contrast to true myasthenia gravis, the condition is only slightly improved by treatment with neostigmine or pyridostigmine, though there may be definite improvement in strength after an injection of edrophonium hydrochloride. However, the tendon reflexes in this condition, unlike those in true myasthenia, are almost always depressed or absent. In contrast to the findings in true myasthenia gravis, repetitive stimulation of motor nerves at tetanic rates usually causes a marked increase in the amplitude of the evoked muscle action potentials and these patients are excessively sensitive to decamethonium. The ultrastructural appearances of the motor end-plates in this condition are also different from those seen in myasthenia gravis (Santa, Engel, and Lambert 1972b). Occasional cases with electrophysiological features of both myasthenia gravis and the myasthenic syndrome occur (Schwartz and Stalberg 1975) but in general the findings are distinctive and tests of neuromuscular transmission (Fig. 19.6) are mandatory whenever this condition is suspected. It now seems that although circulating antibodies against AChR are absent in this condition, there is evidence that an IgG antibody, binding to nerve terminal determinants, may be responsible for the condition which improves with plasma exchange and (in non-neoplastic cases) with prednisone and azathioprine (Lang, Newsom Davis, Wray, Vincent, and Murray 1981). Not only is the progressive potentiation in muscular strength which follows an initial period of fatigue after exercise a distinguishing feature, but the muscular weakness and fatigability may be greatly improved by the administration of guanidine (McQuillen and Johns 1966), which has no convincing effect in true myasthenia gravis. Guanidine hydrochloride is given orally in a total daily dose of 20–50 mg/kg body weight (Lambert 1966; Oh and Kim 1973). 4-aminopyridine in doses varying from 40 to 200 mg daily, has also been found effective in congenital myasthenia and the Eaton–Lambert syndrome, but toxic side-effects (including fits and confusion) severely limit the value of this treatment (Murray and Newsom Davis 1981).

References

Aarli, J. A., Milde, E. -J. and Thunold, S. (1975). Arthritis in myasthenia gravis. *J. Neurol. Neurosurg. Psychiat.* **38**, 1048.

Abramsky, O., Aharonov, A., Teitelbaum, D. and Fuchs, S. (1975). Myasthenia gravis and acetylcholine receptor. *Arch. Neurol., Chicago* **32**, 684.

Aharonov, A., Abramsky, O., Tarrab-Hazdai, R. and Fuchs, S. (1975). Humoral antibodies to acetylcholine receptor in patients with myasthenia gravis. *Lancet* **ii**, 340.

Armstrong, R. M., Nowak, R. M. and Falk, R. E. (1973). Thymic lymphocyte function in myasthenia gravis. *Neurology, Minneapolis* **23**, 1078.

Bach, J. -F., Dardenne, M., Papiernik, M., Barois, A., Levasseur, P. and Le Brigand, H. (1972). Evidence for a serum-factor secreted by the human thymus. *Lancet* **ii**, 1056.

Barwick, D. D. (1981). Clinical electromyography. In *Disorders of voluntary muscle* (ed. J. N. Walton) 4th edn, Ch. 28. Churchill-Livingstone, Edinburgh.

Bergström, K., Franksson, C., Matell, G., Nilsson, B. Y., Persson, A., Von Reis, G. and Stensman, R. (1975). Drainage of thoracic duct lymph in twelve patients with myasthenia gravis. *Eur. Neurol.* **13**, 19.

Bickerstaff, E. R. and Woolf, A. L. (1960). The intramuscular nerve endings in myasthenia gravis. *Brain* **83**, 10.

Bjornskov, E. K., Norris, F. H. and Mower-Kuby, J. (1982). Histochemical staining of the acetylcholine receptor, acetylcholinesterase, and the axon terminal. *Muscle & Nerve* **5**, 140.

Black, J. T., Brati, K. A., DeJesus, P. V., Harner, R. N. and Rowland, L. P. (1973). Myasthenia gravis lacking response to cholinergic drugs. *Neurology, Minneapolis* **23**, 851.

Brown, J. C. and Charlton, J. E. (1975). Study of sensitivity to curare in myasthenic disorders using a regional technique. *J. Neurol. Neurosurg. Psychiat.* **38**, 27.

——, —— and White, D. J. K. (1975). A regional technique for the study of sensitivity to curare in human muscle. *J. Neurol. Neurosurg. Psychiat.* **38**, 18.

—— and Johns, R. J. (1974). Diagnostic difficulties encountered in the myasthenic syndrome sometimes associated with carcinoma. *J. Neurol. Neurosurg. Psychiat.* **37**, 1214.

—— and Wynn Parry, C. B. (1981). Neuromuscular stimulation and transmission. In *Disorders of voluntary muscle* (ed. J. N. Walton) 4th edn, Ch. 26. Churchill-Livingstone, Edinburgh.

Brownell, B., Oppenheimer, D. R. and Spalding, J. M. K. (1972). Neurogenic muscle atrophy in myasthenia gravis. *J. Neurol. Neurosurg. Psychiat.* **35**, 311.

Brumlik, J. and Jacobs, R. S. (1974). Myasthenia gravis associated with diphenylhydantoin therapy for epilepsy. *Can. J. neurol. Sci.* **1**, 127.

Buckingham, J. M., Howard, F. M., Bernatz, P. E., Payne, W. S., Harrison, E. G. Jr., O'Brien, P. C. and Weiland, L. H. (1976). The value of thymectomy in myasthenia gravis: a computer-assisted matched study. *Ann. Surg.* **194**, 453.

Bucknall, R. C., Dixon, A. St. J., Glick, E. N., Woodland, J. and Zutshi, D. W. (1975). Myasthenia gravis associated with penicillamine treatment for rheumatoid arthritis. *Br. med. J.* **1**, 600.

Bundey, S. (1972). A genetic study of infantile and juvenile myasthenia gravis. *J. Neurol. Neurosurg. Psychiat.* **35**, 41.

Campbell, M. J., Simpson, E., Crombie, A. L. and Walton, J. N. (1970). Ocular myasthenia: evaluation of Tensilon, tonography and electronystagmography as diagnostic tests. *J. Neurol. Neurosurg. Psychiat.* **33**, 639.

Cape, C. A. and Utterback, R. A. (1972). Maintenance adrenocorticotropic hormone (ACTH) treatment in myasthenia gravis. *Neurology, Minneapolis* **22**, 1160.

Chou, S. M. (1982). Pathology of intramuscular nerves and nerve terminals. In *Skeletal muscle pathology* (ed. F. L. Mastaglia and J. N. Walton) Ch. 14. Churchill-Livingstone, Edinburgh.

Churchill-Davidson, H. C. and Richardson, A. T. (1952). The action of decamethonium iodide (C.10) in myasthenia gravis. *J. Neurol. Neurosurg. Psychiat.* **15**, 129.

—— and Wise, R. P. (1963). Neuromuscular transmission in the newborn infant. *Anaesthesiology* **24**, 271.

Coërs, C. and Desmedt, J. E. (1959). Mise en évidence d'une malformation caractéristique de la jonction neuromusculaire dans la myasthénie. *Acta neurol. belg.* **59**, 539.

Compston, D. A. S., Vincent, A., Newsom-Davis, J. and Batchelor, J. R. (1980). Clinical, pathological, HLA antigen and immunological evidence for disease heterogeneity in myasthenia gravis. *Brain* **103**, 579.

Dahlbäck, O., Elmqvist, D., Johns, T. R., Radner, S. and Thesleff, S. (1961). An electrophysiologic study of the neuromuscular junction in myasthenia gravis. *J. Physiol., London* **156**, 336.

Dau, P. C., Lindstrom, J. M., Cassel, C. K. and Clark, E. C. (1979). Plasmapheresis in myasthenia gravis and polymyositis. In *Plasmapheresis and the immunobiology of myasthenia gravis* (ed. P. C. Dau) p. 229. Houghton Mifflin, Boston.

Dawkins, R. L., Garlepp, M. and McDonald, B. (1982). Immunopathology of muscle. In *Skeletal muscle pathology* (ed. F. L. Mastaglia and J. N. Walton) Ch. 15. Churchill-Livingstone, Edinburgh.

Decker, D. A. and Fincham, R. W. (1971). Respiratory arrest in myasthenia gravis with colistimethate therapy, *Arch. Neurol., Chicago* **25**, 141.

Desmedt, J. E. (1957). Bases physiopathologiques du diagnostic de la myasthénie par le test de Jolly. *Rev. neurol.* **96**, 505.

—— (1966). Presynaptic mechanisms in myasthenia gravis. *Ann. NY Acad. Sci.* **135**, 209.

—— and Borenstein, S. (1970). The testing of neuromuscular transmission. In *Handbook of clinical neurology* (ed. P. J. Vinken and G. W. Bruyn), Vol. 7, Ch. 4. North-Holland, Amsterdam.

Drachman, D. B. (1978). Myasthenia gravis. *New Engl. J. Med.* **298**, 136.

Engel, A. G. (1984). Myasthenia gravis and myasthenic syndromes. *Ann. Neurol.* **16**, 519.

——, Lambert, E. H. and Gomez, M. R. (1977). A new myasthenic syndrome with end-plate acetylcholinesterase deficiency, small nerve terminals and reduced acetylcholine release. *Ann. Neurol.* **1**, 4.

——, —— and Santa, T. (1973). Study of longterm anticholinesterase therapy: effects on neuromuscular transmission and on motor end-plate fine structure. *Neurology, Minneapolis* **23**, 1273.

——, Tsujihata, M., Lindstrom, J. M. and Lennon, V. A. (1976). The motor end-plate in myasthenia gravis and in experimental autoimmune myasthenia gravis. A quantitative ultrastructural study. *Ann. NY Acad. Sci.* **274**, 60.

Erb, W. H. (1879). Ueber einen eigenthumlichen bulbaren (?) Symptomcomplex. *Arch. Psychiat. Neurol.* **60**, 172.

Fambrough, D. M., Drachman, D. B. and Satyamurti, S. (1973). Neuromuscular function in myasthenia gravis: decreased acetylcholine receptors. *Science* **182**, 293.

Feltkamp, T. E. W., Van Den Berg-Loonen, P. M., Nijenhuis, L. E., Engelfriet, C. P., Van Rossum, A. L., Van Loghem, J. J. and Oosterhuis, H. J. G. H. (1974). Myasthenia gravis, autoantibodies, and HL-A antigens. *Br. med. J.* **1**, 131.

Fenichel, G. M., Gibler, W. B., Olson, W. H. and Dettbarn, W.-D. (1972). Chronic inhibition of cholinesterase as a cause of myopathy. *Neurology, Minneapolis* **22**, 1026.

Ferguson, F. R., Hutchinson, E. C. and Liversedge, L. A. (1955). Myasthenia gravis. Results of medical management. *Lancet* **ii**, 636.

Fraser, D. C., Palmer, A. C., Senior, J. E. B., Parkes, J. D., and Yealland, M. F. T. (1970). Myasthenia gravis in the dog. *J. Neurol. Neurosurg. Psychiat.* **33**, 431.

Fritze, D., Herrmann, C., Naeim, F., Smith, G. S., and Walford, R. L. (1974). HL-A antigens in myasthenia gravis. *Lancet* **i**, 240.

Garlepp, M. J., Dawkins, R. L. and Christiansen, F. T. (1983). HLA antigens and acetylcholine receptor antibodies in penicillamine induced myasthenia gravis. *Br. med. J.* **286**, 338.

Goldman, A. J., Herrmann, C., Keesey, J. C., Mulder, D. G., and Brown, W. J. (1974). Myasthenia gravis and invasive thymoma: a 20-year experience. *Neurology, Minneapolis* **25**, 1021.

Goldstein, G. and Hofmann, W. W. (1968). Electrophysiological changes similar to those of myasthenia gravis in rats with experimental autoimmune thymitis. *J. Neurol. Neurosurg. Psychiat* **31**, 453.

Grob, D. (1953). Course and management of myasthenia gravis. *J. Am. med. Ass.* **153**, 529.

Hansson, O., Johansson, L., Stalberg, E., and Westerholm, C.-J. (1972). Thymectomy in juvenile myasthenia gravis. *Neuropädiatrie* **3**, 429.

Hausmanowa-Petrusewicz, I., Chorzelski, T., and Strugalska, H. (1969). Three-year observation of a myasthenic syndrome concurrent with other autoimmune syndromes in a patient with thymoma. *J. neurol. Sci.* **9**, 273.

Hokkanen, E. (1969). Epidemiology of myasthenia gravis in Finland. *J. neurol. Sci.* **9**, 463.

—— and Toivakka, E. (1969). Streptomycin-induced neuromuscular fatigue in myasthenia gravis. *Ann. clin. Res.* **1**, 220.

Horowitz, S. H., Genkins, G., Kornfeld, P., and Papatestas, A. E. (1975). Regional curare test in evaluation of ocular myasthenia. *Arch. Neurol., Chicago* **32**, 84.

Jacob, A., Clack, E. R., and Emery, A. E. H. (1968). Genetic study of sample of 70 patients with myasthenia gravis. *J. med. Genet.* **5**, 257.

Johns, R. J., Grob, D., and Harvey, A. McG. (1955). Electromyographic changes in myasthenia gravis. *Am. J. Med.* **19**, 679.

——, and —— (1955). Studies in neuromuscular function II. Effects of nerve stimulation on normal subjects and in patients with myasthenia gravis. *Bull. Johns Hopkins Hosp.* **99**, 125.

Johns, T. R. (1977). Treatment of myasthenia gravis: long-term administration of corticosteroids with remarks on thymectomy. In *Advances in neurology*, Vol. 17 (ed. R. C. Griggs and R. T. Moxley) p. 99. Raven Press, New York.

Jolly, F. (1895). Ueber Myasthenia Gravis Pseudoparalytica. *Klin. Wschr.* **32**, 1.

Joseph, B. S. and Johns, T. R. (1973). Recurrence of non-neoplastic thymus after thymectomy for myasthenia gravis. *Neurology, Minneapolis* **23**, 109.

Kornguth, S. E., Hanson, J. C., and Chun, R. W. M. (1970). Anti-neuronal antibodies in patients having myasthenia gravis. *Neurology, Minneapolis* **20**, 749.

Kott, E., Genkins, G. and Rule, A. H. (1973). Leukocyte response to muscle antigens in myasthenia gravis. *Neurology, Minneapolis* **23**, 374.

Kurtzke, J. F. (1978). Epidemiology of myasthenia gravis. In *Neurological epidemiology: principles and clinical applications* (ed. B. S. Schoenberg). *Adv. Neurol.* **19**, 545.

Lambert, E. H. (1966). Defects of neuromuscular transmission in syndromes other than myasthenia gravis. *Ann. NY Acad. Sci.* **135**, 367.

Lang, B., Newsom Davis, J., Wray, D., Vincent, A., and Murray, N. (1981). Autoimmune aetiology for myasthenia (Eaton–Lambert syndrome). *Lancet* **ii**, 224.

Lindstrom, J. (1977). An assay for antibodies to human acetylcholine receptor in serum from patients with myasthenia gravis. *Clin. Immunol. Immunopathol.* **7**, 36.

—— (1978). How the autoimmune response to acetylcholine receptor impairs neuromuscular transmission in myasthenia gravis and its animal mode. *Fed. Proc.* **37**, 2828.

Lisak, R. P. and Barchi, R. L. (1982). *Myasthenia gravis*. Saunders, Philadelphia.

Marshall, A. H. E. and White, R. G. (1961). Experimental thymic lesions resembling those of myasthenia gravis. *Lancet* **i**, 1030.

Martin, L., Herr, J. C., Wanamaker, W., and Kornguth, S. (1974). Demonstration of specific antineuronal nuclear antibodies in sera of patients with myasthenia gravis. *Neurology, Minneapolis* **24**, 680.

Mastaglia, F. L. and Argov, Z. (1981). Drug-induced neuromuscular disorders in man. In *Disorders of voluntary muscle* (ed. J. N. Walton) 4th edn, Ch. 25. Churchill-Livingstone, Edinburgh.

McQuillen, M. P., Cantor, H. E., and O'Rourke, J. R. (1968). Myasthenic syndrome associated with antibiotics. *Arch. Neurol., Chicago* **18**, 402.

—— and Johns, R. J. (1966). The nature of the defect in the Eaton–Lambert syndrome. *Neurology, Minneapolis* **17**, 527.

Murray, N. M. F. and Newsom-Davis, J. (1981). Treatment with oral 4-aminopyridine in disorders of neuromuscular transmission. *Neurology, Minneapolis* **31**, 265.

Nakao, Y., Matsumoto, H., Miyazaki, T., Nishitani, H., Ota, K., Fujita, T., and Tsuji, K. (1980). Gm allotypes in myasthenia gravis. *Lancet* **i**, 677.

Namba, T., Brown, S. B., and Grob, D. (1970). Neonatal myasthenia gravis: report of two cases and review of the literature. *Pediatrics* **45**, 488.

——, Shapiro, M. S., Brunner, N. G., and Grob, D. (1971*a*). Myasthenia gravis occurring in twins. *J. Neurol. Neurosurg. Psychiat.* **34**, 531.

——, Brunner, N. G., Brown, S. B., Muguruma, M., and Grob, D. (1971*b*). Familial myasthenia gravis: report of 27 patients in 12 families and review of 164 patients in 73 families. *Arch. Neurol. Chicago* **25**, 49.

——, ——, Shapiro, M. S. and Grob, D. (1971*c*). Corticotropin therapy in myasthenia gravis: effects, indications, and limitations. *Neurology, Minneapolis* **21**, 1008.

—— and Grob, D. (1966). Autoantibodies and myasthenia gravis, with special reference to muscle ribonucleoprotein. *Ann. NY Acad. Sci.* **135**, 606.

—— and —— (1971). Myasthenia gravis and hyperthyroidism occurring in two sisters, *Neurology, Minneapolis* **21**, 377.

——, Himei, H. and Grob, D. (1967). Complement fixing and tissue binding serum globulins in patients with myasthenia gravis, and their relation to muscle ribonucleoprotein. *J. Lab. clin. Med.* **70**, 258.

Newsom Davis, J. (1979). Antiacetylcholine receptor antibody in myasthenia gravis. In *Clinical neuroimmunology* (ed. F. C. Rose) p. 128. Blackwell, London.

——, Pinching, A. J., Vincent, A., and Wilson, S. G. (1978). Function of circulating antibody to acetylcholine receptor in myasthenia gravis: investigation by plasma exchange. *Neurology, Minneapolis* **28**, 266.

Oh, S. J. (1974). The Eaton–Lambert syndrome in ocular myasthenia gravis. *Arch. Neurol., Chicago* **31**, 183.

—— and Kim, K. W. (1973). Guanidine hydrochloride in the Eaton–Lambert syndrome. *Neurology, Minneapolis* **23**, 1084.

Oosterhuis, H. J. G. H. and Bethlem, J. (1973). Neurogenic muscle involvement in myasthenia gravis. *J. Neurol. Neurosurg. Psychiat.* **36**, 24.

——, —— and Feltkamp, T. E. W. (1968). Muscle pathology, thymoma, and immunological abnormalities in patients with myasthenia gravis. *J. Neurol. Neurosurg. Psychiat.* **31**, 460.

Osserman, K. E. (1958). *Myasthenia gravis*. Grune and Stratton, New York.

—— and Kaplan, L. I. (1953). Studies in myasthenia gravis. Use of edrophonium chloride (Tensilon) in differentiating myasthenic from cholinergic weakness. *Arch. Neurol. Psychiat., Chicago* **70**, 385.

Patrick, J. and Lindstrom, J. (1973). Autoimmune response to acetylcholine receptor. *Science* **180**, 871.

Patten, B. M. (1978). Myasthenia gravis: review of diagnosis and management. *Muscle & Nerve* **1**, 190.

Perlo, V. P., Arnason, B., Poskanzer, D., Castleman, B., Schwab, R. S., Osserman, K. E., Papatestis, A., Alpert, L., and Kark, A. (1971). The role of thymectomy in the treatment of myasthenia gravis. *Ann. NY Acad. Sci.* **183**, 308.

Pinelli, P., Tonali, P. and Scoppetta, C. (1974). Long-term treatment of myasthenia gravis with alternate-day prednisone. *Eur. Neurol.* **12**, 129.

Rooke, E. D., Eaton, L. M., Lambert, E. H., and Hodgson, C. H. (1960). Myasthenia and malignant intrathoracic tumor. *Med. Clin. N. Am.* **44**, 977.

Roses, A. D., Olanow, C. W., McAdams, M. W., and Lane, R. J. M. (1981). No direct correlation between serum antiacetylcholine receptor antibody levels and clinical states of individual patients with myasthenia gravis. *Neurology, Minneapolis 1*, 220.

Rowland, L. P., Lisak, R. P., Schotland, D. L., DeJesus, P. V., and Berg, P. (1973). Myasthenic myopathy and thymoma. *Neurology, Minneapolis* **23**, 282.

Santa, T., Engel, A. G. and Lambert, E. H. (1972a). Histometric study of neuromuscular junction ultrastructure. I. Myasthenia gravis. *Neurology, Minneapolis* **22**, 71.

——, —— and —— (1972b). Histometric study of neuromuscular junction ultrastructure. II. Myasthenic syndrome. *Neurology, Minneapolis* **22**, 370.

Schlezinger, N. S. and Corin, M. S. (1968). Myasthenia gravis associated with hyperthyroidism in childhood. *Neurology, Minneapolis* **18**, 1217.

Schwartz, M. S. and Stalberg, E. (1975). Myasthenia gravis with features of the myasthenic syndrome. *Neurology, Minneapolis* **25**, 80.

Simpson, J. A. (1958). An evaluation of thymectomy in myasthenia gravis. *Brain* **81**, 112.

—— (1960). Myasthenia gravis: a new hypothesis. *Scot. med. J.* **5**, 419.

—— (1971). A morphological explanation of the transmission defect in myasthenia gravis. *Ann. NY Acad. Sci.* **183**, 241.

—— (1981). Myasthenia gravis and myasthenic syndromes. In *Disorders of voluntary muscle* (ed. J. N. Walton) 9th edn, Ch. 16. Churchill-Livingstone, Edinburgh.

Slomić A., Rosenfalck, A., and Buchthal, F. (1968). Electrical and mechanical responses of normal and myasthenic muscle, with particular reference to the staircase phenomenon. *Brain Res.* **10**, 1.

Spector, R. H., Daroff, R. B., and Birkett, J. E. (1975). Edrophonium infra-red optokinetic nystagmography in the diagnosis of myasthenia gravis. *Neurology, Minneapolis* **25**, 317.

Spillane, J. D. (1975). *An atlas of clinical neurology*, 2nd edn. Oxford University Press, London.

Stalberg, E., Trontelj, J., and Schwartz, M. (1976). Single muscle fiber recordings of the jitter phenomenon in patients with myasthenia gravis and in members of their families. *Ann. NY Acad. Sci.* **274**, 189.

Strauss, A. J. L., Segal, B. C., Hsu, K. C., Burkholder, P. M., Nastuk, W. L., and Osserman, K. E. (1960). Immunofluorescence demonstration of a muscle-binding, complement-fixing serum globulin fraction in myasthenia gravis. *Proc. Soc. exp. Biol., NY* **105**, 184.

Szobor, A. (1970). *Crises in myasthenia gravis*. Akadémiai Kiadó, Budapest.

Tarrab-Hazdai, R., Aharonov, A., Silman, I., and Fuchs, S. (1975). Experimental autoimmune myasthenia induced in monkeys by purified acetylcholine receptor. *Nature, London* **256**, 128.

Vetters, J. M., Simpson, J. A., and Folkarde, A. (1969). Experimental myasthenia gravis. *Lancet* **ii**, 28.

Vincent, A., Cull-Candy, S. G., Newsom Davis, J., Trautmann, A., Molenaar, P. C., and Polak, R. L. (1981). Congenital myasthenia: end-plate acetylcholine receptors and electrophysiology in five cases. *Muscle & Nerve* **4**, 306.

—— and Newsom Davis, J. (1979). Absence of antiacetylcholine receptor antibodies in congenital myasthenia gravis. *Lancet* **i**, 441.

Walker, M. B. (1934). Treatment of myasthenia gravis with physostigmine. *Lancet* **i**, 1200.

Warmolts, R. J. and Engel, W. K. (1972). Benefit from alternate-day prednisone in myasthenia gravis. *New Engl. J. Med.* **286**, 17.

Wilks, S. (1877). Bulbar paralysis; fatal; no disease found. *Guy's Hosp. Rep.* **37**, 54.

Wilson, A., Obrist, A. R., and Wilson, H. (1953). Some effects of extracts of thymus glands removed from patients with myasthenia gravis. *Lancet* **ii**, 368.

Wise, G. A. and McQuillen, M. P. (1970). Transient neonatal myasthenia. *Arch. Neurol., Chicago* **22**, 556.

Wray. S. H. and Pavan-Langston, D. (1971). A re-evaluation of edrophonium chloride (Tensilon) tonography in the diagnosis of myasthenia gravis. *Neurology, Minneapolis* **21**, 586.

Endocrine and metabolic myopathies

Endocrine myopathies

Disorders of the thyroid gland

Thyrotoxic myopathy

Chronic thyrotoxic myopathy was first described by Bathurst in 1895 and it is well recognized that, in severe cases of thyrotoxicosis, weakness and wasting of proximal limb muscles, particularly in the upper extremities, may occur and may resolve when the thyroid disease is effectively treated. Ramsay (1965) described clinical and EMG studies carried out on 54 consecutive unselected patients with proven thyrotoxicosis and found that, while few complained of muscular weakness, clinical examination showed demonstrable weakness in over 80 per cent and the EMG a reduced mean action potential duration and an increased percentage of polyphasic potentials in more than 90 per cent of cases. Four months after treatment of the thyrotoxicosis the EMG had returned to normal in most patients. Similar findings were reported by Satoyoshi, Murakami, Kowa, Kinoshita, Noguchi, Hoshina, Nishiyama, and Ito (1963) who also found that weakness sometimes improved when oral potassium was given. Thus in thyrotoxicosis there is almost always a reversible abnormality of muscle function and quantitative electromyography is probably the most sensitive indicator of this change. The cause of the weakness is still unclear; mitochondrial respiratory control is normal (Stocker, Samaha, and De Groat 1968); an abnormally active plasma membrane sodium pump has been postulated (Philipson and Edelman 1977) and it has been suggested that the membrane contains increased catecholamine receptor sites (Williams, Lefkowitz, and Watanabe 1977). Probably several different such factors contribute (Engel 1981).

Exophthalmic ophthalmoplegia (ophthalmic Graves' disease)

Exophthalmic ophthalmoplegia, endocrine exophthalmos, or as it is now more often called, ophthalmic Graves' disease or inflammatory ophthalmopathy, must be mentioned as its principal effect is upon the external ocular muscles, which are greatly increased in bulk, as are the orbital contents as a whole. The subject was reviewed by Brain (1959), Hall, Doniach, Kirkham, and El Kabir (1970) and by Weetman, McGregor, and Hall (1984). The main symptoms are exophthalmos and diplopia and the degree of ophthalmoplegia is usually proportional to the severity of the exophthalmos. Sometimes the latter is so great (Fig. 19.7) that the eyelids cannot be closed and corneal ulceration ensues. Papilloedema may occur and, if not relieved, may progress to optic atrophy and blindness. In severe cases surgical decompression of the orbit is required and measures must be carried out as an emergency (MacCarty, Kenefick, McConahey, and Kearns 1970; Smigiel and MacCarty 1975). Some patients are mildly thyrotoxic, others first develop the syndrome after treatment of thyrotoxicosis, and the condition may occur in association with myxoedema, but most individuals are euthyroid and have a high titre of thyroglobulin antibodies. An exophthalmos-producing substance distinct from the long-acting thyroid stimulator was once thought to be responsible (Hall *et al.* 1970), but recent evidence suggests that the condition is auto-immune and a circulating autoantibody against a human eye muscle soluble antigen can be detected in most cases (Kodama, Sikorska, Bandy-Dafoe, Bayly, and Wall 1982; *The Lancet* 1982). This is an IgG which binds specifically to retro-orbital antigen; it was found by Atkinson, Holcombe, and Kendall-Taylor (1984) in 64 per cent of active untreated cases, 25 per cent of those with active disease receiving prednisone and in 16 per cent of long-standing inactive cases. Hormonal treatment is ineffective, radiotherapy to the orbit has been largely abandoned, but high-dosage steroid treatment or plasmapheresis are most successful in reducing exophthalmos quickly. A recent report suggests that cyclosporin may produce dramatic improvement (Weetman, McGregor, Ludgate, Beck, Mills, Lazarus, and Hall 1983). In mild cases not requiring either steroids or surgery, little can be done and the results of treatment of associated thyrotoxicosis with iodine-131 are unpredictable (Jones, Munro, and Wilson 1969), but the condition is often self-limiting, often improving spontaneously after some years or ultimately becoming stabilized. Guanethidine eye-drops are sometimes useful in reducing lid retraction (Martin and Jay 1969).

In differential diagnosis the orbital pseudotumour syndrome, often due to orbital myositis responsive to prednisone and presumed to be due to a connective-tissue disorder involving orbital muscles (Jellinek 1969) must be considered, as must proptosis, often asymmetrical, due to mucocele of the ethmoid sinus and other orbital lesions (p. 106).

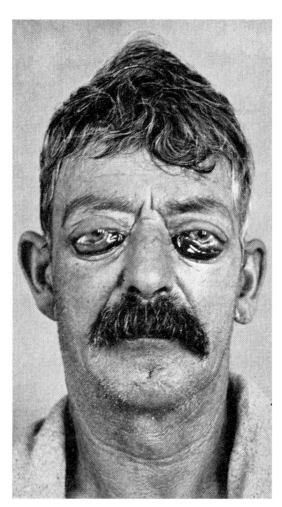

Fig. 19.7. Severe endocrine exophthalmos (ophthalmic Graves' disease).

Thyrotoxicosis and myasthenia gravis

About 5 per cent of myasthenic patients have, or later develop, thyrotoxicosis, another 5 per cent are hypothyroid, and 2 per cent have non-toxic goitre (Engel 1981). Engel (1961) noted that myasthenia may become worse when hyperthyroidism increases. Both conditions must be treated in the usual manner, but it should be noted that the risks of thyroidectomy are often increased in patients suffering from myasthenia gravis.

Thyrotoxic periodic paralysis

An association between thyrotoxicosis and periodic paralysis has been observed, particularly among the Chinese and Japanese, and may be dominantly inherited (McFadzean and Yeung 1969), but 95 per cent of cases are sporadic (Engel 1981). Okinawa, Shizume, Iino, Watanaba, Irie, Noguchi, Kuma, Kuma, and Ito (1957) in a study of 6333 cases of hyperthyroidism, found that 8.9 per cent of the males and 0.4 per cent of the females had had attacks of periodic paralysis which were of hypokalaemic type. Adequate treatment of the hyperthyroidism results in the disappearance of the periodic attacks of weakness or in a marked decrease in their number and severity (Norris, Panner, and Stormont 1968; Brody and Dudley 1969).

Myopathy in hypothyroidism

Muscular hypertrophy with weakness and slowness of muscular contraction and relaxation has been described in children with sporadic cretinism (Debré and Semelaigne 1935; Spiro, Hirano, Beilin, and Finkelstein 1970). When a similar condition occurs in adults it is known as Hoffman's syndrome (Hoffman 1896) and Wilson and Walton (1959) described cases in which the clinical evidence of hypothyroidism was relatively unobtrusive and the muscular symptoms, including muscle pain on exertion, predominated. There is some evidence of impaired glycogenolysis in such cases (McDaniel, Pittman, Oh, and Di Mauro 1977). This syndrome may superficially resemble myotonia and has then been called pseudomyotonia (Crispell and Parson 1954); very rarely hypothyroidism may be superimposed upon a pre-existing and virtually symptomless myotonia congenita (Jarcho and Tyler 1958). Astrom, Kugelberg, and Müller (1961) reported that myxoedema is occasionally associated with a girdle myopathy causing mild proximal weakness and wasting similar to that seen in chronic thyrotoxic myopathy. In their cases improvement was observed on treatment with thyroxin. Salick, Colachis, and Pearson (1968) also reported a case of myxoedematous myopathy and Takamori, Gutmann, Crosby, and Martin (1972) described abnormalities of neuromuscular transmission resembling those of the Eaton–Lambert syndrome in two cases of hypothyroidism.

Disorders of the pituitary and adrenal glands

In acromegaly and pituitary gigantism, generalized muscular weakness may be observed but is rarely striking (Adams 1975). Similarly, widespread weakness with some atrophy may occur in hypopituitarism (Walton 1960), but the exact nature of the myopathic change in such cases is unclear (Engel 1981). However, the clinical, electromyographic, and histological features of the myopathy of acromegaly have been fully elucidated (Mastaglia, Gardner-Medwin, and Hudgson 1971; Pickett, Layzer, Levin, Schneider, Campbell, and Sumner 1975). Muscle pain and proximal weakness predominate with little wasting (Khaleek, Levy, Edwards, McPhail, Mills, Round, and Betteridge 1984). General weakness is also sometimes seen in Addison's disease and probably results from the changes in plasma and muscle water and electrolytes. Treatment leads to a rapid improvement in muscular strength and no permanent muscle changes have been described, though Witts, Lakin, and Thompson (1938) and Thorn (1949) noted contractures at the elbows and knees occurring in occasional cases of Addison's disease and suggested that these were due to changes of unknown nature occurring in the fasciae and tendons.

Cushing's disease and steroid myopathy

In 1959 Müller and Kugelberg (1959) described six patients with Cushing's disease of whom five had weakness of pelvic-girdle and thigh muscles. Electromyography demonstrated myopathic changes in the affected muscles, and in the same year Perkoff, Silber, Tyler, Cartwright, and Wintrobe (1959) reported cases of muscle weakness and wasting occurring in patients under treatment with steroids. Since then both the naturally-occurring myopathy and the iatrogenic disorder have been reported frequently, and the latter is most often caused by steroids such as triamcinolone which have a fluorine atom in the 9α position (Harman 1959; Williams 1959). A similar syndrome has been described in patients receiving dexamethasone and betamethasone (Golding, Murray, Pearce, and Thompson 1961); often in such cases weakness resolved when prednisone was substituted though many cases have been reported (Perkoff et al. 1959; Askari, Vignos, and Maskowitz 1976) in which the latter drug, if given in high dosage, was responsible. Coomes (1965) examined electromyographically 50 patients receiving corticosteroid drugs and compared his findings with those obtained in control individuals. He found that the mean action potential duration of motor action potentials obtained from one deltoid muscle was markedly reduced in patients showing striking side-effects of steroid therapy. He concluded that corticosteroid myopathy is commonest in those patients who show most side-effects of the treatment and that the EMG offers a reliable method of detecting early myopathic change. There is evidence that women are more susceptible than men (Bunch, Worthington, Combs, Ilstrup, and Engel 1980). The myopathy quickly resolves once the steroid treatment is withdrawn and Pleasure, Walsh and Engel (1970) also reported resolution of the myopathy of Cushing's disease after effective treatment. Muscle biopsy typically demonstrates atrophy of Type II muscle fibres in both the naturally occurring and iatrogenic disorders and the potassium content of the muscle is reduced.

Corticotrophin (ACTH) myopathy
Prineas, Hall, Barwick, and Watson (1968) reported proximal muscle weakness and wasting developing in a series of pigmented patients who had undergone adrenalectomy for the treatment of Cushing's disease. Investigation demonstrated that these patients were suffering from a myopathy and muscle biopsy sections showed a striking accumulation of fat within individual muscle fibres. It was concluded that this myopathy was the result of excessive circulating ACTH (corticotrophin) (Nelson's syndrome).

Metabolic myopathies

Myopathy in metabolic bone disease
Prineas, Mason, and Henson (1965) described two patients with chronic muscular weakness, one of whom had a parathyroid adenoma and the other was found to be suffering from osteomalacia and idiopathic steatorrhoea. The main clinical features were proximal muscular wasting and weakness, pain and discomfort on movement, with hypotonia but brisk tendon reflexes. They suggested that in these cases a disturbance of vitamin D metabolism could interfere with the excitation–contraction coupling involving the entry of calcium into the muscle fibre during contraction. There is evidence that deficiency of vitamin D can affect the uptake of calcium by the muscle mitochondria, protein synthesis, ATP stores, and force generation (Pleasure, Wyszynski, Sumner, Schotland, Feldmann, Nugent, Hitz, and Goodman 1979). Similar cases have been described by Smith and Stern (1967). Myopathy in osteomalacia due to anticonvulsant medication has also been described (Marsden, Reynolds, Parsons, Harris, and Duchen 1973) and muscular weakness was also the presenting feature of three cases of hypophosphataemic osteomalacia (Schott and Wills 1975). However, myopathy is not usually a feature of hypoparathyroidism (Engel 1981).

Myopathy in chronic renal failure
Floyd, Ayyar, Barwick, Hudgson, and Weightman (1974) reported 11 cases of proximal myopathy occurring in patients with end-stage renal failure, in four of whom osteomalacia was discovered and in these there was some improvement in muscular

weakness with vitamin D. In the other seven, weakness improved dramatically after renal transplantation or dialysis. In uraemic hyperparathyroidism, metabolic calcification in vessel walls can cause focal cutaneous necrosis, visceral infarcts, and a necrotizing myopathy with myoglobinuria (Goodhue, Davis, and Porro 1972).

Glycogen storage disease of muscle
In 1951 McArdle described the case of a man of 30 who had generalized muscular pain and stiffness which increased during slight exertion. He showed that the blood lactate and pyruvate levels failed to rise after exercise and postulated a defect of glucose utilization. In 1959 two additional cases were reported (Schmid and Mahler 1959; Mommaerts, Illingworth, Pearson, Guillory, and Seraydarian 1959) and one of these also showed myoglobinuria. In both the muscle glycogen content was increased and myophosphorylase activity was absent. Mellick, Mahler, and Hughes (1962) described another case of myophosphorylase deficiency in which there was also muscular weakness in the girdle muscles, and Schmid and Hammaker (1961) described three cases in one family suggesting autosomal recessive inheritance; Adamson, Salter, and Pearce (1967) described three cases of variable severity in a single family and Engel, Eyerman, and Williams (1963) a further two, one of whom had severe muscular weakness and wasting without cramps developing in late life, while a second, also in middle age, developed cramps after exercise without weakness and wasting; both showed a partial defect of muscle phosphorylase activity with a normal total glycogen content in muscle. Thus a partial deficiency of the enzyme may produce a relatively benign disorder of late onset, while at the other extreme, total absence of the enzyme has been reported to cause a severe 'floppy infant' syndrome with death in early infancy (DiMauro and Hartlage 1978). While oral fructose may improve exercise tolerance in some patients, no form of treatment is consistently successful in relieving the symptoms of this usually benign but disabling disorder which is best diagnosed first by estimating lactate in venous blood before and after ischaemic exercise and by muscle biopsy, histochemical staining for phosphorylase, and measurement of the concentration of glycogen and phosphorylase in the sample. Physiological contracture of muscles and myoglobinuria often follow exertion; the mechanism of the contracture is still unexplained (Negel 1981; Pleasure and Bonilla 1982).

It is now well recognized that other forms of muscle glycogenosis, though rare, are more common than was at one time realized. In a child of 4 with a diffuse myopathy, Thomson, MacLaurin, and Prineas (1963) demonstrated a defect of phosphoglucomutase, and more recently DiMauro, Miranda, Olarte, Friedman, and Hays (1982) detected a deficiency of phosphoglycerate mutase in a middle-aged man who had suffered cramps and pigmenturia since adolescence. Tarui, Okuna, Ikura, Tanaka, Suda, and Nishikawa (1965), Layzer, Rowland, and Ranney (1967), Bonilla and Schotland (1970), and Tobin, Huijing, Porro, and Salzman (1973) also described a myopathic disorder closely resembling McArdle's disease clinically and biochemically but which is due to phosphofructokinase deficiency. This condition not only gives muscle pain on exertion and a 'flat' ischaemic lactate test but can also present as a late-onset myopathy (Hays, Hallett, Delfs, Morris, Sotrel, Sheuchuk, and DiMauro 1981). The condition now called limit dextrinosis (Illingworth, Cori, and Cori 1956) gives glycogen storage in liver, skeletal muscle, and in heart and is due to a deficiency of debranching enzyme (amylo-1,6-glucosidase). This condition, however, like Pompe's disease which gives rise to glycogen storage in the heart, skeletal muscles, and central nervous system, and which is due to amylo-1,4-glucosidase (acid maltase) deficiency, is often incompatible with survival beyond the first few years of life. Antenatal diagnosis of Pompe's disease by amniocentesis is now possible (Galjaard, Mekes, De Josselin, De Jong, and Niermeijer 1973)., However, it is now apparent that debranching enzyme deficiency, though usually causing hepatomegaly, growth retardation, fasting hypoglycaemia, and cardiomegaly, can sometimes cause a clinically significant myopathy with muscle aching and fatigue in adolescence or early adult life (Murase, Ikeda, Muro, Nakao, and Sugita 1973). Much more often, acid maltase deficiency is even less grave in its prognosis and many cases are now on record of patients presenting with an apparently progressive myopathy of girdle muscles in late childhood or in adult life (Zellweger, Brown, McCormick, and Tu 1965; Courtecuisse, Royer, Habib, Monnier, and Demos 1965; Hudgson, Gardner-Medwin, Worsfold, Pennington, and Walton 1968; Engel 1970, 1981). Thus the possible diagnosis of glycogen storage disease of muscle must now be considered in all cases of suspected limb-girdle muscular dystrophy arising in middle life, and muscle biopsy may be diagnostic as striking vacuolation of muscle fibres is usually thereby revealed and the vacuoles contain large quantities of glycogen. It seems certain that in years to come, many more specific myopathic disorders related to individual enzyme defects will be defined. Unfortunately none of these conditions yet appears to be amenable to any form of effective treatment; attempts to treat Pompe's disease with liposomes containing purified acid maltase isolated from human placenta have not benefited the human disease; nor has a low-carbohydrate diet combined with epinephrine administration (Rosenow and Engel 1978), although carbohydrate restriction is sensible.

It should also be mentioned that myopathy resulting from severe and prolonged hypoglycaemia has been described in patients suffering from islet-cell adenoma of the pancreas (Mulder, Bastron, and Lambert 1956).

Periodic paralysis syndromes

Hypokalaemic periodic paralysis

The classical hypokalaemic variety of periodic paralysis has been well recognized for many years and has been reviewed by Engel (1981) and Tomé (1982). This condition, usually of dominant inheritance, gives rise to attacks of flaccid weakness of the voluntary muscles but those of speech, swallowing and respiration are usually spared. Attacks most often begin in the second decade and are most frequent in early adult life. Commonly they last for several hours and often start early in the morning on waking, after a period of rest following exertion, or after a heavy carbohydrate meal. During attacks the plasma potassium level is usually found to be low (less than 3 mmol/1); there is a positive balance of potassium and some or all of the retained potassium seems to pass into the muscle cell (Grob, Liljestrand, and Johns 1957; Zierler and Andres 1957). Shy, Wanko, Rowley, and Engel (1961) showed that the resting membrane potential is normal during an attack of paralysis; they also demonstrated that electron microscopy of muscle biopsy specimens taken during an attack shows vacuoles resulting from dilatation of the sarcoplasmic reticulum. It has been suggested that this form of periodic paralysis might be due to intermittent aldosteronism, since patients with primary aldosteronism due to tumours of the adrenal (Conn 1955) do have attacks of muscular weakness. However, aldosteronism can be distinguished from periodic paralysis by the associated hypertension, alkalosis, and hypernatraemia and by the persistence of the hypokalaemia between the attacks; furthermore, in familial periodic paralysis increased aldosterone excretion is not usually found. The many conditions in which prolonged or intermittent muscular weakness can be the result of excessive urinary or gastrointestinal excretion of potassium have been listed by Engel (1981). A similar syndrome has been described in Papua and New Guinea due to dietary potassium/sodium imbalance (Duggin and Price 1974).

Exercise or peripheral-nerve stimulation may abort or postpone attacks of weakness (Campa and Sanders 1974). Potassium chloride, 4–6 g daily, has been used in treating attacks but rarely shortens the episodes of weakness. Spironolactone, 25 mg four times daily, and other aldosterone antagonists were found, however, to reduce greatly their frequency and severity (Poskanzer and Kerr 1961a). Subsequently, acetazolamide 250 mg four times daily was found to be an even more effective prophylactic treatment (Resnick, Engel, Griggs, and Stam 1968), as the metabolic acidosis induced by this drug seems to lower the rate of entry of potassium into the muscle cell (Vroom, Jarrell, and Maren 1975). Occasionally muscular weakness is curiously localized to one or more muscle groups and sometimes after frequent attacks permanent atrophy of muscles develops (Dyken, Zeman, and Rusche 1969), but on the whole the patients tend to improve spontaneously as they grow older.

Hyperkalaemic periodic paralysis (adynamia episodica hereditaria)

In 1951 Tyler, Stephens, Gunn, and Perkoff described a group of cases in which the serum potassium level did not fall during the attacks and the patients were made worse by potassium chloride. Helweg-Larsen, Hauge, and Sagild (1955) described a similar condition and Gamstorp (1956) reported two families and called the condition adynamia episodica hereditaria (hyperkalaemic periodic paralysis is probably a more satisfactory title (Klein, Egan, and Usher 1960). This condition is closely related to paramyotonia (Lundberg, Stalberg, and Thiele 1974) for some of the patients show definite myotonia (Drager, Hamill, and Shy 1958; Van der Meulen, Gilbert, and Kane 1961), though in others the myotonia seems curiously limited to the muscles around the eye and can be evoked by placing ice-bags on the eyelids, a manœuvre which tends to produce striking lid-lag. Van't Hoff (1962) referred to such cases as examples of myotonic periodic paralysis. In affected individuals the attacks are usually shorter in duration than in the hypokalaemic variety, lasting on an average 30–40 minutes, and may be precipitated immediately by exercise. Cardiac arrhythmia is an occasional complication (Lisak, Lebeau, Tucker, and Rowland 1972) and some patients develop muscular wasting (Saunders, Ashworth, Emery, and Benedikz 1968) with histological evidence of myopathy and tubular aggregates on electron microscopy (Macdonald, Rewcastle, and Humphrey 1968). Commonly there is a rise in the serum potassium level, though some patients have severe weakness when the level is no higher than 4 mmol/1, whereas in normal people a level of 7–8 mmol/1 is needed as a rule before weakness develops. Persistent or episodic weakness has been reported in patients with renal or adrenal insufficiency causing hyperkalaemia (secondary hyperkalaemic paralysis). A persistently high serum potassium between attacks of weakness suggests secondary rather than primary hyperkalaemic paralysis (Engel 1981). Abbott, Creutzfeldt, Fowler, and Pearson (1962) and McComas, Mrozek, and Bradley (1968) showed that the muscle fibre membrane potential is lowered during the attacks which may be cut short by the intravenous administration of calcium gluconate or by the inhalation of salbutamol (Wang and Clausen 1976), while acetazolamide, 250 mg two or three times daily, hydrochlorothiazide, 25 two or three times daily, and dichlorphenamide have all been used successfully for prophylaxis (Hoskins, Vroom, and Jarrell 1975).

Sodium-responsive normokalaemic periodic paralysis

The third type of periodic paralysis, the so-called sodium-responsive normokalaemic variety (Poskanzer and Kerr 1961b) is probably a variant of the hyperkalaemic type, but in these cases the attacks occasionally last for days or weeks and often develop at night. Nevertheless the paralysis is always increased by the administration of potassium and improved by large doses of sodium chloride. It was in cases of this type that Shy, Gonatas, and Perez (1966) found increased numbers of mitochondria in muscle biopsy sections examined with the electron microscope and called this change pleoconial myopathy. Meyers, Gilden, Rinaldi, and Hansen (1972) found many tubular aggregates in muscle sections, attributed to proliferation of the sarcoplasmic reticulum.

Poskanzer and Kerr (1961*b*) found that acetazolamide combined with 9-alpha-fluorohydrocortisone, 0.1 mg daily, prevented the attacks.

Clearly, therefore, careful investigation of every case of periodic paralysis is necessary in order to establish the nature of the patient's illness. Attempts to identify a primary enzyme defect or a specific disorder of carbohydrate metabolism in such cases have been unsuccessful, but an abnormality of the plasma membrane seems likely (Engel 1981). Empirical treatment, both given prophylactically or in order to cut short the attacks, is generally successful once the character of the patient's attacks has been carefully defined.

Myoglobinuria

Myoglobin may appear in the urine as a result of acute crush injury of muscle (Bywaters and Stead (1945) and in localized ischaemic muscular necrosis, while, as already mentioned, it can occur in certain acute forms of polymyositis. It has also been described in poisoning as a result of eating quails (Ouzounellis 1968, 1970) and as an occasional consequence of other toxins and drugs as in Haff disease after eating fish or following a bite of the Malayan sea-snake (Rowland, Fahn, Hirschberg, and Harter 1969; Engel 1981).

A specific syndrome of paroxysmal myoglobinuria of unknown aetiology has also been described and is also called idiopathic rhabdomyolysis (Savage, Forbes, and Pearce 1971); this is characterized by acute attacks of severe cramp-like muscle pain and tenderness associated with weakness or paralysis which are accompanied, within a few hours, by myoglobinuria. The condition usually clears up within two to three days with rest, but occasional cases show such severe and widespread muscle damage that death results from renal or respiratory failure (myoglobinuria can cause renal tubular necrosis). Korein, Coddon, and Mowrey (1959) distinguished two types, of which Type I occurred predominantly in males in late adolescence or early adult life; the pain and myoglobinuria followed exercise and sometimes led to permanent weakness and wasting. Some such cases may be due to carnitine palmityl transferase deficiency (Cumming, Hardy, Hudgson, and Walls 1976), or to enzymatic defects in the glycolytic chain (such as McArdle's disease). In cases of Type II, seen particularly in childhood, an acute infection often preceded the muscle pain and myoglobinuria; the attacks were severe, with fever and leucocytosis, but tended to occur at progressively longer intervals and usually cleared up with the passage of time. Further experience has shown that classification into two specific types is not valid as myoglobinuria can be due to muscle trauma, ischaemia, various enzymatic defects, numerous toxins, or a post-infective (possibly auto-immune) process (Engel 1981). Widespread muscle-fibre necrosis and regeneration are usually seen in muscle biopsy sections (Schutta, Kelly, and Zacks 1969).

Malignant hyperpyrexia

This rare condition gives a rapid rise in body temperature during surgical anaesthesia and has often proved fatal. It may be precipitated by many anaesthetic agents, and although it is commonest in patients anaesthetized with halothane and/or suxamethonium, no anaesthetic agent has been shown to be absolutely safe (Harriman, Sumner, and Ellis 1973). The hyperpyrexia is accompanied by extreme muscular rigidity, tachycardia, tachypnoea, cyanosis, and respiratory and metabolic acidosis (King, Denborough, and Zapt 1972). The susceptibility is often dominantly inherited (King *et al.* 1972; Bradley, Ward, Murchison, Hall, and Woolf 1973*a*) and in many affected patients and families evidence of overt or subclinical myopathy is found (Steers, Tallack, and Thompson 1970) and sometimes features superficially resembling dystrophia myotonica or myotonia congenita. A similar condition has been described in Landrace and Pietrain pigs (Hall, Trim, and Woolf 1972; Lister 1973). There is evidence of abnormality of the muscle fibre membrane and sarcoplasmic reticulum in such cases (Harriman *et al.* 1973; Denborough, Warne, Moulds, Tse, and Martin 1974). While the resting activity of creatine kinase in the serum is raised in some susceptible individuals, this alone is insufficient as a predictive screening test, and muscle biopsy under local anaesthesia followed by *in vitro* study of the halothane-induced contracture may be needed to identify the individuals liable to develop the typical reaction to anaesthesia (Ellis, Keaney, Harriman, Sumner, Kyei-Mensah, Tyrrell, Hargreaves, Parikh, and Mulrooney 1972; Ellis, Clarke, Modgill, Currie, and Harriman 1975; Isaacs, Heffron, and Badenhorst 1975; Gronert 1980). Dantrolene sodium, given intravenously (1–2 mg/kg body weight), repeated every 5–10 minutes up to 10 mg/kg, is a specific treatment and is also of prophylactic value (Faust, Gergis, and Sokoll 1979; Engel 1981). A similar syndrome precipitated by fluphenazine in a patient with schizophrenia was controlled by bromocriptine (Granato, Stern, Ringel, Karim, Krumholz, Coyle, and Adler 1983).

Myopathy due to various toxins and drugs

Widespread muscle necrosis leading to renal tubular necrosis is a rare complication of carbon monoxide poisoning (Loughridge, Leader, and Bowen 1958). Severe myalgia and muscular stiffness can occur in patients receiving clofibrate (Smith, MacFie, and Oliver 1970). Among other drugs known to cause myopathy are chloroquine (Hughes, Esiri, Oxbury, and Whitty 1971), emetine (Duane and Engel 1970), epsilon aminocaproic acid (Lane, McLelland, Martin, and Mastaglia 1979), vincristine, lithium, cimetidine, amphotericin B, chloroquine, salbutamol (Mastaglia and Argov 1981), and polymyxin E (Vanhaeverbeek, Ectors, Vanhaelst, and Franken 1974). Severe muscle fibrosis with contractures (myosclerosis) may be rarely seen in spinal muscular atrophy or polymyositis (Bradley, Hudgson, Gardner-Medwin, and Walton 1973*b*) but has also been described as a consequence of the repeated intramuscular injection of meperidine (Aberfeld, Bienenstock, Shapiro, Namba, and Grob 1968), pethidine (Mastaglia *et al.* 1971), and pentazocine (Steiner, Winkelman, and de Jesus 1973). Penicillamine-induced myasthenia gravis is well recognized and disordered neuromuscular transmission can be caused by many antibiotics and anticonvulsant drugs, but penicillamine may also precipitate polymyositis (Mastaglia and Argov 1981).

Alcoholic myopathy

Acute and widespread muscle necrosis with local pain, tenderness, and oedema, sometimes leading to renal damage, myoglobinuria, and oliguria, is now well known to occur in some chronic alcoholic patients following a debauch (Hed, Lundmark, Fahlgren, and Orell 1962; Mastaglia and Argov 1981). In some patients with an acute alcoholic myopathy associated with muscle cramps, impairment of myophosphorylase activity with results of an ischaemic lactate test similar to those observed in McArdle's disease have been described, and myoglobinuria may occur (Perkoff, Dioso, Bleisch, and Klinkerfuss 1967). In addition, however, a subacute, progressive, proximal myopathy has been reported in alcoholic individuals (Hed *et al.* 1962; Klinkerfuss, Bleisch, Dioso, and Perkoff 1967); while undoubtedly some cases so diagnosed have proved to be suffering from alcoholic neuropathy involving motor axons predominantly (Faris and Reyes 1971), the existence of a subacute or chronic myopathy due to alcohol is now well established (Pittman and Decker 1971; Engel 1981) and may be associated with hypokalaemia (Martin, Craig, Eckel, and Munger 1971). Gradual recovery usually follows the withdrawal of alcohol. Cardiomyopathy is also well recognized (*British Medical Journal* 1972).

Xanthinuria

Symptomatic myopathy in a patient with inherited xanthine oxidase deficiency giving rise to xanthinuria was reported by Chalmers and colleagues (Chalmers, Johnson, Pallis, and Watts 1969a; Chalmers, Watts, Bitensky, and Chayen 1969b) and by Parker, Snedden, and Watts (1969) and crystals of xanthine were demonstrated in skeletal muscle by electron microscopy. Similar crystals without clinical evidence of muscle disease may be found in patients with gout treated with allopurinol (Watts, Scott, Chalmers, Bitensky, and Chayen 1971).

Lipid storage myopathy

In 1970 Engel, Vick, Glueck, and Levy described twin 18-year-old sisters who experienced muscle cramps and occasional episodes of myoglobinuria and in whom a defect in the utilization of long-chain fatty acids was demonstrated. Bradley, Hudgson, Gardner-Medwin, and Walton (1969) described a patient with a subacute proximal myopathy associated with the massive deposition of neutral fat in Type I muscle fibres, and Engel and Siekert (1972) reported a similar case in which improvement followed prednisone treatment. It is now known that this condition is due to an inherited deficiency of carnitine (Engel and Angelini 1973; Karpati, Carpenter, Engel, Watters, Allen, Rothman, Klassen, and Mamer 1975; Vandyke, Griggs, Markesbery, and DiMauro 1975) and that in such cases vacuolation of leukocytes may be found (Markesbery, McQuillen, Procopis, Harrison, and Engel 1974). Improvement may follow treatment with carnitine (Karpati et al. 1975; Angelini 1975). While in many cases muscle carnitine deficiency is a relatively benign syndrome, in systemic carnitine deficiency (see Engel 1981) progressive muscular weakness is often accompanied by episodes of acute encephalopathy and hepatic dysfunction and the disease often terminates fatally. A different syndrome which often presents with muscle cramps provoked by exercise and myoglobinuria may result from carnitine palmityl transferase deficiency (Cumming et al. 1976) but in such cases, too, there is often excess lipid storage in type I muscle fibres (Engel, Santa, Stonnington, Jerusalem, Tsujihata, Brownall, Sakatibara, Banker, Sahashi, and Lambert 1979). The enzyme deficiency may be partial or complete and it seems likely that many cases of exercise-induced myoglobinuria reported in the past may have been due to this cause.

AMP deaminase deficiency

AMP deaminase may participate in mechanisms controlling the regulation of adenosine triphosphate (ATP) activity in muscle. Fishbein, Armbrustmacher, and Griffin (1978) found a deficiency of this enzyme in skeletal muscle in young men complaining of muscular cramps and weakness following exercise, but since then, in the light of the clinical heterogeneity of the patients in whom such a deficiency has been reported, the significance of this deficiency has become uncertain (Engel 1981).

Mitochondrial myopathies

This term has been applied to a variety of myopathic disorders in which histochemical staining of muscle biopsy sections has often shown 'ragged-red' Type 1 muscle fibres (Olson, Engel, Walsh, and Einaugler 1972; Tamura, Santa, and Kuroiwa 1974) containing aggregates of dense material shown by electron microscopy to be due to increased numbers of enlarged and abnormal mitochondria, often containing bizarre inclusions. Often in such cases there is also an abnormal accumulation of fat and/or glycogen in the affected fibres. The classification of these conditions has become increasingly complex as new biochemical information has unfolded and the original descriptions of 'megaconial' and 'pleoconial' myopathies in infants or children with congenital hypotonia and myopathy (see below) (Shy and Gonatas 1964; Shy et al. 1966) are now outmoded. In some cases the mitochondrial my-

opathy represents but one facet of a multisystem disease as in the so-called oculocraniosomatic (Kearns–Sayre) syndrome in which there are ocular myopathy, retinal pigmentation, and often cerebellar degeneration and/or cardiomyopathy. Other features shown by many but not all of these conditions include progressive weakness of girdle muscles from early childhood or moderate fatigability and lactic acidaemia (Hudgson, Bradley, and Jenkison 1972; Worsfold, Park, and Pennington 1973; Engel 1981).

Morgan-Hughes, Darveniza, Landon, Land, and Clark (1979) suggested that these disorders could be divided into three principal groups.

1. *Transport or enzymatic defects of mitochondria causing impaired substrate utilization*
These include carnitine deficiency, carnitine palmityl transferase deficiency (see above), pyruvate decarboxylase deficiency, and pyruvate dehydrogenase phosphatase deficiency.

2. *Mitochondrial disorders with defective energy conservation*
The hypermetabolic myopathy described by Ernster, Ikkos, and Luft (1959) and Luft, Ikkos, Palmieri, Ernster, and Afzelius (1962) falls into this category (Afifi, Ibrahim, Bergman, Hayder, Bahuth, and Kaylani 1972; DiMauro, Bonilla, Lee, Schotland, Scarpa, Conn, and Chance 1976). The affected patients are not thyrotoxic but show a very marked increase in basal metabolic rate and their muscle mitochondria are not only morphologically abnormal but also show loose coupling of oxidative phosphorylation. Many other patients, however, including some with subacute ocular or girdle myopathy, show similar loose coupling of oxidative phosphorylation without hypermetabolism (Engel 1981).

3. *Specific deficiencies of one or more enzymatic components of the mitochondrial respiratory chain*
Among the many rare conditions in this group which have been described have been deficiencies of NADH-coenzyme Q reductase, cytochrome b, and cytochrome c, sometimes giving marked muscle weakness increased by exertion as well as lactic acidaemia, and sometimes a severe disorder with death in early life. There are also some mitochondrial myopathies causing lactic acidaemia in which no specific enzymatic defect has yet been identified, some benign, some severe.

References

Abbott, B. C., Creutzfeldt, O., Fowler, B. and Pearson, C. M. (1962). Membrane potentials in human muscles *Fed. Proc.* **21**, 318.
Aberfeld, D. C., Bienenstock, H., Shapiro, M. S., Namba, T. and Grob, D. (1968). Diffuse myopathy related to meperidine addiction in a mother and daughter. *Arch. Neurol., Chicago* **19**, 384.
Adams, R. D. (1975). *Diseases of muscle: a study in pathology*, 3rd edn. Harper and Row, New York.
Adamson, D. C., Salter, R. H. and Pearce, G. W. (1967). McArdle's syndrome (myophosphorylase deficiency). *Quart. J. Med.* **36**, 565.
Afifi, A. K., Ibrahim, M. Z. M., Bergman, R. A., Hayder, N. A., Mire, J., Bahuth, N. and Kaylani, F. (1972). Morphologic features of hypermetabolic mitochondrial disease. A light microscopic, histochemical and electron microscopic study. *J. neurol. Sci.* **15**, 271.
Angelini, C. (1975). Carnitine deficiency. *Lancet* **ii**, 554.
Askari, A., Vignos, P. J. and Moskowitz, R. W. (1976). Steroid myopathy in connective tissue disease. *Am. J. Med.* **61**, 485.
Astrom, K. E., Kugelberg, E. and Müller, R. (1961). Hypothyroid myopathy. *Arch. Neurol., Chicago* **5**, 472.
Atkinson S., Holcombe, M., and Kendall-Taylor, P. (1984). Ophthalmopathic immunoglobulin in patients with Graves' ophthalmopathy. *Lancet* **ii**, 374.
Bathurst, L. W. (1895). A case of Graves' disease associated with idiopathic muscular atrophy. *Lancet* **ii**, 529.
Bonilla, E. and Schotland, D. L. (1970). Histochemical diagnosis of muscle phosphofructokinase deficiency. *Arch. Neurol., Chicago* **22**, 8.
Bradley, W. G., Hudgson, P., Gardner-Medwin, D. and Walton, J. N. (1969). Myopathy associated with abnormal lipid metabolism in skeletal muscle. *Lancet* **i**, 495.
——, ——, —— and —— (1973b). The syndrome of myosclerosis. *J. Neurol. Neurosurg. Psychiat.* **36**, 651.

——, Ward, M., Murchison, D., Hall, L. and Woolf, N. (1973a). Clinical, electrophysiological and pathological studies on malignant hyperpyrexia. *Proc. R. Soc. Med.* **66**, 67.

Brain, W. R. (1959). Pathogenesis and treatment of endocrine exophthalmos. *Lancet* **i**, 109.

British Medical Journal (1972). Alcoholic cardiomyopathy. *Br. med. J.* **2**, 247.

Brody, I. A. and Dudley, A. W. (1969). Thyrotoxic hypokalemic periodic paralysis. *Arch. Neurol., Chicago* **21**, 1.

Bunch, T. W., Worthington, J. W., Combs, J. J., Ilstrup, D. M. and Engel, A. G. 1980). Azathioprine with prednisone for polymyositis. A controlled clinical trial. *Ann. intern. Med.* **92**, 365.

Bywaters, E. G. and Stead, J. K. (1945). Thrombosis of the femoral artery with myoglobinuria and low serum potassium concentration. *Clin. Sci.* **5**, 195.

Campa, J. F. and Sanders, D. B. (1974). Familial hypokalemic periodic paralysis. *Arch. Neurol., Chicago* **31**, 110.

Chalmers, R. A., Johnson, M., Pallis, C., and Watts, R. W. E. (1969a). Xanthinuria with myopathy. *Quart. J. Med.* **38**, 493.

——, Watts, R. W. E., Bitensky, L., and Chayen, J. (1969b). Microscopic studies on crystals in skeletal muscle from two cases of xanthinuria. *J. Path.* **99**, 45.

Conn, J. W. (1955). Primary aldosteronism, a new clinical syndrome. *J. lab. lin. Med.* **45**, 661.

Coomes, E. N. (1965). Corticosteroid myopathy. *Ann. rheum. Dis.* **24**, 465.

Courtecuisse, V., Royer, P., Habib, R., Monnier, C., and Demos, J. (1965). Glycogenose musculaire par déficit d'alpha-1,4-glucosidase simulant une dystrophie musculaire progressive. *Arch. franc. Pédiat.* **22**, 1153.

Crispell, K. R. and Parson, W. (1954). Occurrence of myotonia in 2 patients following thyroidectomy for hyperthyroidism. *Trans. Am. Goiter Ass.* 399.

Cumming, W. J. K., Hardy, M., Hudgson, P., and Wallis, J. (1976). Carnitine-palmityltransferase deficiency. *J. neurol. Sci.* **30**, 247.

Debré, R. and Semelaigne, G. (1935). Syndrome of diffuse muscular hypertrophy in infants causing athletic appearance: its connection with congenital myxedema. *Am. J. Dis. Child.* **50**, 1351.

Denborough, M. A., Warne, G. L., Moulds, R. F. W., Tse, P., and Martin, F. I. R. (1974). Insulin secretion in malignant hyperpyrexia. *Br. med. J.* **3**, 493.

DiMauro, S., Bonilla, E., Lee, C. P., Schotland, D. L. Scarpa, A., Conn, H., and Chance, B. (1976). Luft's disease. Further biochemical and ultrastructural studies of skeletal muscle in the second case. *J. neurol. Sci.* **27**, 217.

—— and Hartlage, P. L. (1978). Fatal infantile form of muscle phosphorylase deficiency. *Neurology, Minneapolis* **28**, 1124.

——, Miranda, A. F., Olarte, M., Friedman, R., and Hays, A. P. (1982). Muscle phosphoglycerate mutase deficiency. *Neurology, Minneapolis* **32**, 584.

Drager, G. A., Hamill, J. F., and Shy, G. M. (1958). Paramyotonia congenita. *Arch. Neurol. Psychiat., Chicago* **80**, 1.

Duane, D. D. and Engel, A. G. (1970). Emetine myopathy. *Neurology, Minneapolis* **20**, 733.

Duggin, G. G. and Price, M. A. (1974). Hypokalaemic muscular paresis in migratory Papua/New Guineans. *Lancet* **i**, 649.

Dyken, M., Zeman, W. and Rusche, T. (1969). Hypokalemic periodic paralysis. *Neurology, Minneapolis* **19**, 691.

Ellis, F. R., Clarke, I. M. C., Modgill, M., Currie, S., and Harriman, D. G. F. (1975). Evaluation of creatine phosphokinase in screening patients for malignant hyperpyrexia. *Br. med. J.* **3**, 511.

——, Keaney, N. P., Harriman, D. G. F., Sumner, D. W., Kyei-Mensah, K., Tyrrell, J. H., Hargreaves, J. B., Parikh, R. K., and Mulrooney, P. L. (1972). Screening for malignant hyperpyrexia. *Br. med. J.* **3**, 559.

Engel, A. G. (1961). Thyroid function and myasthenia gravis. *Arch. Neurol., Chicago* **4**, 663.

—— (1970). Acid maltase deficiency in adults: studies in four cases of a syndrome which may mimic muscular dystrophy or other myopathies. *Brain* **93**, 599.

—— (1981). Metabolic and endocrine myopathies. In *Disorders of voluntary muscle*, 4th edn. (ed. J. N. Walton) Ch. 18. Churchill-Livingstone, Edinburgh.

—— and Angelini, C. (1973). Carnitine deficiency of human skeletal muscle with associated lipid storage myopathy: a new syndrome. *Science* **173**, 899.

——, Santa, T., Stonnington, H. H., Jerusalem, F., Tsujihata, M., Brownell, A. K. W., Sakakibara, H., Banker, B. Q., Sahashi, K., and Lambert, E. H. (1979). Morphometric study of skeletal muscle ultrastructure. *Muscle & Nerve* **2**, 229.

—— and Siekert, R. G. (1972). Lipid storage myopathy responsive to prednisone. *Arch. Neurol., Chicago* **27**, 174.

Engel, W. K., Eyerman, E. L., and Williams, H. E. (1963). Late onset type of skeletal muscle phosphorylase deficiency. A new familial variety with completely and partially affected subjects. *New Engl. J. Med.* **268**, 135.

——, Vick, N. A., Glueck, C. J., and Levy, R. I. (1970). A skeletal-muscle disorder associated with intermittent symptoms and a possible defect of lipid metabolism. *New Engl. J. Med.* **284**, 697.

Ernster, L., Ikkos, D., and Luft, R. (1959). Enzymic activities of human skeletal muscle mitochondria: a tool in clinical metabolic research. *Nature London* **184**, 1851.

Faris, A. A. and Reyes, M. G. (1971). Reappraisal of alcoholic myopathy. *J. Neurol. Neurosurg. Psychiat.* **34**, 86.

Faust, D. K., Gergis, S. D., and Sokoll, M. D. (1979). Management of suspected hyperpyrexia in an infant. *Anesthesia & Analgesia* **58**, 33.

Fishbein, W. N., Armbrustmacher, V. W., and Griffin, J. L. (1978). Myoadenylate deaminase deficiency: a new disease of muscle. *Science* **200**, 545.

Floyd, M., Ayyar, D. R., Barwick, D. D., Hudgson, P., and Weightman, D. (1974). Myopathy in chronic renal failure. *Quart. J. Med.* **43**, 509.

Galjaard, H., Mekes, M., De Josselin De Jong, J. E., and Niermeijer, M. F. (1973). A method for rapid prenatal diagnosis of glycogenosis II (Pompe's disease). *Clin. Chim. Acta* **49**, 361.

Gamstorp, I. (1956). Adynamia episodica hereditaria. *Acta paediat., Uppsala* (Suppl.), **108**, 1.

Golding, D. N., Murray, S., Pearce, G. W., and Thompson, M. (1961). Corticosteroid myopathy. *Ann. phys. Med.* **6**, 171.

Goodhue, W. W., Davis, J. N., and Porro, R. S. (1972). Ischemic myopathy in uremic hyperparathyroidism. *J. Am. med. Ass.* **221**, 911.

Granato, J. E., Stern, B. J., Ringel, A., Karim, A. H., Krumholz, A., Coyle, J., and Adler, S. (1983). Neuroleptic malignant syndrome: successful treatment with dantrolene and bromocriptine. *Ann. Neurol.* **14**, 89.

Grob, D., Liljestrand, A., and Johns, R. J. (1957). Potassium movement in patients with familial periodic paralysis. *Am. J. Med* **23**, 356.

Gronert, G. A. (1980). Malignant hyperthermia. *Anesthesiology* **53**, 395.

Hall, L. W., Trim, C. M., and Woolf, N. (1972). Further studies of porcine malignant hyperthermia. *Br. med. J.* **2**, 145.

Hall, R., Doniach, D., Kirkham, K., and El Kabir, D. (1970). Ophthalmic Graves' disease. *Lancet* **i**, 375.

Harman, J. B. (1959). Muscular wasting and corticosteroid therapy. *Lancet* **i**, 887.

Harriman, D. G. F., Sumner, D. W., and Ellis, F. R. (1973). Malignant hyperpyrexia myopathy. *Quart. J. Med.* **42**, 639.

Hays, A. P., Hallett, M., Delfs, J., Morris, J., Sotrel, A., Shevchuk, M. M., and DiMauro, S. (1981). Muscle phosphofructokinase deficiency: abnormal polysaccharide in a case of late-onset myopathy. *Neurology, Minneapolis* **31**, 1077.

Hed, R., Lundmark, C., Fahlgren, H., and Orell, S. (1962). Acute muscular syndrome in chronic alcoholism. *Acta med. scand.* **171**, 585.

Helweg-Larsen, H. F., Hauge, M., and Sagild, U. (1955). Hereditary transient muscular paralysis in Denmark: genetic aspects of family periodic paralysis and family periodic adynamia. *Acta genet. Basel* **5**, 263.

Hoffman, J. (1896). Ein Fall von Thomsen'scher Krankheit, compliciert durch Neuritis multiplex. *Dtsch Z. Nervelheilk* **9**, 272.

Hoskins, B., Vroom, F. Q., and Jarrell, M. A. (1975). Hyperkalemic periodic paralysis. *Arch. Neurol., Chicago* **33**, 519.

Hudgson, P., Bradley, W. G., and Jenkison, M. (1972). Familial 'mitochondrial' myopathy: a myopathy associated with disordered oxidative metabolism in muscle fibres. Part 1. Clinical, electrophysiological and pathological findings. *J. neurol. Sci.* **16**, 343.

——, Gardner-Medwin, D., Worsfold, M. Pennington, R. J. T., and Walton, J. N. (1968). Adult myopathy in glycogen storage disease due to acid maltase deficiency. *Brain* **91**, 435.

Hughes, J. T., Esiri, M., Oxbury, J. M., and Whitty, C. W. M. (1971). Chloroquine myopathy. *Quart. J. Med* **40**, 85.

Illingworth, B., Cori, G. T., and Cori, C. F. (1956). Amylo-1,6-glucosidase in muscle tissue in generalized glycogen storage disease. *J. biol. Chem.* **218**, 123.

Isaacs, H., Heffron, J. J. A., and Badenhorst, M. (1975). Predictive tests for malignant hyperpyrexia. *Br. J. Anaesth.* **47**, 1075.

Jarcho, L. W. and Tyler, F. H. (1958). Myxoedema, pseudomyotonia and myotonia congenita. *Arch. intern. Med.* **102**, 357.

Jellinek, E. H. (1969). The orbital pseudotumour syndrome and its differentiation from endocrine exophthalmos. *Brain* **92**, 35.

Jones, D. I. R., Munro, D. S., and Wilson, G. M. (1969). Observations on the course of exophthalmos after ^{131}I therapy. *Proc. R. Soc. Med.* **62**, 15.

Karpati, G., Carpenter, S., Engel, A. G., Watters, G., Allen, J., Rothman, S., Klassen, G., and Mamer, O. A. (1975). The syndrome of systemic carnitine deficiency. *Neurology, Minneapolis* **25**, 16.

Khaleeli, A. A., Levy, R. D., Edwards, R. H. T., McPhail, G., Mills, K. R., Round, J. M., and Betteridge, D. J. (1984). The neuromuscular features of acromegaly: a clinical and pathological study. *J. Neurol. Neurosurg. Psychiat.* **47**, 1009.

King, J. O., Denborough, M. A., and Zapf, P. W. (1972). Inheritance of malignant hyperpyrexia. *Lancet* **i**, 365.

Klein, R., Egan, T., and Usher, P. (1960). Changes in sodium, potassium and water in hyperkalaemic periodic paralysis. *Metabolism* **9**, 1005.

Klinkerfuss, G., Bleisch, V., Dioso, M. M., and Perkoff, G. T. (1967). A spectrum of myopathy associated with alcoholism. II. Light and electron microscopic observations. *Ann. intern. Med.* **67**, 493.

Kodama, K., Sikorska, H., Bandy-Dafoe, P., Bayly, R., and Wall, J. R. (1982). Demonstration of a circulating auto-antibody against a soluble eye-muscle antigen in Graves' ophthalmopathy. *Lancet* **ii**, 1353.

Korein, J., Coddon, D. R., and Mowrey, F. H. (1959). The clinical syndrome of paroxysmal paralytic myoglobinuria. *Neurology, Minneapolis* **9**, 767.

The Lancet (1982). Autoimmune endocrine exophthalmos. *Lancet* **ii**, 1378.

Lane, R. J. M., McLelland, N. J., Martin, A. M., and Mastaglia, F. L. (1979). Epsilon aminocaproic acid (EACA) myopathy. *Postgrad. med. J.* **55**, 282.

Layzer, R. B., Rowland, L. P. and Ranney, H. M., (1967). Muscle phosphofructokinase deficiency. *Arch. Neurol., Chicago* **7**, 512.

Lisak, R. P., Lebeau, J., Tucker, S. H., and Rowland, L. P. (1972). Hyperkalemic periodic paralysis and cardiac arrhythmia. *Neurology, Minneapolis* **22**, 810.

Lister, D. (1973). Correction of adverse response to suxamethonium of susceptible pigs. *Br. med. J.* **1**, 208.

Loughbridge, L. W., Leader, L. P., and Bowen, D. A. L. (1958). Acute renal failure due to muscle necrosis in carbon-monoxide poisoning. *Lancet* **ii**, 349.

Luft, R., Ikkos, D., Palmieri, G., Ernster, L., and Afzelius, B. (1962). A case of severe hypermetabolism of nonthyroid origin with a defect in the maintenance of mitochondrial respiratory control: a correlated clinical, biochemical and morphological study. *J. clin. Invest.* **41**, 1776.

Lundberg, P. O., Stalberg, E. and Thiele, B., (1974). Paralysis periodica paramyotonica: a clinical and neurophysiological study. *J. neurol. Sci.* **21**, 309.

MacCarty, C. S., Kenefick, T. P., McDonahey, W. M., and Kearns, T. P. (1970). Ophthalmopathy of Graves' disease treated by removal of roof, lateral walls and lateral sphenoid ridge: review of 46 cases. *Mayo Clin. Proc.* **45**, 488.

Macdonald, R. D., Rewcastle, N. B., and Humphrey, J. G. (1968). The myopathy of hyperkalemic periodic paralysis. *Arch. Neurol., Chicago* **19**, 274.

Markesbery, W. R., McQuillen, M. P., Procopis, P. G., Harrison, A. R., and Engel, A. G. (1974). Muscle carnitine deficiency. *Arch. Neurol., Chicago* **31**, 320.

Marsden, C. D., Reynolds, E. H., Parsons, V., Harris, R., and Duchen, L. (1973). Myopathy associated with anticonvulsant osteomalacia. *Br. med. J.* **4**, 526.

Martin, B. and Jay, B. (1969). Use of guanethidine eye drops in dysthyroid lid retraction. *Proc. R. Soc. Med.* **62**, 18.

Martin, J. B., Craig, J. W., Eckel, R. E., and Munger, J. (1971). Hypokalemic myopathy in chronic alcoholism. *Neurology, Minneapolis* **21**, 1160.

Mastaglia, F. L. and Argov, Z. (1981). Drug-induced neuromuscular disorders in man. In *Disorders of voluntary muscle* (ed. J. N. Walton) 4th edn, Ch. 25. Churchill-Livingstone, Edinburgh.

——, Barwick, D. D. and Hall, R. (1970). Myopathy in acromegaly. *Lancet* **ii**, 907.

——, Gardner-Medwin, D. and Hudgson, P. (1971). Muscle fibrosis and contractures in a pethidine addict. *Br. med. J.* **4**, 532.

McArdle, B. (1951). Myopathy due to a defect in muscle glycogen breakdown. *Clin. Sci.* **10**, 13.

McComas, A. J., Mrozek, K., and Bradley, W. G. (1968). The nature of the electrophysiological disorder in adynamia episodica. *J. Neurol. Neurosurg. Psychiat.* **31**, 448.

McDaniel, H., Pittman, C. S., Oh, S. J., and DiMauro, S. (1977). Carbohydrate metabolism in hypothyroid myopathy. *Metabolism* **26**, 867.

McFadzean, A. J. S. and Yeung, R. (1969). Familial occurrence of thyrotoxic periodic paralysis. *Br. med. J.* **1**, 760.

Mellick, R. S., Mahler, R. F., and Hughes, B. P. (1962). McArdle's syndrome: phosphorylase-deficient myopathy. *Lancet* **i**, 1045.

Meyers, K. R., Gilden, D. H., Rinaldi, C. F., and Hansen, J. L. (1972). Periodic muscle weakness, normokalemia and tubular aggregates. *Neurology, Minneapolis* **22**, 269.

Mommaerts, W. F. H. M., Illingworth, B., Pearson, C. M., Guillory, R. J., and Seraydarian, K. (1959). A functional disorder of muscle associated with the absence of phosphorylase. *Proc. nat. Acad. Sci., Washington* **46**, 791.

Morgan-Hughes, J. A., Darveniza, P., Landon, D. N., Land, J. M., and Clark, J. B. (1979). A mitochondrial myopathy with deficiency of respiratory chain NADH-CoQ reductase activity. *J. neurol. Sci.* **43**, 27.

Mulder, D. W., Bastron, J. A., and Lambert, E. H. (1956). Hyperinsulin neuronopathy. *Neurology, Minneapolis* **6**, 627.

Müller, R. and Kugelberg, E. (1959). Myopathy in Cushing's syndrome. *J. Neurol. Neurosurg. Psychiat.* **22**, 314.

Murase, T., Ikeda, H., Muro, T., Nakao, K., and Sugita, H. (1973). Myopathy associated with type III glycogenosis. *J. neurol. Sci.* **20**, 287.

Norris, F. H., Panner, B. J., and Stormont, B. M. (1969). Thyrotoxic periodic paralysis. *Arch. Neurol., Chicago* **19**, 88.

Okinaka, S., Shizume, K., Jino, S., Watanabe, A., Irie, M., Noguchi, A., Kuma, S., Kuma, K., and Ito, T. (1957). The association of periodic paralysis and hyperthyroidism in Japan. *J. clin. Endocr.* **17**, 1454.

Olson, W., Engel, W. K., Walsh, G. O., and Einaugler, R. (1972). Oculocraniosomatic neuromuscular disease with 'ragged-red' fibres. *Arch. Neurol., Chicago* **26**, 193.

Ouzounellis, T. I. (1968). Myoglobinuries par ingestion de cailles. *Presse Méd.* **76**, 1863.

—— (1970). Some notes on quail poisoning. *J. Am. med. Ass.* **211**, 1186.

Parker, R., Snedden, W. and Watts, R. W. E. (1969). The mass-spectrometric identification of hypoxanthine and xanthine ('oxypurines') in skeletal muscle from two patients with congenital xanthine oxidase deficiency (xanthinuria). *Biochem. J.* **115**, 103.

Perkoff, G. T., Dioso, M. M., Bleisch, V., and Klinkerfuss, G. (1967). A spectrum of myopathy associated with alcoholism, I. Clinical and laboratory findings. *Ann. intern. Med.* **67**, 481.

——, Silber, R., Tyler, F. H., Cartwright, G. E., and Wintrobe, M. M. (1959). Studies in disorders of muscle. XII. Myopathy due to the administration of therapeutic amounts of 17-hydroxycortico-steroids. *Am. J. Med.* **26**, 891.

Philipson, K. D. and Edelman, I. S. (1977). Thyroid hormone control of Na-K-adenosine triphosphatase and K-dependent phosphatase in rat heart. *Am. J. Physiol.* **232**, 196.

Pickett, J. B. E., Layzer, R. B., Levin, S. R., Schneider, V., Campbell, M. J., and Sumner, A. J. (1975). Neuromuscular complications of acromegaly. *Neurology, Minneapolis* **25**, 638.

Pittman, J. G. and Decker, J. W. (1971). Acute and chronic myopathy associated with alcoholism. *Neurology, Minneapolis* **21**, 293.

Pleasure, D. and Bonilla, E. (1982). Skeletal muscle storage diseases: myopathies resulting from errors in carbohydrate and fatty acid metabolism. In *Skeletal muscle pathology* (ed. F. L. Mastaglia and J. N. Walton) Ch. 10. Churchill-Livingstone, Edinburgh.

——, Walsh, G. O. and Engel, W. K. (1970). Atrophy of skeletal muscle in patients with Cushing's syndrome. *Arch. Neurol., Chicago* **22**, 118.

——, Wyszynski, B., Sumner, D., Schotland, D. L., Feldmann, B., Nugent, N., Hitz, K. and Goodman, D. B. P. (1979). Skeletal muscle calcium metabolism and contractile force in vitamin D-deficient chicks. *J. clin. Invest.* **64**, 1157.

Poskanzer, D. C. and Kerr, D. N. S. (1961a). Periodic paralysis with response to spironolactone. *Lancet* **ii**, 511.

—— and —— (1961b). A third type of periodic paralysis with normokalaemia and favourable response to sodium chloride. *Am. J. Med.* **31**, 328.

Prineas, J. W., Hall, R., Barwick, D. D., and Watson, A. J. (1968).

Myopathy associated with pigmentation following adrenalectomy for Cushing's syndrome. *Quart. J. Med.* **37**, 63.

——, Mason, A. S., and Henson, R. A. (1965). Myopathy in metabolic bone disease. *Br. med. J.* **1**, 1034.

Ramsay, I. D. (1965). Electromyography in thyrotoxicosis. *Quart. J. Med.* **34**, 255.

Resnick, J. W., Engel, W. K., Griggs, R. C., and Stam, A. C. (1968). Acetazolamide prophylaxis in hypokalemic periodic paralysis. *New Engl. J. Med.* **278**, 582.

Rosenow, E. C. and Engel, A. G. (1978). Acid maltase deficiency in adults presenting as respiratory failure. *Am. J. Med.* **64**, 85.

Rowland, L. P., Fahn, S., Hirschberg, E., and Harter, D. H. (1964). Myoglobinuria. *Arch. Neurol., Chicago* **10**, 537.

Salick, A. I., Colachis, S. C., and Pearson, C. M. (1968). Myxedema myopathy: clinical, electrodiagnostic, and pathologic findings in advanced cases. *Arch. phys. Med.* **49**, 230.

Satoyoshi, E., Murakami, K., Kowa, H., Kinoshita, M., Noguchi, K., Hoshina, S., Nishiyama, Y., and Ito, K. (1963). Myopathy in thyrotoxicosis. *Neurology, Minneapolis* **13**, 645.

Saunders, M., Ashworth, B., Emery, A. E. H., and Benedikz, J. E. G. (1968). Familial myotonic periodic paralysis with muscle wasting. *Brain* **91**, 295.

Savage, D. C. L., Forbes, M., and Pearce, G. W. (1971). Idiopathic rhabdomyolysis. *Arch. Dis. Childh.* **46**, 594.

Schmid, R. and Hammaker, L. (1961). Hereditary absence of muscle phosphorylase (McArdle's syndrome). *New Engl. J. Med.* **264**, 223.

—— and Mahler, R. (1959). Chronic progressive myopathy with myoglobinuria: demonstration of a glycogenolytic defect in the muscle. *J. clin. Invest.* **38**, 1044.

Schott, G. D. and Wills, M. R. (1975). Myopathy in hypophosphataemic osteomalacia presenting in adult life. *J. Neurol. Neurosurg. Psychiat.* **38**, 297.

Schutta, H. S., Kelly, A. M., and Zacks, S. I. (1969). Necrosis and regeneration of muscle in paroxysmal idiopathic myoglobinuria: electron microscopic observations. *Brain* **92**, 191.

Shy, G. M. and Gonatas, N. K. (1964). Human myopathy with giant abnormal mitochondria. *Science* **145**, 493.

——, —— and Perez, M. C. (1966). Two childhood myopathies with abnormal mitochondria—1. Megaconial myopathy. 2. Pleoconial myopathy. *Brain* **89**, 133.

——, Wanko, T., Rowley, P. T., and Engel, A. G. (1961). Studies in familial periodic paralysis. *Exp. Neurol.* **3**, 53.

Smigiel, M. R. and MacCarty, C. S. (1975). Exophthalmos: the more commonly encountered neurosurgical lesions. *Mayo Clinic Proc.* **50**, 345.

Smith, A. F., MacFie, W. G., and Oliver, M. F. (1970). Clofibrate, serum enzymes, and muscle pain. *Br. med. J.* **2**, 86.

Smith, R. and Stern, G. M. (1967). Myopathy, osteomalacia and hyperparathyroidism. *Brain* **90**, 593.

Spiro, A. J., Hirano, A., Beilin, R. L., and Finkelstein, J. W. (1970). Cretinism with muscular hypertrophy (Kocher–Debré–Semelaigne syndrome). *Arch. Neurol., Chicago* **23**, 340.

Steers, A. J. W., Tallack, J. A., and Thompson, D. E. A. (1970). Fulminating hyperpyrexia during anaesthesia in a member of a myopathic family. *Br. med. J.* **2**, 341.

Steiner, J. C., Winkelman, A. C., and De Jesus, P. V. (1973). Pentazocine-induced myopathy. *Arch. Neurol., Chicago* **28**, 408.

Stocker, W. W., Samaha, F. J., and De Groot, L. J. (1968). Coupled oxidative phosphorylation in muscle of thyrotoxic patients. *Am. J. Med.* **44**, 900.

Takamori, M., Gutmann, L., Crosby, T. S., and Martin, J. D. (1972). Myasthenic syndromes in hypothyroidism: electrophysiological study of neuromuscular transmission and muscle contraction in two patients. *Arch. Neurol., Chicago* **26**, 326.

Tamura, K., Santa, T., and Kuroiwa, Y. (1974). Familial oculocranioskeletal neuromuscular disease with abnormal muscle mitochondria. *Brain* **97**, 665.

Tarui, S., Okuna, G., Ikura, Y., Tanaka, T., Suda, M., and Nishikawa, M. (1965). Phosphofructokinase deficiency in skeletal muscle. A new type of glycogenosis. *Biochem. biophys. Res. Commun.* **19**, 517.

Thomson, W. H. S., MacLaurin, J. C., and Prineas, J. W. (1963). Skeletal muscle glycogenosis; an investigation of two dissimilar cases. *J. Neurol. Neurosurg. Psychiat.* **26**, 60.

Thorn, G. W. (1949). *The diagnosis and treatment of adrenal insufficiency*, p. 144. Thomas, Springfield, Illinois.

Tobin, W. E., Huijing, F., Porro, R. S., and Salzman, R. T. (1973). Muscle phosphofructokinase deficiency. *Arch. Neurol., Chicago* **28**, 128.

Tomé, F. M. S. (1982). Periodic paralysis and electrolyte disorders. In *Skeletal muscle pathology* (ed. F. L. Mastaglia and J. N. Walton) Ch. 8. Churchill-Livingstone, Edinburgh.

Tyler, F. H., Stephens, F. E., Gunn, F. D., and Perkoff, G. T. (1951). Studies on disorders of muscle. VII. Clinical manifestations and inheritance of a type of periodic paralysis without hypopotassaemia. *J. clin. Invest.* **30**, 492.

Van der Meulen, J. P., Gilbert, G. J., and Kane, C. A. (1961). Familial hyperkalaemic paralysis with myotonia. *New Engl. J. Med.* **264**, 1.

Vandyke, D. H., Griggs, R. C., Markesbery, W., and DiMauro, S. (1974). Hereditary carnitine deficiency of muscle. *Neurology, Minneapolis* **25**, 154.

Vanhaeverbeek, M., Ectors, M., Vanhaelst, L., and Franken, L. (1974). Myopathy caused by polymyxin E: functional disorder of the cell membrane. *J. Neurol. Neurosurg. Psychiat.* **37**, 1343.

Van't Hoff, W. (1962). Familial myotonic periodic paralysis. *Quart. J. Med.* **31**, 385.

Vroom, F. Q., Jarrell, M. A., and Maren, T. H. (1975). Acetazolamide treatment of hypokalemic periodic paralysis. *Arch. Neurol., Chicago* **32**, 385.

Walton, J. N. (1960). Muscular dystrophy and its relation to the other myopathies. *Res. Publ. Ass. nerv. ment. Dis.* **38**, 378.

Wang, P. and Clausen, T. (1976). Treatment of attacks in hyperkalaemic familial periodic paralysis by inhalation of salbutamol. *Lancet* **i**, 221.

Watts, R. W. E., Scott, J. T., Chalmers, R. A., Bitensky, L., and Chayen, J. (1971). Microscopic studies on skeletal muscle in gout patients treated with allopurinol. *Quart. J. Med.* **40**, 1.

Weetman, A. P., McGregor, A. M., Ludgate, M., Beck, L., Mills, P. V., Lazarus, J. H., and Hall, R. (1983). Cyclosporin improves Graves' ophthalmopathy. *Lancet* **ii**, 486.

——, ——, and Hall, R. (1984). Ocular manifestations of Graves' disease: a review. *J. R. Soc. Med.* **77**, 936.

Williams, L. T., Lefkowitz, R. J., and Watanabe, A. M. (1977). Thyroid hormone regulation of β-adrenergic receptor number. *J. Biol. Chem.* **252**, 2787.

Williams, R. S. (1959). Triamcinolone myopathy. *Lancet* **2, 698.**

Wilson, J. and Walton, J. N. (1959). Some muscular manifestations of hypothyroidism. *J. Neurol. Neurosurg. Psychiat.* **22**, 320.

Witts, L. J., Lakin, C. E., and Thompson, A. P. (1938). Discussion on Addison's disease at the Association of Physicians. *Quart. J. Med.* **7**, 590.

Worsfold, M., Park, D. C., and Pennington, R. J. (1973). Familial 'mitochondrial' myopathy: a myopathy associated with disordered oxidative metabolism in muscle fibres. Part 2. Biochemical findings. *J. neurol. Sci.* **19**, 261.

Zellweger, H., Brown, B. I., McCormick, W., and Tu, J. B. (1965). A mild form of muscular glycogenosis in two brothers with alpha-1,4-glucosidase deficiency. *Ann. paediat.* **205**, 413.

Zierler, K. L. and Andres, R. (1957). Movement of potassium into skeletal muscle during spontaneous attack in family periodic paralysis. *J. clin. Invest.* **36**, 730.

The floppy infant syndrome

Generalized muscular hypotonia in infancy can be due to many causes. In a survey of 111 floppy infants, Paine (1963) found that 48 were suffering from various forms of cerebral palsy, 28 from mental retardation, 3 from cerebral degenerative disease, and 1 from brain tumour. There were four cases of spinal muscular atrophy and four of myopathy, while 18 were found to have a condition which could only be entitled 'benign congenital hypotonia' (Walton 1956, 1957). Congenital muscular dystrophy as a cause of such a syndrome has already been considered (see p. 556). The term 'benign congenital or infantile hypotonia' can still reasonably be reserved for those floppy infants in whom hypotonia is not shown to be due to any specific metabolic disorder or to be secondary to mental defect or central nervous disease and in whom full investigation, including EMG and muscle biopsy, fails to identify any specific abnormality of the muscle fibres other than, in some cases, an over-all decrease in their diameter, a failure of differentiation into the usual histochemical types or congenital fibre type disproportion (see Dubowitz and Brooke 1973;

Mastaglia and Walton 1982). While recent studies have revealed a remarkable variability in the clinical course of spinal muscular atrophy in infancy and childhood (Byers and Banker 1961; Dubowitz 1964; Gardner-Medwin, Hudgson, and Walton 1967; and see p. 383) it is now apparent that some floppy infants may be suffering from certain apparently specific though benign disorders of muscle which are relatively non-progressive (Gardner-Medwin and Tizard 1981). The syndrome of arthrogryposis multiplex congenita (variable muscular weakness and wasting with contractures, especially in the extremities, present from birth) may be due to congenital muscular dystrophy (p. 556), to denervation due either to failure of development of neurones or fetal spinal muscular atrophy (Bharucha, Pandya, and Dastur 1972; Dastur, Razzak, and Bharucha 1972), or to congenital peripheral neuropathy (Peña, Miller, Budzilovich, and Feigin 1968; Hooshmand, Martinez, and Rosenblum 1971; Yuill and Lynch 1974). Some cases are attributed to excessive intrauterine pressure (Lloyd-Roberts and Lettin 1970). There remain, however, many hypotonic infants who show gradual improvement and in whom no other diagnostic label than one of benign congenital hypotonia can yet be applied, since modern methods of investigation fail to demonstrate any cause for the widespread muscular hypotonia which they manifest. It is, however, clear that this condition is no more than a syndrome, almost certainly of multiple aetiology. Some of the more specific forms of benign and relatively non-progressive myopathy which have been described will now be mentioned.

Central core disease

In 1956 Shy and Magee described a family in which the affected children did not walk until about the age of 4 years. The patients showed profound and widespread muscular hypotonia and muscle biopsy revealed large muscle fibres, most of which showed one or sometimes two central cores which had different staining properties from other fibrils. Further cases were described by Bethlem and Meyjes (1960) and by Engel, Foster, Hughes, Huxley, and Mahler (1961). Dubowitz and Pearse (1960) found the central core to be devoid of oxidative enzymes and of phosphorylase activity and suggested that it was non-functioning. The condition is plainly benign and genetically determined, being probably an autosomal recessive trait, but as in the several other conditions described below, its pathogenesis remains obscure. Muscle cramps after exercise have been described (Bethlem, van Goal, Hülsmann, and Meijer 1966) and multicore formation within a single fibre is not uncommon (Engel, Gomez, and Groover 1971). The finding of multicores in an acquired myopathy beginning in adult life (Bonnette, Roelofs, and Olson 1974) raised some doubts about the specificity of central cores in relation to congenital myopathy, but nevertheless the clinical picture of multicore or 'minicore' disease (Currie, Noronha, and Harriman 1974; Fardeau 1982) is more often one of infantile hypotonia, motor developmental delay, and a non-progressive course with diminished or absent tendon reflexes (Gardner-Medwin and Tizard 1981).

Nemaline myopathy

In 1963 Shy, Engel, Somers, and Wanko described another congenital non-progressive myopathy in which curious collections of rod-shaped bodies were found within the muscle fibres. In some such cases the diagnosis can be suspected clinically as these patients usually show not only evidence of a diffuse myopathy, but also facial weakness, a high arched palate, prognathism of the lower jaw, and skeletal changes resembling those of arachnodactyly, though none of the other stigmata of Marfan's syndrome are present (Conen, Murphy, and Donohue 1963; Engel, Wanko, and Fenichel 1964). Examination of muscle from such cases with the electron microscope (Price, Gordon, Pearson, Munsat, and Blumberg 1965; Hudgson, Gardner-Medwin, Fulthorpe, and Walton 1967; Shafiq, Dubowitz, Peterson, and Milhorat 1967) has shown

that the subsarcolemmal rods appear to be due to a selective swelling and degeneration of Z-bands with consequent destruction of myofilaments in the adjacent part of the muscle fibre. While the condition is often benign and relatively non-progressive, severe cases causing death in infancy have been described (Shafiq et al. 1967), and progressive, ultimately fatal, respiratory failure may occur in the first or second decades (Dubowitz 1978; Gardner-Medwin and Tizard 1981).

The specificity of nemaline rods has been called into question, as these structures may be produced experimentally in muscle by tenotomy (Engel, Brooke, and Nelson 1966) and may be found from time to time in muscle biopsies from patients with a variety of neuromuscular disorders (Karpati, Carpenter, and Eisen 1972). Type I fibre atrophy (Kinoshita and Satoyoshi 1974) and virtual absence of Type II fibres (Karpati, Carpenter, and Andermann 1971) have each been described in association with nemaline bodies and the myopathy which often accompanies the fully developed Marfan syndrome (Goebel, Muller, and De Myer 1973) may not give rise to rod body formation. Nevertheless, the condition is still accepted as a relatively specific variety of congenital myopathy (Fardeau 1982).

Mitochondrial myopathies

These disorders, as a cause of infantile hypotonia or congenital myopathy, were described on p. 579.

Fingerprint body myopathy and other obscure congenital myopathies

In a 5-year-old girl with non-progressive muscular weakness present from infancy, Engel, Angelini, and Gomez (1972) found hypertrophy of Type II muscle fibres and the Type I fibres showed fingerprint-like inclusions clearly demonstrable by electron microscopy. Similar changes were found by Gordon, Rewcastle, Humphrey, and Stewart (1974) in a woman aged 55 years with a history suggesting that she had had a myopathy since birth, but have also been reported in dystrophia myotonica (Tomé and Fardeau 1973). The pathogenesis of this change, and of the crystalline intranuclear inclusions noted by Jenis, Lindquist, and Lister (1969) in another case of congenital myopathy, remain to be determined. Similarly, syndromes of infantile hypotonia due to 'reducing body myopathy' (Brooke and Neville 1972), myopathy with tubular aggregates, sarcotubular myopathy (Jerusalem, Engel, and Gomez 1973), and several other obscure syndromes have yet to be fully characterized (Gardner-Medwin and Tizard 1981; Fardeau 1982).

Myotubular myopathy

In a 9-year-old child with a form of Möbius disease characterized by facial diplegia, external ocular palsies, a decrease in muscle mass, moderate symmetrical muscle weakness, and poor development of all somatic muscles. Spiro, Shy, and Gonatas (1966) found changes which were thought to represent the first example of cellular developmental arrest occurring in man. Most muscle fibres contained central nuclei, often lying in chains, and the appearances were similar to those of myotubes seen in the normal fetus in the early months of intra-uterine life. Subsequent reports, reviewed by Campbell, Rebeiz, and Walton (1969), by van Wijngaarden, Fleury, Bethlem, and Meijer (1969), and by Bradley, Price, and Watanabe (1970) did, however, reveal many differences between these structures and fetal myotubes, so that although the condition is clearly a clinical and morphological entity, its pathogenesis is still a matter of speculation. The central nuclei are confined to the Type I muscle fibres in some cases (Engel, Gold, and Karpati 1968) and some cases are familial. The condition generally runs a benign course and gradual improvement in muscle power usually occurs, but severe cases causing death in infancy, sometimes of X-linked recessive inheritance, have been reported (Engel *et al.* 1968; Barth, van Wijngaarden, and Bethlem 1975). Cardiomyopathy is found in some cases and Type 1 fibre atrophy is common (Shafiq, Sande, Carruthers, Killip, and Milhorat 1972).

Hence, although it is too early to be certain that the syndromes mentioned are all specific disorders of muscle, in the field of benign congenital myopathy new advances are taking place with great rapidity and many interesting histological abnormalities of the muscle fibre are being demonstrated by histochemical, biochemical, and ultrastructural techniques.

References

Barth, P. G., van Wijngaarden, G. K., and Bethlem, J. (1975). X-linked myotubular myopathy with fatal neonatal asphyxia. *Neurology, Minneapolis* **25**, 531.

Bethlem, J. and Meyjes, F. E. P. (1960). Congenital non-progressive central core disease of Shy and Magee. *Psychiat. Neurol. Neurochir., Amsterdam* **63**, 246.

——, van Gool, J., Hulsmann, W. C., and Meijer, A. E. F. H. (1966). Familial non-progressive myopathy with muscle cramps after exercise. *Brain* **89**, 569.

Bharucha, E. P., Pandya, S. S., and Dastur, D. K. (1972). Arthrogryposis multiplex congenita. Part 1: Clinical and electromyographic aspects. *J. Neurol. Neurosurg. Psychiat.* **35**, 425.

Bonnette, H., Roelofs, R., and Olson, W. H. (1974). Multicore disease: report of a case with onset in middle age. *Neurology, Minneapolis* **24**, 1039.

Bradley, W. G., Price, D., and Watanabe, C. K. (1970). Familial centronuclear myopathy. *J. Neurol. Neurosurg. Psychiat.* **32, 687**.

Brooke, M. H. and Neville, H. E. (1972). Reducing body myopathy. *Neurology, Minneapolis* **25**, 531.

Byers, R. K. and Banker, B. Q. (1961). Infantile muscular atrophy. *Arch. Neurol., Chicago* **5**, 140.

Campbell, M. J., Rebeiz, J. J., and Walton, J. N. (1969). Myotubular, centronuclear or pericentronuclear myopathy? *J. neurol. Sci.* **8**, 425.

Conen, P. E., Murphy, E. G., and Donohue, W. L. (1963). Light and electron microscopic studies on 'myogranules' in a child with hypotonia and muscle weakness. *Can. med. Ass. J.* **89**, 983.

Currie, S., Noronha, M., and Harriman, D. (1974). 'Minicore' disease. In *Abstracts of papers presented at the 3rd International Congress of Muscle Diseases*, Newcastle upon Tyne, ICS no. 334, p. 12. Excerpta Medica, Amsterdam.

Dastur, D. K., Razzak, Z. A., and Bharucha, E. P. (1972). Arthrogryposis multiplex congenita. Part 2: Muscle pathology and pathogenesis. *J. Neurol. Neurosurg, Psychiat.* **35**, 435.

Dubowitz, V. (1964). Infantile muscular atrophy. A prospective study with particular reference to a slowly progressive variety. *Brain* **87**, 707.

—— (1978). *Muscle disorders in childhood*. Saunders, London.

—— and Brooke, M. H. (1973). *Muscle biopsy*. Saunders, London.

—— and Pearse, A. G. E. (1960). Oxidative enzymes and phosphorylase in central-core disease of muscle. *Lancet* **ii**, 23.

Engel, A. G., Angelini, C., and Gomez, M. R. (1972). Fingerprint body myopathy: a newly recognized congenital muscle disease. *Mayo Clin. Proc.* **47**, 377.

——, Gomez, M. R. and Groover, R. V. (1971). Multicore disease: a recently recognized congenital myopathy associated with multifocal degeneration of muscle fibers. *Mayo Clin. Proc.* **46**, 666.

Engel, W. K., Brooke, M. H., and Nelson, P. G. (1966). Histochemical studies of denervated or tenotomized cat muscle. *Ann. NY Acad. Sci.* **138**, 160.

——, Foster, J. B., Hughes, B. P., Huxley, H. E., and Mahler, R. (1961). Central core disease—an investigation of a rare muscle cell abnormality. *Brain* **84**, 167.

——, Gold, G. N. and Karpati, G. (1968). Type I fiber hypotrophy and central nuclei. *Arch. Neurol., Chicago* **18**, 435.

——, Wanko, T. and Fenichel, G. M. (1964). Nemaline myopathy: a second case. *Arch. Neurol., Chicago* **11**, 22.

Fardeau, M. (1982). Congenital myopathies. In *Skeletal muscle pathology* (ed. F. L. Mastaglia and J. N. Walton) Ch. 4. Churchill-Livingstone, Edinburgh.

Gardner-Medwin, D., Hudgson, P., and Walton, J. N. (1967). Benign spinal muscular atrophy arising in childhood and adolescence. *J. neurol. Sci.* **5**, 121.

—— and Tizard, J. P. M. (1981). Neuromuscular disorders in infancy and early childhood. In *Disorders of voluntary muscle* (ed. J. N. Walton), 4th edn., Ch. 17. Churchill-Livingstone, Edinburgh.

Goebel, H. H., Muller, J., and DeMyer, W. (1973). Myopathy associated with Marfan's syndrome: fine structural and histochemical observations. *Neurology, Minneapolis* **23**, 1257.

Gordon, A. S., Rewcastle, N. B., Humphrey, J. G., and Stewart, B. M. (1974). Chronic benign congenital myopathy: fingerprint body type. *Can. J. neurol. Sci.* **1**, 106.

Hooshmand, H., Martinez, A. J., and Rosenblum, W. I. (1971). Arthrogryposis multiplex congenita. Simultaneous involvement of peripheral nerve and skeletal muscle. *Arch. Neurol., Chicago* **24**, 561.

Hudgson, P., Gardner-Medwin, D., Fulthorpe, J., and Walton, J. N. (1967). Nemaline myopathy. *Neurology, Minneapolis* **17**, 1125.

Jenis, E. H., Linquist, R. R., and Lister, R. C. (1969). New congenital myopathy with crystalline intranuclear inclusions. *Arch. Neurol., Chicago* **20**, 281.

Jerusalem, F., Engel, A. G., and Gomez, M. R. (1973). Sarcotubular myopathy: a newly recognised, benign, congenital, familial muscle disease. *Neurology, Minneapolis* **23**, 897.

Karpati, G., Carpenter, S., and Andermann, F. (1971). A new concept of childhood nemaline myopathy. *Arch. Ophthalmol.* **85**, 291.

——, —— and Eisen, A. A. (1972). Experimental core-like lesions and nemaline rods. *Arch. Neurol., Chicago* **27**, 237.

Kinoshita, M. and Satoyoshi, E. (1974). Type I fiber atrophy and nemaline bodies. *Arch. Neurol., Chicago* **31**, 423.

Lloyd-Roberts, G. C. and Lettin, A. W. F. (1970). Arthrogryposis multiplex congenita. *J. Bone Jt. Surg.* **52B**, 494.

Mastaglia, F. L. and Walton, J. N. (Eds.) (1982). *Skeletal muscle pathology*. Churchill-Livingstone, Edinburgh.

Paine, R. S. (1963). The future of the 'floppy infant'. *Develop. Med. Child Neurol.* **5**, 115.

Pena, C. E., Miller, F., Budzilovich, G. N., and Feigin, I. (1968). Arthrogryposis multiplex congenita: a report of two cases of a radicular type with familial incidence. *Neurology, Minneapolis* **18**, 926.

Price, H. M., Gordon, G. B., Pearson, C. M., Munsat, T., and Blumberg, J. M. (1965). New evidence for excessive accumulation of Z-band material in nemaline myopathy. *Proc. nat. Acad. Sci., Washington* **54**, 1398.

Shafiq, S. A., Dubowitz, V., Peterson, H. de C., and Milhorat, A. T. (1967). Nemaline myopathy: report of a fatal case, with histochemical and electron microscopic studies. *Brain* **90**, 817.

Shafiq, S. A., Sande, M. A., Carruthers, R. R., Killip, T., and Milhorat, A. T. (1972). Skeletal muscle in idiopathic cardiomyopathy. *J. neurol. Sci.* **15**, 303.

Shy, G. M., Engel, W. K., Somers, J. E., and Wanko, T. (1963). Nemaline myopathy, a new congenital myopathy. *Brain* **86**, 793.

—— and Magee, K. R. (1956). A new congenital non-progressive myopathy. *Brain* **79**, 610.

Spiro, A. J., Shy, G. M. and Gonatas, N. K. (1966). Myotubular myopathy. *Arch. Neurol., Chicago* **14**, 1.

Tomé, F. M. S. and Fardeau, M. (1973). 'Fingerprint inclusions' in muscle fibres in dystrophia myotonica. *Acta neuropath., Berlin* **24**, 62.

Van Wijngaarden, G. K., Fleury, P., Bethlem, J., and Meijer, A. E. F. H. (1969). Familial 'myotubular' myopathy. *Neurology, Minneapolis* **19**, 901.

Walton, J. N. (1956). Amyotonia congenita—a follow-up study. *Lancet* **i**, 1023.

—— (1957). The limp child. *J. Neurol. Neurosurg. Psychiat.* **20**, 144.

Yuill, G. M. and Lynch, P. G. (1974). Congenital non-progressive peripheral neuropathy with arthrogryposis multiplex. *J. Neurol. Neurosurg. Psychiat.* **37**, 316.

Some miscellaneous disorders of muscle

Restless legs

The aetiology of this condition, described and reviewed in detail by Ekbom (1960), is unknown, though pathology in the posterior-nerve roots has been postulated (Nathan 1978). There is no evidence that it is a primary muscular disorder, but it may be seen in uraemic patients with neuropathy (Asbury 1975). It gives unpleasant aching in the muscles of the lower limbs when the patient rests in a chair and the symptoms are often particularly troublesome in bed. They may be associated with cramps and interfere with sleep so that after a period of restless shuffling the patient is compelled to get up and to walk the floor to obtain relief. The syndrome of 'painful legs and moving toes' described by Spillane, Nathan, Kelly, and Marsden (1971) may be an unusually severe variant of this disorder. There are no abnormal physical signs on examination and no lesions within the muscles or peripheral nerves have been discovered (Harriman, Taverner, and Woolf 1970). The aetiology of this troublesome syndrome is totally unexplained, but some patients are greatly helped by treatment with chlorpromazine given in a dosage of 50–100 mg at night, and perhaps 25 mg three times a day as well, while intravenous procaine infusions may also be beneficial (Foster 1981). Diazepam and hydantoinates are sometimes helpful in relieving the associated muscle cramps which occur in some cases.

Tibialis anterior syndrome

Severe boring pain in the tibialis anterior muscle, particularly in adults undertaking unaccustomed exercise, is typical of this syndrome (also called 'shin splints'). The condition is probably due to ischaemia followed by swelling of the tibialis anterior and its associated muscles lying within a tight fascial compartment. In rare cases the pain is intense, and widespread necrosis of the anterior tibial muscles may occur, and can even be fatal as a result of myoglobinuria. In mild chronic cases recurrent pain in the appropriate distribution occurs whenever the patient exerts himself. Relief may then be obtained by means of surgical decompression of the anterior crural compartment (Sirbou, Murphy, and White 1944; British Medical Journal 1974).

Progressive myositis ossificans

Although localized myositis ossificans may occur through ossification of certain muscles as a result of their repeated involvement in the trauma of specific exercises or occupations and may occasionally occur in muscles in the region of the hip joint (particularly the adductors) following paraplegia or paraparesis, as after partial recovery from transverse myelitis, there is a genetically-determined progressive disorder in which widespread ossification of muscles occurs. Most such patients are children who often have associated anomalies of their great toes or other digits and it seems that the ossification in muscle is preceded by sclerosis of intramuscular connective tissue (McKusick 1956). This rare disorder, which is probably transmitted by a dominant gene, often with incomplete penetrance (Tünte, Becker, and Knorre 1967), often begins by giving rise to swelling or swellings in the neck which mimic congenital torticollis and eventually in most cases the muscles of the back, shoulder, and pelvic girdles become ossified. The overlying skin may ulcerate and in the terminal stages aspiration pneumonia and/or asphyxia may occur. There is some evidence that diphosphonate treatment may promote resorption of bone in such cases (Russell, Smith, Bishop, Price, and Squire 1972).

The stiff-man syndrome

In 1956 Moersch and Woltman reported on 14 patients who had suffered progressive fluctuating muscular rigidity and spasm and used the term 'stiff-man syndrome' to describe this condition. The condition predominantly affects male adults who, after a prodromal phase of aching and tightness of the axial muscles, go on to develop symmetrical continuous stiffness of the skeletal muscles upon which painful muscular spasms are superimposed; these may be precipitated by movement. The cause of the condition is unknown but there is evidence to suggest that it may be due to overactivity in a central norepinephrine neuronal system which increases excitability of spinal-cord motor neurones (Schmidt, Stahl, and Spehlmann 1975). Diazepam (Howard 1963) may be remarkably successful in controlling the symptoms, as may baclo-

fen or clonazepam (Martinelli, Pazzaglia, Montagna, Coccagna, Rizzuto, Simonati, and Lugaresi 1978; Foster 1981). It must be distinguished from the syndrome of myokymia with continuous muscle-fibre activity (Isaacs and Heffron 1974; see p. 557) which responds to phenytoin.

References

Asbury, A. K. (1975) Uremic neuropathy. In *Peripheral neuropathy* (ed. P. J. Dyck, P. K. Thomas, and E. H. Lambert) Vol. 2, p. 82. Saunders, Philadelphia.

British Medical Journal (1975). Acute muscle compartment compression syndromes. *Br. med. J.* **3**, 193.

Ekbom, K. A. (1960). Restless legs syndrome. *Neurology, Minneapolis* **10**, 868.

Foster, J. B. (1981). The clinical features of some miscellaneous neuromuscular disorders. In *Disorders of voluntary muscle* (ed. J. N. Walton) 4th edn. Churchill Livingstone, Edinburgh and London.

Harriman, D. G. F., Taverner, D., and Woolf, A. L. (1970). Ekbom's syndrome and burning paraesthesiae. A biopsy study by vital staining and electron microscopy of the intramuscular innervation with a note on age changes in motor nerve endings in distal muscles. *Brain* **93**, 393.

Howard, F. M. (1963). A new and effective drug in the treatment of stiff-man syndrome. *Mayo Clin. Proc.* **38**, 203.

Isaacs, H. and Heferon, J. J. A. (1974). The syndrome of 'continuous muscle-fibre activity' cured: further studies. *J. Neurol. Neurosurg. Psychiat.* **37**, 1231.

Martinelli, P., Pazzaglia, P., Montagna, P., Coccagna, G., Rizzuto, N., Simonati, S., and Lugaresi, E. (1978). Stiff-man syndrome associated with nocturnal myoclonus and epilepsy. *J. Neurol. Neurosurg. Psychiat.* **41**, 458.

McKusick, V. (1956). *Heritable disorders of connective tissue*, p. 184. Mosby, St. Louis, Missouri.

Moersch, F. P. and Woltman, H. W. (1956). Progressive muscular rigidity and spasm (stiff-man syndrome). *Mayo Clin. Proc.* **31**, 421.

Nathan, P. W. (1978). Painful legs and moving toes: evidence on the site of the lesion. *J. Neurol. Neurosurg. Psychiat.* **41**, 934.

Russell, R. G. G., Smith, R., Bishop, M. C., Price, D. A., and Squire, C. M. (1972). Treatment of myositis ossificans progressiva with a diphosphonate. *Lancet* **i**, 10.

Schmidt, R. T., Stahl, S. M., and Spehlmann, R. (1975). A pharmacologic study of the stiff-man syndrome. *Neurology, Minneapolis* **25**, 622.

Sirbou, A. B., Murphy, M. J., and White, A. S. (1944). Soft tissue complications of fractures of the leg. *Calif. west Med.* **60**, 53.

Spillane, J. D., Nathan, P. W., Kelly, R. E., and Marsden, C. D. (1971). Painful legs and moving toes. *Brain* **94**, 541.

Tünte, W., Becker, P. E., and Knorre, G. (1967). Zur Genetik der Myositis ossificans progressiva. *Humangenetik* **4**, 320.

Differential diagnosis

The differential diagnosis of muscle disease depends first upon the clinical history and examination, secondly upon EMG and other neurophysiological evidence, thirdly upon biochemical evidence, and fourthly upon pathological changes in muscle as revealed by biopsy.

Clinical diagnosis

In the characteristic case of muscular dystrophy showing the usual slowly progressive pattern of increasing muscular weakness and selective atrophy of the proximal limb muscles, diagnosis is rarely in doubt. On the other hand, in an infant or child demonstrating relatively diffuse non-progressive atrophy and weakness, the condition may belong to one of the group of benign congenital myopathies. There are, however, some cases in which differential diagnosis between a congenital non-progressive myopathy and progressive muscular dystrophy of early onset may be very difficult on purely clinical grounds and then depends upon ancillary investigations.

If the pattern of muscular weakness and wasting is obscured by subcutaneous fat or when muscular involvement is predominantly distal, as in myotonic dystrophy and distal myopathy, it is not always easy to distinguish muscular dystrophy from neuropathic disorders such as progressive muscular atrophy, polyneuropathy, and peroneal muscular atrophy. Usually, however, the associated neurological signs, including fasciculation, and the sensory abnormalities which generally occur in polyneuropathy and peroneal muscular atrophy are sufficient to clarify the position. In early life, fasciculation is a useful sign, both in the tongue and in limb muscles, which occasionally helps to identify the various forms of spinal muscular atrophy, and the EMG is of particular value in distinguishing the latter disorder from muscular dystrophy, as the classical features of central denervation are almost always found.

Often, therefore, it is comparatively easy to distinguish myopathy from neuropathy on clinical grounds alone, but it can be much more difficult to separate sporadic cases of muscular dystrophy from other forms of myopathy. The possibility of an endocrine cause for the muscular weakness must always be considered, and associated signs of endocrine disease and/or of metabolic bone disease should be sought. And in untreated myasthenia gravis fatigability of muscles is not always immediately apparent, so that in any patient with proximal muscular weakness of comparatively recent onset, even when there is no involvement of ocular and bulbar muscles, a diagnostic injection of edrophonium chloride is indicated. Equivocal improvement following such an injection is sometimes seen in polymyositis and a more definite response may be observed in the myasthenic-myopathic (Eaton–Lambert) syndrome, in which, however, the tendon reflexes are usually absent, whereas in true myasthenia they are brisk, and electrophysiological tests of neuromuscular transmission are usually helpful in making the distinction. It should also be noted that in periodic paralysis and myoglobinuria, permanent muscular atrophy may eventually supervene, though in such cases there is invariably a clear-cut history of episodic attacks of weakness or of muscle pain.

The differential diagnosis between muscular dystrophy and subacute or chronic polymyositis can be extremely difficult. Among the criteria of value in differential diagnosis are first, the rapidity of onset and occasional remissions which occur in polymyositis; secondly, the global weakness and wasting which occur in this disease, unlike the selective pattern which is more characteristic of dystrophy; thirdly, a positive family history, if present, clearly indicates a genetically-determined disorder of muscle; fourthly, the almost constant involvement of neck muscles and the frequent occurrence of dysphagia strongly favour polymyositis, while these features are rare in muscular dystrophy except in the oculopharyngeal variety (it should also be recalled that myasthenia may selectively involve the neck muscles in occasional cases); finally, associated phenomena such as skin changes and the Raynaud phenomenon are found in many cases of polymyositis.

Even with the help of these and other clinical guides, there are very many cases in which diagnosis remains in doubt and depends upon investigative findings.

Electromyography (also see p. 494)

In neuropathic disorders, spontaneous fibrillation potentials can usually be recorded from a muscle undergoing active denervation, while the pattern of motor unit activity on volition, though numbers are reduced, clearly indicates that the surviving motor unit action potentials are either normal or increased in size. Measurement of nerve conduction velocity may assist in identifying the nature and site of a lesion in the motor neurones (p. 496). In myopathic disorders, by contrast, spontaneous activity in the form of fibrillation potentials is uncommon, though fibrillation is found in some cases, being more frequent in polymyositis than in muscular dystrophy (Walton and Adams 1958). In the myotonic disorders a characteristic discharge of chains of oscillations of high frequency is seen. Similar spontaneous discharges evoked by movement of the exploring electrode, which, however, do not show the classical

waxing and waning of the myotonic discharge but which continue at a constant frequency and then cease spontaneously, are recorded in various forms of non-myotonic myopathy including polymyositis and in spinal muscular atrophy and have been called pseudomyotonic or bizarre high-frequency discharges. Volitional activity in the myopathies, and particularly in muscular dystrophy and polymyositis, demonstrates a break-down of the motor unit action potentials corresponding to patchy degeneration of muscle fibres and as a result there is an increase in the proportion of short-duration and polyphasic motor unit action potentials (Kugelberg 1947; Walton 1952). Buchthal, Rosenfalck, and Erminio (1960) showed that a decrease in mean action potential amplitude and duration, together with a reduced motor unit territory and fibre density, is seen particularly often in the Duchenne type of muscular dystrophy. In myotonic dystrophy and polymyositis they found that motor unit territory and the mean duration of the motor unit potentials were similarly reduced, but normal amplitudes were maintained. In polymyositis Buchthal and Pinelli (1953) found that the mean duration of the motor unit action potential was decreased by up to 60 per cent and the incidence of polyphasic potentials was increased three times. In the more benign forms of muscular dystrophy (the limb-girdle and facioscapulohumeral types) similar but less conclusive quantitative changes may be observed (Buchthal 1962; Barwick 1981; Kimura 1983). Changes in the motor unit action potentials similar to those observed in muscular dystrophy are found in thyrotoxic myopathy (Havard, Campbell, Ross, and Spence 1963), in steroid myopathy (Müller and Kugelberg 1959), in the myopathies of Addison's disease and sarcoidosis (Buchthal 1962), and in many other metabolic myopathies. Farmer, Buchthal, and Rosenfalck (1959) found that the absolute refractory period of voluntary muscle was reduced in cases of muscular dystrophy.

More specialized techniques of EMG examination including integration and analysis of the EMG and single-fibre electromyography (see page 496) are reviewed by Lenman (1981) and Kimura (1983) and methods of intracellular recording by McComas and Johns (1981). The electrophysiological technique of estimating the number of functioning motor units in the extensor digitorum brevis muscle of the foot, as developed by McComas, Campbell, and Sica (1971) and later extended to other muscles by others, originally suggested that motor unit dysfunction might play a role in the pathogenesis of muscular dystrophy, but this 'neurogenic hypothesis' was subsequently disproved. Nevertheless, this method of counting functioning motor units has proved to be of considerable diagnostic value (Lenman 1981).

In myasthenia gravis the EMG may be entirely normal, except that a myopathic pattern, as described above, may be obtained from fatigued muscle. A progressive diminution in the amplitude of the action potentials in myasthenic muscle recorded with surface electrodes during supramaximal stimulation of its motor nerve at rates of 3 Hz (Harvey and Masland 1941) is a useful diagnostic sign of myasthenia, but only occurs as a rule in muscles which are clinically affected (Botelho, Deaterly, Austin, and Comroe 1952; Brown 1981). At tetanic rates of stimulation (50 Hz) the amplitude of the evoked muscle action potential usually increases greatly in cases of the myasthenic-myopathic (Eaton–Lambert) syndrome (Lambert, Eaton, and Rooke 1956; Brown 1981) but a similar, though less striking, increment (Simpson 1981) is occasionally seen in myasthenia gravis. Single-fibre EMG (p. 569) has, however, made a major contribution to the diagnosis of myasthenia and other disorders of neuromuscular transmission, just as the technique of 'macro EMG' (see Lenman and Ritchie 1983) which gives considerable information about the numbers, sizes, and remodelling of motor units, has proved very valuable in the diagnosis of spinal muscular atrophy and the other neuropathic disorders. No specific EMG appearances have been described in cases of familial periodic paralysis, but in patients with the various forms of benign congenital myopathy the EMG again reveals a myopathic pattern without any specific features (see Barwick 1981).

Biochemical diagnosis

Many biochemical tests can be employed in differentiating the various forms of myopathy. Thus in the endocrine myopathies tests apposite to the diagnosis of the individual endocrine disorders are required. In the periodic paralysis syndromes, in addition to serial estimations of the serum potassium level and measures designed to precipitate attacks for diagnostic purposes, there are certain cases in which measurement of sodium and potassium output in the urine, and even of sodium and potassium balance, may be needed. In cases of severe generalized muscle pain and weakness, a search for myoglobin in the urine is essential, while in those patients who develop muscle pain after effort it is usually necessary to exclude certain forms of glycogen storage disease by the measurement of lactate in venous blood distal to a tourniquet following a period of ischaemic work; estimation of phosphorylase and of other glycolytic enzymes by histochemical and chemical methods applied to muscle biopsy samples, as well as the estimation of the total glycogen content of muscle, may also be needed (see Engel 1981). In other cases of exercise-induced muscle pain and cramp, it is now also necessary to measure carnitine palmityl transferase and AMP deaminase in biopsy samples, while in cases in which there is evidence of excess lipid storage demonstrated histochemically, especially in Type 1 fibres, measurement of muscle carnitine is now obligatory. And when biopsy in a case of subacute progressive myopathy reveals extensive vacuolation of muscle fibres, shown to be due to glycogen deposition, it will also be necessary to estimate acid maltase and sometimes the branching and debranching enzymes (see above). Similarly, in the presence of lactic acidosis, 'ragged-red' Type 1 fibres, and morphologically abnormal mitochondria, a variety of studies of oxidative phosphorylation in muscle or of enzymes of the electron transport chain will sometimes be required to elucidate the nature of the affliction. A recent important development has been the introduction of topical nuclear magnetic resonance studies, giving an accurate and rapid indication of the concentration of substances such as ATP and ADP within skeletal muscle.

In polymyositis the erythrocyte sedimentation rate is raised in about half the cases and there may be an elevation of the serum gamma-globulin demonstrated by electrophoresis (Barwick and Walton 1963). This is usually mainly IgG but IgM may also be increased, as may be serum C3 complement (Currie 1981). Tests for circulating antibodies in the serum of such patients have been disappointing (Caspary, Gubbay, and Stern 1964). Antimyosin antibody is found not only in some cases of polymyositis and myasthenia gravis, but also in others with muscular dystrophy and neurogenic atrophy and in some normal individuals. Antinuclear factor is present, however, in a higher proportion of cases of polymyositis than of controls. Positive LE-cell preparations are occasionally found (Currie 1981) but such examinations as the latex fixation and Rose-Waaler tests are of little diagnostic value. The more sophisticated immunological methods which may be of value in the diagnosis of polymyositis, myasthenia gravis, and the Guillain–Barré syndrome are respectively reviewed on pages 564, 570, and 527.

The many other relatively non-specific biochemical findings found in cases of myopathy have been reviewed by Pennington (1981). Thus an excessive output of creatine and a diminished creatinuria are common but have little diagnostic significance. Aminoaciduria is also seen in a few cases, while changes observed in serum lipid and protein levels lack specificity. Abnormalities of protein composition and turnover in dystrophic muscle, though of considerable research interest (Rowland, Dunne, Penn, and Maher 1968; Samaha and Gergely 1969; Penn, Cloak, and Rowland 1972; Ionasescu, Zellweger, Shirk, and Conway 1972; Ionasescu, Zellweger, McCormick, and Conway 1973; Samaha 1973),

as well as disorders of carbohydrate metabolism (Ellis and Strickland 1972) do not assist in diagnosis, and nor do studies of erythrocyte deformation, membrane function, or lymphocyte capping (Brown, Chattopadhyay, and Patel 1967; Lumb and Emery 1975; Walton and Gardner-Medwin 1981; and see p. 555). Of much greater diagnostic value have been changes in serum enzyme activities. Sibley and Lehninger (1949) first demonstrated that the serum aldolase level was raised in patients with various muscle diseases including progressive muscular dystrophy. Subsequently many authors showed that the activity of the enzyme in the serum is raised to about 10 times the normal upper limit in early cases of Duchenne type muscular dystrophy, with less striking increases in the more benign varieties. Pearson (1957) found that similar though less striking increases occurred in the serum activity of the transaminases (aminotransferases) and pointed out that a substantial rise in enzyme activity might occur long before overt clinical signs of Duchenne type dystrophy appeared—that is, in the preclinical phase of the disease. In 1959 Ebashi, Toyakura, Momoi, and Sugita reported a pronounced increase in creatine kinase (CK) activity in the serum of patients with muscular dystrophy and demonstrated that in early cases of the Duchenne type this increase might even be three hundredfold. It is now evident that estimation of this serum enzyme is much the most sensitive early diagnostic test for this form of muscular dystrophy, and Pearce, Pennington, and Walton (1964) among others have confirmed the increase in preclinical cases. It is well recognized that the activity of this and other enzymes (see Pennington 1981) which leak out of the diseased muscle into the serum is at its highest in the early stages of all forms of muscle disease and tends to decline as the disease advances. In Duchenne type dystrophy, activity is probably highest at about the second or third year of life and declines progressively thereafter. Similar reductions are seen during the course of limb-girdle and facioscapulohumeral dystrophy and in myotonic dystrophy, although in these three disorders the initial increases are very much less striking. In polymyositis the activity is highest in acute cases before treatment, but a rapid decline occurs following treatment, particularly if it is effective. The activity of this enzyme in the serum has been reported to increase markedly four to six hours after a test dose of prednisone in patients with muscular dystrophy but not in polymyositis (Takahashi, Oimomi, Shinko, Shutta, Matsuo, Takai, and Imura 1975). Estimation of serum CK activity is still the single most useful test for the identification of the carrier state in female relatives of patients suffering from X-linked muscular dystrophy (p. 555), but some have found the estimation of serum pyruvate kinase and of serum myoglobin by radioimmunoassay to be even more sensitive (Pennington 1981).

Histological diagnosis

Traditionally muscle biopsy has been one of the standard methods employed in the differential diagnosis of the various myopathies (Adams, Denny-Brown, and Pearson 1962). Many pathological changes have been described in muscle and detailed reviews have been given by Dubowitz and Brooke (1973), Åstrom and Adams (1981), Hudgson and Mastaglia (1981), Schröder (1982), and Mastaglia and Walton (1981), among others. Percutaneous muscle biopsy of the quadriceps (Edwards 1971) is often useful, especially when repeated biopsy is needed, though the specimen obtained is small. Increasing knowledge has led to decreasing confidence about the specificity of pathological changes seen in muscle biopsy specimens in so far as the differential diagnosis of myopathy is concerned. Although techniques such as intravital staining of the motor end-plates (Coërs 1981; Chou 1982), histochemistry, tissue culture, and electron microscopy have been of considerable interest from the research standpoint, only comparatively recently have they added precision to the histological diagnosis of the myopathies, especially the congenital and metabolic varieties.

Among the most characteristic histological features observed in cases of muscular dystrophy of all types (Adams *et al.* 1962; Pearce and Walton 1962; Pearson 1973) are such changes as marked variations in fibre size, fibre splitting, the central migration of sarcolemmal nuclei (Fig. 19.8), areas of fibre atrophy, the formation of nuclear chains, areas of necrosis with phagocytosis of necrotic sarcoplasm (Fig. 19.9), and basophilia of sarcoplasm with an enlargement of sarcolemmal nuclei (Fig. 19.10) which show prominent nucleoli (changes construed as being due to abortive regeneration); infiltration with fat cells and connective tissue is also observed. Scattered hyaline fibres seen in transverse section with

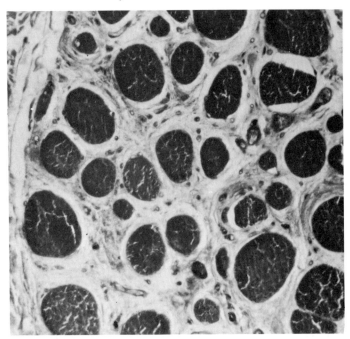

Fig. 19.8. Transverse section of biceps brachii biopsy from a case of advanced limb-girdle dystrophy showing rounding of fibres, random variation in size, central nuclei, fibre-splitting, and infiltration with connective tissue. H & E, × 240.

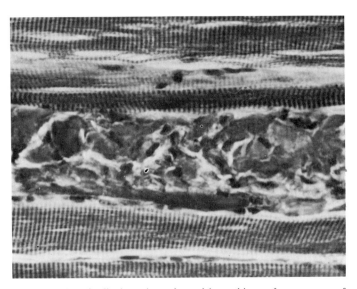

Fig. 19.9. Longitudinal section of quadriceps biopsy from a case of Duchenne type muscular dystrophy demonstrating focal necrosis and phagocytosis of a segment of muscle fibre. Picro-Mallory, × 640.

others which are necrotic, interspersed with clumps of regenerating fibres, are the histological hallmark of Duchenne muscular dystrophy in the early or preclinical stages (Pearson 1962; Cullen

and Fulthorpe 1975). When changes of the type described are uniformly distributed throughout the muscle sections, it is not usually difficult to accept that the diagnosis is one of muscular dystrophy. On the other hand, similar changes may be seen in polymyositis (Walton and Adams 1958; Åstrom and Adams 1981; Mastaglia and Walton 1981), in which condition, however, signs of muscle-fibre destruction and repair (necrosis, phagocytosis, and regenerative activity) are usually more striking and widespread, though they may be surprisingly slight even in acute cases. Most important in the diagnosis of polymyositis, but often scanty and only rarely observed in muscular dystrophy, except in some cases of the facioscapulohumeral syndrome (p. 556), are interstitial, perivascular, or perifascicular infiltrations of inflammatory cells such as lymphocytes and plasma cells (Fig. 19.11). It is also important to note that whereas chronic denervation atrophy, as in the spinal muscular atrophies of childhood, chronic polyneuropathy and motor-neurone disease, usually gives groups of uniformly atrophic fibres lying alongside groups of fibres which are normal in size or even hypertrophied (Fig. 19.12), with so-called 'type-grouping' or large fields of fibres of uniform histochemical type (see Dubowitz and Brooke 1973; Dubowitz 1981; Jennekens 1982; and p. 552), in disseminated neurogenic atrophy the atrophic fibres, often sharply angulated and containing dark pyknotic nuclei, may occur in groups of only four or five fibres and are easily overlooked. Furthermore in chronic denervation many muscles show secondary myopathic change (Drachman, Murphy, Nigam, and Hills 1967; Mastaglia and Walton 1971) with muscle-fibre necrosis, phagocytosis, and regenerative activity so that the unwary may be led to diagnose a primary myopathy. Undoubtedly this error often led in the past to a mistaken diagnosis of muscular dystrophy in patients with spinal muscular atrophy.

If, therefore, in a muscle section there is gross variation in fibre size with fibre-splitting, infiltration with fat and connective tissue, and little phagocytosis or regenerative activity with no evidence of groups of tiny atrophic fibres, one may reasonably assume that the process is probably, but not certainly, dystrophic. If, by contrast, there is widespread necrosis and phagocytosis of muscle fibres with some, though not excessive, variation in fibre size, with profuse regenerative activity and massive infiltration of inflammatory cells between fibres and around blood vessels, it is not difficult to decide that one is probably dealing with a case of polymyositis. Between these two extremes, however, there is considerable overlap in the types of change which may be seen in dystrophy on the one hand and polymyositis on the other. Furthermore, in some cases of myasthenia gravis (Russell 1953) there are degenerative changes within muscle fibres, and lymphorrhages (collections of lymphocytes) may be seen around blood vessels or occasionally between fibres. Changes are often less striking in cases of the myasthenic-myopathic (Eaton–Lambert) syndrome (Croft and Wilkinson 1965), and although the pathological changes in muscle in cases of thyrotoxic and other endocrine myopathies may certainly be construed as being myopathic in the broadest sense, they are often slight and ill-defined.

The finding of striated annulets or so-called ringbinden (Wohlfart 1951; Greenfield, Shy, Alvord, and Berg 1957) in which striated myofibrils encircle muscle fibres cut in transverse section, was often regarded as being diagnostic of myotonic dystrophy (Fig. 19.13), but this is by no means absolute as these abnormalities are occasionally seen in other muscle diseases and are due to the fracture of peripherally-situated myofibrils which then wind around the intact portion of the fibre. In myotonic dystrophy, chains of nuclei within muscle fibres are particularly striking, the nuclei are often small and pyknotic, unlike the large vesicular nuclei occurring in chains which are seen in some cases of Duchenne type dystrophy and of polymyositis and which probably indicate abortive regenerative activity, and there is often selective Type 1 fibre atrophy. Abnormalities of the muscle spindles are often more striking in this condition than in other neuromuscular dis-

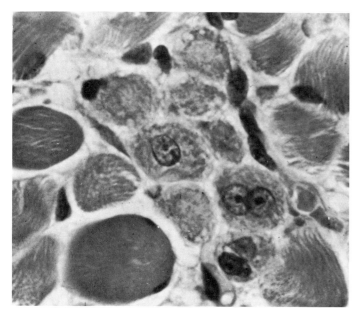

Fig. 19.10. Transverse section of a quadriceps biopsy from a case of preclinical Duchenne type dystrophy. H & E, × 640. Note the group of central fibres with sparse myofibrils and large vesicular nuclei with prominent nucleoli, demonstrating regenerative activity.

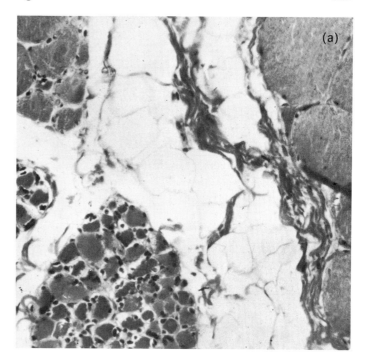

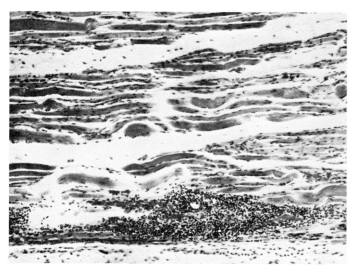

Fig. 19.11. Muscle in acute polymyositis.

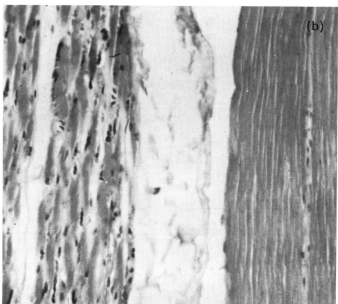

Fig. 19.12. Grouped atrophy of denervation demonstrated in a biopsy of tibialis anterior from a patient with peroneal muscular atrophy. (*a*) Transverse section, H & E, × 640. (*b*) Longitudinal section, H & E, × 640.

eases (Cazzato and Walton 1968; Swash and Fox 1975). Masses of palely-staining homogeneous sarcoplasm lying in the periphery of muscle fibres (so-called sarcoplasmic masses) are also typically seen in myotonic cases (Fig. 19.13). The 'myopathic' changes described can, in the great majority of cases, be readily distinguished from those of denervation atrophy (Fig. 19.12) except, as mentioned above, when secondary myopathic change is widespread and grouped atrophic fibres are few; histochemical studies may be especially useful here, especially when there is 'fibre type grouping', suggesting reinnervation of previously denervated fibres.

Vacuolar change within muscle fibres is another important pathological change. Massive vacuoles within the substance of muscle fibres, often lying in a subsarcolemmal position, and shown by alcoholic PAS staining to contain glycogen, are characteristic of the various forms of glycogen storage disease of muscle (Fig. 19.14) including Pompe's disease (Hudgson, Gardner-Medwin, Worsfold, Pennington, and Walton 1968) and McArdle's disease (Salter, Adamson, and Pearce 1968). Widespread but less

striking vacuolar change is also seen with the light microscope within the muscle fibres of patients with periodic paralysis during attacks, and electron microscopy (Shy, Wanko, Rowley, and Engel 1961) showed that these vacuoles are due to dilatation of the endoplasmic reticulum. Pearson and Yamazaki (1958) found similar vacuolar change in muscle in systemic lupus erythematosus, and comparable histological abnormalities also occur in the myopathy which can result from the long-continued administration of chloroquine (see Kakulas 1981 and Mastaglia and Argov 1981). Vacuolar changes may also be noted with the light microscope in lipid storage myopathy due to carnitine deficiency (Bradley, Hudgson, Gardner-Medwin, and Walton 1969; Engel and Siekert 1972) but this condition is much better identified in frozen sections using stains for neutral fat. Histochemistry is also invalu-

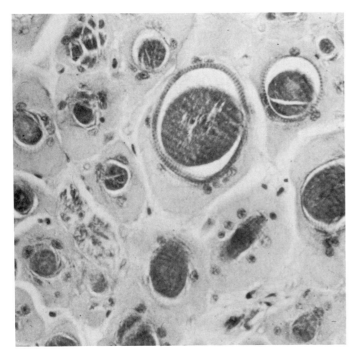

Fig. 19.13. Transverse section of quadriceps, obtained at autopsy from a case of dystrophia myotonica, PTAH, × 480, demonstrating ringbinden and/or sarcoplasmic masses surrounding the transversely-sectioned central myofibrils of virtually every muscle fibre. (By kind permission of Dr G. W. Pearce.)

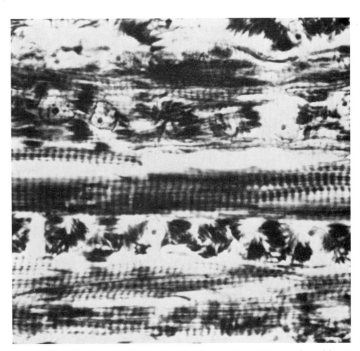

Fig. 19.15. Nemaline myopathy; longitudinal section of biopsy from biceps brachii, PTAH, × 960. Note the collections of rods lying between the fibres. (From Hudgson, Gardner-Medwin, Fulthorpe, and Walton (1967) by kind permission of the editor.)

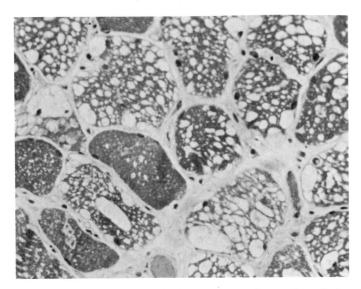

Fig. 19.14. Vacuolar myopathy in glycogen storage disease of muscle due to acid maltase deficiency. Transverse section of quadriceps biopsy. H & E, × 640.

able in the recognition of 'ragged-red' fibres in the mitochondrial myopathies, in confirming the absence of phosphorylase in McArdle's disease, in identifying Type II fibre atrophy in steroid myopathy and many other conditions, or fibre type disproportion in some cases of benign congenital hypotonia, and in demonstrating the 'type-grouping' of many chronic denervating processes, to name only a few of its contributions (see Dubowitz and Brooke 1973; Dubowitz 1981; Mastaglia and Walton 1982). Indeed, histochemical study is now an essential technique in the examination of muscle biopsy specimens and electron microscopy (Cullen and Mastaglia 1982) is also invaluable. It should finally be mentioned that in cases of so-called benign congenital myopathy or hypotonia

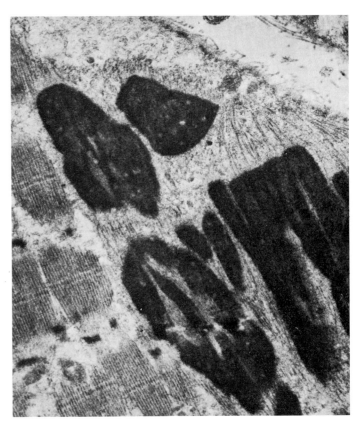

Fig. 19.16. Electron micrograph of longitudinal section of biceps brachii biopsy, × 25,000, demonstrating electron-dense nemaline rods, lying in the sub-sarcolemmal portion of a muscle fibre. (From Hudgson *et al.* (1967) by kind permission of the editor.)

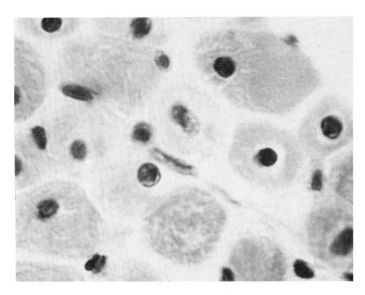

Fig. 19.17. Myotubular or centronuclear myopathy, transverse section of quadriceps biopsy. H & E, × 960. Note the central nuclei surrounded by clear 'halos' in several muscle fibres.

in which myopathic changes have been observed in the EMG, examination of muscle biopsy specimens under the light microscope has been singularly disappointing (Walton 1957), and it is only since particular attention has been paid to these cases, using histochemical stains and electron microscopy, that entities such as central core disease, nemaline myopathy (Fig. 19.15 and 19.16), and myotubular myopathy (Fig. 19.17) and the various mitochondrial myopathies have been recognized and characterized (Fardeau 1982). It is likely that the use of these highly specialized techniques will in the future identify many more specific syndromes within this relatively difficult and little-understood group.

References

Adams, R. D. (1975). *Diseases of muscle*, 3rd edn. Hoeber, New York.

——, Denny-Brown, D. and Pearson, C. M. (1962). *Diseases of muscle, a study in pathology*, 2nd edn. Hoeber, New York.

Åstrom, K. -E. and Adams, R. D. (1981). Pathological reactions of the skeletal muscle fibre in man. In *Disorders of voluntary muscle* (ed. J. N. Walton) 4th edn, Ch. 5. Churchill-Livingstone, Edinburgh and London.

Barwick, D. D. (1981). Clinical electromyography. In *Disorders of voluntary muscle* (ed. J. N. Walton) 4th ed., Ch. 28. Churchill-Livingstone, Edinburgh and London.

—— and Walton, J. N. (1963). Polymyositis. *Am. J. Med.* **35**, 646.

Botelho, S. Y., Deaterly, C. F., Austin, S., and Comroe, J. H. (1952). Evaluation of the electromyogram of patients with myasthenia gravis. *Arch. Neurol. Psychiat., Chicago* **67**, 441.

Bradley, W. G., Hudgson, P., Gardner-Medwin, D., and Walton, J. N. (1969). Myopathy associated with abnormal lipid metabolism in skeletal muscle. *Lancet* **i**, 495.

Brown, H. D., Chattopadhyay, S. K., and Patel, A. B. (1967). Erythrocyte abnormality in human myopathy. *Science* **157**, 1577.

Brown, J. C. (1981). Repetitive stimulation and neuromuscular transmission studies. In *Disorders of voluntary muscle* (ed. J. N. Walton) 4th edn, Ch. 26. Churchill-Livingstone, Edinburgh and London.

Buchthal, F. (1962). The electromyogram. *Wld Neurol.* **3**, 16.

—— and Pinelli, P. (1953). Muscle action potentials in polymyositis. *Neurology, Minneapolis* **3**, 424.

——, Rosenfalck, P. and Erminio, F. (1960). Motor unit territory and fibre density in myopathies. *Neurology, Minneapolis* **10**, 398.

Caspary, E. A., Gubbay, S. S., and Stern, G. M. (1964). Circulating antibodies in polymyositis and other muscle-wasting disorders. *Lancet* **ii**, 941.

Cazzato, G. and Walton, J. N. (1968). The pathology of the muscle spindle: a study of biopsy material in various muscular and neuromuscular diseases. *J. neurol. Sci.* **7**, 15.

Chou, S. M. (1982). Pathology of the neuromuscular junction. In *Skeletal muscle pathology* (ed. F. L. Mastaglia and J. N. Walton), Ch. 14. Churchill-Livingstone, Edinburgh.

Coërs, C. (1981). Pathological anatomy of the intramuscular nerve endings. In *Disorders of voluntary muscle* (ed. J. N. Walton), 4th edn., Ch. 7. Churchill-Livingstone, Edinburgh and London.

Croft, P. B. and Wilkinson, M. (1965). The incidence of carcinomatous neuromyopathy in patients with various types of carcinoma. *Brain* **88**, 427.

Cullen, M. J. and Fulthorpe, J. J. (1975). Stages in fibre breakdown in Duchenne muscular dystrophy. An electron microscopic study. *J. neurol. Sci.* **24**, 179.

—— and Mastaglia, F. L. (1982). Pathological reactions of skeletal muscle. In *Skeletal muscle pathology* (ed. F. L. Mastaglia and J. N. Walton) Ch. 2. Churchill-Livingstone, Edinburgh.

Currie, S. (1981). Inflammatory myopathies: polymyositis and related disorders. In *Disorders of voluntary muscle* (ed. J. N. Walton) 4th edn, Ch. 15, Part 1. Churchill-Livingstone, Edinburgh and London.

Drachman, D. B., Murphy, S. R., Nigam, M. P., and Hills, J. R. (1967). 'Myopathic' changes in chronically denervated muscle. *Arch. Neurol., Chicago* **16**, 14.

Dubowitz, V. (1981). Histochemical aspects of muscle disease. In *Disorders of voluntary muscle* (ed. J. N. Walton) 4th edn. Churchill-Livingstone, Edinburgh and London.

—— and Brooke, M. H. (1973). *Muscle biopsy*. Ch. 8. Saunders, London.

Ebashi, S., Toyokura, Y., Momoi, H., and Sugita, H. (1959). High creatine phosphokinase activity of sera of progressive muscular dystrophy. *J. Biochem., Tokyo* **46**, 103.

Edwards, R. H. T. (1971). Percutaneous needle-biopsy of skeletal muscle in diagnosis and research. *Lancet* **ii**, 593.

Ellis, D. A. and Strickland, J. M. (1972). Differences in the metabolism of glucose between normal and dystrophic human muscle. *Biochem. J.* **130**, 17.

Engel, A. G. and Siekert, R. G. (1972). Lipid storage myopathy responsive to prednisone. *Arch. Neurol., Chicago* **27**, 174.

Fardeau, M. (1982). Congenital myopthies. In *Skeletal muscle pathology* (ed. F. L. Mastaglia and J. N. Walton) Ch. 4. Churchill-Livingstone, Edinburgh.

Farmer, T. W., Buchthal, F. and Rosenfalck, P. (1959). Refractory and irresponsive periods of muscle in progressive muscular dystrophy and paresis due to lower motor neurone involvement. *Neurology, Minneapolis* **9**, 747.

Greenfield, J. G., Shy, G. M., Alvord, E. C., and Berg, L. (1957). *An atlas of muscle pathology in neuromuscular diseases*. Churchill-Livingstone, Edinburgh.

Harvey, A. M. and Masland, R. L. (1941). A method for the study of neuromuscular transmission in human subjects. *Bull. Johns Hopk. Hosp.* **69**, 1.

Havard, C. W. H., Campbell, E. D. R., Ross, H. B., and Spence, A. W. (1963). Electromyographic and histological findings in the muscles of patients with thyrotoxicosis. *Quart. J. Med.* **32**, 145.

Hudgson, P., Gardner-Medwin, D., Fulthorpe, J. J., and Walton, J. N. (1967). Nemaline myopathy. *Neurology, Minneapolis* **17**, 1125.

——, ——, Worsfold, M., Pennington, R. J. T. and Walton, J. N. (1968). Adult myopathy in glycogen storage disease due to acid maltase deficiency. *Brain*, **91**, 435.

—— and Mastaglia, F. L. (1981). Ultrastructural studies of diseased muscle. In *Disorders of voluntary muscle* (ed. J. N. Walton) 4th edn. Churchill-Livingstone, Edinburgh and London.

Ionasescu, V., Zellweger, H., McCormick, W. F., and Conway, T. W. (1973). Comparison of ribosomal protein synthesis in Becker and Duchenne muscular dystrophies. *Neurology, Minneapolis* **23**, 245.

——, ——, Shirk, P. and Conway, T. W. (1972). Abnormal protein synthesis in facioscapulohumeral muscular dystrophy. *Neurology, Minneapolis* **22**, 1286.

Jennekens, F. G. I. (1982). Neurogenic disorders of muscle. In *Skeletal muscle pathology* (ed. F. L. Mastaglia and J. N. Walton) Ch. 22. Churchill-Livingstone, Edinburgh.

Kakulas, B. A. (1981). Experimental myopathies. In *Disorders of voluntary muscle* (ed. J. N. Walton), 4th edn., Ch. 11. Churchill-Livingstone, Edinburgh and London.

Kimura, J. (1983). *Electrodiagnosis in diseases of nerve and muscle: principles and practice*. F. A. Davis, Philadelphia.

Kugelberg, E. (1947). Electromyogram in muscular dystrophy. *J. Neurol. Neurosurg. Psychiat.* **10**, 122.

Lambert, E. H., Eaton, L. M., and Rooke, E. D. (1956). Defect of neuro-muscular conduction associated with malignant neoplasms. *Am. J. Physiol.* **187**, 612.

Lenman, J. A. R. (1981). Integration and analysis of the electromyogram and related techniques. In *Disorders of voluntary muscle* (ed. J. N. Walton) 4th edn, Ch. 29. Churchill-Livingstone, Edinburgh and London.

—— and Ritchie, A. E. (1983). *Clinical electromyography*, 3rd edn. Pitman, London.

Lumb, E. M. and Emery, A. E. H. (1975). Erythrocyte deformation in Duchenne muscular dystrophy. *Br. med. J.* **3**, 467.

Mastaglia, F. L. and Argov, Z. (1981). Drug-induced neuromuscular disorders in man. In *Disorders of voluntary muscle* (ed. J. N. Walton) 4th edn, Ch. 25. Churchill-Livingstone, Edinburgh and London.

—— and Walton, J. N. (1971). Histological and histochemical changes in skeletal muscle from cases of chronic juvenile and early adult spinal muscular atrophy (the Kugelberg–Welander syndrome). *J. neurol. Sci.* **12**, 15.

—— and —— (Eds.) (1982). *Skeletal muscle pathology*. Churchill-Livingstone, Edinburgh.

McComas, A. J., Campbell, M. J. and Sica, R. E. P. (1971). Electrophysiological study of dystrophia myotonica. *J. Neurol. Neurosurg. Psychiat.* **34**, 132.

—— and Johns, R. J. (1981). Potential changes in the normal and diseased muscle cell. In *Disorders of voluntary muscle* (ed. J. N. Walton) 4th edn, Ch. 30. Churchill-Livingstone, Edinburgh and London.

Müller, R. and Kugelberg, E. (1959). Myopathy in Cushing's syndrome. *J. Neurol. Neurosurg. Psychiat.* **22**, 314.

Pearce, G. W. (1965). Histopathology of voluntary muscle. *Postgrad. med. J.* **41**, 294.

—— and Walton, J. N. (1962). Progressive muscular dystrophy: the histopathological changes in skeletal muscle obtained by biopsy. *J. Path. Bact.* **83**, 535.

Pearce, J. M. S., Pennington, R. J. T. and Walton, J. N. (1964). Serum enzyme studies in muscle disease—Part II: Serum creatine kinase activity in muscular dystrophy and in other myopathic and neuropathic disorders. *J. Neurol. Neurosurg. Psychiat.* **27**, 96.

Pearson, C. M. (1957). Serum enzymes in muscular dystrophy and certain other muscular and neuromuscular diseases. I. Serum glutamic oxalecetic transaminase. *New. Engl. J. Med.* **256**, 1069.

—— (1962). Histopathological features of muscle in the preclinical stages of muscular dystrophy. *Brain*, **85**, 109.

—— (1973). *The striated muscle*. Williams and Wilkins, Baltimore.

—— and Yamazaki, J. N. (1958). Vacuolar myopathy in systemic lupus erythematosus. *Am. J. clin. Path.* **29**, 455.

Penn, A. S., Cloak, R. A. and Rowland, . P. (1972). Myosin from normal and dystrophic human muscle. *Arch. Neurol., Chicago* **27**, 159.

Pennington, R. J. T. (1981). Biochemical aspects of muscle disease. In *Disorders of voluntary muscle* (ed. J. N. Walton) 4th edn, Ch. 12. Churchill-Livingstone, Edinburgh and London.

Rowland, L. P., Dunne, P. B., Penn, A. S. and Maher, E. (1968). Myoglobin and muscular dystrophy: electrophoretic and immunochemical study. *Arch. Neurol., Chicago* **18**, 141.

Russell, D. S. (1953). Histological changes in the striped muscles in myasthenia gravis. *J. Path. Bact.* **65**, 279.

Salter, R. H., Adamson, D. G. and Pearce, G. W. (1968). McArdle's syndrome (myophosphorylase deficiency). *Quart. J. Med.* **36**, 565.

Samaha, F. J. (1973). Actomyosin alterations in Duchenne muscular dystrophy. *Arch. Neurol., Chicago* **28**, 405.

—— and Gergely, J. (1969). Biochemistry of normal and myotonic dystrophic human myosin. *Arch. Neurol., Chicago* **21**, 200.

Schröder, J. M. (1982). *Pathologie der Muskulatur*. Springer-Verlag, Berlin.

Shy, G. M., Wanko, T., Rowley, P. T. and Engel, A. G. (1961). Studies in familial periodic paralysis. *Exp. Neurol.* **3**, 53.

Sibley, J. A. and Lehninger, A. L. (1949). Aldolase in the serum and tissues of tumour-bearing animals. *J. nat. Cancer Inst.* **9**, 303.

Simpson, J. A. (1981). Myasthenia gravis and the myasthenic syndromes. In *Disorders of voluntary muscle* (ed. J. N. Walton), 4th edn, Ch. 16. Churchill-Livingstone, Edinburgh and London.

Swash, M. and Fox, K. P. (1975). Abnormal intrafusal muscle fibres in myotonic dystrophy: a study using serial sections. *J. Neurol. Neurosurg. Psychiat.* **38**, 91.

Takahashi, K., Oimomi, M., Shinko, T., Shutta, K., Matsuo, B., Takai, T. and Imura, H. (1975). Response of serum creatine phosphokinase to steroid hormone. *Arch. Neurol., Chicago* **32**, 89.

Walton, J. N. (1952). The electromyogram in myopathy: analysis with the audio-frequency spectrometer. *J. Neurol. Neurosurg. Psychiat.* **14**, 219.

—— (1957). The limp child. *J. Neurol. Neurosurg. Psychiat.* **20**, 144.

—— and Adams, R. D. (1958). *Polymyositis*. Churchill-Livingstone, Edinburgh.

—— and Gardner-Medwin, D. (1981). Progressive muscular dystrophy and the myotonic disorders. In *Disorders of voluntary muscle* (ed. J. N. Walton), 4th edn, Ch 14. Churchill-Livingstone, Edinburgh and London.

Wohlfart, G. (1951). Dystrophia myotonica and myotonia congenita. Histopathological studies with special reference to changes in muscles. *J. Neuropath. exp. Neurol.* **10**, 109.

20

Disorders of the autonomic nervous system

The autonomic nervous system

The 'autonomic' or 'vegetative' nervous system is the part of the nervous system concerned in the innervation of unstriated muscle and many of the secretory glands. Physiologically it is divisible into two parts—the sympathetic and the parasympathetic, which in general are mutually anatagonistic in function and employ anatomically separate pathways.

Anatomy

The brain, hypothalamus and spinal cord

Cerebral control

Parts of the cerebral cortex exercise some control over autonomic activity, but the exact areas of the cortex concerned and the mechanisms by which they produce their effects in man are not fully defined. In fact this subject has become increasingly complex. Detailed reviews of the cerebral control of autonomic and endocrine function have been given by Blackwell and Guillemin (1973), Hayward (1975), Daniel and Prichard (1975), Liddle and Liddle (1981), and Hall (1983). A brief summary of some of the more important points will be given here. Parts of the prefrontal cortex are clearly important. In primates, respiratory and vasomotor changes can be evoked by stimulation of Brodmann's area 13; bilateral excision of the posterior parts of area 14 causes 'sham rage' (see p. 637); and removal of area 24, the anterior cingulate gyrus, renders the animals unusually tame and alters their social adjustment. In man pathways descend to the hypothalamus from the hippocampus, amygdala, prefrontal cortex, and cingulate gyrus, probably concerned with autonomic activity (Jacobson 1972). Lesions of the cingulate gyrus reduce emotional reactions and are sometimes produced therapeutically in the 'psychosurgical' operation of cingulectomy. Stimulation of the prefrontal cortex can produce sweating in the opposite arm and leg. Voluntary evacuation of the bladder and bowels seems to be initiated in the paracentral lobule of the hemisphere. Probably motor impulses from this area, which activate the appropriate parasympathetic nerves, travel downwards with the corticospinal tract. These are but a few examples of cerebral control which almost certainly will be shown to be much more varied and extensive.

Hypothalamic control

The most important cell stations which finally control visceral and other autonomic activity lie in the hypothalamus (Fig. 20.1). Nuclei here receive fibres from the 'visceral' areas of the cerebral cortex mentioned above and in turn give rise to descending pathways which traverse the brainstem and spinal cord. The hypothalamic nuclei not only control autonomic activity but some of them also regulate secretion from the posterior pituitary, to which, through the infundibulum and tuber cinereum, they are closely related anatomically. They also secrete small polypeptide hormones which influence the release of hormones from the anterior pituitary. Thus the cells of the supraoptic nuclei form antidiuretic hormone (ADH) or its precursors, which then travel down the axons into the posterior lobe of the pituitary, to be stored there as neurosecretory granules. Similarly, oxytocin, which stimulates contrac-

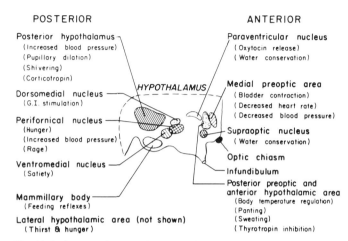

POSTERIOR   ANTERIOR

Posterior hypothalamus
(Increased blood pressure)
(Pupillary dilation)
(Shivering)
(Corticotropin)

Dorsomedial nucleus
(G.I. stimulation)

Perifornical nucleus
(Hunger)
(Increased blood pressure)
(Rage)

Ventromedial nucleus
(Satiety)

Mammillary body
(Feeding reflexes)

Lateral hypothalamic area (not shown)
(Thirst & hunger)

HYPOTHALAMUS

Paraventricular nucleus
(Oxytocin release)
(Water conservation)

Medial preoptic area
(Bladder contraction)
(Decreased heart rate)
(Decreased blood pressure)

Supraoptic nucleus
(Water conservation)

Optic chiasm

Infundibulum

Posterior preoptic and anterior hypothalamic area
(Body temperature regulation)
(Panting)
(Sweating)
(Thyrotropin inhibition)

Fig. 20.1. Autonomic control centres of the hypothalamus. (Reproduced from Guyton (1976) by kind permission of the author and publisher.)

tion of the lactating mammary gland and of the pregnant uterus, is formed in the paraventricular nucleus and is conveyed to the posterior pituitary. Although the anterior pituitary is not under direct nervous control, humoral substances (mainly polypeptides) secreted by hypothalamic neurones are carried to the anterior pituitary through vessels of the hypophysial venous system, thus exciting gonadotrophic, adrenocorticotrophic, somatotrophic, lactogenic, and thyrotrophic secretion. The posterior lobe (the neurohypophysis), unlike the anterior, receives a direct neural input concerned with autonomic activity from the paraventricular nucleus and another from the supraoptic nucleus which is primarily involved in the production of ADH or arginine vasopressin. In each of these ways the hypothalamic nuclei exercise control over the endocrine system. Generally the anterior nuclei are particularly concerned with parasympathetic activity and with control of the pituitary gland. Stimulation in this region may slow the heart rate and increase the antrioventricular conduction time, as well as increasing peristaltic movements in the stomach and bowel and causing contraction of the bladder. Lesions here can cause haemorrhagic erosions of the gastric mucosa. The posterior nuclei, by contrast, influence sympathetic activity. Stimulation here increases the heart rate and blood pressure, dilates the pupils, causes pilo-erection, and inhibits contraction of the gut and bladder. Lesions of this area can cause emotional disturbances such as 'sham rage' in animals or conversely lethargy and hypersomnia. Temperature regulation and control of the emotions and of sleep are also mediated through hypothalamic nuclei. In the anterior hypothalamus there is a centre regulating heat loss so that lesions in this area may cause hypothermia. Yet another centre regulates heat production and conservation, so that lesions here can cause poikilothermia in that the body temperature of the individual matches that of the environment. Glycosuria, often transitory, can also result from lesions of the anterior hypothalamus. Control over the sleep cycle is exerted by virtue of the input to the hypothalamus from the cerebral cortex and its output to the reticular system. In this regard the posterior hypothalamus (Fig. 20.1) is important and lesions here can cause hypersomnia or reversal of the sleep rhythm, while anterior lesions can cause insomnia (Jacobson 1972). The corpora mammillaria, also a part of the hypothalamic system, are important in memory regulation and lesions here may prevent the patient from recording and retaining new information, a feature seen typically in the Korsakow syndrome. The hypothalamus also plays a crucial role in the control of appetite.

The central regulatory neurotransmitters involved in appetite regulation are arranged in a cascade system similar to the . . . system for clotting and complement fixation . . . the similarities between the monoaminergic and peptidergic control of appetite and the central control of analgesia, temperature regulation and gastric acid secretion suggest that there may be a degree of overlap in the control of these closely-related life-sustaining processes (Morley and Levine 1983).

Pathways descend from the hypothalamus to control sympathetic and parasympathetic activity. Sympathetic fibres travel to the dorsal portion of the spinal cord to end in relation to cells in the intermediolateral horn of grey matter. The parasympathetic fibres end in the nuclei of the oculomotor, facial, glossopharyngeal, and vagus nerves, or in the sacral portion of the spinal cord (Table 20.1).

In both sympathetic and parasympathetic nerves two neurones intervene between the central nervous system and the innervated viscus, the efferent path being interrupted at a ganglion. The first neurone, running between the central nervous system and the ganglion, is called preganglionic. The second which runs from the ganglion to the viscus, is termed postganglionic (see Figs. 20.2 and 20.3).

Sympathetic fibres

Efferent paths

The sympathetic outflow from the central nervous system is limited to that part of the spinal cord lying between the first thoracic and the first lumbar segments inclusive, though rarely there are sympathetic nerves arising as high as C8 or as low as L3 (Johnson and Spalding 1974).

Preganglionic fibres. Preganglionic neurones originate in ganglion cells situated in the lateral horn of grey matter of the cord between these levels. Their axons leave the spinal cord by corresponding ventral roots and spinal nerves, from which they pass to the corresponding ganglia of the sympathetic chain. The preganglionic fibres are myelinated, and the root by which they pass from the ventral root to the sympathetic ganglion is known as a white ramus. At the sympathetic ganglion, some preganglionic fibres terminate in the ganglion corresponding to the segment at which they leave the cord. Others pass upwards or downwards in the sympathetic chain, terminating in ganglia above or below. Others again, passing through the ganglia of the sympathetic chain, emerge to terminate in more peripheral ganglia, the collateral sympathetic ganglia, or sympathetic plexuses, which are usually situated in close relationship to blood vessels supplying the principal viscera. The most important such nerves are the splanchnic nerves. The greater splanchnic nerve is derived from the ganglia of the sympathetic chain, from the fifth to the ninth or tenth thoracic segments, and runs to the coeliac plexus; the lesser splanchnic nerve, from the tenth and eleventh thoracic ganglia, goes to the aorticorenal plexus, and the lowest splanchnic nerve, from the eleventh thoracic ganglion, to the renal plexus.

The sympathetic chain. The sympathetic chain, lying close to the vertebral column on either side, consists of several sympathetic ganglia possessing a generally segmental arrangement, linked together by sympathetic fibres. There are three cervical ganglia— superior, middle, and inferior—11 thoracic, four lumbar, and four sacral ganglia, all paired, together with one unpaired coccygeal ganglion. Although all the preganglionic fibres emerge from the thoracic and first lumbar segments of the cord, through the sympathetic chain they are brought into relationship with spinal nerves at every spinal segment.

Postganglionic fibres. The postganglionic sympathetic fibres are unmyelinated. Some arise from ganglion cells in each ganglion of the sympathetic chain and pass to the corresponding spinal nerve by a grey ramus, to be distributed to the tissues innervated by this nerve. Other such fibres arise in collateral ganglia and pass to the various viscera (Fig. 20.2).

Afferent paths

Afferent fibres, both myelinated and unmyelinated, enter the nervous system by the dorsal roots at all levels, having their ganglion cells in the thoracic root ganglia. There has been much dispute about the function of these 'autonomic afferent' fibres (Johnson and Spalding 1974) which travel along the efferent fibres, and their very existence has been called into question, as much autonomic function is affected by activity in somatic afferent fibres. For practical clinical purposes, the autonomic system is best regarded as being wholly efferent.

Parasympathetic fibres

The parasympathetic is also known as the craniosacral autonomic nervous system because its outflow arises in the cranial and sacral regions. Unlike the sympathetic system, the ganglia of the parasympathetic are situated in the immediate neighbourhood of the innervated viscera (Fig. 20.3). Thus the preganglionic fibres are long, and the postganglionic short. The principal cranial preganglionic fibres pass through the third nerve to the ciliary ganglion, through the seventh to the geniculate, pterygopalatine, submaxillary, and otic ganglia, through the ninth to the otic ganglion, and through the vagus to the ganglia of the thoracic and abdominal viscera supplied by this nerve. The vagus is the most important parasympathetic nerve. Its dorsal motor nucleus is the site of origin of the fibres which innervate the viscera it supplies. The sacral autonomic outflow is derived from the second and third sacral segments, and passes to the vesical plexus by the pelvic splanchnic nerves. The sacral parasympathetic outflow also supplies the enteric plexus of the large gut from the splenic flexure to the anus. The principal afferent fibres of the parasympathetic reach the central nervous system through the vagus nerve, having their ganglion cells in the inferior ganglion of that nerve.

Physiology

The autonomic nervous system is largely concerned with controlling visceral activity. It affects the cardiac rhythm and output, respiration, blood-vessel tone, the behaviour of the hollow viscera of the alimentary and urogenital systems, as well as the secretion of the ducted and ductless (endocrine) glands. Many of these activities are in a sense automatic and reflexly controlled, and little influenced by the will. This is fortunate for many of them are too vital to allow of any interference from the capricious behaviour of the mind. The combined activities of the autonomic nerves and of the endocrine glands maintain the constant internal thermal and biochemical environment of the body, a function which Cannon entitled homeostasis.

Activity of the sympathetic system gives dilatation of the pupil and slight protrusion of the eye, increased cardiac output with tachycardia, bronchiolar dilatation, cutaneous vasoconstriction, but dilatation of the coronary and intramuscular arteries, sweating, inhibition of intestinal movement, closure of vesical and rectal sphincters, and erection of hairs (the pilomotor effect) on the skin. It may also raise the blood sugar by liberating glucose from the liver. The animal is prepared for emergency action, termed the 'fight or flight' response. Most terminal sympathetic fibres are adrenergic, i.e.: (a) they produce their effects upon smooth muscle or other tissues by secreting noradrenaline at their nerve endings; and (b) their effects can be largely reproduced by an increase in the amount of circulating adrenaline or noradrenaline in the

Table 20.1. *Summary of the innervation and function of major autonomic effectors**

	Preganglionic neurone	Postganglionic neurone	Function
Head-structures			
Eye: pupillary and ciliary muscles			
Sympathetic	Cord segments T1 to T2	Superior cervical ganglion	Pupillary dilatation (mydriasis); accommodation for far vision
Parasympathetic	Edinger–Westphal nucleus (oculomotor nerve—III)	Ciliary ganglion	Pupillary constriction (miosis); accommodation for near vision
Lacrimal gland			
Sympathetic	Cord segments T1 to T2	Superior cervical ganglion	Vasoconstriction
Parasympathetic	Lacrimal part of superior salivatory nucleus (facial nerve—VII)	Sphenopalatine ganglion	Tear secretion and vasodilatation
Parotid, submandibular, and sublingual salivary glands			
Sympathetic	Upper thoracic cord segments	Superior cervical ganglion	Salivary secretion (mucous, low enzyme, vasoconstriction)
Parasympathetic			
Parotid gland	Inferior salivatory nucleus (glossopharyngeal nerve—IX)	Otic ganglion	Salivary secretion (water, high enzyme, vasodilatation)
Submandibular and sublingual glands	Superior salivatory nucleus (facial nerve—VII)	Submandibular ganglion	Same as above
Thoracic viscera			
Heart			
Sympathetic	Cord segments T1 to T4	Upper thoracic to superior cervical chain ganglia	Acceleration of heart rate and force of contraction; coronary vasodilation
Parasympathetic	Dorsal motor nucleus (vagus nerve—X)	Cardiac plexus	Deceleration of heart rate and force of contraction; coronary vasoconstriction
Oesophagus			
Sympathetic	Thoracic cord segments	Thoracic and cervical chain ganglia	Vasoconstriction
Parasympathetic	Dorsal motor nucleus (vagus nerve—X)	Intramural plexuses	Peristalsis and secretion
Lungs			
Sympathetic	Cord segments T2 to T6	Thoracic chain ganglia	Bronchial dilatation
Parasympathetic	Dorsal motor nucleus (vagus nerve—X)	Pulmonary plexus	Bronchial constriction
Abdominal viscera			
Stomach and intestine			
Sympathetic	Cord segments T5 to T12 (thoracic splanchnic nerves)	Coeliac and superior mesenteric ganglia	Inhibition of peristalsis and secretion; sphincter contraction
Parasympathetic	Dorsal motor nucleus (vagus nerve—X)	Intramural plexuses	Peristalsis and secretion
Adrenal medulla			
Sympathetic	Cord segments T8 to T11 (thoracic splanchnic nerves)	The adrenomedullary cells are derived from neural crests but have no dendrites or axons. They are endocrine cells	Secretion of epinephrine and norepinephrine directly into the blood
Parasympathetic (none)			
Descending colon			
Sympathetic	Cord segments T12 to L2 (lumbar splanchnic nerves)	Inferior mesenteric ganglion	Inhibition of peristalsis and secretion; vasoconstriction
Parasympathetic	Cord segments S2 to S4 (pelvic splanchnic nerves)	Intramural plexuses	Peristalsis and secretion
Pelvic viscera			
Sigmoid colon, rectum and anus, bladder, gonads and associated ducts and organs, and erectile tissue			
Sympathetic	Cord segments T12 to L2 (lumbar splanchnic nerves)	Inferior mesenteric ganglion (hypogastric nerves)	Inhibition of peristalsis and secretion; anal and bladder sphincter contraction; vasoconstriction; ejaculation
Parasympathetic	Cord segments S2 to S4 (pelvic splanchic nerves)	Intramural or specific organ plexuses	Peristalsis and secretion; bladder detrusor muscle contraction; penile and clitoral erection

* Reproduced from Patton, Sundsten, Crill, and Swanson (1976) by kind permission of the authors and publisher.

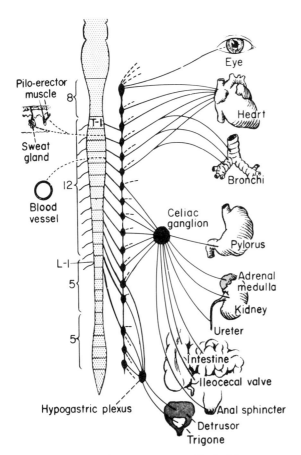

Fig. 20.2. The sympathetic nervous system. Dashed lines represent post-ganglionic fibres in the grey rami leading into the spinal nerves for distribution to blood vessels, sweat glands, and pilo-erector muscles. (Reproduced from Guyton (1976) by kind permission of the author and publisher.)

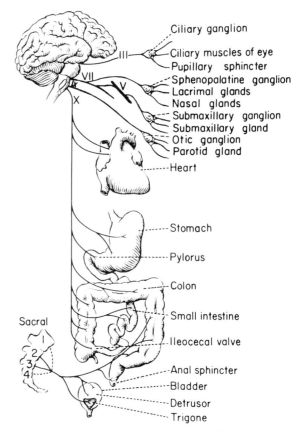

Fig. 20.3. The parasympathetic nervous system. (Reproduced from Guyton (1976) by kind permission of the author and publisher.)

catecholamines released into the CSF may also be important (see p. 71).

Chemical transmission in the autonomic system

Acetylcholine or noradrenaline are normally released locally at autonomic nerve endings. All preganglionic fibres, both sympathetic and parasympathetic, are cholinergic. In addition, as mentioned above, sympathetic activity is influenced by circulating noradrenaline and adrenaline, much of which is secreted by the adrenal medulla. These biogenic amines, and acetylcholine, produce their effects upon the organs whose activities they influence by combining with receptor sites lying in close relationship to the nerve endings. Much recent progress in understanding of autonomic behaviour has resulted from studies of the distribution, function and specificity of these receptors.

Acetylcholine receptors are of two types, identified by their selective responses to two agents: (a) so-called muscarinic receptors which are found in all effector cells stimulated by parasympathetic postganglionic neurones (and in cholinergic endings of the sympathetic system); and (b) nicotinic receptors found especially in the neuromuscular junctions of skeletal muscle but also at synapses in the sympathetic and parasympathetic ganglia themselves. Similarly, adrenergic receptors are of two types: (a) alpha receptors, stimulated mainly by noradrenaline and concerned especially with vasoconstriction, dilatation of the iris, intestinal relaxation, and pilomotor contraction in the skin; and (b) beta receptors, stimulated more particularly by adrenaline and to a lesser extent by noradrenaline, which are responsible for an increased heart rate, vasodilatation of intramuscular blood vessels, intestinal relaxation, uterine relaxation, and bronchodilatation.

The rational use of many therapeutic agents depends upon an understanding of autonomic receptor specificity and function. For

blood. There are exceptions to this rule. Some few sympathetic fibres, particularly those innervating the sweat glands (sudomotor fibres) are cholinergic, i.e. they produce their effects by secreting acetylcholine at the effector organ. In skeletal muscle, there are adrenergic fibres which cause constriction of intramuscular blood vessels and cholinergic fibres which cause dilatation.

Activity of the parasympathetic nervous system is more directly concerned with anabolic, excretory, and reproductive activities; it gives constriction of the pupil, slowing of the heart and a diminished cardiac output, bronchiolar construction, increased intestinal peristalsis, evacuation of the bladder and bowels, and increased secretory activity of the salivary and lacrimal glands. It can also lower the blood sugar by stimulating the production of insulin. Implanted electrodes have been used with appropriate methods of electrical stimulation to empty the bladder and close the urethra in patients with reflex bladder function after spinal injury (Brindley 1977). The parasympathetic system, through the pelvic splanchnic nerves, also controls sexual activity, including erection of the penis and ejaculation in the male and orgasm in the female. Parasympathetic fibres are mainly cholinergic, secreting acetylcholine at their terminals.

Despite the long-held view that intracranial blood vessels are uninfluenced by autonomic activity, there is now evidence that autonomic nerves may have a homeostatic function, particularly in autoregulation, by modulating the myogenic tone of the intracranial vessels in response to altered perfusion pressures and distal circulatory demands (Sundt 1973). Thus a possible role of autonomic dysfunction in causing the arterial spasm which may complicate subarachnoid haemorrhage has been postulated although free example, various parasympathomimetic drugs, such as pilocarpine and methacholine, have a muscarinic effect, while others, such as neostigmine, are essentially nicotinic. Atropine blocks the muscarinic but not the nicotinic effects of such drugs. Similarly, the activities of sympathomimetic drugs, including adrenaline, phenylephrine, and methoxamine, depend upon their relative affinities for alpha and beta receptors. Guanethidine may block the release of noradrenaline from sympathetic nerve terminals. Phenoxybenzamine or phentolamine block the alpha receptors and propranolol blocks beta receptors of the sympathetic nervous system selectively.

Sympathetic denervation of the skin

The sympathetic nerve supply to the skin may be interrupted by lesions or surgical division of the outflow from the spinal cord in the white rami or ganglia, or of the peripheral nerves. In either case the area of denervated skin shows loss of: (1) pilomotor; (2) vasomotor; and (3) sudomotor activity. (1) The pilomotor reflex consists of gooseflesh following the application of cold or the scratch of a pin. (2) Vasomotor paralysis causes flushing, so that the temperature of the denervated area becomes higher than that of the corresponding area on the normal side. This difference may be palpable or may require special techniques of thermometry for its detection. (3) Loss of sweating may also be palpable, but is best investigated by applying to the skin a colour-indicator such as chinizarin 2-6-disulphonic acid. The patient is given 300–600 mg of aspirin and is then warmed. Where sweating occurs the skin becomes violet, the dry areas remaining light. (For details of this test see Guttmann 1940). Alternatively the skin may be painted with a solution of chemically pure iodine in absolute alcohol after which fine rice starch powder is dusted on and the test is continued as above.

Hyperhidrosis

Excessive sweating, e.g. from the palms, may be a congenital abnormality. Localized hyperhidrosis may occur on the face during eating, especially spicy foods—gustatory reflex sweating. Boswell said of Johnson: 'While in the act of eating the veins of his forehead swelled and generally a strong perspiration was visible'. Such gustatory sweating, which may affect only one half of the face, can occur as a congenital abnormality or may sometimes develop for no apparent reason during adult life; it can often be relieved by the use of propantheline. The 'syndrome of crocodile tears', in which lacrimation occurs during eating, may follow facial paralysis and is presumed to be due to aberrant nerve-fibre regeneration, parasympathetic fibres intended for the salivary glands being misdirected to the lacrimal gland. Flushing and hyperhidrosis in the temple may follow injury in the region of the parotid gland—the auriculotemporal syndrome. Hyperhidrosis is also seen in the distribution of a cutaneous nerve which is the site of a partial lesion, as in causalgia. Cerebral lesions causing hemiplegia may lead to excessive sweating on the paralysed half of the body. When necessary, hyperhidrosis can be treated by sympathectomy.

Clinical tests of autonomic function

Tests in common clinical use in order to assess the integrity of the autonomic nervous system are reviewed by Johnson and Spalding (1974) and Bannister (1983). Among those in common use are the following.

Sympathetic nervous system

The sweating response to an induced rise in body temperature is described above; this does not test the afferent side of the reflex arc concerned with sympathetic sudomotor activity and is not a reliable test for integrity of the sympathetic nervous system as a whole as sudomotor activity may be intact when vasomotor activity is impaired and vice versa.

Much more important therefore in determining whether there is widespread reflex vasomotor paralysis are tests involving the accurate measurement of arterial blood pressure and its response to various stresses, including change in posture (in the normal individual the blood pressure usually rises slightly on assuming the erect posture, while in patients with sympathetic denervation there is a marked fall). Valsalva's manoeuvre (a deep inspiration followed by an attempted forcible expiration against a closed glottis) produces a four-phase response in normal individuals; this is blocked and often replaced simply by a temporary fall in blood pressure in patients with autonomic failure (as in orthostatic hypotension—see below).

In attempting to determine whether the afferent or efferent pathways of the sympathetic reflex arc are involved, recording of blood pressure after a sudden loud noise, during intense mental concentration, or after the application of an ice-pack to the skin may sometimes be helpful, as a rise in response to any of these stimuli indicates that the efferent pathway is functioning and that any lesion is likely to be on the afferent side. These tests, however, are not very reliable, as a negative response to each stimulus is sometimes obtained in normal individuals.

The 'flare' response, which is particularly useful in determining the site of the lesion in injury to spinal roots or peripheral nerves, was mentioned on page 493. This test, like the cold vasodilatation response (rapid cooling follows the immersion of normal fingers in water at 5 °C but this is followed by vasodilatation after 5–10 min) depends not on an autonomic reflex but on a sensory-axon reflex. Hence in disease of efferent sympathetic pathways, whether preganglionic or postganglionic, reflex flushing of the skin and sweating are abolished but a flare will develop. Conversely, disease of sensory afferent fibres from an area of skin will abolish the flare and cold vasodilatation responses, leaving sweating intact. Quantitative sudomotor axon reflex tests using acetylcholine electrophoresis have been shown to detect postganglionic sudomotor abnormalities sensitively and reproducibly in patients with autonomic neuropathy (Low, Caskey, Tuck, Fealey, and Dyck 1983)

The absence of finger 'wrinkling' after immersion of the hand in water at 40 °C for 30 min has been thought to be a useful indicator of sympathetic denervation (Bull and Henry 1977). It may also be useful to measure reflex latencies and conduction velocities in sympathetic nerve fibres; these can certainly be measured in normal humans (Fagius and Wallin 1980). Investigation of thermoregulatory mechanisms and especially of bodily adaptation to extremes of heat or cold requires sophisticated equipment and can rarely be utilized in clinical practice.

The parasympathetic nervous system

As the arterial blood pressure rises, the heart rate usually falls due to a parasympathetic baroreceptor reflex and its integrity can be well tested by carrying out Valsalva's manoeuvre (see above) during which the heart rate and blood pressure show an inverse relationship. The integrity of vagal function upon the heart may also be tested by pressure upon the carotid sinus or eyeball which normally produces reflex bradycardia (though these tests must be used with caution as cardiac arrest rarely occurs) or by the use of drugs such as atropine which inhibit vagal activity.

References

Bannister, R. (1983). *Autonomic failure: a textbook of clinical disorders of the autonomic nervous system*. Oxford University Press, Oxford.

Blackwell, R. E. and Guillemin, R. (1973). Hypothalamic control of adenohypophyseal secretions. *Ann. Rev. Physiol.* **35**, 357.

Brindley, G. S. (1977). An implant to empty the bladder or close the urethra. *J. Neurol. Neurosurg. Psychiat.* **40**, 358.

Bull, C. and Henry, J. A. (1977). Finger wrinkling as a test of autonomic function. *Br. med. J.* **1**, 551.

Daniel, P. M. and Prichard, M. M. L. (1975). *Studies of the hypothalamus and the pituitary gland*. Alden Press, Oxford.

Fagius, J. and Wallin, B. G. (1980). Sympathetic reflex latencies and conduction velocities in normal man. *J. neurol. Sci.* **47**, 433.

Guttmann, L. (1940). Topographic studies of disturbances of sweat secretion after complete lesions of peripheral nerves. *J. Neurol. Psychiat.* **3**, 197.

Guyton, A. C. (1976). *Textbook of medical physiology*, 5th edn. Saunders, Philadelphia.

Hall, R. (1983). Pituitary and hypothalamic disorders. In *Oxford textbook of medicine* (ed. D. J. Weatherall, J. G. G. Ledingham, and D. A. Warrell) Section 10. Oxford University Press, Oxford.

Hayward, J. N. (1975). Neural control of the posterior pituitary. *Ann. Rev. Physiol.* **37**, 191.

Jacobson, S. (1972). Hypothalamus and autonomic nervous system in *An introduction to the neurosciences*. (ed. B. A. Curtis, S. Jacobson, and E. M. Marcus) p. 386. Saunders, Philadelphia.

Johnson, R. H. and Spalding, J. M. K. (1974). *Disorders of the autonomic nervous system*. Blackwell, Oxford.

Liddle, G. W. and Liddle, R. A. (1981). Endocrinology, Section VII. In *Pathophysiology*, Vol. 1 of *International textbook of medicine* (ed. L. H. Smith, Jr. and S. O. Thier). Saunders, Philadelphia.

Low, P. A., Caskey, P. E., Tuck, R. R., Fealey, R. D., and Dyck, P. J. (1983). Quantitative sudomotor axon reflex test in normal and neuropathic subjects. *Ann. Neurol.*, **14**, 573.

Morley, J. E. and Levine, A. S. (1983). The central control of appetite. *Lancet*, **i**, 398.

Patton, H. D., Sundsten, J. W., Crill, W. E., and Swanson, P. D. (1976). *Introduction to basic neurology*. Saunders, Philadelphia.

Sundt, T. M. (1973). The cerebral autonomic nervous system: a proposed physiologic function and pathophysiologic response in subarachnoid hemorrhage and in focal cerebral ischemia. *Mayo Clin. Proc.* **48**, 127.

Walton, J. N. (1983). *Introduction to clinical neuroscience*. Baillière Tindall, London.

Disorders of autonomic function

Among the disorders of autonomic function which occur in clinical practice are drug-induced syndromes occurring, for instance, during the treatment of parkinsonism, (page 329), abnormalities of the pupils such as Adie's syndrome (page 104); Horner's syndrome (see p. 103 and Van der Wiel and Van Gijn 1982, 1983) and Raeder's paratrigeminal syndrome (see p. 103 and Mokri 1982); an isolated disturbance of one tympanic nerve after skull fracture giving immediate reduction in the salivary output from the denervated parotid gland followed soon by a massive increase in spontaneous salivation, paradoxically increased, rather than decreased, by atropine (Levin 1983); conditions such as Hirschsprung's disease due to lesions of the myenteric plexus; autonomic manifestations of polyneuropathy including the autonomic neuropathy of diabetes (see p. 538 and Bennett, Hosking, and Hampton 1976) and that of Fabry's disease (see p. 462 and Cable, Kolodny, and Adams 1982); and several specific disorders or phenomena deserving brief attention here, including autonomic dysfunction in lesions of the spinal cord, the role of the autonomic nervous sytem in the mechanisms of referred pain, familial dysautonomia, idiopathic orthostatic hypotension, and acute autonomic neuropathy (also see Bannister 1983).

Disturbances of the functions of the autonomic nervous system after lesions of the spinal cord

Differences in the distribution of the sympathetic and somatic nervous outflow from the spinal cord account for differences in many cases in the distribution of the sympathetic and somatic (motor and sensory) disturbances after spinal-cord lesions. Since the sympathetic outflow to the whole body leaves the cord below the eighth cervical spinal segment, lesions at and above this level may affect sympathetic function over the whole body, though the motor and sensory innervation of the head and neck and of a part of the upper limbs remains undisturbed. At the mid-thoracic level of the cord the upper levels of the sympathetic and somatic disturbances approximately coincide. When the lesion of the cord is situated below the first lumbar spinal segment the somatic innervation is alone affected. The following disturbances of sympathetic function are found in cases of complete transection of the cord and in less severe lesions which interrupt the intraspinal descending sympathetic. The pilomotor reflex elicited by a massive stimulus applied to the skin above the level of the lesion does not extend to areas innervated by parts of the cord below the lesion, but the direct reflex is elicitable by local stimulation in these regions after the spinal shock disappears. The skin temperature over the paralysed parts is higher than in unaffected parts and vasoconstriction in response to exposure of the whole body to cold is diminished below the level of the lesion. Dermographism is diminished at the level of the lesion but usually somewhat increased below. Orthostatic hypotension may occur in cervical-cord lesions but adaptation to repeated changes in posture frequently occurs (Johnson, Smith, and Spalding 1969) (see also the section on compression of the spinal cord, p. 400).

Sweating

Excessive sweating after complete spinal-cord division usually appears over parts of the body which are thus separated from the control of higher autonomic centres. Such sweating develops pari passu with the recovery of other reflex functions in the segments of the cord isolated from cerebral control. It varies in intensity and may be reflexly excited by cutaneous stimuli, flexor spasms, bladder distension and exposure to heat.

Disturbances of sweating are rarely seen after partial cord lesions, except in syringomyelia. In this disease loss of sweating may occur when the sympathetic ganglion cells in the lateral horns of grey matter are destroyed, usually over the face and upper limbs. Excessive sweating of similar distribution may, however, occur, sometimes spontaneously and sometimes being excited reflexly when the patient takes hot or highly seasoned food.

The autonomic nervous system and pain

Referred pain

Since most viscera are innervated only by autonomic nerves it follows that the sensation of visceral pain must be mediated by afferent autonomic fibres, or at least by afferent fibres which travel with them. The remarkable lack of definitive information about the afferent functions of the autonomic nervous system and about the role played by the sympathetic in pain syndromes was underlined by Melzack (1972) who concluded that 'the sympathetic nervous system contributes, in some way, to all of these pain states'. The most potent cause of visceral pain is increased tension in the viscus. Visceral pain is a diffuse and poorly localized sensation, often associated with pain referred to, and tenderness of, the superficial tissues of the body over an area innervated by the same segments of the nervous system as the painful viscus. The physiological explanation of referred pain is uncertain. It has been attributed to heightened excitability or facilitation of synapses concerned in pain conduction in the spinal cord, where impulses from the segments innervating the viscus are received and also to axonal branching with the same fibre supplying both somatic and visceral structures (Sinclair, Weddell, and Feindel 1948). The 'gate theory' (see p. 46) provides an even more plausible explanation but remains unproven. Referred pain may or may not be accompanied by cutaneous hyperpathia. A common example of referred pain is that associated with coronary-artery disease as in angina pectoris.Pain is usually referred into the third, fourth, and fifth cervical and first, second, and third thoracic segments on the left side and often into the same or a somewhat similar area on the right side. Sometimes it is referred to the lower jaw.

The autonomic nervous system sometimes provides an alternative path for painful sensations from areas deprived of their somatic sensory nerves. When pain is evoked in such circumstances the painful impulse may be conducted to the central nervous system by somatic afferents which accompany the autonomic nerves supplying the blood vessels. Certainly the pain sensation which occurs as a consequence of the vasodilatation of intracranial or extracranial arteries (as in migraine) is conveyed by somatic afferent fibres from the walls of the blood vessels. Sympathectomy is also performed for causalgia; the pathogenesis of this disorder is considered on page 498. Similarly, sympathectomy relieves pain in the disorder variously referred to as algodystrophy, 'the shoulder-hand syndrome' or 'reflex dystrophy of the upper extremity'(Pak, Martin, Magness, and Kavanaugh 1970) in which painful swelling of the hand, often with atrophy of bone (Sudeck's atrophy) occurs, usually in association with pericapsulitis of the shoulder joint (a 'frozen shoulder') (also see p. 498).

References

Bannister, R. (1983). *Autonomic failure: a textbook of clinical disorders of the autonomic nervous system.* Oxford University Press, Oxford.

Bennett, T., Hosking, D. J., and Hampton, J. R. (1976). Baroreflex sensitivity and responses to the Valsalva manoeuvre in subjects with diabetes mellitus. *J. Neurol. Neurosurg. Psychiat.* **39**, 178.

Cable, W. J. L., Kolodny, E. H., and Adams, R. D. (1982). Fabry disease: impaired autonomic function. *Neurology, Minneapolis* **32**, 498.

Johnson, R. H., Smith, A. C., and Spalding, J. M. K. (1969). Blood pressure response to standing and to Valsalva's manoeuvre: independence of the two mechanisms in neurological diseases including cervical cord lesions. *Clin. Sci.* **36**, 77.

—— and Spalding, J. M. K. (1974). *Disorders of the autonomic nervous system.* Blackwell, Oxford.

Levin, S. L. (1983). The syndrome of isolated disturbance of the tympanic nerve. *Arch. Neurol., Chicago* **4**, 106.

Melzack, R. (1972). Mechanisms of pathological pain. In *Scientific foundations of neurology* (ed. M. Critchley, J. L. O'Leary, and W. B. Jennett) p. 153. Heinemann, London.

—— (1973). *The puzzle of pain.* Penguin Books, Harmondsworth, Middlesex.

Mokri, B. (1982). Raeder's paratrigeminal syndrome: original concept and subsequent deviations. *Arch. Neurol., Chicago* **39**, 395.

Pak, T. J., Martin, G. M., Magness, J. L., and Kavanaugh, G. L. (1970). Reflex sympathetic dystrophy. Review of 140 cases. *Minn. Med.* **53**, 507.

Sinclair, D. C., Weddell, G., and Feindel, W. H. (1948). Referred pain and associated phenomena. *Brain* **71**, 184.

Van Der Wiel, H. L. and Van Gijn, J. (1982). Horner's syndrome: criteria for oculosympathetic denervation. *J. neurol. Sci.* **56**, 293.

—— and —— (1983). Localization of Horner's syndrome: use and limitations of the hydroxy-amphetamine test. *J. neurol. Sci.* **59**, 229.

Familial dysautonomia and acquired dysautonomia

Familial dysautonomia (the Riley–Day syndrome) is a rare disorder occurring mainly in Jewish children and inherited as an autosomal recessive trait. Clinically it is characterized by defective lacrimation, hyperhidrosis, episodic hypertension, hyperpyrexia and vomiting, and attacks of epilepsy. Most patients also show dysphagia, ageusia, areflexia and relative insensitivity to pain sensation and die as a rule from respiratory infection or uraemia in infancy or childhood. The condition appears to be due to an inborn error of catecholamine metabolism which results in the excretion of homovanillic acid in the urine (Smith, Taylor, and Wortis 1963). The presence of parasympathetic denervation is

confirmed by the instillation of 2.5 per cent methacholine into the eye; this produces miosis (Dancis and Smith 1966). An abnormality of sensory-nerve conduction, with two discrete peaks of differing latency, has been described in such cases (Brown and Johns 1967); on sural-nerve biopsy there is a marked reduction in the number of unmyelinated fibres and of heavily myelinated fibres (Aguayo, Nair, and Bray 1971) and at autopsy there may be focal demyelination in the posterior roots and posterior columns of the spinal cord (Fogelson, Rorke, and Kaye 1967).In affected adults the mean volume of superior cervical sympathetic ganglia is reduced to 34 per cent of normal and the packing density of neurons to 37 per cent of normal (Pearson and Pytel 1978*a*); a similar reduction in neuronal numbers is seen in the sphenopalatine but not in the ciliary ganglia (Pearson and Pytel 1978*b*).

Acquired non-progressive dysautonomia can cause similar symptoms but is a disorder of multiple aetiology, being seen in various generalized neuropathies (as in diabetes mellitus, amyloidosis, or botulism) but sometimes in patients with neoplasms or parkinsonism. In a six-year-old child this syndrome was caused by a ganglioneuroma originating in the sympathetic ganglia and the presenting features were those of sleep apnoea and chronic hypoventilation, manifestations which are only rarely encountered in familial dysautonomia (Frank, Kravath, Inoue, Hirano, Pollak, Rosenberg, and Weitzman 1981).

Other rare syndromes of autonomic failure are being regularly discovered (Bannister 1983); in one such, a *generalized smooth-muscle disease with defective muscarinic-receptor function* (Bannister and Hoyes 1981), the patient had chronic intestinal pseudo-obstruction and in addition defective control of the bladder, pupils, sweating, and cardiovascular function.

References

Aguayo, A. J., Nair, C. P. V., and Bray, G. M. (1971). Peripheral nerve abnormalities in the Riley–Day syndrome. *Arch. Neurol., Chicago* **24**, 106.

Bannister, R. (1983). *Autonomic failure: a textbook of clinical disorders of the autonomic nervous system.* Oxford University Press, Oxford.

—— and Hoyes, A. D. (1981). Generalised smooth-muscle disease with defective muscarinic-receptor function. *Br. med. J.* **282**, 1015.

Brown, J. C. and Johns, R. J. (1967). Nerve conduction in familial dysautonomia (Riley–Day syndrome). *J. Am. med. Ass.* **201**, 200.

Dancis, J. and Smith, A. A. (1966). Familial dysautonomia. *New Engl. J. Med.* **274**, 207.

Fogelson, M. H., Rorke, L. B., and Kaye, R. (1967). Spinal cord changes in familial dysautonomia. *Arch. Neurol., Chicago* **17**, 103.

Frank, Y., Kravath, R. E., Inoue, K., Hirano, A., Pollak, C. P., Rosenberg, R. N., and Weitzman, E. D. (1981). Sleep apnea and hypoventilation syndrome associated with acquired nonprogressive dysautonomia: clinical and pathological studies in a child. *Ann. Neurol.* **10**, 18.

Pearson, J. and Pytel, B. A. (1978*a*). Quantitative studies of sympathetic ganglia and spinal cord intermedio-lateral gray columns in familial dysautonomia. *J. neurol. Sci.* **39**, 47.

—— and —— (1978*b*). Quantitative studies of ciliary and sphenopalatine ganglia in familial dysautonomia. *J. neurol. Sci.* **39**, 123.

Riley, C. M., Day, R. L., Greely, D. M., and Langford, N. S. (1949). Central autonomic dysfunction with defective lacrimation. Report of five cases. *Pediatrics* **3**, 468.

Smith, A. A., Taylor, T., and Wortis, S. B. (1968). Abnormal catecholamine metabolism in familial dysautonomia. *New Engl. J. Med.* **268**, 705.

Idiopathic orthostatic hypotension

This condition was mentioned on page 188. Its most striking clinical manifestations are postural hypotension with syncope on standing and loss of the normal autonomic reflexes (Chokroverty, Barron, Katz, Del Greco, and Sharp 1969; Thomas and Schirger 1970). Anhidrosis, impotence, dysuria, and disorders of bowel function are common (Martin, Travis, and Van den Noirt 1968), there may be undue sensitivity to nicotine (Graham and Oppenheimer 1969), an increased plasma renin accounting for supine hypertension (Love, Brown, Chinn, Johnson, Lever, Park, and Robertson 1971; Mathias, Mathews, and Spalding 1977), and evidence of cerebral dysautoregulation (Meyer, Shimazu, Fukuuchi, Ohuchi, Okamoto, Koto, and Ericsson 1973). It is now customary to distinguish 'pure' progressive autonomic failure in which these manifestations occur without associated evidence of central nervous-system dysfunction (Bannister, Sever, and Gross 1977; Bannister 1979; Bannister, Crowe, Eames, and Burnstock 1981 a) from cases in which these features are associated with typical parkinsonism and others in which there is associated multiple system atrophy (the Shy–Drager syndrome) with cerebellar ataxia, parkinsonian features, and sometimes dementia. In cases of the latter type, vocal-cord paralysis resulting in laryngeal stridor and sleep apnoea is not uncommon (Williams, Hanson, and Calne 1979; Bannister, Gibson, Michaels, and Oppenheimer 1981b) and speech disturbances reflecting impaired laryngeal control are common (Bassich, Ludlow, and Polinsky 1984). In the more 'pure' cases of autonomic failure, periodic respiration in the upright posture is an occasional feature (Chokroverty, Sharp, and Barron 1978). An association with HLA Aw32 has been observed (Bannister, Mowbray, and Sidgwick 1983). The Holmes–Adie syndrome is an occasional accompaniment (Johnson, McLellan, and Love 1971). Pathologically there is degeneration of dorsal vagal nuclei and of the cells of the intermediolateral column in the spinal cord, while Lewy bodies indentical with those seen in idiopathic parkinsonism are sometimes found in the substantia nigra (Vanderhaeghen, Perier, and Sterman 1979; Thapedi, Ashenhurst, and Rozdilsky 1971; Bannister and Oppenheimer 1972) in cases with parkinsonian features and the pathological changes of striatonigral degeneration have also been reported (Schober, Langston, and Forno 1975). Biochemical studies of sympathetic ganglia have shown a fourfold reduction in dopamine β-hydroxylase (Petito and Black 1978), while ultrastructural and catecholamine fluorescence studies have shown reduced numbers of small granular (noradrenergic) vesicles in sympathetic nerves (Bannister et al., 1981a). The numbers of alpha-adrenergic receptors in platelets are increased both in idiopathic orthostatic hypotension and in multiple system atrophy (Kafka, Polinsky, Williams, Kopin, Lake, Elert, and Tokola 1984).

In the treatment of this condition, monoamine oxidase inhibitors increase blood pressure but do not relieve symptoms and are unpredictable (Davies, Bannister, and Sever 1978); levodopa may control the parkinsonism but not the autonomic failure (de Lean and Deck 1976); denervation supersensitivity may prejudice the use of sympathomimetic agents (Polinsky, Kopin, Ebert, and Weise 1981); plasma volume expansion produced by fludrocortisone with or without indomethacin may be helpful, as may be the use of G-suits and other antigravity agents (see The Lancet 1981). Pindolol, a β-adrenoreceptor agonist, given in a dose of 15 mg daily, was found to be helpful by Man in't Veld and Schalekamp (1981) but was ineffective when used by others (The Lancet 1981). An experimental sympathetic neural prosthesis (Polinsky, Samaras, and Kopin 1983) seems a more hopeful prospect.

References

Bannister, R. (1979). Chronic autonomic failure with postural hypotension. Lancet ii, 404.

—— Crowe, R., Eames, R. and Burnstock, G. (1981 a). Adrenergic innervation in autonomic failure. Neurology, Minneapolis 31, 1501.

—— Gibson, W., Michaels, L., and Oppenheimer, D. R. (1981b). Laryngeal abductor paralysis in multiple system atrophy. A report on three necropsied cases, with observations on the laryngeal muscles and the nuclei ambigui. Brain 104, 351.

—— Mowbray, J. and Sidgwick, A. (1983). Genetic control of progressive autonomic failure: evidence for an association with an HLA antigen. Lancet i, 1017.

—— and Oppenheimer, D. R. (1972). Degenerative diseases of the nervous system associated with autonomic failure. Brain 95, 457.

—— Sever, P. and Gross, M. (1977). Cardiovascular reflexes and biochemical responses in progressive autonomic failure. Brain 100, 327.

Bassich, C. J., Ludlow, C. L., and Polinsky, R. J. (1984). Speech symptoms associated with early signs of Shy–Drager syndrome. J. Neurol. Neurosurg. Psychiat. 47, 995.

Chokroverty, S., Barron, K. D., Katz, F. H., Del Greco, F., and Sharp, J. T. (1969). The syndrome of primary orthostatic hypotension. Brain 92, 743.

—— Sharp, J. T. and Barron, K. D. (1978). Periodic respiration in erect posture in Shy–Drager syndrome. J. Neurol. Neurosurg. Psychiat. 41, 980.

Davies, B., Bannister, R., and Sever, P. (1978). Pressor amines and monoamine-oxidase inhibitors for treatment of postural hypotension in autonomic failure: limitations and hazards. Lancet i, 172.

De Lean, J. and Deck, J. H. N. (1976). Shy–Drager syndrome. Neuropathological correlation and response to levodopa therapy. Can. J. neurol. Sci. 3, 167.

Graham, J. G. and Oppenheimer, D. R. (1969). Orthostatic hypotension and nicotine sensitivity in case of multiple system atrophy. J. Neurol. Neurosurg. Psychiat. 32, 28.

Johnson, R. H., McLellan, D. L., and Love, D. R. (1971). Orthostatic hypotension and the Holmes–Adie syndrome. J. Neurol. Neurosurg. Psychiat. 34, 562.

Kafka, M. S., Polinsky, R. J., Williams, A., Kopin, I. J., Lake, C. R., Ebert, M. H., and Tokola, N. S. (1984). Alpha-adrenergic receptors in orthostatic hypotension syndromes. Neurology, Minneapolis 34, 1121.

The Lancet (1981). Management of orthostatic hypotension. Lancet ii, 963.

Love, D. R., Brown, J. J., Chinn, R. H., Johnson, R. H., Lever, A. F., Park, D. M., and Robertson, J. I. S. (1971). Plasma renin in idiopathic orthostatic hypotension: differential response in subjects with probable afferent and efferent autonomic failure. Clin. Sci. 41, 289.

Man in't Veld, A. J. and Schalekamp, M. A. D. H. (1981). Pindolol acts as beta-adrenoceptor agonist in orthostatic hypotension: therapeutic implications. Br. med. J. 282, 929.

Martin, J. B., Travis, R. H., and Van den Noort, S. (1968). Centrally mediated orthostatic hypotension. Arch. Neurol., Chicago 19, 163.

Mathias, C. J., Matthews, W. B., and Spalding, J. M. K. (1977). Postural changes in plasma renin activity and responses to vasoactive drugs in a case of Shy–Drager syndrome. J. Neurol. Neurosurg. Psychiat. 40, 138.

Meyer, J. S., Shimazu, K., Fukuuchi, Y., Ohuchi, T., Okamoto, S., Koto, A., and Ericsson, A. D. (1973). Cerebral dysautoregulation in central neurogenic orthostatic hypotension (Shy–Drager syndrome). Neurology, Minneapolis, 23, 262.

Petito, C. K. and Black, I. B. (1978). Ultrastructure and biochemistry of sympathetic ganglia in idiopathic orthostatic hypotension. Ann. Neurol. 4, 6.

Polinsky, R. J., Kopin, I. J., Ebert, M. H., and Weise, V. (1981). Pharmacologic distinction of different orthostatic hypotension syndromes. Neurology, Minneapolis 31, 1.

—— Samaras, G. M. and Kopin, I. J. (1983). Sympathetic neural prosthesis for managing orthostatic hypotension. Lancet i, 901.

Schober, R., Langston, J. W., and Forno, L. S. (1975). Idiopathic orthostatic hypotension: biochemical and pathologic observations in 2 cases. Eur. Neurol. 13, 177.

Thapedi, I. M., Ashenhurst, E. M., and Rozdilsky, B. (1971). Shy–Drager syndrome: report of an autopsied case. Neurology, Minneapolis 21, 26.

Thomas, J. E. and Schirger, A. (1970). Idiopathic orthostatic hypotension: a study of its natural history in 57 neurologically affected patients. Arch. Neurol., Chicago 22, 289.

Vanderhaeghen, J. J., Perier, O., and Sternon, J. E. (1970). Pathological findings in idiopathic orthostatic hypotension: its relationship with Parkinson's disease. Arch. Neurol., Chicago 22, 207.

Williams, A., Hanson, D., and Calne, D. B. (1979). Vocal cord paralysis in the Shy–Drager syndrome. J. Neurol. Neurosurg. Psychiat. 42, 151.

Acute autonomic neuropathy

This rare, unexplained disorder (Thomashefsky, Horwitz, and Feingold 1972; Hopkins, Neville, and Bannister 1974), has been described as presenting in childhood or adult life with an acute onset and variable features of autonomic paralysis including postural hypotension, paralysis of accommodation, anhidrosis, loss of lacrimation, and urinary and faecal retention. Most reported cases have shown spontaneous recovery after a few weeks or months. Young, Asbury, Corbett, and Adams (1975) described such a case under the title of 'pure pan-dysautonomia with recovery'. Additional cases have been reported by Low, Dyck, Lambert, Brimijoin, Trautmann, Malagelada, Fealey, and Barrett (1983) and Fagius, Westerberg, and Olsson (1983); in addition to pandysautonomia, they described sensory impairment in the limbs and one case was fatal. A resemblance to the Guillain–Barré syndrome was noted.

References

Fagius, J., Westerberg, C.-E., and Olsson, Y. (1983). Acute pandysautonomia and sensory deficit with poor recovery. *J. Neurol. Neurosurg. Psychiat.* **46**, 725.

Hopkins, A., Neville, B., and Bannister, R. (1974). Autonomic neuropathy of acute onset. *Lancet* **i**, 769.

Low, P. A., Dyck, P. J., Lambert, E. H., Brimijoin, W. S., Trautmann, J. C., Malagelada, J. R., Fealey, R. D., and Barrett, D. M. (1983). Acute panautonomic neuropathy. *Ann. Neurol.* **13**, 412.

Thomashefsky, A. J., Horwitz, S. J., and Feingold, M. H. (1972). Acute autonomic neuropathy. *Neurology, Minneapolis* **22**, 251.

Young, R. R., Asbury, A. K., Corbett, J. L., and Adams, R. D. (1975). Pure pandysautonomia with recovery—description and discussion of diagnostic criteria. *Brain* **98**, 613.

Syndromes of the hypothalamus

Adiposity (obesity)

Adiposity, often associated with genital hypoplasia or atrophy, may occur as a symptom of several pathological states involving either the hypothalamus or pituitary, or both of these. The suggestion that obesity is caused by an imbalance in the autonomic nervous system and in particular by autonomic regulation of endocrine pancreatic secretion is probably an oversimplification (Morley and Levine 1983).

The causes of obesity

1. *Chromophobe adenoma or prolactinoma of the pituitary* may produce it (see p. 165).

2. *Tumours above the pituitary*, especially craniopharyngiomas (see p. 165).

3. *Internal hydrocephalus* from any cause may lead to obesity and genital hypoplasia through distension of the third ventricle compressing the sella turcica and the pituitary. In this way the syndrome may result from a tumour remote from the sella turcica, as in the cerebellum. More often, however, it is secondary to aqueduct stenosis or communicating hydrocephalus.

4. The syndrome may be produced by *infective conditions of the nervous system*, especially by encephalitis lethargica and, rarely, basal syphilitic meningitis. Granulomatous meningitis, say in sarcoidosis, may have a similar effect.

5. *Idiopathic adiposogenital dystrophy*. In most cases of this syndrome, including those in which the disturbance of function is most marked, none of the above causes is responsible. The disorder is present from birth, and it is usually noticed at an early age that the child is exceptionally fat. Both sexes are affected, though boys are more often affected than girls. The cheeks are rosy, and the skin is soft and hairless, except on the scalp. Obesity is often associated with skeletal overgrowth, the child being unusually tall as well as exceptionally fat. There is often marked genital hypoplasia, though exceptionally genital function is normal. This is so more often in females than in males. Sugar tolerance is usually increased. Polyuria, lethargy, and narcolepsy are infrequent associated symptoms. There is no evidence of a lesion involving the visual pathways and the sella turcica is radiographically normal. These negative findings, together with the early onset, render

it possible to distinguish the idiopathic variety of adiposogenital dystrophy (Fröhlich's syndrome) from other conditions of which similar disturbances are symptomatic.

Cachexia (diencephalic wasting)

Cachexia is much less often seen as a symptom of a lesion of the hypothalamus than obesity. It is occasionally produced, however, by suprasellar tumours and was common in the advanced stages of parkinsonism due to encephalitis lethargica. A hypothalamic syndrome causing severe wasting in infancy and childhood has also been described (Russell 1951; White and Ross 1963; Gamstorp 1972). Symptoms usually appear in the first two years of life; the child shows rapid longitudinal growth with emaciation and almost total lack of subcutaneous fat despite an adequate food intake and no evidence of malabsorption. The children are alert, often hyperactive, and sometimes euphoric with retraction of the upper eyelids and a 'surprised' expression (Gamstorp 1972). Often the CSF protein content is raised and in most cases a tumour of the diencephalon is found, or an optic-nerve glioma extending posteriorly (Pelc and Flament-Durand 1973), but the syndrome has been reported without a demonstrable tumour (Brain, Darte, Keith, and Kruyff 1966).

Sexual functions

Failure of the sexual functions to develop at the normal age, or retrogression after normal development, may result from lesions either of the hypothalamus or of the pituitary. Sexual infantilism, or, in the adult, impotence or amenorrhoea, according to sex, is then often associated with obesity as described above.

Sexual precocity is much rarer. It may result from either endocrine or nervous disorder. In the endocrine sphere it can be produced by tumours of the ovary, testis, or suprarenal. Pineal tumours cause sexual precocity in some cases, almost always males (see p. 164), but such precocity may also be produced by other tumours of the midbrain and by hydrocephalus from any cause. It has also been reported after encephalitis lethargica and in association with tuberous sclerosis and suprasellar tumours, as well as in rare cases of hypothalamic glioma.

So far we have considered bodily changes in reproductive organs resulting from disease of the nervous system. Loss of sexual desire without such changes may be encountered in patients with a tumour involving the base of the brain and sometimes after head injury, or in association with extensive destructive cerebral lesions of any type. Excessive libido, on the other hand, may be experienced by patients in whom a tumour or more diffuse pathological change, such as early general paresis, diminishes inhibition.

Impotence implies a condition in the male in which sexual desire is normal but the patient cannot achieve an erection of the penis adequate for sexual intercourse. Erection of the penis and ejaculation of semen depend in the first instance upon the integrity of sacral reflex arcs in the spinal cord. Injury to these reflex arcs, as may occur in tabes, spina bifida, or a tumour or injury of the cauda equina, or penile ischaemia, may cause impotence. Since, however, higher centres also play a part in the sexual act, impotence may be produced by lesions of the spinal cord at a higher level, as, for example, in multiple sclerosis. If the nervous system is normal and there is no debilitating general disease, impotence is usually emotional in origin. Simple anxiety may cause it when it may be associated with ejaculatio praecox, explained by the fact that the sympathetic nervous system, which is over–active during anxiety, is inhibitory to erection of the penis but motor to the vesiculae seminales. Usually, however, the causes of neurotic impotence are more complex and often intractable despite psychiatric investigation and treatment.

Diabetes insipidus

Mode of production. It has been shown experimentally that diabetes insipidus follows bilateral destruction of the supra-optic nuclei, or removal of the posterior lobe of the pituitary and its stalk. The antidiuretic hormone (ADH) is produced by the nerve cells of the supra-optic and paraventricular nuclei, and reaches the neurohypophysis by their descending tracts. The hormone is necessary for the resorption of water by the renal tubules. Two separate hormones are secreted by the neurosecretory granules of the posterior pituitary, namely vasopressin and oxytocin. Vasopressin has substantial pressor (blood-pressure raising) and antidiuretic effects and mild oxytocic effects, while oxytocin, as mentioned above, causes ejection of milk from the breast and uterine contraction but is also mildly antidiuretic. The peptide structure of both hormones is now known and both have been synthesized (de Vigneaud 1956). The commercial impure preparation, *Pitressin*, contains several peptides other than lysine vasopressin and arginine vasopressin (ADH), including not only oxytocin, neurophysin, and prolactin, but also a corticotrophin-like peptide (*British Medical Journal* 1977). Strictly, diabetes insipidus means arginine vasopressin (ADH) deficiency.

The secretion of ADH is excited by an increase in plasma osmolality, by a reduction in the circulating blood volume, and by emotional stimuli: it is inhibited by a decrease in plasma osmolality and a rise in circulating blood volume.

Aetiology. Diabetes insipidus may be the result of lesions involving either the tuber cinereum or the neurohypophysis, though in the latter case the polyuria is usually less severe than in the former. However, in 30–50 per cent of cases the condition is idiopathic and usually sporadic, but familial cases are not uncommon. In both familial and idiopathic cases examined at postmortem there is severe loss of neurones in the supraoptic and paraventricular hypothalamic nuclei (Green, Buchan, Alvord, and Swanson 1967). Recent work has strongly suggested an auto-immune aetiology for the idiopathic cases in which serum auto-antibodies to vasopressin-secreting human hypothalamic cells can often be detected by indirect immunofluorescence (Scherbaum and Bottazzo 1983). Tuberal lesions responsible for diabetes insipidus include trauma, ranging from gunshot wounds of the suprahypophysial region to closed head injury with concussion, basal meningitis due to syphilis, sarcoidosis, torula, or a variety of other causes, epidemic encephalitis, cerebral malaria, internal hydrocephalus, and tumours of the third ventricle; and the syndrome may be produced by ischaemia, haemorrhage, primary or secondary neoplasms or tuberculoma of the pituitary. It may also occur in essential xanthomatosis. Chronic sustained hypernatraemia and hypovolaemia without diabetes insipidus can also be a result of hypothalamic tumour (Vejjajiva, Sitprija, and Shuangshoti 1969).

Symptoms and signs Diabetes insipidus causes extreme thirst and the passage of large volumes of urine of low specific gravity, amounting in severe cases to several gallons a day. Sleep is disturbed by thirst and the necessity for frequent micturition. Excessive hunger is a rare accompaniment. There are several tests for diabetes insipidus of which the simplest is that water deprivation does not lead to release of ADH and hence the specific gravity of the urine does not rise above 1 014. Full details of the dehydration test, the vasopressin test, and the hypertonic saline test were given by Dingman and Thorn (1974). The nicotine test, involving assessment of the antidiuretic effect of smoking cigarettes after a period of initial hydration, in order to assess the stimulant effect of nicotine upon the cells of the supraoptic nucleus, is also helpful in some cases.

Diagnosis. The polyuria of diabetes must be distinguished from that occurring in other conditions, especially renal failure, hereditary nephrogenic diabetes insipidus (p. 470), and psychogenic compulsive water-drinking (de Wardener and Barlow 1958). The last is prone to occur in middle-aged women, who show a low plasma osmolality in contrast to the high one of diabetes insipidus, and fail to respond to vasopressin.

Prognosis. The prognosis is related to the nature of the causative lesion. In cases due to inflammatory processes such as sarcoidosis, benefit may follow appropriate treatment. When the cause is tumour or hydrocephalus, relief may follow if the primary disorder can be treated surgically.

Prognosis in traumatic cases is uncertain. Some patients improve or recover after a few months: in others, as in most idiopathic cases, the disorder is permanent.

Treatment. *Pitressin* given as snuff or by injection as the tannate-in-oil was for many years the standard treatment but the injections were painful and often produced antibodies against neurophysin, while the snuff frequently caused rhinitis or allergic pulmonary lesions (*British Medical Journal* 1977). Lysine vasopressin is short-acting and of little value in severe cases but the synthetic analogue L-desamino-8D-arginine vasopressin (DDAVP) given intranasally in a dose of 10–12 μg twice daily in adults or 5 μg twice daily in children has revolutionized treatment. For reasons which remain unclear, hypoglycaemic agents such as chlorpropamide and other drugs including clofibrate and carbamazepine (Wales 1975; *British Medical Journal* 1977) are also effective.

Disturbances of sleep

The role of the hypothalamus in the normal regulation of sleep is still uncertain, but clinical experience shows that lesions in the region of the tuber cinereum may lead either to persistent somnolence or to paroxysmal attacks of hypersomnia similar to idiopathic narcolepsy (see p. 641).

It has been suggested that the syndrome of periodic hypersomnolence and megaphagia which usually occurs in adolescent males (the Kleine–Levin syndrome, see p. 643) is of hypothalamic origin but its aetiology is not yet known. The physiopathology of sleep disorders was reviewed by Dement, Guilleminault, and Zarcone (1975). Sleep-like coma has been reported due to lesions of the posterior hypothalamus (Plum and Posner 1977).

Other hypothalamic disturbances

Sugar metabolism. The disturbances of sugar metabolism which have been produced by experimental hypothalamic lesions find a clinical counterpart in the occurrence of glycosuria as a result of lesions of this part of the brain. It is most often seen in patients with a tumour in the hypothalamus or fourth ventricle and is more often due to a lowered renal threshold than to hyperglycaemia. 'Cerebral glycosuria' may also occur after head injury, subarachnoid haemorrhage, meningitis, and encephalitis.

Temperature regulation. Irregular pyrexia may occur in patients with a lesion in the region of the tuber cinereum, and the hyperpyrexia which not uncommonly follows operations in this region is probably due to impairment of the hypothalamic temperature-regulating mechanism (see p. 593). Urban hypothermia in the elderly is in part due to an age-related decline in the efficiency of cold-defence mechanisms and in part to a reduced ability to detect temperature change (Collins, Exton-Smith, and Doré 1981).

Ulceration of the alimentary canal. Many years ago it was first shown that lesions in the neighbourhood of the hypothalamus were followed by acute ulceration of the upper part of the alimentary canal. Perforating ulcers may thus be produced in the oesophagus, stomach, and duodenum of experimental animals. Cushing drew attention to the occurrence of similar ulceration in man, as a rare sequel of head injury or intracranial injury.

Respiratory disturbances. Abnormalities in the rate and amplitude of respiration may also be produced by hypothalamic lesions and this may well have been the explanation of the respiratory disturbances which were sometimes seen as sequelae of encephalitis lethargica.

Cyclical oedema.

Cyclical oedema. Idiopathic or cyclical oedema, a disorder of unknown cause almost exclusively confined to women, in which intermittent bouts of generalized swelling are aggravated by standing, now seems likely to be due to hypothalamic dysfunction (Young, Brown, John, Chapman, and Lee 1983).

References

Appenzeller, O. (1979). *The autonomic nervous system*. North-Holland, Amsterdam.

Bain, H. W., Darte, J. M. M., Keith, W. S., and Kruyff, E. (1966). The diencephalic syndrome of early infancy due to silent brain tumour. With special reference to treatment. *Pediatrics* **38**, 473.

Bannister, R., Ardill, L., and Fentem, P. (1967). Defective autonomic control of blood vessels in idiopathic orthostatic hypotension. *Brain* **90**, 725.

Beattie, J., Brow, G. R., and Long, C. N. H. (1930). Physiological and anatomical evidence for the existence of nerve tracts connecting the hypothalamus with spinal sympathetic centres. *Proc. R. Soc.* **B106**, 253.

British Medical Journal (1977). Diabetes insipidus—turning off the tap. *Br. med. J.* **1**, 1050.

Clark, W. E. le G. (1948). The connexions of the frontal lobes of the brain. *Lancet* **i**, 353.

Collins, K. J., Exton-Smith, A. N., and Doré, C. (1981). Urban hypothermia: preferred temperature and thermal perception in old age. *Br. med. J.* **282**, 175.

de Vigneaud, V. (1956). Trail of sulfur research: from insulin to oxytocin. *Science* **123**, 967.

de Wardener, H. E. and Barlow, E. D. (1958). Compulsive water-drinking. *Quart. J. Med.* **27**, 567.

Dement, W., Guilleminault, C., and Zarcone, B. (1975). The pathologies of sleep; a case series approach. In *The nervous system*, Vol. 2, *The clinical neurosciences* (ed. T. N. Chase) p. 501. Raven Press, New York.

Dingman, J. F. and Thorn, G. W. (1974). Diseases of the neurohypophysis. In *Harrison's principles of internal medicine*, 7th edn, Chapter 84. McGraw-Hill, New York.

Gamstorp, I. (1972). Neurological disorders and growth disturbances in infancy and childhood. *Eur. Neurol.* **7**, 1.

Green, J. R., Buchan, G. C., Alvord, E. C., Jr, and Swanson, A. G. (1967). Hereditary and idiopathic types of diabetes insipidus. *Brain* **90**, 707.

Haymaker, W., Anderson, E., and Nauta, W. J. H. (1969). *The hypothalamus*. Thomas, Springfield, Illinios.

Head, H. (1893–6). On disturbances of sensation with especial reference to the pain of visceral disease. Part I, *Brain* (1893) **16**, 1; Part II, *Brain* (1894) **17**, 339; Part III, *Brain* (1896) **19**, 153.

Hess, W. R. (1954). *Diencephalon*. Grune and Stratton, New York.

Jacobson, S. (1972). Hypothalamus and autonomic nervous system. In *An introduction to neurosciences* (ed. B. A. Curtis, S. Jacobson, and E. M. Marcus), p. 386. Saunders, Philadelphia.

Le Marquand, H. S. and Russell, D. S. (1934–5). A case of pubertas praecox (macrogenitosomia praecox) in a boy associated with a tumour in the floor of the third ventricle. *Roy. Berks. Hosp. Rep.*, p. 31.

Lewis, T. (1937). The nocifensor system of nerves and its reactions. *Br. med. J.* **1**, 431.

—— (1938). Suggestions relating to the study of somatic pain. *Br. med. J.* **1**, 321.

List, C. F. and Peet, M. M. (1938). Sweat secretion in man. IV. Sweat secretion of the face and its disturbances. *Arch. Neurol. Psychiat.*, Chicago **40**, 442.

Morley, J. E. and Levine, A. S. (1983). The central control of appetite. *Lancet* **i**, 398.

Munch–Peterson, C. J. (1931). Glycosurias of cerebral origin. *Brain* **54**, 72.

Pelc, S. and Flament–Durand, J. (1973). Histological evidence of optic chiasma glioma in the "diencephalic syndrome". *Arch. Neurol.*, Chicago **28**, 139.

Plum, F. and Posner, J. B. (1977). *Diagnosis of stupor and coma*, 3rd edn. Davis, Philadelphia.

Richter, C. P. (1930). Experimental diabetes insipidus. *Brain* **53**, 76.

Russell, A. (1951). A diencephalic syndrome of emaciation in infancy and childhood. *Arch. Dis. Childh.* **26**, 274.

Sachs, E. and Macdonald, M E. (1925). Blood sugar studies in experimental pituitary and hypothalamic lesions, with a review of literature. *Arch. Neurol. Psychiat.*, Chicago **13**, 335.

Scherbaum, W. A. and Bottazzo, G. F. (1983). Autoantibodies to vasopressin cells in idiopathic diabetes insipidus: evidence for an autoimmune variant. *Lancet* **i**, 897.

Sinclair, D. C., Weddell, G., and Feindel, W. H. (1948). Referred pain and associated phenomena. *Brain* **71**, 184.

Vejjajiva, A., Sitprija, V., and Shuangshoti, S. (1969). Chronic sustained hypernatremia and hypovolemia in hypothalamic tumor: a physiologic study. *Neurology, Minneapolis* **19**, 161.

Wales, J. K. (1975). Treatment of diabetes insipidus with carbamazepine. *Lancet* **ii**, 948.

Walker, A. E. (1940). A cyto-architectural study of the prefrontal area of the macaque monkey. *J. comp. Neurol.* **73**, 59.

Wechsler, I. S. (1956). Hypothalamic syndromes. *Br. med. J.* **2**, 375.

White, P. T. and Ross, A. T. (1963). Inanition syndrome in infants with anterior hypothalamic neoplasms. *Neurology, Minneapolis* **13**, 974.

Young, J. B., Brownjohn, A. M., Chapman, C., and Lee, M. R. (1983). Evidence for a hypothalamic disturbance in cyclical oedema. *Br. med. J.* **286**, 1619.

21

Diseases of the bones of the skull

Osteitis deformans

Synonym. Paget's disease.

Definition. A chronic disease of the bones characterized by absorption and new bone formation, often leading to enlargement of the skull, deformity of the vertebral column, bowing of the clavicles and long bones and in some cases to neurological manifestations secondary to the bony changes.

Aetiology and pathology

Osteitis deformans is a rare disease of unknown aetiology developing in middle life and affecting both sexes. It has been estimated to occur in 7 per cent of males and 3.8 per cent of females over the age of 55 years in Britain (Barker, Clough, Guyer, and Gardner 1977). The incidence of the condition varies greatly from country to country, being much lower, for example, in Ireland than in Britain (Detheridge, Barker, and Guyer 1983).

Histologically, the changes in the bones consist of resorption and softening of bone followed by replacement with a poorly mineralized osteoid matrix with increased vascularity, and with extensive fibrosis; enlargement of bones results from the laying down of osteoid both beneath the periosteum and on the inner side of the cortex. Deformities result from bony softening. Often the condition is generalized, if more severe in some bones than others, but in some cases it is restricted, say, to a single vertebral body or to one ilium. The skull, when affected, is thickened, and the distinction between the inner and the outer tables and the diploë is obliterated. The cranial cavity is increased in breadth and to a lesser extent in length, but its vertical diameter is diminished. The base tends to sink relative to the region of the foramen magnum, which is supported by the vertebral column, and platybasia or basilar impression may result (see p. 607). Thickening of the skull also leads to a reduction in size of the vascular and neural foramina and may thus be responsible for symptoms of compression of intracranial structures and cranial nerves. Similar changes in the spine lead to kyphosis and reduction in height, and sometimes to spinal-cord compression. The clavicles and the long bones of the limbs may also become softened, thickened, and bowed. Increased blood flow through newly formed arteriovenous channels may rarely cause high-output cardiac failure.

Osseous symptoms and signs

The onset is insidious, the patient often complaining first of pains in the head and limbs. Gradual enlargement of the skull necessitates an increase in hat size, and deformities of the spine and long bones are noted, together with a resulting loss of height, in extreme cases amounting to as much as 30 cm. The enlarged skull bulges in the frontal and parietal regions. Affected bones often feel warm to the touch. Radiographs show a characteristic appearance, the thickened bone being mottled and 'woolly'; rarely there are large islands of osteoporosis in the skull (Fig. 21.1)

Neurological symptoms and signs

While dementia and epileptic attacks have been thought to occur as a result of compression of the cerebral hemispheres and symptoms of cerebellar deficiency have also been observed as well as

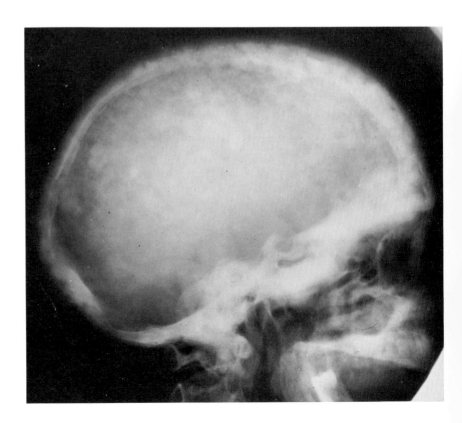

Fig. 21.1. Paget's disease of the skull. Lateral radiograph demonstrating thickening and the typical 'woolly' appearance of the skull vault with some platybasia. (Kindly provided by Dr G. L. Gryspeerdt.)

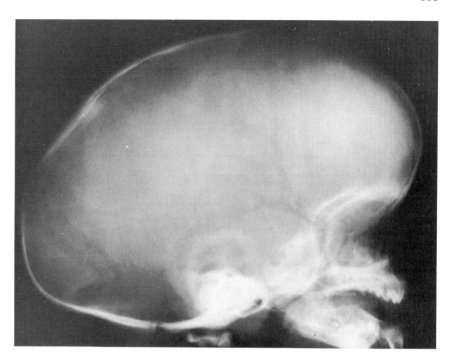

Fig. 21.2. Oxycephaly due to premature synostosis of the sagittal suture; note the abnormal shape of the skull and the thinning of the calvarium.

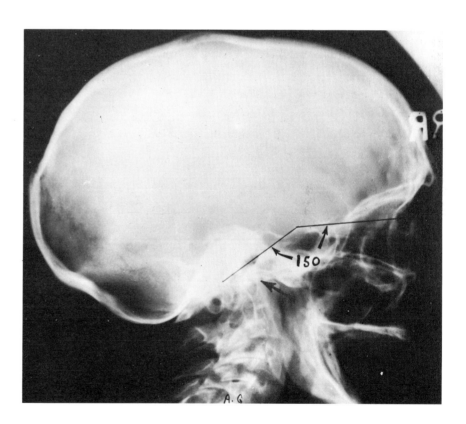

Fig. 21.3. Basilar impression associated with developmental anomalies of the cervical spine. The angle between the basisphenoid and the basilar portion of the occipital bone (small arrows) is 150 degrees, indicating platybasia. The large arrow points to the odontoid peg which is well above Chamberlain's line.

obstructive hydrocephalus (Friedman, Sklaver, and Klawans 1971), Clarke and Harrison (1978) found the evidence of an association with epilepsy or with cerebral or cerebellar dysfunction unconvincing and felt that most if not all of the neurological complications were due to compression of cranial nerves, basilar impression, or spinal-cord compression.

Any of the cranial nerves may be compressed owing to reduction in the calibre of their foramina, the olfactory, optic, and vestibulocochlear nerves being most often affected. Unilateral optic atrophy, paralysis of one lateral rectus, trigeminal neuralgia and

hemifacial spasm have all been described (Friedman *et al.* 1971; Clarke and Harrison 1978) as have dysarthria and dysphagia and other manifestations of basilar impression.

In spite of spinal deformity associated with vertebral collapse, symptoms of compression of spinal roots are rare, but compression of the cord itself is not uncommon and may occur even when a single vertebral body is affected. Symptoms of spinal compression are described on page 402.

A rare familial form has been described in association with retinitis pigmentosa (van Bogaert 1933).

Diagnosis

The diagnosis is readily made by X-ray examination of the bones, and this should always be carried out in middle-aged patients who complain of obscure pains in the head or limbs or exhibit unexplained cranial-nerve palsies or paraplegia. A systolic bruit, due to increased blood flow through the affected bone, may be heard over the skull or spine. The serum alkaline phosphatase is usually raised.

Prognosis

Osteitis deformans is an extremely chronic and slowly progressive disease. Local sarcoma of bone sometimes occurs as a complication.

Rarely, in severe cases, owing to multiple arteriovenous communications in the affected bones, 'high-output' cardiac failure occurs and an association with atheroma and cardiac infarction has been postulated.

Treatment

In the past, treatment with calcium and vitamin D was often recommended, as was mithramycin (Ryan, Schwartz, and Northrop 1970), but no treatment was of proven effectiveness. More recently, however, it has become clear that calcitonin, 50–100 units daily for three months, followed by a similar dose three times weekly for six months or longer, is effective in improving the bone lesions and the neurological complications (de Deuxchaisnes 1983) and is relatively free from side-effects, apart from nausea and flushing which are occasionally troublesome. Nevertheless, when spinal-cord compression or neurological manifestations of basilar impression are severe, surgical decompression is still sometimes needed but may be difficult and hazardous because of vascularity of the bone.

References

Barker, D. J. P., Clough, P. W. L., Guyer, P. B., and Gardner. M. J. (1977). Paget's disease of bone in 14 British towns. *Br. med. J.* **1**, 1181.
Boll, J. (1946–7). Paget's disease of the skull with platybasia. *Proc. R. Soc. Med.* **40**, 85.
Clarke, C. R. A. and Harrison, M. J. G. (1978). Neurological manifestations of Paget's disease. *J. neurol. Sci.* **38**, 171.
de Deuxchaisnes, C. N. (1983). Calcitonin in the treatment of Paget's disease. *Triangle* **22**, 103.
Detheridge, F. M., Barker, D. J. P., and Guyer, P. B. (1983). Paget's disease of bone in Ireland. *Br. med. J.* **287**, 1345.
Friedman, P., Sklaver, N., and Klawans, H. L. (1971). Neurologic manifestations of Paget's disease of the skull. *Dis. nerv. Syst.* **32**, 809.
Grünthal, E. (1931). Über den Hirnbefund bei Pagetscher Krankheit des Schädels. *Z. ges. Neurol. Psychiat.* **136**, 656.
Gurdjian, E. S., Webster, J. E., and Latimer, F. R. (1952). Paget's disease of the spine with compression of the spinal cord. *Trans. Am. neurol. Ass.* **77**, 243.
Paget, J., Fricker, G., and ver Brugghen. A. (1950). Osteitis fibrosa cystica localisata of the skull. *J. Neurosurg.* **7**, 447.
Ryan, W. G., Schwartz, T. B., and Northrop, G. (1970). Experiences in the treatment of Paget's disease of bone with mithramycin. *J. Am. med Ass.* **213**, 1153.
van Bogaert, L. (1933). Über eine hereditäre und familiäre Form der Pagetschen Ostitis deformans mit Chorioretinitis pigmentosa. *Z. ges. Neurol. Psychiat.* **147**, 327.

Leontiasis ossea, polyostotic fibrous dysplasia, and other craniotubular modelling disorders

Leontiasis ossea is characterized by hyperostosis of the bones of the face and skull; sometimes all such bones are involved and the condition is then similar clinically and pathologically to Paget's disease, but in other cases the overgrowth is limited to one or both cranial bones or to one or both jaws. The name of the condition derives from the leonine facial appearance. Unlike typical Paget's disease, the condition, which may give rise to cranial-nerve palsies, usually begins in childhood and is slowly progressive.

Polyostotic fibrous dysplasia (Albright's syndrome) is limited as a rule to young girls; changes in the long bones, cutaneous pigmentation, and precocious puberty may be accompanied by cranial-nerve palsies and/or optic atrophy due to involvement of the bones of the skull base. It is now generally believed that leontiasis ossea is merely a variant of polyostotic fibrous dysplasia in which the bones of the skull and face are selectively involved (Krane 1974). The patches of cutaneous pigmentation often show a jagged outline (coast of Maine) unlike those of smooth outline seen in neurofibromatosis.

The craniotubular modelling disorders (Stein, Witkop, Hill, Fallon, Viernstein, Gucer, McKeever, Long, Altman, Miller, Teitelbaum, and Schlesinger 1983) include sclerosteosis, autosomal recessive and dominant osteopetrosis (Albers–Schonberg disease), cranial metaphyseal dysplasia, Van Buchem's disease, craniodiaphyseal dysplasia, dysosteosclerosis, diaphyseal dysplasia, and hereditary hyperphosphatasia. Most of these disorders, but especially sclerosteosis, are characterized by radiographic abnormalities of the metaphysis or diaphysis of long bones and by cranial-nerve palsies and intracranial hypertension resulting from bony overgrowth of the skull. In addition in sclerosteosis there are prognathism, mandibular thickening, frontal bossing, proptosis, ocular hypertelorism, syndactyly, and increased somatic growth. In infantile osteopetrosis, osteosclerosis, hepatosplenomegaly, and anaemia are prominent but cranial-nerve palsies, macrocephaly, hydrocephalus, mental retardation, and an association with neuronal storage disease have been described (Ambler, Trice, Grauerholz, and O'Shea 1983).

References

Albright, F. (1947). Polyostotic fibrous dysplasia. *J. clin. Endocr.* **7**, 307.
Ambler, M. W., Trice, J., Grauerholz, J. and O'Shea, P. A. (1983). Infantile osteopetrosis and neuronal storage disease. *Neurology, Minneapolis* **33**, 437.
Krane, S. M. (1974). Hyperostosis, neoplasms and other disorders of bone and cartilage. In *Harrison's principles of internal medicine*, 7th edn, Chapter 354. McGraw-Hill, New York.
Smith, A. G. and Zavaleta, A. (1952). Osteoma, ossifying fibroma and fibrous dysplasia of the facial and cranial bones. *Arch. Path.* **54**, 507.
Stein, S. A., Witkop, C., Hill, S., Fallon, M. D., Viernstein, L., Gucer, G., McKeever, P., Long, D., Altman, J., Miller, N. R., Teitelbaum, S. L., and Schlesinger S. (1983). Sclerosteosis: neurogenetic and pathophysiologic analysis of an American kinship. *Neurology, Minneapolis* **33**, 267.

Craniostenosis

Synonyms. Oxycephaly; acrocephaly; turricephaly; tower skull.

Definition. A congenital abnormality of the skull due to premature synostosis of the sutures and characterized by an abnormal shape of the head, exophthalmos, optic atrophy, and symptoms of increased intracranial pressure.

Aetiology and pathology

It is generally agreed that craniostenosis is due to premature synostosis (fusion) of the skull bones. This usually begins in the coronal, sagittal, and lambdoid sutures, but there are many variations, and the synostosis may be asymmetrical. It has been attributed to displacement of the centres of ossification towards the sutures. The condition is congenital and sometimes hereditary. Though the sutures are closed, the brain continues to grow at the usual rate. Compensatory enlargement of the skull occurs through expansion where the sutures are not united and by thinning of the bone—convolutional atrophy—from pressure of the growing brain. The ultimate breakdown of this compensatory process leads to manifestations of increased intracranial pressure. The optic atrophy has been attributed to various causes, including compression of the optic nerves by narrowing of their canals, stretching or compression of the nerves, and papilloedema due to increased intracranial pressure. Probably different factors operate alone or in combination in different cases. The exophthalmos seems to be due to abnormal shallowness of the orbits.

Craniostenosis is also a feature of the acrocephalosyndactyly of Apert, in which oxycephaly is associated with syndactyly, and of craniofacial dysostosis (see below).

Symptoms and signs

Although craniostenosis is a congenital abnormality, the patient may not come under observation until other symptoms, such as headache and failing vision, develop, usually in childhood.

The skull is brachycephalic and dome-shaped, with a high forehead, and there may be flattening of the maxillae or asymmetrical facial deformity. A short upper lip is characteristic. Owing to the shallow orbits the eyes are prominent, and may even become spontaneously dislocated; a divergent squint and nystagmus are common. Papilloedema may be present or optic atrophy, either primary or secondary, with visual impairment leading to blindness if left untreated. Other symptoms due either directly to the bony changes or indirectly to increased intracranial pressure include anosmia and deafness. The mental state is usually normal. Radiographs of the skull show the premature synostosis of the sutures and compensatory enlargement, with marked thinning of the calvarium, especially in the frontal region (Fig. 21.2).

Craniofacial dysostosis. This disorder, described by Crouzon, is related to craniostenosis, and usually hereditary. The forehead recedes to the high, rather pointed vertex—trigonocephaly. There are also hyperplasia of the maxillae and relative prognathism, together with exophthalmos, divergent squint, and in some cases optic atrophy.

Diagnosis

The condition is usually recognized at a glance from the shape of the skull. In microcephaly the abnormally small skull size is secondary to hypoplasia of the brain, and symptoms of increased intracranial pressure are absent. In hydrocephalus the skull is enlarged in all its diameters and its total volume, which in craniostenosis tends to be subnormal, is increased. Craniostenosis is unlikely to be confused with other causes of increased intracranial pressure if the shape of the skull and the X-ray appearances are noted.

Prognosis

In mild cases compensatory enlargement of the skull may be adequate to prevent the development of symptoms. When, however, headache is present or vision is threatened, deterioration is progressive without surgery.

Treatment

Only surgical treatment with opening of the sutures is effective. Since in some cases the optic nerves are directly compressed in their canals, radiographs of the optic foramina should be taken, and surgical decompression may be needed. King (1938) described a new surgical technique, and modern surgical methods have been reviewed by Pemberton and Freeman (1962) and Anderson and Geiger (1965).

References

Anderson, F. M. and Geiger, L. (1965). Craniosynostosis. A survey of 204 cases. *J. Neurosurg.* **22**, 229.

Crouzon, O. (1929). *Études sur les maladies familiales nerveuses et dystrophique.* Masson, Paris.
Davis, F. A. (1925). Tower skull, oxycephalus. *Am. J. Ophthal.* **8**, 513.
King, J. E. J. (1938). Oxycephaly: a new operation and its results. *Arch. Neurol. Psychiat.*, Chicago **40**, 1205.
Pemberton J. W. and Freeman, J. M. (1962). Craniosynostosis. A review of experience with forty patients with particular reference to ocular aspects and comments on operative indications. *Am. J. Ophthal.* **54**, 641.
Saethre, H. (1931). Ueber den Turmschädel, seine Erblichkeit, Pathogenese und neuropsychiatrischen Symptome. *Acta psychiat.*, Kbh. **6**, 405.
Worms, G. and Carillon, R. (1930). Oxycephaly. *Rev. Oto-neuro-ophthal.* **8**, 736.

Cleidocranial dysostosis

In this rare developmental disorder absence of part or the whole of both clavicles is accompanied by an increased width of the forehead. Sometimes one or more shoulder-girdle muscles are absent but there are no associated neurological manifestations except in occasional cases in which there are also congenital malformations of the brain and/or of other parts of the nervous system.

Hypertelorism

In this developmental disorder the distance between the eyes is increased; there is a vertical ridge on the forehead and the bridge of the nose is excessively broad. Usually there is no neurological defect but in occasional rare and severe cases associated maldevelopment of the forebrain gives mental retardation.

References

Currarino, G. and Silverman, F. N. (1960). Orbital hypertelorism, arhinencephaly and trigonocephaly. *Radiology.* **74**, 206.
Klemmer, R. N., Snoke, P. O., and Cooper, H. K. (1931). Cleidocranial dysostosis. *Am. J. Roentgenol.* **25**, 710.

Basilar impression and other craniovertebral anomalies

Basilar impression is an abnormality of the skull base in which the angle between the basisphenoid and the basilar portion of the occipital bone—normally between 110 and 140 degrees—is widened (Fig. 21.3). In the congenital form the foramen magnum is deformed and the medulla is unusually low, so that it and the upper part of the cervical spinal cord may be compressed by the odontoid process of the axis. In a lateral radiograph the line drawn from the posterior end of the hard palate to the posterior lip of the foramen magnum normally lies above the cervical spine, but in basilar impression it crosses the odontoid process at some point (Chamberlain 1939); Bull, Nixon, and Pratt (1955) pointed out that the plane of the axis relative to that of the hard palate is a more reliable guide. Normally these are roughly parallel: in basilar impression they form an acute angle. The condition is often identified, particularly in the American literature, by the term 'platybasia', but the latter term, which simply means a flat base of skull, can equally be applied to the changes which occur, for instance, in Paget's disease. Spillane, Pallis, and Jones (1975) pointed out that basilar impression may be present without platybasia. Basilar impression is the name best reserved for the congenital disorder in which, perhaps because of a congenital abnormality of the occipital bone, the posterior part of the atlas vertebra is partially invaginated into the cranial cavity. De Battersby and Williams (1982) suggest that birth injury with distortion of basicranial synchondroses may be an important aetiological factor.

Basilar impression is therefore congenital and may be associated with fusion of the bodies of some cervical vertebrae—the Klippel–Feil syndrome—or it may be due to osteogenesis imperfecta (Hurwitz and McSwiney 1960). The Klippel–Feil syndrome may, however, occur without associated craniovertebral malformation; some such patients show 'mirror movements' in the upper extremities so that a voluntary movement carried out with one hand is mimicked spontaneously with the other (Gunderson and Solitare 1968).

Basilar impression may lead to hydrocephalus and perhaps to the Arnold–Chiari syndrome (Gustafson and Oldberg 1940), but the latter is more probably an associated congenital abnormality. The spinal cord may show hydromyelia but there is also a clear association with syringomyelia (Foster, Hudgson and Pearce, 1969; Barnett, Foster, and Hudgson 1974). In adults the clinical picture may resemble multiple sclerosis, syringomyelia, or high cervical tumour. The commonest clinical features are those of a spastic tetraparesis with marked impairment of position and joint sense in both hands and to a lesser extent in the legs, but in some cases there are also signs of involvement of lower cranial nerves, cerebellar ataxia, and/or hydrocephalus due to obstruction to the outflow of CSF from the fourth ventricle (O'Connell and Aldren Turner 1950; Michie and Clark 1968). Symptoms suggesting dysfunction of the C8-T1 segments of the spinal cord in some such cases have been attributed to venous obstruction and stagnant hypoxia in the cervical cord (Taylor and Byrnes 1974). The head is sometimes mushroom-shaped and the neck abnormally short, but the diagnosis can only be made by X-ray examination. If symptoms occur the treatment of choice is surgical decompression (Gordon 1969).

Achondroplasia may cause not only spinal-cord compression but also internal hydrocephalus without platybasia or basilar impression, possibly due to shortening of the skull base (Spillane 1952). Symptoms of high cervical-cord compression may result from atlanto-axial subluxation with separation of the odontoid process of the axis; this may be a congenital malformation or the result of trauma but can also occur spontaneously in rheumatoid arthritis (Stevens, Cartlidge, Saunders, Appleby, Hall, and Shaw 1971). It is also an important complication of Down's syndrome (Pueschel 1983). The radiology of the craniovertebral anomalies was reviewed in detail by Wackenheim (1974).

References

Barnett, H. J. M., Foster, J. B., and Hudgson, P. (1974). *Syringomyelia.* Saunders, London.

Bull, J., Nixon, W. L. B., and Pratt, R. T. C. (1955). The radiological criteria and familial occurrence of primary basilar impression *Brain* **78**, 229.

Chamberlain, W. E. (1939). Basilar impression (platybasia). *Yale J. Biol. Med.* **11**, 487.

De Battersby, R. and Williams, B. (1982). Birth injury: a possible contributory factor in the aetiology of primary basilar impression. *J. Neurol. Neurosurg. Psychiat.* **45**, 879.

Foster, J. B., Hudgson, P., and Pearce, G. W. (1969). The association of syringomyelia and congenital cervico-medullary anomalies: pathological evidence. *Brain* **92**, 25.

Gordon, D. S. (1969). Neurological syndromes associated with craniovertebral anomalies. *Proc. R. Soc. Med.* **62**, 725.

Gunderson, C. H. and Solitare, G. B. (1968). Mirror movements in patients with the Klippel-Feil syndrome. *Arch. Neurol., Chicago* **18**, 675.

Gustafson, W. A. and Oldberg, E. (1940). Neurologic significance of platybasia. *Arch. Neurol. Psychiat., Chicago* **44**, 84.

Hurwitz, L. J. and McSwiney, R. R. (1960). Basilar impression and osteogenesis imperfecta in a family. *Brain* **83**, 138.

Michie, I. and Clark, M. (1968). Neurological syndromes associated with cervical and craniocervical anomalies. *Arch. Neurol., Chicago* **18**, 241.

O'Connell, J. E. A. and Aldren Turner, J. W. (1950). Basilar impression of the skull. *Brain* **73**, 405.

Pueschel, S. M. (1983). Atlanto–axial subluxation in Down syndrome. *Lancet* **i**, 980.

Spillane, J. D. (1952). Three cases of achondroplasia with neurological complications. *J. Neurol. Neurosurg. Psychiat.* **15**, 246.

—— Pallis, C. and Jones, A. M. (1957). Developmental abnormalities in the region of the foramen magnum. *Brain* **80**, 11.

Steven, J. C., Cartlidge, N. E., Saunders, M., Appleby, A., Hall, M., and Shaw, D. A. (1971). Atlanto-axial subluxation and cervical myelopathy in rheumatoid arthritis. *Quart. J. Med.* **40**, 391.

Taylor, A. R. and Byrnes, D. P. (1974). Foramen magnum and high cervical cord compression. *Brain* **97**, 473.

Wackenheim, A. (1974). *Roentgen diagnosis of the craniovertebral region.* Springer-Verlag, Berlin.

22

Paroxysmal and convulsive disorders

Epilepsy

Definition. Epilepsy is a paroxysmal and transitory disturbance of the functions of the brain which develops suddenly, ceases spontaneously, and exhibits a conspicuous tendency to recurrence. Though in its most typical forms it is characterized by sudden loss of consciousness, which may or may not be associated with tonic spasm and clonic contractions of the muscles, many varieties of epileptic attack occur, their distinctive features depending upon differences in the site of origin, extent of spread, and nature of the disturbance of function. Epilepsy is thus a symptom. In some cases a local lesion of the brain plays the chief part in causation; in others hereditary predisposition is an important factor: in yet others the cause is unknown. A generalized attack has long been known as 'grand mal', an attack characterized by momentary loss of consciousness only, without falling and without, as a rule, motor accompaniments, as 'petit mal'. However, as will be seen, the term petit mal is best reserved for a specific variety of epilepsy which begins in childhood and there are other varieties of minor epilepsy which are different aetiologically which give only transient impairment of consciousness but yet differ from true petit mal. Attacks of epilepsy are often known as 'fits' or 'seizures'.

The physiological nature of epilepsy

The invention of electroencephalography (see pp. 76 and 618), though it has posed many problems which remain unsolved, threw new light upon the nature of epilepsy. The types of EEG obtained in epilepsy are described in more detail later. For our present purpose it is sufficient to say that epileptic attacks are usually accompanied by changes, which can be recorded, in the electrical potentials of the brain; hence epilepsy was described as 'paroxysmal cerebral dysrhythmia' (Gibbs, Gibbs, and Lennox 1937). However, cortical dysrhythmias similar to those found in epilepsy may be present in EEG recordings from patients with disorders other than epilepsy, and also in non-epileptic relatives of patients with epilepsy. Furthermore, in some undoubted attacks of epilepsy. EEG recordings taken through the intact skull may show no abnormality.

Nevertheless, there is good evidence that the physiological basis of a convulsion is a discharge of neurons rather than a primary impairment or loss of cortical function. Experimentally it can be shown in animals that convulsant drugs induce fits, the pattern of which can be modified by the successful removal of different levels of the nervous system from the cortex downwards. Moreover, electrical stimulation of the cortex in man, as shown initially by Foerster, results in convulsions which can only be satisfactorily interpreted as being the expression of a regional cortical discharge. Transitory post-epileptic symptoms, whether loss or disorder of consciousness, paralysis, or sensory loss, were once thought to be due to temporary exhaustion of neurones which had been the site of discharge. However, Efron (1961) gave cogent reasons for suggesting that an active process of inhibition, resulting from persistent subclinical epileptic discharge, is a more probable explanation for post-epileptic paralysis (Todd's paralysis).

Excitation, however, is not the most likely explanation of loss of consciousness occurring as the sole, or almost the sole, manifestation of epilepsy, as in petit mal. The bilaterally synchronous wave-and-spike cortical discharge which characterizes petit mal seems to originate subcortically, perhaps in the interthalamic nuc-

lei (Jasper and Droogleever-Fortuyn 1947) and the resulting impairment of consciousness was interpreted by Williams (1950) as indicating a blockage of afferent impulses to the cortex. In the light of experimental work and the behaviour of the EEG in man, Gastaut and Fischer-Williams (1960) suggested that 'a grand mal seizure seems to depend on a thalamic discharge which involves the non-specific reticular structures and is projected to the cortex in what may be considered a generalized recruiting response transmitted along the diffuse cortical projection pathways'. They postulated that in grand mal the thalamic discharge was responsible for the loss of consciousness and the discharge of the brainstem reticular formation for the tonic and clonic element in the convulsions. They also explained petit mal (absence seizures) as being the result of a thalamic discharge occurring in a subject with a very effective inhibitory mechanism. The lack of convulsions might then depend on the fact that the reticular formation was rhythmically inhibited. Myoclonic jerks, they noted, were sometimes evoked by sensory stimuli, especially after the administration of convulsant drugs, and seemed to originate in the mesencephalon and thalamus. The disturbances of consciousness, mood, and behaviour which occur as a result of discharges originating in the temporal lobe were thought to indicate dysfunction of the specific integrating role, in relation to consciousness, played by this part of the brain (Penfield and Jasper 1954).

Epilepsy, then, is to be regarded as an uncontrolled neural discharge, that is, as an abnormal conversion of the potential energy of the neurones into kinetic energy. Fundamentally it is a physico-chemical disturbance, and the physico-chemical state of the neurones can be influenced by numerous agencies. Studies of the physiological mechanisms underlying the onset and cessation of a focal attack have helped to elucidate some of these influences. Symonds (1959) suggested that gamma-aminobutyric acid (GABA) may be 'a natural anticonvulsant' formed in the brain. Local lesions might cause seizures either by allowing the local accumulation of an excitatory substance or by depressing the GABA concentration or the tonic inhibitory control of afferent impulses. Later it was shown that the application of acetylcholine (ACh) to the cerebral cortex could provoke focal convulsions, while generalized fits could follow its intravenous or intraventricular injection; thus fits might be due to exogenous or endogenous factors which influenced the local or generalized release of ACh in excess of the quantities normally required for synaptic transmission. GABA and acetylcholine have opposite effects upon neuronal excitability so that an imbalance between these two substances within the brain could be a factor predisposing to seizure production (Jurgelsky and Thomas 1966). The excitability of individual neurones may also be influenced by the activity of the sodium pump which affects the concentration gradient of Na^+ across the neuronal membrane; if the gradient increases the neurone is hyperpolarized and difficult to excite, while if it is diminished neuronal excitability increases. The so-called 'burst' firing patterns of single cortical neurones which may be recorded with microelectrodes in experimental epilepsy in animals and which are presumed to play a part in the genesis of the epileptic spike discharge in the EEG were reviewed by Ward (1972). The balance between ACh (excitatory) and GABA (inhibitory) may be upset, for instance, by pyridoxine deficiency as the latter substance is essential for the synthesis of GABA (see Sutherland and Eadie 1980). Since defects of the GABA inhibitory system were first postulated as being possible causal factors, two important CNS receptor sites have been characterized (see Spero 1982), one a GABA/chloride-ionophor/benzodiazepine-receptor complex, the other a specific phenytoin receptor. Receptor interactions are also clearly important in the pathophysiology of this disorder. These delicate and interrelated factors may be affected not only by the effects of focal cerebral lesions but also by numerous metabolic factors including pyrexia, hypoxia, hypercarbia, hypocalcaemia, hypomagnesaemia, hypoglycaemia, water intoxication, and alkalosis as well as some endocrinopathies and the effects of various drugs and toxins or drug withdrawal. Meldrum (1982), in reviewing the pathophysiology of epilepsy, stressed the importance of such systemic pathological factors. He indicated the concentrations of arterial pO_2, pCO_2, glucose, sodium, calcium, magnesium, urea, and ammonia and the extent of change in serum osmolarity which have been associated with seizure activity in man and in experimental animals and listed 30 exogenous toxins known to produce such attacks. In considering epileptogenesis at the cellular level he stressed the importance of cortical scarring and of cortical irritation produced by blood or its breakdown products in the CSF, as well as enzymatic defects causing deficiency of Na^+-K^+-activated ATPase or of the synthesis of inhibitory transmitter substances. Among the cytological mechanisms of importance are loss of inhibitory interneurones, 'deafferentation', whether due to supersensitivity or loss of dendritic spines, overloading of excitatory synapses, and proliferation of fibrous astrocytes, possibly with inadequate regulation of the extracellular potassium concentration.

During convulsions cerebral metabolism increases and the brain's need for oxygen and glucose increases, while in animals with experimentally induced convulsions brain lactate increases markedly (Posner, Plum, and Poznak 1969; Beresford, Posner, and Plum 1969). Within the first 30 minutes after a generalized seizure, arterial hypertension, a rise in cerebral venous pressure (CVP), an increase in cerebral blood flow (CBF), hyperglycaemia, hyperkalaemia, haemoconcentration, and a low or normal pO_2 with a high arterial pCO_2 are usual, while after 30 minutes there is often arterial hypotension, a raised or normal CVP, a normal CBF, hypoglycaemia (with persisting hyperkalaemia), and secondary hyperpyrexia (Meldrum 1982). Prolactin, LH, and FSH may also rise post-ictally, the latter only in females (Dana-Haeri, Trimble, and Oxley 1983). Low vitamin D and serum calcium levels are often found in institutionalized subjects with chronic epilepsy (Davie, Emberson, Lawson, Roberts, Barnes, Barnes, and Heeley 1983).

It must also be accepted that virtually every individual is potentially epileptic if the provocation, whether physical or pharmacological, is sufficient, but in some, presumed to have a high 'epileptic threshold' this provocation must be intense, while in others in whom seizures occur without apparent precipitating factors the 'convulsive threshold' is presumed to be low. It follows that there is a continuum between the epileptic and normal populations varying between the majority in whom substantial provocation is needed to produce a fit and the severe epileptics who have frequent attacks without evident cause. The margin between the two populations is clearly indistinct.

Aetiology

The following simple and selective classification of some of the principal causes of epilepsy is for convenience arranged schematically, but the precise way in which each cause operates is often obscure and some pathological conditions might well be placed in more than one category.

1. *Local causes*

(*a*) Focal intracranial lesions sometimes associated with increased intracranial pressure:
Intracranial tumour; cerebral abscess; subdural haematoma; angioma or haematoma.

(*b*) Inflammatory and demyelinating conditions:
Meningitis; all forms of acute and subacute encephalitis and many encephalopathies; toxoplasmosis; neurosyphilis; multiple sclerosis; cerebral cysticercosis.

(*c*) Trauma:
Perinatal brain injury and/or haemorrhage; head injuries of childhood and adult life.

(*d*) Congenital abnormalities:
The various forms of cerebral palsy; cerebral malformations.

(*e*) Degenerations and inborn errors of metabolism:
The neuronal storage disorders; diffuse sclerosis and the leukodystrophies; encephalopathies of infancy and childhood, including 'infantile spasms'; tuberous sclerosis and the other phacomatoses; Pick's disease; Alzheimer's disease; progressive myoclonic epilepsy; subacute spongiform encephalopathy; Creutzfeldt–Jakob disease.

(*f*) Vascular disorders:
Cerebral atheroma, intracranial haemorrhage, thrombosis, embolism; eclampsia; hypertensive encephalopathy; cerebral complications of 'connective tissue' or 'collagen' diseases; polycythaemia; intracranial aneurysm; acute cerebral ischaemia from any cause.

2. *General causes*

(*a*) Exogenous poisons:
Alcohol; absinthe; thujone; cocaine; strychnine; lead; chloroform; ether; insulin; amphetamines; camphor; leptazol; picrotoxin; antihistamines; intrathecal penicillin; pyridoxine analogues; some amino acids; local anaesthetics such as cocaine and lignocaine; water-soluble contrast media used intrathecally such as metrizamide; chlorinated hydrocarbon insecticides, organophosphorus and organochlorine compounds used as insecticides, and fluoracetic acid derivatives; amine-oxidase inhibitors, imipramine and its derivatives; and *withdrawal* of alcohol, barbiturates, and other drugs.

(*b*) Anoxia:
Asphyxia; carbon monoxide poisoning; carbon dioxide intoxication; nitrous oxide anaesthesia; profound anaemia.

(*c*) Disordered metabolism:
Uraemia; hepatic failure; water intoxication; high fat intake; porphyria; hypoglycaemia; hyperpyrexia; alkalosis; pyridoxine deficiency.

(*d*) Endocrine disorders:
Parathyroid tetany; idiopathic hypoparathyroidism and pseudohypoparathyroidism; hypo-adrenalism; pituitary dysfunction, including Cushing's disease and hypopituitarism; hyperthyroidism and myxoedema.

(*e*) Sleep deprivation and other disorders of sleep (see Meldrum 1982).

(*f*) Conditions associated particularly with childhood:
Rickets; acute infections ('febrile convulsions').

3. *Psychological factors*
These are relatively unimportant. It is doubtful whether psychological factors alone can ever cause any form of epilepsy. In individuals otherwise predisposed, however, fright or anxiety and many other stress factors (Friis and Lund 1974) may precipitate attacks.

4. *Constitutional epilepsy*
When all the above factors have been excluded there remains a substantial group of patients who suffer from seizures for which no local or general cause can be found (see Laidlaw and Richens 1982; Porter 1984). We must, therefore, regard these individuals as suffering from a predisposition to epilepsy, a predisposition not yet understood, except in terms of the epileptic or convulsive threshold as mentioned above. It is also clear that the distinction between constitutional and symptomatic epilepsy is not clear-cut. There is an intermediate group of patients in whom predisposition determines the development of fits after a focal cerebral lesion such as a head injury. (See Lennox's (1947) study of twin pairs

with seizures.) Thus while a division of cases into symptomatic and idiopathic ('constitutional' or 'cryptogenic' or 'centrencephalic') groups is of some clinical value, a diagnosis of idiopathic epilepsy is, in a sense, a confession of failure as it simply implies that even with modern methods of investigation its cause cannot be demonstrated.

The history of patients suffering from epilepsy

The following questions should be posed to any patient believed to be suffering from fits.

When did the first attack occur? Did it follow an injury or was it associated with an acute illness? How soon was it followed by the second? What is the usual interval between the attacks? Are they increasing in frequency? Do the attacks occur in bouts? Has the patient had a series of attacks without recovering consciousness? Do the attacks occur at any special time of the day? Do they occur only by day or only by night? In the case of a woman, are they related to the menstrual periods? Is any fact known to precipitate the attacks? Does the patient have any warning? If so, what, and by how long does it precede the attack? How does an attack begin? Is its onset local or general, gradual or sudden? Is consciousness lost? Do convulsive movements occur in the attack? If so, are they symmetrical or asymmetrical? Has the patient injured himself in an attack? Does he bite his tongue and pass urine? How long do the attacks last? What is his condition afterwards? Are the attacks followed by headache, sleepiness, paralysis, confusion, or automatism? Is there any weakness of one or more limbs between attacks? What treatment has he had and how has he responded to it? Is he taking any other drugs? Has he at any time suffered from head injury? If the attacks did not begin in infancy, did he suffer from infantile convulsions? Is there a family history of epilepsy, or fainting fits, or of mental illness?

Heredity

Inherited predisposition plays a considerable part in the aetiology. In a series of 200 epileptics studied by Brain there was a positive family history in 28 per cent. We must distinguish, however, between the inheritance of a predisposition and the inheritance of epilepsy. What seems to be inherited is the physical or neurophysiological basis of a 'dysrhythmia', but only a small proportion of those with such a 'dysrhythmia' become epileptic. Lennox, Gibbs, and Gibb (1940) studied the EEG in the parents of epileptics; only in 5 per cent were both normal; in 35 per cent both were abnormal. They found that an abnormal EEG is six times as common among the relatives of epileptics as in controls, and this was true both of 'symptomatic' and 'idiopathic' epileptics. However, a history of epilepsy in other members of the family is obtained twice as often in patients with idiopathic epilepsy as in those with symptomatic seizures. Lennox (1947) believed that the 'dysrhythmia' is inherited as a Mendelian dominant trait and this is now generally agreed although the predisposition is clearly of relatively low penetrance (Brown 1982). For these reasons it is difficult to estimate the risk that an epileptic parent will transmit the disorder to his or her offspring, since it often remains latent and the condition may reappear in a collateral line. Not more than one in 36 of the children of a mixed group of epileptics develops seizures, on average, but in some families the incidence is higher. The risk is greater if there are several cases in the family and if the non-epileptic conjugal partner has a family history of epilepsy or an unstable EEG.

Trauma

The part played by trauma in aetiology is difficult to estimate. Certainly severe head injuries may be followed by epilepsy (p. 232). In adults, post-traumatic epilepsy rarely follows closed head injury unless the latter was severe enough to cause 24 hours of post-traumatic amnesia or unless 'early fits' occurred within the first week after the injury, in which case the development of subsequent post-traumatic epilepsy is much more common (Jennett 1982). The incidence is much greater after penetrating wounds of the brain and in young children or elderly subjects in whom less severe closed head injuries may be followed by fits. After missile injury the incidence rose from 11.4 per cent between one and two years to 33.3 per cent between three and five years in one series (Adelove and Odeku 1971). Jennett, Teather, and Bennie (1973) devised a statistical method of determining the percentage risk in individual cases depending upon such factors as the duration of post-traumatic amnesia, the presence or absence of a dural tear, and the occurrence of early epilepsy. The presence of an acute traumatic intracranial haematoma significantly increases the incidence of both early and late traumatic epilepsy (Jennett 1975). If early epilepsy is defined as one or more fits occurring in the first week, Jennett (1982) concluded that: (a) the overall incidence of epilepsy following missile injury and non-missile depressed fracture is about 30 per cent, fits beginning within the first year in about two-thirds; (b) after severe closed head injury with acute intracranial haematoma the incidence was 35 per cent, without haematoma 3 per cent; in haematoma cases, the incidence was 25 per cent in cases with early epilepsy, 3 per cent without, 17 per cent with depressed fracture, 4 per cent without. In patients with neither haematoma nor depressed fracture, it was 19 per cent with early epilepsy, 1 per cent without. Annegers, Grabow, Groover, Laws, Elveback, and Kurland (1980), in a survey of 2747 patients, found that the incidence of seizures after mild head injury was not significantly greater than in the general population.

One iatrogenic form of post-traumatic epilepsy is that which may follow electroconvulsive therapy (ECT). Patients so treated later demonstrate a five-fold greater tendency to develop spontaneous seizures than a control population, with a greater tendency to recurrence the longer the latency between the treatment and the first attack (Devinsky and Duchowny 1983).

Epilepsy is relatively commoner among firstborn children than among later members of the family, which may be explained by the increased liability of the firstborn to head injury during birth.

Other local cerebral lesions

Many other lesions of the nervous system may cause or predispose to epileptic attacks, for example, infantile hemiplegia. That minor cerebral lesions are also of some importance is indicated by the frequency with which slight pathological changes are found in the nervous system in epileptics. For example, Hodskins and Yakovlev (1930) found that the brain was normal at autopsy in only 17 per cent of 300 epileptics in an institution. In addition to many congenital abnormalities, the effects of perinatal trauma, and lesions caused by encephalitis or encephalopathy in childhood, some other disorders may lead to epilepsy developing in later life. These include eclampsia complicating pregnancy and cortical venous thrombosis complicating otitis media. Among the many lesions described at autopsy in some cases have been 'chronic localized encephalitis' (Rasmussen, Olszewski, and Lloyd-Smith 1958), focal cortical dysplasia (Taylor, Falconer, Bruton, and Corsellis 1971), neuronal heterotopias, hamartomas, meningo-angiomatosis, and other vascular malformations (Matheson 1982; Leblanc, Feindel, and Ethier 1983). However, it must be remembered that the anoxia and other metabolic changes consequent upon repeated convulsions may themselves produce neuropathological abnormalities in the brain (Meldrum and Brierley 1972). Epilepsy is associated with rheumatic heart disease more often than can be explained by chance. In mitral stenosis or valve prolapse small cerebral emboli may cause epilepsy, as may a small asymptomatic infarct due to intracranial atheroma (Dodge, Richardson, and Victor 1954).

Metabolic and endocrine factors

No constant metabolic abnormality is found in epileptic patients, though it is evident that metabolic disturbance often plays a part in the production of fits. Generalized convulsions may occur in tetany due to alkalosis, to destruction of the parathyroids, or to idiopathic hypoparathyroidism, and in epileptics a fit can often be precipitated if alkalosis is induced by over-breathing. There is no evidence, however, that alkalosis is usually responsible for attacks. Attacks are induced in some epileptics by water retention (Ansell and Clarke 1956) or by excessive alcohol consumption. The role of menstruation in precipitating attacks in some women is unexplained, but underlines the importance of hormonal and metabolic factors. Pregnancy may also influence the attacks; some women are free from attacks during pregnancy while others are worse. Schmidt, Canger, Avanzini, Battino, Cusi, Beck-Managetta, Koch, Rating, and Janz (1983) concluded, however, that the course of epilepsy in pregnancy is primarily influenced by non-compliance in drug treatment, sleep deprivation, or inadequate treatment. With good control of anticonvulsant therapy, pregnancy itself has only a minimal influence. Clearly epilepsy may be influenced for better or worse by many different factors.

Febrile convulsions

Convulsions accompanying febrile illnesses in infancy and early childhood are regarded by many authorities as carrying a good prognosis. Certainly some infants have one or two such attacks and no more but many go on to develop spontaneous fits later and some have definite epileptic discharges in the EEG (Frantzen, Lennox-Buchthal, and Nygaard 1968). Boys are more often affected than girls. Often there is a history of similar febrile convulsions occurring in some other member of the family (Frantzen, Lennox-Buchthal, Nygaard, and Stene 1970). Attacks so classified occur only in children of less than nine years of age and almost invariably between 6 months and 5 years of age (Shaw, Gall, and Schuman 1972; Lennox-Buchthal 1974), although fever may occasionally precipitate seizures in adult epileptics (*British Medical Journal* 1972). The attacks are occasionally fatal and if frequent may lead to permanent structural brain damage (*British Medical Journal* 1975 a; Lennox-Buchthal 1982; Gomez and Klass 1983). While many regard febrile convulsions as a specific clinical syndrome, others believe that they constitute merely one form of idiopathic epilepsy of childhood. There has been much dispute about the benefits of prophylactic treatment after the first attack; phenytoin has been found ineffective (Melchior, Buchthal, and Lennox-Buchthal 1971) but many workers recommend phenobarbitone for at least 12 months (Lennox-Buchthal 1974). Various clinical features, including prolonged seizures, focal features, recurrent attacks, early onset, mental retardation, and antecedent brain injury increased the risk of subsequent epilepsy (Lennox-Buchthal 1982). While intravenous diazepam is the drug of choice in an actual attack, sodium valproate (20–30 mg/kg body weight) may prove superior to phenobarbitone for prophylaxis and reduces the incidence of subsequent epilepsy, if started after the first attack, to about 10 per cent (Lennox-Buchthal 1982).

Neonatal fits and benign focal epilepsy of childhood

Neonatal fits may occur in the first 48 hours after birth, usually due to cerebral birth injury, or between the fifth and sixth day when they are generally the result of hypocalcaemia (*British Medical Journal* 1974). Benign focal epilepsy of childhood (Lerman and Kivity 1975; *British Medical Journal* 1975b) is a syndrome in which the patients show typical brief hemifacial seizures which tend to become generalized if they occur during sleep. The EEG usually shows slow, diphasic, high-voltage temporal spikes, often followed by slow waves. In all of a series of 100 cases (Lerman and Kivity 1975) the attacks ceased and the EEG changes disappeared before adult life. More recent reports, reviewed by Gogmez and Klass (1983), have shown that the condition usually develops between four and 10 years, is commoner in boys, often presents with an adversive seizure occurring during sleep or on waking, and that Rolandic as well as midtemporal spike discharges may be

recorded. While some doubt has been cast upon the specificity of this clinical entity, it appears to be a reasonably consistent syndrome which tends to remit with or without treatment.

Migraine

While loss of consciousness in an attack of migraine, often at the height of the headache, is usually syncopal, there is a slightly increased incidence of epilepsy in migraine sufferers, even in those who have no evidence of a cerebral lesion (such as an angioma) of which both the migraine and the epilepsy could be symptomatic. A possible role for tyramine in the physiological mechanism of the two disorders was postulated by Scott, Moffett, and Swash (1972). Cyclical vomiting, often regarded as being a migraine equivalent in childhood, may be a manifestation of simple partial seizures (abdominal epilepsy) (Mitchell, Greenwood, and Messenheimer 1983).

Sex and age incidence and epidemiology

Females were once said to suffer from epilepsy slightly more frequently than males. In Gowers' series of 3000 cases the ratio of females to males was 13:12. However, the sex incidence may be changing; Lennox and Lennox (1960) found that whereas under the age of 5 years there were 105 females for every 100 affected males, over the age of 20 years the male: female incidence was 100:59. The number of epileptics in the United Kingdom has been estimated to be about 300 000 with 35 000 new cases arising annually (Pond, Bidwell, and Stein 1960; Brewis, Poskanzer, Rolland, and Miller 1966; Office of Health Economics 1971). The commonest age of onset is 0–4 years, with the first fit occurring in many more patients between 5 and 24 years of age; the incidence of initial attacks then declines steadily throughout adult life with a further slight peak, especially in males, over the age of 65 years (Office of Health Economics 1971). Similar figures have been reported from many other countries including Switzerland, Holland, and the United States. Incidence rates vary from 20 to 50 per 100 000, prevalence rates from 1.3 per 1000 of the general population to 9.2 in Warsaw and 19.5 in Bogota, Colombia; a reasonable estimate is between 4 and 10 per 1000 world-wide (Zielinsky 1982).

Pathology

No constant pathological change is found in the brains of epileptics, though abnormalities are common. The difficulty is to determine which pathological changes may be the cause of epilepsy and which may have resulted from the seizures which, if severe and frequent, can undoubtedly cause cerebral anoxia. In patients with symptomatic epilepsy secondary to identifiable organic disease of the brain, little difficulty usually arises but the interpretation of minor changes in cases of presumed idiopathic epilepsy is more difficult (Meyer 1963). Probably in most such cases loss of nerve cells in the cortex and cerebellum, a finding often described, is the result, rather than the cause, of the epilepsy but small areas of cortical dysplasia, especially in the temporal lobe, may be causative in some cases (Taylor *et al.* 1971). Other uncommon causes include neuronal heterotopias, polymicrogyria, megalencephaly, areas of glial proliferation (possibly formes frustes of tuberous sclerosis), neurocutaneous melanosis, dermoid and epidermoid cysts, and the vascular malformations mentioned above (Mathieson 1982). Microscopically much attention has been directed to focal lesions in Ammon's horn. When recent these consist of foci of tissue destruction with prominent neuronal loss, especially in Sommer's sector, later followed by gliosis. Such changes may be responsible for temporal-lobe epilepsy in many cases and Earle, Baldwin, and Penfield (1953) suggested that hippocampal herniation at birth is an important aetiological factor. However, similar pathological changes in Ammon's horn and in the region of the amygdala may be due to anoxia and may certainly be the consequence of prolonged or recurrent seizures experimentally induced in animals (Meldrum and Brierley 1972) or of many processes inducing anoxia in man (Corsellis 1957). It now seems possible that in some cases these lesions may result from one or more febrile convulsions in infancy and that the mesial temporal sclerosis so induced then acts as a focus of epileptic discharge resulting in the subsequent development of temporal-lobe (complex partial) epilepsy (Falconer 1974). Perinatal cerebral infarction may be another aetiological factor in some cases (Rémillard, Ethier, and Andermann 1974). Cavanagh (1958) reported eight cases of temporal-lobe epilepsy of many years' standing associated with small tumours, mostly hamartomas, but a few showed early evidence of neoplastic transformation. In a large series of temporal lobes removed from patients with epilepsy, Falconer (1971) found mesial temporal sclerosis in one-half, between one-fifth and a quarter showed hamartomas or developmental anomalies, one-tenth scars or infarcts, and no specific pathological change was found in the remainder.

The clinical classification of seizures

Traditionally (Janz 1969), attacks of epilepsy, whether idiopathic or symptomatic, were divided into major epilepsy (grand mal), minor epilepsy (petit mal), focal epilepsy (Jacksonian epilepsy), temporal-lobe epilepsy (psychomotor epilepsy), and myoclonic attacks, and these traditional terms will be used in this chapter. However, this descriptive classification has become increasingly unsatisfactory for many reasons. Thus there are many forms of minor epilepsy, with or without transient impairment of consciousness, which are not true petit mal; in epilepsy of focal onset, depending upon the site of origin in the brain, a variety of motor, sensory, behavioural, and psychomotor manifestations may be noted but if the epileptic discharge spreads rapidly to become generalized, a major attack may occur and the focal symptoms then constitute merely the aura of the major attack. Temporal-lobe epilepsy is now more generally known as complex partial epilepsy (Penry and Daly 1975). Many new classifications have been proposed, notably by the International League Against Epilepsy (ILAE) (Gastaut 1969) and by Sutherland and Eadie (1980), while Laidlaw and Richens (1982) quote the comprehensive clinical and electroencephalographic classification recommended by the ILAE, the World Federation of Neurology, the World Federation of Neurosurgical Societies, and the International Federation of Societies for Electroencephalography and Clinical Neurophysiology. A simpler working classification, from Marsden and Reynolds (1982), is given in Table 22.1. They point out that it is, and always will be, impossible to create a single code to cover three basically incompatible systems of classification, viz.: one according to the clinical symptoms and signs in the attacks; one relating to the anatomical and physiological evidence as to its source; and one defining aetiology. Thus it is not always profitable to try to force all three systems into a single framework though all three are obviously complementary. The descriptions which follow will therefore be largely clinical, with secondary information included about pathophysiology and aetiology, where relevant, with reference to Table 22.1

Symptoms and signs

Tonic–clonic seizures (major epilepsy or grand mal)

Pre-convulsive symptoms. Epileptic patients sometimes have symptoms before an attack for hours, or even for a day or two, which warn them or those about them that a fit is likely to occur. These vague pre-convulsive symptoms include irritability and depression, abnormal feelings referred to the head, giddiness, and sudden myoclonic twitches.

Precipitating factors. Usually there are none. Rarely the type which more often causes syncope may precipitate a seizure (p. 188). Severe coughing may do so (so-called laryngeal epilepsy). Eating, or drinking alcohol, severe emotional stress, sleep depri-

Table 22.1. Classification of seizures*

1. *Generalized*
   a. Tonic–clonic (grand mal)
   b. Tonic
   c. Atonic
   d. Absence (petit mal)
   e. Atypical absence
   f. Myoclonic

2 *Partial (focal)*
   A. Without impairment of consciousness (simple partial seizures)
   B. With impairment of consciousness (complex partial seizures)
      a. With motor signs (e.g. Jacksonian, versive)
      b. With somato- or special sensory symptoms (e.g. olfactory, visual)
      c. With autonomic features (e.g. epigastric sensations)
      d. With psychic symptoms (e.g. fear, *déjà vu*)
      e. With automatisms (complex partial seizures only)

3. *Partial seizures secondarily generalized*
   i.e. clinical or electrical evidence of focal discharge, during or after the generalized seizure

4. *Unclassifiable*
   Seizures which cannot be classified because of incomplete data.

*From Marsden and Richens (1982).

vation, or various metabolic changes sometimes bring on an attack. There are also many varieties of evoked or reflex epilepsy (see p. 616).

The aura. The aura, or warning of the attack, occurs in up to three-fifths of all seizures. It is a symptom produced by the onset of the epileptic discharge and is perceived by the patient before consciousness is lost. In other cases the patient has no warning, but becomes unconscious at once. In true 'idiopathic' major epilepsy, if such exists, the aura is generally absent or brief and indefinable, but in partial seizures secondarily generalized (Table 22.1) the aura has the typical characteristics of the partial seizure occurring in that patient, before a generalized tonic–clonic fit supervenes. An aura is less common in major seizures than in those with a focal onset. Since the epileptic discharge may originate in many different localities within the brain, many different auras may be experienced. In complex partial seizures it may take the form of mental symptoms, such as a feeling of unreality (*jamais vu*) or, alternatively, of intense familiarity (*déjà vu*), as though events being experienced had happened before. The patient may feel disembodied, or may experience severe but inexplicable fear. This last aura is sometimes associated with running, the patient running several yards before falling unconscious—'cursive epilepsy'. If the discharge begins in the anterior temporal region, olfactory and gustatory hallucinations may occur; if more posterior, there may be visual auras consisting of complex scenes (formed visual hallucinations) or simple flashes of light or balls of fire (crude visual hallucinations); auditory auras may also take the form of systematized hallucinations (hearing actual words or phrases) or may consist merely of crude sounds. Vertigo or subjective giddiness is a common aura. Sensory auras can consist of feelings of numbness, tingling, or electric shocks referred to part of the body, or even a sensation as though a limb were shrivelling up. Painful sensory auras occur, but are rare. Abnormal visceral sensations are common in complex partial attacks, the patient experiencing a peculiar sensation ('butterflies' in the stomach) or sometimes even epigastric pain. Sexual arousal or orgasm sometimes occur (Rémillard, Andermann, Testa, Gloor, Aubé, Martin, Feindel, Guberman, and Simpson 1983). There are many forms of motor aura. A strong impulse to speak can be associated with inability to do so or else there may be chewing or 'smacking' of the lips, again usually in complex partial seizures. The fit may begin with spasm or clonic movement of part of the body, such as turning of the head and eyes to one side (an adversive attack) or flexion of one upper limb, and the patient may be aware of the movement before losing consciousness. Sometimes the whole body is rotated to one side.

Often the aura is brief and is no more than a transient indefinable sensation so that the patient is unable to describe it though he knows that he has a warning of insufficient duration for him to be able to reach a safe place.

The convulsion. The convulsion may begin with the epileptic cry, a harsh scream due to forcible expiration of air through the partly closed vocal cords, but this is more often absent than present. Consciousness is lost either immediately after the aura or at the onset, and the patient falls to the ground. He usually has no recollection of falling. In the fall he may injure himself, and permanent scars on the face, limbs, or trunk are common in epileptics. The first motor manifestation of the convulsion proper is usually a phase of generalized tonic muscular spasm. This is usually symmetrical on both sides of the body, though the head and eyes are sometimes rotated to one side and the mouth is occasionally drawn to one side. The upper limbs are usually adducted at the shoulders and flexed at the elbows and wrists. The fingers are flexed at the metacarpophalangeal and extended at the interphalangeal joints, the thumb being adducted. The lower limbs are usually extended, with the feet inverted. Respiratory and trunk muscles are also affected and respiration is temporarily arrested. The tonic phase may last only a few seconds and rarely for more than half a minute. This phase may be so intense that occasionally compression fracture of the body of one or more thoracic vertebrae can occur in a fit; this should be borne in mind if the patient complains of pain in the back after recovery.

This is followed by the clonic phase, in which sustained tonic contraction of the muscles gives place to sharp, short, interrupted jerks. In the clonic phase the tongue may be bitten if caught between the teeth when the jaw is closed. Foaming at the mouth (salivation) may occur, and the saliva may be blood-stained if the tongue has been bitten. Incontinence of urine often occurs; incontinence of faeces is less common.

At the onset of an epileptic fit the patient may be either pale or flushed. He becomes progressively cyanosed during the arrest of respiration which occurs in the tonic stage, but this passes when breathing is re-established in the clonic stage. Subconjunctival or cutaneous petechial haemorrhages may occur. There is often profuse sweating. The pupils dilate at the beginning of the attack and the reaction to light is usually lost. The corneal reflexes are also lost in a severe attack; the tendon reflexes may be abolished and the plantar reflexes may become extensor for a short time afterwards.

The post-convulsive phase. Towards the end of the clonic phase the intervals between the contractions become longer and the jerks finally cease. The patient remains unconscious for a variable time, usually from a few minutes to half an hour, and on recovering consciousness often sleeps for several hours. Headache is common. Usually after recovering his senses the patient is mentally normal. Exceptionally, however, a convulsion is followed by an abnormal mental state (often simple confusion) lasting for a few minutes or even for several hours. In post-epileptic automatism (usually a feature of complex partial seizures) the patient, though apparently conscious, may carry out a series of complex actions which are often inappropriate to the circumstances and of which he subsequently has no recollection. Sometimes the epileptic attack is followed by a period of hysterical behaviour. Rarely the patient becomes maniacal after a fit. Post-epileptic mental disturbances follow complex partial seizures more often than uncomplicated major fits.

Minor epilepsy

Minor epilepsy is an inclusive term often applied to all mild or brief epileptic attacks in which transient impairment or loss of consciousness is the most prominent feature.

Absence seizures (petit mal)

Whereas some years ago the term petit mal was often used to identify all forms of minor epilepsy unaccompanied by convulsions, the term is now reserved for transient minor 'absences' or 'blank spells' which almost invariably begin in childhood and virtually never in adult life, though in occasional cases, having begun in a child, they may continue for many years (Gibberd 1972). In the present state of knowledge, true petit mal is invariably idiopathic, never symptomatic. The child, without warning, stares blankly into space, the eyes may roll up beneath the upper lids, and for a second or two he will stop talking or whatever he is doing and then will continue with his activity, often unaware that an attack has taken place. Occasionally a single myoclonic twitch of the head and upper limbs may accompany such episodes. Falling does not usually occur and the attacks often occur many times in the day. Some patients with attacks of petit mal also have major seizures or develop these as they grow older. Attacks of true petit mal are usually accompanied by 3 Hz generalized wave-and-spike discharges in the EEG (p. 618). Occasionally the 'petit mal triad' of absences, myoclonic jerking, and drop attacks occurs in such cases but much more often this combination proves to be indicative of one of the forms of progressive myoclonic epilepsy of childhood or of the Lennox–Gastaut syndrome (see below) (Marsden and Reynolds 1982). In occasional cases, too, transient lip-smacking, chewing, or mouthing movements or other brief automatisms are seen in patients with the typical 'petit mal' EEG pattern during the attacks; these have been called complex absences or absences with automatism. Rarely prolonged mental confusion or even stupor in childhood or much less commonly in adult life may result from 'petit mal status' (Brett 1966; Schwartz and Scott 1971; Bateman, O'Grady, Willey, Longley, and Barwick 1983). Very occasionally, in the elderly, psychosis may be simulated (Tivanainen, Bergström, Nuntila, and Vinkari 1984).

An epileptic encephalopathy in childhood characterized by frequent tonic seizures and atypical absences, a low IQ, and an interictal EEG with frequent diffuse spike and slow-wave discharges occurring at 2–2.5 Hz has been called the *Lennox–Gastaut syndrome*, petit mal variant or atypical absence; in such cases benzodiazepine, paradoxically, may precipitate status epilepticus (Tassinari, Gastaut, Dravet, and Roger 1971). It is now evident that this is a syndrome of multiple aetiology, often, but not invariably, associated with progressive organic brain disease. Even if one excludes patients shown eventually to be suffering from a neuronal storage disorder, or tuberous sclerosis, to quote but two examples, the remaining cases are by no means homogeneous. Nevertheless, they share common features including brief atonic, myoclonic, and tonic seizures, an onset usually after two years of age, rarely after seven or eight, a high incidence of mental retardation, slow spike-and-wave discharge in the EEG, and a poor response to treatment (Aicardi 1982). In some cases these features follow a phase of infantile spasms (see below). Possibly most cases of 'petit mal status' are of this type rather than being due to the benign absence syndrome or true petit mal (Brown 1982).

Other forms of minor epilepsy

These can occur at any age and may be idiopathic or symptomatic, the pattern depending upon the origin and spread of the epileptic discharge. Some such attacks, occurring either in childhood or in adult life, are clinically indistinguishable from true petit mal.

The slightest form of minor epilepsy, often described by the patient as a 'sensation', consists of a disturbance of consciousness often similar to the aura of a major attack, and sometimes associated with giddiness. In a 'sensation', consciousness may or may not be completely lost. Next in severity comes complete loss of consciousness, with or without an aura, but the motor and postural functions of the brain are so little affected that the patient remains standing and does not fall. He looks somewhat dazed and stares as in an attack of petit mal. After a few seconds he recovers and may continue what he was doing before the attack. In more severe attacks motor and postural functions are affected, and the patient, besides losing his senses, may fall to the ground or may exhibit slight muscular rigidity or carry out a brief stereotyped movement. Attacks in which falling occurs but in which there are no convulsive movements are often called *akinetic epilepsy*. The term *atonic epilepsy* is sometimes used, alternatively, to describe such attacks or else episodes of inhibitory epilepsy (see below). Akinetic attacks are occasionally due to prolonged episodes of true petit mal; much more often they are properly classifed as minor attacks aetiologically similar to tonic–clonic attacks but without the tonic and clonic contractions. Transitory pallor may occur in minor epilepsy. Incontinence of urine may occur, though it is less frequent than in major attacks. There is usually no post-ictal coma.

Complex partial seizures (temporal-lobe epilepsy).

The clinical picture of complex partial seizures depends upon whether the epileptic discharge remains localized to the temporal lobe (in which case focal features related to temporal-lobe dysfunction are consistently noted), or to the contiguous part of the frontal lobe (Marsden and Reynolds 1982), or whether it spreads rapidly throughout the remainder of the brain, in which case there may be a major fit with a 'temporal-lobe aura' or even a major fit without an aura (*partial seizure secondarily generalized*) which is then indistinguishable from an attack of idiopathic grand mal. The EEG is of considerable value in diagnosis. In these attacks the patient may become confused, often anxious and negativistic, and sometimes carries out movements of a highly organized but semi-automatic character (automatism).

Automatism may take various forms; sometimes it is purposeless, occasionally purposive (e.g. undressing in public or sexual automatisms, including masturbation or pelvic thrusting (Spencer, Spencer, Williamson, and Mattson 1983); and, rarely, aggressive or violent behaviour can occur. In such cases the epileptic discharge seems to originate in the periamygdaloid region (Feindel and Penfield 1954). Only very rarely can violent behaviour occurring during such a period of automatism be accepted as the cause of violent crime (Walton 1963; Gunn and Fenton 1971), but outbursts of rage due to this cause are well documented (Holden 1957). Gelastic epilepsy, in which outbursts of laughing occur during the attack (Gumpert, Hansotia, and Upton 1970), can occur in association with cursive epilepsy (running at the onset) (Chen and Forster 1973); these too are forms of automatism. Attacks may last for only a few seconds or for minutes or longer whether or not a major convulsion follows the aura. Theodore, Porter, and Penry (1983) used videotape analysis and showed that the mean duration of an attack in 163 seizures occurring in 40 patients was 128 seconds. Automatism, usually simple, stereotyped, or aimless, occurred in 97 per cent of seizures, clonic movements of the eyelids in only 19 attacks, and of the extremities in four. Only nine patients had auras. Varied disturbances of the content of consciousness occur in some attacks: these include hallucinations of smell and taste (uncinate epilepsy), vision and hearing, perceptual illusions, disordered sense of reality or of the body, disturbances of memory, and paroxysms of fear. Complex partial status epilepticus, giving fluctuating impairment of consciousness and unsustained responses, is a rare phenomenon which may be confirmed by EEG recording (Shalev and Amir 1983). Recurring nightmares may represent one form of attack (Boller, Wright, Cavalieri, and Mitsumoto 1975). Visual phenomena may include formed hallucinations, macropsia, and micropsia, while depersonalization (*jamais vu* or unreality) suggests to the patient a dream or 'trance-like' state and *déjà vu*, an intense feeling of familiarity, may be accompanied by vivid visual or auditory memory patterns which the patient is subsequently unable to recall, though remembering that they were familiar and a constantly recurring pattern of his attack. Differential diagnosis from the phobic anxiety-depersona-

lization syndrome, often presenting with agaraphobia in middle-aged women ('the house-bound housewife') may give rise to difficulty in differential diagnosis but the EEG can be very helpful (Harper and Roth 1962). Depression is also an occasional feature. Impaired sexual drive is common (Taylor 1969) and hypergraphia (compulsive writing) has been described (Waxman and Geschwind 1974). Uncinate attacks are characterized by hallucinations of smell or taste. They are often accompanied by movements of the lips, tongue, and jaw, for example, those of tasting or chewing, and are commonly associated with a disturbance of memory (Currie, Heathfield, Henson, and Scott 1971). Uncinate attacks are usually the result of organic disease in the region of the uncus (see p. 612).

Jacksonian epilepsy.

Jacksonian epilepsy (motor partial or focal epilepsy) usually begins in one of three foci, the thumb and index finger, the angle of the mouth, or the great toe. A convulsion with such a focal onset and the type of spread described on page 34 is almost always a symptom of organic brain disease in the region of the precentral gyrus. A similar focal onset occasionally occurs in cases in which no such lesion can be demonstrated, especially in benign focal epilepsy of childhood (see p. 612).

Sensory focal epilepsy.

This is the sensory equivalent of motor Jacksonian epilepsy and consists of paraesthesiae, such as tingling or 'electric shocks', less frequently of painful sensation, involving usually a part or the whole of one side of the body. The attacks can occur without loss of consciousness and are usually the result of a lesion in the opposite parietal lobe.

Epilepsia partialis continua.

This is a rare form of focal epilepsy in which Jacksonian attacks, confined to a limited part of the body, continue for hours, days, weeks, or rarely months, without stopping. It is invariably due to a focal cerebral lesion though its nature may not be immediately apparent.

Adversive attacks.

These begin with turning of the head and eyes and sometimes of the body to the opposite side: they originate in front of the precentral gyrus in the region of the so-called frontal eye field (Brodmann's area 8).

Inhibitory or ataxic epilepsy.

This is a very rare form of attack in which transitory loss of power occurs in a limb or in one-half of the body without precedent tonic spasm or clonic movements. It may or may not be associated with impairment or loss of consciousness.

'Drop' attacks.

In these the patient falls to the ground without warning. The only evidence for loss of consciousness is unawareness of the fall itself. The patient can get up at once. There are two varieties: (1) a form of akinetic epilepsy (see above); and (2) sudden falls occurring chiefly in middle-aged or elderly women. It is unlikely that the latter are epileptic; they seem often to be associated with atheromatous ischaemia of the brainstem (vertebro-basilar insufficiency). However, Stevens and Matthews (1983), confirming that this type of attack is almost totally confined to women and that, in contradistinction to akinetic epilepsy, consciousness is fully retained, were not convinced that ischaemia is a satisfactory explanation, but could suggest no satisfactory alternative.

'Tonic epilepsy.'

These attacks consist of episodes of muscular rigidity, usually associated with loss of consciousness, but not followed by clonic movements. Gastaut, Roger, Ouahchi, Timsit, and Broughton (1963) pointed out that these attacks usually last 10–20 seconds, often occur at night, and cause tonic contraction of various combinations of muscle groups, respiratory arrhythmia, tachycardia, mydriasis, flushing, and salivation; some patients have other types of attacks as well and many are mentally retarded. Tonic status epilepticus has been reported to present with a confusional state (Somerville and Bruni 1983). In the usual tonic fit the posture of the body differs from that of the tonic phase of a major seizure. The head is extended, the upper limbs are thrown out in front of the patient, extended at the elbows, internally rotated and hyperpronated, with the fingers somewhat flexed. The lower limbs are extended. This type of fit is usually the result of organic brain disease (see p. 612) but occurs rarely in idiopathic epilepsy. Focal 'tonic fits' in which similar attacks may involve one or two limbs without loss of consciousness have been described in multiple sclerosis and have been attributed to the presence of a brainstem lesion (Matthews 1954).

Diencephalic epilepsy

Epilepsy of diencephalic origin, characterized by many phenomena indicating transient autonomic dysfunction, including spontaneous periodic hypothermia (Fox, Wilkins, Bell, Bradley, Browse, Cranston, Foley, Gilby, Hebden, Jenkins, and Rawlins 1973), has been postulated but there is still controversy as to whether such periodic diencephalic phenomena are truly epileptic.

Vestibular and vestibulogenic attacks. Behrman and Wyke (1958) distinguished two varieties of attack both with an aura of vertigo. They suggested that vestibular attacks originate in the cortical vestibular centre in the midtemporal region and that vestibulogenic attacks are excited by labyrinthine discharge, often from an abnormal labyrinth, which excites discharge from neurones in the brainstem reticular system.

Evoked or reflex epilepsy. Sometimes an attack can be excited by some form of external stimulation (*British Medical Journal* 1975c). This may be a sudden loud noise—*acoustico-motor epilepsy*—or music—*musicogenic epilepsy*—or a visual—*photic*—or cutaneous stimulus. The precipitation of attacks by reading is well recognized ('*reading epilepsy*') (Bingel 1957; Stoupel 1968), but in some cases they are also precipitated by speaking and writing (*language-induced epilepsy*) (Geschwind and Sherwin 1967) or by blinking when starting to speak (Terzano, Parrino, Manzoni, and Mancia 1983). It is uncertain as to whether in reading epilepsy the attacks are precipitated by the written or printed word, by the eye movements involved in reading, or by some other mechanism (Brooks and Jirauch 1971). So-called '*television epilepsy*' has also been increasingly recognized. Both childhood petit mal and more particularly grand mal in children and less commonly in adults may be precipitated by watching television, particularly when the set is flickering or poorly adjusted so that flickering lines appear. Driving along a sunlit road with the sunlight intermittently interrupted by a line of trees is a classical stimulus (Marsden and Reynolds 1982) and in *self-induced epilepsy* children have been observed to produce recurrent attacks, usually of petit mal, by passing their opened fingers rapidly between their eyes and a bright light source, usually the sun (Hutchison, Stone, and Davidson 1958; Whitty 1960; Ames 1971). *Tactile epilepsy* is a form in which attacks, sometimes myoclonic, less often focal or generalized, are induced by touching a limb or by other somatic sensory stimuli. Sometimes a voluntary movement will precipitate an attack. Some such are clearly '*seizures induced by movement*', while other attacks of *paroxysmal kinesogenic choreoathetosis or dystonia*, often of autosomal dominant inheritance (see p. 342) are less clearly epileptic in nature (Lance 1963) but in the light of their response to anticonvulsant drugs are probably related phenomena. In some such cases sudden movement appears to induce a type of 'tonic fit' in the limb which is moved (Lishman, Symons, Whitty, and Willison 1962). Numerous activities which may act in this way were described by Symonds (1959). Coughing may precipitate an attack (*cough seizures*), perhaps through transient reduction in cerebral blood flow due to a reduced venous return to the heart; this is especially liable to occur in patients with overt or unsuspected cerebral vascular disease (Morgan-Hughes 1966), but most such cases are examples of cough syncope. So-called carotid sinus epilepsy (Behrman and Knight 1956) is almost certainly carotid sinus syncope leading to epileptiform manifestations in the attacks.

There may be visceral concomitants; not only may gastric distension precipitate an attack, but in some patients the onset is always associated with diarrhoea.

Reflex inhibition of a fit is an allied phenomenon. When a convulsion has a focal onset and begins with movement, for example, of one limb, a strong stimulus, such as a firm grip, rubbing, or passive movement applied to the limb, will often abort an attack, if it is begun immediately after the onset. Efron (1956, 1957) showed that uncinate attacks may sometimes be arrested by smelling a powerful odour.

Pyknolepsy. Pyknolepsy is a term once applied to a syndrome characterized by very frequent attacks of petit mal. As the condition in no way differs from petit mal the term has now been discarded.

Infantile spasms (West's syndrome)

This name has been given to brief attacks, beginning almost invariably in infants within the first few months of life, in which there is a sudden shock-like flexion of the arms and often flexion of the head, neck, and trunk with drawing up of the knees (so-called salaam attacks). These momentary attacks may occur many times in the day; their development sometimes in infants who appear to be of normal intellect is followed by progressive mental deterioration so that when they eventually cease the child is often left spastic and severely retarded. The incidence is about 0.25–0.35 per 1000 live births, boys are affected more often than girls, and familial occurrence is very rare (Aicardi 1982). The EEG usually shows a pattern of almost continuous irregular slow spike-and-wave activity which has been called hypsarrhythmia (Gibbs and Gibbs 1952; Bower and Jeavons, 1959; Kiloh, McComas, Osselton, and Upton 1981). In many cases coming to autopsy the degenerative changes seen in the cortex and white matter of the cerebrum are non-specific but in some there is evidence of dysmyelination or of other disorders of development, and the syndrome has been observed in children with hypoglycaemia, phenylketonuria, perinatal brain damage, and tuberous sclerosis (della Rovere, Hoare, and Pampiglione 1964). Abnormalities of dendritic development in the pyramidal neurones of the frontal cortex have also been described (Huttenlocher 1974). While anticonvulsants are relatively ineffective (apart from the benzodiazepines which are effective in some cases), ACTH or steroid drugs, if given early enough, sometimes arrest the process. The spasms and the hypsarrhythmic EEG tend to disappear spontaneously before three years of age to be replaced by other types of seizure in about half the patients (Jeavons and Bower 1974). Mental retardation is found in 90 per cent of cases and spastic weakness in about a third. The prognosis is best in idiopathic or cryptogenic cases in which treatment is begun early, and worst in the many in which the spasms are symptomatic of many degenerative brain diseases (Aicardi 1982). The death rate in infancy is between 10 and 20 per cent.

Psychogenic seizures or pseudoseizures

Attacks which can closely simulate epileptic seizures, especially of the akinetic type, may be a manifestation of hysteria, especially in young girls (p. 663) but many forms of psychogenic seizure occur; there has been much recent interest in methods of differentiating between such seizures and true epilepsy; videotape monitoring combined with EEG telemetry is often helpful (Trimble 1983a). While Krumholz and Niedermeyer (1983) found that in 41 patients with well-documented psychogenic seizures, there was evidence of coexisting organic nervous disease in 44 per cent, mental retardation in 17 per cent, and concurrent genuine epilepsy in 37 per cent, Lesser, Lueders, and Dinner (1983), by contrast, found clinical and EEG evidence of epilepsy in only five out of 50 such cases. Appropriate psychotropic drugs, behaviour therapy, relaxation, and biofeedback techniques all have a place in treatment (Trimble 1983a).

Myoclonic epilepsy. See page 630.

The time-relationship of attacks

Individuals differ greatly with respect to the frequency of their attacks. At one extreme are those who have only one, or perhaps two, in a lifetime; at the other, those who convulse several times a day.

As Gowers pointed out, there are three common modes of onset. A child may have petit mal for a long period before beginning to have major fits. Alternatively, the first attack may be a severe one and thereafter major fits may occur at short intervals, with or without attacks of petit mal in addition; or there may be major attacks separated by long intervals of months or even in years. In 76 per cent of Gowers' cases the intervals between attacks were less than one month. Some patients always have attacks in clusters of two or more within a few hours.

Time of day is an important factor. In 42 per cent of a series of cases studied by Brain, attacks occurred by day only, in 24 per cent by night only, and in the remainder both by day and night. When the attacks were confined to the day they occurred only half as often as in the other two groups. 'Nocturnal' attacks can also occur during daytime sleep. Nocturnal fits are most likely to occur shortly after going to sleep and between 4 and 5 a.m., while the commonest time for diurnal attacks is during the first hour after awakening. Gibberd and Bateson (1974), in a review of 645 cases, found that only 38 had attacks which occurred only during sleep; of those beginning with nocturnal attacks only, the proportion who subsequently developed diurnal attacks increased year by year. Sleep deprivation may also precipitate attacks (Gunderson, Dunne, and Feher 1973). Menstruation often influences the occurrence of fits in women. Some have attacks in relation to the menstrual period, usually just before it begins, less often during or immediately after (Laidlaw 1956). 'Long-distance rhythms', i.e. the regular recurrence of attacks at intervals of many months, have also been described.

Status epilepticus.

An epileptic patient may have a succession of fits with recovery of consciousness between them—serial epilepsy. Sometimes however, one attack follows another without any intervening period of consciousness—status epilepticus. Unless the attacks can be arrested, coma deepens, and pyrexia, or even hyperpyrexia, develops, and death occurs. Some patients have a curious liability to develop status epilepticus, and do so on many occasions.

Status epilepticus occurs more often in symptomatic than idiopathic epilepsy; there seems to be an association with frontal-lobe lesions and possibly cerebral oedema (Janz 1964; Oxbury and Whitty 1971). While status in early post-traumatic epilepsy in adults usually implies that the brain injury has been severe, paradoxically it seems to be rare after severe head injury in childhood and much commoner after minor or even trivial injury (Grand 1974). Prolonged confusion due to petit mal status has been described in childhood (Brett 1966) and adult life (p. 614) and subclinical 'electrical status epilepticus' occurring during sleep with almost continuous spike-and-wave discharge which ceases on waking, in mentally retarded children who suffer occasional diurnal petit mal and nocturnal grand mal, has also been reported (Patry, Lyagoubi, and Tassinari 1971). Tonic status and complex partial status, as mentioned above, can also cause prolonged impairment of consciousness, sometimes with automatism or a fugue-like state, in both adults and children (Shalev and Amir 1983; Somerville and Bruni 1983).

Status epilepticus in animals is accompanied first by marked rises in arterial and cerebral venous pressure with severe metabolic and respiratory acidosis, hyperglycaemia, and reduced arteriovenous (AV) differences for oxygen and carbon dioxide. In the later stages blood pressure is low, cerebral AV differences for O_2 and CO_2 are enhanced, and there is usually hyperpyrexia,

hyperkalaemia, and hypoglycaemia (Meldrum and Horton 1973; Meldrum 1982).

Mental and physical abnormalities

No mental or physical abnormalities are constantly associated with epilepsy, and many epileptic patients exhibit neither. Nevertheless, as already indicated, there are many organic or metabolic disorders of the brain which can produce both dementia and epilepsy. Epilepsy is sometimes associated with mental retardation, and one easily recognizable type of retarded, epileptic child is excitable, noisy, destructive, and difficult to control ('the hyperkinetic syndrome'). The cause of the progressive mental deterioration which sometimes accompanies epilepsy is obscure. It may not always be a direct result of the fits, since it can be absent in patients having frequent severe attacks, but recurrent anoxia occurring in major fits and giving rise to progressive brain damage is certainly the cause in many cases.

Behaviour disorders, with aggressive outbursts and paranoid traits, are particularly common in some adults and children with severe temporal-lobe epilepsy (see Gallhofer et al. 1985). Furthermore, epilepsy does occur occasionally in patients suffering from psychotic illnesses, particularly paranoid schizophrenia.

Thus it may be concluded that epilepsy itself does not necessarily *produce* mental changes unless the fits are severe or frequent enought to cause anoxic damage to the brain, when there may be sudden mental deterioration, especially in childhood (Illingworth 1955) or else progressive dementia may develop. Mental dullness and lack of concentration with a deteriorating performance in school or at work is sometimes due to the drugs being given to treat the epilepsy rather than to the condition itself and anticonvulsant-induced folic-acid deficiency has been suggested as a possible aetiological factor (Neubaver 1970). Petit mal and complex partial status should also be excluded (see above). Bourgeois, Prensky, Palkes, Talen, and Busch (1983) have documented a progressive fall in the intelligence quotient in 11 per cent of a series of children whose epilepsy was difficult to control and in whom anticonvulsant blood levels were often found to be in the toxic range. They suggest that, especially in young children, total seizure control should not be achieved at the price of repeated episodes of drug toxicity. Reynolds (1983) and Trimble (1983b) stress that personality disorder is a style of behaviour which encompasses long-lasting personality traits and agree that, especially in patients with temporal-lobe foci of repeated epileptic discharge, there is often a vulnerability to significant personality change. While accepting that this area is still a source of fertile controversy, and while accepting that powerful psychosexual influences as well as the effects of drugs may play a part, they agree that many patients, especially those with poor seizure control, and with medial temporal-lobe lesions, in whom attacks rapidly become generalized and start at about puberty, do develop a psychosis or a subtle organic psychosyndrome with progressive personality change.

Physical signs which were described in some cases of epilepsy in early reports, including nystagmus, dysarthria, and ataxia, were in most instances due to drug treatment rather than to the disease. Other features such as spasticity, cerebellar and other long-tract signs, when present, should invariably suggest that the epilepsy is symptomatic of an underlying organic lesion of the brain.

No constant endocrine abnormality has been found to be associated with epilepsy, though minor disorders of skeletal growth and genital development are common. Some adolescent epileptics are exceptionally tall for their age. Obesity of the hypopituitary and eunuchoid type is sometimes seen, together with a heterosexual distribution of pubic hair, but these changes, as well as coarsening of the facial features (Falconer and Davidson 1973) are more probably due to anticonvulsant therapy, especially with phenytoin. In spite of numerous investigations no constant metabolic abnormality has been identified in cases of 'idiopathic' epilepsy. Frequent major fits, mental backwardness, and tetany, sometimes with intracranial calcification, may occur in cases of idiopathic hypoparathyroidism and in pseudohypoparathyroidism (Simpson 1952; Glaser and Levy 1960); the fits may be improved by treatment with dihydrotachysterol (*A.T. 10*) given in an initial dosage of 1.25 mg three times daily until the serum calcium is normal, and then a smaller maintenance dose is required.

Investigative findings

In 'idiopathic' epilepsy the CSF is normal except that during or after frequent fits or an attack of status there may be a rise in pressure to above 200 mm of fluid and a modest rise in protein content of the fluid. A consistently raised CSF protein and a pleocytosis should suggest that the epilepsy is symptomatic. Pneumoencephalography, sometimes done in the past, usually gave normal findings but in some cases of long-standing epilepsy or epilepsy of late onset signs of ventricular dilatation and cortical atrophy were found (Hunter, Hurwitz, Fullerton, Nieman, and Davies 1962). It was not certain as to whether these findings indicated that the cortical atrophy was the result of frequent fits or whether an unspecified degenerative process causing the cortical atrophy was also the cause of the attacks. The radiological abnormalities resulting from neoplasms, hamartomas, focal scarring, mesial temporal sclerosis, and the other numerous causes of temporal-lobe epilepsy were reviewed by Newcombe and Shah (1975); dilatation of, or a filling defect in, one temporal horn, often requiring tomography for its demonstration, was the commonest finding.

Computerized transaxial tomography (the CT scan p. 80) has been employed increasingly in the investigation of epileptic patients, particularly in adult life, in order to exclude the presence of a cerebral lesion of which the epilepsy may be symptomatic. Bogdanoff, Stafford, Green, and Gonzalez (1975) in a study of 50 unselected cases of focal epilepsy using the CT scan found porencephalic cysts in six, diffuse cerebral atrophy in five, cerebellar hemiatrophy in three, focal cortical atrophy in two, neoplasms in two, hydrocephalus in one, and cerebellar hypoplasia in one. More recently, Guberman (1983), in a study of 196 unselected adult epileptic subjects without abnormal neurological signs, found 16 per cent of abnormal scans, with the highest yield (44 per cent) in patients with partial seizures. In 25 of 51 cases with abnormal scans a specific lesion amenable to treatment was detected including 16 neoplasms and five arteriovenous malformations. Other lesions included focal or diffuse atrophy, infarcts, and tuberous sclerosis. Young, Costanzi, Mohr, and St. Clair Forbes (1982), on the other hand, thought that CT scanning should be reserved for patients showing focal features clinically or in the EEG, but Gilliatt and Shorvon (1983) concluded after finding meningiomas in five out of 80 patients first developing seizures over 40 years of age that CT scanning is obligatory in late-onset epilepsy, i.e. in patients first developing fits after 30 years of age. The scan is also capable of detecting mesial temporal sclerosis in many cases (Wyller and Bolender 1983).

Inter-ictal positron emission tomography (PET scanning) using ^{18}F-fluorodeoxyglucose, is particularly valuable in demonstrating areas of hypometabolism in the cortex in patients with partial seizures (Engel, Brown, Kuhl, Phelps, Mazziotta, and Crandall 1982; Engel, Kuhl, Phelps, and Crandall 1982; Engel, Kuhl, Phelps, and Mazziotta 1982); the EEG is then useful in confirming that the hypometabolic zone is epileptogenic, while the PET scan can be useful in confirming that the epileptic discharge is arising in that zone and is not being conducted from another site (Theodore, Newmark, Sato, Brooks, Patronas, de la Paz, Di Chiro, Kessler, Margolin, Manning, Channing, and Porter 1983); this information is especially valuable in intractable cases of temporal-lobe origin in which surgery is being considered.

Electroencephalography

The diagnostic importance of the EEG in epilepsy lies in the fact that an abnormal inter-ictal record may establish the diagnosis

when this is otherwise in doubt. Further, the effect of different drugs upon the abnormal activity, and the general response to treatment can be studied. It is important to stress the limitations of single routine EEG recordings in the diagnosis of epilepsy. From 10 to 20 per cent of epileptics have a normal EEG, and the percentage is higher in those having grand mal only and after the age of 40. A single normal EEG, therefore, does not exclude epilepsy. Patients with petit mal often show a 3–Hz generalized spike-and-

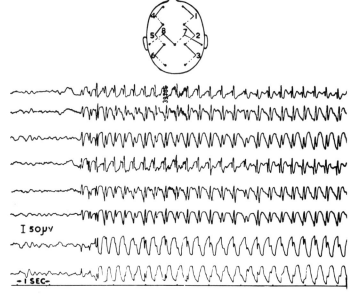

Fig. 22.1. Male, aged 18. Generalized, bilaterally synchronous and symmetrical 3 Hz wave-and-spike discharges during a petit mal (absence) attack.

wave discharge (see Fig. 22.1), but the abnormal activity may be present only after over-breathing. This pattern, however, is not pathognomonic of petit mal, but can occur in other forms of epilepsy. Major (tonic–clonic) seizures are not associated with any single characteristic inter-ictal EEG abnormality, but paroxysmal diffuse multiple spikes in rapid rhythm or isolated generalized paroxysmal outbursts of spike or sharp-wave activity are often associated with grand mal. Temporal-lobe (complex partial) epilepsy is often identified by means of focal spike or sharp-wave discharges arising in one or other temporal region (Fig. 22.2) or by paroxysmal outbursts of rhythmical slow theta activity which are similarly located. These discharges may only become apparent during sleep so that sleep recordings induced by sedative drugs may be helpful. Recording with sphenoidal or pharyngeal electrodes before, during, and after thiopentone-induced sleep is a valuable technique; it often demonstrates focal spikes or sharp waves; the unilateral absence of barbiturate-induced fast activity over one temporal lobe is also a useful guide to the presence of a focal epileptogenic lesion. Focal epileptogenic cortical lesions in other areas are often similarly associated with corresponding focal, abnormal EEG discharges (Fig. 22.3). Photic stimulation with different light sources at varying frequencies (see Fig. 22.4) is often useful in evoking epileptic discharges in the EEG in photosensitive epilepsy (Jeavons 1982a). With the possible exception of the wave-and-spike pattern with its fast and slow variants and focal spike discharges there is no abnormal EEG which is pathognomonic of epilepsy, and non-specific abnormalities may be found in epilepsy, psychoneurosis, psychopathy, or psychosis. It follows that an abnormal EEG can be interpreted only in relation to the clinical history of the patient (Gibbs and Gibbs 1947; Jasper and Kershman 1941; Williams 1941; Kiloh et al, 1981; Driver and McGillivray 1982). Electrocorticography is used for the precise localization of an epileptic focus at operation, and telemetering, a technique by means

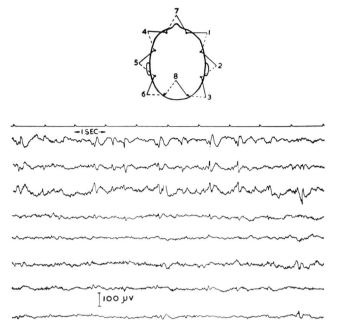

Fig. 22.2. Male, aged 30. Temporal-lobe epilepsy. Focal sharp and slow waves in the right temporal region.

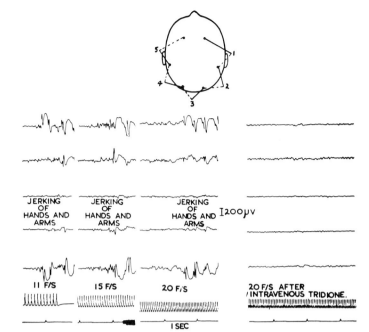

Fig. 22.4. Female, aged 19. Epilepsy, myoclonic. Photo-myoclonic response at various flash frequencies and subsequent effect of intravenous troxidone.

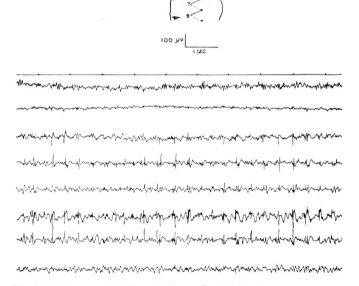

Fig. 22.3. Male, aged 14. Focal epilepsy. Focal spikes in the left temporo-parietal region.

of which the EEG can be conveyed from small transistorized transmitters attached to the mobile patient to a static recorder, can be used for continuous recording during diurnal activity and during sleep. The latter technique, if combined with videotape recording, is particularly useful in relating the patient's behaviour on the one hand to cerebral electrical events on the other. This and related techniques, including continuous recording in the ambulant and/or sleeping patient, using miniaturized tape recorders, are reviewed by Cull, Gilliatt, Willison, and Quy (1982).

Diagnosis

The diagnosis of epilepsy falls into two parts. It is first necessary to distinguish epileptic attacks from other paroxysmal episodes, and secondly, to decide whether the attacks are symptomatic of organic disease or whether the patient is suffering from 'idiopathic' epilepsy.

Diagnosis of the nature of the attack

Both minor and major attacks must be distinguished from *syncope*. Syncope usually occurs in individuals with vasomotor instability or as the result of exhaustion, haemorrhage, an emotional shock, sudden change of posture, standing for long periods, or disease of the autonomic nervous system (see pp. 188 and 599). Both the onset and the cessation of syncopal attacks are usually more gradual than is usually the case in epilepsy and are often preceded by a feeling of faintness. In syncope also the patient is generally limp, whereas muscular rigidity favours epilepsy; on the other hand, transient rigidity and twitching and even incontinence may occur in a severe faint. Perspiration and severe pallor also favour syncope. Nevertheless, in some individuals pressure upon the carotid sinus or circumstances which usually induce syncope can precipitate an epileptic attack. For a discussion of the relationship between syncope and epilepsy, see page 190.

In *narcolepsy* the patient falls asleep, but there are no convulsive movements and the patient, unlike the epileptic, shows all the features of natural sleep and can be immediately roused. In *cataplexy* voluntary power is lost but consciousness is retained.

Aural vertigo may be confused with minor and major epilepsy, in which vertigo may also occur, often as a transient aura. In aural vertigo, however, consciousness is retained and other symptoms of ear disease, such as tinnitus and deafness, are usually present. Though an attack of aural vertigo may be brief, it usually lasts longer than a minor attack or an aura, and passes away more gradually. But the relationship between the labyrinth and epilepsy is complex (see p. 616).

Hysterical fits (psychogenic seizures or pseudoseizures) are usually easily distinguished from epileptic attacks if the patient is seen in an attack. Their onset is usually gradual, and they usually occur only in the presence of an audience. Consciousness is not lost, for the patient can usually be roused by forcible measures, and an attempt to elicit the corneal reflex usually evokes a vigorous contraction of the orbicularis oculi. If the patient cries out in the attack he usually articulates words or phrases, and laughing or crying may occur. The movements of an hysterical convulsion are not clonic jerks as in epilepsy, but such as can be carried out voluntarily, for example, clutching at objects. The tongue is not bitten, nor does incontinence of urine usually occur. However, there is a particular type of hysterical attack which occurs usually in young females, less often in males, in which sudden falling without convulsive movements occurs and the picture may be indistinguishable from that of akinetic epilepsy. After being asked repeatedly by one or more doctors the patient may oblige by passing urine in an attack. These attacks are often very frequent, occur particularly at times of stress, seem to cause the patient little concern, and show virtually no response to anti-convulsant drugs. Diagnostic difficulty is increased by the fact that epileptic and hysterical attacks may coexist in the same individual. A similar type of attack occasionally occurs in a medicolegal context in adults after trivial head injury and then ceases abruptly as a rule after settlement of a compensation claim.

Anxiety attacks are occasionally confused with epilepsy. Consciousness is not lost, but the predominant symptom is an intense sense of anxiety, often associated with feelings of giddiness, palpitation, and sweating.

The *panic attacks* of the phobic anxiety-depersonalization syndrome (Harper and Roth 1962) can be readily confused with temporal-lobe epilepsy as in these episodes mounting panic and angor animi (fear of 'impending doom') are often associated with a sense of intense depersonalization or unreality and if there is associated hyperventilation, syncope sometimes occurs or even tetany. Usually, however, consciousness is unimpaired and there are associated phobias about going out of the house alone (agarophobia), crossing roads, or entering crowded places, which are not a feature of epilepsy. Similar symptoms sometimes occur in depressive illness.

Under the title of *vasovagal attacks*, Gowers (1907) described 'prolonged seizures, the symptoms of which consist chiefly in disturbance of some of the functions of the pneumo-gastric'. The patient complained of gastric, respiratory, or cardiac discomfort, often associated with vasoconstriction and coldness of the extremeties. Women were more subject to these paroxysms than men. They were distinguished from epilepsy by their gradual onset and longer duration, and by the usual retention of consciousness. It is doubtful if they represent a nosological entity; most were probably syncopal, some were due to anxiety, and others were in all probability episodes of temporal-lobe epilepsy, properly falling, as Gowers suggested, into the 'borderland of epilepsy'.

Migraine is a paroxysmal disturbance which rarely simulates epilepsy. The onset of an attack of migraine, however, is gradual. Consciousness is not lost, and headache usually occurs. It must be remembered, however, that the same individual may suffer from both migraine and epilepsy, and that very exceptionally a severe attack of migraine may cause syncope or terminate in an epileptic fit.

Hypoglycaemia (see below) sometimes causes transient episodes of impairment of consciousness, often with pallor or sweating, and severe attacks may lead to an epileptic fit.

When it has been established that a patient suffers from epileptic seizures it remains to exclude the various focal and metabolic causes of convulsions enumerated on page 610.

Diagnosis of the cause

Gross organic lesions such as *hydrocephalus* and *infantile hemiplegia* give rise to no difficulty.

Tuberous sclerosis can be diagnosed as a cause of epilepsy associated with mental defect only when adenoma sebaccum is present, when there are phakomata to be seen in the retina or by the characteristic radiological changes. In atypical absence attacks or infantile spasms in childhood, and indeed in all forms of childhood epilepsy, many *metabolic and degenerative diseases of the brain* must be considered.

Renal disease and *hypertensive encephalopathy* may be excluded by examination of the cardiovascular system, including the blood pressure, and of the urine and the blood urea, but it must be noted that hyperuricaemia with acute renal failure has been described as a sequel of status epilepticus or recurrent major seizures (Warren, Leitch, and Leggett 1975).

The diagnosis of *syphilis* can be established by means of the history, the presence of signs of the infection of the nervous system, and a positive VDRL reaction in the blood or CSF.

When *alcohol* or *drug intoxication* or *withdrawal* is the cause of the convulsions a history of alcoholism or of drug-taking can usually be obtained.

Heart block and other causes of severe cardiogenic syncope offer little difficulty in diagnosis if these possibilities are borne in mind. If an attack is witnessed it is found to coincide with cardiac asystole and flushing usually accompanies the return of consciousness. When complete atrioventricular block is established the pulse rate is usually about 30. Even if the pulse rate is normal between the attacks, impaired conduction in the atrioventricular bundle can usually be demonstrated by an ECG. A 24-hour recording on tape may be useful in demonstrating intermittent heart block or other arrhythmias.

Spontaneous hypoglycaemia may cause syncopal or epileptic attacks, or, in milder cases, fatigability, anxiety, sweating, giddiness, diplopia, or mental confusion. The subject was reviewed by Conn (1947). Apart from gross disease of the liver, hypophysis, or adrenals, the two chief causes are: (1) adenoma, carcinoma, or hyperplasia of the pancreatic islet cells of Langerhans; and (2) reactive hyperinsulinism. The former is the more likely to give rise to epilepsy, which is commonly nocturnal, when the blood sugar is at its lowest. The diagnosis is based upon the low fasting blood sugar in the former, and abnormal sugar tolerance tests and the correlation between the attacks and the low blood sugar in both (Prunty 1944; Conn 1947).

Two common causes of seizures developing after the age of 30 are intracranial tumour and cerebral arteriosclerosis. In *intracranial tumour* fits may precede other symptoms by months or years, and when this is so the cause can often only be suspected. Though the attacks may be generalized, a focal origin should suggest tumour, especially when they are followed by temporary aphasia or paresis. A unilateral bruit over the cranium or neck vessels may suggest an angioma. Sooner or later headache and other symptoms of increased intracranial pressure make their appearance, together with signs of a progressive cerebral lesion. The EEG may suggest the presence of a focal lesion, radiographs of the skull or echo-encephalography may indicate a 'shift' of midline structures and a CT scan or other apppropriate radiological investigations may be required. Indeed many now believe that a CT scan is obligatory in late-onset epilepsy (Gilliatt and Shorvon 1983). Epileptiform attacks due to *cerebral arteriosclerosis* usually occur in late middle life and old age. They may follow upon clinically evident episodes of cerebral infarction (post-hemiplegic epilepsy), but often the cause of the attacks is a previously asymptomatic minor cortical infarct. There may be typical changes in the retinal arteries and the blood pressure may be raised, but usually a CT scan will be needed to identify the cause.

Cysticercosis should be considered when epilepsy begins in adult life in men who have lived abroad, especially in India, and a search should be made for subcutaneous cysts. Calcified cysts may be demonstrated radiographically in the muscles and less often in the brain.

Prognosis

The risk of death occurring during an epileptic attack is relatively slight, except in status epilepticus, in which life is always threatened until consciousness returns, and death may occur even after recovery of consciousness. However, death is well recognized to occur in febrile convulsions in infancy (Lennox-Buchthal 1974) or in accidents due to fits and there have been many reports of unexpected, unexplained death in young and otherwise physically fit epileptic subjects; some are found dead in bed but others die after seizures which were witnessed and showed no unusual characteristics (Hirsch and Martin 1971). Autopsy examination usually fails to demonstrate the cause of death (Terrence, Wisotskey, and Perper 1975). However, some patients are shown to have died from asphyxia due to a nocturnal fit in which the face became buried in a pillow; drowning due to a fit in the bath has also been described. Mortality and morbidity data have been comprehensively reviewed by Kurtzke (1972) and by Zielinsky (1982) who points out that mortality statistics based upon death certification may be open to misinterpretation if symptomatic and idiopathic cases are not separately identified. Age-adjusted annual death rates are usually between 1.0 and 2.0 per 100000 of the population but a figure as high as 4.0 has been reported from Chile. Death from epilepsy is certainly higher in non-whites and in males (Kurtzke 1972).

Minor accidents resulting from the attacks include injuries induced by the fall; these are rarely serious, but shoulder dislocation, produced by muscular contraction, is not uncommon; once having occurred, it is liable to recur in subsequent attacks. The violence of the convulsions may also cause compression fracture of vertebral bodies, usually in the thoracic region, a possibility which always must be considered if a patient complains of pain in the back after a fit. Fractures of limb bones occur less often.

The prognosis as to recovery from the attacks depends upon many factors. To achieve recovery the attacks must be controlled by treatment for a sufficient length of time for the tendency to be permanently suppressed. Early and effective treatment is therefore essential; it must be continued for at least three years after the attacks have ceased and in some cases indefinitely. If it is to be withdrawn, this should be done gradually but even so, fits recur, even after three or more years of freedom in up to 30 per cent of cases. The sooner the treatment can be begun after the first fit, the better the outlook (Shorvon and Reynolds 1982). Holowach, Thurston, and O'Leary (1972) followed up 148 epileptic children, all of whom had been free from attacks for four years on anticonvulsant medication, for 5–12 years after drug withdrawal. Seizures recurred in 24 per cent; there was no relation between relapse on the one hand and sex, race, heredity, puberty, or seizure frequency on the other. With an early onset and prompt control of seizures the relapse rate was only 13 per cent; it was higher in cases of later onset or prolonged duration and in those with neurological, psychological, or marked EEG abnormalities. In adult epileptics, the relapse rate after withdrawal of anticonvulsants is higher, approaching 40 per cent (*The Lancet* 1972a). Individuals suffering from frequent severe attacks are least likely to be completely cured. The outlook is often best when the attacks occur only during sleep, and treatment is most likely to be successful when they take place at a regular time of the day or of the month, so that intensive treatment can be timed so as to avert them. Marked mental deterioration makes the outlook worse. Thus few patients in institutions become free from attacks, and the death rate among institutional epileptics is four times that of the general population. Probably about 30 per cent of non-institutional epileptics are cured, in the sense of remaining free from attacks indefinitely, even after withdrawal of anticonvulsant drugs but in over 60 per cent the attacks can be completely controlled with treatment (Bridge, Kajdi, and Livingston 1947; Frantzen 1961; Rodin 1972).

There has been some controversy about the prognosis of childhood petit mal. Lees and Liversedge (1962) suggested that in many children with typical absence seizures attacks continued into adult life. However, Livingston, Torres, Pauli, and Rider (1965) found that the attacks eventually ceased in adolescence in over three-quarters of their cases, but grand mal eventually developed in 54 per cent of those who started with 'pure' petit mal.

Treatment

General management

Symptomatic epilepsy, resulting, say, from an intracranial tumour, is best treated by curing the condition of which the epilepsy is but a symptom, but this is only rarely possible; hence, in many symptomatic cases, the same treatment as that given for idiopathic epilepsy is needed.

An epileptic patient should as far as possible live a normal life. Children should attend school and should be subjected to normal discipline. Measures useful in the prevention of attacks, of secondary handicaps, and of reducing the stigma which is still too often attached to the diagnosis of epilepsy, were reviewed by Taylor and Bower (1971), vocational and educational problems by Rodin, Rennick, Dennerli, and Lin (1972) and Rodin (1982), and social adjustment by Bagley (1972) and Laidlaw and Laidlaw (1982). Adults should work whenever possible, though certain trades are necessarily ruled out. Occupations involving working at heights, or near dangerous machinery, or driving vehicles are obviously unsuitable, and sufferers from epilepsy were in the past precluded by law from obtaining a driving licence in Great Britain. After a single fit, however, for which investigation demonstrated no obvious cause, many neurologists were prepared to recommend that driving should be banned for one year only and that anticonvulsant drugs should only be taken for the first six months of this period. Maxwell and Leyshon (1971), among others, found that many epileptics had obtained driving licences through false declarations on their application forms. All neurologists are aware of serious, sometimes fatal, road accidents which have presumably occurred as a result of a driver suffering a fit. Now, in the UK, an epileptic patient may, on the presentation of medical evidence, have his driving licence restored after two years of total freedom from attacks, provided he is prepared to continue anticonvulsant therapy indefinitely (Espir 1983; Godwin-Austen and Espir 1983). If he prefers to attempt withdrawal of anticonvulsant drugs, accepting a 40 per cent relapse rate, even after two years of freedom from attacks, one further year of freedom from attacks will normally be required before it is reasonable to certify that the patient no longer suffers from epilepsy and that it is safe for him to drive. However, on this and several other points of importance there is still disagreement and dispute between individual British neurologists (Harvey and Hopkins 1983). Those who wish to attempt withdrawal of treatment should be warned that if a further attack occurs, then another period of two years of freedom from attacks on treatment will be required before driving can be permitted. It is also possible to recommend restoration of a licence to an individual certified, over a three-year period, as suffering from nocturnal attacks only. In general, any history of epilepsy occurring after the age of five years, even if controlled, is sufficient to debar an individual permanently from driving a heavy goods or public service vehicle or from flying an aeroplane. Regulations in various parts if the United States and in other countries vary from state to state and from country to country but are broadly similar (Stock, Burg, Light, and Douglas 1970).

Children should be allowed to take part in sports; an individual decision must be made in every case depending upon the frequency and severity of the attacks but the riding of horses or of bicycles can often be allowed if the attacks are well controlled. Certain risks of everyday life must be explained to the patient and his friends, but it is difficult, if not impossible, to guard against them all. The water in his bath should be shallow, and he should not swim in deep water unaccompanied. Institutional treatment is sometimes necessary for mentally handicapped patients and for those having severe and frequent fits, if adequate home care is not available. Those for whom an ordinary occupation is impossible often do well in special residential centres (Reid 1972). Unfortunately specialized educational, rehabilitative, occupational, and other support services for epileptic patients in the UK remain inadequate, especially when compared to those available in the USA (Shorvon 1983).

No general rule can be laid down concerning marriage. There is no evidence that marriage affects the tendency to fits either beneficially or adversely, though pregnancy may prove either beneficial or the reverse. The risk of transmitting the disorder to children must be individually assessed in each case. This risk is clearly greatest when there is a family history of epilepsy or when an EEG shows that the non-epileptic parent has an abnormal record, and least when a focal lesion of the brain can be held partly responsible for the attacks. Even when the epileptic tendency is inherited it is exceptional for a patient to transmit the disorder as a simple dominant trait, and the chances are 35 to one against any individual child of an epileptic parent developing epilepsy.

Moderate exercise is desirable; attacks rarely occur during such exercise but rarely follow violent exertion. Any factor adversely affecting the general health should receive attention. Alcohol is best avoided, as over-indulgence, or even a modest intake, may precipitate attacks.

Treatment of the epileptic attack

Treatment of a patient in an epileptic attack consists merely in preventing him from injuring himself. A gag should, if possible, be placed between the teeth and an airway maintained. The attack is self-limiting, and no immediate treatment will shorten its course.

Surgical treatment

From the most ancient times trephining the skull played a part in the treatment of epilepsy. Certainly if a surgically accessible intracranial tumour is demonstrated to be the cause, it should be removed. When there is clear evidence of an organic cerebral lesion, especially one of traumatic origin, and the attacks have a focal onset which can be related to the lesion and demonstrated by electrocorticography, excision of the affected area may abolish the attacks (Penfield and Jasper 1954). Hemispherectomy has had a considerable vogue in the management of epilepsy secondary to severe infantile hemiplegia (Krynauw 1950 and see p. 354); it fell temporarily into disfavour because of late complications such as haemosiderosis, but a subtotal operaton which usually avoids such complications is now being widely adopted in appropriate cases (Rasmussen 1983). In other patients with gross destructive cerebral lesions, restricted cortical excisions following upon electrocorticography have sometimes proved beneficial (Rasmussen and Gossman 1963). Surgical division of the corpus callosum has also been effective in some cases of intractable epilepsy in adult life and more especially in childhood (Geoffroy, Lassonde, Delisle, and Décarie 1983). Surgical treatment is, however, indicated only, as a rule, when the attacks are severe and inadequately controlled by drugs (because the surgeon in removing one scar must leave another) and when the lesion is situated in an area of the brain which, when excised, is unlikely to result in permanent and severe neurological deficit. Even in temporal-lobe epilepsy, in which good results, both in respect of seizure control and behavioural improvement, have followed anterior temporal lobectomy in appropriate cases (Penfield and Flanigin 1950; Falconer and Serefitinides 1963; Bengzon, Rasmussen, Gloor, Dussault, and Stephens 1968; Taylor and Falconer 1968; Engel, Driver, and Falconer 1975; Polkey 1982, 1983), probably less than one per cent of cases require, and are suitable for, surgical treatment. The results appear to be best in children in whom mesial temporal

sclerosis (in Ammon's horn) is found at operation (Falconer and Taylor 1968; Falconer 1972; Davidson and Falconer 1975) and in adult patients with attacks of hippocampal origin (Delgado-Escueta and Walsh 1985). However, it is now the general experience in neurological and neurosurgical units that with the increasing efficacy of modern anticonvulsant drugs, fewer patients need surgical treatment.

Cerebellar stimulation

Cooper, Amin, and Gilman (1973) followed by Grabow, Ebersold, Albers, and Schima (1974) showed that repeated electrical stimulation of the cerebellum through electrodes implanted surgically was sometimes very effective in controlling intractable epilepsy and over 700 patients have been so treated (*The Lancet* 1983) with results which have sometimes been dramatic, sometimes disappointing. Technical problems have been substantial and complications not inconsiderable, so that this method, though still promising, remains experimental (Upton 1982).

Treatment with drugs

Many drugs have been found to diminish the severity and frequency of seizures and in favourable cases to abolish them completely (see below). When attacks occur regularly at the same hour of the day or period of the month, the doses can be timed correspondingly so as to produce their maximal effect when the attack is expected. Thus when the attacks are nocturnal or occur in the early morning, a single dose at bedtime may suffice. When they occur only in relation to menstruation, medication can sometimes be increased in the previous and subsequent weeks. When the fits are irregular a dose may be taken two or three times a day but the desirability of giving a single daily dose or divided doses also depends upon the pharmacokinetics of the individual drugs, and upon the differential rates at which they are metabolized in different individuals, since the therapeutic effect depends upon the maintenance of stable blood levels within the therapeutic range (Eadie and Tyrer 1980; Glaser, Penry, and Woodbury 1980; Laidlaw and Richens 1982). Perseverance in treatment is essential, and the patient must continue to take the effective drug for at least three years after the attacks cease, but many patients, especially those whose driving licence has been restored after two years of freedom from attacks, prefer to continue treatment indefinitely to avoid as far as possible any risk of relapse.

Drug treatment

General principles

These are fully reviewed by Glaser *et al.* (1980), Eadie and Tyrer (1980), Calne (1980), Davidson and Lenman (1981) and Porter (1984). It is first important to recognize that one group of drugs, including the barbiturates, hydantoinates, and acetylureas, together with several modern synthetic remedies, are effective in major epilepsy (whether idiopathic or symptomatic) and also in focal epilepsy (including the temporal-lobe or complex partial variety) as well as in some cases of myoclonic epilepsy (see below) but not in petit mal (classical absence seizures). A second group, including the diones and suximides, may control petit mal but have often seemed to make associated major epilepsy worse or to precipitate major attacks in patients with petit mal who had never suffered such episodes before (Gastaut 1964; Wilson 1969). There is also some evidence to indicate that the long-term prognosis of petit mal is better if the child is treated with at least one drug effective in major epilepsy (such as a hydantoin derivative) as well as with one or more of those which are effective in petit mal. That the choice of anticonvulsant in an individual case should be regularly reappraised in the light of new developments in pharmacology, has been underlined by the discovery that sodium valproate, a simple two-chain fatty acid, is much more effective in petit mal than the diones and even the suximides and is also beneficial in focal, complex partial, and major epilepsy (Klawans and

Weiner 1981; Wilder, Ramsay, Murphy, Karas, Marquardt, and Hammond 1983; Turnbull, Howel, Rawlins, and Chadwick 1985). It appears to act by inhibiting GABA transaminase and thus increasing cerebral GABA concentrations. Of the benzodiazepines, which are also being used increasingly, diazepam is most useful in status epilepticus, and clonazepam or clobazam in myoclonic epilepsy, in infantile spasms, and in some cases of major epilepsy, especially when intractable (Richens 1982; Allen, Oxley, Robertson, Trimble, Richens, and Jowad 1983).

In all cases patients or their parents must be warned not to discontinue treatment without medical advice as this may precipitate dangerous episodes of status epilepticus. Difficulties arising in the management of epilepsy represent a major justification for the existence of neurological follow-up clinics, as regular and careful supervision of such patients, with regulation and monitoring of anticonvulsant medication and dosage, may pay considerable dividends. In general, combined tablets, containing more than one drug, are to be condemned, as with these remedies it is not possible to adjust independently the dosage of the individual constituents.

The discovery that the serum levels of many anticonvulsant drugs produced by standard doses vary widely from patient to patient because of individual variations in pharmacokinetics and binding to serum proteins (see Richens 1982) and that low serum levels may be correlated with poor control of seizures and excessively high levels with symptoms of toxicity has been an important development. Patients who are slow inactivators of isoniazid may also have difficulty in metabolizing phenytoin (Brennan, Dehejia, Kutt, Verebely, and McDowell 1970). If serum concentrations of anticonvulsant drugs can be estimated regularly, often with the aid of gas liquid chromatography, the dose can be adjusted to suit the individual in order to achieve better control of the seizures and to lessen side-effects (Gibberd, Dunne, Handley, and Hazleman 1970; Buchanan and Allen 1971; Gardner-Medwin 1973; Richens and Dunlop 1975; Glaser *et al.* 1980). A desirable serum concentration of phenytoin is 60–80 μmol/l (15–20 μg/ml). Richens (1982) concludes that monitoring of blood levels of phenytoin is essential for effective seizure control and that similar monitoring contributes to more effective treatment when using carbamazepine (therapeutic range up to 50 μmol/l), or ethosuximide (up to 700 μmol/l) but is much less useful when using phenobarbitone (up to 170 μmol/l), sodium valproate (up to 700 μmol/l), primidone, or clonazepam. DeMonaco and Lawless (1983) point out that because of the variability of phenytoin protein binding, it is free phenytoin that should be measured. Contrary to the view expressed by Richens (1982), Turnbull, Rawlins, Weightman, and Chadwick (1983) found the monitoring of plasma concentrations of sodium valproate to be useful; there was a close correlation with dosage, and adverse effects were common with concentrations above 700 μmol/l (100 μg/ml) while no tonic–clonic seizures occurred when plasma levels were above 350 μmol/l (50 μg/ml). Thompson and Trimble (1983) sound a note of warning; they found significant deficits in psychological test performance in epileptic patients in whom serum concentrations were towards the upper end of what is normally accepted as the therapeutic range.

Major (tonic–clonic) and focal epilepsy (including complex partial seizures)

General guidelines. The principle must be to give minimum dose of drugs sufficient to control the attacks for as long as may be necessary. Often a single drug suffices but sometimes it is necessary to give a combination of at least two, and rarely of three or more drugs in combination, in order to achieve maximum control, bearing in mind the fact that one drug may potentiate the effect of another, but always remembering that not only are the therapeutic effects of these remedies additive but also that the same may apply to their side-effects. Sometimes, therefore, the addition of a new drug to the patient's existing medication results in psychomotor retardation and a paradoxical increase in the number of fits. Thus

sulthiame added to phenytoin may produce symptoms of phenytoin intoxication (Houghton and Richens 1974). All of the drugs in common use tend to slow the mental processes to a greater or lesser extent but this is particularly true of the barbiturates and some benzodiazepines and occasionally satisfactory control of the attacks is only achieved at the expense of a disabling degree of drowsiness. However, as patients become accustomed to their medication, these side-effects may noticeably diminish so that the initial sedative effects are not invariably an indication for a reduction in treatment if attacks are under control.

Adverse reactions. In addition to sedation, all of the drugs to be considered below, apart from toxic effects specific to the individual remedy, which will be mentioned, can also produce in excessive dosage dysarthria and ataxia, often with nystagmus, blurred vision, and even diplopia. These manifestations often develop relatively suddenly in a patient who has been receiving a stable regimen of treatment for some time; the patient has a 'drugged' and almost drunken appearance which is characteristic but may be misconstrued by the unwary as being due to organic intracranial disease. These toxic effects are particularly common in those taking barbiturates and/or hydantoinates; complete withdrawal of drugs is not necessary, as the level of dosage at which toxic side-effects appear is finely balanced in the individual and a reduction in dosage of a single tablet or capsule per day sometimes results in their rapid amelioration or disappearance, though more often a somewhat greater reduction in daily dosage is required. Estimation of serum levels is of particular value in monitoring the dosage required to abolish side-effects. Tyrer, Eadie, Sutherland, and Hooper (1970) reported an outbreak of phenytoin intoxication resulting from the use of a different excipient in making tablets containing phenytoin; hence factors other than the patient's own ability to absorb and metabolize the drug must be borne in mind. Macrocytic anaemia due to folic-acid deficiency has long been recognized to be an occasional complication of anticonvulsant therapy but Reynolds (1968) suggested that such a deficiency might also account for other side-effects of these drugs and that improvement might follow the regular administration of folic acid, 5 mg daily. Paradoxically, however, this remedy sometimes increases the number of seizures. Hunter, Barnes, and Matthews (1969) found that giving folic acid sometimes reduced the serum vitamin B_{12} levels. The abnormality of folate metabolism, which may be due either to inhibition of intestinal conjugases (Baugh and Krumdieck 1969) or to hepatic enzyme induction (Maxwell, Hunter, Stewart, Ardeman, and Williams 1972), is thought to be one factor accounting for the peripheral neuropathy which occasionally results from long-term phenytoin treatment (Lovelace and Horwitz 1967; Horwitz, Klipstein, and Lovelace 1968; Dam 1982). Hepatic-enzyme induction produced by long-term phenobarbitone or phenytoin treatment can also cause liver damage with rises in serum alkaline phosphatase and alanine aminotransferase activity and an increased prothrombin time, but the incidence of hepatotoxicity which has rarely caused fatal liver failure (Donat, Bocchini, and Gonzalez 1979; Suchy, Balistreri, Buchino, Sondheimer, Bates, Kearns, Stull, and Bove 1979) is significantly higher in patients treated with sodium valproate. The latter drug also causes marked hyperammonaemia in normal humans; this may not be adequately detoxified if there is concomitant liver damage (Warter, Brandt, Marescaux, Rumbach, Michelett, Chabrier, Krieger, and Imler 1983). Troublesome tremor of action type is also seen in up to 10 per cent of patients taking sodium valproate but can be controlled by propranolol (Karas, Wilder, Hammond, and Bauman 1983). Irreversible Purkinje-cell damage with cerebellar ataxia is an occasional complication of severe intoxication (Utterback, Ojeman, and Malek 1958; Hofmann 1958). However, it now seems likely that Purkinje-cell loss and cerebellar ataxia is more often a consequence of the seizures than of phenytoin or carbamazepine treatment (Dam 1982). Drug rashes also occur not infrequently in patients receiving phenobarbitone and hydantoinates; they can sometimes be controlled with antihistamine drugs but more often necessitate withdrawal of the offender and the substitution of another remedy.

Other important side-effects of anticonvulsant drugs, and especially phenytoin, include coarsening of the features, increased body hair, hypertrophy of the gums, Dupuytren's contracture, and a reduction in the serum IgA (see Davies 1981a; Dam 1982), involuntary movements (Ahmad, Laidlaw, Houghton, and Richens 1975), defects of blood coagulation (Solomon, Hilgartner, and Kutt 1972), renal insensitivity to frusemide (Ahmad 1974), disorders of cerebral monoamine metabolism (Chadwick, Jenner, and Reynolds 1975), and disordered calcium metabolism leading to osteomalacia, possibly due to an accelerated breakdown of vitamin D resulting from hepatic enzyme induction (Dent, Richens, Rowe, and Stamp 1970; Richens and Rowe 1970; Christiansen, Kristensen, and Rødbro 1972; *The Lancet* 1972b; Davie, Lawson, Emberson, Barnes, Roberts, and Barnes 1982). Christiansen, Rødbro, and Sjö (1974) suggest that all epileptics receiving anticonvulsant therapy should also be given prophylactic vitamin D. Infants born to epileptic mothers receiving phenobarbitone, a hydantoin, or sodium valproate may show neonatal coagulation defects with spontaneous bleeding. The mothers should be given vitamin K in late pregnancy and the infants should receive intravenous phytomenadione at birth. During episodes of severe anticonvulsant intoxication the CSF protein may be raised (Rawson 1968). Apart from the drowsiness and ataxia referred to above, several anticonvulsants including phenytoin, sodium valproate, and ethosuximide have been reported to cause psychotic behaviour with confusion, hallucinations, and hyperactivity, sometimes, but not invariably due to interaction with isoniazid given concurrently for the treatment of or prophylaxis against tuberculosis (Chadwick, Cummings, Livingstone, and Cartlidge 1979; Valsalan and Cooper 1982; van Wieringen and Vrijlandt 1983). The risk of bone-marrow suppression due to carbamazepine, once thought to be significant, is now known to be slight. However, carbamazepine used in childhood as the initial treatment of tonic–clonic seizures has been reported rarely to precipitate myoclonic, atypical absence and/or atonic seizures (Shields and Saslow 1983).

A possible teratogenic effect of phenytoin has also been postulated. Speidel and Meadow (1972) found that major congenital formations including congenital heart disease, cleft lip and palate, and microcephaly occurred twice as often in the children born to epileptic mothers as would have been expected in the general population, and similar findings were reported by Fedrick (1973) and Loughnan, Gold, and Vance (1973). There is also a slight but significant relationship between the taking of sodium valproate in the first trimester of pregnancy and an incidence of spina bifida of one per cent in the infants of such mothers (Bjerkedal, Czeizel, Goujard, Kallen, Mastroicova, Nevin, Oakley, and Robert 1982; Jeavons 1982b; *The Lancet* 1982). It seems likely that carbamazepine is significantly less teratogenic than phenytoin or sodium valproate (Dam 1982). While most epileptic mothers have normal infants and the effect is not powerful, it clearly warrants further investigation.

The treatment regimen. Whereas in the past phenobarbitone was generally regarded as the initial drug of choice in major or focal epilepsy, the use of barbiturates has declined steadily and the three remedies most often used as the primary medication are phenytoin, carbamazepine, and sodium valproate. Some workers favour giving a single large daily dose of either phenytoin or carbamazepine (Strandjord and Johannessen 1974), but the majority advise giving these drugs in divided doses, usually twice daily (morning and night), rarely more often, beginning with a modest dose but increasing steadily until adequate blood concentrations are achieved and/or the seizures are fully controlled (Richens 1982). Sodium valproate is invariably given at least twice daily.

The total daily dose of phenytoin required to produce adequate blood concentrations and seizure control is usually between 150 and 600 mg daily but few young children require more than 100 mg daily and few adults can tolerate more than 400 mg daily without developing toxic side-effects. Carbamazepine is usually begun, in adults, with a dose of 100 mg twice daily, building up to 400–800 mg a day with proportionally lower doses in childhood, but occasional patients have been known to tolerate, with good effect upon the seizures, as much as 1800 mg daily. The usual starting dose of sodium valproate is 200 mg twice daily with a normal maximum of 1200 mg daily; yet again, a few patients can take as much as 3000 mg a day.

There has been considerable dispute as to whether seizure control is best achieved by a single drug or by combined therapy with two or more remedies. Certainly if the remedy first given is unsuccessful in adequate doses in controlling the seizures, it is reasonable to substitute another by gradual reduction in the dose of the former and a steady increase to optimal dosage levels of the second remedy when the first can then be withdrawn (Shorvon, Chadwick, Galbraith, and Reynolds 1978). Many authorities, however (see Eadie and Tyrer 1980; Glaser *et al.* 1980; Richens 1982) still hold the view that addition of a second anticonvulsant drug, eventually in maximum therapeutic doses, and even very exceptionally of a third, can produce an additive beneficial effect in the control of seizures, though the risk of additive toxic side-effects must also be recognized (also see Mattson 1983). In the treatment of intractable complex partal seizures, Schmidt (1982) found a significant decrease in the number of attacks in only 13 per cent of patients in whom a second drug was added. When carbamazepine given as the initial treatment in 70 adult patients was compared with phenytoin on a double-blind basis, no significant differences were noted in seizure control and/or side-effects (Ramsay, Wildeer, Berger, and Bruni 1983). In patients with complex partial seizures, the addition of sodium valproate to other anticonvulsant drugs produced initially a reduction of seizure frequency of about 50 per cent, but this effect was not sustained (Bruni and Albright 1983). However, when sodium valproate is given with other drugs, especially in childhood, the dose may have to be substantially higher and the drug has to be given more often than in patients taking this remedy alone (Cloyd, Kriel, Fisher, Sawchuk, and Eggerth 1983).

While phenytoin, carbamazepine, and sodium valproate are now the standard remedies, individual variability of response is still such that other anticonvulsant drugs are still widely used, usually with one or more of the above, for their additive effects. These include phenobarbitone (30–60 mg at night) or primidone (250–500 mg twice daily in an adult, 125 mg twice daily in a child). The latter, being metabolized in the body to phenobarbitone, should never be given in combination with phenobarbitone. Methoin (100–200 mg twice daily) is similar in its effect to phenytoin but may cause bone-marrow suppression, while ethotoin (250–500 mg twice daily) is another hydantoin, useful in occasional cases but generally not superior to phenytoin or carbamazepine. Sulthiame (50–100 mg twice daily in children, 200–400 mg twice daily in adults) has been thought to have a valuable adjuvant anticonvulsant effect and to improve behaviour in epileptic children (Liu 1966) but may work simply by increasing phenytoin blood levels (Green, Troupin, Halpern, Friel, and Kanarek 1974). Often used in the past was phenylacetylurea, but this drug is toxic to the blood, liver, and bone marrow and is no longer used. Its chemical derivative, phenylethylacetylurea (200–400 mg twice daily) is much less toxic and is an effective anticonvulsant (Vas and Parsonage 1967); in a double-blind trial it was found to be as effective as phenytoin (Gibberd, Park, Scott, Gawel, Fry, Page, Engler, English, and Rose 1982) but it is no longer available in Britain. Curiously, perhaps, methosuximide, most often used in the treatment of classical absence seizures (see below), may also be of benefit, in combination with other drugs, in refractory complex partial seizures (Browne, Feldman, Buchanan, Allen, Fawcett-Vickers, Szabo, Mattson, Norman, and Greenblatt 1983). Clonazepam (0.5 mg twice daily, increasing up to a maximum of 5–10 mg daily) is sometimes useful but seems more effective in myoclonic epilepsy and in atonic or akinetic seizures. Its newer analogue clobazam is still being tested but in general the benzodiazepines are not as effective as other remedies in the long-term control of tonic–clonic or focal seizures. Beclamide is also a weak anticonvulsant with a minor additive effect (Wilson, Walton, and Newell 1959), now little used, though possibly of value in children with behaviour disorders (Beley, Girard, Leroy, and Pinel 1962; Price and Spencer 1967). The induction of ketosis by a ketogenic diet or by giving medium-chain triglycerides (Huttenlocker, Wilbourn, and Signore 1971), like the use of bromides in epilepsy, is now outmoded.

Classical absence seizures (idiopathic petit mal)
Some authorities still regard ethosuximide, usually given even in young children, in a dose of 250–500 mg twice daily, as the treatment of choice (Browne, Dreifuss, Dyken, Goode, Penry, Porter, White, and White 1975). However, when this drug is used as the initial treatment, it is necessary to give in addition phenytoin or carbamazepine (50–100 mg twice daily) to guard against the immediate or subsequent development of major seizures. Phensuximide (250–500 mg twice daily) and methsuximide (300–600 mg twice daily) are consistently less effective though they seem to be helpful in occasional cases (Richens 1982). Within the last few years, however, it has become apparent that sodium valproate alone is generally superior even to ethosuximide in most cases and has the clear advantage of suppressing not only absences but also the tendency to suffer tonic–clonic seizures (Jeavons, Clark, and Maheshwari 1977). The diones (trimethadione and paramethadione, 600–900 mg daily), which were the first drugs shown to be conclusively effective in petit mal, produced many side-effects and, being significantly less successful than sodium valproate, are virtually no longer used, and chlortetracycline, once helpful in some cases, has also been discarded. However, adjuvant remedies which may be helpful in some cases are acetazolamide (250–500 mg once or twice daily) and clonazepam (1.0–10.0 mg daily; see Dreifuss, Penry, Rose, Kupferberg, Dyken, and Sato 1975). Imipramine, too, which may precipitate major fits in adults but which, paradoxically, sometimes benefits intractable petit mal in a dosage of 1.3mg/kg body weight daily (Fromm, Amores, and Thies 1972) is now little used. Similarly the amphetamines are no longer prescribed in epilepsy but are still occasionally used in hyperkinetic children in whom they have a paradoxical sedative effect, unlike phenobarbitone which may greatly increase hyperkinesis and disordered behaviour.

In the treatment of petit mal, toxic side-effects of medication are in general less of a problem, because of the character of the drugs being used, than in the management of tonic–clonic and focal epilepsy. In all forms of epilepsy, however, the aim must be to achieve a balance between the control of the attacks on the one hand and the preservation of mental capacity, concentration, and alertness on the other.

Treatment of status epilepticus
It has become apparent within the last few years that the benzodiazepines, given by intravenous infusion, are probably the most effective drugs (Delgado-Escueta, Wasterlain, Treiman, and Porter 1983) but the risk of producing prolonged coma with excessive doses must be borne in mind (Richens 1982). Diazepam given in a loading dose of 0.25 mg/kg up to 20 mg followed by 2 mg/min is still the remedy most used and is effective in tonic–clonic and in focal or absence status (Treiman 1983). Clonazepam or lorazepam may ultimately prove even more effective. Occasionally, however, tonic status is precipitated by the use of benzodiazepines (Tassinari, Gastaut, Dravet, and Roger 1972).

For many years paraldehyde was regarded as the most effective drug, being given in doses of 10 ml intramuscularly to an adult and repeated as necessary. In an emergency it could be given by intravenous drip in a dosage of 0.05 to 0.1 ml per kg of body weight in normal saline. Unfortunately the intramuscular injections were painful and occasionally gave abscess formation while phlebitis often followed intravenous administration. However, Curless, Holzman, and Ramsay (1983) found that this drug, given intravenously, is still helpful in some cases of childhood status, in which diazepam, phenytoin, and phenobarbitone have failed. In mild cases the patient may respond to 120–250 mg of phenobarbitone sodium intramuscularly followed by 120 mg every hour for several hours, but this remedy is now used less often than in the past, except when status follows phenobarbitone withdrawal. Intravenous phenytoin given by continuous infusion at a rate not exceeding 50 mg per minute may also be effective, but continuous electrocardiographic monitoring is needed because of the depressant effect of the drug upon cardiac function (Janz and Kautz 1964; Wallis, Kutt, and McDowell 1968). Chlormethiazole, given by intravenous infusion at a rate of 0.7 g/hour, has also been found to control status in some cases (Harvey, Higenbottam, and Loh 1975). General anaesthetics have long been used; thiopentone has been used by intravenous drip (Mortimer 1961) and in severe cases muscle relaxants and positive-pressure respiration have been employed.

Nasal feeding should be used if unconsciousness is prolonged. The patient should be nursed in the semiprone position and endotracheal incubation may be needed.

Petit mal status, which may give prolonged disorientation, accompanied by almost continuous spike-and-wave activity in the child's EEG, is probably best treated by diazepam or clonazepam as the effects of rectal or intravenous sodium valproate are still somewhat unpredictable. Some authorities still use ethosuximide in a dosage of 250 mg four-hourly with phenytoin 50 mg two or three times daily to guard against the development of major seizures, but generally the benzodiazepines are more effective. ACTH has also been recommended in such cases (80 units daily intramuscularly for a week).

Psychotherapy
Epilepsy is not primarily a psychological disorder. In some cases, however, mental stress and emotional difficulties appear to precipitate attacks. Depression, anxiety, and hysterical manifestations may also occur in epileptic individuals. When such contributory causes can be found, benefit may follow the addition of antidepressive and/or tranquillizing remedies to the patient's anticonvulsant medication, always remembering that certain antidepressive drugs (particularly imipramine) may potentiate epileptic discharges, whereas some tranquillizers (e.g. chlordiazepoxide and diazepam) have an anticonvulsant effect.

References

Adeloye, A. and Odeku, E.L. (1971). Epilepsy after missile wounds of the head. *J. Neurol. Neurosurg. Psychiat.* **34**, 98.

Ahmad, S. (1974). Renal insensitivity to frusemide caused by chronic anticonvulsant therapy. *Br. med. J.* **3**, 657.

——, Laidlaw, J., Houghton, G.W., and Richens, A. (1975). Involuntary movements caused by phenytoin intoxication in epileptic patients. *J. Neurol. Neurosurg. Plsychiat.* **38**, 225.

Aicardi, J. (1982). Childhood epilepsies with brief myoclonic, atonic or tonic seizures. In *A textbook of epilepsy* (ed. J. Laidlaw and A. Richens) 2nd edn, p. 88. Churchill-Livingstone, Edinburgh.

Allen, J.W., Oxley, J., Robertson, M.M., Trimble, M.R., Richens, A., and Jawad, S.S.M (1983). Clobazam as adjunctive treatment in refractory epilepsy. *Br. med. J.* **286**, 1246.

Ames, F.R. (1971). 'Self-induction' in photosensitive epilepsy. *Brain* **94**, 781.

Annegers, J.F., Grabow, J.D. Groover, R.V., Laws, E.R., Elveback, L.R., and Kurland, L.T. (1980). Seizures after head trauma: a population study. *Neurology, Minneapolis* **30**, 683.

Ansell, B. and Clarke, E. (1956). Epilepsy and menstruation. The role of water retention. *Lancet* ii, 1232.

Bagley, C (1972). Social prejudice and the adjustment of people with epilepsy. *Epilepsia, Amsterdam* 13, 33.

Baldwin, M. and Bailey, P. (1958). *Temporal lobe epilepsy.* Thomas, Springfield, Illinois.

Bateman, D.E., O'Grady, J.C., Willey, C.J., Longley, B.P., and Barwick, D.D. (1983). De novo minor status epilepticus of late onset presenting as stupor. *Br. med. J.* 287, 1673.

Baugh, C.M. and Krumdieck, C.L. (1969). Effects of phenytoin on folic-acid conjugases in man. *Lancet* ii, 519.

Behrman, S. and Knight, G. (1956). Carotid sinus epilepsy and its treatment by denervation. *Br. med. J.* 2, 1522.

—— and Wyke, B.D. (1958). Vestibulogenic seizures. *Brain* 81, 529.

Beley, A., Girard, C., Leroy, C., and Pinel, J.P. (1962). Studies on the effects of *N*-benzyl-beta-chloropropionamide (Nydrane) in behaviour disorders in children. *Rev. Neuropsychiat. Infantile* 10, 9.

Bengzon, A.R.A., Ramussen, T., Gloor, P., Dussault, J., and Stephens, M. (1968). Prognostic factors in the surgical treatment of temporal lobe epilepsy. *Neurology, Minneapolis* 18, 717.

Beresford, H.R., Posner, J.B., and Plum, F. (1969). Changes in brain lactate during induced cerebral seizures. *Arch. Neurol., Chicago* 20, 243.

Bingel, A. (1957). Reading epilepsy. *Neurology, Minneapolis* 7, 752.

Bird, C.A.K., Griffin, B.P., Miklaszewska, J.M., and Galbraith, A.W. (1966). Tegretol (carbamazepine): a controlled trial of a new anticonvulsant. *Br. J. Psychiat.* 112, 737.

Bjerkedal, T., Czeizel, A., Goujard, J., Kallen, B., Mastroiacova, P., Nevin, N., Oakley, G., and Robert, E. (1982). Valproic acid and spina bifida, *Lancet* ii, 1096.

Bogdanoff, B.M., Stafford, C.R., Green, L., and Gonzalez, C.F. (1975). Computerized transaxial tomography in the evaluation of patients with focal epilepsy. *Neurology, Minneapolis* 25, 1013.

Boller, F., Wright, D.G., Cavalieri, R., and Mitsumoto, H. (1975). Paroxysmal 'nightmares': sequel of a stroke responsive to diphenylhydantoin. *Neurology, Minneapolis* 25, 1026.

Bourgeois, B.F.D., Prensky, A.L., Palkes, H.S., Talent, B.K., and Busch, S.G. (1983). Intelligence in epilepsy: a prospective study in children. *Ann. Neurol.* 14, 438.

Bower, B.D. and Jeavons, P.M. (1959). Infantile spasms and hypsarrhythmia. *Lancet* i, 605.

Brain, W.R. (1925–6). The inheritance of epilepsy. *Quart. J. Med.* 19, 299.

Brennan, R.W., Dehejia, H., Kutt, H., Verebely, K., and McDowell, F. (1970). Diphenylhydantoin intoxication attendant to slow inactivation of isoniazid. *Neurology, Minneapolis* 22, 687.

Brett, E.M. (1966). Minor epileptic status. *J. neurol. Sci.* 3, 52.

Brewis, M., Poskanzer, D.C., Rolland, C., and Miller, H. (1966). Neurological disease in an English city. *Acta neurol. scand.* 42, Suppl. 24.

Bridge, E.M., Kajdi, L., and Livingston, S. (1947). A fifteen year study of epilepsy in children. *Res. Publ. Ass. nerv. ment. Dis.* 26, 451.

British Medical Journal (1972). Febrile convulsions in early childhood. *Br. med. J.* 2, 608.

—— (1974). Fits in the newborn. *Br. med. J.* 1, 127.

—— (1975a). More about febrile convulsions. *Br. med. J.* 1, 591.

—— (1975b). Benign focal epilepsy of childhood. *Br. med. J.* 3, 451.

—— (1975c). 'Reflex' epilepsy. *Br. med. J.* 3, 338.

Brooks, J.E. and Jirauch, P.M. (1971). Primary reading epilepsy: a misnomer. *Arch. Neurol., Chicago* 25, 97.

Brown, J.K. (1982). Fits in children; In *A textbook of epilepsy* (ed. J. Laidlaw and A Richens) 2nd edn, p. 34. Churchill-Livingstone, Edinburgh.

Browne, T.R., Dreifuss, F.E., Dyken, P.R., Goode, D.J., Penry, J.K., Porter, R.J., White, B.G., and White, P.T. (1975). Ethosuximide in the treatment of absence (petit mal) seizures. *Neurology, Minneapolis* 25, 515.

——, Feldman, R.G., Buchanan, R.A., Allen, N.C., Fawcett-Vickers, L., Szabo, G.K., Mattson, G.F., Norman, S.E. and Greenblatt, D.J. (1983). Methsuximide for complex partial seizures: efficacy, toxicity, clinical pharmacology, and drug interactions. *Neurology, Minneapolis* 33, 414.

Bruni, J. and Albright, P. (1983). Valproic acid therapy for complex partial seizures: its efficacy and toxic effects. *Arch. Neurol., Chicago* 40, 135.

Buchanan, R.A. and Allen, R.J. (1971). Dipenylhydantoin (Dilantin) andphenobarbital blood levels in epileptic children. *Neurology, Minneapolis* 21, 866.

Calne, D.B. (1980). *Therapeutics in neurology*, 2nd edn. Blackwell, Oxford.

Cavanagh, J.B. (1958). On certain small tumours—encountered in the temporal lobe. *Brain* 81, 389.

Chadwick, D., Cummings, W.J.K., Livingstone, I. and Cartlidge, N.E.F. (1979). Acute intoxication with sodium valproate. *Ann. Neurol.* 6, 552.

—— Jenner, P. and Reynolds, E.H. (1975). Amines, anticonvulsants, and epilepsy. *Lancet* i, 473.

Chen, R.-C. and Forster, F.M. (1973). Cursive epilepsy and gelastic epilepsy. *Neurology, Minneapolis* 23, 1019.

Christiansen, C., Kristensen, M., and Rødbro, P. (1972). Latent osteomalacia in epileptic patients on anticonvulsants. *Br. med. J.* 3, 738.

——, Rødbro, P. and Sjö, O. (1974). 'Anticonvulsant action' of vitamin D in epileptic patients? A controlled pilot study. *Br. med. J.* 2, 258.

Cloyd, J.C., Kriel, R.L., Fischer, J.H., Sawchuk, R.J., and Eggerth, R.M. (1983). Pharmacokinetics of valproic acid in children: I. Multiple antiepileptic drug therapy. *Neurology, Minneapolis* 33, 185.

Conn, J.W. (1947). The diagnosis and management of spontaneous hypoglycaemia. *J. Am. med. Ass.*, 134, 130.

Cooper, I.S., Amin, I., and Gilman, S. (1973). The effect of chronic stimulation of cerebellar cortex on epilepsy in man. *Trans. Am. Neurol. Ass.* 98, 192.

Corsellis, J.A.N. (1957). The incidence of Ammon's horn sclerosis. *Brain* 80, 193.

Cox, P.J.N. and Martin, E. (1959). Infantile spasms and hypsarrhythmia. *Lancet* i, 1099.

Cull, R., Gilliatt, R.W., Willison, R.G., and Quy, R. (1982). Prolonged observation and EEG monitoring of epileptic patients, in *A textbook of epilepsy* (ed. J. Laidlaw and A. Richens), 2nd edn, p. 211. Churchill-Livingstone, Edinburgh.

Curless, R.G., Holzman, B.H., and Ramsay, R.E. (1983). Paraldehyde therapy in childhood status epilepticus. *Arch. Neurol., Chicago* 40, 477.

Currie, S., Heathfield, K.W.G., Henson, R.A., and Scott, D.F. (1971). Clinical course and prognosis of temporal lobe epilepsy: a survey of 666 patients. *Brain* 94, 173.

Dam, M. (1982). Adverse reactions to anti-epileptic drugs. In *A textbook of epilepsy* (ed J. Laidlaw and A. Richens), 2nd edn, p. 348. Churchill-Livingstone, Edinburgh.

Dana-Haeri, J., Trimble, M.R., and Oxley, J. (1983). Prolactin and gonadotrophin changes following generalised and partial seizures. *J. Neurol. Neurosug. Psychiat.* 46, 331.

Davidson, D.L.W. and Lenman, J.A.R. (1981). *Neurological therapeutics.* Pitman, London.

Davidson, S. and Falconer, M.A. (1985). Outcome of surgery in 40 children with temporal-lobe epilepsy. *Lancet* i, 1260.

Davie, M.W.J., Emberson, C.E., Lawson, D.E.M., Roberts, G.E., Barnes, J.L.C., Barnes, N.D., and Heeley, A.F. (1983). Low plasma 25-hydroxyvitamin D and serum calcium levels in institutionalized epileptic subjects: associated risk factors, consequences and response to treatment with vitamin D. *Quart. J. Med.*, 52, 79.

——, Lawson, D.E.M., Emberson, C., Barnes, J.L.C., Roberts, G.E. and Barnes, N.D. (1982). Vitamin D from skin: contribution to vitamin D status compared with oral vitamin D in normal and anticonvulsant treated subjects. *Clin. Sci.* 63, 461.

Davies, D.M. (1981). *Textbook of adverse drug reactions*, 2nd edn. Oxford University Press, Oxford.

Delgado-Escueta, A.V., Wasterlain, C.G., Treiman, D.M., and Porter, R.J. (Eds.) (1983). *Status epilepticus: mechanisms of brain damage and treatment.* Advances in Neurology, Vol. 34. Raven Press, New York.

——, and Walsh, G.O. (1985). Type 1 complex seizures of hippocampal origin: excellent results of anterior temporal lobectomy. *Neurology, Cleveland* 35, 143.

Della Rovere, M., Hoare, R.D., and Pampiglione, G. (1964). Tuberose sclerosis in children, an E.E.G. study. *Develop. Med. Child Neurol* 6, 149.

DeMonaco, H.J. and Lawless, L.M. (1983). Variability of phenytoin protein binding in epileptic patients, *Arch. Neurol., Chicago* 40, 481.

Dent, C.E., Richens, A., Rowe, D.J.F., and Stamp, T.C.B. (1970). Osteomalacia with long-term anticonvulsant therapy in epilepsy. *Br. med. J.* 4, 69.

Devinsky, O. and Duchowny, M.S. (1983). Seizures after convulsive therapy: a retrospective case survey. *Neurology, Minneapolis* 33, 921.

Dodge, P.R., Richardson, E.P., and Victor, M. (1954). Recurrent convulsive seizures as a sequel to cerebral infarction. *Brain* 77, 610.

Donat, J.F., Bocchini, J.A., and Gonzalez, E. (1979). Valproic acid and fatal hepatitis, *Neurology, Minneapolis* 29, 273.

Dreifuss, F.E., Penry, J.K., Rose, S.W., Kupferberg, H.J., Dyken, P., and Sato, S. (1975). Serum clonazepam concentrations in children with absence seizures. *Neurology, Minneapolis* **25**, 255.

Driver, M.V. and McGillivray, B.B. (1982). Electroencephalography. In *A textbook of epilepsy* (ed. J. Laidlaw, and A. Richens) 2nd edn, p. 155. Churchill-Livingstone, Edinburgh.

Eadie, M.J. and Tyrer, J.H. (1980). *Anticonvulsant therapy*, 2nd edn. Churchill Livingstone, Edinburgh.

Earle, K.M., Baldwin, M., and Penfield, W. (1953). Incisural sclerosis and temporal lobe seizures produced by hippocampal herniation at birth. *Arch. Neurol. Psychiat., Chicago* **69**, 27.

Efron, R. (1956). The effect of olfactory stimuli in arresting uncinate fits. *Brain* **79**, 267.

—— (1957). The conditioned inhibition of uncinate fits. *Brain* **80**, 251.

—— (1961). Post-epileptic paralysis. Theoretical critique and report of a case. *Brain* **84**, 381.

Engel, J., Brown, W.J., Kuhl, D.E., Phelps, M.E., Maziota, J.C., and Crandall, P.H. (1982). Pathological findings underlying focal temporal lobe hypometabolsim in partial epilepsy. *Ann. Neurol.* **12**, 518.

——, Driver, M.V. and Falconer, M.A. (1975). Electrophysiological correlates of pathology and surgical results in temporal lobe epilepsy. *Brain* **98**, 129.

——, Kuhl, D.E., Phelps, M.E. and Crandall, P.H. (1982). Comparative localization of epileptic foci in partial epilepsy by PCT and EEG. *Ann. Neurol.* **12**, 529.

——, ——, —— and Mazzioatta, J.C. (1982). Interictal cerebral glucose metabolism in partial epilepsy and its relation to EEG changes. *Ann. Neurol.* **12**, 510.

Espir, M.L.E. (1983). Fitness to drive. Epilepsy. *Health Trends* **15**, 46.

Falconer, M.A. (1971). Genetic and related aetiological factors in temporal lobe epilepsy. *Epilepsia, Amsterdam* **12**, 13.

—— (1972). Mesial temporal (Ammon's horn) sclerosis as a common cause of epilepsy: aetiology, treatment, and prevention. *Lancet* **ii**, 767.

—— and Davidson, S. (1973). Coarse features in epilepsy as a consequence of anticonvulsant therapy. *Lancet* **ii**, 1112.

—— and Serefitinides, F.A. (1963). A follow-up study in temporal lobe epilepsy. *J. Neurol. Neurosurg. Psychiat.* **26**, 154.

—— and Taylor, D.C. (1968). Surgical treatment of drug-resistant epilepsy due to mesial temporal sclerosis. *Arch. Neurol., Chicago* **19**, 353.

Fazio, C., Manfredi, M., and Piccinelli, A. (1975). Treatment of epileptic seizures with clonazepam. *Arch. Neurol., Chicago* **32**, 304.

Fedrick, J. (1973). Epilepsy and pregnancy: a report from the Oxford record linkage study. *Br. med. J.* **2**, 442.

Feindel, W. and Penfield, W. (1954). Localization of discharge in temporal lobe automatism. *Arch. Neurol. Psychiat., Chicago* **72**, 605.

Fox, R.H., Wilkins, D.C., Bell, J.A., Bradley, R.D., Browse, N.L., Cranston, W.I., Foley, T.H., Gilbey, E.D., Hebden, A., Jenkins, B.S., and Rawlins, M.D. (1973). Spontaneous periodic hypothermia: diencephalic epilepsy. *Br. med. J.* **2**, 693.

Frantzen, E. (1961). An analysis of the results of treatment in epileptics under ambulatory supervision. *Epilepsia, Amsterdam* **2**, 207.

——, Lennox-Buchthal, M. and Nygaard, A. (1969). Longitudinal EEG and clinical study of children with febrile convulsions. *Electroenceph. clin. Neurophysiol.* **24**, 197.

——, ——, and Stene, J. (1970). A genetic study of febrile convulsions. *Neurology, Minneapolis* **20**, 909.

Friis, M.L. and Lund, M. (1974). Stress convulsions. *Arch. Neurol., Chicago* **31**, 155.

Fromm, G.H., Amores, C.Y., and Thies, W. (1972). Imipramine in epilepsy. *Arch. Neurol., Chicago* **27**, 198.

Gallhofer, B., Trimble, M.R., Frackowiak, R., Gibbs, J., and Jones, T. (1985). A study of cerebral blood flow and metabolism in epileptic psychosis. *J. Neurol. Neurosurg. Psychiat.* **48**, 201.

Gardner-Medwin, D. (1973). Why should we measure serum levels of anticonvulsant drugs in epilepsy? *Clin, Electroenceph.* **4**, 132.

Garland, H. and Sumner, D. (1964). Sulthiame in treatment of epilepsy. *Br. med. J.* **1**, 454.

Gastaut, H. (1964). Certain basic concepts concerning the treatment of the epilepsies. *Br. J. clin. Practice* **18**, 26.

—— (1969). Clinical and electroencephalographic classification of epileptic seizures. *Epilepsia, Amsterdam* **10**, Suppl. 1–28.

—— and Fischer-Williams, M. (1960). The physiopathology of epileptic seizures. In *Handbook of physiology* (ed. J. Field) Sect. 1, vol. 1, p. 329. Williams and Wilkins, Baltimore.

——, Naquet, R., Poire, R., and Tassinari, C.A. (1965). Treatment of status epilepticus with diazepam (Valium). *Epilepsia, Amsterdam* **6**, 167.

——, Roger, J., Ouahchi, S., Timsit, M., and Broughton, R. (1963). An electro-clinical study of generalized epileptic seizures of tonic expression. *Epilepsia, Amsterdam* **4**, 15.

Geoffroy, G., Llassonde, M., Delisle, F., and Décarie, M. (1983). Corpus callosotomy for control of intractable epilepsy in children. *Neurology, Minneapolis* **33**, 891.

Geschwind, N. and Sherwin, I. (1967). Language-induced epilepsy. *Arch. Neurol., Chicago* **16**, 25.

Gibberd, F.B. (1972). The prognosis of petit mal in adults. *Epilepsia, Amsterdam* **13**, 171.

—— and Bateson, M.C. (1974). Sleep epilepsy: its pattern and prognosis. *Br. med. J.* **2**, 403.

——, Dunne, J.F., Handley, A.J., and Hazleman, B.L. (1970). Supervision of epilepsy patients taking phenytoin. *Br. med. J.* **1**, 147.

——, Park, D.M., Scott, G., Gawel, M.J., Fry, D.E., Page, N.G.R., Engler, C., English, J.R., and Rose, F.C. (1982). A comparison of phenytoin and pheneturide in patients with epilepsy: a double-blind crossover trial. *J. Neurol. Neurosurg. Psychiat.* **45**, 1113.

Gibbs, E.L. and Gibbs, F.A. (1947). Sleep records in epilepsy. *Res. Publ. Ass. nerv. ment. Dis.* **26**, **26**, 366.

Gibbs, F.A. and Gibbs, E.L. (1952). *Atlas of electroencephalography.* Vol. 2, p. 24. Cambridge, Massachusetts.

——, ——, and Lennox, W.G. (1937), Epilepsy: a paroxysmal cerebral dysrhythmia. *Brain* **60**, 377.

Gilliatt, R.W. and Shorvon, S.D. (1983). Computerised tomography in epilepsy. *Lancet* **i**, 293.

Girdwood, R.H. (1959). The role of folic acid in blood disorders. *Br. med. Bull.* **15**, 17.

Glaser, G.H. and Levy, L.L. (1960). Seizures and idiopathic hypoparathyroidism. *Epilepsia, Amsterdam* **1**, 454.

——, Penry, J.K. and Woodbury, D.M. (Eds.) (1980). *Antiepileptic drugs: mechanisms of action* (Advances in Neurology, Vol. 27). Raven Press, New York.

Godwin-Austen, R.B. and Espir, M.L.E. (1983). *Driving and epilepsy.* Royal Society of Medicine, London.

Gomes, M.R. and Klass, D.W. (1983). Epilepsies of infancy and childhood. *Ann. Neurol.* **13**, 113.

Gowers, W.R. (1901). *Epilepsy and other chronic convulsive diseases.* Aldard, London.

—— (1907). *The borderland of epilepsy.* Adlard, London.

Grabow, J.D., Ebersold, M.J., Albers, J.W. and Schima, E.M. (1974). Cerebellar stimulation for the control of seizures. *Mayo Clin. Proc.* **49**, 759.

Grand, W. (1974). The significance of post-traumatic status epilepticus in childhood. *J. Neurol. Neurosurg. Psychiat.* **37**, 178.

Green, J.R., Troupin, A.S., Halpern, L.M., Friel, P. and Kanarek, P. (1974). Sulthiame: evaluation as an anticonvulsant. *Epilepsia, Amsterdam* **15**, 329.

Guberman, A. (1983). The role of computed cranial tomography (CT) in epilepsy. *Can. J. neurol. Sci*, **10**, 16.

Gumpert, J., Hansotia, P., and Upton, A. (1970). Gelastic epilepsy. *J. Neurol. Neurosurg. Psychiat.* **33**, 479.

Gunderson, C.H., Dunne, P.B., and Feher, T.L. (1973). Sleep deprivation seizures. *Neurology, Minneapolis* **23**, 678.

Gunn, J. and Fenton, G. (1971). Epilepsy, automatism, and crime. *Lancet* **i**, 1173.

Harper, M. and Roth, M. (1962). Temporal lobe epilepsy and the phobic anxiety-depersonalization syndrome. Part I: A comparative study. *Comprehens. Psychiat.* **3**, 129.

Harvey, P. and Hopkins, A. (1983). Views of British neurologists on epilepsy, driving, and the law. *Lancet* **i**, 401.

Harvey, P.K.P., Higenbottam, T.W., and Loh, L. (1975). Chlormethiazole in treatment of status epilepticus. *Br. med. J.* **2**, 603.

Hawkins, C.F. and Meynell, M.J. (1958). Macrocytosis and macrocytic anaemia caused by anti-convulsant drugs. *Quart. J. Med.* **27**, 45.

Hirsch, C.S. and Martin, D.L. (1971). Unexpected death in young epileptics. *Neurology, Minneapolis* **21**, 682.

Hodskins, M.B. and Yakovlev, P.I. (1930). Neurosomatic deterioration in epilepsy. *Arch. Neurol. Psychiat., Chicago* **23**, 986.

Hofmann, W.W. (1958). Cerebellar lesions after parental Dilantin administration. *Neurology, Minneapolis* **8**, 210.

Holden, J.C. (1957). Temporal-lobe epilepsy associated with severe behavioural disturbances. *Lancet* **ii**, 724.

Holowach, J., Thruston, D.L., and O'Leary, J. (1972). Prognosis in childhood epilepsy: follow-up study of 148 cases in which therapy had been suspended after prolonged anticonvulsant control. *New Engl. J. Med.* **286**, 169.

Horwitz, S.J., Klipstein, F.A., and Lovelace, R.E. (1968). Relation of abnormal folate metabolism to neuropathy developing during anticonvulsant drug therapy. *Lancet* i, 563.

Houghton, G.W. and Richens, A. (1974). Phenytoin intoxication induced by sulthiame in epileptic patients. *J. Neurol. Neurosurg. Psychiat.* **37**, 275.

Hunter, R., Barnes, J., and Matthews, D.M. (1969). Effect of folic-acid supplement on serum-vitamin-B$_{12}$ levels in patients on anticonvulsants. *Lancet* ii, 666.

——, Hurwitz, L.J., Fullerton, P.M., Nieman, E.A., and Davies, H. (1962). Unilateral ventricular enlargement. A report of 75 cases. *Brain* **85**, 295.

Hutchison, J.H., Stone, F.H., and Davidson, J.R. (1958). Photogenic epilepsy induced by the patient. *Lancet* i, 243.

Huttenlocher, P.R. (1974). Dendritic development in neocortex of children with mental defect and infantile spasms. *Neurology, Minneapolis* **24**, 203.

——, Wilbourn, A.J. and Signore, J.M. (1971). Medium-chain triglycerides as a therapy for intractable childhood epilepsy. *Neurology, Minneapolis* **21**, 1097.

Iivanainen, M., Bergström, L., Nuutila, A., and Vinkari, M. (1984). Psychosis-like absence status of elderly patients: successful treatment with sodium valproate. *J. Neurol. Neurosurg. Psychiat.* **47**, 965.

Illingworth, R.S. (1955). Sudden mental deterioration with convulsions in infancy. *Arch. Dis. Childh.* **30**, 529.

Jackson, J.H. (1931). Epilepsy and epileptiform convulsions. *Selected writings*, Vol. 1. Staples Press, London.

James, J.L. and Whitty, C.W.M. (1961). The electroencephalogram as a monitor of status epilepticus suppressed peripherally by curarisation. *Lancet* ii, 239.

Janz, D. (1964). Status epilepticus and frontal lobe lesions. *J. neurol. Sci.* **1**, 446.

—— (1969). *Die Epilepsien*. Thieme, Stuttgart.

—— and Kantz, G. (1964). The aetiology and treatment of status epilepticus. *German Medical Monthly* **9**, 451.

Jasper, H.H. and Droogleever-Fortuyn, J. (1947). Experimental studies on the functional anatomy of petit mal epilepsy. *Res. Publ. Ass. nerv. ment. Dis.* **26**, 272.

—— and Kershman, J. (1941). Electro-encephalographic classification of the epilepsies. *Arch. Neurol. Psychiat., Chicago* **45**, 903.

——, P.M. (1982a). Photo-sensitive epilepsy. In *A textbook of epilepsy*. (ed. J. Laidlaw and A. Richens) 2nd edn. Churchill-Livingstone, Edinburgh.

—— (1982b). Sodium valproate and neural tube defects. *Lancet* ii, 1282.

—— and Bower, B.D. (1974). Infantile spasms. In *Handbook of clinical neurology*. (ed P.J. Vinken and G.W. Bruyn) Vol. 15, p. 219. North-Holland, Amsterdam.

—— and Clark, J.E. (1974). Sodium valproate in treatment of epilepsy. *Br. med. J.* **2**, 584.

——, and Maheshwari, M.C. (1977). Treatment of generalised epilepsies of childhood and adolescence with sodium valproate (Epilim). *Develop. Med. Child Neurol.* **19**, 9.

Jennett, W.B. (1975). Epilepsy and acute traumatic intracranial haematoma. *J. Neurol. Neurosurg. Psychiat.* **38**, 378.

Klawans, H.L. and Weiner, W.J. (1981). *Textbook of clinical neuropharmacology*. Raven Press, New York.

—— (1982). Post-traumatic epilepsy. In *A textbook of epilepsy* (ed. J. Laidlaw and A. Richens) 2nd ed, p. 146. Churchill-Livingstone, Edinburgh.

——, Teather, D. and Bennie, S. (1973). Epilepsy after head injury: residual risk after varying fit-free intervals since injury. *Lancet* ii, 652.

Jurgelsky, W. and Thomas, J.A. (1966). The *in vivo* protection of gamma-amino-butyric acid against organic phosphate inhibition of ACHE. *Life Sci.* **5**, 1525.

Karas, B.J., Wilder, B.J., Hammond, E.J. and Bauman, A.W. (1983). Treatment of valproate tremors. *Neurology, Minneapolis* **33**, 1380.

Kiloh, L.G., McComas, A.J., Osselton, J.W., and Upton, A.R.M. (1981). *Clinical electroencephalography*, 4th edn. Butterworth, London.

Krumholz, A. and Niedermeyer, E. (1983). Psychogenic seizures: a clinical study with follow-up data. *Neurology, Minneapolis* **33**, 498.

Krynauw, R.A. (1950). Infantile hemiplegia treated by removing one cerebral hemisphere. *J. Neurol. Neurosurg. Psychiat.* **13**, 243.

Kurtzke, J.F. (1972). Mortality and morbidity data on epilepsy. In *The epidemiology of epilepsy* (ed. M. Alter and W.A. Hauser), NINDS Monograph No. 14, Bethesda, Maryland.

Laidlaw, J. (1956). Catamenial epilepsy. *Lancet* ii, 1235.

—— and Laidlaw, M.V. (1982). People with epilepsy—living with epilepsy. In *A textbook of epilepsy* (ed. J. Laidlaw and A. Richens) 2nd edn, p. 513. Churchill-Livingstone, Edinburgh.

—— and Richens, A. (Eds.) (1982). *A textbook of epilepsy*. 2nd edn. Churchill-Livingstone, Edinburgh.

Lance, J.W. (1963). Sporadic and familial varieties of tonic seizures. *J. Neurol. Neurosurg. Psychiat.* **26**, 51.

The Lancet (1972a). Withdrawal of anticonvulsant drugs in epilepsy. *Lancet* i, 478.

—— (1972b). Anticonvulsant osteomalacia. *Lancet* ii, 805.

—— (1975). Drug levels in epilepsy. *Lancet* ii, 264.

—— (1982). Valproate and malformations, *Lancet* ii, 1313.

—— (1983). Epilepsy, the cerebellum, and cerebellar stimulation. *Lancet* ii, 1122.

Leblanc, R., Feindel, W., and Ethier, R. (1983). Epilepsy from cerebral arteriovenous malformations. *Can. J. neurol. Sci* **10**, 91.

Lees, F. and Liversedge, L.A. (1962). The prognosis of petit mal and minor epilepsy. *Lancet* ii, 797.

Lennox, W.G. (1947). Sixty-six twin pairs affected by seizures. *Res. Publ. Ass. nerv. ment. Dis.* **26**, 11.

——, Gibbs, E.L. and Gibbs, F.A. (1940). The inheritance of epilepsy as revealed by the electroencephalogram, *Arch. Neurol. Psychiat., Chicago* **44**, 1155.

——, and Lennox, M.A. (1960). *Epilepsy and related disorders*. Little Brown, Boston, Massachusetts.

Lennox-Buchthal, M.A. (1974). Febrile convulsions. In *Handbook of clinical neurology* (ed. P.J. Vinken and G.W. Bruyn) Vol. 15, Chapter 12. North-Holland, Amsterdam.

—— (1982). Febrile convulsions. In *A textbook of epilepsy* (ed. J. Laidlaw and A. Richens) 2nd edn, p. 68. Churchill-Livingstone, Edinburgh.

Lerman, P. and Kivity, S. (1975). Benign focal epilepsy of childhood. *Arch. Neurol., Chicago* **32**, 261.

—— and Kivity-Ephraim, S. (1974). Carbamazepine sole anticonvulsant for focal epilepsy of childhood. *Epilepsia, Amsterdam* **15**, 229.

Lesser, R.P., Lueders, H., and Dinner, D.S. (1983). Evidence for epilepsy is rare in patients with psychogenic seizures. *Neurology, Minneapolis* **33**, 502.

Lishman, W.A., Symonds, C.P., Whitty, C.W.M., and Willison, R.G. (1962). Seizures induced by movement. *Brain* **85**, 93.

Liu, M.C. (1966). Clinical experience with sulthiame (Ospolot). *Br. J. Psychiat.* **112**, 621.

Livingston, S., Torres, I., Pauli, L.L., and Rider, R.V. (1965). Petit mal epilepsy. Results of a prolonged follow-up study of 117 patients. *J. Am. med Ass.* **194**, 227.

Loughnan, P.M., Gold, H., and Vance, C.J. (1973). Phenytoin teratogenicity in man. *Lancet* i, 70.

Lovelace, R.E. and Horwitz, S.J. (1967). Peripheral neuropathy in long-term diphenylhydantoin therapy. *Trans. Am. Neurol. Ass.* **92**, 262.

Marsden, C.D. and Reynolds, E.H. (1982). Neurology, In *A textbook of epilepsy* (ed. J. Laidlaw and A. Richens) 2nd edn., p. 132. Churchill-Livingstone, Edinburgh.

Mathieson, G. (1982). Pathology, In *A textbook of epilepsy* (ed. J. Laidlaw and A Richens) 2nd edn, p. 437. Churchill-Livingstone, Edinburgh.

Matthews, W.B. (1954). Tonic seizures in multiple sclerosis. *Brain* **81**, 193.

Mattson, R.H. (1983). The design of clinical studies to assess the efficacy and toxicity of antiepileptic drugs. *Neurology, Minneapolis* **33**, suppl. 1.

Maxwell, J.D., Hunter, J., Stewart, D.A., Ardeman, S., and Williams, R. (1972). Folate deficiency after anticonvulsant drugs: an effect of hepatic enzyme induction? *Br. med. J.* **1**, 297.

Maxwell, R.D.H. and Leyshon, G.E. (1971). Epilepsy and driving. *Br. med. J.* **3**, 12.

Melchior, J.C., Buchthal, F., and Lennox-Buchthal, M. (1971). The ineffectiveness of diphenylhydantoin in preventing febrile convulsions in the age of greatest risk, under three years. *Epilepsia, Amsterdam* **12**, 55.

Meldrum, B.S. (1982). Pathophysiology, In *A textbook of epilepsy*, (ed. J. Laidlaw and A. Richens) 2nd edn, p. 456. Churchill-Livingstone, Edinburgh.

—— and Brierley, J.B. (1972). Neuronal loss and gliosis in the hippocampus following repetitive epileptic seizures induced in adolescent baboons by allyglycine. *Brain Res.* **48**, 361.

—— and Horton, R.W. (1973). Physiology of status epilepticus in primates. *Arch. Neurol., Chicago* **28**, 1.

Meyer, A. (1963). Epilepsy, In *Greenfield's neuropathology*, 2nd edn (ed.

W. Blackwood, W.H. McMenemey, A. Meyer, R.M. Norman and D.S. Russell) Ch. 17. Arnold, London.

Mitchell, W.G., Greenwood, R.S., and Messenheimer, J.A. (1983). Abdominal epilepsy: cyclic vomiting as the major symptom of simple partial seizures. *Arch. Neurol., Chicago* **40**, 251.

Morgan-Hughes, J.A. (1966). Cough seizures in patients with cerebral lesions. *Br. med. J.* **2**, 494.

Mortimer, P.L.F. (1961). The encephalogram as a monitor of status epilepticus. *Lancet* **ii**, 776.

Neubauer, C. (1970). Mental deterioration in epilepsy due to folate deficiency. *Br. med. J.* **2**, 759.

Newcombe, R.L. and Shah, S.H. (1975). Radiological abnormalities in temporal lobe epilepsy with clinicopathological correlations. *J. Neurol. Neurosurg. Psychiat.* **38**, 279.

Norris, J.W. and Pratt, R.F. (1971). A controlled study of folic acid in epilepsy. *Neurology, Minneapolis* **21**, 659.

Office of Health Economics (1971). *Epilepsy in society*. London.

Oxbury, J.M. and Whitty, C.W.M. (1971). Causes and consequences of status epilepticus in adults. *Brain* **94**, 733.

Patry, G., Lyagoubi, S., and Tassinari, A. (1971). Subclinical 'electrical status epilepticus' induced by sleep in children. *Arch. Neurol., Chicago* **24**, 242.

Pedley,T.A. and Meldrum, B.S. (Eds.) (1983). *Recent advances in epilepsy—1*. Churchill-Livingstone, Edinburgh.

Penfield, W. and Flanigin, H. (1950). Surgical therapy of temporal lobe seizures. *Arch. Neurol. Psychiat., Chicago* **64**, 491.

—— and Jasper, H. (1954). *Epilepsy and the functional anatomy of the human brain*. Little Brown, Boston, Massachusetts.

Penry, J.K. and Daly, D.D. (1975). *Complex partial seizures and their treatment*, Advances in Neurology, Vol. 11. Raven Press, New York.

Polkey, C.E. (1982). Neurosurgery. In *A textbook of epilepsy* (ed. J. Laidlaw and A. Richens) 2nd edn. Churchill-Livingstone, Edinburgh.

—— (1983), Effects of anterior temporal lobectomy apart from the relief of seizures: a study of 40 patients. *J. R. Soc. Med.* **76**, 354.

Pond, D.A., Bidwell, B.H., and Stein, L. (1960). A survey of epilepsy in fourteen general practices. I. Demographic and medical data. *Psychiat. Neurol. Neurochir.* **63**, 217.

Porter, R.J. (1984). *Epilepsy: 100 elementary principles*. Saunders, Philadelphia.

Posner, J.B., Plum, F. and Poznak, A. Van (1969). Cerebral metabolism during electrically induced seizures in man. *Arch. Neurol., Chicago* **20**, 388.

Price, S.A. and Spencer, D.A. (1967). A trial of beclamide (Nydrane) in mentally subnormal patients with disorders of behaviour. *J. ment. Subnormal.* **13**, 75.

Prunty, F.T.G. (1944). Reactive hyperinsulinism. *Br. med. J.*, **2**, 398.

Ralston, A.J., Snaith, R.P., and Hinley, J.B. (1970). Effects of folic acid on fit-frequency and behaviour in epileptics on anticonvulsants. *Lancet* **i** 867.

Ramsay, R.E., Wilder, B.J., Berger, J.R., and Bruni, J. (1983). A double-blind study comparing carbamazepine with phenytoin as initial seizure therapy in adults. *Neurology, Minneapolis* **33**. 904.

Rasmussen, T. (1983). Hemispherectomy for seizures revisited. *Can. J. neurol. Sci.*, **10**, 71.

—— and Gossman, H. (1963). Epilepsy due to gross destructive brain lesions. *Neurology, Minneapolis* **13**, 659.

——, Olszewski, J. and Lloyd-Smith, D. (1958). Focal seizures due to chronic localized encephalitis. *Neurology, Minneapolis* **8**, 435.

Rawson, M.D. (1968). Diphenylhydantoin intoxication and cerebrospinal fluid protein. *Neurology, Minneapolis* **18**, 1009.

Reid, J.J.A. (1972). The need for special centres for epilepsy in England and Wales. *Epilpsia, Amsterdam* **13**, 211.

Rémillard, G.M., Andermann, R., Testa, G.F., Gloor, P., Aubé, M., Martin, J.B. Feindel, W., Guberman, A., and Simpson, C. (1983). Sexual ictal manifestations predominate in women with temporal lobe epilepsy: a finding suggesting sexual dimorphism in the human brain. *Neurology, Minneapolis* **33**, 323.

——, Ethier, R. and Andermann, F. (1974). Temporal lobe epilepsy and perinatal occlusion of the posterior cerebral artery. *Neurology, Minneapolis 24*, 1001.

Reynolds, E.H. (1968). Mental effects of anticonvulsants and folic acid metabolism. *Brain* **91**, 197.

—— (1983). Interictal behaviour in temporal lobe epilepsy. *Br. med. J.* **286**, 918.

——, Chanarin, I. and Matthews, D.M. (1968). Neuropsychiatric aspects of anticonvulsant megaloblastic anaemia. *Lancet* **i**, 394.

Richens, A. (1982). Clinical pharmacology and medical treatment. In *A textbook of epilepsy* (ed. J. Laidlaw and A. Richens) 2nd edn, p. 292. Churchill-Livingstone, Edinburgh.

—— and Dunlop, A. (1975) Serum-phenytoin levels in management of epilepsy. *Lancet* **ii**, 247.

—— and Rowe, D.J.F. (1970). Disturbance of calcium metabolism by anticonvulsant drugs. *Br. med. J.* **4**, 73.

Rodin, E.A. (1972). Medical and social prognosis in epilepsy. *Epilepsia, Amsterdam* **13**, 121.

—— (1982). Epilepsy and work. In *A textbook of epilepsy* (ed. J. Laidlaw and A Richens) 2nd edn, p. 496. Churchill-Livingstone, Edinburgh.

——, Rennick, P., Dennerli, R. and Lin, Y. (1972). Vocational and educational problems of epileptic patients. *Epilepsia, Amsterdam* **13**, 149.

Schmidt, D. (1982). Two antiepileptic drugs for intractable epilepsy with complex-partial seizures. *J. Neurol. Neurosurg. Psychiat.* **45**, 1119.

——, Canger, R., Avanzini, G., Battino, D., Cusi, C., Beck-Mannagetta, G., Koch, S., Rating, D., and Janz, D. (1983). Change of seizure frequency in pregnant epileptic women. *J. Neurol. Neurosurg. Psychiat.* **46**, 751.

Schwartz, M.S. and Scott, D.F. (1971). Isolated petit-mal status presenting de novo in middle age. *Lancet* **ii**, 1399.

Scott, D.F., Moffett, A., and Swash, M. (1972). Observations on the relation of migraine and epilepsy. *Epilepsia, Amsterdam* **13**, 365.

Shalev, R.S. and Amir, N. (1983). Complex partial status epilepticus. *Arch. Neurol., Chicago* **40**, 90.

Shaw, R.F., Gall, J.C. Jr., and Schuman, S.H. (1972). Febrile convulsions as a problem in waiting times. *Epilepsia, Amsterdam* **13**, 305.

Shields, W.D. and Saslow, E. (1983). Myoclonic, atonic, and absence seizures following institution of carbamazepine therapy in children. *Neurology, Minneapolis* **33**, 1487.

Shorvon, S.D. (1983). Specialized services for the non-institutionalized patient with epilepsy: developments in the US and the UK. *Health Trends* **15**, 38.

——, Chadwick, D., Galbraith, A.W. and Reynolds, E.H. (1978). One drug for epilepsy. *Br. med. J.* **1**, 474.

—— and Reynolds, E.H. (1982). Early prognosis of epilepsy. *Br. med. J.* **285**, 1699.

Simpson, J.A. (1952). Neurological manifestations of hypoparathyroidism. *Brain* **75**, 76.

Slater, E. and Beard, A.W. (1963). The schizophrenia-like psychoses of epilepsy. *Br. J. Psychiat.*, **109**, 95.

Solomon, G.E., Hilgartner, M.W., and Kutt, H. (1972). Coagulation defects caused by diphenylhydantoin. *Neurology, Minneapolis* **22**, 1165.

Somerville, E.R. and Bruni, J. (1983). Tonic status epilepticus presenting as confusional state. *Ann. Neurol.* **13**, 549.

Speidel, B.D and Meadow, S.R. (1972). Maternal epilepsy and abnormalities of the fetus and newborn. *Lancet* **ii**, 839.

Spencer, S.S., Spencer, D.D., Williamson, P.D., and Mattson, R.H. (1983). Sexual automatisms in complex partial seizures. *Neurology, Minneapolis* **33**, 527.

Spero, L. (1982). Epilepsy. *Lancet* **ii**, 1319.

Stevens, D.L. and Matthews, W.B. (1973). Cryptogenic drop attacks: an affliction of women. *Br. med. J.* **1**, 439.

Stock, M. S., Burg, F. D., Light, W.O., and Douglass, J.M. (1970). Licensing the driver with alterations of consciousness. *Arch. Neurol., Chicago* **23**, 210.

Stoupel, N. (1968). On the reflex epilepsies: epilepsy caused by reading. *Electroenceph. clin. Neurophysiol.* **25**, 416.

Strandjorn, R.E. and Johannessen, S.I. (1974). One daily dose of diphenylhydantoin for patients with epilepsy. *Epilepsia, Amsterdam* **15**, 317.

Suchy, F.J., Balistreri, W.F., Buchino, J.J., Sondheimer, J.M., Bates, S.R., Kearns, G.L., Stull, J.D., and Bove, K.E. (1979). Acute hepatic failure associated with the use of sodium valproate. *New Engl. J. Med.* **300**, 962.

Sutherland, J.M. and Eadie, M.J. (1980). *The epilepsies: modern diagnosis and treatment*, 3rd edn. Churchill-Livingstone, Edinburgh.

Symonds, C. (1959). Excitation and inhibition in epilepsy. *Brain* **82**, 133.

Tassinari, C.A., Dravet, C., Roger, J., Cano, J.P., and Gastaut, H. (1972). Tonic status epilepticus precipitated by intravenous benzodiazepines in five patients with Lennox–Gastaut syndrome. *Epilepsia, Amsterdam* **13**, 421.

——, Gastaut, H., Dravet, C., and Roger, J. (1971). A paradoxical effect:

status epilepticus induced by benzodiazepines. *Electroenceph. clin. Neurophysiol.* **31**, 182.

Taylor, D.C. (1969). Sexual behaviour and temporal lobe epilepsy. *Arch. Neurol., Chicago* **21**, 510.

—— and Bower, B.D. (1971). Prevention in epileptic disorders. *Lancet* **ii**, 1136.

—— and Falconer, M.A. (1968). Clinical, socio-economic, and psychological changes after temporal lobectomy for epilepsy. *Br. J. Psychiat.* **114**, 1247.

——, ——, Bruton, F.J. and Corsellis, J.A.N. (1971). Focal dysplasia of the cerebral cortex in epilepsy. *J. Neurol. Neurosurg. Psychiat.* **34**, 369.

Terrence, C.F. Jr., Wisotzkey, H.M., and Perper, J.A. (1975). Unexpected, unexplained death in epileptic patients. *Neurology, Minneapolis* **25**, 594.

Terzano, M.G., Parrino, L., Manzoni, G.C., and Mancia, D. (1983). Seizures triggered by blinking when beginning to speak. *Arch. Neurol., Chicago* **40**, 103.

Theodore, W.H., Newmark, M.E., Sato, S., Brooks, R., Paronas, N., De La Paz, R., DiChiro, G., Kessler, R.M., Margolin, R., Manning, R.G., Channing, M., and Porter, R.J. (1983). (^{18}F) fluorodeoxyglucose positron emission tomography in refractory complex partial seizures. *Ann. Neurol.* **14**, 429.

——, Porter, R.J. and Penry, J.K. (1983). Complex partial seizures: clinical characteristics and differential diagnosis. *Neurology, Minneapolis* **33**, 1115.

Thompson, P.J. and Trimble, M.R. (1983). Anticonvulsant serum levels: relationship to impairments of cognitive functioning. *J. Neurol. Neurosurg. Psychiat.* **46**, 227.

Treiman, D.M. (1983). General principles of treatment: responsive and intractable status epilepticus in adults. In *Status epilepticus: mechanisms of brain damage and treatment* (ed. A.V. Delgado-Escueta, C.G. Wasterlain, D.M. Treiman and R.J. Porter). Raven Press, New York.

Trimble, M.R. (1983*a*). Pseudoseizures. *Br. J. hosp. Med.* **29**, 326.

—— (1983*b*). Personality disturbances in epilepsy. *Neurology, Minneapolis* **33**, 1332.

Turnbull, D.M., Rawlins, M.D., Weightman, D., and Chadwick, D.W. (1983). Plasma concentrations of sodium valproate: their clinical value. *Ann. Neurol.* **14**, 38.

——, Howel, D., Rawlins, M.D., and Chadwick, D.W. (1985). Which drug for the adult epileptic patient: phenytoin or valproate? *Br. med. J.* **i**, 815.

Tyrer, J.H., Eadie, M.J., Sutherland, J.M., and Hooper, W.D. (1970). Outbreak of anticonvulsant intoxication in an Australian city. *Br. med. J.* **4**, 271.

Upton, A.R.M. (1982). Cerebellar stimulation. In *A textbook of epilepsy* (ed. J. Laidlaw and A Richens) 2nd edn, p. 430. Churchill-Livingstone, Edinburgh.

Utterback, R.A., Ojeman, R., and Malek, J. (1958). Parenchymatous cerebellar degeneration with Dilantin intoxication. *J. Neuropath. exp. Neurol.* **17**, 516.

Valsalan, V.C. and Cooper, G.L. (1982). Carbamazepine intoxication caused by interaction with isoniazid. *Br. med. J.* **285**, 261.

van Wieringen, A. and Vrijlandt, C.M. (1983). Ethosuximide intoxication caused by interaction with isoniazid. *Neurology, Minneapolis* **33**, 1227.

Vas, C.J. and Parsonage, M.J. (1967). Treatment of intractable temporal lobe epilepsy with pheneturide. *Acta neurol. scand.* **43**, 580.

Wallis, W., Kutt, H., and McDowell, F. (1968). Intravenous diphenylhydantoin in treatment of acute repetitive seizures. *Neurology, Minneapolis* **18**, 513.

Walton, J.N. (1963). Some observations on the value of electroencephalography in medico-legal practice. *Medicolegal J.* **31**, 15.

Ward, A.A. Jr. (1982). Basic mechanisms of the epilepsies. In *Scientific foundations of neurology* (ed. M. Critchley, J.L. O'Leary, and W.B. Jennett) p. 91. Heinemann, London.

Warren, D.J., Leitch, A.G., and Leggett, R.J.E. (1975). Hyperuricaemic acute renal failure after epileptic seizures. *Lancet* **ii**, 385.

Warter, J.M., Brandt, C., Marescaux, C., Rumbach, L., Micheletti, G., Chabrier, G., Krieger, J., and Imler, M (1983). The renal origin of sodium valproate-induced hyperammonemia in fasting humans. *Neurology, Minneapolis* **33**, 1136.

Waxman, S.G. and Geschwind, N. (1974). Hypergraphia in temporal lobe epilepsy. *Neurology, Minneapolis* **24**, 629.

Whitty, C.W.M. (1960). Photic and self-induced epilepsy. *Lancet* **i**, 1207.

Wilder, B.J., Ramsay, R.E., Murphy, J.V., Karas, B.J., Marquardt, K., and Hammond, E.J. (1983). Comparison of valproic acid and phenytoin in newly diagnosed tonic–clonic seizures, *Neurology, Minneapolis* **33**, 1474.

Williams, D. (1941). The significance of an abnormal electroencephalogram. *J. Neurol. Psychiat.* **4**, 257.

—— (1950). New orientation in epilepsy. *Br. med. J.* **1**, 685.

Wilson, J. (1969). Drug treatment of epilepsy in childhood. *Br. med. J.* **4**, 475.

——, Walton, J.N. and Newell, D.J. (1959). Beclamide in intractable epilepsy: a controlled trial. *Br. med. J.* **1**, 1275.

Wong, H.B. and Teh, Y.F. (1968). An association between serum-magnesium and tremor and convulsions in infants and children. *Lancet* **ii**, 18.

Wyler, A.R. and Bolender, N.F. (1983). Preoperative CT diagnosis of mesial temporal sclerosis for surgical treatment of epilepsy. *Ann. Neurol.* **13**, 59.

Young, A.C., Costanzi, J.B., Mohr, P.D., and St. Clair Forbes, W. (1982). Is routine computerised axial tomography in epilepsy worth while? *Lancet* **ii**, 1446.

Zielinsky, J.J. (1982). Epidemiology. In *A textbook of epilepsy*, (ed. J. Laidlaw and A Richens) 2nd edn, p. 16. Churchill-Livingstone, Edinburgh.

Myoclonus and the myoclonic epilepsies

The term 'myoclonus' is applied to a brief, shock-like muscular contraction which may involve a whole muscle or is rarely limited to a few muscle fasciculi. It may be confined to a single muscle or may involve many muscles, either successively or simultaneously. Often contractions occur symmetrically in muscles on the opposite sides of the body. The contraction may be too slight to cause movement of a segment of the limb, or can cause such violent movements as to throw the patient to the ground. The contraction does not involve groups of muscles which are normally synergically associated, nor does it usually affect mutually antagonistic muscles.

As Hallett, Chadwick, and Marsden (1979) pointed out, myoclonus is used as a descriptive clinical term which has no physiological, aetiological, or therapeutic implications. They classify this phenomenon into three separate varieties: in 'reticular reflex myoclonus' there is a hyperactive reflex mediated in the brainstem (this is the commonest variety); 'ballistic movement overflow myoclonus' is characterized by widespread synchronous activation of inappropriate muscles during attempted movement; in 'cortical reflex myoclonus', also precipitated by movment but equally often by somatosensory stimulation, each jerk affects only a few contiguous muscles but often involves agonist and antagonist muscles simultaneously and seems to result from hyperactivity of a component of the long-latency stretch reflex. The latter variety is often called 'action myoclonus' and may follow cerebral anoxia (see below); the jerks are often preceded by focal cortical spikes in the EEG.

While myoclonus can occur in association with many varieties of epilepsy, it may also be seen without epilepsy in many degenerative cerebral disorders, especially when these involve the olivodentate system. It may also occur in the absence of any specific pathological change and is then assumed to be a semiphysiological disorder of function. Bradshaw (1954) and Aigner and Mulder (1960) found that no fewer than 30 different entities had then been described in which myoclonus might occur.

The causes of myoclonus

While the sharp, transient muscular contractions or 'jerks' which constitute myoclonus are in most cases accepted as representing a type of transient epileptic discharge arising in cerebral or brainstem neurones, other forms of epilepsy are not invariably associated with myoclonus. Myoclonic jerks which occur on falling asleep in the 'drifting' stage are physiological and probably depend upon a transient reactivation of reticular system neurones. When, however, nocturnal myoclonus continues during sleep, major tonic–clonic fits, possibly nocturnal, often eventually occur in such cases and this syndrome is undoubtedly a form of epilepsy.

Recurrent myoclonic jerks in the early morning after waking, causing the patient to spill the breakfast tea or coffee or even to 'throw' cutlery across the room, are not infrequently seen in some children with idiopathic epilepsy, and a single myoclonic jerk in the upper limbs occasionally occurs in an attack of petit mal. Jeavons (1977) identified as a distinctive disorder eyelid myoclonus with absence seizures, responding usually to sodium valproate but not to ethosuximide, and also a benign myoclonic epilepsy of adolescence (see below). 'Jerking' or 'jumping' of the limbs and trunk in response to a sudden noise may sometimes be so intense as to be undoubtedly pathological. It has been called hyperekplexia or the 'essential startle disease' (Gastaut and Villeneuve 1967; Andermann, Keene, Andermann, and Quesney 1980; Kurczynski 1983), is occasionally familial, and may be indistinguishable from myoclonus, except that it is always precipitated by noise. Physiological evidence which suggests that evoked potentials may easily be recorded in scalp EEG recordings as a result of peripheral sensory stimuli suggests that often in patients with the benign forms of myoclonus, inhibitory mechanisms in the brainstem reticular substance are defective.

In Unverricht's progressive myoclonic epilepsy degenerative changes and Lafora bodies are found in cortical ganglion cells and in cerebellar dentate nuclei. Myoclonus may also occur in encephalitis lethargica, in many forms of encephalopathy, subacute sclerosing panencephalitis, and many neuronal storage disorders. Jones and Nevin (1954) described it as a symptom of subacute spongiform encephalopathy and it is now accepted as a common manifestation of Creutzfeldt–Jakob disease (see p. 379). The olivodentate form may be the result of a degenerative process of unknown cause, as in Hunt's dyssynergia cerebellaris myoclonica (p. 366), or of vascular lesions, tumours, and multiple sclerosis. Action myoclonus may be a sequel of cerebral anoxia (see below). Myoclonus in the legs has been described as a result of pathological changes in the spinal cord (Campbell and Garland 1956).

Myoclonus is thus a manifestation of many different lesions, processes, and pathophysiological mechanisms; often the nature of the underlying disorder of function is obscure. The clinical classification of varieties of myoclonus is, therefore, still somewhat arbitrary.

Varieties of myoclonus

Facial myoclonus

This name has been given, erroneously, by some authors to hemifacial spasm (see p. 116).

Myoclonus in encephalitis and myelitis

Myoclonus was an uncommon symptom of encephalitis lethargica, occurring with special frequency in some epidemics (see p. 275). It is seen less often in viral and demyelinating forms of encephalitis and encephalopathy. It is common in subacute sclerosing panencephalitis and in Creutzfeldt–Jakob disease.

Spinal myoclonus

Myoclonus in neck and shoulder and muscles has been reported in cervical herpes zoster. Rhythmical jerking in one upper limb has also been described as the result of a cervical-cord tumour (Garcin, Rondot, and Guiot 1968). Campbell and Garland (1956) reported a condition which they called progressive myoclonic spinal neuronitis in which myoclonic jerking in the lower limbs was followed by the development of a progressive paraplegia. Rhythmical myoclonus in the lower part of the body, sometimes involving the abdominal wall, coming on acutely and resolving after diazepam treatment, was thought by Hopkins and Michael (1974) possibly to be due to viral invasion of the spinal cord, and White-

ley, Swash, and Urich (1976) described two patients with encephalomyelitis giving rise to rigidity and stimulus-sensitive muscular spasms of the lower limbs. The latter authors postulated a possible relationship between spinal myoclonus and the 'stiffman' syndrome. In one case of spinal myoclonus presumed to be due to viral neuronitis the condition resolved spontaneously, and in another it was due to spinal-cord ischaemia and was thought, on the basis of pathological findings, to be due to abnormal activity of alpha motor neurones released from control by spinal internuncial neurones (Davis, Murray, Diengdoh, Galea-Debono, and Kocen 1981). Other causes have included cord compression, meningomyelocele, syringomyelia, and an arteriovenous malformation of the cord (Levy, Plassche, Riggs, and Shoulsson 1983); in the latter the myoclonus was controlled by clonazepam.

Palato-pharyngo-laryngo-oculo-diaphragmatic myoclonus

This syndrome is characterized by synchronous rhythmical myoclonus of the soft palate, pharynx, larynx, eyes, and diaphragm, and sometimes of other muscles. The jerking may be unilateral or bilateral. The palatal movement was once called 'nystagmus of the soft palate'. The rate of the movements varies from 80 to 180 to the minute, and is usually about 120 to 130. It is usually uninfluenced by drugs, and apparently by sleep, but may be inhibited at first by voluntary effort, and disappears if paralysis supervenes in the affected muscles. It appears to be due to a degenerative process of unknown cause involving the olivary nuclei in most cases, but has been seen in multiple sclerosis and brainstem infarction. The disorder appears to be one of the olivo-cerebellar modulatory projection on to the rostral brainstem (Herrmann and Brown 1967).

Benign (hereditary) essential myoclonus

Friedreich in 1881 described a condition characterized by the onset during adult life of frequent myoclonic muscular contractions. These are most often seen in the facial muscles and in the biceps, triceps, and brachioradialis in the upper limbs and in the quadriceps, and to a lesser extent in hip adductors and thigh extensors in the lower limbs. The contractions involve the whole muscle or groups of muscles and occur regularly with a frequency varying from 10 to 50 times a minute. The jerking movements are increased by tension and anxiety and may be inhibited by volitional contraction; though they may affect symmetrically muscles on both sides of the body, these do not contract synchronously. The movements disappear during sleep. Sensation is unimpaired, and the only associated abnormality is some briskness of tendon reflexes. The disorder is a benign but chronic one and sometimes resolves spontaneously. These patients do not as a rule develop epileptic seizures, dementia, or ataxia; no consistent pathological changes have been discovered in the brain in this condition, which Freidreich called paramyoclonus multiplex, or myoclonus simplex; Mahloudji and Pikielny (1967) suggested that it should be called 'hereditary essential myoclonus' though not all cases are familial. There is recent evidence to suggest that clonazepam may be the most effective remedy.

Myoclonic epilepsy of adolescence

This condition (Jeavons 1977) usually begins at about puberty, rarely before the age of nine years, with myoclonic jerks involving the head, arms, and upper trunk. The single jerks often recur over a 30-minute period, especially on waking, and in girls are common before or during menstruation. Tonic–clonic attacks are rare, especially during the day, but when they do occur are often preceded by an exacerbation of myoclonus. Sodium valproate is the drug of choice but clonazepam is also effective (Jeavons 1982).

Baltic myoclonus epilepsy

This benign form of myoclonic epilepsy is very similar to the adolescent form described above, save that in the countries bordering the Baltic Sea, especially Finland, it is usually hereditary (probably autosomal recessive) and both clinically and electroencephalographically there is marked photosensitivity. The condition is made much worse by phenytoin which may induce ataxia and dementia, but is usually well controlled by sodium valproate and/or clonazepam and then runs a benign course (Eldridge, Iivanainen, Stern, Koeber, and Wilder 1983).

Action myoclonus

In 1963 Lance and Adams described a syndrome of action myoclonus occurring as a sequel of hypoxic encephalopathy. They said that 'The essential clinical picture was that of an arrhythmic fine or coarse jerking of a muscle or group of muscles in disorderly fashion, excited mainly by muscular activity particularly when a conscious attempt at precision was required, worsened by emotional arousal, suppressed by barbiturates and superimposed upon a mild cerebellar ataxia'. Many additional cases have now been reported and diazepam was shown to control the jerking (Lance 1968; Sherwin and Redmon 1969). Clonazepam, which raises brain levels of serotonin (Chadwick, Harris, Jenner, Reynolds, and Marsden 1975) is even more effective (Hallett *et al.* 1979).

Infantile myoclonic encephalopathy (polymyoclonia)

This rare condition, also described under the heading of dancing eyes and dancing feet (Dyken and Kolář 1968), was mentioned on page 305. It begins suddenly in infancy with opsoclonus, limb myoclonus, and irritability and runs a protracted but relatively non-progressive course with exacerbations and remissions. It appears to be due to an auto-immune demyelinating encephalopathy.

Progressive familial myoclonic epilepsy

Myoclonic jerks often occur in patients suffering from tonic–clonic epilepsy, occurring between the attacks and sometimes becoming more frequent before the attack occurs. In addition major seizures also occur rarely in patients regarded as suffering from essential myoclonus, though it is difficult to say on what grounds such cases are distinguished from idiopathic epilepsy with myoclonus. The term 'progressive familial myoclonus epilepsy' is best reserved for the rare but well-defined syndrome first described by Unverricht in 1891, and later carefully studied by Lundborg (1903). More recent reports are by Harriman and Millar (1955), Noad and Lance (1960). Harenko and Toivakka (1961), and Rallo, Martin, Infante, Beuamanoir, and Klein (1968). Myoclonus epilepsy thus defined often occurs in several sibs, being inherited as an autosomal recessive trait.

One distinctive pathological feature is the presence of inclusion bodies in the cytoplasm of the nerve cells. Harriman and Millar described two types: (1) Lafora bodies staining like amyloid; and (2) less specific lipid inclusions. The most stiking pathological changes are found in cerebral cortical neurones and in the dentate nuclei of the cerebellum. Millar and Neill (1959) found an abnormal mucoprotein in the serum in many such cases. Yokoi, Austin, Witmer, and Sakai (1968) showed that isolated Lafora bodies contain insoluble aggregates of an unusual polyglucosan and suggested that progressive myoclonic epilepsy should be regarded as a 'glycogen deposition disease'. Ultrastructural changes were described by Brown, Kotorii, and Riehl (1968) and Ter Harn (1974). In many cases typical Lafora bodies, identifiable as membrane-bound spaces containing mucopolysaccharide, may be demonstrated in muscle biopsy sections examined with the electron microscope (Carpenter, Karpati, Andermann, Jacob, and Andermann 1974; Neville, Brooke, and Austin 1974; Coleman,

Gambetti, di Mauro, and Blume 1974). Liver biopsy may also be diagnostic, even in presymptomatic children (Baumann, Kocoshis, and Wilson 1983). Lafora body disease has also been shown rarely to give a syndrome resembling presenile dementia in adult life (Suzuki, David, and Kutschman 1971).

The onset of symptoms occurs as a rule between the ages of 6 and 16, usually when the patient is about 10, development up to that point having been normal. Generalized tonic–clonic attacks with loss of consciousness appear first, and, to begin with, often occur only at night. After several years the characteristic myoclonic jerks develop. These are shock-like muscular contractions simultaneously involving symmetrical muscles on both sides of the body, sufficiently strong to produce movements of the limb segments. They involve the muscles of the face, trunk, and of both upper and lower limbs. They disappear during sleep and are intensified by emotional excitement. They often increase in severity before a generalized seizure but are not attended by loss of consciousness. Myoclonus may occur in the ocular muscles, the lips, and the tongue, interfering with speech and with swallowing. In the limbs the flexors are more often attacked than the extensors. Writing may become impossible, and sudden contractions of the flexors of the lower limbs when the patient is standing or walking may throw him violently to the ground. After some years, during which myoclonic and tonic–clonic attacks continue, a progressive dementia develops, and the patient passes into the third stage of the disease, in which the major attacks tend to disappear, though myoclonus continues. Dysarthria and dysphagia increase, and death follows progressive cachexia. Noad and Lance (1960) reported a family with signs of cerebellar ataxia. The EEG usually shows bilaterally synchronous sharp waves occurring repetitively in time with the myoclonic jerks resembling the waves seen in the lipidoses.

The relationship of this condition to Hunt's dyssynergia cerebellaris myoclonica (p. 366) is uncertain but in the latter disorder myoclonus and cerebellar ataxia, rather than major fits and dementia, predominate. The two disorders also differ pathologically (de Barsy, Myle, Troch, Matthys, and Martin 1969) in that no Lafora bodies are seen in the Ramsay Hunt syndrome and the changes are those of dentatorubral atrophy. Cases of 'progressive myoclonic epilepsy without Lafora bodies' (Matthews, Howell, and Stevens 1969) may have been of the latter type (also see below).

Treatment is merely palliative. The usual anticonvulsant drugs may partially control the generalized seizures, but have less influence upon the myoclonus. Clonazepam may have a temporary beneficial effect upon the myoclonus but not upon the progressive dementia.

Other forms of myoclonic epilepsy

Hereditary dentatorubral-pallidoluysian atrophy

This condition, which appears to be of autosomal dominant inheritance, gives rise to myoclonus, major tonic–clonic seizures, cerebellar ataxia, progressive dementia, and choreoathetosis due to degeneration of the dentatorubral and pallidoluysian systems but without Lafora bodies (Naito and Oyanagi 1982).

Myoclonic epilepsy with mitochondrial disorder

Many recent reports have appeared of muscular atrophy with mitochondrial myopathy (see p. 579) occurring in a number of patients with symptoms resembling those of progressive myoclonic epilepsy or of the Ramsay Hunt syndrome (see above). In one recent case (Sasaki, Ruzuhara, Kanazawa, Nakanishi, and Ogata 1983) the patient had action myoclonus, cerebellar ataxia, axonal neuropathy, mitochondrial myopathy, and ACTH deficiency.

Myoclonic dystonia

The term 'hereditary myoclonic dystonia' was first used by Davidenkow (1926) to describe an association between dystonia of trunk and neck muscles and myoclonic jerking of facial and neck muscles in two middle-aged sibs. Obeso, Rothwell, Land, and Marsden (1983) point out that associated localized or more generalized myoclonic jerks are an occasional accompaniment of either generalized or segmental dystonia and can give rise to diagnostic difficulty.

References

Aigner, B.R. and Mulder, D.W. (1960). Myoclonus. *Arch. Neurol., Chicago* **2**, 600.

Andermann, F., Keene, D.L., Andermann, E., and Quesney, L.F. (1980). Startle disease or hyperekplexia: further delineation of the syndrome. *Brain* **103**, 985.

Baumann, R.J., Kocoshis, S.A., and Wilson, D. (1983). Lafora disease: liver histopathology in presymptomatic children. *Ann. Neurol.* **14**, 86.

Bradshaw, J.P.P. (1954). A study of myoclonus. *Brain* **77**, 138.

Brown, W.J., Kotorii, K. and Riehl, J.-L. (1968). Ultrastructural studies in myoclonus epilepsy. *Neurology, Minneapolis* **18**, 427.

Campbell, A.M.G. and Garland, H.G. (1956). Progressive myoclonic spinal neuronitis. *J. Neurol. Neurosurg. Psychiat.* **19**, 268.

Carpenter, S., Karpati, G., Andermann, F., Jacob, J.C., and Andermann, E. (1974). Lafora's disease: peroxisomal storage in skeletal muscle. *Neurology, Minneapolis* **24**, 531.

Chadwick, D., Harris, R., Jenner, P., Reynolds, E.H., and Marsden, C.D. (1975). Manipulation of brain serotonin in the treatment of myoclonus. *Lancet* ii, 434.

Coleman, D.L., Gambetti, P., Di Mauro, S., and Blume, R.E. (1974). Muscle in Lafora disease. *Arch. Neurol., Chicago* **31**, 396.

Davidenkow, S. (1926). Auf hereditär-abiotophischer Grundlage akut auftretende, regressierende unde episodische Erkrankungen des Nervensystems und Bemerkungen uber die familiäre subakute, myoklonische Dystonie. *Z. ges. Neurol. Psychiat.* **104**, 596.

Davis, S.M., Murray, N.M.F., Diengdoh, J.V., Galea-Debono, A., and Kocen, R.S. (1981). Stimulus-sensitive spinal myoclonus. *J. Neurol. Neurosurg. Psychiat.* **44**, 884.

de Barsy, T., Myle, G., Troch, C., Matthys, R. and Martin, J.J. (1969). La dyssynergie cérébelleuse myoclonique (R. Hunt): affection autonome ou variante du type dégénératif de l'épilepsie myoclonique progressive (Unverricht–Lundborg) (approche anatomo-chimique). *J. neurol. Sci.* **8**, 111.

Dyken, P. and Kolář, O. (1968). Dancing eyes, dancing feet: infantile polymyoclonia. *Brain* **91**, 305.

Eldridge, R., Iivanainen, M., Stern, R., Koerber, T., and Wilder, B.J. (1983). 'Baltic' myoclonus epilepsy: hereditary disorder of childhood made worse by phenytoin. *Lancet* ii, 838.

Garcin, R., Rondot, P., and Guiot, G. (1968). Rhythmic myoclonus of the right arm as the presenting symptom of a cervical cord tumour. *Brain* **91**, 75.

Gastaut, H. and Villeneuve, A. (1967). The startle disease or hyperekplexia. *J. neurol. Sci.* **5**, 423.

Guillain, G. (1937–8). The syndrome of synchronous and rhythmic palato-pharyngo-laryngo-oculo-diaphragmatic myoclonus. *Proc. R. Soc. Med.* **31**, 1031.

Hallett, M., Chadwick, D., and Marsden, C.D. (1979). Cortical reflex myoclonus. *Neurology, Minneapolis* **29**, 1107.

Harenko, A. and Toivakka, E.I. (1961). Myoclonus epilepsy (Unverricht–Lundborg) in Finland. *Acta neurol. scand.* **37**, 282.

Harriman, D.G.F. and Millar, J.H.D. (1955). Progressive familial myoclonic epilepsy in three families; its clinical features and pathological basis, *Brain* **78**, 325.

Hermann, C., Jr. and Brown, J.W. (1967). Palatal myoclonus: a reappraisal. *J. neurol. Sci.* **5**, 473.

Hopkins, A.P. and Michael, W.F. (1974). Spinal myoclonus. *J. Neurol. Neurosurg. Psychiat.* **37**, 1112.

Jeavons, P.M. (1977). Nosological problems of myoclonic epilepsies in childhood and adolescence. *Develop. Med. Child Neurol.* **19**, 3.

—— (1982), Photosensitive epilepsy. In *A textbook of epilepsy* (ed. J. Laidlaw and A. Richens) 2nd edn. Churchill-Livingstone, Edinburgh.

Jones, D.P. and Nevin, S. (1954). Rapidly progressive cerebral degeneration (subacute vascular encephalopathy with mental disorder, focal disturbances, and myoclonic epilepsy). *J. Neurol. Neurosurg. Psychiat.* **17**, 148.

Kurczynski, T.W. (1983) Hyperekplexia. *Arch. Neurol., Chicago* **40**, 246.

Lance, J.W. (1968). Myoclonic jerks and falls: aetiology, classification and treatment. *Med. J. Aust.* **1**, 113.

—— and Adams, R.D. (1963). The syndrome of intention or action myoclonus as a sequel to hypoxic encephalopathy. *Brain*, **86**, 111.

Levy, R., Plassche, W., Riggs, J., and Shoulson, I. (1983). Spinal myoclonus related to an arteriovenous malformation: response to clonazepam therapy. *Arch. Neurol., Chicago* **40**, 254.

Lundborg, H. (1903). *Die progressive Myoklonus-Epilepsie*. Almquist and Wiksell, Uppsala.

Mahloudji, M. and Pikielny, R.T. (1967). Hereditary essential myoclonus. *Brain* **90**, 669.

Matthews, W.B., Howell, D.A., and Stevens, D.L. (1969). Progressive myoclonus epilepsy without Lafora bodies. *J. Neurol. Neurosurg. Psychiat.* **32**, 116.

Millar, J.H.D. and Neill, D.W. (1959). Serum mucoproteins in progressive familial myoclonic epilepsy. *Epilepsia, Amsterdam* **1**, 115.

Maito, H. and Oyanagi, S. (1982). Familial myoclonus epilepsy and choreoathetosis: hereditary dentatorubral-pallidoluysian atrophy. *Neurology, Minneapolis* **32**, 798.

Neville, H.E., Brooke, M.H., and Austin, J.H. (1974). Studies in myoclonus epilepsy (Lafora body form). IV. Skeletal muscle abnormalities. *Arch. Neurol., Chicago* **30**, 466.

Noad, K.B. and Lance, J.W. (1960). Familial myoclonic epilepsy and its association with cerebellar disturbance. *Brain* **83**, 618.

Obesu, JA. Rothwell, J.C., Lang, A.E., and Marsden, C.D. (1983). Myoclonic dystonia. *Neurology, Minneapolis* **33**, 825.

Ralo, E., Martin, F., Infante, F., Beaumanoir, A., and Klein, D. (1968). Epilepsie myoclonique progressive maligne (maladie de Lafora). *Acta neurol. belg.* **68**, 356.

Sasaki, H., Kuzuhara, S., Kanazawa, I., Nakanishi, T., and Ogata, T. (1983). Myoclonus, cerebellar disorder, neuropathy, mitochondrial myopathy, and ACTH deficiency. *Neurology, Minneapolis* **33**, 1288.

Sherwin, I. and Redmon, W. (1969). Successful treatment in action myoclonus. *Neurology, Minneapolis* **19**, 846.

Suzuki, K., David, E., and Kutschman, B. (1971). Presenile dementia with 'Lafora-like' intraneuronal inclusions. *Arch. Neurol., Chicago* **25**, 69.

Ter Harn, M.W. van Hercop (1974). Lafora disease, In *Handbook of clinical neurology*, Vol. 15 (ed. P.J. Vinken and G.W. Bruyn) Chapter 22. North-Holland, Amsterdam.

Unverricht, H. (1891). *Die Myoclonie*. Franz Deutsche, Leipzig.

Whiteley, A.M., Swash, M., and Urich, H. (1976). Progressive encephalomyelitis with rigidity: its relation to subacute myoclonic spinal neuronitis and to the stiff-man syndrome. *Brain* **99**, 27.

Yokoi, S., Austin, J., Witmer, F. and Sakai, M. (1968). Studies in myoclonus epilepsy (Lafora body form). *Arch. Neurol., Chicago* **19**, 15.

Tetany

Definition. Tetany, or carpopedal spasm, is a form of muscular spasm beginning in, and sometimes remaining limited to, peripheral limb muscles which is associated with increased excitability of the neuromuscular apparatus to all forms of stimuli. It is a symptom of many disorders which either reduce the calcium content of the blood or increase its alkalinity.

Aetiology

The two principal causes of tetany are hypocalcaemia and alkalosis, but it may occur less often in potassium or magnesium deficiency. Alkalosis, as after hyperventilation, can alter the protein binding of calcium so that the ionized calcium fraction is decreased, causing hypocalcaemic tetany even while the total plasma calcium is normal. The causes of hypocalcaemia include low plasma albumin (in malnutrition, liver disease, and chronic diarrhoea or malabsorption), vitamin D deficiency or resistance, chronic renal disease, hypoparathroidism and related disorders, acute pancreatitis, the administration of drugs such as calcitonin, phosphate, or diphosphonates, and carcinoma, especially of the prostate (see Kanis 1983). Tetany may, in fact, occur rarely in metabolic acidosis if there are associated hyperphosphataemia and hypocalcaemia; if bicarbonate is given to correct the acidosis this may precipitate tetany due to the associated hypocalcaemia but this complication can usually be prevented by giving calcium gluconate (see Welt 1974). The diagnosis of alkalotic tetany can be confirmed by the finding of an increase in plasma bicarbonate with an alkalotic urine.

Conditions characterized by hypocalcaemia

Parathyroid deficiency. The important role of the parathyroids in the metabolism of calcium is well recognized. Hyperparathyroidism due to a parathyroid tumour causes the blood calcium content to rise above its normal figure of 2.12–2.60 mmol (0.9–1.1g)/l. Hypoparathyroidism leads to a subnormal blood-calcium which may be as low as 1.1–1.4 mmol (0.4–0.5 g)/l, and in such cases tetany may occur—tetania parathyreopriva. Hypoparathyroidism, which is rare, is usually the result of accidental removal of the parathyroid glands during thyroidectomy but may rarely follow ^{131}I treatment of thyrotoxicosis, presumably as a result of irradiation of the parathyroids (see Pots 1974). Tetany may also occur in idiopathic hypoparathyroidism (probably an auto-immune disorder) and pseudohypoparathyroidism (due to a deficient end-organ response to endogenous parathyroid hormone).

Defective intestinal calcium absorption. Fatty diarrhoea, when severe and of long duration, can reduce the blood calcium sufficiently to cause tetany. Thus it may occur in sprue, in idiopathic steatorrhoea, and, exceptionally, in tuberculous enteritis. The low blood calcium in such cases, once attributed to loss of calcium from the intestine, is more probably due to poor absorption of vitamin D (Hunter 1930). No hard and fast line can be drawn between defective absorption and excessive loss. Tetany is also an occasional manifestation of acute pancreatitis; the hypocalcaemia which rarely occurs in this condition is unexplained (see Snodgrass 1974).

Rickets and osteomalacia. In the past, dietary deficiency of vitamin D or lack of exposure to sunlight was the commonest cause of rickets which often gave rise to infantile tetany (spasmophilia). About 10 per cent of such infants also developed epileptic seizures. The widespread use of vitamin supplements in infancy has virtually abolished rickets due to dietary deficiency but a number of forms of vitamin-D resistant rickets have been described; in one of these, hypophosphatasia, a single enzyme defect has been identified (Fraser 1957; Krane 1974). Some cases of adult osteomalacia are due to an inadequate dietary intake of calcium and vitamin D (Dent and Smith 1969), but there are many other causes (Kanis 1983).

Increased demand for calcium. Pregnancy and lactation cause tetany, owing to the increased demand which they make upon the calcium resources of the mother. The likelihood of this occurring is much increased when the intake of vitamin D and calcium is subnormal, as in osteomalacia.

High urinary calcium loss. Chronic renal failure may lead to tetany through hypocalcaemia with a raised serum phosphate, present also in hypoparathyroidism, but this complication is rare, presumably because of the associated acidosis. A raised blood potassium may be a contributory factor.

Conditions characterized by alkalosis

Alkalosis occurs when the ratio of acid to base in the blood is diminished, with the result that the pH, normally between 7.3 and 7.5, rises, as does the serum bicarbonate. This may occur in the following conditions:

Excessive ingestion of alkali. Overdosage with sodium bicarbonate and other alkalis used in the treatment of dyspepsia may cause alkalosis and hence tetany, especially if renal disease impairs the ability of the kidneys to excrete alkali.

Hyperventilation. Overbreathing, by washing out CO_2 from the blood, may lead to alkalosis and hence to tetany. Tetany may thus be induced by voluntary or hysterical overbreathing, or by central hyperpnoea due to dysfunction of the respiratory centre, as in encephalitis.

High intestinal obstruction. It has long been known that tetany may complicate disorders associated with repeated vomiting—gastric tetany—and McCallum suggested that in such cases alkalosis was produced by a loss of acid from the body in the vomit. Since, however, alkalosis may occur in cases of pyloric obstruction due to carcinoma of the stomach, in which the vomit may be free from acid, this hypothesis cannot be the whole explanation. High intestinal obstruction in itself leads to a fall in the chloride content and a rise in the bicarbonate content of the blood.

Other causes of tetany

So-called idiopathic tetany was once described in an epidemic form in some countries of central Europe, usually in the spring months. Tetany also occurs rarely in association with a low blood potassium, e.g. in hyperaldosteronism or after the prolonged administration of corticosteroids. Normocalcaemic tetany, presumed to be genetically determined, without any abnormality of serum calcium, magnesium or potassium, without alkalosis, and with a normal parathormone concentration, has been described in a child with neonatal and childhood seizures (Isgreen 1976); an abnormal response of neural membranes was postulated.

Pathophysiology

The pathophysiology of tetany was reviewed by Alajouanine, Contamin, and Cathala (1958). They considered it to be a functional disorder of peripheral sensorimotor nerve fibres resulting from hypocalcaemia. Electrically the nerves show hyperexcitability, diminished capacity for accommodation, and a tendency to show repetitive responses to single stimuli. McComas (1977) suggested that in addition the muscle fibres are hyperexcitable and may then fire impulses spontaneously or after mechanical or electrical stimuli which are normally ineffective. Kimura (1983) points out that decreased extracellular calcium increases sodium (Na^+) conductance leading to membrane depolarization and repetitive nerve firing; the EMG may then show grouped motor unit action potentials which fire asynchronously at 4–5 per second, separated by intervals of comparative silence.

Symptoms and signs

An attack of tetany is usually preceded by tingling sensations in the extremities, especially in the hands, and there are often similar paraesthesiae and a sense of stiffness in the lips and tongue. The attack itself consists of muscular spasm which develops spontaneously, but its intensity may be increased by external stimuli, such as passive movement of the limbs. In mild cases the spasm is confined to the hands and feet, or even to the hands. The tonic contraction of the interossei of the hands leads to a typical attitude—*le main d'accoucheur*. The fingers are slightly flexed at the metacarpophalangeal joints and extended at the interphalangeal joints. They are strongly adducted, and the thumb is similarly adducted and usually extended. Why the muscular spasm is limited in mild cases to the hands is unknown. Exceptionally the fingers become flexed at all joints. The characteristic attitude of the feet is one of plantar-flexion at the ankle and adduction of the toes.

In severe attacks the muscular spasm spreads more proximally. In the upper limbs it usually predominates in the elbow flexors and shoulder adductors. In the lower limbs the knees are usually extended and the hips adducted. The muscles of the head may also go into spasm, with trismus and retraction of the angles of the mouth (*risus sardonicus*). The eyes may be partly closed (blepharospasm) and the bulbar muscles may also be affected, especially those of the larynx. Laryngospasm with resultant stridor was once common in children with rickets (laryngismus stridulus), but is now rare. Dysarthria and dyspnoea may thus be produced. Spasm of the trunk muscles can also occur, leading to slight opisthotonos. Tonic–clonic seizures have been described, especially in childhood.

Though slight attacks of tetany are painless, severe cramp-like pain attends the more violent spasms. Sweating and tachycardia and even pyrexia may occur in severe attacks.

The increased neuromuscular excitability is demonstrable by certain tests, even in the absence of actual attacks of tetany. *Chvostek's sign* consists of a brisk contraction of the facial muscles in response to a light tap over the facial nerve in front of the ear. Pressure upon the main artery supplying a limb or upon the peripheral nerves produced by the inflated cuff of a sphygmomanometer may precipitate an attack of tetany—*Trousseau's sign*. Electrophysiological changes are discussed above.

In hypoparathyroidism generalized tonic–clonic seizures may occur, but are rare except in children with idiopathic hypoparathyroidism in whom mental retardation is also usual (p. 470). Confusion and intellectual impairment may occur in acquired hypoparathyroidism, while papilloedema may develop, with or without cataract, in the idiopathic form. The EEG may show spikes and slow waves in the frontal areas. X-rays of the skull may demonstrate calcification in the basal ganglia and dentate nuclei (Roberts 1959; Glaser and Levy 1960).

Diagnosis

The clinical manifestations of tetany are so striking as to be unmistakable. The onset of the muscular spasm in the hands and feet and the associated signs of increased neuromuscular excitability are pathognomonic. Tetanus is distinguished by the fact that in this disease muscular spasm, though subject to exacerbations, is constant and not, as in tetany, intermittent. Moreover, in tetanus the *main d'accoucheur* attitude does not occur and trismus usually develops early, whereas in tetany this is a late symptom occurring only in severe attacks. Hysteria may be associated with tetany when produced by hysterical hyperventilation. In addition hysterical muscular rigidity may simulate tetany. Other hysterical features, such as anaesthesia, are usually found in such cases, and the patient's emotional reaction is often characteristic.

In every case of tetany the underlying cause must be ascertained. This is usually easy if the common causes are born in mind and appropriate tests are performed. It is always desirable that the pH and bicarbonate content of the plasma and the calcium and phosphate content of the serum should be ascertained in order to determine whether the condition is due to a low blood calcium or alkalosis.

Prognosis

Recovery from an attack of tetany is almost invariable, though death rarely occurs in a severe attack, owing to laryngeal or bronchial spasm. The outlook with respect to cessation of the attacks depends upon the cause and the efficacy of treatment.

Treatment

In hypocalcaemic tetany the blood calcium may be raised by giving effervescent calcium tablets along with calciferol in a dose appropriate to the individual. Dihydrotachysterol (*A.T. 10*), has a more rapid effect and is given in a dosage of 1.25 mg three times daily until the serum calcium is normal, after which a single daily maintenance dose may suffice. A severe attack may be cut short by slowly injecting 20 ml of a 5 per cent solution of calcium gluconate intravenously.

In tetany due to steatorrhoea, the malabsorption syndrome should be treated appropriately and the patient should be given calciferol. This vitamin, with or without irradiation with ultraviolet light, is all that is required in the treatment of tetany associated with rickets; the same treatment should be given in osteomalacia and also when tetany occurs in pregnancy, together with calcium by mouth and a calcium-rich diet. Parathyroid extract is contraindicated in these conditions, as it raises the blood calcium by withdrawing calcium from the bones.

When tetany is due to vitamin-resistant rickets or some other inborn error of metabolism the appropriate treatment will depend upon the identification of the underlying biochemical disorder.

References

Ajajouanine, T., Contamin, F., and Cathala, H.P. (1958). *Le syndrome tetanie*. Masson, Paris.

Dent, C.E. and Smith, R. (1969). Nutritional osteomalacia. *Quart. J. Med.* **38**, 195.

Foley, J. (1951). Calcification in a family. *J. Neurol. Neurosurg. Psychiat.* **14**, 253.

Fraser, D. (1957). Hypophosphatasia. *Am. J. Med.* **22**, 730.

Glaser, G.H. and Levy, L.L. (1960). Seizures and idiopathic hypoparathyroidism. *Epilepsia, Amsterdam* **1**, 454.

Grant, D.K. (1953). Papilloedema and fits in hypoparathyroidism. *Quart. J. Med.* **22**, 243.

Hunter, D. (1930). Goulstonian Lectures. The significance to clinical medicine of studies in calcium and phosphorus metabolism. *Lancet* **i**, 897, 947, 999.

Isgreen, W.P. (1976). Normocalcemic tetany: a problem of erethism. *Neurology, Minneapolis* **26**, 825.

Kanis, J.A. (1983). Disorders of calcium metabolism. In *Oxford textbook of medicine*. (ed. D.J. Weatherall, J.G.G. Ledingham, and D.A. Warrell), Vol. 1, Chapter 10, p. 10.41. Oxford University Press, Oxford.

Kimura, J. (1983). *Electrodiagnosis in disease of nerve and muscle*. Davis, Philadelphia.

Krane, S.M. (1974). Metabolic bone disease. In *Harrison's principles of internal medicine*, 7th edn, Chapter 352, McGraw-Hill, New York.

McComas, A.J. (1977). *Neuromuscular function and disorders*. Butterworths, London.

Potts, J.T. Jr. (1974). Disorders of parathyroid glands. In *Harrison's principles of internal medicine*, 7th edn, Chapter 350. McGraw-Hill, New York.

Roberts, P.D. (1959). Familial calcification of the basal ganglia and its relation to hypoparathyroidism. *Brain* **82**, 599.

Snodgrass, P.J. (1974). Diseases of the pancreas, in *Harrison's principles of internal medicine*, 7th edn, Chapter 302. McGraw-Hill, New York.

Welt, LG. (1974). Acidosis and alkalosis. in *Harrison's principles of internal medicine*, 7th edn, Chapter 265. McGraw-Hill, New York.

West, R. (1935). Studies in the neurological mechanism of parathyroid tetany. *Brain* **58**, 1.

23

Psychological aspects of neurology (including consideration of memory, sleep, coma, and the dementias)

Developments in psychology and psychiatry have made it necessary to restrict the scope of the psychological section of a textbook of neurology. Much of psychiatry now falls outside the province of the neurologist. Nevertheless, as the brain is the organ of the mind the neurologist has many opportunities of observing the effects of nervous disease on mental function and of studying disorders of perception, memory, and emotion. He is also concerned with the psychoses and psychoneuroses in considering the differential diagnosis of organic nervous disease. This section, therefore, deals with psychological medicine primarily from the standpoint of the neurologist. But neurologists, like all doctors, see many patients suffering from emotional symptoms; hence some consideration of the relationships between neurology and psychiatry is needed.

Anatomy and physiology

General considerations

The principal difference between the human and the subhuman brain lies in the great development of the cerebral cortex in man. The cortex is, in the first instance, an end-station which receives nervous impulses derived from the eyes, ears, and other sensory organs. The corresponding cortical regions are linked by association paths through which the sensations which form the raw material of perception evoke memories and become enriched with meaning, which can be communicated to others by means of speech, writing, and gesture (Critchley 1975). The function of the cerebral cortex, therefore is primarily discriminative, and the massive development of man's cortex when compared with that of lower animals is paralleled by the great enhancement of the range of his discriminative faculties, which has occurred despite there having been little improvement, and in some cases an actual regression, of his sensory acuity.

By contrast there is far less difference between man and lower animals in the development of subcortical centres, and in particular of the thalamus and hypothalamus. It is these regions of the brain, basal alike in situation and in function, which are intimately concerned with the affective element in feeling, with emotional and instinctive life, the regulation of the autonomic nervous system and to some extent of metabolic and endocrine function. The brain, however, works as a whole and there is a constant interplay between cortical and subcortical activity. Perception evokes emotion and, conversely, emotion provides the interest which activates perception.

There is another aspect, however, of the relationship between cortical and subcortical functions. Discrimination, the function of the cortex, implies inhibition, for, if an organism is to react appropriately to a stimulus, inappropriate reactions must be simultaneously inhibited. This is true even of a simple reflex arc; it is much more necessary when the range both of potential stimuli and of potential reactions has been so greatly enlarged by the development of the cerebral cortex. The cortex, therefore, acquires inhibitory functions as the complement of its discriminative functions.

Anatomy and physiology of the diencephalon

The thalamus is in many ways both physiologically and anatomically concerned with the organization of animal behaviour. The dorsal thalamus consists of an external portion and an internal core, each with nuclei which receive impulses from outside the thalamus and other nuclei which, as far as is known, do not. These are distinguished as extrinsic and intrinsic nuclei. The extrinsic nuclei of the external division receive the somatic sensory tracts, and the optic and auditory pathways: the intrinsic nucleus is the posterior nucleus. The extrinsic nuclei of the internal core receive impulses from the posterior hypothalamus and the central reticular formation: the intrinsic nucleus is the medial. The extrinsic nuclei of the external portion project to the primary sensory cortical areas concerned with somatic sensibility, hearing, and vision in the parietal, temporal, and occipital lobes, while the intrinsic, posterior, nucleus projects to the rest of the parieto-temporo-occipital cortex. The extrinsic nuclei of the internal core project to the limbic areas of the medial aspect of the frontal and parietal lobes and to the anterior rhinencephalon and the basal ganglia, while the medial, the intrinsic, nucleus projects to the antero-frontal cortex. There is an important corticofugal pathway (the medial forebrain bundle) running from the mediobasal part of the frontal lobe to the thalamus and the hypothalamic nuclei, including the corpora mammillaria.

Experimental stimulation and destruction of these regions in animals leads to the following conclusions. The projections from the extrinsic nuclei of the external part of the dorsal thalamus are the familiar sensory afferent pathways, and interference with them causes sensory loss in the corresponding modalities. Damage to the parts of the cerebral cortex supplied by the projections from the intrinsic nuclei of the external part leads to a failure to differentiate and respond to patterns of sensory stimuli—a condition resembling agnosia in man. These nuclei, their projections, and the corresponding cortical areas must therefore be regarded as constituting a higher-level perceptual discriminative mechanism.

On the other hand, ablation or electrical stimulation of the anatomical systems represented by the nuclei of the internal core of the thalamus, and their projections through the medial and basal telencephalon, affects feeding (eating and drinking), fighting and aggression, fleeing and avoidance, mating, and maternal behaviour: they are therefore concerned with what may broadly be termed instinctive behaviour. All such activities in man are linked with emotion to a greater or a lesser extent, and it seems a reasonable inference that the same is true of animals.

The role of various hypothalamic nuclei in controlling the activity of the autonomic nervous system has already been described (pp. 593–4); emotional disorders and altered autonomic activity are closely interlinked and it is now apparent that the hypothalamus, brainstem reticular system, parts of the thalamus, the nucleus accumbens, the hippocampus, amygdala, fornix, and, in particular, the cingulate gyrus are closely interlinked and play a fundamental integrating role in controlling emotion as well as memory and behaviour (Trimble 1981). Even though in anatomical terms, parts of the hypothalamus and brainstem reticular substance are not strictly part of the limbic system, functionally they are so closely related that all of these structures may be regarded as forming the limbic brain (Fig. 23.1). It has also become apparent that the basal ganglia, while primarily concerned with the modulation of motor activity (see pp. 322–5) possess certain behavioural functions; this is particularly true of the nucleus accumbens which is closely related anatomically to the striatum

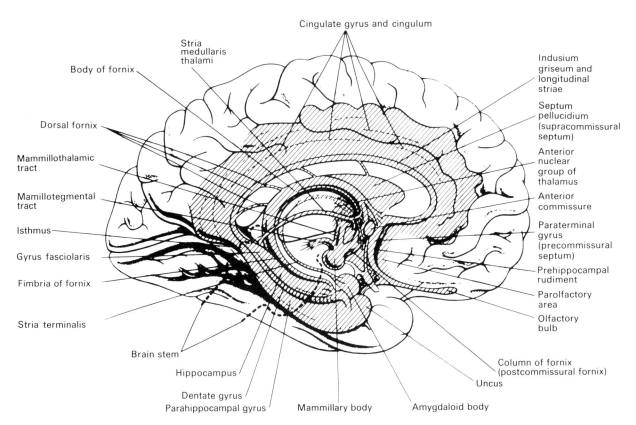

Cingulate gyrus and cingulum

Stria medullaris thalami

Body of fornix

Indusium griseum and longitudinal striae

Septum pellucidium (supracommissural septum)

Dorsal fornix

Anterior nuclear group of thalamus

Mammillothalamic tract

Anterior commissure

Mamillotegmental tract

Paraterminal gyrus (precommissural septum)

Isthmus

Prehippocampal rudiment

Gyrus fasciolaris

Parolfactory area

Fimbria of fornix

Olfactory bulb

Stria terminalis

Brain stem

Column of fornix (postcommissural fornix)

Hippocampus

Uncus

Dentate gyrus

Parahippocampal gyrus   Mammillary body   Amygdaloid body

Fig. 23.1. Anatomy of the limbic system illustrated by the shaded areas of the figure. (Reproduced from Warwick and Williams (1973) by kind permission of the editors and publisher.)

and which appears to act as a 'bridge', bringing limbic influences to bear on motor function (Trimble 1981). The respective roles of the various neurotransmitters (acetylcholine, dopamine, serotonin, catecholamines, substance P, endorphins, and many more) were considered on pp. 8–9. It is now well known that increased serotonin activity leads to psychomotor retardation and that serotonin antagonist drugs have a stimulant and antidepressive effect. Drugs which diminish catecholamine activity decrease spontaneous locomotion and inhibit conditioned responses and exploratory behaviour, while dopamine agonists can cause stereotyped behaviour. Adrenergic and noradrenergic activity play an important part in pleasure and reward, and in hypothalamic function (see below). By contrast, the mesolimbic dopamine system seems to be related to motivational arousal, and that of the striatum to motor arousal so that the proper functioning of these systems is needed for the integration of sensory inputs, memory, motivation, and motor expression (Iversen 1977; Kupferman 1981).

In the hypothalamus, in addition to the anterior and posterior nuclei concerned with temperature and cardiovascular control and with endocrine activity, and the supraoptic nucleus which produces ADH, the perifornical nucleus, when stimulated, causes hunger, increased blood pressure and sometimes rage, the ventromedial nucleus satiety, the lateral hypothalamic area thirst and hunger, and the mammillary body feeding reflexes (see Lishman 1978; Guyton 1981). Many of these functions seem to be mediated through the brainstem reticular formation.

The limbic system: behavioural functions

Neurophysiological studies in primates have shown that many hypothalamic and other limbic centres are especially concerned with sensations which have an emotional content and are either pleasant (rewarding) or painful, probably in an emotional rather than a physical sense (punishment or aversion). Thus centres in the septum, nucleus accumbens, hypothalamic ventromedial nuclei, and medial forebrain bundle may produce such a feeling of reward on stimulation that if an indwelling electrode is inserted and the animal can then apply stimuli himself he will do so repeatedly. By contrast, stimulation of the perifornical nucleus of the hypothalamus and of the mesencephalic central grey matter gives manifestations suggestive of pain, displeasure, and punishment, and will outweigh the effects of simultaneous stimulation of a reward centre (Herd 1972; Isaacson 1974; Weil 1974), while in man stimulation of the hippocampus and amygdala are also unpleasant (Trimble 1981). Physiologically, both habituation (diminishing response) and reinforcement have been shown with different stimulus patterns; pharmacologically both reward and punishment can be suppressed by various tranquillizing drugs (Cooper, Bloom, and Roth 1974). Perhaps much of human behaviour is dependent upon the balance of activity in reward and punishment centres.

In animals it has also been shown that intense stimulation of the punishment centres (e.g. the perifornical nucleus) may produce a rage response, while stimulation more rostrally gives manifestations of fear and anxiety; by contrast, repeated stimulation of reward centres gives docility and tranquillity. The influence of the hypothalamus upon the reticular system in relation to sleep and waking is shown by the fact that stimulation dorsal to the mammillary bodies gives excessive wakefulness and excitement with sympathetic overactivity, while stimulation in parts of the septum, anterior hypothalamus, or in some parts of the thalamic reticular nuclei causes somnolence and sometimes actual sleep (see Guyton 1981).

The limbic lobe and emotion

Psychophysiologically, emotion implies a number of factors: there is (1) some external object which excites it; (2) there are specific feelings characteristic of particular emotions; and (3) the emotion tends to find expression in some characteristic action. Accompanying the feelings and the motor activities there are: (4) certain other physiological states in which the autonomic nervous system and endocrine activity play an important part. And, finally, there is often: (5) a pre-existing physiological state which is necessary if the appetite, or emotional need, is to be experienced. This is most obvious in the case of hunger, thirst, and the sexual impulse.

Papez in 1937 suggested that the cortical control of emotional processes began in the hippocampus and that the information was then transferred via the fornix to the mammillary body and anterior thalamic nuclei. This 'Papez circuit' (Fig. 23.1), as Smythies (1966) showed, was the forerunner conceptually of the limbic system which controls not only the emotions but also memory and much of behaviour. Unfortunately, however, these functions are often so subjective that the functions of many parts of the limbic system are poorly understood and what little we know has been largely derived from experiments involving electrical stimulation.

Stimulation of the *amygdala* (Smythies 1970; Isaacson 1974) can cause changes in heart rate and blood pressure, defaecation and micturition, pupillary dilatation, and an increased output of various anterior pituitary hormones. In other areas stereotyped behaviour and/or involuntary movements (tonic or circling movements, chewing or lip-smacking) may be elicited or alternatively an arrest reaction, in which the animal 'freezes' in one posture. Yet other areas, if stimulated, give manifestations of rage, fear, reward, or punishment as described above, while elsewhere stimuli produce sexual activity including erection, ejaculation, copulatory movements, ovulation, or uterine contraction. Thus many of the emotional and behavioural manifestations of temporal-lobe epilepsy, including fear (Williams 1956) or hypersexuality (Green 1958) may be reproduced. The part played by the amygdala in the control of aggressive behaviour can be shown by the fact that destruction of the ventromedial nucleus of the hypothalamus leads to a lowered threshold for aggressive behaviour occurring in response to appropriate stimuli, but this is abolished by destruction of the amygdala (Trimble 1981).

The *hippocampus* distributes many outgoing signals to the hypothalamus and other parts of the limbic system via the fornix (Guyton 1981). Apart from its olfactory function, its other major role is related to memory (see below). Stimulation of other parts of the limbic cortex (the cingulate gyrus and orbitofrontal cortex) can affect the respiratory and cardiac rate and blood pressure, facilitate movements induced by cortical stimulation elsewhere, and can produce licking, swallowing, changes in gastrointestinal motility and secretion, and various affective reactions (e.g. rage or docility, increased or diminished awareness). Ablation of the cingulate gyri may give tameness in animals and suppression of previous rage reactions, while bilateral ablations of the orbitofrontal cortex may cause insomnia and motor restlessness (Hyvarinen 1973). In man, cingulectomy and various other ablations of limbic cortex have been used as psychosurgical procedures for the treatment of obsessional states, hypersexuality, and other behaviour disorders (Winter 1971; Lishman 1981; Trimble 1981).

Memory

Clinical, behavioural, and neuropathological evidence clearly indicates, as mentioned above, that the recording of and registration of information occurs in the hippocampus and its connections (Barbizet 1963; Lance and McLeod 1981) but the storage of the memory trace or engram plainly involves a considerable part of the limbic system. In clinical practice, memory is often divided into short-term, long-term, and secondary varieties (p. 653). Severe loss of recent memory with inability to record and retain new impressions occurs as a consequence of lesions of the mammillary bodies in the Wernicke–Korsakoff syndrome or after surgery (Kahn and Crosby 1972). Remote memory is sometimes impaired in these subjects to a greater extent than is generally

realized (Sanders and Warrington 1971). However, division of the fornix (Whitty 1962) and extensive bilateral frontal-lobe damage (Denny-Brown 1951) do not as a rule affect memory, while bilateral anterior cingulectomy produces only transient memory impairment (Whitty and Lewin 1960); however, the effects of bilateral lesions of the thalamic dorsomedial nuclei in animals upon learning tasks may be more profound (Schulman 1964). Sweet, Talland, and Erwin (1959) reported a case in which memory was impaired as a result of surgical division of the anterior pillars of the fornix during removal of a colloid cyst of the third ventricle, but it is possible that structures other than the fornix were also damaged. In the 'split-brain' animal each hemisphere can be trained to store information, so that the corpus callosum is not essential for information processing, storage, and retrieval (Sperry 1961). However, after commissurotomy in man (Zaidel and Sperry 1974), some defects of memory were found, suggesting that 'processes mediating the initial encoding of engrams and the retrieval and read-out of contralateral engram elements involve interhemispheric cooperation'. Work carried out in flatworms (McConnell 1962) suggested that cellular RNA was concerned in the memory process and that acquired information could be transferred to another worm which ingested the RNA derived from one which had succeeded in learning a task. Much more work upon the transfer of memory by such chemical means has been done, with results which have often been conflicting. As Cooper *et al.* (1974) said, 'There is evidence that protein and RNA synthesis may occur along with learning but the experiment has yet to be designed which explicitly relates these two events'. For the present, therefore, we should still regard memory as being a process which can be explained and controlled by neurophysiological mechanisms and disordered by many diseases which affect the structure and/or function of the brain.

Much information has now accumulated to indicate that in clinical practice it is lesions of the anterior temporal lobe and particularly of the hippocampus which most often impair memory. The so-called Kluver–Bucy syndrome, resulting from bilateral anterior temporal lobectomy in cats, usually involving the amygdala in whole or in part, gives loss of fear, tameness, and diminished aggression and a change in dietary habits, sexual overactivity, and sometimes 'psychic blindness', but, contrary to a widely held belief, no impairment of memory (see Guyton 1981). In human subjects, however, in whom a superficially similar syndrome can result from bilateral temporal-lobe damage due to head injury, Alzheimer's disease, or herpes simplex encephalitis, memory loss is invariable (Lilly, Cummings, Benson, and Frankel 1983). Penfield and Jasper (1954) and Penfield (1958), in the course of their investigations of temporal-lobe epilepsy, showed that memories could be evoked by hippocampal stimulation, and Bickford, Mulder, Dodge, Svien, and Rome (1958) produced a temporary loss of memory for recent events by electrical stimulation in this region. Scoville and Milner (1957) observed persistent, profound, and generalized loss of recent memory in 10 cases of bilateral hippocampal excision, the amnesia being unrelated to any deterioration of the intellect or personality of the subject and de Jong, Itabashi, and Olson (1969) described such a case following bilateral hippocampal infarction. Milner (1958, 1966) and Walker (1957) both reported cases of recent memory impairment after *unilateral* temporal-lobe lesions. It was suggested that in such cases the corresponding area on the opposite side must previously have been damaged, and in fact, recent neuropathological studies (Brierley 1966; van Buren and Borke 1972; Penfield and Mathieson 1974) have confirmed this hypothesis. However, the use of more precise techniques of assessing cognitive function, involving dichotic learning tasks and other methods of assessing auditory inattention (*British Medical Journal* 1972; Heilman, Watson, and Schulman 1974) have shown that a unilateral defect of 'auditory memory' may follow unilateral anterior temporal lobectomy performed for temporal-lobe epilepsy (Blakemore and Falconer

1967). Hence there is no doubt that bilateral hippocampal lesions are likely to cause permanent and continuing loss of memory for recent events; this was noted by Rose and Symonds (1960) and by Brierley, Corsellis, Hierons, and Nevin (1960) in patients who had suffered from encephalitis, which had selectively damaged the limbic brain, including the hippocampus. The important area seems to lie from 5.5 cm to 8 cm behind the tip of the temporal lobe. Such memory loss may be particularly prominent after recovery from herpes simplex encephalitis (p. 280). Recent work on the neuroanatomy of memory is reviewed by Horel (1978) (who stresses the importance of the 'temporal stem', the fibre tract connecting the mesial temporal cortex to the amygdala) and by Young (1979).

The syndrome of *transient global amnesia*, which gives a sudden impairment of recent memory, often with retrograde amnesia for several days or weeks which subsequently is reduced to an hour or two at most after recovery, and which usually occurs in a few hours (Steinmetz and Vroom 1972), is described along with other disorders of memory, on pp. 653–5. All available evidence suggests that this syndrome, which may recur, usually results from bilateral temporal-lobe ischaemia due to atherosclerosis (Heathfield, Croft, and Swash 1973).

The functions of the frontal lobe

In animals experimental damage to the frontal cortex, which derives its thalamic input from the medial nuclear group, affects the ability of the animal to solve problems which depend upon the use of past experience. It has long been believed that the frontal lobes play an important part in the control of intellect, initiative, personality, and social consciousness. Penfield and Evans (1935) found that amputation of one frontal lobe produced little change except for some impairment of those processes necessary for planned initiative, and Jefferson (1937) concluded from eight cases of unilateral frontal lobectomy that the role of the frontal lobes was quantitative rather than qualitative. Rylander (1939) reported 32 cases of operation on the frontal lobe. Emotional changes consisted of disinhibition and a tendency to euphoria, less often to depression. Changes in psychomotor activity took the form either of restlessness or lack of initiative and interest. The more automatic forms of intelligence were relatively well preserved, together with attention and memory, but higher forms of reasoning, thinking in symbols, and judgment had deteriorated. All of these features were noted in Brickner's (1939) patient who was observed for eight years after bilateral frontal lobectomy.

The operation of prefrontal leucotomy or lobotomy threw new light upon the functions of the frontal lobes which may be summarized as follows: 'According to Freeman and Watts, the prefrontal regions in man are concerned with foresight, imagination and the apperception of the self. These psychological functions are invested with emotion by way of the association fibres that link the hippocampus and cingulate gyrus with the thalamus and the hypothalamus. It would seem, then, that the functions of the prefrontal lobes are concerned with the adjustment of the personality as a whole to future contingencies. The imagination, therefore, in the pure sense of the term, may be said to reside in the prefrontal areas. Pure intellection in the sense of analysis, synthesis, and selectivity does not appear to require the integrity of the frontal and prefrontal areas to the extent that was previously thought necessary' (Brain and Strauss 1945). This view was supported by the observations of Hebb and Penfield (1940) and Hebb (1941) that extensive resection of one or both frontal lobes is not necessarily followed by intellectual deterioration, though Penfield (1948) in a later study found a slight drop in general intelligence after frontal gyrectomy and lobotomy, which he attributed to greater distractibility. But, as Smythies (1966) pointed out, despite much speculation and the virtual certainty that the frontal lobe is concerned with certain social behaviour patterns, its exact functions are still poorly understood (Meyer 1974). Disturbances of micturi-

tion, including frequency, urgency, and incontinence, result from some bifrontal lesions (Andrew and Nathan 1964) and less often from unilateral frontal tumours (Maurice-Williams 1974). However, it is reasonable to infer that the frontal lobes possess a regulating function, shaping the development of intellectual resources and the pursuit of long-term goals (Humphrey 1972). The effect upon personality of massive bifrontal lesions was well demonstrated by the celebrated case of Phineas Gage who in 1848 had a crowbar driven through the front of his skull. He was described as 'fitful, irreverent, indulging at times in the greatest profanity . . . manifesting but little deference for his fellows, impatient of restraint or advice when it conflicts with his desires, at times pertinaciously obstinate, yet capricious and vacillatory'. Thus, a 'frontal-lobe syndrome' has come to be recognized; an affected individual previously capable of judgment and sustained application and organization of his life, may become aimless and improvident, with loss of tact, sensitivity, and self-control and with impulsiveness and a failure to appreciate the consequences of reckless behaviour.

Destruction of the dorsomedial nuclei of the thalamus may produce similar effects to those of frontal leucotomy and the syndrome can follow stereotaxic surgery for parkinsonism. Since the efferent frontothalamic pathways are comparatively scanty it has been suggested that leucotomy works by interrupting afferent pathways from the dorsomedial nuclei to the frontal cortex and from the anteromedial nuclei to the cingulate gyri. Because the standard prefrontal operation all too often relieved stress at the cost of lethargy, social incompetence, and other manifestations of the frontal-lobe syndrome (Partridge 1950) it has been discarded in favour of more selective procedures such as undercutting of the orbital cortex, cingulectomy, frontal tractotomy, and various stereotaxic techniques (Knight 1964; Bond 1972; Trimble 1981) which aim to produce relief of emotional tension, obsessions, or behaviour disorder with minimal effects upon intellect and personality.

References

Andrew, J. and Nathan, P. W. (1964). Lesions of the anterior frontal lobes and disturbances of micturition and defaecation. *Brain* **87**, 233.

Barbizet, J. (1963). Defect of memorizing of hippocampal-mammillary origin: a review. *J. Neurol. Neurosurg. Psychiat.* **26**, 127.

Bard, P. (1928). A diencephalic mechanism for the expression of rage with special reference to the sympathetic nervous system. *Am. J. Physiol.* **84**, 490.

Bickford, R. C., Mulder, D. W., Dodge, H. W., Jr., Svien, H. J., and Rome, H. P. (1958). Changes in memory function induced by electrical stimulation of the temporal lobe in man. *Res. Publ. Ass. nerv. ment. Dis.* **36**, 227.

Blakemore, C. F. and Falconer, M. A. (1967). Long-term effects of anterior temporal lobectomy on certain cognitive functions. *J. Neurol. Neurosurg. Psychiat.* **30**, 364.

Bond, M. R. (1972). Psychosurgery. In *Scientific foundations of neurology* (ed. M. Critchley, J. L. O'Leary, and W. B. Jennett), p. 227. Heinemann, London.

Brain, W. R. and Strauss, E. B. (1945). *Recent advances in neurology and neuropsychiatry*. Churchill, London.

Brickner, R. M. (1939). Bilateral frontal lobectomy. Follow-up report of case. *Arch. Neurol. Psychiat., Chicago* **41**, 580.

Brierley, J. B. (1966). The neuropathology of amnesic states. In *Amnesia* (ed. C. W. M. Whitty and O. L. Zangwill) p. 15. Butterworths, London.

—— and Beck, E. (1958). The effects upon behaviour of lesions in the dorsomedial and anterior thalamic nuclei of car and monkey. *Ciba Foundation Symposium on the neurological basis of behaviour*, p. 90. Ciba Foundation, London.

——, Corsellis, J. A. N., Hierons, R., and Nevin, S. (1960). Subacute encephalitis of later life *Brain* **83**, 357.

British Medical Journal (1972). Auditory inattention. *Br. med. J.* **2**, 178.

Cooper, J. B., Bloom, F. E., and Roth, R. H. (1974). *The biochemical basis of neuropharmacology*, 2nd edn. Oxford University Press, Oxford.

Critchley, M. (1975). *Silent language*. Butterworths, London.

deJong, R. N., Itabashi, H. H., and Olson, J. R. (1969). Memory loss due to hippocampal lesions. *Arch. Neurol., Chicago* **20**, 339.

Denny-Brown, D. (1951). The frontal lobes and their functions. In *Modern trends in neurology* (ed. A. Feiling) p. 13. Butterworths, London.

—— and Chambers, R. A. (1958). The parietal lobe and behavior. *Res. Publ. Ass. nerv. ment. Dis.* **36**, 35.

Green, J. D. (1958). The rhinencephalon and behaviour. *Ciba Foundation Symposium on the neurological basis of behaviour*, p. 222. Ciba Foundation, London.

Guyton, A. C. (1981). *Textbook of medical physiology*, 6th edn. Saunders, Philadelphia.

Heathfield, K. W. G., Croft, P. B., and Swash, M. (1973). The syndrome of transient global amnesia. *Brain* **96**, 729.

Hebb, D. O. (1941). Human intelligence after removal of cerebral tissue from the right frontal lobe. *J. genet. Psychol.* **25**, 257.

—— and Penfield, W. (1940). Human behaviour after extensive bilateral removal from the frontal lobes. *Arch. Neurol. Psychiat., Chicago* **44**, 421.

Heilman, K. M., Watson, R. T., and Schulman, H. M. (1974). A unilateral memory defect. *J. Neurol. Neurosurg. Psychiat.* **37**, 790.

Herd, J. A. (1972). Physiology of strong emotions. *Physiologist* **17**, 5.

Horel, J. A. (1978). The neuroanatomy of amnesia: a critique of the hippocampal memory hypothesis. *Brain* **101**, 403.

Humphrey, M. E. (1972). Personality. In *Scientific foundations of neurology* (ed. M. Critchley, J. L. O'Leary, and W. B. Jennett). Heinemann, London.

Hyvarinen, J. (1973). CNS: afferent mechanisms with emphasis on physiological and behavioral correlations. *Ann. Rev. Physiol.* **35**, 243.

Isaacson, R. L. (1974). *The limbic system*. Plenum, New York.

Iversen, S. D. (1977). Striatal function and stereotyped behavior. In *Psychobiology of the striatum* (ed. A. R. Cools, R. H. M. Lohman, and J. H. L. van der Becken) p. 99. Elsevier, Holland.

Jefferson, G. (1937). Removal of right and left frontal lobes in man. *Br. med. J.* **2**, 199.

Kahn, E. A. and Crosby, E. C. (1972). Korsakoff's syndrome associated with surgical lesions involving the mammillary bodies. *Neurology, Minneapolis* **22**, 117.

Kandel, E. R. and Schwartz, J. H. (Eds.) (1981). *Principles of neural science*. Arnold, London.

Klüver, H. (1958). 'The temporal lobe syndrome' produced by bilateral ablations. *Ciba Foundation Symposium on the neurological basis of behaviour*, p. 175. Ciba Foundation, London.

Knight, G. (1964). The orbital cortex as an objective in the surgical treatment of mental illness. *Br. J. Surg.* **51**, 114.

Kupferman, I. (1981). Hypothalamus and limbic system I and II. In *Principles of neural science* (ed. E. R. Kandel and J. H. Schwartz). Arnold, London.

Lance, J. W. and McLeod, J. G. (1981). *A physiological approach to clinical neurology*, 3rd edn. Butterworth, London.

Lilly, R., Cummings, J. L., Benson, F., and Frankel, M. (1983). The human Klüver–Bucy syndrome, *Neurology, Minneapolis* **33**, 1141.

Lishman, W. A. (1978). *Organic psychiatry*. Blackwell, Oxford.

Maurice-Williams, R. S. (1974). Micturition symptoms in frontal tumours. *J. Neurol. Neurosurg. Psychiat.* **37**, 431.

McConnell, J. V. (1962). Memory transfer through cannibalism in planarians. *J. Neuropsychiat.* **3**, Suppl. 1, 42.

Meyer, A. (1974). The frontal lobe syndrome, the aphasias and related conditions—a contribution to the history of cortical localization. *Brain* **97**, 565.

Milner, B. (1958). Psychological defects produced by temporal lobe excision. *Res. Publ. Ass. nerv. ment. Dis.* **36**, 244.

—— (1966). Amnesia following operations on the temporal lobe. In *Amnesia* (ed. C. W. M. Whitty and O. L. Zangwill). p. 109. Butterworths, London.

Papez, J. W. (1937). A proposed mechanism of emotion. *Arch. Neurol. Psychiat., Chicago* **38**, 725.

Partridge, M. A. (1950). *Prefrontal leucotomy*. Oxford Medical, Oxford.

Penfield, W. (1948). Bilateral frontal gyrectomy and postoperative intelligence. *Res. Publ. Ass. nerv. ment. Dis.* **27**, 519.

—— (1958). The role of the temporal cortex in the recall of past experience and interpretation of the present. *Ciba Foundation Symposium on the neurological basis of behaviour*, p. 149. Ciba Foundation, London.

—— and Evans, J. (1935). The frontal lobes in man. A clinical study of maximum removals. *Brain* **58**, 115.

—— and Jasper, H. (1954). *Epilepsy and the functional anatomy of the human brain*. Little Brown, Boston.

—— and Mathieson, G. (1974). Memory. Autopsy findings and comments on the role of hippocampus in experiential recall. *Arch. Neurol., Chicago* **31**, 145.

Pribram, K. (1958). Comparative neurology and the evolution of behavior. In *Behavior and evolution* (ed. A. Roe and G. G. Simpson). Yale University, New Haven.

Rose, F. C. and Symonds, C. P. (1960). Persistent memory defect following encephalitis. *Brain* **83**, 195.

Rylander, G. (1939). *Personality changes after operations on the frontal lobes*. Munksgaard, Copenhagen.

Sanders, H. I. and Warrington, E. K. (1971). Memory for remote events in amnesic patients. *Brain* **94**, 661.

Schulman, S. (1964). Impaired delayed response from thalamic lesions. *Arch. Neurol., Chicago* **11**, 477.

Scoville, W. B. and Milner, B. (1957). Loss of recent memory after bilateral hippocampal lesions. *J. Neurol. Neurosurg. Psychiat.* **20**, 11.

Smythies, J. R. (1966). *The neurological foundations of psychiatry*. Blackwell, Oxford.

—— (1970). *Brain mechanisms and behavior*. Academic Press, New York.

Sperry, R. W. (1961). Cerebral organization and behaviour. *Science* **133**, 1749.

Steinmetz, E. F. and Vroom, F. Q. (1972). Transient global amnesia. *Neurology, Minneapolis* **22**, 1193.

Sweet, W. H., Talland, G. A., and Erwin, F. R. (1959). Loss of recent memory following section of the fornix. *Trans. Am. neurol. Ass.* **84**, 76.

Talland, G. A. (1959). The interference theory of forgetting and the amnesic syndrome. *J. abnorm. soc. Psychol.* **59**, 10.

Trimble, M. R. (1981). *Neuropsychiatry*. Wiley, Chichester.

Van Buren, J. M. and Borke, R. C. (1972). The mesial temporal substratum of memory. *Brain* **95**, 599.

Walker, A. E. (1957). Recent memory impairment in unilateral temporal lobe lesions. *Arch. Neurol. Psychiat., Chicago* **78**, 543.

Warwick, R. and Williams, D. L. (Eds.) (1973). *Gray's anatomy*, 35th British edn. Longman Group Ltd, London.

Weil, J. L. (1974). *A neurophysiological model of emotional and intentional behavior*. Thomas, Springfield, Illinois.

Whitty, C. W. M. (1962). The neurological basis of memory. In *Modern trends in neurology—3*, p. 314. Butterworths, London.

—— and Lewin, W. (1960). A Korsakoff syndrome in the post-cingulectomy confusional state. *Brain* **83**, 648.

Williams, D. (1956). The structure of emotions reflected in epileptic experiences. *Brain* **79**, 29.

Winter, A. (Ed.) (1971). *The surgical control of behavior*. Thomas, Springfield, Illinois.

Young, J. Z. (1979). Memory and its models. In *Scientific models and man* (ed. H. Harris), Chapter 3. Clarendon Press, Oxford.

Zaidel, D. and Sperry, R. W. (1974). Memory impairment after commissurotomy in man. *Brain* **97**, 263.

Consciousness and unconsciousness

The neural basis of consciousness

Consciousness is a primary element in experience and cannot be defined in terms of anything else. Neurology lends support to the distinction between the content of consciousness and the state of consciousness itself. The content of consciousness consists of sensations, emotions, images, memories, ideas, and similar experiences, and these depend upon the activities of the cerebral cortex and thalamus and their interrelationship, in the sense that lesions of these structures alter the content of consciousness without as a rule changing the state of consciousness as such. However, other structures, particularly that part of the central reticular formation of the brainstem known as the ascending reticular activating system, which extends at least from the lower border of the pons to the ventromedial thalamus, profoundly influence the state of consciousness. The cells of this system occupy a paramedian area in the brainstem from the lower part of the pons to a rostral level including the posterior hypothalamus, the thalamic intralaminar nuclei, and the septal area. Magoun and his collaborators

(Magoun 1952), and Gellhorn (1954) showed that, in Gellhorn's words, 'the cortex receives at least two kinds of afferent impulses, those which alter the activity of the greater part or the whole of the cortex and those which activate specific cortical projection areas (visual, auditory, etc.)', and that 'destruction of the reticulo-hypothalamic system does not interfere with the action of the sensory impulses on a specific projection area, but it eliminates the tonic impulses from the hypothalamic-reticular system on the cortex as a whole. Under these conditions no conscious processes are elicited.' Drugs which tend to produce unconsciousness, such as anaesthetics and hypnotics, selectively depress the ascending reticular alerting system, while those which cause wakefulness have the opposite, facilitating effect upon it.

In valuable reviews, Plum (1972) and Plum and Posner (1980) summarized the position as follows:

1. Lesions which destroy the reticular formation below the lower third of the pons do not produce coma.

2. Above this level a lesion must destroy both sides of the paramedian reticulum to interrupt consciousness.

3. The arousal effects of reticular stimulation upon behaviour and the EEG are separable in that bilateral lesions of the pontine tegmentum producing coma may be associated with a normal 'waking' EEG.

4. Sleep is an active physiological process, not a mere failure of arousal and is clearly separable from stupor and coma.

5. Sleeping and waking can occur in man even after total bilateral destruction of the cerebral hemispheres.

Hence a lesion or dysfunction of the reticular system will only produce stupor or coma if it:

(*a*) affects both sides of the brainstem;

(*b*) is located between the lower third of the pons and the posterior diencephalon; and

(*c*) is either of acute onset or large in its extent.

Sleep

Sleep is a periodic physiological depression of function of those parts of the brain concerned with consciousness, induced by the appropriate state of the reticulo-hypothalamic system. Electro-encephalography shows that as sleep deepens there is a transition from normal alpha waves to a phase of bursts of more rapid waves (spindles) and then the development of slow random waves. Dreams are associated with a burst of alpha waves during paradoxical sleep (see below). As Plum and Posner (1980) and Kelly (1981) point out, sleep is an active physiological process during which some neurones show decreased activity while in others activity is increased. Normal sleep has been shown to have several stages, one of which is the so-called 'rapid eye-movement' (REM) phase during which most dreams occur. This phase, also called 'paradoxical sleep', occurs shortly after falling asleep and again shortly before waking and seems to be the most important stage of sleep in relieving fatigue. Paradoxical sleep occupies in total about 20–25 per cent of a night's sleep in the healthy adult and itself possesses tonic and phasic features. The tonic features include an EEG of fairly low voltage, devoid of spindles and slow waves, penile erection, and loss of muscle tone. Phasic features include changes in blood pressure, heart rate, and respiration, increased cerebral blood flow, occasional myoclonic jerks, and bursts of conjugate eye movement (Oswald 1972, 1985). While severe night mares usually occur during paradoxical sleep, sleep walking, enuresis, and night terrors in childhood more often occur during orthodox (slow-wave) sleep. A disordered relationship between the REM and non-REM phases of sleep may occur in various disorders of brain function (Jouvet 1962). Insomnia, particularly in the elderly, is usually associated with brief awakenings and with a reduced proportion of paradoxical sleep (Kales 1969). In drug-withdrawal syndromes (e.g. delirium tremens), the patient tends

to alternate between wakefulness and fitful sleep of which up to 100 per cent is paradoxical (Oswald 1972). Barbiturate anaesthetics produce EEG changes similar to those of normal sleep. Though sleep-like states can be induced by electrical stimulation of nuclei in the median raphe of the medulla, it is an oversimplification to regard this as a 'sleep centre'. The nuclei of the sleep-inducing area of the medullary raphe are rich in serotonin but it is not possible as yet to conclude that serotonin release induces sleep and at least two sleep-inducing peptides (DSIP and SPS) have been isolated which induce slow-wave sleep (Kelly 1981). Whatever the exact neurophysiological and pharmacological facts prove to be, sleep clearly results from complex processes whereby, facilitated by fatigue, the withdrawal of afferent impulses leads to a reversible depression of the alerting system, thus inactivating the cerebral cortex (Wolstenholme and O'Connor 1961).

During sleep not only is consciousness lost, but other physical changes occur. The pulse rate, blood pressure, and the respiratory rate generally fall in orthodox sleep but rise in the paradoxical phase; the eyes deviate upwards, the pupils are contracted, but usually react to light, though slowly; the tendon reflexes are abolished and the plantar reflexes may become extensor. There is also a fall in cerebral blood flow with reduced vasomotor responsiveness to carbon dioxide (Sakai, Meyer, Karacan, Derman, and Yamamoto 1980).

Narcolepsy and other sleep disturbances

Narcolepsy is sleep which is abnormal as its onset is often irresistible, though the circumstances may be inappropriate and excessive fatigue is absent. The patient can be roused from the narcoleptic attack as from normal sleep.

It is necessary to consider with narcolepsy several other forms of sleep disturbance which, as they may be associated with narcolepsy or with each other in the same patient, are closely related to one another. These are cataplexy, sleep paralysis, hallucinatory states associated with sleep, 'idiopathic' hypersomnolence, sleep apnoea, and somnambulism. The first case of narcolepsy was probably described by Westphal in 1877, but the title was first used by Gélineau (1880).

Narcolepsy

The irresistible attacks of sleep characteristic of narcolepsy may be very numerous, occurring many times a day. It has been estimated that there may be 100 000 narcoleptics in the United States (Guilleminault, Wilson, and Dement 1974; *British Medical Journal* 1975b). In the attacks the patient quickly falls asleep but can be aroused immediately by appropriate stimuli. The attacks are most likely to occur in circumstances normally conducive to drowsiness, such as after a heavy meal, during a lecture, in the cinema, in church, or during a monotonous occupation, especially when driving a car. They are usually worse in the afternoon. They are occasionally precipitated by strong emotion. The sleep is usually brief, lasting only for seconds or minutes, but if the patient remains undisturbed he may sleep for hours. Typically in such cases the patient lapses at once into paradoxical sleep for about 15 minutes in contrast to the course of events in normal sleep (Roth, Bruhová, and Lehovsky; 1969; Kales, Cadieux, Soldatos, Bixler, Schweitzer, Prey, and Vela-Bueno); vivid dreams are common even in very brief episodes. Nocturnal recordings from such patients often show an abnormal relationship between REM and non-REM (orthodox) sleep (Dement, Rechtschaffen, and Gulevich 1966). Measurement of pupillary size correlates with degrees of wakefulness and is a useful means of assessing the response of narcoleptic subjects to treatment (Yoss, Moyer, and Ogle 1969). Birchfield, Sieker, and Heyman (1958) found mild hypoxia and hypercapnia in narcoleptic subjects when awake, comparable to the findings in normal subjects during sleep. Acceptable diagnostic criteria for distinguishing narcolepsy from 'idiopathic' day-time sleepiness or hypersomnolence (see below) include an association with cataplexy, hypnagogic hallucinations or sleep paralysis, immediate REM sleep, and short sleep latency (Faull, Guilleminault, Berger, and Barchas 1983). Biogenic amines such as dopamine and its metabolites are increased in the CSF both in patients with narcolepsy and hypersomnolence, suggesting an association between pathological sleepiness and increased dopamine turnover in the central nervous system (Parkes, Fenton, Struthers, Curzon, Kantamaneni, Buxton, and Record 1974; Montplaisir, de Champlain, Young, Missala, Sourkes, Walsh and Rémillard 1982; Faull *et al.* 1983). The condition is strongly familial, probably due to a gene on the short arm of chromosome 6 and there is a virtually 100 per cent association with HLA DR 2 (Langdon, Welsh, van Dam, Vaughan, and Parkes 1984). Psychosocial consequences of the disorder include driving accidents due to falling asleep at the wheel, accidents at home or at work, sometimes induced by smoking, loss of employment, marital disharmony, and other deleterious effects upon education, recreation, and personality (Broughton, Ghanem, Hishikawa, Sugita, Nevsimalova, and Roth 1981; Kales *et al.* 1982a; Kales, Soldatos, Bixler, Caldwell, Cadieux, Verrechio, and Kales 1982b).

Cataplexy

A cataleptic attack is one to which sufferers from narcolepsy are liable, but which differs from sleep in that, though the patient suddenly loses all power of movement and of maintaining posture, consciousness is preserved. Sometimes head tremor or muscular twitching also occurs, but these are more often absent. The patient sinks limply to the ground with the eyes closed. The muscles are hypotonic, the pupils may fail to react to light, the tendon reflexes may be diminished or lost, and during attacks the plantar reflexes may be extensor. Though transiently unable to move or to utter a sound, the patient is fully aware of all that is happening. Cataplectic attacks usually last less than a minute and recovery is rapid. They are commonly precipitated by strong emotion, pleasurable or otherwise, especially by laughter or excitement, and the patient may be unable to move until he has controlled his emotion (Guilleminault *et al.* 1974). Experimental cataplexy in dogs is suppressed more by inhibition of the uptake of norepinephrine than of serotonin, suggesting a disorder of aminergic–cholinergic interaction; most drugs which control cataplexy also suppress REM sleep (Foutz, Delashaw, Guilleminault, and Dement 1981).

Sleep paralysis

Sleep paralysis resembles cataplexy except that instead of being precipitated by emotional stimuli when awake, it usually occurs during the period of falling asleep or of awakening. The patient, though fully conscious, is unable to move hand or foot and often experiences intense anxiety. A touch rapidly relieves the paralysis. So-called 'night-nurse's paralysis' is undoubtedly a similar phenomenon.

Hallucinatory states associated with sleep

Sufferers from narcolepsy sometimes experience vivid hallucinations. These, more often visual than auditory, usually occur as the patient is falling asleep, and are then called hypnagogic hallucinations. Rarely, they occur during the night, when the patient seems partially awake. These hallucinations are often elaborate and terrifying, and though they seem real at the time their true character is readily recognized when the patient is fully awake. The night-terrors of childhood appear to be of a similar nature.

Idiopathic hypersomnolence

This condition, which may be familial or sporadic, is characterized by recurring daytime sleepiness but the desire to sleep is not as irresistible as in narcolepsy. Periods of daytime sleep are often prolonged, preceded by long periods of drowsiness, and not

refreshing; if sleep is resisted, automatism can occur due to 'microsleeps' (Roffwarg 1979). Sleep is, at least initially, of non-REM or orthodox type, there is no association with cataplexy, hypnagogic hallucinations, sleep paralysis, or sleep apnoea and many patients on waking exhibit drowsiness and unsteadiness for a time ('sleep drunkenness'); they also sleep heavily at night, as though, both by day and by night, the 'set' of their reticular activating system is abnormally and predominantly inhibitory.

Sleep apnoea

Many years ago, the Pickwickian syndrome was identified and was attributed to hypothalamic dysfunction, being characterized by obesity, daytime hypersomnolence (orthodox sleep), and nocturnal periodic breathing with hypercapnia (Kuhlo 1968). It has since become apparent that sleep apnoea (*The Lancet* 1979; Apps 1983), defined as cessation of airflow at the nostrils and mouth lasting for at least 10 seconds, may occur up to 10 times a night in normal subjects but only during REM sleep. In patients with sleep apnoea syndromes the episodes are more prolonged and frequent (at least 30 during a seven-hour nocturnal sleep) (Guilleminault and Dement 1978). Sleep apnoea can result from neurological disorders associated with alveolar hypoventilation (such as muscular dystrophy or motor-neurone disease), autonomic dysfunction (the Shy–Drager syndrome), brainstem lesions (such as bulbar poliomyelitis or encephalitis), or Ondine's curse, in which primary insensitivity of the respiratory centre of unknown cause impairs respiratory reflex drive so that breathing becomes almost wholly voluntary and no longer automatic. In the primary apnoea syndrome, not secondary to overt neurological dysfunction (Chokroverty and Sharp 1981), the condition may be essentially obstructive with continuation of abdominal and thoracic inspiratory movements despite occlusion of the upper airway, or central due to transient cessation of respiratory motor activity, or a combination of the two (*The Lancet* 1981). Some patients with the obstructive form have large adenoids or tonsils or laryngeal stenosis but in many the pharynx fails to open on inspiration during sleep and many are obese. Commonly there is severe nocturnal snoring, accentuated by alcohol (Issa and Sullivan 1982) and daytime hypersomnolence (usually orthodox sleep), but an association with true narcolepsy is uncommon (Parkes 1981). Central apnoea is sometimes associated with chronic respiratory insufficiency and CO_2 retention and this may be accentuated by nocturnal sedation (Rudolf, Geddes, Turner, and Saunders 1978). Regional cerebral blood-flow studies show that brainstem functional activity is low while awake but critically reduced during sleep (Meyer, Sakai, Karacan, Derman, and Yamamoto, 1980) while cyclic AMP and 5-HIAA may be increased in the CSF (Cramer, Warter, Renaud, Krieger, Marescaux, and Hammers 1981).

Somnambulism

Somnambulism can perhaps be regarded as a reciprocal of cataplexy in that the patient, though partly asleep, is able to stand and walk in an automatic fashion. It is rarely associated with narcolepsy, usually occurs during orthodox sleep in adolescents who are anxious but otherwise normal. It can occur as an isolated incident after exposure to unusual stress (e.g. during examinations).

The nature of narcolepsy and allied disorders

Contrary to the views once proposed these phenomena are clearly unrelated to epilepsy. Narcolepsy is paradoxical sleep of sudden and irresistible onset, and cataplexy a form of localized sleep affecting centres concerned in movement and posture only. Sleep paralysis, also associated with paradoxical sleep, is due to a failure of uniform spread of sleep over the reticular system, the parts concerned with consciousness remaining awake while those concerned with motor and postural control have fallen asleep, or, conversely, have awakened before them. Hypnagogic hallucinations seem to be the product of a dissociation of the consciousness, akin to dreaming, or to the evocation of memory engrams when the subject is partially awake; and somnambulism, associated with orthodox rather than paradoxical sleep, can be regarded as a condition in which the highest levels are asleep, but lower levels concerned with the control of organized movement are awake. Thus an imbalance of activity in the parts of the reticular activating mechanism can be postulated.

The causes of hypersomnolence and related disorders

True narcolepsy is always idiopathic but abnormal daytime hypersomnolence may not only be due to the idiopathic condition described above but can also follow head injury or result from cerebral arteriosclerosis, neurosyphilis, encephalitis, or intracranial tumour involving the posterior part of the hypothalamus (Guilleminault, Faull, Miles, and Van den Hoed 1983). It can also result from insomnia, sometimes due to nocturnal myoclonus or restless legs and many other causes (Parkes 1981). Cataplexy is very rarely symptomatic but has been described in association with attacks resembling narcolepsy and sleep paralysis in a patient with a glioblastoma of the midbrain (Stahl, Layzer, Aminoff, Townsend, and Feldon 1980). Males are more subject to idiopathic narcolepsy than females and the onset usually occurs during adolescence or, at any rate, under the age of 30. It can probably be regarded in the true sense as a functional disorder, that is, a disturbance of function consisting of a exaggeration of a normal tendency to drowsiness.

Diagnosis

Both narcolepsy and cataplexy are so distinctive that diagnosis usually presents no difficulty. Narcolepsy is distinguished from both epilepsy and syncope by the circumstances in which the attacks occur and by the ease of arousal, cataplexy by the preservation of consciousness. As idiopathic or symptomatic hypersomnolence is sometimes difficult to distinguish from idiopathic narcolepsy, however, it may be useful to record the EEG and eye movements during sleep and it is also wise to exclude organic disease involving the brainstem or hypothalamus by skull X-ray and CT scan.

Prognosis

The disorder does not threaten life unless the patient is unfortunate enough to have an attack in a dangerous situation as when driving a vehicle. The response to treatment is sometimes disappointing and the attacks often continue idefinitely, though occasionally they cease spontaneously.

Treatment

The sufferer from narcolepsy is necessarily debarred from occupations in which an attack of sleep may endanger him or others, and should usually be banned from driving if his attacks are severe or uncontrolled. Traditionally amphetamine and its derivatives were often recommended for the treatment of both narcolepsy and cataplexy. While barbiturates reduce selectively the proportion of paradoxical sleep but prolong orthodox sleep, amphetamines reduce the duration of both and doses of dextroamphetamine sulphate or methylphenidate given on waking and again at midday, graduated according to need, have certainly controlled narcolepsy in many cases. When narcolepsy or cataplexy by day are associated with disturbances of nocturnal sleep it may be wise to give a nightly dose of nitrazepam. With increasing concern being expressed about the illegal use of amphetamines and their analogues, and evidence that clomipramine 75 mg daily is often effective in both narcolepsy and cataplexy (Guilleminault *et al.* 1974; *British Medical Journal* 1975 *a, b*) many regard the latter as the drug of choice in most cases; it is also helpful in controlling hypnagogic hallucinations. Certainly it seems to be superior to imipramine and desimipramine, once widely used (Hishikawa, Ida,

Nakai, and Kaneko 1966). Other remedies found to be of value include propranolol 20 mg four times daily (Kales, Cadieux, Soldatos, and Tan 1979), mazindol 3–8 mg daily (in narcolepsy, not cataplexy) (Parkes and Schachter 1979), fluvoxamine 25–200 mg daily (especially in cataplexy) (Schachter and Parkes 1980; Thompson, Schachter, and Parkes 1982), codeine and pentazocine (not to be recommended because of the danger of addiction) (Harper 1981), and nocturnal gamma-hydroxybutyrate (1.5–4.0 g) (Broughton and Mamelak 1979, 1980). Sleep apnoea has been relieved by protriptyline (5–20 mg at night) (Clark, Schmidt, Schaal, Boudoulas, and Schuller 1979). Idiopathic hypersomnolence does not usually respond as well to these remedies but can be relieved by serotonin antagonists such as methysergide 3–6 mg daily and perhaps even more satisfactorily by pizotifen, cyproheptadine, or mianserin, though not all workers have found these remedies effective (Parkes 1981).

Periodic somnolence and morbid hunger

Kleine (1925) and Levin (1936) described a rare disorder characterized by periodic attacks of excessive appetite (bulimia) followed by profound sleepiness which may last for days. During this phase the patient's personality may be profoundly altered, but in the intervals between the attacks he is usually normal. In the attacks of prolonged somnolence the patient awakens only as a rule to eat ravenously (often of a wide variety of unusual foods) and abnormal sexual behaviour with frequent masturbation and hypersexuality may be seen (Critchley 1962; Garland, Sumner, and Fourman 1965). The condition occurs almost invariably in adolescent males but a case in a young female has been described (Duffy and Davison 1968). Depression, delusions, and amnesia may be noted temporarily after an attack. The cause is unknown and no physical abnormality, clinical, biochemical, or electroencephalographic, can generally be discovered during the attack. Amphetamine was used with some success (Gallinek 1954) in treatment and Duffy and Davison (1968) found that intravenous methedrine cut short the attacks. Imipramine and its derivatives, especially clomipramine (Parkes, Fenton, Struthers, Curzon, Kantamaneni, Buxton, and Record 1974), now appear to be the treatment of choice. In one fatal case (death in an attack is very rare and most patients ultimately recover) the findings at autopsy raised the possibility of a viral cause but were inconclusive (Carpenter, Yassa, and Ochs 1982).

References

Apps, M. C. P. (1983). Sleep-disordered breathing. *Br. J. hosp. Med.* **30**, 339.

Birchfield, R. I., Sieker, H. O., and Heyman, A. (1958). Alterations in blood gases during natural sleep and narcolepsy. *Neurology, Minneapolis* **8**, 107.

Brain, W. R. (1939). Sleep normal and pathological. *Br. med. J.* **2**, 51.

—— (1958). The physiological basis of consciousness, *Brain* **81**, 426.

British Medical Journal (1975*a*). Treatment of cataplexy. *Br. med. J.* **1**, 233.

—— (1975*b*). Narcolepsy. *Br. med. J.* **1**, 477.

Broughton, R., Ghanem, Q., Hishikawa, Y., Sugita, Y., Nevsimalova, S., and Roth, D. (1981). Life effects of narcolepsy in 180 patients from North America, Asia and Europe compared to matched controls. *Can. J. neurol. Sci.* **8**, 299.

—— and Mamelak, M. (1979). The treatment of narcolepsy–cataplexy with nocturnal gamma-hydroxybutyrate. *Can. J. neurol. Sci.* **6**, 1.

—— and —— (1980). Effects of nocturnal gamma-hydroxybutyrate on sleep/waking patterns in narcolepsy–cataplexy. *Can. J. neurol. Sci.* **7**, 23.

Cairns, H. (1952). Disturbances of consciousness with lesions of the brainstem and diencephalon. *Brain* **75**, 109.

Carpenter, S., Yassa, R., and Ochs, R. (1982). A pathologic basis for Kleine–Levin syndrome. *Arch. Neurol., Chicago* **39**, 25.

Chokroverty, S. and Sharp, J. T. (1981). Primary sleep apnoea syndrome. *J. Neurol. Neurosurg. Psychiat.* **44**, 970.

Clark, R. W., Schmidt, H. S., Schaal, S. F., Boudoulas, H., and Schuller, D. E. (1979). Sleep apnea: treatment with protriptyline. *Neurology, Minneapolis* **29**, 1287.

Cramer, H., Warter, J. M., Renaud, B., Krieger, J., Marescaux, C. H. R., and Hammers, R. (1981). Cerebrospinal fluid adenosine 3',5'-monophosphate, 5-hydroxyindoleacetic acid and homovanillic acid in patients with sleep apnoea syndrome. *J. Neurol. Neurosurg. Psychiat.* **44**, 1165.

Critchley, M. (1962). Periodic hypersomnia and megaphagia in adolescent males. *Brain* **85**, 627.

Daniels, L. E. (1934). Narcolepsy. *Medicine, Baltimore* **13**, 1.

Dement, W., Rechtshaffen, A., and Gulevich, G. (1966). The nature of the narcoleptic sleep attack. *Neurology, Minneapolis* **16**, 18.

Duffy, J. P. and Davison, K. (1968). A female case of the Kleine–Levin syndrome. *Br. J. Psychiat.* **114**, 77.

Faull, K. F., Guilleminault, C., Berger, P. A., and Barchas, J. D. (1983). Cerebrospinal fluid monoamine metabolites in narcolepsy and hypersomnia. *Ann. Neurol.* **13**, 258.

Foutz, A. S., Delashaw, J. B., Guilleminault, C., and Dement, W. C. (1981). Monoaminergic mechanisms and experimental cataplexy. *Ann. Neurol.* **10**, 369.

Gallinek, A. (1954). The syndrome of episodes of hypersomnia, bulimia and abnormal mental states. *J. Am. med. Ass.* **154**, 1081.

Garland, H., Sumner, D., and Fourman, P. (1965). The Kleine–Levin syndrome. Some further observations. *Neurology, Minneapolis* **15**, 1161.

Gélineau, Dr. (1880). De la narcolepsie. *Gaz. Hôp., Paris* **53**, 626, 635.

Gellhorn, E. (1954). Physiological processes related to consciousness and perception. *Brain* **67**, 401.

Guilleminault, C. and Dement, W. C. (Eds.) (1978). *Sleep apnea syndromes*. A. R. Liss, New York.

——, Faull, K. F., Miles, L., and Van den Hoed, J. (1983). Posttraumatic excessive daytime sleepiness: a review of 20 patients. *Neurology, Minneapolis* **33**, 1584.

——, Wilson, R. A., and Dement, W. C. (1974). A study on cataplexy. *Arch. Neurol., Chicago* **31**, 255.

Harper, J.M. (1981). Gelineau's narcolepsy relieved by opiates. *Lancet* **i**, 92.

Hishikawa, Y., Ida, H., Nakai, K., and Kaneko, Z. (1966). Treatment of narcolepsy with imipramine (Tofranil) and desmethylimipramine (Pertofran). *J. neurol. Sci.* **3**, 453.

Issa, F. G. and Sullivan, C. E. (1982). Alcohol, snoring and sleep apnoea. *J. Neurol. Neurosurg. Psychiat.* **45**, 353.

Jouvet, M. (1962). Recherches sur les structures nerveuses et les mécanismes responsables des différentes phases du sommeil physiologique. *Arch. ital. Biol.* **100**, 125.

Kales, A. (Ed.) (1969). *Sleep: physiology and pathology*. Saunders, Philadelphia.

Kales, A., Cadieux, R., Soldatos, C. R., and Tan, T.-L. (1979). Successful treatment of narcolepsy with propranolol: a case report. *Arch. Neurol., Chicago* **36**, 650.

——, ——, ——, Bixler, E. O., Schweitzer, P. K., Prey, W. T., and Vela-Bueno, A. (1982a). Narcolepsy–cataplexy: I. Clinical and electrophysiologic characteristics. *Arch. Neurol., Chicago* **39**, 164.

——, Soldatos, C. R., Bixler, E. O., Caldwell, A., Cadieux, R. J., Verrechio, J. M., and Kales, J. D. (1982b). Narcolepsy–cataplexy: II. Psychosocial consequences and associated psychopathology. *Arch. Neurol., Chicago* **39**, 169.

Kelly, D. D. (1981). Physiology of sleep and dreaming. In *Principles of neural science* (ed. E. R. Kandel and J. H. Schwartz) Chapter 40. Elsevier North-Holland, Amsterdam.

Kleine, W. (1925). Periodische Schlafsucht. *Mschr. Psychiat. Neurol.* **57**, 285.

Kuhlo, W. (1968). Neurophysiologische und klinische Untersuchungen beim Pickwick-Syndrome. *Arch. Psychiat. Neurol.* **211**, 170.

The Lancet (1979). Sleep apnea syndromes. *Lancet*, **i**, 25.

—— (1981). To sleep, perchance to breathe. . . . *Lancet* **ii**, 670.

Langdon, N., Welsh K. I., van Dam, M., Vaughan, R. W., and Parkes, D. (1984). Genetic markers in narcolepsy. *Lancet* **ii**, 1178.

Levin, M. (1932). Cataplexy. *Brain* **55**, 397.

—— (1936). Periodic somnolence and morbid hunger: a new syndrome. *Brain* **59**, 494.

Magoun, H. W. (1952). The ascending reticular activating system. *Res. Publ. Ass. nerv. ment. Dis.* **30**, 480.

Meyer, J. S., Sakai, F., Karacan, I., Derman, S., and Yamamoto, M. (1980). Sleep apnea, narcolepsy, and dreaming: regional cerebral hemodynamics. *Ann. Neurol.* **7**, 479.

Montplaisir, J., de Champlain, J., Young, S. N., Missala, K., Sourkes, T. L., Walsh, J., and Rémillard, G. (1982). Narcolepsy and idiopathic hypersomnia: biogenic amines and related compounds in CSF. *Neurology, Minneapolis* **32**, 1299.

Oswald, I. (1972). Sleep. In *Scientific foundations of neurology* (ed. M. Critchley, J. L. O'Leary, and W. B. Jennett) p. 190. Heinemann, London.

—— (1985). Sleep. In *Oxford companion to medicine* (ed. J. Walton, P. B. Beeson, and R. Bodley Scott). Oxford University Press, Oxford. (In press)

Parkes, J. D. (1981). Day-time drowsiness. *Lancet* **ii**, 1213.

——, Fenton, G., Struthers, G., Curzon, G., Kantamaneni, B. D., Buxton, B. H., and Record, C. (1974). Narcolepsy and cataplexy. Clinical features, treatment and cerebrospinal fluid findings. *Quart. J. Med.* **43**, 525.

—— and Schachter, M. (1979). Mazindol in the treatment of narcolepsy. *Acta neurol. scand.* **60**, 250.

Plum, F. (1972). Organic disturbances of consciousness. In *Scientific foundations of neurology* (ed. M. Critchley, J. L. O'Leary, and W. B. Jennett) p. 192. Heinemann, London.

—— and Posner, J. B. (1980). *Stupor and coma*, 3rd edn. Davis, Philadelphia.

Ranson, S. W. (1939). Somnolence caused by hypothalamic lesions in the monkey. *Arch. Neurol. Psychiat., Chicago* **41**, 1.

Roffwarg, H. P. (1979). Classification of sleep and arousal disorders. *Sleep* **2**, 1.

Roth, B., Bruhová, S., and Lehovsky, M. (1969). REM sleep and NREM sleep in narcolepsy and hypersomnia. *Electroenceph. clin. Neurophysiol.* **26**, 176.

Rudolf, M., Geddes, W. M., Turner, J. A. M., and Saunders, K. B. (1978). Depression of central respiratory drive by nitrazepam. *Thorax* **33**, 97.

Sakai, F., Meyer, J. S., Karacan, I., Derman, S., and Yamamoto, M. (1980). Normal human sleep: regional cerebral hemodynamics. *Ann. Neurol.* **4**, 471.

Schachter, M. and Parkes, J. D. (1980). Fluvoxamine and clomipramine in the treatment of cataplexy. *J. Neurol. Neurosurg. Psychiat.* **43**, 171.

Stahl, S. M., Layzer, R. B., Aminoff, M. J., Townsend, J. J., and Feldon, S. (1980). Continuous cataplexy in a patient with a midbrain tumor: the limp man syndrome. *Neurology, Minneapolis* **30**, 1115.

Thompson, C., Schachter, M., and Parkes, J. D. (1982). Drugs for cataplexy. *Ann. Neurol.* **12**, 62.

Wilson, S. A. K. (1928). The narcolepsies. *Brain* **51**, 63.

Wolstenholme, G. and O'Connor, M. (1961). *Ciba Foundation Symposium on the nature of sleep*. Ciba Foundation, London.

Yoss, R. E., Moyer, N. J., and Ogle, K. N. (1969). The pupillogram and narcolepsy. *Neurology, Minneapolis* **19**, 921.

Stupor and coma

Between full consciousness and pathological complete unconsciousness or coma there exist many states which differ not only in degree but also in quality, and especially in the nature of the impairment of consciousness and of the content of such consciousness as remains. It is convenient to distinguish broadly two different states of impaired consciousness, namely, coma and stupor. In coma as once defined the patient could not be aroused by any stimulus, however vigorous and painful. Semicoma was then defined as complete loss of consciousness with a response only at the reflex level, while less severe degrees of impairment of consciousness were entitled severe, moderate, and mild confusion (Medical Research Council 1941). However, in modern parlance the term semicoma is little used and coma is defined as 'a state of unarousable psychological unresponsiveness in which the subjects lie with eyes closed . . . they show no psychologically understandable response to external stimulus or inner need' (Plum and Posner 1980). The term *confusion* is still widely used, however, to identify impairment of consciousness with lack of clarity of mental processes (an obtunded state) short of stupor or coma, while *delirium* is confusion with an overlay of excitement. The Glasgow coma scale (Teasdale and Jennett 1974; Teasdale, Knill-Jones, and Van der Sande 1978), in which four grades of eye opening, five of the 'best verbal response' and five of the 'best motor response' are charted in individual cases, has been found to be of great practical value in assessing grades of impairment of consciousness. By contrast to coma, lethargy is a state of drowsiness and indifference in which increased stimulation may be needed to obtain a response, while stupor is a term used to define a state 'from which the subject can only be aroused by vigorous and continuous external stimulation' (Plum and Posner 1980). Hypersomnia is sometimes so severe that it may be regarded as one variety of stupor. *Akinetic mutism*, another state of stupor described by Cairns, resembled sleep in being associated with general muscular relaxation, but differed from sleep in that, although the patient's eyes remained apparently alert to moving objects, strong afferent stimuli were incapable of arousing him. According to Plum and Posner (1980), in akinetic mutism the patient, though usually lying with his eyes closed, retains cycles of self-sustained arousal, giving the appearance of vigilance but vocalizing little or not at all. He is totally incontinent and makes only the most rudimentary movements even in response to noxious stimuli. The state is thus one of 'motionless, mindless wakefulness' or one cause of 'mute of malady' (*British Medical Journal* 1973) and despite the patient's immobility there are few signs of damage to descending motor pathways. Plum and Posner (1980) suggest that this, and the very closely related if not identical states which have been called 'persistent vegetative state', 'coma vigil', or 'the apallic syndrome' (most often seen as a sequel of severe head injury or cerebral anoxia) must be distinguished from coma.

Also different is the so-called de-efferented state or '*locked-in syndrome*' in which the patient is fully aware of his surroundings and is conscious and alert, but usually tetraplegic, aphonic, and anarthric so that he can communicate only through blinking or by carrying out various ocular movements voluntarily (Nordgren, Markesbery, Fukuda and Reeves 1971; Feldman 1971; Hawkes 1974; Bauer, Gerstenbrand, and Rumpl 1979). It is therefore most important to distinguish this state, in which the patient can hear and respond, despite extensive paralysis, from akinetic mutism. The EEG may be helpful, showing a reactive alpha or theta rhythm consistent with consciousness (Hawkes and Bryan-Smith 1974). So-called 'alpha coma' (with a responsive alpha rhythm) is common in drug intoxication (Carroll and Mastaglia 1979).

Lesions responsible for stupor and coma
The clinico-pathological studies of Cairns (1952) and French (1952) established that *stupor or coma* usually resulted from lesions involving the central portion of the brainstem between the anterior end of the third ventricle and the lower pons, while extensive bilateral destruction of the cerebral cortex did not necessarily cause unconsciousness. Many pathological processes can therefore be responsible, the chief of which are head injury, tumour, vascular and inflammatory lesions, and it seems that toxic and metabolic states usually lead to unconsciousness primarily through their effect upon this part of the brain. In 500 cases of stupor or coma, initially of unknown aetiology, 101 proved to be due to supratentorial lesions (probably producing their effects by indirect action upon the brainstem), 65 to subtentorial lesions, and 326 to diffuse or metabolic brain dysfunction, while there were eight cases of psychiatric 'coma', four due to conversion reactions (hysteria), two to depression, and two to catatonic stupor (Plum and Posner 1980).

In Cairns' (1952) original description, *akinetic mutism* resulted from a craniopharyngioma compressing the walls of the third ventricle. Skultety (1968), as a result of experimental work in animals and clinicopathological observations in man, found that bilateral lesions of the periaqueductal grey matter of the upper brainstem

were alone insufficient to cause this state and Plum and Posner (1980) review reports of its developing as a consequence of bilateral frontal-lobe infarction, diffuse cortical or white-matter damage due to anoxia, hypoglycaemia, head injury or demyelination, hydrocephalus, bilateral destruction of the corpus striatum, globus pallidus or thalamus, paramedian lesions of the brainstem reticular substance, and brainstem compression secondary to cerebellar haemorrhage. Nevertheless, dysfunction of the reticular system or of its afferent or efferent connections was probably a common factor.

The *locked-in syndrome*, by contrast, is clearly related to bilateral destruction of the medulla or basis pontis with sparing of the tegmentum, usually as a consequence of demyelination (e.g. in central pontine myelinolysis) or ventral pontine infarction (Adams, Victor, and Mancall 1959; Kemper and Romanul 1967), generally due to basilar artery occlusion (McCusker, Rudick, Honch, and Griggs 1982). However, it has been described as a consequence of bilateral infarction of the lateral two-thirds of the cerebral peduncles (Karp and Hurtig 1974).

The causes of stupor and coma

This section will discuss the principal causes of impairment of consciousness as a necessary preliminary to considering how to identify the cause in any particular case. Even though the causes will be described in general terms, it is often impossible to determine precisely how each cause operates.

Cerebral vascular lesions

A cerebral vascular lesion is a common cause of coma. Usually the impairment of consciousness is due to the fact that the cerebral vascular lesion directly or indirectly interferes with the functions of the ascending reticular alerting formation (see Johnson, Sambre, and Spalding 1984). Ischaemia of this structure may result from either increased intracranial pressure, local pressure upon the diencephalon or brainstem, or impairment of blood supply due to atheroma of the relevant arteries. Alternatively, median raphe haemorrhages in the brainstem due to venous engorgement resulting from tentorial herniation can have a similar effect. The conditions most likely to produce these changes are: (1) a massive subarachnoid haemorrhage; (2) a subarachnoid haemorrhage invading one cerebral hemisphere; (3) a large intracerebral or intracerebellar haemorrhage, or one rupturing into a cerebral ventricle; (4) an area of cerebral infarction in one hemisphere large enough to cause considerable oedema of the hemisphere; (5) brainstem haemorrhage or infarction due to vertebrobasilar atheroma; and (6) hypertensive encephalopathy. The symptomatology of these lesions is described elsewhere, but in general a vascular cause for coma is suggested by the presence of severe atheroma or hypertension, a sudden or relatively sudden onset of symptoms, focal signs suggesting a vascular lesion, or signs of meningeal irritation of sudden onset. A CT scan is usually diagnostic; lumbar puncture, once almost universally used for diagnosis in such cases, is now used much more sparingly to identify the presence of blood or xanthochromia in the CSF when no focal intracranial collection of blood is shown by scanning.

Space-occupying lesions

Coma due to intracranial tumour or abscess usually comes on much more slowly than that due to a cerebral vascular lesion, though occasionally haemorrhage into a tumour or the sudden development of oedema or of tentorial or cerebellar herniation may cause rapid loss of consciousness. A history of symptoms of increased intracranial pressure, especially headache increasing in severity, is usually obtainable, and papilloedema is often present. Signs of vascular disease are usually absent, but clinical diagnosis may be difficult when a tumour develops late in life in a patient with hypertension or atheroma. Subdural haematoma most often occurs in the middle-aged or elderly, in whom it may develop without evident cause or insidiously after minor head injury. Headache is usually prominent, but not always, and impairment of consciousness, when it develops, often fluctuates strikingly. Papilloedema and signs of focal cerebral compression are only rarely present.

Head injury

When coma is due to head injury, there is usually a clear history of the injury, and there may be bruising of the scalp or signs of fracture of the vault or base of the skull. However, a patient who loses his senses from some other cause may injure his head in falling, while an injury to the head may affect the brain indirectly, for example, by leading to thrombosis of one internal carotid artery. Traumatic intracranial arterial haemorrhage leads to progressively deepening coma, ultimately with signs of a focal lesion of one hemisphere, often beginning with convulsions and later producing hemiplegia. Before these late signs appear, herniation of the medial portion of the temporal lobe through the tentorial hiatus often causes compression of the third nerve as it crosses the free border of the tentorium; as a result the pupil on the same side becomes fixed and dilated and other signs of a third-nerve palsy on the same side may develop later. By contrast, cerebellar tonsillar herniation due to a space-occupying lesion (whether haemorrhage, tumour, or abscess) in the posterior fossa usually gives occipital headache and neck stiffness, possibly with bradycardia and depression of respiration due to brainstem compression. However, it may be impossible clinically to distinguish between traumatic intracranial arterial haemorrhage (which is usually extradural) and an acute subdural haematoma which generally results from cerebral laceration.

Meningitis and encephalitis

When meningitis causes coma, the onset of symptoms is usually subacute, and before losing consciousness the patient complains of intense headache, associated with fever and neck stiffness. The diagnosis is confirmed by identifying the characteristic changes in the CSF, from which it may be possible to isolate the causal organism. The onset of encephalitis is also usually subacute, and often associated with fever and/or seizures, though herpes simplex encephalitis (p. 280) may be explosive in onset, leading to coma within a few hours. The physical signs are those of more or less diffuse damage to the brain, and in many cases also the spinal cord, the precise distribution and character varying in relation to the aetiology. Signs of meningeal irritation are present in some but not all cases, and there is often, but not invariably, a CSF pleocytosis.

Other brain diseases

Among the many other diseases which may from time to time cause coma and which must be distinguished by their age of onset and specific clinical features are the leukodystrophies and cerebral storage disorders, multiple sclerosis with extensive cerebral demyelination (rarely), central pontine myelinolysis, deficiency disorders such as Wernicke's encephalopathy, many degenerative or toxic encephalopathies, and slow virus disorders such as multifocal leukoencephalopathy or Creutzfeldt–Jacob disease.

Metabolic disorders

Uraemic coma. Uraemic coma may occur in acute or chronic renal failure. The metabolic changes so produced are complex, and the raised blood urea (or non-protein nitrogen), though providing a useful index of severity, is not alone responsible for loss of consciousness. There is usually metabolic acidosis, accompanied by complex electrolyte disturbances. Water intoxication, due to fluid retention, with a serum osmolality of less than 260 mOsm/l, is a factor in some cases. The blood calcium may be subnormal and the administration of alkalis to correct the acidosis may precipitate tetany. There is usually a raised blood pyruvate, and the cerebral consumption of oxygen is reduced. Headache, vomiting, dyspnoea, mental confusion, drowsiness or restlessness, and insomnia are early symptoms, and later muscular twitchings or generalized convulsions are likely to precede the coma. The raised blood urea establishes the diagnosis, but differentiation from hypertensive encephalopathy, often accompanied by azotaemia, is not always easy (Plum and Posner 1980). A fatal encephalopathy of undetermined cause, often associated with spongiform change in the brain, giving rise to progressive dysarthria, mental changes, an abnormal EEG, and often ultimately seizures, myoclonus, asterixis, apraxia, and focal neurological signs with eventual coma has been described in patients with renal failure under treatment with chronic haemodialysis (Burks, Alfrey, Huddlestone, Norrenberg, and Lewin 1976). In fact, since 1976 the dialysis dysequilibrium syndrome, which is commoner in children and during rapid changes in blood solutes, has been separately identified as a temporary disorder, often associated with cerebral sodium loss, which is correctable by careful control of serum electrolytes and osmolality during dialysis (see Plum and Posner 1980). Progressive dialysis encephalopathy (dialysis dementia) is a different condition, usually if not invariably due to aluminium in the water supply used for dialysis (p. 660).

Diabetic coma. Diabetic coma is usually associated with ketoacidosis, a blood sugar greater than 40 mmol/l, and massive ketonuria. However, lactic acidosis without ketonuria is an occasional cause of metabolic acidosis in diabetic subjects, especially after treatment with hypoglycaemic agents, and must be distinguished from that which can result from severe anoxia or from poisoning with methyl alcohol or paraldehyde. Hyperosmolality due to hyperglycaemia (hyperglycaemic nonketotic diabetic coma) is also common (Gerich, Martin, and Recant 1971; Gordon and Kibadi 1976) and a similar syndrome has been described in non-diabetic patients with severe burns (Rosenberg, Brief, Kinney, Herrera, Wilson, and Moore 1965). The patient is usually wasted, pale, and dehydrated. Both the rate and amplitude of respiration are increased, and the ocular tension is low. The pulse is rapid and feeble, and the blood pressure tends to fall. The tendon reflexes are sometimes depressed due to an associated diabetic neuropathy but may be normal, and the plantar responses are usually flexor until the patient is actually comatose. The breath may have the characteristic odour of acetone. Large quantities of sugar and acetone are demonstrable in the urine in ketotic cases, and the blood sugar is much raised. Because there is a high incidence of vascular disease in diabetic subjects, cerebral infarction or haemorrhage and hypertensive or uraemic encephalopathy (secondary to diabetic renal disease) must also be considered, as must coma due to syncope, hypoxia, or hypotension secondary to diabetic autonomic neuropathy (Page and Watkins 1978).

Hypoglycaemic coma. Hypoglycaemic coma is not difficult to recognize if due to an overdose of insulin or another hypoglycaemic agent which the patient is known to be taking. Glycosuria does not exclude this, since the urine may have been excreted before the patient became hypoglycaemic. Spontaneous hypoglycaemia sufficient to cause coma is usually the result in an adult of the excessive production of insulin by a tumour arising from cells of the pancreatic islets of Langerhans. In such cases convulsions or periods of confusion or disordered behaviour may precede the onset of coma by weeks or months. On the other hand, the coma can occur without warning in a patient apparently previously healthy, and the patient may then live on in coma for weeks or months. Hypoglycaemia may also occur spontaneously in early infancy and can then be responsible for severe brain damage if not recognized and treated early, and in adult life it can also arise spontaneously in patients with liver disease, in alcoholism, hypopituitarism, and Addison's disease. At the onset the hypoglycaemic patient sweats profusely, the pupils are dilated, the tendon reflexes increased, and the plantar reflexes may be extensor. Hypothermia sometimes occurs; in occasional cases there are symptoms and signs of focal cerebral dysfunction (a 'stroke-like' presentation) (Montgomery and Pinner 1964). The diagnosis is made by estimating the blood sugar, which is found to be very low in an attack, in the region of 1.5–2.5 mmol/l or even much lower.

Unless treated promptly and effectively, hypoglycaemia can result in irreversible brain damage and the pathological changes, affecting the cerebellar Purkinje cells, the cerebral cortex, basal ganglia, and hippocampus, are similar to those of severe anoxia. Dementia and cerebellar ataxia are the main clinical features of this syndrome.

Heat stroke. After prolonged exertion in hot surroundings (as in racing cyclists) the normal rise in body temperature with profuse sweating can be followed by an ominous clinical picture of hyperpyrexia, an abrupt cessation of sweating, the rapid onset of coma, convulsions, and death. The condition may be precipitated by the use of amphetamine or other stimulant drugs. Hyperpyrexia may also be seen in tetanus and as a result of lesions involving the floor of the third ventricle (such as intraventricular haemorrhage) or pons (e.g. pontine haemorrhage). Many patients who survive heat stroke are left with permanent neurological sequelae including paraparesis, cerebellar ataxia, or dementia (Salem 1966). Malignant hyperpyrexia (p. 578) is a rare complication of general anaesthesia in susceptible individuals.

Hypothermia. An abnormally low body temperature may give rise to deepening coma. While hypothermia can occur in cases of myxoedema and hypopituitarism (see below), accidental hypothermia can result from a failure of the normal temperature-regulating mechanism of the body, the reverse of that seen in heat stroke. It can result from prolonged exposure in cold conditions (as in mountaineers or fell-walkers) and has also been described in elderly patients, often suffering from disorders such as arthritis or parkinsonism which reduce mobility, who live in unheated rooms in winter conditions (Rosin and Exton-Smith 1964). Drugs such as chlorpromazine may also precipitate hypothermic coma which can be fatal. Often there is generalized rigidity and muscle fasciculation may be seen but true shivering is absent; hypoxia and CO_2 retention are common (McNicol and Smith 1964). The mortality rate is high but in those patients who respond to gradual warming (and treatment for hypothyroidism when appropriate) complete recovery is usual. Spontaneous periodic hypothermia (Shapiro's syndrome) is a rare syndrome of recurrent hypothermia, usually occurring in association with agenesis of the corpus callosum, polydipsia, polyuria, and hyponatraemia (Mooradian, Morley, McGeachie, Lundgren, and Morley 1984).

Hepatic coma. The cause of hepatic coma is still incompletely understood (see p. 451). The diagnosis is not usually difficult when the patient is known to be suffering from liver failure. Jaundice, however, may be absent. In patients with liver disease coma tends to be precipitated by gastrointestinal haemorrhage, hypotension, infection, the rapid removal of large quantities of ascitic fluid, the use of certain diuretics, the administration of some sedatives, particularly morphine, general anaesthesia, and the ingestion of high protein foods or ammonium compounds. Except when

it is of sudden onset, hepatic coma is usually preceded by the neurological symptoms of hepatic insufficiency, especially asterixis or flapping tremor. Otherwise the diagnosis rests upon the presence of physical signs of liver disease, including hepatic foetor, and biochemical evidence of disturbed liver function.

Pancreatic encephalopathy. Episodic stupor or coma is well-recognized to occur in chronic relapsing pancreatitis and is also seen, though less often, in acute pancreatitis, usually beginning between the second and fifth days and characterized by agitated delirium, hallucinations, focal or generalized convulsions, and often signs of bilateral corticospinal-tract dysfunction (Plum and Posner 1980). The cause is unknown.

Porphyria. Porphyria is an occasional cause of coma, especially after the administration of barbiturates in a susceptible individual.

Pulmonary disease. Hypoventilation due to chronic pulmonary disease may give an encephalopathy leading ultimately to coma, especially in patients with cor pulmonale in whom coma may occasionally follow the prolonged administration of oxygen. The syndrome of alveolar hypoventilation (p. 472) is usually characterized by dull headache followed by drowsiness and, if unchecked, the patient may ultimately lapse into coma. Hypoxia is accompanied by hypercarbia (see below) with a chronic insensitivity of the respiratory centre. Asterixis and myoclonus are not uncommon in such cases (Plum and Posner 1980).

Anoxia. Apart from that which may result from carbon monoxide poisoning, cerebral anoxia may result from suffocation, drowning, severe anaemia, ischaemia due to cardiac arrest, complications of open-heart surgery, heart disease, pulmonary embolism, fat embolism (after severe limb fractures), or diffuse embolism or other disease of the large cerebral arteries or smaller cerebral vessels (as in thrombotic microangiopathy or disseminated intravascular coagulation), to name but a few causes. Plum and Posner (1980) divide anoxia into the anoxic, anaemic, and ischaemic varieties (see p. 440). Cerebral malaria is a rare cause of ischaemic anoxia.

Disorders of osmolality. Hyponatraemia or water intoxication has been increasingly recognized as a cause of delirium, leading often to coma. It is most often due to inappropriate ADH secretion, due to bronchial carcinoma, or to organic lesions in the region of the hypothalamus and/or pituitary, but sometimes occurring without evident cause (Goldberg 1963). Sometimes it results from compulsive water drinking in psychotic or alcoholic individuals or it may complicate chronic renal failure.

Hypernatraemia may cause delirium, less often coma, and is seen in children with severe diarrhoea, or adults with diabetes insipidus, but can also be iatrogenic due to excess saline administration. These causes of delirium, drowsiness, or coma are recognized by measurement of the serum osmolality.

Coma of endocrine origin

This may present diagnostic difficulty when developing in patients in whom the pre-existing endocrine disease has not been recognized.

Hypopituitary coma. In hypopituitarism, coma is the result of complex interacting factors, of which the most important are hypoglycaemia, hypotension, impaired adrenal cortical function and occasionally hypothermia. The onset may be sudden, as when precipitated by infection or by narcotic drugs. The patient is often a woman with the typical endocrine changes of hypopituitarism. The blood pressure and blood sugar are usually low, and the body temperature is often subnormal. The urinary excretion of 17-ketosteroids and the serum cortisol are very low. The syndrome of pituitary apoplexy (p. 165) must be remembered as a possible cause of sudden collapse and coma in patients with pituitary neoplasms who may also exhibit signs of hypopituitarism.

Coma in myxoedema. A myxoedematous patient may gradually become comatose, more often in the winter months. The characteristic feature is profound hypothermia, temperatures of 26–31 °C being by no means uncommon. A low-reading thermometer must be used to record these and on suspicion the temperature must be taken rectally. The patient presents the usual clinical and biochemical features of myxoedema.

Adrenal cortical failure. Coma from this cause is difficult to recognize if it occurs suddenly as a response to stress, for example, in a patient not known to be suffering from Addison's disease. The hypotension and electrolyte disturbances, however, are characteristic. Mild delirium is not uncommon in untreated Addison's disease, but as Plum and Posner (1980) point out, stupor and coma only occur as a rule in Addisonian crises. Papilloedema resulting from cerebral oedema has been described (Jefferson 1956). Acute adrenal failure due to meningococcal septicaemia (the Fredericksen–Waterhouse syndrome), once relatively common, is now a rare cause of sudden collapse and coma in infants and young children.

Abnormalities of blood calcium. Hypercalcaemia as a cause of mental confusion or coma may be missed if the blood calcium is not routinely examined. Hypercalcaemia may be due to parathyroid tumour, carcinoma, with or without bone secondaries, myelomatosis, vitamin D intoxication, or sarcoidosis (Lemann and Donatelli 1964; Watson 1963; Dent and Watson 1964). Hypocalcaemia, due to idiopathic or acquired hypoparathyroidism, may also cause coma, but much less often (Plum and Posner 1980); tetany and/or convulsions are the more usual manifestations but cerebral oedema with papilloedema has been reported (Grant 1953).

Carbon dioxide intoxication

Carbon dioxide retention may be the result of acute or chronic pulmonary disease, or respiratory failure of neuromuscular origin in, for example, motor-neurone disease, poliomyelitis, polyneuritis, myopathy, and myasthenia. It causes a fall in the pH and a rise in the pCO_2 in the blood. Though the patient is hypoxic, the state of consciousness is related to the level of CO_2 in the blood. In chronic CO_2 retention the respiratory centre fails to react to the raised level of CO_2 and respiration is then maintained by the receptors which respond to oxygen lack. Consequently, administering oxygen to such patients may remove the stimulus to respiration, raise the blood CO_2 still further, and precipitate coma. The same result may be produced by sedatives, particularly morphine, or even by barbiturates. Milder degrees of CO_2 intoxication cause drowsiness and confusion. In some cases there is papilloedema due to cerebral oedema. Estimation of the pCO_2 in arterial blood will usually confirm the diagnosis.

Carbon monoxide intoxication

In carbon monoxide intoxication there is almost always a history of exposure to coal-gas or the exhaust fumes of a motor-car, or some other source of carbon monoxide, such as combustion of a gas, paraffin, or solid-fuel stove or water heater in an inadequately ventilated room. In doubtful cases the diagnosis can be made by the spectroscopic examination of the blood.

Narcotic and sedative drugs

Drug or alcohol intoxication is now the commonest cause of coma in hospital casualty departments or emergency rooms (Plum and Posner 1980). Possession of a supply of the drug, the finding of an empty container, medical records, history from a relative or friend may all give invaluable clues. Narcotic overdose is often readily identified by the pin-point pupils, shallow respiration, and needle marks on the skin. Whereas in the past the drugs most often used in suicidal attempts were aspirin and barbiturates, and narcotics such as pethidine, methadone, morphia, or heroin were less often used, the drugs most often responsible for coma due to overdose now are the tranquillizers and/or antidepressive remedies, paracetamol, and the anticonvulsants.

When alcohol is the cause of coma, this can usually be established from the history; the face is flushed, the conjunctivae congested, the pulse rapid, and the blood pressure low. The size of the pupils varies according to the agent: they are often dilated in alcoholic coma, contracted in coma due to opiates, but in the case of other drugs are intermediate in size. The reaction to light is often sluggish, and sometimes absent. The tendon reflexes tend to be diminished or lost, and the plantar reflexes are often extensor. Respiration is shallow, and the pulse rapid. The drug responsible should be sought in the stomach washings and in blood and urine.

Epilepsy

In post-epileptic coma there is usually a history of epilepsy, or at least of the attack which preceded the coma. In the absence of this information, scars on the face or a bitten tongue may provide a clue. Focal signs of a cerebral lesion are usually absent, but the plantar reflexes may be extensor. After a single seizure the period of unconsciousness is usually short, not more than 30–60 min, but status epilepticus can be followed by prolonged coma. Prolonged drowsiness or confusion can rarely result from petit mal or complex partial status in childhood, less often in adults (p. 614). In elderly patients with symptomatic epilepsy due to cerebral scarring resulting, for instance, from previous infarction, post-epileptic stupor and subsequent delirium may be unusually prolonged due to the cerebral metabolic demand consequent upon one or more prolonged seizures as well as the resultant hypoxia.

Hysteria

In hysterical trance ('psychogenic unresponsiveness'—Plum and Posner 1980), the patient, though apparently unconscious, usually shows some response to external stimuli. For example, an attempt to elicit the corneal reflex may cause a vigorous contraction of the orbicularis oculi. Marked resistance to passive movement of the limbs may be present, and signs of organic disease are absent. The caloric and optokinetic responses and the EEG are all generally normal. The diagnosis of catatonic stupor as a cause of psychogenic unresponsiveness may be more difficult as in such cases the EEG is often abnormal (Plum and Posner 1980); catatonia (the limbs maintain a posture passively imposed by the examiner) may be a helpful sign in such cases.

The investigation of the unconscious patient

The patient in coma requires a most detailed and systematic examination, as the clue to the cause of the unconsciousness may lie in any system.

The head

The head should be examined for evidence of injury indicated by cuts or abrasions. The skull should be palpated for a depressed fracture, and the ears and nose examined for haemorrhage and leakage of CSF. The ears should also be examined for signs of infection. Scars on the face may point to injuries received in previous epileptic seizures, and the tongue should be examined to see if it has been recently bitten or is the site of similar scars.

The breath

The smell of the breath may be invaluable; thus in alcoholic intoxication the characteristic odour of alcohol can be detected, and that of acetone in diabetic coma. In hepatic coma there is a characteristic foetor, but the smell of the breath in uraemia may be simulated by that present in many unconscious patients with oral infection.

The neck

An attempt should be made gently to flex the cervical spine. Neck stiffness may indicate meningitis or subarachnoid haemorrhage. Inequalities in the pulsation of the carotid arteries or bruits may suggest arterial stenosis or thrombosis as a possible cause of cerebral ischaemia or infarction.

The skin

Cyanosis may be present when coma is due to CO_2 intoxication, while carbon monoxide poisoning causes a cherry-red colour, though this is more evident after death. Patients with Addison's disease often show the characteristic pigmentation. Multiple telangiectases are found in hereditary telangiectasia, in which condition a cerebral telangiectasis may rarely cause cerebral haemorrhage, while spider naevi over the upper part of the body are characteristic of hepatic disease. Purpura may be associated with an intracranial haemorrhage in thrombocytopenic purpura or other haemorrhagic disorders, with cerebral embolism in subacute infective endocarditis, and also with meningococcal meningitis. The characteristic skin changes of myxoedema and hypopituitarism (with loss of body hair) will be present in patients suffering from coma due to those conditions. The scars of injections may be found in diabetics and drug addicts.

Respiration

After voluntary hyperventilation patients with diffuse metabolic or structural brain disease may demonstrate post-hyperventilation apnoea (Plum and Posner 1980) but the performance of this test demands that the patient should be sufficiently conscious to be able to perform it. Periodic (Cheyne–Stokes) respiration, in which hyperpnoea alternates with apnoea, usually occurs in patients with central cerebral or high brainstem lesions. Central neurogenic hyperventilation (Plum and Swanson 1959) has been described in patients with dysfunction of the brainstem tegmentum. It is a syndrome comprising elevated arterial oxygen tension (pO_2), decreased arterial carbon dioxide tension (pCO_2) and respiratory alkalosis in the absence of any evidence of pulmonary congestion. Most such patients have brainstem tumours, and most, but not all (Rodriguez, Baele, Marsh, and Okazaki 1982) are in coma, but sometimes the condition complicates hepatic encephalopathy (Plum 1982). Rapid regular respiration without the other defining features of central neurogenic hyperventilation as described is also common in comatose patients (Leigh and Shaw, 1976). Brainstem lesions may also give apneustic breathing (a pause at full inspiration—Plum and Alvord 1964) or ataxic, irregular respiration with random deep and shallow breaths; the latter pattern occurs particularly with medullary lesions (Plum and Swanson 1958). At its worst, in some medullary lesions, the respiratory centre becomes so insensitive to normal chemical stimuli, but conversely so sensitive to sedative drugs, that the patient, who can breathe adequately when commanded to do so, hypoventilates progressively and may even stop breathing completely when asleep (Plum and Posner 1980). Autonomous breathing (Newsom Davis 1974) is a rare syndrome which may occur as a consequence of a lesion at the cervicomedullary junction giving paralysis of the chest and limbs but with retention of spontaneous breathing; however, the patient is unable to take a breath or to stop breathing voluntarily.

The pupils

Plum and Posner (1980) summarized the pupillary changes found in comatose patients. Midbrain tectal lesions give round, regular, medium-sized pupils which do not react to light but may show hippus; nuclear midbrain lesions also as a rule give medium-sized pupils, fixed to all stimuli, which are often irregular and unequal. A third-nerve lesion distal to the nucleus gives a fixed, dilated pupil on the side of the lesion. Tegmental lesions in the pons give bilaterally small pupils which in pontine haemorrhage may be pin-

point. A lateral medullary lesion can give an ipsilateral Horner's syndrome, while the pupil on the side of an occluded carotid artery causing cerebral infarction is often small. Bilateral pupillary dilatation during neck flexion can be a sign of uncal herniation (Norris and Fawcett 1965). Drugs such as atropine, and cerebral anoxia, dilate the pupils, morphine constricts, and many metabolic encephalopathies give small pupils with a normal light reflex.

Ocular movements

In unconscious patients with bilateral or diffuse disorders of the cerebrum the eyes look straight ahead, oculocephalic movements (on head rotation) are brisk, and caloric stimulation gives sustained deviation of the eyes. A frontal-lobe lesion may cause deviation of the eyes towards the side of the lesion, while, conversely, a lateral pontine lesion can cause conjugate deviation to the opposite side with absence of oculocephalic and caloric responses. Skew deviation results from a dorsolateral pontine lesion. Conjugate deviation downwards means a midbrain lesion, while disconjugate ocular deviation means a structural brainstem lesion if strabismus can be excluded. Oculocephalic and caloric responses are normal in metabolic disorders unless severe (Plum and Posner 1980). Total absence of the caloric and oculocephalic reflexes is one important criterion of an irreversible brainstem lesion and of brain death (see below).

Blink (facial) reflexes

Recording of the R1 (early) and R2 (late) components of the blink reflexes has also been shown to be of value in the assessment of brainstem function in severe traumatic coma and in assessing outcome (Buonaguidi, Rossi, Sartucci, and Ravelli 1979).

Other systems

The examination of other parts of the nervous system is of special importance in view of the many nervous disorders which give rise to coma. Special attention should be paid to the fundi where papilloedema may indicate increased intracranial pressure, or may be associated with the other vascular changes of hypertensive retinopathy. The cardiovascular system may yield evidence of hypertension, atheroma, or mitral stenosis and atrial fibrillation, a common cause of cerebral embolism. The prolapsing mitral valve and atrial myxoma are much less common. The lungs may reveal the cause of CO_2 retention. X-ray of the chest is always necessary to help to exclude primary or secondary carcinoma. The abdomen may show the venous congestion and hepatomegaly of chronic liver disease, or the renal enlargement of polycystic kidneys, or one of the abdominal or pelvic organs may be the site of a neoplasm.

Laboratory investigations

Routine studies of urine and blood should be carried out and screening for drugs or other poisons is particularly important. In addition, the blood sugar and blood urea should always be examined, and the blood electrolytes, calcium, osmolality, pO_2, and pCO_2 will also need to be investigated if it is thought that the coma could be the result of hypoxia or CO_2 retention, or alternatively in order to monitor ventilation in the management of the unconscious patient. Provided there is no contraindication such as the risk of uncal or cerebellar herniation (and here a CT scan may be invaluable), examination of the CSF may be indicated. This is essential to establish the diagnosis of meningitis or subarachnoid haemorrhage.

Other investigations

Other investigations, indicated in many cases, include X-rays of the skull, electroencephalography, computerized transaxial tomography, cerebral angiography, electrocardiography, and/or echocardiography.

The EEG in coma

The EEG may be of value in the diagnosis of coma in several ways: (1) it may suggest the presence of a focal lesion as opposed to a diffuse inflammatory or metabolic cause; (2) it may provide some evidence as to the probable nature of the focal lesion, as described elsewhere; (3) if there is a diffuse disturbance, the EEG may throw some light on its nature, distinguishing, for example, between some forms of encephalitis, epilepsy, and metabolic disorders; and (4) changes in the degree of abnormality, particularly in metabolic disorders, may provide evidence of improvement or deterioration in the patient's condition. Nevertheless, though useful and totally without risk, the EEG remains an imprecise method and the superior information derived from CT scanning, and more recently from NMR scanning, has meant that its usefulness in investigating coma is declining.

The diagnosis of brain death

This problem has assumed increasing importance in recent years, first because of the increasing difficulty of deciding in patients with brain damage whether it is justifiable to maintain life indefinitely with assisted respiration and other supportive means, and secondly because of the difficult question of deciding when it may be concluded that the cerebral lesion is irreversible, that death is imminent, and that preparations may be made to remove viable organs, especially the corneas, kidneys, liver, lungs, and heart, for subsequent transplantation. Plum (1972) identified the clinical criteria used to diagnose brain death at the Cornell-New York Hospital Medical Centre; while this question continues to be a fertile source of ethical and medicolegal controversy, these represent a reasonable guide to modern practice:

1. **The nature and duration of coma**

   (a) The cause must be unequivocally structural disease (e.g. trauma, neoplasm, etc.) or of clearly known anoxic origin.

   (b) There must be no chance that depressant drugs or hypothermia contribute to the clinical picture.

   (c) Signs of absent brain function must persist at least 12 hours under direct observation.

2. **Cerebral cortical function must be absent**

   (a) Behavioural or reflex responses above the foramen magnum level must be lacking to noxious stimuli applied anywhere on the body.

   (b) The EEG properly recorded must be isoelectric for 60 min at an amplitude of 50 μV/cm.

3. **Brainstem function must be absent**

   (a) The pupils must be fixed to a strong light stimulus and without evidence of peripheral third-nerve injury.

   (b) Oculovestibular responses must be absent.

   (c) There must be no motor activity whatever in structures innervated by cranial nerves.

   (d) Spontaneous respiration must be absent. If the patient is on a respirator, there must be no breathing movements despite being removed from the respirator for 3 min (receiving diffusion oxygen) and having a normal arterial pCO$_2$ at the start.

   (e) The circulation may be intact.

   (f) Purely spinal reflex responses may be retained.

   In the United Kingdom, considerable controversy was engendered in 1980 by a BBC television programme (*The Lancet* 1980) which questioned the validity of the criteria used in the diagnosis of brain death and which were based upon those published in 1976 by the Conference of Medical Royal Colleges and Faculties of the UK. *The Lancet* (1981a) commented that over 30 sets of criteria had been published from many parts of the world and in the last few years many additional methods over and above the clinical criteria listed above have been proposed, including, among others, cerebral angiography, common carotid-artery velocity waveform

analysis, CT scanning, auditory and somatosensory evoked potential recording, and cerebral blood-flow measurement (Pearson, Korein, Harris, Wichter, and Braunstein 1977; Goldie, Chiappa, Young, and Brooks 1981; Kreutzer, Rutherford, and Lehman 1982). In fact, the British criteria in current use correspond almost exactly to those listed above, save that in the UK the clinical tests must now be carried out independently by two medical practitioners with expertise in the field, the tests should be repeated with consistent results, and an EEG is not regarded as essential (Robson 1981; Pallis 1983). Current practice in the USA relies upon similar clinical criteria but requires an EEG and a precise technique of defining aponea after the cessation of artificial ventilation (Schafer and Caronna 1978; President's Commission 1981; Molinari 1982). The British criteria have been found reliable in clinical practice in that not one of 1003 survivors of severe head injury, for example, would have been suspected of being brain-dead (Jennett, Gleave, and Wilson 1981).

Predicting the outcome

Much work has been done of late to try to identify the factors that may be helpful in predicting outcome in patients becoming comatose other than as a result of head injury or drugs. Bates, Caronna, Cartlidge, Knill-Jones, Levy, Shaw, and Plum (1977) studied 310 patients in an international co-operative trial and found that 16 per cent of the patients achieved an independent existence within a month; severe disability or a persistent vegetative state developed in 25 per cent of those who were comatose for six hours and in 79 per cent of those still in coma after a week. Absence of pupillary light and corneal reflexes six hours after the onset of coma due to cardiopulmonary arrest is generally incompatible with survival (Snyder, Gumnit, Leppik, Hauser, Loewenson, and Ramirez-Lassepas 1981). While recovery from the 'locked-in syndrome' has been reported very rarely (McCusker *et al.* 1982), a partial return of cognition or even restoration to partial independence may occur equally rarely in individuals in a prolonged vegetative state (Rosenberg, Johnson, and Brenner 1977; Shuttleworth 1983), and dopamine agonists may be of some benefit in occasional cases of akinetic mutism (Ross and Stewart 1981), deep and prolonged coma carries a universally poor prognosis. Whether the coma is due to head injury (Jennett, Teasdale, Braakman, Minderhoud, Heiden, and Kurze 1979) or is nontraumatic, absent pupillary, light, corneal, caloric, and oculocephalic reflexes in the first 24 hours carry only a one in 20 chance of recovery and no patient recovered in one series in whom these reflexes were still absent and there was no motor response to painful stimuli, or an extensor posture persisted after three days (Levy, Bates, Caronna, Cartlidge, Knill-Jones, Lapinsk, Singer, Shaw, and Plum 1981). Generally, too, the outlook is worse when coma is due to a destructive cerebral lesion than when it results from ischaemia or a metabolic encephalopathy. Conversely, independent recovery is likely in patients who, at the end of the first day, speak a few words, open their eyes in response to noise, have spontaneous eye movements, nystagmus in response to caloric stimulation, preserved oculocephalic reflexes, or purposive responses to commands (*The Lancet* 1981b; *British Medical Journal* 1981).

The management of the unconscious patient

Improvements in the technique of dealing with the unconscious patient have recently been so great that it is now possible to maintain unconscious patients in a condition of otherwise good health indefinitely.

Nursing. The unconscious patient should be nursed on his side without a pillow, and turned at least every two hours, the usual attention being paid to the care of the skin, especially the pressure areas. If the foot of the bed is raised 15–22 cm so that the trachea is horizontal, the need for tracheostomy (see below) may be reduced (Atkinson 1970).

The respiratory tract. The mouth and pharynx should be cleansed regularly with a swab held in forceps, and mucus and saliva are prevented from accumulating in the pharynx by clearing the mouth periodically with a soft rubber catheter attached to a mechanical sucker. Regular turning of the patient will improve pulmonary ventilation, and a physiotherapist should where necessary supervise postural drainage. If there are signs of pulmonary collapse, the patient will require bronchoscopy to clear an obstructed bronchus. An oral airway is always required in a comatose patient, and, if there is severe respiratory insufficiency or apnoea, artificial respiration will also be necessary. This is usually best carried out by a positive-pressure mechanical respirator combined with tracheal intubation at first and later tracheostomy if unconsciousness is likely to last more than 24 hours; a cuffed tracheostomy tube has the advantage of preventing the aspiration of food or saliva. The blood gases must be checked regularly to be sure that ventilation is satisfactory. The role of artificial ventilation in neurological disease has been reviewed by Douglas, Fergusson, Crompton, and Grant (1983). Penicillin should be given regularly as a prophylactic against pneumonia, but if chest infection occurs a broad-spectrum antibiotic should be substituted.

Feeding. A patient who is unconscious for more than a few hours requires both food and drink, and since he cannot swallow this must be given by oesophageal tube. This, however, is not a complete safeguard against the aspiration of food, since a feed may be regurgitated and vomiting may occur. These risks reinforce the need for tracheostomy in most cases. Many nutritious commercial preparations are available for tube feeding, providing not only an adequate fluid and calorie intake but also the necessary vitamin and mineral supplements.

The blood electrolytes. There are several ways in which the blood electrolytes may become disordered in the unconscious patient. When coma is itself the result of a metabolic disorder, the biochemical changes which that produces will be present. The blood biochemistry may also be disordered as the result of an excessive or inadequate intake of water, or an excessive amount of protein in the diet. A cerebral lesion may itself lead to hypernatraemia or, alternatively, to hyponatraemia unresponsive to corticosteroids; the latter is often due to inappropriate secretion of antidiuretic hormone (ADH). The fluid intake and output of the unconscious patient should therefore be carefully recorded, and from time to time also the serum osmolality, blood urea, sodium, potassium, chloride, glucose, and other solutes.

The sphincters. The unconscious patient will have retention or incontinence of urine, and this is best dealt with by the use of a self-retaining catheter which should be changed every few days. The urine should be examined regularly for signs of infection. Constipation is best dealt with by enemas.

External stimulation

There is increasing evidence to suggest that when signs of recovery from coma begin to appear, regular repetitive stimulation of each of the special senses with stereotyped and graded stimuli applied by nurses or even family members under supervision, and passive limb movements, followed by active willed movement under the supervision of a physiotherapist, are helpful in speeding recovery.

Hallucinations and allied disorders of perception

Hallucinations may be defined as mental impressions of sensory vividness occurring without external stimulus, but appearing to be located, or to possess a cause located, outside the subject. An illusion is defined as a misinterpretation of an external stimulus, but illusions in some cases are closely related to hallucinations and can occur as symptoms of hallucinatory states. A delusion, by contrast, is an idea or thought (such as a false concept of persecution) which has no substance in fact; in contrast to visual and auditory hallucinations, it is purely a thought process with no sensory content, but hallucinations and delusions may occur together in various toxic/confusional states and in psychotic illnesses such as schizophrenia. Psychophysiologically, though hallucinations manifest themselves as changes in the content of consciousness, there is considerable evidence that they are often the result of disordered function of the reticulohypothalamic and associated pathways concerned with the state of consciousness as a whole.

The principal circumstances in which hallucinations may occur are: (1) in dreaming and the hypnagogic state; (2) in pathological disorders of sleep; (3) as a result of organic disease of the sense organs or of the central nervous system (including focal epilepsy); (4) in states of intoxication, particularly after the administration of certain drugs such as mescaline and lysergic acid or after withdrawal of alcohol, amphetamines, barbiturates, or other psychotropic drugs; and (5) in certain psychoses.

Lhermitte (1951) reviewed the subject of hallucinations with particular reference to those resulting from nervous disease. Visual hallucinations can occur in patients suffering from severe visual loss as a result of disease of the eyes, or with lesions in any part of the visual pathways as well as elsewhere in the nervous system. Crude hallucinations (e.g. flashes of light) may be due to irritation of such pathways, whereas formed hallucinations more often arise in the visual association areas of the cortex. When a hemianopia is present, the hallucinations may be seen in the normal half fields or in the blind half fields. Lhermitte himself described what he termed peduncular hallucinosis, namely the occurrence of hallucinations, especially visual hallucinations, as a result of lesions of the upper part of the brainstem. He interpreted these hallucinations as expressing a dissociation of the state of sleep in which, although bodily activity remains awake, mental processes are disturbed or memory engrams are evoked permitting the appearance of images analogous to those which normally occur only in dreams. There have also been recent reports of hallucinations resulting from brainstem compression (Dunn, Weisberg, and Nadell 1983). Clearly any explanation of hallucinations occurring in association with organic lesions of the sense organs or the central nervous system must also take into account the mental state of the patient as a whole; thus they are common in delirium but then have no localizing value.

Hallucinations involving various sensory modalities, together with perceptual illusions and other disorders of consciousness, are particularly liable to occur as a result of lesions of the temporal lobes. The perceptual illusions include disordered visual perception, for example macropsia or micropsia and a similar alteration in auditory perception, feelings of unreality of the self or the surroundings, and disturbances of awareness of the body. Visual hallucination of the self has been described in which the individual feels that he is observing his own body from outside his physical self; this unusual phenomenon has some affinities with sensations of intense depersonalization or unreality. Visual hallucinations also sometimes occur as a result of epileptic discharge arising in the posterior part of the temporal lobe or in the parieto-occipital region and, when 'formed', invariably indicate the presence of a focal cortical lesion when toxic causes can be excluded. Agitated delirium and visual impairment may, for example, result from medial temporo-occipital infarction (Medina, Chokroverty, and Rubino 1977).

References
Adams, R. D., Victor, M., and Mancall, E. L. (1959). Central pontine myelinolysis. *Arch. Neurol. Psychiat.* **81**, 154.

Atkinson, W. J. (1970). Posture of the unconscious patient. *Lancet* **i**, 404.

Bates, D., Caronna, J. J., Cartlidge, N. E. F., Knill-Jones, R. P., Levy, D. E., Shaw, D. A., and Plum, F. (1977). A prospective study of non-traumatic coma: methods and results in 310 patients. *Ann. Neurol.* **2**, 211.

Bauer, G., Gerstenbrand, F., and Rumpl, E. (1979). Varieties of the locked-in syndrome. *J. Neurol.* **221**, 77.

Brain, W. R. (1947). Some observations on visual hallucinations and central metamorphopsia. *Acta psychiat. scand.*, Suppl. 46.

British Medical Journal (1973). Mute of malady. *Br. med. J.* **1**, 755.

—— (1981). Outcome of non-traumatic coma. *Br. med. J.*, **283**, 3.

Buonaguidi, R., Rossi, B., Sartucci, F., and Ravelli, V. (1979). Blink reflexes in severe traumatic coma. *J. Neurol. Neurosurg. Psychiat.* **42**, 470.

Burks, J. S., Alfrey, A. C., Huddlestone, J., Norrenberg, M. D., and Lewin, E. (1976). A fatal encephalopathy in chronic haemodialysis patients. *Lancet* **i**, 764.

Cairns, H. (1952). Disturbances of consciousness with lesions of the brainstem and diencephalon. *Brain* **75**, 109.

Carroll, W. M. and Mastaglia, F. L. (1979). Alpha and beta coma in drug intoxication uncomplicated by cerebral hypoxia. *Electroenceph. clin. Neurophysiol.* **46**, 95.

Conference of Medical Royal Colleges and Faculties of the United Kingdom (1976). Diagnosis of brain death. *Lancet* **ii**, 1069.

Dent, C. E. and Watson, L. C. A. (1964). Hyperparathyroidism and cancer. *Br. med. J.* **2**, 218.

Douglas, J. G., Fergusson, R. J., Crompton, G. K., and Grant, I. W. B. (1983). Artificial ventilation for neurological disease: retrospective analysis 1972–81. *Br. med. J.* **286**, 1943.

Dunn, D. W., Weisberg, L. A., and Nadell, J. (1983). Peduncular hallucinations caused by brainstem compression. *Neurology, Minneapolis* **33**, 1360.

Feldman, M. H. (1971). Physiological observations in a chronic case of 'locked-in' syndrome. *Neurology, Minneapolis* **21**, 459.

French, J. B. (1952). Brain lesions associated with prolonged unconsciousness. *Arch. Neurol. Psychiat., Chicago* **68**, 727.

Gerich, J. E., Martin, M. M., and Recant, L. (1971). Clinical and metabolic characteristics of hyperosmolar nonketotic coma. *Diabetes* **20**, 228.

Goldberg, M. (1963). Hyponatraemia and the inappropriate secretion of antidiuretic hormone. *Am. J. Med.* **35**, 293.

Goldie, W. D., Chiappa, K. H., Young, R. R., and Brooks, E. B. (1981). Brainstem auditory and short-latency somatosensory evoked responses in brain death. *Neurology, Minneapolis* **31**, 248.

Gordon, E. E. and Kibadi, U. M. (1976). The hyperglycaemic, hyperosmolar syndrome. *Am. J. Med. Sci.* **271**, 252.

Grant, D. K. (1953). Papilloedema and fits in hypoparathyroidism. *Quart. J. Med.* **22**, 243.

Hawkes, C. H. (1974). 'Locked-in' syndrome: report of seven cases. *Br. med. J.* **4**, 379.

—— and Bryan-Smith, L. (1974). The electroencephalogram in the 'locked-in' syndrome. *Neurology, Minneapolis* **24**, 1015.

Jefferson, A. (1956). Clinical correlation between encephalopathy and papilloedema in Addison's disease. *J. Neurol. Neurosurg. Psychiat.* **19**, 21.

Jennett, B., Gleave, J., and Wilson, P. (1981). Brain death in three neurosurgical units. *Br. med. J.* **282**, 533.

——, Teasdale, G., Braakman, R., Minderhoud, J., Heiden, J., and Kurze, T. (1979). Prognosis of patients with severe head injury. *Neurosurgery* **4**, 283.

Johnson, R. H., Sambre, D. G., and Spalding, J. M. K. (1984). *Neurocardiology*. Saunders, London.

Karp, J. S. and Hurtig, H. I. (1974). 'Locked-in' state with bilateral midbrain infarcts. *Arch. Neurol., Chicago* **30**, 176.

Kemper, T. L. and Romanul, F. C. A. (1967). State resembling akinetic mutism in basilar artery occlusion. *Neurology, Minneapolis* **17**, 74.

Kreutzer, E. W., Rutherford, R. B., and Lehman, R. A. W. (1982). Diagnosis of brain death by common carotid artery velocity waveform analysis. *Arch. Neurol., Chicago* **39**, 136.

The Lancet (1980). Death and the brainstem. *Lancet* **ii** 1286.

—— (1981*a*). Brain death. *Lancet* **i**, 363.

—— (1981*b*). Outcome of non-traumatic coma. *Lancet* **ii**, 507.

Leigh, R. J. and Shaw, D. A. (1976). Rapid regular respiration in unconscious patients. *Arch. Neurol., Chicago* **33**, 356.

—— and Zee, D. S. (1983). *The neurology of eye movements*. Davis, Philadelphia.

Lemann, J. and Donatelli, A. A. (1964). Calcium intoxication due to primary hyperparathyroidism: a medical and surgical emergency. *Ann. intern. Med.* **60**, 447.

Levy, D. E., Bates, D., Caronna, J. J., Cartlidge, N. E. F., Knill-Jones, R. P., Lapinsk, R. H., Singer, B. H., Shaw, D. A., and Plum, F. (1981). Prognosis in non-traumatic coma. *Ann. intern. Med.* **94**, 293.

Lhermitte, J. (1951). *Les hallucinations*. Masson, Paris.

McCusker, E. A., Rudick, R. A., Honch, G. W., and Griggs, R. C. (1982). Recovery from the 'locked-in' syndrome. *Arch. Neurol., Chicago* **39**, 145.

McNicol, M. W. and Smith, R. (1964). Accidental hypothermia. *Br. med. J.* **1**, 19.

Medical Research Council (1941). *A glossary of psychological terms commonly used in cases of head injury*. HMSO, London.

Medina, J. L., Chokroverty, S., and Rubino, F. A. (1977). Syndrome of agitated delirium and visual impairment: a manifestation of medial temporo-occipital infarction. *J. Neurol. Neurosurg. Psychiat.* **40**, 861.

Molinari, G. F. (1982). Brain death, irreversible coma, and words doctors use. *Neurology, Minneapolis* **32**, 400.

Montgomery, B. M. and Pinner, C. A. (1964). Transient hypoglycaemic hemiplegia. *Arch. intern. Med.* **114**, 680.

Mooradian, A. D., Morley, G. K., McGeachie, R., Lundgren, S., and Morley, J. E. (1984). Spontaneous periodic hypothermia. *Neurology, Minneapolis* **34**, 79.

Newsom Davis, J. (1974). Autonomous breathing. *Arch. Neurol., Chicago* **30**, 480.

Nordgren, R. E., Markesbery, W. R., Fukuda, K., and Reeves, A. G. (1971). Seven cases of cerebromedullospinal disconnection: the 'locked-in' syndrome. *Neurology, Minneapolis* **21**, 1140.

Norris, F. H. and Fawcett, J. (1965). A sign of intracranial mass with impending uncal herniation. *Arch. Neurol., Chicago* **12**, 381.

Page, M. M. and Watkins, P. J. (1978). Cardiorespiratory arrest and diabetic autonomic neuropathy. *Lancet* **i**, 14.

Pallis, C. (1983). ABC of brainstem death. *Articles from the British Medical Journal*. British Medical Journal, London.

Pearson, J., Korelin, J., Harris, J. H., Wichter, M., and Braunstein, P. (1977). Brain death: II. Neuropathological correlation with the radioisotopic bolus technique for evaluation of critical deficit of cerebral blood flow. *Ann. Neurol.* **2**, 206.

Plum, F. (1972). Organic disturbances of consciousness. In *Scientific foundations of neurology* (ed. M. Critchley, J. L. O'Leary, and W. B. Jennett) p. 193. Heinemann, London.

—— (1982). Mechanisms of 'central' hyperventilation. *Ann. Neurol.* **11**, 636.

—— and Alvord, E. C. Jr. (1964). Apneustic breathing in man. *Arch. Neurol., Chicago* **10**, 101.

—— and Posner, J. B. (1980). *Stupor and coma*, 3rd edn. Davis, Philadelphia.

—— and Swanson, A. G. (1958). Abnormalities in the central regulation of respiration in acute and convalescent poliomyelitis. *Arch. Neurol. Psychiat., Chicago* **80**, 267.

—— and —— (1959). Central neurogenic hyperventilation in man. *Arch. Neurol. Psychiat., Chicago* **81**, 535.

President's Commission for the Study of Ethical Problems in Medicine and Biochemical and Behavioral Research (1981). Guidelines for the determination of death: report of the medical consultants on the diagnosis of death. *J. Am. med. Ass.* **246**, 2184.

Robson, J. G. (1981). Brain death. *Lancet* **ii**, 365.

Rodriguez, M., Baele, P. L., Marsh, H. M., and Okazaki, H. (1982). Central neurogenic hyperventilation in an awake patient with brainstem astrocytoma. *Ann. Neurol.* **11**, 625.

Rosenberg, G. A., Johnson, S. F., and Brenner, R. P. (1977). Recovery of cognition after prolonged vegetative state. *Ann. Neurol.* **2**, 167.

Rosenberg, S. A., Brief, D. K., Kinney, J. M., Herrera, M. G., Wilson, R. E., and Moore, F. D. (1965). The syndrome of dehydration, coma and severe hyperglycaemia without ketosis in patients convalescing from burns. *New Engl. J. Med.* **272**, 931.

Rosin, A. J. and Exton-Smith, A. N. (1964). Clinical features of accidental hypothermia, with some observations on thyroid function. *Br. med. J.* **1**, 16.

Ross, E. D. and Stewart, R. M. (1981). Akinetic mutism from hypothalamic damage: successful treatment with dopamine agonists. *Neurology, Minneapolis* **31**, 1435.

Salem, S. N. (1966). Neurological complications of heat stroke in Kuwait. *Ann. trop. Med. Parasitol.* **60**, 393.

Schafer, J. A. and Caronna, J. J. (1978). Duration of apnea needed to confirm brain death. *Neurology, Minneapolis* **28**, 661.

Shuttleworth, E. (1983). Recovery to social and economic independence from prolonged postanoxic vegetative state. *Neurology, Minneapolis* **33**, 372.

Skultety, F. M. (1968). Clinical and experimental aspects of akinetic mutism. *Arch. Neurol., Chicago* **19**, 1.

Snyder, B. D., Gumnit, R. J., Leppik, I. E., Hauser, W. A., Loewenson, R. B., and Ramirez-Lassepas, M. (1981). Neurologic prognosis after cardiopulmonary arrest: IV. Brainstem reflexes. *Neurology, Minneapolis* **31**, 1092.

Teasdale, G. and Jennett, W. B. (1974). Assessment of coma and impaired consciousness. *Lancet* ii, 81.

——, Knill-Jones, R., and Van der Sande, J. (1978). Observer variability in assessing impaired consciousness and coma. *J. Neurol. Neurosurg. Psychiat.* **41**, 603.

Watson, L. C. A. (1963). Hypercalcaemia and cancer. *Postgrad. med. J.* **39**, 646.

Disorders of memory

Memory may be defined as the power to retain and recall past experiences; as thus defined, however, it clearly includes functions of differing complexity. Perhaps the simplest form is that involved in remembering a series of digits or a short phrase. In such an act of recollection or mechanical memory there is little emphasis upon the 'pastness' of what is recollected. The emphasis is rather upon the persistence into the present of items which have been recorded or 'learned', perhaps through repetition. In such an act of remembering there is nothing more than the three fundamental elements of memory—registration, retention, and recall. Compare this, however, with the recollection, evoked by a place or a scent, of a single past experience fraught with emotion. Recall is then initiated by an associative process and there is much emphasis upon the 'pastness' of the experience by contrast with a present in which it is no longer occurring. Moreover, one of two such past episodes is remembered as having been experienced before the other, so that arising out of the memory function is the experience of a personal past time as an extended dimension in which past experiences bear a constant and linear relation to each other. Furthermore, these experiences are recognized as being those of a single person; hence it follows that memory is essential to the experience of personal identity.

There is another function of memory which seems to be intermediate between the mechanical reproduction of words or digits and the recollection of an isolated incident. This is the recall of an image built up as a result of repeated experiences as, for example, that of a house or a person with whom one is familiar. A similar function of remembering enters not only into the act of representing to oneself the familiar house or face in its absence, but also into the act of recognizing it when it is presented again.

In clinical practice it is now customary to regard *sensory memory* as the ability to retain recorded signals in the sensory or receptive areas of the brain for a very short period of time after they have been received. *Short-term (or primary) memory* is the ability to retain facts, words, numbers, or letters (such as telephone numbers or a name and address) for a few seconds or minutes combined with ability to recall the information at will. *Long-term memory* is the storage in the brain of information which can be recalled minutes, hours, days, months, or years later. *Secondary memories* are those long-term memories which are stored in the form of relatively weak memory traces so that the information can only be recalled for a few days or is difficult to remember at all. *Tertiary memories*, by contrast, are so deeply imprinted (such as the individual's name, the letters of the alphabet) that they can be recalled at will throughout life. The recall mechanism is attributed to activity in precisely defined reverberating neuronal circuits, long-term memory to progressive synaptic facilitation; Repetition of information (rehearsal) and the codifying of sensory stimuli into different classes of information assist in the consolidation of long-term memories and the transfer of sensory into long-term memory (Walton 1982). Loss of memory is called amnesia.

The anatomical and physiological basis of memory
This is discussed on page 638.

Tests of memory
Clearly, the function of remembering cannot adequately be tested by using simple tests which merely investigate the patient's power to retain and recall a series of digits or words. One must also assess the patient's power to recall events from his past life, both remote and recent, as well as his capacity for mechanical memory as illustrated by the recollection of digits, sentences, or passages learnt by heart (see p. 657). A useful battery of clinical bedside tests is described by Strub and Black (1981) who also reviewed the use of more precise psychometric techniques.

Some organic causes of amnesia
The importance of the temporal lobe in memory mechanisms has already been stressed (p. 638); it is well recognized that bilateral temporal-lobe disease or resection may seriously impair memory. Among the conditions which can cause severe memory loss, characterized particularly by an inability to record, retain, and recall recent impressions with, as a rule, relative sparing of memory for remote events, are inflammatory and degenerative diseases of the brain which cause dementia (including general paresis, the presenile and senile dementias, and multi-infarct dementia), temporal-lobe tumours, herpes simplex encephalitis, severe anoxia or hypoglycaemia, severe head injury with diffuse brain damage, chronic alcoholism and, in some cases, bilateral rostral leucotomy (Whitty and Lishman 1966). Severe memory loss has also been observed as a feature of limbic encephalitis in association with carcinoma (Henson and Urich 1982) and as a presumed paraneoplastic phenomenon (the 'Ophelia syndrome') in Hodgkin's disease (Carr 1982). Transient amnesia can also occur as a result of various toxic confusional states, milder anoxic episodes, concussion, acute alcoholic or drug intoxication, encephalitis and meningitis, epilepsy (particularly of the temporal-lobe or complex partial type), migraine and other forms of cerebral ischaemia, and a variety of deficiency disorders (particularly of thiamine, giving the Korsakow syndrome—see below). There is some evidence that certain drugs, such as piracetam (Dimond and Brouwers 1976) and many others, but especially cholinergic preparations such as physostigmine and lecithin (Goldberg, Gerstman, Mattis, Hughes, Bilder, and Sirio 1982; *The Lancet* 1982) may enhance verbal memory in normal human subjects and in some individuals with various defects of memory such as post-traumatic amnesia. For this reason it is suggested that anticholinergic drugs are best avoided in elderly or demented subjects with failing memory.

Transient global amnesia
This syndrome, believed to be due to transient ischaemia in one or both temporal lobes, as it usually occurs in middle-aged or elderly individuals with evidence of cerebral atherosclerosis, is a disorder of sudden onset (Fisher and Adams 1958). It has been reported to follow intense emotion, sexual intercourse, intense pain, and exposure to cold (Fisher 1982), the ingestion of clioquinol (Mumenthaler, Kaeser, Meyer, and Hess 1979), cerebral angiography (Cochran, Morrell, Huckman, and Cochran 1982), polycythaemia vera, recurrent cerebral embolism or other 'risk factors' for stroke (Shuping, Rollinson, and Toole 1980), and left temporal haemorrhage (Landi, Giusti, and Guidotti 1982); the syndrome has also been described in four brothers (Corston and Godwin-Austen 1982). CT scanning sometimes shows unilateral, rarely bilateral, temporal lesions and is often negative (Ladurner,

Skvarc, and Sager 1982). It has already been mentioned on page 639 that memory loss for recent events develops rapidly and in the attacks, despite their inability to register new impressions, the patients retain their personal identity, show no abnormality of behaviour apart from anxiety and no evidence of impaired perception. Even virtuoso musical performance may be unimpaired (Byer and Crowley 1980). Retrograde amnesia can be striking in an attack (Gordon and Marin 1979). Recovery is usually complete within a few hours, and retrograde amnesia shrinks rapidly, usually leaving the patient with no disability other than amnesia for the events occurring in the attack itself (Fogelholm, Kivalo, and Bergström 1975). Ponsford and Donnan (1980) found no lasting memory impairment on follow-up but Mazzucchi, Moretti, Caffarra, and Parma (1980), by contrast, identified lasting defects of verbal long-term memory in many of their cases.

Hysterical amnesia

This is considered on page 662.

Korsakow's syndrome

The single most characteristic feature of Korsakow's syndrome or psychosis is a specific form of amnesia. The patient has a gross defect of memory for recent events so that he has no recollection of what has happened even half an hour previously. He is disorientated in space and time and he fills the gaps in his memory by confabulating, that is, by giving imaginary accounts of his activities. Thus a bedridden patient may describe a walk which he asserts he has just taken. Berlyne (1972) defined confabulation as 'the falsification of memory occurring in a clear consciousness in association with an organically derived amnesia'. Stuss, Alexander, Lieberman, and Levine (1978) suggest that spontaneous confabulation requires a deficit of frontal-lobe function as well as amnesia. Shapiro, Alexander, Gardner, and Mercer (1981) found that confabulation could be mild or severe; when severe it was often associated with perseveration, impaired self-monitoring, and failure to inhibit incorrect responses.

The amnesia of Korsakow's syndrome appears to be due to a lesion in the mammillary bodies and in other parts of the limbic system (see below). There is also a reduced capacity for retention and a disturbance of perception except for the immediate apprehension of spatially and temporally unitary patterns (Talland 1958, 1959; Talland and Ekdahl 1959). Lidz (1942) found that in this 'amnestic syndrome' the patient could neither evoke the past nor relate his current experience to it. However, Seltzer and Benson (1974), who compared, by means of a multiple-choice questionnaire based upon well-known events of the past 50 years, the performance of 11 alcoholic subjects with Korsakow's syndrome with that of 50 control subjects, found in the patients a severe defect of recent memory but almost normal recall of events occurring in the remote past. The defective appreciation of time relationships is secondary to the amnesia.

Korsakow's psychosis is seen typically in chronic alcoholism, almost always with Wernicke's encephalopathy, so that the Korsakow–Wernicke syndrome is spoken of (also see Perkin and Handler 1983). The lesions involve the medial parts of the medial, dorsal pulvinar, and antero-ventral thalamic nuclei, the mammillary bodies, and the terminal portions of the fornices, and consist of loss of medullated fibres and nerve cells, large numbers of adventitial histiocytes and microglia, proliferation of capillaries, and in a few cases haemorrhages.

Korsakow's syndrome can also result from other lesions involving the same structures, e.g. head injury, anoxia, carbon monoxide poisoning, epilepsy, electroconvulsive therapy, acute encephalitis, general paresis, other forms of dementia, intracranial tumour, cerebral arteriosclerosis, cerebral sarcoidosis and other forms of granulomatous meningitis, subarachnoid haemorrhage, and the operation of cingulectomy. It has also been described as a sequel of gastrectomy, malnutrition, malabsorption, and pancreatitis (Pallis and Lewis 1974).

References

Berlyne, N. (1972). Confabulation. *Br. J. Psychiat.* **120**, 31.

Byer, J. A. and Crowley, W. J., Jr (1980). Musical performance during transient global amnesia. *Neurology, Minneapolis* **30**, 80.

Carr, I. (1982). The Ophelia syndrome: memory loss in Hodgkin's disease. *Lancet* **i**, 844.

Cochran, J. W., Morrell, F., Huckman, M. S., Cochran, E. J. (1982). Transient global amnesia after cerebral angiography: report of seven cases. *Arch. Neurol., Chicago* **39**, 593.

Corston, R. N. and Godwin-Austen, R. B. (1982). Transient global amnesia in four brothers. *J. Neurol. Neurosurg. Psychiat.* **45**, 375.

Dimond, S. J. and Brouwers, E. Y. M. (1976). Increase in the power of human memory in normal man through the use of drugs. *Psychopharmacology* **49**, 307.

Fisher, C. M. (1982). Transient global amnesia: precipitating activities and other observations. *Arch. Neurol., Chicago* **39**, 605.

—— and Adams, R. D. (1958). Transient global amnesia. *Trans. Am. neurol. Ass.* **83**, 143.

Fogelholm, R., Kivalo, E., and Bergström, L. (1975). The transient global amnesia syndrome. *Eur. Neurol.* **13**, 72.

Goldberg, E., Gerstman, L. J., Mattis, S., Hughes, J. E. O., Bilder, R. M. Jr., and Sirio, C. A. (1982). Effects of cholinergic treatment on post-traumatic anterograde amnesia. *Arch. Neurol., Chicago* **39**, 581.

Gordon, B. and Marin, O. S. M. (1979). Transient global amnesia: an extensive case report. *J. Neurol. Neurosurg. Psychiat.* **42**, 572.

Henson, R. A. and Urich, H. (1982). *Cancer and the nervous system.* Blackwell, Oxford.

Ladurner, G., Skvarc, A., and Sager, W. D. (1982). Computer tomography in transient global amnesia. *Eur. Neurol.* **21**, 34.

The Lancet (1982). Drugs and memory. *Lancet* **ii**, 474.

Landi, G., Giusti, M. C., and Guidotti, M. (1982). Transient global amnesia due to left temporal haemorrhage. *J. Neurol. Neurosurg. Psychiat.* **45**, 1062.

Lidz, T. (1942). The amnestic syndrome. *Arch. Neurol. Psychiat., Chicago* **47**, 588.

Mazzucchi, A., Moretti, G., Caffarra, P., and Parma, M. (1980). Neuropsychological functions in the follow-ups of transient global amnesia. *Brain,* **103**, 161.

Mumenthaler, M., Kaeser, H. E., Meyer, A., and Hess, T. (1979). Transient global amnesia after clioquinol: five personal observations from outside Japan. *J. Neurol. Neurosurg. Psychiat.* **42**, 1084.

Pallis, C. A. and Lewis, P. D. (1974). *The neurology of gastrointestinal disease.* Saunders, London.

Perkin, G. D. and Handler, C. E. (1983). Wernicke–Korsakoff syndrome. *Br. J. hosp. Med.* **30**, 331.

Ponsford, J. L. and Donnan, G. A. (1980). Transient global amnesia—a hippocampal phenomenon? *J. Neurol. Neurosurg. Psychiat.* **43**, 285.

Rosenbaum, M. and Merritt, H. H. (1939). Korsakoff's syndrome. Clinical study of the alcoholic form, with special regard to prognosis. *Arch. Neurol. Psychiat., Chicago* **51**, 978.

Seltzer, B. and Benson, D. F. (1974). The temporal pattern of retrograde amnesia in Korsakoff's disease. *Neurology, Minneapolis* **24**, 527.

Shapiro, B. E., Alexander, M. P., Gardner, H., and Mercer, B. (1981). Mechanisms of confabulation. *Neurology, Minneapolis* **31**, 1070.

Shuping, J. R., Rollinson, R. D., and Toole, J. F. (1980). Transient global amnesia. *Ann. Neurol.* **7**, 281.

Strub, R. L. and Black, F. W. (1981). *Organic brain syndromes: an introduction to neurobehavioral disorders.* Davis, Philadelphia.

Stuss, D. T., Alexander, M. P., Lieberman, A., and Levine, H. (1978). An extraordinary form of confabulation. *Neurology, Minneapolis* **28**, 1166.

Talland, G. A. (1958). Psychological studies in Korsakow's psychosis. II. Perceptual functions. *J. nerv. ment. Dis.* **127**, 197.

—— (1959). The interference theory of forgetting and the amnesic syndrome. *J. abnorm. soc. Psychol.* **59**, 10.

—— and Ekdahl, M. (1959). Psychological studies of Korsakow's psychosis. IV. The note and mode of forgetting narrative material. *J. nerv. ment. Dis.* **129**, 391.

Walton, J. N. (1982). *Essentials of neurology*, 5th edn. Pitman, London.

Whitty, C. W. M. and Lishman, W. A. (1966). Amnesia in cerebral disease. In *Amnesia* (ed. C. W. M. Whitty and O. L. Zangwill) p. 92. Butterworths, London.

Disorders of mood

The neural basis of registration of emotion and the integration of the accompanying physical changes have been discussed on page 637. It is to disorders of these mechanisms and of their relationship with higher levels of the nervous system that we must look for explanations of mood disorders occurring as a result of organic nervous disease. For more detailed commentaries upon disorders of mood and emotion consequent upon affective and psychotic disorders the reader is referred to textbooks of psychiatry (see Gelder, Gath, and Mayou 1983); such conditions will only be mentioned here in so far as they enter into the differential diagnosis of those mood changes which occur in organic nervous disease. In passing, it is important to note that the borderland between neurology and psychiatry is becoming less well defined. Thus, to quote but a few examples, there is evidence that depression is associated with dysfunction of the hypothalamic–pituitary–adrenal axis (*British Medical Journal* 1981) and with a reduced availability of monoamines, principally noradrenaline and serotonin, at several cerebral receptor sites (*The Lancet* 1982; van Praag 1982), while many of the physical accompaniments of anxiety are related to neurotransmitter release and can be relieved at least in part by β-adrenergic blockade (Braestrup and Nielsen 1982). And in schizophrenia (Bird, Barnes, Iversen, Spokes, Mackay, and Shepherd 1977; Crow 1980) and schizophrenia-like psychoses (Pepplinkhuizen, Blom, Bruinvels, and Moleman 1980) increased cerebral dopamine receptors and reduced glutamic acid decarboxylase activity, to mention but two abnormalities, have been reported, although PET scanning has been disappointingly negative in such cases (Sheppard, Manchanda, Gruzelier, Hirsch, Wise, Frackowiak, and Jones 1983). Thus it seems evident that neuropharmacological studies (see Bloom 1985) will cast increasing light in the future upon the pathogenesis of major psychiatric syndromes and upon the means by which organic disease of the nervous system causes mental symptoms.

Emotional instability

Emotional instability or lability is a common symptom of nervous diseases, especially of those in which cerebral lesions are diffuse. The patient is easily moved by almost any form of emotion. He is quickly irritated or angered, easily becomes apprehensive, is readily depressed or reduced to tears. Less often, he experiences pleasurable emotion with abnormal facility and is readily moved to laughter. Emotional instability of this kind is common after head injury, after massive cerebral infarction, and in patients with diffuse cerebral arteriosclerosis. It is often present in early dementia, however caused, and is also common in advanced multiple sclerosis. This exaggerated emotional reaction common to so many disorders appears to be due to impairment of the control which higher levels of the nervous system normally exercise over the thalamus and hypothalamus.

Impulsive disorders of conduct

Emotional instability as described above does not usually lead to disordered behaviour, perhaps because conduct is normally more strongly inhibited than emotion. Exceptionally, however, impairment of higher control releases emotions which pass into action. This most often occurs in children or adolescents in whom the control of impulsive action, through education and increasing maturity, is as yet incomplete. The antisocial behaviour and even acts of violence sometimes committed by children and adolescents who have had encephalitis lethargica or other disorders causing diffuse brain damage are examples of this, and are similar to the behaviour seen in aggressive psychopaths, and rarely in epileptics, either before a complex partial seizure or in a phase of post-epileptic automatism or, even more rarely, in the intervals between attacks.

Emotional apathy

A general loss of emotional responsiveness without proportionate intellectual deterioration was once commonly seen in association with parkinsonism due to encephalitis lethargica. In view of the known predilection of the agent of this disease for the diencephalic grey matter, it was reasonable to attribute the apathy to injury to the posterior hypothalamus. A similar picture is seen in the later stages of dementia from any cause. Here it is likely that the apathy is in part, at least, secondary to deterioration of thought and perception. However, apathy is also seen in many forms of organic encephalopathy, degenerative brain disease, and in some psychotic disorders, especially severe depression and schizophrenia. The apathetic patient loses all his former interests and affections and, lacking the drive of the instinctive life, becomes incapable of effort, and sinks into a vegetative existence.

Euphoria

Euphoria (or elation) is a term used to indicate a mood characterized by feelings of cheerfulness and happiness, a sense of exceptional mental well-being. Transitory euphoria is induced in many people by alcohol. As a prevailing mood, it is sometimes seen in multiple sclerosis. Some sufferers from this disease remain serene and happy in spite of their increasing physical disabilities though others become depressed. Euphoria is also encountered occasionally in patients with intracranial tumours, especially when situated in the temporal lobe or, less often, in the frontal lobe or corpus callosum. Euphoria is also common in general paresis and is the predominating emotional state in milder cases of mania. Its psychophysiological basis is little understood.

Excitement

Excitement is a term somewhat loosely applied to several forms of mental over-activity, which may predominantly involve the intellectual, emotional, or psychomotor spheres. All three may be affected together, as in acute mania, characterized by flight of ideas, elation, and psychomotor restlessness. Delusional ideas may be linked with excitement in some delirious and confusional states, and in catatonic schizophrenia. Delirium has been defined as confusion with an overlay of excitement. It can occur as a result of head injury, diffuse inflammation of the brain or in a variety of toxic and metabolic confusional states, including those resulting from drug withdrawal. Psychomotor restlessness is associated with anxiety in agitated depression; and the prevailing mood may be one of rage in the outbursts of aggressive psychopaths. Meyer (1944) showed that states of excitement may be caused by lesions of the anterior hypothalamus.

Depression

Depression can be regarded as the opposite of euphoria. It is a mood of dejection and gloom for which often the patient can offer no explanation. It is encountered in a variety of states. It sometimes follows infections, especially influenza, and the use of certain drugs, such as sulphonamides. It may be a reaction to an adequate external cause, such as failure or bereavement, or a neurotic reaction to personal difficulties (reactive depression). In sufferers from cyclothymia, depression is liable to occur as a recurrent disorder of mood, sometimes alternating with phases of excitement, though often these are no more than a mild general sense of elation. In cyclothymic individuals the depressive phase is often associated with psychomotor retardation, causing difficulty in concentrating, often with insomnia and loss of appetite. Such patients typically wake early and feel at their worst in the early part of the day. Depression also occurs as the predominant feature of endogenous depression or involutional melancholia, in which it may be associated with agitation. Patients suffering from such psychotic depression in a severe form often have delusions of guilt or of a hypochondriacal nature. Often, too, they have physical symptoms including headache, fatigue, and facial and/or limb or low back pain with the typical pattern of early-morning waking. Depression is also common in patients suffering from organic brain disease. This may be in part a natural reaction to illness or disability and it is most prominent in individuals of cyclothymic temperament in whom the physical ilness appears to release a pre-existing tendency to depression. Thus depression is not uncommon after head injury, in some patients suffering from multiple sclerosis, and sometimes in those with intracranial tumour, general paresis, parkinsonism, and many other neurological disorders.

Anxiety

Fear is an emotional reaction to imminent danger; anxiety is the reaction to a possible future danger—fear linked with anticipation. Anxiety may be produced in many ways and is often a perfectly natural emotional reaction. It may also be the effect of certain toxins, many of which have a sympathomimetic effect, such as adrenaline, ephedrine, amphetamine, nicotine, and thyroxine. Anxiety may be the prevailing mood in patients suffering from organic disease of the brain as, for example, after head injury, and is then probably in part the outcome of diminished control of emotional reactions by higher centres, and in part a reaction to the disability produced by the injury or disease. Fear may be very evident in delirious states, when it appears as a reaction to terrifying hallucinations, and it can be linked with depression in involutional melancholia. In very many cases, however, anxiety is neurotic—that is, it is the abnormal and excessive product of unconscious mental processes.

References

Agranoff, B. W. (1975). Biochemical strategies in the study of memory formation. In *Nervous system* (ed. D. B. Tower), Vol. 1, *The basic neurosciences* (ed. R. O. Brady) p. 585. Raven Press, New York.

Bird, E. D., Barnes, J., Iversen, L. L., Spokes, E. G., Mackay, A. V. P., and Shepherd, M. (1977). Increased brain dopamine and reduced glutamic acid decarboxylase and choline acetyl transferase activity in schizophrenia and related psychoses. *Lancet* ii, 1157.

Bloom, F. (1985). Neurotransmitter diversity and its functional significance. *J. R. Soc. med.* 78, 189.

Braestrup, C. and Nielsen, M. (1982). Anxiety. *Lancet* ii, 1030.

British Medical Journal (1981). The new psychiatry. *Br. med. J.* 283, 513.

Cottrell, S. S. and Wilson, S. A. K. (1926). The affective symptomatology of disseminated sclerosis. *J. Neurol. Psychopath.* 7, 1.

Crow, T. J. (1980). Molecular pathology of schizophrenia: more than one disease process? *Br. med. J.* 1, 66.

Fulton, J. F. and Ingraham, F. D. (1929). Emotional disturbances following experimental lesions of the base of the brain (pre-chiasmal). *J. Phyisoll., London* 67, 27.

Gelder, M., Gath, D., and Mayou, R. (1983). *Oxford textbook of psychiatry*. Oxford University Press, Oxford.

The Lancet (1982). α₂-adrenergic receptors in depression. *Lancet* i, 781.

Meyer, A. (1944). The Wernicke syndrome. *J. Neurol. Neurosurg. Psychiat.* 7, 66.

Pepplinkhuizen, L., Blom, W., Bruinvels, J., and Moleman, P. (1980). Schizophrenia-like psychosis caused by a metabolic disorder. *Lancet* i, 454.

Reitan, R. M. and Davison, L. A. (Eds.) (1974). *Clinical neuropsychology: current status and applications*. Winston, Wiley, Washington, D.C.

Sheppard, G., Manchanda, R., Gruzelier, J., Hirsch, S. R., Wise, R., Frackowiak, R., and Jones, T. (1983). ¹⁵O positron emission tomographic scanning in predominantly never-treated acute schizophrenic patients. *Lancet* ii, 1448.

Smythies, J. R. (1966). *The neurological foundations of psychiatry*. Blackwell, Oxford.

van Praag, H. M. (1982). Depression. *Lancet* ii, 1259.

The investigation of mental changes after cerebral lesions

Much attention has been devoted to the psychological investigation of patients with cerebral lesions (neuropsychology), and the Second World War gave a great impetus to this discipline. Numerous tests and several batteries of tests have been employed (Babcock 1930; Wechsler 1941; Reynell 1944; Klein and Mayer-Gross 1957; Reitan and Davison 1974; Heilman and Valenstein 1979; Strub and Black 1981; Wallesch, Kornhuber, Kunz, and Brunner 1983). Though much of theoretical interest can be learned from patients in states of confusion, the chief practical importance of psychometric studies lies in the diagnosis of dementia, and in the assessment of the nature and severity of residual psychological changes after head injury or other cerebral lesions with particular reference to prognosis and rehabilitation.

Specific defects of speech and perception

It is first necessary to recognize specific perceptual or cognitive defects, such as aphasia, acalculia, and the various forms of apraxia and agnosia. Two types of defect are of special importance, as emphasized by Zangwill (1945). Minor degrees of aphasia, which can prevent a patient from formulating and expressing his thoughts with fluency, may be identified only by special tests of high-grade comprehension and reasoning. And disorders of spatial judgment and manipulative skill—minor degrees of spatial agnosia or constructional apraxia—can interfere with the performance of skilled and semi-skilled manual occupations. These disorders are discussed elsewhere (see pp. 55 and 62 and Geschwind 1974). The Wechsler intelligence scale for children (W.I.S.C.) is particularly useful in childhood, when a discrepancy between the results obtained on the verbal and performance scales may indicate a specific inability to carry out certain performance tasks (motor skills) thus indicating some degree of apraxia (Gubbay 1975). The assessment of Schonell's 'reading age' is also valuable in the assessment of suspected dyslexia. Similar tests are available for adults; thus the Wechsler Adult Intelligence Scale (W.A.I.S.) is widely employed; Critchley (1972) and Rosenfield and Kinsbourne (1981) describe current techniques for assessing disorders of communication.

Intellectual deficits

The study of intellectual deficits by using appropriate tests has shown that after damage to the brain 'certain abilities or attainments, such as vocabulary, general information, and powers of comprehension suffer less in deterioration than do such capacities as reasoning ability, attention, recent memory, and "relational thinking"' (Reynell 1944). Babcock's and Reynell's batteries were designed to detect such differences. But the functions which suffer are themselves complex. Trist and Trist (1942–3) found Weigl's 'form-colour sorting test' of special value as a test of conceptual thought. Piercy (1964) and Oldfield (1972) gave valuable reviews of current methods, and Allison (1962) described techniques of particular value in the elderly. A simple test commonly employed is to ask the patient to subtract serial sevens from 100 aloud (the 100–7 test); the patient's performance may be impaired as a consequence of dementia but also by acalculia. In this and other tests it is important as far as possible to ascertain and bear in mind the patient's premorbid intellectual and educational status. Many of the psychometric methods commonly employed (e.g. the W.A.I.S. and W.I.S.C.) are capable of demonstrating not only intellectual impairment but also allow assessment of the premorbid intelligence quotient. The Halstead–Reitan battery may be even more sensitive in adults (Lehman, Chelune, and Heaton 1979). It is also useful on occasion to test the patient's powers of abstract thought by asking him to interpret proverbs such as 'People who live in glass houses should not throw stones'. A concrete interpretation ('They would break the glass') may occur in dementia but is more often a consequence of thought disorder such as schizophrenia.

Defects of memory

Memory defects are common after cerebral lesions and are often, but not invariably associated with defects of intellect (Newcombe 1972). Inquiry should first be made about everyday events in the patient's immediate past. His memory for remote events is also tested. He should be asked to name notable personalities (e.g. the last three prime ministers or American presidents). Digit retention and recall tests are also useful. Zangwill (1942–3) first ascertained the normal span, i.e. the number of digits which the patient could repeat correctly after one hearing, and then the number of hearings necessary for correct repetition when one more digit was added. The deteriorated patient can repeat fewer than normal (7) and may exhibit a sharp threshold, i.e. he may fail completely to remember one more. Reynell scored the total number of digits repeated forwards correctly and then the number repeated backwards, the average being 7 +5. It is also customary to use the name, address, and flower test, in which the patient is given a name, an address, and the name of a flower to recall several minutes later after other tests have been interposed. Also commonly used is one of the Babcock Sentences, No. 23, which runs as follows: 'One thing a nation must have to become rich and great is a large, secure supply of wood.' The observer ascertains the number of hearings necessary before the patient can repeat it correctly. More than three is abnormal.

Emotional factors and personality changes

Psychometric tests are also useful in distinguishing between failures of performance due to intellectual defects and those resulting from emotional disturbance. Thus Zangwill (1942–3) found the 'organic' reaction-type characterized by impairment of learning capacity and the 'neurotic' reaction-type by exaggerated variability of response and a tendency to fail on easy tasks. Tests such as the Minnesota Personality Inventory (M.M.P.I.) and many others are helpful in assessing personality traits and alterations consequent upon disease (Humphrey 1972). The importance of personality change, consequent upon organic cerebral lesions, needs no emphasis. It can only be interpreted in the light of the patient's previous personality, of which the new personality is often a 'caricature' (Patterson 1942); i.e. previous trends are exaggerated. In other cases the change is an inversion, and the previously cheerful, sociable, alert person may become depressed, antisocial, and lacking in initiative. Many depression rating scales such as that defined by Hamilton are useful. After brain damage the distinction made by Zangwill between 'organic' and 'neurotic' would perhaps be better described as between intellectual and emotional; for it is artificial to distinguish between organic and psychogenic symptoms in such patients: we are again dealing with a brain-mind unity.

References

Allison, R. S. (1962). *The senile brain*. Arnold, London.

Babcock, H. (1930). An experiment in the measurement of mental deterioration. *Arch. Psych.* **117**, 5.

Critchley, M. (1972). Communication: recognition of its minimal impairment. In *Scientific foundations of neurology* (ed. M. Critchley, J. L. O'Leary, and W. B. Jennett) p. 221. Heinemann, London.

Geschwind, N. (1974). *Selected papers on language and the brain*. Reidel, Dordrecht, Holland.

Gubbay, S. S. (1975). *Clumsy children*. Saunders, London.

Heilman, K. M. and Valenstein, E. (1979). *Clinical neuropsychology*. Oxford University Press, New York.

Humphrey, M. E. (1972). Intelligence. In *Scientific foundations of neurology* (ed. M. Critchley, J. L. O'Learly, and W. B. Jennett) p. 221. Heinemann, London.

Klein, R. and Mayer-Gross, W. (1957). *The clinical examination of patients with organic cerebral disease*. Cassell, London.

Lehman, R. A. W., Chelune, G. J., and Heaton, R. K. (1979). Level and variability of performance on neuropsychological tests. *J. clin. Psychol.* **35**, 358.

Newcombe, F. (1972). Memory. In *Scientific foundations of neurology* (ed. M. Critchley, J. L. O'Leary, and W. B. Jennett) p. 205. Heinemann, London.

Oldfield, R. C. (1972). Intelligence. In *Scientific foundations of neurology* (ed. M. Critchley, J. L. O'Leary, and W. B. Jennett) p. 201. Heinemann, London.

Patterson, A. (1942). Emotional and cognitive changes in the post-traumatic confusional state. *Lancet*, **ii**, 717.

Piercy, M. (1964). The effects of cerebral lesions on intellectual function: a review of current research trends. *Br. J. Psychiat.* **110**, 310.

Rapaport, D. (1945). *Diagnostic psychological testing*. Year Book, Chicago.

Reitan, R. M. and Davison, L. A. (Eds.) (1974). *Clinical neuropsychology: current status and applications*. Winston, Wiley, Washington, DC.

Reynell, W. R. (1944). A psychometric method of determining intellectual loss following head injury. *J. ment. Sci.* **90**, 710.

Rosenfield, D. B. and Kinsbourne, M. (1981). Neurologic aspects of behaviour. In *Current neurology* (ed. S. Appel), Chapter 17. Wiley, New York.

Strub, R. L. and Black, F. W. (1981). *Organic brain syndromes: an introduction to neurobehavioral disorders*. Davis, Philadelphia.

Trist, E. L. and Trist, V. (1942–3). Discussion on the quality of mental test performance in intellectual deterioration. *Proc. R. Soc. Med.* **36**, 243.

Wallesch, C. W., Kornhuber, H. H., Kunz, T., and Brunner, R. J. (1983). Neuropsychological deficits associated with small unilateral thalamic lesions. *Brain* **106**, 141.

Wechsler, D. (1941). *Measurement of adult intelligence*. Williams and Wilkins, Baltimore.

Zangwill, O. L. (1942–3). Clinical tests of memory impairment. *Proc. R. Soc. Med.* **36**, 576.

—— (1945). A review of psychological work at the brain injuries unit. Edinburgh, 1941–5. *Br. med. J.* **2**, 248.

Dementia

Dementia is a term applied to a diffuse deterioration in mental functions, resulting from organic disease of the brain and manifesting itself primarily in disorders of thought and memory and secondarily of feeling and conduct. It may be produced by many pathological processes and the clinical picture varies somewhat according to the previous temperament of the patient, the age of onset, and to the localization, rate of progress, and nature of the causal pathological change.

Symptoms

Judgement and reasoning

The earliest disability is often an impairment of judgment and reasoning manifesting itself in a failure to grasp the meaning of a situation as a whole and hence to react to it appropriately. At this stage, for example, the patient's business, academic, or social judgement begins to fail, though in the semi-automatic activities of life no defect may be immediately apparent.

Memory

Memory becomes impaired, the recollection of recent events (short-term memory) suffering more than remote (see p. 653). Even when both are grossly defective, mechanical memory (immediate recall) may be preserved for a time. In more severe dementia, defective memory linked with defective perception leads to disorientation in space and time.

The emotional life

Although in some patients emotional life is little disturbed, in others impairment of higher control leads to emotional instability causing irritability and impulsive conduct. Acts of violence, alcoholic excess, and sexual aberrations are thus explained. The prevailing mood may be one of euphoria, with hilariousness and hyperactivity, or of depression, anxiety, or maniacal excitement, but is, to some extent, influenced by the pre-existing psychological constitution. In the late stages the patient is apathetic.

Delusions

Delusions are comparatively uncommon, but can occur, for instance, in the fatuous euphoric state which sometimes results from general paresis and occasionally from other conditions; when they do occur they are usually associated with impaired judgement and defective appreciation of reality. Delusions centred on the self are likely to be grandiose in a state of euphoria and self-condemnatory or hypochondriacal in a state of depression. Delusions regarding others are often hostile and express fear, suspicion, or jealousy.

Care of the person

In the later stages of dementia the patient becomes careless in dress and in personal cleanliness, and finally incontinent. This can be attributed at first to a progressive decay in self-regard and later also to lack of perception and insight and frontal-lobe damage.

Speech

In the later stages also, speech sometimes undergoes progressive disintegration. Though each of the forms of aphasia caused by focal lesions of the brain can develop in dementia, there may also be destruction of speech function as a whole, so that it becomes increasingly meaningless and ends in jargon or isolated words or phrases, 'logoclonia'. Agnosia and apraxia may also be seen.

Physical concomitants

The presence or absence of physical signs depends upon the nature of the causal disorder and the distribution of the pathological changes, but, whatever the cause, there is usually a general physical deterioration with loss of weight, and depression of endocrine function. Whatever the cause also, extensor plantar responses are common in the later stages.

Aetiology

The more important causes of dementia, many of which have already been considered in detail in earlier chapters, are:

1. Syphilis—general paresis, cerebral meningovascular syphilis, etc.

2. Cerebral arteriosclerosis and other vascular disorders (multi-infarct dementia), including Binswanger's disease.

3. The presenile and senile dementias—a mixed group of degenerative diseases of unknown origin—Pick's disease, Alzheimer's disease, Huntington's chorea, and other degenerative diseases, including progressive multisystem degeneration (the Shy–Drager syndrome).

4. Intracranial tumour, carcinomatous meningitis, reticulosis and dementia in paraneoplastic neurological syndromes (non-metastatic) complications of malignant disease.

5. Communicating 'low-pressure' or obstructive hydrocephalus.

6. Non-syphilitic inflammatory diseases—encephalitis (various forms), intracranial abscess, meningitis, sarcoidosis, granulomatous angiitis, and other collagen diseases, crytococcosis and slow virus infections including Creutzfeldt–Jakob disease, and progressive multifocal leukoencephalopathy.

7. Intoxications and deficiency diseases—alcoholism, drug addiction, chronic exposure to heavy metals and numerous drugs or toxins, carbon monoxide poisoning, uraemia, vitamin B_{12} neuropathy, pellagra, Wernicke's encephalopathy, myxoedema, liver failure, dialysis dementia.

8. Dementia supervening in chronic psychotic states.

9. Miscellaneous demyelinating and metabolic disorders, including multiple sclerosis, the diffuse cerebral scleroses and leukodystrophies, the lipidoses, and other storage diseases, many of which may cause dementia in childhood.

10. Severe head injury.

11. Severe and diffuse brain damage due to anoxia (as in some cases of intractable epilepsy), hypoglycaemia, or heat stroke.

12. Dementia in tuberous sclerosis and neurofibromatosis (the phacomatoses) and in the hereditary ataxias (some forms).

Since in most of these disorders the dementia is an inconstant or even a rare manifestation, accounts must be sought in the appropriate sections of this book. The presenile and senile dementias, however, which, with the exception of Huntington's chorea, normally present with disorders of memory, intellect, and personality, are most conveniently considered at this point, and also provide an opportunity of considering the differential diagnosis of dementia.

The presenile and senile dementias

Alzheimer's disease

Alzheimer's disease is a progressive cerebral degeneration, in many ways comparable to accelerated cerebral ageing, occurring in middle or late life. It is probably the commonest cause of progressive dementia in the middle-aged and elderly population; of about 1.3 million demented patients in the United States, some 50–60 per cent suffer from Alzheimer's disease (Terry and Katzman 1983). Although a familial incidence is relatively uncommon and the condition has been reported in one monozygotic twin (Hunter, Dayan, and Wilson 1972), there is increasing evidence of a significant genetic factor and in one series secondary cases of dementia were found in 25 per cent of families (Heyman, Wilkinson, Hurwitz, Schmechel, Sigmon, Weinberg, Helms, and Swift 1983). There is also clear evidence that Alzheimer's disease commonly supervenes in adult cases of Down's syndrome, but parental age at birth does not appear otherwise to be a significant risk factor (Corkin, Growdon, and Rasmussen 1983).

In the past it was customary to distinguish between presenile dementia (occurring in those under 65 years of age) and senile dementia developing in the over-65s, but this distinction is now generally accepted as being artificial (Mayeux and Rosen 1983). Nevertheless, there is evidence that Alzheimer's disease developing insidiously in old age (AD-1) may differ from the more rapidly progressive variety (AD-2) which runs a more rapid course and begins in middle age (Bondareff, 1983). Pathologically, in both varieties the principal pathological changes are, first, a profusion of senile plaques (see p. 9) throughout the cerebral cortex, especially, but by no means exclusively in the frontal lobes, and generally sparing the basal ganglia and cerebellum, associated with intraneuronal fibrillary tangles. These tangles are most numerous in various basal nuclei and the thalamus, less widespread in the lenticular nuclei and pons. Granulovacuolar degeneration in the nerve cells of the hippocampal pyramidal layer is even more specific (Woodard 1962) but amyloid accumulation is probably less so (Somerville 1985). The olfactory bulbs are also affected (Esiri and Wilcock 1984). Severe cell loss has also been found in the nucleus basalis and nucleus locus coeruleus (the origin of the adrenergic projection to the cerebral cortex) (Bondareff, Mountjoy, and Roth 1982; Tagliavini and Pilleri 1983; Mann, Yates, and Marcyniuk 1984) and all of these changes, along with cerebral cortical atrophy, ventricular enlargement, and clinical signs of parietal-lobe involvement have been found to be much more striking in AD-2 (Bondareff 1983).

Similar changes are seen in many other degenerative brain diseases but in a different distribution. Thus in progressive supranuclear palsy, neurofibrillary tangles, by contrast, are found especially in the subthalamic nuclei, globus pallidus, midbrain reticular formation, and pontine nuclei (Ishino and Otsuki 1975). Ultrastructural studies have shown that senile plaques are composed of degenerating neuronal terminals with 'twisted tubules', amyloid, and reactive cells (microglia, macrophages, and astrocytes) and three varieties of plaque have been characterized (Wisniewski and Terry 1973). Neurochemical studies have shown that the plaques consistently contain certain combinations of amino acids and that their cones also contain phosphorus and sulphur (Nikaido, Austin, Rinehart, Truebb, Hutchinson, Stukenbrok, and Miles 1971), while neurofibrillary tangles appear to show an increased content of silicon (Nikaido, Austin, and Rinehart 1972) and silicon may be increased in the CSF (Hershey, Hershey, Varnes, Vibhakar, Lavin, and Strain 1983). Neurofibrillary tangles are of neurofilament origin (see Bowen and Davison 1984). Immunocytochemical studies of neuronal perikarya have shown that the tangles and antigenic neurofilament triplet protein probably contain related antigenic determinants (Elovaara, Paetau, Lehto, Dahl, Virtanen, and Palo 1983). Tomlinson, Blessed, and Roth (1968) showed that all of the changes described, with the possible exception of granulo-vacuolar degeneration, can be found in the brains of non-demented elderly people, but there is a quantitative relationship between the severity of dementia and the severity and ubiquity of the pathological changes described (Roth, Tomlinson, and Blessed 1966; Tomlinson, Blessed, and Roth 1970).

Biochemical research in the last few years has moved apace. Crapper, Krishnan, and Quittkat (1976) found an increased concentration of aluminium in the brains of affected patients but this has not been confirmed by others and it is now uncertain whether trace-element intoxication plays a significant role. However, a major advance was the discovery that acetylcholine (ACh) and choline acetyltransferase (CAT) activity are markedly reduced in the cerebral cortex (Bowen, Smith, White, Davison 1976; Davies and Maloney 1976; Perry, Perry, Blessed, and Tomlinson 1978). Subsequently, extensive research has amply confirmed this finding and studies of many other neuropeptides have also shown reduced somatostatin in the cortex; variations are also beginning to emerge in respect of the biochemical changes found in different cortical areas and basal nuclei (Besson 1983; Deakin 1983). While it is reasonable to regard the disease as being a 'disorder of cortical cholinergic innervation' (Coyle, Prince, and DeLong 1983), there is no evidence to show whether the condition is due to an 'abiotrophy' in the traditional sense, to a slow virus infection, or to disordered auto-immunity. The possibility of intoxication with trace elements such as aluminium which increase the permeability of the blood–brain barrier also continues to be raised (Banks and Kastin 1983). The significance of a reduced CSF vasopressin concentration (Sørensen, Hammer, Vorstrup, and Gjerris 1983) is also unclear.

Alzheimer's disease can develop at any time after the age of 40, very rarely before. The symptoms are generally those of a progressive dementia, often with apraxia and speech disturbances. The onset is insidious but, as mentioned above, more rapid in AD-2.

In the early stages the patient suffers from loss of memory, becomes careless in dress and conduct and more and more neglectful of work and family responsibility. Epileptic seizures may occur but are uncommon. Speech becomes slurred, and there is difficulty in recalling words. A variant entitled hereditary dysphasic dementia has been defined (Morris, Cole, Banker, and Wright 1984). As the disease progresses there is complete disorientation. The patient recognizes none of his friends, becomes restless, and may wander about. A progressive deterioration takes place in the faculty of speech, which, from paraphasic talkativeness, becomes reduced to isolated words and phrases. Movements become stereotyped and the snout, sucking, or rooting or even grasp reflexes are often elicitable in the late stages. Spastic paralysis of the limbs and even contracture occasionally develop. The duration of the disease is from one and a half to 15 years.

Following the discovery that 'low-pressure hydrocephalus' (p. 140) can give rise to dementia and that the condition may be relieved by venticulo-atrial shunting, there were reports suggesting that this operation might be beneficial in Alzheimer's disease (Appenzeller and Salmon 1967) and that CSF hydrodynamics might be abnormal (Sohn, Siegel, Gado, and Torack 1973). However, in a comprehensive study Coblentz, Mattis, Zingesser, Kasoff, Wisniewski, and Katzman (1973) concluded that the abnormalities of CSF dynamics reported were due to misleading radiological findings and that shunting was of no benefit. More recently, in the light of the finding of diminished cortical CT activitty, numerous cholinergic agents and ACh precursors, including choline, lecithin, and physostigmine, have been tried, but any benefit has been either transient or insignificant (Jotkowitz 1983; Castleden 1984); however, co-dergocrine mesylate, which acts in a regulatory manner at both dopaminergic and serotoninergic sites and decreases the cyclic AMP response to noradrenaline (see Castleden 1984) seems to confer consistent modest benefit but is still under trial. The management of dementia at home and/or in hospital also presents major nursing and social problems (see Mayeux and Rosen 1983).

Pick's disease

Synonym. Circumscribed cortical or lobar atrophy.

This condition, which is much less common than Alzheimer's disease, is characterized by circumscribed atrophy of the cerebral cortex, usually confined to the frontal and temporal regions. The upper three cortical layers are principally affected, exhibiting chromatolysis and disappearance of ganglion cells. There is some glial increase in the atrophic areas. On light microscopy, cortical neurones show typical amphophilic and argentophilic Pick bodies with ballooning and central chromatolysis; senile plaques are relatively infrequent and neurofibrillary tangles are absent. The senile plaques are typical save for the fact that the twisted tubules seen in Alzheimer's disease are absent (Wisniewski, Coblentz, and Terry 1972). The Pick bodies are made up of filaments, ribosomes, vesicles, and lipochrome and occasional tubules; there is thus a clear difference between the histological changes observed in Alzheimer's disease and Pick's disease, in that in the former lesions of the so-called twisted tubule type predominate, while the latter shows predominantly neurofilamentary changes (Brion, Mikol, and Psimaras 1973). Exceptionally, the changes of both Pick's and Alzheimer's disease may be found in a single individual (Smith and Lantos 1983). As in Alzheimer's disease, neurones in the nucleus basalis of Meynert may be reduced (Uhl, Hilt, Hedreen, Whitehouse, and Price 1983), but neither CAT nor somatostatin are reduced in the cortex, in contrast to Alzheimer's disease (Wood, Etienne, Lal, Nair, Finlayson, Gauthier, Palo, Haltia, Paetau, and Bird 1983). A suggestion that zinc is elevated in the cortex has not been confirmed (Ehmann, Alauddin, Hossain, and Markesbery 1984).

The cause of the disease is unknown. It appears to be a form of primary degeneration developing in middle life. Multiple cases have often been described in one sibship. The age of onset is usually between 50 and 60, and the disease has a duration of from three to 12 years, always terminating fatally. Females are said to be affected more often than males. It is characterized by a progressive dementia and often aphasia. Restlessness and loss of normal inhibitions are prominent in the early stages. The patient is often voluble and tends to make jokes and puns. At first the more abstract intellectual functions suffer, but the more concrete type of behaviour is well preserved and the patient is emotionally accessible. Later, apathy becomes pronounced and epileptic attacks may occur. Speech is reduced to a few stereotyped phrases. In the terminal stages there is much loss of weight, and the patient becomes bed-ridden, and tends to develop contractures. The condition is uninfluenced by treatment.

The diagnosis of the cause of dementia

The cause of dementia is sometimes obvious, as when the condition follows head injury, acute encephalitis, severe anoxia, or chronic alcoholism. Luetic dementia, whether due to general paresis or meningovascular syphilis, is associated with characteristic serological reactions and usually with abnormal neurological signs. In cases of intracranial tumour the history is usually short, and the course of the dementia steadily progressive. The diagnosis is easy if symptoms and signs of increased intracranial pressure are present. In their absence full investigation, especially with computerized transaxial tomography (Roberts and Caird 1976; de Leon and George 1983) and/or other specialized neuroradiological studies will be necessary. Electroencephalography often shows marked slowing of the dominant rhythms in the presenile and senile dementias but rarely gives specific or diagnostic findings except in Creutzfeldt–Jakob disease or subacute sclerosing panencephalitis. Air encephalography can be diagnostic (if CT scanning is equivocal) in cases of low-pressure or communicating hydrocephalus which may present with fluctuating confusion, dementia, and ataxia. Air outlines the dilated ventricles but none passes over the cortex and clinical deterioration often follows the procedure. Isotope encephalography may confirm the diagnosis but false positive results are not uncommon and the findings must be interpreted with care (Coblentz *et al.* 1973). Very exceptionally, brain biopsy may be justified to confirm the exact nature of the pathological change; the indications for this procedure were reviewed by Pearce and Miller (1973). Arteriosclerotic (multi-infarct) dementia is usually encountered after the age of 60. The onset is usually insidious, and there is almost always a history of focal lesions due to minor 'strokes'. Evidence of arteriosclerosis is usually found as a rule in the retinal and peripheral circulation, with or without high blood pressure. In fact, atherosclerotic dementia is uncommon, even in old age, and cerebral softening must be severe and widespread (and is usually easily identified by CT scanning) if it is to cause multi-infarct dementia (Tomlinson *et al.* 1968; Hachinski, Lassen, and Marshall 1974; Brust 1983). Psychometric testing with the Wechsler Adult Intelligence Scale (W.A.I.S.) has been shown to give a consistently poorer performance on tests of cognitive and intellectual ability in patients with Alzheimer's disease than in those with multi-infarct dementia (Perez, Rivera, Meyer, Gay, Taylor, and Mathew 1975). Indeed, detailed psychometric testing is invariably indicated in cases of suspected dementia. Measurement of regional cerebral blood flow and PET scanning may also be helpful (Simard, Olesen, Paulson, Lassen, and Skinhøj 1971; Ferris, de Leon, Wolf, George, Reisberg, Christman, Yonekura, and Fowler 1983) as these usually give relatively normal findings in Alzheimer's disease but are much more abnormal in patients with cerebrovascular disease.

Differentiation of the primary presenile and senile dementias may be much more difficult. These usually begin between 45 and 60. Other common causes of dementia can readily be excluded. CT scanning (or pneumoencephalography, now much less often performed) usually demonstrates some general dilatation of the cerebral ventricles and/or cortical atrophy, especially over the anterior part of the hemispheres in Pick's disease, but more diffuse in Alzheimer's disease. Guidelines relating to the clinical diagnosis of Alzheimer's disease have been published by McKhann, Drachman, Folsten, Katzman, Price, Stadlan (1984). Early psychomotor restlessness and jocularity and a family history of presenile dementia would favour Pick's disease as against Alzheimer's disease. In Huntington's chorea the involuntary movements are usually diagnostic but occasionally dementia antedates the chorea; then the family history, if known, is all-important. Clinical features of parkinsonism may raise the possibility of progressive multi-system degeneration (p. 599) or, in an appropriate setting, the parkinsonism–dementia complex (p. 331), and many other degenerative diseases of the nervous system, including, for example, some hereditary ataxias and progressive myoclonic epilepsy are often associated with dementia. Presenile dementia and motor neurone disease often coexist in Japan (Mitsuyama 1984)

The possibility of a metabolic or endocrine cause for dementia must always be borne in mind. In vitamin B_{12} deficiency, dementia may antedate symptoms and signs of anaemia and spinal-cord involvement and estimation of the serum B_{12} or a Schilling test may be necessary for diagnosis. The cause of 'dialysis dementia', due to chronic intoxication by aluminium in the water supply (Mahurkar, Salta, Smith, Dhar, Meyers, and Dunea 1973; Lederman and Henry 1978; Parkinson, Feest, Ward, Fawcett, and Kerr 1979; European Dialysis and Transplant Association 1980) is self-evident. It reduces GABA in both brain and CSF (Sweeney, Perry, Price, Reeve, Godolphin, and Kish 1985). The condition is becoming much less common since deionized water has been used, but desferrioxamine may be helpful in treating established cases (Milen Sharf, Bell, and Meyers 1982). Myxoedema will usually be apparent clinically, if considered. The fluctuating confusion of subdural haematoma is sometimes mistaken for dementia, but there is often associated drowsiness and headache and CT scanning or angiography are diagnostic.

It must also be remembered that retardation in severe endogenous depression may be misconstrued as being due to dementia, while some patients with receptive aphasia due to focal cerebral lesions are wrongly regarded as suffering from dementia in view of their failure to communicate; a similar error is not uncommon in patients with delirium and/or toxic confusional states, or with specific disturbances of memory such as Korsakow's syndrome or transient global amnesia (Pearce and Miller 1973). Impairment of memory without change in personality or intellectual function, like psychomotor retardation alone, gives insufficient grounds for the diagnosis of dementia. Hysteria in young patients and hysterical 'pseudodementia' in adults, sometimes arising as a result of desire for financial compensation after minor head injury, can also give difficulty. Marsden and Harrison (1972) found that of 106 patients admitted to hospital with a presumptive diagnosis of dementia, 15 had some other condition, usually depressive illness, and 15 a disorder which was amenable to treatment. Among the 84 patients shown to have impairment of intellect and/or learning capacity and memory, several proved to have intracranial mass lesions, diffuse arterial disease, or alcoholism as the presumptive cause.

References

Allison, R. S. (1962). *The senile brain*. Arnold, London.

Appenzeller, O. and Salmon, J. H. (1967). Treatment of parenchymatous degeneration of the brain by ventriculoatrial shunting of the cerebrospinal fluid. *J. Neurosurg.* **26**, 478.

Banks, W. A. and Kastin, A. J. (1983). Aluminium increases permeability of the blood–brain barrier to labelled DSIP and β-endorphin: possible implications for senile and dialysis dementia. *Lancet* **ii**, 1227.

Besson, J. (1983). Dementia: biological solution still a long way off. *Br. med. J.* **287**, 926.

Bondareff, W. (1983). Age and Alzheimer disease. *Lancet* **i**, 1447.

——, Mountjoy, C. Q., and Roth, M. (1982). Loss of neurons of origin of the adrenergic projection to cerebral cortex (nucleus locus ceruleus) in senile dementia. *Neurology, Minneapolis* **32**, 164.

Bowen, D. M. and Davison, A. N. (1984). Dementia in the elderly: biochemical aspects. *J. R. Coll. Physcns.* **18**, 25.

——, Smith, C. B., White, P., and Davison, A. N. (1976). Neurotransmitter-related enzymes and indices of hypoxia in senile dementia and other abiotrophies. *Brain* **99**, 459.

Brion, S., Mikol, J., and Psimaras, A. (1973). Recent findings in Pick's disease. In *Progress in neuropathology*, Vol. II (ed. H. M. Zimmerman) p. 421. Grune and Stratton, New York.

Brust, J. C. M. (1983). Dementia and cerebrovascular disease. In *The dementias* (ed. R. Mayeux and W. G. Rosen), p. 131. Raven Press, New York.

Castleden, C. M. (1984). Therapeutic possibilities in patients with senile dementia. *J. R. Coll. Physcns.* **18**, 28.

Coblentz, J. M., Mattis, S., Zingesser, L. H., Kasoff, S. S., Wisniewski,

H. M., and Katzman, R. (1973). Presenile dementia. Clinical aspects and evaluation of cerebrospinal fluid dynamics. *Arch. Neurol., Chicago* **29**, 299.

Constantinidis, J. (1971). Demence presenile d'Alzheimer et demence senile alzheimerisée. Étude statistique des correlations anatomocliniques. In *Psychiatry*, International Congress Series No. 274, p. 84. Excerpta Medica, Amsterdam.

Corkin, S., Growdon, J. H., and Rasmussen, S. L. (1983). Parental age as a risk factor in Alzheimer's disease. *Ann. Neurol.* **13**, 674.

Coyle, J. T., Prince, D. L., and DeLong, M. R. (1983). Alzheimer's disease: a disorder of cortical cholinergic innervation. *Science* **219**, 1184.

Crapper, D. R., Krishnan, S. S., and Quittkat, S. (1976). Aluminium, neurofibrillary degenration and Alzheimer's disease. *Brain* **99**, 67.

Davies, P. and Maloney, A. F. J. (1976). Selective loss of central cholinergic neurons in Alzheimer's disease. *Lancet* **ii**, 1403.

Deakin, J. F. W. (1983). Alzheimer's disease: recent advances and future prospects. *Br. med. J.* **287**, 1323.

de Leon, M. J. and George, A. E. (1983). Computed tomography in aging and senile dementia of the Alzheimer type. In *The dementias* (ed. R. Mayeux and W. G. Rosen), p. 103. Raven Press, New York.

Ehmann, W. D., Alauddin, M., Hossain, T. I. M., and Markesbery, W. R. (1984). Brain trace elements in Pick's disease. *Ann. Neurol.* **15**, 102.

Elovaara, I., Paetau, A., Lehto, V.-P., Dahl, D., Virtanen, I., and Palo, J. (1983). Immunocytochemical studies of Alzheimer neuronal perikarya with intermediate filament antisera. *J. neurol. Sci.* **62**, 315.

Esiri, M. M. and Wilcock, G. K. (1984). The olfactory bulbs in Alzheimer's disease. *J. Neurol. Neurosurg. Psychiat.* **47**, 56.

European Dialysis and Transplant Association (1980). Dialysis dementia in Europe. *Lancet* **ii**, 190.

Ferris, S. H., de Leon, M. J., Wolf, A. P., George, A. E., Reisberg, B., Christman, D. R., Yonekura, Y., and Fowler, J. S. (1983). Positron emission tomography in dementia. In *The dementias* (ed. R. Mayeux and W. G. Rosen) p. 123. Raven Press, New York.

Hachinski, V. C., Lassen, N. A., and Marshall, J. (1974). Multi-infarct dementia. A cause of mental deterioration in the elderly. *Lancet* **ii**, 207.

Hershey, C. O., Hershey, L. A., Varnes, A., Vibhakar, S. D., Lavin, P., and Strain, W. H. (1983). Cerebrospinal fluid trace element content in dementia: clinical, radiologic, and pathologic correlations. *Neurology, Minneapolis* **33**, 1350.

Heyman, A., Wilkinson, W. E., Hurwitz, B. J., Schmechel, D., Sigmon, A. H., Weinberg, T., Helms, M. J., and Swift, M. (1983). Alzheimer's disease: genetic aspects and associated clinical disorders. *Ann. Neurol.* **14**, 507.

Hunter, R., Dayan, A. D., and Wilson, J. (1972). Alzheimer's disease in one monozygotic twin. *J. Neurol. Neurosurg. Psychiat.* **35**, 707.

Ishino. H. and Otsuki, S. (1975). Distribution of Alzheimer's neurofibrillary tangles in the basal ganglia and brainstem of progressive supranuclear palsy and Alzheimer's disease. *Folia Psychiat. Neurol. Japonica* **29**, 179.

Jotkowitz, S. (1983). Lack of clinical efficacy of chronic oral physostigmine in Alzheimer's disease. *Ann. Neurol.* **14**, 690.

Larsson, T., Sjögren, T., and Jacobson, G. (1963). Senile dementia. *Acta psychiat., Kbh.* **39**, Suppl. 167.

Lederman, R. J. and Henry, C. E. (1978). Progressive dialysis encephalopathy. *Ann. Neurol.* **4**, 199.

Mahurkar, S. D., Salta, R., Smith, E. C., Dhar, S. K., Meyers, L. Jr, and Dunea, G. (1973). Dialysis dementia. *Lancet* **i**, 1412.

Mann, D. M. A., Yates, P. O., and Marcyniuk, B. (1984). A comparison of changes in the nucleus basalis and locus caeruleus in Alzheimer's disease. *J. Neurol. Neurosurg. Psychiat.* **47**, 201.

Marsden, C. D. and Harrison, M. J. G. (1972). Outcome of investigation of patients with presenile dementia. *Br. med. J.* **2**, 249.

Mayeux, R. and Rosen, W. G. (Eds.) (1983). *The dementias*. Raven Press, New York.

McKhann, G., Drachman, D., Folstein, M., Katzman, R., Price, D., and Stadlan, E. M. (1984). Clinical diagnosis of Alzheimer's disease. *Neurology, Minneapolis* **34**, 939.

McMenemey, W. H. (1958). In *Neuropathology* (ed. J. G. Greenfield, W. Blackwood, W. H. McMenemey, A. Meyer, and R. M. Norman) p. 475. Arnold, London.

Milne, F. J., Sharf, B., Bell, P. D., and Meyers, A. M. (1982). Low aluminium water, desferrioxamine, and dialysis encephalopathy. *Lancet* **ii**, 502.

Mitsuyama, Y. (1984). Presenile dementia with motor neurone disease in Japan: clinico-pathological review of 26 cases. *J. Neurol. Neurosurg. Psychiat.* **47**, 953.

Morris, J. C., Cole, M., Banker, B. Q., and Wright, D. (1984). Heredi-

tary dysphasic dementia and the Pick-Alzheimer spectrum. *Ann. neurol.* **16**, 455.

Nikaido, T., Austin, J., Rinehart, R., Truebb, L., Hutchinson, J., Stukenbrok, H., and Miles, B. (1971). Studies in ageing of the brain. I. Isolation and preliminary characterization of Alzheimer plaques and cores. *Arch. Neurol., Chicago* **25**, 198.

——, ——, and —— (1972). Studies in ageing of the brain. II. Microchemical analyses of the nervous system in Alzheimer patients. *Arch. Neurol., Chicago* **27**, 549.

Parkinson, I. S., Feest, T. G., Ward, M. K., Fawcett, P. R. W., and Kerr, D. N. S. (1979). Fracturing dialysis osteodystrophy and dialysis encephalopathy: an epidemiological survey. *Lancet* **i**, 406.

Pearce, J. and Miller, E. (1973). *Clinical aspects of dementia*. Baillière-Tindall, London.

Perez, F. I., Rivera, V. M., Meyer, J. S., Gay, J. R. A., Taylor, R. L., and Mathew, N. T. (1975). Analysis of intellectual and cognitive performance in patients with multi-infarct dementia, vertebrobasilar insufficiency with dementia, and Alzheimer's disease. *J. Neurol. Neurosurg. Psychiat.* **38**, 533.

Perry, E. K., Perry, R. H., Blessed, G., and Tomlinson, B. E. (1978). Changes in brain cholinesterases in senile dementia of Alzheimer's type. *Neuropathol. appl. Neurobiol.* **4**, 273.

Roberts, M. A. and Caird, F. I. (1976). Computerised tomography and intellectual impairment in the elderly. *J. Neurol. Neurosurg. Psychiat.* **39**, 986.

Roth, M., Tomlinson, B. E., and Blessed, G. (1966). Correlation between scores for dementia and counts of 'senile plaques' in cerebral grey matter of elderly subjects. *Nature, London* **209**, 109.

Simard, D., Olesen, J., Paulson, O. B., Lassen, N. A., and Skinhøj, E. (1971). Regional cerebral blood flow and its regulation in dementia. *Brain* **94**, 273.

Sjögren, T., Sjögren, H., and Lindgren, A. G. H. (1952). Morbus Alzheimer and Morbus Pick. *Acta psychiat. scand.* Suppl. 82.

Smith, D. A. and Lantos, P. L. (1983). A case of combined Pick's disease and Alzheimer's disease. *J. Neurol. Neurosurg. Psychiat.* **46**, 675.

Sohn, R. S., Siegel, B. A., Gado, M., and Torack, R. M. (1973). Alzheimer's disease with abnormal cerebrospinal fluid flow. *Neurology, Minneapolis* **23**, 1058.

Sørensen, P.S., Hammer, M., Vorstrup, S., and Gjerris, F. (1983). CSF and plasma vasopressin concentrations in dementia. *J. Neurol. Neurosurg. Psychiat.* **46**, 911.

Somerville, R. A. (1985). Ultrastructural links between scrapie and Alzheimer's disease. *Lancet* **i**, 504.

Sweeney, V. P., Perry, T. L., Price, J. D. E., Reeve, C. E., Godolphin, W. J. and Kish, S. J. (1985). Brain γ-aminobutyric acid deficiency in dialysis encephalopathy. *Neurology, Cleveland* **35**, 180.

Tagliavini, F. and Pilleri, G. (1983). Basal nucleus of Meynert. A neuropathological study in Alzheimer's disease, simple senile dementia, Pick's disease and Huntington's chorea. *J. neurol. Sci.* **62**, 243.

Terry, R. D. and Katzman, R. (1983). Senile dementia of the Alzheimer type. *Ann. Neurol.* **14**, 497.

Tomlinson, B. E., Blessed, G., and Roth, M. (1968). Observations on the brains of non-demented old people. *J. neurol. Sci.* **7**, 331.

——, ——, and —— (1970). Observations on the brains of demented old people. *J. neurol. Sci.* **11**, 205.

Uhl, G. R., Hilt, D. C., Hedreen, J. C., Whitehouse, P. J., and Price, D. L. (1983). Pick's disease (lobar sclerosis): depletion of neurons in the nucleus basalis of Meynert. *Neurology, Minneapolis* **33**, 1470.

Wisniewski, H. M., Coblentz, J. M., and Terry, R. D. (1972). Pick's disease. A clinical and ultrastructural study. *Arch. Neurol., Chicago* **26**, 97.

—— and Terry, R. D. (1973). Re-examination of the pathogenesis of the senile plaque. In *Progress in neuropathology*, Vol. II (ed. H. M. Zimmerman) p. 1. Grune and Stratton, New York.

Wood, P. L., Etienne, P., Lal, S., Nair, N. P. V., Finlayson, M. H., Gauthier, S., Palo, J., Haltia, M., Paetau, A., and Bird, E. D. (1983). A post-mortem comparison of the cortical cholinergic system in Alzheimer's disease and Pick's disease. *J. neurol. Sci.* **62**, 211.

Woodard, J. S. (1962). Clinico-pathological significance of granulo-vacuolar degeneration in Alzheimer's disease. *J. Neuropath. exp. Neurol.* **21**, 85.

Hysteria

Definition. A disorder characterized by dissociation of the personality due to subconscious motivation, sometimes causing amnesia, but more often somatic symptoms such as 'fits', paralysis, and sensory disturbances in the absence of organic disease of the nervous system.

Aetiology

In hysteria the type of abnormal reaction exhibited by the patient is determined by the striking tendency of the hysterical personality to dissociation. In response to emotional stress (as described later), certain psychophysiological features become separated from the conscious life. In general, all hysterical syndromes can be regarded as representing the subconscious results of an attempt to escape from a stressful situation. In the most severe cases the dissociation is so striking that the patient seems at different times almost to be under the control of different personalities, which exhibit differences in temperament and which may or may not have access to each other's memories. A similar profound mental dissociation is responsible for the state known as hysterical fugue, in which the patient disappears from home and wanders in a random manner, having lost his sense of identity. During the period of fugue he has no access to the memories of his normal personality, and on recovery may have no recollection of the events of his fugue. Such profound degrees of dissociation are, however, uncommon, and usually the dissociation occurs in a sense at the physiological level, part of the body being functionally cut off in a way from conscious volition, so that the patient is unable to move it or to feel with it, hysterical paralysis or anaesthesia resulting.

The nature of hysterical dissociation is little understood. The poverty of the affective reactions of many such individuals is well known—*la belle indifférence* of Janet—and Golla showed that in spite of the severity of their somatic reactions the psycho-galvanic response to noxious stimuli is greatly depressed in hysterical patients. However, many psychiatrists now believe that *la belle indifférence* is an unreliable diagnostic sign and that hysterical patients frequently show evidence of overt anxiety (Merskey 1982; Roy 1982). The underlying abnormality which finds expression in hysteria may well in many cases be inborn and certainly often develops at an early age. But certain organic nervous diseases seem to predispose to hysterical reactions, especially multiple sclerosis, and symptoms characteristic of hysteria sometimes occur in patients with a focal lesion of one temporal lobe, suggesting that hysterical dissociation may sometimes have an organic basis. Women suffer from hysteria more frequently than men.

It is also important to recognize that when hysterical manifestations first develop in adult life, unless there is some obvious motive (such as, for instance, escape from exceptional stress, or desire for material gain such as compensation after injury), they may be due either to an underlying organic disorder (such as early dementia) or to a masked affective disorder (such as endogenous depression). Slater (1965) drew attention to the frequency with which symptoms regarded by experienced clinicians as being due to hysteria often conceal evidence of underlying organic disease of the nervous system. He suggested that all too often this diagnosis is 'a disguise for ignorance and a fertile source of clinical error'. His warning that overt hysterical phenomena sometimes imply the presence of, as yet, unrecognized organic disease, was timely but Carter (1972) later argued cogently that hysteria, nevertheless, deserves continuing recognition as a disease entity in which patients respond to stress by converting their emotional problems into physical disabilities.

The mode of production of hysterical symptoms

The hysterical symptom is at one and the same time: (1) a product of suggestion; (2) the expression of an idea in the patient's mind; and (3) a means to achieve a purpose.

1. The precise nature of a hysterical symptom in a given case is usually, even perhaps always, determined by suggestion. The suggestion sometimes originates in an organic disorder from which the patient actually suffers. Thus laryngitis can lead to aphonia,

which is then perpetuated as a hysterical symptom. Accidents of all kinds (p. 228) are also apt to cause hysterical symptoms which perpetuate or exaggerate the disabilities caused by an injury. A doctor, nurse, or friend of the patient may unwittingly evoke such a symptom by seeming to imply that a disability is to be expected. There are also 'fashions' in hysterical symptoms which seem partly to be determined by the expectations of doctors interested in the subject at the time. Finally, the symptom may be an imitation of an organic disorder in a person whom the patient knows and with whom for some reason he identifies himself.

2. Suggestion operates through the patient's acceptance or belief on irrational grounds of the idea that he is suffering from a certain symptom or disease. Thus hysterical aphonia expresses the idea 'I have lost my voice', hysterical paralysis the idea 'I cannot move my limb', and so on. This is of great diagnostic importance, as it is unlikely, except in doctors and nurses, in whom diagnosis may present exceptional difficulties, that the patient's idea of a symptom will correspond with similar symptoms and signs produced by organic disease. The resulting discrepancies greatly facilitate diagnosis of one from the other.

3. The purposive character of hysterical symptoms is important in relation to treatment. Its purpose can usually be expressed as an unconscious solution, however unsatisfactory, of a mental conflict. The patient finds himself in a situation in which a course of action which he wishes to follow conflicts with his sense of duty or self-respect. The hysterical symptom unconsciously solves this conflict, though at the price of a neurotic disability. For example, a girl was compelled to give up her work to look after her invalid mother. She developed a hysterical paralysis of her right hand which prevented her from doing housework, and assistance had to be obtained to look after both her mother and herself. Her hysterical illness saved her from her unpleasant duty and also preserved her self-respect, since she felt that no one could blame her for being ill. At the same time she ceased to do any work at all, unconsciously revenged herself on her exacting parent, and became an object of sympathy to those with whom she came in contact. Hysteria may also fulfil other purposes than the solution of such a conflict, and a symptom may achieve more than one objective. The symptom frequently expresses a demand for sympathy, especially when the patient feels neglected or insufficiently appreciated. Tyrannical parents and unfaithful spouses excite such a demand directly, while invalid parents or other ailing relatives evoke it competitively. The hysterical symptom often, too, assumes symbolic significance, thus expressing the patient's feelings. One example is the adoption of a crucifixion attitude in a hysterical fit.

The patient suffering from hysteria is thus an individual who is often confronted with a mental conflict between two opposing wishes. While in this mental state, he (or she) conceives subconsciously a suggestion of continuing ill health precipitated either by an actual organic illness or by some outside source. He accepts this suggestion with relief and then manifests hysterical symptoms which provide a solution, even if a pathological and unsatisfactory one, to his difficulty, and may also express his emotional reaction in symbolic form.

Symptoms and signs

Amnesia and dissociation of the personality

Loss of memory and personality dissociation are among the most striking symptoms of hysteria, but in florid form are rare. The commonest example is the hysterical fugue, in which the patient disappears from home and wanders about, having lost his sense of identity. This state may last for hours, days, or even months, and on recovery the patient usually has no recollection of the events of this period. During the fugue he may be dazed and confused or more often apparently normal, living as a normal individual, carrying on an occupation but often with a mode of life different from his usual one. Hysterical amnesias and fugues are usually reactions to difficulties which render normal life intolerable. A wife has been known to react in this way to the infidelity of her husband and to adopt during her fugue the name of his mistress. A patient already in financial difficulties had a quantity of uninsured stock stolen from his car. He drove for miles in a state of fugue, subsequently returning home exhausted and without any recollection of the events of the day, including the theft. In such a case the fugue and the amnesia offered an escape from an unbearable situation which so dominated the patient's life that he could only escape from it by suppressing a large field of consciousness. Amnesia may also occur in association with hysterical fits, the events of the attack being subsequently forgotten. Patients suffering from hysterical fugue can justly be regarded as examples of dissociated personality, since they have alternating phases of awareness with mutually isolated memories. More complicated cases of 'multiple personality' have been described in which more than two sub-personalities alternated or coexisted, some having access to the memories of the others. It is occasionally possible to reproduce personality dissociations, by hypnotic suggestion, and the experiences of a period of hysterical amnesia can often be recalled under hypnosis.

Only a few cases of 'loss of memory' are hysterical in origin (p. 653). There are many other causes of mental confusion or impairment of memory such that the patient may wander and be unable to give an account of himself. And, in addition, hysterical amnesia may be feigned, as in certain notable criminal cases in which the accused claimed memory loss in a deliberate attempt to escape the consequences of his actions. Distinction between such conscious motivation and true subconscious motivation can be a matter of very great difficulty; indeed the dividing line, in some cases, is indistinct and impossible to define.

Pseudodementia

Hysterical pseudodementia, or the Ganser syndrome, is characterized by failure of memory and by acting out of the patient's idea of a psychosis, i.e. bizarre behaviour, excitement, or stupor.

Hysterical 'fits'

It is sometimes difficult to decide from the history whether attacks are hysterical or epileptic, but the question is usually resolved if the doctor is able to witness a fit. The attack is often a dramatic performance appropriately staged and hence does not occur when the patient is alone or at least out of reach of an audience. Often it is directly precipitated by emotional stress. The onset is usually gradual without the fulminating suddenness of an epileptic fit. Whereas the epileptic often falls precipitately to the ground and may injure himself, the hysteric subsides more often with some care, leaning, for example, against a wall or slipping slowly from a chair on to the ground. The tonic–clonic epileptic fit follows a more or less stereotyped course as described on p. 614 with a series of phases often ending in post-convulsive coma of variable length, sometimes followed by automatism. In hysterical fits these phases do not occur. Crying-out often occurs during the attack, but unlike the occasional convulsive cry of the epileptic, which is merely an inarticulate phonation, consists of emotional reactions, e.g. laughing and crying, or the articulate utterance of words or sentences. The movements of the hysterical fit are not of a low order like the clonic movements of epilepsy, but are co-ordinated and purposive. The hysteric clutches at surrounding objects, struggles, and may attempt to fall out of bed or to tear off his clothes. Opisthotonos is common, and bizarre attitudes may be adopted. The tongue is not bitten in a hysterical convulsion, and incontinence of urine does not usually occur, but if the patient learns that micturition is typical of epileptic attacks, this symptom may be produced. Some hysterical 'fits', particularly in adolescent girls, are not accompanied by movements, and the patient simply slumps to the floor and gets up again a few seconds or minutes

later. These attacks can be difficult to distinguish from akinetic epilepsy but usually occur at work or at school, do not cause injury, and are uninfluenced by anticonvulsant drugs. Similar attacks, occurring sometimes very frequently, may occur in adults after trivial head injury in a compensation setting and resolve after financial settlement. In tonic–clonic epileptic seizures consciousness is lost at the onset, so that the patient during and immediately after the fit shows no response to external simuli. The hysteric when in a 'fit', though often in a dissociated or trance-like state, is not completely unconscious and can sometimes be roused by firm handling, as through the time-honoured practice of administering a douche of cold water. The corneal reflex is often absent in an epileptic during a fit and in the post-convulsive phase. This reflex may seem to be absent in hysteria, but an attempt to elicit it during a hysterical fit often evokes violent contraction of the orbicularis oculi. The hysterical 'fit', unlike the epileptic, has no well-defined end but often fades away with sighs, groans, and restlessness. After the attack the patient, though seemingly shaken and exhausted, does not usually show the tendency to sleep which follows many epileptic fits. The plantar reflexes are for a time extensor after some epileptic fits. Flexor responses after an attack do not exclude epilepsy, but extensor responses do exclude hysteria as the cause, provided there is no coexisting corticospinal-tract lesion to which they are attributed and provided the patient has not learned, as in some cases of the 'Munchausen syndrome' (p. 666), to simulate the response.

Paralysis

Hysterical paralysis can affect any part of the body normally under voluntary control. Most often it involves one limb or part of a limb, the movements at one joint being alone affected. Less frequently more than one limb is affected, as in hysterical hemiplegia, paraplegia, or diplegia. The paralysis may seem to be accompanied by flaccidity or rigidity, or there may be no overt disturbance of muscle tone. Hysterical paralysis of the face and tongue is rare and is often associated with spasm of corresponding muscles on the opposite side. The diagnosis of hysterical paralysis rests upon the following points:

Anomalies of distribution. Since the paralysis corresponds to the patient's subconscious concept of what form it should take, there are inevitably discrepancies between hysterical paralysis and that produced by organic lesions of the nervous system (except, perhaps, in those with anatomical knowledge, such as doctors or nurses). The distribution of the weakness is often anomalous. Thus in hysterical hemiplegia there is no weakness of the face. Paralysis affecting only movements at a single joint is almost unknown in organic disease.

Contraction of antagonistic muscles. It is very common in hysterical paralysis to find that when the patient attempts to move an affected limb the antagonistic muscles as well as the prime movers contract. Thus elbow extension is associated with active contraction of the biceps, flexion of the knee with contraction of quadriceps. Such antagonistic contractions can easily be detected if the examiner places a finger upon the biceps tendon and patella respectively. Electromyography can give useful confirmation. Such a disorder of movement in a sense expresses mental conflict at a physiological level, giving simultaneous contraction of muscles which would carry out a movement and of those which would prevent it. Antagonistic contraction is, however, absent when the paralysis is so severe that the prime movers hardly contract at all. It is characteristic of hysterical weakness or paralysis that the patient demonstrates a massive expenditure of effort in attempts to move the paralysed member, but to little effect.

Muscular wasting and contractures. These are absent except in long-standing cases, in which these phenomena may supervene due to prolonged disuse and postural abnormality. Thus when hysterical flexion of the fingers (which may literally dig into the palm) (Fig. 23.2) or hysterical inversion of the foot, say, has been present for months or years, shortening of tendons and muscles may eventually occur. Even so, considerable relaxation and a much improved range of movement may still be achieved by electrical stimulation of antagonistic muscles or under anaesthesia.

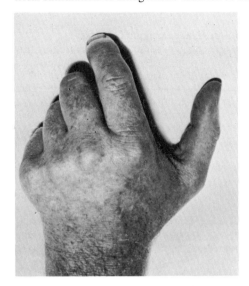

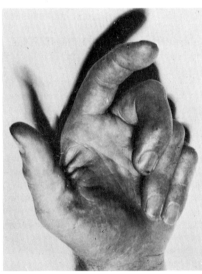

Fig. 23.2. Hysterical contracture of the middle, ring, and little fingers following upon a trivial industrial injury (photograph kindly supplied by Dr J. D. Spillane).

The reflexes. The tendon reflexes in hysteria depend upon variable factors. They are often symmetrically and moderately exaggerated. Extreme rigidity can make them difficult to elicit. Moderate unilateral rigidity may cause them to appear exaggerated on the affected side, but if adequate muscular relaxation can be obtained they are never asymmetrical, and never diminished. The same is true of the abdominal reflexes, and the plantar reflexes are flexor unless the patient has learned the pathological significance and characteristic features of an extensor plantar response. Even so, the simulated extensor plantar response is much more likely to be due to conscious motivation (as in malingering, or the Munchausen syndrome—see below) than to the true subconscious motivation of hysteria. True ankle clonus does not occur, though a few clonic jerks may be evoked if the lower limb is incompletely relaxed.

Gait

Hysterical disorders of gait may be associated with hysterical weakness of one or both lower limbs, and sometimes seem to represent an exaggeration of the normal instability which occurs on first getting out of bed after an illness. A hysterical gait is usually easy to recognize because of its bizarre character and lack of resemblance to any disorder of gait produced by organic disease. In hysterical hemiplegia the affected lower limb is ostentatiously dragged along the ground and not circumducted, as in hemiplegia due to a corticospinal lesion. Exaggerated stiffness or alternatively gross pseudo-ataxia are also common. Often a patient who, while lying in bed, shows normal power and co-ordination, walks with the greatest difficulty, clinging to and staggering from the bed to other furniture. Falling is common, especially when other patients are present, but the fall does not cause injury. In severe cases even two persons may have difficulty in supporting the patient, for whereas a patient with organic disease causing difficulty in walking does his best to support himself, the unconscious efforts of the hysterical patient seem directed to falling. It is, of course, important to recall that truncal ataxia due to dysfunction of midline cerebellar structures is not associated with the classical signs of neocerebellar lesions or even overt incoordination in the recumbent patient, while the bizarre gait of early torsion dystonia (p. 339), especially in childhood, is not uncommonly misconstrued by the inexperienced observer as being hysterical because of the lack of other convincing physical signs.

Rigidity

Hysterical rigidity can be localized to a paralysed limb, or more generalized, as in hysterical trance. Trismus is also an occasional manifestation. The rigidity of hysteria increases in proportion to the effort made by the observer to move the rigid part passively, whereas in organic nervous disease the rigidity is a definite quantum which can be overcome by the exercise of a slightly greater force. Moreover, in hysteria a successful attempt to break down the rigidity almost always leads to an intense emotional reaction in the patient.

Involuntary movements

Tremor is a common hysterical phenomenon. It may be fine, but is more often coarse and variable in frequency and amplitude, whether generalized or localized. A coarse tremor is often associated with hysterical paralysis, being intensified when the patient attempts to move the paralysed limb. It is increased when attention is directed to it, and may be absent in movements carried out when the attention is distracted. Hysterical involuntary movements can also simulate chorea, though not sufficiently so to deceive the skilled observer. In such cases movements do not usually involve the face. However, blepharospasm, increasing when an attempt is made passively to open the eyes (see below), is sometimes hysterical but must be distinguished from Meige's syndrome (p. 349).

Sensory symptoms and signs

Hysterical sensory impairment is common. It is most often confined to a limb affected by other hysterical symptoms, such as weakness or paralysis. It occasionally affects only some modalities, especially appreciation of light touch and cutaneous pain, but more often all forms are lost. When cutaneous sensibility is lost over the periphery of the limb, the anaesthetic area is demarcated from the area of normal sensation by a sharp upper border which encircles the limb and usually coincides with a joint. Sensation may be lost over half of the body, and in such cases there may be loss of smell and taste on the same side as well. Anaesthesia of the whole body is less frequent. Apparent anaesthesia of the cornea, palate, and pharynx, with loss of the corresponding reflexes, is an unexplained symptom of hysteria, and may be present without other sensory disturbances.

Hysterical sensory loss is distinguished from that due to organic disease of the nervous system by its failure to correspond to that resulting from lesions of the sensory tracts, spinal segments, or peripheral nerves. Anaesthesia of 'glove and stocking' distribution may simulate that found in sensorimotor or sensory neuropathy, but in these disorders the transition from impaired to normal sensation is usually gradual. Hysterical patients often exhibit striking discrepancies in their sensory symptoms which are incompatible with an organic origin. Thus co-ordination may be perfect in spite of apparent complete loss of position and joint sense in a limb. Or a patient with hysterical hemianaesthesia may state that he is unable to feel a vibrating tuning-fork placed over the affected half of the sternum or skull, although the bone conducts the stimulus perfectly to the opposite side. In hysterical persons sensory loss can readily be, and perhaps always is, produced by suggestion; it may be possible to 'find' islands of normal sensation within an anaesthetic area by suggesting to an observer, in the patient's hearing, that such findings are common.

Deafness. There is little difficulty in detecting hysterical deafness when examination shows that the ears and vestibular reactions are normal, but the diagnosis is more difficult when hysterical deafness is superimposed upon impaired hearing due to organic disease. Hysterical deafness may disappear during sleep, so that the patient can be aroused by sounds, and the blink reflex on auditory stimulation may be preserved. When Bárány's noise-box is used, a patient suffering from hysterical deafness will raise his voice, but this does not occur when deafness is due to disease of the ear. Hysterical vertigo is rare, but feelings of giddiness, instability, and depersonalization are common.

Pain. There has been much discussion as to whether hysterical pain is qualitatively the same as that caused by organic disease, and this has been denied on the ground that the hysterical patient, though complaining of severe pain, usually shows none of the physical reactions associated with organic pain and presents an appearance which belies his allegations of intense suffering. Hysterical pain is especially common in the face and head. The recognition of its nature depends upon the absence of symptoms and/or signs of organic disease sufficient to expain it, its failure to respond to powerful analgesic drugs, or to local anaesthetic block of the nerves innervating the affected region, and upon the mental state of the patient. Walters (1961) preferred the title 'psychogenic regional pain' to 'hysterical pain'. Among common syndromes of psychogenic pain, discussed elsewhere in this volume, are headache, atypical facial neuralgia, chest pain in the effort syndrome, low back pain as a consequence of anxiety and depression, proctalgia fugax (attacks of anal pain often wakening the patient from sleep), and many other varieties. Methods of management of psychogenic pain were discussed by Bonica (1974).

Ocular symptoms
Hysterical blindness can be unilateral or bilateral; it may be complete or can consist merely of a reduction of visual acuity. Bilateral blindness may be a perpetuation of the transitory visual impairment associated with syncope or head injury. Unilateral blindness may be associated with hysterical hemianaesthesia on the same side. In hysterical blindness the optic discs and the pupillary reactions to light are normal, and it may be possible to evoke blinking by a sudden feint with the hand towards the eyes. Moreover, the blind hysteric when walking will avoid obstacles in his path, but so, too, may the patient with visual agnosia due to organic brain disease. There are several useful tests for the detection of unilateral hysterical blindness. Diplopia may be produced by covering one eye with an appropriate prism, or one eye may be covered with a red, and the other with a green glass, the patient being then asked to read a word-test of alternate red and green letters. Since one colour is invisible to each eye, if all the letters are read the patient must be using both eyes. Visual-field defects are also com-

mon in hysteria and usually result from suggestion at the time of examination. The commonest type is a concentric defect of the field which takes the form of a spiral with the field progressively diminishing with each circuit of the test object but 'tubular vision' may also occur.

Disturbances of ocular movement include spasm of convergence, which is almost always hysterical, and may be associated with spasm of accommodation. Defects and dissociation of conjugate ocular movements in the lateral and vertical planes may be produced by spasm of the ocular muscles, and a coarse pseudonystagmus may occur. Hysterical ptosis is the result of spasm of the palpebral fibres of the orbicularis oculi, and when the lid is passively raised this spasm can be felt to increase. Blepharospasm is similarly produced.

Symptoms referred to the alimentary canal
Hysterical dysphagia is rare, but air-swallowing is common. It can lead to extreme gastric distension. Globus hystericus, described as a sensation of constriction or a lump in the throat, is sometimes but by no means always the result of air-swallowing. It must be distinguished from the similar sensation which can occur in some patients with hiatus hernia.

Hysterical vomiting when mild may lead to no loss of weight; when severe it may cause marked acidosis and emaciation. Cyclical vomiting in childhood is often psychogenic. It is usually symbolic of an intense aversion to some task or situation, of which the patient is literally, as well as metaphorically, sick. However, self-induced vomiting in women can be a feature of anorexia nervosa (see below) but is even more common in bulimia nervosa, a syndrome described relatively recently in which patients have powerful and intractable urges to overeat; they also have a morbid fear of becoming fat and seek to avoid the 'fattening' effects of food by induced vomiting or abusing purgatives, or both (Fairburn and Cooper 1982).

Hysterical anorexia—'anorexia nervosa'—can arise as a primary hysterical reaction to the patient's emotional difficulties, or may be secondary to other hysterical symptoms referred to the alimentary canal, and which the patient believes are exacerbated by taking food. It occurs in adolescent girls and young women, and can lead to extreme emaciation, and to amenorrhoea. It often follows a period of dieting in order to lose weight, leading to an aversion to food, and the affected girls may go to remarkable lengths to avoid eating and find many methods of disposing secretly of the food they are given. Hirsutism is common and the latency of the tendon reflexes may be prolonged (Fowler, Banim, and Ikram 1972). The many endocrine and metabolic abnormalities observed in such cases are secondary to caloric deficit and carbohydrate deprivation (Kanis, Brown, Fitzpatrick, Hibbert, Horn, Nairn, Shirling, Strong, and Walton 1974). Wernicke's encephalopathy may result (Handler and Perkin 1982).

Hysterical diarrhoea and constipation may occur, and many abdominal and pelvic symptoms, including the spastic-colon or irritable-bowel syndrome, are clearly stress-related and largely emotionally induced. Among the many forms of *epidemic hysteria* which have been described, abdominal pain, sometimes with vomiting and diarrhoea, fainting, and/or overbreathing occurring in schoolchildren, mainly girls, is one variety (*British Medical Journal* 1979). And many believe that several epidemics of benign myalgic encephalomyelitis (p. 259) fall into the same category.

Cardiac symptoms
Tachycardia and palpitation are prominent symptoms of cardiac neurosis (effort syndrome). In hysteria, however, such symptoms may occur in a patient who is outwardly placid. The recognition of their nature is important, lest sufferers should be restricted in their activity for long periods with a mistaken diagnosis of organic heart disease.

Respiratory symptoms

Respiratory tics have already been described. Hysterical hyperventilation is sometimes seen and usually follows exceptional stress. It also occurs in some panic attacks of the phobic anxiety-depersonalization syndrome and indeed there is evidence that hyperventilation sometimes causes the panic attacks and that there may be underlying beta-adrenergic supersensitivity (Hibbert 1984). The excessive pulmonary ventilation may lead to pulmonary tetany and even syncope. The hysterical nature of the symptom can usually be detected by the fact that the hyperventilation disappears or is much diminished when the patient is engaged in conversation, whereas talking increases the dyspnoea due to organic disease.

Urinary symptoms

Nocturnal enuresis in childhood is the perpetuation of, or a reversion to, the infantile lack of control over the bladder. Its motive is frequently a desire to attract attention, and the symptom tends to be reinforced by punishment or admonition. Pathological polyuria and organic causes of enuresis, especially spinal dysraphism, must be excluded, but psychogenic polydipsia (compulsive water-drinking) is occasionally a contributory factor. Hysterical retention of urine occasionally occurs in young girls.

The skin

'Dermatitis artefacta' is a term applied to cutaneous lesions voluntarily produced by a hysterical patient, either by scratching, abrading, or deliberate bruising, or by the use of external agents, including corrosives. These lesions are usually easily recognized by their appearance and by the fact that they quickly heal when covered by an occlusive dressing. Pruritus is often a hysterical symptom, though atopic eczema is also stress-related. Cyanosis and oedema may occur in a limb affected by hysterical paralysis and has been observed as a result of the purposive use of tight elastic bands applied around a limb by the hysterical patient. Here again the boundary between true hysteria (subconscious motivation) and deliberate self-injury (rarely mutilation) in the sympathy-craving, attention-seeking, individual with a 'desire to be ill' (see below) is indistinct.

The spine

The spine may also be affected by hysterical pain and tenderness, and occasionally remarkable deformities occur in hysteria, sometimes leading to a grossly flexed or otherwise bizarre posture.

Pyrexia

Probably in most cases of factitious pyrexia occuring in hysteria, the thermometer is manipulated by the patient. This source of error can readily be detected by adequate supervision when the temperature is taken rectally. Rarely, however, it seems that an actual rise of body temperature may occur as a hysterical manifestation. The 'desire to be ill' is classified by some authorities as a condition which shows some affinities with hysteria though it would appear that many of the affected individuals have serious personality defects (Bayliss 1984). Not only may the patients feign pyrexia by manipulation of clinical thermometers but some may actually produce illness in themselves by injecting themselves with insulin or with their own bath water. *E. coli* arthritis is invariably due to this cause. This type of phenomenon is most often seen in nurses, doctors, or other health-care professionals.

The 'Munchausen syndrome'

The 'Munchausen syndrome' (Asher 1951; O'Shea, McGennis, Gahill, and Falvey 1984) is a name given to a group of patients with a related syndrome who move from hospital to hospital, cleverly feigning physical illness, including cardiac infarction, renal colic, perforated peptic ulcer, or even cerebral vascular accidents.

One well-known British patient, an ex-male-nurse, cleverly feigned a pontine lesion by using eye drops to dilate one pupil and constrict the other, while demonstrating convincing evidence of a hemiplegia and hemianalgesia with an extensor plantar response on the affected side. Many other such cases have been reported. While some such individuals are addicted to morphine or pethidine and simply seek injections of the appropriate drugs and others seek nothing more than a bed for the night, most undertake these activities for complex psychological reasons (Mayer-Gross, Slater, and Roth 1960). While patients with factitious pyrexia and other forms of illness as mentioned above are mostly young women, those with the Munchausen syndrome are nearly always men of relatively low socio-economic status, often with a lifelong pattern of social maladjustment (Bayliss 1984).

Speech

Hysterical speech disturbances—mutism and aphonia—are described elsewhere (pp. 54–5).

Diagnosis

The diagnosis of individual hysterical symptoms has already been considered. In general the diagnosis depends upon the presence of positive signs of hysteria as described above and never solely upon the absence of signs of organic disease. It is also helpful, whenever possible, to identify a motive. Hence, in every case, both the nervous system and other systems to which symptoms may be referred must be thoroughly examined. One organic nervous disease often confused with hysteria is multiple sclerosis, on account of the transitory occurrence in its early stages of weakness and sensory phenomena. Examination of such patients, however, will often reveal signs of organic neurological disease, the commonest of which are pallor of the optic discs, nystagmus, diminution or absence of the abdominal reflexes, and extensor plantar responses. Visual and/or somatosensory evoked potential recording is often useful in doubtful cases, just as electromyography is of great value in patients with presumed hysterical paralysis. The possibility that overt hysterical manifestations may be superimposed upon the subclinical features of an underlying organic disease such as intracranial neoplasia or dementia or a psychotic depression must also be considered. Undoubtedly some such symptoms are in a sense iatrogenic in that they may be exaggerated or distorted by emotional factors in patients who find themselves unable to persuade a doctor that they are genuinely ill. And in patients with physical disease, including the many disorders generally acknowledged to be psychosomatic, it is not uncommon to find that a vicious-circle mechanism operates in which physical symptoms cause anxiety which in turn breeds tension and increases the severity of the initial physical symptoms, thus creating a 'functional' or even, in some severe cases, a hysterical overlay which markedly distorts the manifestations of the primary organic condition.

The distinction between hysteria (subconscious motivation) and malingering (conscious motivation) may be a matter of considerable difficulty in individuals who seek compensation after injury or in others accused of criminal offences (who may feign amnesia) as the clinical manifestations of the two conditions are outwardly similar. Unfortunately we have no definitive objective tests to help us in making this distinction (Miller 1966).

Prognosis

The prognosis in relation to individual symptoms of hysteria is good in most cases, though relapses are frequent unless the patient can readjust psychologically or unless the causal stress can be abolished or modified substantially. Chronic cases are common in which a single symptom persists for years, often because it is the patient's reaction to a domestic situation which also continues unchanged. Some victims of chronic hysteria are those in whom the expectation of compensation for an injury or the receipt of a pension puts a premium upon the persistence of their disability.

Treatment

General considerations

When a hysterical symptom is a neurotic solution of a mental conflict, symptomatic treatment alone is inadequate. It is essential, if possible, that the cause of the conflict should be exposed and removed. Analytical psychological methods, however, are often rendered difficult by lack of intelligence or by resistance in the patient, and in severely dissociated individuals with amnesia, drug-induced abreaction, hypnosis, or narco-analysis may be needed. When the cause of the symptom has been revealed and, where possible, removed, treatment may then be directed towards relief of the symptom itself. A detailed physical examination and laboratory tests giving negative results may convince the patient that no organic cause for the disability exists. In many cases recovery is best effected by a gradual and prolonged process of suggestion, persuasion, and re-education. Some, however, prefer to try to remove the symptom at one sitting. This method requires great tact, patience, and skill and is not without risk, since failure of a protracted attempt to cure will only reinforce the patient's belief in the intractable nature of his disorder. The removal of a symptom by hypnotic suggestion is sometimes undesirable in adult patients, as it tends to strengthen the abnormal suggestibility which is an undesirable characteristic of the hysterical personality. This method, however, is much more admissible in dealing with children, in whose education suggestion plays a legitimate part.

The management of hysteria, especially if symptoms are intractable or recurrent, is often extremely difficult, and some cases are in effect incurable. Psychotropic drugs are useful in some cases especially in eradicating associated symptoms of anxiety and/or depression. While the measures mentioned here and below are often effective in promoting the resolution of some hysterical phenomena, long-term psychiatric support and supervision is generally needed in more intractable cases (see Gelder, Gath, and Mayou 1983).

Treatment of individual symptoms

Hysterical 'fits'. A hysterical attack can usually be quickly controlled by firm handling, especially if the patient is isolated from a sympathetic audience. Firm but sympathetic reassurance is often effective, too, in terminating hysterical hyperventilation and associated panic attacks.

Paralysis and rigidity. These manifestations often occur together, and, as they depend in part upon involuntary muscular contraction of agonists, the patient is taught to relax the muscles of the affected region and is told that when they relax movement will be easy. Electrical stimulation will show that the affected muscles can contract; the patient is then persuaded to imitate the movements excited electrically.

Hysterical gait. This is one phenomenon which can sometimes be cured at a single treatment. The patient is first encouraged to walk with adequate support from the doctor or physiotherapist. The support is gradually diminished until the patient realizes that he is walking or even eventually running alone.

Enuresis. Before accepting an emotional cause for enuresis in childhood, urinary-tract infection, polyuria, or organic lesions which impair sphincter control, especially spinal dysraphic syndromes, must be excluded. An attempt should be made to identify the cause, which is sometimes insecurity, conflict with a sib, or simply a desire to attract attention or affection. Both the parents and the patient must be encouraged to expect a cure, and neither punishment nor admonition for lapses should be permitted. Propantheline or ephedrine in appropriate doses given before retiring may be used to depress reflex evacuation of the bladder until the habit of continence is established. Alternatively, drugs such as imipramine given to lighten sleep have been found helpful in some cases. Hypnotic suggestion or various deconditioning techniques will often bring about cure in hitherto intractable cases (Kolvin, MacKeith, and Meadow 1973).

Vomiting. The psychological cause of the vomiting must first be ascertained and discussed with the patient, who requires reassurance that no organic cause for it exists. Special diets, alkalies, and other drugs which have been prescribed should be discontinued. The patient should then be persuaded to eat a light meal with firm reassurance that no vomiting will follow. Hysterical vomiting is occasionally curable at one sitting but sometimes more prolonged psychotherapy is needed; a cure, once effected, is usually permanent.

Anorexia nervosa. The patient should be interviewed apart from relatives and friends and the cause of the anorexia can usually be ascertained. It is often necessary to explain that those symptoms which the patient attributes to taking food are really the result of taking too little. In severe cases admission to hospital is usually required and many feeding regimens, however slow to have an effect, have proved helpful. Chlorpromazine or other phenothiazines are helpful in some cases; for details the reader is referred to textbooks of psychiatry.

Occupational cramps or neuroses

Synonyms. Craft palsy.

Definition. A functional nervous disorder prone to afflict those whose occupation entails the persistent use of finely co-ordinated movements, especially of the hand; it is characterized by a progressive occupational disability, due to spasm of the muscles employed, which are often the site of pain and sometimes of tremor.

Aetiology

Occupational neurosis was once attributed to fatigue of cortical ganglion cells or to a disorder of the basal ganglia. Most authorities now take the view, however, that it is primarily psychogenic. However, this view has been vigorously and cogently disputed by Sheehy and Marsden (1982) who, after studying 29 subjects with writers' cramp (and four with typists' and one with pianists' cramp) divided their cases into two major groups, simple and dystonic. They claim to have found subtle physical signs also found in other basal ganglia diseases in patients with the simple form and other evidence of segmental or even generalized dystonia in patients with the dystonic form. They therefore concluded that the condition is undoubtedly organic and that it is a focal dystonia. *The Lancet* (1982), too, concluded that 'few neurologists nowadays would regard writers' cramp, or the comparable musicians' cramps, as psychogenic'.

While there can be no doubt that localized or generalized dystonia may cause difficulty in writing and that that difficulty is in some respects comparable to the phenomenon of simple writers' cramp, like Hudgson (1982), I find the conclusions of Sheehy and Marsden inherently implausible and unacceptable. In my experience even subtle physical signs are absent in the many 'simple' cases that I have seen and neither focal dystonia nor any other organic disorder could in my view impair movements *only* when they take part in one co-ordinated act while leaving totally unaffected all other precise and complex voluntary actions involving the affected member. One patient of mine, a professional oboeist, became incapable of playing the oboe because of spasm of the lips but had no difficulty with the flute. The muscular spasm evoked by an attempt to carry out the act involves both prime movers and their antagonists, thus resembling the disorder of function seen in hysterical paralysis. The disability may also be influenced by external factors in a manner which would be inexplicable if it were organic. For example, a lawyer who suffered from severe writers' cramp was almost totally unable to write when sitting, but could do so when standing. Occupational neurosis, moreover, may be associated with other hysterical symptoms and sometimes has an overt psychological cause. Thus a woman who developed writers' cramp after an unhappy marriage also had vaginismus. Admittedly Sheehy and Marsden (1982) were unable to detect neurotic or hysterical traits on psychometric testing of their patients and many affected individuals show no overt psychopathology. However, simple writers' cramp and other occupational cramps show various analogies with stammering, another functional disorder of finely co-ordinated movements; indeed, it is like a manual stammer. It must be conceded, however, that sufferers from occupational cramps may have a physiological predisposition which determines the character of their symptoms, just as, for example, left-handedness seems sometimes to predispose to stammering.

Fatigue and the effort to carry out accurate work against a deadline are important precipitating factors, and as in most cases the sufferer's livelihood depends upon his speed and accuracy, impaired efficiency evokes anxiety, which probably plays a part in psychogenesis. Numerous occupational neuroses have been described, writers', telegraphists', goldbeaters', violinists', and piano-players' cramps being the most familiar, but there is probably no occupation involving repetitive fine movements which is immune. Both sexes are affected, but males more so than females.

Symptoms and signs

The features of writers' cramp only will be described, since the disorder is essentially similar in other occupations. The onset is gradual, and the condition reveals itself at first only when the patient is fatigued, when difficulty in controlling the pen leads to inaccurate writing. When the condition is well developed, any attempt to write evokes a spasm of the muscles concerned in holding and moving the pen, and this may spread to the whole upper limb which thus becomes rigid, so that the act is brought to an abrupt stop. More often the attempt to write leads to jerky and incoordinate finger movements, so that the writing is completely illegible. The pen may be driven into the paper. In some cases a tremor of the hand develops. No two patients present precisely the same disorder of function. An attempt is often made to circumvent the disability by various tricks and unusual methods of holding the pen. Once writing stops the muscular spasm disappears. After attempting to write, the patient complains of a sense of fatigue or of aching pain in the muscles, not only of the upper limb but sometimes also of the neck. Muscular wasting, sensory loss, and reflex changes are absent and all other fine finger movements are normal. In the early stages the disability is limited to the single act which precipitates it. Later it may extend to other similar acts carried out by the same hand. Thus the woman already mentioned, after developing writers' cramp, learned to type. Her disability then extended to typing and finally to the use of a paint-brush in water-colour sketching. The sufferer from writers' cramp who learns to write with the left hand may develop the same disorder in this.

Diagnosis

Occupational cramp must be distinguished from organic disorders of the nervous system, such as focal or more generalized dystonia, which may lead to difficulty in performing fine movements. A careful history and physical examination usually render the diagnosis easy, since in such cases signs of organic disease are detectable and the disability usually involves other finely co-ordinated acts, and not just writing, from the beginning.

Prognosis

The prognosis of occupational neurosis is usually poor, as in many cases the disability is progressive, though recovery is rarely seen and some patients struggle on in their occupation despite their disability. Others find a change of occupation to one not involving writing (or the activity precipitating a specific cramp) helpful.

Treatment

Prolonged rest from the occupation is occasionally helpful but rarely practicable. The way in which muscular spasm interferes with the act should be explained and the patient should be taught muscular relaxation under skilled supervision. This may later be combined with re-educational exercises for the affected limb, with a gradual return to work, but these measures are usually ineffectual. Learning to write with the other hand, or using a typewriter may help, but not infrequently the second hand, and even the movements involved in typewriting, are later affected. Liversedge and Sylvester (1955) devised a method of 'deconditioning' the patient with electrical stimuli and this was helpful in some cases. Some patients obtain benefit from the use of drugs such as chlordiazepoxide (*Librium*), 10 mg three or four times a day, or diazepam (*Valium*), 2–5 mg three or four times daily, but while these may partially relieve muscular spasms they are in no sense curative and their effect is usually transient.

References

Asher, R. (1951). Munchausen's syndrome. *Lancet* **ii,** 239.

Bayliss, R. I. S. (1984). The deceivers. *Br. med. J.* **288,** 583.

Bonica, J. J. (Ed.) (1974). *Pain.* Raven Press, New York.

British Medical Journal (1979). Epidemic hysteria. *Br. med. J.* **2,** 408.

Carter, A. B. (1972). A physician's view of hysteria. *Lancet* **ii,** 1241.

Eysenck, H. J. (1960). *Handbook of abnormal psychology.* Pitman, London.

Fairburn, C. G. and Cooper, P. J. (1982). Self-induced vomiting and bulimia nervosa: an undetected problem. *Br. med. J.* **284,** 1153.

Fowler, P. B. S., Banim, S. O., and Ikram, H. (1972). Prolonged ankle reflex in anorexia nervosa. *Lancet* **ii,** 307.

Gelder, M., Gath, D., and Mayou, R. (1983). *Oxford textbook of psychiatry.* Oxford University Press, Oxford.

Handler, C. E. and Perkin, G. D. (1982). Anorexia nervosa and Wernicke's encephalopathy: an underdiagnosed association. *Lancet* **ii,** 771.

Hibbert, G. A. (1984). Hyperventilation as a cause of panic attacks. *Br. med. J.* **288,** 263.

Hudson, P. (1983). Writers' cramp. *Br. med. J.* **286,** 585.

Kanis, J. A., Brown, P., Fitzpatrick, K., Hibbert, D. J., Horn, D. B., Nairn, I. M., Shirling, D., Strong, J. A., and Walton, H. J. (1974). Anorexia nervosa: a clinical, psychiatric, and laboratory study. *Quart. J. Med.* **43,** 321.

Kolvin, I., MacKeith, R. C., and Meadow, S. R. (Eds.) (1973). *Bladder control and enuresis.* Clinics in Developmental Medicine, Nos. 48/49. Heinemann, London.

The Lancet (1982). Writers' cramp. *Lancet* **ii,** 969.

Liversedge, L. R. and Sylvester, J. D. (1955). Conditioning techniques in the treatment of writer's cramp. *Lancet* **i,** 1147.

Mayer-Gross, W., Slater, E., and Roth, M. (1960). *Clinical psychiatry,* 2nd edn. Cassell, London.

Merskey, H. (1982). *The analysis of hysteria.* Ballière Tindall, London.

Miller, H. (1966). Mental sequelae of head injury. *Proc. R. Soc. Med.* **59,** 257.

O'Shea, B., McGennis, A., Cahill, M., and Falvey, J. (1984). Munchausen's syndrome. *Br. J. hosp. Med.* **31,** 269.

Roy, A. (1982). *Hysteria.* Wiley, Chichester.

Sheehy, M. P. and Marsden, C. D. (1982). Writers' cramp—a focal dystonia. *Brain* **105,** 461.

Slater, E. (1965). Diagnosis of 'hysteria'. *Br. med. J.* 1395.

Walters, A. (1961). Psychogenic regional pain alias hysterical pain. *Brain* **84,** 1.

Index

Abbreviations

CSF   cerebrospinal fluid
CT   computerized tomography
EEG   electroencephalography
EMG   electromyography

GABA   γ-aminobutyric acid
ICP   increased intracranial pressure
NMR   nuclear magnetic resonance

abdominal reflexes 50
abducens nerve (6th cranial) 107
  paralysis 107
    benign unilateral 108
    causes 107–8
    in brain stem tumour 167
    in eighth nerve tumour 167
    south east Asian 108
    treatment 108
aberration, chromatic/spherical 84
abetalipoproteinaemia (Bassen–Kornzweig
    syndrome) 464, 482
absinthe drinkers 428
acalculia 57, 163
acanthocytosis of red cells 482–3
accessory nerve (11th cranial) 133
  lesions 133
accident neurosis 228
accommodation 83
acetazolamide
  for: hypokalaemic periodic paralysis 577
    hyperkalaemic periodic paralysis 577
acetylcholine 4, 6, 7–8, 551, 552
  electrophoresis 597
  denervation hypersensitivity to 25
  neuromuscular junction effect 27
  receptors 7, 596
  release 25, 596
acetylcholinesterase 552
achondroplasia 608
achromatopsia 62
acid maltase deficiency 577
acoustic neuroma (8th nerve tumour) 167, 170
  canal paresis 123
  CT scan 156, 157 (fig.)
  pneumoencephalogram 160 (fig.)
  surgical treatment 171
acquired non-progressive dysautonomia 599
acrocephalosyndactyly of Apert 607
acrocephaly (craniostenosis; oxycephaly;
    turricephaly; tower skull) 136, 606–7
acrodermatitis chronica atrophicans 548
acrodynia (pink disease; erythroedema
    polyneuritis) 542
acrodystrophic (hereditary sensory)
    neuropathy 45, 414
acromegaly 164, 470
  polyneuropathy 541
acrylamide neuropathy 534
actinomycosis 248
actinomycosis of muscle 563
acupuncture, β-endorphin increase in CSF 47
acquired immune deficiency syndrome
    (AIDS) 294
ACTH, see corticotrophin
acyclovir
  for: herpes simplex encephalitis 280
    herpes zoster 293

Addison's disease 470
  coma due to 648
  EMG 586
  muscle disorder in 575
  papilloedema in 648
Addison–Schilder's disease
    (adrenoleucodystrophy) 320–1
adenine arabinoside (vidarabine)
  for: herpes simplex encephalitis 280
    herpes zoster 293
adenoma sebaceum 358
adenomas, multiple, in pituitary tumour 164
adenosine 6, 9
adenosine triphosphate (ATP) 5
adiposity (obesity) 601
adiposogenital dystrophy, idiopathic (Fröhlich's
    syndrome) 601
adrenal cortical failure 648
adrenal hypercorticism 489
adrenaline 8, 597
adrenergic receptors 596
adrenoleucodystrophy (Addison–Schilder's
    disease) 320–1
adversive attacks 161
adynamia episodica hereditaria (hyperkalaemic
    periodic paralysis) 577
affective responses 38
ageusia 129, 229
agnosia (mind-blindness) 62–3
  auditory 62–3
  developmental 63
  finger 163
  tactile 63
  topographical 64
  visual 62, 163
agraphia 57, 163
agyria (lissencephaly) 357
Aicardi's syndrome 357
air embolism 200
air encephalography 80
  in: brain injury 229
    dementia 660
    syringomyelia 414
akinesia 324, 328
akinetic mutism 645, 650
akinetic-rigid syndromes 322
akithisia 328
Albers–Schonberg disease (autosomal
    recessive/dominant osteoporosis) 606
Albright's syndrome (polyostotic fibrous
    dysplasia) 606
alcohol
  for benign familial tremor 330
  intrathecal injection, for flexor spasms 395
alcohol addiction 426–31
  aetiology 426
  beriberi in 474
  blood disorders 428

brain damage 426
  CSF acidosis 428
  CT scan of brain 426
  definition (WHO) 426
  diagnosis 428–9
  epilepsy 428
  fetal malformations 426
  hyponatraemia 428
  incidence 15
  pellagra-associated 476
  prognosis 429
  subdural haematoma-associated 232
  treatment 429–30
  withdrawal 427
  see also specific alcoholic syndromes
alcoholic cardiomyopathy 428, 578
alcoholic cerebellar degeneration 428, 429
  prognosis 429
alcoholic dementia 428, 429
alcoholic hallucinations, acute 427
  treatment 430
alcoholic intoxication, acute 427, 648
alcoholic myopathy 428, 429, 578
  prognosis 429
alcoholic polyneuropathy 531–2
  treatment 430
alcoholic pseudoparesis 268
Alcoholics Anonymous 429
aldolase, serum/CSF, in stroke 197
aldose reductase inhibitor, for diabetic
    neuropathy 539
Alexander's disease 463
alexia 57, 163
  pure, without agraphia (subcortical
    word-blindness; visual aphasia) 57
  with agraphia (visual asymbolia; cortical
    word-blindness; Dejerine's first
    type) 57
  without agraphia (Dejerine's second type) 57
algodystrophy (shoulder–hand syndrome; reflex
    dystrophy of upper extremity) 498–9,
    508
Alpers' disease (progressive cerebral
    poliodystrophy) 468
alpha coma 645
alpha neurone, see lower motor neurone
aluminium encephalopathy 438
alveolar hypoventilation syndrome 472, 647
Alzheimer's disease 658–9, 660
  Down's syndrome associated 471
amantidine hydrochloride
  for: Creutzfeldt–Jacob disease 379
    herpes zoster 293
    parkinsonism 332
    subacute sclerosing panencephalitis 280
    torticollis 341
amaurosis fugax 92, 193
  treatment 199

amaurotic family idiocy, infantile
(cerebromacular degeneration;
Tay–Sachs disease; Sandhoff's
disease) 93, 455–6
amaurotic family idiocy,
late-infantile/juvenile/late-onset 456
ambenonium hydrochloride (Mytelase), for
myasthenia gravis 571
amblyopia 100
concomitant squint-associated 96
nutritional 92
nystagmus-associated 100
paraplegia-associated 478
tobacco–alcohol 92, 428
in tropical ataxic syndrome 92
West Indian 478
amino-acid disorders 453–4
aminoaciduria 453
γ-aminobutyric acid (GABA) 324
in Huntington's chorea 346, 347
natural convulsant 609
transmitter, in neurones of substantia
nigra 17
4-aminopyridine
for: congenital myasthenia 572
Eaton–Lambert syndrome 572
amitriptyline 8
for: lumbar disc lesions 518
migraine 181
heat stroke precipitated by 444
amnesia
hysterical 662
in: alcoholism 428, 653
Alzheimer's disease 659
brain injury 653
dementia 653, 657
Korsakov's syndrome 427–8
temporal lobe lesions 653
toxic/confusional states 653
neuropathology 638–9
organic causes 653
post-traumatic 227
retrograde 227
transient 653
transient global 639, 653–4
amoebic meningoencephalitis 249
AMP deaminase deficiency 579
amphetamine 8
for: cataplexy 643
narcolepsy 643
periodic somnolence and morbid
hunger 643
heat stroke precipitated by 444
amphetamine addiction 434
cerebral arteritis 221
necrotizing angiitis 544
amphotericin B
for: amoebic meningoencephalitis 249
coccidiomycosis 248
Cryptococcus neoformans meningitis 248
fungal meningitis 249
ampicillin
for: intracranial abscess 252
meningitis 244
amusia 57
amygdala 638
amyloidosis 484
neuropathy 541–2
peripheral-nerve entrapment 520
amyotonia congenita 383
amyotrophic lateral sclerosis, *see* motor-neurone
disease
anaemia, syncope due to 189
anaesthesia, hysterical 664
anaesthesia dolorosa 112
anaesthetic agents, addiction to 434

analgesia 44
analgesics
addiction 431; *see also* drug addiction
for headache 177
anal reflex 51
anencephaly 356, 418
aneurysm, intracranial 206–8
anterior communicating artery 212 (fig.)
atheromatous 208
berry (congenital) 206–7
symptoms before rupture 207
treatment 212
see also subarachnoid haemorrhage
carotico-cavernous-sinus aneurysm
(fistula) 208
cerebellar arteries 207
embolic (mycotic) 207–8
infraclinoid 207
oculomotor nerve paralysis 107
polyarteritis nodosa 208
space-occupying lesions 170
syphilitic 208
vertebral artery 207
angina of effort 47
angioblastoma 143
angioendotheliosis 484
angiokeratoma corporis diffusum (Fabry's
disease) 462, 548
angiography 80
aortic arch catheterization 156, 197
arteriovenous angioma 208
berry aneurysm, unruptured 207
brain injury 229
brain stem tumour 168
carotid 156
cerebral atheroma 193, 197
frontal lobe glioma 158 (fig.)
intracranial abscess 252
intracranial tumour 154, 156–8
metastatic 158
spinal cord compression 406
temporal lobe glioma 158 (fig.)
stroke 197
subdural haematoma 232
venous sinus thrombosis 224
vertebral 156
angioma 143, 155, 170, 180
angiography 158 (fig.)
surgical treatment 171
angiomatous malformations 149
angiostrongylus infection 261
angiotensin, for Shy–Drager syndrome 189
anisocoria 103
ankle clonus 49
ankle jerk 50
anorexia nervosa 665
treatment 667
anosmia 83, 229
anosognosia 64
anoxia
anaemic 441
coma due to 647
ischaemic 441
anoxic-ischaemic brain injury 188, 441
Antabuse, *see* disulfiram
antecollis 341
anterior cerebral artery 183
developmental anomaly 183
occlusion 195
anterior choroidal artery 184
anterior communicating artery aneurysm 212
(fig.)
anterior inferior cerebellar artery 184
anterior internuclear ophthalmoplegia (ataxic
nystagmus; Ham's sign) 98, 311
anterior interosseous nerve 30 (fig.), 32 (table)

lesions 504
muscles supplied by 30, 32 (table)
anterior spinal artery 184, 390
occlusion (spinal stroke) 391, 423
anterior tibial nerve 510
antibiotics
for: brain trauma 230
infective thrombophlebitis 224
intracranial abscess 252
meningitis 244–5
venous sinus thrombosis 224
myasthenia induced by 568
anticholinesterase drugs, for myasthenia
gravis 571
anticoagulants
for: cerebral embolism prevention 200
ischaemic stroke 199
thrombophlebitis 224
anticonvulsants 622–3
adverse effects 434, 623–5
folate deficiency due to 482, 623
for: acute toxic encephalopathy 254
multiple sclerosis 314
glare phenomenon 94
serum concentrations 623
suicide with 434
antidepressants 8
action on pupil/accommodation 103
for: epilepsy 625
lumbar disc lesions 518
migraine 181
parkinsonism 332
MAO inhibitors 8
tricyclic 8, 332
adverse effects 434
antidiuretic hormone (ADH) 593, 602
antihistamines for migraine 180
antimyosin antibody 587
antinuclear factor 587
antisocial behaviour 655
antiviral agents 280
Anton's syndrome 64
anxiety 656
aortic-arch catheterization 193, 197
apallic syndrome 645
Apert's syndrome (acrocephalosyndactyly) 607
Apgar score 236
aphasia 55–9
aphasia
acquired, with convulsive disorder 57
auditory (pure/subcortical word-deafness) 56
causes 57–8
classification 55–6
conduction 56, 161
developmental expressive 59
developmental receptive (congenital
word–deafness; congenital auditory
imperception) 59–60, 60
examination of patient 57
expressive (Broca's) 56, 161
global 56
historical survey 55
in: left transverse sinus thrombosis 223
meningovascular syphilis 264
migraine 179
temporal lobe tumour 162
jargon 56
nature 55
nominal (amnestic; anomia) 56–7, 161
posterior association 56–7
prognosis 58
syndrome of isolated speech area 56
tactile 57
treatment 58
visual (alexia without agraphia; subcortical
word-blindness) 57

Wernicke's 56, 161
aphonia 55
apiol poisoning 55
apneustic (ataxic) breathing 136, 649
apoplectiform episodes (congestive attacks) 267
apoplexy 193
appetite, hypothalamic control of 594
apraxia 62
  constructional (optical) 62
  developmental 63
  dressing 62
  gait 62
  ideational 62
  ideomotor 62
  in: corpus callosum tumour 162
    precentral tumour 162
aqueduct stenosis 138, 141 (fig.)
arachidonic acid deficiency 459
arachnoid 237
arachnoidal cyst 151, 169, 402
arachnoiditis 401
  lumbo-sacral 401
archicortex 12
arecoline 8
argininaemia 452
arginine vasopressin 593
arginosuccinicaciduria 452
Argyll Robertson pupil 103, 104
  in: facial hemiatrophy 388
    general paresis 267
    progressive hypertrophic
      polyneuropathy 546
    tabes dorsalis 270
Arnold–Chiari malformation 138, 417, 608
  hydrocephalus-associated 138
  spina bifida-associated 418
arsenical polyneuropathy 533
arteriovenous angioma 208
arteriovenous malformations 149
artery of Adamkiewicz 390, 423
arthrogryposis multiplex congenita 384, 583
arylsulphatase A deficiency 460
arylsulphatase B deficiency 460
ascending reticular activating system 640–1
aspartic acid 6, 9
aspartylglucosaminuria 466–7
aspergillosis 249
aspirin
  for: amaurosis fugax 199
    ischaemic stroke prevention 199
    poliomyelitis 284
    transient ischaemic attacks 199
astereognosis 45, 63
asterixis 331
astigmatism 84
astroblastoma 145
  spinal 401
astrocyte 4
  fibrous 4, 6 (fig.)
  protoplasmic 4, 6 (fig.)
astrocytoma 145, 147 (figs.), 166, 170
  angiography 158
  corpus callosum invasion 163
  epilepsy due to 153
  pontine 167
  prognosis 171
  radiotherapy 171
  secretions 143
  surgical treatment 171
  third ventricle 163
ataxia 35–6
  cerebellar: acute, of infancy/childhood 304–5
    Harding's 366
    in ocular myopathy 557
    post heat stroke 444
  Ferguson–Critchley type 365 6

Friedreich's 363 4, 367
  frontal lobe 161
  Harding's cerebellar 366
  hereditary 331, 362–7
    clinical varieties 363–7
    diagnosis 367
    optic atrophy 93
    polyneuropathy 548
    rare 366–7
    retinal lesions 90
    treatment 367
  hereditary paroxysmal (periodic) 366
  in: Arnold Chiari malformation 417
    cerebellar tumour 166, 167
    general paresis 267
    gliomatosis cerebri 169
    Refsum's disease 462
    vitamin B_{12} neuropathy 480
    Wernicke's encephalopathy 476
  Marie's spastic 365
  nerve deafness–mental–retardation–motor
    neurone lesion syndrome 366
  nystagmus–vestibulo ocular reflex
    abnormality syndromes 366
  Sanger–Brown's spinocerebellar 365
  sensory 36
  in: centrum semiovale tumour 163
    parietal lobe tumour 162
    tabes dorsalis 269
  truncal (central) 36
    in cerebellar tumour 166
ataxia telangiectasia (Louis–Bar syndrome) 362
ataxic (apneustic) breathing 136, 649
ataxic cerebral palsy 352
ataxic nystagmus (anterior internuclear
    ophthalmoplegia; Ham's sign) 98, 311
atenolol, for benign familial tremor 330
atheroma (atherosclerosis) 192; see also
    cerebral atheroma
athetosis 75, 322, 323, 342–3
  bilateral 342
  post-cerebral haemorrhage 217
  unilateral 342
atlanto-axial subluxation 406, 608
atrial myxoma 200
atropine 8, 597
  action on pupil 103
  for: carotid sinus syncope 190
    organophosphorus poisoning 439
  vagal inhibition by 597
atypical facial neuralgia 111, 176, 521
audiometry 120
auditory evoked potentials 121
auditory function tests 120–1
auditory imperception, congenital
    (developmental receptive aphasia;
    congenital auditory imperception) 59
auditory memory 638
auditory neglect 64
auditory nerve, see vestibulocochlear nerve
auditory ossicles 118
auditory pathways, central 120
aural vertigo 619
auriculotemporal syndrome 597
Australian X disease (Japanese type B
    encephalitis) 277–8
auto-immune disease
  non-organ-specific 564
  polyneuropathy 544–5
automatism
  during complex partial seizure 615
  post-epileptic 614
autonomic nervous system 593–8
  anatomy 593 4
  cerebral control 593
  chemical transmission in 596–7

  function disorders 598
    post-spinal lesions 598
    sweating 598
  homeostatic function 596
  hypothalamic control 593–4
  innervation/function of autonomic effectors
    595 (table)
  pain and 598–9
  parasympathetic system, see parasympathetic
    system
  physiology 594–6
  sympathetic system, see sympathetic system
autonomic neuropathy, acute 600–1
autonomous breathing 649
autotopagnosia 64
Avellis' syndrome (palatopharyngeal
    paralysis) 132, 196
avoiding reflexes 52
axillary (circumflex) nerve 30 (fig.), 32 (fig.)
  lesions 503
  muscle supplied by 30 (fig.)
axon 3
  cellular sheath 3
  conduction along 5–6
  demyelination 9–10
  myelin sheath 3–4
  Wallerian degeneration 9–10
axonotmesis 492, 493, 525 (fig.)
azathioprine
  for: Eaton–Lambert syndrome 572
    Guillain–Barré syndrome 529
    myasthenia gravis 571
    polyneuropathy 529
    recurrent/relapsing 531
Azorean disease (Joseph disease, Machado
    disease) 366

Babcock's battery 656
Babinski–Nageotte syndrome 196
baclofen
  for: congenital diplegia/quadriplegia 353
    multiple sclerosis 313
    muscular spasms/spasticity 395
    trigeminal neuralgia 112
BAL (dimercaprol) 338
  for: lead poisoning 437
    manganese poisoning 437
    mercury poisoning 438
Bannwarth's syndrome 528
Baràny's pointing test 36
barbiturate(s)
  anaesthesia 641
  poisoning 432–3
    chronic 432
  for: cerebral oedema 137
    ischaemic stroke 199
    Reye's syndrome 254
barbiturate addiction 432
Bardet–Bell syndrome 93
basal exit foramina tumour 168
basal ganglia 17–18
  behavioural functions 636–7
  blood supply 184
  calcification 367
  connections 17
  disorders 322–5
  familial calcification (Fahr's disease) 366–7
  familial degeneration and acanthocytosis 348
  function 17–18, 29
  massive lesions 323–4
  neurotransmitter anatomy 325 (fig.)
  pathophysiology 324–5
  status dysmelinatus (état marbré) 351
  status marmoratus 351
  symptom-lesion relationship 323–4
  tumour 163

basilar artery 184
  aneurysm 207
  occlusion 195–6
    post-electric shock 443
    thrombosis in 192
    top of the basilar syndrome 195
basilar impression 605 (fig.) 607–8
Bassen–Kornzweig syndrome
    (abetalipoproteinaemia) 464, 482
Batten–Bielschowsky's amaurotic family
    idiocy 457
battered baby syndrome 231
B cells 296
Becker muscular dystrophy 55
beclamide, for epilepsy 625
Behçet's disease 259–60
Behr's syndrome 93, 366
Bell's palsy (facial paralysis) 114–16
  aetiology 114
  diagnosis 115
  pathology 114–15
  prognosis 115
  recurrent idiopathic 115
  symptoms and signs 115
  treatment 115–16
Bell's phenomenon 115
Benedikt's syndrome 46, 196
benign coital cephalalgia 176–7
benign congenital hypotonia 383, 385–6, 582
benign exertional headache 182
benign IgG paraproteinaemia neuropathy 545
benign intracranial hypertension (toxic
    hydrocephalus) 140, 169
    treatment 142
benign myalgic encephalomyelitis (epidemic
    neuromyasthenia) 259
benign positional vertigo (nystagmus)
    syndrome 124
benzhexol
  for: athetosis 343
    parkinsonian syndrome 332
  toxic effects 332
benzodiazepines 8
  adverse effects 432
  for: delirium tremens 429
    petit mal status 625
    status epilepticus 625
  tonic status due to 625
benztropine (Cogentin) 332
  toxic effects 332
benzylpenicillin (penicillin G)
  for: meningitis 244
    meningovascular syphilis 266
    Whipple's disease 262
Berg–Neel syndrome 485
beriberi 474–5
betamethasone
  for: benign intracranial hypertension 142
    cerebral oedema 137
bethanecol, for retention of urine 394
Betz cells 13, 15
biceps jerk 50
bicuculline 9
bilharzia (schistosomiasis) 261
Binswanger's disease (chronic progressive
    subcortical encephalopathy) 218
biogenic amines 8–9
birth injuries, intracranial 235–6
bismuth poisoning 438
Bjerrum's screen 87
blastomycosis 249
bladder
  care of, in paraplegia 395
  disturbances of function 393
    treatment 394
  innervation, anatomy/physiology 393

investigations of function 393
blepharospasm 116
  hysterical 664, 665
blepharospasm–oromandibular dystonia
    (Meige's syndrome; Brueghel's
    syndrome) 349
blindness
  hysterical 665
  in: amaurotic family idiocy 457
    Behçet's disease 260
    brain trauma 229
    carbon monoxide poisoning 442
    chiasm lesions 88, 165
    herpes zoster 292
    hydrocephalus 139
    hypertensive encephalopathy 205
    meningococal meningitis 241
    multiple sclerosis 310
    optic nerve glioma 166
    pituitary tumour 165
    Tay–Sachs disease 456
    temporal arteritis 220
  transient cortical 89
  see also optic atrophy
blind spot enlargement 87
blink (facial) reflexes 113
  unconscious patient 649
blood–brain barrier 186
blood–CSF barrier 65
blood pressure, cerebral tumour effect on 153
blood-vessel tumours/malformations 149–50
bobble-head doll syndrome 140
body-image disorders 63–4
  parietal lobe lesion-induced 163
body of Luys (subthalamic nucleus) 17, 324
  infarction 195
Bornholm disease (epidemic pleurodynia;
    epidemic myalgia) 290, 563
botulinum toxin 27
botulism 447–8
  infant 447
Bourneville's disease (tuberous sclerosis;
    epiloia; Brushfield–Wyatt disease) 143,
    358–9
boutons de passage 4
boutons terminaux 3, 4
brachial neuralgia 400
brachial plexus 29 (fig.), 32 (table), 499–500
  lesions 500
    diagnosis of site 501
    lower plexus paralysis
        (Dejerine–Klumpke) 500
    total paralysis 500
    upper plexus paralysis
        (Erb–Duchenne) 500
  lesions of cords 500–1
    inner medial cord 501
    lateral cord 500
    middle plexus paralysis 500–1
    posterior cord 500
  muscles supplied by 32 (table)
  post-fixed type 499
  prefixed type 499
  traction injuries 500
    treatment 498
bradycardia, in increased intracranial
    pressure 136
brain injury
  coma due to 646
  concussion, see concussion
  non-penetrating 226–36
    aetiology 226
    diagnosis 229–30
    investigations 229
    pathology 226
    symptoms and signs 227–9

treatment 230–1
  nuclear ophthalmoplegia 99
brain oedema, see cerebral oedema
brain death 650
    EEG 78, 630
brainstem 19
  abscess 251
  blood supply 184
  compression: by 8th nerve tumour 167
    hallucinations due to 651
  glioma, ventriculogram 161 (fig.)
  infarction 196
  lateral tegmental haemorrhage 216
  nuclear ophthalmoplegia due to lesions 99
  perinatal damage 352
  sensory abnormalities due to lesions 45–6
  transitory ischaemia 126
  tumours 161 (fig.), 167–8
  vertigo due to lesions 126
brainstem encephalitis 487
  brain swelling, see cerebral oedema
Brazilian spotted fever 256
Brill's disease 256
Broca's aphasia 56, 195
Brodman's area 8
  lesion of 33
bromide intoxication, chronic 433
bromide test 243
bromocriptine 8
  for: malignant hyperpyrexia 578
    parkinsonism 333
        benserazide and 333
        carbidopa and 333
        domperidone and 333
        levodopa and 333
    pituitary tumour 172
    spasmodic torticollis 342
    torsion dystonia 340
bronchus, carcinoma of 484, 486
Brown's syndrome 99
Brown–Séquard syndrome 45
  partial, in multiple sclerosis 310, 312
brucellosis 247–8
Brudzinski's sign 239
Brueghel's syndrome
    (blepharospasm–oromandibular
    dystonia; Meige's syndrome) 349
bruit
  carotico-cavernous-sinus
    aneurysm/fistula 208
  cervical 193
  cranial 154
  spinal angioma 402, 403
  tinnitus associated 121
Brushfield–Wyatt disease (tuberous sclerosis;
    epiloia; Bourneville's disease) 143,
    358–9
buckthorn neuropathy 538
Buerger's disease (thromboangiitis
    obliterans) 220
bulbar palsy
  acute thyrotoxic 568
  dysarthria 54
bulbar paralysis
  in acute lymphocytic choriomeningitis 288
bulbocavernous reflex 51
bulimia 643
bulimia nervosa 665
α-bungarotoxin 7
bunyavirus, California arthropod-borne 279
butyrophenones 8
  adverse effects 432

cachexia (diencephalic wasting) 601
  in third ventricle tumour 163
caisson disease, see decompression sickness

calcification, intracranial, radiographic
        appearance 79
calcinosis universalis 565
calcitonin, for osteitis deformans 606
calcium, for tetany 635
calcium carbimide (Abstem) 429
calcium gluconate
    for: hyperkalaemic periodic paralysis 577
        tetany 635
calcium versenate 338
    for: heavy metal naturopathy 533
        lead poisoning 437, 533
calf muscle
    contracture 418
    hypertrophy 554
cAMP (cyclic adenosine 3,5-monophosphate) 9
caloric test 122–4
    in unconscious patient 649
canal paresis 123
Canavan's diffuse sclerosis (van
        Bogaert–Bertrand syndrome) 463
canine distemper virus 301
Cannabis indica (marihuana; hashish)
        habituation 433–4
capillary angioma (telangiectasis) 149
carbachol, for retention of urine 394
carbamazepine (Tegretol)
    adverse effects 435, 624
    for: diabetes insipidus 602
        epilepsy 624, 625
            serum concentration 623
        glossopharyngeal neuralgia 128
        herpes zoster 293
        multiple sclerosis 314
        palatal myoclonus 349
        tabetic pain 271
        tinnitus 121
        torsion dystonia 340
        trigeminal neuralgia 111–12
carbon dioxide intoxication 472, 648
carbon monoxide intoxication 188, 441–2, 648
carbon tetrachloride 534
carcinoma, intramedullary metastases 401
carcinomatous motor-neurone disease 487
carcinomatous neuropathy 486–8
    clinical features 487–8
        encephalitic form 487
        myasthenic (Eaton-Lambert)
                syndrome 488
        myelopathy (myelitis) 487–8
        myopathy 488
        neuromyopathy 488
        polyneuropathy 488
        sensory neuropathy 488
        subacute cerebellar degeneration 488
        subacute necrotizing myelopathy 488
    CSF 487
    pathology 487
cardiac arrest 188
cardiac centre 19
cardiac disorders, syncope due to 189
cardiac neurosis (effort syndrome) 665
cardiomyopathy, alcoholic 428
carmustine (BCNU) 172
carnitine deficiency
    inherited 579, 589
    systemic 469
carnitine acetyltransferase deficiency 459, 469
carnitine palmityl transferase deficiency 469,
        578
carnosinaemia 454
carnosinase deficiency 454
carotico-cavernous-sinus aneurysm (fistula) 208
carotid arteritis 354
carotid angiography 194
    venous sinus thrombosis 224

carotid endarterectomy 199
carotid sinus syncope 189–90
carpal tunnel syndrome 505
    myeloma-induced 484
    in myxoedema 541
carpopedal spasm, see tetany
cassava root, cyanide in 92
cataplexy 642
    treatment 643
catatonia 161, 648
catatonic stupor 648
catechol-o-methyltransferase 8
cauda equina 22
    blood supply 390, 423
    compression 407
        lymphoma-induced 486
        myeloma-induced 484
    infarction 423–4
    injuries 397
    ischaemia 424
        intermittent claudication due to 424
        transient 424
    radiculitis 519
    tumours, back pain due to 402
cauda equina syndrome 401
caudal dysplasia (sacral agenesis) 417
caudate nucleus 17
    blood supply 184
causalgia 498
cavernous haemangioma 149, 400
cavernous sinus 222
    thrombosis 223, 224
    3rd, 4th, 6th cranial nerve damage 108
central (truncal) ataxia 36
central core disease 583, 589
central neurogenic respiration 136, 649
central pontine myelinolysis 319, 428, 470
    prognosis 429
central retinal artery occlusion 195
centrum semiovale tumour 163
cephalosporium infection 249
cerebellum 18–19
    abscess 251
    angioma, haemorrhage from 216
    ataxia, acute, of infancy/childhood 304–5
    atrophy, delayed cortical 365–6
    birth injury 236
    blood supply 184
    cells 18
    cerebral palsy due to lesions 352
    compression by 8th nerve tumour 167
    degeneration 364–6
        alcoholic 428
        primary parenchymatous 365
        subacute 488
    diplegia 352
    dysarthria due to lesions 54
    dysfunction 35–6
        in cerebellar tumour 166
    function 18–19
    haemorrhage into 216
    pressure cone (tonsillar herniation) 66, 136
    sensory supply to 41
    tumours 166–7
        hemisphere 166
        midline 166–7
cerebral abscess 169, 251
    actinomycosis 248
    EEG 78
    papilloedema due to 90
    typhoid 255
cerebral anoxia 440–1
cerebral arteries syndromes 194–7
    intracranial tumour-resembling 169
cerebral arteritis, in drug addicts 221
cerebral atheroma (atherosclerosis) 185

diagnosis 197–8
diffuse 197
investigations 197
lacunar infarction 196–7
prognosis 198
syncope 190
    see also cerebral ischaemia
cerebral atrophy, in boxers 228
cerebral circulation
    arterial 183–6
        anomalies 185
    brainstem centre control 186
    collateral channels 184–5
    disorders 183–225
    measurement of blood flow 185
    metabolism and 185–6
    vascular disease effects 185
    venous 221–4
cerebral compression, acute traumatic 228
    prognosis 230
cerebral contusion 226–7, 227
    headache 177
cerebral cortex 12–15
    electrical activity 14
    end-station 636
    functions 636
    layers 14
    lesions 34
    neurones 13–14
    precentral, see precentral cortex
    prefrontal, autonomic system control by 593
    primary sensory 41, 42
        lesions, Jacksonian epilepsy due to 46
    somatosensory 41–2
    visual, see visual cortex
cerebral dominance 53
cerebral dysfunction, effects on bladder 393
cerebral embolism 200–1
    aetiology 200
    diagnosis 200
    paradoxical 200
    pathology 200
    prognosis 200–1
    symptoms 200
    treatment 201
cerebral endarteritis 264
cerebral gigantism 468
cerebral glycosuria 602
cerebral haemorrhage 214–17
    aetiology 214–15
    corpus striatum 215
    diagnosis 216–17
    internal capsule 215
    intraventricular 216
        neonatal 216
    investigations 216
    lobar 215
    pathology 214–15
    pontine 215–16
    prognosis 217
    symptoms/signs 215–16
    thalamic 215
    treatment 217
cerebral hemispheres 12–15
cerebral hypoxia 440–1
cerebral infarction 192–4
    aetiology 192
    in migraine 177
    luxury perfusion syndrome 186
    non-embolic 193
    pathology 192
cerebral irritation (traumatic delirium) 228
cerebral ischaemia 185, 188–90
    post-open heart surgery 188
    prognosis 196
    treatment 185, 198–200

cerebral ischaemia—*cont.*
    see also cerebral atheroma; transient cerebral
        ischaemic attack
cerebral laceration 227
cerebral leptomeningitis 264
cerebral malformation 356
cerebral metabolism 185–6
    brainstem centre control 186
cerebral metastatic neoplasms 484
cerebral leucodystrophy 169
cerebral oedema (brain oedema, swelling) 137
    in: brain injury 227
        intracranial tumour 153
        stroke 198
    papilloedema due to 90, 91
cerebral palsy 351–4
    aetiology 351
    diagnosis 352–3
    extrapyramidal 352
    mental retardation associated 352
    pathology 351–2
    prognosis 353
    symptoms and signs 352–3
    treatment 353
cerebral tumour, *see* intracranial tumours *and*
        specific tumours
cerebral vascular resistance 185
cerebral veins 222–3
    thrombosis 223–4
cerebral white matter hypoplasia 357
cerebro-hepatorenal syndrome 465
cerebromacular degeneration (infantile
        amaurotic family idiocy; Tay–Sachs
        disease; Sandhoff's disease) 93, 455–6
cerebro-oculorenal syndrome (Lowe's
        syndrome; oculo-cerebral
        dystrophy) 454
cerebrospinal epidermoid (cholesteatoma) 143,
        151
cerebrospinal fluid (CSF) 64–72
    absorption 64
    appearance 65, 68–9
        blood 68–9
        fibrin clot 68
        turbidity 68
        xanthochromia 69, 70
    cells 69
        abnormalities 69
    chemical composition 65, 69–71
        acid–base balance 71
        amino acids 71
        biogenic amines 71
        creatine kinase 71
        2′,3′-cyclic nucleotide
            3′-phosphohydrolase 71
        electrolytes 70–1
        enzymes 71
        esterases, non-specific 71
        fractionation of proteins 70
        GABA 71
        glucose 70
        glutamic-oxalacetic transaminase
            (aspartate aminotransferase) 71
        glutamine 71
        homovanillic acid 71
        5-hydroxyindole acetic acid 71
        5-hydroxytryptamine (serotonin) 71
        keratin 71
        lactic dehydrogenase 71
        protein 69–70
        proteinases, acid/alkali 71
        phospholipids 70
        sterols 71
    circulation 64
    examination 68–71
    fistulae 71–2

formation 64–5
    functions 66
    in meningitis 69
    intracranial tumour 154
    methods of obtaining 66–8
        cisternal puncture 67
        lateral cervical puncture 67–8
        lumbar puncture 66–7
        ventricular puncture 67
    microbiological examination 71
    neoplastic cells in 484
    pressure 68
        pathological variations 68
        Queckenstedt's test 68
        Tobey–Ayer test 68
    rate of formation 64
    volume 65
cerebrospinal rhinorrhoea 140, 231
cerebrotendinous xanthomatosis 461
cerebrovascular disease
    classification 191
    radiation-induced 218–19
    without brain changes 219
    see also cerebral haemorrhage; cerebral
        infarction
cervical-cord lesions, orthostatic hypotension
        due to 598
cervical disc lesions 515–16
    brachial radiculopathy due to 515–16
cervical pachymeningitis 265
cervical rib 501–2
cervical rigidity (neck stiffness)
    in: acute pyogenic meningitis 238–9
        Eastern encephalomyelitis 279
        epidemic encephalitis 277
        increased intracranial pressure 136
        post-vaccinal encephalomyelitis 302
        subarachnoid haemorrhage 209
cervical spinal atrophy, congenital 418
cervical spondylosis 400, 516
cervical tabes 269
Chaddock's reflex (external malleolar sign) 51
Chagas' disease 257
Charcot–Marie–Tooth disease, *see* peroneal
        muscular atrophy 380
Charcot's joint 269, 270
    in: diabetic neuropathy 539
        spina bifida 419
        syringomyelia 414
    treatment 272
Chediak–Hegashi syndrome 464
chelating agents
    for: lead poisoning 438
        manganese poisoning 438
        mercury poisoning 438
chemoreceptors 7
cherry-red spot, macular 456, 458
cherry-red spot–myoclonus syndrome (sialidosis
        type 1) 459
Cheyne–Stokes breathing
    in: acute pyogenic meningitis 238
        cerebral haemorrhage 215
Chiari malformation, nystagmus 100
Chiari type I malformation
    spina bifida associated 418
    syringomyelia associated 412, 415
Chiari type II malformation, *see* Arnold–Chiari
        malformation
chloral hydrate addiction/habituation 432
chloramphenicol
    for meningitis 245
    optic nerve damage due to 92
chlordecone 439
chlordiazepoxide (Librium)
    for: athetosis 343
        clonic facial spasm 116

delirium tremens 429
        migraine 181
        torticollis 341
chlordiazepoxide habituation 432
chlormethiazole, for status epilepticus 625
chloroquine 440
    neuromyopathy 536
    optic nerve damage due to 92
chlorpromazine
    for: heat stroke 444
        Huntington's chorea 347
        Ménière's syndrome 127
        porphyria 45
        restless legs 585
        subarachnoid haemorrhage 211
        Sydenham's chorea 345
        tetanus 446
chlorpropamide, for diabetes insipidus 602
chlorthalidone, for benign intracranial
        hypertension 142
cholecystokinin 324
cholesteatoma (cerebrospinal epidermoid) 143,
        151
choline, for Friedreich's ataxia 364
chondrodystrophic myotonia (Schwartz–Jampel
        syndrome) 559
chondroma 400
chordoma 151, 158, 401
    radiotherapy 171
    surgical treatment 171
chorea 322, 323, 343–9
    congenital, with hemiatrophy 349
    dominantly inherited, without dementia 348
    familial, with myoclonic epilepsy 348
    gravidarum 344, 345
    Huntington's, *see* Huntington's chorea
    in: alcohol withdrawal 349
        congenital heart disease 349
        hypernatraemia 349
        oral contraceptive medication 349
        polycythaemia 349
    maniacal 344, 345
    post-cerebral haemorrhage 217
    senile 348
    Sydenham's, *see* Sydenham's chorea
chorea-acanthocytosis (familial dengeneration
        of basal ganglia and acanthocytosis) 348
choreiform syndrome 356
choreoathetosis 322
    familial paroxysmal dystonic 342
    in Hallervorden–Spatz disease 339
    paroxysmal kinesogenic 342
choriomeningitis, acute lymphocytic 288
choroid plexus 64
    papilloma 151, 209
        surgical treatment 171
chromatolysis 9
chromosomal anomalies 471
Chvostek's sign 635
chymopopain 518–19
cigarette smoking 434
    carbon monoxide inhalation 441
    polyneuropathy due to 549
cimetidine 440
cingulate gyrus lesions 593
cingulectomy 593, 638
ciliary ganglion 104
ciliospinal reflex 103
circle of Willis 184–5
circulatory arrest, complete 188
circumflex nerve, *see* axillary nerve
cirrhosis of liver, in Wilson's disease 337
cisternal puncture 67
cisternography, metrizamide 160
citrullinaemia 452
Claude's syndrome 196

claustrum 17
cleidocranial dysostosis 607
clindamycin, for meningitis 245
clioquinol
    optic nerve damage due to 92
    poisoning 439–40
clobazepam, for epilepsy 623, 625
clofibrate
    for: diabetes insipidus 602
        hypercholesterolaemia 199
clomipramine
    for: cataplexy 643
        hypnagogic hallucinations 643
        narcolepsy 643
        nocturnal enuresis 394
        periodic somnolence and morbid
            hunger 643
clonazepam
    for: epilepsy 623, 625
        familial paroxysmal dystonic
            choreoathetosis 342
        Gilles de la Tourette syndrome 350
        petit mal status 625
        status epilepticus 625
clonic facial spasm (hemifacial spasm) 116
    in herpes zoster 292
clonidine
    for: drug addiction 432
        Gilles de la Tourette syndrome 350
        migraine 181
clumsiness 44
clumsy children 63, 365
clonus 31, 49
cluster headache (migrainous neuralgia) 111
cocaine, action on pupil 103
cocaine addiction 432
coccidiomycosis 248
cochlea 118
Cockayne's syndrome 464, 548
codeine, for narcolepsy 643
codeine addiction 431; see also drug addiction
coeliac disease (non-tropical sprue),
        neurological complications 469
coenures cerebralis (Multiceps multiceps
        infestation) 260
colistemethate, myasthenia induced by 568
collagen disease
    muscle involvement 563
    neuropathy 544–5
Colorado tick fever virus 279
colour blindness 85
colour vision 85
colpocephaly 357
coma 644–8
    alpha 645
    EEG 78, 650
    hyperosmolal 470
    hypoglycaemic 646–7
    in: adrenal cortical failure 648
        alcohol intoxication 648
        anoxia 647
        brain disease 646
        carbon dioxide intoxication 648
        carbon monoxide intoxication 648
        cerebral vascular lesions 645
        diabetes mellitus 646
        disseminated intravascular
            coagulation 221
        drug intoxication 648
        encephalitis 646
        epilepsy 648
        head injury 646
        heat stroke 647
        hypercalcaemia 648
        hypernatraemia 647
        hypocalcaemia 648

hypoglycaemia 646–7
hyponatraemia (water intoxication) 647
hypopituitarism 647
hypothermia 647
hysteria 648
liver disease 647
meningitis 646
myxoedema 648
pancreatic encephalopathy 647
porphyria 450, 647
post-circulatory arrest 188
pulmonary disease 647
space-occupying lesions 645–6
subarachnoid haemorrhage 209
uraemia 646
investigation, see unconscious patient,
    investigation
prognosis 650
pupil in 649
sleep-like 602
coma vigil 645
combined system disease, see vitamin B₁₂
    neuropathy
common carotid artery
    atheroma 193
    blood flow in 186
common peroneal (lateral popliteal) nerve 31
    (fig.), 32 (table)
    lesions 510
        treatment 510–11
    muscles supplied by 31 (fig.), 32 (table)
compound nerve action potential 24–5
compression myelitis 402
compulsive water drinking 647
computerized transaxial tomography (CT) 80,
    81 (fig.)
    acoustic neuroma 156, 157 (fig.)
    arteriovenous angioma 208
    berry aneurysm, unruptured 207
    Binswanger's disease 218
    boxing injuries 228
    carbon monoxide intoxication 441
    cerebellar infarction 196
    cerebral atrophy, marihuana-induced 433–4
    cerebral haemorrhage 215, 216
    cerebral metastases 484
    disseminated intravascular coagulation 221
    glioblastoma 156
    glioma 156, 177 (figs.)
    Huntington's chorea 347
    hypertensive encephalopathy 205
    intracranial abscess 252
    intracranial birth injuries 236
    intracranial tumour 154, 156, 157 (figs.)
    lateral tegmental brainstem
        haemorrhages 216
    Leigh's disease 466
    meningioma 156, 157, (figs.)
    migraine 178
    Minimata disease 438
    multiple sclerosis 312
    presenile dementia 198
    spina bifida 419
    spinal cord compression 400, 405, 406
    subarachnoid haemorrhage 210–11
    subdural haematoma 232
    venous sinus thrombosis 224
concussion, 226, 227–8
    headache 177
    nystagmus 100
    prognosis 230
confusion 644
    in: alveolar hypoventilation 472
        porphyria 450
        typhoid fever 255
        vitamin B₁₂ deficiency 480

congenital auditory imperception 59
congenital benign myopathy 586–7
congenital cervical spinal atrophy 418
congenital diplegia and quadriplegia (congenital
        spastic paralysis; Little's disease) 351–3
    aetiology 351
    diagnosis 352–3
    pathology 351–2
    prognosis 353
    treatment 353
    see also cerebral palsy
congenital extradural cyst (intraspinal
        meningocele) 401
congenital hypomyelination neuropathy 546
congenital insensitivity to pain 548
congenital muscular dystrophy 556
congenital spastic paralysis, see congenital
        diplegia and quadriplegia
congestive attacks (apoplectiform episodes)
    267
conjunctivitis, acute haemorrhagic 290
connective-tissue disease, muscle
        involvement 563
consciousness 640–1
constitution 2
contralateral hemianaesthesia 195
contre-coup injury to brain 226, 227
conus medullaris 22
    multiple sclerosis of 312
convergence, ocular 83
convulsions, see epilepsy
coonhound paralysis 527
corneal reflex 48–9, 113
    loss of: in brainstem tumour 167
        in eighth nerve tumour 167
coronary artery bypass surgery, peripheral nerve
        lesions 501
corpora mammillaria 593–4
corpus callosum 12
    agenesis 357
    division of 53, 622
    tumours 151, 155, 163, 170
corpus striatum 17
    haemorrhage into 215
cortical evoked potentials 392
cortical word-blindness (alexia with agraphia;
        visual asymbolia; Dejerine's first type of
        alexia) 57
corticospinal/corticobulbar (pyramidal)
        tract 15–16
    in: centrum semiovale tumour 163
        corpus calosum tumour 163
        midbrain tumour 164
        precentral tumour 162
        prefrontal tumour 161
        third ventricle tumour 163
    localization of lesions 34–5
        cortical 34
        medulla oblongata 34
        midbrain 34
        pons 34–5
        subcortical 34
corticosteroids, see steroids
corticostriatonigral degeneration 331
corticotrophin (ACTH)
    for: Guillain–Barré syndrome 528–9
        myasthenia gravis 571
        petit mal status 625
        polyneuropathy 526
        disseminated myelitis and optic
            neuritis 306
    in basophil adenoma 165
    hypersecretion by pituitary basophil
        adenoma 165
    myopathy 576
    serum measurement 165

cortisone
  for: Bell's palsy 115
      Guillain–Barré syndrome 528–9
Costen's syndrome 111, 176, 521
costoclavicular syndromes 501–2
cough headache 177
cough syncope 189
Coxsackie viruses 289–90
  B5 encephalitis 280
  muscle infection 563
cranial (temporal, giant cell) arteritis 108, 194,
  220
cranial metaphyseal dysplasia 606
cranial metastases 484
cranial nerves 19
  examination of 75
  multiple recurrent palsies 108
  nuclei 20–1 (fig.)
  nutritional disorders 478
  palsies (paralysis)
    in: hydrocephalus 140
      meningovascular syphilis 264
      mumps 289
      tabes dorsalis 270
      traumatic 229
  see also specific cranial nerves
cranial polyneuritis (polyneuritis cranialis) 108,
  528, 549–50
craniodiaphyseal dysplasia 606
craniofacial dysostosis 607
craniopharyngioma 143, 150, 165–6
  optic chiasm lesion 88
  obesity due to 601
  parkinsonism due to 163
  radiographic appearance 155 (fig.), 166
  surgical treatment 171
craniostenosis (oxycephaly; acrocephaly;
  turricephaly; tower skull) 606–7
craniotubular modelling disorders 606
cranium, see skull
creatine kinase, serum/CSF, in stroke 197
cremasteric reflex 50
cretinism, endemic 469, 470
Creutzfeldt–Jakob disease (subacute spongiform
  encephalopathy of man) 274, 294, 379
  EEG 78
cri du chat syndrome 471
crocodile tears syndrome 115, 597
cryoglobulinaemia 485
  neuropathy 545
cryptococcosis 489
cuneate nucleus 19
cuneocerebellar tract 19
curare 552
Cushing's disease 165, 470, 489
  steroid myopathy 575–6
  treatment 172
cutaneous hyperpathia 598
cyclic adenosine 3, 5-monophosphate (cAMP) 9
cyclic idiopathic oedema 603
cyclical vomiting 179, 612
cyclophosphamide, for myasthenia gravis 571
cyclopia 357
cyclosporin, for exophthalmic ophthalmoplegia
cyclothymia 655
cyproheptadine, for idiopathic
  hypersomnolence 643
cyst
  congenital extradural (intraspinal
    meningocele) 401
  dermoid 401
  dorsal neurenteric 401
  hydatid (echinococcosis) 261
  intraspinal epidermoid 401
  parasitic cerebral 143, 152, 170–1
cysticercosis 260

epilepsy due to 620
  of muscle 563
cysticercus cellulosae 152
cystic fibrosis, degeneration of posterior spinal
  column in 469
cystometrogram 393
cystometry 393
cytomegalovirus infection 293, 489
cytosine arabinoside, for herpes simplex
  encephalitis 280
cytotoxic drugs 172

Dandy–Walker syndrome 138
dantrolene sodium
  for: congenital diplegia/quadriplegia 353
    malignant hyperpyrexia 578
    multiple sclerosis 313
    muscular spasms/spasticity 395
deafness
  hereditary 121
  hysterical 665
  in: compression of lateral meniscus 164
    congenital neurosyphilis 272
    eighth nerve tumour 167
    Friedreich's ataxia 364
    Guillain–Barré syndrome 528
    herpes zoster 292
    kernicterus 356
    Ménière's disease 127
    meningococcal meningitis 246
    multiple sclerosis 311
    mumps 289
  Refsum's disease 462
  lesions causing 121
  mental illness induced by 121
deanol, for Meige's syndrome 349
debranching enzyme deficiency 576–7
decamethonium 27, 552
decarboxylase inhibitors 333
decerebrate rigidity 31
decompression sickness (caisson disease) 200,
  442–3
  paraplegia 396, 424
  spinal cord dysfunction 424
deep pressure testing 39
deficiency disorders 473–83
degeneration in nervous system 9–10
Degos disease (malignant atrophic
  papillosis) 218, 367
Dejerine's first type of alexia (alexia with
  agraphia; visual asymbolia; cortical
  word-blindness) 57
Dejerine's second type of alexia (alexia without
  agraphia) 57
Dejerine–Klumpke paralysis 500
Dejerine–Sottas disease 546
de Lange syndrome 471
delayed cortical cerebellar atrophy 365–6
delirium 644
  in: heat stroke 444
    hyponatraemia 647
    poliomyelitis 283
delirium tremens 427
  treatment 429–30
delusions 651
  in dementia 658
dementia 657–61
  aetiology 658
  alcoholic 428, 429
  diagnosis of cause 660
  dialysis (progressive dialysis
    encephalopathy) 646, 660
  EEG 78, 660
  in: alcoholism 428, 429
    Behçet's disease 259
    corpus callosum tumour 163

encephalitis lethargica 276
  Friedreich's ataxia 364
  general paresis 267
  gliomatosis cerebri 169
  glycoprotein storage disease 465
  Hallervorden–Spatz disease 339
  Huntington's chorea 346
  Hurler's disease 467
  hydrocephalus 140
  metachromatic leucodystrophy 460
  motor neurone disease 374
  multi-infarct 197, 198
  olivopontocerebellar atrophy 365
  pellagra 477
  subacute sclerosing panencephalitis 280
  syphilitic leptomeningitis 264
  third ventricle tumour 163
  vitamin B_{12} deficiency 480
  post-heat stroke 444
  presenile 658
  symptoms 657–8
  see also Alzheimer's disease; Pick's disease
demyelinating diseases, classification 298–9
demyelination 9–10
dendrites 3
  morphological states 3 (fig.)
denervation supersensitivity 189
depolarization block 27
deprenyl, for parkinsonism 333
depression 655–6
  in: migraine 180
    parkinsonian state 329
dermatitis artefacta 666
dermatome 23, 42
dermoid cyst 151
1-desamino-8D-arginine vasopressin (DDAVP),
  for diabetes insipidus 602
desimipramine 8
  for nocturnal enuresis 394
desmosterol 154
developmental dysarthria 60
developmental dyslexia 60
Devic's disease (disseminated myelitis with optic
  neuritis; acute disseminated myelitis;
  diffuse myelitis with optic neuritis;
  neuromyelitis optica;
  ophthalmoneuromyelitis) 92, 306
dexamethasone
  for: acute cerebral malaria 256
    acute toxic encephalopathy 254
    benign intracranial hypertension 142
    cerebral oedema 137
    cysticercosis 260
    intracranial abscess 252
    intracranial tumour 171
    ischaemic stroke 198
    lead encephalopathy 437
    raised intracranial pressure 171
    spinal cord trauma 397
    venous sinus thrombosis 224
dextran
  for: cerebral embolism 201
    ischaemic stroke 198–9
    venous sinus thrombosis 224
dextroamphetamine sulphate, for
  narcolepsy 643
diabetes insipidus 470, 602
  in: congenital neurosyphilis 272
    Hand–Schüller–Christian disease 461
    third ventricle tumour 163
  nephrogenic 470
diabetes mellitus
  in: craniopharyngioma 166
    Friedreich's ataxia 364
    pituitary gland tumour 164
diabetic amyotrophy 539

diabetic coma 646
  hyperglycaemic non-ketotic 646
diabetic polyneuropathy 538–40
  acute painful 539
  autonomic 539
  pure sensory 539
diabetic pseudotabes 271, 539
diabetic thoracic radiculopathy 539
diacetylmorphine (heroin) addiction 431;
  see also drug addiction
dialysis dementia (progressive dialysis
    encephalopathy) 438–9, 646, 660
dialysis dysequilibrium syndrome 646
diaphyseal dysplasia 606
diastematomyelia 416, 417 (fig.), 419
diazepam (Valium)
  dependence 432
  for: clonic facial spasm 116
    congenital diplegia/quadriplegia 353
    delirium tremens 430
    heat stroke 444
    lumbar disc lesions 518
    motor neurone disease 375
    multiple sclerosis 313
    muscular spasms/spasticity 395
    occupational cramp 668
    petit mal status 625
    poliomyelitis 284
    restless legs 585
    status epilepticus 623, 625
    Sydenham's chorea 345
    tetanus 446
    torsion dystonia 340
    torticollis 341
dichlorphenamide, for hyperkalaemic periodic
    paralysis 577
dichromats 85
diencephalic syndrome of infancy
    (wasting) 168, 470, 601
diencephalic wasting (cachexia) 601
diencephalon 636–7
diffuse sclerosis (Schilder's disease) 319–20
digital-nerve neuropathy 507
digit retention/recall tests 657
dihydroergotamine
  for: migraine 180–1
    periodic migrainous neuralgia 182
dihydromorphinone addiction 431; *see also* drug
    addiction
dihydrotachysterol (A.T.10), for tetany 635
diisopropyl phosphofluoridate 8
dimenhydrinate
  for: benign paroxysmal vertigo 127
    Ménière's syndrome 127
dimercaprol (BAL) 338
dimethysergide
  for: migraine 180
    periodic migrainous neuralgia 182
dimethyl sulphoxide, for spinal cord trauma 397
dipercaprol, for heavy metal neuropathy 533
diphenylhydantoin neuropathy 537
diphtheria
  hemiplegia 543, 544
  neuropathy 524 (fig.), 543–4
  pseudotabetic 544
  spasmodic 544
diplegia 29
  cerebellar 352
  congenital, *see* congenital diplegia and
    quadriplegia
  hysterical 663–4
diploic veins 223
diplopia 96–7
  concomitant squint associated 96
  diminution by prism 108
  in: Arnold–Chiari malformation 417

botulism 447
brainstem tumour 167
  eighth nerve tumour 167
  exophthalmic ophthalmoplegia 574
  migraine 179
  multiple sclerosis 311
  ocular myopathy 557
  pellagra 477
  Schilder's diffuse sclerosis 320
  spinocerebellar ataxia 365
  tabes dorsalis 270
dipsomania 427
dipyridamole
  for: ischaemic stroke prevention 199
    transient ischaemic attacks 199
disodium calcium
    ethylene-diamine-tetra-acetate
    (CaEDTA; Versene) 437
disseminated intravascular coagulation 221
disseminated sclerosis, *see* multiple sclerosis
distal muscular dystrophy 557
distigmine (Ubretid), for retention of urine 394
disulfiram (Antabuse) 429
  neuropathy 537
  optic nerve damage due to 92
diuretics, for benign intracranial
    hypertension 142
dizziness, psychogenic 126
doll's head phenomenon (oculocephalic
    reflex) 49, 98
dominant spino-pontine atrophy 365
domperidone 333
  and bromocriptine 333
Donohue's syndrome (leprechaunism) 471
dopamine 4, 6, 8
  for carbon monoxide intoxication 442
  in parkinsonism 17, 324
dopamine agonists 333
dopamine-β-hydroxylase 8
Doppler ultrasonography, extracranial
    arteries 186, 194–5, 197
dorsal neurenteric cysts 401
dorsal root ganglia degeneration, sensory
    neuropathy due to 514
dorsal scapular nerve compression 502
Down's syndrome (mongolism) 471
drop attacks 615
  third ventricle colloid cyst-induced 163
drugs
  anticholinergic, action on pupils 103
  anti-platelet aggregation 199
  beta-blockers plus hydrallazine and diuretics
    for hypertensive encephalopathy 206
  hypotensive, for
    hypertensive encephalopathy 206
    stroke 199
  optic nerve damage-inducing 92, 94
  tinnitus-inducing 121
  vertigo-inducing 126
  see also specific drugs
drug addiction 431–5
  cerebral arteritis 221
  opiates 431
  symptoms 431
  synthetic analgesics 431
  treatment 432
  withdrawal (abstinence) symptoms 431–2
drug habituation 431
drug intoxication, coma due to 648
Duane's syndrome 99, 107
Duchenne muscular dystrophy, *see* muscular
    dystrophy
dura mater 237
dysaesthesiae 44
dysarthria 54
  post-heat stroke 444

dysarthria–clumsy hand syndrome 196, 197
dysautonomia
  acquired non-progressive 599
  familial (Riley–Day syndrome) 599
dysdiadochokinesis 36
dyskinesias 322
dyslalia 60
dyslexia
  developmental 60
  treatment 60
  word-form (spelling) 57
dysmyelinating disorders 298, 299
dysmetria 36
dysosteosclerosis 606
dysphagia
  in: Arnold–Chiari malformation 417
    eighth nerve tumour 167
dysphasia 54; *see also* aphasia
dyssynergia cerebellaris myoclonica
    (Ramsay–Hunt syndrome) 114, 266, 631
dystonia 323
dystonia musculorum deformans (torsion
    spasm) 31, 323, 324, 339–40
dystrophia myotonica (myotonia
    atrophica) 558–9
  alveolar hypoventilation in 472
  muscle biopsy 588, 590 (fig.)
  treatment 560

ear 118; *see also* internal ear
Eaton–Lambert syndrome
    (myasthenic–myopathic syndrome) 488,
    564, 570 (fig.), 571–2
  diagnosis 586
  muscle biopsy 588
echinococcosis (hydatid cysts) 261
  of muscle 563
echo-encephalography 78
  brain injury 229
  intracranial abscess 252
  intracranial tumour 154
Echo viruses 290
  infection of muscle 563
eclampsia 611
ectopic spinal cord 418
edrophonium hydrochloride (Tensilon) 569,
    571
effort syndrome (cardiac neurosis) 665
Ehlers–Danlos syndrome 218
ejaculatio praecox 601
elation (euphoria) 655
electric shock 443
electrocardiogram (ECG), subarachnoid
    haemorrhage 210
electroconvulsive therapy (ECT)
  epilepsy after 611
  unilateral 53
electrocorticography 15, 618
electroencephalography (EEG) 76–8
  acute necrotizing (herpetic) encephalitis 78
  brain trauma 229
  comatose patient 650
  dementia 78, 660
  diffuse encephalopathy 78
  dystrophia myotonica 559
  epilepsy 77, 618–19
  hepatic failure 78, 451
  herpes simplex encephalitis 280
  Huntington's chorea 347
  hypoparathyroidism 635
  hypsarrhythmia 358
  infantile neuroaxonal dystrophy 468
  intracranial abscess 252
  intracranial tumour 78, 154
  leucodystrophies 456
  locked-in coma 645

electroencephalography—*cont.*
  migraine 179
  multiple sclerosis 78
  myoclonus 630
  parkinsonism 78
  Pelizaeus–Merzbacher disease 463
  phenylketonuria 453
  progressive familial myoclonic epilepsy 632
  Schilder's disease 456
  sleep 641
  subacute sclerosing panencephalitis 78
  subarachnoid haemorrhage 210
  subdural haematoma 78
  syncope 190
  Tay–Sachs disease 456
  tetanus 446
  tuberous sclerosis 358
  unconscious patient 650
  vitamin B_{12} deficiency 480
electrogustrometry 128
electromyography (EMG) 494–6, 551, 586–7
  automatic frequency analysis 494
  Bell's palsy 115
  benign congenital hypotonia 386
  benign myalgic encephalomyelitis 259
  completely denervated muscle 494
  dystrophia myotonica 559
  familial periodic paralysis 586
  floppy infant syndrome 582
  hysterical paralysis 663
  macro EMG 586
  motor neurone disease 374
  myasthenia gravis 586
  myasthenic syndrome 488
  myopathy 488, 495
    benign congenital 586–7
    metabolic 586
    steroid 586
    thyrotoxic 586
  myotonia 495
  normal muscle 494
  partially denervated muscle 495
    fasciculation potentials 495
  peripheral nerve lesions 493
  peroneal muscular atrophy 381
  polymyositis 586
  single fibre 496
  spinal muscular atrophy 384
  syringomyelia 414
  tetanus 446
  tetany 634
  thyrotoxic myopathy 574
  torsion dystonia 340
electroretinogram 87
emepromium
  for: frequency, urgency, precipitance of
    micturition 394
    nocturnal enuresis 394
emission computerized tomography 80
  intracranial tumour 154
emotion, limbic lobe role 637–8
emotional apathy 655
emotional stability 655
emphysema, papilloedema due to 91
encephalitis
  acute haemorrhagic 354
  brainstem 487
  California bunyavirus 279
  chronic localized 611
  Colorado tick fever 279
  coma due to 646
  Coxsackie virus 290
  cytomegalovirus 293
  Echo virus 290
  epidemic, *see* epidemic encephalitis
  Far Eastern tick-borne 277

herpes simplex 169, 280
herpes zoster 292
lethargica, *see* epidemic encephalitis
    lethargica
limbic 280, 487
measles 290
  pseudotumoural picture 169
  Russian autumnal 277
  subclinical lethargic 326
  suppurative 250; *see also* intracranial abscess
  West Nile 277
  Venezuelan 279
  see also encephalomyelitis; encephalopathy
encephalography, *see* isotope encephalography
encephalomalacia
  neonatal polycystic 351
  periventricular 351
encephalomyelitis 300–5
  acute disseminated (acute perivascular
    myelinoclasis) 29 (table)
    aetiology 301
    pathology 300
  auto-immune 11
  chickenpox-complicating 304
  Coxsackie 290
  diagnosis 305
  Eastern (equine) 278–9
  experimental allergic 301
  measles 303
  mumps 289
  post-infective 11, 354
  post-rabies vaccination 301
  post-vaccinal 302
  prognosis 305
  progressive and rigidity 290
  rubella-complicating 304
  smallpox-complicating 303
  spontaneous acute disseminated 304
  treatment 305
  Western (equine) 278–9
encephalomyelopathy, acute toxic 238, 254
encephalomyelopathy, subacute necrotizing
    (Leigh's disease) 466
encephalomyocarditis of new-born 290
encephalopathy
  acute toxic 238, 254
  alcoholic 428, 429
  aluminium 438
  chronic progressive subcortical 218
  dialysis 438–9
  cystic multilocular 351
  diffuse, EEG 78
  glycine (non-ketotic hyperglycinaemia) 453
  hepatic 428
  hexachlorophene-induced 440
  in: hypoglycaemia 466
    hypoventilation 647
    inappropriate ADH secretion 647
    Minimata disease 438
    pellagra 477
    systemic carnitive deficiency 469
  lead: acute 436
    chronic 436
    treatment 436–7
  multilocular cystic 351
  necrotizing, methotrexate-induced 485
  pancreatic 647
  papilloedema due to 91
  phenytoin-induced 623
  post-anoxic 442
  post-pertussis inoculation 255
  post-vaccinal 302
  rejection 439
  subacute myoclonic, of infants 305
  sub-acute spongiform, of man, *see*
    Creutzfeldt–Jakob disease

Wernicke's 430, 475–6
endocarditis, bacterial 200
  mute juvenile 200
β-endorphin (C-fragment of β-lipoprotein) 47
enkephalin 47
enophthalmos 106
enteroviruses, polio-like syndromes 283
entrapment neuropathies 499
eosinophilic inclusion (Lewy bodies) 323, 326
ependymal cells 4–5
ependymoma 146, 147 (fig.)
  fourth ventricle 168
    radiotherapy 171
    surgical treatment 171
    ventriculogram 160 (fig.)
  spinal 401
ephedrine, for diabetic neuropathic oedema 539
epicritic sensation, recovery of 497
epidemic cervical myalgia 521
epidemic encephalitis, Japanese type B 277–8
epidemic encephalitis, Murray Valley type
    (Australian X disease) 277–8
epidemic encephalitis, St. Louis type 277–8
epidemic encephalitis lethargica (epidemic
    encephalitis type A; sleepy
    sickness) 275–7
  aetiology 275
  diagnosis 277
  cachexia (diencephalic wasting) 601
  obesity 601
  parkinsonism due to 329–30
  pathology 275
  prognosis 277
  symptoms and signs 275–7
  treatment 277
epidemic myalgia (pleurodynia; Bornholm
    disease) 290, 563
epidemic neuromyasthenia (benign myalgic
    encephalomyelitis) 259
epidemic pleurodynia (Bornholm disease) 290,
    563
epilepsia partialis continua 116, 161, 615
  measles encephalitis induced 290
epilepsy 609–30
  abdominal 612
  absence seizures (petit mal) 614
    drug treatment 622, 625
    EEG 77
    triad 614
  absence status 614, 615
    drowsiness/confusion following 648
    treatment 625
  acoustic-motor 616
  adversive 615
  aetiology 610–12
    age incidence 612
    cerebral tumour 153
    endocrine factors 611–12
    firstborn children 611
    heredity 611
    hydrocephalus 139
    local cerebral lesions 611
    menstruation 617
    metabolic factors 611–12
    migraine 612
    post-electroconvulsive therapy 611
    pregnancy 612
    rheumatic heart disease 611
    sex incidence 612
    trauma 232–3, 611
  akinetic 189, 615
  alcohol-induced 428
  ataxic (inhibitory) 615
  atonic 615
  automatism: during complex partial
    seizure 615

post-epileptic 614
benign focal, of childhood 612
carotid sinus 616
classification 610–11, 613
coma, post-convulsion 648
complex partial seizures (temporal-lobe
    epilepsy) 162, 615
    lobectomy, auditory memory defect
        after 638
    personality disorder 617
    surgical treatment 622
complex partial status 615
    drowsiness/confusion following 648
cough 616
constitutional 610–11
cursive 613, 615
diagnosis: cause 620
    nature of attack 619–20
diencephalic 616
differential diagnosis 169
drop attacks 615
epidemiology 612
evoked (reflex) 616
febrile convulsions 612
gelastic 615
grand mal, *see below* tonic–clonic seizures
hyperkinetic syndrome associated 617
in: amaurotic family idiocy 457
    carbon monoxide intoxication 442
    cerebral malformations 356–7
    corpus callosum tumour 163
    cysticercosis 260
    eighth nerve tumour 167
    encephalomyelitis 302, 303, 304
    ergotism 448–9
    Gaucher's disease 458
    general paresis 267
    gliomatosis cerebri 169
    Hallevorden–Spatz disease 339
    hereditary spastic paraplegia 363
    hypertensive encephalopathy 205
    hypoparathyroidism 635
    influenzal meningitis 238
    intracranial tumour 153
    Leigh's disease 466
    lithium poisoning 439
    metachromatic leucodystrophy 460
    Niemann–Pick disease 458
    oast-house disease 453
    occipital lobe tumour 163
    polyneuritis nodosa 219
    porphyria 450
    prefrontal tumour 161
    Schilder's diffuse sclerosis 320
    subacute sclerosing panencephalitis 280
    suprasellar meningioma 166
    Tay–Sachs disease 456
    toxocara infection 261
    transverse sinus thrombosis 223
    triethyl tin poisoning 438
    tuberous sclerosis 358
    Western encephalomyelitis 279
infantile spasms (West's syndrome) 616
inhibitory (ataxic) 615
investigation 618–19
    CSF 618
    CT 618
    EEG 77–8, 618–19
    positron emission tomography 618
Jacksonian 34, 615
    in: acute pyogenic meningitis 239
        glioma 198
        precentral tumour 161, 162
    sensory focal 46, 162, 615
    serial 161
    status 161

language-induced 616
laryngeal 613
Lennox–Gastaut syndrome 614
major, *see below* tonic–clonic seizures
mental abnormalities 617
migraine associated 178, 612
minor 614–15
    sensation 614–15
    see also absence seizures *above*
motor vehicle driving regulations 621
movement-induced seizures 616
musicogenic 616
myoclonic, *see* myoclonic epilepsy
neonatal 612
oral contraceptive induced 440
paroxysmal kinesogenic choreoathetosis
    (dystonia) 616
partial seizure secondarily generalized 615
pathology 612–13
patient's history 611
personality disorder 617
petit mal, *see* absence seizures *above*
photic 616
physical abnormalities 617
physiological nature 609–10
pleural 189
post-epileptic automatism 614
post-hemiplegic 217
post-traumatic 232–3, 611
prognosis 621
psychogenic (pseudoseizures; hysterical
    fits) 616, 619–20
psychological factors 610
reading 616
reflex (evoked) 616
reflex inhibition of fit 616
serial 617
status epilepticus, *see* status epilepticus
television 616
temporal lobe, *see* complex partial seizures
    above
threshold 610
time relationship of attacks 617
tonic 615–16
    in cerebellar tumour 166
    status 615
tonic–clonic seizures (major epilepsy; grand
    mal) 613–14
    aura 613–14
    convulsion 614
    drug treatment 623–5;
    see also anticonvulsants *and specific drugs*
    EEG 77, 618–19
    post-convulsive phase 614
    precipitating factors 613
    pre-convulsive symptoms 613
treatment 621–5
    attack 622
    cerebellar stimulation 622
    drug 622–5;
    see also anticonvulsants *and specific drugs*
    general management 621–2
    psychotherapy 625
    surgical 622
uncinate 162, 615
vasovagal attacks 620
vestibular/vestibulogenic 616
voluntary movement precipitated 616
West's syndrome (infantile spasms) 616
epiloia (tuberous sclerosis; Bourneville's
    disease; Brushfield–Wyatt disease) 143,
    358–9
epineurium 25
epsilon aminocaproic acid (EΛCΛ) 211–12
Erb–Duchenne paralysis 500
Erb's syphilitic spastic paraplegia 265

ergotamine tartrate
    for: migraine 180
        periodic migrainous neuralgia 182
ergot derivatives, for migraine 177
ergotism 448–9
erythrocyte-UFA mobility test 312
erythroedema polyneuritis (pink disease;
    acrodynia) 542
erythromycin
    for: meningitis 244
        meningovascular syphilis 266
eserine (physostigmine) 8, 27
essential startle disease (hyperekplexia) 631
ethambutol
    neuropathy 537
    optic nerve damage due to 92
ethmoid sinus mucocele 180
ethosuximide
    adverse effects 624
    for epilepsy 622
        serum concentration 623
ethotoin, for epilepsy 624
euphoria (elation) 655
evoked potentials 41, 78
examination of patient 74–6
    consciousness, state of 74
    cranial nerves 75
    emotional state 75
    gait 75
    intellectual and memory functions 74–5
    limbs and trunk 75
    muscular power and co-ordination 75–6
    reflexes 76
    sensation 76
    skull and skeleton 75
    speech and articulation 75
    sphincters 76
    trophic disturbances 76
excitatory postsynaptic potential 6
excitement 655
exophthalmic ophthalmoplegia (ophthalmic
    Graves' disease) 574–5
exophthalmos 106
external auditory canal 118
external carotid steal 185
external malleolar sign (Chaddock's reflex) 51
exteroceptors 4, 38
extracerebral/cranial arteries
    blood flow in 186
    dilatation in migraine 178
extracranial–intracranial anastomosis 199
extradural abscess 251
extradural venography 406
extrapyramidal lesions
    dysarthria 54
extrapyramidal syndromes 322–50
    in encephalitis lethargica 276
    symptoms and signs 322–4
extrapyramidal system 324
eye, skew deviation 36
eyelids
    innervation 105
    ptosis 105–6
    retraction of upper lid 105

Fabry's disease (angiokeratoma corporis
    diffusum) 462, 548
facial (tardive) dyskinesia 9, 349
facial hemiatrophy (Parry–Romberg
    syndrome) 387–8
facial muscles, primary dysfunction of 114
facial myokymia 116
    unilateral 167
facial naevus 154
facial nerve (7th cranial) 113–16
    injury 229

mimic paralysis 114
paralysis, *see* Bell's palsy; facial paralysis
reflexes 113
facial neuralgia, atypical 111
facial paralysis 114–15
in: acute lymphocytic choriomeningitis 288
birth injury 114
epidemic encephalitis 278
herpes zoster 292
leukaemia 485
malaria 256
Melkersson's syndrome 114, 550
mumps 289
Ramsay Hunt syndrome 114
syphilis 264
infranuclear 141
primary degeneration/disorder of facial
muscle 114
supranuclear 114
see also Bell's palsy
facial (blink) reflexes 49
unconscious patient 649
facial spasm 116
facio-pharyngo-glosso-masticatory diplegia
(Foux–Chavany–Marie syndrome) 195
facioscapulohumeral muscular atrophy 557
facioscapulohumeral muscular dystrophy 556–7
Fahr's disease (familial calcification of basal
ganglia) 155, 366–7
failure to thrive 168
failure to thrive–retinitis
pigmentosa–deafness–mental
retardation–spinal muscular
atrophy–hepatosplenomegaly–
adrenocortical
deficiency syndrome 459
fainting, *see* syncope
falx
calcification 237
meningioma 391
familial agenesis of vermis 366
familial cerebral amyloid angiopathy 218
familial cerebral amyloidosis 379–80
familial dysautonomia (Riley–Day
syndrome) 599
familial neurovisceral lipidosis (generalized
GM$_1$ gangliosidosis; pseudoHurler's
disease) 456–7
familial paroxysmal dystonic
choreoathetosis 342
familial periodic paralysis, EMG 586
familial syncope 188
Fanconi syndrome 454
Farber's disease (lipogranulomatosis) 461
fasciculation 35
in: motor neurone disease 372–3
Werdnig–Hoffman disease 384
fat embolism 200
febrile convulsions 612
Fechner's law 39
femoral nerve 31 (fig.), 32 (table)
lesions 509
muscles supplied by 31 (fig.), 32 (table)
Ferguson-Critchley ataxia 365–6
ferrocalcinosis 367
fetal alcohol syndrome 426
fibrillation, muscular 35
fibroblastoma, perineural, *see* acoustic neuroma
fibroma, cutaneous 360
fibromatosis, *see* neurofibromatosis
filum terminale 19–20
ependymoma 401
finger drop
in: lead neuropathy 436, 437
radial nerve paralysis 503
finger–nose test 75

parietal lobe tumour effect on 162
fingerpoint body neuropathy 583
finger wrinkling test 597
fits, *see* epilepsy
flapping tremor (asterixis) 451
flare response 597
flexion-adduction sign 521
flexion dystonia 324
flexor withdrawal reflex 391–2
floppy infant syndrome 342, 576, 582–3
flucytosine, for *Cryptococcus neoformans*
meningitis 248
fludrocortisone
for: idiopathic orthostatic hypotension 600
Shy–Drager syndrome 189
flufenamic acid, for migraine 180
flunarizine, in open heart surgery 188
fluorescent treponemal antibody absorption test
(FTA-ABS) 263
fluoride 440
5-fluorocytosine, for *Cryptococcus neoformans*
meningitis 248
fluvoxamine
for: cataplexy 643
narcolepsy 643
folate deficiency 482, 623
folic acid 623
foot drop, in lead neuropathy 436
foramen magnum tumour 168
Forbes–Albright syndrome 165
forced groping (instinctive grasp reaction) 51
form–colour sorting test 656
fortification spectra 179
Foster Kennedy syndrome 136, 153, 161
fourth ventricle tumours 168
Foux–Chavany–Marie syndrome
(facio-pharyngo-glosso-masticatory
diplegia) 195
Foville's syndrome 35, 196
Fredericksen-Waterhouse syndrome 648
Friedreich's ataxia 363–4, 367
Fröhlich's syndrome (idiopathic adiposogenital
dystrophy) 601
Froin's syndrome 70
frontal lobe
abscess 251
ataxia 161
bilateral infarction 197
functions 639
tumours 160–2
frontal-lobe syndrome 639
frozen shoulder, *see* pericapsulitis of shoulder
joint
fructose intolerance 465
fructosuria 465–6
frusemide
for: benign intracranial hypertension 142
cerebral oedema 137
functional disorders 2
fusiform cells 13
fusimotor system 27–8

GABA, *see* γ-aminobutyric acid
gait
examination of 75
festinant 328
hysterical 664
in: cerebellar tumour 166, 167
congenital diplegia/quadriplegia 352
parkinsonism 328
torsion dystonia 339-40
scissors 352
stepping 532
see also ataxia
galactosaemia 465
galactosylceramide lipidosis (Krabbe's disease;

globoid-cell leucodystrophy) 459–60
gallamine 552
gamma-encephalography 78
cerebral atheroma 197
intracranial tumour 154
spinal cord compression 406
gamma-hydroxybutyrate, for narcolepsy 643
gammopathies, benign monoclonal 485
gangliocytoma 146
ganglioglioma 146
ganglioneuroblastoma 146
ganglioneuroma 143
spinal 401
gangrene
in: diabetic neuropathy 539
ergotism 449
spina bifida 419
Ganser syndrome (pseudodementia) 660, 663
gargoylism (Hurler's syndrome) 467
gastrectomy, neurological complications 469
gastric crisis, in tabes dorsalis 270
gastrointestinal disease, neurological
complications 469
Gaucher's disease 458–9
gene(s), immune response 296–7
generalized GM$_1$ gangliosidosis (familial
neurovisceral lipidosis; pseudoHurler's
disease) 456–7
generalized smooth-muscle disease with
defective muscarinic-receptor
function 599
general paresis (dementia paralytica; general
paralysis of the insane; GPI) 267-8
congenital 272
tremor in 331
geniculate bodies 19
geniculate ganglion, herpes zoster of 292
geniculocalcarine pathway 86, 89 (fig.)
genito-femoral nerve lesions 509
gentamicin
for: brucellosis 248
intracranial abscess 252
meningitis 244
Gerstmann syndrome 356
constructional (optical) apraxia 62
developmental form 63
finger agnosia 64
giant axonal neuropathy 548
giant-cell (temporal, cranial) arteritis 108, 194,
220
giant motor units 495
giddiness
in: cerebellar tumour 166
eighth nerve tumour 167
gigantism 164, 541
Gilles de la Tourette syndrome 350
ginger paralysis 535
girdle (root) pain 269, 522
gitter cells 7 (fig.) 11, 192
glabellar tap reflex 113, 327
in parkinsonism 327
Glasgow Coma Scale 227 (table), 645
Glasgow Outcome Scale 230
glioblastoma
angiography 158
CT scan 156
epilepsy due to 153
multifocal 143
prognosis 171
radiotherapy 171
surgical treatment 171
glioblastoma multiforme 144, 146 (fig.), 170
glioma 143, 144–6
brainstem, ventriculogram 161 (fig.)
CT scan 156, 157 (figs.)
frontal lobe, angiography 158 (fig.)

optic chiasm 88, 166
optic nerve 166
pontine, radiotherapy 171
radiotherapy 171
surgical treatment 171
temporal, angiography 158 (fig.)
temporo-occipital, visual fields 89 (fig.)
gliomatosis cerebri, 144, 169
gliosis 4
global contralateral hemianaesthesia 64
globoid-cell leucodystrophy (Krabbe's disease;
    galactosylceramide lipidosis) 459–60
globus hystericus 665
globus pallidus (pallidum) 17, 324
    blood supply 184
globus tumour 151, 168
    radiotherapy 171
glossopharyngeal nerve (9th cranial) 128
    unilateral paralysis 168
glossopharyngeal neuralgia 128
glue-sniffing 434
    neuropathy 534
glutamic acid 6, 9
glutaric acidaemia 342, 453
gluteal nerves 31 (fig.), 32 (table)
    muscles supplied by (fig.), 32 (table)
gluteal reflex 50
gluten sensitivity 549
glutethimide addiction 432
glycerol, for ischaemic stroke 198–9
glycine encephalopathy (non-ketotic
    hyperglycinaemia) 453
glycogen storage disease 465
    of muscle 576–7
        vacuolar myopathy 589, 590 (fig.)
glycoprotein storage disease (polyglucosan body
    disease) 465
glycosuria
    in: cerebral tumour 153
        third ventricle tumour 163
gnathostoma infection 261
Golgi (–Massoni) tendon organs 27, 38
Gordon's (paradoxical flexor) reflex 51
Gowers, Paton, and Foster Kennedy's
    syndrome 90
Gowers' sign 554
grab reflexes 52
gracile nucleus 19
Gradenigo's syndrome 108, 110, 224
granulomatous angiitis 220, 221
graphaesthesia 39
grasp reflex
    foot 51–2, 161
    hand 51, 161
    in corpus callosum tumour 163
Graves' disease, ophthalmic 108
great-toe reflex 517
ground substance 5
growth, abnormal, in pineocytoma 164
guanethidine 597
    eye drops 575
guanidine hydrochloride 27, 552
    for Eaton Lambert syndrome 572
Guillain-Barré syndrome (acute post-infective
    polyradiculoneuropathy) 526–30
    aetiology 527
    cytomegalovirus-induced 293
    diagnosis 528
    herpes zoster-induced 292
    immunoregulation in 297
    Landry's paralysis due to 423
    pathology 527
    prognosis 528
    sensory disturbances 45
    symptoms and signs 527–8
    treatment 528–9

gumma
    cerebral 152, 264–5
    spinal cord 401
gustatory reflex sweating 597
haemangioblastoma 149–50, 166, 170
    angiogram 158, 159 (fig.)
    coincidental abnormalities 150
    cystic 166
    genetic factor 143
    radiotherapy 171
    ventriculogram 150
haemangiopericytoma 148
haematin, for porphyria 450
haematological disorders, neurological
    complications 379–83
haematomyelia 398–9, 507
haemoglobinopathies 482
haemophilia 482
haemosiderosis, superficial, of nervous
    system 211
Hallervorden–Spatz disease 339
Hallgren's syndrome 367
hallucinations 651
    auditory, temporal lobe tumour-induced 121,
        162
    hypnagogic 642–3
        treatment 643
    in: chronic bromide intoxication 433
        delirium tremens 427
        occipital tumour 163
        rabies 287
        temporal lobe tumour 427
    marihuana-induced 433
    olfactory, uncal lesion-induced 83
hallucinogenic agents 9, 434
hallucinogenic fungi 434
hallucinosis, acute alcoholic 427
haloperidol
    for: Gilles de la Tourette syndrome 350
        Meige's syndrome 349
        subarachnoid haemorrhage 211
        Sydenham's chorea 345
        torticollis 341
    parkinsonism induced by 327
    toxic effects 432
Halstead–Reitan battery 656
handedness 53
hand muscles, see muscles of hand
Hand–Schüller–Christian disease 461
Harding's cerebellar ataxia 366
Harris's sign (anterior internuclear
    ophthalmoplegia; ataxic nystagmus) 98,
    311
Hartnup disease 453–4
hashish (marihuana; Cannabis indica)
    habituation 433–4
headache 175–7
    benign exertional 182
    causes 176–7
    cluster (migrainous neuralgia) 111, 182
    cough 177
    'hangover' 176
    histamine 182
    in: alveolar hypoventilation 472
        Arnold–Chiari malformation 417
        cerebellar tumour 167
        concussion 177
        craniopharyngioma 166
        eighth nerve tumour 167
        fourth ventricle tumour 168
        gliomatosis cerebri 169
        hypertensive encephalopathy 205
        increased intracranial pressure 136
        intracranial tumour 152
        meningitis 238

tuberculous 242
    midbrain tumour 164
    multiple sclerosis 311
    pituitary tumour 165
    subarachnoid haemorrhage 209
    third ventricle tumour 163
    trauma 177
    low intracranial pressure 177
    meningeal irritation 176
    mode of production 176
    nitrite 176
    occipital 176
    psychogenic 177
    referred pain 176
    treatment 177
    vascular origin 176–7
head injury, see brain injury
head retraction 239
hearing 117–21
    tests 120–1
heart block 620
heart stroke 444, 647
heavy metal polyneuropathy 533
Heerfordt's syndrome 114
Heine–Medin disease, see poliomyelitis
hemianaesthesia, global contralateral 64
hemianopia 87
    binasal 87, 88
    bitemporal 87, 88
    in: craniopharyngioma 166
        pituitary tumour 165
    crossed, in aneurysm of posterior cerebral
        artery 207
    homonymous 87
        congruous/incongruous 87
    in: centrum semiovale tumour 163
        cortical lesions 88
        migraine 179, 180
        multiple sclerosis 310
        occipital lobe tumour 163
        pituitary tumour 165
    quadrantic (quadrantopia) 87
hemiballismus 323, 349
    contralateral 195
    post-haemorrhage in region of subthalamic
        nucleus 217
hemichorea 344
hemifacial spasm (clonic facial spasm) 116
    in Paget's disease 605
hemihypertrophy 388–9
hemiparesis and ataxia 196
hemiplegia (hemiparesis) 28–9, 33
    associated reactions 51
    congenital 354–5
    hysterical 663–4
    in: brainstem tumour 167
        cerebral haemorrhage 215
        corpus callosum tumour 163
        diphtheria 544
        ergotism 449
        general paralysis 267
        gliomatosis cerebri 169
        internal carotid artery occlusion 194
        transverse sinus thrombosis 223
    infantile 354–5
    non-progressive athetoid 342
    pure motor 195, 196–7
    spinal 35
    stuttering 194
    young adults 264
hemiplegic spasticity 33
hemispherectomy 355, 622
Hennebert's sign 126
heparin, for transient ischaemic attacks
    199
hepatic cirrhosis, neuropathy 541

hepatic coma 647
  EEG 78
hepatic encephalopathy 428
hepatic failure, neurological
    manifestations 451–2
hepatitis, active, chronic neuropathy in 541
hepatitis, infective 257
hepatolenticular degeneration, *see* Wilson's
    disease
hereditary areflexia with distal amyotrophy and
    ataxia (Roussy-Lévy syndrome) 266
hereditary ataxia 331
hereditary dentatorubral–pallidoluysian
    atrophy 366, 632
hereditary distal myopathy 381–2
hereditary haemorrhagic telangiectasia 482
hereditary hyperphosphatasia 606
hereditary myoclonic dystonia 632–3
hereditary neuropathy plus liability to pressure
    palsy 520
hereditary paroxysmal (periodic) ataxia 366
hereditary sensory neuropathy (acrodystrophic
    neuropathy) 414, 514, 548
hereditary spastic paraplegia 363
heredity 2
heredopathia atactica polyneuritiformis, *see*
    Refsum's disease
heroin (diacetylmorphine) addiction 431; *see
    also* drug addiction
herpangina 290
herpes simplex 489
  encephalitis 280
herpes zoster (shingles) 291–3, 489
  aetiology 291
  complications 291, 292
  diagnosis 292
  encephalitic 292
  generalised 292
  geniculate 292
  in tabes dorsalis 270
  limbs and trunk 291
  meningitic 292
  myelitic 292
  ophthalmic 291–2
    granulomatous arteritis 221
  pathology 291
  polyneuritic 292
  post-subarachnoid bleeding 210
  prognosis 292
  symptoms and signs 291–2
  treatment 292–3
Heubner's artery 183
  occlusion 195
hexachlorophene 440
hexachlorophene neuropathy 533
n-hexane neuropathy 534
hippocampus 638
  bilateral excision 638
  infarction 638
hippus 103
histamine headache 183
history
  family 74
  present illness 73–4
  previous illness 74
  social 74
HLA DR2 642
Hodgkin cycle 6
Hoffmann's reflex 49–50
Holmes–Adie syndrome (tonic pupils and
    absent tendon reflexes) 104–5
  Shy–Drager syndrome associated 189
holoprosencephaly 356–7
homatropine, action on pupil 103
homocystinuria 454
homonymous hemianopia 97

homovanillic acid 325, 332
horizontal cells 13
Horner's syndrome 35, 103, 106
  in: facial hemiatrophy 388
    internal carotid artery dissection 194
    lateral medullary syndrome of
        Wallenberg 196
    post-ophthalmoplegic migraine 179
    post-periodic migrainous neuralgia 182
house-bound housewife syndrome 615
H reflex 49, 324, 392
Hughlings Jackson's syndrome 132, 134, 196
human tetanus immune globulin 446
Hunter syndrome 467
Huntington's chorea 345–8
  aetiology 346
  biochemical abnormalities 346
  diagnosis 346–7
  pathology 345–6
  predictive tests 347
  prognosis 347
  symptoms and signs 346
  treatment 347
  tremor 328 (fig.), 346
Hurler's disease (gargoylism) 467
Hutchinson pupil 228
hyaline-membrane disease 351
hydatid cysts (echinococcosis) 261
hydrocephalus 137–42
  aetiology 137–8
    impaired absorption of CSF 138
    increased formation of CSF 137–8
    obstructed circulation 138
  benign intracranial hypertension (toxic
      hydrocephalus) 140–1, 142, 169
  classification 138–9
  communicating 138–9
  CSF changes 140
  dementia due to 153
  diagnosis 140
  hypertensive 137
  in: eighth nerve tumour 167
    meningococcal meningitis 241
    meningovascular syphilis 264
    medbrain tumour 164
    pineal body tumour
    third ventricle tumour 163
  incidence 139
  internal, obesity due to 601
  intracranial tumour-resembling 170
  low-pressure 139, 140, 170
  obstructive 138
  otitic 141, 224
  papilloedema due to 90
  pathology 139
  post-cerebral injury 227
  prognosis 141
  radiology 79, 140
  symptoms and signs 139–40
    infantile hydrocephalus 139–40
    post-infantile hydrocephalus 140
  toxic, *see* benign intracranial hypertension
  treatment: in infantile hydrocephalus 141
    post-infantile hydrocephalus 141–2
hydrochlorothiazide, for hyperkalaemic periodic
    paralysis 577
hydrophobia (rabies) 286–7
hydroxocobalamin
  for Leber's optic atrophy 93
γ-hydroxybutyrate 9
hydroxymethylglutamyl-coenzyme A lyase
    deficiency 453
5-hydroxytryptamine (serotonin) 6, 8, 324
  in: CSF 71
    migraine 178
  increased activity effects 637

hypaesthesia 44
hypalgesia 44
hyperglycinaemias 453
  non-ketotic (glycine encephalopathy) 453
hyperkinetic syndrome 355, 617
  amphetamines for 625
hypermetropia (hyperopia) 84
hypernatraemia in infancy 470
hyperopia (hypermetropia) 84
hyperornithaemia 452
hyperosmolal coma 470
hyperostosis of frontal bone 79
hyperoxaluria, primary, neuropathy 536
hyperpathia 44, 493, 497
hypersomnia, in congenital neurosyphilis 272
hypersomnolence, idiopathic 642, 645
  treatment 643
hypertelorism 607
hypertension, cerebral blood flow in 185
hypertensive encephalopathy 205–6
  aetiology 205
  diagnosis 205
  pathology 205
  prognosis 206
  symptoms 205
  treatment 206
hypertonia 29
  extrapyramidal 31
hyperuricaemia (Lesch–Nyhan
    syndrome) 464–5, 620
hyperventilation
  central neurogenic 153, 649
  hypocapnia due to 186, 189
  hysterical 666
hypervitaminosis A 141
hypnotics, habituation to 432
hypo-alpha-lipoproteinaemia (Tangier
    disease) 464, 548
hypocalcaemia 648
hypocapnia, hyperventilation-induced 186,
    189
hypoglossal nerve (12th cranial) 133–4
  lesions 134
hypoglycaemia 466, 489
  spontaneous 620
hypoglycaemic coma 646–7
hypoglycaemic neuropathy 540–1
hypoglycinaemia, episodic 466
hypokalaemic periodic paralysis 577
hyponatraemia (water intoxication) 470, 489,
    647
  in beer drinkers 428
hypo-osmolality 470
hypoparathyroidism, idiopathic 470, 634
  tonic–clonic seizures 635
hypopituitarism 153, 164, 165, 470
  treatment 172
hypopituitary coma 647
hypotension
  chronic orthostatic, *see* Shy–Drager syndrome
  postural 188
hypothalamus
  antidiuretic hormone production 593
  autonomic control centres 593–4
  functions 637
  nuclei 593, 636, 637
  syndromes 601–3
    adiposity (obesity) 601
    alimentary canal ulceration 602
    cachexia (diencephalic wasting) 601
    cyclical oedema 603
    diabetes insipidus 602
    respiratory disturbances 602–3
    sexual dysfunction 601
    sleep disturbances 602
    sugar metabolism disturbances 602

hypothermia 647
  accidental 444, 602, 647
  for cerebral embolism 201
  in hypoglycaemic coma 647
    Wernicke's encephalopathy 476
  spontaneous periodic (Shapiro's
    syndrome) 647
hypothyroidism, myopathy in 575
hypotonia 32–3
  cerebellar 36
  generalised muscular, in infancy 582–3
  in tabes dorsalis 269
  hypoxic–ischaemic leukoencephalopathy 441
hypsarrhythmia 78
hysteria 661–7
  aetiology 662
  diagnosis 666
  epidemic 665
  prognosis 666–7
  rabies-simulating 287
  symptoms and signs 662–6
    amnesia 662–3
    anorexia nervosa 665
    aphonia 55
    blepharospasm 664, 665
    cardiac 665
    constipation 665
    contraction of antagonistic muscles 663
    contractures 663–4
    cutaneous 666
    diarrhoea 665
    dissociation of personality 662–3
    dysphagia 665
    fits (psychogenic; pseudoseizures) 616,
      619–20, 663
    fugue 662–3
    gait 664
    involuntary movements 664
    Munchausen syndrome 666
    muscular wasting 663–4
    mutism 54
    nystagmus-like movements 101
    ocular 665
    opisthotonus 663
    pain 665
    paralysis 663–4
    production of 662
    pseudodementia (Ganser syndrome) 660,
      663
    pyrexia 666
    recurrent fainting in girls 189
    respiratory 666
    rigidity 664
    sensory 46, 664–5
    spinal 666
    tendon reflexes 664
    trance (psychogenic
      unresponsiveness) 648
    urinary 666
    vomiting 665
  treatment 667

ibuprofen, optic nerve damage due to 92
idiopathic adiposogenital dystrophy (Fröhlich's
    syndrome) 601
idiopathic hypersomnolence 642
  treatment 643
idiopathic (cyclical) oedema 603
idiopathic orthostatic hypotension 598, 599–600
idiopathic regressing arteriography 218
idiopathic rhabdomyolysis 578
idoxuridine, for herpes simplex encephalitis 280
IgM plasma-cell dyscrasia neuropathy 545
ilioinguinal nerve lesions 508–9
illusion 651

imipramine 8
  for: absence seizures 625
    nocturnal enuresis 394
    parkinsonism 332
    periodic somnolence and morbid
      hunger 643
immune response genes 296–7
immunity, disordered,
    neurological/neuromuscular diseases
    associated 295
immunoregulation 295–7
  B cells 296
  Guillain–Barré syndrome 297
  immune response genes 296–7
  multiple sclerosis 297
  myasthenia gravis 297
  network hypothesis 296
  polymyositis 297
  T cells 296
immunosuppressive drugs
  for: Guillain–Barré 529
    myasthenia gravis 571
    pulseless disease 221
  virus activation by 290
impotence 601
  in: motor-neurone disease 374
    multiple sclerosis 311, 312
    prolactinoma 165
    spina bifida 419
    tabes dorsalis 270
    vitamin B$_{12}$ neuropathy 480
impulsive disorders of conduct 655
inappropriate ADH secretion 647
inborn errors of metabolism 452–69
inclusion body myositis 565–6
incontinence of faeces, in multiple sclerosis 312
incontinence of urine, in multiple sclerosis 312
inco-ordination 35–6
increased intracranial pressure (ICP) 135–7
  continuous monitoring 135
  effects 135–7
  on: cerebral circulation 135–6
    heart rate 136
    respiration 136
    skull rigidity 136
  false localizing signs 136
  headache 136
  infratentorial lesions 136–7
  papilloedema 90, 136
  subfalcial herniation 136
  tentorial herniation 136
  tonsillar herniation (cerebellar pressure
    cone) 136
  vomiting 136
  see also intracranial tumour
indomethacin
  for: benign exertional headache 182
    periodic migrainous headache 182
    Shy–Drager syndrome 189
infantile amaurotic family idiocy
    (cerebromacular degeneration;
    Tay–Sachs disease; Sandhoff's
    disease) 455–6
infantile myoclonic encephalopathy
    (polymyoclonia) 632
infantile neuroaxonal dystrophy 468
infantile osteoporosis 606
infantile paralysis, see poliomyelitis
infantile spasms (West's syndrome) 616
infantile spinal muscular atrophy 383
infectious mononucleosis 258, 482
infective hepatitis 257
inferior colliculus 120
inferior olivary nuclei 19
inferior sagittal sinus 222
influenza 257

infra-orbital nerve injection 521
infratentorial lesions 136–7
inhibitory postsynaptic potential 6
inosiplex (isosiplex), for subacute sclerosing
    panencephalitis 280
instinctive grasp reaction (forced groping) 51
insular sclerosis, see multiple sclerosis
intention tremor 36, 310
intercostal nerve injection 522
intercostal neuropathy 522
interferon
  for: recurrent/relapsing polyneuropathy 530
    subacute sclerosing panencephalitis 280
intermittent claudication, ischaemia of spinal
    cord/cauda equina 424
internal auditory artery 184
  occlusion 196
internal capsule
  blood supply 184
  haemorrhage into 215
internal carotid artery 183
  fibromuscular hyperplasia of wall 194
  kinked 194
  occlusion 194–5
    by suprasellar meningioma 166
    cerebral blood flow effect 185
    CO$_2$ inhalation 185–6
  stenosis 192, 193, 194
    treatment 199
  thrombosis 192, 354
internal ear 118–19
  cochlear mechanisms 119
  function 119
  organ of Corti 118, 119
    degeneration 121
interoceptors 4
intervertebral-disc disease 80, 514–15
intracerebral steal syndrome 186
intracranial abscess 250–2
  aetiology 250–1
  diagnosis 252
  investigations 252
  otitic 250
  pathology 250
  prognosis 252
  symptoms and signs 251–2
  treatment 252
  see also cerebral abscess
intracranial aerocele (traumatic
    pneumocephalus) 231
intracranial birth injuries 236
intracranial haemorrhage, traumatic 227
intracranial sinuses 221–2
  thrombophlebitis in pregnancy 224
  thrombosis 224
    diagnosis 224
    in Behçet's disease 259
    investigations 224
    prognosis 224
    symptoms 224
    treatment 224
intracranial tumours 143–72
  aetiology 143
  basal exit foramina 168
  basal ganglia 163
  centrum semiovale 163
  cerebellar, see cerebellum
  CSF 154
  diagnosis of nature of tumour 170–1
  EEG 78, 154
  examination of head 154
  false localizing signs 153
  foramen magnum 168
  fourth ventricle 168
  frontal lobe 160–2
  histological classification 145 (table)

intracranial tumours—*cont.*
  incidence 143–4
  infective 152
  management of suspect 154–60
    cerebral angiography 154, 156–8
    CT scan 154, 156, 157 (figs.)
    echoencephalogram 154
    EEG 154
    emission brain tomography 154
    lumbar puncture 154
    metrizamide cisternography 160
    pneumoencephalography 154, 158–9
    positron emission tomography 154
    radiography of chest 154
    radiography of skull 155
    ventriculography 154, 159–60, 161 (figs.)
  metastatic 151–2, 157 (fig.), 170
    angiography 158
    radiotherapy 171
  midbrain 164
  mode of onset 152
  neoplastic invasion of basal meninges/skull
    base 168–9
  occipital lobe 163
  oculomotor nerve paralysis 107
  parasellar 164
  parietal lobe 162–3
  pathogenesis 143
  pathology 144
  pineal body 164
  pituitary, *see* pituitary gland tumour
  pontine 167–8
  precentral 161–2
  prefrontal 160–1
  prognosis 171
  sudden death 171
  symptoms/signs of raised intracranial
    pressure 152–3
    blood pressure disturbance 153
    epilepsy 153
    glycosuria 153
    headache 152
    hypopituitarism 153
    mental symptoms 153
    papilloedema 90, 152–3
    pulse rate disturbance 153
    respiratory rate disturbance 153
    somnolence 153
    vertigo 153
    vomiting 153
  temporal lobe 162
  third ventricle 163
  treatment 171–2
    chemotherapy 172
    radiation 171–2
    surgery 171
  see also specific tumours
intraspinal meningocele (congenital extradural
  cyst) 401
inverted reflexes 50
investigation of mental changes after cerebral
  lesions 656–7
  emotional factors 657
  intellectual deficits 656–7
  memory defects 657
  personality changes 657
  specific defects of speech/perception 656
investigation of patient 76–81
involuntary movements 75
  in: congenital diplegia 352
    encephalitis lethargica 276
    hysteria 664
    striatal disorders 322–3
  post-cerebral haemorrhage 217
involutional melancholia 656
iodine deficiency 469

iodopsin 84
iodoquinolone derivatives, optic nerve damage
  due to 92
isolated speech area syndrome 56
isoniazid
  for: Huntington's chorea 347
    tuberculous meningitis 245
  neuropathy 532
isoprinosine (inosiplex), for subacute sclerosing
  panencephalitis 280
isotope encephalography
  CSF leakage, post-skull fracture 229
  intracranial abscess 252
  presenile dementia 198
isotope ventriculography 78–9
isovaleric acidaemia 453

Jacksonian epilepsy, *see* epilepsy, Jacksonian
Jackson's law of dissolution 33
Jakob–Creutzfeldt disease, *see*
  Creutzfeldt–Jakob disease
jaw reflex 49
Jendrassik's manoeuvre (reinforcement) 29, 49,
  324
joint sense testing 39
Joseph disease (Machado disease; Azorean
  disease) 366
jugular foramen syndrome 132, 168

kanamycin
  for: brucellosis 248
    meningitis 244
  myasthenia gravis induced by 568
Kayser–Fleischer ring 337
Kearns–Sayre (oculocraniosomatic)
  syndrome 90, 557,579
Kenya fever 256
keratoconjunctivitis sicca (Sjögren's
  syndrome) 112
kernicterus 351, 356
Kernig's sign 239
  in: Eastern encephalomyelitis 279
    meningeal irritation 176, 239
    poliomyelitis 283
    post-vaccinal encephalomyelitis 302
    subarachnoid haemorrhage 209
    venous sinus thrombosis 224
Kernohan's sign (Kernohan–Woltman
  syndrome) 136, 153,167
β-ketothiolase deficiency 453
kinesia paradoxica 328
Kleine–Levin syndrome (periodic
  hypersomnolence and megaphagia) 602
Klinefelter's syndrome 471
Klippel–Feil syndrome 79, 608
Kluver–Bucy syndrome 638
knee-jerk 50
Köhlmeier–Degos disease (malignant atrophic
  papillosis) 218, 367
Korsakow-like syndrome, in third ventricle
  tumour 163
Korsakow's syndrome 426, 427–8, 429, 654
  in: arsenical poisoning 533
    syphilitic meningitis 264
    vitamin B_{12} deficiency 480
  prognosis 429
  treatment 430
Korsakow–Wernicke syndrome 654
Krabbe's disease (globoid-cell leucodystrophy;
  galactosylceramide lipidosis) 459–60
Krause's bulbs 38
Kufs' disease 457
Kugelberg–Welander syndrome
  (pseudomyopathic spinal muscular
  atrophy) 384–5

kuru 274, 294
kwashiorkor 469

labyrinthine dysfunction 36
labyrinthitis, acute 126
lactic dehydrogenase, serum/CSF, in stroke 197
lacunar infarction 196–7
laevulose, for porphyria 450
Landry's paralysis 421, 423
Lange's colloidal gold reaction 70
laryngeal crisis, in tabes dorsalis 270
laryngeal paralysis 130–1
  bilateral 131–2
  infranuclear lesions-induced 131
  in lead poisoning 436
  nuclear lesion–induced 131
  speech in 132
  supranuclear lesion-induced 131
  unilateral 131
Lasègue's sign 517
lateral cervical puncture 67–8
lateral cutaneous nerve of thigh lesions 508
lateral geniculate body 86
lateral medullary syndrome of Wallenberg 46,
  124 (fig.), 176, 196
lateral popliteal nerve, *see* common peroneal
  nerve
lateral spinothalamic tract 40–1
lateral vestibulospinal tract 17
lathyrism 478
Laurence–Moon–Biedl syndrome 93
lead poisoning 435–7
  aetiology 435–6
  diagnosis 436
  mental retardation 436
  neuropathy 534
  pathology 436
  prognosis 436–7
  symptoms and signs 436–7
  treatment 437
  urinary screen tests 436
  see also encephalopathy, lead
lead tetra-ethyl 435, 436
Leber's optic atrophy 93
lecithin, memory enhancement by 653
left handedness 53
Leigh's disease (subacute necrotizing
  encephalomyelopathy) 466
lengthening reaction 323
Lennox–Gaustaut syndrome 614
lentiform nucleus 17
leontiasis ossea 606
leprous neuritis 545–6
leptomeningitis, *see* meningitis
Lesch–Nyhan syndrome
  (hyperuricaemia) 464–5, 620
leucodystrophies, polyneuropathy 548
leuco-encephalitis, acute haemorrhagic (acute
  necrotizing haemorrhagic
  leucoencephalopathy) 305–6
leucoencephalopathy, acute necrotizing
  haemorrhagic (acute haemorrhagic
  leuco-encephalitis) 305–6
leucoencephalopathy, hypoxic–ischaemic 441
leucoencephalopathy, progressive
  multifocal 143, 485, 486
leukaemia 485–6
  acute lymphoblastic, radiotherapy for 171
  spinal cord/spinal extradural space
    deposits 401
levator palpebrae paralysis 106
levodopa 8, 324
  benserazide and 333
  bromocriptine and 333
  carbidopa and 333
  drug holiday 333

for: athetoid cerebral palsy 353
    manganese poisoning 437
    parkinsonism 332–3
    Shy–Drager syndrome 189
    spasmodic torticollis 342
    torsion dystonia 340
  side effects 324, 332
levodopa syndrome 333
levorphan addiction 431; *see also* drug addiction
Lewy bodies (eosinophilic inclusions) 323, 326
Lhermitte's sign 44, 310, 403
libido, excessive 601
Librium, see chlordiazepoxide
lightning pains 289
lightning stroke 443
lignocaine, for tinnitus 121
limb-girdle muscular dystrophy 555–6
limbic encephalitis 280, 487
limbic system 12
  ablation of cortex 638
  anatomy 637 (fig.)
  behavioural functions 637
  emotional activity 637–8
limit dextrinosis 576
lincomycin, for meningitis 245
Lindau's disease 150
  retinal angioblastoma 90
linear scleroderma (morphoea), muscle
    abnormalities 564
lipid proteinosis (Urbach–Weithe's disease) 468
lipid storage myopathy 579
lipogranulomatosis (Farber's disease) 461
lipoidoses (lipid storage diseases) 455–64
  classification 455 (table)
  EEG 78
lipoma, spinal 401
β-lipoprotein, C-fragment (β-endorphin) 47
lipoprotein disorders 464
lissencephaly (agyria) 357
listerosis 242
lisuride
  for: Meige's syndrome 349
    parkinsonism 333
lithium, for torsion dystonia 340
lithium poisoning 439
Little's disease, *see* congenital diplegia and
    quadriplegia
locked-in coma (syndrome) 196, 251, 528, 645
  prognosis 650
locomotor ataxia, *see* tabes dorsalis
logoclonia 658
lomustine (CCNU) 172
long-loop reflexes 324
long thoracic nerve lesions 502
lorazepam, for status epilepticus 625
loudness recruitment 120
Louis–Bar syndrome (ataxia telangiectasia) 362
louping-ill 277, 288
lower motor neurone (alpha neurone) 16, 23–4,
  25
lower motor neurone lesion 35
  differential diagnosis 35
  dysarthria 54
Lowe's syndrome (oculo-cerebral dystrophy;
    cerebro-oculorenal syndrome) 454
lumbar canal stenosis 517
lumbar disc lesions 516–19
  aetiology 516
  diagnosis 517–18
  prognosis 518
  symptoms and signs 516–17
  treatment 518–19
    chemonucleolysis 518–19
    lumbar extradural injection 518
    physiotherapy 519
    sacral epidural injection 518

X-ray examination 517
lumbar discography 406
lumbar puncture 66–7
  intracranial tumour suspect 154
  sequelae 67
lumbo–sacral arachnoiditis 401
lumbo–sacral joint, congenital
    abnormalities 517
lumbo-sacral plexus 508
  ischaemia 492
  neuritis 521
lung disease, chronic, of prematurity 351
luxury perfusion syndrome 186
lymphocytic choriomeningitis, acute 288
lymphomas 486
lysergic acid diethylamide (LSD) 9, 434
lysine vasopressin, for diabetes insipidus 602
lysosomal storage diseases 455; *see also*
    lipoidoses

McArdle's disease 589
Machado disease (Joseph disease; Azorean
    disease) 366
macrocephaly 357
macroglia 4
macroglobulinaemia (Waldenström's
    syndrome) 485
macroglobulinaemia neuropathy 545
macrogyria (pachygyria) 357
macrosaccadic oscillations 101
macula
  cherry red spot 90, 93
  sparing 88
main d'accoucheur 634
main succulente 414
malabsorption syndromes, neurological
    complications 469
malaria 256–7, 647
malignant atrophic papillosis (Degos disease;
    Köhlmeier–Degos disease) 218, 367
malignant hyperpyrexia 578, 647
mammillary bodies 637
mandibular nerve 109
manganese poisoning 339, 437
mania, acute 655
mannitol, for cerebral oedema 137
maple-syrup disease 453
marche à petits pas 328
Marchiafava–Bignami disease 428, 429
  prognosis 429
Marcus Gunn jaw-winking phenomenon 106
Marcus Gunn response (retrobulbar pupil
    reaction) 92, 104
Marie's spastic ataxia 365
marihuana (hashish; Cannabis indica)
    habituation 433–4
Marinesco–Sjögren syndrome 366
Maroteaux–Lamy syndrome 460
Marsden's automatic response 324
Martinotti cells 13–14
mass reflex 392
maxillary nerve 109
mazindol, for narcolepsy 643
measles 489
medial forebrain bundle 636
medial geniculate body 120
medial longitudinal fasciculus (posterior
    longitudinal bundle) 98
medial popliteal nerve, *see* tibial nerve
medial vestibulospinal tract 17
median nerve 30 (fig.), 32 (table), 504
  lesions 504–5
  muscles supplied by 30 (fig.), 32 (table)
medulla oblongata 19
  lesions 35
  tumours 167–8

see also brainstem
medulloblastoma 144, 146 (fig.), 166, 170
  prognosis 171
  radiotherapy 171
  spinal 401
  ventriculogram 160 (fig.)
megalencephaly 357
Meige's syndrome
    (blepharospasm–oromandibular
    dystonia; Brueghel's syndrome) 349
Meissner's corpuscles 38
Melkersson's syndrome 114, 550
memory 638–9, 653
  auditory, unilateral defect of 638
  defects after cerebral lesions 657
    investigation 657
  disorders, *see* amnesia
  drugs enhancing 653
  effects of cerebral surgery 638
  long-term 653
  secondary 653
  sensory 653
  short-term (primary) 653
  in 'split-brain' animal 638
  tertiary 653
  tests of 653
  verbal, drugs enhancing 653
menace reflex 87
Ménière's disease 126–7
  canal paresis 123
meningeal cry 238, 242
meninges
  anatomy 237
  carcinomatosis 168–9
  disease 237–49
  irritation 176
  neoplastic infiltration 107, 168–9
meningioma 146–8, 170
  anosmia due to 83
  CT scan 156, 157 (fig.)
  en plaque 148
  epilepsy due to 153
  frontal, dementia due to 153
  jugular foramen, near 168
  multiple 148
  optic chiasm lesion 88
  parasagittal 148, 162, 391
  psammomatous 148 (fig.)
  recurrence after apparent removal 171
  spinal 401
  subfrontal, angioplasty 159 (fig.)
  suprasellar 148, 166
  surgical treatment 171
meningism 238, 239
meningitis 237–47
  acute 237
    aetiology 237–8
    organisms causing 238
    treatment 244–5
  acute aseptic 288
  acute benign lymphocytic 288
  acute pyogenic 238–40
    CSF 239
    diagnosis 239
    electrolyte/metabolic disturbances 239
    papilloedema due to 91
    pathology 238
    prognosis 240
    sixth nerve paralysis 107
    symptoms and signs 238–9
    treatment 244–5
  aseptic 279, 289–90
  carcinomatous 484
  coma due to 646
  Coxsackie 289–90
  cryptococcal, 3rd nerve paralysis 107

meningitis—*cont.*
  Cryptococcus neoformans 248
  CSF in 69
  cytomegalovirus 293
  Echo virus 290
  epidemic serous 288
  fungal 249
  granulomatous, obesity due to 601
  in: brucellosis 247
    coccidiomycosis 248
    herpes zoster 292
    infectious mononucleosis 258
    mumps 289
    typhoid fever 255
  leptospiral 247
  listerial 242
  lymphomatous 486
  meningococcal 240–1
    adrenal type 241
    aetiology 240
    chronic meningococcaemia 241
    chronic posterior basic 241
    complications 241
    fulminating cerebral 241
    investigations 241
    pathology 240
    prophylaxis 241
    symptoms and signs 240–1
    treatment 244–5
  Mollaret's 247
  organisms causing 238
  spinal 265, 401
    tuberculous 265, 401
  treatment 244–5
  tuberculous 242–3
    aetiology 242
    CSF 242–3
    diagnosis 243
    oculomotor nerve paralysis 107
    pathology 242
    prognosis 243
    retinal tubercles 90
    spinal 265, 401
    symptoms and signs 242
    transient aseptic 242
    treatment 245
    tuberculoma associated 242
  viral 288
meningococcaemia, chronic 241
meningococcal septicaemia, acute adrenal
      failure due to (Fredericksen–Waterhouse
      syndrome) 648
meningoencephalitis, amoebic 249
meningomyelitis
  syphilitic 265
  tuberculous 401, 421
meningomyelocele 418
Menkes' kinky-hair disease
      (trichopoliodystrophy) 467–8
mental retardation
  endocrine causes 470–1
  in kernicterus 356
  non-metabolic causes 471
  non-specific 471–2
  undetermined cause 471–2
  see also specific syndromes
mental symptoms
  in: corpus callosum tumour 163
    encephalitis lethargica 276
    general paresis 267
    hypertensive encephalopathy 205
    parkinsonian syndrome 329
mephenesin carbamate, for muscular
      spasms/spasticity 395
meprobamate habituation 432
meralgia paraesthetica 508

mercury
  in: Minimata disease 438
    pink disease 542
mercury poisoning 438, 543
Merkel's disease 38
mescaline 434
mesencephalic artery syndrome 196
metachromatic leucodystrophy (sulphatide
      lipidosis) 460–1
metastases
  cerebral 484
    in fourth ventricle 168
    of medulloblastoma 144
  cranial 484
  extradural 168–9
  in sella turcica 166
  spinal 400, 408, 409
metazoal infections 260–1
metenkephalin 324
methacholine 597
methadone, for drug addiction 432
methadone addiction 431; *see also* drug
      addiction
methaqualone 535
methedrine, for periodic somnolence plus
      morbid hunger 643
methicillin, for meningitis 244
methixene (Tremonil) 332
  toxic effects 332
methoin, for epilepsy 624
methosuximide, for epilepsy 624
methotrexate 172, 440
  necrotizing encephalopathy due to 485
methoxamine 597
methsuximide 625
methyl alcohol poisoning 92, 427
methyl-n-butyl ketone 534
methylmalonic acidaemia 453
methylphenidate 8
  for narcolepsy 643
methylprednisolone, lumbar extradural
      injection 518
methysergide, for idiopathic
      hypersomnolence 643
metoclopramide, torticollis due to 341
metrizamide cisternography 160
mianserin, for idiopathic hypersomnolence 643
miconazole, for *Cryptococcus neoformans*
      meningitis 248
microangiopathy 482
microcephaly 357
microglia 4, 7 (fig.)
micrographia, in parkinsonism 328
micropolygyria 357
microsleeps 642
micturition disturbances 393–4
micturition syncope 188
midbrain 19
  contusion 229
  lesions 34
    pupillary effect 104
  tumours 164
  see also brainstem
middle cerebral artery 183
  occlusion 185, 195
middle fossa syndrome 168
migraine 177–82
  aetiology 177–8
  complicated 179
  complications 180
  course 180
  diagnosis 169, 180
  EEG 179
  epilepsy associated 178, 612
  equivalents 179
  facioplegic 179

  hemiplegic 179
  inheritance 178
  menstrual 178
  ophthalmoplegic 107, 179
  oral contraceptive induced 440
  pathology 177–8
  prodromal phase, internal carotid artery
        circulation reduced 185
  prognosis 180
  retinal 179–80
  status hemicranialis 180
  symptomatic 180
  symptoms 178–9
  treatment 180–1
  varieties 179–80
migrainous neuralgia (cluster headache) 111,
      182
Millard–Gubler syndrome 35, 196
Miller Fisher syndrome 108, 528, 530
Minamata disease 438
mind-blindness, *see* agnosia
minimal brain dysfunction 63, 355–6
minipolymyoclonus 385
Minnesota Personality Inventory
      (M.M.P.I.) 657
miosis 84
mirror writing 53, 60
misonidazole neuropathy 536–7
mitochondrial disorders 459
mitochondrial myopathies 579, 589
mitral-valve leaflet prolapse 193–4, 200
Moebius syndrome 107, 114
Mollaret's meningitis 247
Monge's disease (mountain sickness) 443
mongolism (Down's syndrome) 471
monoamine oxidase 8
monoamine oxidase inhibitors 8
  for idiopathic orthostatic hypotension 600
  toxic effects 176, 434
monochromats 85
monoclonal gammopathy neuropathy 545
mononeuritis multiplex 520, 544
mononeuropathy 520
mononucleosis, infectious 258, 482
monoparesis 28
monoplegia 28
  faciobrachial 224
  in precentral tumour 162
mood disorders 655–6
morbid hunger and periodic somnolence 643
morphine 47, 103
  receptors 47
Morvan's syndrome 45, 414, 514
motor end plate 24, 25 (fig.)
motor-neurone disease (amyotrophic lateral
      sclerosis; progressive muscular atrophy;
      progressive bulbar palsy; motor system
      disease) 370–9
  aetiology 371–2
  alveolar hypoventilation in 472
  diagnosis 374–5
  electrodiagnostic findings 373–4
    EMG 374
    motor nerve conduction 373–4
  pathology 370–1
  post-poliomyelitis 284
  prognosis 375
  pseudopolyneuritic form 373
  reflexes 374
  serum enzymes 374
  symptoms and signs 372–4
    lower motor-neurone degeneration
        372–3
    upper motor-neurone degeneration 374
  treatment 375–6
motor system 15–37

motor-system disease, *see* motor-neurone
    disease
motor unit 24, 25
mountain sickness (Monge's disease) 443
movement disorders classification 322 (table)
movement organization 15, 17
moxalactam, for meningitis 245
Moyamoya disease 192–3, 209
mucopolysaccharide metabolism disorders 467
mucopolysaccharidosis, peripheral-nerve
    entrapment 520
mucormycosis 249
Muller's law 38
Multiceps multiceps infestation (coenures
    cerebralis) 260
multiple myelomatosis 152
multiple sclerosis (disseminated sclerosis;
    insular sclerosis) 307–14
  acute 312
  aetiology 308–9
    as astrocytic lesion 299
    distribution, age, sex 309
    inherited predisposition 308
    precipitating factors 308–9
    subacute fat embolism 299
  brainstem form 312
  cerebellar form 312
  cerebral form 312
  cerebral-tumour resembling 169
  Charcot's triad 312
  CSF 311–12
  diagnosis 312–13
  diagnostic tests 78, 311–12
  EEG 78
  facial myokymia 116
  generalized form 312
  immunoregulation in 297
  mode of onset 309
  ocular symptoms onset 312
  pathology 307–8
  pregnancy and 309, 313
  prognosis 313
  sensory form 312
  spinal form 312
  symptom complexes 312
  symptoms and signs 309–11
    aphasia 310
    auditory 311
    autonomic dysfunction 311
    dysarthria 310
    headache 311
    inco-ordination 310
    intention tremor 310, 331
    mental 311
    motor 309–10
    nystagmus 310, 311
    ocular movement disorders 310–11
    optic neuritis 91–2, 310
    paroxysmal 311
    pupillary abnormalities 311
    pyrexia 311
    reflex changes 311
    retrobulbar neuritis 310
    sensory 45, 310
    sphincter control impairment 311
    trigeminal neuralgia 110, 111, 310
    vestibular 311
    visual 310–11
  treatment 313–14
mumps, nervous complications of 289
Munchausen syndrome 666
muscle 25–7
  A-bands 551
  anatomy 551–2
  antagonists 16
  continuous fibre activity 557–8

contraction 551
crush injuries 578
depolarization block 552
fixators 16
inflammatory disorders 563–7
innervation/organization in trunk and
    limbs 28
motor unit action potentials 551
muscle fibre types 26–7
neoplastic invasion 484
pain/cramp, exercise-induced, biochemical
    diagnosis 587
parasitic infestations 563
passive stretching effects 27–8
physiology 551–2
prime movers (agonists) 16
'ragged-red' fibres 557, 579, 589
specific infections 563
synergists 16
T system of tubules 551
type I/II fibres 551–2
type-grouping 552, 588, 589
ultrastructure 26
vacuolar change 589
viral infections 563
weakness/paralysis 28–9
Z-line 551
muscle biopsy 587–9
  in: Duchenne dystrophy 588, 589 (fig.)
    facioscapulohumeral dystrophy 586
    limb-girdle dystrophy 588 (fig.)
    muscular dystrophy 588
    myasthenia gravis 588
    myopathy 587–9
    polymyositis 588
    Pompe's disease 589
    striated annulets (*ringbinden*) 588, 590 (fig.)
muscle carnitine deficiency 579
muscle disorders 553–92
  biochemical diagnosis 587
  classification 553
  differential diagnosis 585–9
  electromyography 586–7
  histological diagnosis 587–9
  NMR 587
  see also specific disorders
muscles of hand wasting 507–8
  electrodiagnosis 508
  in: algodystrophy 508
    anterior horn lesions: acute 507
      slow onset 507
    arachnoiditis 507
    carpal tunnel syndrome 505
    cervical rib 501, 507
    costoclavicular syndromes 501, 507
    Déjerine–Klumpke birth palsy 507
    Guillain–Barré syndrome 507
    haematomyelia 507
    herpes zoster 507
    ischaemia/ischaemic contracture 508
    medial cord of brachial plexus lesions 507
    median nerve lesions 504, 507–8
    motor neurone disease 373, 507
    multiple sclerosis 310
    muscular dystrophy 508
    peroneal muscular atrophy 507–8
    polyneuropathy 507
    spinal cord lesions 507
    spinal cord tumour 507
    spinal muscular atrophy 385, 507
    Sudeck's atrophy 508
    syphilitic meningomyelitis 507
    trophic disorders 508
    ulnar nerve lesions 505, 506, 507–8
    vascular lesions of spinal cord 507
    ventral roots lesion 507

muscle spindles (stretch receptors) 16, 27
muscle tone 29
  postural 29
muscular dystrophy 553–7
  alveolar hypoventilation in 472
  benign X-linked (Becker) 555
  biochemical diagnosis 587
  childhood, with autosomal recessive
    inheritance 556
  classification 553–4
  clinical features 554
  congenital 556
  dysarthria in 54
  EMG 586
  facioscapulohumeral 556–7
    EMG 586
    muscle biopsy 588
  limb-girdle 555–6
    EMG 586
    muscle biopsy 588 (fig.)
  muscle biopsy 588
  ocular myopathy 557
  oculopharyngeal 557
  severe X-linked (Duchenne) type 554–5
    biochemical diagnosis 587
    EMG 586
    identification of carriers 587
    muscle biopsy 588, 589 (fig.)
    muscle fibre plasma membrane defect 553
    treatment 559–60
  X-linked scapuloperoneal 555
  treatment 559–60
muscular wasting
  in: chronic spinal muscular atrophy 384–5
    Creutzfeldt–Jakob disease 379
    motor neurone disease 403
    multiple sclerosis 309–10
    myasthenia gravis 568
    peroneal muscular atrophy 381
    scapulohumeral muscular atrophy 385
    spinal cord compression 403
    Werdnig–Hoffman disease 384
  see also muscular dystrophy; muscles of hand
musculocutaneous nerve 30 (fig.), 32 (table)
  lesions 503–4
  muscles supplied by 30 (fig.), 32 (table)
musculospinal nerve, *see* radial nerve
musician's cramp 667–8
mussel poisoning 448
mutism 54
  akinetic 280, 645, 650
  elective (voluntary) 54
  hysterical 54
myasthenia gravis 567–70
  aetiology 570–1
  alveolar hypoventilation in 472
  anti-AChR antibody measurement 569
  benign thymic hyperplasia associated 570
  classification 567
  diagnosis 569–70, 586
  dysarthria in 54
  edrophonium hydrochloride test 569
  EMG 586
  immunoregulation in 297
  incidence 568
  malignant thymoma associated 570
  muscle biopsy 588
  natural history 568
  neonatal 568
  penicillamine-induced 578
  symptoms and signs 568
  thyrotoxicosis associated 568, 575
  treatment 571
myasthenic crisis 568
myasthenic–myopathic syndrome, *see*
    Eaton–Lambert syndrome

myasthenic syndrome, drug-induced 568
myatonia 383
mycoplasma infection 258
myelin 24, 298
 amino-aciduria-induced abnormalities 454
 basic protein measurement 229
myelinoclasis, acute perivascular, *see*
  encephalomyelitis, acute disseminated
myelitis (myelopathy) 420–2
 acute transverse 421, 423
 aetiology 420–1
 compression 402
 diagnosis 421
 herpes zoster 292
 pathology 421
 prognosis 421
 symptoms and signs 421
 treatment 422
myelitis, acute disseminated (disseminated
  myelitis with optic neuritis; neuromyelitis
  optica; ophthalmoneuromyelitis; Devic's
  disease) 92, 306
myelitis, diffuse, with optic neuritis
  (disseminated myelitis with optic neuritis;
  neuromyelitis optica; ophthalmomyelitis;
  Devic's disease) 92, 306
myelitis, disseminated, with optic neuritis (acute
  disseminated myelitis; diffuse myelitis
  with optic neuritis; neuromyelitis optica;
  ophthalmoneuromyelitis; Devic's
  disease) 92, 306
myelitis, subacute necrotic 422
myelodysplasia (spinal dysraphism) 416–17
myelography 80
 cervical disc prolapse 515
 cervical spondylosis 516
 diastematomyelia 419
 lumbar disc prolapse 517
 myelodysplasia 417
 spina bifida 419
 spinal cord compression 400, 404–5
 spinal subarachnoid haemorrhage 211
 syringomyelia 414, 415 (fig.)
myeloma (plasmacytoma) 152, 484–5
 vertebral body 400
myelomalacia 421
myelo-optico-neuropathy, subacute
  (SMON) 439–40
myelopathy
 acute necrotic 423
 radiation 422
 subacute necrotic 422, 488
 see also myelitis
myeloscintography 406
myoclonic dystonia 632
myoclonic epilepsy
 adolescent 631
 Baltic 632
 familial chorea associated 348
 mitochondrial disorder associated 632
 progressive familial 632
 progressive without Lafora bodies 632
 Unverricht's progressive 631
myoclonic spinal neuronitis, subacute 290
myoclonus 75, 630–3
 action 630, 632
 ballistic movement overflow 630
 benign (hereditary) essential 631
 causes 630–1
 cortical reflex 630
 early morning 631
 EEG 630
 eyelid, with absence seizures 631
 facial 631
 in: Creutzfeldt–Jakob disease 631
   encephalitis 631

myelitis 631
 Niemann–Pick disease 458
 subacute sclerosing panencephalitis 279
 nocturnal 630
 palatal 349
 palato-pharyngo-laryngo-oculo-
   diaphragmatic 631
 post-anoxic 442
 reticular reflex 630
 spinal 290, 631
myoglobinuria 578
 in: alcoholic myopathy 578
   carnitine palmityl transferase
     deficiency 469, 578
   crush injury 578
   glycogen storage disease of muscle 576
   polymyositis 565
   tibialis anterior syndrome 585
 paroxysmal 578
 toxin-induced 578
myo-inositol, for diabetic polyneuropathy 539
myokymia 35, 557
myopathy
 alcoholic 428, 429, 578
   prognosis 429
 benign congenital, EMG 586–7
 biochemical diagnosis 587
 carcinomatous 488, 564
 corticotrophin (ACTH) 576
 definition of term 553
 drug-induced 578
 dysarthria in 54
 EMG, *see* electromyography
 endocrine 574–6
 fingerprint body 583
 in: acid maltase deficiency 577
   acromegaly 470
   carbon monoxide poisoning 578
   chronic renal failure 576
   Cushing's syndrome 575–6
   hypoparathyroidism 576
   hypothyroidism 575
   islet-cell adenoma of pancreas 577
   metabolic bone disease 576
   osteomalacia 576
   post-adrenalectomy syndrome 576
   thalassaemia 482
   xanthinuria 579
 lipid storage 579
 metabolic 576–9
   EMG 586
 mitochondrial 579, 589
 muscle biopsy 587–9
 myotubular 583–4, 589
 necrotizing inflammatory 563
 nemaline 583, 589, 591 (figs.)
 obscure congenital 583
 ocular 557
 reducing body 583
 steroid 575–6
   EMG 586
 subacute progressive, biochemical
   investigation 587
 thyrotoxic 574
   EMG 586
myopia 84
myositis
 acute suppurative 563
 inclusion body 565–6
 influenzal 563
 localized nodular 565
 tropical (staphylococcal pyomyositis) 563
myotome 23
myotonia 557
 symptomatic 558
 treatment 560

myotonia atrophica (dystrophia myotonia) 558,
  560
myotonia congenita 558
myotonia paradoxa 558
myotonic disorders 557–9
myotubular myopathy 583–4, 589
myxoedema 470
 carpal tunnel syndrome 541
 coma 648
 polyneuropathy 541
myxoedematous madness 470

naloxone, for spinal cord trauma 397
narcolepsy 641, 642–3
 diagnosis 643
 HLA DR2 642
 treatment 643
nasolacrimal reflex 113
nasomental reflex 113
nasopharyngeal carcinoma, skull base
  invasion 168 (fig.)
 radiotherapy 171
Navajo children, hereditary syndrome in 548
neck stiffness, *see* cervical rigidity
neck–tongue syndrome 521
Nelson's syndrome 165, 576
nemaline myopathy 583, 589, 591 (fig.)
neocerebellum 19
neocortex 12
neomycin, for Reye's syndrome 254
neonatal intraventricular haemorrhage 216
neoplasms arising outside nervous system
 neurological manifestations 484–91
 types of 'neuromyopathy' 486 (table)
neoplastic disorders, pathology 11
neostigmine 8, 27, 552, 597
 for: motor neurone disease 375
   myasthenia gravis 571
nerve conduction velocity measurement 496–7
nerve impulse 7
nerve plexuses, neoplastic invasion 484
neuralgia 176
 ciliary 176
 migrainous (cluster headache) 111, 182
 periodic migrainous 182
 sphenopalatine (Sluder's) 176
neuralgic amyotrophy (shoulder–girdle
  neuritis) 508, 521–2
neural progressive muscular atrophy, *see*
  peroneal muscular atrophy
neurapraxia 492, 493
neuraxonal dystrophy 548
neurilemma 5
neuroblastoma 146
neuroeffectors 4
neurofibrillary tangles
 in: Alzheimer's disease 658, 659
   parkinsonism 326
neurofibroma 360
 spinal 401
 visceral 361
neurofibromatosis (neurofibroblastomatosis;
  von Recklinghausen's disease) 143,
  359–61
 aetiology 360
 complications 361
 diagnosis 361
 pathology 359–60
 peroneal muscular atrophy, deafness,
   albinism, Axenfeld's defect and 367
 phakoma 90
 prognosis 361
 symptoms and signs 360–1
 treatment 361
neuroglia 4–5
neuroimmunology 295–7

neuroma, plexiform 360–1
neurometabolic disorders,
    neoplasm-associated 488–9
neuromuscular junction (end-plate) 24
  drug effect on 27
neuromuscular system
  segmental/peripheral organization 28
neuromuscular transmission 25
neuromyelitis optica (disseminated myelitis with
    optic neuritis; acute disseminated
    myelitis; diffuse myelitis with optic
    neuritis; ophthalmoneuromyelitis;
    Devic's disease) 92, 306
neuromyopathy, carcinomatous 488
neuromyositis 564
neuromyotonia 525, 557
neuronal ceroid lipofuscinosis 457
neuronal intranuclear inclusion disease 339
neurone 2–3, 5–6
  alpha motor 23
  axon 3
  cell body 2
  dendrites 3
  gamma motor 23
  internuncial 38, 40
  physiology 5–7
  primary afferent 23
  saltatory jumps (conduction) 3, 5
  spindle-shaped 3 (fig.)
neuronitis, subacute myoclonic spinal 290
neuronophagia 9
neuropathic keratitis 110
neuropathy (polyneuropathy;
    polyneuritis) 522–49
  acrodermatitis chronica atrophicans 548
  acrodystrophic (hereditary sensory
     neuropathy) 45, 414
  acrylamide 534
  aetiology 522–3
  alcoholic 531–2
    treatment 430
  amyloid 541–2
  brachial, post-electric shock 443
  buckthorn 538
  carcinomatous 488
  chloroquine 536
  chronic progressive 549
  cold injury 549
  congenital hypomyelination 546
  diabetic, see diabetic polyneuropathy
  diagnosis 524 6
  diphenylhydantoin 537
  diphtheritic 524 (fig.), 543–4
  distal sensorimotor 544
  disulfiram (Antabuse) 537
  dying-back 522
  ethambutol 537
  face, neck scalp 520–1
  giant axonal 548
  hereditary, with liability to pressure palsy 520
  hexachlorophene 533
  history 522
  hypertrophic 525 (figs.)
  hypoglycaemic 540–1
  in: acromegaly 541
    arsenical poisoning 533
    autoimmune diseases 544–5
    beriberi 474–5
    carbon monoxide poisoning 442
    Cockayne's syndrome 548
    collagen diseases 544–5
    gigantism 541
    glue-sniffers 534
    heavy metal poisoning 533
    hereditary ataxias 548
    herpes zoster 292

Krabbe's disease 548
lead poisoning 435, 436, 534
leucodystrophy 548
lipid metabolism disorders 548
liver disease 541
malaria 256
mercury poisoning 543
metachromatic leukodystrophy 548
mumps 289
myxoedema 541
necrotizing angiitis 544
neuroaxonal dystrophy 548
peroneal muscular atrophy 548
polyarteritis nodosa 544
porphyria 450, 548
pregnancy 538
primary hyperoxaluria 536
rheumatoid arthritis 544–5
sarcoidosis 544–5
scleroderma 544–5
systemic lupus erythematosus 220, 544–5
Tangier disease (alpha-lipoprotein
  deficiency) 548
temporal arteritis 220
thyrotrophic hormone deficiency 541
Wernicke's encephalopathy 476
xanthomatosis 541
inherited 546–9
intercostal 522
ischaemic monomelic 492, 520
isoniazid 532
misonidazole 536–7
nitrofurantoin 535
non-hereditary sensory 548
nutritional: in former prisoners of war 477
  of obscure origin 477–8
organic chlorine compounds
    (insecticides) 533–4
organic solvents 534
panautonomic 549
parathion 533
pathology 523–4
perhexilene 537
post-electric shock 443
post-heat stroke 444
post-typhoid/paratyphoid 255
progressive hypertrophic 546–8
radiation injury 549
recurrent relapsing 530–1
sensory abnormalities 45
sodium cyanate 537–8
steroid-induced 544
subacute retrobulbar 478
thalidomide 535
tomaculous 520, 524
tropical ataxia 477–8
treatment 526
triorthocresylphosphate 535
uraemic 535–6
vincristine 536
neurosyphilis 10–11, 263–73
Argyll Robertson pupil 104
symptomatic 264
basal meningitis, obesity due to 601
cerebral 264–5
  CSF 265
  diagnosis 265
  endarteritis 264
  leptomeningitis 264
  pathology 264
  prognosis 265
  symptoms and signs 264–5
  treatment 266
congenital 272
general paresis 267–8
  congenital 272

gumma: of brain 152, 264–5
    of spinal cord 401
incidence 263
intracranial aneurysm 208
meningovascular 264–6
  congenital 272
  oculomotor nerve paralysis 107
  treatment 266
  tumour resembling 169
ophthalmoplegia 99
optic atrophy 93
pachymeningitis 237, 264, 265
radiculitis 265, 266
reflex iridoplegia 169, 264
secondary syphilis 263
  CSF 264
spinal 265–6
  cervical pachymeningitis 265
  CSF 266
  diagnosis 266
  endarteritis 265, 266
  meningomyelitis 265, 265–6
  pachymeningitis 265
  prognosis 266
  radiculitis 265, 266
  treatment 266
tabes dorsalis 268–72; see also tabes dorsalis
neurotendinous endings (Golgi organs) 27
neurotmesis 492, 492–3
neurotonia 524
nicotinic acid deficiency 473
Niemann–Pick disease 458
nifurtimox, for trypanosomiasis 257
night-nurse's paralysis 642
nitrate, headache produced by 176
nitrofurantoin neuropathy 535
nociceptors 38
nodes of Ranvier 3, 4, 24
nocardiosis 249
nocturnal enuresis 393, 666
  treatment 394, 667
non-progressive athetoid hemiplegia 342
nontropical sprue (coeliac disease), neurological
    complications 469
noradrenaline 468
  release at autonomic nerve-endings 596
nuclear magnetic resonance (NMR) 80
  intracranial tumour 154
  multiple sclerosis 312
  muscle disorders 587
nucleus accumbens 636–7
nucleus cuneatus (of Burdach) 40
nucleus gracilis (of Goll) 40
numb chin syndrome 484
numbness 42–4
nystagmus 99–101
  ataxic (anterior internuclear
    ophthalmoplegia; Harris's sign) 98
  causes 99–100
  central 122
  congenital 101
  degrees of 99
  familial 101
  horizontal pursuit defect 100
  hysterical 101
  in: acute lymphocytic choriomeningitis 288
    alcoholic neuropathy 522
    Arnold–Chiari malformation 417
    brainstem tumour 167
    cerebellar lesion 36
    cerebellar tumours 166, 166–7
    diffuse sclerosis 320
    eighth nerve tumour 167
    epidemic encephalitis 278
    Friedreich's ataxia 364
    hydrocephalus 140

nystagmus—*cont.*
  in: acute lymphocytic choriomeningitis—*cont.*
    multiple sclerosis 310
    neuronal intranuclear inclusion
      disease 339
    Schilder's diffuse sclerosis 320
    spinal cord lesion 100
    syringomyelia 413
    vitamin B_{12} neuropathy 480
    Wernicke's encephalopathy 476
  labyrinthine 100
  miner's 100
  optokinetic 100
  pendular 310
  periodic alternating 100
  phasic 99
  positional 99, 100, 124
  primary position upbeat 100
  rebound 100
  retinal origin 100
  see-saw 100–1
  toxic 101
  vertical 417, 476
  voluntary 101

oast-house syndrome 453
obesity (adiposity) 601
  in chromophobe adenoma 165
obturator nerve 31 (fig.), 32 (table)
  lesions 508
  muscles supplied by 31 (fig.), 32 (table)
occipital-condyle syndrome 168
occipital lobe tumours 163
occipital nerve injection 521
occipito-mesencephalic pathways 97
occipito-pretectal pathways 97
occupational cramps (neuroses; craft
    palsy) 667–8
ocular bobbing 101
ocular flutter 101
ocular motor apraxia 98
ocular movements, external 95–101
  congenital defects 99
  conjugate (version) 97
  cortical centre 97
  defective 96
  disconjugate (vergence) 97
  dissociation of conjugate lateral
    movement 98
  internuclear lesion 98
  internuclear pathways 97–8
  paralysis, *see* ophthalmoplegia
  reflex 98
  saccadic 97
    cerebellar lesion-inducing 98
  skew deviation 98
  slow-pursuit 97
  spasmodic conjugate lateral movement 98
  spasmodic conjugate vertical movement 98
  supranuclear lesions 98
  supranuclear pathway 97–8
  unconscious patient 649
ocular muscles, external 95–6
  nuclei 95
  paralysis, *see* ophthalmoplegia
  see also ocular movement
ocular myopathy 557
oculocephalic reflex (doll's head
    phenomenon) 49, 98
  absence, in unconscious patient 649
oculo-cerebral dystrophy (Lowe's syndrome;
    cerebro-oculorenal syndrome) 454
oculocraniosomatic (Kearns–Sayre)
    syndrome 90, 557, 579
oculogyric crises 276, 330, 339
oculomotor nerve (3rd cranial) 106, 107–8

compression by temporal lobe tumour 162
paralysis 106
  causes 107–8
  congenital unilateral 99
  in: cavernous sinus thrombosis 223
    cerebral aneurysm 207
    syphilitic meningitis 264
  treatment 108
  viral 108
  pupillary effect of lesion 104
  south east Asian palsy 108
  vascular lesion 108
oculopharyngeal muscular dystrophy 557
oculovestibular calorific reflex 49
odontoid process separation 400, 608
oedema
  idiopathic (cyclical) 603
  of brain, *see* cerebral oedema
olfactory nerve (1st cranial) 83
  pressure on 83, 161
oligodendrocyte 4
  interfascicular 4
oligodendroglioma 146, 147, 155 (fig.)
  spinal 401
  treatment 171
olivopontocerebellar atrophy 98, 365
olivorubrocerebellar atrophy 365
Ondine's curse 472, 642
Onufrowicz nucleus 392
Opalski cell 336
open-heart surgery, neurological
    complications 188
Ophelia syndrome 653
ophthalmic artery occlusion 195
ophthalmic Graves' disease (exophthalmic
    ophthalmoplegia) 574–5
ophthalmic nerve 109
ophthalmoneuromyelitis (disseminated myelitis
    with optic neuritis; acute disseminated
    myelitis; diffuse myelitis with optic
    neuritis; neuromyelitis optica; Devic's
    disease) 92, 306
ophthalmoplegia (ocular muscle
    paralysis) 96–7, 106–8
  acute idiopathic 99
  anterior internuclear (Harris's sign, ataxic
    nystagmus) 98
  erroneous projection of visual field 96
  exophthalmic 574–5
  external 99
  diplopia due to 96–7; *see also* diplopia
  in: Behçet's disease 259
    botulism 447
    carcinomatous neuropathy 487
    cerebellar atrophy 366
    craniostenosis 607
    diabetes mellitus 539
    diphtheria 543
    encephalitis lethargica 276
    Guillain–Barré syndrome 528
    herpes zoster 292
    midbrain tumour 164
    multiple sclerosis 311
    myasthenia gravis 568
    ocular myopathy 557
    Paget's disease 605
    pituitary tumour 165
    spinocerebellar ataxia 365
    tetanus, cephalic 445
    Wernicke's encephalopathy 476
  nuclear 99
  of conjugate lateral movement 98
  of conjugate vertical deviation 98
  of convergence 98
  painful (superior orbital fissure
    syndrome) 108

position of false image 97
posterior internuclear 98
progressive 99
squint 96
syphilitic 99
total 99
ophthalmoplegia plus 557
ophthalmoplegic migraine 107
ophthalmoscopy 89–90
opiates, addiction to 431; *see also* drug
    addiction
opipramol, for migraine 181
opisthotonus 31
  in: diphtheria 544
    hysteria 663
    midbrain tumour 164
    tetanus 445
    tetany 635
Oppenheim's reflex 51
opsoclonus 101
  in polymyoclonia 632
optic atrophy 93–4
  causes 93–4
  dominant 93
  heredofamilial (Behr's syndrome) 366
  in: cerebellar ataxia 366
    cerebral palsy 352
    craniostenosis 607
    diabetes mellitus 539
    diffuse sclerosis 320
    Friedreich's ataxia 364
    general paresis 267
    hereditary spastic paraplegia 363
    Hurler's disease 467
    infantile neuroaxonal dystrophy 468
    Krabbe's disease 459
    lead poisoning 436
    Leigh's disease 466
    lipoidoses 456, 457
    metachromatic leucodystrophy 460
    migraine 180
    multiple sclerosis 91, 310
    mumps 289
    neurofibromatosis 361
    neurosyphilis 93
      congenital 272
    Paget's disease 605
    subacute myelo-optico-neuropathy 440
    suprasellar meningioma 166
    tabes dorsalis 268, 270
    Tay–Sachs disease 456
    tropical ataxic neuropathy 477
    vitamin B_{12} deficiency 480
  Leber's 93
  pressure-induced 94
  primary 93
  prognosis 94
  secondary 93
  trauma-induced 94
  toxic 93–4
  visual fields in 94
optic chiasm 86
  compression by: craniopharyngioma 166
          pituitary tumour 165
  glioma 166
  lesions 88
  tumours in region of 164
optic fundus
  abnormalities 90
  examination (ophthalmoscopy) 89–90
optic nerve (2nd cranial) 86
  hypoplasia 93
  lesions 87, 90–4
  pupillary effects 104
optic neuritis, *see* optic neuropathy
optic neuropathy (neuritis) 91–2

aetiology 91
clinical features 92
in: multiple sclerosis 91–2, 310
    mumps 289
    serum neuropathy 538
    systemic lupus erythematosus 220
metabolic, nutritional, toxic causes 92
prognosis 94
terminology 91
vascular causes 92
optic radiation 86
blood supply 184
lesions 88
optic tract 86
lesions 88
    pupillary effect 104
oral contraceptives
cerebral embolism due to 200
side effects 440
vertebral artery atheroma associated 196
orbital pseudotumour syndrome 108, 574
orbital syndrome 168
orbital tumour 108
organic acidaemias 453
organic chloride compounds (insecticides),
    neuropathy/retrobulbar neuritis due
    to 533–4
organic solvents, neuropathy due to 534
organochlorine poisoning 439
organ of Corti 118
organophosphorus poisoning 439
demyelination 299
ornithine transcarbamoylase deficiency 452
orphenadrine hydrochloride (Disipal) 332
orthoptic exercises 108
orthostatic hypotension, chronic (progressive
    multisystem degeneration;
    Shy–Drager syndrome) 188–9, 331
oscillopsia 99, 310
in Arnold–Chiari malformation 417
osteitis deformans (Paget's disease) 604–6
osteochondroma 151
osteogenesis imperfecta 608
osteoma 151–400
osteopetrosis
autosomal recessive/dominant
    (Albers–Schonberg disease) 606
infantile 606
otolith function tests 124
ovarian dysgenesis (Turner's syndrome) 471
oxotremorine 8
oxycephaly (craniostenosis; acrocephaly;
    turricephaly; tower skull) 136, 606–7
oxytocin 593, 602

pachygyria (macrogyria) 357
pachymeningitis 237
cranial (syphilitic) 264
pachymeningitis cervicalis hypertrophica 265
Pacinian corpuscles 38
Paget's disease (osteitis deformans) 604–6
pain 44, 46–7
assessment 44
cerebral cortex role 46
cervical (glossopharyngeal neuralgia) 128
congenital indifference (pain asymbolia) 63
diaphragmatic 47
gate theory 46, 589
impairment of sensibility, in tabes
    dorsalis 269
in trigeminal area 110, 111; *see also*
    trigeminal neuralgia
modulation 46–7
muscular 47
neuropharmacology 47
occipital, in eighth nerve tumour 167

post-cerebral haemorrhage 217
pseudovisceral 47
psychogenic 521
recording 46–7
referred 47, 598–9
spontaneous 44
tabetic, *see* tabes dorsalis
thalamic 44, 46
threshold 46
transmission in peripheral nerves 39–40, 46–7
types 47
visceral 47
painful feet 477
painful legs and moving toes syndrome 525
palatal myoclonus 349
palatal paralysis 130
palatal reflex 49
palatopharyngeal paralysis (Avellis'
    syndrome) 132, 196
paleocortex 12
palilalia 54, 327
palmomental reflex 50
palsy 29
panautonomic neuropathy 549
pancreatic encephalopathy 647
pandysautonomia 528
panencephalitis, subacute sclerosing 169,
    279–80, 303
    EEG 78
Papez circuit 638
papilloedema (choked disc) 90
in: acute lymphocytic choriomeningitis 288
    Addison's disease 648
    alveolar hypoventilation 472
    Behçet's syndrome 259
    cavernous sinus thrombosis 223
    cerebellar tumour 152, 167
    cerebral abscess 90
    cerebral oedema 90, 91, 648
    cerebral tumour 152–3
    craniostenosis 607
    Devic's disease 306
    eighth nerve tumour 167
    emphysema 91
    encephalopathy 91
    exophthalmic ophthalmoplegia 574
    fourth ventricle tumour 168
    gliomatosis cerebri 169
    Guillain–Barré syndrome 528
    hydrocephalus 90
    hypertensive encephalopathy 205
    intracranial abscess 251
    intracranial sinus thrombosis 91
    intracranial tumour 90, 152
    meningitis 91
    meningovascular syphilis 264
    midbrain tumour 164
    raised intracranial pressure 90, 136
    secondary syphilis 263
    schistosomiasis 261
    subarachnoid haemorrhage 91, 209
    superior sagittal sinus thrombosis 223
    temporal arteritis 220
    transverse sinus thrombosis 223
ophthalmoscopic appearance 91
pseudopapilloedema compared 91
visual fields in 91
paracentral artery occlusion 195
paradoxical embolism 200
paradoxical flexor (Gordon's) reflex 51
paraesthesiae 44
in: acromegaly 164
    alcoholic polyneuropathy 532
    cervical rib 501, 502
    cord compression 402
    eighth nerve tumour 167

haematomyelia 399
migraine 179
multiple sclerosis 310
parietal lobe tumour 162
saxitonin poisoning 448
spinal cord compression 402
tabes dorsalis 269
tetany 634
third ventricle tumour 163
ulnar nerve lesions 506
vitamin B_{12} neuropathy 480
parageusia 129
paraldehyde, for status epilepticus 625
paralysis agitans (Parkinson's disease) 329
treatment: medical 332–3
          surgical 333
see also Parkinsonian syndrome
paramedian arteries 184
paramyotonia congenita 559
treatment 560
paranasal sinuses
carcinoma 108
sinusitis 108
paraneoplastic neurological syndromes 486
paraparesis, spastic
in: fructosuria 466
    pellagra 477
    tropical ataxic neuropathy 477
paraplegia 29, 391–2
amblyopia-associated 478
hysterical 391, 392, 663–4
in: electric shock 443
    ergotism 449
    hypertensive encephalopathy 205
    malaria 256
    multiple sclerosis 309–10
    spinal syphilis 265, 266
Jamaican 478
patient care 394–6
psychotherapy 396
spastic, in prisoners of war 478
paraplegia-in-extension 33, 391–2
paraplegia-in-flexion 33, 391–2
parasellar region
lesions 170
tumours 164
parasellar syndrome 168
parasitic cysts, cerebral 143, 152, 170–1
parasympathetic system 594
clinical tests 597
see also autonomic nervous system
parasympathomimetic drugs 597
parathion polyneuropathy 533
paratyphoid fever 255
paresis 28–9
parietal lobe tumour 162–3
Parinaud's syndrome 98, 164
Parkinsonian syndrome (Parkinsonism) 325–36
aetiology 326–7
akinesia 327–8
akithisia 328
atherosclerotic 197, 198, 327, 329, 330
attitude 327
autonomic symptoms 329
biochemical changes 326
bradykinesia 327–8
cholinergic activation in thalamostriate
    neurones 324
diagnosis 330–1
dopamine concentration in basal ganglia 324
drug-induced 326–7
EEG 78
facies 327
familial fatal 327
gait 328
gamma innervation disorder 324

Parkinsonian syndrome
  (Parkinsonism)—*cont.*
  glabellar tap sign 49, 327
  hemiplegic 327
  in: Behçet's disease 259
    craniopharyngioma 163
    encephalitis 276
    manganese poisoning 437
    olivopontocerebellar atrophy 365
  mental state 329
  micrographia 328
  movement disorders 327–8
  oculogyric crises 330
  ocular manifestations 327
  pathology 325–6
  pill-rolling movement 328
  post-carbon monoxide poisoning 442
  post-encephalitis lethargica 329–30
  reflexes 329
  rigidity 323, 328
  symptoms and signs 327–9
    sensory 329
  treatment: medical 332–3
      surgical 333
  tremor 323, 328
    static 328
parkinsonism-dementia complex 327, 329, 331
Parkinson's disease, *see* paralysis agitans
parosmia 83
paroxysmal cerebral dysrhythmia 609
paroxysmal kinesogenic choreoathetosis
  (dystonia) 342, 616
paroxysmal nocturnal haemoglobinuria 482
Parry–Romberg syndrome (facial
  hemiatrophy) 387–8
PAS, for meningitis 245
past-pointing 36
pathological drunkenness 427
pathological reactions in nervous system 10–11
patient-operated selector mechanisms
  (POSSUM) 396
peduncular hallucinosis 651
Pelizaeus–Merzbacher disease 463
pellagra 476–7
pendular reflex 344
penicillamine 338
  for heavy metal neuropathy 533
  myasthenia gravis induced by 578
  polymyositis induced by 578
  side effects 338
penicillin
  for: general paralysis 268
    leptospiral meningitis 247
    meningovascular syphilis 266
penicillin G *see* benzylpenicillin
pentazocine, for narcolepsy 643
pentazocine addiction 431; *see also* drug
  addiction
pentolinium, for hypertensive
  encephalopathy 206
pentoxifylline
  for: ischaemic stroke prevention 199
    transient ischaemic attacks 199
perforating ulcer
  in: peroneal muscular atrophy 381
    tabes dorsalis 270
pergolide 333
perhexilene neuropathy 537
periarteritis nodosa (polyarteritis nodosa) 219
pericapsulitis of shoulder joint (frozen
  shoulder) 493, 503
  in algodystrophy 499
  sympathectomy 599
perifornical nucleus 637
perimetry
  confrontation 87

mechanical 87
perinatal trauma 236
perineuritis, inflammatory sensory 544
perineurium 25
periodic hypersomnolence and megaphagia
  (Kleine–Levin syndrome) 602
periodic migrainous neuralgia 182
periodic paralysis
  biochemical diagnosis 587
  hyperkalaemic (adynamia episodica
    hereditaria) 577
  hypokalaemic 577
  sodium-responsive normokalaemic 557–8
  thyrotoxic 575
periodic somnolence and morbid hunger 643
peripheral nerves 24–5, 492–550
  cutaneous areas 43 (fig.)
  neoplastic invasion 484
  sensory abnormalities 45
  traumatic (and allied) lesions 492–8
    diagnosis of nature of 493–7
    electrophysiological techniques 494
    EMG 494–5
    ischaemic 492
    myelography 493
    nerve conduction velocity
      measurement 496–7
    pressure neuropathy 492
    procaine nerve-block 494
    recovery 497
    sweating responses 494
    tests 493–7
    treatment 497–8
  tumours 492
  see also neuropathy
periventricular encephalomalacia 351
pernicious anaemia 479, 480, 481; *see also*
  vitamin B_{12} neuropathy
peroneal muscular atrophy (neural progressive
  muscular atrophy; Charcot–Marie–Tooth
  disease) 380–3
  aetiology 381
  diagnosis 381–2
  pathology 380–1
  polyneuropathy 548
  prognosis 382
  symptoms and signs 381
  treatment 382
peroneal nerves 31 (fig.)
  muscles supplied by 31 (fig.)
persistent vegetative state 228, 230, 645
  prognosis 650
personality
  assessment 657
  change: in brain damage 639
    gliomatosis cerebri 169
  frontal lobes and 639
pes cavus, in spina bifida 418
pethidine (meperidine)
  for: headache 177, 211
    tabetic crisis 272
pethidine (meperidine) addiction 431; *see also*
  drug addiction
petrosal sinuses 222
  thrombophlebitis 224
phaeochromocytoma 205
phakoma 90, 361
phantom limb 44, 63–4
pharyngeal plexus 129
pharyngeal reflex 49
pharyngeal spasm, in rabies 287
pharynx 130
  paralysis 130
phenazocine addiction 431; *see also* drug
  addiction
phencyclidine 434

phenelzine, for migraine 181
phenobarbitone
  adverse reactions 435, 623
  for: athetosis 343
    epilepsy 622, 624
      serum concentration 623
    status epilepticus 625
    Sydenham's chorea 345
phenol intrathecal injection
  for: flexor spasms 395
    spasticity 353
phenothiazines 8, 324
  for subarachnoid haemorrhage 211
  parkinsonism due to 327
phenoxybenzamine 393, 597
  for: cerebral embolism 201
    retention of urine 394
phensuximide 625
phentolamine 597
phenylephrine 597
phenylethylacetylurea, for epilepsy 624
phenylketonuria 453
phenytoin sodium (Epanutin; Dilantin)
  adverse effects 435, 623, 624
  for: epilepsy 623, 624, 625
    serum concentration 623
    muscular dystrophy 560
    status epilepticus 625
    tinnitus 121
  myasthenia induced by 568
  teratogenic effect 624
phobic anxiety depersonalization syndrome 620
phosphofructokinase deficiency 576
phosphoglucomutase defect 576
phosphoglycerate mutase deficiency 576
phrenic nerve 499
  irritation 499
  paralysis 499
physostigmine (eserine) 8, 27, 552
  action on pupil 103
  for Friedreich's ataxia 364
  memory enhancement by 653
pia mater 237
Pick's disease 659, 660
Pickwickian syndrome 472, 642
pill-rolling movement 328
pilocarpine 103, 597
pindolol
  for: benign familial tremor 330
    chronic orthostatic hypotension 189
    idiopathic orthostatic hypotension 600
pineal body 155
  tumours 164
pinealoma 151, 171
pineoblastoma 164
pineocytoma 164
ping-pong gaze 98
pink disease (erythroedema polyneuritis;
  acrodynia) 542–3
piracetam, memory enhancement by 653
pitressin, for diabetes insipidus 602
pituitary apoplexy 165, 647
pituitary disease, muscle disorders in 575–6
pituitary tumours 150–1, 164–5
  adenocarcinoma 151
  basophil adenoma 165
  chromophobe adenoma 165
    obesity due to 601
    pneumoencephalogram 159 (fig.)
    third-nerve paralysis 107
    visual effects 88 (fig.)
  growth hormone-secreting 164–5
  pressure symptoms 165
  prolactinoma 165
    obesity due to 601
  radiographic appearance 165

treatment 171, 172
pizotifen
 for: benign recurrent vertigo 127
  idiopathic hypersomnolence 643
  migraine 180
plantar interdigital nerves 510
plantar nerves 510
plantar reflex (response) 50–1
 equivocal 51
 extensor 51
 flexor 50–1
plasmacytoma (myeloma) 152, 484–5
plasmapheresis
 for: myasthenia gravis 571
  polyneuropathy 529
   recurrent/relapsing 531
platybasia 607
pleural epilepsy 189
pleurodynia (epidemic myalgia; Bornholm
  disease) 290
pneumocephalus, traumatic (intracranial
  aerocele) 231
pneumococci, resistant 244
pneumoencephalography 158–9
 cerebral atrophy, marihuana-induced 433
 Huntington's chorea 347
 intracranial tumour 154, 158–9
 normal appearance 159 (fig.)
 pituitary chromophobe adenoma 159 (fig.)
 presenile dementia 198
 tuberous sclerosis 358
pneumonitis (atypical pneumonia), in acute
  lymphocytic choriomeningitis 288
podophyllum 440
polar spongioblastoma 145
poliodystrophy, progressive 467
polioencephalitis 282, 283
 treatment 285
poliomyelitis (infantile paralysis; Heine–Medin
  disease) 282
 aetiology 282
 brainstem form (polioencephalitis) 283
 CSF 283
 diagnosis 283–4
 epidemiology 282–3
 motor-neurone disease following 284
 pathology 282
 prognosis 284
 prophylaxis 285
 second attacks 284
 subacute 485
 symptoms and signs 283
 treatment 284–5
polyarteritis nodosa (periarteritis nodosa) 219
 muscle infarction 563–4
 neuropathy 544
polycythaemia vera 482
 cerebral blood flow in 185
 syncope due to 189
polyglucosan body disease (glycoprotein storage
  disease) 465
polyinosinic-polycytidylic acid poly-L-lysine 531
polymyalgia rheumatica 566
polymyoclonia (progressive myoclonic
  encephalopathy) 632
polymyositis 564–5
 acrosclerosis, dysphagia, Raynaud's
  syndrome and 564
 acute/fulminant 563, 589 (fig.)
 aetiology 564
 antinuclear factor 587
 biochemical diagnosis 587
 classification 564
 clinical manifestations 565
 dysarthria in 54
 EMG 586

erythrocyte sedimentation rate 587
gamma-globulin, serum 587
immunoregulation in 297
incidence 564–5
muscle biopsy 588
penicillamine-precipitated 578
positive LE-cell preparations 587
prognosis 565
treatment 565
polymixin B, for meningitis 244
polyneuritis, see neuropathy
polyneuritis cranialis (cranial polyneuritis) 108,
  528, 549–50
polyneuropathy, see neuropathy
polyoma virus 485
polyostotic fibrous dysplasia (Albright's
  syndrome) 606
polyradiculoneuropathy, see Guillain–Barré
  syndrome
Pompe's disease (glycogenosis) 465
 antenatal diagnosis 576
 muscle biopsy 589
 treatment 577
pons 19
 blood supply 184
 haemorrhage into 215
 lacunar infarcts 196
 lesions 34
 tumours 167–8
  radiotherapy 171
 see also brainstem
porencephaly 351
porphyria 449–51, 548, 647
positional tests 124
positron emission tomography (PET) 80
 cerebral blood flow 185
 intracranial tumour 154
post-adrenalectomy syndrome 576
post-asthmatic pseudopolio syndrome 284
post-concussional syndrome 228
posterior cerebral artery 184
 developmental anomaly 183
 occlusion 89, 195
posterior choroidal arteries 184
posterior communicating artery 195
 developmental anomaly 183
 occlusion 195
posterior inferior cerebellar artery 184
posterior interosseous nerve 30 (fig.), 32 (table)
 lesions 503
 muscles supplied by 30 (fig.), 32 (table)
posterior longitudinal bundle (medial
  longitudinal fasciculus) 98
posterior longitudinal ligament, lumbar,
  protrusion of 517
posterior spinal arteries 390
 occlusion 424
 thrombosis 423
posterior thalamo-subthalamic paramedian
  artery occlusion 196
posterior tibial nerve lesions 510
posterolateral sclerosis, see vitamin B$_{12}$
  neuropathy
post-herpetic neuralgia 111, 291, 292
 treatment 293
postsynaptic membranes 4
postural hypotension 188
postural reflexes 51
 associated reactions 51
postural sensibility in toes, loss of, paracentral
  tumour-induced 162
potassium, high serum, Landry's paralysis
  associated 423
Prader–Willi syndrome 471
pralidoxine, for organophosphorus
  poisoning 439

prandial syncope 188
precentral cortex
 lesions causing micturition disturbances 393
 representation in 15
precentral tumours 161–2
prednisone
 for: Bell's palsy 115–16
  chronic progressive polyneuropathy 549
  Cryptococcus neoformans meningitis 248
  disseminated myelitis and optic
   neuritis 306
  Eaton–Lambert syndrome 572
  myasthenia gravis 571
  sarcoidosis 258
  tabetic pains 271
  temporal arteritis 220
pregnancy
 beriberi in 474
 carpal tunnel syndrome in 55
 epilepsy in 612
 multiple sclerosis in 309, 313
 neuropathy in 538
 tetany in 634
 thrombophlebitis in 224
presbyopia 84
presenile dementia 658
presenile polioencephalopathy, subacute 379
pressure-sores, treatment of 395
presynaptic inhibition 6
primary carpal stenosis 505
primidone
 for benign familial tremor 330
 toxic effects 435
procainamide for mystonia 560
procaine for restless legs 585
procaine penicillin, for meningovascular
  syphilis 266
prochlorperazine
 for: Ménière's syndrome 127
  migraine 180
proctalgia fugax 665
progressive bulbar palsy, see motor-neurone
  disease
progressive cerebral poliodystrophy (Alper's
  disease) 468
progressive dialysis encephalopathy (dialysis
  dementia) 646
progressive hypertrophic polyneuropathy 546–8
progressive lenticular degeneration, see Wilson's
  disease
progressive multifocal
  leuco-encephalopathy 485, 486
progressive multisystem degeneration, see
  Shy–Drager syndrome
progressive muscular atrophy, see
  motor-neurone disease
progressive myoclonic spinal neuronitis 631
progressive myositis ossificans 585
progressive spinal muscular atrophy, acute, of
  infancy (Werdnig–Hoffman
  disease) 383–4, 384–5
progressive supranuclear degeneration 99
progressive supranuclear palsy 331 (fig.), 332
progressive systemic sclerosis, muscle
  involvement 564
prolactinoma 165, 601
promethazine, for Ménière's syndrome 127
pronator sign 344
propantheline bromide
 action on pupil 103
 for: carotid sinus syncope 190
  frequency, urgency, precipitancy of
   micturition 394
  motor-neurone disease 375
  nocturnal enuresis 394
  syncope 190

prophenazine, heat stroke precipitated by 444
propionic acidaemia 453
d-propoxyphene addiction 431; see also drug
          addiction
propranolol 597
   for: benign familial tremor 330
          benign recurrent vertigo 127
          cataplexy 643
          migraine 181
          narcolepsy 643
          parkinsonism 332
proprioceptors 4, 38
prosopagnosia 62, 163
prostacyclin, in open-heart surgery 188
prostaglandins 9
protein-calorie malnutrition, infantile 469
protopathic pain (hyperpathia) 44, 493, 497
protriptyline, for sleep apnoea 643
pseudoathetosis 44, 162, 269
pseudobulbar palsy 197
pseudodementia (Ganser syndrome) 660, 663
pseudoHurler's disease (generalized GM$_1$
          gangliodosis; familial neurovisceral
          lipidosis) 456–7
pseudohypoparathyroidism 155, 470
pseudomyopathic spinal muscular atrophy
          (Kugelberg–Welander syndrome) 384–5
pseudomyotonia 547, 558
pseudonystagmus 101
pseudopapilloedema 91
pseudopolio syndrome, post-asthmatic 284
pseudoseizures 616
pseudo-tetanus 446
pseudoxanthoma elasticum 218
psychic blindness 638
psychogenic dizziness 126
psychogenic regional pain 665
psychogenic unresponsiveness (hysterical
          trance) 648
psychomotor restlessness 655
ptosis 105–6
   hysterical 665
   in: Friedreich's ataxia 364
          multiple sclerosis 311
          myasthenia gravis 568
          ocular myopathy 557
          pineal body tumour 164
          third nerve palsy 106
          tabes dorsalis 270
pubertal delay, in pineocytoma 164
pulseless disease (Takayashu's disease) 198, 221
pulse rate, cerebral tumour effect on 153
punch-drunkenness 228
pupil 102–5
   accommodation paralysis 103
   Argyll Robertson, see Argyll Robertson pupil
   Behr's 104
   ciliary fibres 102–3
   ciliospinal reflex 103
   comatose patient 649
   dilator pupillae paralysis 103
   drug action on 103
   fixed dilated, temporal-lobe tumour
                induced 162
   in: botulism 447
          coma 649
          diabetic neuropathy 539
          general paresis 267
          midbrain tumour 164
          multiple sclerosis 311
          narcolepsy 641
          peroneal atrophy 381
          tabes dorsalis 270
          third nerve paralysis 106
   inequality 103
   innervation 102–3

iridoconstrictor fibres 102
iridodilator fibres 102
light reflex 103
   ocular-sympathetic paralysis 103
   pinpoint 215
   reaction on accommodation/convergence 103
   size 103
   sphincter pupillae paralysis 103
   tonic, with absent tendon
             reflexes (Holmes–Adie syndrome)
             104–5
pure motor hemiplegia 195, 196–7
pure pan-dysautonomia with recovery 601
pure sensory stroke (contralateral
          hemianaesthesia) 195
pure word-dumbness 56
purine metabolism disorders 464–5
Purkinje cells, degeneration 487
Purkinje shift 84
purpura, thrombotic thrombocytopenic 221
putamen 17, 324
   blood supply 184
pyknolepsy 616
pyramidal cells 3 (fig.), 13
pyramidal (corticospinal/corticobulbar)
          system 15–16
pyridostigmine (Mestinon) 8
   for myasthenia gravis 571
pyridoxine deficiency 473–4, 609
pyrimethamine, for toxoplasmosis 259
pyruvate decarboxylase deficiency 466
   brain-restricted 467

Q fever 256
quadrantic hemianopia (quadrantanopia) 87
quadriplegia (tetraplegia; tetraparesis) 29, 352,
          399
quail poisoning 578
Queckenstedt's test 68, 252, 404
quinine, for acute cerebral malaria 256
quintothalamic tract 41

rabies (hydrophobia) 286–7
radial (musculospinal) nerve 30 (fig.), 32 (table)
   lesions 503
   muscles supplied by 30 (fig.), 32 (table)
radial reflex (supinator-jerk) 50
   inversion 403
radiation-induced cerebrovascular
          disease 218–19
radiation myelopathy 422
radiculitis, syphilitic 265, 266
radiography 78–80
   acoustic neuroma 167
   basilar impression 608
   berry aneurysm, calcified 207
   brain trauma 229
   cervical disc prolapse 515
   cervical spondylosis 516
   craniopharyngioma 166
   craniostenosis 607
   dementia 660
   epilepsy 618
   Hand–Schüller–Christian disease 461
   head injury 229
   hydrocephalus 140
   intracranial tumour 155
   lumbar disc lesions 517
   meningioma 166
   optic chiasm glioma 166
   Paget's disease 604
   pituitary tumours 165
   skull 79
   spinal column 79–80
   spinal cord compression 404
   subarachnoid haemorrhage 210

syringomyelia 414
   unconscious patient 649
radiotherapy
   Cushing's disease 172
   exophthalmic ophthalmoplegia 574
   intracranial tumours 171–2
   leukaemia 171
   myelopathy following 422
   post-herpetic neuralgia 293
   spinal metastases 409
   spinal tumour 410
   syringomyelia 415
   vertebral metastases 409
Raeder's paratrigeminal syndrome 103, 207
raised intracranial pressure, see increased
          intracranial pressure
Ramsay Hunt syndrome (dyssynergia
          cerebellaris syndrome) 114, 366, 631
rape-seed oil 440
Raynaud's syndrome, in polymyositis 565
reading age 656
receptors 4
   adaptation 7
   adrenergic 8
   cholinergic opiate 8
   physiology 6–7
   sensory 38
          proprioceptive 38
rectal crisis, in tabes dorsalis 270
rectum
   care of, in paraplegia 395
   innervation 394
recurrent laryngeal nerves 129–30
   lesions 132
   recovery from paralysis 132
   superior 133
red nucleus 17, 19
reducing body myopathy 583
referred pain 176, 598–9
   facial 111
   gate theory 46, 598
   in head and neck 176
reflex(es) 48–52
   abdominal 50
   anal 50
   ankle-jerk 50
   avoiding 52
   biceps-jerk 50
   blink (facial) 49, 113, 649
   bulbocavernous 51
   Chaddock's (external malleolar sign) 51
   ciliospinal 103
   corneal 48–9
   cremasteric 50
   cutaneous 50–1
   examination of 76
   excretory, in paraplegia-in-flexion 392
   facial (blink) 49, 113, 649
   flexor finger-jerk 50
   flexor withdrawal 391–2
   glabellar tap 113, 327
          in parkinsonism 327
   gluteal 50
   Gordon's (paradoxical flexor) 51
   grab 52
   grasp: foot 51–2, 161
          hand 51, 161
   great toe 517
   groping 51
   H 49, 324, 392
   Hoffman's 49–50
   inverted 50
   jaw 49
   knee-jerk 50
   long-loop 324
   mass 392

naso-lacrimal 113
nasomental 113
oculocephalic (doll's head phenomenon) 49, 98
oculovestibular caloric 49
Oppenheim's 51
palatal 49
palmomental 50
pendular 344
pharyngeal 49
plantar 50–1
    equivocal 51
    extensor 51
    flexor 50–1
postural 51
    associated reactions 51
radial (supinator jerk) 50
    inversion 403
rooting 49
sexual, in paraplegia-in-flexion 392
snout 49
stapedius 113
stretch 392
sucking (rooting) 49
tendon 49–50
    spread of 50
tonic neck 32, 51
tonic stretch 28
triceps-jerk 50
reflex bradycardia 597
reflex dystrophy of upper extremity (algodystrophy; shoulder–hand syndrome) 498–9, 508
reflex iridoplegia 104
in neurosyphilis 169, 264
refraction 83
Refsum's disease (heredopathia atactica polyneuritiformis) 93, 462–3
regeneration in nervous system 9–10
reinforcement (Jendrassik's manœuvre) 29
rejection encephalopathy 439
Remak cells 3
renal transplantation, intracranial tumour after 143
Renshaw cells 23, 29
reserpine 8, 324, 326
    migraine precipitated by 178
    toxic effects 432
respiration
    cerebral tumour effect on 153
    intracranial pressure effect on 136
respiratory centre 19
restless legs 535, 584
retention of faeces
    in: post-vaccinal encephalomyelitis 302
        spinal cord compression 407
retention of urine
    in: acute lymphocytic choriomeningitis 288
        multiple sclerosis 311
        parasagittal meningioma 162
        post-vaccinal encephalomyelitis 302
        spinal cord compression 403, 407
    treatment 394
reticular formation 19
reticuloses 148, 485–6
reticulospinal tract 17, 29
    disorders 33
reticulum-cell sarcoma 143
retina 84–5
    function 84–5
        colour vision 85
        dark/light adaptation 84
        photochemical/electrophysiological mechanisms 84
        visual sensitivity/acuity 85
    structure 84

retinal artery
    occlusion 177
    spasm 178
    thrombosis 179–80
retinitis pigmentosa 90, 93
    in: ocular myopathy 557
        osteitis deformans 605
        Refsum's disease 462
retrobulbar neuritis 91, 92
    in: hyperemesis gravidarum 538
        multiple sclerosis 310
        post-infective polyneuritis 528
    intracranial tumour-resembling 169
    scotoma due to 87 (fig.)
    see also optic neuropathy
retrobulbar pupil reaction (Marcus Gunn response) 92, 104
retrocollis 341
Rett's syndrome 357
Reye's syndrome 254, 451
Reynell's battery 656
rheumatoid arthritis
    myositis 563
    neuropathy 544–6
rheumatoid cervical myelopathy 400
rhinencephalon 12
rhodopsin 84
riboflavine deficiency 473
rib-tip syndrome 522
ricketsial infections 356
right handedness 53
rigidity 323
    clasp-knife 31
    cog-wheel 31, 323, 328
    decerebrate 31
    hysterical 332
    in: arthritis 332
        corticospinal tract lesions 332
        parkinsonism 323, 328
    plastic (lead-pipe) 31, 328
    see also hypertonia
Riley–Day syndrome (familial dysautonomia) 599
Rinne's test 120
risus sardonicus 445, 634
Rocky Mountain spotted fever 256
Rocky Mountain wood tick toxin 423
Romberg's sign 44, 269
rooting (sucking) reflex 49
rooting (girdle) pains 269
Roussy–Lévy syndrome (hereditary areflexia and distal amyotrophy and ataxia) 366
rubella, congenital 293–4
rubrospinal tract 16–17
Ruffini's corpuscles 38

saccule 122
sacral agenesis (caudal dysplasia) 417
sacral nerve roots, cysts on 517
sacral reflex arc 393
    lesions involving 393
sagittal sinus thrombosis 141, 487
St. Vitus' dance, see Sydenham's chorea
salbutamol, for hyperkalaemic periodic paralysis 577
Salk vaccine 283, 285
Salla disease 459
Sandhoff's disease (infantile amaurotic family idiocy); cerebromacular degeneration; Tay–Sachs disease) 93, 455–6
Sanger-Brown's spinocerebellar ataxia 365
saphenous nerve lesions 509
sarcoidosis 258
    muscle involvement 563
    neuropathy 544
    oculomotor nerve paralysis 107

sensory perineuritis 544
sarcoma 400
sarcosporidiosis of muscle 563
saxitoxin poisoning 448
scalenus anterior syndrome 501
scaphocephaly 605 (fig.)
scapuloperoneal muscular dystrophy 385, 555
scarlet fever 255
Scarpa's ganglion 122
Schilder's disease (diffuse sclerosis) 319–20
Schistosoma japonicum infestation of brain 152
schistosomiasis (bilharzia) 261
schizencephaly 357
schizophrenia 655
    in Friedreich's ataxia 364
Schmidt-Lantermann incisures 24
Schmidt's syndrome 132, 196
Schonell's reading age test 656
Schwann cells 3, 4
Schwannoma 148
Schwartz–Jampel syndrome (chondrodystrophic myotonia) 559
sciatica 516; see also lumbar disc lesions
sciatic nerve 31 (fig.), 32 (table), 509
    lesions 509–10
        treatment 510–11
    muscles supplied by 31 (fig.), 32 (table)
scleroderma, neuropathy 544–5
sclerosing panencephalitis, subacute 279–80
sclerosteosis 606
scopolamine 8
scorpion venoms 448
scotoma 87
    charting with Bjerrum's screen 87
scrapie 274, 294
scrub typhus (Tsutsugamushi disease) 256
sea anemone venoms 448
sedatives, addiction to 432–3
seizures induced by movement 616
sella turcica
    ballooning 155
    empty 136, 165
    J-shaped 166
    radiographic appearance 79
semicircular canals 122
semicoma 644
sensory ataxia 36, 44
sensory evoked potentials 14, 405
sensory inattention 44
sensory spots, cutaneous 38
sensory system 37–48
    abnormalities of sensation 42–6
        clinical significance 45–6
        pathophysiology 45–6
        signs 44–5
        symptoms 42–4
        see also pain
    affective responses 38
    cortex, see cerebral cortex
    cutaneous segmentation 42
    examination 39
    measurement 39
    modalities, simpler 39
    motor responses 37
    organization 38
    receptors 38
        proprioceptive 38
    sensory parameters 38–9
        duration 38
        intensity 38
        localization 38
        quality (modality) 38
        temporal 38
    sensory pathways 39–41
    sensory responses 37
septum pellucidum hypoplasia 93

serial sevens (100–7) test 656
serotonin *see* 5-hydroxytryptamine
serum neuropathy 538
serum protein abnormalities, neuropathy
    associated 545
sexual desire, loss of 601
sexual function disturbance 601
sexual infantilism 601
sexual precocity
  in: hypothalamic syndromes 601
      pineolcytoma 164
sexual regression 593
sham rage 593
shape appreciation 39
Shapiro's syndrome (spontaneous periodic
    hypothermia) 647
shin splints (tibialis anterior syndrome) 585
shock
  cerebral 1, 32, 33
  spinal 1, 32
shoulder-girdle neuritis (neuralgic
    amyotrophy) 508, 521–2
shoulder–hand syndrome (algodystrophy; reflex
    dystrophy of upper extremity) 498–9,
    508, 599
  sympathectomy for 599
shuddering attacks 330
Shy–Drager syndrome (progressive multisystem
    degeneration; chronic orthostatic
    hypotension) 188–9, 331
  sleep apnoea 472
sialidosis
  type I (cherry-red spot–myoclonus
    syndrome) 459
  type II 459
sickle-cell disease 482
single-photon emission computed tomography
    (SPECT), cerebral blood flow 185
sinuses, intracranial 221–2
  thrombosis 233–4
    papilloedema due to 91
sinusitis
  frontal 111
  maxillary 111
size appreciation 39
Sjögren–Larsson syndrome 366
Sjögren's syndrome (keratoconjunctivitis
    sicca) 112
skew deviation of eyes 98
skin, sympathetic denervation of 597
skull
  diseases 604–8
  metastases in 176
  neoplastic invasion of base 168–9
  osteitis of 107–8, 176
  syphilitic 176
sleep 641
  hallucinatory states associated 642
  hypothalamic control 593
  paradoxical (rapid eye-movement phase) 641
sleep disturbances 602, 641–3
sleep drunkenness 642
sleep-inducing peptides 641
sleep paralysis 642
sleepy sickness, *see* epidemic encephalitis
    lethargica
slow virus infections 294, 301
Sluder's (sphenopalatine) neuralgia 176
smell 83
  loss, uncal lesion induced 162
snake bite 444
snout reflex 49
sodium amylobarbitone, intracarotid
    injection 53
sodium cyanate neuropathy 537–8
sodium nitroprusside, for hypertensive

encephalopathy 206
sodium-responsive normokalaemic periodic
    paralysis 577–8
sodium valproate
  adverse reactions 435, 623
  for: epilepsy 622, 623, 624, 625
      serum concentration 623
      petit mal status 625
solanine 440
somatosensory potentials, evoked 41, 496–7
somnambulism 642, 643
somnolence
  in: centrum semiovale tumour 163
  hydrocephalus 153
  hypothalamic tumour 153
  third ventricle tumour 163
somnolence syndrome 486
solatol, for benign familial tremor 330
sound waves 117
spasm, recruitment 445
spasmodic torticollis (wry neck) 323, 341–2
spasticity 29–31
  hemiplegic 33
  in centrum ovale tumour 163
spastic paraplegia
  hereditary 363
  nutritional 478
speech 52–62
  anatomy 52–4
  disorders 54–62
    developmental *see below*
  in: dementia 658
    Friedreich's ataxia 364
    general paresis 267
    laryngeal paralysis 132
    motor neurone disease 373
    multiple sclerosis 310
    myasthenia gravis 568
    neuronal intranuclear inclusion
      disease 339
    parkinsonism 327
    primary parenchymatous degeneration of
      cerebellum 365
    Wilson's disease 337
  physiology 52–4
  psychology 52–3
speech disorders, developmental 59–60
  developmental dysarthria 60
  developmental dyslexia 60
  developmental expressive aphasia 59
  developmental receptive aphasia (congenital
    word-deafness; congenital auditory
    imperception) 59–60, 60
  dyslalia 60
  mirror-writing 53, 60
Spielmeyer–Vogt's amaurotic family idiocy 457
spina bifida 418–20
  aetiology 418
  diagnosis 419
    antenatal 419
  pathology 418
  prognosis 419
  symptoms and signs 418–19
  tests: CSF 419
    CT scan 419
    radiography 419
  treatment 419–20
spinal accessory nerve 32 (table)
  trapezius muscle supplied by 32 (table)
  unilateral paralysis 168
spinal artery steal phenomenon 423
spinal cord
  acute transverse lesion 33
  blood supply 423
  central softening (haemorrhagic necrosis) 398
  compression, *see* spinal cord compression

dysfunction 392
  ectopic 418
  embolism 424
  gray matter 22
  infarction 423–4
  injuries 396–8
    aetiology 396
    concussion/contusion 396
    diagnosis 397
    laceration 397
    pathology 396–7
    prognosis 397
    symptoms and signs 397
    treatment 397
  ischaemia 390–1, 424
    intermittent claudication due to 424
  lesion, micturition disturbances 393
  motor organization 23–4
  oedema, in radiation myelopathy 422
  repair 392
  segment 22
  segmental–vertebral relationship 22
  sensory abnormalities 45
  sensory organization 23–4
  transection of dorsal column 40
  transient ischaemia 424
  venous drainage 391
spinal cord compression 400–12
  causes 400–2
    achondroplasia 401
    arachnoidal cysts 402
    arachnoiditis 401–2
    cervical-disc lesion 515
    ectopic calcification in
      pseudoparathyroidism 470
    epidural abscess 401
    epidural haematoma 400
    extradural abscess 400, 401
    intervertebral-disc protusion 400
    intramedullary abscess 401
    kyphoscoliosis 401
    lymphoma 486
    myeloma 484
    neoplasms of vertebral column 400
    odontoid-process separation 400
    osteitis deformans 400
    parasitic cysts 402
    progressive hypertrophic
      polyneuropathy 547
    spinal tumour 401
    subdural haematoma 400
    syphilitic spinal osteitis 400
    thalassaemia 400
    tuberculous osteitis 400
    vertebral-column disease 400–1
  diagnosis 407–8
    causal 408
    differential 407
    localization of segmental level 407–8
    relationship of source of compression to
      cause 408
  effects on cord 402
  prognosis 408–9
    acute intervertebral disc prolapse 409
    arachnoidal cyst 409
    arachnoiditis 409
    cervical spondylosis 409
    secondary carcinoma 409
    spinal tumour 409
    tuberculous disease 408–9
  symptoms and signs 402–3
    autonomic 403
    cervical 5th–6th segments 406
    cervical 8th–thoracic 1st 406
    exacerbation after lumbar puncture 404
    lumbar 3rd–4th segments 407

mid-thoracic region 406
mode of onset 402–3
motor 403
papilloedema 402
reflexes 403
sacral 1st–2nd segments 407
sacral 3rd–4th segments 407
sensory 403
sphincters 403
spine 403
thoracic 9th–10th segments 406
thoracic 12th–lumbar 1st segments 407
upper cervical region 406
tests 403–6
angiography 406
CSF 403–4
CT scan 400, 405, 406
electromanometry 404
electrophysiological studies 405–6
extradural venography 406
gamma-encephalography 406
lumbar discography 406
manometry 404
myelography 404
myeloscintography 406
Queckenstedt's test 404
radiography 404
treatment 409–10
achondroplasia 409
arachnoiditis 410
cervical spondylosis 409
extradural abscess 410
granulomatous meningitis 410
kyphoscoliosis 409
lumbar spondylosis 409
Paget's disease 409
secondary carcinoma of vertebrae 409
spinal tumour 410
spondylolisthesis 409
tuberculous disease 409
vertebral haemangioma 409
spinal dysraphism (myelodysplasia) 416–17,
418–19
spinal endarteritis 265, 266
spinal epidural abscess 401
spinal epidural haematoma 400
spinal evoked potentials 392
spinal extradural abscess 400, 401
spinal intramedullary abscess 401
spinal ganglia 22–3
spinal hemiplegia 35
spinal metastases 400, 408, 409
spinal muscular atrophy, chronic, of childhood,
adolescence, early adult life 384–5
spinal myoclonus 290, 631
spinal nerves 22–3, 28
cutaneous areas 43 (fig.)
spinal pachymeningitis 265
spinal radiculitis 514
spinal radiculopathy 514
brachial, cervical-disc lesion-induced 515–16
acute 515–16
chronic 515
intervertebral-disc lesion-induced 514–15
spinal roots compression
in: lymphoma 486
myeloma 484
spinal segmental relationship to vertebrae 408
spinal shock, in multiple sclerosis 312
spinal stroke (anterior spinal artery
occlusion) 391, 423
spinal subdural haematoma 400
spinal tenderness, to pressure/percussion 403
spinal tumours 401
spinal veins 391
spinocerebellar tracts 19

spino-pontine atrophy, dominant 365
spinothalamic tracts 40–1
spiramycin, for toxoplasmosis 259
spongiform encephalopathy, subacute 379
spongioblastoma
polar 145
spinal 401
spontaneous periodic hypothermia (Shapiro's
syndrome) 647
Spurling's sign 515
squint (strabismus) 96; see also
ophthalmoplegia
stammering (stuttering) 60–1
stapedius reflex 113
staphylococcal pyomyositis (tropical
myositis) 563
Stargardt's disease 93
static vestibular receptors (tonus elements) 122
status epilepticus 617
absence seizures 614, 615
treatment 625
complex partial seizures 615
electrical 617
hyperuricaemia following 620
in: brain injury 233
general paresis 267
meningitis 245
porphyria 450
tuberous sclerosis 358
Jacksonian 161
metabolic changes in 617
treatment 625
status hemicranialis 180
steeplechase jockeys, brain injuries in 228
stellate (granule) cells 13
stereoanaesthesia 45, 162
sternomastoid paralysis 133
steroids
for: acute cerebral malaria 256
Behçet's disease 260
benign intracranial hypertension 142
cerebral haemorrhage 217
cerebral oedema 137
Cryptococcus neoformans meningitis 248
granulomatous angiitis 220
intracranial abscess 252
intracranial tumour 171
ischaemic stroke 198
Leber's optic atrophy 93
polyarteritis nodosa 219
polymyalgia rheumatica 566
polyneuropathy 529
chronic progressive 549
relapsing/recurrent 531
pulseless disease 221
raised intracranial pressure 171
sarcoidosis 258
tabetic pains 271
temporal arteritis 220
thrombotic thrombocytopenic
purpura 221
lumbar extradural injection 518
polyneuropathy induced by 544
stiff-man syndrome 585, 631
stiff neck 521
Stokes–Adams syndrome 189
strabismus (squint) 96
Strachan's syndrome 478
streptomycin
adverse effects 126, 245
for tuberculous meningitis 245
myasthenia induced by 568
stretch receptors (muscle spindles) 16
stretch reflex 392
stretch syncope 189
striatal disorders, symptoms and signs 322–3

stroke
clinical features 193
epidemiology 191
incidence 191–2
prognosis 198
pure sensory 195, 197
rehabilitation after 199–200
stuttering 193
treatment 198–200
undetermined aetiology 219
see also cerebral haemorrhage; cerebral
infarction; cerebral thrombosis
stroke-in-evolution 193,194
strychnine poisoning 448
stupor 644–8
catatonic 648
causes 645
brain disease 646
cerebral vascular lesions 645
encephalitis 646
head injury 646
meningitis 646
pancreatic encephalopathy 647
porphyria 450
space-occupying lesions 646–6
Sturge–Weber syndrome 79, 150
stuttering (stammering) 60–1
stuttering hemiplegia 194
stuttering stroke 193
subacute combined degeneration of brain/spinal
cord, see vitamin B_{12} neuropathy
subacute myelo-optico-neuropathy
(SMON) 439–40
subacute necrotizing encephalomyelopathy
(Leigh's disease) 466
subacute necrotizing myelopathy 488
subacute 'poliomyelitis' 485
subarachnoid abscess 251–2
subarachnoid haemorrhage 208–12
aetiology 208–9
CSF: blood 68–9
xanthochromia 69
diagnosis 211
haemosiderosis, superficial, as
complication 211
incidence 209
investigations 210–11
CSF 210
radiology 210–11
papilloedema due to 91, 209
prognosis 211
spinal 209, 210, 401
symptoms and signs 209–10
focal 210
treatment 211–12
surgical 212
subclavian artery
aneurysmal dilatation 501
compression of 501
subclavian steal syndrome 185, 190, 196
treatment 199
subcortical lesions 34
subdural abscess/empyema 251
subdural haematoma 231–2
chronic, intracranial tumour-resembling 169
EEG 78
subfalcial herniation 136
substance P 9, 324
substantia gelatinosa 23, 38
central dysfunction in 111
internuncial neurones 38, 40
substantia nigra 17, 19, 326 (fig.)
subthalamic nucleus (body of Luys) 17, 324
infarction 195
sucking (rooting) reflex 49
sudden infarct/adult death 472

Sudeck's atrophy 508
sudomotor axon reflex tests 597
sulphadiazine, for toxoplasmosis 259
sulphatide lipidosis (metachromatic
    leucodystrophy) 460–1
sulphinpyrazone
  for: ischaemic stroke prevention 199
      transient ischaemic attacks 199
sulpiride, for facial (tardive) dyskinesia 349
sulthiame, for epilepsy 624
superior cerebellar artery 184
  occlusion 196
superior colliculus 86, 97
superior laryngeal nerve 133
superior orbital fissure syndrome (painful
    ophthalmoplegia) 108
superior sagittal sinus 222
  thrombosis 222–3, 224
supinator-jerk (radial reflex) 50
supranuclear pseudo-ophthalmoplegia 98
supra-optic nucleus 637
supra-orbital nerve injection 521
suprascapular nerve lesions 503
suxamethonium 8, 27, 552
swallow syncope 189
swayback disease of sheep 299
sweating, excessive, post-spinal cord lesions 598
Sydenham's chorea 343–5
  aetiology 343–4
  diagnosis 344–5
  pathology 343
  prognosis 345
  symptoms and signs 3444
  thyrotoxicosis associated 344
  treatment 345
sympathectomy
  causalgia 498
  hyperhidrosis 597
  pain relief by 599
  shoulder–hand syndrome 599
sympathetic nervous system
  chain 594
  fibres 594
  ocular, paralysis, in brainstem tumour 167
  see also autonomic nervous system
sympathomimetic drugs 597
synapses 4, 6, 7–9
syncope (fainting) 188–9, 619
  carotid sinus 189–90
  cough 189
  diagnosis 190
  EEG 190
  familial 188
  micturition 188
  physical causes 189–90
  prandial 188
  prognosis 190
  proneness 188
  psychological causes 189
  swallow 189
  symptoms 190
  treatment 190
syphilis
  neurosyphilis, *see* neurosyphilis
  secondary 263
    paresis of vertical gaze 263
  tests 263
syringobulbia 414, 415
  neuralgia of face/scalp 176
  ophthalmoplegia 99
syringomyelia 412–16
  aetiology 413
  associated abnormalities 414
  communicating 412, 415 (fig.)
  diagnosis 414–15
  non-communicating 412–13

pathogenesis 412–13
  pathology 412
  prognosis 415
  symptoms and signs 413–14, 415 (fig.)
    motor 413
    sensory 45, 413
    trophic 413–14
  tests: CSF 414
    electromyography 414
    myelography 414, 415 (fig.)
    radiology 414
  thermo-anaesthesia 413
  traumatic 397
  treatment 415–16
systemic lupus erythematosus 219–20
  muscle involvement 564
  neuropathy 544
  vacuolar myopathy 589

tabes dorsalis (locomotor ataxia) 268–72
  aetiology 268
  cervical 269
  complications 271
  congenital 272
  crisis 270, 271
  CSF 270–1
  paroxysmal facial pain 111
  pathology 268–9
  prognosis 271
  symptoms and signs 45, 269–70
  treatment 271–2
taboparesis 267, 269
tache cérébrale 239, 241, 242
tachistoscopy 87
tactile discrimination (two-point) 38, 39
  loss of, in parietal lobe tumour 163
tactile inattention 39
  contralateral 163
Taenia solium infestation (cysticercosis) 260
Takayashu's disease (pulseless disease) 198, 221
Tangier disease
    (hypo-alpha-lipoproteinaemia) 464, 548
tardive (facial) dyskinesia 9, 349
tardy ulnar palsy 506
tarsal tunnel syndrome
  anterior 510
  posterior 510
taste 128
  fibres 129
  hallucinations 129
  loss of 83, 129
    in: clonic facial spasm 116
    uncal lesion 162
Tay–Sachs disease (infantile amaurotic family
    idiocy; cerebromacular degeneration;
    Sandhoff's disease) 93, 455–6
T cells 296
  in multiple sclerosis 307
teichopsia 179
telangiectasis (capillary angioma) 149
telemetry 618–19
temporal (giant cell, cranial) arteritis 108, 194,
    220
temporal lobe
  abscess 251
  tinnitus 121
  tumour 162
temporal stem 639
tendon reflexes 49–50
  spread of 50
tennis elbow syndrome 503
tentorial herniation 136
teratoma, spinal 401
testicular sensation loss, in tabes dorsalis 269
tetanoid chorea, *see* Wilson's disease
tetanus 444–7

aetiology 444–5
  autonomic manifestations 445
  cephalic 445
  diagnosis 446
  incubation period 445
  local 445
  modified 446
  neonatorum 445
  pathology 445
  prognosis 446
  splanchnic 445
  symptoms 445–6
  treatment 446
tetanus antitoxin 446
tetany (carpopedal spasm) 633–5
  aetiology 633–4
  causes 634–5
  diagnosis 635
  normocalcaemic 634
  pathophysiology 634
  prognosis 635
  symptoms and signs 634–5
  treatment 635
tetrabenazine
  for: athetosis 343
    facial (tardive) dyskinesia 349
    Huntington's chorea 347
    spasmodic torticollis 342
  parkinsonism induced by 327
tetracycline
  benign intrcranial hypertension due to 141
  for: brucellosis 248
    Whipple's disease 262
tetramisole, optic nerve damage due to 92
tetraplegia (tetraparesis; quadriplegia) 29, 399
tetrodotoxin 448
texture appreciation 39
thalamic over-reaction 162
thalamic syndrome (pain) 44, 46
  posterior cerebral artery occlusion 195
thalamus 17, 41, 636
  blood supply 184
  haemorrhage into 215
  nuclei 636
    damage 636
    destruction of dorsomedial 639
thalassaemia 482
thalidomide neuropathy 535
thallium poisoning 439
thermal sensation testing 39
thermoanaesthesia 44, 413
thiamine (vitamin B_1)
  deficiency 473
  for: alcoholic polyneuropathy 532
    beriberi 475
thiethylperazine maleate, for Ménière's
    syndrome 127
thiopentone, for status epilepticus 625
thiopropazate (Dartalan)
  for: athetosis 343
    facial (tardive) dyskinesia 349
    Huntington's chorea 347
thioxanthenes 8
third ventricle
  colloid cyst 151, 160 (fig), 163
    surgical treatment 171
  tumour 163
thromboangiitis obliterans (Buerger's
    disease) 220
thrombocytopenic purpura 482
thrombotic thrombocytopenic purpura 221
thujone 428
thumb, weakness of, in precentral tumour 162
thymectomy 565, 571
thyrotoxic myopathy 574
thyrotoxic periodic paralysis 575

thyrotoxicosis 470
  myasthenia gravis associated 568, 575
thyrotrophic hormone deficiency, neuropathy
    due to 541
tibialis anterior syndrome (skin splints) 585
tibial (medial popliteal) nerve 31 (fig), 32
    (table)
  lesions 510
  muscles supplied by 31 (fig), 32 (table)
tic 75
tic douloureux, *see* trigeminal neuralgia
Tinel's sign 44, 497
tinnitus 121
  in: eighth nerve tumour 167
    Ménière's disease 126–7
    temporal lobe tumour 162
tin (organic) poisoning 438
tobacco–alcohol amblyopia 92, 428
Tobey–Ayer test 68, 224
Todd's (post-epileptic) paralysis 162, 609
Tolosa–Hunt syndrome 108, 170
tongue
  fasciculation, in motor neurone disease 373
  hemiatrophy 134
  in: hemiplegia 33
    syringomyelia 413
  paralysis 134
    in precentral tumour 162
    unilateral 134
tongue-biting, in epilepsy 614
tonic innervation (perserveration) 161
tonic neck reflexes 32, 51
tonic seizures 311
tonic stretch reflex 28
tonsillar herniation (cerebellar pressure
    cone) 136
tonus elements (static vestibular receptors) 122
top of the basilar syndrome 195
torsion dystonia (dystonia musculorum
    deformans) 31, 323, 324, 339–40
torticollis
  congenital 341
  in post-encephalitic Parkinsonism 277
  spasmodic (wry neck) 323, 341–2
touch testing 39
tourniquet paralysis 492
tower skull (craniostenosis; acrocephaly;
    oxicephaly; turricephaly) 136, 606–07
toxic encephalomyopathy, acute 238, 254
toxic hydrocephalus, *see* benign intracranial
    hypertension
toxocara infection 261
toxoplasmosis 258–9, 489
  of muscle 563
tranexamic acid (AMCA) 211–12
tranquillisers 8
  for: epilepsy 625
    lumbar disc lesions 518
    migraine 181
    tension headache 177
transient cerebral ischaemic attack 193–4, 194
  internal carotid artery occlusion 195
  middle cerebral artery stenosis 195
  treatment 199
transient global amnesia 639
  in hippocampal tumour 162
transmitters 4
transverse sinuses 222
  thrombosis 141, 223, 224
traumatic encephalopathy 228
  prognosis 230
traumatic pneumocephalus (intracranial
    aerocele) 231
traumatic porencephaly 229
Treacher Collins syndrome 471
tremor 323

action, post-cerebral haemorrhage 217
  benign (essential) familial 323, 328 (fig), 330
  extrapyramidal 323
  flapping (wing-beating; asterixis) 331
  in: acute anxiety 331
    general paresis 331
    hereditary ataxia 331
    hyperthyroidism 331
    hysteria 330–1. 664
    multiple sclerosis 331
    parkinsonism 217, 328
    Wilson's disease 337
  intention (kinetic) 36, 323, 328 (fig.)
    in multiple sclerosis 310, 331
  senile 330
  sodium valproate-induced 623
  titubating 36
  toxic 331
trench fever 256
treponemal immobilisation test (TPI) 263
triceps-jerk 50
trichinosis 261, 563
trichlorethylene 534
trichopoliodystrophy (Menkes' kinky-hair
    disease) 467–8
trichromats 85
triethyl tetramine 338
trifluoperazine, for migraine 181
trigeminal artery 183
trigeminal nerve (5th cranial) 109–10
  central connections 109–10
  descending root 41
  Gasserian ganglion: alcohol injection 108
    compression 162, 165
    herpes zoster 176
  injury 229
  lesions: central 110
    peripheral 110
  mandibular branch 109
  maxillary branch 109
  motor root 109
  ophthalmic branch 109
  peripheral distribution 42, 109
  sensory pathways 41
  unilateral pain, pressure-induced 152, 176
trigeminal neuralgia (tic douloureux) 110–12
  aetiology 110
  diagnosis 111
  in: malaria 256
    Paget's disease 605
  incidence 110
  pathology 110–11
  prognosis 111
  symptoms 111
  treatment 111–12
  trigger zones 111
trigeminal neuropathy 112, 521
  in multiple sclerosis 312
trigeminothalamic tract 41
triglycerides, serum, in stroke 197
trigonocephaly 607
triorthocresylphosphate neuropathy 535
trismus 446
  in: acute toxic encephalopathy 254
    hysteria 446, 666
    post-vaccinal encephalomyelitis 302
    rabies 287
    tetanus 445
trisomy E (17–18) syndrome 471
trochlear nerve (4th cranial)
  paralysis 106–7
    causes 107–8
    orbital lesions 108
    south-east Asian 108
trophic changes
  in: Morvan's syndrome 414

myelodysplasia 416
  spina bifida 419
  syringomyelia 413–14
  tabes dorsalis 270
tropical ataxic neuropathy 92, 477–8
troxidone, glare phenomenon 94
Trousseau's sign 635
truncal (central) ataxia, *see* ataxia, truncal
trypanosomiasis 257, 563
Tsutsugamushi disease (scrub typhus) 256
tuberculoma 143, 152, 170
  meningitis associated 242
  spinal 401
  surgical treatment 171
tuberculosis, miliary, retinal tubercles in 90
tuberculous meningitis, *see* meningitis,
    tuberculous
tuberculous spinal disease 408, 408–9
tuberous sclerosis (epiloia; Bourneville's
    disease; Brushfield–Wyatt disease) 143,
    358–9
  phakoma 90
tubocurarine 8, 552
  for tetanus 446
tunnel vision 94
Turner's syndrome (ovarian dysgenesis) 471
turricephaly (craniostenosis; oxycephaly;
    acrocephaly; tower skull) 136, 606–7
two-point discrimination 38, 39
typhoid fever 255
typhus fever 256
tyramine, for Shy-Drager syndrome 189
tyrosine 8
tyrosine hydroxylase deficiency 327

Uhthoff's symptom 91
ulegyria 351, 354
ulnar nerve 30 (fig.), 505
  lesions 505–7
  muscles supplied by 30 (fig.), 32 (fig.)
uncinate fits
  in: suprasellar meningioma 166
    temporal lobe tumour 162
unconscious patient
  investigation 648–9
    abdomen 649
    blink (facial) reflexes 649
    breath 648
    cardiovascular system 649
    EEG 650
    fundi 649
    head 648
    laboratory investigations 649
    neck 649
    ocular movements 649
    pupils 649
    respiration 649
    skin 649
    special investigations 649
  management 650–1
uncus
  lesions 83, 162
  tumour 162
upper motor neurone 15–16
upper motor neurone lesion 33–4
  causes 34
  differential diagnosis 34
  dysarthria 54
uraemic coma 646
uraemic polyneuropathy 535–6
Urbach–Wiethe's disease (lipoid
    proteinosis) 468
urea-cycle disorders 452–3
uric acid, serum, in stroke 197
useless hand syndrome 44, 309

Usher's syndrome 367
utricle 122

vagus nerve (10th cranial) 129–33
  lesions 130–3
    laryngeal paralysis, see laryngeal paralysis
    nuclear 132
    palatal paralysis 130
    pharyngeal paralysis 130
    posterior fossa 132
  peripheral distribution 129–30
  trunk 129
    lesions 132
  unilateral paralysis 168
  visceral function 132
  see also recurrent laryngeal nerve
Valsalva's manœuvre 597
van Bogært–Bertrand syndrome (Canavan's
    diffuse sclerosis) 463
van Buchem's disease 606
vancomycin, for meningitis 245
varicella-zoster virus 291
vasa nervorum 25
  occlusion 219
vascular disorders, pathology 11
vasopressin 602
vasovagal attacks 620
VDRL flocculation test 263
venography, extradural 406
venous sinuses, see intracranial sinuses
ventral spinothalamic tract 40–1
ventricles, cerebral
  dilatation, angiography 158 (fig.)
  haemorrhage into 216
    neonatal 216
ventricular puncture 67
ventriculography 80
  brainstem glioma 161 (fig.)
  intracranial abscess 252
  intracranial tumour 154, 159–60, 161 (figs.)
  medulloblastoma 160 (fig.)
vermis, familial agenesis of 366
Vernet's (jugular foramen) syndrome 132
vertebrae–spinal segment relationship 408
vertebral artery 184
  atheroma 193
  compression during childbirth 352
  developmental anomaly 183
  kinking 192
  occlusion 195–6
  stenosis 193
  thrombosis 192
vertebro-basilar insufficiency 193, 196, 406
vertical gaze paresis 263
vertigo 36, 125–7
  aural 126
  benign paroxysmal, of childhood 127
  benign positional 126
  benign recurrent 127
  causes 125
  cerebellar origin 126
  epidemic 126
  in: brainstem lesion 126
    cerebral tumour 153
    cortical disturbance 126
    eighth nerve lesion 126
    intracranial tumour 153
  ocular origin 126
vestibular neuronitis 126
  canal paresis 123
vestibular system 122
  dysfunction, induced manifestation 122
    caloric test 122–4
    positional tests 124
  function examination 122

vestibulocochlear nerve (8th cranial) 117,
    119–20
  tumours, see acoustic neuroma
  see also vestibular system
vibration sense testing 39
vidarabine (adenine arabinoside)
  for: herpes simplex encephalitis 280
    herpes zoster 293
vinca alkaloids, recurrent laryngeal nerve
    paralysis due to 132
vincristine 172
vincristine neuromyopathy 536
viruses 274
  immunosuppressive agent activation 290
  neurotropic 10
virus infections 274–94
  'slow virus' 294, 301
  tests 274
vision 83–4
visual acuity 85
  disorders 85
  testing 85
visual asymbolia (alexia with agraphia; cortical
    word-blindness; Déjerine's first type of
    alexia) 57
visual cortex 86
  association cortex irritation 87
  blood supply 89
  lesions 88, 89
visual disorientation 87
visual evoked response 87, 312
visual fields
  abnormalities 87
  charting 86–7
  erroneous projection 96
  in: chiasmal lesions 165
    diffuse sclerosis 320
    migraine 177, 179
    multiple sclerosis 310
    neuromyelitis optica 92, 306
    occipital tumour 163
    optic atrophy 94
    optic radiation lesions 88
    papilloedema 91, 153
    parietal tumour 163
    pituitary tumour 165
    tabes dorsalis 270
    temporal lobe tumour 162
    visual pathway lesion 87–9
visual impairment
  in: Arnold–Chiari malformation 417
    multiple sclerosis 309, 310
    Schilder's diffuse sclerosis 320
visual inattention 87
  contralateral 163
visual pathways 85–9
vitamin A
  deficiency 137–8, 473
  excess 473
vitamin B group deficiency 373–4
vitamin B$_1$ deficiency 92
vitamin B$_{12}$
  congenital malabsorption 480
  deficiency 92
vitamin B$_{12}$ neuropathy (subacute combined
    degeneration of spinal cord/brain;
    posterolateral sclerosis; combined system
    disease) 479–82
  aetiology 479–80
  diagnosis 480–1
  pathology 479
  prognosis 481
  symptoms and signs 45, 480
  treatment 481
vitamin D
  deficiency 473

excess 473
vitamin E deficiency 384, 474
vocal-cord paralysis, in distal spinal muscular
    atrophy 385
Vogt–Koyanagi–Harada syndrome 290
volatile inhalants, addiction to 434
Volkmann's ischaemic paralysis 492
vomiting
  in: cerebellar tumour 167
    craniopharyngioma 166
    eighth nerve tumour 167
    fourth ventricle tumour 168
    hydrocephalus 139
    hysteria 665
    increased intracranial pressure 136
    intracranial tumour 152
    midbrain tumour 164
    pituitary tumour 165
    transverse sinus thrombosis 223
von Gierke's disease 465
von Graefe's sign 105
von Hippel's disease 150
von Recklinghausen's disease, see
    neurofibromatosis

Waldenström's syndrome
    (macroglobulinaemia) 485
Wallenberg's (lateral medullary) syndrome 46,
    176, 196
Wartenberg's sign 33
Waterhouse–Friderichsen syndrome 241
water intoxication, see hyponatraemia
Weber's law 39
Weber's syndrome 34, 196
Weber's test 120
Wechsler Adult Intelligence Scale
    (W.A.I.S.) 656, 660
Wechsler Intelligence Scale for Children
    (W.I.S.C.) 656
Wegener's granulomatosis 219
weight appreciation 39
Weigl's form–colour sorting test 656
Weil's disease 247
Werding–Hoffman disease (progressive spinal
    muscular atrophy) 383–4, 384–5
Wernicke–Korsakow syndrome 426
Wernicke's aphasia 56, 195
Wernicke's encephalopathy 426, 475–6
  treatment 430
Wernicke's hemianopic reaction 104
West Indian amblyopia 478
West's syndrome (infantile spasms) 616
whiplash injury 399
Whipple's disease 261–2, 469
white asphyxia in newborn 236
whooping cough 255
  encephalopathy following inoculation 255
Wilson's disease (tetanoid chorea;
    pseudosclerosis; progressive lenticular
    degeneration; hepatolenticular
    degeneration) 336–8
  aetiology 337
  biochemical changes 337
  diagnosis 337–8
  pathology 336–7
  prognosis 338
  radiology 337
  symptoms and signs 337
  treatment 338
winging of scapula 502
Wolman's disease 461
word-blindness, subcortical (alexia without
    agraphia; visual aphasia) 57
word-deafness
  congenital (congenital auditory imperception;
    developmental receptive

aphasia) 59–60, 60
  subcortical (auditory aphasia) 56
wrist-drop
  in: lead neuropathy 436, 437
    radial nerve paralysis 503
writer's cramp 667–8
wry neck (spasmodic torticollis) 323, 341–2

xanthinuria 579
xanthochromia of CSF 69
  Froin's syndrome 70
xanthomatosis 461, 541
xanthopsia 94
xeroderma pigmentosum 367
X-linked infantile progressive bulbar palsy 385

X-linked recessive gene 472
X-linked syndrome, Menkes' kinky-hair syndrome-resembling 468
xylocaine, injection and alcohol, for paraplegia 395

zebra bodies 455
zoster-varicella virus 291

Susan D. Pe
233 Bluewing C
Worthington, Ohio
43c

431-0120